IV Incompatibilities/
Compatibilities presen[t]
important information fo[r]
IV drugs.

rigidity, peripheral circulatory collapse, cardiac arrest, anaphylactoid effects).
**Storage** • Store at room temperature.

**Epidural, Liposomal**
• May give either diluted or undiluted. • Do not use an in-line filter. • Store solution in refrigerator/do not freeze. May store at room temperature for 7 days. • Following withdrawal from vial, use within 4 hrs. • Gently invert vial to resuspend drug; avoid aggressive agitation.

**⚠ IV INCOMPATIBILITIES**
Amphotericin B complex (Abelcet, AmBisome, Amphotec), cefepime (Maxipime) doxorubicin (Doxil), lipids, phenytoin (Dilantin), thiopental.

**⚠ IV COMPATIBILITIES**
Amiodarone (Cordarone), atropine, bumetanide (Bumex), bupivacaine (Marcaine, Sensorcaine), diltiazem (Cardizem), diphenhydramine (Benadryl), dobutamine (Dobutrex), dopamine (Intropin), glycopyrrolate (Robinul), heparin, hydroxyzine (Vistaril), lidocaine, lorazepam (Ativan), magnesium, midazolam (Versed), milrinone (Primacor), nitroglycerin, potassium, propofol (Diprivan), total parenteral nutrition (TPN).

**INDICATIONS/ROUTES/DOSAGE**
◄ALERT► Dosage should be titrated to desired effect.
*Analgesia*
**PO (IMMEDIATE-RELEASE): ADULTS, ELDERLY:** 10–30 mg q3–4h as needed. **CHILDREN:** 0.15–0.3 mg/kg q3–4h as needed.
**PO (EXTENDED-RELEASE [AVINZA]): ADULTS, ELDERLY:** Dosage requirement should be established using promptrelease formulations and is based on total daily dose. Avinza is given once a day only.
**PO (EXTENDED-RELEASE [KADIAN]): ADULTS, ELDERLY:** Dosage requirement should be established using promptrelease formulations and is based on total daily dose. Dose is given once a day or divided and given q12h.

*Patient-Controlled Analgesia (PCA)*
**IV: ADULTS, ELDERLY: Loading dose:** 5–10 mg. **Intermittent bolus:** 0.5–3 mg. **Lockout interval:** 5–12 min. **Continuous infusion:** 1–10 mg/hr. **4-hr limit:** 20–30 mg.

**SIDE EFFECTS**
**Frequent:** Sedation, decreased B/P (including orthostatic hypotension), diaphoresis, facial flushing, constipation, dizziness, drowsiness, nausea, vomiting. **Occasional:** Allergic reaction (rash, pruritus), dyspnea, confusion, palpitations, tremors, urinary retention, abdominal cramps, vision changes, dry mouth, headache, decreased appetite, pain/burning at injection site. **Rare:** Paralytic ileus.

**ADVERSE EFFECTS/ TOXIC REACTIONS**
Overdose results in respiratory depression, skeletal muscle flaccidity, cold/clammy skin, cyanosis, extreme drowsiness progressing to seizures, stupor, coma. Tolerance to analgesic effect, physical dependence may occur with repeated use.

**NURSING CONSIDERATIONS**

**BASELINE ASSESSMENT**
Pt should be in recumbent position before drug is given by parenteral route. Assess onset, type, location, duration of pain.

**INTERVENTION/EVALUATION**
Monitor vital signs 5–10 min after IV administration, 15–30 min after subcutaneous, IM. Be alert for decreased respirations, B/P. Check for adequate voiding. Monitor daily pattern of **bowel activity and stool consistency.** Avoid constipation.

**PATIENT/FAMILY TEACHING**
• Discomfort may occur with injection. • Change positions slowly to avoid orthostatic hypotension. • Avoid tasks that require alertness, motor skills until response to drug is established. • Avoid alcohol, CNS depressants.

Side Effects section in each drug monograph specifies the frequency of particular side effects.

Adverse Reactions highlight the particularly dangerous side effects.

**M**

◆ Canadian trade name     Non-Crushable Drug     High Alert drug

New to this Edition!
• 29 drugs recently approved by the FDA
• Hundreds of updates and revisions
• Over 270 updated Black Box Alerts

High Alert drugs are shaded in blue for easy identification.

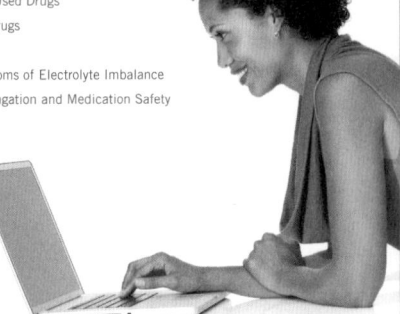

# Saunders

# NURSING DRUG HANDBOOK 2018

**ROBERT J. KIZIOR, BS, RPh**
Department of Pharmacy
Alexian Brothers Medical Center
Elk Grove Village, Illinois

**Keith J. Hodgson, RN, BSN, CCRN**
Staff Nurse, Intensive Care Unit
Former Staff Nurse, Emergency Department
St. Joseph's Hospital
Tampa, Florida

ELSEVIER

# ELSEVIER

3251 Riverport Lane
St. Louis, Missouri 63043

SAUNDERS NURSING DRUG HANDBOOK 2018

ISBN: 978-0-323-52509-1
ISSN: 1098-8661

---

## NOTICES

Knowledge and best practice in this field are constantly changing. As new research and experience broaden our understanding, changes in research methods, professional practices, or medical treatment may become necessary.

Practitioners and researchers must always rely on their own experience and knowledge in evaluating and using any information, methods, compounds, or experiments described herein. In using such information or methods, they should be mindful of their own safety and the safety of others, including parties for whom they have a professional responsibility.

With respect to any drug or pharmaceutical products identified, readers are advised to check the most current information provided (i) on procedures featured or (ii) by the manufacturer of each product to be administered, to verify the recommended dose or formula, the method and duration of administration, and contraindications. It is the responsibility of practitioners, relying on their own experience and knowledge of their patients, to make diagnoses, to determine dosages and the best treatment for each individual patient, and to take all appropriate safety precautions.

To the fullest extent of the law, neither the Publisher nor the authors, contributors, or editors, assume any liability for any injury and/or damage to persons or property as a matter of products liability, negligence or otherwise, or from any use or operation of any methods, products, instructions, or ideas contained in the material herein.

---

ISBN: 978-0-323-52509-1

*Executive Content Strategist:* Sonya Seigafuse
*Content Development Manager:* Billie Sharp
*Publishing Services Manager:* Julie Eddy
*Project Manager:* Mike Sheets
*Design Direction:* Paula Catalano

Printed in the United States of America

Last digit is the print number: 9 8 7 6 5 4 3 2 1

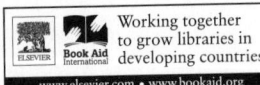

Working together
to grow libraries in
developing countries

www.elsevier.com • www.bookaid.org

# CONTENTS

# AUTHOR BIOGRAPHIES

## Robert (Bob) J. Kizior, BS, RPh

Bob graduated from the University of Illinois School of Pharmacy and is licensed to practice in the state of Illinois. He has worked as a hospital pharmacist for more than 40 years at Alexian Brothers Medical Center in Elk Grove Village, Illinois—a suburb of Chicago. Bob is the Pharmacy Surgery Coordinator for the Department of Pharmacy, where he participates in educational programs for pharmacists, nurses, physicians, and patients. He plays a major role in coordinating pharmacy services in the OR satellite. Bob is a former adjunct faculty member at William Rainey Harper Community College in Palatine, Illinois.

An avid sports fan, Bob also has eclectic tastes in music that range from classical, big band, rock 'n' roll, and jazz to country and western. Bob spends much of his free time reviewing the professional literature to stay current on new drug information.

## Keith J. Hodgson, RN, BSN, CCRN

Keith was born into a loving family in Chicago, Illinois. His mother, Barbara B. Hodgson, was an author and publisher of several medication products, and her work has been a part of his life since he was a child. By the time he was 4 years old, Keith was already helping his mother with the drug cards by stacking the draft pages that were piled up throughout their home.

Because of his mother's influence, Keith contemplated becoming a nurse in college, but his mind was fully made up after he shadowed his sister in the Emergency Department. Keith received his Associates Degree in Nursing from Hillsborough Community College and his Bachelor of Science in Nursing from the University of South Florida in Tampa, Florida. Keith started his career in the Emergency Department and now works in the Trauma/Neurological/Surgical Intensive Care Unit at St. Joseph's Hospital in Tampa, Florida.

Keith's favorite interests include music, reading, Kentucky basketball, and, if he gets the chance, watching every minute of the Olympic Games.

# REVIEWERS

**James Graves, PharmD**
St. Mary Health Center
Jefferson City, Missouri

**Sarah E. Heeter, RN, BSN**
Barnes-Jewish St. Peters Hospital
St. Peters, Missouri

**Randolph E. Regal, BS, PharmD**
Clinical Associate Professor
Adult Internal Medicine/Gastroenterology
University of Michigan College of Pharmacy and
 Hospitals
Ann Arbor, Michigan

**Travis Sonnett, PharmD**
Inpatient Pharmacy Supervisor/Adjunct Faculty
Mann-Grandstaff VA Medical Center
Washington State University College of Pharmacy
Spokane, Washington

# CONSULTANTS*

**Katherine B. Barbee, MSN, ANP, F-NP-C**
Kaiser Permanente
Washington, District of Columbia

**Marla J. DeJong, RN, MS, CCRN, CEN, Capt**
Wilford Hall Medical Center
Lackland Air Force Base, Texas

**Diane M. Ford, RN, MS, CCRN**
Andrews University
Berrien Springs, Michigan

**Denise D. Hopkins, PharmD**
College of Pharmacy
University of Arkansas
Little Rock, Arkansas

**Barbara D. Horton, RN, MS**
Arnot Ogden Medical Center School of Nursing
Elmira, New York

**Mary Beth Jenkins, RN, CCRN, CAPA**
Elliott One Day Surgery Center
Manchester, New Hampshire

**Kelly W. Jones, PharmD, BCPS**
McLeod Family Medicine Center
McLeod Regional Medical Center
Florence, South Carolina

**Linda Laskowski-Jones, RN, MS, CS, CCRN, CEN**
Christiana Care Health System
Newark, Delaware

**Jessica K. Leet, RN, BSN**
Cardinal Glennon Children's Hospital
St. Louis, Missouri

**Denise Macklin, BSN, RNC, CRNI**
President, Professional Learning Systems, Inc.
Marietta, Georgia

**Judith L. Myers, MSN, RN**
Health Sciences Center
St. Louis University School of Nursing
St. Louis, Missouri

**Kimberly R. Pugh, MSEd, RN, BS**
Nurse Consultant
Baltimore, Maryland

**Regina T. Schiavello, BSN, RNC**
Wills Eye Hospital
Philadelphia, Pennsylvania

**Gregory M. Susla, PharmD, FCCM**
National Institutes of Health
Bethesda, Maryland

---

*The author acknowledges the work of the consultants in previous edition(s).

## ACKNOWLEDGMENTS

I would like to thank my co-author Bob Kizior for his knowledge, experience, support, and friendship. We would like to give special thanks to Sonya Seigafuse, Jean Fornango, Charlene Ketchum, Julie Eddy, Mike Sheets, and the entire Elsevier team for their superior dedication, hard work, and belief in us. We gratefully acknowledge Evelyn Dayringer and the staff at Graphic World for their tenacious attention to detail and work. We would also like to thank Jim Witmer, RN, BSN, for his support, attention to detail, and knowledge. Without this wonderful team, none of this would be possible.

**Keith J. Hodgson, RN, BSN, CCRN**

## DEDICATION

I dedicate my work to the practicing nurse, those aspiring to become nurses, and to all health care professionals who are dedicated to the art and science of healing.

**Bob Kizior, BS, RPh**

I dedicate this work to my sister, Lauren, a foundation for our family; my sister, Kathryn, for her love and support; my father, David Hodgson, the best father a son could have; my brothers-in-law, Andy and Jim, great additions to the family; the grandchildren, Paige Olivia, Logan James, Ryan James, and Dylan Boyd; to Jen Nicely for always being there; and to my band of brothers, Peter, Jamie, Miguel, Ritch, George, Jon, Domingo, Ben, Craig, Pat, and Shay.

We also make a special dedication to Barbara B. Hodgson, RN, OCN. She truly was a piece of something wonderful. Barbara often gave her love and support without needing any in return, and would do anything for a smile. Not only was she a colleague and a friend, she was also a small business owner, an artist, a dreamer, and an innovator. We hope the pride we offer in her honor comes close to what she always gave us. Her dedication and perseverance lives on.

**Keith J. Hodgson, RN, BSN, CCRN**

## BIBLIOGRAPHY

Briggs GG, Freeman RK, Yaffe SJ: *Drugs in Pregnancy and Lactation: A Reference Guide to Fetal and Neonatal Risk,* ed 9, Philadelphia, 2011, Lippincott Williams & Wilkins.

*Drug Facts and Comparisons 2016,* Philadelphia, 2016, Lippincott Williams & Wilkins.

Lacy CF, Armstrong LL, Goldman MP, Lance LL: *Lexi-Comp's Drug Information Handbook,* ed 25, Hudson, OH, 2016–2017, Lexi-Comp.

Takemoto CK, Hodding JH, Kraus DM: *Lexi-Comp's Pediatric Dosage Handbook,* ed 21, Hudson, OH, 2015–2016, Lexi-Comp.

Trissel LA: *Handbook of Injectable Drugs,* ed 19, Bethesda, MD, 2016, American Society of Health-System Pharmacists.

## ILLUSTRATION CREDITS

Kee JL, Hayes ER, McCuiston LE (eds): *Pharmacology: A Nursing Process Approach,* ed 7, Philadelphia, 2012, Saunders.

*Mosby's GenRx,* ed 12, St. Louis, 2004, Mosby.

# PREFACE

Nurses are faced with the ever-challenging responsibility of ensuring safe and effective drug therapy for their patients. Not surprisingly, the greatest challenge for nurses is keeping up with the overwhelming amount of new drug information, including the latest FDA-approved drugs and changes to already approved drugs, such as new uses, dosage forms, warnings, and much more. Nurses must integrate this information into their patient care quickly and in an informed manner.

**Saunders Nursing Drug Handbook 2018** is designed as an easy-to-use source of current drug information to help the busy nurse meet these challenges. What separates this book from others is that it guides the nurse through patient care to better practice and better care.

This handbook contains the following:

1. **An IV compatibility chart.** This handy chart is bound into the handbook to prevent accidental loss.
2. **The Drug Classifications section.** The action and uses for some of the most common clinical and pharmacotherapeutic classes are presented. Unique to this handbook, each class provides an at-a-glance table that compares all the generic drugs within the classification according to product availability, dosages, side effects, and other characteristics. Its half-page color tab ensures you can't miss it!
3. **An alphabetical listing of drug entries by generic name.** Blue letter thumb tabs help you page through this section quickly. Information on medications that contain a Black Box Alert is an added feature of the drug entries. This alert identifies those medications for which the FDA has issued a warning that the drugs may cause serious adverse effects. Tall Man lettering, with emphasis on certain syllables to avoid confusing similar sounding/looking medications, is shown in slim blue capitalized letters (e.g., *aceta**ZOLAMIDE***). High Alert drugs with a blue icon 〖HIGH ALERT〗 are considered dangerous by The Joint Commission and the Institute for Safe Medication Practices (ISMP) because if they are administered incorrectly, they may cause life-threatening or permanent harm to the patient. The entire High Alert generic drug entry sits on a blue-shaded background so that it's easy to spot! To make scanning pages easier, each new entry begins with a shaded box containing the generic name, pronunciation, trade name(s), fixed combination(s), and classification(s).
4. **A comprehensive reference section.** Appendixes include vital information on calculation of doses; controlled drugs; chronic wound care; drugs of abuse; equianalgesic dosing; herbals: common natural medicines; lifespan, cultural aspects, and pharmacogenomics of drug therapy; normal laboratory values; cytochrome P450 enzymes; poison antidotes; preventing medication errors; parenteral fluid administration; and Common Terminology Criteria for Adverse Events (CTCAE).
5. **Drugs by Disorder.** You'll find Drugs by Disorder in the front of the book for easy reference. It lists common disorders and the drugs most often used for treatment.
6. **The index.** The comprehensive index is located at the back of the book on light blue pages. Undoubtedly the best tool to help you navigate the handbook, the comprehensive index is organized by showing generic drug names in **bold**, trade names in regular type, classifications in *italics,* and the page number of the main drug entry listed first and in **bold**.

## A DETAILED GUIDE TO THE SAUNDERS NURSING DRUG HANDBOOK

An intensive review by consultants and reviewers helped us to revise the **Saunders Nursing Drug Handbook** so that it is most useful in both educational and clinical practice. The main objective of the handbook is to provide essential drug information in a user-friendly format. The bulk of the handbook contains an alphabetical listing of drug entries by generic name.

To maintain the portability of this handbook and meet the challenge of keeping content current, we have also included additional information for some medications on the Evolve® Internet site. Users can also choose from 100 monographs for the most commonly used medications and customize and print drug cards. Evolve® also includes drug alerts (e.g., medications removed from the market) and drug updates (e.g., new drugs, updates on existing entries). Information is periodically added, allowing the nurse to keep abreast of current drug information.

We have incorporated the IV Incompatibilities/Compatibilities ▓ heading. The drugs listed in this section are compatible or incompatible with the generic drug when administered directly by IV push, via a Y-site, or via IV piggyback. We have highlighted the intravenous drug administration and handling information with a special heading icon ▯ and have broken it down by Reconstitution, Rate of Administration, and Storage.

We present entries in an order that follows the logical thought process the nurse undergoes whenever a drug is ordered for a patient:

- What is the drug?
- How is the drug classified?
- What does the drug do?
- What is the drug used for?
- Under what conditions should you **not** use the drug?
- How do you administer the drug?
- How do you store the drug?
- What is the dose of the drug?
- What should you monitor the patient for once he or she has received the drug?
- What do you assess the patient for?
- What interventions should you perform?
- What should you teach the patient?

The following are included within the drug entries:

**Generic Name, Pronunciation, Trade Names.** Each entry begins with the generic name and pronunciation, followed by the U.S. and Canadian trade names. Exclusively Canadian trade names are followed by a blue maple leaf ♣. Trade names that were most prescribed in the year 2015 are underlined in this section.

**Black Box Alert.** This feature highlights drugs that carry a significant risk of serious or life-threatening adverse effects. Black Box Alerts are ordered by the FDA.

**Do Not Confuse With.** Drug names that sound similar to the generic and/or trade names are listed under this heading to help you avoid potential medication errors.

**Fixed-Combination Drugs.** Where appropriate, fixed-combinations, or drugs made up of two or more generic medications, are listed with the generic drug.

**Pharmacotherapeutic and Clinical Classification Names.** Each entry includes both the pharmacotherapeutic and clinical classifications for the generic drug.

**Action/Therapeutic Effect.** This section describes how the drug is predicted to behave, with the expected therapeutic effect(s) under a separate heading.

**Pharmacokinetics.** This section includes the absorption, distribution, metabolism, excretion, and half-life of the medication. The half-life is bolded in blue for easy access.

**Uses/Off-Label.** The listing of uses for each drug includes both the FDA uses and the off-label uses. The off-label heading is shown in bold blue for emphasis.

**Precautions.** This heading incorporates a discussion about when the generic drug is contraindicated or should be used with caution. The cautions warn the nurse of specific situations in which a drug should be closely monitored.

**Lifespan Considerations** ⏳. This section includes lactation data and age-specific information concerning children and elderly people.

**Interactions.** This heading enumerates drug, food, and herbal interactions with the generic drug. As the number of medications a patient receives increases, awareness of drug interactions becomes more important. Also included is information about therapeutic and toxic blood levels in addition to the altered lab values that show what effects the drug may have on lab results.

**Product Availability.** Each drug monograph gives the form and availability of the drug. The icon 🍃 identifies noncrushable drug forms.

**Administration/Handling.** Instructions for administration are given for each route of administration (e.g., IV, IM, PO, rectal). Special handling, such as refrigeration, is also included where applicable. The routes in this section are always presented in the order IV, IM, SQ, and PO, with subsequent routes in alphabetical order (e.g., Ophthalmic, Otic, Topical). **IV administration** 🍃 is broken down by reconstitution, rate of administration (how fast the IV should be given), and storage (including how long the medication is stable once reconstituted).

**IV Incompatibilities/IV Compatibilities** 🔲. These sections give the nurse the most comprehensive compatibility information possible when administering medications by direct IV push, via a Y-site, or via IV piggyback.

**Indications/Routes/Dosage.** Each entry provides specific dosing guidelines for adults, elderly, children, and patients with renal and/or hepatic impairment. Dose modification for toxicity has been added where applicable. Dosages are clearly indicated for each approved indication and route.

**Side Effects.** Side effects are defined as those responses that are usually predictable with the drug, are **not** life-threatening, and may or may not require discontinuation of the drug. Unique to this handbook, side effects are grouped by frequency listed from highest occurrence percentage to lowest so that the nurse can focus on patient care without wading through myriad signs and symptoms of side effects.

**Adverse Effects/Toxic Reactions.** Adverse effects and toxic reactions are very serious and often life-threatening undesirable responses that require prompt intervention from a health care provider.

**Nursing Considerations.** Nursing considerations are organized as care is organized. That is:

- What needs to be assessed or done before the first dose is administered? (Baseline Assessment)
- What interventions and evaluations are needed during drug therapy? (Intervention/Evaluation)
- What explicit teaching is needed for the patient and family? (Patient/Family Teaching)

**Saunders Nursing Drug Handbook** is an easy-to-use source of current drug information for nurses, students, and other health care providers. It is our hope that this handbook will help you provide quality care to your patients.

We welcome any comments you may have that would help us to improve future editions of the handbook. Please contact us via the publisher at *http://evolve.elsevier.com/SaundersNDH.*

**Robert J. Kizior, BS, RPh**
**Keith J. Hodgson, RN, BSN, CCRN**

# NEWLY APPROVED MEDICATIONS

| Name | Indications |
|------|-------------|
| Alectinib (Alecensa) | An oral kinase inhibitor for certain types of non–small-cell lung (NSCL) cancer. |
| Atezolizumab (Tecentriq) | A programmed death-ligand 1 (PD-L 1) blocking antibody for treatment of advanced urothelial carcinoma (bladder cancer) |
| Brivaracetam (Briviact) | A selective, high-affinity synaptic vesicle protein 2A ligand for treatment of partial onset seizures |
| Cabozantinib (Cabometyx) | A tyrosine kinase inhibitor for treatment of advanced renal cell carcinoma |
| Cobimetinib (Cotellic) | An oral kinase inhibitor for advanced melanoma |
| Daclizumab (Zinbryta) | An interleukin-2 receptor blocking antibody indicated for relapsing forms of multiple sclerosis |
| Daratumumab (Darzalex) | A monoclonal antibody for multiple myeloma |
| Elbasvir and grazoprevir (Zepatier) | Combination NS5A replication complex inhibitor and NS3/4A protease inhibitor for treatment of chronic hepatitis C virus (HCV) genotypes 1 and 4 infections. |
| Elotuzumab (Empliciti) | An immune system activator for multiple myeloma |
| Ikekizumab (Taltz) | A humanized interleukin-17A antagonist for treatment of adults with moderate to severe plaque psoriasis |
| Ixazombi (Ninlaro) | An oral proteasome inhibitor for multiple myeloma |
| Lixisenatide (Adylyxin) | A glucagon receptor agonist used as an adjunct to diet and exercise to improve glycemic control in type 2 diabetes |
| Mepolizumab (Nucala) | A monoclonal antibody for add-on maintenance treatment of severe asthma |
| Necitumumab (Portrazza) | An epidermal growth factor receptor antagonist for metastatic squamous non–small-cell lung (NSCL) cancer |
| Osimertinib (Tagrisso) | An oral kinase inhibitor for metastatic non–small-cell lung (NSCL) cancer |
| Patiromer (Veltassa) | An oral potassium binder for hyperkalemia |
| Pimavanserin (Nuplazid) | An atypical antipsychotic for Parkinson's disease psychosis |

*Continued*

| Name | Indications |
|------|-------------|
| Reslizumab (Cinqair) | An interleukin-5 antagonist for add-on maintenance treatment of severe asthma |
| Sofosbuvir/velpatasvir (Epclusa) | Fixed-dose combination for treatment of chronic hepatitis C |
| Trabectedin (Yondelis) | An alkylating agent for advanced soft tissue sarcomas |
| Venetoclax (Venelexta) | A BCL-2 inhibitor for chronic lymphocytic leukemia |

# DRUGS BY DISORDER

**Note: Not all medications appropriate for a given condition are listed, nor are those not listed inappropriate.**
Generic names appear first, followed by brand names in parentheses.

**Alcohol dependence**
Acamprosate (Campral)
Disulfiram (Antabuse)
Naltrexone (Depade, ReVia, Vivitrol)

**Allergic rhinitis**
Azelastine (Astepro)
Azelastine/fluticasone (Dymista)
Beclomethasone (Beconase AQ)
Budesonide (Rhinocort Aqua)
Ciclesonide (Omnaris)
Flunisolide (Nasarel)
Fluticasone (Flonase)
Mometasone (Nasonex)
Olopatadine (Patanase)
Triamcinolone (Nasacort)

**Allergy**
Beclomethasone (Beclovent, Vanceril)
Betamethasone (Celestone)
Budesonide (Pulmicort, Rhinocort)
Cetirizine (Zyrtec)
Clemastine (Tavist)
Cyproheptadine (Periactin)
Desloratadine (Clarinex)
Dexamethasone (Decadron)
Dimenhydrinate (Dramamine)
Diphenhydramine (Benadryl)
Epinephrine (Adrenalin)
Fexofenadine (Allegra)
Flunisolide (AeroBid, Nasalide)
Fluticasone (Flovent)
Hydrocortisone (Solu-Cortef)
Levocetirizine (Xyzal)
Loratadine (Claritin)
Prednisolone (Prelone)
Prednisone (Deltasone)
Promethazine (Phenergan)
Triamcinolone (Kenalog)

**Alzheimer's disease**
Donepezil (Aricept, Aricept ODT)
Galantamine (Razadyne, Razadyne ER)
Memantine (Namenda, Namenda XR)
Rivastigmine (Exelon, Exelon Patch)

**Angina**
Amlodipine (Norvasc)
Atenolol (Tenormin)
Diltiazem (Cardizem, Dilacor)
Isosorbide (Imdur, Isordil)
Metoprolol (Lopressor)
Nadolol (Corgard)
Nicardipine (Cardene)
Nifedipine (Adalat, Procardia)
Nitroglycerin
Propranolol (Inderal)
Verapamil (Calan, Isoptin)

**Anxiety**
Alprazolam (Xanax)
Buspirone (BuSpar)
Diazepam (Valium)
Hydroxyzine (Atarax, Vistaril)
Lorazepam (Ativan)
Oxazepam (Serax)
Paroxetine (Paxil)
Trazodone (Desyrel)
Venlafaxine (Effexor)

**Arrhythmias**
Adenosine (Adenocard)
Amiodarone (Cordarone, Pacerone)
Digoxin (Lanoxin)
Diltiazem (Cardizem, Dilacor)
Disopyramide (Norpace)
Dofetilide (Tikosyn)
Dronedarone (Multaq)
Esmolol (Brevibloc)
Flecainide (Tambocor)

Ibutilide (Corvert)
Lidocaine
Metoprolol (Lopressor)
Mexiletine (Mexitil)
Propafenone (Rythmol)
Propranolol (Inderal)
Sotalol (Betapace)
Verapamil (Calan, Isoptin)

**Arthritis, rheumatoid (RA)**
Abatacept (Orencia)
Adalimumab (Humira)
Anakinra (Kineret)
Azathioprine (Imuran)
Certolizumab (Cimzia)
Etanercept (Enbrel)
Golimumab (Simponi)
Hydroxychloroquine (Plaquenil)
Infliximab (Remicade)
Leflunomide (Arava)
Methotrexate
Prednisone (Deltasone)
Rituximab (Rituxan)
Sulfasalazine (Azulfidine-EN)
Tocilizumab (Actemra)
Tofacitinib (Xeljanz)

**Asthma**
Albuterol (Proventil, Ventolin)
Aminophylline (Theophylline)
Arformoterol (Brovana)
Beclomethasone (Beclovent, Vanceril)
Budesonide (Pulmicort)
Ciclesonide (Alvesco)
Cromolyn (Crolom, Intal)
Epinephrine (Adrenalin)
Flunisolide (AeroBid)
Fluticasone (Flovent)
Hydrocortisone (Solu-Cortef)
Ipratropium (Atrovent)
Levalbuterol (Xopenex)
Mepolizumab (Nucala)
Metaproterenol (Alupent)
Methylprednisolone (Solu-Medrol)
Mometasone (Asmanex)
Montelukast (Singulair)
Prednisolone (Prelone)
Prednisone (Deltasone)
Reslizumab (Cinqair)
Salmeterol (Serevent)
Terbutaline (Brethine)

Theophylline (Slo-Bid)
Zafirlukast (Accolate)

**Attention-deficit hyperactivity disorder (ADHD)**
Atomoxetine (Strattera)
Clonidine (Catapres, Kapvay)
Desipramine (Norpramin)
Dexmethylphenidate (Focalin, Focalin XR)
Dextroamphetamine (Dexedrine, Dextrostat)
Guanfacine (Intuniv)
Lisdexamfetamine (Vyvanse)
Methylphenidate (Concerta, Daytrana, Focalin, Methylin, Ritalin)
Mixed amphetamine (dextroamphetamine and amphetamine salts) (Adderall, Adderall XR)

**Benign prostatic hypertrophy (BPH)**
Alfuzosin (Uroxatral)
Doxazosin (Cardura)
Dutasteride (Avodart)
Finasteride (Proscar)
Mirabegron (Myrbetriq)
Silodosin (Rapaflo)
Tadalafil (Cialis)
Tamsulosin (Flomax)
Terazosin (Hytrin)

**Bipolar disorder (mania)**
Carbamazepine (Tegretol)
Lamotrigine (Lamictal)
Lithium (Lithobid)
Oxcarbazepine (Trileptal)
Quetiapine (Seroquel)
Valproic acid (Depakene, Depakote)

**Bladder hyperactivity**
Darifenacin (Enablex)
Oxybutynin (Ditropan, Gelnique)
Solifenacin (VESIcare)
Tolterodine (Detrol)
Trospium (Sanctura)

**Bronchospasm**
Albuterol (Proventil, Ventolin)
Bitolterol (Tornalate)
Levalbuterol (Xopenex)
Metaproterenol (Alupent)

Salmeterol (Serevent)
Terbutaline (Brethine)

**Cancer**
Abarelix (Plenaxis)
Abiraterone (Zytiga)
Ado-trastuzumab (Kadcyla)
Afatinib (Gilotrif)
Aldesleukin (Proleukin)
Alemtuzumab (Campath)
Alitretinoin (Panretin)
Altretamine (Hexalen)
Anastrozole (Arimidex)
Arsenic trioxide (Trisenox)
Asparaginase (Elspar)
Atezolizumab (Tecentriq)
Axitinib (Inlyta)
Azacitidine (Vidaza)
BCG (TheraCys, Tice BCG)
Belinostat (Beleodaq)
Bendamustine (Treanda)
Bevacizumab (Avastin)
Bexarotene (Targretin)
Bicalutamide (Casodex)
Bleomycin (Blenoxane)
Blinatumomab (Blincyto)
Bortezomib (Velcade)
Bosutinib (Bosulif)
Brentuximab (Adcetris)
Busulfan (Myleran)
Cabazitaxel (Jevtana)
Cabozantinib (Cabometyx)
Capecitabine (Xeloda)
Carboplatin (Paraplatin)
Carfilzomib (Kyprolis)
Carmustine (BiCNU)
Ceritinib (Zykadia)
Cetuximab (Erbitux)
Chlorambucil (Leukeran)
Cisplatin (Platinol)
Cladribine (Leustatin)
Clofarabine (Clolar)
Cobimetinib (Cotellic)
Crizotinib (Xalkori)
Cyclophosphamide (Cytoxan)
Cytarabine (Ara-C, Cytosar)
Dabrafenib (Tafinlar)
Dacarbazine (DTIC)
Dactinomycin (Cosmegen)
Daratumumab (Darzalex)
Dasatinib (Sprycel)

Daunorubicin (Cerubidine, DaunoXome)
Degarelix (Firmagon)
Denileukin (Ontak)
Dinutuximab (Unituxin)
Docetaxel (Taxotere)
Doxorubicin (Adriamycin, Doxil)
Elotuzumab (Empliciti)
Enzalutamide (Xtandi)
Epirubicin (Ellence)
Eribulin (Halaven)
Erlotinib (Tarceva)
Estramustine (Emcyt)
Etoposide (VePesid)
Everolimus (Afinitor)
Fludarabine (Fludara)
Fluorouracil
Flutamide (Eulexin)
Fulvestrant (Faslodex)
Gefitinib (Iressa)
Gemcitabine (Gemzar)
Goserelin (Zoladex)
Hydroxyurea (Hydrea)
Ibritumomab (Zevalin)
Ibrutinib (Imbruvica)
Idarubicin (Idamycin)
Idelalisib (Zydelig)
Ifosfamide (Ifex)
Imatinib (Gleevec)
Interferon alfa-2b (Intron A)
Ipilimumab (Yervoy)
Irinotecan (Camptosar)
Ixabepilone (Ixempra)
Ixazombi (Ninlaro)
Lapatinib (Tykerb)
Letrozole (Femara)
Leuprolide (Lupron)
Levatinib (Lenvima)
Lomustine (CeeNU)
Mechlorethamine (Mustargen)
Megestrol (Megace)
Melphalan (Alkeran)
Mercaptopurine (Purinethol)
Methotrexate
Mitomycin (Mutamycin)
Mitotane (Lysodren)
Mitoxantrone (Novantrone)
Necitumumab (Portrazza)
Nelarabine (Arranon)
Nilotinib (Tasigna)
Nilutamide (Nilandron)

Nivolumab (Opdivo)
Obinutuzumab (Gazyva)
Ofatumumab (Arzerra)
Olaparib (Lynparza)
Omacetaxine (Synribo)
Osimertinib (Tagrisso)
Oxaliplatin (Eloxatin)
Paclitaxel (Taxol)
Palbociclib (Ibrance)
Panitumumab (Vectibix)
Panobinostat (Farydak)
Pazopanib (Votrient)
Pegaspargase (Oncaspar)
Pembrolizumab (Keytruda)
Pemetrexed (Alimta)
Pentostatin (Nipent)
Pertuzumab (Perjeta)
Plicamycin (Mithracin)
Pomalidomide (Pomalyst)
Ponatinib (Iclusig)
Pralatrexate (Folotyn)
Procarbazine (Matulane)
Ramucirumab (Cyramza)
Rasburicase (Elitek)
Regorafenib (Stivarga)
Rituximab (Rituxan)
Romidepsin (Istodax)
Sipuleucel-T (Provenge)
Sonidegib (Odomzo)
Sorafenib (Nexavar)
Streptozocin (Zanosar)
Sunitinib (Sutent)
Tamoxifen (Nolvadex)
Temozolomide (Temodar)
Temsirolimus (Torisel)
Teniposide (Vumon)
Thioguanine
Thiotepa (Thioplex)
Tipifarnib (Zarnestra)
Tipiracil/trifluridine (Lonsurf)
Topotecan (Hycamtin)
Toremifene (Fareston)
Tositumomab (Bexxar)
Trabectedin (Yondelis)
Trametinib (Mekinist)
Trastuzumab (Herceptin)
Tretinoin (ATRA, Vesanoid)
Valrubicin (Valstar)
Vandetanib (Caprelsa)
Vemurafenib (Zelboraf)
Venetoclax (Venclexta)

Vinblastine (Velban)
Vincristine (Oncovin)
Vinorelbine (Navelbine)
Vismodegib (Erivedge)
Vorinostat (Zolinza)

**Cerebrovascular accident (CVA)**
Aspirin
Clopidogrel (Plavix)
Heparin
Nimodipine (Nimotop)
Prasugrel (Effient)
Warfarin (Coumadin)

**Chronic obstructive pulmonary disease (COPD)**
Aclidinium (Tudorza)
Albuterol (Proventil HFA, Ventolin HFA)
Aminophylline (Theophylline)
Arformoterol (Brovana)
Budesonide (Pulmicort)
Budesonide/formoterol (Symbicort)
Indacaterol (Arcapta)
Ipratropium (Atrovent HFA)
Levalbuterol (Xopenex)
Olodaterol (Striverdi Respimat)
Pirbuterol (Maxair)
Roflumilast (Daliresp)
Salmeterol (Serevent)
Salmeterol/fluticasone (Advair)
Theophylline (Theochron, Theo ZY)
Tiotropium (Spiriva)
Umeclidinium (Incruse Ellipta)

**Constipation**
Bisacodyl (Dulcolax)
Docusate (Colace)
Lactulose (Kristalose)
Lubiprostone (Amitiza)
Methylcellulose (Citrucel)
Milk of magnesia (MOM)
Polyethylene glycol (MiraLAX)
Psyllium (Metamucil)
Senna (Senokot)
Tegaserod (Zelnorm)

**Deep vein thrombosis (DVT)**
Dalteparin (Fragmin)
Edoxaban (Savaysa)
Enoxaparin (Lovenox)
Heparin

Tinzaparin (Innohep)
Warfarin (Coumadin)

**Depression**
Amitriptyline (Elavil, Endep)
Brexpiprazole (Rexulti)
Bupropion (Aplenzin, Wellbutrin)
Citalopram (Celexa)
Desipramine (Norpramin)
Desvenlafaxine (Khedezla, Pristiq)
Doxepin (Sinequan)
Duloxetine (Cymbalta)
Escitalopram (Lexapro)
Fluoxetine (Prozac)
Fluvoxamine (Luvox)
Levomilnacipran (Fetzima)
Imipramine (Tofranil)
Mirtazapine (Remeron)
Nortriptyline (Aventyl, Pamelor)
Paroxetine (Paxil)
Selegiline (Emsam)
Sertraline (Zoloft)
Trazodone (Desyrel)
Venlafaxine (Effexor)
Vilazodone (Viibryd)
Vortioxetine (Brintellix)

**Diabetes mellitus**
Acarbose (Precose)
Albiglutide (Tanzeum)
Alogliptin (Nesina)
Bromocriptine (Cycloset)
Canagliflozin (Invokana)
Colesevelam (Welchol)
Dapagliflozin (Farxiga)
Dulaglutide (Trulicity)
Empagliflozin (Jardiance)
Exenatide (Byetta)
Glimepiride (Amaryl)
Glipizide (Glucotrol)
Glyburide (Micronase)
Insulin preparations (see Classification section)
Linagliptin (Tradjenta)
Liraglutide (Victoza)
Lixisenatide (Adlyxin)
Metformin (Glucophage)
Nateglinide (Starlix)
Pioglitazone (Actos)
Pramlintide (Symlin)
Repaglinide (Prandin)

Rosiglitazone (Avandia)
Saxagliptin (Onglyza)
Sitagliptin (Januvia)

**Diabetic peripheral neuropathy**
Amitriptyline (Elavil)
Bupropion (Wellbutrin)
Capsaicin (Trixaicin)
Carbamazepine (Tegretol)
Citalopram (Celexa)
Desipramine (Norpramin)
Duloxetine (Cymbalta)
Gabapentin (Neurontin)
Lamotrigine (Lamictal)
Lidocaine patch (Lidoderm)
Nortriptyline (Pamelor)
Oxcarbazepine (Trileptal)
Oxycodone (OxyContin)
Paroxetine (Paxil)
Pregabalin (Lyrica)
Tramadol (Ultram)
Valproic acid (Depakote)
Venlafaxine, extended-release (Effexor XR)

**Diarrhea**
Bismuth subsalicylate (Pepto-Bismol)
Diphenoxylate and atropine (Lomotil)
Fidaxomicin (Dificid)
Kaolin-pectin (Kaopectate)
Loperamide (Imodium)
Octreotide (Sandostatin)
Rifaximin (Xifaxan)

**Edema**
Amiloride (Midamor)
Bumetanide (Bumex)
Chlorthalidone (Hygroton)
Ethacrynic acid (Edecrin)
Furosemide (Lasix)
Hydrochlorothiazide (HydroDIURIL)
Indapamide (Lozol)
Metolazone (Zaroxolyn)
Spironolactone (Aldactone)
Torsemide (Demadex)
Triamterene (Dyrenium)

**Epilepsy**
Brivaracetam (Briviact)
Carbamazepine (Tegretol)
Clobazam (Onfi)
Clonazepam (Klonopin)

Clorazepate (Tranxene)
Diazepam (Valium)
Eslicarbazepine (Aptiom)
Ethosuximide (Zarontin)
Ezogabine (Potiga)
Fosphenytoin (Cerebyx)
Gabapentin (Neurontin)
Lacosamide (Vimpat)
Lamotrigine (Lamictal, Lamictal ODT, Lamictal XR)
Levetiracetam (Keppra)
Lorazepam (Ativan)
Midazolam (Versed)
Oxcarbazepine (Trileptal)
Perampanel (Fycompa)
Phenobarbital
Phenytoin (Dilantin)
Pregabalin (Lyrica)
Primidone (Mysoline)
Rufinamide (Banzel)
Tiagabine (Gabitril)
Topiramate (Qudexy XR, Topamax Trokendi XR)
Valproic acid (Depakene, Depakote)
Vigabatrin (Sabril)
Zonisamide (Zonegran)

**Esophageal reflux, esophagitis**
Cimetidine (Tagamet)
Dexlansoprazole (Dexilant)
Esomeprazole (Nexium)
Famotidine (Pepcid)
Lansoprazole (Prevacid)
Nizatidine (Axid)
Omeprazole (Prilosec)
Pantoprazole (Protonix)
Rabeprazole (AcipHex)
Ranitidine (Zantac)

**Fever**
Acetaminophen (Tylenol)
Aspirin
Ibuprofen (Advil, Caldolor, Motrin)
Naproxen (Aleve, Anaprox, Naprosyn)

**Fibromyalgia**
Acetaminophen (Tylenol)
Amitriptyline (Elavil)
Carisoprodol (Soma)
Citalopram (Celexa)
Cyclobenzaprine (Flexeril)

Duloxetine (Cymbalta)
Fluoxetine (Prozac)
Gabapentin (Neurontin)
Milnacipran (Savella)
Paroxetine (Paxil)
Pregabalin (Lyrica)
Tramadol (Ultram)
Venlafaxine (Effexor)

**Gastric/Duodenal Ulcer**
Cimetidine (Tagamet)
Esomeprazole (Nexium)
Famotidine (Pepcid)
Lansoprazole (Prevacid)
Nizatidine (Axid)
Omeprazole (Prilosec)
Pantoprazole (Protonix)
Rabeprazole (AcipHex)
Ranitidine (Zantac)
Sucralfate (Carafate)

**Gastritis**
Cimetidine (Tagamet)
Famotidine (Pepcid)
Nizatidine (Axid)
Ranitidine (Zantac)

**Gastroesophageal reflux disease (GERD)**
Cimetidine (Tagamet)
Dexlansoprazole (Dexilant)
Esomeprazole (Nexium)
Famotidine (Pepcid)
Lansoprazole (Prevacid)
Nizatidine (Axid)
Omeprazole (Prilosec)
Pantoprazole (Protonix)
Rabeprazole (AcipHex)
Ranitidine (Zantac)

**Glaucoma**
Acetazolamide (Diamox)
Apraclonidine (Iopidine)
Betaxolol (Betoptic)
Bimatoprost (Lumigan)
Brimonidine (Alphagan)
Brinzolamide (Azopt)
Carbachol
Dorzolamide (Trusopt)
Echothiophate iodide (Phospholine)
Latanoprost (Xalatan)

Levobunolol (Betagan)
Pilocarpine (Isopto Carpine)
Tafluprost (Zioptan)
Timolol (Timoptic)
Travoprost (Travatan)
Unoprostone (Rescula)

**Gout**
Allopurinol (Zyloprim)
Colchicine (Colcrys)
Febuxostat (Uloric)
Ibuprofen (Motrin)
Indomethacin (Indocin)
Naproxen (Naprosyn)
Pegloticase (Krystexxa)
Piroxicam (Feldene)
Probenecid (Benemid)
Sulindac (Clinoril)

**Heart failure (HF)**
Bisoprolol (Zebeta)
Bumetanide (Bumex)
Candesartan (Atacand)
Captopril (Capoten)
Carvedilol (Coreg)
Digoxin (Lanoxin)
Dobutamine (Dobutrex)
Dopamine (Intropin)
Enalapril (Vasotec)
Eplerenone (Inspra)
Fosinopril (Monopril)
Furosemide (Lasix)
Hydralazine (Apresoline)
Isosorbide (Isordil)
Ivabradine (Corlanor)
Lisinopril (Prinivil, Zestril)
Losartan (Cozaar)
Metoprolol (Lopressor)
Milrinone (Primacor)
Nitroglycerin
Quinapril (Accupril)
Ramipril (Altace)
Sacubitril/valsartan (Entresto)
Spironolactone (Aldactone)
Torsemide (Demadex)
Valsartan (Diovan)

**Hepatitis B**
Adefovir (Hepsera)
Entecavir (Baraclude)
Lamivudine (Epivir)

Peginterferon alpha-2a
 (Pegasys)
Telbivudine (Tyzeka)
Tenofovir (Viread)

**Hepatitis C**
Daclatasvir (Daklinza)
Elbasvir/Grazoprevir (Zepatier)
Ledipasvir/Safosbuvir (Harvoni)
Ombitasvir/paritaprevir/ritonavir
 (Technivie)
Ombitasvir/paritaprevir/ritonavir/
 dasabuvir (Viekira Pak)
Peginterferon alfa-2a (Pegasys)
Peginterferon alfa-2b (Pegintron)
Ribavirin (Copegus, Rebetol,
 Ribasphere)
Simeprevir (Olysio)
Sofosbuvir (Sovaldi)
Sofosbuvir/Velpatasvir (Epclusa)

**Human immunodeficiency
virus (HIV)**
Abacavir (Ziagen)
Atazanavir (Reyataz)
Cobicistat (Tybost)
Darunavir (Prezista)
Delavirdine (Rescriptor)
Didanosine (Videx)
Dolutegravir (Tivicay)
Efavirenz (Sustiva)
Elvitegravir (Vitekta)
Emtricitabine (Emtriva)
Enfuvirtide (Fuzeon)
Etravirine (Intelence)
Fosamprenavir (Lexiva)
Indinavir (Crixivan)
Lamivudine (Epivir)
Lopinavir/ritonavir (Kaletra)
Maraviroc (Selzentry)
Nelfinavir (Viracept)
Nevirapine (Viramune)
Raltegravir (Isentress)
Rilpivirine (Edurant)
Ritonavir (Norvir)
Saquinavir (Invirase)
Stavudine (Zerit)
Tenofovir (Viread)
Tesamorelin (Egrifta)
Tipranavir (Aptivus)
Zidovudine (AZT, Retrovir)

**Hypercholesterolemia**
Alirocumab (Praluent)
Atorvastatin (Lipitor)
Cholestyramine (Questran)
Colesevelam (Welchol)
Colestipol (Colestid)
Evolocumab (Repatha)
Ezetimibe (Zetia)
Fenofibrate (Antara, Lofibra, Tricor)
Fenofibric Acid (Trilipix)
Fish oil (Lovaza)
Fluvastatin (Lescol)
Gemfibrozil (Lopid)
Lomitapide (Juxtapid)
Lovastatin (Altoprev, Mevacor)
Mipomersen (Kynamro)
Niacin (Niaspan, Slo-Niacin)
Pitavastatin (Livalo)
Pravastatin (Pravachol)
Rosuvastatin (Crestor)
Simvastatin (Zocor)

**Hyperphosphatemia**
Aluminum salts
Calcium salts
Ferric Citrate (Auryxia)
Lanthanum (Fosrenol)
Sevelamer (Renagel)

**Hypertension**
Aliskiren (Tekturna)
Amlodipine (Norvasc)
Atenolol (Tenormin)
Azilsartan (Edarbi)
Benazepril (Lotensin)
Bisoprolol (Zebeta)
Candesartan (Atacand)
Captopril (Capoten)
Clonidine (Catapres)
Diltiazem (Cardizem, Dilacor)
Doxazosin (Cardura)
Enalapril (Vasotec)
Eplerenone (Inspra)
Eprosartan (Teveten)
Felodipine (Plendil)
Fosinopril (Monopril)
Hydralazine (Apresoline)
Hydrochlorothiazide (HydroDIURIL)
Indapamide (Lozol)
Irbesartan (Avapro)
Isradipine (DynaCirc)

Labetalol (Normodyne, Trandate)
Lisinopril (Prinivil, Zestril)
Losartan (Cozaar)
Metolazone (Diulo, Zaroxolyn)
Metoprolol (Lopressor)
Minoxidil (Loniten)
Moexipril (Univasc)
Nadolol (Corgard)
Nebivolol (Bystolic)
Nicardipine (Cardene)
Nifedipine (Adalat, Procardia)
Nitroglycerin
Nitroprusside (Nipride)
Olmesartan (Benicar)
Perindopril (Aceon)
Pindolol (Visken)
Prazosin (Minipress)
Propranolol (Inderal)
Quinapril (Accupril)
Ramipril (Altace)
Spironolactone (Aldactone)
Telmisartan (Micardis)
Terazosin (Hytrin)
Trandolapril (Mavik)
Valsartan (Diovan)
Verapamil (Calan, Isoptin)

**Hypertriglyceridemia**
Atorvastatin (Lipitor)
Colesevelam (Welchol)
Fenofibrate (Tricor)
Fluvastatin (Lescol)
Gemfibrozil (Lopid)
Icosapent (Vascepa)
Lovastatin (Mevacor)
Niacin (Niaspan)
Omega-3 acid ethyl esters (Lovaza)
Pravastatin (Pravachol)
Rosuvastatin (Crestor)
Simvastatin (Zocor)

**Hyperuricemia**
Allopurinol (Zyloprim)
Febuxostat (Uloric)
Pegloticase (Krystexxa)
Probenecid (Benemid)

**Hypotension**
Dobutamine (Dobutrex)
Dopamine (Intropin)
Ephedrine

Epinephrine
Norepinephrine (Levophed)
Phenylephrine (Neo-Synephrine)

**Hypothyroidism**
Levothyroxine (Levoxyl, Synthroid)
Liothyronine (Cytomel)
Thyroid

**Idiopathic thrombocytopenic purpura (ITP)**
Cyclophosphamide (Cytoxan)
Dexamethasone (Decadron)
Hydrocortisone (Solu-Cortef)
Immune globulin intravenous
Methylprednisolone (Solu-Medrol)
Prednisone
$Rh_o(D)$ immune globulin (RhoGAM)
Rituximab (Rituxan)

**Insomnia**
Diphenhydramine (Benadryl)
Estazolam (ProSom)
Eszopiclone (Lunesta)
Flurazepam (Dalmane)
Ramelteon (Rozerem)
Suvorexant (Belsomra)
Temazepam (Restoril)
Zaleplon (Sonata)
Zolpidem (Ambien, Edluar)

**Inflammatory bowel disease (Crohn's disease, ulcerative colitis)**
Adalimumab (Humira)
Azathioprine (Imuran)
Balsalazide (Colazal, Giazo)
Budesonide (Entocort EC, Uceris)
Certolizumab (Cimzia)
Cyclosporine (Sandimmune)
Golimumab (Simponi)
Hydrocortisone (Colocort, Cortifoam)
Infliximab (Remicade)
Mercaptopurine (Purinethol)
Mesalamine (Apriso, Asacol HD, Delzicol, Lialda, Pentasa)
Methotrexate (Otrexup, Rasuvo)
Olsalazine (Dipentum)
Prednisone
Sulfasalazine (Azulfidine)
Tacrolimus (Prograf)
Vedolizumab (Entyvio)

**Migraine headaches**
Almotriptan (Axert)
Amitriptyline (Elavil, Endep)
Diclofenac (Cambia)
Dihydroergotamine
Eletriptan (Relpax)
Ergotamine (Ergomar)
Frovatriptan (Frova)
Naratriptan (Amerge)
Propranolol (Inderal)
Rizatriptan (Maxalt)
Sumatriptan (Imitrex)
Zolmitriptan (Zomig)

**Multiple sclerosis (MS)**
Alemtuzumab (Lemtrada)
Daclizumab (Zinbryta)
Dalfampridine (Ampyra)
Dimethyl fumarate (Tecfidera)
Fingolimod (Gilenya)
Glatiramer (Copaxone)
Interferon beta-1a (Avonex, Rebif)
Interferon beta-1b (Betaseron, Extavia)
Peginterferon beta-la (Plegridy)
Mitoxantrone (Novantrone)
Natalizumab (Tysabri)
Teriflunomide (Aubagio)

**Myelodysplastic syndrome**
Azacitidine (Vidaza)
Clofarabine (Clolar)
Decitabine (Dacogen)
Lenalidomide (Revlimid)

**Myocardial infarction (MI)**
Alteplase (Activase)
Aspirin
Atenolol (Tenormin)
Captopril (Capoten)
Clopidogrel (Plavix)
Dalteparin (Fragmin)
Diltiazem (Cardizem, Dilacor)
Enalapril (Vasotec)
Enoxaparin (Lovenox)
Heparin
Lidocaine
Lisinopril (Prinivil, Zestril)
Metoprolol (Lopressor)
Morphine
Nitroglycerin
Propranolol (Inderal)

Quinapril (Accupril)
Ramipril (Altace)
Reteplase (Retavase)
Warfarin (Coumadin)

**Nausea**
Aprepitant (Emend)
Chlorpromazine (Thorazine)
Dexamethasone (Decadron)
Dimenhydrinate (Dramamine)
Dronabinol (Marinol)
Droperidol (Inapsine)
Fosaprepitant (Emend)
Granisetron (Kytril)
Hydroxyzine (Vistaril)
Lorazepam (Ativan)
Meclizine (Antivert)
Metoclopramide (Reglan)
Nabilone (Cesamet)
Ondansetron (Zofran)
Palonosetron (Aloxi)
Prochlorperazine (Compazine)
Promethazine (Phenergan)
Rolapitant (Varubi)

**Obesity**
Benzphetamine (Didrex)
Bupropion (Wellbutrin)
Bupropion/naltrexone (Contrave)
Diethylpropion (Tenuate)
Exenatide (Bydureon, Byetta)
Lorcaserin (Belviq)
Methamphetamine (Desoxyn)
Orlistat (Alli, Xenical)
Phendimetrazine (Bontril)
Phentermine (Ionamin)
Phentermine and topiramate (Qsymia)

**Obsessive-compulsive disorder (OCD)**
Citalopram (Celexa)
Clomipramine (Anafranil)
Escitalopram (Lexapro)
Fluoxetine (Prozac)
Fluvoxamine (Luvox)
Paroxetine (Paxil)
Sertraline (Zoloft)

**Organ transplant, rejection prophylaxis**
Azathioprine (Imuran)

Basiliximab (Simulect)
Belatacept (Nulojix)
Cyclophosphamide (Cytoxan, Neosar)
Cyclosporine (Sandimmune)
Daclizumab (Zenapax)
Everolimus (Zortress)
Mycophenolate (CellCept)
Sirolimus (Rapamune)
Tacrolimus (Prograf)

**Osteoarthritis**
Acetaminophen (Tylenol)
Celecoxib (Celebrex)
Diclofenac (Cataflam, Pennsaid, Voltaren)
Duloxetine (Cymbalta)
Etodolac (Lodine)
Flurbiprofen (Ansaid)
Ibuprofen (Motrin)
Ketoprofen (Orudis)
Meloxicam (Mobic)
Nabumetone (Relafen)
Naproxen (Naprosyn)
Sulindac (Clinoril)
Tramadol (Ultram)

**Osteoporosis**
Alendronate (Fosamax)
Calcitonin (Miacalcin)
Calcium salts
Conjugated estrogens/bazedoxifene (Duavee)
Denosumab (Prolia)
Ibandronate (Boniva)
Raloxifene (Evista)
Risedronate (Actonel)
Teriparatide (Forteo)
Vitamin D
Zoledronic acid (Reclast)

**Paget's disease**
Alendronate (Fosamax)
Calcitonin (Miacalcin)
Etidronate (Didronel)
Pamidronate (Aredia)
Risedronate (Actonel)
Tiludronate (Skelid)
Zoledronic acid (Reclast)

**Pain, mild to moderate**
Acetaminophen (Tylenol)
Aspirin

Celecoxib (Celebrex)
Codeine
Diclofenac (Cataflam, Voltaren, Zipsor)
Diflunisal (Dolobid)
Etodolac (Lodine)
Flurbiprofen (Ansaid)
Ibuprofen (Advil, Caldolor, Motrin)
Ketorolac (Toradol)
Naproxen (Anaprox, Naprosyn)
Salsalate (Disalcid)
Tramadol (Ultram)

**Pain, moderate to severe**
Butorphanol (Stadol)
Fentanyl (Onsolis, Sublimaze)
Hydromorphone (Dilaudid)
Methadone (Dolophine)
Morphine (MS Contin)
Morphine/naltrexone (Embeda)
Nalbuphine (Nubain)
Oxycodone (OxyFast, Roxicodone)
Oxymorphone (Opana)
Ziconotide (Prialt)

**Panic attack disorder**
Alprazolam (Xanax)
Clonazepam (Klonopin)
Paroxetine (Paxil)
Sertraline (Zoloft)
Venlafaxine (Effexor)

**Parkinsonism**
Apomorphine (Apokyn)
Carbidopa/levodopa (Sinemet,
    Sinemet CR)
Entacapone (Comtan)
Pimavanserin (Nuplazid)
Pramipexole (Mirapex)
Rasagiline (Azilect)
Ropinirole (Requip)
Rotigotine (Neupro)
Selegiline (Eldepryl, Zelapar)
Tolcapone (Tasmar)

**Peptic ulcer disease**
Cimetidine (Tagamet)
Dexlansoprazole (Dexilant)
Esomeprazole (Nexium)
Famotidine (Pepcid)
Lansoprazole (Prevacid)
Nizatidine (Axid)

Omeprazole (Prilosec)
Pantoprazole (Protonix)
Rabeprazole (AcipHex)
Ranitidine (Zantac)
Sucralfate (Carafate)

**Pneumonia**
Amoxicillin (Amoxil)
Amoxicillin/clavulanate (Augmentin)
Ampicillin (Polycillin)
Azithromycin (Zithromax)
Cefaclor (Ceclor)
Cefpodoxime (Vantin)
Ceftriaxone (Rocephin)
Cefuroxime (Kefurox, Zinacef)
Clarithromycin (Biaxin)
Co-trimoxazole (Bactrim, Septra)
Erythromycin
Gentamicin (Garamycin)
Levofloxacin (Levaquin)
Linezolid (Zyvox)
Moxifloxacin (Avelox)
Piperacillin/tazobactam (Zosyn)
Tobramycin (Nebcin)
Vancomycin (Vancocin)

**Pneumonia, *Pneumocystis jiroveci***
Atovaquone (Mepron)
Clindamycin (Cleocin)
Co-trimoxazole (Bactrim, Septra)
Pentamidine (Pentam)
Trimethoprim (Proloprim)

**Post-traumatic stress disorder**
Amitriptyline (Elavil)
Aripiprazole (Abilify)
Citalopram (Celexa)
Escitalopram (Lexapro)
Fluoxetine (Prozac)
Imipramine (Tofranil)
Lamotrigine (Lamictal)
Olanzapine (Zyprexa)
Paroxetine (Paxil)
Phenelzine (Nardil)
Prazosin (Minipress)
Propranolol (Inderal)
Quetiapine (Seroquel)
Risperidone (Risperdal)
Sertraline (Zoloft)
Topiramate (Topamax)
Valproic acid (Depakote)

Venlafaxine (Effexor)
Ziprasidone (Geodon)

**Pruritus**
Amcinonide (Cyclocort)
Cetirizine (Zyrtec)
Clemastine (Tavist)
Clobetasol (Temovate)
Cyproheptadine (Periactin)
Desloratadine (Clarinex)
Desonide (Tridesilon)
Desoximetasone (Topicort)
Diphenhydramine (Benadryl)
Fluocinolone (Synalar)
Fluocinonide (Lidex)
Halobetasol (Ultravate)
Hydrocortisone (Cort-Dome, Hytone)
Hydroxyzine (Atarax, Vistaril)
Prednisolone (Prelone)
Prednisone (Deltasone)
Promethazine (Phenergan)

**Psychosis**
Aripiprazole (Abilify)
Asenapine (Saphris)
Brexpiprazole (Rexulti)
Cariprazine (Vraylar)
Chlorpromazine (Thorazine)
Clozapine (Clozaril)
Fluphenazine (Prolixin)
Haloperidol (Haldol)
Iloperidone (Fanapt)
Loxapine (Adasuve)
Lurasidone (Latuda)
Olanzapine (Zyprexa)
Quetiapine (Seroquel, Seroquel XR)
Risperidone (Risperdal)
Thioridazine (Mellaril)
Thiothixene (Navane)
Ziprasidone (Geodon)

**Pulmonary arterial hypertension**
Ambrisentan (Letairis)
Bosentan (Tracleer)
Epoprostenol (Flolan)
Iloprost (Ventavis)
Macitentan (Opsumit)
Riociguat (Adempas)
Sildenafil (Revatio)
Tadalafil (Adcirca)
Treprostinil (Remodulin, Tyvaso)

**Respiratory distress syndrome (RDS)**
Beractant (Survanta)
Calfactant (Infasurf)
Poractant alfa (Curosurf)

**Restless legs syndrome**
Cabergoline (Dostinex)
Carbidopa/levodopa (Sinemet)
Clonazepam (Klonopin)
Gabapentin (Horizant, Neurontin)
Levodopa
Oxycodone (Roxicodone)
Pramipexole (Mirapex)
Ropinirole (Requip)
Rotigotine (Neupro)
Tramadol (Ultram)
Zaleplon (Sonata)
Zolpidem (Ambien)

**Schizophrenia**
Aripiprazole (Abilify)
Asenapine (Saphris)
Brexpiprazole (Rexulti)
Cariprazine (Vraylar)
Chlorpromazine (Thorazine)
Clozapine (Clozaril)
Fluphenazine (Prolixin)
Haloperidol (Haldol)
Iloperidone (Fanapt)
Lurasidone (Latuda)
Olanzapine (Zyprexa)
Paliperidone (Invega, Invega Sustenna)
Quetiapine (Seroquel, Seroquel XR)
Risperidone (Risperdal)
Thioridazine (Mellaril)
Thiothixene (Navane)
Ziprasidone (Geodon)

**Smoking cessation**
Bupropion (Zyban)
Clonidine (Catapres)
Nicotine (NicoDerm, Nicotrol)
Nortriptyline (Pamelor)
Varenicline (Chantix)

**Thrombosis**
Apixaban (Eliquis)
Dalteparin (Fragmin)
Edoxaban (Savaysa)
Enoxaparin (Lovenox)
Fondaparinux (Arixtra)

Heparin
Tinzaparin (Innohep)
Warfarin (Coumadin)

**Thyroid disorders**
Levothyroxine (Levoxyl, Synthroid)
Liothyronine (Cytomel)
Thyroid

**Transient ischemic attack (TIA)**
Aspirin
Clopidogrel (Plavix)
Prasugrel (Effient)
Warfarin (Coumadin)

**Tremor**
Atenolol (Tenormin)
Chlordiazepoxide (Librium)
Diazepam (Valium)
Lorazepam (Ativan)
Metoprolol (Lopressor)
Nadolol (Corgard)
Propranolol (Inderal)

**Tuberculosis (TB)**
Bedaquiline (Sirturo)
Cycloserine (Seromycin)
Ethambutol (Myambutol)
Isoniazid (INH)
Pyrazinamide
Rifabutin (Mycobutin)
Rifampin (Rifadin)
Rifapentine (Priftin)

**Urticaria**
Cetirizine (Zyrtec)
Cimetidine (Tagamet)
Clemastine (Tavist)
Cyproheptadine (Periactin)
Diphenhydramine (Benadryl)
Hydroxyzine (Atarax, Vistaril)
Loratadine (Claritin)

Promethazine (Phenergan)
Ranitidine (Zantac)

**Vertigo**
Dimenhydrinate (Dramamine)
Diphenhydramine (Benadryl)
Meclizine (Antivert)
Scopolamine (Trans-Derm Scop)

**Vomiting**
Aprepitant (Emend)
Chlorpromazine (Thorazine)
Dexamethasone (Decadron)
Dimenhydrinate (Dramamine)
Dronabinol (Marinol)
Droperidol (Inapsine)
Fosaprepitant (Emend)
Granisetron (Kytril)
Hydroxyzine (Vistaril)
Lorazepam (Ativan)
Meclizine (Antivert)
Metoclopramide (Reglan)
Nabilone (Cesamet)
Ondansetron (Zofran)
Palonosetron (Aloxi)
Prochlorperazine (Compazine)
Promethazine (Phenergan)
Rolapitant (Varubi)
Scopolamine (Trans-Derm Scop)
Trimethobenzamide (Tigan)

**Zollinger-Ellison syndrome**
Aluminum salts
Cimetidine (Tagamet)
Esomeprazole (Nexium)
Famotidine (Pepcid)
Lansoprazole (Prevacid)
Omeprazole (Prilosec)
Pantoprazole (Protonix)
Rabeprazole (AcipHex)
Ranitidine (Zantac)

# DRUG CLASSIFICATION CONTENTS

# Allergic Rhinitis Nasal Preparations

## USES

Relieve symptoms associated with allergic rhinitis. These symptoms include rhinorrhea, nasal congestion, pruritus, sneezing, postnasal drip, nasal pain.

Allergic rhinitis or hay fever is an inflammation of the nasal airways occurring when an allergen (e.g., pollen) is inhaled. This triggers antibody production. The antibodies bind to mast cells, which contain histamine. Histamine is released, causing symptoms of allergic rhinitis.

## ACTION

**Intranasal corticosteroids:** Depress migration of polymorphonuclear leucocytes and fibroblasts, reverse capillary permeability, and stabilize nasal membranes to prevent/control inflammation.

**Intranasal antihistamines:** Reduce histamine-mediated symptoms of allergic rhinitis, including pruritus, sneezing, rhinorrhea, watery eyes.

**Intranasal mast cell stabilizers:** Inhibit the mast cell release of histamine and other inflammatory mediators.

**Intranasal anticholinergics:** Block acetylcholine in the nasal mucosa. Effective in treating rhinorrhea associated with allergic rhinitis.

**Intranasal decongestants:** Vasoconstrict the respiratory mucosa, provide short-term relief of nasal congestion.

## CORTICOSTEROIDS

| Generic (Brand) | Adult Dose | Pediatric Dose | Side Effects |
|---|---|---|---|
| **Beclomethasone (Beconase AQ) (Qnasl)** | Beconase AQ: 1–2 sprays in each nostril 2 times/day<br>Qnasl: 80 mcg/spray: 2 sprays in each nostril once daily | Beconase AQ: 6–12 yrs: 1–2 sprays in each nostril 2 times/day<br>Qnasl: 4–11 yrs: 40 mcg/spray: 1 spray in each nostril once daily | Altered taste and smell, epistaxis, burning, stinging, headache, nasal septum perforation |
| **Budesonide (Rhinocort Allergy Spray, Rhinocort Aqua)** | Rhinocort Aqua: 1–4 sprays in each nostril daily<br>Rhinocort Allergy Spray: 1–2 sprays in each nostril once daily | Rhinocort Allergy Spray, Rhinocort Aqua: 6–11 yrs: 1–2 sprays in each nostril daily | Bronchospasm, cough, epistaxis, nasal/throat irritation |
| **Ciclesonide (Omnaris, Zetonna)** | Omnaris: 2 sprays in each nostril daily<br>Zetonna: 1 spray in each nostril daily | Omnaris: 6–11 yrs: 2 sprays in each nostril daily (seasonal allergic rhinitis only) | Fever, headache, nausea, cough, epistaxis, nasal septum disorder |

| Generic (Brand) | Adult Dose | Pediatric Dose | Side Effects |
| --- | --- | --- | --- |
| **Flunisolide (Nasalide)** | 2 sprays in each nostril 2 or 3 times/day (maximum: 8 sprays in each nostril daily) | 6–14 yrs: 2 sprays in each nostril 2 times/day or 1 spray in each nostril 3 times/day (maximum: 4 sprays in each nostril daily) | Nasal burning/stinging, nasal dryness/irritation |
| **Fluticasone (Flonase, Flonase Allergy Relief)** | Flonase, Flonase Allergy Relief: 1–2 sprays in each nostril once daily | Flonase: 4–17 yrs: 1–2 sprays in each nostril daily; Flonase Allergy Relief: 4–11 yrs: 1 spray in each nostril once daily | Dizziness, fever, headache, nausea, cough, epistaxis |
| **Fluticasone/Azelastine (Dymista)** | 1 spray in each nostril 2 times/day | Not indicated in children younger than 6 yrs | Same as fluticasone and azelastine |
| **Fluticasone (Flonase Sensimist, Veramyst)** | 1–2 sprays in each nostril daily | 2–11 yrs: 1–2 sprays in each nostril daily | Same as fluticasone |
| **Mometasone (Nasonex)** | 2 sprays in each nostril daily | 2–11 yrs: 1 spray in each nostril daily | Headache, nasopharyngitis, sinusitis |
| **Triamcinolone (Nasacort Allergy 24 HR, Nasacort AQ)** | 1–2 sprays in each nostril daily | 2–5 yrs: 1 spray in each nostril once daily; 6–11 yrs: 1–2 sprays in each nostril daily | Bronchitis, chest congestion, cough, epistaxis, pharyngitis, sinusitis |

## ANTIHISTAMINES

| Generic (Brand) | Adult Dose | Pediatric Dose | Side Effects |
| --- | --- | --- | --- |
| **Azelastine (Astelin) Astepro 0.15%** | Astelin: 1–2 sprays in each nostril 2 times/day Astepro 0.15%: 1–2 sprays in each nostril two times/day or 2 sprays each nostril once daily (for seasonal allergic rhinitis) | Astelin: 5–11 yrs: 1 spray in each nostril 2 times/day | Sedation, epistaxis, nasal irritation |
| **Azelastine/Fluticasone (Dymista)** | 1 spray in each nostril 2 times/day | Not approved for children younger than 6 yrs | Same as azelastine and fluticasone |
| **Olopatadine (Patanase)** | 2 sprays in each nostril 2 times/day | 6–11 yrs: 1 spray in each nostril 2 times/day | Same as azelastine |

## MAST CELL STABILIZERS

| Generic (Brand) | Adult Dose | Pediatric Dose | Side Effects |
|---|---|---|---|
| **Cromolyn** (Nasalcrom) | 1 spray in each nostril 3–6 times/day | 2–11 yrs: 1 spray in each nostril 3–6 times/day | Nasal irritation, unpleasant taste |

## ANTICHOLINERGICS

| Generic (Brand) | Adult Dose | Pediatric Dose | Side Effects |
|---|---|---|---|
| **Ipratropium** (Atrovent) 0.03% | 2 sprays in each nostril 2–3 times/day | 6–12 yrs: 2 sprays in each nostril 2–3 times/day | Nasal irritation, epistaxis, dizziness, headache, blurry vision |
| **Ipratropium** (Atrovent) 0.06% | 2 sprays in each nostril 3–4 times/day | 5–12 yrs: 2 sprays in each nostril 3 times/day | Same as ipratropium 0.03% |

## DECONGESTANTS

| Generic (Brand) | Adult Dose | Pediatric Dose | Side Effects |
|---|---|---|---|
| **Oxymetazoline** (Afrin) | 2–3 drops or sprays 2 times/day | 2–3 drops or sprays 2 times/day | Insomnia, tachycardia, nervousness, nausea, vomiting, transient burning, headache, rebound congestion if used longer than 72 hrs |
| **Phenylephrine** (Neo-Synephrine) | 2–3 drops or 1–2 sprays q4h as needed (0.25% or 0.5%) | 6–11 yrs: 2–3 drops (0.25%) q4h as needed; 1–5 yrs: 2–3 drops (0.125%) q4h as needed | Restlessness, nervousness, headache, rebound nasal congestion, burning, stinging, dryness |

# Angiotensin-Converting Enzyme (ACE) Inhibitors

## USES

Treatment of hypertension (HTN), adjunctive therapy for heart failure (HF).

## ACTION

*Antihypertensive:* Inhibits angiotensin-converting enzyme (ACE). ACE catalyzes conversion of angiotensin I to angiotensin II, a potent vasoconstrictor that also stimulates aldosterone secretion by adrenal cortex. Beneficial effects in HTN/HF appear to be suppression of the renin-angiotensin-aldosterone system. Reduces peripheral arterial resistance.

*HF:* Decreases peripheral vascular resistance (afterload), pulmonary capillary wedge pressure (preload); improves cardiac output, exercise tolerance.

## ACE INHIBITORS

| Name | Availability | Uses | Dosage Range (per day) | Side Effects |
|------|-------------|------|------------------------|--------------|
| **Benazepril (Lotensin)** | **T:** 5 mg, 10 mg, 20 mg, 40 mg | HTN | **HTN:** Initially, 10 mg/day. Usual dose: 10–40 mg/day. | Headaches, dizziness, fatigue, cough |
| **Captopril (Capoten)** | **T:** 12.5 mg, 25 mg, 50 mg, 100 mg | HTN<br>HF | **HTN:** Initially, 12.5–25 mg 2–3 times/day. Usual dose: 50–100 mg 2 times/day.<br>**HF:** Initially, 6.25 mg 3 times/day. Target: 50 mg 3 times/day. | Insomnia, headaches, dizziness, fatigue, GI complaints, cough, rash |
| **Enalapril (Vasotec)** | **T:** 2.5 mg, 5 mg, 10 mg, 20 mg<br>**IV:** 1.25 mg/ml | HTN<br>HF | **HTN:** Initially, 2.5–5 mg/day; may increase at 1–2 wk intervals. Usual dose: 10–40 mg/day.<br>**HF:** Initially, 2.5 mg 2 times/day, may increase at 1–2 wk intervals. Target: 20 mg/day in 1–2 divided doses. | Chest pain, hypotension, headaches, fatigue, dizziness |
| **Fosinopril (Monopril)** | **T:** 10 mg, 20 mg, 40 mg | HTN<br>HF | **HTN:** Initially, 10 mg/day. Usual dose: 10–40 mg/day.<br>**HF:** Initially, 5–10 mg/day. Target: 10–40 mg/day. | Hypotension, nausea, vomiting, cough |

*Continued*

## ACE INHIBITORS—cont'd

| Name | Availability | Uses | Dosage Range (per day) | Side Effects |
|---|---|---|---|---|
| Lisinopril (Prinivil, Zestril) | **T:** 2.5 mg, 5 mg, 10 mg, 20 mg, 40 mg | HTN HF | **HTN:** Initially, 5–10 mg/day. Usual dose: 10–40 mg/day. **HF:** Initially, 2.5–5 mg/day. Target: 20–40 mg/day. | Chest pain, hypotension, headaches, dizziness, fatigue, diarrhea |
| Moexipril (Univasc) | **T:** 7.5 mg, 15 mg | HTN | **HTN:** Initially, 3.75–7.5 mg/day. Usual dose: 7.5–30 mg/day in 1–2 divided doses. | Dizziness, fatigue, diarrhea, cough |
| Perindopril (Aceon) | **T:** 2 mg, 4 mg, 6 mg | HTN | **HTN:** Initially, 4 mg/day. May increase at 1–2 wk intervals. Usual dose: 4–8 mg/day. | Hypotension, dizziness, fatigue, syncope, cough |
| Quinapril (Accupril) | **T:** 5 mg, 10 mg, 20 mg, 40 mg | HTN HF | **HTN:** Initially, 10–20 mg once daily. Usual dose: 10–40 mg once daily. **HF:** Initially, 5 mg 2 times/day. Titrate to 20–40 mg/day in 2 divided doses. | Chest pain, hypotension, headaches, dizziness, fatigue, diarrhea, nausea, vomiting, cough |
| Ramipril (Altace) | **C:** 1.25 mg, 2.5 mg, 5 mg, 10 mg | HTN HF | **HTN:** Initially, 2.5 mg once daily. Usual dose: 5–10 mg/day. **HF:** Initially, 1.25–2.5 mg once daily. Target: 10 mg once daily. | Hypotension, headaches, dizziness, cough |
| Trandolapril (Mavik) | **T:** 1 mg, 2 mg, 4 mg | HTN HF | **HTN:** Initially, 1–2 mg once daily. Usual dose: 2–8 mg/day. **HF:** Initially, 1 mg once daily. Target: 4 mg once daily. | Dizziness, dyspepsia, cough, asthenia (loss of strength, energy), syncope, myalgia |

*C*, Capsules; *HF*, heart failure; *HTN*, hypertension; *T*, tablets.

# Angiotensin II Receptor Antagonists

## USES

Treatment of hypertension (HTN) alone or in combination with other antihypertensives. Treatment of heart failure (HF).

## ACTION

Angiotensin II receptor antagonists (AIIRA) block vasoconstrictor and aldosterone-secreting effects on angiotensin II by selectively blocking the binding of angiotensin II

to $AT_1$ receptors in vascular smooth muscle and the adrenal gland, causing vasodilation and a decrease in aldosterone effects.

## ANGIOTENSIN II RECEPTOR ANTAGONISTS

| Name | Availability | Uses | Dosage Range (per day) | Side Effects |
|---|---|---|---|---|
| Azilsartan (Edarbi) | T: 40 mg, 80 mg | HTN | 40–80 mg once daily | Diarrhea, hypotension, muscle spasms, weakness |
| Candesartan (Atacand) | T: 4 mg, 8 mg, 16 mg, 32 mg | HTN HF | Initially, 16 mg once daily. Usual dose: 8–32 mg in 1–2 divided doses Initially 4–8 mg once daily. Double dose at 2 wk intervals. Target: 32 mg once daily. | Headaches, upper respiratory tract infection, pain, dizziness |
| Eprosartan (Teveten) | T: 400 mg, 600 mg | HTN | Initially, 600 mg/day. Usual dose: 600–800 mg in 1–2 divided doses | Headaches, upper respiratory tract infection, myalgia |
| Irbesartan (Avapro) | T: 75 mg, 150 mg, 300 mg | HTN Nephropathy | 150–300 mg once daily 300 mg once daily | Headaches, upper respiratory tract infection |
| Losartan (Cozaar) | T: 25 mg, 50 mg, 100 mg | HTN Nephropathy | Initially, 50 mg once daily. Usual dose: 25–100 mg/day. Initially, 50 mg/day; may increase to 100 mg/day. | Dizziness, headaches, upper respiratory tract infection, diarrhea, fatigue, cough |

*Continued*

## ANGIOTENSIN II RECEPTOR ANTAGONISTS—cont'd

| Name | Availability | Uses | Dosage Range (per day) | Side Effects |
|---|---|---|---|---|
| **Olmesartan (Benicar)** | **T:** 5 mg, 20 mg, 40 mg | HTN | Initially, 20 mg once daily. May increase to 40 mg once daily after 2 wks. | Headaches, upper respiratory tract infection, flu-like symptoms, dizziness, bronchitis, rhinitis, back pain, pharyngitis, sinusitis, diarrhea, peripheral edema |
| **Telmisartan (Micardis)** | **T:** 40 mg, 80 mg | HTN | Initially 40 mg once daily. Usual dose: 40–80 mg once daily. | Upper respiratory tract infection, dizziness, back pain, sinusitis, diarrhea |
| | | CV risk reduction | 80 mg once daily | |
| **Valsartan (Diovan)** | **T:** 80 mg, 160 mg | HTN | Initially, 80 or 160 mg once daily. Usual dose: 80–320 mg once daily | Dizziness, headaches, upper respiratory tract infection, diarrhea, fatigue |
| | | HF | Initially 20–40 mg 2 times/day. Titrate to 80–160 mg 2 times/day. | |
| | | Post MI | Initially, 20 mg 2 times/day. Titrate to target of 160 mg 2 times/day | |

*CV,* Cardiovascular; *HF,* heart failure; *HTN,* hypertension; *MI,* myocardial infarction; *T,* tablets.

# Antacids

## USES

Relief of symptoms associated with hyperacidity (e.g., heartburn, acid indigestion, sour stomach), hyperacidity associated with gastric/duodenal ulcers, treatment of pathologic gastric hypersecretion associated with Zollinger-Ellison syndrome, symptomatic treatment of gastroesophageal reflux disease (GERD), prevention and treatment of upper GI stress-induced ulceration and bleeding (esp. in intensive care unit [ICU]).

Aluminum hydroxide in conjunction with a low-phosphate diet to reduce elevated phosphate in pts with renal insufficiency. Calcium for calcium deficiency; magnesium for magnesium deficiency.

## ACTION

Antacids act primarily in the stomach to neutralize gastric acid (increase pH) and reduce the amount of acid refluxed into the esophagus or emptied into the duodenum. Antacids do not have a direct effect on acid output. The ability to increase pH depends on the dose, dosage form used, presence or absence of food in the stomach, and acid-neutralizing capacity (ANC). ANC is the number of mEq of hydrochloric acid that can be neutralized by a particular weight or volume of antacid.

Antacids reduce elevated phosphate by binding with phosphate in the intestine to form an insoluble complex, which is then eliminated.

## ANTACIDS

| Antacid | Brand Names | Availability | Dosage Range | Side Effects |
|---|---|---|---|---|
| **Aluminum** | | | | |
| **Hydroxide** | Amphojel, Alternagel | L: 320 mg/5 ml | **C:** 300–900 mg between meals and at bedtime. **A:** 600–1,200 mg between meals and at bedtime | Chalky taste, mild constipation, abdominal cramps, nausea, fecal discoloration, vomiting, hypophosphatemia, aluminum toxicity, osteomalacia |

*Continued*

**ANTACIDS—cont'd**

| Antacid | Brand Names | Availability | Dosage Range | Side Effects |
|---|---|---|---|---|
| **Calcium** | | | | |
| **Carbonate** | Tums, Caltrate 600 | **T (chewable):** 500 mg, 750 mg, 1,000 mg<br>**T:** 1,250 mg, 1,500 mg | **C:** (2–4 yrs): 375–400 mg/day. **Maximum:** 1,500 mg; (5–11 yrs): 750–800 mg/day. **Maximum:** 3,000 mg.<br>**C:** (>12 yrs), A: **Maximum:** 8,000 mg/day. | Abdominal pain, acid rebound, constipation, nausea, vomiting, xerostomia, milk-alkali syndrome (with chronic high doses or renal failure) |
| **Magnesium** | | | | |
| **Hydroxide** | Milk of Magnesia | **T (chewable):** 400 mg<br>**L:** 400 mg/5 ml, 1,200 mg/5 ml | **Liquid:**<br>**C:** 2.5–5 ml up to 4 times/day<br>**A:** 5–15 ml up to 4 times/day<br>**Tablet:**<br>**C:** 1 tablet up to 4 times/day<br>**A:** 2–4 tablets up to 4 times/day | Chalky taste, diarrhea, laxative effect, electrolyte imbalance (dizziness, irregular heartbeat, fatigue) |
| **Oxide** | Mag-Ox 400 | **T:** 400 mg | 400–800 mg/day | Diarrhea with excessive doses |

*A,* Adults; *C,* children *L,* liquid; *T,* tablets.

# Antianxiety Agents

## USES

Treatment of anxiety including generalized anxiety disorder (GAD), panic disorder, obsessive-compulsive disorder (OCD), social anxiety disorder (SAD), post-traumatic stress disorder (PTSD), and acute stress disorder. In addition, some benzodiazepines are used as hypnotics, anticonvulsants to prevent delirium tremors during alcohol withdrawal, and as adjunctive therapy for relaxation of skeletal muscle spasms. Midazolam, a short-acting benzodiazepine, is used for preop sedation and relief of anxiety for short diagnostic/endoscopic procedures (see individual monograph for midazolam).

## ACTION

Benzodiazepines are the largest and most frequently prescribed group of antianxiety agents. The exact mechanism is unknown, but they may increase the inhibiting effect of gamma-aminobutyric acid (GABA), which inhibits its nerve impulse transmission by binding to specific benzodiazepine receptors in various areas of the central nervous system (CNS).

◄**ALERT**► Refer to individual entries of nonbenzodiazepine drugs for more information on uses and actions.

## ANTIANXIETY AGENTS

| Name | Availability | Uses | Dosage | Side Effects |
|---|---|---|---|---|
| **Benzodiazepine** | | | | |
| **Alprazolam (Xanax)** | **T:** 0.25 mg, 0.5 mg, 1 mg, 2 mg<br>**S:** 1 mg/ml<br>**ER:** 0.5 mg, 1 mg, 2 mg, 3 mg<br>**ODT:** 0.25 mg, 0.5 mg, 1 mg, 2 mg | Anxiety, panic disorder | Initially, 0.25–0.5 mg 3 times/day. May increase every 3–4 days. Maximum: 4 mg/day. | Drowsiness, weakness, fatigue, ataxia, slurred speech, confusion, lack of coordination, impaired memory, paradoxical agitation, dizziness, nausea |

*Continued*

## ANTIANXIETY AGENTS—cont'd

| Name | Availability | Uses | Dosage | Side Effects |
|---|---|---|---|---|
| **Chlordiazepoxide (Librium)** | **C:** 5 mg, 10 mg, 25 mg<br>**T:** 10 mg, 25 mg<br>**I:** 100 mg | Anxiety, alcohol withdrawal | Anxiety: 5–10 mg 3–4 times/day up to 20–25 mg 3–4 times/day.<br>Alcohol withdrawal:<br>Initially, 50–100 mg. May increase to 300 mg/24 hrs. | Drowsiness, fatigue, ataxia, memory impairment |
| **Clorazepate (Tranxene)** | **T:** 3.75 mg, 7.5 mg, 15 mg<br>**SD:** 11.25 mg, 22.5 mg | Anxiety, alcohol withdrawal, anticonvulsant | 7.5–15 mg 2–4 times/day. | Hypotension, drowsiness, fatigue, ataxia, memory impairment, headache, nausea |
| **Diazepam (Valium)** | **T:** 2 mg, 5 mg, 10 mg<br>**S:** 5 mg/5 ml<br>**I:** 5 mg/ml | Anxiety, alcohol withdrawal, anticonvulsant, muscle relaxant | 2–10 mg, 2–4 times/day. | Hypotension, ataxia, drowsiness, fatigue, vertigo |
| **Lorazepam (Ativan)** | **T:** 0.5 mg, 1 mg, 2 mg<br>**S:** 2 mg/ml<br>**I:** 2 mg/ml, 4 mg/ml | Anxiety, alcohol withdrawal | Initially, 2–3 mg/day in 2–3 divided doses. Usual dose: 2–6 mg/day in divided doses. | Sedation, respiratory depression, ataxia, dizziness, headache |
| Nonbenzodiazepine | | | | |
| **Buspirone (BuSpar)** | **T:** 5 mg, 7.5 mg, 10 mg, 15 mg, 30 mg | Anxiety | Initially, 7.5 mg 2 times/day. May increase every 2–3 days by 2.5 mg bid. Maximum: 30 mg 2 times/day. | Dizziness, light-headedness, headaches, nausea, restlessness |
| **Hydroxyzine (Atarax, Vistaril)** | **T:** 10 mg, 25 mg, 50 mg<br>**C:** 25 mg, 50 mg, 100 mg<br>**S:** 10 mg/5 ml | Anxiety | 50–100 mg 4 times/day | Drowsiness; dry mouth, nose, and throat |

| | | | | |
|---|---|---|---|---|
| **Paroxetine (Paxil)** | **S:** 10 mg/5 ml<br>**T:** 10 mg, 20 mg, 30 mg, 40 mg<br>**T (CR):** 12.5 mg, 25 mg, 37.5 mg | Anxiety, depression, obsessive-compulsive disorder, panic disorder | Initially, 20 mg once daily. May increase by 10 mg/day at 1 wk intervals up to 50 mg/day.<br>**CR:** Initially, 12.5 mg/day. May increase by 12.5 mg/day at 1 wk intervals up to 37.5 mg/day. | Drowsiness; dry mouth, nose, and throat; dizziness, diarrhea, diaphoresis, constipation, vomiting, tremors |
| **Venlafaxine (Effexor)** | **C (ER):** 37.5 mg, 75 mg, 150 mg<br>**T (ER):** 37.5 mg, 75 mg, 150 mg | Anxiety, depression | Initially 37.5–75 mg once daily. May increase by 75 mg/day at least every 4 days up to 225 mg/day. | Drowsiness, nausea, headaches, dry mouth |

*C,* Capsules; *CR,* controlled-release; *ER,* extended-release; *I,* injection; *ODT,* orally disintegrating tablet; *S,* solution; *SD,* single dose; *T,* tablets.

# Antiarrhythmics

## USES

Prevention and treatment of cardiac arrhythmias, such as premature ventricular contractions, ventricular tachycardia, premature atrial contractions, paroxysmal atrial tachycardia, atrial fibrillation and flutter.

## ACTION

The antiarrhythmics are divided into four classes based on their effects on certain ion channels and/or receptors located on the myocardial cell membrane. Class I is further divided into three subclasses (IA, IB, IC) based on electrophysiologic effects.

*Class I:* Blocks cardiac sodium channels and slows conduction velocity, prolonging refractory period and decreasing automaticity of sodium-dependent tissue.

*Class IA:* Blocks sodium and potassium channels.

*Class IB:* Shortens the repolarization phase.

*Class IC:* No effect on repolarization phase, but slows conduction velocity.

*Class II:* Slows sinus and atrioventricular (AV) nodal conduction.

*Class III:* Blocks cardiac potassium channels, prolonging the repolarization phase of electrical cells.

*Class IV:* Inhibits the influx of calcium through its channels, causing slower conduction through the sinus and AV nodes.

## ANTIARRHYTHMICS

| Name | Availability | Uses | Dosage Range | Side Effects |
|---|---|---|---|---|
| **Class IA** | | | | |
| **Disopyramide** (Norpace, Norpace CR) | **C:** 100 mg, 150 mg **C (ER):** 100 mg, 150 mg | AF, WPW, PSVT, PVCs, VT | **C:** 100–200 mg q6h. **ER:** 200–400 mg q12h. | Dry mouth, blurred vision, urinary retention, HF, proarrhythmia, heart block, nausea, vomiting, diarrhea, hypoglycemia, nervousness |
| **Procainamide** (Procan-SR, Pronestyl) | **I:** 100 mg/ml, 500 mg/ml | AF, WPW, PVCs, VT | Loading dose: 15–18 mg/kg over 20–30 min. Maintenance dose: 1–4 mg/min as a continuous infusion. | Hypotension, fever, agranulocytosis, SLE, headaches, proarrhythmia, confusion, disorientation, GI symptoms, hypotension |

| | | | | |
|---|---|---|---|---|
| **Quinidine (Quinaglute, Quinidex)** | **T:** 200 mg, 300 mg **T (ER):** 300 mg, 324 mg **I:** 80 mg/ml | AF, WPW, PVCs, VT | **A (PO):** 400 mg q6h **(ER):** 300–q8–12h or 648 mg q8h. | Diarrhea, hypotension, nausea, vomiting, cinchonism, fever, bitter taste, heart block, thrombocytopenia, proarrhythmia |
| Class IB | | | | |
| **Lidocaine (Xylocaine)** | **I:** 300 mg for IM **IV Infusion:** 2 mg/ml, 4 mg/ml | PVCs, VT, VF | **IV:** Initially, 1–1.5 mg/kg. May repeat 0.5–0.75 mg/kg q5–10 min. Maximum cumulative dose: 3 mg/kg, then 1–4 mg/min infusion | Drowsiness, agitation, muscle twitching, seizures, paresthesia, proarrhythmia, slurred speech, tinnitus, cardiac depression, bradycardia, asystole |
| **Mexiletine (Mexitil)** | **C:** 150 mg, 200 mg, 250 mg | PVCs, VT, VF | **A:** Initially, 200 mg q8h. Adjust every 2–3 days in 50–100 mg increments. Maximum: 1,200 mg/day. | Drowsiness, agitation, muscle twitching, seizures, paresthesia, proarrhythmia, nausea, vomiting, blood dyscrasias, hepatitis, fever |
| Class IC | | | | |
| **Flecainide (Tambocor)** | **T:** 50 mg, 100 mg, 150 mg | AF, PSVT, life-threatening ventricular arrhythmias | **A:** Initially, 100 mg q12h. May increase by 50 mg q12h at 4 day intervals. Maximum: 400 mg/day. | Dizziness, tremors, bradycardia, heart block, HF, GI upset, neutropenia, flushing, blurred vision, metallic taste, proarrhythmia |
| **Propafenone (Rythmol)** | **T:** 150 mg, 225 mg, 300 mg **ER:** 225 mg, 325 mg, 425 mg | PAF, WPW, life-threatening ventricular arrhythmias | **A: T:** Initially, 150 mg q8h. May increase at 3–4 day intervals up to 300 mg q8h. **ER:** Initially, 225 mg q12h. May increase at a minimum of 5 days up to 425 mg q12h. | Dizziness, blurred vision, altered taste, nausea, exacerbation of asthma, proarrhythmia, bradycardia, heart block, HF, GI upset, bronchospasm, hepatotoxicity |

*Continued*

## ANTIARRHYTHMICS—cont'd

| Name | Availability | Uses | Dosage Range | Side Effects |
|---|---|---|---|---|
| **Class II (Beta-Blockers)** | | | | |
| **Acebutolol (Sectral)** | **C:** 100 mg, 200 mg, 400 mg | Ventricular arrhythmias | **A:** Initially, 200 mg 2 times/day. Maintenance: 600–1200 mg/day in divided doses. | Bradycardia, hypotension, depression, nightmares, fatigue, sexual dysfunction, SLE, arthritis, myalgia |
| **Esmolol (Brevibloc)** | **I:** 10 mg/ml | Supraventricular tachycardia | **A:** 50–200 mcg/kg/min | Hypotension, heart block, HF, bronchospasm |
| **Propranolol (Inderal)** | **T:** 10 mg, 20 mg, 40 mg | Tachyarrhythmias | **A:** Initially, 10–30 mg 3–4 times/day Maintenance: 10–40 mg 3–4 times/day | Bradycardia, hypotension, depression, nightmares, fatigue, sexual dysfunction, heart block, bronchospasm |
| **Class III** | | | | |
| **Amiodarone (Cordarone, Pacerone)** | **T:** 100 mg, 200 mg, 400 mg **I:** 50 mg/ml | AF, PAF, PSVT, life-threatening ventricular arrhythmias | **A (PO):** 800–1,600 mg/day in divided doses for 1–3 wks, then 600–800 mg/day in divided doses **(IV):** 150 mg bolus, then 900 mg over 18 hrs | Blurred vision, photophobia, constipation, ataxia, proarrhythmia, pulmonary fibrosis, bradycardia, heart block, hyperthyroidism or hypothyroidism, peripheral neuropathy, GI upset, blue-gray skin, optic neuritis, hypotension |
| **Dofetilide (Tikosyn)** | **C:** 125 mcg, 250 mcg, 500 mcg | AF, A flutter | **A:** Individualized | Torsades de pointes, hypotension |
| **Dronedarone (Multaq)** | **T:** 400 mg | AF, A flutter | **A (PO):** 400 mg 2 times/day | Diarrhea, nausea, abdominal pain, vomiting, asthenia |

| | | | |
|---|---|---|---|
| **Ibutilide (Corvert)** | **I:** 0.1 mg/ml | AF, A flutter | **A (greater than 60 kg):** 1 mg over 10 min; **(less than 60 kg):** 0.01 mg/kg over 10 min | Torsades de pointes |
| **Sotalol (Betapace)** | **T:** 80 mg, 120 mg, 160 mg | AF, PAF, PSVT, life-threatening ventricular arrhythmias | **A:** Initially, 80 mg 2 times/day. May increase at 3 day intervals up to 160 mg 2 times/day. | Fatigue, dizziness, dyspnea, bradycardia, proarrhythmia, heart block, hypotension, bronchospasm |
| **Class IV (Calcium Channel Blockers)** | | | | |
| **Diltiazem (Cardizem)** | **I:** 25 mg/ml vials<br>**Infusion:** 1 mg/ml | AF, A flutter, PSVT | **A (IV):** 20–25 mg bolus, then infusion of 5–15 mg/hr | Hypotension, bradycardia, dizziness, headaches, heart block, asystole, HF |
| **Verapamil (Calan, Isoptin)** | **I:** 5 mg/2 ml | AF, A flutter, PSVT | **A (IV):** 5–10 mg | Hypotension, bradycardia, dizziness, headaches, constipation, heart block, HF, asystole, fatigue, edema, nausea |

*A,* Adults; *AF,* atrial fibrillation; *A flutter,* atrial flutter; *C,* capsules; *HF,* heart failure; *ER,* extended-release; *I,* injection; *PAF,* paroxysmal atrial fibrillation; *PSVT,* paroxysmal supraventricular tachycardia; *PVCs,* premature ventricular contractions; *SLE,* systemic lupus erythematosus; *SR,* sustained-release; *T,* tablets; *VT,* ventricular tachycardia; *WPW,* Wolff-Parkinson-White syndrome.

# Antibiotics

## USES

Treatment of wide range of gram-positive or gram-negative bacterial infections, suppression of intestinal flora before surgery, control of acne, prophylactically to prevent rheumatic fever, prophylactically in high-risk situations (e.g., some surgical procedures or medical conditions) to prevent bacterial infection.

## ACTION

Antibiotics are natural or synthetic compounds that have the ability to kill or suppress the growth of microorganisms.

One means of classifying antibiotics is by their anti-microbial spectrum. Narrow-spectrum agents are effective against few microorganisms (e.g., aminoglycosides are effective against gram-negative aerobes), whereas broad-spectrum agents are effective against a wide variety of microorganisms (e.g., fluoroquinolones are effective against gram-positive cocci and gram-negative bacilli).

Antimicrobial agents may also be classified based on their mechanism of action.

- Agents that inhibit cell wall synthesis or activate enzymes that disrupt the cell wall, causing a weakening in the cell, cell lysis, and death. Include penicillins, cephalosporins, vancomycin, imidazole antifungal agents.
- Agents that act directly on the cell wall, affecting permeability of cell membranes, causing leakage of intracellular substances. Include antifungal agents amphotericin and nystatin, polymyxin, colistin.

- Agents that bind to ribosomal subunits, altering protein synthesis and eventually causing cell death. Include aminoglycosides.
- Agents that affect bacterial ribosome function, altering protein synthesis and causing slow microbial growth. Do not cause cell death. Include chloramphenicol, clindamycin, erythromycin, tetracyclines.
- Agents that inhibit nucleic acid metabolism by binding to nucleic acid or interacting with enzymes necessary for nucleic acid synthesis. Inhibit DNA or RNA synthesis. Include rifampin, metronidazole, fluoroquinolones (e.g., ciprofloxacin).
- Agents that inhibit specific metabolic steps necessary for microbial growth, causing a decrease in essential cell components or synthesis of nonfunctional analogues of normal metabolites. Include trimethoprim, sulfonamides.
- Agents that inhibit viral DNA synthesis by binding to viral enzymes necessary for DNA synthesis, preventing viral replication. Include acyclovir, vidarabine.

## SELECTION OF ANTIMICROBIAL AGENTS

The goal of therapy is to achieve antimicrobial action at the site of infection sufficient to inhibit the growth of the microorganism. The agent selected should be the most active against the most likely infecting organism, least likely to cause toxicity or allergic reaction. Factors to consider in selection of an antimicrobial agent include the following:

- Sensitivity pattern of the infecting microorganism
- Location and severity of infection (may determine route of administration)
- Pt's ability to eliminate the drug (status of renal and hepatic function)
- Pt's defense mechanisms (includes both cellular and humoral immunity)
- Pt's age, pregnancy status, genetic factors, allergies, CNS disorder, preexisting medical problems

## CATEGORIZATION OF ORGANISMS BY GRAM STAINING

| Gram-Positive Cocci | Gram-Negative Cocci | Gram-Positive Bacilli | Gram-Negative Bacilli |
|---|---|---|---|
| **Aerobic** | **Aerobic** | **Aerobic** | **Aerobic** |
| *Staphylococcus aureus* | *Neisseria gonorrhoeae* | *Listeria monocytogenes* | *Escherichia coli* |
| *Staphylococcus epidermidis* | *Neisseria meningitidis* | *Bacillus anthracis* | *Klebsiella pneumoniae* |
| *Streptococcus pneumoniae* | *Moraxella catarrhalis* | *Corynebacterium diphtheriae* | *Proteus mirabilis* |
| *Streptococcus pyogenes* | | **Anaerobic** | *Serratia marcescens* |
| *Viridans streptococci* | | *Clostridium difficile* | *Acinetobacter* spp. |
| *Enterococcus faecalis* | | *Clostridium perfringens* | *Pseudomonas aeruginosa* |
| *Enterococcus faecium* | | *Clostridium tetani* | *Enterobacter* spp. |
| **Anaerobic** | | *Actinomyces* spp. | *Haemophilus influenzae* |
| *Peptostreptococcus* spp. | | | *Legionella pneumophila* |
| *Peptococcus* spp. | | | **Anaerobic** |
| | | | *Bacteroides fragilis* |
| | | | *Fusobacterium* spp. |

# Antibiotic: Aminoglycosides

## USES

Treatment of serious infections when other less-toxic agents are not effective, are contraindicated, or require adjunctive therapy (e.g., with penicillins or cephalosporins). Used primarily in the treatment of infections caused by gram-negative microorganisms, such as those caused by *Proteus, Klebsiella, Pseudomonas, Escherichia coli,* *Serratia,* and *Enterobacter.* Inactive against most gram-positive microorganisms. Not well absorbed systemically from GI tract (must be administered parenterally for systemic infections). Oral agents are given to suppress intestinal bacteria.

## ACTION

Bactericidal. Transported across bacterial cell membrane; irreversibly bind to specific receptor proteins of bacterial ribosomes. Interfere with protein synthesis, preventing cell reproduction and eventually causing cell death.

## ANTIBIOTIC: AMINOGLYCOSIDES

| Name | Availability | Dosage Range | Side Effects |
|---|---|---|---|
| **Amikacin** | **I:** 50 mg/ml, 250 mg/ml | **A:** 5–7.5 mg/kg q8h or 15–20 mg/kg once daily <br> **C:** 5–7.5 mg/kg q8h | Nephrotoxicity, neurotoxicity, ototoxicity (both auditory and vestibular), hypersensitivity (skin itching, redness, rash, swelling) |
| **Gentamicin** | **I:** 10 mg/ml, 40 mg/ml | **A:** 4–7 mg/kg once daily or 1–2.5 mg/kg q8–12h <br> **C:** 2–2.5 mg/kg q8h | Same as amikacin |
| **Tobramycin** | **I:** 10 mg/ml, 40 mg/ml | **A:** 5–7 mg/kg once daily or 1–2.5 mg/kg q8h <br> **C:** 2–2.5 mg/kg q8h | Same as amikacin |

*A,* Adults; *C (dosage),* children; *I,* injection; *T,* tablets.

# Antibiotic: Cephalosporins

## USES

Broad-spectrum antibiotics, which, like penicillins, may be used in a number of diseases, including respiratory diseases, skin and soft tissue infection, bone/joint infections, genitourinary infections, prophylactically in some surgical procedures.

*First-generation cephalosporins* have activity against gram-positive organisms (e.g., streptococci and most staphylococci) and activity against most gram-negative organisms, including *Escherichia coli, Klebsiella pneumoniae, Proteus mirabilis, Salmonella,* and *Shigella.*

## ACTION

*Second-generation cephalosporins* have same effectiveness as first-generation and increased activity against gram-negative organisms, including *Haemophilus influenzae, Neisseria, Enterobacter,* and several anaerobic organisms.

*Third-generation cephalosporins* are less active against gram-positive organisms but more active against the Enterobacteriaceae with some activity against *Pseudomonas aeruginosa, Serratia* spp., and *Acinetobacter* spp.

*Fourth-generation cephalosporins* have good activity against gram-positive organisms (e.g., *Staphylococcus*

*aureus*) and gram-negative organisms (e.g., *Pseudomonas aeruginosa, E. coli, Klebsiella,* and *Proteus*).

*Fifth-generation cephalosporins* have good activity against gram-positive organisms (e.g., *Staphylococcus aureus, Streptococcus* spp.) and gram-negative organisms (e.g., *E. coli, Klebsiella* spp.).

Cephalosporins inhibit cell wall synthesis or activate enzymes that disrupt the cell wall, causing cell lysis and cell death. May be bacteriostatic or bactericidal. Most effective against rapidly dividing cells.

## ANTIBIOTIC: CEPHALOSPORINS

| Name | Availability | Dosage Range | Side Effects |
|---|---|---|---|
| **First-Generation** | | | |
| **Cefadroxil (Duricef)** | **C:** 500 mg<br>**T:** 1 g<br>**S:** 125 mg/5 ml, 250 mg/5 ml, 500 mg/5 ml | **A:** 500 mg–1 g<br>**C:** 15 mg/kg q12h | Abdominal cramps/pain, fever, nausea, vomiting, diarrhea, headaches, oral/vaginal candidiasis |
| **Cefazolin (Ancef)** | **I:** 500 mg, 1 g, 2 g | **A:** 500 mg–2 g q6–8h<br>**C:** 25–100 mg/kg/day divided q6–8h | Fever, rash, diarrhea, nausea, pain at injection site |

*Continued*

## ANTIBIOTIC: CEPHALOSPORINS—cont'd

| Name | Availability | Dosage Range | Side Effects |
|---|---|---|---|
| **Cephalexin (Keflex, Keftab)** | **C:** 250 mg, 500 mg<br>**T:** 250 mg, 500 mg, 1 g | **A:** 250 mg–1 g q6–12h<br>**C:** 25–100 mg/kg/day divided q6–8h | Headache, abdominal pain, diarrhea, nausea, dyspepsia |
| Second-Generation | | | |
| **Cefaclor (Ceclor)** | **C:** 250 mg, 500 mg<br>**T (ER):** 500 mg<br>**S:** 125 mg/5 ml, 187 mg/5 ml, 250 mg/5 ml, 375 mg/5 ml | **A:** 250–500 mg q8h<br>**ER:** 500 mg q12h<br>**C:** 20–40 mg/kg/day q8–12h | Rash, diarrhea, increased transaminases<br>May have serum sickness–like reaction |
| **Cefotetan** | **I:** 1 g, 2 g | **A:** 500 mg–3 g q12h<br>**C:** 20–40 mg/kg q12h | Diarrhea, increased AST, ALT, hypersensitivity reactions |
| **Cefoxitin (Mefoxin)** | **I:** 1 g, 2 g | **A:** 1–2 g q6–8h<br>**C:** 80–160 mg/kg/day divided q6h | Diarrhea |
| **Cefprozil (Cefzil)** | **T:** 250 mg, 500 mg<br>**S:** 125 mg/5 ml, 250 mg/5 ml | **A:** 500 mg q12–24h<br>**C:** 7.5–15 mg/kg q12h | Dizziness, abdominal pain, diarrhea, nausea, increased AST, ALT |
| **Cefuroxime (Ceftin, Kefurox, Zinacef)** | **T:** 125 mg, 250 mg, 500 mg<br>**S:** 125 mg/5 ml, 250 mg/5 ml<br>**I:** 750 mg, 1.5 g | **A (PO):** 125–500 mg q12h<br>**(IM/IV):** 750 mg–1.5 g q8–12h<br>**C (PO):** 10–15 mg/kg q12h<br>**(IM/IV):** 75–150 mg/kg/day divided q8h | Diarrhea, nausea, vomiting, thrombophlebitis, increased AST, ALT |
| Third-Generation | | | |
| **Cefdinir (Omnicef)** | **C:** 300 mg<br>**S:** 125 mg/5 ml | **A:** 300 mg q12h or 600 mg once daily<br>**C:** 7 mg/kg q12h or 14 mg/kg once daily | Headache, hyperglycemia, abdominal pain, diarrhea, nausea |

| Drug | | Dosage | Adverse effects |
|---|---|---|---|
| Cefditoren (Spectracef) | T: 200 mg, 400 mg | A: 200–400 mg q12h<br>C: (>11 yrs): 200–400 mg q12h | Diarrhea, nausea |
| Cefotaxime (Claforan) | I: 500 mg, 1 g, 2 g | A: 1–2 g q4–12h<br>C: 50–300 mg/kg/day divided q4-6h | Rash, diarrhea, nausea, pain at injection site |
| Cefpodoxime (Vantin) | T: 100 mg, 200 mg<br>S: 50 mg/5 ml, 100 mg/5 ml | A: 100–400 mg q12h<br>C: 5 mg/kg q12h | Rash, diarrhea, nausea |
| Ceftazidime (Fortaz, Tazicef, Tazidime) | I: 500 mg, 1 g, 2 g | A: 500 mg–2 g q8–12h<br>C: 30–50 mg/kg q8h | Diarrhea, pain at injection site |
| Ceftibuten (Cedax) | C: 400 mg<br>S: 90 mg/5 ml, 180 mg/5 ml | A: 400 mg once daily<br>C: 4.5 mg/kg bid or 9 mg/kg once daily | Headache, nausea, diarrhea |
| Ceftriaxone (Rocephin) | I: 250 mg, 500 mg, 1 g, 2 g | A: 1–2 g q12–24h<br>C: 50–100 mg/kg/day divided q12–24h | Rash, diarrhea, eosinophilia, increased AST, ALT |
| **Fourth-Generation** | | | |
| Cefepime (Maxipime) | I: 1 g, 2 g | A: 1–2 g q8–12h<br>C: 50 mg/kg q8–12h | Rash, diarrhea, nausea; increased AST, ALT |
| **Fifth-Generation** | | | |
| Ceftaroline (Teflaro) | I: 400 mg, 600 mg | A: 600 mg q12h | Headache, insomnia, rash, pruritus, diarrhea, nausea |
| **Fixed-Combinations** | | | |
| Ceftazidime/avibactam (Avycaz) | I: 2 g ceftazidime/0.5 g avibactam | A: 2.5 g q8h | Nausea, vomiting, constipation, anxiety |
| Ceftolozane/tazobactam (Zerbaxa) | I: 1 g ceftolozane/0.5 g tazobactam | A: 1.5 g q8h | Nausea, diarrhea, headache, pyrexia |

*A,* Adults; *C,* capsules; *C (dosage),* children; *ER,* extended-release; *I,* injection; *S,* suspension; *T,* tablets.

# Antibiotic: Fluoroquinolones

## USES

Fluoroquinolones act against a wide range of gram-negative and gram-positive organisms. They are used primarily in the treatment of lower respiratory infections, skin/skin structure infections, urinary tract infections, and sexually transmitted diseases.

## ACTION

Bactericidal. Inhibit DNA gyrase in susceptible microorganisms, interfering with bacterial DNA replication and repair.

## ANTIBIOTIC: FLUOROQUINOLONES

| Name | Availability | Dosage Range | Side Effects |
|---|---|---|---|
| **Ciprofloxacin (Cipro)** | **T:** 100 mg, 250 mg, 500 mg, 750 mg<br>**S:** 250 mg/5 ml, 500 mg/5 ml<br>**I:** 200 mg, 400 mg | **A (PO):** 250–750 mg q12h;<br>**(IV):** 200–400 mg q12h | Dizziness, headaches, anxiety, drowsiness, insomnia, abdominal pain, nausea, diarrhea, vomiting, phlebitis (parenteral) |
| **Gemifloxacin (Factive)** | **T:** 320 mg | **A:** 320 mg once daily | Headache, dizziness, rash, diarrhea, nausea |
| **Levofloxacin (Levaquin)** | **T:** 250 mg, 500 mg, 750 mg<br>**I:** 250 mg, 500 mg, 750 mg<br>**OS:** 250 mg/10 ml | **A (PO/IV):** 250–750 mg/day as single dose | Headache, insomnia, dizziness, rash, nausea, diarrhea, constipation |
| **Moxifloxacin (Avelox)** | **T:** 400 mg<br>**I:** 400 mg | **A:** 400 mg/day | Headache, dizziness, insomnia, nausea, diarrhea |
| **Ofloxacin** | **T:** 300 mg, 400 mg | **A:** 200–400 mg q12h | Dizziness, headache, insomnia, abdominal cramps, diarrhea, nausea |

*A*, Adults; *I*, injection; *OS*, oral solution; *PO*, oral; *S*, suspension; *T*, tablets.

# Antibiotic: Macrolides

## USES

Macrolides act primarily against most gram-positive microorganisms and some gram-negative cocci. Azithromycin and clarithromycin appear to be more potent than erythromycin. Macrolides are used in the treatment of pharyngitis/tonsillitis, sinusitis, chronic bronchitis, pneumonia, uncomplicated skin/skin structure infections.

## ACTION

Bacteriostatic or bactericidal. Reversibly binds to the P site of the 50S ribosomal subunit of susceptible organisms, inhibiting RNA-dependent protein synthesis.

## ANTIBIOTIC: MACROLIDES

| Name | Availability | Dosage Range | Side Effects |
|---|---|---|---|
| **Azithromycin (Zithromax)** | **T:** 250 mg, 600 mg<br>**S:** 100 mg/5 ml, 200 mg/5 ml, 1-g packet<br>**I:** 500 mg | **A (PO):** 500 mg once, then 250 mg once daily<br>**(IV):** 500 mg/day<br>**C (PO/IV):** 5–10 mg/kg once daily | **PO:** Nausea, diarrhea, vomiting, abdominal pain<br>**IV:** Pain, redness, swelling at injection site |
| **Clarithromycin (Biaxin)** | **T:** 250 mg, 500 mg<br>**T (XL):** 500 mg<br>**S:** 125 mg/5 ml | **A:** 250–500 mg q12h (or XL 1,000 mg once daily)<br>**C:** 7.5 mg/kg q12h | Headaches, loss of taste, nausea, vomiting, diarrhea, abdominal pain/discomfort |
| **Erythromycin**<br>**(EES, Eryc, EryPed,**<br>**Ery-Tab, Erythrocin, PCE)** | **T:** 200 mg, 250 mg, 333 mg, 400 mg, 500 mg<br>**C:** 250 mg<br>**S:** 100 mg/2.5 ml, 125 mg/5 ml, 200 mg/5 ml, 250 mg/5 ml, 400 mg/5 ml | **A (PO):** 250–500 mg q6h<br>**(IV):** 500 mg–1 g q6h<br>**C (PO):** 7.5 mg/kg q6h<br>**(IV):** 15–20 mg/kg/day in divided doses q6h | **PO:** Nausea, vomiting, diarrhea, abdominal pain<br>**IV:** Inflammation, phlebitis at injection site |

*A*, Adults; *C*, capsules; *C (dosage)*, children; *I*, injection; *S*, suspension; *T*, tablets; *XL*, long-acting.

# Antibiotic: Penicillins

## USES

Penicillins (also referred to as beta-lactam antibiotics) may be used to treat a large number of infections, including pneumonia and other respiratory diseases, urinary tract infections, septicemia, meningitis, intra-abdominal infections, gonorrhea and syphilis, bone/joint infection.

Penicillins are classified based on an antimicrobial spectrum:

*Natural penicillins* are very active against gram-positive cocci but ineffective against most strains of *Staphylococcus aureus* (inactivated by enzyme penicillinase).

*Penicillinase-resistant penicillins* are effective against penicillinase-producing *Staphylococcus aureus* but are less effective against gram-positive cocci than the natural penicillins.

*Broad-spectrum penicillins* are effective against gram-positive cocci and some gram-negative bacteria (e.g., *Haemophilus influenzae, Escherichia coli, Proteus mirabilis, Salmonella,* and *Shigella*).

*Extended-spectrum penicillins* are effective against gram-negative organisms, including *Pseudomonas aeruginosa, Enterobacter, Proteus* spp*., Klebsiella, Serratia* spp*.,* and *Acinetobacter* spp.

## ACTION

Penicillins inhibit cell wall synthesis or activate enzymes, which disrupt the bacterial cell wall, causing cell lysis and cell death. May be bacteriostatic or bactericidal. Most effective against bacteria undergoing active growth and division.

## ANTIBIOTIC: PENICILLINS

| Name | Availability | Dosage Range | Side Effects |
|---|---|---|---|
| **Natural** | | | |
| **Penicillin G benzathine (Bicillin, Bicillin LA)** | **I:** 600,000 units, 1.2 million units, 2.4 million units | **A:** 1.2–2.4 million units as single dose<br>**C:** 25,000–50,000 units/kg as single dose | Mild diarrhea, nausea, vomiting, headaches, sore mouth/tongue, vaginal itching/discharge, allergic reaction (including anaphylaxis, skin rash, urticaria, pruritus) |

| | | |
|---|---|---|
| **Penicillin G potassium (Pfizerpen)** | **I:** 1, 2, 3, 5 million-unit vials | **A:** 2–4 million units q4h<br>**C:** 100,000–400,000 units/kg/day divided q4–6h | Rash, injection site reaction, phlebitis |
| **Penicillin V potassium (Apo-Pen-VK)** | **T:** 250 mg, 500 mg<br>**S:** 125 mg/5 ml, 250 mg/5 ml | **A:** 250–500 mg q6–8h<br>**C:** 25–50 mg/kg/day in divided doses q6–8h | Diarrhea, nausea, vomiting |
| Penicillinase-Resistant | | |
| **Dicloxacillin (Dynapen, Pathocil)** | **C:** 125 mg, 250 mg, 500 mg<br>**S:** 62.5 mg/5 ml | **A:** 125–500 mg q6h<br>**C:** 25–50 mg/kg/day divided q6h | Abdominal pain, diarrhea, nausea |
| **Nafcillin (Unipen)** | **I:** 500 mg, 1 g, 2 g | **A (IV):** 500 mg–2 g q4–6h<br>**C (IV):** 50–200 mg/kg/day in divided doses q4–6h | Inflammation, pain, phlebitis<br>Increased risk of interstitial nephritis |
| **Oxacillin (Bactocill)** | **C:** 250 mg, 500 mg<br>**S:** 250 mg/5 ml<br>**I:** 250 mg, 500 mg, 1 g, 2 g | **A (IV):** 1–2 g q4–6h<br>**C (IV):** 25–50 mg/kg q6h | Diarrhea, nausea, vomiting<br>Increased risk of hepatotoxicity, interstitial nephritis |
| Broad-Spectrum | | |
| **Amoxicillin (Amoxil, Trimox)** | **T:** 125 mg, 250 mg, 500 mg, 875 mg<br>**C:** 250 mg, 500 mg<br>**S:** 200 mg/5 ml, 400 mg/5 ml, 125 mg/5 ml, 250 mg/5 ml | **A:** 250–500 mg q8h or 500–875 g q12h<br>**C:** 20–90 mg/kg/day divided q8–12h | Diarrhea, colitis, nausea |
| **Amoxicillin/clavulanate (Augmentin)** | **T:** 250 mg, 500 mg, 875 mg<br>**T (chewable):** 125 mg, 200 mg, 250 mg, 400 mg<br>**S:** 125 mg/5 ml, 200 mg/5 ml, 250 mg/5 ml, 400 mg/5 ml | **A:** 875 mg q12h or 250–500 mg q8h<br>**C:** 25–90 mg/kg/day divided q12h | Diarrhea, rash, nausea, vomiting |

*Continued*

## ANTIBIOTIC: PENICILLINS—cont'd

| Name | Availability | Dosage Range | Side Effects |
|---|---|---|---|
| **Ampicillin (Principen)** | **C:** 250 mg, 500 mg<br>**S:** 125 mg/5 ml, 250 mg/5 ml<br>**I:** 125 mg, 250 mg, 500 mg, 1 g, 2 g | **A (PO):** 250–500 mg q6h<br>**(IV):** 500 mg–2 g q6h<br>**C (PO):** 12.5–50 mg/kg q6h<br>**(IV):** 25–50 mg/kg q6h | Nausea, vomiting, diarrhea |
| **Ampicillin/sulbactam (Unasyn)** | **I:** 1.5 g, 3 g | **A:** 1.5–3 g q6h<br>**C:** 25–50 mg/kg q6h | Local pain at injection site, rash, diarrhea |
| Extended-Spectrum | | | |
| **Piperacillin/tazobactam (Zosyn)** | **I:** 2.25 g, 3.375 g, 4.5 g | **A:** 3.375 g q6h or 4.5 g q6–8h<br>**C:** 240–300 mg/kg/day divided q8h | Diarrhea, insomnia, headache, fever, rash |

*A,* Adults; *C,* capsules; *C (dosage),* children; *I,* injection; *PO,* oral; *S,* suspension; *T,* tablets.

# Anticoagulants/Antiplatelets/Thrombolytics

## USES

Treatment and prevention of venous thromboembolism, acute MI, acute cerebral embolism; reduce risk of acute MI; reduction of total mortality in pts with unstable angina; prevent occlusion of saphenous grafts following open heart surgery; prevent embolism in select pts with atrial fibrillation, prosthetic heart valves, valvular heart disease, cardiomyopathy. Heparin also used for acute/chronic consumption coagulopathies (disseminated intravascular coagulation).

## ACTION

*Anticoagulants:* Inhibit blood coagulation by preventing the formation of new clots and extension of existing ones *but do not dissolve formed clots.* Anticoagulants are subdivided. *Heparin* (including low molecular weight heparin): Indirectly interferes with blood coagulation by blocking the conversion of prothrombin to thrombin and fibrinogen to fibrin. *Coumarin:* Acts indirectly to prevent synthesis in the liver of vitamin K–dependent clotting factors. *Direct Thrombin Inhibitors:* Inhibit thrombin from converting fibrinogen to fibrin. *Factor Xa Inhibitors:* Inhibits platelet activation and fibrin clot formation.

*Antiplatelets:* Interfere with platelet aggregation. Effects are irreversible for life of platelet. Medications in this group act by different mechanisms. Aspirin irreversibly inhibits cyclo-oxygenase and formation of thromboxane $A_2$. Clopidogrel, dipyridamole, prasugrel, and ticlopidine have similar effects as aspirin and are known as adenosine diphosphate (ADP) inhibitors. Abciximab, eptifibatide, and tirofiban block binding of fibrinogen to the glycoprotein IIb/IIIa receptor on platelet surface (known as platelet glycoprotein IIb/IIIa receptor antagonists).

*Thrombolytics:* Act directly or indirectly on fibrinolytic system to dissolve clots (converting plasminogen to plasmin, an enzyme that digests fibrin clot).

## ANTICOAGULANTS/ANTIPLATELETS/THROMBOLYTICS

| Name | Availability | Uses | Side Effects |
|---|---|---|---|
| **Anticoagulants** | | | |
| Direct Thrombin Inhibitors | | | |
| **Argatroban** | I: 100 mg/ml | Prevent/treat VTE in pts with HIT or at risk for HIT undergoing PCI | Bleeding, hypotension, hematuria |

*Continued*

## ANTICOAGULANTS/ANTIPLATELETS/THROMBOLYTICS—cont'd

| Name | Availability | Uses | Side Effects |
|---|---|---|---|
| Bivalirudin (Angiomax) | I: 250-mg vials | Pts with unstable angina undergoing PTCA | Bleeding, hypotension, pain, headache, nausea, back pain |
| Dabigatran (Pradaxa) | C: 75 mg, 110 mg, 150 mg | Reduce risk for stroke/embolism with nonvulvular atrial fibrillation, prevent/treat DVT/PE, postoperative prophylaxis of DVT/PE following hip replacement | Bleeding, gastritis, dyspepsia |
| Desirudin (Iprivask) | I: 15 mg | Prophylaxis of DVT following hip surgery | Bleeding |
| **Heparin, Low Molecular Weight Heparins** | | | |
| Dalteparin (Fragmin) | I: 2,500 units, 5,000 units, 7,500 units, 10,000 units | Prevent DVT following hip surgery, abdominal surgery, unstable angina or non–Q-wave MI | Bleeding, hematoma, increased ALT, AST, pain at injection site, bruising |
| Enoxaparin (Lovenox) | I: 30 mg, 40 mg, 60 mg, 80 mg, 100 mg, 120 mg, 150 mg | Prevent DVT following hip surgery, knee surgery, abdominal surgery, unstable angina or non–Q-wave MI, acute illness | Bleeding, thrombocytopenia, hematoma, increased ALT, AST, nausea, bruising |
| Heparin | I: 1,000 units/ml, 2,500 units/ml, 5,000 units/ml, 7,500 units/ml, 10,000 units/ml, 20,000 units/ml | Prevent/treat VTE | Bleeding, thrombocytopenia, skin rash, itching, burning |
| Tinzaparin (Innohep) | I: 10,000 units/ml, 20,000 units/ ml vials | Treat DVT/PE, prevent VTE following surgery | Bleeding, thrombocytopenia, increased ALT, injection site hematoma |
| **Factor Xa Inhibitor** | | | |
| Apixaban (Eliquis) | T: 2.5 mg, 5 mg | Reduce risk of stroke/embolism in nonvalvular atrial fibrillation Prevent VTE post hip/knee replacement surgery, prevent/treat recurrence | Bleeding, nausea, anemia |

| | | | |
|---|---|---|---|
| **Edoxaban (Savaysa)** | **T:** 15 mg, 30 mg, 60 mg | Prevent thromboembolism in nonvalvular atrial fibrillation, treat DVT/PT | Bleeding, anemia, rash, abnormal liver function tests |
| **Fondaparinux (Arixtra)** | **I:** 2.5 mg, 5 mg, 7.5 mg, 10 mg | Prophylaxis of DVT following hip fracture, abdominal surgery, hip surgery, knee surgery, treat DVT/PE | Bleeding, thrombocytopenia, hematoma, fever, nausea, anemia |
| **Rivaroxaban (Xarelto)** | **T:** 10 mg | Prevent DVT post knee, hip replacement Prevent thromboembolism in atrial fibrillation. Prevent/treat DVT/PE | Bleeding |
| Coumarin | | | |
| **Warfarin (Coumadin)** | **PO:** 1 mg, 2 mg, 2.5 mg, 3 mg, 4 mg, 5 mg, 6 mg, 7.5 mg, 10 mg **I:** 5 mg | Prevent/treat VTE in pts; prevent systemic embolism in pts with heart valve replacement, valve heart disease, MI, atrial fibrillation | Bleeding, skin necrosis, anorexia, nausea, vomiting, diarrhea, rash, abdominal cramps, purple toe syndrome, drug interactions (see individual monograph) |
| Antiplatelets | | | |
| **Abciximab (ReoPro)** | **I:** 2 mg/ml | Adjunct to PCI to prevent acute cardiac ischemic complications (with heparin and aspirin) | Bleeding, hypotension, nausea, vomiting, back pain, allergic reactions, thrombocytopenia |
| **Aspirin** | **PO:** 81 mg, 165 mg, 325 mg, 500 mg, 650 mg | TIA acute MI, chronic stable/unstable angina, revascularization procedures Prevent reinfarction and thromboembolism post MI | Tinnitus, dizziness, hypersensitivity, dyspepsia, minor bleeding, GI ulceration |
| **Clopidogrel (Plavix)** | **PO:** 75 mg | Reduce risk of stroke, MI, or vascular death in pts with recent MI, noncardioembolic stroke, peripheral artery disease. Reduce CV death, MI, stroke, reinfarction in pts with non-STEMI/STEMI | Bleeding, rash, pruritus, bruising, epistaxis |

*Continued*

## ANTICOAGULANTS/ANTIPLATELETS/THROMBOLYTICS—cont'd

| Name | Availability | Uses | Side Effects |
|---|---|---|---|
| **Cangrelor (Kengreal)** | **I:** 50 mg | Adjunct to PCI to reduce risk of MI, repeat coronary revascularization, stent thrombosis | Bleeding |
| **Eptifibatide (Integrilin)** | **I:** 0.75 mg/ml, 2 mg/ml | Treat acute coronary syndrome | Bleeding, hypotension |
| **Prasugrel (Effient)** | **PO:** 5 mg, 10 mg | Reduce thrombotic cardiovascular events in pts with ACS to be managed with PCI (including stenting) | Bleeding, hypotension |
| **Ticagrelor (Brilinta)** | **PO:** 60 mg, 90 mg | Reduce thrombotic cardiovascular events in pts with ACS | Bleeding, dyspnea |
| **Tirofiban (Aggrastat)** | **I:** 50 mcg/ml, 250 mcg/ml | Treat acute coronary syndrome | Bleeding, thrombocytopenia, bradycardia, pelvic pain |
| **Vorapaxar (Zontivity)** | **T:** 2.08 mg | Reduce thrombotic cardiovascular events (e.g., MI, stroke) in pts with history of MI or peripheral arterial disease | Bleeding |
| **Thrombolytics** | | | |
| **Alteplase (Activase)** | **I:** 50 mg, 100 mg | Acute MI, acute ischemic stroke, pulmonary embolism | Bleeding, epistaxis |
| **Tenecteplase (TNKase)** | **I:** 50 mg | Acute MI | Bleeding, hematuria |

*ACS,* Acute coronary syndrome; *DTV,* deep vein thrombosis; *HIT,* heparin-induced thrombocytopenia; *I,* injection; *MI,* myocardial infarction; *PCI,* percutaneous coronary intervention; *PO,* oral; *PTCA,* percutaneous transluminal coronary angioplasty; *STEMI,* ST segment elevation MI; *T,* tablet; *TIA,* transient ischemic attack; *VTE,* venous thromboembolism.

# Anticonvulsants

## USES

Anticonvulsants are used to treat seizures. Seizures can be divided into two broad categories: partial seizures and generalized seizures. *Partial seizures* begin focally in the cerebral cortex, undergoing limited spread. Simple partial seizures do not involve loss of consciousness but may evolve secondarily into generalized seizures. Complex partial seizures involve impairment of consciousness.

*Generalized seizures* may be convulsive or nonconvulsive and usually produce immediate loss of consciousness.

## ACTION

Anticonvulsants can prevent or reduce excessive discharge of neurons with seizure foci or decrease the spread of excitation from seizure foci to normal neurons. The exact mechanism is unknown but may be due to (1) suppressing sodium influx, (2) suppressing calcium influx, or (3) increasing the action of gamma-aminobutyric acid (GABA), which inhibits neurotransmitters throughout the brain.

## ANTICONVULSANTS

| Name | Availability | Uses | Dosage Range | Side Effects |
|------|-------------|------|-------------|-------------|
| **Carbamazepine (Carbatrol, Carnexiv, Epitol, Tegretol, Tegretol XR)** | S: 100 mg/5 ml<br>T (chewable): 100 mg<br>T: 200 mg<br>T (ER): 100 mg, 200 mg, 400 mg<br>C (ER): 100 mg, 200 mg, 300 mg<br>I: 10 mg/ml | Complex partial, tonic-clonic, mixed seizures; trigeminal neuralgia | **Note:** Refer to monograph for IV dosage<br>A: Initially, 400 mg/day in 2 divided doses. May increase up to 200 mg/day at weekly intervals up to 800–1,600 mg/day in 2–3 doses.<br>C: Initially, 200 mg/day in 2 divided doses. May increase by 100 mg/day at weekly intervals up to 400–800 mg/day in 3–4 doses. | Dizziness, diplopia, leukopenia, drowsiness, blurred vision, headache, ataxia, nausea, vomiting, hyponatremia |
| **Clonazepam (Klonopin)** | T: 0.5 mg, 1 mg, 2 mg | Petit mal, akinetic, myoclonic, absence seizures | A: Initially, not to exceed 1.5 mg in 3 divided doses. May increase q3days up to 2–8 mg/day in 1–2 divided doses. | CNS depression, sedation, ataxia, confusion, depression, behavior disorders, respiratory depression |

*Continued*

ANTICONVULSANTS—cont'd

| Name | Availability | Uses | Dosage Range | Side Effects |
|------|-------------|------|--------------|--------------|
| **Ezogabine** (Potiga) | **T:** 50 mg, 200 mg, 300 mg, 400 mg | Partial onset seizures | **A:** Initially, 100 mg 3 times/day. May increase at weekly intervals up to 150 mg/day. Usual dose: 200–400 mg 3 times/day. | Dizziness, somnolence, fatigue, confusion, vertigo, tremor, balance disorder, urinary retention |
| **Fosphenytoin** (Cerebyx) | **I:** 50 mg PE/ml | Status epilepticus, seizures occurring during neurosurgery | **A:** 15–20 mg PE/kg bolus, then 4–6 mg PE/kg/day maintenance. | Burning, itching, paresthesia, nystagmus, ataxia |
| **Gabapentin** (Neurontin) | **C:** 100 mg, 300 mg, 400 mg **S:** 250 mg/5 ml | Partial and generalized seizures | **A:** 300 mg 3 times/day. Usual dose: 900–1,800 mg/day in 3 doses. | CNS depression, fatigue, drowsiness, dizziness, ataxia, nystagmus, blurred vision, confusion; may cause weight gain |
| **Lacosamide** (Vimpat) | **T:** 50 mg, 100 mg, 150 mg, 200 mg **S:** 10 mg/ml **I:** 10 mg/ml | Adjunctive therapy, partial seizures | **A:** Monotherapy: Initially, 100 mg 2 times/day. May increase at weekly intervals by 50 mg 2 times/day. Maintenance: 150–200 mg 2 times/day. Adjunctive: Initially, 50 mg 2 times/day. May increase by 50 mg 2 times/day. Maintenance: 100–200 mg 2 times/day. | Diplopia, headache, dizziness, nausea |
| **Lamotrigine** (Lamictal) | **T:** 25 mg, 100 mg, 150 mg, 200 mg **T (ER):** 25 mg, 50 mg, 100 mg, 200 mg, 250 mg, 300 mg **T (ODT):** 25 mg, 50 mg, 100 mg, 200 mg **T (Chew):** 5 mg, 25 mg | Partial seizures, primary generalized tonic-clonic seizures, generalized seizures of Lennox-Gastaut syndrome | **A:** Refer to individual monograph. | Dizziness, ataxia, drowsiness, diplopia, nausea, rash, headache, vomiting, insomnia, incoordination |

| | | | |
|---|---|---|---|
| **Levetiracetam (Keppra)** | **T:** 250 mg, 500 mg, 750 mg, 1,000 mg<br>**S:** 100 mg/ml<br>**T(ER):** 500 mg, 750 mg | Adjunctive therapy, partial seizures, primary tonic-clonic seizures, myoclonic seizures | **A: T:** Initially, 500 mg 2 times/day. May increase q2wks by 500mg/dose. Usual dose: 1,500 mg 2 times/day.<br>**ER:** Initially, 1,000 mg once daily. May increase q2wks by 1,000 mg/day up to 3,000 mg once daily. | Dizziness, drowsiness, weakness, irritability, hallucinations, psychosis |
| **Oxcarbazepine (Trileptal)** | **T:** 150 mg, 300 mg, 600 mg<br>**T(ER):** 150 mg, 300 mg, 600 mg | Partial seizures | **A: T:** 600 mg/day in 2 divided doses. May increase by 600 mg/day at weekly intervals up to 1,200 mg/day in 2 divided doses.<br>**ER:** 600 mg once daily. May increase by 600 mg/day at weekly intervals up to 1,200–2,400 mg/day. | Drowsiness, dizziness, headaches, diplopia, ataxia, nausea, vomiting, hyponatremia, skin reactions |
| **Phenobarbital** | **T:** 30 mg, 60 mg, 100 mg<br>**I:** 65 mg, 130 mg | Tonic-clonic, partial seizures; status epilepticus | **A (PO):** 100–300 mg/day;<br>**(IM/IV):** 200–600 mg.<br>**C (PO):** 3–5 mg/kg/day;<br>**(IM/IV):** 100–400 mg. | CNS depression, sedation, paradoxical excitement and hyperactivity, rash |
| **Phenytoin (Dilantin)** | **C:** 30 mg, 100 mg<br>**T (chewable):** 50 mg<br>**S:** 125 mg/5 ml<br>**I:** 50 mg/ml | Tonic-clonic, psychomotor seizures | **A:** Initially, 100 mg 3 times/day. May increase at 7–10 days intervals. Usual dose: 400 mg/day. **C:** Initially, 5 mg/kg/day in 2–3 divided doses. May increase at 7–10 days intervals. Usual dose: 4–8 mg/kg/day in 1–3 doses. | Nystagmus, ataxia, hypertrichosis, gingival hyperplasia, rash, osteomalacia, lymphadenopathy |
| **Pregabalin (Lyrica)** | **C:** 25 mg, 50 mg, 75 mg, 100 mg, 150 mg, 200 mg, 225 mg, 300 mg | Adjunctive therapy, partial seizures | **A:** Initially 150 mg/day (75 mg 2 times/day or 50 mg 3 times/day) up to 600 mg/day in 2 or 3 doses. | Confusion, drowsiness, dizziness, ataxia, weight gain, dry mouth, blurred vision, peripheral edema, myopathy, angioedema, decreased platelet count |

*Continued*

ANTICONVULSANTS—cont'd

| Name | Availability | Uses | Dosage Range | Side Effects |
|---|---|---|---|---|
| **Primidone (Mysoline)** | **T:** 50 mg, 250 mg | Complex partial, akinetic, tonic-clonic seizures | **A:** 750–1250 mg/day in 3–4 doses<br>**C:** 10–25 mg/kg/day | CNS depression, sedation, paradoxical excitement and hyperactivity, rash, dizziness, ataxia |
| **Rufinamide (Banzel)** | **S:** 40 mg/ml<br>**T:** 200 mg, 400 mg | Lennox-Gastaut syndrome (adjunct) | **A:** Initially, 400–800 mg/day in 2 divided doses. May increase by 400–800 mg/day every other day<br>**C:** Initially, 10 mg/kg/day in 2 divided doses. May increase by 10 mg/kg/day every other day up to 45 mg/kg/day. **Maximum:** 3,200 mg/day. | Fatigue, dizziness, headache, nausea, drowsiness |
| **Tiagabine (Gabitril)** | **T:** 4 mg, 12 mg, 16 mg, 20 mg | Partial seizures | **A:** Initially, 4 mg up to 56 mg/day in 2–4 doses. May increase by 4–8 mg/day at weekly intervals<br>**C:** Initially, 4 mg up to 32 mg/day in 2–4 doses. May increase by 4–8 mg/day at weekly intervals. | Dizziness, asthenia, nervousness, anxiety, tremors, abdominal pain |
| **Topiramate (Topamax)** | **T:** 25 mg, 100 mg, 200 mg<br>**C (Sprinkle):** 15 mg, 25 mg<br>**C (ER 24 HR Sprinkle):**<br>(Qudexy XR): 25 mg,<br>50 mg, 100 mg, 150 mg<br>**C XR (Trokendi XR):** 25 mg,<br>50 mg, 100 mg, 200 mg | Partial seizures, Lennox-Gastaut syndrome | See individual monograph. | Drowsiness, dizziness, headache, ataxia, confusion, weight loss, diplopia |
| **Valproic acid (Depakene, Depakote)** | **C:** 250 mg<br>**S:** 250 mg/5 ml<br>**Sprinkles:** 125 mg<br>**T:** 125 mg, 250 mg, 500 mg<br>**T (ER):** 500 mg<br>**I:** 100 mg/ml | Complex partial, absence seizures | **A, C:** Initially, 15 mg/kg/day. May increase by 5–10 mg/kg/day at weekly intervals up to 60 mg/kg/day. | Nausea, vomiting, tremors, thrombocytopenia, hair loss, hepatic dysfunction, weight gain, decreased platelet function |

| **Vigabatrin (Sabril)** | T: 500 mg<br>PS: 500 mg | Infantile spasms, refractory complex partial seizures | **A:** Initially, 500 mg 2 times/day. May increase by 500 mg increments at weekly intervals up to 1,500 mg 2 times/day.<br>**C:** Initially, 250 mg 2 times/day. May increase by 500 mg/day at weekly intervals up to 1,000 mg 2 times/day. | Vision changes, eye pain, abdominal pain, agitation, confusion, mood/mental changes, abnormal coordination, weight gain |
| **Zonisamide (Zonegran)** | C: 100 mg | Partial seizures | **A:** Initially, 100 mg/day. May increase to 200 mg/day after 2 wks, then 300 mg/day up to 400 mg/day at 2 wk intervals. | Drowsiness, dizziness, anorexia, diarrhea, weight loss, agitation, irritability, rash, nausea, cognitive side effects, kidney stones |

*A,* Adults; *C,* capsules; *C (dosage),* children; *ER,* extended-release; *I,* injection; *ODT,* orally disintegrating tablets; *PE,* phenytoin equivalent; *PO,* oral; *PS,* powder sachet; *S,* suspension; *T,* tablets.

# Antidepressants

## USES

Used primarily for the treatment of depression. Depression can be a chronic or recurrent mental disorder presenting with symptoms such as depressed mood, loss of interest or pleasure, guilt feelings, disturbed sleep/appetite, low energy, and difficulty in thinking. Depression can also lead to suicide.

## ACTION

Antidepressants include tricyclics, monoamine oxidase inhibitors (MAOIs), selective serotonin reuptake inhibitors (SSRIs), serotonin-norepinephrine reuptake inhibitors (SNRIs), and other antidepressants. Depression may be due to reduced functioning of monoamine neurotransmitters (e.g., norepinephrine, serotonin [5-HT], dopamine) in the CNS (decreased amount and/or decreased effects at the receptor sites). Antidepressants block metabolism, increase amount/effects of monoamine neurotransmitters, and act at receptor sites (change responsiveness/sensitivities of both presynaptic and postsynaptic receptor sites).

## ANTIDEPRESSANTS

| Name | Availability | Uses | Dosage Range (per day) | Side Effects |
|---|---|---|---|---|
| **Tricyclics** | | | | |
| **Amitriptyline (Elavil)** | **T:** 10 mg, 25 mg, 50 mg, 75 mg, 100 mg, 150 mg | Depression, neuropathic pain | Initially, 25–100 mg at bedtime or in divided doses. Usual dose: 100–300 mg/day. | Drowsiness, blurred vision, constipation, confusion, postural hypotension, cardiac conduction defects, weight gain, seizures, dry mouth |
| **Desipramine (Norpramin)** | **T:** 10 mg, 25 mg, 50 mg, 75 mg, 100 mg, 150 mg | Depression, neuropathic pain | Initially, 25–100 mg at bedtime or in divided doses. Usual dose: 100–300 mg/day. | Dizziness, drowsiness, fatigue, headache, anorexia, diarrhea, nausea |
| **Imipramine (Tofranil)** | **T:** 10 mg, 25 mg, 50 mg **C:** 75 mg, 100 mg, 125 mg, 150 mg | Depression, enuresis, neuropathic pain, panic disorder, ADHD | Initially, 25–100 mg at bedtime or in divided doses. Usual dose: 100–300 mg/day. | Dizziness, fatigue, headache, vomiting, xerostomia |
| **Nortriptyline (Aventyl, Pamelor)** | **C:** 10 mg, 25 mg, 50 mg, 75 mg **S:** 10 mg/5 ml | Depression, neuropathic pain, smoking cessation | Initially, 50–100 mg once daily. Usual dose: 50–150 mg once daily. | Dizziness, fatigue, headache, anorexia, xerostomia |
| **Selective Serotonin Reuptake Inhibitors** | | | | |
| **Citalopram (Celexa)** | **T:** 10 mg, 20 mg, 40 mg **ODT:** 40 mg **S:** 10 mg/5 ml | Depression, OCD, panic disorder | 20–40 mg | Insomnia or sedation, nausea, agitation, headaches |
| **Escitalopram (Lexapro)** | **T:** 5 mg, 10 mg, 20 mg **S:** 5 mg/5 ml | Depression, GAD | 10–20 mg | Insomnia or sedation, nausea, agitation, headaches |

| | | | | |
|---|---|---|---|---|
| **Fluoxetine (Prozac)** | **C:** 10 mg, 20 mg, 40 mg<br>**C (DR):** 90 mg<br>**T:** 10 mg, 20 mg<br>**S:** 20 mg/5 ml | Depression, OCD, panic disorder, anorexia, bulimia, bipolar disorder, premenstrual syndrome | Initially, 10–20 mg once daily. Usual dose: 20 mg once daily.<br>**DR:** 90 mg once weekly. | Akathisia, sexual dysfunction, skin rash, urticaria, pruritus, decreased appetite, asthenia, diarrhea, drowsiness, headaches, diaphoresis, insomnia, nausea, tremors |
| **Paroxetine (Paxil)** | **T:** 10 mg, 20 mg, 30 mg, 40 mg<br>**S:** 10 mg/5 ml<br>**ER:** 12.5 mg, 25 mg, 37.5 mg | Depression, OCD, panic attack, SAD | Initially/usual dose: 20 mg daily.<br>**ER:** Initially, 12.5–25 mg once daily. Usual dose: 25 mg once daily. | Asthenia, constipation, diarrhea, diaphoresis, insomnia, nausea, sexual dysfunction, tremors, vomiting, urinary frequency or retention |
| **Sertraline (Zoloft)** | **T:** 25 mg, 50 mg, 100 mg<br>**S:** 20 mg/ml | Depression, OCD, panic attack | 50–200 mg | Sexual dysfunction, dizziness, drowsiness, anorexia, diarrhea, nausea, dry mouth, abdominal cramps, decreased weight, headaches, increased diaphoresis, tremors, insomnia |
| **Vortioxetine (Trintellix)** | **T:** 5 mg, 10 mg, 15 mg, 20 mg | Depression | Initially, 10 mg once daily. Usual dose: 10–20 mg once daily. | Nausea, constipation |
| Serotonin-Norepinephrine Reuptake Inhibitors | | | | |
| **Desvenlafaxine (Pristiq)** | **T:** 25 mg, 50 mg, 100 mg | Depression | 50–100 mg | Nausea, dizziness, insomnia, hyperhidrosis, constipation, drowsiness, decreased appetite, anxiety, male sexual function disorders |
| **Duloxetine (Cymbalta)** | **C:** 20 mg, 30 mg, 60 mg | Depression, fibromyalgia, neuropathic pain | Initially, 30–60 mg once daily. Usual dose: 60 mg once daily or 2 divided doses. | Nausea, dry mouth, constipation, decreased appetite, fatigue, diaphoresis |

*Continued*

## ANTIDEPRESSANTS—cont'd

| Name | Availability | Uses | Dosage Range (per day) | Side Effects |
|---|---|---|---|---|
| **Venlafaxine (Effexor)** | **T:** 25 mg, 37.5 mg, 50 mg, 75 mg, 100 mg, 150 mg, 225 mg **T (ER):** 37.5 mg, 75 mg, 150 mg | Depression, anxiety | Initially, 25 mg 3 times or **(ER):** 37.5 mg once daily. Usual dose: 75 mg 3 times/day or **(ER)** 75–225 mg once daily. | Increased blood pressure, agitation, sedation, insomnia, nausea |
| **Other** | | | | |
| **Brexpiprazole (Rexulti)** | **T:** 0.25 mg, 0.5 mg, 1 mg, 2 mg, 3 mg, 4 mg | Depression | Initially, 0.5–1 mg/day. May increase at weekly interval to 1 mg/day. **Maximum:** 3 mg/day. | Weight gain, akathisia |
| **Bupropion (Wellbutrin)** | **T:** 75 mg, 100 mg **SR:** 100 mg, 150 mg, 200 mg | Depression, smoking cessation, ADHD, bipolar disorder | Initially, 100 mg 2 times/day. Usual dose: 100 mg 3 times/day. **SR:** Initially, 150 mg once daily. Usual dose: 150 mg 2 times/day. | Insomnia, irritability, seizures |
| **Mirtazapine (Remeron)** | **T:** 7.5 mg, 15 mg, 30 mg, 45 mg | Depression | Initially, 15 mg once at bedtime. Usual dose: 30–45 mg once daily. | Sedation, dry mouth, weight gain, agranulocytosis, hepatic toxicity |
| **Trazodone (Desyrel)** | **T:** 50 mg, 100 mg, 150 mg, 300 mg **ER:** 150 mg, 300 mg | Depression | Initially, 75 mg 2 times/day or **(ER):** 150 mg once daily. Usual dose: 150 mg bid or **(ER):** 150–375 mg once daily. | Sedation, orthostatic hypotension, priapism |
| **Vilazodone (Viibryd)** | **T:** 10 mg, 20 mg, 40 mg | Depression | Initially, 10 mg once daily. Usual dose: 40 mg once daily. | Diarrhea, nausea, dizziness, dry mouth, insomnia, vomiting, decreased libido |

**ADHD,** Attention-deficit hyperactivity disorder; **C,** capsules; **DR,** delayed-release; **ER,** extended-release; **GAD,** generalized anxiety disorder; **OC,** oral concentrate; **OCD,** obsessive-compulsive disorder; **ODT,** orally disintegrating tablets; **S,** suspension; **SAD,** social anxiety disorder; **SR,** sustained-release; **T,** tablets.

# Antidiabetics

## USES

*Insulin:* Treatment of insulin-dependent diabetes (type 1) and non–insulin-dependent diabetes (type 2). Also used in acute situations such as ketoacidosis, severe infections, major surgery in otherwise non–insulin-dependent diabetics. Administered to pts receiving parenteral nutrition. Drug of choice during pregnancy. All insulins, including long-acting insulins, can cause hypoglycemia and weight gain.

*Alpha-glucosidase inhibitors:* Adjunct to diet and exercise for management of type 2 diabetes mellitus.

*Biguanides:* Adjunct to diet and exercise for management of type 2 diabetes mellitus.

*Dipeptidyl peptidase 4 inhibitors (DPP-4):* Adjunct to diet and exercise for management of type 2 diabetes mellitus.

*Meglitinide:* Adjunct to diet and exercise for management of type 2 diabetes mellitus.

*Sulfonylureas:* Adjunct to diet and exercise for management of type 2 diabetes mellitus.

*Thiazolidinediones:* Adjunct to diet and exercise for management of type 2 diabetes mellitus.

*Sodium-glucose co-transporter 2 (SGLT2):* Adjunct to diet and exercise for management of type 2 diabetes mellitus.

## ACTION

*Insulin:* A hormone synthesized and secreted by beta cells of Langerhans' islet in the pancreas. Controls storage and utilization of glucose, amino acids, and fatty acids by activated transport systems/enzymes. Inhibits breakdown of glycogen, fat, protein. Insulin lowers blood glucose by inhibiting glycogenolysis and gluconeogenesis in liver; stimulates glucose uptake by muscle, adipose tissue. Activity of insulin is initiated by binding to cell surface receptors.

*Alpha-glucosidase inhibitors:* Work locally in small intestine, slowing carbohydrate breakdown and glucose absorption.

*Biguanides:* Inhibit hepatic gluconeogenesis, glycogenolysis; enhance insulin sensitivity in muscle and fat.

*DPP-4:* Inhibit degradation of endogenous incretins, which increases insulin secretion, decreases glucagon secretion.

*Meglitinide:* Stimulates pancreatic insulin secretion.

*Sulfonylureas:* Stimulate release of insulin from beta cells of the pancreas.

*Thiazolidinediones:* Enhance insulin sensitivity in muscle and fat.

*SGLT2:* Reduces reabsorption of filtered glucose, lowers renal threshold for glucose, increases urinary glucose excretion.

## ANTIDIABETICS

### Insulin

| Type | Onset | Peak | Duration | Comments |
|---|---|---|---|---|
| **Rapid-Acting** | | | | |
| **Apidra, glulisine** | 10–15 min | 1–1.5 hrs | 3–5 hrs | Stable at room temp for 28 days<br>Can mix with NPH |
| **Humalog, lispro** | 15–30 min | 0.5–2.5 hrs | 6–8 hrs | Stable at room temp for 28 days<br>Can mix with NPH |
| **Novolog, aspart** | 10–20 min | 1–3 hrs | 3–5 hrs | Stable at room temp for 28 days<br>Can mix with NPH |
| **Short-Acting** | | | | |
| **Humulin R, Novolin R, regular** | 30–60 min | 1–5 hrs | 6–10 hrs | Stable at room temp for 28 days<br>Can mix with NPH |
| **Intermediate-Acting** | | | | |
| **Humulin N, Novolin N, NPH** | 1–2 hrs | 6–14 hrs | 16–24 hrs | Stable at room temp for 28 days<br>Can mix with aspart, lispro, glulisine |
| **Long-Acting** | | | | |
| **Lantus, glargine** | 1.1 hrs | No significant peak | 24 hrs | Do NOT mix with other insulins<br>Stable at room temp for 28 days |
| **Levemir, detemir** | 0.8–2 hrs | No significant peak | 12–24 hrs<br>(dose dependent) | Do NOT mix with other insulins<br>Stable at room temp for 42 days |
| **Toujeo, glargine** | Over 6 hrs | No significant peak | Longer than 24 hrs | Do NOT mix with other insulins<br>Stable at room temp for 28 days |
| **Tresiba, degludec** | 0.5–1.5 hrs | 12 hrs | 42 hrs | Do NOT mix with other insulins<br>Stable at room temp for 56 days |

**ORAL AGENTS**

| Name | Availability | Dosage Range | Side Effects |
|------|-------------|--------------|--------------|
| Sulfonylureas | | | |
| **Glimepiride (Amaryl)** | **T:** 1 mg, 2 mg, 4 mg | Initially, 1–2 mg/day. May increase by 1–2 mg q1–2 weeks. **Maximum:** 8 mg/day | Hypoglycemia, dizziness, headache, nausea, flu-like syndrome |
| **Glipizide (Glucotrol)** | **T:** 5 mg, 10 mg<br>**T (XL):** 5 mg | **T:** Initially, 5 mg/day. May increase by 2.5–5 mg q3–4 days. **(XL):** Initially, 5 mg/day. **Maximum:** 20 mg/day | Dizziness, nervousness, anxiety, diarrhea, tremor |
| **Glyburide (DiaBeta, Micronase)** | **T:** 1.25 mg, 2.5 mg, 5 mg<br>**PT:** 1.5 mg, 3 mg | **T:** Initially, 2.5–5 mg/day. May increase by 2.5 mg/day at weekly intervals up to 20 mg/day<br>**PT:** Initially, 1.5–3 mg/day. May increase by 1.5 mg at weekly intervals up to 12 mg/day | Dizziness, headache, nausea |
| Alpha-Glucosidase Inhibitors | | | |
| **Acarbose (Precose)** | **T:** 25 mg, 50 mg, 100 mg | Initially, 25 mg 3 times/day. May increase at 4–8 wk intervals. Usual dose: 50–100 mg 3 times/day | Flatulence, diarrhea, abdominal pain, increased risk of hypoglycemia when used with insulin or sulfonylureas |
| **Miglitol (Glyset)** | **T:** 25 mg, 50 mg, 100 mg | Initially, 25 mg 3 times/day. May increase at 4–8 wk intervals to 50 mg 3 times/day, then 100 mg 3 times/day | Flatulence, diarrhea, abdominal pain, rash |

*Continued*

**ANTIDIABETICS—cont'd**

| Name | Availability | Dosage Range | Side Effects |
|---|---|---|---|
| **Dipeptidyl Peptidase Inhibitors** | | | |
| **Alogliptin (Nesina)** | **T:** 6.25 mg, 12.5 mg, 25 mg | 6.25–25 mg/day | Nasopharyngitis, cough, headache, upper respiratory tract infections |
| **Linagliptin (Tradjenta)** | **T:** 5 mg | 5 mg/day | Arthralgia, back pain, headache |
| **Saxagliptin (Onglyza)** | **T:** 2.5 mg, 5 mg | 2.5–5 mg/day | Upper respiratory tract infection, urinary tract infection, headache |
| **Sitagliptin (Januvia)** | **T:** 25 mg, 50 mg, 100 mg | 25–100 mg/day | Nasopharyngitis, upper respiratory tract infection, headaches, modest weight gain, increased incidence of hypoglycemia when added to a sulfonylurea |
| **Biguanides** | | | |
| **Metformin (Glucophage)** | **T:** 500 mg, 850 mg, 1,000 mg<br>**XR:** 500 mg, 750 mg, 1,000 mg | **T:** Initially, 500 mg 2 times/day or 850 mg once daily. May increase by 500 mg/day at weekly intervals up to 2,550 mg/day<br>**(XR):** Initially, 500–1,000 mg/day. May increase by 500 mg/day at weekly intervals up to 2,500 mg/day | Nausea, vomiting, diarrhea, loss of appetite, metallic taste, lactic acidosis (rare but potentially fatal complication) |
| **Glucagon-Like Peptide-1 (GLP-1)** | | | |
| **Albiglutide (Tanzeum)** | **I:** 30 mg, 50 mg | 30–50 mg once weekly | Diarrhea, nausea, upper respiratory tract infection, injection site reaction |
| **Exenatide (Byetta)** | **I:** 5 mcg, 10 mcg | 5–10 mcg 2 times/day | Diarrhea, dizziness, dyspnea, headaches, nausea, vomiting |

| Exenatide extended-release (Bydureon) | I: 2 mg | 2 mg once weekly | Diarrhea, nausea, headache |
|---|---|---|---|
| Liraglutide (Victoza) | I: 0.6 mg, 1.2 mg, 1.8 mg (6 mg/ml) | Initially, 0.6 mg/day. May increase at weekly intervals up to 1.2 mg/day, then 1.8 mg/day | Headache, nausea, diarrhea |
| Meglitinides | | | |
| Nateglinide (Starlix) | T: 60 mg, 120 mg | 60–120 mg 3 times/day | Hypoglycemia, upper respiratory infection, dizziness, back pain, flu-like syndrome |
| Repaglinide (Prandin) | T: 0.5 mg, 1 mg, 2 mg | 0.5–1 mg with each meal. Usual dose: 0.5–4 mg/day (**Maximum:** 16 mg/day) | Headache, hypoglycemia, upper respiratory infection |
| SGLT2 | | | |
| Canagliflozin (Invokana) | T: 100 mg, 300 mg | 100–300 mg/day | Increased urination, genital yeast infections, urticaria, rash, pruritus |
| Dapagliflozin (Farxiga) | T: 5 mg, 10 mg | 5–10 mg/day | Genital yeast infections, nasopharyngitis, urinary tract infections |
| Empagliflozin (Jardiance) | T: 10 mg, 25 mg | 10–25 mg/day | Female genital mycotic infections, urinary tract infections |
| Thiazolidinediones | | | |
| Pioglitazone (Actos) | T: 15 mg, 30 mg, 45 mg | 15–30 mg/day | Mild to moderate peripheral edema, weight gain, increased risk of HF, associated with reduced bone mineral density and increased incidence of fractures |

*Continued*

## ANTIDIABETICS—cont'd

| Name | Availability | Dosage Range | Side Effects |
|---|---|---|---|
| Rosiglitazone (Avandia) | **T:** 2 mg, 4 mg, 8 mg | Initially, 4 mg/day. May increase at 8–12 weeks to 8 mg/day as a single or 2 divided doses | Increased cholesterol, weight gain, back pain, upper respiratory tract infection |
| *Miscellaneous* | | | |
| Bromocriptine (Cycloset) | **T:** 0.8 mg | 1.6–4.8 mg/day | Nausea, fatigue, dizziness, vomiting |
| Colesevelam (Welchol) | **T:** 625 mg **S:** 1.875 g, 3.75 g packet | 3.75 g/day | Constipation, dyspepsia, nausea |
| Pramlintide (Symlin) | **I:** 1,500 mcg/1.5 ml, 2,700 mcg/2.7 ml | Type I: 15–60 mcg immediately prior to meals Type 2: 60–120 mcg immediately prior to meals | Abdominal pain, anorexia, headaches, nausea, vomiting, severe hypoglycemia may occur when used in combination with insulin (reduction in dosages of short-acting, including premixed, insulins recommended) |

*HF*, Heart failure; *I*, injection; *PT*, prestab; *S*, suspension; *T*, tablets; *XL*, extended-release; *XR*, extended-release.

# Antidiarrheals

## USES

Acute diarrhea, chronic diarrhea of inflammatory bowel disease, reduction of fluid from ileostomies.

## ACTION

*Systemic agents:* Act as smooth muscle receptors (enteric) disrupting peristaltic movements, decreasing GI motility, increasing transit time of intestinal contents.

*Local agents:* Adsorb toxic substances and fluids to large surface areas of particles in the preparation. Some of these agents coat and protect irritated intestinal walls. May have local anti-inflammatory action.

## ANTIDIARRHEALS

| Name | Availability | Type | Dosage Range |
|------|-------------|------|-------------|
| **Bismuth (Pepto-Bismol)** | **T:** 262 mg<br>**C:** 262 mg<br>**L:** 130 mg/15 ml, 262 mg/15 ml, 524 mg/15 ml | Local | **A:** 2 T or 30 ml<br>**C (9–12 yrs):** 1 T or 15 ml<br>**C (6–8 yrs):** 2/3 T or 10 ml<br>**C (3–5 yrs):** 1/3 T or 5 ml |
| **Diphenoxylate with atropine (Lomotil)** | **T:** 2.5 mg<br>**L:** 2.5 mg/5 ml | Systemic | **A:** 5 mg 4 times/day<br>**C:** 0.3–0.4 mg/kg/day in 4 divided doses **(L)** |
| **Loperamide (Imodium)** | **C:** 2 mg<br>**T:** 2 mg<br>**L:** 1 mg/5 ml, 1 mg/ml | Systemic | **A:** Initially, 4 mg **(Maximum: 16 mg/day)**<br>**C (9–12 yrs):** 2 mg 3 times/day<br>**C (6–8 yrs):** 2 mg 2 times/day<br>**C (2–5 yrs):** 1 mg 3 times/day **(L)** |

*A,* Adults; *C,* capsules; *C (dosage),* children; *L,* liquid; *S,* suspension; *T,* tablets.

# Antifungals: Systemic Mycoses

Systemic mycoses are subdivided into opportunistic infections (candidiasis, aspergillosis, cryptococcosis, and mucormycosis) that are seen primarily in debilitated or immunocompromised hosts and nonopportunistic infections (blastomycosis, histoplasmosis, and coccidioidomycosis) that occur in any host. Treatment can be difficult because these infections often resist treatment and may require prolonged therapy.

## ANTIFUNGALS: SYSTEMIC MYCOSES

| Name | Indications | Side Effects |
|---|---|---|
| **Amphotericin B** | Potentially life-threatening fungal infections, including aspergillosis, blastomycosis, coccidioidomycosis, cryptococcosis, histoplasmosis, systemic candidiasis | Fever, chills, headache, nausea, vomiting, nephrotoxicity, hypokalemia, hypomagnesemia, hypotension, dyspnea, arrhythmias, abdominal pain, diarrhea, increased hepatic function tests |
| **Amphotericin B lipid complex (Abelcet)** | Invasive fungal infections | Chills, fever, hypotension, headache, nausea, vomiting |
| **Amphotericin B liposomal (AmBisome)** | Empiric therapy for presumed fungal infections in febrile neutropenic pts, treatment of cryptococcal meningitis in HIV-infected pts, treatment of *Aspergillus, Candida, Cryptococcus* infections, treatment of visceral leishmaniasis | Peripheral edema, tachycardia, hypotension, chills, insomnia, headache |
| **Amphotericin B colloidal dispersion (Amphotec)** | Invasive *Aspergillus* | Hypotension, tachycardia, chills, fever, vomiting |
| **Anidulafungin (Eraxis)** | Candidemia, esophageal candidiasis | Diarrhea, hypokalemia, increased hepatic function tests, headache |
| **Caspofungin (Cancidas)** | Candidemia, invasive aspergillosis, empiric therapy for presumed fungal infections in febrile neutropenic pts | Headache, nausea, vomiting, diarrhea, increased hepatic function tests |
| **Fluconazole (Diflucan)** | Treatment of vaginal candidiasis; oropharyngeal, esophageal candidiasis; and cryptococcal meningitis. Prophylaxis to decrease incidence of candidiasis in pts undergoing bone marrow transplant receiving cytotoxic chemotherapy and/or radiation | Nausea, vomiting, abdominal pain, diarrhea, dysgeusia, increased hepatic function tests, liver necrosis, hepatitis, cholestasis, headache, rash, pruritus, eosinophilia, alopecia |
| **Isavuconazonium (Cresemba)** | Treatment of invasive aspergillosis, invasive mucormycosis | Nausea, vomiting, diarrhea, increased hepatic enzymes, hypokalemia, constipation, dyspnea, cough, peripheral edema, back pain |

| | | |
|---|---|---|
| **Itraconazole (Sporanox)** | Blastomycosis, histoplasmosis, aspergillosis, onychomycosis, empiric therapy of febrile neutropenic pts with suspected fungal infections, treatment of oropharyngeal and esophageal candidiasis | Congestive heart failure, peripheral edema, nausea, vomiting, abdominal pain, diarrhea, increased hepatic function tests, liver necrosis, hepatitis, cholestasis, headache, rash, pruritus, eosinophilia |
| **Ketoconazole (Nizoral)** | Candidiasis, chronic mucocutaneous candidiasis, oral thrush, candiduria, blastomycosis, coccidioidomycosis | Nausea, vomiting, abdominal pain, diarrhea, gynecomastia, increased LFT, liver necrosis, hepatitis, cholestasis, headache, rash, pruritus, eosinophilia |
| **Micafungin (Mycamine)** | Esophageal candidiasis, *Candida* infections, prophylaxis in pts undergoing hematopoietin stem cell transplantation | Fever, chills, hypokalemia, hypomagnesemia, hypocalcemia, myelosuppression, thrombocytopenia, nausea, vomiting, abdominal pain, diarrhea, increased LFT, dizziness, headache, rash, pruritus, pain or inflammation at injection site, fever |
| **Posaconazole (Noxafil)** | Prevent invasive aspergillosis and *Candida* infections in pts 13 yrs and older who are immunocompromised, treatment of oropharyngeal candidiasis | Fever, headaches, nausea, vomiting, diarrhea, abdominal pain, hypokalemia, cough, dyspnea |
| **Voriconazole (Vfend)** | Invasive aspergillosis, candidemia, esophageal candidiasis, serious fungal infections | Visual disturbances, nausea, vomiting, abdominal pain, diarrhea, increased LFT, liver necrosis, hepatitis, cholestasis, headache, rash, pruritus, eosinophilia |

# Antifungals: Topical

## USES

Treatment of tinea infections, cutaneous candidiasis (moniliasis) due to *Candida albicans*.

## ACTION

Exact mechanism unknown. May deplete essential intracellular components by inhibiting transport of potassium, other ions into cells; alter membrane permeability, resulting in loss of potassium, other cellular components.

## ANTIFUNGALS: TOPICAL

| Name | Availability | Dosage Range | Side Effects |
|---|---|---|---|
| **Butenafine (Mentax)** | C: 1% | 2 times/day | Burning, stinging, pruritus, contact dermatitis, erythema |
| **Ciclopirox (Loprox)** | C: 1%<br>L: 1% | 2 times/day | Irritation, pruritus, redness |
| **Clotrimazole<br>(Lotrimin, Mycelex)** | C: 1%<br>L: 1%<br>S: 1% | 2 times/day | Erythema, stinging, blistering, edema, pruritus |
| **Efinaconazole (Jublia)** | S: 10% | Once daily | Application site dermatitis/vesicles |
| **Ketoconazole (Nizoral)** | C: 2% | 1–2 times/day | Irritation, pruritus, stinging |
| **Miconazole<br>(Micatin, Monistat)** | C: 2%<br>P: 2% | 2 times/day | Irritation, burning, allergic contact dermatitis |
| **Nystatin (Mycostatin, Nilstat)** | C: 100,000 g<br>O: 100,000 g<br>P: 100,000 g | 2–3 times/day | Irritation |
| **Oxiconazole (Oxistat)** | C: 1%<br>L: 1% | 1–2 times/day | Pruritus, burning, stinging, irritation, pain, tingling |
| **Sertaconazole (Ertaczo)** | C: 2% | 2 times/day | Dry skin, burning, pruritus, erythema |
| **Tavaborole (Kerydin)** | S: 5% | Once daily | Ingrown toenails, exfoliation, erythema, dermatitis |
| **Terbinafine (Lamisil)** | C: 1%<br>G: 10 mg | 1–2 times/day | Irritation, burning, pruritus, dryness |
| **Tolnaftate (Tinactin)** | C: 1%<br>G: 1%<br>S: 1% | 2 times/day | Mild irritation |

*C,* Cream; *G,* gel; *L,* lotion; *O,* ointment; *P,* powder; *S,* solution.

# Antiglaucoma Agents

## USES

Reduction of elevated intraocular pressure (IOP) in pts with open-angle glaucoma and ocular hypertension.

## ACTION

Medications decrease IOP by two primary mechanisms: decreasing aqueous humor (AH) production or increasing AH outflow.

- *Miotics (direct acting and indirect acting):* Constrict pupils, opening channels in the trabecular meshwork, reducing resistance to outflow of AH.
- *Alpha₂ agonists:* Activate receptors in ciliary body, inhibiting aqueous secretion and increasing uveoscleral aqueous outflow.
- *Beta blockers:* Reduce production of aqueous humor.
- *Carbonic anhydrase inhibitors:* Decrease production of AH by inhibiting enzyme carbonic anhydrase.
- *Prostaglandins:* Increase outflow of aqueous fluid through uveoscleral route.

## ANTIGLAUCOMA AGENTS

| Name | Availability | Dosage Range | Side Effects |
|---|---|---|---|
| **Miotics** | | | |
| **Carbachol** (Isopto-Carbachol) | **S:** 1.5%, 3% | 1 drop qid | Brow ache, corneal toxicity, conjunctival inflammation, transient myopia, blurred vision, retinal detachment |
| **Pilocarpine** (Isopto Carpine Pilopine HS [Gel]) | **G:** 4% **S:** 1%, 2%, 4% | **S:** 1 drop qid **G:** 1 drop HS | Same as carbachol |
| **Alpha₂ Agonists** | | | |
| **Apraclonidine** (Iopidine) | **S:** 0.5%, 1% | 1 drop tid | Fatigue, somnolence, local allergic reaction, dry eyes, stinging |

*Continued*

## ANTIGLAUCOMA AGENTS—cont'd

| Name | Availability | Dosage Range | Side Effects |
|---|---|---|---|
| **Brimonidine (Alphagan HP)** | S: 0.1%, 0.15%, 0.2% | 1 drop tid | Same as apraclonidine |
| *Prostaglandins* | | | |
| **Bimatoprost (Lumigan)** | S: 0.01% | 1 drop daily in evening | Conjunctival hyperemia; darkening of iris, eyelids; increase in length, thickness, and number of eyelashes; local irritation; itching; dryness; blurred vision |
| **Latanoprost (Xalatan)** | S: 0.005% | 1 drop daily in evening | See bimatoprost |
| **Tafluprost (Zioptan)** | S: 0.0015% | 1 drop daily in evening | See bimatoprost |
| **Travoprost (Travatan)** | S: 0.004% | 1 drop daily in evening | See bimatoprost |
| *Beta Blockers* | | | |
| **Betaxolol (Betoptic, Betoptic-S)** | Suspension (Betoptic-S): 0.25% S (Betoptic): 0.5% | Betoptic-S: 1 drop 2 times/day Betoptic: 1–2 drops 2 times/day | Fatigue, dizziness, bradycardia, respiratory depression, mask symptoms of hypoglycemia, block effects of beta agonists in treatment of asthma |
| **Carteolol (Ocupress)** | S: 1% | 1 drop 2 times/day | Same as betaxolol |
| **Levobunolol (Betagan)** | S: 0.25% 0.5% | 1 drop 1–2 times/day | Same as betaxolol |
| **Metipranolol (OptiPranolol)** | S: 0.3% | 1 drop 2 times/day | Same as betaxolol |
| **Timolol (Betimol, Istalol, Timoptic, Timoptic XE)** | S: 0.25%, 0.5% G, Timoptic XE: 0.25%, 0.5% | S: 1 drop 2 times/day (Istalol): 1 drop daily G: 1 drop daily | Same as betaxolol |
| *Carbonic Anhydrase Inhibitors* | | | |
| **Brinzolamide (Azopt)** | Suspension: 1% | 1 drop 3 times/day | Bitter taste, stinging, redness, burning, conjunctivitis, dry eyes, blurred vision |

| Dorzolamide (Trusopt) | S: 2% | 1 drop 3 times/day | Same as brinzolamide |
|---|---|---|---|
| Combinations | | | |
| **Brimonidine/timolol (Combigan)** | 0.2%/0.5% | 1 drop bid | See individual agents |
| **Brinzolamide/ brimonidine (Simbrinza)** | 1%/0.2% | 1 drop tid | See individual agents |
| **Timolol/dorzolamide (Cosopt)** | 0.5%/2% | 1 drop bid | See individual agents |

*C,* Capsules; *G,* gel; *O,* ointment; *S,* solution; *T,* tablets.

# Antihistamines

## USES

Symptomatic relief of upper respiratory allergic disorders. Allergic reactions associated with other drugs respond to antihistamines, as do blood transfusion reactions. Used as a second-choice drug in treatment of angioneurotic edema. Effective in treatment of acute urticaria and other dermatologic conditions. May also be used for preop sedation, Parkinson's disease, and motion sickness.

## ACTION

Antihistamines ($H_1$ antagonists) inhibit vasoconstrictor effects and vasodilator effects on endothelial cells of histamine. They block increased capillary permeability, formation of edema/wheal caused by histamine. Many antihistamines can bind to receptors in CNS, causing primarily depression (decreased alertness, slowed reaction times, drowsiness) but also stimulation (restlessness, nervousness, inability to sleep). Some may counter motion sickness.

## ANTIHISTAMINES

| Name | Availability | Dosage Range | Side Effects |
|---|---|---|---|
| **Cetirizine (Zyrtec)** | **T:** 5 mg, 10 mg<br>**C:** 5 mg, 10 mg<br>**T (chew):** 5 mg/10 mg<br>**S:** 5 mg/5 ml | **A:** 5–10 mg/day<br>**C (6–12 yrs):** 5–10 mg/day<br>**C (2–5 yrs):** 2.5–5 mg/day | Headache, somnolence, fatigue, abdominal pain, dry mouth |
| **Desloratadine (Clarinex)** | **T:** 5 mg<br>**ODT:** 2.5 mg, 5 mg<br>**S:** 0.5 mg/ml | **A, C (12 yrs and older):** 5 mg/day<br>**C (6–11 yrs):** 2.5 mg/day<br>**C (1–5 yrs):** 1.25 mg/day<br>**C (6–11 mos):** 1 mg/day | Dizziness, fatigue, headache, nausea |
| **Dimenhydrinate (Dramamine)** | **T:** 50 mg<br>**T (chew):** 25 mg, 50 mg | **A:** 50–100 mg q4–6h<br>**C:** 12.5–50 mg q6–8h | Dizziness, drowsiness, headache, nausea |
| **Diphenhydramine (Benadryl)** | **T:** 25 mg, 50 mg<br>**C:** 25 mg, 50 mg<br>**L:** 12.5 mg/5 ml | **A:** 25–50 mg q6–8h<br>**C (6–11 yrs):** 12.5–25 mg q4–6h<br>**C (2–5 yrs):** 6.25 mg q4–6h | Chills, confusion, dizziness, fatigue, headache, sedation, nausea |
| **Fexofenadine (Allegra)** | **T:** 30 mg, 60 mg, 180 mg<br>**ODT:** 30 mg<br>**S:** 30 mg/5 ml | **A:** 60 mg q12h or 180 mg/day<br>**C (2–11 yrs):** 30 mg q12h, **(6–23 mos):** 15 mg bid | Headache, vomiting, fatigue, diarrhea |
| **Hydroxyzine (Atarax)** | **T:** 10 mg, 25 mg, 50 mg<br>**C:** 25 mg, 50 mg, 100 mg<br>**S:** 10 mg/5 ml | **A:** 25 mg q6–8h<br>**C:** 2 mg/kg/day in divided doses q6–8h | Dizziness, drowsiness, fatigue, headache |
| **Levocetirizine (Xyzal)** | **T:** 5 mg<br>**S:** 2.5 mg/ml | **A, C (12 yrs and older):** 5 mg once daily in evening<br>**C (6–11 yrs):** 2.5 mg once daily in evening<br>**(6 mos–5 yrs):** 1.25 mg once daily | Fatigue, fever, somnolence, vomiting |

| Loratadine (Claritin) | ODT: 10 mg<br>T (chewy): 5 mg<br>T: 10 mg<br>S: 1 mg/ml | **A:** 10 mg/day<br>**C (6–12 yrs):** 10 mg/day **(2–5 yrs):** 5 mg/day | Fatigue, headache, malaise, somnolence, abdominal pain |
| Promethazine (Phenergan) | T: 12.5 mg, 25 mg, 50 mg<br>S: 6.25 mg/5 ml | **A:** 25 mg at bedtime or 12.5 mg q8h<br>**C:** 0.5 mg/kg at bedtime or 0.1 mg/kg q6–8h | Confusion, dizziness, drowsiness, fatigue, constipation, nausea, vomiting |

*A,* Adults; *C,* capsules; *C (dosage),* children; *L,* liquid; *ODT,* orally disintegrating tablet; *S,* syrup; *SR,* sustained-release; *T,* tablets.

# Antihyperlipidemics

## USES

Cholesterol management.

## ACTION

*Bile acid sequestrants:* Bind bile acids in the intestine; prevent active transport and reabsorption and enhance bile acid excretion. Depletion of hepatic bile acid results in the increased conversion of cholesterol to bile acids.

*HMG-CoA reductase inhibitors (statins):* Inhibit HMG-CoA reductase, the last regulated step in the synthesis of cholesterol. Cholesterol synthesis in the liver is reduced.

*Niacin (nicotinic acid):* Reduces hepatic synthesis of triglycerides and secretion of very low density lipoprotein (VLDL) by inhibiting the mobilization of free fatty acids from peripheral tissues.

*Fibric acid:* Increases the oxidation of fatty acids in the liver, resulting in reduced secretion of triglyceride-rich lipoproteins, and increases lipoprotein lipase activity and fatty acid uptake.

*Cholesterol absorption inhibitor:* Acts in the gut wall to prevent cholesterol absorption through the intestinal villi.

*Omega fatty acids:* Exact mechanism unknown. Mechanisms may include inhibition of acyl-CoA, decreased lipogenesis in liver, increased lipoprotein lipase activity.

*PCSK9 inhibitors:* Binds with high-affinity and specificity to LDL cholesterol receptors, promoting their degradation.

## ANTIHYPERLIPIDEMICS

| Name | Primary Effect | Dosage | Comments/Side Effects |
|---|---|---|---|
| **Bile Acid Sequestrants** | | | |
| **Cholestyramine (Prevalite, Questran)** | Decreases LDL<br>Increases HDL, TG | 4 g 1–2 times/day<br>May increase over 1 mo interval. Usual dose: 8–16 g/day in 2 divided doses | May bind drugs given concurrently. Take at least 1 hr before or 4–6 hrs after cholestyramine.<br>**Side Effects:** Constipation, heartburn, nausea, vomiting, stomach pain |
| **Colesevelam (Welchol)** | Decreases LDL<br>Increases HDL, TG | 3.75 g once daily or 1.875 g 2 times/day | Take with food.<br>**Side Effects:** Constipation, dyspepsia, weakness, myalgia, pharyngitis |
| **Colestipol (Colestid)** | Decreases LDL<br>Increases TG | **G:** Initially, 5 g once or twice daily. May increase by 5 g/day q1–2 mos. Maintenance: 5–30 g/day.<br>**T:** Initially, 2 g once or twice daily. May increase by 2 g 2 times/day at 1–2 mo intervals. Maintenance: 2–16 g/day | Do not crush tablets. May bind drugs given concurrently. Take at least 1 hr before or 4–6 hrs after colestipol.<br>**Side Effects:** Constipation, headache, dizziness, anxiety, vertigo, drowsiness, nausea, vomiting, diarrhea, flatulence |
| **Cholesterol Absorption Inhibitor** | | | |
| **Ezetimibe (Zetia)** | Decreases LDL<br>Increases HDL<br>Decreases TG | 10 mg once daily | Administer at least 2 hrs before or 4 hrs after bile acid sequestrants.<br>**Side Effects:** Dizziness, headache, fatigue, diarrhea, abdominal pain, arthralgia, sinusitis, pharyngitis |

## Fibric Acid

| Name | Action | Dose | Notes |
|---|---|---|---|
| **Fenofibrate (Antara, Lofibra, Tricor, Triglide)** | Decreases TG, Decreases LDL, Increases HDL | **Antara:** 43–130 mg/day<br>**Lofibra:** 67–200 mg/day<br>**Tricor:** 48–145 mg/day<br>**Triglide:** 50–160 mg/day<br>**Fenoglide:** 40–120 mg/day<br>**Lipofen:** 50–150 mg/day | May increase levels of ezetimibe. Concomitant use of statins may increase rhabdomyolysis, elevate CPK levels, and cause myoglobinuria.<br>**Side Effects:** Abdominal pain, constipation, diarrhea, respiratory complaints, headache, fever, flu-like syndrome, asthenia |
| **Fenofibric acid (Fibricor, Trilipix)** | Decreases TG, LDL, Increases HDL | **Trilipix:** 45–135 mg/day<br>**Fibricor:** 35–105 mg/day | May give without regard to meals. Concomitant use of statins may increase rhabdomyolysis.<br>**Side Effects:** Headache, upper respiratory tract infection, pain, nausea, dizziness, nasopharyngitis |
| **Gemfibrozil (Lopid)** | Decreases TG, Increases HDL | 600 mg 2 times/day | Give 30 min before breakfast and dinner. Concomitant use of statins may increase rhabdomyolysis, elevate CPK levels, and cause myoglobinuria.<br>**Side Effects:** Fatigue, vertigo, headache, rash, eczema, diarrhea, abdominal pain, nausea, vomiting, constipation |

## Niacin

| Name | Action | Dose | Notes |
|---|---|---|---|
| **Niacin, nicotinic acid (Niacor, Niaspan)** | Decreases LDL, TG, Increases HDL | **Regular-release (Niacor):**<br>1 g tid<br>**Extended-release (Niaspan):**<br>1 g at bedtime | Diabetics may experience a dose-related elevation in glucose.<br>**Side Effects:** Increased LFT, hyperglycemia, dyspepsia, itching, flushing, dizziness, insomnia |

*Continued*

## ANTIHYPERLIPIDEMICS—cont'd

| Name | Primary Effect | Dosage | Comments/Side Effects |
|------|---------------|--------|----------------------|
| **Statins** | | | |
| Atorvastatin (Lipitor) | Decreases LDL, TG Increases HDL | Initially, 10–20 mg/day. Range: 10–80 mg/day | May interact with CYP3A4 inhibitors (e.g., amiodarone, diltiazem, cyclosporine, grapefruit juice) increasing risk of myopathy. **Side Effects:** Myalgia, myopathy, rhabdomyolysis, headache, chest pain, peripheral edema, dizziness, rash, abdominal pain, constipation, diarrhea, dyspepsia, nausea, flatulence, increased LFT, back pain, sinusitis |
| Fluvastatin (Lescol) | Decreases LDL, TG Increases HDL | 40–80 mg/day | Primarily metabolized by CYP2C9 enzyme system. May increase levels of phenytoin, rifampin. May lower fluvastatin levels. **Side Effects:** Headache, fatigue, dyspepsia, diarrhea, nausea, abdominal pain, myalgia, myopathy, rhabdomyolysis |
| Lovastatin (Mevacor) | Decreases LDL, TG Increases HDL | Initially, 20 mg/day. Adjust at 4 wk intervals. **Maximum:** 80 mg/day | May interact with CYP3A4 inhibitors (e.g., amiodarone, diltiazem, cyclosporine, grapefruit products) increasing risk of myopathy. **Side Effects:** Increased CPK levels, headache, dizziness, rash, constipation, diarrhea, abdominal pain, dyspepsia, nausea, flatulence, myalgia, myopathy, rhabdomyolysis |
| Pitavastatin (Livalo) | Decreases LDL, TG Increases HDL | Initially, 2 mg/day. May increase at 4 wk intervals to 4 mg/day | Erythromycin, rifampin may increase concentration. **Side Effects:** Myalgia, back pain, diarrhea, constipation, pain in extremities |
| Pravastatin (Pravachol) | Decreases LDL, TG Increases HDL | Initially, 40 mg/day. Titrate to response. Range: 10–80 mg/day | May be less likely to be involved in drug interactions. Cyclosporine may increase pravastatin levels. **Side Effects:** Chest pain, headache, dizziness, rash, nausea, vomiting, diarrhea, increased LFTs, cough, flu-like symptoms, myalgia, myopathy, rhabdomyolysis |

| Rosuvastatin (Crestor) | Decreases LDL, TG<br>Increases HDL | , Initially, 10–20 mg/day.<br>Titrate to response.<br>Range: 5–40 mg/day | May be less likely to be involved in drug interactions. Cyclosporine may increase rosuvastatin levels.<br>**Side Effects:** Chest pain, peripheral edema, headache, rash, dizziness, vertigo, pharyngitis, diarrhea, nausea, constipation, abdominal pain, dyspepsia, sinusitis, flu-like symptoms, myalgia, myopathy, rhabdomyolysis |
| --- | --- | --- | --- |
| Simvastatin (Zocor) | Decreases LDL, TG<br>Increases HDL | 5–40 mg/day | May interact with CYP3A4 inhibitors (e.g., amiodarone, diltiazem, cyclosporine, grapefruit products) increasing risk of myopathy.<br>**Side Effects:** Constipation, flatulence, dyspepsia, increased LFTs, increased CPK, upper respiratory tract infection |
| Omega Fatty Acids | | | |
| Icosapent (Vascepa) | Decreases TG | 2 g 2 times/day | **Side Effects:** Arthralgia |
| Lovaza | Decreases TG<br>Increases LDL, HDL | 2 g 2 times/day or 4 g once daily | Use with caution with fish or shellfish allergy.<br>**Side Effects:** Eructation, dyspepsia, taste perversion |
| PCSK9 Inhibitors | | | |
| Alirocumab (Praluent) | Decreases LDL | **SQ:** 75 mg q2wks | **Side Effects:** Hypersensitivity reactions (e.g., rash), nasopharyngitis, injection site reactions, influenza |
| Evolcumab (Repatha) | Decreases LDL | **SQ:** 140 mg q2wks or 420 mg qmo | **Side Effects:** Nasopharyngitis, upper respiratory tract infection, influenza, back pain, injection site reactions |

*CPK,* Creatine phosphokinase; *G,* granules; *HDL,* high-density lipoprotein; *LDL,* low-density lipoprotein; *SQ,* subcutaneous; *T,* tablets; *TG,* triglycerides.

# Antihypertensives

## USES

Treatment of mild to severe hypertension.

## ACTION

Many groups of medications are used in the treatment of hypertension.

*ACE inhibitors:* Decrease conversion of angiotensin I to angiotensin II, a potent vasoconstrictor, reducing peripheral vascular resistance and B/P.

*Alpha agonists (central action):* Stimulate alpha₂-adrenergic receptors in the cardiovascular centers of the CNS, reducing sympathetic outflow and producing an antihypertensive effect.

*Alpha antagonists (peripheral action):* Block alpha₁-adrenergic receptors in arterioles and veins, inhibiting vasoconstriction and decreasing peripheral vascular resistance, causing a fall in B/P.

*Angiotensin receptor blockers:* Block vasoconstrictor effects of angiotensin II by blocking the binding of angiotensin II to AT1 receptors in vascular smooth muscle, helping blood vessels to relax and reduce B/P.

*Beta blockers:* Decrease B/P by inhibiting beta₁-adrenergic receptors, which lowers heart rate, heart workload, and the heart's output of blood.

*Calcium channel blockers:* Reduce B/P by inhibiting flow of extracellular calcium across cell membranes of vascular tissue, relaxing arterial smooth muscle.

*Diuretics:* Inhibit sodium (Na) reabsorption, increasing excretion of Na and water. Reduce plasma, extracellular fluid volume, and peripheral vascular resistance.

*Renin inhibitors:* Directly inhibit renin, decreasing plasma renin activity (PRA), inhibiting conversion of angiotensinogen to angiotensin, producing antihypertensive effect.

*Vasodilators:* Directly relax arteriolar smooth muscle, decreasing vascular resistance. Exact mechanism unknown.

## ANTIHYPERTENSIVES

| Name | Availability | Dosage Range | Side Effects |
|---|---|---|---|
| **(ACE) Inhibitors** | | | |
| **Benazepril (Lotensin)** | **T:** 5 mg, 10 mg, 20 mg, 40 mg | 20–80 mg/day as single or 2 divided doses | Postural dizziness, headache, cough |
| Captopril | **T:** 12.5 mg, 25 mg, 50 mg, 100 mg | 25–50 mg 2–3 times/day | Rash, cough, hyperkalemia |
| Enalapril (Vasotec) | **T:** 2.5 mg, 5 mg, 10 mg, 20 mg | 2.5–40 mg/day in 1–2 divided doses | Hypotension, chest pain, syncope, headache, dizziness, fatigue |
| Fosinopril | **T:** 10 mg, 20 mg, 40 mg | 10–80 mg/day | Dizziness, cough, hyperkalemia |
| Lisinopril (Prinivil, Zestril) | **T:** 2.5 mg, 5 mg, 10 mg, 20 mg, 30 mg, 40 mg | 10–40 mg/day | Hypotension, headache, fatigue, dizziness, hyperkalemia, cough |
| Quinapril | **T:** 5 mg, 10 mg, 20 mg, 40 mg | 10–40 mg/day | Hypotension, dizziness, fatigue, headache, myalgia, hyperkalemia |
| Ramipril (Altace) | **T or C:** 1.25 mg, 2.5 mg, 5 mg, 10 mg | 2.5–20 mg/day | Cough, hypotension, angina, headache, dizziness, hyperkalemia |
| **Alpha Agonists: Central Action** | | | |
| Clonidine (Catapres) | **T:** 0.1 mg, 0.2 mg, 0.3 mg **P:** 0.1 mg/hr, 0.2 mg/hr, 0.3 mg/hr | **PO:** 0.1–0.8 mg/day **Topical:** 0.1–0.6 mg/wk | Sedation, dry mouth, constipation, sexual dysfunction, bradycardia, xerostomia, drowsiness, headache |
| **Alpha Agonists: Peripheral Action** | | | |
| Doxazosin (Cardura) | **T:** 1 mg, 2 mg, 4 mg, 8 mg | **PO:** 2–16 mg/day | Dizziness, vertigo, headaches |
| Prazosin (Minipress) | **C:** 1 mg, 2 mg, 5 mg | **PO:** 6–20 mg/day | Dizziness, light-headedness, headaches, drowsiness |
| Terazosin (Hytrin) | **C:** 1 mg, 2 mg, 5 mg, 10 mg | **PO:** 1–20 mg/day | Dizziness, headaches, asthenia (loss of strength, energy) |
| **Angiotensin Receptor Blockers** | | | |
| Azilsartan (Edarbi) | **T:** 40 mg, 80 mg | 40–80 mg/day | Diarrhea, hypotension, nausea, cough |

*Continued*

ANTIHYPERTENSIVES—cont'd

| Name | Availability | Dosage Range | Side Effects |
|---|---|---|---|
| **Candesartan (Atacand)** | **T:** 4 mg, 8 mg, 16 mg, 32 mg | 8–32 mg/day | Hypotension, dizziness, headache, hyperkalemia |
| **Eprosartan (Teveten)** | **T:** 400 mg, 600 mg | 400–800 mg/day | Headache, cough, dizziness |
| **Irbesartan (Avapro)** | **T:** 75 mg, 150 mg, 300 mg | 150–300 mg/day | Fatigue, diarrhea, cough |
| **Losartan (Cozaar)** | **T:** 25 mg, 50 mg, 100 mg | 25–100 mg/day | Chest pain, fatigue, hypoglycemia, weakness, cough, hypotension |
| **Olmesartan (Benicar)** | **T:** 5 mg, 20 mg, 40 mg | 20–40 mg/day | Dizziness, headache, diarrhea, flu-like symptoms |
| **Valsartan (Diovan)** | **T:** 80 mg, 160 mg, 320 mg | 80–320 mg/day | Dizziness, fatigue, increased BUN |
| **Beta Blockers** | | | |
| **Atenolol (Tenormin)** | **T:** 25 mg, 50 mg, 100 mg | 25–100 mg/day | Fatigue, bradycardia, reduced exercise tolerance, increased triglycerides, bronchospasm, sexual dysfunction, masked hypoglycemia |
| **Bisoprolol (Zebeta)** | **T:** 5 mg, 10 mg | 2.5–10 mg/day | Fatigue, insomnia, diarrhea, arthralgia, upper respiratory infections |
| **Metoprolol (Lopressor)** | **T:** 25 mg, 50 mg, 100 mg | 50–100 mg/day | Hypotension, bradycardia, fatigue, 1st degree heart block, dizziness |
| **Metoprolol XL (Toprol XL)** | **T:** 25 mg, 50 mg, 100 mg, 200 mg | 50–100 mg/day | Same as metoprolol |
| **Calcium Channel Blockers** | | | |
| **Amlodipine (Norvasc)** | **T:** 2.5 mg, 5 mg, 10 mg | 2.5–10 mg/day | Headache, fatigue, peripheral edema, flushing, worsening heart failure |
| **Diltiazem CD (Cardizem CD)** | **C:** 120 mg, 180 mg, 240 mg, 300 mg | 180–420 mg/day | Dizziness, headache, bradycardia, heart block, worsening heart failure, edema, constipation |
| **Felodipine (Plendil)** | **T:** 2.5 mg, 5 mg, 10 mg | 2.5–20 mg/day | Headache, flushing, peripheral edema |

| | | |
|---|---|---|
| **Nifedipine XL**<br>(Adalat CC,<br>Procardia XL) | **T:** 30 mg, 60 mg, 90 mg | 90–120 mg/day | Flushing, peripheral edema, headache, dizziness, nausea |
| **Verapamil SR**<br>(Calan SR) | **T:** 120 mg, 180 mg, 240 mg<br>**T (Sustained-Release):** 120 mg,<br>180 mg | **T (Immediate-<br>Release):**<br>80–320 mg/day<br>**T (Sustained-Release):**<br>120–480 mg/day | Headache, gingival hyperplasia, constipation |
| Diuretics | | | |
| **Chlorthalidone**<br>(Hygroton) | **T:** 25 mg, 50 mg | 12.5–25 mg/day | Same as hydrochlorothiazide |
| **Hydrochlorothiazide**<br>(Hydrodiuril) | **T:** 25 mg, 50 mg | 12.5–50 mg/day | Hypokalemia, hyperuricemia, hypomagnesemia, hyperglycemia |
| Renin Inhibitor | | | |
| **Aliskiren** (Tekturna) | **T:** 150 mg, 300 mg | **PO:** 150–300 mg/day | Diarrhea, dyspepsia, headache, dizziness, fatigue, upper<br>respiratory tract infection |
| Vasodilators | | | |
| **Hydralazine**<br>(Apresoline) | **T:** 10 mg, 25 mg, 50 mg, 100 mg | **PO:** 40–300 mg/day | Anorexia, nausea, diarrhea, vomiting, headaches, palpitations |
| **Minoxidil** (Loniten) | **T:** 2.5 mg, 10 mg | **PO:** 10–40 mg/day | Rapid/irregular heartbeat, hypertrichosis, peripheral edema |

*C,* Capsules; *P,* patch; *T,* tablets.

# Antimigraine (Triptans)

## USES

Treatment of migraine headaches with or without aura in adults 18 yrs and older.

## ACTION

Triptans are selective agonists of the serotonin (5-HT) receptor in cranial arteries, which cause vasoconstriction and reduce inflammation associated with antidromic neuronal transmission correlating with relief of migraine headache.

## TRIPTANS

| Name | Availability | Dosage Range | Contraindications | Common Side Effects |
|------|--------------|--------------|-------------------|---------------------|
| **Almotriptan (Axert)** | **T:** 6.25 mg, 12.5 mg | 6.25–12.5 mg; may repeat after 2 hrs | Ischemic heart disease, angina pectoris, arrhythmias, previous MI, uncontrolled hypertension, hemiplegic or basilar migraine, peripheral vascular disease | Drowsiness, dizziness, paresthesia, nausea, vomiting, headache, xerostomia |
| **Eletriptan (Relpax)** | **T:** 20 mg, 40 mg | **A:** 20–40 mg; may repeat after 2 hrs (**Maximum:** 60 mg/day) | Same as almotriptan | Chest pain, dizziness, drowsiness, headache, paresthesia, nausea, xerostomia, weakness |
| **Frovatriptan (Frova)** | **T:** 2.5 mg | 2.5 mg; may repeat after 2 hrs; no more than 3 **T**/day | Same as almotriptan | Hot/cold sensations, dizziness, fatigue, headaches, skeletal pain, dyspepsia, flushing, paresthesia, drowsiness, xerostomia, nausea |
| **Naratriptan (Amerge)** | **T:** 1 mg, 2.5 mg | 1–2.5 mg; may repeat once after 4 hrs | Same as almotriptan plus severe renal/hepatic disease | Neck pain, pain, nausea, fatigue |

| | | | |
|---|---|---|---|
| **Rizatriptan (Maxalt, Maxalt-MLT)** | **T:** 5 mg, 10 mg, **DT:** 5 mg, 10 mg | 5 or 10 mg; may repeat after 2 hrs | Same as almotriptan | Chest pain, drowsiness, xerostomia, weakness, paresthesia, nausea, dizziness, drowsiness, fatigue |
| **Sumatriptan (Imitrex, Sumavel DosePro, Onzetra, Xsail, Zecuity)** | **T:** 25 mg, 50 mg, 100 mg **NS:** 5 mg, 10 mg, 20 mg **I:** 4 mg, 6 mg **NP:** 8 pouches of 2 nose pieces each 11 mg/piece **Transdermal:** 6.5 mg/4 hrs | **PO:** 25–100 mg; may repeat after 2 hrs **NS:** 5–20 mg; may repeat after 2 hrs **Subcutaneous:** 4–6 mg; may repeat after 1 hr **NP:** 22 mg; may repeat after 2 hrs | Same as almotriptan plus severe hepatic dysfunction | *Oral:* Hot/cold flashes, flushing, malaise, fatigue *Injection:* Atypical sensations, flushing, chest pain/discomfort, injection site reaction, dizziness, vertigo, paresthesia, dizziness; bleeding, bruising, swelling, erythema at injection site *Nasal:* Discomfort, nausea, vomiting, altered taste *Transdermal:* Localized pain, skin discoloration, allergic contact dermatitis, pruritis, local irritation |
| **Zolmitriptan (Zomig, Zomig-ZMT)** | **T:** 2.5 mg, 5 mg **DT:** 2.5 mg, 5 mg **NS:** 5 mg/0.1 ml | 2.5–5 mg; may repeat after 2 hrs **NS:** 1 spray (5 mg) at onset of migrane headache; may repeat after 2 hrs | Same as almotriptan plus symptomatic Wolff-Parkinson-White syndrome | Atypical sensations, pain, nausea, dizziness, asthenia, drowsiness |

*A,* Adults; *DT,* disintegrating tablets; *I,* injection; *NP,* nasal powder; *NS,* nasal spray; *T,* tablets.

# Antipsychotics

## USES

Antipsychotics are primarily used in managing schizophrenia. They may also be used in treatment of bipolar disorder, schizoaffective disorder, and irritability associated with autism. The goals in treating schizophrenia include targeting symptoms, preventing relapse, and increasing adaptive functioning. Use of antipsychotic medications is the mainstay of schizophrenia management.

## ACTION

The precise mechanism of action of antipsychotic medications is unknown, but they have been categorized into two groups:

*Typical (traditional):* Associated with high dopamine antagonism and low serotonin antagonism.

*Atypical:* Those having moderate to high dopamine antagonism and high serotonin antagonism and those having low dopamine antagonism and high serotonin antagonism.

## SIDE EFFECTS (Please refer to individual monographs)

*Typical versus atypical:* Typical antipsychotics are associated with a greater risk of extrapyramidal side effects, and atypicals are associated with a greater risk of weight gain.

*Endocrine:* Hyperprolactinemia, weight gain, increased risk of diabetes.

*Cardiovascular:* Orthostatic hypotension, electrocardiographic changes.

*Lipids:* Increased triglycerides, cholesterol.

*Central nervous system:* Dystonic reactions, akathisia, pseudo-parkinsonism, tardive dyskinesia, sedation, risk of seizures.

## TYPICAL ANTIPSYCHOTICS

| Name | Uses | Dosage (Oral) |
|------|------|---------------|
| **Fluphenazine** | Adult psychosis | 1–5 mg/day |
| **Haloperidol (Haldol)** | Adult and child psychosis | 1–15 mg/day |
| **Thioridazine** | Adult, adolescent, child schizophrenia and psychosis | 200–800 mg/day |
| **Thiothixene (Navane)** | Adult and adolescent schizophrenia | Moderate: 15 mg/day<br>Severe: 20–30 mg/day |

## ATYPICAL ANTIPSYCHOTICS

| Name | Uses | Dosage |
|------|------|--------|
| **Aripiprazole (Abilify)** | Adult and adolescent schizophrenia; adult and child bipolar I disorder; adult major depressive disorder; irritability with adolescent autism | 10–15 mg/day |
| **Brexipiprazole (Rexulti)** | Adult schizophrenia; adult major depressive disorder | 2–4 mg/day |
| **Cariprazine (Vraylar)** | Adult schizophrenia, bipolar I disorder (manic or mixed episodes) | 1.5–6 mg/day |
| **Clozapine (Clozaril)** | Schizophrenia; suicidal behavior in adult schizophrenia and schizoaffective disorder | 300–450 mg/day |
| **Iloperidone (Fanapt)** | Adult schizophrenia | 12–24 mg/day |
| **Lurasidone (Latuda)** | Adult schizophrenia, bipolar I disorder (manic or mixed episodes) | 40–160 mg/day |
| **Olanzapine (Zyprexa)** | Adult, adolescent, and child schizophrenia; adult, adolescent mania in bipolar I disorder | 10–20 mg/day |
| **Paliperidone (Invega)** | Adult and adolescent schizophrenia; adult schizoaffective disorder | 3–12 mg/day |
| **Quetiapine (Seroquel)** | Adult and adolescent schizophrenia; adult, adolescent, and child bipolar I disorder | 400–800 mg/day |
| **Risperidone (Risperdal)** | Adult and adolescent schizophrenia; adult, adolescent, and child bipolar I disorder; irritability with adolescent and child autism | 4–8 mg/day |
| **Ziprasidone (Geodon)** | Adult schizophrenia; manic or mixed episodes associated with adult bipolar I disorder | 40–160 mg/day |

# Antivirals

## USES

Treatment of HIV infection. Treatment of cytomegalovirus (CMV) retinitis in pts with AIDS, acute herpes zoster (shingles), genital herpes (recurrent), mucosal and cutaneous herpes simplex virus (HSV), chickenpox, and influenza A viral illness.

## ACTION

Effective antivirals must inhibit virus-specific nucleic acid/protein synthesis. Possible mechanisms of action of antivirals used for non-HIV infection may include interference with viral DNA synthesis and viral replication, inactivation of viral DNA polymerases, incorporation and termination of the growing viral DNA chain, prevention of release of viral nucleic acid into the host cell, or interference with viral penetration into cells.

## ANTIVIRALS

| Name | Availability | Uses | Side Effects |
|---|---|---|---|
| **Abacavir (Ziagen)** | **T:** 300 mg<br>**OS:** 20 mg/ml | HIV infection | Nausea, vomiting, loss of appetite, diarrhea, headaches, fatigue, hypersensitivity reactions |
| **Acyclovir (Zovirax)** | **T:** 400 mg, 800 mg<br>**C:** 200 mg<br>**I:** 50 mg/ml | Mucosal/cutaneous HSV-1 and HSV-2, varicella-zoster (shingles), genital herpes, herpes simplex, encephalitis, chickenpox | Malaise, anorexia, nausea, vomiting, light-headedness |
| **Adefovir (Hepsera)** | **T:** 10 mg | Chronic hepatitis B | Asthenia, headaches, abdominal pain, nausea, diarrhea, flatulence, dyspepsia |
| **Amantadine (Symmetrel)** | **T:** 100 mg<br>**C:** 100 mg<br>**S:** 50 mg/5 ml | Influenza A | Anxiety, dizziness, headaches, nausea, loss of appetite |
| **Cidofovir (Vistide)** | **I:** 75 mg/ml | CMV retinitis | Decreased urination, fever, chills, diarrhea, nausea, vomiting, headaches, loss of appetite |

| | | | |
|---|---|---|---|
| **Darunavir (Prezista)** | **T:** 75 mg, 150 mg, 400 mg, 600 mg, 800 mg | HIV infection | Diarrhea, nausea, vomiting, headaches, skin rash, constipation |
| **Delavirdine (Rescriptor)** | **T:** 100 mg, 200 mg | HIV infection | Diarrhea, fatigue, rash, headaches, nausea |
| **Didanosine (Videx)** | **C:** 125 mg, 200 mg, 250 mg, 400 mg<br>**Powder for suspension:** 2 g, 4 g | HIV infection | Peripheral neuropathy, anxiety, headaches, rash, nausea, diarrhea, dry mouth |
| **Efavirenz (Sustiva)** | **C:** 50 mg, 200 mg<br>**T:** 600 mg | HIV infection | Diarrhea, dizziness, headaches, insomnia, nausea, vomiting, drowsiness |
| **Etravirine (Intelence)** | **T:** 25 mg, 100 mg, 200 mg | HIV infection | Rash, nausea, abdominal pain, vomiting |
| **Famciclovir (Famvir)** | **T:** 125 mg, 250 mg, 500 mg | Herpes zoster, genital herpes, herpes labialis, mucosal/cutaneous herpes simplex | Headaches, nausea |
| **Foscarnet (Foscavir)** | **I:** 24 mg/ml | CMV retinitis, HSV infections | Decreased urination, abdominal pain, nausea, vomiting, dizziness, fatigue, headaches |
| **Ganciclovir (Cytovene)** | **I:** 500 mg | CMV retinitis, CMV disease | Sore throat, fever, unusual bleeding/bruising |
| **Indinavir (Crixivan)** | **C:** 200 mg, 400 mg | HIV infection | Blood in urine, weakness, nausea, vomiting, diarrhea, headaches, insomnia, altered taste |
| **Lamivudine (Epivir)** | **T:** 100 mg, 150 mg, 300 mg<br>**OS:** 5 mg/ml, 10 mg/ml | HIV infection, chronic hepatitis B | Nausea, vomiting, abdominal pain, paresthesia |
| **Lopinavir/ritonavir (Kaletra)** | **T:** 100 mg/25 mg, 200 mg/50 mg<br>**OS:** 80 mg/20 mg per ml | HIV infection | Diarrhea, nausea |

*Continued*

## ANTIVIRALS—cont'd

| Name | Availability | Uses | Side Effects |
|---|---|---|---|
| **Maraviroc (Selzentry)** | **T:** 150 mg, 300 mg | HIV infection | Cough, pyrexia, upper respiratory tract infection, rash, musculoskeletal symptoms, abdominal pain, dizziness |
| **Nelfinavir (Viracept)** | **T:** 250 mg, 625 mg | HIV infection | Diarrhea |
| **Oseltamivir (Tamiflu)** | **C:** 30 mg, 45 mg, 75 mg<br>**S:** 6 mg/ml | Influenza A or B | Diarrhea, nausea, vomiting |
| **Raltegravir (Isentress)** | **T:** 400 mg<br>**T (chew):** 25 mg, 100 mg | HIV infection | Nausea, headache, diarrhea, pyrexia |
| **Ribavirin (Virazole)** | **Aerosol:** 6 g<br>**OS:** 40 mg/ml<br>**T:** 200 mg, 400 mg, 600 mg | Lowers respiratory infections in infants, children due to respiratory syncytial virus (RSV), chronic hepatitis C | Anemia |
| **Ritonavir (Norvir)** | **C:** 100 mg **T:** 100 mg<br>**OS:** 80 mg/ml | HIV infection | Weakness, diarrhea, nausea, decreased appetite, vomiting, altered taste |
| **Saquinavir (Invirase)** | **C:** 200 mg<br>**T:** 500 mg | HIV infection | Weakness, diarrhea, nausea, oral ulcers, abdominal pain |
| **Stavudine (Zerit)** | **C:** 15 mg, 20 mg, 30 mg, 40 mg<br>**OS:** 1 mg/ml | HIV infection | Paresthesia, decreased appetite, chills, fever, rash |
| **Tenofovir (Viread)** | **T:** 150 mg, 200 mg, 250 mg, 300 mg<br>**Powder (oral):** 40 mg/g | HIV infection | Diarrhea, nausea, pharyngitis, headaches |

| Valacyclovir (Valtrex) | T: 500 mg, 1 g | Herpes zoster, genital herpes, herpes labialis, chickenpox | Headaches, nausea |
| Valganciclovir (Valcyte) | T: 450 mg, OS: 50 mg/ml | CMV retinitis | Anemia, abdominal pain, diarrhea, headaches, nausea, vomiting, paresthesia |
| Zanamivir (Relenza) | Inhalation: 5 mg | Influenza A and B | Cough, diarrhea, dizziness, headaches, nausea, vomiting |
| Zidovudine (Retrovir) | C: 100 mg, S: 50 mg/5 ml, I: 10 mg/ml | HIV infection | Fatigue, fever, chills, headaches, nausea, muscle pain |

*C,* Capsules; *I,* injection; *OS,* oral solution; *S,* syrup; *T,* tablets.

# Beta-Adrenergic Blockers

## USES

Management of hypertension, angina pectoris, arrhythmias, hypertrophic subaortic stenosis, migraine headaches, MI (prevention), glaucoma.

## ACTION

Beta-adrenergic blockers competitively block beta-adrenergic receptors, located primarily in myocardium, and beta$_1$-adrenergic receptors, located primarily in bronchial and vascular smooth muscle. By occupying beta-receptor sites, these agents prevent naturally occurring or administered epinephrine/norepinephrine from exerting their effects. The results are basically opposite to those of sympathetic stimulation.

Effects of beta$_1$ blockade include slowing heart rate, decreasing cardiac output and contractility; effects of beta$_2$ blockade include bronchoconstriction, increased airway resistance in pts with asthma or COPD. Beta blockers can affect cardiac rhythm/automaticity (decrease sinus rate, SA/AV conduction; increase refractory period in AV node); decrease systolic and diastolic B/P; exact mechanism unknown but may block peripheral receptors, decrease sympathetic outflow from CNS, or decrease renin release from kidney. All beta blockers mask tachycardia that occurs with hypoglycemia. When applied to the eye, reduce intraocular pressure and aqueous production.

## BETA-ADRENERGIC BLOCKERS

| Name | Availability | Indication | Dosage Range |
|------|--------------|------------|--------------|
| **Acebutolol** (Sectral) | **C:** 200 mg, 400 mg | HTN, ventricular arrhythmia | **HTN:** Initially, 400 mg once daily or 2 divided doses. Usual dose: 400–800 mg/day. **Arrhythmia:** Initially, 200 mg 2 times/day. Gradually increase to 300–600 mg 2 times/day |
| **Atenolol** (Tenormin) | **T:** 25 mg, 50 mg, 100 mg | HTN, angina, MI | **Angina:** Initially, 50 mg once daily. May increase to 100 mg once daily after one wk. **HTN:** Initially, 50 mg once daily. May increase to 100 mg once daily after 2 wks. **MI:** 50 mg bid or 100 mg once daily |

| Drug | Availability | Uses | Dosage |
|---|---|---|---|
| **Bisoprolol** (Zebeta) | T: 5 mg, 10 mg | HTN | Initially, 5 mg once daily. May increase to 10 mg/day, then 20 mg/day. Usual dose: 5–10 mg/day |
| **Carvedilol** (Coreg) | T: 3.125 mg, 6.25 mg, 12.5 mg, 25 mg<br>C (SR): 10 mg, 20 mg, 40 mg, 80 mg | HF, LVD after MI, HTN | **Immediate-Release HF:** Initially, 3.25 mg 2 times/day. May increase at 2 wk intervals to 6.25 mg 2 times/day, then 12.5 mg 2 times/day, then 25 mg 2 times/day. **LVD after MI:** Initially, 6.25 mg 2 times/day. May increase q3–10 days to 12.5 mg 2 times/day, then 25 mg 2 times/day. **HTN:** Initially, 6.25 mg 2 times/day. May increase q7–14 days to 12.5 mg 2 times/day, then 25 mg 2 times/day. **Extended-Release HF:** 10–80 mg once daily. **LVD after MI:** 10–80 mg once daily. **HTN:** 20–80 mg once daily |
| **Labetalol** (Trandate) | T: 100 mg, 200 mg, 300 mg | HTN | Initially, 100 mg 2 times/day. May increase q2–3 days in 100 mg 2 times/day increments. Usual dose: 200 mg 2 times/day |
| **Metoprolol** (Lopressor [IR], Toprol XL [SRI]) | T (IR): 50 mg, 100 mg<br>T (SR): 25 mg, 50 mg | HTN, angina, HF, MI | **IR:** **Angina:** Initially, 50 mg 2 times/day. May increase up to 400 mg/day. **HTN:** Initially, 100 mg once daily. May increase at weekly intervals up to 450 mg/day. **Post-MI:** 100 mg bid. **SR:** **Angina:** 100–400 mg once daily. **HF:** 12.5–200 mg once daily. **HTN:** 25–400 mg once daily |
| **Nadolol** (Corgard) | T: 20 mg, 40 mg, 80 mg | HTN, angina | **Angina, HTN:** Initially, 40 mg once/day. Usual dose: 40–80 mg once daily |

Continued

## BETA-ADRENERGIC BLOCKERS—cont'd

| Name | Availability | Indication | Dosage Range |
|---|---|---|---|
| **Nebivolol (Bystolic)** | **T:** 2.5 mg, 5 mg, 10 mg, 20 mg | HTN | Initially, 5 mg once daily. May increase at 2 wk intervals up to 40 mg/day |
| **Pindolol (Visken)** | **T:** 5 mg, 10 mg | HTN | Initially, 5 mg 2 times/day. May increase to 10–40 mg/day. **Maximum:** 60 mg/day |
| **Propranolol (Inderal)** | **T (IR):** 10 mg, 20 mg, 40 mg, 60 mg, 80 mg<br>**C (SR):** 60 mg, 80 mg, 120 mg, 160 mg<br>**S:** 4 mg/ml, 8 mg/ml<br>**I:** 1 mg/ml | HTN, angina, MI, arrhythmias, migraine, essential tremor, hypertrophic subaortic stenosis | **IR:**<br>**Angina:** 80–320 mg/day in 2–4 divided doses<br>**Arrhythmias:** 10–30 mg 3–4 times/day<br>**HTN:** 40 mg bid up to 240 mg/day in 2–3 divided doses<br>**Hypertrophic subaortic stenosis:** 20–40 mg 3–4 times/day<br>**Post-MI:** 180–240 mg/day in 2–4 divided doses<br>**Migraine:** Initially, 80 mg/day. May increase gradually up to 240 mg/day in divided doses<br>**Tremor:** Initially, 40 mg 2 times/day. Usual dose: 120–320 mg/day<br>**SR:**<br>**Angina:** Initially, 80 mg once daily. May increase q3–7days up to 320 mg/day<br>**HTN:** 80–120 mg once daily<br>**Migraine:** Initially, 80 mg once daily. Gradually increase up to 240 mg once daily<br>**Hypertrophic subaortic stenosis:** 80–160 mg once daily |

*C,* Capsules; *HF,* heart failure; *HTN,* hypertension; *I,* injection; *LVD,* left ventricular dysfunction; *S,* solution; *SR,* sustained-release; *T,* tablets.

# Bronchodilators

## USES

Relief of bronchospasm occurring during anesthesia and in bronchial asthma, bronchitis, emphysema.

## ACTION

*Inhaled corticosteroids:* Exact mechanism unknown. May act as anti-inflammatories, decrease mucus secretion.

*Beta₂-adrenergic agonists:* Stimulate beta receptors in lung, relax bronchial smooth muscle, increase vital capacity, decrease airway resistance.

*Anticholinergics:* Inhibit cholinergic receptors on bronchial smooth muscle (block acetylcholine action).

*Leukotriene modifiers:* Decrease effect of leukotrienes, which increase migration of eosinophils, producing mucus/edema of airway wall, causing bronchoconstriction.

*Methylxanthines:* Directly relax smooth muscle of bronchial airway, pulmonary blood vessels (relieve bronchospasm, increase vital capacity). Increase cyclic 3,5-adenosine monophosphate.

## BRONCHODILATORS

| Name | Availability | Dosage Range | Side Effects |
|---|---|---|---|
| **Anticholinergics** | | | |
| **Aclidinium (Tudorza)** | **Inhalation powder:** 400 mcg/actuation | **A:** 400 mcg 2 times/day | Headache, nasopharyngitis, cough |
| **Ipratropium (Atrovent)** | **NEB:** 0.02% (500 mcg) **MDI:** 17 mcg/actuation | **A (NEB):** 500 mcg q6–8h **A (MDI):** 2 puffs 4 times/day | Upper respiratory tract infection, bronchitis, sinusitis, headache, dyspnea |
| **Tiotropium (Spiriva, Spiriva Respimat)** | **Inhalation powder:** 18 mcg/capsule **Aerosol Solution:** 1.25 mcg/inhalation | **A:** Once/day (inhaled twice) **Aerosol Solution:** 2 inhalations once daily | Xerostomia, upper respiratory tract infection, sinusitis, pharyngitis |
| **Umeclidinium (Incruse Ellipta)** | **Inhalation powder:** 62.5 mcg/blister | **A:** One inhalation once daily | Nasopharyngitis, upper respiratory tract infection, cough, arthralgia |

*Continued*

## BRONCHODILATORS—cont'd

| Name | Availability | Dosage Range | Side Effects |
|---|---|---|---|
| Bronchodilators | | | |
| **Albuterol**<br>**(ProAir HFA, ProAir**<br>**Respiclick Proventil**<br>**HFA, Ventolin HFA)** | **DPI:** 90 mcg/actuation<br>**MDI:** 90 mcg/actuation<br>**NEB:** 2.5 mg/3 ml,<br>2.5 mg/0.5 ml,<br>0.63–1.25 mg/3 ml | **DPI:** 1–2 inhalations q4–6h as needed<br>**MDI:** 2 inhalations q4–6h as needed<br>**NEB:** 1.25–5 mg q4–6h as needed | Tachycardia, skeletal muscle tremors, muscle cramping, palpitations, insomnia, hypokalemia, increased serum glucose |
| **Albuterol/ipratropium**<br>**(Combivent Respimat,**<br>**DuoNeb)** | **MDI:** 90 mcg albuterol/<br>18 mcg ipratropium/<br>actuation<br>**NEB:** 2.5 mg albuterol/<br>0.5 mg ipratropium/3 ml | **MDI:** 1 inhalation 4 times/day as needed<br>**NEB:** 2.5 mg/0.5 mg 4 times/day as needed | Same as individual listing for albuterol and ipratropium |
| **Formoterol**<br>**(Foradil, Perforomist)** | **DPI:** 12 mcg/capsule<br>**NEB:** 20 mcg/2 ml | **DPI:** 12 mcg q12h<br>**NEB:** 20 mcg q12h | Diarrhea, nausea, asthma exacerbation, bronchitis, infection |
| **Formoterol/budesonide**<br>**(Symbicort)** | **MDI:** 80, 160 mcg/<br>4.5 mcg/inhalation | **MDI:** 2 inhalations 2 times/day | Same as individual listing for formoterol and budesonide |
| **Formoterol/mometasone**<br>**(Dulera)** | **MDI:** 5 mcg/100 mcg,<br>5 mcg/200 mcg | **MDI:** 2 inhalations 2 times/day | Same as individual listing for formoterol and beclomethasone |
| **Indacaterol (Arcapta)** | **DPI:** 75 mcg/capsule | **DPI:** 75–300 mcg once daily | Cough, oropharyngeal pain, nasopharyngitis, headache, nausea |
| **Levalbuterol (Xopenex)** | **MDI:** 45 mcg/actuation<br>**NEB:** 0.31, 0.63, 1.25 mg/<br>3 ml, 1.25 mg/0.5 ml | **MDI:** 2 inhalations q4–6h as needed<br>**NEB:** 0.31–1.25 mg q6–8h | Tremor, rhinitis, viral infection, headache, nervousness, asthma, pharyngitis, rash |

| Drug | Formulation | Dosage | Side Effects |
|---|---|---|---|
| Olodaterol (Striverdi Respimat) | MDI: 2.5 mcg/actuation | MDI: 2 inhalations once daily | Nasopharyngitis, rash, dizziness, cough, bronchitis, upper respiratory tract infections |
| Olodaterol/tiotropium (Stiolto Respimat) | MDI: 2.5 mcg/2.5 mcg | MDI: 2 inhalations once daily | Nasopharyngitis, cough, back pain |
| Salmeterol (Serevent Diskus) | DPI: 50 mcg/blister | DPI: 50 mcg q12h | Headache, pain, throat irritation, nasal congestion, bronchitis, pharyngitis |
| Salmeterol/fluticasone (Advair Diskus, Advair HFA) | DPI: 100, 250, 500 mcg/ 50 mcg/blister MDI: 45, 115, 230 mcg/ 21 mcg/inhalation | DPI: 1 inhalation 2 times/day MDI: 2 inhalations 2 times/day | Same as individual listing for salmeterol and fluticasone |
| Vilanterol/umeclidinium (Anoro) | DPI: 25 mcg/62.5 mcg | DPI: Once daily | Pharyngitis, sinusitis, lower respiratory tract infections, constipation, diarrhea, muscle spasms, neck/chest pain |
| Inhaled Corticosteroids | | | |
| Beclomethasone (Qvar) | MDI: 40, 80 mcg/inhalation | MDI: 40–320 mcg 2 times/day | Cough, hoarseness, headache, pharyngitis |
| Budesonide (Pulmicort Flexhaler, Pulmicort Respules) | DPI: (Flexhaler): 90, 180 mcg/inhalation DPI: (Turbuhaler): 200 mcg/inhalation NEB: (Respules): 0.25, 0.5 mg/2 ml | DPI: (Flexhaler): 180–720 mcg 2 times/day DPI: (Turbuhaler): 400–2,400 mcg/day in 2–4 divided doses NEB: (Respules): 250–500 mcg 1–2 times/day or 1 mg once daily | Headache, nausea, respiratory infection, rhinitis |
| Ciclesonide (Alvesco HFA) | HFA: 80, 160 mcg/inhalation | HFA: 80–640 mcg 2 times/day | Headache, nasopharyngitis, upper respiratory infection, epistaxis, nasal congestion, sinusitis |

*Continued*

## BRONCHODILATORS—cont'd

| Name | Availability | Dosage Range | Side Effects |
|---|---|---|---|
| Fluticasone (Arnuity Ellipta, Flovent Diskus, Flovent HFA) | **DPI: (Flovent Diskus):** 50, 100, 250 mcg/blister (Arnuity Ellipta): 100 mcg, 200 mcg/activation **MDI: (Flovent HFA):** 44, 110, 220 mcg/inhalation | **DPI: (Flovent Diskus):** 100–1,000 mcg 2 times/day (Arnuity Ellipta): 100–200 mcg once daily **MDI: (Flovent HFA):** 88–880 mcg 2 times/day | Headache, nasal congestion, pharyngitis, sinusitis, respiratory infections |
| Formoterol/budesonide (Symbicort) | **MDI:** 80, 160 mcg/4.5 mcg/inhalation | **MDI:** 2 inhalations 2 times/day | Same as individual listing for formoterol and budesonide |
| Mometasone (Asmanex Twisthaler) | **DPI:** 110–220 mcg/inhalation | **DPI:** 220–880 mcg once daily in evening or 220 mcg bid | Same as beclomethasone |
| Salmeterol/fluticasone (Advair Diskus, Advair HFA) | **DPI:** 100, 250, 500 mcg 50 mcg/blister **MDI:** 45, 115, 230 mcg/ 21 mcg/inhalation | **DPI:** 1 inhalation 2 times/day **MDI:** 2 inhalations 2 times/day | Same as individual listing for salmeterol and fluticasone |
| Vilanterol/fluticasone (Breo Ellipta) | **DPI:** 25 mcg/100 mcg; 25 mcg/200mcg | **DPI:** 1 inhalation once daily | Nasopharyngitis, upper respiratory infection, headache, oral candidiasis |
| **Leukotriene Modifiers** | | | |
| Montelukast (Singulair) | **T:** 4 mg, 5 mg, 10 mg | **A:** 10 mg/day **C (6–14 yrs):** 5 mg/day **C (2–5 yrs):** 4 mg/day | Dyspepsia, increased LFT, cough, nasal congestion, headache, dizziness, fatigue |
| Zafirlukast (Accolate) | **T:** 10 mg, 20 mg | **A, C (12 yrs and older):** 20 mg 2 times/day **C (5–11 yrs):** 10 mg 2 times/day | Headache, nausea, diarrhea, infection |
| **PDE-4 Inhibitor** | | | |
| Roflumilast (Daliresp) | **T:** 500 mcg | **A:** 500 mcg once daily | Headache, dizziness, insomnia |

*A*, Adults; *C (dosage)*, children; *DPI*, dry powder inhaler; *HFA*, hydrofluoroalkane; *MDI*, metered dose inhaler; *NEB*, nebulization; *T*, tablets.

# Calcium Channel Blockers

## USES

Treatment of essential hypertension, treatment of and prophylaxis of angina pectoris (including vasospastic, chronic stable, unstable), prevention/control of supraventricular tachyarrhythmias, prevention of neurologic damage due to subarachnoid hemorrhage.

## ACTION

Calcium channel blockers inhibit the flow of extracellular $Ca^{2+}$ ions across cell membranes of cardiac cells, vascular smooth muscle tissue. They relax arterial smooth muscle, depress the rate of sinus node pacemaker, slow AV conduction, decrease heart rate, produce negative inotropic effect (rarely seen clinically due to reflex response). Calcium channel blockers decrease coronary vascular resistance, increase coronary blood flow, reduce myocardial oxygen demand. Degree of action varies with individual agent.

## CALCIUM CHANNEL BLOCKERS

| Name | Availability | Indications | Dosage Range | Side Effects |
|---|---|---|---|---|
| **Amlodipine (Norvasc)** | **T:** 2.5 mg, 5 mg, 10 mg | HTN, angina | **HTN:** Initially, 2.5–5 mg once daily. May titrate q7–14 days up to 10 mg/day<br>**Angina:** 5–10 mg once daily | Abdominal pain, flushing, headaches, peripheral edema |
| **Diltiazem (Cardizem)** | **T:** 30 mg, 60 mg, 90 mg, 120 mg **(ER):** 120 mg, 180 mg, 240 mg, 300 mg, 360 mg, 420 mg<br>**C (SR-12HR):** 60 mg, 90 mg, 120 mg, **(ER-24HR):** 120 mg, 180 mg, 240 mg, 300 mg, 360 mg, 420 mg<br>**I:** 5 mg/ml | **PO:** HTN, angina<br>**IV:** Arrhythmias | **See monograph**<br>**HTN:** 120–540 mg/day<br>**Angina:** 120–480 mg/day<br>**I:** 20–25 mg IV bolus, then 5–15 mg/hr infusion | Dizziness, drowsiness, edema, headache |
| **Felodipine (Plendil)** | **T:** 2.5 mg, 5 mg, 10 mg | HTN | Initially, 5 mg/day. May increase q2wks. Usual dose: 5–10 mg/day | Peripheral edema, headaches |

*Continued*

## CALCIUM CHANNEL BLOCKERS—cont'd

| Name | Availability | Indications | Dosage Range | Side Effects |
|------|-------------|-------------|--------------|--------------|
| Isradipine | **C:** 2.5 mg, 5 mg | HTN | Initially, 2.5 mg 2 times/day. May increase at 2–4 wk intervals at 2.5–5 mg increments. Usual dose: 5–10 mg 2 times/day | Headaches |
| **Nicardipine** (Cardene) | **C (IR):** 20 mg, 30 mg<br>**C (ER):** 30 mg, 45 mg, 60 mg<br>**I:** 2.5 mg/ml | HTN, angina | **Angina/HTN:** Initially, 20–30 mg 3 times/day. May increase q3days. Usual dose: 20–40 mg 3 times/day | Flushing, peripheral edema, headache, dizziness |
| **Nifedipine** (Adalat, Procardia) | **C (IR):** 10 mg, 20 mg<br>**T (ER):** 30 mg, 60 mg, 90 mg | HTN, angina | **HTN (ER):** Initially, 30–60 mg once daily. Usual dose: 90–120 mg once daily<br>**Angina (IR):** 10–20 mg tid or **(ER):** Initially, 30–60 mg once daily. Titrate up to 90 mg daily. **Maximum:** 120 mg | Peripheral edema, dizziness, flushed face, headaches, nausea |
| **Nimodipine** (Nimotop, Nymalize) | **C:** 30 mg<br>**S:** 60 mg/20 ml | Prevent neurologic damage following subarachnoid hemorrhage | 60 mg q4h for 21 days | Nausea, reduced B/P, headache, rash, diarrhea |
| **Verapamil** (Calan, Isoptin) | **T (IR):** 40 mg, 80 mg, 120 mg<br>**T (SR):** 120 mg, 180 mg, 240 mg | HTN, angina | **Angina (IR):** Initially, 40–120 mg 3 times/day. Usual dose: 80–160 mg tid or **(SR):** Initially, 180 mg at HS. May increase at weekly intervals up to 480 mg/day<br>**HTN (IR):** Initially, 80 mg 3 times/day. Usual dose: 240–480 mg/day in divided doses **(SR):** Initially, 120–180 mg/day. May increase at weekly intervals to 240 mg/day, then 180 mg 2 times/day. **Maximum:** 240 mg 2 times/day | Nausea, gingival hyperplasia, headache, fatigue, dizziness |

*C,* Capsules; *CR,* controlled-release; *ER,* extended-release; *HTN,* hypertension; *I,* injection; *S,* solution; *SR,* sustained-release; *T,* tablets.

# Chemotherapeutic Agents

## USES

Treatment of a variety of cancers; may be palliative or curative. Treatment of choice in hematologic cancers. Often used as adjunctive therapy (e.g., with surgery or irradiation); most effective when tumor mass has been removed or reduced by radiation. Often used in combinations to increase therapeutic results, decrease toxic effects. Certain agents may be used in nonmalignant conditions: polycythemia vera, psoriasis, rheumatoid arthritis, or immunosuppression in organ transplantation (used only in select cases that are severe and unresponsive to other forms of therapy). Refer to individual monographs.

## ACTION

Most antineoplastics can be divided into alkylating agents, antimetabolites, anthracyclines, plant alkaloids, and topoisomerase inhibitors. These agents affect cell division or DNA synthesis. Newer agents (monoclonal antibodies and tyrosine kinase inhibitors) directly target a molecular abnormality in certain types of cancer. Hormones modulate tumor cell behavior without directly attacking those cells. Some agents are classified as miscellaneous.

## CHEMOTHERAPEUTIC AGENTS

| Name | Availability | Category | Side Effects |
|------|--------------|----------|--------------|
| **Abiraterone (Zytiga)** | **T:** 250 mg | Antiandrogen | Joint swelling, hypokalemia, edema, muscle discomfort, hot flashes, diarrhea, UTI, cough, hypertension, arrhythmia, dyspepsia, upper respiratory tract infection |
| **Aldesleukin (Proleukin)** | **I:** 22 million units | Biologic response modifier | Hypotension, sinus tachycardia, nausea, vomiting, diarrhea, renal impairment, anemia, rash, fatigue, agitation, pulmonary congestion, dyspnea, fever, chills, oliguria, weight gain, dizziness |
| **Alectinib (Alecensa)** | **C:** 150 mg | Kinase inhibitor | Constipation, fatigue, edema, myalgia |

*Continued*

# CHEMOTHERAPEUTIC AGENTS—cont'd

| Name | Availability | Category | Side Effects |
|---|---|---|---|
| **Anastrozole (Arimidex)** | T: 1 mg | Aromatase inhibitor | Peripheral edema, chest pain, nausea, vomiting, diarrhea, constipation, abdominal pain, anorexia, pharyngitis, vaginal hemorrhage, anemia, leukopenia, rash, weight gain, diaphoresis, increased appetite, pain, headaches, dizziness, depression, paresthesia, hot flashes, increased cough, dry mouth, asthenia, dyspnea, phlebitis |
| **Arsenic trioxide (Trisenox)** | I: 10 mg/ml | Miscellaneous | AV block, GI hemorrhage, hypertension, hypoglycemia, hypokalemia, hypomagnesemia, neutropenia, oliguria, prolonged QT interval, seizures, sepsis, thrombocytopenia |
| **Asparaginase (Elspar)** | I: 10,000 units | Miscellaneous | Anorexia, nausea, vomiting, hepatic toxicity, nephrotoxicity, clotting factor abnormalities, malaise, confusion, lethargy, EEG changes, respiratory distress, fever, hyperglycemia, depression, stomatitis, allergic reactions, drowsiness |
| **Atezolizumab (Tecentriq)** | I: 60 mg/ml | Miscellaneous | Fatigue, decreased appetite, nausea, urinary tract infections, constipation, pyrexia |
| **Axitinib (Inlyta)** | T: 1 mg, 5 mg | Kinase inhibitor | Diarrhea, hypertension, fatigue, decreased appetite, nausea, dysphoria, vomiting, asthenia, constipation |
| **Azacitidine (Vidaza)** | I: 100 mg | DNA methylation inhibitor | Edema, hypokalemia, weight loss, myalgia, cough, dyspnea, upper respiratory tract infection, back pain, pyrexia, weakness |
| **BCG (TheraCys, Tice BCG)** | I: 50 mg, 81 mg | Biologic response modulator | Nausea, vomiting, anorexia, diarrhea, dysuria, hematuria, cystitis, urinary urgency, anemia, malaise, fever, chills |
| **Belinostat (Beleodaq)** | I: 500 mg | Miscellaneous | Nausea, fatigue, pyrexia, anemia, vomiting |
| **Bendamustine (Treanda)** | I: 100 mg | Alkylating agent | Neutropenia, pyrexia, thrombocytopenia, nausea, anemia, leukopenia, vomiting |
| **Bevacizumab (Avastin)** | I: 25 mg/ml | Monoclonal antibody | Increased B/P, fatigue, blood clots, diarrhea, decreased WBCs, headaches, decreased appetite, stomatitis |
| **Bexarotene (Targretin)** | C: 75 mg Gel: 1% | Miscellaneous | Anemia, dermatitis, fever, hypercholesterolemia, infection, leukopenia, peripheral edema |

| | | | |
|---|---|---|---|
| **Bicalutamide** (Casodex) | **T:** 50 mg | Antiandrogen | Gynecomastia, hot flashes, breast pain, nausea, diarrhea, constipation, nocturia, impotence, pain, muscle pain, asthenia, abdominal pain |
| **Bleomycin** (Blenoxane) | **I:** 15 units, 30 units | Antibiotic | Nausea, vomiting, anorexia, stomatitis, hyperpigmentation, alopecia, pruritus, hyperkeratosis, urticaria, pneumonitis progression to fibrosis, weight loss, rash |
| **Blinatumomab** (Blincyto) | **I:** 35 mcg | Miscellaneous | Pyrexia, headache, peripheral edema, febrile neutropenia, nausea, hypokalemia, tremor, rash, constipation |
| **Bortezomib** (Velcade) | **I:** 3.5 mg | Proteasome inhibitor | Anxiety, dizziness, headaches, insomnia, peripheral neuropathy, pruritus, rash, abdominal pain, decreased appetite, constipation, diarrhea, dyspepsia, nausea, vomiting, arthralgia, dyspnea, asthenia, edema, pain |
| **Bosutinib** (Bosulif) | **T:** 100 mg, 500 mg | Kinase inhibitor | Nausea, diarrhea, thrombocytopenia, vomiting, abdominal pain, anemia, fever, fatigue |
| **Brentuximab** (Adcetris) | **I:** 50 mg | Miscellaneous | Neutropenia, peripheral sensory neuropathy, fatigue, nausea, anemia, upper respiratory tract infection, diarrhea, pyrexia, thrombocytopenia, cough, vomiting |
| **Busulfan** (Myleran) | **T:** 2 mg | Alkylating agent | Nausea, vomiting, hyperuricemia, myelosuppression, skin hyperpigmentation, alopecia, anorexia, weight loss, diarrhea, stomatitis |
| **Cabazitaxel** (Jevtana) | **I:** 60 mg/1.5 ml | Microtubule inhibitor | Neutropenia, anemia, leukopenia, thrombocytopenia, diarrhea, fatigue, nausea, vomiting, constipation, asthenia, abdominal pain, hematuria, anorexia, peripheral neuropathy, dyspnea, alopecia |
| **Cabozantinib** (Cabometyx) | **T:** 20 mg, 40 mg, 60 mg | Kinase inhibitor | Diarrhea, fatigue, nausea, decreased appetite, palmar-plantar erythrodysesthesia, hypertension, decreased weight, constipation, vomiting |
| **Capecitabine** (Xeloda) | **T:** 150 mg, 300 mg | Antimetabolite | Nausea, vomiting, diarrhea, stomatitis, myelosuppression, palmar-plantar erythrodysesthesia syndrome, dermatitis, fatigue, anorexia |
| **Carboplatin** (Paraplatin) | **I:** 50 mg, 150 mg, 450 mg | Alkylating agent | Nausea, vomiting, nephrotoxicity, myelosuppression, alopecia, peripheral neuropathy, hypersensitivity, ototoxicity, asthenia, diarrhea, constipation |
| **Carfilzomib** (Kyprolis) | **I:** 60 mg | Proteasome inhibitor | Anemia, fatigue, nausea, thrombocytopenia, dyspnea, diarrhea, pyrexia |
| **Carmustine** (BiCNU) | **I:** 100 mg | Alkylating agent | Anorexia, nausea, vomiting, myelosuppression, pulmonary fibrosis, pain at injection site, diarrhea, skin discoloration |

*Continued*

## CHEMOTHERAPEUTIC AGENTS—cont'd

| Name | Availability | Category | Side Effects |
|---|---|---|---|
| **Ceritinib (Zykadia)** | C: 150 mg | Kinase inhibitor | Diarrhea, nausea, increased LFTs, vomiting, abdominal pain, fatigue, decreased appetite, constipation |
| **Cetuximab (Erbitux)** | I: 2 mg/ml | Monoclonal antibody | Dyspnea, hypotension, acne-like rash, dry skin, weakness, fatigue, fever, constipation, abdominal pain |
| **Chlorambucil (Leukeran)** | T: 2 mg | Alkylating agent | Myelosuppression, dermatitis, nausea, vomiting, hepatic toxicity, anorexia, diarrhea, abdominal discomfort, rash |
| **Cisplatin (Platinol-AQ)** | I: 50 mg, 100 mg | Alkylating agent | Nausea, vomiting, nephrotoxicity, myelosuppression, neuropathies, ototoxicity, anaphylactic-like reactions, hyperuricemia, hypomagnesemia, hypophosphatemia, hypokalemia, hypocalcemia, pain at injection site |
| **Cladribine (Leustatin)** | I: 1 mg/ml | Antimetabolite | Nausea, vomiting, diarrhea, myelosuppression, chills, fatigue, rash, fever, headaches, anorexia, diaphoresis |
| **Cobimetinib (Cotellic)** | T: 20 mg | Kinase inhibitor | Diarrhea, photosensitivity reaction, nausea, vomiting, pyrexia, increased ALT, AST, alkaline phosphatase |
| **Crizotinib (Xalkori)** | C: 200 mg, 250 mg | Tyrosine kinase inhibitor | Vision disorders, nausea, vomiting, diarrhea, edema, constipation |
| **Cyclophosphamide (Cytoxan)** | I: 100 mg, 200 mg, 500 mg, 1 g, 2 g<br>T: 25 mg, 50 mg | Alkylating agent | Nausea, vomiting, hemorrhagic cystitis, myelosuppression, alopecia, interstitial pulmonary fibrosis, amenorrhea, azoospermia, diarrhea, darkening skin/fingernails, headaches, diaphoresis |
| **Cytarabine (Ara-C, Cytosar)** | I: 100 mg, 500 mg, 1 g, 2 g | Antimetabolite | Anorexia, nausea, vomiting, stomatitis, esophagitis, diarrhea, myelosuppression, alopecia, rash, fever, neuropathies, abdominal pain |
| **Dacarbazine (DTIC)** | I: 200 mg | Alkylating agent | Nausea, vomiting, anorexia, hepatic necrosis, myelosuppression, alopecia, rash, facial flushing, photosensitivity, flu-like symptoms, confusion, blurred vision |
| **Daratumumab (Darzalex)** | I: 20 mg/ml | Monoclonal antibody | Fatigue, nausea, infusion reactions, back pain, pyrexia, nausea, upper respiratory tract infections |
| **Dasatinib (Sprycel)** | T: 20 mg, 50 mg, 70 mg | Tyrosine kinase inhibitor | Pyrexia, pleural effusion, febrile neutropenia, GI bleeding, pneumonia, thrombocytopenia, dyspnea, anemia, cardiac failure, diarrhea |
| **Daunorubicin (Cerubidine)** | I: 20 mg | Anthracycline | HF, nausea, vomiting, stomatitis, mucositis, diarrhea, hematuria, myelosuppression, alopecia, fever, chills, abdominal pain |

| | | | |
|---|---|---|---|
| **Daunorubicin liposomal (DaunoXome)** | I: 50 mg | Anthracycline | Nausea, diarrhea, abdominal pain, anorexia, vomiting, stomatitis, myelosuppression, rigors, back pain, headaches, neuropathy, depression, dyspnea, fatigue, fever, cough, allergic reactions, diaphoresis |
| **Denileukin (Ontak)** | I: 300 mcg/2 ml | Miscellaneous | Hypersensitivity reaction, back pain, dyspnea, rash, chest pain, tachycardia, asthenia, flu-like symptoms, chills, nausea, vomiting, infection |
| **Dinutuximab (Unituxin)** | I: 3.5 mg/ml | Monoclonal antibody | Pain, arthralgia, myalgia, neuralgia, pyrexia, hypotension, vomiting, diarrhea, urticaria, hypoxia |
| **Docetaxel (Taxotere)** | I: 20 mg, 80 mg | Antimicrotubular | Hypotension, nausea, vomiting, diarrhea, mucositis, myelosuppression, rash, paresthesia, hypersensitivity, fluid retention, alopecia, asthenia, stomatitis, fever |
| **Doxorubicin (Adriamycin)** | I: 10 mg, 20 mg, 50 mg, 75 mg, 150 mg, 200 mg | Anthracycline | Cardiotoxicity, including HF; arrhythmias, nausea, vomiting, stomatitis, esophagitis, GI ulceration, diarrhea, anorexia, hematuria, myelosuppression, alopecia, hyperpigmentation of nail beds and skin, local inflammation at injection site, rash, fever, chills, urticaria, lacrimation, conjunctivitis |
| **Doxorubicin liposomal (Doxil)** | I: 20 mg, 50 mg | Anthracycline | Neutropenia, palmar-plantar erythrodysesthesia syndrome, cardiomyopathy, HF |
| **Elotuzumab (Empliciti)** | I: 300 mg, 400 mg | Immunostimulatory antibody | Fatigue, diarrhea, pyrexia, constipation, cough, peripheral neuropathy, naso-pharyngitis, decreased appetite, upper respiratory tract infections, pneumonia |
| **Enzalutamide (Xtandi)** | C: 40 mg | Antiandrogen | Fatigue, weakness, back pain, diarrhea, tissue swelling, musculoskeletal pain, headache, upper respiratory tract infections, blood in urine, spinal cord compression |
| **Epirubicin (Ellence)** | I: 2 mg/ml | Anthracycline | Anemia, leukopenia, neutropenia, infection, mucositis |
| **Erlotinib (Tarceva)** | T: 25 mg, 100 mg, 150 mg | Tyrosine kinase inhibitor | Diarrhea, rash, nausea, vomiting |
| **Estramustine (Emcyt)** | C: 140 mg | Alkylating agent | Increased risk of thrombosis, gynecomastia, nausea, vomiting, diarrhea, thrombocytopenia, peripheral edema |
| **Etoposide (VePesid)** | I: 20 mg/ml C: 50 mg | Podophyllotoxin derivative | Nausea, vomiting, anorexia, myelosuppression, alopecia, diarrhea, drowsiness, peripheral neuropathies |

*Continued*

## CHEMOTHERAPEUTIC AGENTS—cont'd

| Name | Availability | Category | Side Effects |
|------|-------------|----------|-------------|
| Everolimus (Afinitor, Zortress) | **T (Afinitor):** 5 mg, 10 mg **T (Zortress):** 0.25 mg, 0.5 mg, 0.75 mg | mTOR kinase inhibitor | Stomatitis, infections, asthenia, fatigue, cough, diarrhea |
| Exemestane (Aromasin) | **T:** 25 mg | Aromatase inactivator | Dyspnea, edema, hypertension, mental depression |
| Fludarabine (Fludara) | **I:** 50 mg | Antimetabolite | Nausea, diarrhea, stomatitis, bleeding, anemia, myelosuppression, skin rash, weakness, confusion, visual disturbances, peripheral neuropathy, coma, pneumonia, peripheral edema, anorexia |
| Fluorouracil (Adrucil, Efudex) | **I:** 50 mg/ml **Cream:** 1%, 5% **Solution:** 1%, 2%, 5% | Antimetabolite | Nausea, vomiting, stomatitis, GI ulceration, diarrhea, anorexia, myelosuppression, alopecia, skin hyperpigmentation, nail changes, headaches, drowsiness, blurred vision, fever |
| Flutamide (Eulexin) | **C:** 125 mg | Antiandrogen | Hot flashes, nausea, vomiting, diarrhea, hepatitis, impotence, decreased libido, rash, anorexia |
| Fulvestrant (Faslodex) | **I:** 125 mg/2.5 ml, 250 mg/5 ml syringes | Estrogen receptor antagonist | Asthenia, pain, headaches, injection site pain, flu-like symptoms, fever, nausea, vomiting, constipation, anorexia, diarrhea, peripheral edema, dizziness, depression, anxiety, rash, increased cough, UTI |
| Gefitinib (Iressa) | **T:** 250 mg | Tyrosine kinase inhibitor | Diarrhea, rash, acne, nausea, dry skin, vomiting, pruritus, anorexia |
| Gemcitabine (Gemzar) | **I:** 200 mg, 1 g | Antimetabolite | Increased LFT, nausea, vomiting, diarrhea, stomatitis, hematuria, myelosuppression, rash, mild paresthesia, dyspnea, fever, edema, flu-like symptoms, constipation |
| Goserelin (Zoladex) | **I:** 3.6 mg, 10.8 mg | Hormone agonist | Hot flashes, sexual dysfunction, erectile dysfunction, gynecomastia, lethargy, pain, lower urinary tract symptoms, headaches, nausea, depression, diaphoresis |
| Hydroxyurea (Hydrea) | **C:** 500 mg | Antimetabolite | Anorexia, nausea, vomiting, stomatitis, diarrhea, constipation, myelosuppression, fever, chills, malaise |
| Ibritumomab (Zevalin) | Injection kit | Monoclonal antibody | Neutropenia, thrombocytopenia, anemia, infection, asthenia, abdominal pain, fever, pain, headaches, nausea, peripheral edema, allergic reaction, GI hemorrhage, apnea |

| Idarubicin (Idamycin PFS) | I: 5 mg, 10 mg, 20 mg | Anthracycline | HF, arrhythmias, nausea, vomiting, stomatitis, myelosuppression, alopecia, rash, urticaria, hyperuricemia, abdominal pain, diarrhea, esophagitis, anorexia |
| Idelalisib (Zydelig) | T: 100 mg, 150 mg | Kinase inhibitor | Diarrhea, pyrexia, fatigue, nausea, cough, abdominal pain, pneumonia, increased ALT/AST |
| Ifosfamide (Ifex) | I: 1 g, 3 g | Alkylating agent | Nausea, vomiting, hemorrhagic cystitis, myelosuppression, alopecia, lethargy, drowsiness, confusion, hallucinations, hematuria |
| Imatinib (Gleevec) | C: 100 mg | Tyrosine kinase inhibitor | Nausea, fluid retention, hemorrhage, musculoskeletal pain, arthralgia, weight gain, pyrexia, abdominal pain, dyspnea, pneumonia |
| Interferon alfa-2b (Intron-A) | I: 3 million units, 5 million units, 10 million units, 18 million units, 25 million units, 50 million units | Miscellaneous | Mild hypotension, hypertension, tachycardia with high fever, nausea, diarrhea, altered taste, weight loss, thrombocytopenia, myelosuppression, rash, pruritus, myalgia, arthralgia associated with flu-like symptoms |
| Ipilimumab (Yervoy) | I: 5 mg/ml | Miscellaneous | Fatigue, diarrhea, pruritus, rash, colitis |
| Irinotecan (Camptosar) | I: 40 mg, 100 mg | Camptothecin | Diarrhea, nausea, vomiting, abdominal cramps, anorexia, stomatitis, increased AST, severe myelosuppression, alopecia, diaphoresis, rash, weight loss, dehydration, increased serum alkaline phosphatase, headaches, insomnia, dizziness, dyspnea, cough, asthenia, rhinitis, fever, back pain, chills |
| Ixabepilone (Ixempra) | I: 15 mg, 45 mg | Antimicrotubular | Peripheral sensory neuropathy, fatigue, myalgia, alopecia, nausea, vomiting, stomatitis, diarrhea, anorexia, abdominal pain |
| Ixazomib (Ninlaro) | C: 2.3 mg, 3 mg, 4 mg | Proteasome inhibitor | Diarrhea, constipation, thrombocytopenia, peripheral neuropathy, nausea, peripheral edema, back pain, vomiting |
| Lapatinib (Tykerb) | T: 250 mg | Tyrosine kinase inhibitor | Diarrhea, palmar-plantar erythrodysesthesia, nausea, rash, vomiting, fatigue |
| Lenvatinib (Lenvima) | C: 4 mg, 10 mg | Kinase inhibitor | Hypertension, fatigue, diarrhea, arthralgia, decreased weight, nausea, stomatitis, headache, vomiting, proteinuria, abdominal pain |

*Continued*

# CHEMOTHERAPEUTIC AGENTS—cont'd

| Name | Availability | Category | Side Effects |
|------|-------------|----------|--------------|
| Letrozole (Femara) | T: 2.5 mg | Aromatase inhibitor | Hypertension, nausea, vomiting, constipation, diarrhea, abdominal pain, anorexia, rash, pruritus, musculoskeletal pain, arthralgia, fatigue, headaches, dyspnea, coughing, hot flashes |
| Leuprolide (Lupron) | I: 3.75 mg, 5 mg, 7.5 mg, 11.25 mg, 15 mg, 22.5 mg, 30 mg | Hormone agonist | Hot flashes, gynecomastia, nausea, vomiting, constipation, anorexia, dizziness, headaches, insomnia, paresthesia, bone pain |
| Lomustine (CeeNU) | C: 10 mg, 40 mg, 100 mg | Alkylating agent | Anorexia, nausea, vomiting, stomatitis, hepatotoxicity, nephrotoxicity, myelosuppression, alopecia, confusion, slurred speech |
| Mechlorethamine (Mustargen) | I: 10 mg/ml | Alkylating agent | Severe nausea and vomiting, metallic taste, diarrhea, myelosuppression, alopecia, phlebitis, vertigo, tinnitus, hyperuricemia, infertility, azoospermia, anorexia, headaches, drowsiness, fever |
| Megestrol (Megace) | T: 20 mg, 40 mg Suspension: 40 mg/ml | Hormone | Deep vein thrombosis, Cushing-like syndrome, alopecia, carpal tunnel syndrome, weight gain, nausea |
| Melphalan (Alkeran) | T: 2 mg | Alkylating agent | Anorexia, nausea, vomiting, myelosuppression, diarrhea, stomatitis |
| Mercaptopurine (Purinethol) | T: 50 mg | Antimetabolite | Anorexia, nausea, vomiting, stomatitis, hepatic toxicity, myelosuppression, hyperuricemia, diarrhea, rash |
| Methotrexate (Rheumatrex) | T: 2.5 mg, 5 mg, 7.5 mg, 10 mg, 15 mg I: 5 mg, 50 mg, 100 mg, 200 mg, 250 mg | Antimetabolite | Nausea, vomiting, stomatitis, GI ulceration, diarrhea, hepatic toxicity, renal failure, cystitis, myelosuppression, alopecia, urticaria, acne, photosensitivity, interstitial pneumonitis, fever, malaise, chills, anorexia |
| Mitomycin (Mutamycin) | I: 20 mg, 40 mg | Antibiotic | Anorexia, nausea, vomiting, stomatitis, diarrhea, renal toxicity, myelosuppression, alopecia, pruritus, fever, hemolytic uremic syndrome, weakness |

| | | | |
|---|---|---|---|
| **Mitotane (Lysodren)** | **T:** 500 mg | Miscellaneous | Anorexia, nausea, vomiting, diarrhea, skin rashes, depression, lethargy, drowsiness, dizziness, adrenal insufficiency, blurred vision, impaired hearing |
| **Mitoxantrone (Novantrone)** | **I:** 20 mg, 25 mg, 30 mg | Anthracenedione | HF, tachycardia, EKG changes, chest pain, nausea, vomiting, stomatitis, mucositis, myelosuppression, rash, alopecia, urine discoloration (bluish green), phlebitis, diarrhea, cough, headaches, fever |
| **Necitumumab (Portrazza)** | **I:** 16 mg/ml | Epidermal growth factor receptor (EGFR) antagonist | Rash, hypomagnesemia |
| **Nelarabine (Arranon)** | **I:** 5 mg/ml | Antimetabolite | Anemia, neutropenia, thrombocytopenia, nausea, vomiting, diarrhea, fatigue, fever, dyspnea, severe neurologic events (convulsions, peripheral neuropathy) |
| **Nilotinib (Tasigna)** | **C:** 200 mg | Tyrosine kinase inhibitor | Rash, pruritus, nausea, fatigue, headache, constipation, diarrhea, vomiting, thrombocytopenia, neutropenia |
| **Nilutamide (Nilandron)** | **T:** 50 mg | Antiandrogen | Hypertension, angina, hot flashes, nausea, anorexia, increased hepatic enzymes, dizziness, dyspnea, visual disturbances, impaired adaptation to dark, constipation, decreased libido |
| **Nivolumab (Opdivo)** | **I:** 10 mg/ml | Miscellaneous | Fatigue, dyspnea, musculoskeletal pain, decreased appetite, cough, nausea, constipation |
| **Olaparib (Lynparza)** | **C:** 50 mg | Miscellaneous | Anemia, fatigue, nausea, vomiting, diarrhea, dysgeusia, dyspepsia, headache, decreased appetite |
| **Osimertinib (Tagrisso)** | **T:** 40 mg, 80 mg | Kinase inhibitor | Diarrhea, rash, dry skin, nail toxicity |
| **Oxaliplatin (Eloxatin)** | **I:** 50 mg, 100 mg | Alkylating agent | Fatigue, neuropathy, abdominal pain, dyspnea, diarrhea, nausea, vomiting, anorexia, fever, edema, chest pain, anemia, thrombocytopenia, thromboembolism, altered hepatic function tests |
| **Paclitaxel (Taxol)** | **I:** 30 mg, 100 mg | Antimicrotubular | Hypertension, bradycardia, EKG changes, nausea, vomiting, diarrhea, mucositis, myelosuppression, alopecia, peripheral neuropathies, hypersensitivity reaction, arthralgia, myalgia |

*Continued*

**CHEMOTHERAPEUTIC AGENTS—cont'd**

| Name | Availability | Category | Side Effects |
|---|---|---|---|
| **Palbociclib (Ibrance)** | C: 75 mg, 100 mg, 125 mg | Kinase inhibitor | Neutropenia, leukopenia, fatigue, anemia, upper respiratory tract infection, nausea, stomatitis, alopecia, diarrhea, thrombocytopenia, decreased appetite, vomiting, asthenia, peripheral neuropathy, epistaxis |
| **Panitumumab (Vectibix)** | I: 20 mg/ml | Monoclonal antibody | Pulmonary fibrosis, severe dermatologic toxicity, infusion reactions, abdominal pain, nausea, vomiting, constipation, skin rash, fatigue |
| **Panobinostat (Farydak)** | C: 10 mg, 15 mg, 20 mg | Miscellaneous | Diarrhea, fatigue, nausea, peripheral edema, decreased appetite, pyrexia, vomiting |
| **Pegaspargase (Oncaspar)** | I: 750 international units/ml | Miscellaneous | Hypotension, anorexia, nausea, vomiting, hepatotoxicity, pancreatitis, depression of clotting factors, malaise, confusion, lethargy, EEG changes, respiratory distress, hypersensitivity reaction, fever, hyperglycemia, stomatitis |
| **Pemetrexed (Alimta)** | I: 500 mg | Antimetabolite | Anorexia, constipation, diarrhea, neuropathy, anemia, chest pain, dyspnea, rash, fatigue |
| **Pentostatin (Nipent)** | I: 10 mg | Antibiotic | Nausea, vomiting, hepatic disorders, elevated hepatic function tests, leukopenia, anemia, thrombocytopenia, rash, fever, upper respiratory infection, fatigue, hematuria, headaches, myalgia, arthralgia, diarrhea, anorexia |
| **Pertuzumab (Perjeta)** | I: 420 mg/14 ml | HERZ/neu receptor antagonist | Alopecia, diarrhea, nausea, neutropenia, rash, fatigue, peripheral neuropathy |
| **Procarbazine (Matulane)** | C: 50 mg | Alkylating agent | Nausea, vomiting, stomatitis, diarrhea, constipation, myelosuppression, pruritus, hyperpigmentation, alopecia, myalgia, paresthesia, confusion, lethargy, mental depression, fever, hepatic toxicity, arthralgia, respiratory disorders |
| **Ramucirumab (Cyramza)** | I: 100 mg, 500 mg | Miscellaneous | Diarrhea, hypertension |
| **Rituximab (Rituxan)** | I: 100 mg, 500 mg | Monoclonal antibody | Hypotension, arrhythmias, peripheral edema, nausea, vomiting, abdominal pain, leukopenia, thrombocytopenia, neutropenia, rash, pruritus, urticaria, angioedema, myalgia, headaches, dizziness, throat irritation, rhinitis, bronchospasm, hypersensitivity reaction |

| | | | |
|---|---|---|---|
| **Sipuleucel-T (Provenge)** | **I:** Minimum of 50 million autologous CD54+ cells in lactated Ringer's | | Chills, fatigue, fever, back pain, nausea, headache, joint ache |
| **Sonidegib (Odomzo)** | **C:** 200 mg | Hedgehog pathway inhibitor | Muscle spasms, alopecia, dysgeusia, fatigue, nausea, diarrhea, decreased weight, musculoskeletal pain, myalgia, headache, abdominal pain, vomiting, pruritus |
| **Sorafenib (Nexavar)** | **T:** 200 mg | Tyrosine kinase inhibitor | Fatigue, alopecia, nausea, vomiting, anorexia, constipation, diarrhea, neuropathy, dyspnea, cough, asthenia, pain |
| **Sunitinib (Sutent)** | **C:** 12.5 mg, 25 mg, 50 mg | Tyrosine kinase inhibitor | Hypotension, edema, fatigue, headache, fever, dizziness, rash, hyperpigmentation, diarrhea, nausea, dyspepsia, altered taste, vomiting, neutropenia, thrombocytopenia, increased ALT/AST |
| **Tamoxifen (Nolvadex-D)** | **T:** 10 mg, 20 mg | Estrogen receptor antagonist | Skin rash, nausea, vomiting, anorexia, menstrual irregularities, hot flashes, pruritus, vaginal discharge or bleeding, myelosuppression, headaches, tumor or bone pain, ophthalmic changes, weight gain, confusion |
| **Temozolomide (Temodar)** | **C:** 5 mg, 20 mg, 100 mg, 250 mg | Alkylating agent | Amnesia, fever, infection, leukopenia, neutropenia, peripheral edema, seizures, thrombocytopenia |
| **Temsirolimus (Torisel)** | **I:** 25 mg/ml | mTOR kinase inhibitor | Rash, asthenia, mucositis, nausea, edema, anorexia, thrombocytopenia, leukopenia |
| **Thioguanine (Tabloid)** | **T:** 40 mg | Antimetabolite | Anorexia, stomatitis, myelosuppression, nausea, vomiting, diarrhea |
| **Thiotepa (Thioplex)** | **I:** 15 mg | Alkylating agent | Anorexia, nausea, vomiting, mucositis, myelosuppression, amenorrhea, reduced spermatogenesis, fever, hypersensitivity reactions, pain at injection site, headaches, dizziness, alopecia |
| **Tipiracil/trifluridine (Lonsurf)** | **T:** 6.14 mg/15 mg; 8.19 mg/20 mg | Miscellaneous | Asthenia, fatigue, nausea, diarrhea, vomiting, decreased appetite, pyrexia, abdominal pain |
| **Topotecan (Hycamtin)** | **I:** 4 mg | Camptothecin | Nausea, vomiting, diarrhea, constipation, abdominal pain, stomatitis, anorexia, neutropenia, leukopenia, thrombocytopenia, anemia, alopecia, headaches, dyspnea, paresthesia |

*Continued*

## CHEMOTHERAPEUTIC AGENTS—cont'd

| Name | Availability | Category | Side Effects |
|---|---|---|---|
| **Toremifene (Fareston)** | **T:** 60 mg | Estrogen receptor antagonist | Elevated hepatic function tests, nausea, vomiting, constipation, skin discoloration, dermatitis, dizziness, hot flashes, diaphoresis, vaginal discharge or bleeding, ocular changes, cataracts, anxiety |
| **Trabectedin (Yondelis)** | **I:** 1 mg | Alkylating agent | Nausea, vomiting, fatigue, diarrhea, decreased appetite, peripheral edema, dyspnea, headache; increased ALT, AST, alkaline phosphatase; neutropenia, thrombocytopenia, anemia |
| **Trastuzumab (Herceptin)** | **I:** 440 mg | Monoclonal antibody | HF, heart murmur ($S_3$ gallop), nausea, vomiting, diarrhea, abdominal pain, anorexia, rash, peripheral edema, back or bone pain, asthenia (loss of strength, energy), headaches, insomnia, dizziness, cough, dyspnea, rhinitis, pharyngitis |
| **Tretinoin (Vesanoid)** | **C:** 10 mg | Miscellaneous | Flushing, nausea, vomiting, diarrhea, constipation, dyspepsia, mucositis, leukocytosis, dry skin/mucous membranes, rash, pruritus, alopecia, dizziness, anxiety, insomnia, headaches, depression, confusion, intracranial hypertension, agitation, dyspnea, shivering, fever, visual changes, earaches, hearing loss, bone pain, myalgia, arthralgia |
| **Valrubicin (Valstar)** | **I:** 200 mg/5 ml | Anthracycline | Dysuria, hematuria, urinary frequency/incontinence/urgency |
| **Vandetanib (Caprelsa)** | **T:** 100 mg, 300 mg | Tyrosine kinase inhibitor | Diarrhea, rash, acne, nausea, hypertension, headache, fatigue, decreased appetite, abdominal pain |
| **Venetoclax (Venclexta)** | **T:** 10 mg, 50 mg, 100 mg | BCL-2 inhibitor | Diarrhea, neutropenia, anemia, nausea, upper respiratory tract infections, thrombocytopenia, fatigue |
| **Vinblastine (Velban)** | **I:** 10 mg | Vinca alkaloid | Nausea, vomiting, stomatitis, constipation, myelosuppression, alopecia, peripheral neuropathy, loss of deep tendon reflexes, paresthesia, diarrhea |
| **Vincristine (Oncovin)** | **I:** 1 mg, 2 mg, 3 mg | Vinca alkaloid | Nausea, vomiting, stomatitis, constipation, pharyngitis, polyuria, myelosuppression, alopecia, numbness, paresthesia, peripheral neuropathy, loss of deep tendon reflexes, headaches, abdominal pain |
| **Vincristine liposomal (Marqibo)** | **I:** 5 mg/31 ml | Vinca alkaloid | Constipation, nausea, pyrexia, fatigue, peripheral neuropathy, febrile neutropenia, diarrhea, anemia, reduced appetite, insomnia |

| | | |
|---|---|---|
| Vinorelbine (Navelbine) | I: 10 mg, 50 mg | Vinca alkaloid | Elevated LFT, nausea, vomiting, constipation, ileus, anorexia, stomatitis, myelosuppression, alopecia, vein discoloration, venous pain, phlebitis, interstitial pulmonary changes, asthenia, fatigue, diarrhea, peripheral neuropathy, loss of deep tendon reflexes |
| Vismodegib (Erivedge) | C: 150 mg | Hedgehog pathway inhibitor | Alopecia, muscle spasms, dysgensia, weight loss, fatigue, nausea, diarrhea, reduced appetite, vomiting, arthralgia |
| Vorinostat (Zolinza) | C: 100 mg | Histone deacetylase inhibitor | Diarrhea, fatigue, nausea, thrombocytopenia, anorexia, dysgeusia |
| ziv-aflibercept (Zaltrap) | I: 25 mg/ml | Miscellaneous | Leukopenia, neutropenia, diarrhea, proteinuria, increased ALT/AST, stomatitis, thrombocytopenia, hypertension, epistaxis, headache, abdominal pain |

*AV,* Atrioventricular; *C,* capsules; *EEG,* electroencephalogram; *EKG,* electrocardiogram; *GI,* gastrointestinal; *HF,* heart failure; *I,* injection; *LFT,* liver function test; *T,* tablets; *UTI,* urinary tract infection.

# Contraception

## ACTION

Combination oral contraceptives decrease fertility primarily by inhibition of ovulation. In addition, they can promote thickening of the cervical mucus, thereby creating a physical barrier for the passage of sperm. Also, they can modify the endometrium, making it less favorable for nidation.

## CLASSIFICATION

Oral contraceptives either contain both an estrogen and a progestin (combination oral contraceptives) or contain only a progestin (progestin-only oral contraceptives). The combination oral contraceptives have three subgroups:

*Monophasic:* Daily estrogen and progestin dosage remains constant.

*Biphasic:* Estrogen remains constant, but the progestin dosage increases during the second half of the cycle.

*Triphasic:* Progestin changes for each phase of the cycle.

*Four-phasic:* Contains four progestin/estrogen dosing combinations during the 20-day cycle.

Over the past several years, options have expanded to include a combined hormonal patch (Ortho Evra), vaginal ring (NuvaRing), and extended cycle contraceptives (e.g., Loestrin-24 FE, Seasonale, Seasonique, Yaz). The latest oral contraceptive, Natazia, is a four-phase dosing regimen (estradiol steps down and dienogest, a progestin, steps up during the cycle to help avoid breakthrough bleeding).

## COMMON COMPLAINTS WITH ORAL CONTRACEPTIVES

| | |
|---|---|
| Too much estrogen | Nausea, bloating, breast tenderness, increased B/P, melasma, headache |
| Too little estrogen | Early or midcycle breakthrough bleeding, increased spotting, hypomenorrhea |
| Too much progestin | Breast tenderness, headache, fatigue, changes in mood |
| Too little progestin | Late breakthrough bleeding |
| Too much androgen | Increased appetite, weight gain, acne, oily skin, hirsutism, decreased libido, increased breast size, breast tenderness, increased LDL cholesterol, decreased HDL cholesterol |

*B/P,* Blood pressure; *HDL,* high-density lipoprotein; *LDL,* low-density lipoprotein.

## CONTRACEPTIVES

| Name | Estrogen Content | Progestin Content |
|---|---|---|
| **Low-Dose Monophasic Pills** | | |
| Aubra | EE 20 mcg | Levonorgestrel 0.1 mg |
| Aviane | | |
| Falmina | | |
| Lessina | | |
| Lutera | | |
| Orsythia | | |
| Sronyx | | |
| Gildess 1/20 | EE 20 mcg | Norethindrone 1 mg |
| Junel 1/20 | | |
| Junel Fe 1/20 | | |
| Loestrin Fe 1/20 | | |
| Microgestin Fe 1/20 | | |
| Tarina Fe 1/20 | | |

*Continued*

| | | |
|---|---|---|
| Altavera<br>Levora<br>Marlissa<br>Portia-28 | EE 30 mcg | Levonorgestrel 0.15 mg |
| Cryselle-28<br>Lo/Ovral-28<br>Low-Ogestrel, -28 | EE 30 mcg | Norgestrel 0.3 mg |
| Gildess 1.5/30<br>Junel 1.5/30<br>Junel Fe 1.5/30<br>Larin 1.5/30<br>Loestrin Fe 1.5/30<br>Microgestin 1.5/30<br>Microgestin Fe 1.5/30 | EE 30 mcg | Norethindrone acetate 1.5 mg |
| Apri<br>Desogen<br>Ortho-Cept<br>Reclipsen | EE 30 mcg | Desogestrel 0.15 mg |
| Yasmin<br>Ocella<br>Syeda | EE 30 mcg | Drospirenone 3 mg |
| Kelnor 1/35<br>Zovia 1/35 | EE 35 mcg | Ethynodiol diacetate 1 mg |
| Ortho-Cyclen<br>Mononessa<br>Previfem<br>Sprintec | EE 35 mcg | Norgestimate 0.25 mg |
| Necon 1/50<br>Norinyl 1+50 | Mestranol 50 mcg | Norethindrone 1 mg |

## CONTRACEPTIVES—cont'd

| Name | Estrogen Content | Progestin Content |
|------|------------------|-------------------|
| Balziva<br>Femcon Fe<br>Gildagia<br>Zenchent | EE 35 mcg | Norethindrone 0.4 mg |
| Brevicon-28<br>Modicon<br>Necon 0.5/35<br>Nortrel 0.5/35 | EE 35 mcg | Norethindrone 0.5 mg (total of 10.5 mg/cycle) |
| Necon 1/35-28<br>Norinyl 1+35<br>Nortrel 1/35<br>Ortho-Novum 1/35-28 | EE 35 mcg | Norethindrone 1 mg (total of 21 mg/cycle) |
| **High-Dose Monophasic Pills** | | |
| Zovia 1/50-28 | EE 50 mcg | Ethynodiol diacetate 1 mg |
| Ogestrel 0.5/50-28 | EE 50 mcg | Norgestrel 0.5 mg |
| **Biphasic Pills** | | |
| Azurette<br>Kariva<br>Mircette | EE 20 mcg × 21 days, placebo × 2 days,<br>10 mcg × 5 days | Desogestrel 0.15 mg × 21 days |
| Necon 10/11 | EE 35 mcg | Norethindrone 0.5 mg × 10 days, 1 mg × 11 days |
| **Triphasic Pills** | | |
| Tilia<br>Tri-Legest Fe | EE 20 mcg × 5 days, 30 mcg × 7 days,<br>35 mcg × 9 days | Norethindrone 1 mg × 21 days |
| Ortho Tri-Cyclen Lo | EE 25 mcg × 21 days | Norgestimate 0.18 mg × 7 days, 0.215 mg × 7 days, 0.25 mg × 7 days |

| | | |
|---|---|---|
| Caziant<br>Cyclessa<br>Velivet | EE 25 mcg × 21 days | Desogestrel 0.1 mg × 7 days, 0.125 mg × 7 days, 0.15 mg × 7 days |
| Enpresse<br>Trivora | EE 30 mcg × 6 days, 40 mcg × 5 days, 30 mcg × 10 days | Levonorgestrel 0.05 mg × 6 days, 0.075 mg × 5 days, 0.125 mg × 10 days |
| Ortho Tri-Cyclen<br>Trinessa<br>Tri-Previfem<br>Tri-Sprintec | EE 35 mcg × 21 days | Norgestimate 0.18 mg × 7 days, 0.215 mg × 7 days, 0.25 mg × 7 days |
| Aranelle<br>Leena<br>Tri-Norinyl | EE 35 mcg × 21 days | Norethindrone 0.5 mg × 7 days, 1 mg × 9 days, 0.5 mg × 5 days |
| Ortho-Novum 7/7/7<br>Nortrel 7/7/7<br>Necon 7/7/7 | EE 35 mcg × 21 days | Norethindrone 0.5 mg × 7 days, 0.75 mg × 7 days, 1 mg × 7 days |
| **Four Phasic** | | |
| Natazia | Estradiol 3 mg × 2 days, then 2 mg × 2 days, then 1 mg × 2 days, then 2-day pill-free interval | Dienogest none × 2 days, then 2 mg × 5 days, then 3 mg × 17 days, then none for 4 days |
| **Extended-Cycle Pills** | | |
| Loestrin FE | EE 20 mcg × 24 days | Norethindrone 1 mg × 24 days |
| Jolessa | EE 30 mcg × 84 days | Levonorgestrel 0.15 mg × 84 days |
| Quartette<br>Quasense | EE 20 mcg × 42 days, 25 mcg × 21 days, 30 mcg × 21 days, then 10 mcg × 7 days | Levonorgestrel 0.15 mg × 84 days |

*Continued*

## CONTRACEPTIVES—cont'd

| Name | Estrogen Content | Progestin Content |
|---|---|---|
| Seasonique | EE 30 mcg × 84 days, 10 mcg × 7 days | Levonorgestrel 0.15 mg × 84 days |
| Yaz | EE 20 mcg × 24 days | Drospirenone 3 mg × 24 days |
| Gianvi | | |
| **Continuous Cycle Pill** | | |
| Amethyst | EE 20 mcg | Levonorgestrel 90 mcg |
| **Progestin-Only Pills** | | |
| Camila | N/A | Norethindrone 0.35 mg |
| Errin | | |
| Jolivette | | |
| Nor-QD | | |
| Nora-BE | | |
| **Emergency Contraception** | | |
| Plan B | N/A | Levonorgestrel 0.75-mg tablets taken 12 hrs apart |
| Next Choice | | |
| Ella | N/A | Ulipristal 30 mg one time within 5 days after unprotected intercourse |
| **Hormonal Alternative to Oral Contraception** | | |
| Depo-Provera CI | None | Medroxyprogesterone 150 mg |
| Medroxyprogesterone Acetate | | |
| Depo-SubQ Provera 104 | None | Medroxyprogesterone 104 mg |
| Implanon | None | Etonogestrel (release rate varies over time) |
| Mirena | None | Levonorgestrel 20 mcg/day for 5 yrs |
| NuvaRing | Ethinyl estradiol 15 mcg/day | Etonogestrel 0.12 mg/day |
| Ortho Evra | Ethinyl estradiol 20 mcg/day | Norelgestromin 200 mcg/day |

*EE,* ethinyl estradiol.

# Corticosteroids

## USES

Replacement therapy in adrenal insufficiency, including Addison's disease. Symptomatic treatment of multiorgan disease/conditions. Rheumatoid arthritis (RA), osteoarthritis, severe psoriasis, ulcerative colitis, lupus erythematosus, anaphylactic shock, acute exacerbation of asthma, status asthmaticus, organ transplant.

## ACTION

Suppress migration of polymorphonuclear leukocytes (PML) and reverse increased capillary permeability by their anti-inflammatory effect. Suppress immune system by decreasing activity of lymphatic system.

## CORTICOSTEROIDS

| Name | Availability | Route of Administration | Side Effects |
|---|---|---|---|
| **Beclomethasone** (Beconase, Qnasl, QVAR) | **Aerosol (oral inhalation), QVAR:** 40 mcg/inhalation, 80 mcg/inhalation **Aerosol (spray, intranasal), Qnasl:** 80 mcg/inhalation **Suspension (intranasal), Beconase:** 42 mcg/inhalation | Inhalation, intranasal | **I:** Cough, dry mouth/throat, headaches, throat irritation, increased blood glucose **Nasal:** Headaches, sore throat, intranasal ulceration, increased blood glucose |
| **Betamethasone** (Celestone) | **I:** 6 mg/ml | IV, intralesional, intra-articular | |
| **Budesonide** (Pulmicort, Rhinocort) | **Nasal:** 32 mcg/spray **Suspension for nebulization:** 250 mcg, 500 mcg | Intranasal | Nausea, vomiting, increased appetite, weight gain, insomnia, increased blood glucose Headaches, sore throat, intranasal ulceration, increased blood glucose |
| **Cortisone** (Cortone) | **T:** 5 mg, 10 mg, 25 mg | PO | Insomnia, nervousness, increased appetite, indigestion, increased blood glucose |

*Continued*

## CORTICOSTEROIDS—cont'd

| Name | Availability | Route of Administration | Side Effects |
|------|-------------|------------------------|--------------|
| **Dexamethasone (Decadron)** | **T:** 0.5 mg, 1 mg, 4 mg, 6 mg<br>**OS:** 0.5 mg/5 ml<br>**I:** 4 mg/ml, 10 mg/ml | PO, parenteral | Insomnia, weight gain, increased appetite, increased blood glucose |
| **Fludrocortisone (Florinef)** | **T:** 0.1 mg | PO | Edema, headache, peptic ulcer, increased blood glucose |
| **Flunisolide (Nasalide)** | **Nasal:** 25 mcg/spray | Inhalation, intranasal | Headache, nasal congestion, pharyngitis, upper respiratory infections, altered taste/smell, increased blood glucose |
| **Fluticasone (Flonase, Flovent)** | **Inhalation:** 44 mcg, 110 mcg, 220 mcg<br>**Nasal:** 50 mg, 100 mcg | Inhalation, intranasal | Headache, burning/stinging, nasal congestion, upper respiratory infections, increased blood glucose |
| **Hydrocortisone (Solu-Cortef)** | **T:** 5 mg, 10 mg, 25 mg<br>**I:** 100 mg, 250 mg, 500 mg, 1 g | PO, parenteral | Insomnia, headache, nausea, vomiting, increased blood glucose |
| **Methylprednisolone (Solu-Medrol)** | **T:** 4 mg<br>**I:** 40 mg, 125 mg, 500 mg, 1 g, 2 g | PO, parenteral | Headache, insomnia, nervousness, increased appetite, nausea, vomiting, increased blood glucose |
| **Prednisolone (Prelone)** | **T:** 5 mg<br>**OS:** 5 mg/5 ml, 15 mg/5 ml | PO | Headache, insomnia, weight gain, nausea, vomiting, increased blood glucose |
| **Prednisone** | **T:** 1 mg, 2.5 mg, 5 mg, 10 mg, 20 mg, 50 mg | PO | Headache, insomnia, weight gain, nausea, vomiting, increased blood glucose |
| **Triamcinolone (Kenalog, Nasacort AQ)** | **Injection, suspension:** 10 mg/ml, 40 mg/ml<br>**Intranasal, suspension:** 55 mcg/inhalation | IM, inhalation (nasal) | **PO:** Insomnia, increased appetite, nausea, vomiting, increased blood glucose<br>**I:** Cough, dry mouth/throat, headaches, throat irritation, increased blood glucose |

*I,* Injection; *OS,* oral suspension; *T,* tablets.

# Corticosteroids: Topical

## USES

Provide relief of inflammation/pruritus associated with corticosteroid-responsive disorders (e.g., contact dermatitis, eczema, insect bite reactions, first- and second-degree localized burns/sunburn).

## ACTION

Diffuse across cell membranes, form complexes with cytoplasm. Complexes stimulate protein synthesis of inhibitory enzymes responsible for anti-inflammatory effects (e.g., inhibit edema, erythema, pruritus, capillary dilation, phagocytic activity).

Topical corticosteroids can be classified based on potency:

May use for facial and intertriginous application for only limited time.

*High potency:* For more severe inflammatory conditions (e.g., lichen simplex chronicus, psoriasis). May use for facial and intertriginous application for short time only. Used in areas of thickened skin due to chronic conditions.

*Low potency:* Modest anti-inflammatory effect, safest for chronic application, facial and intertriginous application, with occlusion, for infants/young children.

*Medium potency:* For moderate inflammatory conditions (e.g., chronic eczematous dermatoses).

*Very high potency:* Alternative to systemic therapy for local effect (e.g., chronic lesions caused by psoriasis). Increased risk of skin atrophy. Used for short periods on small areas. Avoid occlusive dressings.

## CORTICOSTEROIDS: TOPICAL

| Name | Availability | Potency | Side Effects |
|------|-------------|---------|--------------|
| **Alclometasone (Aclovate)** | **C, O:** 0.05% | Low | Skin atrophy, contact dermatitis, stretch marks on skin, enlarged blood vessels in the skin, hair loss, pigment changes, secondary infections |
| **Amcinonide (Cyclocort)** | **C, O, L:** 0.1% | High | Same as alclometasone |

*Continued*

## CORTICOSTEROIDS: TOPICAL—cont'd

| Name | Availability | Potency | Side Effects |
|---|---|---|---|
| **Betamethasone dipropionate** | **C, O, G, L:** 0.05% | High | Same as alclometasone |
| **Betamethasone valerate** | **C:** 0.01%, 0.05%, 0.1%<br>**O:** 0.1%<br>**L:** 0.1% | High | Same as alclometasone |
| **Clobetasol (Temovate)** | **C, O:** 0.05% | High | Same as alclometasone |
| **Desonide (Tridesilon)** | **C, O, L:** 0.05% | Low | Same as alclometasone |
| **Desoximetasone (Topicort)** | **C:** 0.25%, 0.5%<br>**O:** 0.25%<br>**G:** 0.05% | High | Same as alclometasone |
| **Fluocinolone (Synalar)** | **C:** 0.01%, 0.025%, 0.2%<br>**O:** 0.025% | High | Same as alclometasone |
| **Fluocinonide (Lidex)** | **C, O, G:** 0.05% | High | Same as alclometasone |
| **Flurandrenolide (Cordran)** | **C, O, L:** 0.025%, 0.05% | Medium | Same as alclometasone |
| **Fluticasone (Cutivate)** | **C:** 0.05%<br>**O:** 0.005% | Medium | Same as alclometasone |
| **Halobetasol (Ultravate)** | **C, O:** 0.05% | High | Same as alclometasone |
| **Hydrocortisone (Hytone)** | **C, O:** 0.5%, 1%, 2.5% | Medium | Same as alclometasone |
| **Mometasone (Elocon)** | **C, O, L:** 0.1% | Medium | Same as alclometasone |
| **Prednicarbate (Dermatop)** | **C:** 0.1% | Medium | Same as alclometasone |
| **Triamcinolone (Aristocort, Kenalog)** | **C, O, L:** 0.025%, 0.1%, 0.5% | Medium | Same as alclometasone |

*C,* Cream; *G,* gel; *L,* lotion; *O,* ointment.

# Diuretics

## USES

*Thiazides:* Management of edema resulting from a number of causes (e.g., HF, hepatic cirrhosis); hypertension either alone or in combination with other antihypertensives.

*Loop:* Management of edema associated with HF, cirrhosis of the liver, and renal disease. Furosemide used in treatment of hypertension alone or in combination with other antihypertensives.

*Potassium-sparing:* Adjunctive treatment with thiazides; loop diuretics in treatment of HF and hypertension.

## ACTION

Increase the excretion of water/sodium and other electrolytes via the kidneys. Exact mechanism of antihypertensive effect unknown; may be due to reduced plasma volume or decreased peripheral vascular resistance. Subclassifications of diuretics are based on their mechanism and site of action.

*Thiazides:* Act at cortical diluting segment of nephron, block reabsorption of Na, Cl, and water; promote excretion of Na, Cl, K, and water. *Loop:* Act primarily at the thick

ascending limb of Henle's loop to inhibit Na, Cl, and water absorption.

*Potassium-sparing:* Spironolactone blocks aldosterone action on distal nephron (causes K retention, Na excretion). Triamterene, amiloride act on distal nephron, decreasing Na reuptake, reducing K secretion.

## DIURETICS

| Name | Availability | Dosage Range | Side Effects |
|---|---|---|---|
| Thiazide, Thiazide-related | | | |
| **Chlorothiazide (Diuril)** | **T:** 250 mg, 500 mg<br>**S:** 250 mg/5 ml<br>**I:** 500 mg | **Edema:** 500–1,000 mg 1–2 times/day<br>**HTN:** 500–2,000 mg/day in 1–2 divided doses | Confusion, fatigue, muscle cramps, abdominal discomfort |

Continued

## DIURETICS—cont'd

| Name | Availability | Dosage Range | Side Effects |
|---|---|---|---|
| Chlorthalidone | **Hygroton:** 25 mg, 50 mg, 100 mg | **Edema:** Initially, 50–100 mg once daily or 100 mg every other day. **Maximum:** 200 mg/day | Same as chlorothiazide |
| Hydrochlorothiazide | **T:** 12.5 mg, 25 mg, 50 mg **C:** 12.5 mg | **Edema:** 25–100 mg/day in 1–2 divided doses **HTN:** Initially, 12.5–25 mg once daily. May increase up to 50 mg/day in 1 or 2 divided doses | Orthostatic hypotension, photosensitivity, hypokalemia, anorexia, epigastric distress, increased blood glucose |
| Indapamide (Lozol) | **T:** 1.25 mg, 2.5 mg | **Edema:** Initially, 2.5 mg/day. May increase after 1 wk to 5 mg/day **HTN:** Initially, 2.5 mg/day. May increase q4wks to 2.5, then to 5 mg/day | Loss of appetite, diarrhea, headaches, dizziness, light-headedness, insomnia, upset stomach |
| Metolazone (Zaroxolyn) | **T:** 2.5 mg, 5 mg, 10 mg | **Edema:** 2.5–20 mg once daily **HTN:** 2.5–5 mg once daily | Orthostatic hypotension, dizziness, hypokalemia, nausea, diarrhea, abdominal pain |
| **Loop** | | | |
| Bumetanide (Bumex) | **T:** 0.5 mg, 1 mg, 2 mg **I:** 0.25 mg/ml | **Edema:** Initially, 0.5–2 mg/dose 1–2 times/day. **Maximum:** 10 mg/day | Orthostatic hypotension, cramps or pain, hypokalemia (dry mouth, fatigue, muscle cramps), blurred vision, headaches |
| Furosemide (Lasix) | **T:** 20 mg, 40 mg, 80 mg **OS:** 10 mg/ml, 40 mg/5 ml **I:** 10 mg/ml | **HTN:** 20–80 mg/day in 2 divided doses **Edema: PO:** 20–80 mg/dose. May increase by 20–40 mg/dose up to 600 mg/day. **IV:** 20–40 mg/dose. May increase by 20 mg/dose. **Maximum:** 200 mg/dose | Orthostatic hypotension, cramps or pain, hypokalemia (dry mouth, fatigue, muscle cramps), blurred vision, headaches |

| | | | |
|---|---|---|---|
| **Torsemide (Demadex)** | **T:** 5 mg, 10 mg, 20 mg, 100 mg<br>**I:** 10 mg/ml | **Edema:** 10–200 mg/day<br>**HTN:** Initially, 5 mg/day. May increase after 4–6 wks to 10 mg/day | Constipation, dizziness, upset stomach, headache, hypokalemia (dry mouth, fatigue, muscle cramps) |
| Potassium-sparing | | | |
| **Amiloride (Midamor)** | **T:** 5 mg | **HF/Edema:** Initially, 5 mg/day. May increase to 10 mg/day | Hyperkalemia, nausea, abdominal pain, diarrhea |
| **Eplerenone (Inspra)** | **T:** 25 mg, 50 mg | **HF:** Initially, 25 mg/day, titrate to 50 mg once daily<br>**HTN:** Initially, 50 mg/day. May increase to 50 mg 2 times/day | Hyperkalemia, hypertriglyceridemia |
| **Spironolactone (Aldactone)** | **T:** 25 mg, 50 mg, 100 mg | **Edema:** 25–200 mg/day in 1 or 2 divided doses<br>**HTN:** 50–100 mg/day in 1 or 2 divided doses<br>**Hypokalemia:** 25–100 mg/day<br>**HF:** Initially, 12.5–25 mg once daily.<br>**Maximum:** 50 mg/day | Hyperkalemia, nausea, vomiting, abdominal cramps, diarrhea |
| **Triamterene (Dyrenium)** | **C:** 50 mg, 100 mg | **Edema, HTN:** 100–300 mg/day in 1–2 divided doses | Same as amiloride |

*C,* Capsules; *HF,* heart failure; *HTN,* hypertension; *I,* injection; *OS,* oral solution; *S,* suspension; *T,* tablets.

# H₂ Antagonists

## USES

Short-term treatment of duodenal ulcer (DU), active benign gastric ulcer (GU), maintenance therapy of DU, pathologic hypersecretory conditions (e.g., Zollinger-Ellison syndrome), gastroesophageal reflux disease (GERD), and prevention of upper GI bleeding in critically ill pts.

## ACTION

Inhibit gastric acid secretion by interfering with histamine at the histamine H₂ receptors in parietal cells. Also inhibit acid secretion caused by gastrin. Inhibition occurs with basal (fasting), nocturnal, food-stimulated, or fundic distention secretion. H₂ antagonists decrease both the volume and H₂ concentration of gastric juices.

## H₂ ANTAGONISTS

| Name | Availability | Dosage Range | Side Effects |
|------|-------------|--------------|--------------|
| Cimetidine (Tagamet) | **T:** 200 mg, 300 mg, 400 mg, 800 mg<br>**L:** 300 mg/5 ml | **Treatment of DU:** 800 mg at bedtime, 400 mg 2 times/day or 300 mg 4 times/day<br>**Maintenance of DU:** 400 mg at bedtime<br>**Treatment of GU:** 800 mg at bedtime or 300 mg 4 times/day<br>**GERD:** 400 mg 4 times/day or 800 mg 2 times/day<br>**Hypersecretory:** 300 mg 4 times/day.<br>**Maximum:** 2,400 mg/day | Headaches, fatigue, dizziness, confusion, diarrhea, gynecomastia |
| Famotidine (Pepcid) | **T:** 10 mg, 20 mg, 40 mg<br>**OS:** 40 mg/5 ml<br>**I:** 10 mg/ml | **Treatment of DU:** 40 mg/day in 1 or 2 divided doses<br>**Maintenance of DU:** 20 mg/day<br>**Treatment of GU:** 40 mg/day at bedtime<br>**GERD:** 20 mg 2 times/day for 6 wks<br>**Hypersecretory:** Initially, 20 mg q6h. May increase up to 160 mg q6h | Headaches, dizziness, diarrhea, constipation, abdominal pain, tinnitus |

| | | | |
|---|---|---|---|
| **Nizatidine (Axid)** | **OS:** 15 mg/ml<br>**C:** 75 mg, 150 mg, 300 mg | **Treatment of GU:** 300 mg at hs or 150 mg 2 times/day<br>**GERD:** 150 mg 2 times/day<br>**Treatment of DU:** 300 mg at hs or 150 mg 2 times/day<br>**Maintenance of DU:** 150 mg/day at bedtime | Fatigue, urticaria, abdominal pain, constipation, nausea |
| **Ranitidine (Zantac)** | **T:** 75 mg, 150 mg, 300 mg<br>**C:** 150 mg, 300 mg<br>**Syrup:** 15 mg/ml<br>**I:** 25 mg/ml | **Treatment of DU:** 300 mg at hs or 150 mg 2 times/day<br>**Maintenance of DU:** 150 mg/day at bedtime<br>**Treatment of GU:** 150 mg 2 times/day<br>**GERD:** 150 mg 2 times/day<br>**Hypersecretory:** 150 mg 2 times/day.<br>**Maximum:** 6 g/day.<br>**Erosive Esophagitis:** Treatment: 150 mg 4 times/day. Maintenance: 150 mg 2 times/day | Blurred vision, constipation, nausea, abdominal pain |

*C,* Capsules; *DT,* disintegrating tablets; *DU,* duodenal ulcer; *GERD,* gastroesophageal reflux disease; *GU,* gastric ulcer; *I,* injection; *L,* liquid; *OS,* oral suspension; *T,* tablets.

# Hepatitis C Virus

Hepatitis C virus (HCV) is the leading blood borne infection in the US. HCV is transmitted by exposure to infected blood products. Risk factors for acquiring HCV include injection drug use, receiving contaminated blood products, needle sticks, and vertical transmission. If untreated, HCV may progress to chronic HCV and long-term sequelae including cirrhosis and hepatocellular carcinoma. There are seven known genotypes of HCV (genotypes 1-7) which impact the selection of initial therapy and treatment response. Genotype 1 is the most common and is further subtyped into genotypes 1a and 1b.

Currently, there are two indirect-acting antivirals and seven direct-acting antivirals approved for the treatment of chronic HCV.

## ACTION

### Indirect Acting Antivirals (IAA)

*Alpha Interferons (peg-interferons)*: Induces immune response against HCV, inhibiting viral replication

*Ribavirin*: Exact mechanism unknown but has activity against several RNA and DNA viruses

### Direct Acting Antivirals (DAA)

*NS3/4A Protease Inhibitors (PIs)*: Targets the serine protease NS3/NS4 that is responsible for processing HCV polyprotein and producing new viruses.

*Nonstructural Protein 5A (NS5A) Inhibitors*: Suppress the NS5A protein, that is essential for viral assembly and replication.

*Nonstructural Protein 5B (NS5B) Inhibitors*: Suppress the NS5B RNA-dependent RNA polymerase that is responsible for HCV replication.

## ANTI-HEPATITIS C VIRUS PREPARATIONS

| Name | Type | Genotype | Dosage | Side Effects |
|---|---|---|---|---|
| **Elbasvir, grazoprevir (Zepatier)** | DAA NS5A/NS3/4A protease inhibitor | 1, 4 | **Genotype 1a:** One tablet daily for 12 wks (16 wks with baseline NS5A polymorphins) **Genotype 1b:** One tablet daily for 12 wks **Genotype 4:** One tablet daily for 12 wks (16 wks peginterferon/ribavirin experienced) | Fatigue, headache, nausea |
| **Simeprevir (Olysio)** | DAA (NS3/4A-PI) | 1, 4 | 150 mg once daily plus peginterferon and ribavirin for 12 wks, then additional 12–36 wks of peginterferon and ribavirin) 150 mg once daily plus sofosbuvir for 12 wks without cirrhosis or 24 wks with cirrhosis | (With peginterferon, ribavirin): rash, itching, nausea, photosensitivity (With sofosbuvir): fatigue, headache, nausea, insomnia, pruritus, rash, dizziness, diarrhea |
| **Sofosbuvir (Sovaldi)** | DAA (NS5B) | 1, 2, 3, 4 | **Genotypes 1, 4:** 400 mg once daily plus peginterferon and ribavirin for 12 wks 400 mg once daily plus simeprevir for 12 wks without cirrhosis or 24 wks with cirrhosis **Genotypes 2, 3:** 400 mg once daily plus ribavirin for 12 wks for genotype 2 or 24 wks for genotype 3 | (With peginterferon, ribavirin): Fatigue, headache, nausea, insomnia, anemia (With simeprevir): fatigue, headache, nausea, insomnia, pruritus, rash, dizziness, diarrhea |
| **Ledipasvir, Sofosbuvir (Harvoni)** | DAA (NS5A/NS5B) | 1, 4, 5, 6 | **Genotype 1:** One tablet (90 mg/400 mg) for 12 wks in treatment-naïve pt with or without cirrhosis and treatment-experienced pt without cirrhosis; for 24 wks for treatment experienced pts with cirrhosis **Genotypes 4, 5, 6:** One tablet daily for 12 wks | Fatigue, headache, nausea, diarrhea, insomnia; elevations in bilirubin, lipase, and creatinine kinase |

*Continued*

# ANTI-HEPATITIS C VIRUS PREPARATIONS—cont'd

| Name | Type | Genotype | Dosage | Side Effects |
|------|------|----------|--------|--------------|
| **Ombitasvir, Paritaprevir, Ritonavir, Dasabuvir (Viekira Pak)** | DAA (NS5A/protease inhibitor/CYP3A inhibitor/polymerase inhibitor) | 1 | Two ombitasvir, paritaprevir, ritonavir tablets (12.5 mg, 75 mg, 50 mg) once daily in the morning plus one dasabuvir 250 mg tablet 2 times/day. Patients with **genotype 1a or 1b with cirrhosis** will also receive ribavirin for 12 wks (genotype 1a with cirrhosis: 12–24 wks based on treatment history; liver transplant pts: 24 wks) | (With ribavirin): fatigue, nausea, itching, insomnia (Without ribavirin): nausea, itching, insomnia |
| **Peginterferon alfa 2a (Pegasys)** | IAA (Interferon) | 1, 2, 3, 4 | 180 mcg SQ wkly for 12–48 wks based on antiviral regimen, pt history, response | (With ribavirin): fatigue, weakness, fever, myalgia, headache |
| **Peginterferon alfa 2b (PegIntron)** | IAA (Interferon) | 1, 2, 3, 4 | 1.5 mcg/kg SQ wkly for 12–48 wks based on antiviral regimen, pt history, response | (With ribavirin): injection site reaction, fatigue, weakness, headache, rigors, fever, nausea, myalgia, insomnia, mood instability, hair loss |
| **Ribavirin (Copegus, Ribasphere)** | IAA (Nucleoside analogue) | 1, 2, 3, 4 | **Genotypes 2, 3**: 400 mg 2 times/day (with peginterferon) **Genotypes 1, 4**: <75 kg: 400 mg qam and 600 mg qpm 75kg or greater: 600 mg 2 times/day | (With peginterferon): fatigue, weakness, headache, rigors, fever, nausea, myalgia, insomnia, mood instability, hair loss |
| **Daclatasvir (Daklinza)** | DAA (NS5A) | 3 | 60 mg once daily with sofosbuvir for 12 wks | Headache, fatigue |
| **Ombitasvir, paritaprevir, ritonavir (Technivie)** | DAA (NS5A/protease Inhibitor/CYP3A inhibitor) | 4 | Two tablets once daily with ribavirin for 12 wks | Asthenia, fatigue, nausea, insomnia |
| **Sofosbuvir/velpatasvir (Epclusa)** | DAA (NS5B/NS5A) | 1, 2, 3, 4, 5, 6 | One tablet daily for 12 wks | Insomnia, anemia, headache, fatigue, nausea, diarrhea |

# Hormones

## USES

Functions of the body are regulated by two major control systems: the nervous system and the endocrine (hormone) system. Together they maintain homeostasis and control different metabolic functions in the body.

Hormones are concerned with control of different metabolic functions in the body (e.g., rates of chemical reactions in cells, transporting substances through cell membranes, cellular metabolism [growth/secretions]). By definition, a hormone is a chemical substance secreted into body fluids by cells and has control over other cells in the body.

Hormones can be local or general:

- *Local hormones* have specific local effects (e.g., acetylcholine, which is secreted at parasympathetic and skeletal nerve endings).

- *General hormones* are mostly secreted by specific endocrine glands (e.g., epinephrine/norepinephrine are secreted by the adrenal medulla in response to sympathetic stimulation), transported in the blood to all parts of the body, causing many different reactions.

Some general hormones affect all or almost all cells of the body (e.g., thyroid hormone from the thyroid gland increases the rate of most chemical reactions in almost all cells of the body); other general hormones affect only specific tissue (e.g., ovarian hormones are specific to female sex organs and secondary sexual characteristics of the female).

## ACTION

Endocrine hormones almost never directly act intracellularly affecting chemical reactions. They first combine with hormone receptors either on the cell surface or inside the cell (cell [cytoplasm or nucleus]). The combination of hormone and receptors alters the function of the receptor, and the receptor is the direct cause of the hormone effects.

*Altered receptor function* may include the following:

*Altered cell permeability,* which causes a change in protein structure of the receptor, usually opening or closing a channel for one or more ions. The movement of these ions causes the effect of the hormone.

*Activation of intracellular enzymes* immediately inside the cell membrane (e.g., hormone combines with receptor that then becomes the activated enzyme adenyl cyclase, which causes formation of cAMP).

◄**ALERT▶** cAMP has effects inside the cell. It is not the hormone but cAMP that causes these effects.

Regulation of hormone secretion is controlled by an internal control system, the negative feedback system:

- Endocrine gland oversecretes.
- Hormone exerts more and more of its effect.
- Target organ performs its function.

*Continued*

# Hormones—cont'd

## ACTION—cont'd

- Too much function in turn feeds back to endocrine gland to decrease secretory rate.

The endocrine system contains many glands and hormones. A summary of the important glands and their hormones secreted are as follows:

The pituitary gland (hypophysis) is a small gland found in the sella turcica at the base of the brain. The pituitary is divided into two portions physiologically: the anterior pituitary (adenohypophysis) and the posterior pituitary (neurohypophysis). Six important hormones are secreted from the anterior pituitary and two from the posterior pituitary.

Anterior pituitary hormones:
- Growth hormone (GH)
- Adrenocorticotropin (corticotropin)
- Thyroid-stimulating hormone (thyrotropin) (TSH)
- Follicle-stimulating hormone (FSH)
- Luteinizing hormone (LH)
- Prolactin

Posterior pituitary hormones:
- Antidiuretic hormone (vasopressin)
- Oxytocin

Almost all secretions of the pituitary hormones are controlled by hormonal or nervous signals from the hypothalamus. The hypothalamus is a center of information concerned with the well-being of the body, which in turn is used to control secretions of the important pituitary hormones just listed. Secretions from the posterior pituitary are controlled by nerve signals originating in the hypothalamus; anterior pituitary hormones are controlled by hormones secreted within the hypothalamus. These hormones are as follows:

- Thyrotropin-releasing hormone (TRH) releasing thyroid-stimulating hormone
- Corticotropin-releasing hormone (CRH) releasing adrenocorticotropin
- Growth hormone–releasing hormone (GHRH) releasing growth hormone and growth hormone inhibitory hormone (GHIH) (same as somatostatin)
- Gonadotropin-releasing hormone (GnRH) releasing the two gonadotropic hormones LH and FSH
- Prolactin inhibitory factor (PIF) causing inhibition of prolactin and prolactin-releasing factor

### ANTERIOR PITUITARY HORMONES

All anterior pituitary hormones (except growth hormone) have as their principal effect stimulating target glands.

### GROWTH HORMONE (GH)

Growth hormone affects almost all tissues of the body. GH (somatotropin) causes growth in almost all tissues of the body (increases cell size, increases mitosis with increased number of cells, and differentiates certain types of cells). Metabolic effects include increased rate of protein synthesis, mobilization of fatty acids from adipose tissue, decreased rate of glucose utilization.

### THYROID-STIMULATING HORMONE (TSH)

Thyroid-stimulating hormone controls secretion of the thyroid hormones. The thyroid gland is located immediately below the larynx on either side of and anterior to the trachea and secretes two significant hormones, thyroxine ($T_4$) and triiodothyroxine ($T_3$), which have a profound effect on increasing the metabolic rate of the body. The thyroid gland also secretes calcitonin, an important hormone for calcium metabolism. Calcitonin promotes deposition of calcium in the bones, which decreases calcium concentration in the extracellular fluid.

### ADRENOCORTICOTROPIN

Adrenocorticotropin causes the adrenal cortex to secrete adrenocortical hormones. The adrenal glands lie at the superior poles of the two kidneys. Each gland is composed of two distinct parts: the adrenal medulla and the cortex. The adrenal medulla, related to the sympathetic nervous system, secretes the hormones epinephrine and norepinephrine. When stimulated, they cause constriction of blood vessels, increased activity of the heart, inhibitory effects on the GI tract, and dilation of the pupils. The adrenal cortex secretes corticosteroids, of which there are two major types: mineralocorticoids and glucocorticoids. Aldosterone, the principal mineralocorticoid, primarily affects electrolytes of the extracellular fluids. Cortisol, the principal glucocorticoid, affects glucose, protein, and fat metabolism.

### LUTEINIZING HORMONE (LH)

Luteinizing hormone plays an important role in ovulation and causes secretion of female sex hormones by the ovaries and testosterone by the testes.

### FOLLICLE-STIMULATING HORMONE (FSH)

Follicle-stimulating hormone causes growth of follicles in the ovaries before ovulation and promotes formation of sperm in the testes.

Ovarian sex hormones are estrogens and progestins. Estradiol is the most important estrogen; progesterone is the most important progestin.

*Estrogens* mainly promote proliferation and growth of specific cells in the body and are responsible for development of most of the secondary sex characteristics. Primarily cause cellular proliferation and growth of tissues of sex organs/other tissue related to reproduction. Ovaries, fallopian tubes, uterus, vagina increase in size. Estrogen initiates growth of breast and milk-producing apparatus, external appearance.

*Progesterone* stimulates secretion of the uterine endometrium during the latter half of the female sexual cycle, preparing the uterus for implantation of the fertilized ovum. Decreases the frequency of uterine contractions (helps prevent expulsion of the implanted ovum). Progesterone promotes development of breasts, causing alveolar cells to proliferate, enlarge, and become secretory in nature.

*Testosterone* is secreted by the testes and formed by the interstitial cells of Leydig. Testosterone production increases under the stimulus of the anterior pituitary gonadotropic hormones. It is responsible for distinguishing characteristics of the masculine body (stimulates the growth of male sex organs and promotes the development of male secondary sex characteristics, e.g., distribution of body hair, effect on voice, protein formation, and muscular development).

### PROLACTIN

Prolactin promotes the development of breasts and secretion of milk.

## POSTERIOR PITUITARY HORMONES

### ANTIDIURETIC HORMONE (ADH) (VASOPRESSIN)

ADH can cause antidiuresis (decreased excretion of water by the kidneys). In the presence of ADH, the permeability of the renal-collecting ducts and tubules to water increases, which allows water to be absorbed, conserving water in the body. ADH in higher concentrations is a very potent vasoconstrictor, constricting arterioles everywhere in the body, increasing B/P.

### OXYTOCIN

Oxytocin contracts the uterus during the birthing process, esp. toward the end of the pregnancy, helping expel the baby. Oxytocin also contracts myoepithelial cells in the breasts, causing milk to be expressed from the alveoli into the ducts so that the baby can obtain it by suckling.

## PANCREAS

The pancreas is composed of two tissue types: *acini* (secrete digestive juices in the duodenum) and *islets of Langerhans* (secrete insulin/glucagons directly into the blood). The islets of Langerhans contain three cells: alpha, beta, and delta. Alpha cells secrete glucagon, beta cells secrete insulin, and delta cells secrete somatostatin.

*Continued*

# Hormones—cont'd

## ACTION—cont'd

*Insulin* promotes glucose entry into most cells, thus controlling the rate of metabolism of most carbohydrates. Insulin also affects fat metabolism.

*Glucagon* effects are opposite those of insulin, the most important of which is increasing blood glucose concentration by releasing it from the liver into the circulating body fluids.

*Somatostatin* (same chemical as secreted by the hypothalamus) has multiple inhibitory effects: depresses secretion of insulin and glucagon, decreases GI motility, decreases secretions/absorption of the GI tract.

# Human Immunodeficiency Virus (HIV) Infection

## USES

*Antiretroviral agents* are used in the treatment of HIV infection.

## ACTION

*Nucleoside reverse transcriptase inhibitors (NRTIs)* compete with natural substrates for formation of proviral DNA by reverse transcriptase inhibiting viral replication.

*Nucleotide reverse transcriptase inhibitors (NtRTIs)* inhibit reverse transcriptase by competing with the natural substrate deoxyadenosine triphosphate and by DNA chain termination.

*Non-nucleoside reverse transcriptase inhibitors (NNRTIs)* directly bind to reverse transcriptase and block RNA-dependent and DNA-dependent DNA polymerase activities by disrupting the enzyme's catalytic site.

*Protease inhibitors (PIs)* bind to the active site of HIV-1 protease and prevent the processing of viral gag and gag-pol polyprotein precursors resulting in immature, noninfectious viral particles.

*Fusion inhibitors* interfere with the entry of HIV-1 into cells by inhibiting fusion of viral and cellular membranes.

*CCR5 co-receptor antagonist* selectively binds to human chemokine receptor CCR5 present on cell membrane preventing HIV-1 from entering cells.

*Integrase inhibitor* inhibits catalytic activity of HIV-1 integrase, an HIV-1 encoded enzyme required for viral replication.

ANTIRETROVIRAL AGENTS FOR TREATMENT OF HIV INFECTION

| Name | Availability | Dosage Range | Side Effects |
|---|---|---|---|
| Nucleoside Analogues | | | |
| **Abacavir (Ziagen)** | **T:** 300 mg<br>**OS:** 20 mg/ml | **A:** 300 mg 2 times/day or 600 mg once daily | Nausea, vomiting, malaise, rash, fever, headaches, asthenia, fatigue, hypersensitivity reactions |
| **Didanosine (Videx EC)** | **DR:** 125 mg, 200 mg, 250 mg, 400 mg<br>**OS:** 2 g/bottle, 4 g/bottle | **DR (weighing 60 kg or more):** 400 mg once daily; **(weighing 25–59 kg):** 250 mg once daily; **(weighing 20–24 kg):** 200 mg once daily<br>**OS (weighing more than 60 kg):** 200 mg q12h or 400 mg once daily; **(weighing less than 60 kg):** 125 mg q12h or 250 mg once daily | Peripheral neuropathy, pancreatitis, diarrhea, nausea, vomiting, headaches, insomnia, rash, hepatitis, seizures |
| **Emtricitabine (Emtriva)** | **C:** 200 mg<br>**OS:** 10 mg/ml | **A:** 200 mg/day **(C)**<br>240 mg/day **(OS)** | Headaches, insomnia, depression, diarrhea, nausea, vomiting, rhinitis, asthenia, rash |
| **Lamivudine (Epivir)** | **T:** 100 mg, 150 mg, 300 mg<br>**OS:** 5 mg/ml, 10 mg/ml | **A:** 150 mg 2 times/day or 300 mg once daily<br>**C:** 4 mg/kg 2 times/day | Diarrhea, malaise, fatigue, headaches, nausea, vomiting, abdominal pain, peripheral neuropathy, arthralgia, myalgia, skin rash |
| **Stavudine (Zerit)** | **C:** 15 mg, 20 mg, 30 mg, 40 mg<br>**OS:** 1 mg/ml | **A (weighing more than 60 kg):** 40 mg 2 times/day (20 mg 2 times/day if peripheral neuropathy occurs); **(weighing 60 kg or less):** 30 mg 2 times/day (15 mg 2 times/day if peripheral neuropathy occurs) | Peripheral neuropathy, anemia, leukopenia, neutropenia |
| **Zidovudine (Retrovir)** | **C:** 100 mg<br>**T:** 300 mg<br>**Syrup:** 50 mg/5 ml, 10 mg/ml | **A:** 300 mg 2 times/day | Anemia, granulocytopenia, myopathy, nausea, malaise, fatigue, insomnia |

Continued

## ANTIRETROVIRAL AGENTS FOR TREATMENT OF HIV INFECTION—cont'd

| Name | Availability | Dosage Range | Side Effects |
|------|-------------|--------------|--------------|
| **Nucleotide Analogues** | | | |
| **Tenofovir TAF (Vemlidy)** | **T:** 25 mg | **A:** 25 mg once daily | Headache, abdominal pain, fatigue, cough, nausea, back pain |
| **Tenofovir TDF (Viread)** | **T:** 300 mg | **A:** 300 mg once daily | Nausea, vomiting, diarrhea, headache, fatigue |
| **Non-nucleoside Analogues** | | | |
| **Delavirdine (Rescriptor)** | **T:** 100 mg, 200 mg | **A:** 200 mg 3 times/day for 14 days, then 400 mg 3 times/day | Rash, nausea, headaches, elevated hepatic function tests |
| **Efavirenz (Sustiva)** | **C:** 50 mg, 200 mg **T:** 600 mg | **A:** 600 mg/day **C:** 200–600 mg/day based on weight | Headaches, dizziness, insomnia, fatigue, rash, nightmares |
| **Etravirine (Intelence)** | **T:** 100 mg, 200 mg | **A:** 200 mg 2 times/day | Skin reactions (e.g., Stevens-Johnson syndrome, erythema multiforme), nausea, abdominal pain, vomiting |
| **Nevirapine (Viramune, Viramune XR)** | **T:** 200 mg **T (ER):** 400 mg **S:** 50 mg/ml | **A:** 200 mg/day for 14 days, then (if no rash) 200 mg 2 times/day | Rash, nausea, fatigue, fever, headaches, abnormal hepatic function tests |
| **Rilpivirine (Edurant)** | **T:** 25 mg | **A:** 25 mg once daily with a meal | Depression, insomnia, headache, rash |
| **Protease Inhibitors** | | | |
| **Atazanavir (Reyataz)** | **C:** 100 mg, 150 mg, 200 mg, 300 mg | **A:** 400 mg/day or 300 mg (with 100 mg ritonavir) once daily | Headaches, diarrhea, abdominal pain, nausea, rash |
| **Darunavir (Prezista)** | **T:** 400 mg, 600 mg | **A:** 600 mg 2 times/day (with ritonavir 100 mg) or 800 mg once daily with ritonavir 100 mg | Diarrhea, nausea, vomiting, headaches, skin rash, constipation |
| **Fosamprenavir (Lexiva)** | **T:** 700 mg **OS:** 50 mg/ml | **A:** 1,400–2,800 mg/day with 100 mg ritonavir | Headaches, fatigue, rash, nausea, diarrhea, vomiting, abdominal pain |
| **Indinavir (Crixivan)** | **C:** 200 mg, 400 mg | **A:** 800 mg q8h or 800 mg 2 times/day with ritonavir 100 mg | Nephrolithiasis, hyperbilirubinemia, abdominal pain, asthenia, fatigue, flank pain, nausea, vomiting, diarrhea, headaches, insomnia, dizziness, altered taste |

| | | |
|---|---|---|
| **Lopinavir/ritonavir (Kaletra)** | **C:** 133/33 mg<br>**OS:** 80/20 mg | **A:** 400 mg/100 mg 2 times/day or 800 mg/200 mg once daily<br>**C (4–12 yrs):** 10–13 mg/kg 2 times/day | Diarrhea, nausea, vomiting, abdominal pain, headaches, rash |
| **Nelfinavir (Viracept)** | **T:** 250 mg<br>**Oral Powder:** 50 mg/g | **A:** 750 mg q8h or 1,250 mg 2 times/day<br>**C:** 20–25 mg/kg q8h | Diarrhea, fatigue, asthenia, headaches, hypertension, impaired concentration |
| **Ritonavir (Norvir)** | **C:** 100 mg<br>**OS:** 80 mg/ml | **A:** Titrate up to 800 mg/day based on protease inhibitor | Nausea, vomiting, diarrhea, altered taste, fatigue, elevated LFT and triglyceride levels |
| **Saquinavir (Invirase)** | **C:** 200 mg<br>**T:** 500 mg | **A:** 1,000 mg 2 times/day with ritonavir 100 mg | Diarrhea, elevated LFTs, hypertriglycerides, cholesterol, abnormal fat accumulation, hyperglycemia |
| **Tipranavir (Aptivus)** | **C:** 250 mg<br>**OS:** 100 mg/ml | **A:** 500 mg (with 200 mg ritonavir) 2 times/day | Diarrhea, nausea, fatigue, headaches, vomiting |
| Fusion Inhibitors | | |
| **Enfuvirtide (Fuzeon)** | **I:** 108 mg (90 mg when reconstituted) | **Subcutaneous:** 90 mg 2 times/day | Insomnia, depression, peripheral neuropathy, decreased appetite, constipation, asthenia, cough |
| CCR5 Antagonists | | |
| **Maraviroc (Selzentry)** | **T:** 150 mg, 300 mg | **A:** 300 mg 2 times/day<br>**CYP3A4 inducers:** 600 mg 2 times/day<br>**CYP3A4 inhibitors:** 150 mg 2 times/day | Cough, pyrexia, upper respiratory tract infections, rash, musculoskeletal symptoms, abdominal pain, dizziness |
| Integrase Inhibitor | | |
| **Raltegravir (Isentress)** | **T:** 400 mg | **A:** 400 mg 2 times/day | Nausea, headache, diarrhea, pyrexia |
| **Dolutegravir (Tivicay)** | **T:** 50 mg | **A:** 50 mg once daily or 50 mg bid (with CYP3A inducers or resistance) | Insomnia, headache |

*A,* Adults; *C,* capsules; *C (dosage),* children; *DR,* delayed-release; *ER,* extended-release; *I,* injection; *OS,* oral solution; *S,* suspension; *T,* tablets; *TAF,* tenofovir alafenamide; *TDF,* tenofovir disoproxil fumarate.

## FIXED-COMBINATION THERAPIES

| Brand Name | Generic Name | Dosage |
|---|---|---|
| Atripla | Efavirenz 600 mg<br>Emtricitabine 200 mg<br>Tenofovir (TDF) 300 mg | 1 tablet once daily |
| Combivir | Lamivudine 150 mg<br>Zidovudine 300 mg | 1 tablet twice daily |
| Complera | Emtricitabine 200 mg<br>Rilpivirine 27.5 mg<br>Tenofovir (TDF) 300 mg | 1 tablet once daily |
| Descovy | Emtricitabine 200 mg<br>Tenofovir (TAF) 25 mg | 1 tablet once daily |
| Epzicom | Abacavir 600 mg<br>Lamivudine 300 mg | 1 tablet once daily |
| Evotaz | Atazanavir 300 mg<br>Cobicistat 150 mg | 1 tablet once daily |
| Genvoya | Cobicistat 150 mg<br>Elvitegravir 150 mg<br>Emtricitabine 200 mg<br>Tenofovir (TAF) 10 mg | 1 tablet once daily |
| Odefsey | Emtricitabine 200 mg<br>Rilpivirine 25 mg<br>Tenofovir (TAF) 25 mg | 1 tablet once daily |
| Prezcobix | Cobicistat 150 mg<br>Darunavir 800 mg | 1 tablet once daily |

| | | |
|---|---|---|
| Stribild | Cobicistat 150 mg<br>Elvitegravir 150 mg<br>Emtricitabine 200 mg<br>Tenofovir (TDF) 300 mg | 1 tablet once daily |
| Triumeq | Abacavir 600 mg<br>Dolutegravir 50 mg<br>Lamivudine 300 mg | 1 tablet once daily |
| Trizivir | Abacavir 300 mg<br>Lamivudine 150 mg<br>Zidovudine 300 mg | 1 tablet twice daily |
| Truvada | Emtricitabine 200 mg<br>Tenofovir (TDF) 300 mg | 1 tablet once daily |

*TAF,* tenofovir alafenamide; *TDF,* tenofovir disoproxil fumarate.

# Immunosuppressive Agents

## USES

Improvement of both short- and long-term allograft survivals.

## ACTION

*Basiliximab:* An interleukin-2 (IL-2) receptor antagonist inhibiting IL-2 binding. This prevents activation of lymphocytes, and the response of the immune system to antigens is impaired.

*Cyclosporine:* Inhibits production and release of IL-2.

*Daclizumab:* An IL-2 receptor antagonist inhibiting IL-2 binding.

*Mycophenolate:* A prodrug that reversibly binds and inhibits inosine monophosphate dehydrogenase (IMPD), resulting in inhibition of purine nucleotide synthesis; inhibiting DNA and RNA synthesis and subsequent synthesis of T and B cells.

*Sirolimus:* Inhibits IL-2–stimulated T-lymphocyte activation and proliferation, which may occur through formation of a complex.

*Tacrolimus:* Inhibits IL-2–stimulated T-lymphocyte activation and proliferation, which may occur through formation of a complex.

## IMMUNOSUPPRESSIVE AGENTS

| Name | Availability | Dosage | Side Effects |
|------|--------------|--------|--------------|
| Basiliximab (Simulect) | **I:** 10 mg, 20 mg | 20 mg for 2 doses (on day of transplant, then 4 days after transplantation) | Abdominal pain, asthenia, cough, dizziness, dyspnea, dysuria, edema, hypertension, infection, tremors |
| Cyclosporine (Neoral, Sandimmune) | **C:** 25 mg, 50 mg, 100 mg<br>**S:** 100 mg/ml<br>**I:** 50 mg/ml | Dose dependent on type of transplant and formulation | Hypertension, hyperkalemia, nephrotoxicity, coarsening of facial features, hirsutism, gingival hyperplasia, nausea, vomiting, diarrhea, hepatotoxicity, hyperuricemia, hypertriglyceridemia, hypercholesterolemia, tremors, paresthesia, seizures, risk of infection/malignancy |
| Mycophenolate (CellCept, Myfortic) | **Cellcept:**<br>**C:** 250 mg<br>**I:** 500 mg<br>**S:** 200 mg/ml<br>**T:** 500 mg<br>**Myfortic:**<br>**T(DR):** 180 mg, 320 mg | **Cellcept:**<br>1–1.5 g 2 times/day based on type of transplant<br>**Myfortic:**<br>**Renal:** 720 mg 2 times/day | Diarrhea, vomiting, leukopenia, neutropenia, infections |
| Sirolimus (Rapamune) | **S:** 1 mg/ml<br>**T:** 0.5 mg, 1 mg, 2 mg | 2–6 mg/day | Dyspnea, leukopenia, thrombocytopenia, hyperlipidemia, abdominal pain, acne, arthralgia, fever, diarrhea, constipation, headaches, vomiting, weight gain |
| Tacrolimus (Prograf) | **C:** 0.5 mg, 1 mg, 5 mg<br>**I:** 5 mg/ml<br>**C(ER):** 0.5 mg, 1 mg, 5 mg<br>**T(ER):** 0.75 mg, 1 mg, 4 mg | **Heart:** 0.075 mg/kg/day in 2 divided doses q12h<br>**Kidney:** 0.1–0.2 mg/kg/day in 2 divided doses q12h<br>**Liver:** 0.1–0.15 mg/kg/day in 2 divided doses q12h | Nephrotoxicity, neurotoxicity, hyperglycemia, nausea, vomiting, photophobia, infections, hypertension, hyperlipidemia |

*C,* Capsules; *DR,* Delayed release; *ER,* extended release; *I,* injection; *S,* oral solution or suspension; *T,* tablets.

# Laxatives

## USES

Short-term treatment of constipation; colon evacuation before rectal/bowel examination; prevention of straining (e.g., after anorectal surgery, MI); to reduce painful elimination (e.g., episiotomy, hemorrhoids, anorectal lesions); modification of effluent from ileostomy, colostomy; prevention of fecal impaction; removal of ingested poisons.

## ACTION

Laxatives ease or stimulate defecation. Mechanisms by which this is accomplished include (1) attracting, retaining fluid in colonic contents due to hydrophilic or osmotic properties; (2) acting directly or indirectly on mucosa to decrease absorption of water and NaCl; or (3) increasing intestinal motility, decreasing absorption of water and NaCl by virtue of decreased transit time.

*Bulk-forming:* Act primarily in small/large intestine. Retain water in stool, may bind water, ions in colonic lumen (soften feces, increase bulk); may increase colonic bacteria growth (increases fecal mass). Produce soft stool in 1–3 days.

*Osmotic agents:* Act in colon. Similar to saline laxatives. Osmotic action may be enhanced in distal ileum/colon by bacterial metabolism to lactate, other organic acids. This decrease in pH increases motility, secretion. Produce soft stool in 1–3 days.

*Saline:* Acts in small/large intestine, colon (sodium phosphate). Poorly, slowly absorbed; causes hormone cholecystokinin release from duodenum (stimulates fluid secretion, motility); possesses osmotic properties; produces watery stool in 2–6 hrs (small doses produce semifluid stool in 6–12 hrs).

*Stimulant:* Acts in colon. Enhances accumulation of water/electrolytes in colonic lumen, enhances intestinal motility. May act directly on intestinal mucosa. Produces semifluid stool in 6–12 hrs.

**◄ALERT►** Bisacodyl suppository acts in 15–60 min.

*Stool softener:* Acts in small/large intestine. Hydrates and softens stools by its surfactant action, facilitating penetration of fat and water into stool. Produces soft stool in 1–3 days.

## LAXATIVES

| Name | Onset of Action | Uses | Side Effects/Precautions |
|---|---|---|---|
| **Bulk-forming** | | | |
| **Methylcellulose (Citrucel)** | 12–24 hrs up to 3 days | Treatment of constipation for postpartum women, elderly, pts with diverticulosis, irritable bowel syndrome, hemorrhoids | Gas, bloating, esophageal obstruction, colonic obstruction, calcium and iron malabsorption |
| **Psyllium (Metamucil)** | Same as methylcellulose | Treatment of chronic constipation and constipation associated with rectal disorders; management of irritable bowel syndrome | Diarrhea, constipation, abdominal cramps, esophageal/colon obstruction, broncho-spasm |
| **Stool Softener** | | | |
| **Docusate (Colace, Surfak)** | 1–3 days | Treatment of constipation due to hard stools, in painful anorectal conditions, and for those who need to avoid straining during bowel movements | Stomachache, mild nausea, cramping, diarrhea, irritated throat (with liquid and syrup dose forms) |
| **Saline** | | | |
| **Magnesium citrate (Citrate of Magnesia, Citro-Mag)** | 30 min–3 hrs | Bowel evacuation prior to certain surgical and diagnostic procedures | Hypotension, abdominal cramping, diarrhea, gas formation, electrolyte abnormalities |
| Magnesium hydroxide | 30 min–3 hrs | Short-term treatment of occasional constipation | Electrolyte abnormalities can occur; use caution in pts with renal or cardiac impairment; diarrhea, abdominal cramps, hypotension |
| **Sodium phosphate (Fleet Phospho-Soda)** | 2–15 min | Relief of occasional constipation; bowel evacuation prior to certain surgical and diagnostic procedures | Electrolyte abnormalities; do not use for pts with HF, severe renal impairment, ascites, GI obstruction, active inflammatory bowel disease |

*Continued*

## LAXATIVES—cont'd

| Name | Onset of Action | Uses | Side Effects/Precautions |
|------|-----------------|------|--------------------------|
| **Osmotic** | | | |
| **Lactulose (Kristalose)** | 24–48 hrs | Short-term relief of constipation | Nausea, vomiting, diarrhea, abdominal cramping, bloating, gas |
| **Polyethylene glycol (MiraLax)** | 24–48 hrs | Short-term relief of constipation | Bitter taste, diarrhea |
| **Stimulant** | | | |
| **Bisacodyl (Dulcolax)** | **PO:** 6–12 hrs **Rectal:** 15–60 min | Short-term relief of constipation | Elecrolyte imbalance, abdominal discomfort, gas, potential for overuse/abuse |
| **Senna (Senokot)** | 6–12 hrs | Short-term relief of constipation | Abdominal discomfort, cramps |

*GI,* Gastrointestinal; *HF,* heart failure.

# Nonsteroidal Anti-Inflammatory Drugs (NSAIDs)

| USES | ACTION |
|------|--------|
| Provide symptomatic relief from *pain/inflammation* in the treatment of musculoskeletal disorders (e.g., rheumatoid arthritis [RA], osteoarthritis, ankylosing spondylitis), *analgesic* for low to moderate pain, *reduction in fever* (many agents not suited for routine/prolonged therapy due to toxicity). By virtue of its action on platelet function, aspirin is used in treatment or prophylaxis of diseases associated with hypercoagulability (reduces risk of stroke/heart attack). | Exact mechanism for anti-inflammatory, analgesic, antipyretic effects unknown. Inhibition of enzyme cyclo-oxygenase, the enzyme responsible for prostaglandin synthesis, appears to be a major mechanism of action. May inhibit other mediators of inflammation (e.g., leukotrienes). Direct action on hypothalamus heat-regulating center may contribute to antipyretic effect. |

## NSAIDs

| Name | Availability | Dosage Range | Side Effects |
|------|-------------|--------------|--------------|
| **Aspirin** | **Caplet:** 500 mg<br>**Suppository:** 300 mg, 600 mg<br>**T:** 325 mg<br>**T (EC):** 81 mg, 325 mg<br>**T (chew):** 81 mg | **Analgesic/antipyretic:** 325–650 mg q4–6h prn or 975 mg q6h prn or 500–1000 mg q4–6h prn | GI discomfort, dizziness, headaches, increased risk of bleeding |
| **Celecoxib (Celebrex)** | **C:** 50 mg, 100 mg, 200 mg, 400 mg | 200 mg q12h (**Maximum:** 600 mg day 1, then 400 mg/day) | Diarrhea, back pain, dizziness, heartburn, headaches, nausea, abdominal pain |
| **Diclofenac (Voltaren, Zipsor, Zorvolex)** | **T:** 25 mg, 50 mg, 75 mg<br>**C (Zipsor):** 25 mg<br>**C (Zorvolex):** 18 mg, 35 mg | 50 mg tid<br>(**Zipsor**): 25 mg 4 times/day<br>(**Zorvolex**): 18–35 mg 3 times/day | Indigestion, constipation, diarrhea, nausea, headaches, fluid retention, abdominal cramps |

*Continued*

## NSAIDs—cont'd

| Name | Availability | Dosage Range | Side Effects |
|---|---|---|---|
| **Diflunisal (Dolobid)** | T: 500 mg | **Arthritis:** 0.5–1 g/day in 2 divided doses<br>**Maximum:** 1.5 g/day<br>**P:** 500 mg once, then 250 mg q8–12h | Headaches, abdominal cramps, indigestion, diarrhea, nausea |
| **Etodolac (Lodine)** | **T:** 400 mg, 500 mg<br>**T (ER):** 400 mg, 500 mg, 600 mg<br>**C:** 200 mg, 300 mg | **Arthritis:** 400 mg 2 times/day or 300 mg 2–3 times/day or 500 mg 2 times/day. **(ER):** 400 mg up to 1,000 mg once daily<br>**P:** 200–400 mg q6–8h as needed | Indigestion, dizziness, headaches, bloated feeling, diarrhea, nausea, weakness, abdominal cramps |
| **Fenoprofen (Nalfon)** | **C:** 200 mg, 400 mg<br>**T:** 600 mg | **Arthritis:** 400–600 mg 3–4 times/day<br>**P:** 200 mg q4–6h as needed | Nausea, indigestion, anxiety, constipation, shortness of breath, heartburn |
| **Ibuprofen (Advil, Caldolor, Motrin)** | **I:** 100 mg/ml<br>**T:** 100 mg, 200 mg, 400 mg, 600 mg, 800 mg<br>**T (chewable):** 50 mg, 100 mg<br>**C:** 200 mg<br>**S:** 100 mg/5 ml | **Inflammatory disease:** 400–800 mg/dose 3–4 times/day<br>**P:** 200–400 mg/dose q4–6h as needed | Dizziness, abdominal cramps, abdominal pain, heartburn, nausea |
| **Indomethacin (Indocin, Tivorbex)** | **(Tivorbex)** 20 mg, 40 mg<br>**C:** 25 mg, 50 mg<br>**C (SR):** 75 mg<br>**S:** 25 mg/5 ml | **Arthritis:** 25–50 mg/dose 2–3 times/day<br>**Maximum:** 200 mg/day<br>**P: (Tivorbex only):** 20 mg 3 times/day or 40 mg 2–3 times/day | Fluid retention, dizziness, headaches, abdominal pain, indigestion, nausea |
| **Ketoprofen (Orudis KT)** | **C:** 25 mg, 50 mg<br>**C (ER):** 200 mg | **Arthritis:** 50 mg 4 times/day or 75 mg 3 times/day<br>**ER:** 200 mg once daily<br>**P:** 25–50 mg q6–8h as needed | Headaches, anxiety, abdominal pain, bloated feeling, constipation, diarrhea, nausea |

| | | | |
|---|---|---|---|
| Ketorolac (Toradol) | T: 10 mg<br>I: 15 mg/ml, 30 mg/ml | **P: (PO):** 10 mg q4–6h as needed;<br>**(IM/IV):** 60–120 mg/day in divided doses | Fluid retention, abdominal pain, diarrhea, dizziness, headaches, nausea |
| Meloxicam (Mobic, Vivlodex) | **C: (Vivlodex):** 5 mg, 10 mg<br>**T: (Mobic):** 7.5 mg, 15 mg<br>**S:** 7.5 mg/5 ml | **Arthritis: (Mobic):** 7.5–15 mg once daily<br>**(Vivlodex):** 5–10 mg once daily | Heartburn, indigestion, nausea, diarrhea, headaches |
| Nabumetone (Relafen) | T: 500 mg, 750 mg | **Arthritis:** 1–2 g/day in 1–2 divided doses | Fluid retention, dizziness, headaches, abdominal pain, constipation, diarrhea, nausea |
| Naproxen (Anaprox, Naprosyn) | T: 250 mg, 375 mg, 500 mg<br>T (CR): 375 mg, 500 mg<br>S: 125 mg/5 ml | **Arthritis:** 500–1,000 mg/day in 2 divided doses<br>**Maximum:** 1,500 mg/day<br>**P:** 500 mg once, then 500 mg q12h or 250 mg q6–8h as needed | Tinnitus, fluid retention, shortness of breath, dizziness, drowsiness, headaches, abdominal pain, constipation, heartburn, nausea |
| Oxaprozin (Daypro) | C: 600 mg<br>T: 600 mg | **Arthritis:** 600–1,200 mg once daily | Constipation, diarrhea, nausea, indigestion |
| Piroxicam (Feldene) | C: 10 mg, 20 mg | **Arthritis:** 10–20 mg/day in 1–2 divided doses | Abdominal pain, stomach pain, nausea |
| Sulindac (Clinoril) | T: 150 mg, 200 mg | **Arthritis:** 150 mg bid | Dizziness, abdominal pain, constipation, diarrhea, nausea |

*A,* Adults; *C,* capsules; *CR,* controlled-release; *ER,* extended-release; *I,* injection; *P,* pain; *S,* suspension; *SR,* sustained-release; *T,* tablets.

# Nutrition: Enteral

Enteral nutrition (EN), also known as *tube feedings*, provides food/nutrients via the GI tract using special formulas, delivery techniques, and equipment. All routes of EN consist of a tube through which liquid formula is infused.

## INDICATIONS

Tube feedings are used in pts with major trauma, burns; those undergoing radiation and/or chemotherapy; pts with hepatic failure, severe renal impairment, physical or neurologic impairment; preop and postop to promote anabolism; prevention of cachexia, malnutrition; dysphagia, pts requiring mechanical ventilation.

## ROUTES OF ENTERAL NUTRITION DELIVERY

**NASOGASTRIC (NG):**

**INDICATIONS:** Most common for short-term feeding in pts unable or unwilling to consume adequate nutrition by mouth. Requires at least a partially functioning GI tract.

**ADVANTAGES:** Does not require surgical intervention and is fairly easily inserted. Allows full use of digestive tract. Decreases abdominal distention, nausea, vomiting that may be caused by hyperosmolar solutions.

**DISADVANTAGES:** Temporary. May be easily pulled out during routine nursing care. Has potential for pulmonary aspiration of gastric contents, risk of reflux esophagitis, regurgitation.

**NASODUODENAL (ND), NASOJEJUNAL (NJ):**

**INDICATIONS:** Pts unable or unwilling to consume adequate nutrition by mouth. Requires at least a partially functioning GI tract.

**ADVANTAGES:** Does not require surgical intervention and is fairly easily inserted. Preferred for pts at risk for aspiration. Valuable for pts with gastroparesis.

**DISADVANTAGES:** Temporary. May be pulled out during routine nursing care. May be dislodged by coughing, vomiting. Small lumen size increases risk of clogging when medication is administered via tube, more susceptible to rupturing when using infusion device. Must be radiographed for placement, frequently extubated.

**GASTROSTOMY:**

**INDICATIONS:** Pts with esophageal obstruction or impaired swallowing; pts in whom NG, ND, or NJ not feasible; when long-term feeding indicated.

**ADVANTAGES:** Permanent feeding access. Tubing has larger bore, allowing noncontinuous (bolus) feeding (300–400 ml over 30–60 min q3–6h). May be inserted endoscopically using local anesthetic (procedure called *percutaneous endoscopic gastrostomy* [PEG]).

**DISADVANTAGES:** Requires surgery; may be inserted in conjunction with other surgery or endoscopically (see ADVANTAGES). Stoma care required. Tube may be inadvertently dislodged. Risk of aspiration, peritonitis, cellulitis, leakage of gastric contents.

**JEJUNOSTOMY:**

**INDICATIONS:** Pts with stomach or duodenal obstruction, impaired gastric motility; pts in whom NG, ND, or NJ not feasible; when long-term feeding indicated.

**ADVANTAGES:** Allows early postop feeding (small bowel function is least affected by surgery). Risk of aspiration reduced. Rarely pulled out inadvertently.

**DISADVANTAGES:** Requires surgery (laparotomy). Stoma care required. Risk of intraperitoneal leakage. Can be dislodged easily.

## INITIATING ENTERAL NUTRITION

With continuous feeding, initiation of isotonic (about 300 mOsm/L) or moderately hypertonic feeding (up to 495 mOsm/L) can be given full strength, usually at a slow rate (30–50 ml/hr) and gradually increased (25 ml/hr q6–24h). Formulas with osmolality greater than 500 mOsm/L are generally started at half strength and gradually increased in rate, then concentration. Tolerance is increased if the rate and concentration are not increased simultaneously.

*Continued*

# Nutrition: Enteral—cont'd

## SELECTION OF FORMULAS

*Protein:* Has many important physiologic roles and is the primary source of nitrogen in the body. Provides 4 kcal/g protein. Sources of protein in enteral feedings: sodium caseinate, calcium caseinate, soy protein, dipeptides.

*Carbohydrate (CHO):* Provides energy for the body and to maintain body temperature. Provides 3.4 kcal/g carbohydrate. Sources of CHO in enteral feedings: corn syrup, cornstarch, maltodextrin, lactose, sucrose, glucose.

*Fat:* Provides concentrated source of energy. Referred to as *kilocalorie dense* or *protein sparing.* Provides 9 kcal/g fat. Sources of fat in enteral feedings: corn oil, safflower oil, medium-chain triglycerides.

*Electrolytes, vitamins, trace elements:* Contained in formulas (not found in specialized products for renal/hepatic insufficiency).

All products containing protein, fat, carbohydrate, vitamin, electrolytes, trace elements are nutritionally complete and designed to be used by pts for long periods.

## COMPLICATIONS

**MECHANICAL:** Usually associated with some aspect of the feeding tube.

*Aspiration pneumonia:* Caused by delayed gastric emptying, gastroparesis, gastroesophageal reflux, or decreased gag reflex. May be prevented or treated by reducing infusion rate, using lower-fat formula, feeding beyond pylorus, checking residuals, using small-bore feeding tubes, elevating head of bed 30–45 degrees during and for 30–60 min after intermittent feeding, and regularly checking tube placement.

*Esophageal, mucosal, pharyngeal irritation, otitis:* Caused by using large-bore NG tube. Prevented by use of small bore whenever possible.

*Irritation, leakage at ostomy site:* Caused by drainage of digestive juices from site. Prevented by close attention to skin/stoma care.

*Tube, lumen obstruction:* Caused by thickened formula residue, formation of formula-medication complexes. Prevented by frequently irrigating tube with clear water (also before and after giving formulas/medication), avoiding instilling medication if possible.

**GASTROINTESTINAL:** Usually associated with formula, rate of delivery, unsanitary handling of solutions or delivery system.

*Diarrhea:* Caused by low-residue formulas, rapid delivery, use of hyperosmolar formula, hypoalbuminemia, malabsorption, microbial contamination, or rapid GI transit time. Prevented by using fiber supplemented formulas, decreasing rate of delivery, using dilute formula, and gradually increasing strength.

*Cramps, gas, abdominal distention:* Caused by nutrient malabsorption, rapid delivery of refrigerated formula. Prevented by delivering formula by continuous methods, giving formulas at room temperature, decreasing rate of delivery.

*Nausea, vomiting:* Caused by rapid delivery of formula, gastric retention. Prevented by reducing rate of delivery, using dilute formulas, selecting low-fat formulas.

*Constipation:* Caused by inadequate fluid intake, reduced bulk, inactivity. Prevented by supplementing fluid intake, using fiber-supplemented formula, encouraging ambulation.

**METABOLIC:** Fluid/serum electrolyte status should be monitored. Refer to monitoring section. In addition, the very young and very old are at greater risk of developing complications such as dehydration or overhydration.

## MONITORING

*Daily:* Estimate nutrient intake, fluid intake/output, weight of pt, clinical observations.

*Weekly:* Serum electrolytes (potassium, sodium, magnesium, calcium, phosphorus), blood glucose, BUN, creatinine, hepatic function tests (e.g., AST, ALT, alkaline phosphatase), 24-hr urea and creatinine excretion, total iron-binding capacity (TIBC) or serum transferrin, triglycerides, cholesterol.

*Monthly:* Serum albumin.

*Other:* Urine glucose, acetone (when blood glucose is greater than 250), vital signs (temperature, respirations, pulse, B/P) q8h.

### DRUG THERAPY: DOSAGE FOR SELECTION/ ADMINISTRATION:

Drug therapy should not have to be compromised in pts receiving enteral nutrition:

- Temporarily discontinue medications not immediately necessary.
- Consider an alternate route for administering medications (e.g., transdermal, rectal, intravenous).

- Consider alternate medications when current medication is not available in alternate dosage forms.

### ENTERAL ADMINISTRATION OF MEDICATIONS:

Medications may be given via feeding tube with several considerations:

- Tube type
- Tube location in the GI tract
- Site of drug action
- Site of drug absorption
- Effects of food on drug absorption
- Use of liquid dosage forms is preferred whenever possible; many tablets may be crushed; contents of many capsules may be emptied and given through large-bore feeding tubes.
- Many oral products should not be crushed (e.g., sustained-release, enteric coated, capsule granules).
- Some medications should not be given with enteral formulas because they form precipitates that may clog the feeding tube and reduce drug absorption.
- Feeding tube should be flushed with water before and after administration of medications to clear any residual medication.

*Continued*

# Nutrition: Parenteral

Parenteral nutrition (PN), also known as *total parenteral nutrition* (TPN) or *hyperalimentation* (HAL), provides required nutrients to pts by IV route of administration. The goal of PN is to maintain or restore nutritional status caused by disease, injury, or inability to consume nutrients by other means.

## INDICATIONS

Conditions when pt is unable to use alimentary tract via oral, gastrostomy, or jejunostomy route. Impaired absorption of protein caused by obstruction, inflammation, or antineoplastic therapy. Bowel rest necessary because of GI surgery or ileus, fistulas, or anastomotic leaks. Conditions with increased metabolic requirements (e.g., burns, infection, trauma). Preserve tissue reserves (e.g., acute renal failure). Inadequate nutrition from tube feeding methods.

## COMPONENTS OF PN

To meet IV nutritional requirements, six essential categories in PN are needed for tissue synthesis and energy balance.

*Protein:* In the form of crystalline amino acids (CAA), primarily used for protein synthesis. Several products are designed to meet specific needs for pts with renal failure (e.g., NephrAmine), hepatic disease (e.g., HepatAmine), stress/trauma (e.g., Aminosyn HBC), use in neonates and pediatrics (e.g., Aminosyn PF, TrophAmine). Calories: 4 kcal/g protein.

*Energy:* In the form of dextrose, available in concentrations of 5%—70%. Dextrose less than 10% may be given peripherally; concentrations greater than 10% must be given centrally. Calories: 3.4 kcal/g dextrose.

*IV fat emulsion:* Available in 10% and 20% concentrations. Provides a concentrated source of energy/calories (9 kcal/g fat) and is a source of essential fatty acids. May be administered peripherally or centrally.

*Electrolytes:* Major electrolytes (calcium, magnesium, potassium, sodium; also acetate, chloride, phosphate). Doses of electrolytes are individualized, based on many factors (e.g., renal/hepatic function, fluid status).

*Vitamins:* Essential components in maintaining metabolism and cellular function; widely used in PN.

*Trace elements:* Necessary in long-term PN administration. Trace elements include zinc, copper, chromium, manganese, selenium, molybdenum, iodine.

*Miscellaneous:* Additives include insulin, albumin, heparin, and H₂ blockers (e.g., cimetidine, ranitidine, famotidine). Other medication may be included, but compatibility for admixture should be checked on an individual basis.

## ROUTE OF ADMINISTRATION

PN is administered via either peripheral or central vein.

*Peripheral:* Usually involves 2–3 L/day of 5%–10% dextrose with 3%–5% amino acid solution along with IV fat emulsion. Electrolytes, vitamins, trace elements are added according to pt needs. Peripheral solutions provide about 2,000 kcal/day and 60–90 g protein/day.

**ADVANTAGES:** Lower risks vs. central mode of administration.

**DISADVANTAGES:** Peripheral veins may not be suitable (esp. in pts with illness of long duration); more susceptible to phlebitis (due to osmolalities greater than 600 mOsm/L); veins may be viable only 1–2 wks; large volumes of fluid are needed to meet nutritional requirements, which may be contraindicated in many pts.

*Central:* Usually utilizes hypertonic dextrose (concentration range of 15%–35%) and amino acid solution of 3%–7% with IV fat emulsion. Electrolytes, vitamins, trace elements are added according to pt needs. Central solutions provide 2,000–4,000 kcal/day. Must be given through large central vein with high blood flow, allowing rapid dilution, avoiding phlebitis/thrombosis (usually through percutaneous insertion of catheter into subclavian vein, then advancement of catheter to superior vena cava).

**ADVANTAGES:** Allows more alternatives/flexibility in establishing regimens; allows ability to provide full nutritional requirements without need of daily fat emulsion; useful in pts who are fluid restricted (increased concentration), those needing large nutritional requirements (e.g., trauma, malignancy), or those for whom PN indicated more than 7–10 days.

**DISADVANTAGES:** Risk with insertion, use, maintenance of central line; increased risk of infection, catheter-induced trauma, and metabolic changes.

*Continued*

# Nutrition: Parenteral—cont'd

## MONITORING

May vary slightly from institution to institution.

*Baseline:* CBC, platelet count, prothrombin time (PT), weight, body length/head circumference (in infants), serum electrolytes, glucose, BUN, creatinine, uric acid, total protein, cholesterol, triglycerides, bilirubin, alkaline phosphatase, lactate dehydrogenase (LDH), AST, albumin, prealbumin, other tests as needed.

*Daily:* Weight, vital signs (temperature, pulse, respirations [TPR]), nutritional intake (kcal, protein, fat), serum electrolytes (potassium, sodium chloride), glucose (serum, urine), acetone, BUN, osmolarity, other tests as needed.

*2–3 times/wk:* CBC, coagulation studies (PT, partial thromboplastin time [PTT]), serum creatinine, calcium, magnesium, phosphorus, acid-base status, other tests as needed.

*Weekly:* Nitrogen balance, total protein, albumin, prealbumin, transferrin, hepatic function tests (AST, ALT), serum alkaline phosphatase, LDH, bilirubin, Hgb, uric acid, cholesterol, triglycerides, other tests as needed.

## COMPLICATIONS

*Mechanical:* Malfunction in system for IV delivery (e.g., pump failure; problems with lines, tubing, administration sets, catheter). Pneumothorax, catheter misdirection, arterial puncture, bleeding, hematoma formation may occur with catheter placement.

*Infectious:* Infections (pts often more susceptible to infections), catheter sepsis (e.g., fever, shaking, chills, glucose intolerance where no other site of infection is identified).

*Metabolic:* Includes hyperglycemia, elevated serum cholesterol and triglycerides, abnormal serum hepatic function tests.

*Fluid, electrolyte, acid-base disturbances:* May alter serum potassium, sodium, phosphate, magnesium levels.

*Nutritional:* Clinical effects seen may be due to lack of adequate vitamins, trace elements, essential fatty acids.

## DRUG THERAPY/ADMINISTRATION METHODS:

Compatibility of other intravenous medications pts may be administered while receiving parenteral nutrition is an important concern.

Intravenous medications usually are given as a separate admixture via piggyback to the parenteral nutrition line, but in some instances may be added directly to the parenteral nutrition solution. Because of the possibility of incompatibility when adding medication directly to the parenteral nutrition solution, specific criteria should be considered:

- Stability of the medication in the parenteral nutrition solution
- Properties of the medication, including pharmacokinetics that determine if the medication is appropriate for continuous infusion
- Documented chemical and physical compatibility with the parenteral nutrition solution

In addition, when medication is given via piggyback using the parenteral nutrition line, important criteria should include the following:

- Stability of the medication in the parenteral nutrition solution
- Documented chemical and physical compatibility with the parenteral nutrition solution

# Obesity Management

## USES

Adjunct to diet and physical activity in the treatment of chronic, relapsing obesity.

## ACTIONS

Two categories of medications are used for weight control.

*Appetite suppressants:* Block neuronal uptake of norepinephrine, serotonin, dopamine, causing a feeling of fullness or satiety.

*Digestion inhibitors:* Reversible lipase inhibitors that block the breakdown and absorption of fats, decreasing appetite and reducing calorie intake.

## ANOREXIANTS

| Name | Availability | Dosage | Side Effects |
|---|---|---|---|
| **Diethylpropion (Tenuate, Tenuate Dospan)** | **T:** 25 mg, **T (CR):** 75 mg | 25 mg 3–4 times/day or 75 mg daily in midmorning | Headaches, euphoria, palpitations, hypertension, pulmonary hypertension, valvular heart disease, seizures, bone marrow depression, dependence, withdrawal psychosis |
| **Liraglutide (Victoza)** | **I:** 18 mg/3 ml | **SQ:** Initially, 0.6 mg/day. May increase by 0.6 mg/day weekly up to 3 mg/day | Diarrhea, constipation, dyspepsia, fatigue, vomiting, increased heart rate, renal impairment |
| **Lorcaserin (Belviq, Belviq XR)** | **C:** 10 mg **T:** 20 mg | (Belviq) 10 mg 2 times/day (Belviq XR) 20 mg once daily | Nausea, headache, dizziness, fatigue, dry mouth, diarrhea, constipation, hypoglycemia, hallucinations, decreased white/red blood cells, euphoria, cognitive impairment |
| **Naltrexone/ bupropion (Contrave)** | **T:** 8 mg/90 mg | Titrate weekly up to 2 tablets 2 times/day (1 tablet once daily, then 1 tablet 2 times/day, then 2 tablets in AM and 1 in PM, then 2 tablets 2 times/day) | Suicidal ideation, mood changes, seizures, increased HR with or without B/P, allergic reactions, hepatic toxicity, nausea, vomiting, headache, dizziness, dry mouth, angle closure glaucoma |

*Continued*

## ANOREXIANTS—cont'd

| Name | Availability | Dosage | Side Effects |
|------|-------------|--------|--------------|
| **Orlistat** (Alli, Xenical) | **C:** 60 mg, 120 mg | **Alli:** 60 mg up to tid with meals **Xenical:** 120 mg tid with each meal containing fat | Flatulence, rectal incontinence, oily stools, cholelithiasis, abdominal/rectal pain, hepatitis, pancreatitis, nausea |
| **Phenteramine** (Apidex-P, Suprenza) | **C:** 15 mg, 30 mg, 37.5 mg **T:** 37.5 mg **T (ODT):** 15 mg, 30 mg, 37.5 mg | 15–37.5 mg/day in 1 or 2 divided doses **ODT:** 15–37.5 mg once daily in morning | Headaches, euphoria, palpitations, hypertension, pulmonary hypertension, valvular heart disease, tremor, dependence, withdrawal psychosis, CNS stimulation, GI complaints |
| **Phenteramine/ topiramate (Qsymia)** | **C:** 13.75 mg/ 23 mg | 3.75 mg/23 mg to 15 mg/92 mg once daily in the morning | Paresthesia, dizziness, insomnia, depression, tachycardia, cognitive impairment, angle-closure glaucoma, hypokalemia, metabolic acidosis, constipation, dry mouth, suicidal ideation, kidney stones |

*AS*, Appetite suppressant; *B/P*, blood pressure; *C*, capsules; *CNS*, central nervous system; *CR*, controlled-release; *DI*, digestion inhibitor; *GI*, gastrointestinal; *HR*, heart rate; *I*, injection; *ODT*, orally disintegrating tablets; *SQ*, subcutaneously; *T*, tablets.

# Osteoporosis

## HISTORY

Osteoporosis is a bone disease that can lead to fractures. Bone mineral density (BMD) is reduced, bone microarchitecture is disrupted, and the amount and variety of proteins in bone are altered. Osteoporosis primarily affects women after menopause (postmenopausal osteoporosis) but may develop in men, in anyone in the presence of particular hormonal disorders (e.g., parathyroid glands), after overconsumption of dietary proteins, or as a result of medications (e.g., glucocorticoids). Several pharmacologic options, along with lifestyle changes, that can be used to prevent and/or treat osteoporotic fractures include bisphosphonates, selective estrogen receptor modulator (SERM), parathyroid hormone (PTH), calcitonin, and monoclonal antibodies.

## ACTION

*Bisphosphonates:* Inhibit bone resorption via actions on osteoclasts or osteoclast precursors, decrease rate of bone resorption, leading to an indirect increase in BMD.

*Selective estrogen receptor modulator (SERM):* Decreases bone resorption, increasing BMD and decreasing the incidence of fractures.

*Parathyroid hormone:* Stimulates osteoblast function, increasing gastrointestinal calcium absorption and increasing renal tubular reabsorption of calcium. This increases BMD, bone mass, and strength, resulting in a decrease in osteoporosis-related fractures.

*Calcitonin:* Inhibitor of bone resorption. Efficacy not observed in early postmenopausal women and is used only in women with osteoporosis who are at least 5 yrs beyond menopause.

*Monoclonal antibody:* Inhibits the RANK ligand (RANKL), a cytokine member of the tumor necrosis factor family. This inhibits osteoclast formation, function, and survival, which decreases bone resorption and increases bone mass and strength in cortical and trabecular bone.

## BISPHOSPHONATES

| Name | Availability | Dosage | Side Effects |
|---|---|---|---|
| **Alendronate** (Binosto, Fosamax) | **T:** 5 mg, 10 mg, 35 mg, 40 mg, 70 mg **S:** 70 mg/75ml | **Prevention:** 5 mg/day or 35 mg/wk **Treatment:** 10 mg/day or 70 mg/wk | Transient, mild hypocalcemia, hypophosphatemia, dysphagia, esophagitis, esophageal and gastric ulcer, abdominal pain, diarrhea, musculoskeletal pain |
| **Ibandronate** (Boniva) | **T:** 150 mg **I:** 1 mg/ml | **Prevention and treatment:** 150 mg/mo **IV Injection:** Treatment: 3 mg/3 mos | Dyspepsia, back pain, dysphagia, esophagitis, esophageal and gastric ulcer, abdominal pain, diarrhea, musculoskeletal pain |
| **Risedronate** (Actonel) | **T:** 5 mg, 30 mg, 35 mg, 150 mg **T (DR):** 35 mg | **Prevention and treatment:** 5 mg/day, 35 mg/wk, or 150 mg/mo | Hypertension, headache, rash, dysphagia, esophagitis, esophageal and gastric ulcer, abdominal pain, diarrhea, musculoskeletal pain |
| **Zoledronic acid** (Reclast) | **I:** 5 mg | **Prevention: IV:** 5 mg every 2 yrs **Treatment: IV:** 5 mg every yr | Hypertension, pain, fever, headache, chills, fatigue, nausea, musculoskeletal pain |

## SERM

| Name | Availability | Dosage | Side Effects |
|---|---|---|---|
| **Raloxifene** (Evista) | **T:** 60 mg | **Prevention and treatment:** 60 mg/day | Peripheral edema, hot flashes, arthralgia, leg cramps, muscle spasms, flu syndrome, infection |

## PARATHYROID HORMONE

| Name | Availability | Dosage | Side Effects |
|---|---|---|---|
| **Teriparatide** (Forteo) | **I:** 250 mcg/ml syringe delivers 20 mcg/dose | **Treatment:** 20 mcg subcutaneously once daily | Hypercalcemia, muscle cramps, nausea, dizziness, headache |

## CALCITONIN

| Name | Availability | Dosage | Side Effects |
|------|-------------|--------|--------------|
| Calcitonin (Fortical, Miacalcin) | I (Miacalcin): 200 units/ml Nasal (Fortical, Miacalcin): 200 units/activation | **Treatment: IM/Subcutaneous** (Miacalcin): 100 units every other day **Nasal:** 200 units in 1 nostril daily | Rhinitis, local nasal irritation. **Injection:** nausea, local inflammation, flushing of face, hands |

## MONOCLONAL ANTIBODY RANKL INHIBITOR

| Name | Availability | Dosage | Side Effects |
|------|-------------|--------|--------------|
| Denosumab (Prolia) | I: 60 mg/ml | **Subcutaneous:** 60 mg once every 6 mos | Back pain, pain in extremity, hypercholesterolemia, musculoskeletal pain, cystitis |

*DR,* Delayed-release; *I,* injection; *S,* solution (oral); *T,* tablet.

# Parkinson's Disease Treatment

| USES | ACTION |
|------|--------|
| To slow or stop clinical progression of Parkinson's disease and to improve function and quality of life in pts with Parkinson's disease, a progressive neurodegenerative disorder. | Normal motor function is dependent on the synthesis and release of dopamine by neurons projecting from the substantia nigra to the corpus striatum. In Parkinson's disease, disruption of this pathway results in diminished levels of the neurotransmitter dopamine. Medication is aimed at providing improved function using the lowest effective dose. |

## TYPES OF MEDICATIONS FOR PARKINSON'S DISEASE
## DOPAMINE PRECURSOR

**Levodopa/carbidopa:**

**Levodopa:** Dopamine precursor supplementation to enhance dopaminergic neurotransmission. A small amount of levodopa crosses the blood-brain barrier and is decarboxylated to dopamine, which is then available to stimulate dopaminergic receptors.

**Carbidopa:** Inhibits peripheral decarboxylation of levodopa, decreasing its conversion to dopamine in peripheral tissues, which results in an increased availability of levodopa for transport across the blood-brain barrier.

## COMT INHIBITORS

**Entacapone, tolcapone:** Reversible inhibitor of catechol-*O*-methyltransferase (COMT). COMT is responsible for catalyzing levodopa. In the presence of a decarboxylase inhibitor (carbidopa), COMT becomes the major metabolizing enzyme for levodopa in the brain and periphery. By inhibiting COMT, higher plasma levels of levodopa are attained, resulting in more dopaminergic stimulation in the brain and lessening the symptoms of Parkinson's disease.

## DOPAMINE RECEPTOR AGONISTS

**Bromocriptine:** Stimulates postsynaptic dopamine type 2 receptors in the neostriatum of the CNS.

**Pramipexole:** Stimulates dopamine receptors in the striatum of the CNS.

**Ropinirole:** Stimulates postsynaptic dopamine D2 type receptors within the caudate putamen in the brain.

## MONOAMINE OXIDASE B INHIBITORS

**Rasagiline, Selegiline:** Increase dopaminergic activity due to irreversible inhibition of monoamine oxidase type B (MAO B). MAO B is involved in the oxidative deamination of dopamine in the brain.

# Parkinson's Disease Treatment

## MEDICATIONS FOR TREATMENT OF PARKINSON'S DISEASE

| Name | Type | Availability | Dosage | Side Effects |
|---|---|---|---|---|
| **Amantadine** | Dopamine agonist | **C:** 100 mg<br>**Syrup:** 10 mg/ml<br>**T:** 100 mg | 100 mg 2 times/day. May increase up to 400 mg/day in divided doses | Cognitive impairment, confusion, insomnia, hallucinations, levido reticularis |
| **Carbidopa/levodopa (Parcopa, Rytary, Sinemet, Sinemet CR)** | Dopamine precursor | **OD (Parcopa):** 10/100 mg, 25/100 mg, 25/250 mg<br>**Immediate-release (Sinemet):** 10/100 mg, 25/100 mg, 25/250 mg<br>**Extended-release (Sinemet CR):** 25/100 mg, 50/200 mg<br>**(Rytary):** 23.75 mg/95 mg, 36.25 mg/145 mg, 48.75 mg/195 mg, 61.25 mg/245 mg | **Parcopa:** 300–1,500 mg levodopa in divided doses<br>**Sinemet:** 300–1,500 mg levodopa in divided doses<br>**Sinemet CR:** Initially, 400 mg/day in 2 divided doses. May increase up to 1,600 mg levodopa in divided doses<br>**Rytary:** Initially, 23.75 mg/95 mg 3 times/day. May increase up to 612.5 mg/2,450 mg per day in divided doses | Anorexia, nausea, orthostatic hypotension initially; hallucinations, confusion, sleep disturbances with chronic use, constipation, dry mouth, headache, dyskinesia |
| **Entacapone (Comtan)** | COMT inhibitor | **T:** 200 mg | 200 mg 3–4 times/day up to **maximum** of 8 times/day (1,600 mg) | Dyskinesias, nausea, diarrhea, urine discoloration |
| **Pramipexole (Mirapex, Mirapex ER)** | Dopamine agonist | **T:** 0.125 mg, 0.25 mg, 0.5 mg, 0.75 mg, 1 mg, 1.5 mg<br>**ER:** 0.375 mg, 0.75 mg, 1.5 mg, 2.25 mg, 3 mg, 3.75 mg, 4.5 mg | **T:** Initially, 0.125 mg 3 times/day. May increase q5–7 days. Usual dose: 0.5–1.5 mg 3 times/day<br>**ER:** Initially, 0.375 mg once daily. May increase q5–7 days by 0.75 mg/dose up to 4.5 mg once daily | Nausea, drowsiness, lower extremity edema, postural hypotension, confusion, toxic psychosis (avoid use in pts with dementia) |

*Continued*

## MEDICATIONS FOR TREATMENT OF PARKINSON'S DISEASE—cont'd

| Name | Type | Availability | Dosage | Side Effects |
|---|---|---|---|---|
| **Rasagiline** (Azilect) | MAO B inhibitors | T: 0.5 mg, 1 mg | 0.5–1 mg once daily | Nausea, orthostatic hypotension |
| **Ropinirole** (Requip, Requip XL) | Dopamine agonist | T: 0.25 mg, 0.5 mg, 1 mg, 2 mg, 3 mg, 4 mg, 5 mg XL: 2 mg, 4 mg, 6 mg, 8 mg, 12 mg | T: Initially, 0.25 mg 3 times/day. May increase at weekly intervals to 0.5 mg 3 times/day, then 0.75 mg 3 times/day, then 1 mg 3 times/day. May then increase by 1.5 mg/day up to 9 mg/day, then by 3 mg/day up to total dose of 24 mg/day in divided doses XL: Initially, 2 mg/day for 1–2 wks, then increase by 2 mg/day at weekly intervals | Nausea, drowsiness, lower extremity edema, postural hypotension, confusion, toxic psychosis (avoid use in pts with dementia) |
| **Rotigotine** (Neupro) | Dopamine agonist | Transdermal patch: 1 mg/24 hrs, 2 mg/24 hrs, 3 mg/24 hrs, 4 mg/24 hrs, 6 mg/24 hrs, 8 mg/24 hrs | Early stage: Initially, 2 mg/24 hrs up to 6 mg/24 hrs Advanced stage: Initially, 4 mg/24 hrs up to 8 mg/24 hrs | Peripheral edema, dizziness, fatigue, application site reactions, sleep disturbances, dyskinesia, nausea, arthralgia |
| **Selegiline** (Eldepryl, Zelapar) | MAO B inhibitor | C (Eldepryl): 5 mg OD (Zelapar): 1.25 mg | C: 5 mg with breakfast and lunch OD: 1.25–2.5 mg daily in the morning | Nausea, orthostatic hypotension |
| **Tolcapone** (Tasmar) | COMT inhibitor | T: 100 mg | Initially, 100 mg 3 times/day. May increase to 200 mg 3 times/day | Dyskinesias, nausea, diarrhea, urine discoloration |

*C,* Capsules; *COMT,* catechol-*O*-methyltransferase; *ER,* extended-release; *I,* injection; *MAO B,* monoamine oxidase B; *OD,* orally disintegrating; *T,* tablets; *XL,* extended-release.

# Proton Pump Inhibitors

## USES

Treatment of various gastric disorders, including gastric and duodenal ulcers, gastroesophageal reflux disease (GERD), pathologic hypersecretory conditions.

## ACTION

Suppresses gastric acid secretion by specific inhibition of the hydrogen-potassium-adenosine triphosphatase ($H^+/K^+$ ATPase) enzyme system, which transports the acid at the gastric parietal cells. These agents do not have anticholinergic or histamine receptor antagonistic properties.

## PROTON PUMP INHIBITORS

| Name | Availability | Indications | Usual Dosage | Side Effects |
|---|---|---|---|---|
| **Dexlansoprazole** (Dexilant) | **C:** 30 mg, 60 mg | Erosive esophagitis, heartburn associated with nonerosive GERD | 30–60 mg/day | Diarrhea, abdominal pain, nausea, upper respiratory tract infection, vomiting, flatulence |
| **Esomeprazole** (Nexium) | **C:** 20 mg, 40 mg **I:** 20 mg, 40 mg | *Helicobacter pylori* eradication, GERD, erosive esophagitis | 20–40 mg/day | Headaches, diarrhea, abdominal pain, nausea |
| **Lansoprazole** (Prevacid) | **C:** 15 mg, 30 mg **T (ODT):** 15 mg, 30 mg | Duodenal ulcer, gastric ulcer, NSAID-associated gastric ulcer, hypersecretory conditions, *H. pylori* eradication, GERD, erosive esophagitis | 15–30 mg/day | Diarrhea, skin rash, pruritus, headaches |
| **Omeprazole** (Prilosec) | **C:** 10 mg, 20 mg, 40 mg | Duodenal ulcer, gastric ulcer, hypersecretory conditions, *H. pylori* eradication, GERD, erosive esophagitis | 20–40 mg/day | Headaches, diarrhea, abdominal pain, nausea |
| **Omeprazole and Sodium Bicarbonate** (Zegerid) | **P:** 20 mg, 40 mg | Duodenal ulcer, benign gastric ulcer, GERD, erosive esophagitis | 20–40 mg/day | Headaches, abdominal pain, diarrhea, nausea |
| **Pantoprazole** (Protonix) | **T:** 20 mg, 40 mg **I:** 40 mg | Erosive esophagitis, hypersecretory conditions | 40 mg/day | Diarrhea, headaches |
| **Rabeprazole** (Aciphex) | **T:** 20 mg **S:** 5 mg, 10 mg | Duodenal ulcer, hypersecretory conditions, *H. pylori* eradication, GERD, erosive esophagitis | 20 mg/day | Headaches |

*C,* Capsules; *GERD,* gastroesophageal reflux disease; *I,* injection; *NSAID,* nonsteroidal anti-inflammatory drug; *ODT,* orally disintegrating tablets; *P,* powder for suspension; *S,* sprinkles; *T,* tablets.

# Rheumatoid Arthritis

Rheumatoid arthritis (RA) is an autoimmune disease associated with progressive disability, systemic complications, early death, and socioeconomic costs. RA affects most joints and their surrounding tissues. RA is characterized by synovial inflammation and hyperplasia, autoantibody production (e.g., rheumatoid factor), cartilage and bone destruction, and systemic features (e.g., cardiovascular, pulmonary, psychological, skeletal disorders). The clinical hallmark of RA is polyarticular synovial inflammation of peripheral joints (typically in the hands, resulting in pain, stiffness, and some degree of irreversible joint damage; deformity; and disability).

Medications used in RA include disease-modifying antirheumatic drugs (DMARDS) and biologic agents, including tumor necrosis factor (TNF) inhibitors.

## DMARDS

| Name | Dosage | Side Effects/Comments |
|---|---|---|
| Hydroxychloroquine (Plaquenil) | Induction: 400–600 mg/day for 4–12 wks<br>Maintenance: 200–400 mg/day | **Side Effects:** nausea, epigastric pain, hemolysis may occur in pts with G6PD deficiency, retinal toxicity with long-term use |
| Leflunomide (Arava) | Induction: 100 mg/day × 3 days<br>Maintenance: 10–20 mg/day | **Side Effects:** diarrhea, respiratory tract infection, hypertension, headache, reversible alopecia, rash, myelosuppression, and/or elevated hepatic enzymes<br>**Comments:** contraindicated for use during pregnancy |
| Methotrexate (oral) (Rheumatrex, Trexall)<br>Methotrexate (injectable) Otrexup, Rasuvo | Induction: 7.5–10 mg PO once/wk<br>Maintenance: 7.5–25 mg PO once wkly<br>Induction: 7.5 PO once wkly<br>Maintenance: 10–25 mg IM or SQ once wkly | **Side Effects:** stomatitis, anorexia, nausea, vomiting, diarrhea, abdominal cramps, hepatic enzyme elevations, thrombocytopenia<br>**Comments:** not recommended in pts with CrCl <30 ml/min; should not be prescribed for women who are or may become pregnant |
| Sulfasalazine (Azulfidine) | Induction: 3–4 g/day in divided doses<br>Maintenance: 2 g/day in divided doses | **Side Effect:** headache, nausea, anorexia, rash, hemolysis may occur in pts with G6PD deficiency |

## BIOLOGIC AGENTS

### TNF INHIBITORS

| Name | Dosage | Side Effects/Comments |
|---|---|---|
| Adalimumab (Humira) | 40 mg SQ once wkly or q2wks | **Side Effects:** headache, skin rash, positive ANA titer, antibody development, injection site reaction (erythema, itching, pain, swelling), upper respiratory tract infection<br>**Comments:** increased risk for serious infections (e.g., tuberculosis, invasive fungal infections), avoid use in pts with recent history of malignancy or pre-existing demyelinating disorders |
| Certolizumab (Cimzia) | Induction: 400 mg SQ at 0, 2, 4 wks<br>Maintenance: 200 mg SQ every other week or 400 mg q4wks | **Side Effects:** nausea, infection, upper respiratory tract infection, skin rash<br>**Comments:** see adalimumab |
| Etanercept (Enbrel) | 25 mg SQ 2 times/wk or 50 mg SQ once/wk | **Side Effects:** headache, skin rash, diarrhea, injection site reactions (e.g., erythema, swelling), upper respiratory tract infection, rhinitis<br>**Comments:** see adalimumab |
| Golimumab (Simponi, Simponi Aria) | Simponi: 50 mg SQ once monthly<br>Simponi Aria:<br>Induction: 2 mg/kg IV at 0 and 4 wks<br>Maintenance: 2 mg/kg IV q8wks | **Side Effects:** positive ANA titer, upper respiratory tract infection (e.g., nasopharyngitis, rhinitis)<br>**Comments:** see adalimumab |
| Infliximab (Remicade) | Induction: 3 mg/kg IV at 0, 2, and 6 wks<br>Maintenance: 3 mg/kg IV q8wks | **Side Effects:** nausea, diarrhea, abdominal pain, increased ANA titer, upper respiratory tract infection, sinusitis, cough, pharyngitis<br>**Comments:** see adalimumab |

## OTHER BIOLOGIC AGENTS

| Name | Dosage | Side Effects/Comments |
|---|---|---|
| Abatacept (Orencia) | **IV:** 500 mg, 750 mg, or 1,000 mg IV at 0, 2, and 4 wks, then q4wks<br>**SQ:** 125 mg SQ once/wk | **Side Effects:** nausea, UTIs, acute exacerbation of COPD, hypertension, headache, dizziness<br>**Comments:** may increase risk of serious infections (e.g., pneumonia, pyelonephritis, cellulitis, diverticulitis) |
| Rituximab (Rituxan) | 1,000 mg IV twice, 2 wks apart | **Side Effects:** hypotension, peripheral edema, abdominal pain anemia, arthralgia, infusion site reactions<br>**Comments:** Pts at high risk for hepatitis B virus infection should be screened before beginning therapy |
| Tocilizumab (Actemra) | **IV:** Induction: 4 mg/kg IV q4wks<br>Maintenance: 8 mg/kg q4 wks<br>**SQ:** Induction: 162 mg SQ every other week<br>Maintenance: 162 mg once wkly | **Side Effects:** hypertension, upper abdominal pain, increased ALT/AST, injection site reactions, neutropenia, dyslipidemia<br>**Comments:** severe complications including GI perforation and hypersensitivity with anaphylaxis have been reported |
| Tofacitinib (Xeljanz) | 5 mg PO bid | **Side Effects:** diarrhea, nasopharyngitis, upper respiratory infections, headache hypertension, increased LFT, dyslipidemia, cytopenias have been reported<br>**Comments:** screening for tuberculosis recommended, increased incidence of solid cancers detected |

*ANA,* Antinuclear antibodies; *CNS,* central nervous system; *COPD,* chronic obstructive pulmonary disease; *GI,* gastrointestinal; *UTI,* urinary tract infection.

# Sedative-Hypnotics

## USES

Treatment of insomnia (i.e, difficulty falling asleep initially, frequent awakening, awakening too early).

## ACTION

*Benzodiazepines* are the most widely used agents and largely replace barbiturates due to greater safety, lower incidence of drug dependence. Benzodiazepines nonselectively bind to at least three receptor subtypes accounting for sedative, anxiolytic, relaxant, and anticonvulsant properties. Benzodiazepines enhance the effect of the inhibitory neurotransmitter gamma-aminobutyric acid (GABA), which inhibits impulse transmission in the CNS reticular formation in brain. Benzodiazepines decrease sleep latency, number of nocturnal awakenings, and time spent in awake stage of sleep; increase total sleep time. The *nonbenzodiazepines* zaleplon and zolpidem preferentially bind with one receptor subtype, reducing sleep latency and nocturnal awakenings and increasing total sleep time. Ramelteon is a selective agonist of melatonin receptors (responsible for determining circadian rhythms and synchronizing sleep-wake cycles).

## SEDATIVE-HYPNOTICS

| Name | Availability | Dosage Range | Side Effects |
|---|---|---|---|
| **Benzodiazepines** | | | |
| **Estazolam** | **T:** 1 mg, 2 mg | **A:** 1–2 mg <br> **E:** 0.5–1 mg | Daytime sedation, memory and psychomotor impairment, tolerance, withdrawal reactions, rebound insomnia, dependence |
| **Flurazepam** | **C:** 15 mg, 30 mg | **A/E:** 15–30 mg <br> **E:** 15 mg | Headaches, unpleasant taste, dry mouth, dizziness, anxiety, nausea |
| **Temazepam (Restoril)** | **C:** 7.5 mg, 15 mg, 30 mg | **A:** 15–30 mg <br> **E:** 7.5–15 mg | Same as flurazepam |

*Continued*

## SKELETAL MUSCLE RELAXANTS—cont'd

| Name | Availability | Dosage Range | Side Effects |
|------|-------------|-------------|-------------|
| Nonbenzodiazepines | | | |
| Eszopiclone (Lunesta) | T: 1 mg, 2 mg, 3 mg | A: 1–3 mg<br>E: 1–2 mg | Headaches, unpleasant taste, dry mouth, dizziness, anxiety, nausea |
| Ramelteon (Rozerem) | T: 8 mg | A, E: 8 mg | Headaches, dizziness, fatigue, nausea |
| Suvorexant (Belsomra) | T: 5 mg, 10 mg, 15 mg, 20 mg | A, E: 10–20 mg | Next day somnolence, leg weakness |
| Zaleplon (Sonata) | C: 5 mg, 10 mg | A: 10–20 mg<br>E: 5 mg | Headaches, dizziness, myalgia, drowsiness, asthenia, abdominal pain |
| Zolpidem (Ambien, Ambien CR, Edluar, Intermezzo, Zolpimist) | T: 5 mg, 10 mg<br>CR: 6.25 mg, 12.5 mg<br>SL (Edluar): 5 mg,<br>10 mg (Intermezzo):<br>1.75 mg, 3.5 mg<br>OS: 5 mg/actuation | OS, T, SL (Edluar): 5 mg (females, elderly); 5–10 mg (males) (Intermezzo): 1.75 mg (females, elderly); 3.5 mg (males)<br>CR: 6.25 mg (females, elderly); 6.25–12.5 mg (males) | Dizziness, daytime drowsiness, headaches, confusion, depression, hangover, asthenia |

*A,* Adults; *C,* capsules; *CR,* controlled-release; *E,* elderly; *OS,* oral solution; *SL,* sublingual; *T,* tablets.

# Skeletal Muscle Relaxants

| USES | ACTION |
|---|---|
| *Central acting muscle relaxants:* Adjunct to rest, physical therapy for relief of discomfort associated with acute, painful musculoskeletal disorders (i.e., local spasms from muscle injury). | *Central acting muscle relaxants:* Exact mechanism unknown. May act in CNS at various levels to depress polysynaptic reflexes; sedative effect may be responsible for relaxation of muscle spasm. |
| *Baclofen, dantrolene, diazepam:* Treatment of spasticity characterized by heightened muscle tone, spasm, loss of dexterity caused by multiple sclerosis, cerebral palsy, spinal cord lesions, CVA. | *Baclofen, diazepam:* May mimic actions of gamma-aminobutyric acid on spinal neurons; do not directly affect skeletal muscles. |
| | *Dantrolene:* Acts directly on skeletal muscle, relieving spasticity. |

## SKELETAL MUSCLE RELAXANTS

| Name | Indication | Dosage Range | Side Effects/Comments |
|---|---|---|---|
| **Baclofen (Lioresal)** | Spasticity associated with multiple sclerosis, spinal cord injury | Initially 5 mg 3 times/day<br>Increase by 5 mg 3 times/day q3days<br>**Maximum:** 20 mg 4 times/day | Drowsiness, dizziness, GI effects<br>Caution with renal impairment, seizure disorders<br>Withdrawal syndrome (e.g., hallucinations, psychosis, seizures) |

*Continued*

## SKELETAL MUSCLE RELAXANTS—cont'd

| Name | Indication | Dosage Range | Side Effects/Comments |
|---|---|---|---|
| **Carisoprodol (Rela)** | Discomfort due to acute, painful, musculoskeletal conditions | 250–350 mg 4 times/day | Drowsiness, dizziness, GI effects<br>Hypomania at higher than recommended doses<br>Withdrawal syndrome<br>Hypersensitivity reaction (skin reaction, bronchospasm, weakness, burning eyes, fever) or idiosyncratic reaction (weakness, visual or motor disturbances, confusion) usually occurring within first 4 doses |
| **Chlorzoxazone (Lorzone)** | Discomfort due to acute, painful, musculoskeletal conditions | Initially 250–500 mg 3–4 times/day<br>**Maximum:** 750 mg 3–4 times/day | Drowsiness, dizziness, GI effects, rare hepatotoxicity<br>Hypersensitivity reaction (urticaria, itching)<br>Urine discoloration to orange, red, or purple |
| **Cyclobenzaprine (Flexeril)** | Muscle spasm, pain, tenderness, restricted movement due to acute, painful, musculoskeletal conditions | Initially 5–10 mg 3 times/day | Drowsiness, dizziness, GI effects<br>Anticholinergic effects (dry mouth, urinary retention)<br>Quinidine-like effects on heart (QT prolongation)<br>Long half-life |
| **Dantrolene (Dantrium)** | Spasticity associated with multiple sclerosis, cerebral palsy, spinal cord injury | Initially 25 mg/day for 1 wk, then 25 mg 3 times/day for 1 wk, then 50 mg 3 times/day for 1 wk, then 100 mg 3 times/day<br>**Maximum:** 100 mg 4 times/day | Drowsiness, dizziness, GI effects<br>Contraindicated with hepatic disease<br>Dose-dependent hepatotoxicity<br>Diarrhea that is dose dependent and may be severe, requiring discontinuation |
| **Diazepam (Valium)** | Spasticity associated with cerebral palsy, spinal cord injury; reflex spasm due to muscle, joint trauma or inflammation | 2–10 mg 3–4 times/day | Drowsiness, dizziness, GI effects<br>Abuse potential |

| | | | |
|---|---|---|---|
| **Metaxalone** (Skelaxin) | Discomfort due to acute, painful, musculoskeletal conditions | 800 mg 3–4 times/day | Drowsiness (low risk), dizziness, GI effects Paradoxical muscle cramps Mild withdrawal syndrome Contraindicated in serious hepatic or renal disease |
| **Methocarbamol** (Robaxin) | Discomfort due to acute, painful, musculoskeletal conditions | Initially 1,500 mg 4 times/day **Maintenance:** 1,000 mg 4 times/day | Drowsiness, dizziness, GI effects Urine discoloration to brown, brown-black, or green |
| **Orphenadrine** (Norflex) | Discomfort due to acute, painful, musculoskeletal conditions | 100 mg 2 times/day | Drowsiness, dizziness, GI effects Long half-life Anticholinergic effects (dry mouth, urinary retention) Rare aplastic anemia Some products may contain sulfites |
| **Tizanidine** (Zanaflex) | Spasticity | Initially 4 mg q6–8h (**maximum** 3 times/day), may increase by 2–4 mg as needed/tolerated **Maximum:** 36 mg (limited information on doses greater than 24 mg) | Drowsiness, dizziness, GI effects Hypotension (20% decrease in B/P) Hepatotoxicity (usually reversible) Withdrawal syndrome (hypertension, tachycardia, hypertonia) Effect is short lived (3–6 hrs) Dose cautiously with creatinine clearance less than 25 ml/min |

*B/P,* Blood pressure; *GI,* gastrointestinal.

# Smoking Cessation Agents

Tobacco smoking is associated with the development of lung cancer and chronic obstructive pulmonary disease. Smoking is harmful not just to the smoker but also to family members, coworkers, and others breathing cigarette smoke.

Quitting smoking decreases the risk of developing lung cancer, other cancers, heart disease, stroke, and respiratory illnesses. Several medications have proved useful as smoking cessation aids. Nausea and light-headedness are possible signs of overdose of nicotine warranting a reduction in dosage.

## SMOKING CESSATION AGENTS

| Name | Availability | Dose Duration | Cautions/Side Effects | Comments |
|------|-------------|---------------|----------------------|----------|
| **Bupropion (Zyban)** | **T:** 150 mg | 150 mg every morning for 3 days, then 150 mg 2 times/day Start 1–2 wks before quit date **Duration:** 7–12 wks up to 6 mos for maintenance | History of seizure, eating disorder, use of MAOI within previous 14 days, bipolar disorder **Side Effects:** Insomnia, dry mouth, tremor, rash | Stop smoking during second wk of treatment and use counseling support services along with medication |
| **Clonidine (Catapres, Catapres-TTS)** | **T:** 0.1 mg, 0.2 mg **Patch:** 0.1 mg/24 hrs, 0.2 mg/24 hrs, 0.3 mg/24 hrs | **Oral:** 0.15–0.75 mg/day **Patch:** 0.1–0.2 mg daily **Duration:** 3–10 wks | Rebound hypertension. **Side Effects:** Dry mouth, drowsiness, dizziness, sedation, constipation | Abrupt discontinuation can result in anxiety, agitation, headaches, tremors accompanied or followed by rapid rise in B/P |

| | | | |
|---|---|---|---|
| **Nicotine gum (Nicorette)** | **Squares:** 2 mg, 4 mg | 1 gum q1–2h for 6 wks, then q2–4h for 3 wks then q4–8h for 3 wks<br>**Maximum:** 24 pieces/day<br>**Duration:** up to 12 wks | Recent MI (within 2 wks), serious arrhythmias, serious or worsening angina pectoris<br>**Side Effects:** Dyspepsia, mouth soreness, hiccups | 2 mg recommended for pts smoking less than 25 cigarettes/day, 4 mg for pts smoking 25 or more cigarettes/day<br>Chew until a peppery or minty taste emerges and then "park" between cheek and gums to facilitate nicotine absorption through oral mucosa<br>Chew slowly and intermittently to avoid jaw ache and achieve maximum benefit<br>Only water should be taken 15 min before and during chewing |
| **Nicotine inhaler (Nicotrol)** | **Cartridge:** 10 mg (delivers 4 mg nicotine) | 4–16 cartridges daily; taper frequency of use over the last 6–12 wks<br>**Duration:** up to 6 mos | Recent MI (within 2 wks), serious arrhythmias, serious or worsening angina pectoris<br>**Side Effects:** Local irritation of mouth and throat, coughing, rhinitis | Use at or above room temperature (cold temperatures decrease amount of nicotine inhaled) |
| **Nicotine lozenge (Nicorette Lozenges)** | **Lozenges:** 2 mg, 4 mg | One lozenge q1–2h for 6 wks, then q2–4h for 3 wks, then q4–8h for 3 wks<br>**Duration:** 12 wks<br>**Maximum:** 5 lozenges in 6 hrs; 20 lozenges in 1 day | Recent MI (within 2 wks), serious arrhythmias, serious or worsening angina pectoris<br>**Side Effects:** Local skin reaction, insomnia, nausea, sore throat | First cigarette smoked within 30 min of waking, use 4 mg; after 30 min of waking, use 2 mg<br>Use at least 9 lozenges/day first 6 wks<br>Only 1 lozenge at a time, 5 per 6 hrs and 20 per 24 hrs<br>Do not chew or swallow |
| **Nicotine nasal spray (Nicotrol NS)** | 10 mg/ml (delivers 0.5 mg/spray) | 8–40 doses/day<br>A dose consists of one 0.5 mg delivery to each nostril; initial dose is 1–2 sprays/hr, increasing as needed<br>**Duration:** 3–6 mos | Recent MI (within 2 wks), serious arrhythmias, serious or worsening angina pectoris<br>**Side Effects:** Nasal irritation | Do not sniff, swallow, or inhale through nose while administering nicotine doses (may increase irritation)<br>Tilt head back slightly for best results |

*Continued*

## SMOKING CESSATION AGENTS—cont'd

| Name | Availability | Dose Duration | Cautions/Side Effects | Comments |
|---|---|---|---|---|
| **Nicotine patch (NicoDerm CQ)** | **Nicoderm CQ:** 7 mg/24 hrs, 14 mg/24 hrs, 21 mg/24 hrs **Nicotrol:** 5 mg/16 hrs, 10 mg/16 hrs, 15 mg/16 hrs | Apply upon waking on quit date: **Nicoderm CQ (greater than 10 cigarettes/day):** 21 mg/24 hrs for 4 wks, then 14 mg/24 hrs for 2 wks, then 7 mg/24 hrs for 2 wks **(10 or fewer cigarettes/day):** 14 mg/24 hrs for 6 wks, then 7 mg/24 hrs for 2 wks | Recent MI (within 2 wks), serious arrhythmias, serious or worsening angina pectoris **Side Effects:** Local skin reaction, insomnia | The 16- and 24-hr patches are of comparable efficacy Begin with a lower-dose patch in pts smoking 10 or fewer cigarettes/day Place new patch on relatively hair-free location, usually between neck and waist, in the morning If insomnia occurs, remove the 24-hr patch prior to bedtime or use the 16-hr patch Rotate patch site to diminish skin irritation |
| **Nortriptyline (Pamelor)** | **T:** 25 mg, 50 mg, 75 mg, 100 mg | Initially 25 mg/day, increasing gradually to target dose of 75–100 mg/day 10–28 days prior to selected "quit" date, continue for 12 wks or more after "quit" day **Duration:** up to 12 wks | Risk of arrhythmias **Side Effects:** Sedation, dry mouth, blurred vision, urinary retention, light-headedness, shaky hands | Initiate therapy 10–28 days before the quit date to allow steady state of nortriptyline at target dose |
| **Varenicline (Chantix)** | **T:** 0.5 mg, 1 mg | **Days 1–3:** 0.5 mg daily; **days 4–7:** 0.5 mg 2 times/day; **day 8 to end of treatment:** 1 mg 2 times/day **Duration:** begin 1 wk before set quit date, continue for 12 wks. May use additional 12 wks if failed to quit after first 12 wks | **Side Effects:** Nausea; sleep disturbances; headaches; may impair ability to drive, operate machinery; depressed mood; altered behavior; suicidal ideation reported | Use lower dosage if not able to tolerate nausea and vomiting Use counseling support services along with medication |

*B/P,* Blood pressure; *MAOI,* monoamine oxidase inhibitor; *MI,* myocardial infarction; *T,* tablets.

# Vitamins

## INTRODUCTION

Vitamins are organic substances required for growth, reproduction, and maintenance of health and are obtained from food or supplementation in small quantities (vitamins cannot be synthesized by the body or the rate of synthesis is too slow/inadequate to meet metabolic needs). Vitamins are essential for energy transformation and regulation of metabolic processes. They are catalysts for all reactions using proteins, fats, carbohydrates for energy, growth, and cell maintenance.

## WATER SOLUBLE

Water-soluble vitamins include vitamin C (ascorbic acid), $B_1$ (thiamine), $B_2$ (riboflavin), $B_3$ (niacin), $B_5$ (pantothenic acid), $B_6$ (pyridoxine), folic acid, $B_{12}$ (cyanocobalamin). Water-soluble vitamins act as coenzymes for almost every cellular reaction in the body. B-complex vitamins differ from one another in both structure and function but are grouped together because they first were isolated from the same source (yeast and liver).

## FAT SOLUBLE

Fat-soluble vitamins include vitamins A, D, E, and K. They are soluble in lipids and are usually absorbed into the lymphatic system of the small intestine and then into the general circulation. Absorption is facilitated by bile. These vitamins are stored in the body tissue when excessive quantities are consumed. May be toxic when taken in large doses (see sections on individual vitamins).

## VITAMINS

| Name | Uses | Deficiency | Side Effects |
|------|------|-----------|--------------|
| Vitamin A (Aquasol A) | Required for normal growth, bone development, vision, reproduction, maintenance of epithelial tissue | Dry skin, poor tooth development, night blindness | **High dosages:** Hepatotoxicity, cheilitis, facial dermatitis, photosensitivity, mucosal dryness |
| Vitamin $B_1$ (thiamine) | Important in red blood cell formation, carbohydrate metabolism, neurologic function, myocardial contractility, growth, energy production | Fatigue, anorexia, growth retardation | **Large parenteral doses:** May cause pain on injection |
| Vitamin $B_2$ (riboflavin) | Necessary for function of coenzymes in oxidation-reduction reactions, essential for normal cellular growth, assists in absorption of iron and pyridoxine | Numbness in extremities, blurred vision, photophobia, cheilosis | Orange-yellow discoloration in urine |

*Continued*

## VITAMINS—cont'd

| Name | Uses | Deficiency | Side Effects |
|------|------|-----------|-------------|
| **Vitamin B₃ (niacin)** | Coenzyme for many oxidation-reduction reactions | Pellegra, headache, anorexia, memory loss, insomnia | **High dosages (more than 500 mg):** Nausea, vomiting, diarrhea, gastritis, hepatotoxicity, skin rash, facial flushing, headaches |
| **Vitamin B₅ (pantothenic acid)** | Precursor to coenzyme A; important in synthesis of cholesterol, hormones, fatty acids | Natural deficiency unknown | Occasional GI disturbances (e.g., diarrhea) |
| **Vitamin B₆ (pyridoxine)** | Enzyme cofactor for amino acid metabolism, essential for erythrocyte production, Hgb synthesis | Neuritis, anemia, lymphopenia | **High dosages:** May cause sensory neuropathy |
| **Vitamin B₁₂ (cyanocobalamin)** | Coenzyme in cells, including bone marrow, CNS, and GI tract, necessary for lipid metabolism, formation of myelin | Gastrointestinal disorders, anemias, poor growth | Skin rash, pain at injection site |
| **Vitamin C (ascorbic acid)** | Cofactor in various physiologic reactions, necessary for collagen formation, acts as antioxidant | Poor wound healing, bleeding gums, scurvy | **High dosages:** May cause calcium oxalate crystalluria, esophagitis, diarrhea |
| **Vitamin D (Calciferol)** | Necessary for proper formation of bone, calcium, mineral homeostasis, regulation of parathyroid hormone, calcitonin, phosphate | Rickets, osteomalacia | Hypercalcemia, kidney stones, renal failure, hypertension, psychosis, diarrhea, nausea, vomiting, anorexia, fatigue, headaches, altered mental status |
| **Vitamin E (Aquasol E)** | Antioxidant, promotes formation, functioning of red blood cells, muscle, other tissues | Red blood cell breakdown | **High dosages:** GI disturbances, malaise, headaches |

*CNS*, Central nervous system; *F*, females; *GI*, gastrointestinal; *M*, males.

# abacavir

a-**bak**-a-veer
(Ziagen)

■ **BLACK BOX ALERT** ■ Serious, sometimes fatal hypersensitivity reactions, lactic acidosis, severe hepatomegaly with steatosis (fatty liver) have occurred.

### FIXED-COMBINATION(S)

**Epzicom:** abacavir/lamivudine (antiretroviral): 600 mg/300 mg. **Triumeq:** abacavir/dolutegravir (integrase inhibitor)/lamivudine (antiretroviral): 600 mg/50 mg/300 mg. **Trizivir:** abacavir/lamivudine (antiretroviral)/zidovudine (antiretroviral): 300 mg/150 mg/300 mg.

### ◆CLASSIFICATION

**PHARMACOTHERAPEUTIC:** Antiretroviral agent. **CLINICAL:** Antiviral.

## USES

Treatment of HIV infection, in combination with at least two other antiretroviral agents.

## PRECAUTIONS

**Contraindications:** Hypersensitivity to abacavir (do **not** rechallenge). Pts testing positive for the HLA-B *5701 allele are at increased risk for hypersensitivity reaction. Moderate or severe hepatic impairment. **Cautions:** Mild hepatic disease. Pts at risk for coronary heart disease (e.g., hypertension, hyperlipidemia, diabetes, smoking). Pts at risk for hepatotoxicity (e.g., female gender, obesity), pts with plasma HIV RNA levels greater than 100,000 copies/ml.

## ACTION

Interferes with HIV viral RNA-dependent DNA polymerase. **Therapeutic Effect:** Inhibits/prevents HIV replication in infected cells.

## PHARMACOKINETICS

Rapidly absorbed after PO administration. Widely distributed, including to cerebrospinal fluid (CSF) and erythrocytes. Metabolized in liver. Protein binding: 50%. Primarily excreted in urine. Unknown if removed by hemodialysis. **Half-life:** 1.5 hrs.

## ⧖ LIFESPAN CONSIDERATIONS

**Pregnancy/Lactation:** Unknown if excreted in breast milk. Breastfeeding not recommended (may increase potential for HIV transmission, adverse effects). **Children:** Safety and efficacy not established in pts less than 3 mos of age. **Elderly:** No age-related precautions noted.

## INTERACTIONS

**DRUG: Alcohol** may increase concentration, risk of toxicity. **HERBAL:** None significant. **FOOD:** None known. **LAB VALUES:** May increase serum amylase, ALT, AST, CPK, GGT, blood glucose, triglycerides. May decrease Hgb, leukocytes, lymphocytes.

## AVAILABILITY (Rx)

**Solution, Oral:** 20 mg/ml. **Tablets:** 300 mg.

## ADMINISTRATION/HANDLING

**PO**
• May give without regard to food. • Oral solution may be refrigerated. Do not freeze.

## INDICATIONS/ROUTES/DOSAGE

**HIV Infection (in Combination with Other Antiretrovirals)**
**PO: ADULTS:** 300 mg twice daily or 600 mg once daily. **CHILDREN 3 MOS–16 YRS:** 8 mg/kg twice daily. **Maximum:** 300 mg twice daily. (Alternative dosing) **CHILDREN 14 KG OR GREATER:** 14–19 kg: 150 mg (½ tab) twice daily. 20–24 kg: 150 mg (½ tab) in AM 300 mg (1 tab) in PM. 25 kg or greater: 300 mg (1 tab) twice daily.

**Dosage in Renal Impairment**
No dose adjustment.

**Dosage in Hepatic Impairment**
**Mild Impairment:** 200 mg twice daily (oral solution recommended). **Moderate to Severe Impairment:** Not recommended (contraindicated by manufacturer).

## SIDE EFFECTS

**ADULT: Frequent (47%–11%):** Nausea, nausea with vomiting, diarrhea, decreased appetite. **Occasional (39%–11%):** Insomnia (7%). **CHILDREN: Frequent:** Nausea with vomiting, fever, headache, diarrhea, rash. **Occasional:** Decreased appetite (9%).

## ADVERSE EFFECTS/ TOXIC REACTIONS

Hypersensitivity reaction may be life-threatening. Signs and symptoms include fever, rash, fatigue, intractable nausea/vomiting, severe diarrhea, abdominal pain, cough, pharyngitis, dyspnea. Life-threatening hypotension may occur. Lactic acidosis, severe hepatomegaly with steatosis may occur.

## NURSING CONSIDERATIONS

### BASELINE ASSESSMENT

Obtain CBC, LFT before beginning therapy and at periodic intervals during therapy. Question history of hypersensitivity reaction. Question for possibility of pregnancy. Increased risk of sensitivity (cutaneous, GI, pulmonary) in those with positive HLA-B*5701 genotype status. Offer emotional support.

### INTERVENTION/EVALUATION

Stop abacavir if 3 or more of the following occur: rash, fever, GI disturbances (diarrhea, nausea, vomiting), flu-like symptoms, respiratory difficulty. Assess for nausea, vomiting. Monitor daily pattern of bowel activity, stool consistency. Assess dietary pattern; monitor for weight loss. Monitor lab values, hepatic function.

### PATIENT/FAMILY TEACHING

• Immediately report allergic reaction of any kind. • Do not take any medications, including OTC drugs, without consulting physician. • Small, frequent meals may offset anorexia, nausea. • Abacavir is not a cure for HIV infection, nor does it reduce risk of transmission to others. • Pt must continue practices to prevent HIV transmission.

---

## abatacept

a-**bay**-ta-sept
(Orencia)
**Do not confuse Orencia with Oracea.**

### ◆ CLASSIFICATION

**PHARMACOTHERAPEUTIC:** Selective T-cell costimulation modulator. **CLINICAL:** Rheumatoid arthritis agent.

### USES

Reduction of signs and symptoms, progression of structural damage in adults with moderate to severe rheumatoid arthritis (RA) alone or in combination with other disease-modifying antirheumatic medications. Treatment of moderate to severe active polyarticular juvenile idiopathic arthritis in pts 6 yrs and older. May use alone or in combination with methotrexate. NOTE: Do not use with anakinra or tumor necrosis factor [TNF] antagonists.

### PRECAUTIONS

**Contraindications:** Hypersensitivity to abatacept. **Cautions:** Chronic, latent, or localized infection; conditions predisposing to infections; COPD (higher incidence of adverse effects); elderly, hx recurrent infections.

### ACTION

Inhibits T-lymphocyte activation, necessary in the inflammatory cascade leading to joint inflammation and destruction. Blocks production of inflammatory mediators. **Therapeutic Effect:** Induces positive clinical response in adult pts with moderate to severely active RA or juvenile idiopathic arthritis.

### PHARMACOKINETICS

Higher clearance with increasing body weight. Age, gender do not affect clearance. **Half-life:** 8–25 days.

---

## ⧖ LIFESPAN CONSIDERATIONS

**Pregnancy/Lactation:** Crosses placenta; unknown if distributed in breast milk. **Children:** Safety and efficacy not established in pts younger than 6 yrs. **Elderly:** Cautious use due to increased risk of serious infection and malignancy.

## INTERACTIONS

**DRUG:** May increase risk of infection, decrease efficacy of immune response associated with **live vaccines** (do not give concurrently or within 2 mos of stopping abatacept). **Tumor necrosis factor (TNF) antagonists (adalimumab, etanercept, infliximab)** may increase risk of infection. **HERBAL:** Echinacea may decrease concentration/effects. **FOOD:** None known. **LAB VALUES:** None significant.

## AVAILABILITY (Rx)

**Injection, Powder for Reconstitution:** 250 mg. **Injection, Solution:** 125 mg/ml single-dose prefilled syringe.

## ADMINISTRATION/HANDLING

 IV

**Reconstitution •** Reconstitute each vial with 10 ml Sterile Water for Injection using the silicone-free syringe provided with each vial and an 18- to 21-gauge needle. • Rotate solution gently to prevent foaming until powder is completely dissolved. • From a 100-ml 0.9% NaCl infusion bag, withdraw and discard an amount equal to the volume of the reconstituted vials (for 2 vials remove 20 ml, for 3 vials remove 30 ml, for 4 vials remove 40 ml) resulting in final volume of 100 ml. • Slowly add the reconstituted solution from each vial into the infusion bag using the same syringe provided with each vial. • Concentration in the infusion bag will be 10 mg/ml or less abatacept.

**Rate of Administration •** Infuse over 30 min using a 0.2- to 1.2-micron low protein-binding filter.

**Storage •** Store vials in refrigerator. • Any reconstitution that has been prepared by using siliconized syringes will develop translucent particles and must be discarded. • Solution should appear clear and colorless to pale yellow. Discard if solution is discolored or contains precipitate. • Solution is stable for up to 24 hrs after reconstitution. • Reconstituted solution may be stored at room temperature or refrigerated.

**Subcutaneous**

• Store prefilled syringes in refrigerator. Allow to warm to room temperature (30–60 min). • Inject in front of thigh, outer areas of upper arms, or abdomen. • Avoid areas that are tender, bruised, red, scaly, or hard. • Do not rub injection site.

## ▦ IV INCOMPATIBILITY

Do not infuse concurrently in same IV line as other agents.

## INDICATIONS/ROUTES/DOSAGE

**Note:** Discontinue in pts developing serious infection.

**Rheumatoid Arthritis (RA)**

**IV: BODY WEIGHT 101 KG OR MORE:** 1 g (4 vials) given as a 30-min infusion. Following initial therapy, give at 2 wks and 4 wks after first infusion, then q4wks thereafter. **BODY WEIGHT 60–100 KG:** 750 mg (3 vials) given as a 30-min infusion. Following initial therapy, give at 2 wks and 4 wks after first infusion, then q4wks thereafter. **BODY WEIGHT 59 KG OR LESS:** 500 mg (2 vials) given as a 30-min infusion. Following initial therapy, give at 2 wks and 4 wks after first infusion, then q4wks thereafter.

**Subcutaneous:** Following a single IV infusion, 125 mg given within a day, then 125 mg once a week (may be initiated without an IV loading dose).

**Juvenile Idiopathic Arthritis**

**IV: CHILDREN 6 YRS AND OLDER, WEIGHING LESS THAN 75 KG:** 10 mg/kg. **CHILDREN WEIGHING 75 KG OR MORE:** Refer to adult dosing. **Maximum:** 1,000 mg. Following initial therapy, give 2 wks and 4 wks after first infusion, then q4wks thereafter.

**Dosage Adjustment for Toxicity**
Discontinue in pts developing a serious infection.

**Dosage in Renal/Hepatic Impairment**
No dose adjustment.

## SIDE EFFECTS

**Frequent (18%):** Headache. **Occasional (9%–6%):** Dizziness, cough, back pain, hypertension, nausea.

## ADVERSE EFFECTS/ TOXIC REACTIONS

Upper respiratory tract infection, nasopharyngitis, sinusitis, UTI, influenza, bronchitis occur in 5% of pts. Serious infections manifested as pneumonia, cellulitis, diverticulitis, acute pyelonephritis occur in 3% of pts. Hypersensitivity reaction (rash, urticaria, hypotension, dyspnea) occurs rarely. May increase risk of malignancies.

## NURSING CONSIDERATIONS

### BASELINE ASSESSMENT

Assess onset, type, location, duration of pain/inflammation. Inspect appearance of affected joint for immobility, deformities, skin condition. Screen for latent TB infection prior to initiating therapy.

### INTERVENTION/EVALUATION

Assess for therapeutic response: relief of pain, stiffness, swelling; increased joint mobility; reduced joint tenderness; improved grip strength. Monitor for hypersensitivity reaction.

### PATIENT/FAMILY TEACHING

• Consult physician if infection, hypersensitivity reaction, infusion-related reaction occurs. • Do not receive live vaccines during treatment or within 3 mos of its discontinuation. • COPD pts must report worsening of respiratory symptoms.

# *abciximab*

ab-**sik**-si-mab
(ReoPro)

## ◆ CLASSIFICATION

**PHARMACOTHERAPEUTIC:** Glycoprotein IIb/IIIa receptor inhibitor. **CLINICAL:** Antiplatelet; antithrombotic.

## USES

Adjunct to aspirin and heparin therapy to prevent cardiac ischemic complications in pts undergoing percutaneous coronary intervention (PCI) and those with unstable angina not responding to conventional medical therapy when PCI is planned within 24 hrs. **OFF-LABEL:** Support PCI during ST-segment elevation myocardial infarction (STEMI).

## PRECAUTIONS

**Contraindications:** Hypersensitivity to abciximab. Active internal bleeding, arteriovenous malformation or aneurysm, CVA with residual neurologic deficit, history of CVA (within the past 2 yrs) or oral anticoagulant use within the past 7 days unless PT is less than 1.2 times control, history of vasculitis, hypersensitivity to murine proteins, intracranial neoplasm, prior IV dextran use before or during percutaneous transluminal coronary angioplasty (PTCA), recent surgery or trauma (within the past 6 wks), recent GI or GU bleeding (within the past 6 wks), thrombocytopenia (less than 100,000/ mm³), and severe uncontrolled hypertension. Concomitant use of another glycoprotein IIb/IIIa inhibitor. **Cautions:** Increased risk of bleeding in pts who weigh less than 75 kg; pts older than 65 yrs; pts with history of GI disease; pts receiving thrombolytics; PTCA in less than 12 hrs of onset of symptoms for acute MI; prolonged PTCA (longer than 70 min); failed PTCA.

## ACTION

Binds to GP IIb/IIIa receptor sites on platelets. **Therapeutic Effect:** Inhibits platelet aggregation.

## PHARMACOKINETICS

Rapidly cleared from plasma. Initial-phase half-life is less than 10 min; second-phase half-life is 30 min.

## ⏳ LIFESPAN CONSIDERATIONS

**Pregnancy/Lactation:** Unknown if distributed in breast milk. **Children:** Safety and efficacy not established. **Elderly:** Increased risk of major bleeding.

## INTERACTIONS

**DRUG:** Alteplase, apixaban, argatroban, aspirin, clopidogrel, dipyridamole, ibuprofen, naproxen, rivaroxaban, warfarin may increase risk of bleeding. **HERBAL:** None significant. **FOOD:** None known. **LAB VALUES:** Increases activated clotting time (ACT), prothrombin time (PT), activated partial thromboplastin time (aPTT); decreases platelet count.

## AVAILABILITY (Rx)

**Injection Solution:** 2 mg/ml (5-ml vial).

## ADMINISTRATION/HANDLING

 IV

**Reconstitution • Bolus dose:** Withdraw bolus dose into syringe using a 0.2- or 0.5-micron low protein-binding filter. • **Continuous infusion:** Withdraw dose through a 0.2- or 0.5-micron low protein-binding filter and further dilute into 250 ml D₅W or 0.9% NaCl. **Rate of Administration •** Bolus given over 1 min.

**Administration Precautions •** Give in separate IV line; do not add any other medication to infusion. • For bolus injection and continuous infusion, use sterile, nonpyrogenic, low protein-binding 0.2- or 0.22-micron filter.

**Storage •** Store vials in refrigerator. • Solution appears clear, colorless. • Do not shake. • Prepared solution is stable for 12 hrs. Discard any unused portion left in vial or if preparation contains opaque particles.

## 🔷 IV INCOMPATIBILITY

Administer in separate line; no other medication should be added to infusion solution.

## 🔷 IV COMPATIBILITIES

Adenosine (Adenocard), argatroban, atropine sulfate, bivalirudin (Angiomax), diphenhydramine (Benadryl), fentanyl (Sublimaze), metoprolol (Lopressor), midazolam (Versed).

## INDICATIONS/ROUTES/DOSAGE

**Percutaneous Coronary Intervention (PCI)**
**IV Bolus: ADULTS:** 0.25 mg/kg 10–60 min before PCI, then 12-hr IV infusion of 0.125 mcg/kg/min. **Maximum:** 10 mcg/min.

**PCI (Unstable Angina)**
**IV Bolus: ADULTS:** 0.25 mg/kg, followed by 18- to 24-hr infusion of 10 mcg/min, ending 1 hr after procedure.

**Dosage in Renal/Hepatic Impairment**
No dose adjustment.

## SIDE EFFECTS

**Frequent (16%–12%):** Nausea, hypotension. **Occasional (9%):** Vomiting. **Rare (3%):** Bradycardia, confusion, dizziness, pain, peripheral edema, UTI.

## ADVERSE EFFECTS/ TOXIC REACTIONS

Major bleeding complications may occur; stop infusion immediately. Hypersensitivity reaction may occur. Atrial fibrillation or flutter, pulmonary edema, complete AV block occur occasionally.

## NURSING CONSIDERATIONS

### BASELINE ASSESSMENT

Concomitant heparin gtt should be discontinued 4 hrs before arterial sheath removal (or per facility protocol). Maintain pt on bed rest for 6–8 hrs following sheath removal or drug discontinuation, whichever is later. Check platelet count, PT, aPTT, PFA, before infusion (assess for preexisting blood abnormalities), 2–4 hrs following treatment, and at 24 hrs or before discharge, whichever is first. Check insertion site, distal pulse of affected limb while femoral artery sheath is in place, and then routinely for 6 hrs following femoral artery sheath removal. Minimize need for injections, blood draws, catheters, other invasive procedures.

### INTERVENTION/EVALUATION

Monitor ACT, PT, aPTT, platelet count, Hgb, Hct. Stop abciximab and/or heparin infusion if serious bleeding occurs that is uncontrolled by pressure. Observe for mental status changes. Assess skin for ecchymosis, petechiae, particularly at femoral arterial access, also at catheter insertion, arterial and venous puncture, cutdown, needle sites. Handle pt carefully and as infrequently as possible to prevent bleeding. Do not obtain B/P in lower extremities (possible deep vein thrombi). Assess for decrease in B/P, increase in pulse rate, complaint of abdominal or back pain, severe headache, evidence of GI hemorrhage. Question for increase in discharge during menses. Assess urinary output for hematuria. Monitor for hematoma. Use care in removing any dressing, tape.

### PATIENT/FAMILY TEACHING

• Assess skin for bruising up to 3 days after infusion. • Report signs of bleeding.

## abiraterone  TOP 100

a-bir-a-ter-one
(Zytiga)
**Do not confuse Zytiga with Zetia or Zyrtec.**

### ◆CLASSIFICATION

**PHARMACOTHERAPEUTIC:** Androgen biosynthesis inhibitor. **CLINICAL:** Antineoplastic.

### USES

Treatment of metastatic castration-resistant prostate cancer in combination with prednisone.

### PRECAUTIONS

**Contraindications:** Hypersensitivity to abiraterone. Use in women who are pregnant or may become pregnant. **Cautions:** History of cardiovascular disease (especially HF, recent MI, or ventricular arrhythmia) due to potential for hypertension, hypokalemia, fluid retention; moderate hepatic impairment, adrenal insufficiency. Avoid use with strong CYP3A4 inducers.

### ACTION

Inhibits androgen production in adrenal gland, testes, and prostate tumors. Inhibits formation of testosterone precursors. **Therapeutic Effect:** Lowers serum testosterone to castrate levels.

### PHARMACOKINETICS

Protein binding: 99%. Primarily excreted in feces. **Peak plasma concentration:** 2 hrs. **Half-life:** 12 hrs (up to 19 hrs with hepatic impairment).

### ⏳ LIFESPAN CONSIDERATIONS

**Pregnancy/Lactation:** Contraindicated in women who are or may become pregnant. **Children:** Safety and efficacy not established. **Elderly:** No age-related precautions noted.

## INTERACTIONS

**DRUG:** May increase concentration/toxicity of **silodosin, tamoxifen, thioridazine, topotecan.** May decrease effect of **clopidogrel, tramadol. CYP3A4 inhibitors** (e.g., **clarithromycin, ketoconazole**) may increase concentration. **CYP3A4 inducers** (e.g., **carbamazepine**) may decrease concentration. **HERBAL:** None significant. **FOOD:** Do not give with **food** (no **food** should be consumed for at least 2 hrs before or 1 hr after dose). **LAB VALUES:** May increase serum ALT, AST, bilirubin, triglycerides. May decrease potassium, phosphate.

## AVAILABILITY (Rx)

**Tablets:** 250 mg.

## ADMINISTRATION/HANDLING

### PO

• Give on empty stomach only (at least 1 hr before or 2 hrs after food). • Give with water. • Administer whole. Do not break, crush, dissolve, or divide tablets. Women who are or may become pregnant should wear gloves if handling the tablets.

## INDICATIONS/ROUTES/DOSAGE

◄**ALERT**► Consider increased dosage of prednisone during unusual stress or infection. Interrupting prednisone therapy may induce adrenocorticoid insufficiency.

**Metastatic Castration-Resistant Prostate Cancer**
**PO: ADULTS, ELDERLY:** 1,000 mg once daily (with prednisone 5 mg 2 times/day).

**Dosage Modification**

**Hepatic Enzymes Greater Than Upper Limit of Normal (ULN) (During Treatment)**

| Lab Values | Recommendation |
| --- | --- |
| ALT, AST elevations greater than 5 × ULN or bilirubin greater than 3 × ULN with 1,000 mg | Interrupt treatment and restart at 750 mg once ALT, AST less than 2.5 × ULN or bilirubin less than 1.5 × ULN. |
| ALT, AST elevations greater than 5 × ULN or bilirubin greater than 3 × ULN with 750 mg | Interrupt treatment and restart at 500 mg once ALT, AST less than 2.5 × ULN or bilirubin less than 1.5 × ULN. |

If hepatotoxicity occurs at reduced dose of 500 mg daily, discontinue treatment.

**Dosage Adjustment for Concomitant Strong CYP3A4 Inducers**
Increase abiraterone dose to 1,000 mg twice daily.

**Dosage in Renal Impairment**
No dose adjustment.

**Dosage in Hepatic Impairment**
**Mild Impairment:** No dosage adjustment necessary. **Moderate Impairment:** Reduce dose to 250 mg daily. Discontinue if ALT, AST greater than 5 times ULN or bilirubin greater than 3 times ULN. **Severe Impairment:** Avoid use.

## SIDE EFFECTS

**Frequent (30%–26%):** Joint swelling/discomfort, peripheral edema, muscle spasm, musculoskeletal pain, hypokalemia. **Occasional (19%–6%):** Hot flashes, diarrhea, UTI, cough, hypertension, urinary frequency, nocturia. **Rare (less than 6%):** Heartburn, upper respiratory tract infection.

## ADVERSE EFFECTS/ TOXIC REACTIONS

Mineralocorticoid excess (severe fluid retention, hypokalemia, hypertension) may compromise pts with prior cardiovascular history. Safety not established in

---

✦ Canadian trade name       🥄 Non-Crushable Drug       🔲 High Alert drug pts with left ventricular ejection fraction less than 50%. Tachycardia, atrial fibrillation, supraventricular tachycardia, atrial flutter, complete AV block, bradyarrhythmia reported in 7% of pts. Chest pain, unstable angina, HF reported in less than 4% of pts. Stress, infection, or interruption of daily steroids may cause adrenocortical insufficiency. Hepatotoxicity (ALT, AST greater than 5 times ULN) reported in 2% of pts. Pts with hepatic impairment are more likely to develop hepatotoxicity.

## NURSING CONSIDERATIONS

### BASELINE ASSESSMENT

Obtain baseline BMP, LFT. Evaluate history of HF, myocardial infarction, arrhythmias, angina pectoris, peripheral edema, hepatic impairment, adrenal or pituitary abnormalities, left ventricular ejection fraction if applicable. Question possibility of pregnancy before treatment (Pregnancy Category X). Question history of corticosteroid intolerance if applicable.

### INTERVENTION/EVALUATION

Assess for peripheral edema behind medial malleolus (sacral area in bedridden patients). Monitor BMP, LFT. Monitor for mineralocorticoid excess (hypokalemia, hypertension, fluid retention) at least once monthly. Assess for cardiac arrhythmia if hypokalemia occurs. Obtain EKG for palpitations, dyspnea, dizziness. Monitor for signs and symptoms of adrenocortical insufficiency during prednisone interruption, periods of stress, infection. Measure ALT, AST, alkaline phosphatase, bilirubin every 2 wks for 3 mos, then monthly. If hepatotoxicity occurs, dosage modification will be necessary. Pts with moderate hepatic impairment must have hepatic function tests every wk for first month, then every 2 wks for 2 mos, then monthly. If ALT, AST above 5 times ULN or bilirubin above 3 times ULN, treatment should be discontinued.

### PATIENT/FAMILY TEACHING

• Must be taken on empty stomach (no food 2 hrs before and 1 hr after dose). • If taken with food, toxic levels may result. • Sexually active men must wear condom during treatment and for 1 wk after treatment. • Women who are pregnant or are planning pregnancy may not touch medication without gloves. • Dizziness, palpitations, headache, confusion, muscle weakness, leg swelling/discomfort may become more apparent during periods of unusual stress, infection, or interruption of prednisone therapy. • Blood tests will be performed routinely. • Report signs of liver problems (yellowing of skin, bruising, light-colored stool, right upper quadrant pain), chest pain, palpitations. • An increase in urinary frequency or nocturia is expected as treatment becomes therapeutic. • Do not chew, crush, dissolve, or divide tablets.

## acetaminophen    TOP 100

a-**seet**-a-**min**-oh-fen
(Abenol ✦, Acephen, Apo-Acetaminophen ✦, Atasol ✦, Feverall, Mapap, Ofirmev, Tempra ✦, Tylenol, Tylenol Arthritis Pain, Tylenol Children's Meltaways, Tylenol Junior Meltaways, Tylenol Extra Strength)
■ **BLACK BOX ALERT** ■ Potential for severe liver injury. Acetaminophen injection associated with acute liver failure.
**Do not confuse Acephen with Aciphex, Feverall with Fiberall, Fioricet with Fiorinal, Percocet with Percodan, Tylenol with atenolol, timolol, Tylenol PM, or Tylox, or Vicodin with Hycodan.**

### FIXED-COMBINATION(S)

**Capital with Codeine, Tylenol with Codeine:** acetaminophen/codeine: 120 mg/12 mg per 5 ml. **Endocet:** acetaminophen/oxycodone:

---

325 mg/5 mg, 325 mg/7.5 mg, 325 mg/10 mg. **Fioricet:** acetaminophen/caffeine/butalbital: 325 mg/40 mg/50 mg. **Hycet:** acetaminophen/hydrocodone: 325 mg/7.5 mg per 15 ml. **Norco:** acetaminophen/hydrocodone: 325 mg/5 mg, 325 mg/7.5 mg, 325 mg/10 mg. **Percocet, Roxicet:** acetaminophen/oxycodone: 325 mg/5 mg. **Tylenol with Codeine:** acetaminophen/codeine: 300 mg/15 mg, 300 mg/30 mg, 300 mg/60 mg. **Ultracet:** acetaminophen/tramadol: 325 mg/37.5 mg. **Vicodin:** acetaminophen/hydrocodone: 300 mg/5 mg. **Vicodin ES:** acetaminophen/hydrocodone: 300 mg/7.5 mg. **Vicodin HP:** acetaminophen/hydrocodone: 300 mg/10 mg. **Xartemis XR:** acetaminophen/oxycodone: 325 mg/7.5 mg. **Xodol:** acetaminophen/hydrocodone: 300 mg/5 mg, 300 mg/7.5 mg, 300 mg/10 mg.

### ◆CLASSIFICATION

**PHARMACOTHERAPEUTIC:** Central analgesic. **CLINICAL:** Non-narcotic analgesic, antipyretic.

### USES

Relief of mild to moderate pain, fever. **IV:** (Additional) Management of moderate to severe pain when combined with opioid analgesia.

### PRECAUTIONS

**Contraindications:** Hypersensitivity to acetaminophen. (Ofirmev): severe hepatic impairment or severe active liver disease. **Cautions:** Sensitivity to acetaminophen; severe renal impairment; alcohol dependency, hepatic impairment, or active hepatic disease; chronic malnutrition and hypovolemia (Ofirmev); G6PD deficiency (hemolysis may occur). Limit dose to less than 4 g/day.

### ACTION

Appears to inhibit prostaglandin synthesis in the CNS and, to a lesser extent, block pain impulses through peripheral action. Acts centrally on hypothalamic heat-regulating center, producing peripheral vasodilation (heat loss, skin erythema, diaphoresis). **Therapeutic Effect:** Results in antipyresis. Produces analgesic effect.

### PHARMACOKINETICS

| Route | Onset | Peak | Duration |
|---|---|---|---|
| PO | Less than 60 min | 1–3 hrs | 4–6 hrs |

Rapidly, completely absorbed from GI tract; rectal absorption variable. Protein binding: 20%–50%. Widely distributed to most body tissues. Metabolized in liver; excreted in urine. Removed by hemodialysis. **Half-life:** 1–4 hrs (increased in pts with hepatic disease, elderly, neonates; decreased in children).

### ⌛ LIFESPAN CONSIDERATIONS

**Pregnancy/Lactation:** Crosses placenta; distributed in breast milk. Routinely used in all stages of pregnancy, appears safe for short-term use. **Children/Elderly:** No age-related precautions noted.

### INTERACTIONS

**DRUG: Alcohol** (chronic use), **hepatotoxic medications** (e.g., phenytoin), **hepatic enzyme inducers** (e.g., phenytoin, rifampin) may increase risk of hepatotoxicity with prolonged high dose or single toxic dose. May increase risk of bleeding with **warfarin** with chronic, high-dose use. **HERBAL: St. John's wort** may decrease blood levels. **FOOD: Food** may decrease rate of absorption. **LAB VALUES:** May increase serum ALT, AST, bilirubin, prothrombin levels (may indicate hepatotoxicity).

## AVAILABILITY (OTC)

**Caplets (Tylenol):** 325 mg, 500 mg, 650 mg. **Elixir:** 160 mg/5 ml. **Injection, Solution (Ofirmev):** 1,000 mg/100 ml glass vial. **Liquid (Oral [Tylenol Extra Strength]):** 160 mg/5 ml, 500 mg/5 ml, 500 mg/15 ml. **Solution (Oral Drops [Mapap]):** 80 mg/0.8 ml. **Suppository (Acephen, Feverall):** 80 mg, 120 mg, 325 mg, 650 mg. **Suspension (Mapap):** 160 mg/5 ml. **Tablets (Mapap, Tylenol):** 325 mg, 500 mg. **Tablets (Chewable [Mapap]):** 80 mg. **Tablets (Orally Disintegrating):** 80 mg, 160 mg.

 **Caplets: (Extended-Release [Tylenol Arthritis Pain]):** 650 mg.

## ADMINISTRATION/HANDLING

### IV

**Reconstitution** • Does not require further dilution. • Store at room temperature. • Withdraw doses less than 1,000 mg. • Place in separate empty, sterile container. **Rate of Administration** • Infuse over 15 min. **Stability** • Once opened or transferred, stable for 6 hrs at room temperature.

### PO

• Give without regard to meals. • Tablets may be crushed. • Do not crush extended-release caplets. • Suspension: Shake well before use. • Take with full glass of water.

### Rectal

• Moisten suppository with cold water before inserting well up into rectum. • Do not freeze suppositories.

## INDICATIONS/ROUTES/DOSAGE

**Note:** Over-the-counter (OTC) use of acetaminophen should be limited to 3,000 mg/day.

### Analgesia and Antipyresis

**IV: ADULTS, ADOLESCENTS WEIGHING 50 KG OR MORE:** 1,000 mg q6h or 650 mg q4h. **Maximum single dose:** 1,000 mg; **maximum total daily dose:** 4,000 mg. **ADULTS, ADOLESCENTS WEIGHING LESS THAN 50 KG:** 15 mg/kg q6h or 12.5 mg/kg q4h.

**Maximum single dose:** 750 mg; **maximum total daily dose:** 75 mg/kg/day (3,750 mg). **CHILDREN 2–12 YRS:** 15 mg/kg q6h or 12.5 mg/kg q4h. **Maximum single dose:** 750 mg. **Maximum:** 75 mg/kg/day, not to exceed 3,750 mg/day. **INFANTS AND CHILDREN LESS THAN 2 YRS:** 7.5–15 mg/kg q6h. **Maximum:** 60 mg/kg/day. **NEONATES:** (Limitied data available) Loading dose: 20 mg/kg. **PMA 37 or greater than 37 wks:** 10 mg/kg/dose q6h. **Maximum:** 40 mg/kg/day. PMA 33–36 wks: 10 mg/kg/dose q8h. **Maximum:** 40 mg/kg/day. **PMA 28–32 wks:** 10 mg/kg/dose q12h. **Maximum:** 22.5 mg/kg/day.

**PO: ADULTS, ELDERLY, CHILDREN 13 YRS AND OLDER:** 325–650 mg q4–6h or 1 g 3–4 times/day. **Maximum:** 4 g/day. **CHILDREN 12 YRS AND YOUNGER:** 10–15 mg/kg/dose q4–6h as needed. **Maximum:** 5 doses/24 hrs or 75 mg/kg/day. Do not exceed 4,000 mg/day. **NEONATES:** Term: 10–15 mg/kg/dose q4–6h. **Maximum:** 90 mg/kg/day. **GA 33–37 wks or term less than 10 days:** 10–15 mg/kg/dose q6h. **Maximum:** 60 mg/kg/day. **GA: 28–32 wks:** 10–12 mg/kg/dose q6–8h. **Maximum:** 40 mg/kg/day.

**Rectal: ADULTS:** 325–650 mg q4–6h. **Maximum:** 4 g/24 hrs. **CHILDREN:** 10–20 mg/kg/dose q4–6h as needed. **Maximum:** 5 doses/24 hrs. **NEONATES:** Term: Initially, 30 mg/kg/once, then 20 mg/kg/dose q6–8h. **Maximum:** 90 mg/kg/day. **GA 33–37 wks or term less than 10 days:** Initially, 30 mg/kg once, then 15 mg/kg/dose q8h. **Maximum:** 60 mg/kg/day. **GA: 28–32 wks:** 20 mg/kg/dose q12h. **Maximum:** 40 mg/kg/day.

### Dosage in Renal Impairment

| Creatinine Clearance | Frequency |
| --- | --- |
| **Oral** | |
| 10–50 ml/min | q6h |
| Less than 10 ml/min | q8h |
| Continuous renal replacement therapy | q6h |
| **IV** | |
| 30 ml/min or less (use caution, decrease daily dose, extend dosing interval) | |

**Dosage in Hepatic Impairment**
Use with caution. IV contraindicated with severe impairment.

## SIDE EFFECTS

**Rare:** Hypersensitivity reaction.

## ADVERSE EFFECTS/ TOXIC REACTIONS

**Early Signs of Acetaminophen Toxicity:** Anorexia, nausea, diaphoresis, fatigue within first 12–24 hrs. **Later Signs of Toxicity:** Vomiting, right upper quadrant tenderness, elevated LFTs within 48–72 hrs after ingestion. **Antidote:** Acetylcysteine (see Appendix J for dosage).

## NURSING CONSIDERATIONS

### BASELINE ASSESSMENT

If given for analgesia, assess onset, type, location, duration of pain. Effect of medication is reduced if full pain response recurs prior to next dose. Assess for fever. Assess alcohol usage.

### INTERVENTION/EVALUATION

Assess for clinical improvement and relief of pain, fever. **Therapeutic serum level:** 10–30 mcg/ml; **toxic serum level:** greater than 200 mcg/ml. Do not exceed maximum daily recommended dose: 4 g/day.

### PATIENT/FAMILY TEACHING

• Consult physician for use in children younger than 2 yrs, oral use longer than 5 days (children) or longer than 10 days (adults), or fever lasting longer than 3 days. • Severe/recurrent pain or high/continuous fever may indicate serious illness. • Advise not to take more than 4 g/24-hr period. Many nonprescription combination products contain acetaminophen. Avoid alcohol.

# acetylcysteine (*N*-acetylcysteine)

a-**seet**-il-**sis**-teen
(Acetadote, Cetylev, Mucomyst ✦, Parvolex ✦)
**Do not confuse acetylcysteine with acetylcholine, or Mucomyst with Mucinex.**

## ◆ CLASSIFICATION

**PHARMACOTHERAPEUTIC:** Respiratory inhalant, intratracheal. **CLINICAL:** Mucolytic, antidote.

## USES

**Inhalation:** Adjunctive treatment for abnormally viscid mucous secretions present in acute and chronic bronchopulmonary disease and pulmonary complications of cystic fibrosis and surgery, diagnostic bronchial studies. **Injection, PO:** Antidote in acute acetaminophen toxicity.

## PRECAUTIONS

**Contraindications:** Hypersensitivity to acetylcysteine. **Cautions:** Pts with bronchial asthma; debilitated pts with severe respiratory insufficiency (increases risk of anaphylactoid reaction).

## ACTION

Mucolytic splits linkage of mucoproteins, reducing viscosity of pulmonary secretions. Acetaminophen toxicity: Hepatoprotective by restoring hepatic glutathione and enhancing nontoxic conjugation of acetaminophen. **Therapeutic Effect:** Facilitates removal of pulmonary secretions by coughing, postural drainage, mechanical means. Protects against acetaminophen overdose-induced hepatotoxicity.

## INTERACTIONS

**DRUG:** None significant. **HERBAL:** None significant. **FOOD:** None known. **LAB VALUES:** None significant.

---

 Canadian trade name      Non-Crushable Drug     High Alert drug

## AVAILABILITY (Rx)

**Inhalation Solution (Mucomyst):** 10% (100 mg/ml), 20% (200 mg/ml). **Injection Solution (Acetadote):** 20% (200 mg/ml). **Tablets, Effervescent:** 500 mg, 2.5 g.

## ADMINISTRATION/HANDLING

 IV

The total dose is 300 mg/kg administered over 21 hrs. Dose preparation is based on pt weight. Total volume administered should be adjusted for pts less than 40 kg and for pts requiring fluid restriction. Store unopened vials at room temperature. Following dilution in D$_5$W, stable for 24 hrs at room temperature. Color change of opened vials may occur (does not affect potency).

**Three-Bag Method (as Antidote):**
**Loading, Second, and Third Doses**
**Pts Greater Than or Equal to 40 kg:**
Loading dose: 150 mg/kg in 200 ml of diluent administered over 60 min.
Second dose: 50 mg/kg in 500 ml of diluent administered over 4 hrs.
Third dose: 100 mg/kg in 1,000 ml of diluent administered over 16 hrs.

**Pts Greater Than 20 kg but Less Than 40 kg:**
Loading dose: 150 mg/kg in 100 ml of diluent administered over 60 min.
Second dose: 50 mg/kg in 250 ml of diluent administered over 4 hrs.
Third dose: 100 mg/kg in 500 ml of diluent administered over 16 hrs.

**Pts Less Than or Equal to 20 kg:**
Loading dose: 150 mg/kg in 3 ml/kg of body weight of diluent administered over 60 min.
Second dose: 50 mg/kg in 7 ml/kg of body weight of diluent administered over 4 hrs.
Third dose: 100 mg/kg in 14 ml/kg of body weight of diluent administered over 16 hrs.

**PO**
• For treatment of acetaminophen overdose. • Give as 5% solution. • Dilute 20% solution 1:3 with cola, orange juice, other soft drink. • Give within 1 hr of preparation.

**Inhalation, Nebulization**
• 20% solution may be diluted with 0.9% NaCl or sterile water; 10% solution may be used undiluted.

## ▦ IV COMPATIBILITIES

Cefepime (Maxipime), ceftazidime (Fortaz).

## INDICATIONS/ROUTES/DOSAGE

**Bronchopulmonary Disease**
*Inhalation, Nebulization*
◄**ALERT**► Bronchodilators should be given 10–15 min before acetylcysteine.
**ADULTS, ELDERLY, CHILDREN:** 3–5 ml (20% solution) 3–4 times/day or 6–10 ml (10% solution) 3–4 times/day. Range: 1–10 ml (20% solution) q2–6h or 2–20 ml (10% solution) q2–6h. **INFANTS:** 1–2 ml (20%) or 2–4 ml (10%) 3–4 times/day.
**Intratracheal: ADULTS, CHILDREN:** 1–2 ml of 10% or 20% solution instilled into tracheostomy q1–4h.

**Acetaminophen Overdose**
◄**ALERT**► It is essential to initiate treatment as soon as possible after overdose and, in any case, within 24 hrs of ingestion.
**PO *(Effervescent Tablets, Oral Solution 5%)*: ADULTS, ELDERLY, CHILDREN:** Loading dose of 140 mg/kg, followed in 4 hrs by maintenance dose of 70 mg/kg q4h for 17 additional doses (or until acetaminophen assay reveals nontoxic level). Repeat dose if emesis occurs within 1 hr of administration.
**IV: ADULTS, ELDERLY, CHILDREN:** (Consists of 3 doses. Total Dose: 300 mg/kg.) 150 mg/kg infused over 60 min, then 50 mg/kg infused over 4 hrs, then 100 mg/kg infused over 16 hrs (see Administration/Handling for dilution). **GREATER THAN**

**100 KG:** (Consists of 3 doses. Total Dose: 30 g.) 15 g over 60 min; 5 g over 4 hrs; 10 g over 16 hrs. Duration of administration may vary depending on acetaminophen levels and LFTs obtained during treatment. Pts who still have detectable levels of acetaminophen or elevated LFT results continue to benefit from additional acetylcysteine administration beyond 24 hrs.

**Diagnostic Bronchial Studies**
**Inhalation, Nebulization: ADULTS:** 1–2 ml of 20% solution or 2–4 ml of 10% solution 2–3 times before the procedure.

## SIDE EFFECTS

**IV: (10%):** Nausea, vomiting. **(7%–6%):** Acute flushing, erythema. **(4%):** Pruritus. **Frequent: Inhalation:** Stickiness on face, transient unpleasant odor. **Occasional: Inhalation:** Increased bronchial secretions, throat irritation, nausea, vomiting, rhinorrhea. **Rare: Inhalation:** Rash. **PO:** Facial edema, bronchospasm, wheezing, nausea, vomiting.

## ADVERSE EFFECTS/ TOXIC REACTIONS

Large doses may produce severe nausea/vomiting. **(Less than 2%):** Serious anaphylactoid reactions including cough, wheezing, stridor, respiratory distress, bronchospasm, hypotension, and death have been known to occur with IV administration.

## NURSING CONSIDERATIONS

### BASELINE ASSESSMENT

**Mucolytic:** Assess pretreatment respirations for rate, depth, rhythm. **IV antidote:** Obtain baseline labs and drug screen. For use as antidote, obtain acetaminophen level to determine need for treatment with acetylcysteine.

### INTERVENTION/EVALUATION

If bronchospasm occurs, discontinue treatment, notify physician; bronchodilator may be added to therapy. Monitor rate, depth, rhythm, type of respiration (abdominal, thoracic). Observe sputum for color, consistency, amount. **IV antidote:** Administer within 8 hrs of acetaminophen ingestion for maximal hepatic protection; ideally, within 4 hrs after immediate-release and 2 hrs after liquid acetaminophen formulations.

### PATIENT/FAMILY TEACHING

• Slight, disagreeable sulfuric odor from solution may be noticed during initial administration but disappears quickly. • Adequate hydration is important part of therapy. • Follow guidelines for proper coughing and deep breathing techniques.

# aclidinium

a-kli-**din**-ee-um
(Tudorza)

◆**CLASSIFICATION**

**PHARMACOTHERAPEUTIC:** Long-acting antimuscarinic, anticholinergic. **CLINICAL:** Bronchodilator.

## USES

Long-term maintenance treatment of airflow obstruction in pts with chronic obstructive pulmonary disease (COPD), including chronic bronchitis and emphysema.

## PRECAUTIONS

◀**ALERT**▶ Not indicated for use as a rescue medication. Contact physician if paradoxical bronchospasm, worsening of narrow-angle glaucoma, urinary retention, or immediate hypersensitivity occurs. **Contraindications:** Hypersensitivity to aclidinium. **Cautions:** Prostatic hyperplasia, urinary retention, bladder-neck obstruction, narrow-angle glaucoma, hypersensitivity to milk proteins, atropine.

## ACTION

Inhibits $M_1$ to $M_5$ muscarinic receptors in smooth muscle of airway, preventing

acetylcholine-induced bronchospasm.
**Therapeutic Effect:** Bronchodilation.

## PHARMACOKINETICS

Peak plasma levels noted within 10 min following inhalation. Extensively metabolized via hydrolysis, both chemically and enzymatically by esterases. Primarily eliminated in urine, with a smaller amount excreted in feces. **Half-life:** 5–8 hrs.

## ⧗ LIFESPAN CONSIDERATIONS

**Pregnancy/Lactation:** May produce teratogenic effects. May be excreted in breast milk; do not breastfeed. **Children:** Safety and efficacy not established. **Elderly:** No age-related precautions noted.

## INTERACTIONS

**DRUG:** May increase effects of **anticholinergic agents** (e.g., **atropine, glycopyrrolate**). **HERBAL:** None significant. **FOOD:** None known. **LAB VALUES:** None known.

## AVAILABILITY (Rx)

**Powder for Inhalation:** 400 mcg/inhalation.

## ADMINISTRATION/HANDLING

**Inhalation**
• Remove inhaler from pouch; allows 60 doses for oral inhalation. • The inhaler is a white and green device with a dose indicator, a storage unit containing drug product formulation, and a mouthpiece covered by a green protective cap. • Each actuation delivers 375 mcg of medication from the mouthpiece. • Follow manufacturer guidelines for assembly of plastic dosing mechanism and proper use of inhaler.
**Storage** • Store pouch at room temperature; inhaler should be stored inside the sealed pouch and only be opened immediately before use. • Discard inhaler 45 days after opening the pouch, after the marking "0" with a red background shows in middle of dose indicator, or when the device locks out, whichever comes first.

## INDICATIONS/ROUTES/DOSAGE

**Maintenance Therapy:**
**Inhalation: ADULTS, ELDERLY:** 400 mcg twice daily.

## SIDE EFFECTS

**Occasional (7%–3%):** Headache, nasopharyngitis, cough, diarrhea. **Rare (2%–1%):** Sinusitis, rhinitis, toothache, vomiting.

## ADVERSE EFFECTS/ TOXIC REACTIONS

Severe dyspnea may indicate paradoxical bronchospasm. Acute narrow-angle glaucoma (eye pain or discomfort, blurred vision, visual halos, or colored images in association with red eyes from conjunctival congestion and corneal edema) occur rarely. Signs and symptoms of prostatic hyperplasia or bladder-neck obstruction (difficulty passing urine, painful urination) have been observed. Hypersensitivity reaction has been noted rarely.

## NURSING CONSIDERATIONS

### BASELINE ASSESSMENT

Assess rate, depth, rhythm, type of respirations. Obtain EKG, serum potassium, ABG determinations, $O_2$ saturation, pulmonary function test. Assess lung sounds for wheezing (bronchoconstriction), rales. Receive full medication history and screen for possible drug interactions.

### INTERVENTION/EVALUATION

Assess lung sounds. Observe for sudden shortness of breath, wheezing (pulmonary bronchospasm). Routinely monitor BMP, blood glucose, $O_2$ saturation. Evaluate EKG for palpitation, tachycardia. Monitor for hypokalemia. Monitor for acute urinary retention. Question for eye pain or discomfort, changes in vision, conjunctival congestion (worsening of narrow-angle glaucoma).

### PATIENT/FAMILY TEACHING

• The inhaler contains 60 doses of medication, with the number 60 on dose indicator. • As each dose is used, the dose indicator will display down in intervals of 10. • The marking "0" with a red background shows in the middle of the dose indicator. • Discard pouch after 45 days, after the marking "0" with a red background shows in the middle of the dose indicator, or when device locks out, whichever comes first. • Increase fluid intake (decreases lung secretion viscosity). • Report difficulty breathing, painful or difficulty passing urine, visual changes.

# acyclovir

a-**sye**-klo-veer
(Apo-Acyclovir ✤, Zovirax)
**Do not confuse acyclovir with ganciclovir, Retrovir, or valacyclovir, or Zovirax with Doribax, Valtrex, Zithromax, Zostrix, Zyloprim, or Zyvox.**

### FIXED-COMBINATION(S)

**Liposivir:** acyclovir/hydrocortisone (a steroid): 5%/1%.

## ◆CLASSIFICATION

**PHARMACOTHERAPEUTIC:** Synthetic nucleoside. **CLINICAL:** Antiviral.

## USES

**Parenteral**
Treatment of initial and prophylaxis of recurrent mucosal and cutaneous herpes simplex virus (HSV-1 and HSV-2) in immunocompromised pts. Treatment of severe initial episodes of herpes genitalis in immunocompetent pts. Treatment of herpes simplex encephalitis including neonatal herpes simplex virus. Treatment of varicella-zoster virus (VZV) infections in immunocompetent pts.

**Oral**
Treatment of initial episodes and prophylaxis of recurrent herpes simplex (HSV-2 genital herpes). Treatment of chickenpox (varicella). Acute treatment of herpes zoster (shingles). Management of initial genital herpes.
**OFF-LABEL:** (Parenteral/Oral): Prevention of HSV reactivation in HIV-positive pts; hematopoietic stem cell transplant (HSCT); during periods of neutropenia in pts with cancer; prevention of VZV reactivation in allogenic HSCT; treatment of disseminated HSC or VZV in immunocompromised pts with cancer; empiric treatment of suspected encephalitis in immunocompromised pts with cancer; treatment of initial and prophylaxis of recurrent mucosal and cutaneous herpes simplex infections in immunocompromised pts.

**Topical**
**Cream:** Treatment of recurrent herpes labialis (cold sores). **Ointment:** Treatment of mucocutaneous HSV in immunocompromised pts.

## ⌛ PRECAUTIONS

**Contraindications:** Use in neonates when acyclovir is reconstituted with Bacteriostatic Water for Injection containing benzyl alcohol. Hypersensitivity to acyclovir, valacyclovir. **Cautions:** Immunocompromised pts (thrombocytopenic purpura/hemolytic uremic syndrome reported); elderly, renal impairment, use of other nephrotoxic medications. IV Use: Pts with underlying neurologic abnormalities, serious hepatic/electrolyte abnormalities, substantial hypoxia.

## ACTION

Converts to acyclovir triphosphate, which competes for viral DNA polymerase, becoming part of DNA chain. **Therapeutic Effect:** Interferes with DNA synthesis and viral replication. Virustatic.

## PHARMACOKINETICS

15%–30% absorbed from GI tract. Bioavailability: 10%–20%; minimal absorption following topical application. Protein binding: 9%–36%. Widely distributed. Partially metabolized in liver.

---

✤ Canadian trade name     🮲 Non-Crushable Drug     🮖 High Alert drug

Excreted primarily in urine. Removed by hemodialysis. **Half-life:** 2.5 hrs (increased in renal impairment).

## ⏳ LIFESPAN CONSIDERATIONS

**Pregnancy/Lactation:** Crosses placenta; distributed in breast milk. **Children:** Safety and efficacy not established in pts younger than 2 yrs (younger than 1 yr for IV use). **Elderly:** Age-related renal impairment may require decreased dosage. May experience more neurologic effects (e.g., agitation, confusion, hallucinations).

## INTERACTIONS

**DRUG:** None significant. **HERBAL:** None significant. **FOOD:** None known. **LAB VALUES:** May increase serum ALT, AST, BUN, creatinine.

## AVAILABILITY (Rx)

**Cream:** 5%. **Injection, Powder for Reconstitution:** 500 mg, 1,000 mg. **Injection, Solution:** 50 mg/ml. **Ointment:** 5%. **Suspension, Oral:** 200 mg/5 ml. **Tablets:** 400 mg, 800 mg. **Tablet (buccal):** 50 mg.

💊 **Capsules:** 200 mg.

## ADMINISTRATION/HANDLING

 IV

**Reconstitution** • Add 10 ml Sterile Water for Injection to each 500-mg vial (50 mg/ml). Do not use Bacteriostatic Water for Injection containing benzyl alcohol or parabens (will cause precipitate). • Shake well until solution is clear. • Further dilute with at least 100 ml D₅W or 0.9 NaCl. Final concentration should be 7 mg/ml or less. (Concentrations greater than 10 mg/ml increase risk of phlebitis.)
**Rate of Administration** • Infuse over at least 1 hr (nephrotoxicity due to crystalluria and renal tubular damage may occur with too-rapid rate). • Maintain adequate hydration during infusion and for 2 hrs following IV administration. **Storage** • Store vials at room temperature. • Solutions of 50 mg/ml stable

for 12 hrs at room temperature; may form precipitate if refrigerated. • IV infusion (piggyback) stable for 24 hrs at room temperature.

**PO**
• May give without regard to food.
• Do not crush/break capsules. • Store capsules at room temperature.

**Topical**
(Ointment): • Avoid contact with eye.
• Use finger cot/rubber glove to prevent autoinoculation.
(Cream): • Apply to only cover cold sores or area with symptoms. • Rub until it disappears.

## ▦ IV INCOMPATIBILITIES

Aztreonam (Azactam), diltiazem (Cardizem), dobutamine (Dobutrex), dopamine (Intropin), levofloxacin (Levaquin), meropenem (Merrem IV), ondansetron (Zofran), piperacillin and tazobactam (Zosyn).

## ▦ IV COMPATIBILITIES

Allopurinol (Alloprim), amikacin (Amikin), ampicillin, cefazolin (Ancef), cefotaxime (Claforan), ceftazidime (Fortaz), ceftriaxone (Rocephin), cimetidine (Tagamet), clindamycin (Cleocin), diphenhydramine (Benadryl), famotidine (Pepcid), fluconazole (Diflucan), gentamicin, heparin, hydromorphone (Dilaudid), imipenem (Primaxin), lorazepam (Ativan), magnesium sulfate, methylprednisolone (Solu-Medrol), metoclopramide (Reglan), metronidazole (Flagyl), morphine, multivitamins, potassium chloride, propofol (Diprivan), ranitidine (Zantac), vancomycin.

## INDICATIONS/ROUTES/DOSAGE

**Genital Herpes (Initial Episode)**
**IV: ADULTS, ELDERLY, CHILDREN 12 YRS AND OLDER:** 5 mg/kg q8h for 5–7 days or 5–10 mg/kg q8h for 2–7 days.
**PO: ADULTS, ELDERLY, CHILDREN 12 YRS AND OLDER:** 200 mg q4h 5 times/day for 10 days or 400 mg 3 times/day for 7–10 days.

**CHILDREN YOUNGER THAN 12 YRS:** 40–80 mg/kg/day in 3–4 divided doses for 5–10 days. **Maximum:** 1 g/day.

**Topical: ADULTS:** (Ointment) ½ inch for 4-inch square surface q3h (6 times/day) for 7 days.

**Genital Herpes (Recurrent)**
**Intermittent Therapy**
**PO: ADULTS, ELDERLY, CHILDREN 12 YRS AND OLDER:** 200 mg q4h 5 times/day for 5 days or 400 mg 3 times/day for 5–10 days or 800 mg 2 times/day for 5 days or 800 mg 3 times/day for 2 days.

**Chronic Suppressive Therapy**
**PO: ADULTS, ELDERLY, CHILDREN 12 YRS AND OLDER:** 400 mg twice/day or 200 mg 3–5 times/day for up to 12 mos. **CHILDREN YOUNGER THAN 12 YRS:** 40–80 mg/kg/day in 3 divided doses. **Maximum:** 1 g/day.

**Herpes Simplex Mucocutaneous**
**PO: ADULTS, ELDERLY:** 400 mg 5 times/day for 7–14 days.
**IV: ADULTS, ELDERLY, CHILDREN 12 YRS AND OLDER:** 5 mg/kg/dose q8h for 7–14 days. **CHILDREN YOUNGER THAN 12 YRS:** 10 mg/kg q8h for 7–14 days.
**Topical: ADULTS:** (Ointment) ½ inch for 4-inch square surface q3h (6 times/day) for 7 days.

**Herpes Simplex Encephalitis**
**IV: ADULTS, ELDERLY, CHILDREN 12 YRS AND OLDER:** 10 mg/kg q8h for 10 days. **CHILDREN 3 MOS–YOUNGER THAN 12 YRS:** 20 mg/kg q8h for 10 days.

**Herpes Zoster (Shingles)**
**IV: ADULTS, CHILDREN 12 YRS AND OLDER:** (immunocompromised) 10 mg/kg/dose q8h for 7–10 days. **CHILDREN YOUNGER THAN 12 YRS:** (immunocompromised) 10 mg/kg/dose q8h for 7–10 days.
**PO: ADULTS, ELDERLY, CHILDREN 12 YRS AND OLDER:** 800 mg q4h 5 times/day for 7–10 days.

**Herpes Labialis (Cold Sores)**
**Topical: ADULTS, ELDERLY, CHILDREN 12 YRS AND OLDER:** Apply to affected area

5 times/day for 4 days. **Buccal Tablet:** 50 mg as a single dose to upper gum region.

**Varicella-Zoster (Chickenpox)**
**◄ ALERT ►** Begin treatment within 24 hrs of onset of rash.
**PO: ADULTS, ELDERLY, CHILDREN OLDER THAN 12 YRS AND CHILDREN 2–12 YRS, WEIGHING 40 KG OR MORE:** 800 mg 4 times/day for 5 days. **CHILDREN 2–12 YRS, WEIGHING LESS THAN 40 KG:** 20 mg/kg 4 times/day for 5 days. **Maximum:** 800 mg/dose.

**Usual Neonatal Dosage**
**HSV (treatment) (IV):** 20 mg/kg/dose q8h for 14–21 days.
**HSV (chronic suppression) (PO):** 300 mg/m²/dose q8h following IV therapy for 6 mos.
**Varicella-Zoster (IV):** 10–15 mg/kg/dose q8h for 5–10 days.

**Dosage in Renal Impairment**
Dosage and frequency are modified based on severity of infection and degree of renal impairment.
**PO:** Normal dose 200 mg q4h, 200 mg q8h, or 400 mg q12h.
**Creatinine clearance 10 ml/min and less:** 200 mg q12h.
**PO:** Normal dose 800 mg q4h.
**Creatinine clearance greater than 25 ml/min:** Give usual dose and at normal interval, 800 mg q4h. **Creatinine clearance 10–25 ml/min:** 800 mg q8h. **Creatinine clearance less than 10 ml/min:** 800 mg q12h.
**IV:**

| Creatinine Clearance | Dosage |
| --- | --- |
| Greater than 50 ml/min | 100% of normal q8h |
| 25–50 ml/min | 100% of normal q12h |
| 10–24 ml/min | 100% of normal q24h |
| Less than 10 ml/min | 50% of normal q24h |
| Hemodialysis (HD) | 2.5–5 mg/kg q24h (give after HD) |
| Peritoneal dialysis (PD) | 50% normal dose q24h |
| Continuous renal replacement therapy (CRRT) | 5–10 mg/kg q12–24h (q12h for viral meningoenphalitis/ VZV infection) |

**Dosage in Hepatic Impairment**

**Mild to Moderate Impairment:** No dose adjustment. **Severe Impairment:** Use caution.

## SIDE EFFECTS

**Frequent: Parenteral (9%–7%):** Phlebitis or inflammation at IV site, nausea, vomiting. **Topical (28%):** Burning, stinging. **Occasional: Parenteral (3%):** Pruritus, rash, urticaria. **PO (12%–6%):** Malaise, nausea. **Topical (4%):** Pruritus. **Rare: PO (3%–1%):** Vomiting, rash, diarrhea, headache. **Parenteral (2%–1%):** Confusion, hallucinations, seizures, tremors. **Topical (less than 1%):** Rash.

## ADVERSE EFFECTS/ TOXIC REACTIONS

Rapid parenteral administration, excessively high doses, or fluid and electrolyte imbalance may produce renal failure. Toxicity not reported with oral or topical use.

## NURSING CONSIDERATIONS

### BASELINE ASSESSMENT

Question for history of allergies, esp. to acyclovir. Assess herpes simplex lesions before treatment to compare baseline with treatment effect.

### INTERVENTION/EVALUATION

Assess IV site for phlebitis (heat, pain, red streaking over vein). Evaluate cutaneous lesions. Ensure adequate ventilation. Manage chickenpox and disseminated herpes zoster with strict isolation. Encourage fluid intake.

### PATIENT/FAMILY TEACHING

• Drink adequate fluids. • Do not touch lesions with bare fingers to prevent spreading infection to new site. • **Genital Herpes:** Continue therapy for full length of treatment. • Space doses evenly. • Use finger cot/rubber glove to apply topical ointment. • Avoid sexual intercourse during duration of lesions to prevent infecting partner. • Acyclovir does not cure herpes infections. • Pap smear should be done at least annually due to increased risk of cervical cancer in women with genital herpes.

## adalimumab                      TOP 100

a-da-**lim**-ue-mab
(Humira)

■ **BLACK BOX ALERT** ■ Increased risk for serious infections. Tuberculosis, invasive fungal infections, other opportunistic infections have occurred. Test for tuberculosis prior to and during treatment. Lymphoma, other malignancies reported in children/adolescents. Hepatosplenic T-cell lymphoma reported primarily in pts with Crohn's disease or ulcerative colitis and concomitant azathioprine or mercaptopurine.
**Do not confuse Humira with Humalog or Humulin, or adalimumab with belimumab or ipilimumab.**

## ◆CLASSIFICATION

**PHARMACOTHERAPEUTIC:** Monoclonal antibody. **CLINICAL:** Rheumatoid arthritis agent.

## USES

Reduces signs/symptoms, progression of structural damage and improves physical function in adults with moderate to severe RA. May be used alone or in combination with other disease-modifying antirheumatic drugs. First-line treatment of moderate to severe RA, treatment of psoriatic arthritis, treatment of ankylosing spondylitis, to induce/maintain remission of moderate to severe active Crohn's disease, moderate to severe plaque psoriasis in pts 6 yrs of age and older. Reduces signs and symptoms of moderate to severe active polyarticular juvenile rheumatoid arthritis in pts 2 yrs and older. Treatment of active ulcerative colitis in pts unresponsive to immunosuppressants. Treatment of moderate to severe hidradentis suppurativa. Treatment of uveitis (non-infectious intermediate, posterior and panuveitis) in adults.

## PRECAUTIONS

**Contraindications:** Hypersensitivity to adalimumab. Severe infections (e.g., sepsis, TB). **Cautions:** Pts with chronic infections (e.g., diabetes), elderly, predisposition to infections, decreased left ventricular function, HF, demyelinating disorders, invasive fungal infections.

## ACTION

Binds specifically to tumor necrosis factor (TNF) alpha cell, blocking its interaction with cell surface TNF receptors. **Therapeutic Effect:** Decreases signs/symptoms of RA, psoriatic arthritis, ankylosing spondylitis, Crohn's disease, ulcerative colitis. Inhibits progression of rheumatoid and psoriatic arthritis. Reduces epidermal thickness, inflammation of plaque psoriasis.

## PHARMACOKINETICS

**Half-life:** 10–20 days.

## ⌛ LIFESPAN CONSIDERATIONS

**Pregnancy/Lactation:** Unknown if distributed in breast milk. **Children:** Safety and efficacy not established. **Elderly:** Cautious use due to increased risk of serious infection and malignancy.

## INTERACTIONS

**DRUG: Abatacept, anakinra, immunosuppressive therapy** may increase risk of infections. May decrease efficacy of immune response with **live vaccines** (should not give concurrently). **HERBAL:** Echinacea may decrease effects. **FOOD:** None known. **LAB VALUES:** May increase serum cholesterol, other lipids, alkaline phosphatase.

## AVAILABILITY (Rx)

**Injection Solution:** 20 mg/0.4 ml, 40 mg/0.8 ml in prefilled syringes.

## ADMINISTRATION/HANDLING

**Subcutaneous**
• Refrigerate; do not freeze. • Discard unused portion. • Rotate injection sites. Give new injection at least 1 inch from an old site and never into area where skin is tender, bruised, red, or hard. • Give in thigh or lower abdomen. • Avoid areas within 2 inches of navel.

## INDICATIONS/ROUTES/DOSAGE

**Rheumatoid Arthritis (RA)**
**Subcutaneous: ADULTS, ELDERLY:** 40 mg every other wk. Dose may be increased to 40 mg/wk in pts not taking methotrexate.

**Ankylosing Spondylitis, Psoriatic Arthritis**
**Subcutaneous: ADULTS, ELDERLY:** 40 mg every other wk.

**Crohn's Disease**
**Subcutaneous: ADULTS, ELDERLY, CHILDREN 6 YRS AND OLDER WEIGHING 40 KG OR MORE:** Initially, 160 mg given as 4 injections on day 1 or 2 injections/day over 2 days, then 80 mg 2 wks later (day 15). **Maintenance:** 40 mg every other wk beginning at day 29. **CHILDREN 6 YRS AND OLDER WEIGHING 17–39 KG:** 80 mg (2 40-mg injections on day 1), then 40 mg 2 wks later. **Maintenance:** 20 mg every other wk beginning at day 29.

**Plaque Psoriasis, Uveitis**
**Subcutaneous: ADULTS, ELDERLY:** Initially, 80 mg as a single dose, then 40 mg every other wk starting 1 wk after initial dose.

**Juvenile Rheumatoid Arthritis**
**Subcutaneous: CHILDREN 2 YRS AND OLDER, WEIGHING 10–14 KG:** 10 mg every other wk. **WEIGHING 15–29 KG:** 20 mg every other wk. **WEIGHING 30 KG OR MORE:** 40 mg every other wk.

**Ulcerative Colitis**
**Subcutaneous: ADULTS, ELDERLY:** Initially, 160 mg (4 injections in 1 day or 2 injections over 2 days) then 80 mg 2 wks later (day 15), then 40 mg every other wk beginning on day 29.

**Hidradentis Suppurativa**
**Subcutaneous: ADULTS, ELDERLY:** Initially, 160 mg (4 injections day 1) or 80 mg (2 injections on days 1 and 2), then 80 mg 2 wks later (day 15), then 40 mg weekly beginning day 29.

**Dosage in Renal/Hepatic Impairment**
No dose adjustment.

## SIDE EFFECTS

**Frequent (20%):** Injection site erythema, pruritus, pain, swelling. **Occasional (12%–9%):** Headache, rash, sinusitis, nausea. **Rare (7%–5%):** Abdominal or back pain, hypertension.

## ADVERSE EFFECTS/ TOXIC REACTIONS

Hypersensitivity reactions (rash, urticaria, hypotension, dyspnea), infections (primarily upper respiratory tract, bronchitis, urinary tract) occur rarely. May increase risk of serious infections (pneumonia, tuberculosis, cellulitis, pyelonephritis, septic arthritis).

## NURSING CONSIDERATIONS

### BASELINE ASSESSMENT

Assess onset, type, location, duration of pain or inflammation. Inspect appearance of affected joints for immobility, deformities, skin condition. If pt is to self-administer, instruct on subcutaneous injection technique, including areas of the body acceptable for injection sites.

### INTERVENTION/EVALUATION

Monitor lab values, particularly CBC. Assess for therapeutic response: relief of pain, stiffness, swelling; increased joint mobility; reduced joint tenderness; improved grip strength.

### PATIENT/FAMILY TEACHING

• Injection site reaction generally occurs in first month of treatment and decreases in frequency during continued therapy. • Do not receive live vaccines during treatment. Report rash, nausea.

# adefovir

a-**def**-o-veer
(Hepsera)
■ **BLACK BOX ALERT** ■ May cause HIV resistance in unrecognized or untreated HIV infection. Lactic acidosis, severe hepatomegaly with steatosis (fatty liver), acute exacerbation of hepatitis have occurred. Use with caution in pts with renal dysfunction or in pts at risk for renal toxicity.

## ◆CLASSIFICATION

**PHARMACOTHERAPEUTIC:** Antiviral. **CLINICAL:** Hepatitis B agent.

## USES

Treatment of chronic hepatitis B virus infection in adults with evidence of active viral replication based on persistent elevations of serum ALT or AST or histologic evidence.

## PRECAUTIONS

**Contraindications:** Hypersensitivity to adefovir. **Cautions:** Pts with known risk factors for hepatic disease (female gender, obesity, prolonged treatment), renal impairment, elderly. Concurrent administration with tenofovir-containing products.

## ACTION

Interferes with hepatitis B viral RNA-dependent DNA polymerase, an enzyme, causing DNA chain termination after its incorporation into viral DNA. **Therapeutic Effect:** Prevents viral cell replication.

## PHARMACOKINETICS

Rapidly converted to adefovir in intestine. Binds to proteins after PO administration. Protein binding: less than 4%. Excreted in urine. **Half-life:** 7 hrs (increased in renal impairment).

## ⌛ LIFESPAN CONSIDERATIONS

**Pregnancy/Lactation:** Unknown if drug crosses placenta or is distributed in breast milk. **Children:** Safety and efficacy not established. **Elderly:** Age-related renal impairment, decreased cardiac function requires cautious use.

## INTERACTIONS

**DRUG: Nephrotoxic agents, (e.g., IV contrast dye, vancomycin), NSAIDs** may increase risk of renal toxicity. May alter effects of **tenofovir** (avoid concomitant use). **HERBAL:** None significant. **FOOD: Alcohol** may increase risk of hepatotoxicity. **LAB VALUES:** May increase serum ALT, AST, amylase.

## AVAILABILITY (Rx)

**Tablets:** 10 mg.

## ADMINISTRATION/HANDLING

**PO**
• Give without regard to food.

## INDICATIONS/ROUTES/DOSAGE

**Chronic Hepatitis B (Normal Renal Function)**
**PO: ADULTS, ELDERLY, CHILDREN 12 YRS AND OLDER:** 10 mg once daily.

**Chronic Hepatitis B (Impaired Renal Function)**
**PO: ADULTS, ELDERLY WITH CREATININE CLEARANCE 20–49 ML/MIN:** 10 mg q48h. **ADULTS, ELDERLY WITH CREATININE CLEARANCE 10–19 ML/MIN:** 10 mg q72h. **ADULTS, ELDERLY ON HEMODIALYSIS:** 10 mg every 7 days following dialysis.

**Dosage in Hepatic Impairment**
No adjustment needed.

## SIDE EFFECTS

**Frequent (13%):** Asthenia. **Occasional (9%–4%):** Headache, abdominal pain, nausea, flatulence. **Rare (3%):** Diarrhea, dyspepsia.

## ADVERSE EFFECTS/ TOXIC REACTIONS

Nephrotoxicity, characterized by increased serum creatinine and decreased serum phosphorus levels, is treatment-limiting toxicity of adefovir therapy. Lactic acidosis, severe hepatomegaly occur rarely, particularly in female pts.

## NURSING CONSIDERATIONS

### BASELINE ASSESSMENT

Obtain baseline renal function lab values before therapy begins and routinely thereafter. Pts with renal insufficiency, preexisting or during treatment, may require dose adjustment. HIV antibody testing should be performed before therapy begins (unrecognized or untreated HIV infection may result in emergence of HIV resistance).

### INTERVENTION/EVALUATION

Monitor I&O. Closely monitor for adverse reactions in those taking other medications that are excreted renally or with other drugs known to affect renal function.

### PATIENT/FAMILY TEACHING

• Report nausea, vomiting, abdominal pain. • Avoid alcohol.

# adenosine

ah-**den**-oh-seen
(Adenocard, Adenoscan)

## ◆CLASSIFICATION

**PHARMACOTHERAPEUTIC:** Cardiac agent, diagnostic aid. **CLINICAL:** Antiarrhythmic.

## USES

**Adenocard:** Treatment of paroxysmal supraventricular tachycardia (PSVT), including pts associated with accessory bypass tracts (Wolff-Parkinson-White syndrome). **Adenoscan:** Adjunct in diagnosis in myocardial perfusion imaging or stress echocardiography. **OFF-LABEL:** Acute vasodilator testing in pulmonary artery hypertension.

## PRECAUTIONS

**Contraindications:** Hypersensitivity to adenosine. Second- or third-degree AV block, symptomatic bradycardia, sick sinus syndrome (except in pts with functioning pacemaker). Bronchoconstrictive or bronchospastic lung disease, asthma.

**Cautions:** Pts with first-degree AV block, bundle branch block; concurrent use of drugs that slow AV conduction (e.g., digoxin, verapamil); autonomic dysfunction, pericarditis, pleural effusion, carotid stenosis, uncorrected hypovolemia; elderly, pts with bronchoconstriction.

## ACTION

Slows impulse formation in SA node and conduction time through AV node. Acts as a diagnostic aid in myocardial perfusion imaging or stress echocardiography by causing coronary vasodilation and increased blood flow. **Therapeutic Effect:** Restores normal sinus rhythm.

## INTERACTIONS

**DRUG: Methylxanthines (e.g., theophylline)** may decrease effect. **Dipyridamole, nicotine** may increase effect. **Carbamazepine** may increase degree of heart block caused by adenosine. **HERBAL:** None significant. **FOOD:** Avoid **caffeine** (may decrease effect). **LAB VALUES:** None significant.

## AVAILABILITY (Rx)

**Injection Solution (Adenocard):** 3 mg/ml in 2-ml, 4-ml vials. **Injection Solution (Adenoscan):** 3 mg/ml in 20-ml, 30-ml vials.

## ADMINISTRATION/HANDLING

 **IV**

**Rate of Administration** • Administer very rapidly (over 1–2 sec) undiluted directly into vein, or if using IV line, use closest port to insertion site. If IV line is infusing any fluid other than 0.9% NaCl, flush line first. • After rapid bolus injection, follow with 0.9% NaCl rapid flush.
**Storage** • Store at room temperature. Solution appears clear. • Crystallization occurs if refrigerated; if crystallization occurs, dissolve crystals by warming to room temperature. • Discard unused portion.

## ▦ IV INCOMPATIBILITIES

Any drug or solution other than 0.9% NaCl, $D_5W$, Ringer's lactate, or abciximab.

## INDICATIONS/ROUTES/DOSAGE

**Paroxysmal Supraventricular Tachycardia (PSVT) (Adenocard)**
**Rapid IV Bolus: ADULTS, ELDERLY, CHILDREN WEIGHING 50 KG OR MORE:** Initially, 6 mg given over 1–2 sec. If first dose does not convert within 1–2 min, give 12 mg; may repeat 12-mg dose in 1–2 min if no response has occurred. Follow each dose with 20 ml 0.9% NaCl by rapid IV push. **CHILDREN WEIGHING LESS THAN 50 KG:** Initially 0.05–0.1 mg/kg. If first dose does not convert within 1–2 min, may increase dose by 0.05–0.1 mg/kg. May repeat until sinus rhythm is established or up to a maximum single dose of 0.3 mg/kg or 12 mg. Follow each dose with 5–10 ml 0.9% NaCl by rapid IV push.

**Diagnostic Testing (Adenoscan)**
**IV Infusion: ADULTS:** 140 mcg/kg/min for 6 min using syringe or infusion pump. Total dose: 840 mcg/kg. Thallium is injected at midpoint (3 min) of infusion.

**Dosage in Renal/Hepatic Impairment**
No dose adjustment.

## SIDE EFFECTS

**Frequent (18%–12%):** Facial flushing, dyspnea. **Occasional (7%–2%):** Headache, nausea, light-headedness, chest pressure. **Rare (1% or less):** Paresthesia, dizziness, diaphoresis, hypotension, palpitations; chest, jaw, or neck pain.

## ADVERSE EFFECTS/ TOXIC REACTIONS

Frequently produces transient, short-lasting heart block.

## NURSING CONSIDERATIONS

### BASELINE ASSESSMENT

Identify arrhythmia per cardiac monitor, 12-lead EKG, and assess apical pulse.

### INTERVENTION/EVALUATION

Assess cardiac performance per continuous EKG. Monitor B/P, apical pulse (rate, rhythm, quality). Auscultate pt breath sounds for clarity. Monitor respiratory rate. Monitor I&O; assess for fluid retention. Monitor serum electrolytes.

### PATIENT/FAMILY TEACHING

• May induce feelings of impending doom, which resolves quickly. • Flushing/headache may occur temporarily following administration. • Report continued chest pain, lightheadedness, head or neck pain, difficulty breathing.

# ado-trastuzumab

ado-tras-**tooz**-oo-mab
(Kadcyla)

■ **BLACK BOX ALERT** ■ Do not substitute ado-trastuzumab for trastuzumab. Hepatotoxicity, hepatic failure may lead to death. Monitor hepatic function prior to each dose. May decrease left ventricular ejection fraction (LVEF). Embryo-fetal toxicity may result in birth defects and/or fetal demise.

**Do not confuse ado-trastuzumab with trastuzumab.**

## ◆CLASSIFICATION

**PHARMACOTHERAPEUTIC:** HER2-targeted antibody and microtubule inhibitor conjugate. **CLINICAL:** Antineoplastic.

## USES

Treatment of HER2-positive, metastatic breast cancer in pts who have previously received trastuzumab and a taxane agent separately or in combination, or pts who have developed recurrence within 6 mos of completing adjuvant therapy.

## PRECAUTIONS

**Contraindications:** Hypersensitivity to trastuzumab. **Cautions:** History of cardiomyopathy, HF, MI, arrhythmias, hepatic disease, thrombocytopenia, pulmonary disease, peripheral neuropathy, pregnancy.

## ACTION

Inhibits proliferation of tumor cells that overexpress human epidermal growth factor receptor 2 (HER2). Promotes cellular death (apoptosis) by mediating release of cytotoxic catabolytes. Disrupts cellular microtubule networks. **Therapeutic Effect:** Inhibits tumor cell survival in HER2-positive breast cancer.

## PHARMACOKINETICS

Metabolized in liver. Protein binding: 93%. Peak plasma concentration: 30–90 min. **Half-life:** 4 days.

## ⌛ LIFESPAN CONSIDERATIONS

**Pregnancy/Lactation:** May cause fetal harm. Use contraception during treatment and up to 6 mos after discontinuation. Unknown if distributed in breast milk. Do not breastfeed. **Children:** Safety and efficacy not established. **Elderly:** No age-related precautions noted.

## INTERACTIONS

**DRUG:** CYP3A4 inhibitors (e.g., ketoconazole, ritonavir) may increase concentration/effect. **HERBAL:** None significant. **FOOD:** None known. **LAB VALUES:** May increase serum ALT, AST, bilirubin. May decrease platelets, serum potassium.

## AVAILABILITY (Rx)

**Lyophilized Powder for Injection:** 100-mg vial, 160-mg vial.

## ADMINISTRATION/HANDLING

◀**ALERT**▶ Use 0.22-micron in-line filter. Do not administer IV push or bolus.

🖐 IV

**Reconstitution** • Use proper chemotherapy precautions. • Slowly inject 5 ml of Sterile Water for Injection into 100 mg vial or 8 ml Sterile Water for Injection for 160 mg vial. • Final concentration: 20 mg/ml. • Gently swirl until completely dissolved. • Do not shake. • Inspect for particulate

---

matter/discoloration. • Calculate dose from 20 mg/ml vial. • Further dilute in 250 ml of 0.9% NaCl only. • Invert bag to mix (do not shake).

**Rate of Administration** • Infuse using 0.22-micron in-line filter. • Infuse initial dose over 90 min. • Infuse subsequent doses over 30 min. • Slow or interrupt infusion rate if hypersensitivity reaction occurs.

**Storage** • Refrigerate unused vials. • Reconstituted vials, diluted solutions should be used immediately (may be refrigerated for up to 24 hrs).

### ▨ IV INCOMPATIBILITIES

Do not use dextrose-containing solutions.

### INDICATIONS/ROUTES/DOSAGE

**Note:** Do not substitute with conventional trastuzumab (Herceptin).

**Metastatic Breast Cancer**
**IV Infusion: ADULTS/ELDERLY:** 3.6 mg/kg every 3 wks until disease progression or unacceptable toxicity.

**Dose Modification**
*Reduction Schedule for Adverse Effects:*
Initial dose: 3.6 mg/kg. First reduction: 3 mg/kg. Second reduction: 2.4 mg/kg. **Increased ALT, AST:** If less than 5 times upper limit of normal (ULN), continue same dose. If 5–20 times ULN, hold until less than 5 times ULN and reduce by one dose level. If greater than 20 times ULN, discontinue. **Increased Bilirubin:** Hold until less than 1.5 times ULN, then continue same dose. If 3–10 times ULN, hold until less than 1.5 times ULN, then reduce by one dose level. If greater than 10 times ULN, discontinue. **Left Ventricular Dysfunction:** If LVEF greater than 45%, continue same dose. If LVEF 40%–45% with a decrease less than 10% from baseline, continue dose (or reduce) and repeat LVEF in 3 wks. If LVEF 40%–45% with decrease greater than 10% from baseline, hold and repeat assessment in 3 wks. Discontinue therapy if no recovery within 10% of baseline, LVEF less than 40%, or symptomatic HF. **Thrombocytopenia:**

If platelet count is 25,000 mm³–50,000 mm³, hold until level greater than 75,000 mm³ and then continue same dose. If platelet count is less than 25,000 mm³, hold until level greater than 75,000 mm³ and reduce one dose level.

**Dosage in Renal/Hepatic Impairment**
No dose adjustment.

### SIDE EFFECTS

**Frequent (40%–21%):** Nausea, fatigue, musculoskeletal pain, headache, constipation, diarrhea. **Occasional (19%–7%):** Abdominal pain, vomiting, pyrexia, arthralgia, asthenia, cough, dry mouth, stomatitis, myalgia, insomnia, rash, dizziness, dyspepsia, chills, dysgeusia, peripheral edema. **Rare (6%–3%):** Pruritus, blurry vision, dry eye, conjunctivitis, lacrimation.

### ADVERSE EFFECTS/ TOXIC REACTIONS

Hepatotoxicity may include elevated transaminase, nodular regenerative hyperplasia, portal hypertension. Left ventricular dysfunction reported in 1.8% of pts. Interstitial lung disease (ILD), including pneumonitis, may lead to ARDS. Hypersensitivity reactions reported in 1.4% of pts. Thrombocytopenia (34% of pts) may increase risk of bleeding. Peripheral neuropathy observed rarely. Approx. 5.3% of pts tested positive for anti–ado-trastuzumab antibodies (immunogenicity).

### NURSING CONSIDERATIONS

#### BASELINE ASSESSMENT

Obtain baseline CBC, BMP, PT/INR if on anticoagulants. Confirm HER2-positive titer. Screen for baseline HF, hepatic impairment, peripheral edema, pulmonary disease, thrombocytopenia. Obtain negative pregnancy test before initiating treatment. Question current breastfeeding status. Obtain baseline echocardiogram for LVEF status.

#### INTERVENTION/EVALUATION

Observe for hypersensitivity reactions during infusion. Monitor LFT, potassium levels before and during treatment. Obtain LVEF q3mos or with any dose reduction regarding LVEF status. Assess for bruising, jaundice, right upper quadrant (RUQ) abdominal pain. Obtain anti–ado-trastuzumab antibody titer if immunogenicity suspected. Obtain stat EKG for palpitations or irregular pulse, chest X-ray for difficulty breathing, cough, fever. Monitor for neurotoxicity (peripheral neuropathy).

### PATIENT/FAMILY TEACHING

• Blood levels will be monitored routinely. • Avoid pregnancy. • Contraception should be used during treatment and up to 6 mos after discontinuation. • Report black/tarry stools, RUQ abdominal pain, nausea, bruising, yellowing of skin or eyes, difficulty breathing, palpitations, bleeding. • Avoid alcohol. • Treatment may reduce the heart's ability to pump; expect routine echocardiograms. • Report bleeding of any kind or extremity numbness, tingling, weakness, pain.

# afatinib

a-**fa**-ti-nib
(Gilotrif)
**Do not confuse afatinib with ibrutinib, dasatinib, gefitinib, or sunitinib.**

### ◆ CLASSIFICATION

**PHARMACOTHERAPEUTIC:** Kinase inhibitor. **CLINICAL:** Antineoplastic.

## USES

First-line treatment of metastatic non–small cell lung cancer (NSCLC) in pts with epidermal growth factor (EDGF) exon 19 deletions or exon 21 (L858R) substitution mutations. Treatment of metastatic, squamous NSCLC progressing after platinum-based chemotherapy.

## PRECAUTIONS

**Contraindications:** Hypersensitivity to afatinib. **Cautions:** Hepatic impairment; severe renal impairment; pts with hx of keratitis, severe dry eye, ulcerative keratitis, or wearing contact lens; hypovolemia; pulmonary disease; ulcerative lesions. Patients with GI disorders associated with diarrhea (e.g., Crohn's disease), cardiac risk factors, and/or decreased left ventricular ejection fraction.

## ACTION

Highly selective blocker of ErbB family (e.g., HER2), irreversibly binds to intracellular tyrosine kinase domain. **Therapeutic Effect:** Inhibits tumor growth, causes tumor regression.

## PHARMACOKINETICS

Readily absorbed following PO administration. Enzymatic metabolism is minimal. Protein binding: 95%. Peak plasma concentration: 2–5 hrs. Excreted in feces (85%), urine (4%). **Half-life:** 37 hrs.

## ⧗ LIFESPAN CONSIDERATIONS

**Pregnancy/Lactation:** May cause fetal harm. Unknown if distributed in breast milk. Must either discontinue drug or discontinue breastfeeding. Contraception recommended during treatment and up to 2 wks after discontinuation. **Children:** Safety and efficacy not established. **Elderly:** No age-related precautions noted.

## INTERACTIONS

**DRUG: P-glycoprotein inhibitors (e.g., amiodarone, cyclosporine, ketoconazole)** may increase concentration/effect. **P-glycoprotein inducers (e.g., carbamazepine, rifampin)** may decrease concentration/effect. **HERBAL:** None significant. **FOOD: High-fat meals** may decrease absorption. **LAB VALUES:** May increase serum ALT, AST. May decrease serum potassium.

## AVAILABILITY (Rx)

**Tablets:** 20 mg, 30 mg, 40 mg.

---

## ADMINISTRATION/HANDLING

### PO

• Give at least 1 hr before or 2 hrs after meal. Do not take missed dose within 12 hrs of next dose.

## INDICATIONS/ROUTES/DOSAGE

### Non–Small Cell Lung Cancer

**PO: ADULTS/ELDERLY:** Initially, 40 mg once daily until disease progression or no longer tolerated. Do not take missed dose within 12 hrs of next dose.

### Dose Modification

**Chronic Use of P-glycoprotein (P-gp) Inhibitors:** Reduce daily dose by 10 mg if tolerated. Resume previous dose after discontinuation of inhibitor if tolerated. **Chronic Use of P-glycoprotein Inducers:** Increase daily dose by 10 mg if tolerated. May resume initial dose 2–3 days after discontinuation of P-gp inducer. **Moderate to Severe Diarrhea (more than 48 hrs):** Withhold dose until resolution to mild diarrhea. **Moderate Cutaneous Skin Reaction (more than 7 days):** Withhold dose until reaction resolves, then reduce dose appropriately. **Suspected Keratitis:** Withhold until appropriately ruled out. If keratitis confirmed, continue only if benefits outweigh risks.

### Permanent Discontinuation

Discontinue if persistent severe diarrhea, respiratory distress, severe dry eye, or life-threatening bullous, blistering, exfoliating lesions, persistent ulcerative keratitis, interstitial lung disease, symptomatic left ventricular dysfunction occurs.

### Dosage in Renal/Hepatic Impairment

No dose adjustment. **Severe Impairment:** Avoid use.

## SIDE EFFECTS

**Frequent (96%–58%):** Diarrhea, rash, dermatitis, stomatitis, paronychia (nail infection). **Occasional (31%–11%):** Dry skin, decreased appetite, pruritus, epistaxis, weight loss, cystitis, pyrexia, cheilitis (lip inflammation), rhinorrhea, conjunctivitis.

## ADVERSE EFFECTS/ TOXIC REACTIONS

Diarrhea may lead to severe, sometimes fatal, dehydration or renal impairment. Bullous and exfoliative skin lesions occur rarely. Rash, erythema, acneiform lesions occur in 90% of pts. Palmar-plantar erythrodysesthesia syndrome (PPES), a chemotherapy-induced skin condition that presents with redness, swelling, numbness, skin sloughing of the hands and feet, has been reported. Interstitial lung disease (ILD), including pulmonary infiltration, pneumonitis, ARDS, allergic alveolitis, reported in 2% of pts. Hepatotoxicity reported in 10% of pts. Keratitis such as eye inflammation, lacrimation, light sensitivity, blurred vision, red eye occur in 1% of pts.

## NURSING CONSIDERATIONS

### BASELINE ASSESSMENT

Obtain baseline CBC, BMP, visual acuity. Obtain negative pregnancy test before initiating therapy. Question current breastfeeding status. Screen for history/co-morbidities, contact lens use. Receive full medication history including herbal products. Assess skin for lesions, ulcers, open wounds.

### INTERVENTION/EVALUATION

Monitor renal/hepatic function tests, urine output. Encourage PO intake. Assess for hydration status. Offer antidiarrheal medication for loose stool. Report oliguria, dark or concentrated urine. Immediately report skin lesions, vision changes, dry eye, severe diarrhea. Obtain chest X-ray if ILD suspected.

### PATIENT/FAMILY TEACHING

• Most pts experience diarrhea and severe cases may lead to dehydration or kidney failure; maintain adequate hydration. • Avoid pregnancy; contraception should be used during treatment and up to 2 wks after discontinuation. • Report any yellowing of skin or eyes, abdominal pain, bruising, black/tarry stools, dark urine, decreased urine output. • Minimize exposure to sunlight. • Immediately report eye problems (pain, swelling, blurred vision, vision changes) or skin blistering/redness. • Do not eat 1 hr before or 2 hrs after dose. • Do not wear contact lenses (may increase risk of keratitis).

# albiglutide

al-bi-**gloo**-tide
(Tanzeum)

■ **BLACK BOX ALERT** ■ Thyroid C-cell tumors have occurred in animal studies with glucagon-like peptide-1 (GLP-1) receptor agonists; unknown if relevant in humans.
**Do not confuse albiglutide with exenatide, dulaglutide, or liraglutide.**

## ◆CLASSIFICATION

**PHARMACOTHERAPEUTIC:** Glucagon-like peptide-1 (GLP-1) receptor agonist. **CLINICAL:** Antidiabetic.

## USES

Adjunct to diet and exercise to improve glycemic controls in pts with type 2 diabetes mellitus.

## PRECAUTIONS

**Contraindications:** Personal/family history of medullary thyroid carcinoma. Pts with multiple endocrine neoplasia syndrome type 2. Hypersensitivity to albiglutide. **Cautions:** Pts with hx pancreatitis, renal impairment. Not recommended in pts with preexisting severe GI disease, diabetic ketoacidosis; type 1 diabetes mellitus; pancreatitis; or as a first-line treatment regimen.

## ACTION

Agonist of human glucagon-like peptide-1 (GLP-1). Increases glucose-dependent insulin secretion, decreases inappropriate glucagon secretion. Slows gastric emptying. **Therapeutic Effect:** Augments glucose-dependent insulin secretion.

## PHARMACOKINETICS

Metabolized by protein degradation into small peptides, amino acids by proteolytic enzymes. Protein binding: Not specified. Peak plasma concentration: 3–5 days. Steady state reached in 4–5 wks. **Half-life:** 5 days.

## ⧗ LIFESPAN CONSIDERATIONS

**Pregnancy/Lactation:** Likely distributed in breast milk; drug is albumin-based protein therapeutic. Must either discontinue drug or discontinue breastfeeding. Due to extended clearance period, recommend discontinuation of therapy at least 1 mo before planned pregnancy. **Children:** Safety and efficacy not established in pts younger than 18 yrs. **Elderly:** No age-related precautions noted.

## INTERACTIONS

**DRUG: Insulin, metformin, sulfonylureas** may increase hypoglycemic effect. May decrease effect of **PO drugs requiring rapid onset** due to delayed gastric emptying. **HERBAL:** Fenugreek, flaxseed, ginseng, gotu kola may increase risk of hypoglycemia. **FOOD:** None known. **LAB VALUES:** Expended to decrease serum glucose, Hgb A1c. May increase serum ALT, GGT.

## AVAILABILITY (Rx)

**Pre-filled Injector Pens:** 30 mg, 50 mg.

## ADMINISTRATION/HANDLING
### Subcutaneous

• Administer any time of day, without regard to meals, on same day each week. May change administration day if last dose was given more than 4 days ago. If dose is missed, administer within 3 days of missed dose. If more than 3 days pass after missed dose, wait until next regularly scheduled dose. • If refrigerated, allow pen to sit at room temperature for 15 min before using.

---

✦ Canadian trade name     🗡 Non-Crushable Drug     🔲 High Alert drug

**Reconstitution** • Hold pen body with clear cartridge pointing up to see the [1] in number window. • Check expiration date. • Twist clear cartridge on pen in direction of arrow until pen is felt/heard to "click" into place and the [2] is seen in number window; this will mix diluent and lyophilized powder.

**Patient Instruction for Reconstitution** • Slowly and gently rock pen side to side 5 times to mix. • Avoid shaking; may cause foaming and alter desired dose. • Wait 15 min for 30-mg pen or 30 min for 50-mg pen to ensure solution is mixed. • After waiting, slowly and gently rock pen side-to-side 5 additional times to finalize full reconstitution. • Visually inspect solution for particulate matter in viewing window.

**Professional Healthcare Instruction for Reconstitution:** • Hold pen with clear cartridge pointing up and maintain upward orientation throughout reconstitution. • Gently swirl pen in small circular motion for at least 1 min. • Avoid shaking; may cause foaming and alter desired dose. • Inspect solution and, if needed, continue to gently swirl pen until fully dissolved and free of all particles (2–5 min for 30-mg pen or 7–10 min for 50-mg pen). • A small amount of foaming on top of solution at end of reconstitution is normal. • Verify solution is yellow in color.

**Preparation**
• Holding pen upright, attach needle • Gently tap clear cartridge to bring large bubbles to top. • Remove air bubbles by slowly twisting pen until the [3] is seen in number window. • At same time, injection button will automatically release from bottom of pen.

**Administration**
• Subcutaneously insert needle into abdomen, thigh, or upper arm region. • Press injection button until "click" is heard, then hold button for additional 5 sec to deliver full dose. • Do not reuse needle. • Rotate injection sites.

**Storage**
• Mixed solution should appear yellow; free of all particles. • Use within 8 hrs of reconstitution. • Once needle is attached, use immediately; product can clog needle if allowed to dry after priming. • Refrigerate unused pens; do not freeze. • Once dispensed, may store pen at room temperature up to 4 wks.

## INDICATIONS/ROUTES/DOSAGE

**Type 2 Diabetes Mellitus**
**Subcutaneous: ADULTS/ELDERLY:** 30 mg once weekly into abdomen, thigh, or upper arm region. May increase to 50 mg once weekly if glycemic response inadequate. **Missed Dose:** Administer within 3 days after missed dose, then resume on usual day of administration. If longer than 3 days, skip missed dose and resume administration on next regular weekly dose.

*Dose Modification*
**Concomitant Use with Insulin Secretagogue (e.g., Sulfonylurea) or Insulin:** Consider reduced dose based on glycemic goal.

**Dosage in Renal/Hepatic Impairment**
No dose adjustment.

## SIDE EFFECTS

**Occasional (14%–5%):** Upper respiratory tract infection, diarrhea, nausea, injection site reactions (hematoma, erythema, rash), cough, back pain, arthralgia, sinusitis, influenza. **Rare (3%–2%):** Dyspepsia, vomiting, gastric reflux.

## ADVERSE EFFECTS/TOXIC REACTIONS

May increase risk of acute renal failure or worsening of chronic renal impairment (esp. with dehydration), severe gastroparesis, thyroid C-cell tumors. May increase risk of hypoglycemia when used with other hypoglycemic agents or insulin. Dyspnea, pruritus, rash may indicate hypersensitivity reaction. Other adverse events include appendicitis (0.3% of pts), atrial fibrillation/flutter (1% of pts), pancreatitis

(0.3% of pts), pneumonia (1.8% of pts). Immunogenicity (anti-alglutide antibody formation) reported in 5.5% of pts. Some pts with antibody formation also tested positive for antibodies to GLP-1 and human albumin. May cause increased risk of hepatic injury (elevated LFT).

## NURSING CONSIDERATIONS

### BASELINE ASSESSMENT

Obtain baseline fasting glucose level, Hgb A1c; BMP, LFT if applicable. Question history of medullary thyroid carcinoma, multiple neoplasia syndrome type 2, pancreatitis. Receive full medication history including herbal products. Screen for use of other hypoglycemic agents or insulin. Assess pt's understanding of diabetes management, routine home glucose monitoring. Assess hydration status.

### INTERVENTION/EVALUATION

Monitor capillary blood glucose levels, Hgb A1c; hepatic/renal function in pts with renal impairment reporting severe gastrointestinal reactions including gastroparesis, vomiting, diarrhea. Screen for thyroid tumors (dysphagia, dyspnea, persistent hoarseness, neck mass). If tumor is suspected, consider endocrinologist consultation. Clinical significance of serum calcitonin level or thyroid ultrasound with GLP-1-associated thyroid tumors is debated/unknown. Assess for hypoglycemia, hyperglycemia, hypersensitivity/allergic reaction. Screen for glucose-altering conditions: fever, stress, surgical procedures, trauma. Obtain dietary consult for nutritional education. Encourage PO intake.

### PATIENT/FAMILY TEACHING

• Diabetes mellitus requires lifelong control. Diet and exercise are principal parts of treatment; do not skip or delay meals. Test blood sugar regularly. • When taking additional medications to lower blood sugar or when glucose demands are altered (fever, infection, stress trauma), have low blood sugar treatment available (glucagon, oral dextrose). • Monitor daily calorie intake. • Report suspected pregnancy or plans of breastfeeding. • Therapy may increase risk of thyroid cancer; report lumps or swelling of the neck, hoarseness, trouble swallowing, shortness of breath. • Persistent, severe abdominal pain that radiates to the back (with or without vomiting) may indicate acute pancreatitis. • Rash, itching, hives may indicate allergic reaction.

# albumin, human

al-**bue**-min
(Albuked-5, Albuked-25, Albuminar-5, Albuminar-25, AlbuRx, Albutein, Buminate, Flexbumin, Plasbumin-5, Plasbumin-25)
**Do not confuse albumin with albuterol, or Buminate with bumetanide.**

## ◆CLASSIFICATION

**PHARMACOTHERAPEUTIC:** Plasma protein fraction. **CLINICAL:** Blood derivative.

## USES

Hypovolemia plasma volume expansion, maintenance of cardiac output in treatment of shock or impending shock. May be useful in treatment of severe burns, adult respiratory distress syndrome (ARDS), cardiopulmonary bypass, hemodialysis. **OFF-LABEL:** Large-volume paracentesis. In cirrhotics, with diuretics to help facilitate diuresis.

## PRECAUTIONS

**Contraindications:** Hypersensitivity to albumin. Pts at risk for volume overload (e.g., severe anemia, HF). Dilution with sterile water for injection. **Cautions:** Pts for whom sodium restriction is necessary, hepatic/renal failure (added protein load). Avoid 25% concentration in preterm infants (risk of intraventricular hemorrhage).

---

✦ Canadian trade name          ⚒ Non-Crushable Drug          🔲 High Alert drug

## ACTION

Blood volume expander. **Therapeutic Effect:** Provides increase in intravascular oncotic pressure, mobilizes fluids into intravascular space.

## PHARMACOKINETICS

| Route | Onset | Peak | Duration |
|-------|-------|------|----------|
| IV | 15 min (in well-hydrated pt) | N/A | Dependent on initial blood volume |

Distributed throughout extracellular fluid. **Half-life:** 15–20 days.

## ☒ LIFESPAN CONSIDERATIONS

**Pregnancy/Lactation:** Unknown if drug crosses placenta or is distributed in breast milk. **Children/Elderly:** No age-related precautions noted.

## INTERACTIONS

**DRUG:** None significant. **HERBAL:** None significant. **FOOD:** None known. **LAB VALUES:** May increase serum alkaline phosphatase.

## AVAILABILITY (Rx)

**Injection Solution: (5%):** 50 ml, 250 ml, 500 ml. **(25%):** 20 ml, 50 ml, 100 ml.

## ADMINISTRATION/HANDLING

 IV

**Reconstitution** • A 5% solution may be made from 25% solution by adding 1 volume 25% to 4 volumes 0.9% NaCl (NaCl preferred). Do not use Sterile Water for Injection (life-threatening hemolysis, acute renal failure can result).
**Rate of Administration** • Give by IV infusion. Rate is variable, depending on use, blood volume, concentration of solute. 5%: Do not exceed 2–4 ml/min in pts with normal plasma volume, 5–10 ml/min in pts with hypoproteinemia. 25%: Do not exceed 1 ml/min in pts with normal plasma volume, 2–3 ml/min in pts with hypoproteinemia. 5% is administered undiluted; 25% may be administered undiluted or

diluted in 0.9% NaCl. • May give without regard to pt blood group or Rh factor.
**Storage** • Store at room temperature. Appears as clear, brownish, odorless, moderately viscous fluid. • Do not use if solution has been frozen, appears turbid, contains sediment, or if not used within 4 hrs of opening vial.

## ▩ IV INCOMPATIBILITIES

Lipids, micafungin (Mycamine), midazolam (Versed), vancomycin (Vancocin), verapamil (Isoptin).

## ▩ IV COMPATIBILITIES

Diltiazem (Cardizem), lorazepam (Ativan).

## INDICATIONS/ROUTES/DOSAGE

◀ **ALERT** ▶ 5% should be used in hypovolemic or intravascularly depleted pts. 25% should be used in pts in whom fluid and sodium intake must be minimized.

**Usual Dosage**
**IV: ADULTS, ELDERLY:** Initially, 25 g; may repeat in 15–30 min.

**Hypovolemia**
**IV: ADULTS, ELDERLY, ADOLESCENTS:** 5% albumin: 0.5–1 g/kg/dose, repeat as needed. **CHILDREN:** 0.5–1 g/kg/dose (10–20 ml/kg/dose of 5% albumin). Repeat in 30 min intervals as needed.

**Hemodialysis**
**IV: ADULTS, ELDERLY:** 50–100 ml (12.5–25 g) of 25% albumin as needed.

**Dosage in Renal/Hepatic Impairment**
No dose adjustment.

## SIDE EFFECTS

**Occasional:** Hypotension. **Rare:** High dose in repeated therapy: altered vital signs, chills, fever, increased salivation, nausea, vomiting, urticaria, tachycardia.

## ADVERSE EFFECTS/ TOXIC REACTIONS

Fluid overload may occur, marked by increased B/P, distended neck veins.

Pulmonary edema may occur, evidenced by labored respirations, dyspnea, rales, wheezing, coughing. Neurologic changes that may occur include headache, weakness, blurred vision, behavioral changes, incoordination, isolated muscle twitching.

## NURSING CONSIDERATIONS

### BASELINE ASSESSMENT

Obtain B/P, pulse, respirations immediately before administration. Adequate hydration required before albumin is administered.

### INTERVENTION/EVALUATION

Monitor B/P for hypotension/hypertension. Assess frequently for evidence of fluid overload, pulmonary edema (see Adverse Effects/Toxic Reactions). Check skin for flushing, urticaria. Monitor I&O ratio (watch for decreased output). Assess for therapeutic response (increased B/P, decreased edema).

---

# albuterol

al-**bue**-ter-ol
(Airomir ✦, Apo-Salvent ✦, PMS-Salbutamol ✦, ProAir HFA, ProAir RespiClick, Proventil HFA, Ventolin HFA, VoSpire ER)
**Do not confuse albuterol with Albumin or atenolol, Proventil with Bentyl, Prilosec, or Prinivil, or Ventolin with Benylin or Vantin.**

## FIXED-COMBINATION(S)

**Combivent Respimat:** albuterol/ipratropium (a bronchodilator): 100 mcg/20 mcg per actuation. **DuoNeb:** albuterol/ipratropium 3 mg/0.5 mg.

## ◆CLASSIFICATION

**PHARMACOTHERAPEUTIC:** Sympathomimetic (adrenergic agonist). **CLINICAL:** Bronchodilator.

## USES

Treatment or prevention of bronchospasm due to reversible obstructive airway disease, prevention of exercise-induced bronchospasm.

## PRECAUTIONS

**Contraindications:** Hypersensitivity to albuterol. Severe hypersensitivity to milk protein (powder for inhalation). **Cautions:** Hypertension, cardiovascular disease, hyperthyroidism, diabetes mellitus, HF, convulsive disorders, glaucoma, hypokalemia, arrhythmias.

## ACTION

Stimulates beta₂-adrenergic receptors in lungs, resulting in relaxation of bronchial smooth muscle. **Therapeutic Effect:** Relieves bronchospasm and reduces airway resistance.

## PHARMACOKINETICS

| Route | Onset | Peak | Duration |
|---|---|---|---|
| PO | 15–30 min | 2–3 hrs | 4–6 hrs |
| PO (extended-release) | 30 min | 2–4 hrs | 12 hrs |
| Inhalation | 5–15 min | 0.5–2 hrs | 2–5 hrs |

Rapidly, well absorbed from GI tract; rapidly absorbed from bronchi after inhalation. Metabolized in liver. Primarily excreted in urine. **Half-life:** 3.8–6 hrs.

## ⌛ LIFESPAN CONSIDERATIONS

**Pregnancy/Lactation:** Appears to cross placenta; unknown if distributed in breast milk. May inhibit uterine contractility. **Children:** Safety and efficacy not established in pts younger than 2 yrs (syrup) or younger than 6 yrs (tablets). **Elderly:** May be more sensitive to tremor or tachycardia due to age-related increased sympathetic sensitivity.

## INTERACTIONS

**DRUG: Beta-adrenergic blocking agents (e.g., labetolol, metoprolol)** antagonize effects. May produce bronchospasm.

---

✦ Canadian trade name  🟢 Non-Crushable Drug  🔲 High Alert drug

**Atomoxetine, MAOIs, tricyclic antidepressants** may potentiate cardiovascular effects. May increase effects of **loop diuretics (e.g., furosemide)** (produce hypokalemia), **sympathomimetics** (increase CNS stimulation). **HERBAL: St. John's wort** may decrease level/effects. **Ephedra, yohimbe** may cause CNS stimulation. **FOOD:** Limit caffeine (may cause CNS stimulation). **LAB VALUES:** May increase blood glucose level. May decrease serum potassium level.

## AVAILABILITY (Rx)

**Inhalation Aerosol (ProAir HFA, ProAir RespiClick, Proventil HFA, Ventolin HFA):** 90 mcg/spray. **Solution for Nebulization:** 0.63 mg/3 ml (0.021%), 1.25 mg/3 ml (0.042%), 2.5 mg/3 ml (0.084%), 5 mg/ml (0.5%). **Syrup:** 2 mg/5 ml. **Tablets:** 2 mg, 4 mg.

Tablets (Extended-Release [VoSpire ER]): 4 mg, 8 mg.

## ADMINISTRATION/HANDLING

**PO**
• Do not break, crush, dissolve, or divide extended-release tablets. • Administer with food.

**Inhalation Aerosol**
• Shake container well before inhalation. • Wait 2 min before inhaling second dose (allows for deeper bronchial penetration). • Rinse mouth with water immediately after inhalation (prevents mouth/throat dryness).

**Nebulization**
• Administer over 5–15 min.

## INDICATIONS/ROUTES/DOSAGE

**Acute Bronchospasm**
**Inhalation: ADULTS, ELDERLY, CHILDREN OLDER THAN 12 YRS:** (Acute, Severe): 4–8 puffs q20min up to 4 hrs, then q1–4h as needed. *(Quick Relief):* 2 inhalations q4–6h. **CHILDREN 12 YRS AND YOUNGER:** (Acute, Severe): 4–8 puffs q20min for

3 doses, then q1–4h as needed. **(Quick Relief):** 2 puffs q4–6h as needed.
**Nebulization: ADULTS, ELDERLY, CHILDREN OLDER THAN 12 YRS:** (Acute, Severe): 2.5–5 mg q20min for 3 doses, then 2.5–10 mg q1–4h or 10–15 mg/hr continuously. **(Quick Relief):** 1.25–5 mg q4–8h as needed. **CHILDREN 12 YRS AND YOUNGER:** 0.15 mg/kg q20min for 3 doses (minimum: 2.5 mg), then 0.15–0.3 mg/kg q1–4h as needed. **Maximum:** 10 mg q1–4h as needed or 0.5 mg/kg/hr by continuous infusion. **CHILDREN 5–11 YRS:** (Quick Relief): 1.25–5 mg q4–8h as needed; **CHILDREN 4 YRS OR YOUNGER:** (Quick Relief): 0.63–2.5 mg q4–6hr as needed.

**Chronic Bronchospasm**
**PO: ADULTS, CHILDREN OLDER THAN 12 YRS:** 2–4 mg 3–4 times/day. **Maximum:** 8 mg 4 times/day. **ELDERLY:** 2 mg 3–4 times/day. **Maximum:** 8 mg 4 times/day. **CHILDREN 6–12 YRS:** 2 mg 3–4 times/day. **Maximum:** 24 mg/day. **CHILDREN 2–5 YRS:** 0.1–0.2 mg/kg/dose 3 times/day. **Maximum:** 4 mg 3 times/day.
**PO** *(Extended-Release)*: **ADULTS, CHILDREN OLDER THAN 12 YRS:** 4–8 mg q12h. **Maximum:** 32 mg/day. **CHILDREN 6–12 YRS:** 4 mg q12h. **Maximum:** 24 mg/day. **Nebulization: ADULTS, ELDERLY, CHILDREN 12 YRS AND OLDER:** 2.5 mg 3–4 times/day as needed. Children 2–11 yrs: 0.63–1.25 mg 3–4 times/day as needed. **Inhalation: ADULTS, ELDERLY, CHILDREN:** 2 puffs q4–6h.

**Exercise-Induced Bronchospasm**
**Inhalation: ADULTS, ELDERLY, CHILDREN 5 YRS AND OLDER:** 2 puffs 5 min before exercise. **CHILDREN 4 YRS AND YOUNGER:** 1–2 puffs 5 min before exercise.

**Usual Neonatal Dosage**
**Nebulization:** 1.25–2.5 mg q8h.
**Inhalation:** (mechanically ventilated) 90 mcg/spray, 1–2 sprays q6h.

**Dosage in Renal/Hepatic Impairment**
No dose adjustment.

## SIDE EFFECTS

**Frequent (27%–4%):** Headache, restlessness, nervousness, tremors, nausea, dizziness, throat dryness and irritation, pharyngitis, B/P changes including hypertension; heartburn, transient wheezing. **Occasional (3%–2%):** Insomnia, asthenia, altered taste. **Inhalation:** Dry, irritated mouth or throat; cough, bronchial irritation. **Rare:** Drowsiness, diarrhea, dry mouth, flushing, diaphoresis, anorexia.

## ADVERSE EFFECTS/ TOXIC REACTIONS

Excessive sympathomimetic stimulation may produce palpitations, exectopy, tachycardia, chest pain, slight increase in B/P followed by substantial decrease, chills, diaphoresis, blanching of skin. Too-frequent or excessive use may lead to decreased bronchodilating effectiveness and severe, paradoxical bronchoconstriction.

## NURSING CONSIDERATIONS

### BASELINE ASSESSMENT

Assess lung sounds, pulse, B/P, color, character of sputum noted. Offer emotional support (high incidence of anxiety due to difficulty in breathing and sympathomimetic response to drug).

### INTERVENTION/EVALUATION

Monitor rate, depth, rhythm, type of respiration; quality and rate of pulse; EKG; serum potassium, glucose; ABG determinations. Assess lung sounds for wheezing (bronchoconstriction), rales.

### PATIENT/FAMILY TEACHING

• Follow guidelines for proper use of inhaler. • Increase fluid intake (decreases lung secretion viscosity). • Do not take more than 2 inhalations at any one time (excessive use may produce paradoxical bronchoconstriction or decreased bronchodilating effect). • Rinsing mouth with water immediately after inhalation may prevent mouth/throat dryness. • Avoid excessive use of caffeine derivatives (chocolate, coffee, tea, cola, cocoa).

# alectinib

al-**ek**-ti-nib
(Alecensa)
**Do not confuse alectinib with afatinib, ibrutinib, imatinib, or gefitinib.**

## ◆CLASSIFICATION

**PHARMACOTHERAPEUTIC:** Kinase inhibitor. **CLINICAL:** Antineoplastic.

## USES

Treatment of pts with anaplastic lymphoma kinase (ALK)–positive metastatic non–small cell lung cancer (NSCLC) who have progressed or are intolerant to crizotinib.

## PRECAUTIONS

**Contraindications:** Hypersensitivity to alectinib. **Cautions:** Baseline anemia, leukopenia; bradycardia, bradyarrhythmias, chronic edema, diabetes, dehydration, electrolyte imbalance, hepatic/renal impairment, HF, ocular disease, pulmonary disease, history of thromboembolism.

## ACTION

Inhibits tyrosine kinase activity and tumor cell proliferation. Inhibits autophosphorylation of ALK and ALK-dependent signaling proteins. **Therapeutic Effect:** Inhibits lung cancer growth and metastasis.

## PHARMACOKINETICS

Metabolized in liver. Protein binding: Greater than 99%. Peak plasma concentration: 4 hrs. Steady state reached in 7 days. Eliminated in feces (98%), urine (less than 0.5%). **Half-life:** 33 hrs.

## ⌛ LIFESPAN CONSIDERATIONS

**Pregnancy/Lactation:** Avoid pregnancy; may cause fetal harm. Females of reproductive potential should use effective contraception during treatment and for at least 1 wk after discontinuation. Unknown

---

if distributed in breast milk. Breastfeeding not recommended during treatment and for at least 1 wk after discontinuation. Males with female partners of reproductive potential must use barrier methods during treatment and up to 3 mos after discontinuation. **Children:** Safety and efficacy not established. **Elderly:** Safety and efficacy not established.

## INTERACTIONS

**DRUG:** None significant. **HERBAL:** None significant. **FOOD:** **High-fat, high-calorie meals** increase absorption/exposure. **LAB VALUES:** May increase serum alkaline phosphatase, ALT, AST, bilirubin, CPK, creatinine, glucose. May decrease serum calcium, potassium, phosphate, sodium; Hgb, Hct, lymphocytes, RBCs.

## AVAILABILITY (Rx)

Capsules: 150 mg.

## ADMINISTRATION/HANDLING

**PO**
• Give with food. • Administer whole; do not break, crush, cut, or open capsules. • If a dose is missed or vomiting occurs during administration, give next dose at regularly scheduled time.

## INDICATIONS/ROUTES/DOSAGE

**Non–Small Cell Lung Cancer**
**PO: ADULTS, ELDERLY:** 600 mg twice daily until disease progression or unacceptable toxicity occurs.

**Dose Reduction Schedule**
**First dose reduction:** 450 mg twice daily. **Second dose reduction:** 300 mg twice daily. Permanently discontinue if unable to tolerate 300 mg twice daily.

**Dose Modification**
*Bradycardia*
**Symptomatic bradycardia:** Withhold treatment until recovery to asymptomatic bradycardia or to a heart rate of 60 bpm or greater, then resume at reduced dose level (if pt not taking concomitant medications known to cause bradycardia).

**Symptomatic bradycardia in pts taking concomitant medications known to cause bradycardia:** Withhold treatment until recovery to asymptomatic bradycardia or heart rate of 60 bpm or greater. If concomitant medication can be adjusted or discontinued, then resume at same dose. If concomitant medication cannot be adjusted or discontinued, then resume at reduced dose level. **Life-threatening bradycardia in pts who are not taking concomitant medications known to cause bradycardia:** Permanently discontinue. **Life-threatening bradycardia in pts who are taking concomitant medications known to cause bradycardia:** Withhold treatment until recovery to asymptomatic bradycardia or heart rate of 60 bpm or greater. If concomitant medication can be adjusted or discontinued, then resume at reduced dose level with frequent monitoring. Permanently discontinue if bradycardia recurs despite dose reduction.

**CPK Elevation**
**CPK elevation greater than 5 times upper limit of normal (ULN):** Withhold treatment until recovery to baseline or less than or equal to 2.5 times ULN, then resume at same dose. **CPK elevation greater than 10 times ULN or second occurrence of CPK elevation greater than 5 times ULN:** Withhold treatment until recovery to baseline or less than or equal to 2.5 times ULN, then resume at reduced dose level.

**Hepatotoxicity**
**ALT or AST elevation greater than 5 times ULN with total bilirubin less than or equal to 2 times ULN:** Withhold treatment until recovery to baseline or less than or equal to 3 times ULN, then resume at reduced dose level. **ALT or AST elevation greater than 3 times ULN with total bilirubin greater than 2 times ULN in the absence of cholestasis or hemolysis:** Permanently discontinue. **Total bilirubin elevation greater than 3 times ULN:** Withhold

treatment until recovery to baseline or less than or equal to 1.5 times ULN, then resume at reduced dose level.

**Pulmonary**
**Any grade treatment-related interstitial lung disease/pneumonitis:** Permanently discontinue.

**Dosage in Renal Impairment**
**Mild to moderate impairment:** No dose adjustment. **Severe impairment:** Not specified; use caution.

**Dosage in Hepatic Impairment**
**Mild impairment:** No dose adjustment. **Moderate to severe impairment:** Not specified; use caution.

## SIDE EFFECTS

**Frequent (41%–19%):** Fatigue, asthenia, constipation, edema (peripheral, generalized, eyelid, periorbital), myalgia, musculoskeletal pain, cough, generalized rash, papular rash, pruritus, macular rash, maculopapular rash, acneiform dermatitis, erythema, nausea. **Occasional (18%–10%):** Headache, diarrhea, dyspnea, back pain, vomiting, increased weight, blurred vision, vitreous floaters, visual impairment, reduced visual acuity, asthenopia, diplopia, photosensitivity.

## ADVERSE EFFECTS/TOXIC REACTIONS

Approx. 23% of pts required at least one dose reduction. Median time to first dose reduction was 48 days. Decreased Hgb levels were reported in 56% of pts. Drug-induced hepatotoxicity with elevations of serum ALT/AST greater than 5 times ULN reported in 4%–5% of pts. Most reported cases of hepatotoxicity occurred during first 2 mos of therapy. Common Terminology Criteria for Adverse Events (CT-CAE) grade 3 interstitial lung disease occurred in less than 1% of pts. Symptomatic bradycardia reported in 7.5% of pts. Severe myalgia, musculoskeletal pain occurred in 29% of pts. CPK elevation occurred in 43% of pts. Other serious adverse effects may include endocarditis, hemorrhage (unspecified), intestinal perforation, pulmonary embolism.

## NURSING CONSIDERATIONS

### BASELINE ASSESSMENT
Obtain baseline CBC, CPK, BMP, LFT; serum ionized calcium, phosphate; capillary blood glucose, urine pregnancy, vital signs. Obtain baseline EKG in pts with history of arrhythmias, HF, concurrent use of medications known to bradycardia. Question possibility of pregnancy or plans of breastfeeding. Question history of hepatic/renal impairment, pulmonary embolism, diabetes, cardiac/pulmonary disease. Screen for medication known to cause bradycardia. Assess visual acuity. Verify ALK-positive NSCLC test prior to initiation.

### INTERVENTION/EVALUATION
Monitor CBC routinely; LFTs q2wks during first 2 mos of treatment, then periodically thereafter (or more frequently in pts with hepatic impairment). Obtain BMP, serum ionized calcium, magnesium if arrhythmia or severe dehydration occurs. Monitor vital signs (esp. heart rate). Obtain EKG for bradycardia, chest pain, dyspnea. Worsening cough, fever, dyspnea may indicate interstitial lung disease/pneumonitis. Monitor for hepatotoxicity, hyperglycemia, vision changes, myalgia, musculoskeletal pain.

### PATIENT/FAMILY TEACHING
• Blood levels, EKGs will be monitored routinely. • Report history of heart problems including extremity swelling, HF, slow heart rate. Therapy may decrease your heart rate; report dizziness, chest pain, palpitations, or fainting. • Worsening cough, fever, or shortness of breath may indicate severe lung inflammation. • Avoid pregnancy; contraception recommended during treatment and for up to 7 days after final dose. Do not breastfeed. Males with female partners of reproductive potential should use

condoms during sexual activity during treatment and up to 3 mos after final dose. • Blurry vision, confusion, frequent urination, increased thirst, fruity breath may indicate high blood sugar levels. • Report any yellowing of skin or eyes, upper abdominal pain, bruising, black/tarry stools, dark urine. • Do not take newly prescribed medication unless approved by doctor who originally started treatment. • Avoid prolonged sun exposure/tanning beds. Use high SPF sunscreen and lip balm to protect against sunburn. • Take with food. • Avoid alcohol.

# alendronate

a-**len**-dro-nate
(Apo-Alendronate ✤, Binosto, Fosamax)
**Do not confuse alendronate with risedronate, or Fosamax with Flomax.**

## FIXED-COMBINATION(S)

**Fosamax Plus D:** alendronate/cholecalciferol (vitamin D analogue): 70 mg/2,800 international units, 70 mg/5,600 international units.

## ◆CLASSIFICATION

**PHARMACOTHERAPEUTIC:** Bisphosphonate. **CLINICAL:** Bone resorption inhibitor, calcium regulator.

## USES

**Fosamax:** Treatment of osteoporosis in men. Treatment of glucocorticoid-induced osteoporosis in men and women with low bone mineral density who are receiving at least 7.5 mg prednisone (or equivalent), treatment and prevention of osteoporosis in males and postmenopausal women, treatment of Paget's disease. **Binosto:** Treatment of osteoporosis in males and postmenopausal women.

## PRECAUTIONS

**Contraindications:** Hypocalcemia, abnormalities of the esophagus, inability to stand or sit upright for at least 30 min, sensitivity to alendronate or other bisphosphonates; oral solution or effervescent tablet should not be used in pts at risk for aspiration. **Cautions:** Renal impairment, dysphagia, esophageal disease, gastritis, ulcers, or duodenitis.

## ACTION

Inhibits bone resorption via actions on osteoclasts or osteoclast precursors. **Therapeutic Effect:** Leads to increased bone mineral density. **Paget's disease:** Decreases bone formation, but bone has a more normal architecture.

## PHARMACOKINETICS

Poorly absorbed after PO administration. Protein binding: 78%. After PO administration, rapidly taken into bone, with uptake greatest at sites of active bone turnover. Excreted in urine, feces (as unabsorbed drug). **Terminal half-life:** Greater than 10 yrs (reflects release from skeleton as bone is resorbed).

## ⧗ LIFESPAN CONSIDERATIONS

**Pregnancy/Lactation:** Possible incomplete fetal ossification, decreased maternal weight gain, delay in delivery. Unknown if distributed in breast milk. Breastfeeding not recommended. **Children:** Safety and efficacy not established. **Elderly:** No age-related precautions noted.

## INTERACTIONS

**DRUG: Calcium, antacids** may decrease absorption. **Aspirin, NSAIDs** may increase risk of ulcers, upper GI adverse effects. **HERBAL:** None significant. **FOOD:** Concurrent **beverages, dietary supplements, food** may interfere with absorption. **Caffeine** may reduce efficacy. **LAB VALUES:** Reduces serum calcium, phosphate concentrations. Significant decrease in serum alkaline phosphatase noted in pts with Paget's disease.

## AVAILABILITY (Rx)

**Solution, Oral:** 70 mg/75 ml. **Tablets:** 5 mg, 10 mg, 35 mg, 40 mg, 70 mg. **Tablets, Effervescent:** (**Binosto**): 70 mg.

## ADMINISTRATION/HANDLING

### PO
• Give at least 30 min before first food, beverage, or medication of the day. • **Tablets:** Give with 6–8 oz plain water only (mineral water, coffee, tea, juice will decrease absorption). • **Tablets, Effervescent:** Dissolve in 4 oz water. Wait at least 5 min after effervescence stops. Stir for 10 sec and drink. **Oral Solution:** Follow with at least 2 oz of water.

## INDICATIONS/ROUTES/DOSAGE

**Note:** Consider discontinuing after 3–5 yrs for osteoporosis in pts at low risk for fractures.

### Osteoporosis (in Men)
**PO: ADULTS, ELDERLY:** 10 mg once daily in the morning or 70 mg weekly.

### Glucocorticoid-Induced Osteoporosis
**PO: ADULTS, ELDERLY:** 5 mg once daily in the morning. **POSTMENOPAUSAL WOMEN NOT RECEIVING ESTROGEN:** 10 mg once daily in the morning.

### Postmenopausal Osteoporosis
**PO** *(Treatment):* **ADULTS, ELDERLY:** 10 mg once daily in the morning or 70 mg weekly. **PO** *(Prevention):* **ADULTS, ELDERLY:** 5 mg once daily in the morning or 35 mg weekly.

### Paget's Disease
**PO: ADULTS, ELDERLY:** 40 mg once daily in the morning for 6 mos.

### Dosage in Renal Impairment
Not recommended with creatinine clearance less than 35 ml/min.

### Dosage in Hepatic Impairment
No dose adjustment.

## SIDE EFFECTS

**Frequent (8%–7%):** Back pain, abdominal pain. **Occasional (3%–2%):** Nausea, abdominal distention, constipation, diarrhea, flatulence. **Rare (less than 2%):** Rash; severe bone, joint, muscle pain.

## ADVERSE EFFECTS/ TOXIC REACTIONS

Overdose produces hypocalcemia, hypophosphatemia, significant GI disturbances. Esophageal irritation occurs if not given with 6–8 oz of plain water or if pt lies down within 30 min of administration. May increase risk of osteonecrosis of the jaw.

## NURSING CONSIDERATIONS

### BASELINE ASSESSMENT
Obtain baseline serum calcium, phosphate, alkaline phosphatase. Hypocalcemia, vitamin D deficiency must be corrected before therapy.

### INTERVENTION/EVALUATION
Monitor chemistries (esp. serum calcium, phosphorus, alkaline phosphatase levels).

### PATIENT/FAMILY TEACHING
• Expected benefits occur only when medication is taken with full glass (6–8 oz) of plain water, first thing in the morning and at least 30 min before first food, beverage, or medication of the day is taken. Any other beverage (mineral water, orange juice, coffee) significantly reduces absorption of medication. • Do not lie down for at least 30 min after taking medication (potentiates delivery to stomach, reducing risk of esophageal irritation). • Report if swallowing difficulties develop, pain when swallowing, chest pain, new/worsening heartburn. • Consider weight-bearing exercises, modify behavioral factors (e.g., cigarette smoking, alcohol consumption). • Supplemental calcium and vitamin D should be taken if dietary intake inadequate.

---

## alfuzosin

al-fue-**zoe**-sin
(Apo-Alfuzosin ✷, Uroxatral,
Xatral ✷)

### ◆CLASSIFICATION

**PHARMACOTHERAPEUTIC:** Alpha₁-adrenergic blocker. **CLINICAL:** Benign prostatic hyperplasia agent.

### USES

Treatment of signs and symptoms of benign prostatic hyperplasia (BPH). **OFF-LABEL:** Facilitates expulsion of ureteral stones.

### PRECAUTIONS

**Contraindications:** Hypersensitivity to alfuzosin. Moderate to severe hepatic impairment; concurrent use of strong CYP3A4 inhibitors (e.g., ketoconazole) or other alpha-adrenergic blockers. **Cautions:** Pts with known QT interval prolongation (congenital or acquired). Severe renal or mild hepatic impairment.

### ACTION

Blocks adrenoreceptors of lower urinary tract (e.g., prostate, bladder neck). **Therapeutic Effect:** Relaxes smooth muscle; improves urinary flow, symptoms of prostatic hyperplasia.

### PHARMACOKINETICS

Readily absorbed (decreased under fasting conditions). Protein binding: 90%. Metabolized in liver. Primarily excreted in urine. **Half-life:** 10 hrs.

### ⌛ LIFESPAN CONSIDERATIONS

**Pregnancy/Lactation:** Not indicated for use in this pt population. **Children:** Not indicated for use in this pt population. **Elderly:** No age-related precautions noted.

### INTERACTIONS

**DRUG:** **Other alpha-blocking agents (e.g., doxazosin, prazosin, tamsulosin, terazosin)** may have additive effect. **CYP3A4 inhibitors (e.g., ritonavir, ketoconazole) PDE5 inhibitors (e.g., sildenafil)** may increase level/effects. **HERBAL: St. John's wort** may decrease level/effects. **FOOD: Food** increases absorption. **LAB VALUES:** None significant.

### AVAILABILITY (Rx)

▨ Tablets (Extended-Release): 10 mg.

### ADMINISTRATION/HANDLING

**PO**
• Give immediately after the same meal each day. • Swallow whole; do not break, crush, dissolve, or divide extended-release tablets.

### INDICATIONS/ROUTES/DOSAGE

**Benign Prostatic Hyperplasia**
**PO: ADULTS:** 10 mg once daily, after same meal each day.

**Dosage in Renal/Hepatic Impairment**
See Precautions.

### SIDE EFFECTS

**Frequent (7%–6%):** Dizziness, headache, malaise. **Occasional (4%):** Dry mouth. **Rare (3%–2%):** Nausea, dyspepsia (heartburn, epigastric discomfort), diarrhea, orthostatic hypotension, tachycardia, drowsiness.

### ADVERSE EFFECTS/ TOXIC REACTIONS

Ischemia-related chest pain may occur rarely (2% of pts). Priapism has been reported.

### NURSING CONSIDERATIONS

#### BASELINE ASSESSMENT

Question for sensitivity to alfuzosin, use of other alpha-blocking agents (doxazosin, prazosin, tamsulosin, terazosin). Obtain B/P.

### INTERVENTION/EVALUATION

Assist with ambulation if dizziness occurs. Report headache. Monitor for hypotension. Question for improvement in urine flow, hesitancy.

### PATIENT/FAMILY TEACHING

• Take after the same meal each day. • Avoid tasks that require alertness, motor skills until response to drug is established. • Do not chew, crush, dissolve, or divide extended-release tablets.

# alirocumab

al-i-**rok**-ue-mab
(Praluent)
**Do not confuse alirocumab with adalimumab or raxibacumab.**

## ◆CLASSIFICATION

**PHARMACOTHERAPEUTIC:** Proprotein convertase subtilisin kexin 9 (PCSK9) inhibitor, monoclonal antibody. **CLINICAL:** Antihyperlipidemic.

## USES

Adjunct to diet and maximally tolerated statin therapy for the treatment of adults with heterozygous familial hypercholesterolemia or clinical atherosclerotic cardiovascular disease who require additional lowering of low-density lipoprotein cholesterol (LDL-C).

## PRECAUTIONS

**Contraindications:** Severe hypersensitivity to alirocumab. **Cautions:** Hepatic impairment.

## ACTION

Prevents binding of PCSK9 to LDL receptors on hepatocytes. Increases hepatic uptake of LDL. **Therapeutic Effect:** Decreases serum cholesterol levels.

## PHARMACOKINETICS

Distributed primarily in circulatory system. Metabolized by protein degradation into small peptides, amino acids. Peak plasma concentration: 3–7 days. Steady state reached by 2–3 doses. **Half-life:** 17–20 days.

## LIFESPAN CONSIDERATIONS

**Pregnancy/Lactation:** May cross placental barrier, esp. during second and third trimesters. Unknown if distributed in breast milk. Human immunoglobulin G is present in breast milk. **Children:** Safety and efficacy not established. **Elderly:** No age-related precautions noted.

## INTERACTIONS

**DRUG:** None known. **HERBAL:** None significant. **FOOD:** None known. **LAB VALUES:** Expected to decrease serum LDL-C levels. May increase serum ALT, AST.

## AVAILABILITY (Rx)

**Injection Solution:** 75 mg/ml, 150 mg/ml in single-dose, prefilled syringe or pen.

## ADMINISTRATION/HANDLING

 SQ

• Visually inspect for particulate matter or discoloration. Solution should appear clear, colorless to pale yellow. • Allow pen/syringe to warm to room temperature for 30–40 min prior to use. • Subcutaneously insert needle into abdomen, thigh, or upper arm region and inject solution. It may take up to 20 sec to fully inject dose. • Do not inject into areas of active skin disease or injury such as sunburns, skin rashes, inflammation, or skin infections. • Rotate injection sites.

### Storage

• Refrigerate unused pens/syringes in outer carton. • Do not freeze. • Discard if pen/syringe has been at room temperature more than 24 hrs or longer. • Protect from light.

## INDICATIONS/ROUTES/DOSAGE

**Heterozygous Familial Hypercholesterolemia**
**SQ: ADULTS, ELDERLY:** 75 mg once every 2 wks. May increase to maximum dose of 150 mg once every 2 wks if response

inadequate. If a dose is missed, administer within 7 days of scheduled dose, then resume normal schedule. If missed dose is not within 7 days, wait until next scheduled dose.

**Dosage in Renal Impairment**
No dose adjustment.

**Dosage in Hepatic Impairment**
**Mild to Moderate Impairment:** No dose adjustment. **Severe Impairment:** Use caution.

## SIDE EFFECTS

**Occasional (11%–7%):** Nasopharyngitis, injection site reactions (e.g., erythema, itching, swelling, pain/tenderness, bruising/contusion). **Rare (5%–2%):** Diarrhea, bronchitis, myalgia, muscle spasm, sinusitis, cough, musculoskeletal pain.

## ADVERSE EFFECTS/TOXIC REACTIONS

Serious hypersensitivity reactions (e.g., pruritus, rash, urticaria), including some serious events (e.g., hypersensitivity vasculitis, hypersensitivity reactions requiring hospitalization) have been reported. Infections such as UTI (5% of pts), influenza (6% of pts) have occurred. Neurologic events such as confusion, memory impairment reported in less than 1% of pts. Immunogenicity (anti-alirocumab antibodies) reported in 5% of pts. Pts who developed neutralizing antibodies had a higher incidence of injection site reactions.

## NURSING CONSIDERATIONS

### BASELINE ASSESSMENT

Obtain baseline LDL-C level, LFT. Question history of hypersensitivity reaction, hepatic impairment. Assess skin for sunburns, skin rashes, inflammation, or skin infections.

### INTERVENTION/EVALUATION

Obtain LDL-C level within 4–8 wks after treatment initiation or with any dose titration. Monitor for hypersensitivity reactions.

If hypersensitivity reaction occurs, discontinue therapy and treat symptoms accordingly; monitor until symptoms resolve. Monitor for infections including UTI, influenza.

### PATIENT/FAMILY TEACHING

• Provide proper injection techniques to pts and caregivers. • Treatment may cause serious allergic reactions such as itching, hives, rash, or more serious reactions requiring hospitalization. If allergic reaction occurs, immediately seek medical attention. • Do not reuse prefilled pens/syringes.

## *aliskiren*     HIGH ALERT

a-lis-**kye**-ren
(Rasilez ✤, Tekturna)

■ **BLACK BOX ALERT** ■ May cause fetal injury, mortality. Discontinue as soon as possible once pregnancy detected.
**Do not confuse Tekturna with Valturna.**

### FIXED-COMBINATION(S)

**Amturnide:** aliskiren/amlodipine (a calcium channel blocker)/ hydrochlorothiazide (a diuretic): 150 mg/5 mg/12.5 mg, 300 mg/ 5 mg/12.5 mg, 300 mg/5 mg/25 mg, 300 mg/10 mg/12.5 mg, 300 mg/ 10 mg/25 mg. **Tekamlo:** aliskiren/ amlodipine (a calcium channel blocker): 150 mg/5 mg, 150 mg/ 10 mg, 300 mg/5 mg, 300 mg/ 10 mg. **Tekturna HCT:** aliskiren/ hydrochlorothiazide (a diuretic): 150 mg/12.5 mg, 150 mg/25 mg, 300 mg/12.5 mg, 300 mg/25 mg. **Valturna:** aliskiren/valsartan (an angiotensin II receptor antagonist): 150 mg/160 mg, 300 mg/320 mg.

### ◆CLASSIFICATION

**PHARMACOTHERAPEUTIC:** Renin-angiotensin system antagonist. **CLINICAL:** Antihypertensive.

## USES

Treatment of hypertension. May be used alone or in combination with other antihypertensives.

## PRECAUTIONS

**Contraindications:** Hypersensitivity to aliskiren. Concurrent use with ACE inhibitor or Angiotensin II Receptor Blockers in pts with diabetes. **Cautions:** Severe renal impairment. History of angioedema, dialysis, nephrotic syndrome, renovascular hypertension. Concurrent use with P-glycoprotein inhibitors (e.g., cyclosporine).

## ACTION

Direct renin inhibitor. Decreases plasma renin activity (PRA), inhibiting the conversion of angiotensinogen to angiotensin I, decreasing the formation of angiotensin II. **Therapeutic Effect:** Reduces B/P.

## PHARMACOKINETICS

Peak plasma concentration reached within 1–3 hrs. Protein binding: 49%. Metabolized in liver. Minimally excreted in urine. Peak plasma steady-state levels reached in 7–8 days. **Half-life:** 24 hrs.

## ⧗ LIFESPAN CONSIDERATIONS

**Pregnancy/Lactation:** Carcinogenic potential to fetus. May cause fetal/neonatal morbidity, mortality. Unknown if distributed in breast milk. **Children:** Safety and efficacy not established. **Elderly:** No age-related precautions noted.

## INTERACTIONS

**DRUG: Cyclosporine, itraconazole** may increase concentration/effect. **HERBAL: Ephedra, ginseng, yohimbe** may worsen hypertension. **Garlic, black cohosh** may increase antihypertensive effect. **FOOD: High-fat meals** substantially decrease absorption. **Grapefruit products** may reduce antihypertensive effects. Separate by 4 hrs. **LAB VALUES:** May increase serum BUN, creatinine, uric acid, creatinine kinase, potassium. May decrease Hgb, Hct.

## AVAILABILITY (Rx)

🔖 **Tablets, Film-Coated:** 150 mg, 300 mg.

## ADMINISTRATION/HANDLING

**PO**
- High-fat meals substantially decrease absorption. • Consistent administration with regard to meals is recommended.
- Do not break, crush, dissolve, or divide film-coated tablets.

## INDICATIONS/ROUTES/DOSAGE

**Hypertension**
**PO: ADULTS, ELDERLY:** Initially, 150 mg/day. May increase to 300 mg/day.

**Dosage in Renal Impairment**
**Mild to moderate impairment:** No dose adjustment. **Severe impairment:** Use caution.

**Dosage in Hepatic Impairment**
No dose adjustment.

## SIDE EFFECTS

**Rare (2%–1%):** Diarrhea, particularly in women, elderly (older than 65 yrs), gastroesophageal reflux, cough, rash.

## ADVERSE EFFECTS/ TOXIC REACTIONS

Angioedema, periorbital edema, edema of hands, generalized edema have been reported.

## NURSING CONSIDERATIONS

### BASELINE ASSESSMENT

Correct hypovolemia in pts on concurrent diuretic therapy. Obtain B/P and apical pulse immediately before each dose, in addition to regular monitoring (be alert to fluctuations). If excessive reduction in B/P occurs, place pt in supine position, feet slightly elevated.

### INTERVENTION/EVALUATION

Assess for edema. Monitor I&O; weigh daily. Monitor B/P, renal function tests, potassium, Hgb, Hct.

---

 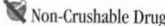

## PATIENT/FAMILY TEACHING

• Pregnant pts should avoid second- and third-trimester exposure to aliskiren. • Report if swelling of face/lips/tongue, difficulty breathing occur. • Avoid strenuous exercise during hot weather (risk of dehydration, hypotension). • Do not chew, crush, dissolve, or divide film-coated tablets.

# allopurinol

al-oh-**pure**-i-nol
(Aloprim, Apo-Allopurinol ✦, Zyloprim)
**Do not confuse allopurinol with Apresoline or haloperidol, or Zyloprim with Zorprin or Zovirax.**

## ◆CLASSIFICATION

**PHARMACOTHERAPEUTIC:** Xanthine oxidase inhibitor. **CLINICAL:** Antigout.

## USES

**PO:** Management of primary or secondary gout (e.g., acute attack, nephropathy). Treatment of secondary hyperuricemia that may occur during cancer treatment. Management of recurrent uric acid and calcium oxalate calculi. **Injection:** Management of elevated uric acid in cancer treatment for leukemia, lymphoma, or solid tumor malignancies.

## PRECAUTIONS

**Contraindications:** Severe hypersensitivity to allopurinol. **Cautions:** Renal/hepatic impairment, pts taking diuretics, mercaptopurine or azathioprine, other drugs causing myelosuppression. Do not use in asymptomatic hyperuricemia.

## ACTION

Decreases uric acid production by inhibiting xanthine oxidase, an enzyme responsible for converting xanthine to uric acid. **Therapeutic Effect:** Reduces uric acid concentrations in serum and urine.

## PHARMACOKINETICS

| Route | Onset | Peak | Duration |
|-------|-------|------|----------|
| PO, IV | 2–3 days | 1–3 wks | 1–2 wks |

Well absorbed from GI tract. Widely distributed. Protein binding: less than 1%. Metabolized in liver. Excreted primarily in urine. Removed by hemodialysis. **Half-life:** 1–3 hrs; metabolite, 12–30 hrs.

## ⌛ LIFESPAN CONSIDERATIONS

**Pregnancy/Lactation:** Unknown if drug crosses placenta or is distributed in breast milk. **Children/Elderly:** No age-related precautions noted.

## INTERACTIONS

**DRUG: Loop or thiazide diuretics (e.g., furosemide, hydrochlorothiazide)** may increase level/effect. May increase effect of **oral anticoagulants (e.g., warfarin).** May increase concentration, toxicity of **azathioprine, mercaptopurine. Amoxicillin, ampicillin** may increase incidence of rash. **HERBAL:** None significant. **FOOD:** None known. **LAB VALUES:** May increase serum BUN, alkaline phosphatase, ALT, AST, creatinine.

## AVAILABILITY (Rx)

**Injection, Powder for Reconstitution (Aloprim):** 500 mg. **Tablets (Zyloprim):** 100 mg, 300 mg.

## ADMINISTRATION/HANDLING

 **IV**

**Reconstitution** • Reconstitute 500-mg vial with 25 ml Sterile Water for Injection (concentration of 20 mg/ml). • Further dilute with 0.9% NaCl or D₅W (50–100 ml) to a concentration of 6 mg/ml or less. **Rate of Administration** • Infuse over 15–60 min. Daily doses can be given as a single infusion or in equally divided doses at 6-, 8-, or 12-hr intervals. **Storage** • Solution should appear clear and colorless. • Store unreconstituted vials at room temperature. • Do not refrigerate reconstituted and/or diluted solution. Must administer within 10 hrs of preparation. • Do not use if precipitate forms or solution is discolored.

**PO**

• Give after meals with plenty of fluid. • Fluid intake should yield slightly alkaline urine and output of approximately 2 L in adults. • Dosages greater than 300 mg/day to be administered in divided doses.

## ▓ IV INCOMPATIBILITIES

Amikacin (Amikin), carmustine (BiCNU), cefotaxime (Claforan), clindamycin (Cleocin), cytarabine (Ara-C), dacarbazine (DTIC), diphenhydramine (Benadryl), doxorubicin (Adriamycin), doxycycline (Vibramycin), gentamicin, haloperidol (Haldol), hydroxyzine (Vistaril), idarubicin (Idamycin), imipenem-cilastatin (Primaxin), methylprednisolone (Solu-Medrol), metoclopramide (Reglan), ondansetron (Zofran), streptozocin (Zanosar), tobramycin, vinorelbine (Navelbine).

## ▓ IV COMPATIBILITIES

Bumetanide (Bumex), calcium gluconate, furosemide (Lasix), heparin, hydromorphone (Dilaudid), lorazepam (Ativan), morphine, potassium chloride.

## INDICATIONS/ROUTES/DOSAGE

◀ALERT▶ Doses greater than 300 mg given in divided doses.

**Gout**
PO: **ADULTS, CHILDREN OLDER THAN 10 YRS:** Initially, 100 mg/day. Increase at weekly intervals needed to achieve desired serum uric acid level. **(Mild):** 200–300 mg/day. **(Moderate to Severe):** 400–600 mg/day in 2–3 divided doses. **Maximum:** 800 mg/day.

**Secondary Hyperuricemia Associated with Chemotherapy**
PO: **ADULTS, CHILDREN OLDER THAN 10 YRS:** 600–800 mg/day in 2–3 divided doses for 2–3 days starting 1–2 days before chemotherapy. **CHILDREN 6–10 YRS:** 300 mg/day

in 2–3 divided doses. **CHILDREN YOUNGER THAN 6 YRS:** 150 mg/day in 3 divided doses.
◀ALERT▶ IV: Daily dose can be given as single infusion or at 6-, 8-, or 12-hr intervals.
IV: **ADULTS, ELDERLY, CHILDREN 10 YRS OR OLDER:** 200–400 mg/m²/day beginning 24–48 hrs before initiation of chemotherapy. **CHILDREN YOUNGER THAN 10 YRS:** 200 mg/m²/day beginning 24–48 hrs before initiation of chemotherapy. **Maximum:** 600 mg/day.

**Recurrent Uric Acid Calcium Oxalate Calculi**
PO: **ADULTS:** 200–300 mg/day in single or divided doses.

**Dosage in Renal Impairment**
Dosage is modified based on creatinine clearance. PO: Removed by hemodialysis. Administer dose posthemodialysis or administer 50% supplemental dose.

**IV/PO**

| Creatinine Clearance | Dosage |
|---|---|
| 10–20 ml/min | 200 mg/day |
| 3–9 ml/min | 100 mg/day |
| Less than 3 ml/min | 100 mg at extended intervals |
| HD | 100 mg q48h (increase cautiously to 300 mg) |

**Dosage in Hepatic Impairment**
No dose adjustment.

## SIDE EFFECTS

**Occasional: PO:** Drowsiness, unusual hair loss. **IV:** Rash, nausea, vomiting. **Rare:** Diarrhea, headache.

## ADVERSE EFFECTS/ TOXIC REACTIONS

Pruritic maculopapular rash, possibly accompanied by malaise, fever, chills, joint pain, nausea, vomiting should be considered a toxic reaction. Severe hypersensitivity reaction may follow appearance of rash. Bone marrow depression, hepatotoxicity, peripheral neuritis, acute renal failure occur rarely.

## NURSING CONSIDERATIONS

### BASELINE ASSESSMENT

Obtain baseline BMP, LFT. Instruct pt to drink minimum of 2,500–3,000 ml of fluid daily while taking medication.

### INTERVENTION/EVALUATION

Discontinue medication immediately if rash or other evidence of allergic reaction occurs. Monitor I&O (output should be at least 2,000 ml/day). Assess serum chemistries, uric acid, hepatic function. Assess urine for cloudiness, unusual color, odor. **Gout:** Assess for therapeutic response: relief of pain, stiffness, swelling; increased joint mobility; reduced joint tenderness; improved grip strength.

### PATIENT/FAMILY TEACHING

• May take 1 wk or longer for full therapeutic effect. • Maintain adequate hydration; drink 2,500–3,000 ml of fluid daily while taking medication. • Avoid tasks that require alertness, motor skills until response to drug is established. • Avoid alcohol (may increase uric acid).

## almotriptan

al-moe-**trip**-tan
(Axert)
**Do not confuse almotriptan with alvimopan, or Axert with Antivert.**

### ◆CLASSIFICATION

**PHARMACOTHERAPEUTIC:** Serotonin receptor agonist (5-HT$_{1B}$). **CLINICAL:** Antimigraine.

### USES

Acute treatment of migraine headache with or without aura in adults. Acute treatment of migraine headache in adolescents 12–17 yrs with history of migraine with or without aura and having attacks usually lasting 4 or more hrs when left untreated.

### PRECAUTIONS

**Contraindications:** Hypersensitivity to almotriptan. Cerebrovascular disease (e.g., stroke, transient ischemic attacks), peripheral vascular disease (e.g., ischemic bowel disease), hemiplegic or basilar migraine, ischemic heart disease (including angina pectoris, history of MI, silent ischemia, and Prinzmetal's angina), uncontrolled hypertension, use within 24 hrs of ergotamine-containing preparations or another 5-HT$_{1B}$ agonist. **Cautions:** Mild to moderate renal or hepatic impairment, pt profile suggesting cardiovascular risks, controlled hypertension; history of CVA, sulfonamide allergy.

### ACTION

Binds selectively to serotonin receptors in cranial arteries producing a vasoconstrictive effect. Decreases inflammation associated with relief of migraine. **Therapeutic Effect:** Produces relief of migraine headache.

### PHARMACOKINETICS

Well absorbed after PO administration. Protein binding: 35%. Metabolized by liver. Primarily excreted in urine. **Half-life:** 3–4 hrs.

### ⌛ LIFESPAN CONSIDERATIONS

**Pregnancy/Lactation:** Unknown if distributed in breast milk. **Children:** Safety and efficacy not established in pts younger than 12 yrs. **Elderly:** No age-related precautions noted.

### INTERACTIONS

**DRUG:** Ergotamine-containing drugs may produce vasospastic reaction. **MAOIs** may increase concentration. Combined use of **SSRIs** or **SNRIs** (e.g., **fluoxetine, fluvoxamine, paroxetine, sertraline**) may produce weakness, hyperreflexia, incoordination. **CYP3A4 inhibitors** (e.g., **erythromycin, itraconazole, ketoconazole, ritonavir**) may increase plasma concentration/effect. **HERBAL:** None significant. **FOOD:** None known. **LAB VALUES:** None significant.

## AVAILABILITY (Rx)

Tablets: 6.5 mg, 12.5 mg.

## ADMINISTRATION/HANDLING

### PO

• Swallow whole; do not break, crush, dissolve, or divide tablets. • Take with full glass of water. • May give without regard to food.

## INDICATIONS/ROUTES/DOSAGE

### Migraine Headache

**PO: ADULTS, ELDERLY, ADOLESCENTS 12–17 YRS:** Initially, 6.25–12.5 mg as a single dose. If headache returns, dose may be repeated after 2 hrs. **Maximum:** 2 doses/24 hrs (25 mg).

### Concurrent Use of CYP3A4 Inhibitors

**ADULTS, ELDERLY:** Recommended initial dose is 6.25 mg, maximum daily dose is 12.5 mg. Avoid use in pts with renal or hepatic impairment AND use of CYP3A4 inhibitors.

### Dosage in Renal Impairment

**CrCl 30 ml/min or less:** Initially, 6.25 mg in a single dose. **Maximum:** 12.5 mg/day.

### Dosage in Hepatic Impairment

Initially, 6.25 mg in a single dose. **Maximum:** 12.5 mg/day.

## SIDE EFFECTS

**Rare (2%–1%):** Nausea, dry mouth, headache, dizziness, somnolence, paresthesia, flushing.

## ADVERSE EFFECTS/ TOXIC REACTIONS

Excessive dosage may produce tremor, redness of extremities, decreased respirations, cyanosis, seizures, chest pain. Serious arrhythmias occur rarely but particularly in pts with hypertension, diabetes, obesity, smokers, and those with strong family history of coronary artery disease.

## NURSING CONSIDERATIONS

### BASELINE ASSESSMENT

Question for history of peripheral vascular disease, cardiac conduction disorders. Question pt regarding onset, location, duration of migraine, and possible precipitating factors.

### INTERVENTION/EVALUATION

Evaluate for relief of migraine headache and associated photophobia, phonophobia (sound sensitivity), nausea, vomiting.

### PATIENT/FAMILY TEACHING

• Take a single dose as soon as symptoms of an actual migraine attack appear. • Medication is intended to relieve migraine, not to prevent or reduce number of attacks. • Lie down in quiet, dark room for additional benefit after taking medication. • Avoid tasks that require alertness, motor skills until response to drug is established. • Report immediately if palpitations, pain or tightness in chest or throat, or pain or weakness of extremities occurs. • Swallow whole; do not chew, crush, dissolve, or divide tablets.

# alogliptin

al-oh-**glip**-tin
(Nesina)
**Do not confuse alogliptin with linagliptin, saxagliptin, or sitagliptin.**

## FIXED COMBINATION(S)

**Kazano:** alogliptin/metformin (an antidiabetic): 12.5 mg/500 mg, 12.5 mg, 1,000 mg. **Oseni:** alogliptin/pioglitazone (an antidiabetic): 12.5 mg/15 mg, 12.5 mg/30 mg, 12.5 mg/45 mg, 25 mg/15 mg, 25 mg/30 mg, 25 mg/45 mg.

## ◆CLASSIFICATION

**PHARMACOTHERAPEUTIC:** Dipeptidyl peptidase-4 (DDP-4) inhibitor. **CLINICAL:** Antidiabetic.

## USES

Adjunctive treatment to diet and exercise to improve glycemic control in pts with type 2 diabetes mellitus.

## PRECAUTIONS

**Contraindications:** Hypersensitivity to alogliptin, other DD4 inhibitors. **Cautions:** Concurrent use of other hypoglycemic medication, cholelithiasis, hepatic or renal impairment. History of pancreatitis. Not to be used in type 1 diabetes or ketoacidosis. Possible increased risk for HF.

## ACTION

Slows inactivation of incretin hormones by inhibiting DDP-4 enzyme. **Therapeutic Effect:** Incretin hormones increase insulin synthesis/release from pancreas and decrease glucagon secretion. Lowers serum glucose levels.

## PHARMACOKINETICS

Rapidly absorbed following PO administration. Metabolized in liver. Protein binding: 20%. Minimal metabolism (60%–70% excreted unchanged). Peak plasma concentration: 1–2 hrs. Primarily excreted in urine. **Half-life:** 21 hrs.

## ⧗ LIFESPAN CONSIDERATIONS

**Pregnancy/Lactation:** Unknown if distributed in breast milk. **Children:** Safety and efficacy not established. **Elderly:** May have increased risk of hypoglycemia.

## INTERACTIONS

**DRUG: Insulin, oral hypoglycemics** may increase risk of hypoglycemia. **HERBAL:** Herbal supplements having hypoglycemic effects may increase risk of hypoglycemia. **FOOD:** None known. **LAB VALUES:** May decrease serum glucose. May increase serum ALT, AST.

## AVAILABILITY (Rx)

**Tablets:** 6.25 mg, 12.5 mg, 25 mg.

## ADMINISTRATION/HANDLING

PO
• May give without regard to food.

## INDICATIONS/ROUTES/DOSAGE

**Type 2 Diabetes Mellitus**
**PO: ADULTS/ELDERLY:** 25 mg once daily.

**Dosage in Renal Impairment**
**Creatinine clearance 30–59 ml/min:** 12.5 mg once daily. **Creatinine clearance less than 30 ml/min:** 6.25 mg once daily.

**Dosage in Hepatic Impairment**
No dose adjustment.

## SIDE EFFECTS

**Occasional (4%):** Nasopharyngitis, cough, headache, upper respiratory tract infections.

## ADVERSE EFFECTS/ TOXIC REACTIONS

Hypoglycemia reported in 1.5% of pts (5% specifically in elderly). Concomitant use of hypoglycemic medication may increase hypoglycemic risk. Pancreatitis reported in less than 1%. Hypersensitivity reactions including angioedema (tongue/lip swelling), urticaria, bronchospasm occur rarely. Hepatic failure (fatal vs. nonfatal) reported in less than 2% of pts.

## NURSING CONSIDERATIONS

### BASELINE ASSESSMENT

Obtain baseline serum chemistries, capillary blood glucose, Hgb A1c level. Assess pt's understanding of diabetes management, routine home glucose monitoring. Receive full medication history, including herbal products. Question history of co-morbidities, esp. alcohol dependency, renal or hepatic impairment.

### INTERVENTION/EVALUATION

Monitor blood glucose, Hgb A1c level, hepatic/renal function tests. Assess for hypoglycemia, hyperglycemia, hypersensitivity reaction. Screen for glucose-altering conditions: fever, increased activity or stress, surgical procedures. Obtain dietary consult for nutritional education. Severe abdominal pain, nausea may indicate pancreatitis.

• Diabetes mellitus requires lifelong control. Diet and exercise are principal parts of treatment; do not skip or delay meals. • Test blood glucose regularly. • When taking combination drug therapy or when glucose demands are altered (e.g., fever, infection, trauma, stress, heavy physical activity), have hypoglycemic treatment (glucagon, oral dextrose) available. • Report suspected pregnancy or plans of breastfeeding. • Monitor daily calorie intake. • Avoid alcohol. • Report abdominal pain, yellowing of the skin or eyes, fatigue, loss of appetite, dark urine, or decreased urine output.

# *ALPRAZolam

al-**praz**-oh-lam
(Alprazolam Intensol, Alprazolam XR, Apo-Alpraz ✱, Niravam, Xanax, Xanax XR)
**Do not confuse alprazolam with lorazepam, or Xanax with Tenex, Tylox, Xopenex, Zantac, or Zyrtec.**

## ◆CLASSIFICATION

**PHARMACOTHERAPEUTIC:** Benzodiazepine **(Schedule IV). CLINICAL:** Antianxiety.

## USES

Management of generalized anxiety disorders (GAD). Short-term relief of symptoms of anxiety, panic disorder, with or without agoraphobia. Anxiety associated with depression. **OFF-LABEL:** Anxiety in children. Preoperative anxiety.

## PRECAUTIONS

**Contraindications:** Hypersensitivity to alprazolam. Acute narrow angle-closure glaucoma, concurrent use with ketoconazole or itraconazole. **Cautions:** Renal/hepatic impairment, predisposition to urate nephropathy, obese pts. Concurrent use of CYP3A4 inhibitors/inducers and major CYP3A4 substrates; debilitated pts, respiratory disease, depression (esp. suicidal risk), elderly (increased risk of severe toxicity).

## ACTION

Enhances the inhibitory effects of the neurotransmitter gamma-aminobutyric acid in the brain. **Therapeutic Effect:** Produces anxiolytic effect due to CNS depressant action.

## PHARMACOKINETICS

Well absorbed from GI tract. Protein binding: 80%. Metabolized in liver. Primarily excreted in urine. Minimal removal by hemodialysis. **Half-life:** 6–27 hrs.

## ⧗ LIFESPAN CONSIDERATIONS

**Pregnancy/Lactation:** Crosses placenta; distributed in breast milk. Chronic ingestion during pregnancy may produce withdrawal symptoms, CNS depression in neonates. **Children:** Safety and efficacy not established. **Elderly:** Use small initial doses with gradual increase to avoid ataxia (muscular incoordination) or excessive sedation.

## INTERACTIONS

**DRUG:** Potentiated effects when used with **other CNS depressants (including alcohol).** CYP3A4 inhibitors **(e.g., antifungal agents [azole], olanzapine, protease inhibitors, SSRIs)** may increase CNS effect. **CYP3A4 inducers (e.g., carbamazepine, rifampin)** may decrease effect. **HERBAL: Gotu kola, kava kava, St. John's wort, valerian** may increase CNS depressant effect. **St. John's wort, yohimbe** may decrease effectiveness. **FOOD: Grapefruit products** may increase level, effects. **LAB VALUES:** None significant.

## AVAILABILITY (Rx)

**Solution, Oral (Alprazolam Intensol):** 1 mg/ml. **Tablets (Orally Disintegrating [Niravam]):** 0.25 mg, 0.5 mg, 1 mg, 2 mg. **Tablets (Immediate-Release [Xanax]):** 0.25 mg, 0.5 mg, 1 mg, 2 mg.

 Tablets (Extended-Release [Xanax XR]): 0.5 mg, 1 mg, 2 mg, 3 mg.

## ADMINISTRATION/HANDLING

### PO, Immediate-Release
• May give without regard to meals.
• Tablets may be crushed. • If oral intake is not possible, may be given sublingually.

### PO, Extended-Release
• Administer once daily. • Do not break, crush, dissolve, or divide extended-release tablets. Swallow whole.

### PO, Orally Disintegrating
• Place tablet on tongue, allow to dissolve. • Swallow with saliva. • Administration with water not necessary. • If using ½ tab, discard remaining ½ tab.

## INDICATIONS/ROUTES/DOSAGE

### Anxiety Disorders
**PO** *(Immediate-Release)*: **ADULTS:** Initially, 0.25–0.5 mg 3 times/day. May titrate q3–4days. **Maximum:** 4 mg/day in divided doses. **CHILDREN, YOUNGER THAN 18 YRS:** 0.125 mg 3 times/day. May increase by 0.125–0.25 mg/dose. **Maximum:** 0.06 mg/kg/day or 0.02 mg/kg/dose. Range: 0.375–3 mg/day. **ELDERLY, DEBILITATED PTS, PTS WITH HEPATIC DISEASE OR LOW SERUM ALBUMIN:** Initially, 0.25 mg 2–3 times/day. Gradually increase to optimum therapeutic response.
**PO** *(Orally Disintegrating)*: **ADULTS:** 0.25–0.5 mg 3 times/day. **Maximum:** 4 mg/day in divided doses.

### Anxiety with Depression
**PO: ADULTS:** (average dose required) 2.5–3 mg/day in divided doses.

### Panic Disorder
**PO** *(Immediate-Release)*: **ADULTS:** Initially, 0.5 mg 3 times/day. May increase at 3- to 4-day intervals in increments of 1 mg or less a day. Range: 5–6 mg/day.

**Maximum:** 10 mg/day. **ELDERLY:** Initially, 0.125–0.25 mg twice daily. May increase in 0.125-mg increments until desired effect attained.

### PO *(Extended-Release)*:
◀**ALERT**▶ To switch from immediate-release to extended-release form, give total daily dose (immediate-release) as a single daily dose of extended-release form.
**ADULTS:** Initially, 0.5–1 mg once daily. May titrate at 3- to 4-day intervals. Range: 3–6 mg/day. **ELDERLY:** Initially, 0.5 mg once daily.
**PO** *(Orally Disintegrating)*: **ADULTS:** Initially, 0.5 mg 3 times/day. May increase at 3- to 4-day intervals. Range: 5–6 mg/day.

### Dosage in Renal Impairment
No dose adjustment.

### Dosage in Hepatic Impairment
**Severe Disease: Immediate-Release:** 0.25 mg 2–3 mg times/day. **Extended-Release:** 0.5 mg once daily.

## SIDE EFFECTS

**Frequent (41%–20%):** Ataxia, light-headedness, drowsiness, slurred speech (particularly in elderly or debilitated pts). **Occasional (15%–5%):** Confusion, depression, blurred vision, constipation, diarrhea, dry mouth, headache, nausea. **Rare (4% or less):** Behavioral problems such as anger, impaired memory; paradoxical reactions (insomnia, nervousness, irritability).

## ADVERSE EFFECTS/ TOXIC REACTIONS

Abrupt or too-rapid withdrawal may result in restlessness, irritability, insomnia, hand tremors, abdominal/muscle cramps, diaphoresis, vomiting, seizures. Overdose results in drowsiness, confusion, diminished reflexes, coma. Blood dyscrasias noted rarely. **Antidote:** Flumazenil (see Appendix K for dosage).

---

*"Tall Man" lettering                    underlined – top prescribed drug

## NURSING CONSIDERATIONS

### BASELINE ASSESSMENT

Assess degree of anxiety; assess for drowsiness, dizziness, light-headedness. Assess motor responses (agitation, trembling, tension), autonomic responses (cold/clammy hands, diaphoresis).

### INTERVENTION/EVALUATION

For pts on long-term therapy, perform hepatic/renal function tests, CBC periodically. Assess for paradoxical reaction, particularly during early therapy. Evaluate for therapeutic response: calm facial expression, decreased restlessness, insomnia. Monitor respiratory and cardiovascular status.

### PATIENT/FAMILY TEACHING

• Drowsiness usually disappears during continued therapy. • If dizziness occurs, change positions slowly from recumbent to sitting position before standing. • Avoid tasks that require alertness, motor skills until response to drug is established. • Smoking reduces drug effectiveness. • Sour hard candy, gum, sips of water may relieve dry mouth. • Do not abruptly withdraw medication after long-term therapy. • Avoid alcohol. • Do not take other medications without consulting physician.

## alteplase

HIGH ALERT

al-te-plase
(Activase, Cathflo Activase)
**Do not confuse alteplase or Activase with Altace, or Activase with Cathflo Activase.**

### ◆CLASSIFICATION

**PHARMACOTHERAPEUTIC:** Tissue plasminogen activator (tPA). **CLINICAL:** Thrombolytic.

## USES

Treatment of ST-elevation MI for lysis of thrombi in coronary arteries, acute ischemic stroke, acute massive pulmonary embolism. Treatment of occluded central venous catheters. **OFF-LABEL:** Acute peripheral occlusive disease, prosthetic valve thrombosis. Acute ischemic stroke presenting 3–4½ hrs after onset of symptoms.

## PRECAUTIONS

**Contraindications:** Hypersensitivity to alteplase. Active internal bleeding, AV malformation or aneurysm, bleeding diathesis CVA, intracranial neoplasm, intracranial or intraspinal surgery or trauma, recent (within past 2 mos), severe uncontrolled hypertension, suspected aortic dissection. **Cautions:** Recent (within 10 days) major surgery or GI bleeding, OB delivery, organ biopsy, recent trauma or CPR, left heart thrombus, endocarditis, severe hepatic disease, pregnancy, elderly, cerebrovascular disease, diabetic retinopathy, thrombophlebitis, occluded AV cannula at infected site.

## ACTION

Binds to fibrin in a thrombus and converts entrapped plasminogen to plasmin, initiating fibrinolysis. **Therapeutic Effect:** Degrades fibrin clots, fibrinogen, other plasma proteins.

## PHARMACOKINETICS

Rapidly metabolized in liver. Primarily excreted in urine. **Half-life:** 35 min.

## ☒ LIFESPAN CONSIDERATIONS

**Pregnancy/Lactation:** Use only when benefit outweighs potential risk to fetus. Unknown if drug crosses placenta or is distributed in breast milk. **Children:** Safety and efficacy not established. **Elderly:** May have increased risk of bleeding; monitor closely.

## INTERACTIONS

**DRUG:** Heparin, **low molecular weight heparins, medications altering platelet function (e.g., clopidogrel, NSAIDs, thrombolytics), oral anticoagulants (e.g., warfarin)** increase risk of hemorrhage. **HERBAL:** Cat's claw, dong quai, evening primrose,

**feverfew, garlic, ginkgo, ginseng, green tea, horse chestnut, red clover** may increase risk of bleeding due to antiplatelet activity. **FOOD:** None known. **LAB VALUES:** Decreases plasminogen, fibrinogen levels during infusion, decreases clotting time (confirms the presence of lysis). May decrease Hgb, Hct.

## AVAILABILITY (Rx)

**Injection, Powder for Reconstitution:** 2 mg (Cathflo Activase), 50 mg (Activase), 100 mg (Activase).

## ADMINISTRATION/HANDLING

 IV

**Reconstitution • Activase:** Reconstitute immediately before use with Sterile Water for Injection. • Reconstitute 100-mg vial with 100 ml Sterile Water for Injection (50-mg vial with 50 ml sterile water) without preservative to provide a concentration of 1 mg/ml. **Activase Cathflo:** Add 2.2 ml Sterile Water for Injection to provide concentration of 1 mg/ml. • Avoid excessive agitation; gently swirl or slowly invert vial to reconstitute.
**Rate of Administration • Activase:** Give by IV infusion via infusion pump (see Indications/Routes/Dosage). • If minor bleeding occurs at puncture sites, apply pressure for 30 sec; if unrelieved, apply pressure dressing. • If uncontrolled hemorrhage occurs, discontinue infusion immediately (slowing rate of infusion may produce worsening hemorrhage). • Avoid undue pressure when drug is injected into catheter (can rupture catheter or expel clot into circulation). **Activase Cathflo:** Instill dose into occluded catheter. • After 30 min, assess catheter function by attempting to aspirate blood. • If still occluded, let dose dwell an additional 90 min. • If function not restored, a second dose may be instilled.
**Storage • Activase:** Store vials at room temperature. • After reconstitution, solution appears colorless to pale

yellow. • Solution is stable for 8 hrs after reconstitution. Discard unused portions. • **Activase Cathflo:** Refrigerate vials.

## 🔲 IV INCOMPATIBILITIES

Dobutamine (Dobutrex), dopamine (Intropin), heparin.

## 🔲 IV COMPATIBILITIES

Lidocaine, metoprolol (Lopressor), morphine, nitroglycerin, propranolol (Inderal).

## INDICATIONS/ROUTES/DOSAGE

**Acute MI**
**IV Infusion: ADULTS WEIGHING MORE THAN 67 KG: Total dose:** 100 mg over 90 min, starting with 15-mg bolus over 1–2 min, then 50 mg over 30 min, then 35 mg over 60 min. **ADULTS WEIGHING 67 KG OR LESS: Total dose:** Start with 15-mg bolus over 1–2 min, then 0.75 mg/kg over 30 min (**maximum:** 50 mg), then 0.5 mg/kg over 60 min (**maximum:** 35 mg). **Maximum total dose:** 100 mg.

**Acute Pulmonary Emboli**
**IV Infusion: ADULTS:** 100 mg over 2 hrs. May give as a 10-mg bolus followed by 90 mg over 2 hrs. Institute or reinstitute heparin near end or immediately after infusion when activated partial thromboplastin time (aPTT) or thrombin time (TT) returns to twice normal or less.

**Acute Ischemic Stroke**
◄**ALERT**► Dose should be given within the first 3 hrs of the onset of symptoms. Recommended total dose: 0.9 mg/kg. **Maximum:** 90 mg.
**IV Infusion: ADULTS WEIGHING 100 KG OR LESS:** 0.09 mg/kg as IV bolus over 1 min, then 0.81 mg/kg as continuous infusion over 60 min. **WEIGHING GREATER THAN 100 KG:** 9 mg bolus over 1 min, then 81 mg as continuous infusion over 60 min.

**Central Venous Catheter Clearance**
**IV: ADULTS, ELDERLY:** Up to 2 mg; may repeat after 2 hrs. If catheter functional, withdraw 4–5 ml blood to remove drug and residual clot.

**Usual Neonatal Dosage**
**Occluded IV Catheter:** Use 1 mg/ml conc (**maximum:** 2 mg/2 ml) leave in lumen up to 2 hrs, then aspirate.
**Systemic Thrombosis:** 0.1–0.6 mg/kg/hr for 6 hrs.

**Dosage in Renal/Hepatic Impairment**
No dose adjustment.

## SIDE EFFECTS

**Frequent:** Superficial bleeding at puncture sites, decreased B/P. **Occasional:** Allergic reaction (rash, wheezing, bruising).

## ADVERSE EFFECTS/ TOXIC REACTIONS

Severe internal hemorrhage may occur. Lysis of coronary thrombi may produce atrial or ventricular arrhythmias or stroke.

## NURSING CONSIDERATIONS

### BASELINE ASSESSMENT

Assess for contraindications to therapy. Obtain baseline B/P, apical pulse. Record weight. Evaluate 12-lead EKG, cardiac enzymes, electrolytes. Assess Hct, platelet count, thrombin time (TT), prothrombin time (PT), activated partial thromboplastin time (aPTT), fibrinogen level before therapy is instituted. Type, crossmatch, hold blood.

### INTERVENTION/EVALUATION

Perform continuous cardiac monitoring for arrhythmias. Check B/P, pulse, respirations q15min until stable, then hourly. Check peripheral pulses, heart and lung sounds. Monitor for chest pain relief and notify physician of continuation or recurrence (note location, type, intensity). Assess for bleeding: overt blood, occult blood in any body substance. Monitor aPTT per protocol. Maintain B/P; avoid any trauma that might increase risk of bleeding (e.g., injections, shaving). Assess neurologic status frequently.

# amikacin

am-i-**kay**-sin
Amikin ✦

■ **BLACK BOX ALERT** ■ May cause neurotoxicity, nephrotoxicity, and/ or neuromuscular blockade and respiratory paralysis. Ototoxicity usually is irreversible; nephrotoxicity usually is reversible.
**Do not confuse amikacin or Amikin with Amicar, or amikacin with anakinra.**

## ◆CLASSIFICATION

**PHARMACOTHERAPEUTIC:** Aminoglycoside. **CLINICAL:** Antibiotic.

## USES

Treatment of serious infections due to *Pseudomonas,* other gram-negative organisms (*Proteus, Serratia,* other gram-negative bacilli) including biliary tract, bone and joint, CNS, intra-abdominal, skin and soft tissue, urinary tract. Treatment of bacterial pneumonia, septicemia. **OFF-LABEL:** *Mycobacterium avium* complex (MAC).

## PRECAUTIONS

**Contraindications:** Hypersensitivity to amikacin, other aminoglycosides. **Cautions:** Preexisting renal impairment, auditory or vestibular impairment, hypocalcemia, elderly, pts with neuromuscular disorder, dehydration, concomitant use of neurotoxic or nephrotoxic medications.

## ACTION

Inhibits protein synthesis in susceptible bacteria by binding to 30S ribosomal unit. **Therapeutic Effect:** Interferes with protein synthesis of susceptible microorganisms.

## PHARMACOKINETICS

Rapid, complete absorption after IM administration. Protein binding: 0%–10%. Widely distributed (penetrates blood-brain barrier when meninges are inflamed). Excreted unchanged in urine.

---

Removed by hemodialysis. **Half-life:** 2–4 hrs (increased in renal impairment, neonates; decreased in cystic fibrosis, burn pts, febrile pts).

## ⏳ LIFESPAN CONSIDERATIONS

**Pregnancy/Lactation:** Readily crosses placenta; small amounts distributed in breast milk. May produce fetal nephrotoxicity. **Children:** Neonates, premature infants may be more susceptible to toxicity due to immature renal function. **Elderly:** Higher risk of toxicity due to age-related renal impairment, increased risk of hearing loss.

## INTERACTIONS

**DRUG: Nephrotoxic and ototoxic medications** may increase toxicity. May increase effects of **cyclosporine, neuromuscular blocking agents. HERBAL:** None significant. **FOOD:** None known. **LAB VALUES:** May increase serum creatinine, BUN, ALT, AST, bilirubin, LDH. May decrease serum calcium, magnesium, potassium, sodium. **Therapeutic levels:** Peak: life-threatening infections: 25–40 mcg/ml; serious infections: 20–25 mcg/ml; urinary tract infections: 15–20 mcg/ml. **Trough:** Less than 8 mcg/ml. **Toxic levels:** Peak: greater than 40 mcg/ml; **trough:** greater than 10 mcg/ml.

## AVAILABILITY (Rx)

**Injection Solution:** 250 mg/ml.

## ADMINISTRATION/HANDLING
🔲 IV

**Reconstitution** • Dilute to concentration of 0.25–5 mg/ml in 0.9% NaCl or D₅W.
**Rate of Administration** • Infuse over 30–60 min.
**Storage** • Store vials at room temperature. • Solution appears clear but may become pale yellow (does not affect potency). • Intermittent IV infusion (piggyback) is stable for 24 hrs at room temperature, 2 days if refrigerated. • Discard if precipitate forms or dark discoloration occurs.

**IM**
• To minimize discomfort, give deep IM slowly. • Less painful if injected into gluteus maximus rather than in lateral aspect of thigh.

## ▦ IV INCOMPATIBILITIES

Amphotericin, azithromycin (Zithromax), propofol (Diprivan).

## ▦ IV COMPATIBILITIES

Amiodarone (Cordarone), aztreonam (Azactam), calcium gluconate, cefepime (Maxipime), cimetidine (Tagamet), ciprofloxacin (Cipro), clindamycin (Cleocin), dexmedetomidine (Precedex), diltiazem (Cardizem), diphenhydramine (Benadryl), enalapril (Vasotec), esmolol (BreviBloc), fluconazole (Diflucan), furosemide (Lasix), levofloxacin (Levaquin), lorazepam (Ativan), magnesium sulfate, midazolam (Versed), morphine, ondansetron (Zofran), potassium chloride, ranitidine (Zantac), vancomycin.

## INDICATIONS/ROUTES/DOSAGE

**Usual Parenteral Dosage**
**IV, IM: ADULTS, ELDERLY, CHILDREN, INFANTS:** 5–7.5 mg/kg/dose q8h. **NEONATES:** 15 mg/kg/dose q12–48h (based on wgt).

**Dosage in Renal Impairment**
Dosage and frequency are modified based on degree of renal impairment and serum drug concentration. After a loading dose of 5–7.5 mg/kg, maintenance dose and frequency are based on serum creatinine levels and creatinine clearance.

| Creatinine Clearance | Dosing Interval |
| --- | --- |
| 60 ml/min or greater | q8h |
| 40–59 ml/min | q12h |
| 20–39 ml/min | q24h |
| Less than 20 ml/min | Loading dose, monitor levels |
| Hemodialysis | q48–72h (give after HD on dialysis days) |
| Continuous renal replacement therapy (CRRT) | Initially, 10 mg/kg, then 7.5 mg/kg q24–48h |

**Dosage in Hepatic Impairment**
No dose adjustment.

## SIDE EFFECTS

**Frequent:** Phlebitis, thrombophlebitis. **Occasional:** Rash, fever, urticaria, pruritus. **Rare:** Neuromuscular blockade (difficulty breathing, drowsiness, weakness).

## ADVERSE EFFECTS/ TOXIC REACTIONS

Serious reactions include nephrotoxicity (increased thirst, decreased appetite, nausea, vomiting, increased BUN and serum creatinine levels, decreased creatinine clearance); neurotoxicity (muscle twitching, visual disturbances, seizures, paresthesia); ototoxicity (tinnitus, dizziness, loss of hearing).

## NURSING CONSIDERATIONS

### BASELINE ASSESSMENT

Dehydration must be treated prior to aminoglycoside therapy. Establish baseline hearing acuity before beginning therapy. Question for history of allergies, esp. to aminoglycosides and sulfite. Obtain specimen for culture, sensitivity before giving first dose (therapy may begin before results are known).

### INTERVENTION/EVALUATION

Monitor I&O (maintain hydration), urinalysis. Monitor results of serum peak/ trough levels. Be alert to ototoxic, neurotoxic, nephrotoxic symptoms (see Adverse Effects/Toxic Reactions). Check IM injection site for pain, induration. Evaluate IV site for phlebitis. Assess for skin rash, diarrhea, superinfection (particularly genital/anal pruritus), changes of oral mucosa. When treating pts with neuromuscular disorders, assess respiratory response carefully. **Therapeutic levels:** Peak: life-threatening infections: 25–40 mcg/ml; serious infections: 20–25 mcg/ ml; urinary tract infections: 15–20 mcg/ ml. **Trough:** Less than 8 mcg/ml. **Toxic levels:** Peak: greater than 40 mcg/ml; **trough:** greater than 10 mcg/ml.

## PATIENT/FAMILY TEACHING

• Continue antibiotic for full length of treatment. • Space doses evenly. • IM injection may cause discomfort. • Report any hearing, visual, balance, urinary problems, even after therapy is completed. • Do not take other medications without consulting physician.

## amiodarone HIGH ALERT

a-mi-**oh**-da-rone
(Apo-Amiodarone ✚, Cordarone, Nexterone, Pacerone)

■ **BLACK BOX ALERT** ■ Pts should be hospitalized when amiodarone is initiated. Alternative therapies should be tried first before using amiodarone. Only indicated for pts with life-threatening arrhythmias due to risk of toxicity. Pulmonary toxicity may occur without symptoms. Hepatotoxicity is common, usually mild (rarely possible). Can exacerbate arrhythmias.

**Do not confuse amiodarone with amiloride, or Cordarone with Cardura.**

## ◆CLASSIFICATION

**PHARMACOTHERAPEUTIC:** Cardiac agent. **CLINICAL:** Antiarrhythmic.

## USES

Management of life-threatening recurrent ventricular fibrillation, hemodynamically unstable ventricular tachycardia (VT) unresponsive to other therapy. **OFF-LABEL:** Treatment of atrial fibrillation, paroxysmal supraventricular tachycardia (SVT); ventricular tachyarrhythmias.

## PRECAUTIONS

**Contraindications:** Hypersensitivity to amiodarone, iodine. Bradycardia-induced syncope (except in the presence of a pacemaker), second- and third-degree AV block (except in presence of a pacemaker); severe sinus node dysfunction, causing marked sinus bradycardia; cardiogenic

 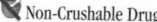

shock. **Cautions:** May prolong QT interval. Thyroid disease, electrolyte imbalance, hepatic disease, hypotension, left ventricular dysfunction, pulmonary disease. Pts taking warfarin, surgical pts.

## ACTION

Prolongs duration of myocardial cell action potential and refractory period by acting directly on all cardiac tissue. Decreases AV and sinus node function. **Therapeutic Effect:** Suppresses arrhythmias.

## PHARMACOKINETICS

| Route | Onset | Peak | Duration |
|-------|-------|------|----------|
| PO | 3 days–3 wks | 1 wk–5 mos | 7–50 days after discontinuation |

Slowly, variably absorbed from GI tract. Protein binding: 96%. Extensively metabolized in liver. Excreted via bile; not removed by hemodialysis. **Half-life:** 26–107 days; metabolite, 61 days.

## ⏳ LIFESPAN CONSIDERATIONS

**Pregnancy/Lactation:** Crosses placenta; distributed in breast milk. May adversely affect fetal development. **Children:** Safety and efficacy not established. **Elderly:** May be more sensitive to effects on thyroid function. May experience increased incidence of ataxia, other neurotoxic effects.

## INTERACTIONS

**DRUG: Sofosbuvir** may cause severe bradycardia. May increase **thioridazine** concentration and produce additive prolongation of QT interval. May increase cardiac effects with **other antiarrhythmics.** May increase effect of **beta blockers (e.g., labetolol, metoprolol), oral anticoagulants (e.g., warfarin).** May increase concentration, toxicity of **aripiprazole, colchicine, digoxin, phenytoin.** May increase risk of **simvastatin** toxicity, myopathy, rhabdomyolysis. **HERBAL: St. John's wort** may decrease effect. **Ephedra** may

worsen arrhythmia. **FOOD: Grapefruit products** may alter effect. Avoid use during therapy. **LAB VALUES:** May increase serum ALT, AST, alkaline phosphatase, ANA titer. May cause changes in EKG, thyroid function test results. **Therapeutic serum level:** 0.5–2.5 mcg/ml; toxic serum level not established.

## AVAILABILITY (Rx)

**Infusion (Pre-Mix):** Nexterone: 150 mg/100 ml; 360 mg/200 ml. **Injection, Solution (Cordarone IV):** 50 mg/ml. **Tablets:** 100 mg (Pacerone), 200 mg (Cordarone, Pacerone), 400 mg (Pacerone).

## ADMINISTRATION/HANDLING

 **IV**

**Reconstitution** • Infusions longer than 2 hrs must be administered/diluted in glass or polyolefin bottles. • Dilute loading dose (150 mg) in 100 ml D₅W (1.5 mg/ml). • Dilute maintenance dose (900 mg) in 500 ml D₅W (1.8 mg/ml). Concentrations greater than 3 mg/ml cause peripheral vein phlebitis.
**Rate of Administration** • Does not need protection from light during administration. • Administer through central venous catheter (CVC) if possible, using in-line filter. • Bolus over 10 min (15 mg/min) not to exceed 30 mg/min; then 1 mg/min over 6 hrs; then 0.5 mg/min over 18 hrs. • Infusions longer than 1 hr, concentration not to exceed 2 mg/ml unless CVC used.
**Storage** • Store at room temperature. • Stable for 24 hrs when diluted in glass or polyolefin containers; stable for 2 hrs when diluted in PVC containers.

### PO
• Give consistently with regard to meals to reduce GI distress. • Tablets may be crushed • Do not give with grapefruit products.

## ▨ IV INCOMPATIBILITIES

Cefazolin (Ancef), heparin, sodium bicarbonate.

---

<u>underlined</u> – top prescribed drug

## ▧ IV COMPATIBILITIES

Dexmedetomidine (Precedex), dobutamine (Dobutrex), dopamine (Intropin), furosemide (Lasix), insulin (regular), labetalol (Normodyne), lidocaine, lorazepam (Ativan), midazolam (Versed), morphine, nitroglycerin, norepinephrine (Levophed), phenylephrine (Neo-Synephrine), potassium chloride, vancomycin.

## INDICATIONS/ROUTES/DOSAGE

### Ventricular Arrhythmias

**PO: ADULTS, ELDERLY:** Initially, 800–1,600 mg/day in 1–2 divided doses for 1–3 wks. After arrhythmia is controlled or side effects occur, reduce to 600–800 mg/day for 4 wks. **Maintenance:** 400 mg/day.

**IV Infusion: ADULTS, ELDERLY:** Initially, 1,050 mg over 24 hrs; 150 mg over 10 min, then 360 mg over 6 hrs; then 540 mg over 18 hrs. May continue at 0.5 mg/min. After first 24 hrs, infuse 720 mg/24 hrs (0.5 mg/min) with a concentration of 1–6 mg/ml.

### Dosage in Renal Impairment

No dose adjustment.

### Dosage in Hepatic Impairment

Use caution.

## SIDE EFFECTS

**Expected:** Corneal microdeposits noted in almost all pts treated for more than 6 mos (can lead to blurry vision). **Occasional (greater than 3%): PO:** Constipation, headache, decreased appetite, nausea, vomiting, paresthesia, photosensitivity, muscular incoordination. **Parenteral:** Hypotension, nausea, fever, bradycardia. **Rare (less than 3%): PO:** Bitter or metallic taste, decreased libido, dizziness, facial flushing, blue-gray coloring of skin (face, arms, and neck), blurred vision, bradycardia, asymptomatic corneal deposits, rash, visual disturbances, halo vision.

## ADVERSE EFFECTS/TOXIC REACTIONS

Serious, potentially fatal pulmonary toxicity (alveolitis, pulmonary fibrosis, pneumonitis, acute respiratory distress syndrome) may begin with progressive dyspnea and cough with crackles, decreased breath sounds, pleurisy, HF, or hepatotoxicity. May worsen existing arrhythmias or produce new arrhythmias.

## NURSING CONSIDERATIONS

### BASELINE ASSESSMENT

Obtain baseline ALT, AST, alkaline phosphatase, EKG; pulmonary function tests, CXR in pts with pulmonary disease. Assess B/P, apical pulse immediately before drug is administered (if pulse is 60/min or less or systolic B/P is less than 90 mm Hg, withhold medication, contact physician).

### INTERVENTION/EVALUATION

Monitor for symptoms of pulmonary toxicity (progressively worsening dyspnea, cough). Dosage should be discontinued or reduced if toxicity occurs. Assess pulse for quality, rhythm, bradycardia. Monitor EKG for cardiac changes (e.g., widening of QRS, prolongation of PR and QT intervals). Notify physician of any significant interval changes. Assess for nausea, fatigue, paresthesia, tremor. Monitor for signs of hypothyroidism (periorbital edema, lethargy, pudgy hands/feet, cool/pale skin, vertigo, night cramps) and hyperthyroidism (hot/dry skin, bulging eyes [exophthalmos], frequent urination, eyelid edema, weight loss, difficulty breathing). Monitor serum ALT, AST, alkaline phosphatase for evidence of hepatic toxicity. Assess skin, cornea for bluish discoloration in pts who have been on drug therapy longer than 2 mos. Monitor thyroid function test results. If elevated hepatic enzymes occur, dosage reduction or discontinuation is necessary. Monitor for therapeutic serum level (0.5–2.5 mcg/ml). Toxic serum level not established.

---

✢ Canadian trade name      Non-Crushable Drug     ▦▦ High Alert drug

## PATIENT/FAMILY TEACHING

• Protect against photosensitivity reaction on skin exposed to sunlight. • Bluish skin discoloration gradually disappears when drug is discontinued. • Report shortness of breath, cough. • Outpatients should monitor pulse before taking medication. • Do not abruptly discontinue medication. • Compliance with therapy regimen is essential to control arrhythmias. • Restrict salt, alcohol intake. • Avoid grapefruit products. • Recommend ophthalmic exams q6mos. • Report any vision changes, signs/symptoms of cardiac arrhythmias.

---

# amitriptyline

a-mi-**trip**-ti-leen
(Apo-Amitriptyline ✲, Elavil ✲, Levate ✲, Novo-Tryptyn ✲)

■ **BLACK BOX ALERT** ■ Increased risk of suicidal thinking and behavior in children, adolescents, young adults 18–24 yrs with major depressive disorder, other psychiatric disorders.

**Do not confuse amitriptyline with aminophylline, imipramine, or nortriptyline, or Elavil with Eldepryl, enalapril, Equanil, or Mellaril.**

## FIXED-COMBINATION(S)

**Limbitrol:** amitriptyline/chlordiazepoxide (an antianxiety): 12.5 mg/5 mg, 25 mg/10 mg.

## ◆CLASSIFICATION

**PHARMACOTHERAPEUTIC:** Tricyclic. **CLINICAL:** Antidepressant, antineuralgic, antibulimic.

## USES

Treatment of depression. **OFF-LABEL:** Neuropathic pain, related to diabetic neuropathy or postherpetic neuralgia; treatment of migraine. Treatment of depression in children, post-traumatic stress disorder (PTSD).

## PRECAUTIONS

**Contraindications:** Hypersensitivity to amitriptyline. Acute recovery period after MI, use within 14 days of MAOIs. **Cautions:** Prostatic hypertrophy, history of urinary retention or obstruction, narrow-angle glaucoma, diabetes mellitus, seizures, hyperthyroidism, cardiac/hepatic/renal disease, schizophrenia, xerostomia, visual problems, constipation or bowel obstruction, elderly, increased intraocular pressure (IOP), hiatal hernia, suicidal ideation.

## ACTION

Blocks reuptake of neurotransmitters (norepinephrine, serotonin) at presynaptic membranes, increasing availability at postsynaptic receptor sites. Strong anticholinergic activity. **Therapeutic Effect:** Antidepressant effect.

## PHARMACOKINETICS

Rapidly and well absorbed from GI tract. Protein binding: 90%. Metabolized in liver. Primarily excreted in urine. Minimal removal by hemodialysis. **Half-life:** 10–26 hrs.

## ⧗ LIFESPAN CONSIDERATIONS

**Pregnancy/Lactation:** Crosses placenta; minimally distributed in breast milk. **Children:** More sensitive to increased dosage, toxicity, increased risk of suicidal ideation, worsening of depression. **Elderly:** Increased risk of toxicity. Increased sensitivity to anticholinergic effects. Caution in pts with cardiovascular disease.

## INTERACTIONS

**DRUG:** CNS depressants (e.g., **alcohol, anticonvulsants, barbiturates, phenothiazines, sedative-hypnotics**) may increase sedation, respiratory depression, hypotensive effect. **Dronedarone, thioridazine, toremefine, ziprasidone** levels may be increased. **Quetiapine** may increase level/effect. May increase risk of hypertensive crisis, hyperpyresis, seizures with **MAOIs.** **HERBAL:** St. John's wort may decrease levels. **Gotu kola, kava kava, St. John's wort, valerian** may increase CNS depression. **FOOD:** None known. **LAB VALUES:** May alter EKG readings (flattened T wave), serum glucose (increase or decrease). **Therapeutic serum level:** Peak: 120–250 ng/ml; **toxic serum level:** greater than 500 ng/ml.

## AVAILABILITY (Rx)

**Tablets:** 10 mg, 25 mg, 50 mg, 75 mg, 100 mg, 150 mg.

## ADMINISTRATION/HANDLING

**PO**

• Give with food or milk if GI distress occurs.

## INDICATIONS/ROUTES/DOSAGE

**Depression**

**PO: ADULTS:** Initially, 25–50 mg/day as a single dose at bedtime, or in divided doses. May gradually increase up to 100–300 mg/day. Titrate to lowest effective dosage. **ELDERLY:** 10 mg 3 times/day and 20 mg at bedtime.

**Pain Management**

**PO: ADULTS, ELDERLY:** 25–50 mg at bedtime. May increase to 150 mg/day. **ADOLESCENTS:** 10 mg 3 times/day and 20 mg at bedtime. **CHILDREN:** Initially, 0.1 mg/kg. May increase over 2 wks to 0.5–2 mg/kg at bedtime.

**Dosage in Renal/Hepatic Impairment**
Use with caution.

## SIDE EFFECTS

**Frequent:** Dizziness, drowsiness, dry mouth, orthostatic hypotension, headache, increased appetite, weight gain, nausea, unusual fatigue, unpleasant taste. **Occasional:** Blurred vision, confusion, constipation, hallucinations, delayed micturition, eye pain, arrhythmias, fine muscle tremors, parkinsonian syndrome, anxiety, diarrhea, diaphoresis, heartburn, insomnia. **Rare:** Hypersensitivity, alopecia, tinnitus, breast enlargement, photosensitivity.

## ADVERSE EFFECTS/ TOXIC REACTIONS

Overdose may produce confusion, seizures, severe drowsiness, changes in cardiac conduction, fever, hallucinations, agitation, dyspnea, vomiting, unusual fatigue, weakness. Abrupt withdrawal after prolonged therapy may produce headache, malaise, nausea, vomiting, vivid dreams. Blood dyscrasias, cholestatic jaundice occur rarely.

## NURSING CONSIDERATIONS

### BASELINE ASSESSMENT

Observe and record behavior. Assess psychological status, thought content, suicidal ideation, sleep patterns, appearance, interest in environment. For pts on long-term therapy, hepatic/renal function tests, blood counts should be performed periodically.

### INTERVENTION/EVALUATION

Supervise suicidal-risk pt closely during early therapy (as depression lessens, energy level improves, increasing suicide potential). Assess appearance, behavior, speech pattern, level of interest, mood. Monitor B/P for hypotension, pulse, arrhythmias. **Therapeutic serum level:** Peak: 120–250 ng/ml; **toxic serum level:** greater than 500 ng/ml.

### PATIENT/FAMILY TEACHING

• Go slowly from lying to standing. • Tolerance to postural hypotension, sedative and anticholinergic effects usually develop during early therapy. • Maximum therapeutic effect may be noted in 2–4 wks. • Sensitivity to sun may occur. • Report visual disturbances. • Do not abruptly discontinue medication. • Avoid tasks that require alertness, motor skills until response to drug is established. • Avoid alcohol. • Sips of water may relieve dry mouth.

---

✦ Canadian trade name    🦺 Non-Crushable Drug    📋 High Alert drug

# *amLODIPine    TOP 100

am-**loe**-di-peen
(Apo-Amlodipine ✦, Norvasc)
**Do not confuse amlodipine
with amiloride, or Norvasc with
Navane or Vascor.**

## FIXED-COMBINATION(S)

**Anturnide:** amlodipine/aliskiren (a
renin inhibitor)/hydrochlorothiazide
(a diuretic): 5 mg/150 mg/12.5 mg,
5 mg/300 mg/12.5 mg, 5 mg/300
mg/25 mg, 10 mg/300 mg/12.5 mg,
10 mg/300 mg/25 mg. **Azor:** amlo-
dipine/olmesartan (an angiotensin II
receptor antagonist): 5 mg/20 mg, 10
mg/20 mg, 5 mg/40 mg, 10 mg/40
mg. **Caduet:** amlodipine/atorvastatin
(hydroxamethylglutaryl-CoA [HMG-
CoA] reductase inhibitor): 2.5 mg/
10 mg, 2.5 mg/20 mg, 2.5 mg/40 mg,
5 mg/10 mg, 10 mg/10 mg, 5 mg/
20 mg, 10 mg/20 mg, 5 mg/40 mg,
10 mg/40 mg, 5 mg/80 mg, 10 mg/80
mg. **Exforge:** amlodipine/valsartan
(an angiotensin II receptor antagonist): 5 mg/160 mg, 10 mg/160 mg,
5 mg/320 mg, 10 mg/320 mg. **Exforge HCT:** amlodipine/valsartan/
hydrochlorothiazide (a diuretic):
5 mg/160 mg/12.5 mg, 5 mg/160 mg/
25 mg, 10 mg/160 mg/12.5 mg, 10 mg/
160 mg/25 mg, 10 mg/320 mg/25 mg.
**Lotrel:** amlodipine/benazepril (an
angiotensin-converting enzyme [ACE]
inhibitor): 2.5 mg/10 mg, 5 mg/
10 mg, 5 mg/20 mg, 5 mg/40 mg, 10
mg/20 mg, 10 mg/40 mg. **Prestalia:**
amlodipine/perindopril (an ACE inhibitor): 2.5 mg/3.5 mg; 5 mg/7 mg;
10 mg/14 mg. **Tekamlo:** amlodipine/
aliskiren (a renin inhibitor): 5 mg/
150 mg, 5 mg/300 mg, 10 mg/150 mg,
10 mg/300 mg. **Tribenzor:** amlodip-
ine/olmesartan/hydrochlorothiazide:
5 mg/20 mg/12.5 mg, 5 mg/
40 mg/12.5 mg, 5 mg/40 mg/25 mg,
10 mg/40 mg/12.5 mg, 10 mg/

40 mg/25 mg. **Twynsta:** amlodipine/
telmisartan (an angiotensin II receptor antagonist): 5 mg/40 mg, 5 mg/80
mg, 10 mg/40 mg, 10 mg/80 mg.

## ◆CLASSIFICATION

**PHARMACOTHERAPEUTIC:** Calcium
channel blocker. **CLINICAL:** Antihypertensive, antianginal.

## USES

Management of hypertension, coronary artery disease (chronic stable angina, vasospastic [Prinzmetal's or variant] angina).

## PRECAUTIONS

**Contraindications:** Hypersensitivity    to
amlodipine. **Cautions:** Hepatic impairment, severe aortic stenosis, hypertophic
cardiomyopathy with outflow tract obstruction.

## ACTION

Inhibits calcium movement across cardiac and vascular smooth muscle cell
membranes. **Therapeutic Effect:** Dilates coronary arteries, peripheral
arteries/arterioles. Decreases total peripheral vascular resistance and B/P by
vasodilation.

## PHARMACOKINETICS

| Route | Onset | Peak | Duration |
|-------|-------|------|----------|
| PO | 0.5–1 hr | N/A | 24 hrs |

Slowly absorbed from GI tract. Protein
binding: 95%–98%. Metabolized in liver.
Excreted primarily in urine. Not removed
by hemodialysis. **Half-life:** 30–50 hrs
(increased in elderly, pts with hepatic
cirrhosis).

## ⧖ LIFESPAN CONSIDERATIONS

**Pregnancy/Lactation:** Unknown if drug
crosses placenta or is distributed in breast
milk. **Children:** Safety and efficacy not
established. **Elderly:** Half-life may be
increased, more sensitive to hypotensive
effects.

## INTERACTIONS

**DRUG:** May increase level of **simvastatin. Azole antifungals, cyclosporine, protease inhibitors** may increase concentration. **Carbamazepine, rifampin** may decrease level/effect. **HERBAL: St. John's wort** may decrease concentration. **Ephedra, yohimbe** may worsen hypertension. **Garlic** may increase antihypertensive effect. **FOOD: Grapefruit products** may increase concentration, hypotensive effects. **LAB VALUES:** May increase hepatic enzyme levels.

## AVAILABILITY (Rx)

**Tablets:** 2.5 mg, 5 mg, 10 mg.

## ADMINISTRATION/HANDLING

**PO**
• May give without regard to food.

## INDICATIONS/ROUTES/DOSAGE

**Hypertension**
**PO: ADULTS:** Initially, 5 mg/day as a single dose. May titrate every 7–14 days. **Maximum:** 10 mg/day. **SMALL-FRAME, FRAGILE, ELDERLY:** 2.5 mg/day as a single dose. May titrate q7–14 days. **Maximum:** 10 mg/day. **CHILDREN 6–17 YRS:** 2.5–5 mg/day.

**CAD**
**PO: ADULTS:** 5–10 mg/day as a single dose. **ELDERLY, PTS WITH HEPATIC INSUFFICIENCY:** 5 mg/day as a single dose.

**Dosage in Renal Impairment**
No dose adjustment.

**Dosage in Hepatic Impairment**
**ADULTS, ELDERLY:** (Hypertension) Initially, 2.5 mg/day. (Angina) Initially, 5 mg/day. Titrate slowly in pts with severe impairment.

## SIDE EFFECTS

**Frequent (greater than 5%):** Peripheral edema, headache, flushing. **Occasional (5%–1%):** Dizziness, palpitations, nausea, unusual fatigue or weakness (asthenia). **Rare (less than 1%):** Chest pain, bradycardia, orthostatic hypotension.

## ADVERSE EFFECTS/ TOXIC REACTIONS

Overdose may produce excessive peripheral vasodilation, marked hypotension with reflex tachycardia, syncopy.

## NURSING CONSIDERATIONS

### BASELINE ASSESSMENT

Assess baseline renal/hepatic function tests, B/P, apical pulse.

### INTERVENTION/EVALUATION

Assess B/P (if systolic B/P is less than 90 mm Hg, withhold medication, contact physician). Assess for peripheral edema behind medial malleolus (sacral area in bedridden pts). Assess skin for flushing. Question for headache, asthenia.

### PATIENT/FAMILY TEACHING

• Do not abruptly discontinue medication. • Compliance with therapy regimen is essential to control hypertension. • Avoid tasks that require alertness, motor skills until response to drug is established. • Do not ingest grapefruit products.

# amoxicillin

a-**mox**-i-sil-in
(Apo-Amoxi ✦, Moxatag, Novamoxin ✦)
**Do not confuse amoxicillin with amoxapine or Atarax.**

## ◆CLASSIFICATION

**PHARMACOTHERAPEUTIC:** Penicillin. **CLINICAL:** Antibiotic.

## USES

Treatment of susceptible infections due to streptococci, *E. coli, E. faecalis, P. mirabilis, H. influenzae, N. gonorrhoeae* including ear, nose, and throat; lower respiratory tract; skin and skin structure; UTIs; acute uncomplicated gonorrhea; *H. pylori.* **OFF-LABEL:** Treatment of Lyme disease and typhoid fever.

 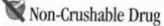

Postexposure prophylaxis for anthrax exposure.

## PRECAUTIONS

**Contraindications:** Hypersensitivity to amoxicillin. **Cautions:** History of allergies (esp. cephalosporins), infectious mononucleosis, renal impairment, asthma.

## ACTION

Inhibits bacterial cell wall synthesis. **Therapeutic Effect:** Bactericidal in susceptible microorganisms.

## PHARMACOKINETICS

Well absorbed from GI tract. Protein binding: 20%. Partially metabolized in liver. Primarily excreted in urine. Removed by hemodialysis. **Half-life:** 1–1.3 hrs (increased in renal impairment).

## ⧗ LIFESPAN CONSIDERATIONS

**Pregnancy/Lactation:** Crosses placenta, appears in cord blood, amniotic fluid. Distributed in breast milk in low concentrations. May lead to allergic sensitization, diarrhea, candidiasis, skin rash in infant. **Children:** Immature renal function in neonate/young infant may delay renal excretion. **Elderly:** Age-related renal impairment may require dosage adjustment.

## INTERACTIONS

**DRUG: Allopurinol** may increase incidence of rash. **Probenecid** may increase concentration, toxicity risk. May decrease effect of **oral contraceptives. HERBAL:** None significant. **FOOD:** None known. **LAB VALUES:** May increase serum ALT, AST, bilirubin, BUN, creatinine, LDH. May cause positive Coombs' test.

## AVAILABILITY (Rx)

**Capsules:** 250 mg, 500 mg. **Powder for Oral Suspension:** 125 mg/5 ml, 200 mg/5 ml, 250 mg/5 ml, 400 mg/5 ml. **Tablets:** 500 mg, 875 mg. **Tablets (Chewable):** 125 mg, 250 mg. **Tablets, Extended-Release (Moxatag):** 775 mg.

## ADMINISTRATION/HANDLING

**PO**

• Give without regard to meals. • Instruct pt to chew/crush chewable tablets thoroughly before swallowing. • Oral suspension dose may be mixed with formula, milk, fruit juice, water, cold drink. • Give immediately after mixing. • After reconstitution, oral suspension is stable for 14 days at either room temperature or refrigerated. **Moxatag:** Take within 1 hr of finishing a meal.

## INDICATIONS/ROUTES/DOSAGE

**Susceptible Infections**
**PO: ADULTS, ELDERLY:** 250–500 mg q8h or 500–875 mg q12h or 775 mg (Moxatag) once daily. **CHILDREN OLDER THAN 3 MOS:** 25–50 mg/kg/day in divided doses q8h. Maximum single dose: 500 mg. **CHILDREN 3 MOS AND YOUNGER:** 25–50 mg/kg/day in divided doses q8h. **NEONATE:** 20–30 mg/kg/day in divided doses q12h.

**Lower Respiratory Tract Infection**
**PO: ADULTS, ELDERLY:** 500 mg q8h or 875 mg q12h. **CHILDREN:** 45 mg/kg/day in divided doses q12h or 40 mg/kg/day in divided doses q8h.

**H. Pylori Infection**
**PO: ADULTS, ELDERLY:** 1 g twice daily in combination with at least 1 other antibiotic and an acid-suppressing agent (proton pump inhibitor or $H_2$ antagonist).

**Otitis Media**
**PO: CHILDREN:** 80–90 mg/kg/day in 2 divided doses. **NEONATES:** 30–40 mg/kg/day in divided doses q8h.

**Dosage in Renal Impairment**
◀**ALERT**▶ Immediate-release 875-mg tablet or 775-mg extended-release tablet should not be used in pts with creatinine clearance less than 30 ml/min. Dosage interval is modified based on creatinine clearance. **Creatinine clearance 10–30 ml/min:** 250–500 mg q12h. **Creatinine**

clearance less than 10 ml/min: 250–500 mg q24h.

**Dosage in Hepatic Impairment**
No dose adjustment.

## SIDE EFFECTS

**Frequent:** GI disturbances (mild diarrhea, nausea, vomiting), headache, oral/vaginal candidiasis. **Occasional:** Generalized rash, urticaria.

## ADVERSE EFFECTS/ TOXIC REACTIONS

Antibiotic-associated colitis, other super-infections (abdominal cramps, severe watery diarrhea, fever) may result from altered bacterial balance of GI tract. Severe hypersensitivity reactions, including anaphylaxis, acute interstitial nephritis, occur rarely.

## NURSING CONSIDERATIONS

### BASELINE ASSESSMENT

Question for history of allergies, esp. penicillins, cephalosporins, renal impairment.

### INTERVENTION/EVALUATION

Promptly report rash, diarrhea (fever, abdominal pain, mucus and blood in stool may indicate antibiotic-associated colitis). Be alert for superinfection: fever, vomiting, diarrhea, anal/genital pruritus, black "hairy" tongue, oral mucosal changes (ulceration, pain, erythema). Monitor renal/hepatic function tests.

### PATIENT/FAMILY TEACHING

• Continue antibiotic for full length of treatment. • Space doses evenly. • Take with meals if GI upset occurs. • Thoroughly crush or chew the chewable tablets before swallowing. • Report rash, diarrhea, other new symptoms.

# amoxicillin/ clavulanate

a-**mox**-i-sil-in/**klav**-yoo-la-nate
(Amoclan, Apo-Amoxi-Clav ✤, Augmentin, Augmentin ES 600, Augmentin XR, Clavulin ✤, Novo-Clavamoxin ✤)
**Do not confuse Augmentin with amoxicillin or Azulfidine.**

## ◆CLASSIFICATION

**PHARMACOTHERAPEUTIC:** Penicillin. **CLINICAL:** Antibiotic.

## USES

Treatment of susceptible infections due to *streptococci, E. coli, E. faecalis, P. mirabilis,* beta-lactamase producing *H. influenzae, Klebsiella* spp., *M. catarrhalis,* and *S. aureus* (not methicillin-resistant *Staphylococcus aureus* [MRSA]) including lower respiratory, skin and skin structure, UTIs, otitis media, sinusitis. **OFF-LABEL:** Chronic antimicrobial suppression of prosthetic joint infection.

## PRECAUTIONS

**Contraindications:** Hypersensitivity to amoxicillin, clavulanate, any penicillins; history of cholestatic jaundice or hepatic impairment with amoxicillin/clavulanate therapy. Augmentin XR (additional): Severe renal impairment, hemodialysis pt. **Cautions:** History of allergies, esp. cephalosporins; renal impairment, infectious mononucleosis.

## ACTION

Amoxicillin inhibits bacterial cell wall synthesis. Clavulanate inhibits bacterial beta-lactamase. **Therapeutic Effect:** Amoxicillin is bactericidal in susceptible microorganisms. Clavulanate protects amoxicillin from enzymatic degradation.

## PHARMACOKINETICS

Well absorbed from GI tract. Protein binding: 20%. Partially metabolized in liver. Primarily excreted in urine. Removed by hemodialysis. **Half-life:** 1–1.3 hrs (increased in renal impairment).

## ⏳ LIFESPAN CONSIDERATIONS

**Pregnancy/Lactation:** Crosses placenta, appears in cord blood, amniotic fluid. Distributed in breast milk in low concentrations. May lead to allergic sensitization, diarrhea, candidiasis, skin rash in infant. **Children:** Immature renal function in neonate/young infant may delay renal excretion. **Elderly:** Age-related renal impairment may require dosage adjustment.

## INTERACTIONS

**DRUG: Allopurinol** may increase incidence of rash. **Probenecid** may increase concentration, toxicity risk. May decrease effect of **oral contraceptives. HERBAL:** None significant. **FOOD:** None known. **LAB VALUES:** May increase serum ALT, AST. May cause positive Coombs' test.

## AVAILABILITY (Rx)

**Powder for Oral Suspension (Amoclan, Augmentin):** 125 mg–31.25 mg/5 ml, 200 mg–28.5 mg/5 ml, 250 mg–62.5 mg/5 ml, 400 mg–57 mg/5 ml, 600 mg–42.9 mg/5 ml. **Tablets (Augmentin):** 250 mg–125 mg, 500 mg–125 mg, 875 mg–125 mg. **Tablets (Chewable [Augmentin]):** 200 mg–28.5 mg, 400 mg–57 mg.

 **Tablets (Extended-Release [Augmentin XR]):** 1,000 mg–62.5 mg.

## ADMINISTRATION/HANDLING

**PO**

• Store tablets at room temperature. • After reconstitution, oral suspension is stable for 10 days but should be refrigerated. • May mix dose of suspension with milk, formula, or juice and give immediately. • Give without regard to meals. • Give with food to increase absorption, decrease stomach upset. • Instruct pt to chew/crush chewable tablets thoroughly before swallowing. • Do not break, crush, dissolve, or divide extended-release tablets.

## INDICATIONS/ROUTES/DOSAGE

**Note:** Dosage based on amoxicillin component.

**Usual Adult Dosage**
**PO: ADULTS, ELDERLY:** 250 mg q8h or 500 mg q8–12h or 875 mg q12h or 2,000 mg q12h.

**Usual Pediatric Dosage**
**PO: CHILDREN OLDER THAN 3 MOS, WEIGHING 40 KG OR MORE: (Mild-Moderate):** 500 mg q12h or 250 mg q8h. **(Severe):** 875 mg q12h or 500 mg q8h. **(Extended-Release):** 2,000 mg q12h. **WEIGHING LESS THAN 40 KG: (Mild-Moderate):** 25 mg/kg/day in 2 divided doses or 20 mg/kg/day in 3 divided doses. **(Severe):** 45 mg/kg/day in 2 divided doses or 40 mg/kg/day in 3 divided doses. **Maximum Single Dose:** 500 mg. **LESS THAN 3 MOS:** Amoxicillin 30 mg/kg/day divided q12h using 125 mg/5ml suspension only.

**Usual Neonate Dosage**
**PO: NEONATES, CHILDREN YOUNGER THAN 3 MOS:** 30 mg/kg/day (125 mg/5 ml suspension) in divided doses q12h.

**Dosage in Renal Impairment**
◀**ALERT**▶ Do not use 875-mg tablet or extended-release tablets for creatinine clearance less than 30 ml/min. Dosage and frequency are modified based on creatinine clearance. **Creatinine clearance 10–30 ml/min:** 250–500 mg q12h. **Creatinine clearance less than 10 ml/min:** 250–500 mg q24h. **HD:** 250–500 mg q24h, give dose during and after dialysis. **PD:** 250 mg q12h.

**Dosage in Hepatic Impairment**
No dose adjustment (see Contraindications).

## SIDE EFFECTS

**Occasional (9%–4%):** Diarrhea, loose stools, nausea, skin rashes, urticaria. **Rare (less than 3%):** Vomiting, vaginitis, abdominal discomfort, flatulence, headache.

## ADVERSE EFFECTS/ TOXIC REACTIONS

Antibiotic-associated colitis, other superinfections (abdominal cramps, severe watery diarrhea, fever) may result from altered bacterial balance. Severe hypersensitivity reactions, including anaphylaxis, acute interstitial nephritis, occur rarely.

## NURSING CONSIDERATIONS

### BASELINE ASSESSMENT

Question for history of allergies, esp. penicillins, cephalosporins, renal impairment.

### INTERVENTION/EVALUATION

Promptly report rash, diarrhea (fever, abdominal pain, mucus and blood in stool may indicate antibiotic-associated colitis). Be alert for signs of superinfection including fever, vomiting, diarrhea, black "hairy" tongue, ulceration or changes of oral mucosa, anal/genital pruritus. Monitor renal/hepatic tests with prolonged therapy.

### PATIENT/FAMILY TEACHING

• Continue antibiotic for full length of treatment. • Space doses evenly. • Take with meals if GI upset occurs. • Thoroughly crush or chew the chewable tablets before swallowing. • Notify physician if rash, diarrhea, other new symptoms occur.

---

## amphotericin B   HIGH ALERT

am-foe-**ter**-i-sin
(Abelcet, AmBisome,
Amphotec, Fungizone ✦)

■ **BLACK BOX ALERT** ■ (Nonliposomal) To be used primarily for pts with progressive, potentially fatal fungal infection. Not to be used for noninvasive forms of fungal disease (oral thrush, vaginal candidiasis).

### ◆CLASSIFICATION

**PHARMACOTHERAPEUTIC:** Polyene antifungal. **CLINICAL:** Antifungal, antiprotozoal.

## USES

**Abelcet:** Treatment of aspergillosis or any type of invasive fungal infections refractory or intolerant to Fungizone. **AmBisome:** Empiric treatment of fungal infection in febrile neutropenic pts. *Aspergillus, Candida* species, *Cryptococcus* infections refractory to Fungizone or pt with renal impairment or toxicity with Fungizone. Treatment of cryptococcal meningitis in HIV-infected pts. Treatment of visceral leishmaniasis. **Amphotec:** Treatment of invasive aspergillosis in pts with renal impairment or toxicity or prior treatment failure with Fungizone. **Fungizone:** Treatment of life-threatening fungal infections caused by susceptible fungi including *Candida* spp., *Histoplasma, Cryptococcus, Aspergillus, Blastomyces.* **OFF-LABEL:** **Abelcet, Amphotec:** Serious *Candida* infections. **AmBisome:** Treatment of systemic histoplasmosis infection.

## PRECAUTIONS

**Contraindications:** Hypersensitivity to amphotericin B. **Cautions:** Concomitant use with other nephrotoxic drugs; renal impairment.

## ACTION

Generally fungistatic but may become fungicidal with high dosages or very susceptible microorganisms. Binds to sterols in fungal cell membrane. **Therapeutic Effect:** Alters fungal cell membrane permeability, allowing loss of potassium, other cellular components, resulting in cell death.

## PHARMACOKINETICS

Protein binding: 90%. Widely distributed. Metabolic fate unknown. Cleared by nonrenal pathways. Minimal removal by hemodialysis. Amphotec and Abelcet are not dialyzable. **Half-life:** Fungizone, 24 hrs (increased in neonates and children); Abelcet, 7.2 days; AmBisome, 100–153 hrs; Amphotec, 26–28 hrs.

---

✦ Canadian trade name          ✔ Non-Crushable Drug          ▦ High Alert drug

## LIFESPAN CONSIDERATIONS

**Pregnancy/Lactation:** Crosses placenta; unknown if distributed in breast milk. **Children:** Safety and efficacy not established, but use the least amount for therapeutic regimen. **Elderly:** No age-related precautions noted.

## INTERACTIONS

**DRUG: Antineoplastic agents** may increase potential for bronchospasm, renal toxicity, hypotension. **Steroids** may cause severe hypokalemia. May increase **digoxin** toxicity (due to hypokalemia). **Nephrotoxic medications (e.g., cyclosporine, IV contrast dye, vancomycin)** may increase nephrotoxicity. **HERBAL:** None significant. **FOOD:** None known. **LAB VALUES:** May increase serum ALT, AST, alkaline phosphatase, BUN, creatinine. May decrease serum calcium, magnesium, potassium.

## AVAILABILITY (Rx)

**Injection, Powder for Reconstitution:** 50 mg (AmBisome, Amphotec, Fungizone), 100 mg (Amphotec). **Injection, Suspension (Abelcet):** 5 mg/ml.

## ADMINISTRATION/HANDLING

 **IV**

• Use strict aseptic technique; no bacteriostatic agent or preservative is present in diluent.

### Reconstitution

**ABELCET**

• Shake 20-ml (100-mg) vial gently until contents are dissolved. Withdraw required dose using 5-micron filter needle (supplied by manufacturer). • Dilute with $D_5W$ to 1–2 mg/ml.

**AMBISOME**

• Reconstitute each 50-mg vial with 12 ml Sterile Water for Injection to provide concentration of 4 mg/ml. • Shake vial vigorously for 30 sec. Withdraw required dose and inject syringe contents through a 5-micron filter into an infusion of $D_5W$ to provide final concentration of 1–2 mg/ml

(0.2–0.5 mg/ml for infants and small children).

**AMPHOTEC**

• Add 10 ml Sterile Water for Injection to each 50-mg vial to provide concentration of 5 mg/ml. Shake gently. • Further dilute **only** with $D_5W$ to a concentration of 0.1–2 mg/ml.

**FUNGIZONE**

• Add 10 ml Sterile Water for Injection to each 50-mg vial. • Further dilute with 250–500 ml $D_5W$. • Final concentration should not exceed 0.1 mg/ml (0.25 mg/ml for central infusion).

### Rate of Administration

• Give by slow IV infusion. Infuse conventional amphotericin over 4–6 hrs; Abelcet over 2 hrs (shake contents if infusion longer than 2 hrs); Amphotec over minimum of 2 hrs (avoid rate faster than 1 mg/kg/hr); AmBisome over 1–2 hrs.

### Storage

**ABELCET**

• Refrigerate unreconstituted solution. Reconstituted solution is stable for 48 hrs if refrigerated, 6 hrs at room temperature.

**AMBISOME**

• Refrigerate unreconstituted solution. Reconstituted vials are stable for 24 hrs when refrigerated. Concentration of 1–2 mg/ml is stable for 6 hrs.

**AMPHOTEC**

• Refrigerate unused vials. • Reconstituted solution is stable for 24 hrs if refrigerated.

**FUNGIZONE**

• Refrigerate unused vials. • Once reconstituted, vials stable for 24 hrs at room temperature, 7 days if refrigerated. • Diluted solutions stable for 24 hrs at room temperature, 2 days if refrigerated.

## IV INCOMPATIBILITIES

**Note:** Abelcet, AmBisome, Amphotec: Do not mix with any other drug, diluent, or solution. Fungizone: Allopurinol (Aloprim), aztreonam (Azactam), calcium gluconate, cefepime (Maxipime), cimetidine (Tagamet), ciprofloxacin (Cipro), dexmedetomidine (Precedex), diphenhydramine

(Benadryl), dopamine (Intropin), enalapril (Vasotec), filgrastim (Neupogen), fluconazole (Diflucan), foscarnet (Foscavir), magnesium sulfate, meropenem (Merrem IV), ondansetron (Zofran), piperacillin and tazobactam (Zosyn), potassium chloride, propofol (Diprivan).

## ⬛ IV COMPATIBILITY

Lorazepam (Ativan).

## INDICATIONS/ROUTES/DOSAGE

**Usual Abelcet Dose**

**IV Infusion** *(Abelcet)*: ADULTS, CHILDREN: 2.5–5 mg/kg/day at rate of 2.5 mg/kg/hr.

**Usual AmBisome Dose**

**IV Infusion** *(Ambisome)*: ADULTS, CHILDREN: 3–6 mg/kg/day over 2 hrs.

**Usual Amphotec Dose**

**IV Infusion** *(Amphotec)*: ADULTS, CHILDREN: 3–4 mg/kg/day at rate no faster than 1 mg/kg/hr. **Maximum:** 6 mg/kg/day.

**Fungizone, Usual Dose**

**IV Infusion:** ADULTS, ELDERLY: Dosage based on pt tolerance and severity of infection. Initially, 1-mg test dose is given over 20–30 min. If tolerated, usual dose is 0.3–1.5 mg/kg/day or 1–1.5 mg/kg q48h. **Maximum:** 1.5 mg/kg/day. **CHILDREN:** Test dose of 0.1 mg/kg/dose (**maximum:** 1 mg) is infused over 30–60 min. If test dose is tolerated, usual dose is 0.25–1 mg/kg/day or 1–1.5 mg/kg q48h. **NEONATES:** Initially, 0.5 mg/kg/dose once daily. May gradually increase by 0.25–0.5 mg/kg each day to maximum of 1.5 mg/kg/day. **Maintenance dose:** 0.25–1 mg/kg/day or 1–1.5 mg/kg/dose every other day.

**Dosage in Renal/Hepatic Impairment**
No dose adjustment.

## SIDE EFFECTS

**Frequent (greater than 10%): Abelcet:** Chills, fever, increased serum creatinine, multiple organ failure. **AmBisome:** Hypokalemia, hypomagnesemia, hyperglycemia, hypocalcemia, edema, abdominal pain, back pain, chills, chest pain, hypotension, diarrhea, nausea, vomiting, headache, fever, rigors, insomnia, dyspnea, epistaxis, increased hepatic/renal function test results. **Amphotec:** Chills, fever, hypotension, tachycardia, increased serum creatinine, hypokalemia, bilirubinemia. **Amphocin:** Fever, chills, headache, anemia, hypokalemia, hypomagnesemia, anorexia, malaise, generalized pain, nephrotoxicity.

## ADVERSE EFFECTS/ TOXIC REACTIONS

Cardiovascular toxicity (hypotension, ventricular fibrillation), anaphylaxis occur rarely. Altered vision/hearing, seizures, hepatic failure, coagulation defects, multiple organ failure, sepsis may occur. Each alternative formulation is less nephrotoxic than conventional amphotericin (Amphocin).

## NURSING CONSIDERATIONS

### BASELINE ASSESSMENT

Obtain baseline BMP, LFT, serum magnesium, ionized calcium. Question for history of allergies, esp. to amphotericin B, sulfite. Avoid, if possible, other nephrotoxic medications. Obtain premedication orders to reduce adverse reactions during IV therapy (antipyretics, antihistamines, antiemetics, corticosteroids).

### INTERVENTION/EVALUATION

Monitor B/P, temperature, pulse, respirations; assess for adverse reactions (fever, tremors, chills, anorexia, nausea, vomiting, abdominal pain) q15min twice, then q30min for 4 hrs of initial infusion. If symptoms occur, slow infusion, administer medication for symptomatic relief. For severe reaction, stop infusion and notify physician. Evaluate IV site for phlebitis. Monitor I&O, renal function tests for nephrotoxicity. Monitor

CBC, BMP (esp. potassium), LFT, serum magnesium.

**PATIENT/FAMILY TEACHING**

• Prolonged therapy (wks or mos) is usually necessary. • Fever reaction may decrease with continued therapy. • Muscle weakness may be noted during therapy (due to hypokalemia).

# ampicillin

am-pi-**sil**-in
(Apo-Ampi ✦, Novo-Ampicillin ✦, Nu-Ampi ✦)
**Do not confuse ampicillin with aminophylline.**

◆**CLASSIFICATION**

**PHARMACOTHERAPEUTIC:** Penicillin.
**CLINICAL:** Antibiotic.

## USES

Treatment of susceptible infections due to streptococci, *S. pneumoniae,* staphylococci (non–penicillinase producing), meningococci, *Listeria,* some *Klebsiella, E. coli, H. influenzae, Salmonella, Shigella* including GI, GU, respiratory infections, meningitis, endocarditis prophylaxis. **OFF-LABEL:** Surgical prophylaxis for liver transplantation.

## PRECAUTIONS

**Contraindications:** Hypersensitivity to ampicillin or any penicillin. Infections caused by penicillinase-producing organisms. **Cautions:** History of allergies, esp. cephalosporins, renal impairment, asthmatic pts, infectious mononucleosis.

## ACTION

Inhibits cell wall synthesis in susceptible microorganisms. **Therapeutic Effect:** Bactericidal in susceptible microorganisms.

## PHARMACOKINETICS

Moderately absorbed from GI tract. Protein binding: 15%–25%. Widely distributed. Partially metabolized in liver. Primarily excreted in urine. Removed by hemodialysis. **Half-life:** 1–1.5 hrs (increased in renal impairment).

## ⌛ LIFESPAN CONSIDERATIONS

**Pregnancy/Lactation:** Crosses placenta; appears in cord blood, amniotic fluid. Distributed in breast milk in low concentrations. May lead to allergic sensitization, diarrhea, candidiasis, skin rash in infant. **Children:** Immature renal function in neonates/young infants may delay renal excretion. **Elderly:** Age-related renal impairment may require dosage adjustment.

## INTERACTIONS

**DRUG: Allopurinol** may increase incidence of rash. **Probenecid** may increase concentration, toxicity risk. May decrease effects of **oral contraceptives.** May increase level/effect of **methotrexate. HERBAL:** None significant. **FOOD:** None known. **LAB VALUES:** May increase serum ALT, AST. May cause positive Coombs' test.

## AVAILABILITY (Rx)

**Capsules:** 250 mg, 500 mg. **Injection, Powder for Reconstitution:** 125 mg, 250 mg, 500 mg, 1 g, 2 g. **Powder for Oral Suspension:** 125 mg/5 ml, 250 mg/5 ml.

## ADMINISTRATION/HANDLING

 **IV**

**Reconstitution** • For IV injection, dilute each vial with 5 ml Sterile Water for Injection or 0.9% NaCl (10 ml for 1- and 2-g vials). **Maximum concentration:** 100 mg/ml for IV push. • For intermittent IV infusion (piggyback), further dilute with 50–100 ml 0.9% NaCl. **Maximum concentration:** 30 mg/ml.
**Rate of Administration** • For IV injection, give over 3–5 min (125–500 mg) or over 10–15 min (1–2 g). For

intermittent IV infusion (piggyback), infuse over 15–30 min. • Due to potential for hypersensitivity/anaphylaxis, start initial dose at few drops per min, increase slowly to ordered rate; stay with pt first 10–15 min, then check q10min.
**Storage** • IV solution, diluted with 0.9% NaCl, is stable for 8 hrs at room temperature or 2 days if refrigerated. • If diluted with D₅W, is stable for 2 hrs at room temperature or 3 hrs if refrigerated. • Discard if precipitate forms.

**IM**
• Reconstitute each vial with Sterile Water for Injection or Bacteriostatic Water for Injection (consult individual vial for specific volume of diluent). • Stable for 1 hr. • Give deeply in large muscle mass.

**PO**
• Oral suspension, after reconstitution, is stable for 7 days at room temperature, 14 days if refrigerated. • Shake oral suspension well before using. • Give orally 1–2 hrs before meals for maximum absorption.

### ▦ IV INCOMPATIBILITIES

Diltiazem (Cardizem), midazolam (Versed), ondansetron (Zofran).

### ▦ IV COMPATIBILITIES

Calcium gluconate, cefepime (Maxipime), dexmedetomidine (Precedex), dopamine (Intropin), famotidine (Pepcid), furosemide (Lasix), heparin, hydromorphone (Dilaudid), insulin (regular), levofloxacin (Levaquin), lipids, magnesium sulfate, morphine, multivitamins, potassium chloride, propofol (Diprivan).

### INDICATIONS/ROUTES/DOSAGE

**Usual Dosage**
**PO: ADULTS, ELDERLY:** 250–500 mg q6h. **CHILDREN:** 50–100 mg/kg/day in divided doses q6h. **Maximum:** 2–4 g/day.
**IV, IM: ADULTS, ELDERLY:** 1–2 g q4–6h or 50–250 mg/kg/day in divided doses. **Maximum:** 12 g/day. **CHILDREN:** 25–200 mg/kg/day in divided doses q6h.

**Maximum:** 12 g/day. **NEONATES:** 50 mg/kg/dose q6–12h.

**Dosage in Renal Impairment**

| Creatinine Clearance | Dosage |
|---|---|
| 10–50 ml/min | Administer q6–12h |
| Less than 10 ml/min | Administer q12–24h |
| Hemodialysis | 1–2 g q12–24h |
| Peritoneal dialysis | 250 mg q12h |
| Continuous renal replacement therapy (CRRT) | 2g, then 1–2 g q6–8h |

**Dosage in Hepatic Impairment**
No dose adjustment.

### SIDE EFFECTS

**Frequent:** Pain at IM injection site, GI disturbances (mild diarrhea, nausea, vomiting), oral or vaginal candidiasis. **Occasional:** Generalized rash, urticaria, phlebitis, thrombophlebitis (with IV administration), headache. **Rare:** Dizziness, seizures (esp. with IV therapy).

### ADVERSE EFFECTS/ TOXIC REACTIONS

Antibiotic-associated colitis, other superinfections (abdominal cramps, severe watery diarrhea, fever) may result from altered bacterial balance in GI tract. Severe hypersensitivity reactions, including anaphylaxis, acute interstitial nephritis occur rarely.

### NURSING CONSIDERATIONS

**BASELINE ASSESSMENT**
Question for history of allergies, esp. penicillins, cephalosporins; renal impairment.

**INTERVENTION/EVALUATION**
Promptly report rash (although common with ampicillin, may indicate hypersensitivity) or diarrhea (fever, abdominal pain, mucus and blood in stool may indicate antibiotic-associated colitis). Evaluate IV site for phlebitis. Check IM injection site for pain, induration. Monitor I&O,

urinalysis, renal function tests. Be alert for superinfection: fever, vomiting, diarrhea, anal/genital pruritus, oral mucosal changes (ulceration, pain, erythema).

### PATIENT/FAMILY TEACHING

• Continue antibiotic for full length of treatment. • Space doses evenly. • More effective if taken 1 hr before or 2 hrs after food/beverages. • Discomfort may occur with IM injection. • Report rash, diarrhea, or other new symptoms.

---

# ampicillin/ sulbactam

amp-i-**sil**-in/sul-**bak**-tam (Unasyn)

## ◆CLASSIFICATION

**PHARMACOTHERAPEUTIC:** Penicillin. **CLINICAL:** Antibiotic.

## USES

Treatment of susceptible infections, including intra-abdominal, skin/skin structure, gynecologic infections, due to beta-lactamase-producing organisms including *H. influenzae, E. coli, Klebsiella, Acinetobacter, Enterobacter, S. aureus,* and *Bacteroides* spp. **OFF-LABEL:** Endocarditis, community-acquired pneumonia, surgical prophylaxis, pelvic inflammatory disease.

## PRECAUTIONS

**Contraindications:** Hypersensitivity to ampicillin, any penicillins, or sulbactam. Hx of cholestatic jaundice, hepatic impairment associated with ampicillin/sulbactam. **Cautions:** History of allergies, esp. cephalosporins, renal impairment, infectious mononucleosis, asthmatic pts.

## ACTION

Ampicillin inhibits bacterial cell wall synthesis. Sulbactam inhibits bacterial beta-lactamase. **Therapeutic Effect:** Ampicillin is bactericidal in susceptible microorganisms. Sulbactam protects ampicillin from enzymatic degradation.

## PHARMACOKINETICS

Protein binding: 28%–38%. Widely distributed. Partially metabolized in liver. Primarily excreted in urine. Removed by hemodialysis. **Half-life:** 1–1.3 hrs (increased in renal impairment).

## ⏳ LIFESPAN CONSIDERATIONS

**Pregnancy/Lactation:** Crosses placenta; appears in cord blood, amniotic fluid. Distributed in breast milk in low concentrations. May lead to allergic sensitization, diarrhea, candidiasis, skin rash in infant. **Children:** Safety and efficacy not established in pts younger than 1 yr. **Elderly:** Age-related renal impairment may require dosage adjustment.

## INTERACTIONS

**DRUG: Allopurinol** may increase incidence of rash. **Probenecid** may increase concentration, toxicity risk. May decrease effect of **oral contraceptives.** May increase level/effect of **methotrexate. HERBAL:** None significant. **FOOD:** None known. **LAB VALUES:** May increase serum ALT, AST, alkaline phosphatase, LDH, creatinine. May cause positive Coombs' test.

## AVAILABILITY (Rx)

**Injection, Powder for Reconstitution:** 1.5 g (ampicillin 1 g/sulbactam 500 g), 3 g (ampicillin 2 g/sulbactam 1 g).

## ADMINISTRATION/HANDLING
 IV

**Reconstitution** • For IV injection, dilute with Sterile Water for Injection to provide concentration of 375 mg/ml. • For intermittent IV infusion (piggyback), further dilute with 50–100 ml 0.9% NaCl. **Rate of Administration** • For IV injection, give slowly over minimum of 10–15 min. • For intermittent IV infusion (piggyback), infuse over 15–30 min. • Due to potential for hypersensitivity/anaphylaxis, start initial dose at few drops per min, increase slowly to ordered rate; stay with pt first 10–15 min, then check q10min.

**Storage** • IV solution, diluted with 0.9% NaCl, is stable for up to 72 hrs if refrigerated (4 hrs if diluted with D₅W). • Discard if precipitate forms.

**IM**
• Reconstitute each 1.5-g vial with 3.2 ml Sterile Water for Injection or lidocaine to provide concentration of 250 mg ampicillin/125 mg sulbactam/ml. • Give deeply into large muscle mass within 1 hr after preparation.

### ▓ IV INCOMPATIBILITIES

Amiodarone (Cordarone), diltiazem (Cardizem), idarubicin (Idamycin), ondansetron (Zofran).

### ▓ IV COMPATIBILITIES

Famotidine (Pepcid), heparin, insulin (regular), morphine.

### INDICATIONS/ROUTES/DOSAGE

**Usual Dosage Range**
**IV, IM: ADULTS, ELDERLY, CHILDREN 13 YRS AND OLDER:** 1.5–3 g q6h. **Maximum:** 12 g/day. **IV: CHILDREN 12 YRS AND YOUNGER:** 100–200 mg ampicillin/kg/day in divided doses q6h. **Maximum:** 12 g/day (Unasyn). 8 g/day (ampicillin). **NEONATES:** 100 mg (ampicillin)/kg/day in divided doses q8–12h.

**Dosage in Renal Impairment**
Dosage and frequency are modified based on creatinine clearance and severity of infection.

| Creatinine Clearance | Dosage |
|---|---|
| Greater than 30 ml/min | No dose adjustment |
| 15–30 ml/min | 1.5–3 g q12h |
| 5–14 ml/min | 1.5–3 g q24h |
| Hemodialysis | 1.5–3 g q12–24h (after HD on dialysis days) |
| Peritoneal dialysis | 1.5-3 g q12–24h |
| Continuous renal replacement therapy (CRRT) | 3 g, then 1.5–3 g q6–12h |

**Dosage in Hepatic Impairment**
No dose adjustment.

### SIDE EFFECTS

**Frequent:** Diarrhea, rash (most common), urticaria, pain at IM injection site, thrombophlebitis with IV administration, oral or vaginal candidiasis. **Occasional:** Nausea, vomiting, headache, malaise, urinary retention.

### ADVERSE EFFECTS/ TOXIC REACTIONS

Antibiotic-associated colitis, other superinfections (abdominal cramps; severe, watery diarrhea; fever) may result from altered bacterial balance in GI tract. Severe hypersensitivity reactions, including anaphylaxis, acute interstitial nephritis, blood dyscrasias may occur. High dosage may produce seizures.

### NURSING CONSIDERATIONS

**BASELINE ASSESSMENT**
Question for history of allergies, esp. penicillins, cephalosporins; renal impairment.

**INTERVENTION/EVALUATION**
Promptly report rash (although common with ampicillin, may indicate hypersensitivity) or diarrhea (fever, abdominal pain, mucus and blood in stool may indicate antibiotic-associated colitis). Evaluate IV site for phlebitis. Check IM injection site for pain, induration. Monitor I&O, urinalysis, renal function tests. Be alert for superinfection: fever, vomiting, diarrhea, anal/genital pruritus, oral mucosal changes (ulceration, pain, erythema).

**PATIENT/FAMILY TEACHING**
• Take antibiotic for full length of treatment. • Space doses evenly. • Discomfort may occur with IM injection. • Report rash, diarrhea, or other new symptoms.

## anastrozole

<sub></sub> **HIGH ALERT**

an-**as**-troe-zole
Apo-Anastrozole ✦
(Arimidex)
**Do not confuse anastrozole with letrozole, or Arimidex with Imitrex.**

### ◆CLASSIFICATION

**PHARMACOTHERAPEUTIC:** Aromatase inhibitor. **CLINICAL:** Antineoplastic hormone.

## USES

Treatment of advanced breast cancer in postmenopausal women who have developed progressive disease while receiving tamoxifen therapy. First-line therapy in advanced or metastatic breast cancer in postmenopausal women. Adjuvant treatment in early hormone receptor–positive breast cancer in postmenopausal women. **OFF-LABEL:** Treatment of recurrent or metastatic endometrial or uterine cancers; treatment of ovarian cancer.

## PRECAUTIONS

**Contraindications:** Hypersensitivity to anastrozole. Pregnancy, women who may become pregnant. **Cautions:** Preexisting ischemic cardiac disease, osteopenia (higher risk of developing osteoporosis), hyperlipidemia.

## ACTION

Decreases circulating estrogen level by inhibiting aromatase, the enzyme that catalyzes the final step in estrogen production. **Therapeutic Effect:** Inhibits growth of breast cancers that are stimulated by estrogens by lowering serum estradiol concentration.

## PHARMACOKINETICS

Well absorbed into systemic circulation (absorption not affected by food). Protein binding: 40%. Extensively metabolized in liver. Eliminated by biliary system and, to a lesser extent, kidneys. **Mean half-life:** 50 hrs in postmenopausal women. Steady-state plasma levels reached in about 7 days.

## ⏳ LIFESPAN CONSIDERATIONS

**Pregnancy/Lactation:** Crosses placenta; may cause fetal harm. Unknown if distributed in breast milk. **Children:** Safety and efficacy not established. **Elderly:** No age-related precautions noted.

## INTERACTIONS

**DRUG: Estrogen therapies** may reduce concentration/effects. **Tamoxifen** may reduce plasma concentration. **HERBAL:** Avoid **black cohosh, dong quai, licorice, red clover. FOOD:** None known. **LAB VALUES:** May elevate serum GGT level in pts with liver metastases. May increase serum ALT, AST, alkaline phosphate, total cholesterol, LDL.

## AVAILABILITY (Rx)

**Tablets:** 1 mg.

## ADMINISTRATION/HANDLING

**PO**
• Give without regard to food.

## INDICATIONS/ROUTES/DOSAGE

**Breast Cancer (Advanced)**
**PO: ADULTS, ELDERLY:** 1 mg once daily (continue until tumor progresses).

**Breast Cancer (Early, Adjuvant)**
**PO: ADULTS, ELDERLY:** 1 mg once daily.

**Dosage in Renal/Hepatic Impairment**
No dose adjustment.

## SIDE EFFECTS

**Frequent (16%–8%):** Asthenia, nausea, headache, hot flashes, back pain, vomiting, cough, diarrhea. **Occasional (6%–4%):** Constipation, abdominal pain, anorexia, bone pain, pharyngitis, dizziness, rash, dry mouth, peripheral edema, pelvic pain, depression, chest pain, paresthesia. **Rare (2%–1%):** Weight gain, diaphoresis.

## ADVERSE EFFECTS/ TOXIC REACTIONS

Thrombophlebitis, anemia, leukopenia occur rarely. Vaginal hemorrhage occurs rarely (2%).

## NURSING CONSIDERATIONS

### INTERVENTION/EVALUATION

Monitor for asthenia, dizziness; assist with ambulation if needed. Assess for headache, pain. Offer antiemetic for nausea, vomiting. Monitor for onset of diarrhea; offer antidiarrheal medication.

### PATIENT/FAMILY TEACHING

• Notify physician if nausea, asthenia (loss of strength, energy), hot flashes become unmanageable.

# anidulafungin

a-**nid**-ue-la-**fun**-jin
(Eraxis)

## ◆ CLASSIFICATION

**PHARMACOTHERAPEUTIC:** Echinocandin. **CLINICAL:** Antifungal.

## USES

Treatment of candidemia, other forms of *Candida* infections (e.g., intra-abdominal abscess, peritonitis), esophageal candidiasis.

## PRECAUTIONS

**Contraindications:** Hypersensitivity to anidulafungin, other echinocandins. **Cautions:** Hepatic impairment.

## ACTION

Inhibits synthesis of the enzyme glucan, (vital component of fungal cell formation), preventing fungal cell wall formation. **Therapeutic Effect:** Fungistatic.

## PHARMACOKINETICS

Distributed in tissue. Moderately bound to albumin. Protein binding: 84%–99%. Slow chemical degradation; 30% excreted in feces over 9 days. Not removed by hemodialysis. **Half-life:** 40–50 hrs.

##  LIFESPAN CONSIDERATIONS

**Pregnancy/Lactation:** May be embryotoxic. Crosses placental barrier. Unknown if distributed in breast milk. **Children:** Safety and efficacy not established. **Elderly:** No age-related precautions noted.

## INTERACTIONS

**DRUG:** None significant. **HERBAL:** None significant. **FOOD:** None known. **LAB VALUES:** May increase serum alkaline phosphatase, amylase, ALT, AST, bilirubin, calcium, creatinine, CPK, LDH, lipase. May decrease serum albumin, bicarbonate, magnesium, protein, potassium, Hgb, Hct, WBCs, neutrophils, platelet count. May prolong prothrombin time (PT).

## AVAILABILITY (Rx)

**Injection, Powder for Reconstitution:** 50-mg vial, 100-mg vial.

## ADMINISTRATION/HANDLING

IV

**Reconstitution** • Reconstitute each 50-mg vial with 15 ml Sterile Water for Injection (100 mg with 30 ml). Swirl, do not shake. • Further dilute 50 mg with 50 ml D₅W or 0.9% NaCl (100 mg with 100 ml, 200 mg with 200 ml).
**Rate of Administration** • Do not exceed infusion rate of 1.1 mg/min. Not for IV bolus injection.
**Storage** • Refrigerate unreconstituted vials. Reconstituted vials are stable for 24 hrs at room temperature. Infusion solution is stable for 48 hrs at room temperature.

## ▧ IV INCOMPATIBILITIES

Amphotericin B (Abelcet, AmBisome), ertapenem (Invanz), sodium bicarbonate.

## ▧ IV COMPATIBILITIES

Dexamethasone (Decadron), famotidine (Pepcid), furosemide (Lasix), hydromorphone (Dilaudid), lorazepam (Ativan), methylprednisolone (Solu-Medrol), morphine. Refer to IV Compatibility Chart in front of book.

## INDICATIONS/ROUTES/DOSAGE

◀ALERT▶ Duration of treatment based on pt's clinical response. In general, treatment is continued for at least 14 days after last positive culture.

**Candidemia, Other Candida Infections**
**IV: ADULTS, ELDERLY:** Give single 200-mg loading dose on day 1, followed by 100 mg/day thereafter for at least 14 days after last positive culture.

**Esophageal Candidiasis**
**IV: ADULTS, ELDERLY:** Give single 100-mg loading dose on day 1, followed by 50 mg/day thereafter for a minimum of 14 days and for at least 7 days following resolution of symptoms.

**Dosage in Renal/Hepatic Impairment**
No dose adjustment.

## SIDE EFFECTS

**Rare (3%–1%):** Diarrhea, nausea, headache, rigors, peripheral edema.

## ADVERSE EFFECTS/ TOXIC REACTIONS

Hypokalemia occurs in 4% of pts. Hypersensitivity reaction characterized by facial flushing, hypotension, pruritus, urticaria, rash occurs rarely. Hepatitis, elevated LFT, hepatic failure was reported.

## NURSING CONSIDERATIONS

### BASELINE ASSESSMENT

Obtain baseline CBC, BMP, LFT. Obtain specimens for fungal culture prior to therapy. Treatment may be instituted before results are known.

### INTERVENTION/EVALUATION

Monitor for evidence of hepatic dysfunction, hypokalemia. Monitor daily pattern of bowel activity, stool consistency. Assess for rash, urticaria.

### PATIENT/FAMILY TEACHING

• For esophageal candidiasis, maintain diligent oral hygiene.

# antihemophilic factor (factor VIII, AHF)

an-tee-hee-moe-**fil**-ik **fak**-tor
(**Antihemophilic Factor/von Willebrand Factor Complex:** Alphanate, Humate-P, Wilate. **Human:** Hemofil M, Koate-DVI, Monoclate-P. **Recombinant:** Advate, Eloctate, Kogenate FS, Recombinate, Xyntha)

## ◆ CLASSIFICATION

**PHARMACOTHERAPEUTIC:** Antihemophilic agent. **CLINICAL:** Hemostatic.

## USES

**Human:** Prevention/treatment of hemorrhagic episodes, perioperative management of hemophilia A. **Alphanate, Humate-P, Wilate:** Prevention/treatment of hemorrhagic episodes in pts with hemophilia A. Prophylaxis with surgical/invasive procedures, treatment of bleeding in pts with von Willebrand disease (vWD) when desmopressin is known or suspected to be inadequate. **Recombinant:** Management of hemophilia A, prevention and control of bleeding episodes, perioperative management of hemophilia A, prophylaxis of joint bleeding and reduce risk of joint damage in children with hemophilia A.

## PRECAUTIONS

**Contraindications:** Hypersensitivity to any component of product. **Cautions:** Hepatic disease, pts with blood types A, B, AB (progressive anemia, intravascular hemolysis may occur).

## ACTION

Assists in conversion of prothrombin to thrombin, essential for blood coagulation.

Replaces missing clotting factor VIII. **Therapeutic Effect:** Produces hemostasis; corrects or prevents bleeding episodes.

## PHARMACOKINETICS

**Half-life:** 8–27 hrs.

## ⧗ LIFESPAN CONSIDERATIONS

**Pregnancy/Lactation:** Unknown if drug crosses placenta or is distributed in breast milk. **Children:** Safety and efficacy not established. **Elderly:** No age-related precautions noted.

## INTERACTIONS

**DRUG:** None significant. **HERBAL:** None significant. **FOOD:** None known. **LAB VALUES:** None significant.

## AVAILABILITY (Rx)

**Human: Injection, Powder for Reconstitution (Hemofil M, Koate-DVI, Monoclate-P):** Actual number of units listed on each vial. **Alphanate:** 250 units, 500 units, 1,000 units, 1,500 units. **Eloctate:** 250 units, 500 units, 750 units, 1,000 units, 1,500 units, 2,000 units, 3,000 units. **Humate-P:** 250 units, 500 units, 1,000 units. **Recombinant: Injection, Powder for Reconsitution: Advate:** 250 units, 500 units, 1,000 units, 1,500 units, 2,000 units, 3,000 units. **Kogenate, Recombinate:** 250 units, 500 units, 1,000 units. **Xyntha:** 250 units, 500 units, 1,000 units, 2,000 units.

## ADMINISTRATION/HANDLING

 IV

**Reconstitution** • Warm concentrate and diluent to room temperature. • Using needle supplied by the manufacturer, add diluent to powder to dissolve, gently agitate or rotate. Do not shake vigorously. Complete dissolution may take 5–10 min. • Use second filtered needle supplied by the manufacturer, and add to infusion bag.
**Rate of Administration** • **Advate:** Over 5 min or less. **Maximum:** 10 ml/min. • **Hexilate FS, Kogenate FS:** Over 1–15 min based on pt tolerance. • **Xyntha:** Over several min. • **Hemofil M,** **Koate-DVI:** Over 5–10 min. **Maximum:** 10 ml/min. • **Monoclate-P:** Infuse at 2 ml/min. • **Alphanate:** 10 ml/min. **Humate-P:** 4 ml/min.

**Administration Precautions** • Check pulse rate prior to and following administration. If pulse rate increases, reduce or stop administration. • After administration, apply prolonged pressure on venipuncture site. • Monitor IV site for oozing q5–15min for 1–2 hrs following administration.

**Storage** • May refrigerate or store at room temperature. • See individual products for specific storage durations.

## ⊞ IV INCOMPATIBILITIES

Do not mix with other IV solutions or medications.

## INDICATIONS/ROUTES/DOSAGE

**Hemophilia A, Von Willebrand Disease**
**IV: ADULTS, ELDERLY, CHILDREN:** Dosage is highly individualized and is based on pt's weight, severity of bleeding, coagulation studies.

**Dosage in Renal/Hepatic Impairment**
No dose adjustment.

## SIDE EFFECTS

**Occasional:** Allergic reaction, including fever, chills, urticaria, wheezing, hypotension, nausea, feeling of chest tightness, stinging at injection site, dizziness, dry mouth, headache, altered taste.

## ADVERSE EFFECTS/ TOXIC REACTIONS

Risk of transmitting viral hepatitis. Intravascular hemolysis may occur if large or frequent doses are used with blood group A, B, or AB.

## NURSING CONSIDERATIONS

### BASELINE ASSESSMENT

Question history of hepatic disease, prior hypersensitivity reaction. When monitoring B/P, avoid overinflation of cuff to prevent trauma, bleeding. Remove adhesive tape from any pressure dressing carefully and slowly.

### INTERVENTION/EVALUATION

Following IV administration, apply prolonged pressure on venipuncture site. Monitor IV site for oozing q5–15 min for 1–2 hrs following administration. Assess for allergic reaction. Immediately report any evidence of hematuria or change in vital signs. Assess for decreases in B/P, increased pulse rate, complaint of abdominal or back pain, severe headache (may be evidence of hemorrhage). Question for increased discharge during menses. Assess skin for bruises, petechiae. Check for excessive bleeding from minor cuts, scratches. Assess gums for erythema, gingival bleeding. Assess urine for hematuria. Evaluate for therapeutic relief of pain, reduction of swelling, restricted joint movement.

### PATIENT/FAMILY TEACHING

• Use electric razor, soft toothbrush to prevent bleeding. • Report any sign of bleeding, including red or dark urine, black/red stool, coffee-ground vomitus, blood-tinged mucus from cough. • Wear identification indicating a hemolytic condition. • Bring adequate supply of agent when traveling.

# apixaban

a-**pix**-a-ban
(Eliquis)
**Do not confuse apixaban with rivaroxaban, argatroban, or dabigatran.**

■ **BLACK BOX ALERT** ■ Discontinuation in absence of alternative anticoagulation increases risk for thrombotic events. Spinal or epidural hematoma resulting in paralysis may occur with neuraxial anesthesia or spinal/epidural puncture.

### ◆CLASSIFICATION

**PHARMACOTHERAPEUTIC:** Factor Xa inhibitor. **CLINICAL:** Anticoagulant.

## USES

Reduces risk for stroke, systemic embolism in pts with nonvalvular atrial fibrillation. Prophylaxis of DVT following hip or knee replacement surgery. Treatment of DVT and PE. Reduces risk of recurrent DVT/PE following initial therapy.

## PRECAUTIONS

**Contraindications:** Severe hypersensitivity to apixaban. Active pathologic bleeding. **Cautions:** Mild to moderate hepatic impairment, severe renal impairment (may increase bleeding risk). Avoid use in pts with severe hepatic impairment, prosthetic heart valve, significant rheumatic heart disease.

## ACTION

Selectively blocks active site of factor Xa, a key factor in the intrinsic and extrinsic pathway of blood coagulation cascade. **Therapeutic Effect:** Inhibits clot-induced platelet aggregation, fibrin clot formation.

## PHARMACOKINETICS

Readily absorbed after PO administration. Peak plasma concentration: 3–4 hrs. Protein binding: 87%. Metabolized in liver. Excreted primarily in urine, feces. **Half-life:** 12 hrs.

## 🕱 LIFESPAN CONSIDERATIONS

**Pregnancy/Lactation:** Unknown if distributed in breast milk. **Children:** Safety and efficacy not established. **Elderly:** No age-related precautions noted.

## INTERACTIONS

**DRUG:** CYP3A4 inducers (e.g., **carbamazepine, rifampin**) may decrease level/effect. **Aspirin, NSAIDs, warfarin, heparin, antiplatelet agents, CYP3A4 inhibitors,** (e.g., **ketoconazole, clarithromycin**) may increase concentration, bleeding risk. **HERBAL: St. John's wort** may decrease level/effect. **Flaxseed, garlic, ginger, ginko biloba, ginseng, Omega-3** may increase risk of bleeding. **FOOD: Grapefruit products** may increase level/adverse effects. **LAB VALUES:** May decrease platelet count, Hgb, LFT.

## AVAILABILITY (Rx)

Tablets: 2.5 mg, 5 mg.

## ADMINISTRATION/HANDLING

◀**ALERT**▶ Discontinuation in absence of alternative anticoagulation increases risk for thrombotic events.

**PO**
• Give without regard to meals. • If elective surgery or invasive procedures with moderate or high risk for bleeding, discontinue apixaban at least 24–48 hrs prior to procedure.

## INDICATIONS/ROUTES/DOSAGE

**NonValvular Atrial Fibrillation**
**PO: ADULTS, ELDERLY:** 5 mg twice daily. In pts with at least 2 of the following characteristics: age 80 yrs or older, body weight 60 kg or less, serum creatinine 1.5 mg/dL or greater, concurrent use with CYP3A4, or P-gp inhibitors (e.g., ketoconazole, ritonavir), reduce dose to 2.5 mg twice daily.

**DVT/PE Treatment**
**PO: ADULTS/ELDERLY:** 10 mg twice daily for 7 days, then 5 mg twice daily.

**DVT Prophylaxis (Hip/Knee Replacement)**
**Note:** Begin 12–24 hrs postoperatively. **ADULTS, ELDERLY:** 2.5 mg twice daily (35 days for hip; 12 days for knee).

**DVT Prophylaxis, Reduce Risk Recurrent DVT/PE**
**PO: ADULTS, ELDERLY:** 2.5 mg twice daily (after at least 6 mos of treatment).

**Dosage in Renal Impairment**
**DVT/PE/Reduce Risk Recurrent DVT, Postoperative:** No adjustment. **Nonvalvular A-fib, HD:** SCr < 1.5: No adjustment. **SCr 1.5 or greater, age older than 80 yrs, weight 60 kg or less:** 2.5 mg 2 times/day.

**Dosage in Hepatic Impairment**
**Mild Impairment:** No dose adjustment. **Moderate Impairment:** Use caution. **Severe Impairment:** Not recommended.

## SIDE EFFECTS

**Rare (3%–1%):** Nausea, ecchymosis.

## ADVERSE EFFECTS/ TOXIC REACTIONS

Increased risk for bleeding/hemorrhagic events. May cause serious, potentially fatal, bleeding, accompanied by one or more of the following: a decrease in Hgb of 2 g/dL or more; a need for 2 or more units of packed RBCs; bleeding occurring at one of the following sites: intracranial, intraspinal, intraocular, pericardial, intra-articular, intramuscular with compartment syndrome, retroperitoneal. Serious reactions include jaundice, cholestasis, cytolytic hepatitis, Stevens-Johnson syndrome, hypersensitivity reaction, anaphylaxis.

## NURSING CONSIDERATIONS

### BASELINE ASSESSMENT

Obtain baseline CBC. Question history of bleeding disorders, recent surgery, spinal punctures, intracranial hemorrhage, bleeding ulcers, open wounds, anemia, hepatic impairment. Obtain full medication history including herbal products.

### INTERVENTION/EVALUATION

Periodically monitor CBC, stool for occult blood. Be alert for complaints of abdominal/back pain, headache, confusion, weakness, vision change (may indicate hemorrhage). Question for increased menstrual bleeding/discharge. Assess for any sign of bleeding: bleeding at surgical site, hematuria, blood in stool, bleeding from gums, petechiae, ecchymosis.

### PATIENT/FAMILY TEACHING

• Do not take/discontinue any medication except on advice from physician. • Avoid alcohol, aspirin, NSAIDs. • Consult physician before surgery, dental work. • Use

---

electric razor, soft toothbrush to prevent bleeding. • Report blood-tinged mucus from coughing, heavy menstrual bleeding, headache, vision problems, weakness, abdominal pain, frequent bruising, bloody urine or stool, joint pain or swelling.

# apremilast

a-**pre**-mi-last
(Otezla)
**Do not confuse apremilast with roflumilast.**

## ◆CLASSIFICATION

**PHARMACOTHERAPEUTIC:** Phosphodiesterase 4 (PDE4) inhibitor. **CLINICAL:** Anti–psoriatic arthritis agent.

## USES

Treatment of adult pts with active psoriatic arthritis, moderate to severe plaque psoriasis.

## PRECAUTIONS

**Contraindications:** Hypersensitivity to apremilast. **Cautions:** History of depression, severe renal impairment, suicidal ideation. Pts with latent infections (e.g., TB, viral hepatitis).

## ACTION

Selectively inhibits PDE4, increasing cyclic AMP (cAMP) and inflammatory mediators. **Therapeutic Effect:** Reduces psoriatic arthritis exacerbations.

## PHARMACOKINETICS

Readily absorbed after PO administration. Protein binding: 68%. Peak plasma concentration: 2.5 hrs. Metabolized in liver. Eliminated in urine (58%), feces (39%). **Half-life:** 6–9 hrs.

## ⧗ LIFESPAN CONSIDERATIONS

**Pregnancy/Lactation:** Unknown if distributed in breast milk. Not recommended for nursing mothers. **Children:** Safety and efficacy not established in pts younger than 18 yrs. **Elderly:** No age-related precautions noted.

## INTERACTIONS

**DRUG: Strong CYP450 inducers (carbamazepine, phenobarbital, phenytoin, rifampin)** may decrease concentration/effect. **HERBAL: St. John's wort** may decrease concentration/effect. **FOOD:** None significant. **LAB VALUES:** None known.

## AVAILABILITY (Rx)

▧ **Tablets:** 10 mg, 20 mg, 30 mg.

## ADMINISTRATION/HANDLING

**PO**
• Give without regard to meal. Administer whole; do not crush, cut, dissolve, or divide.

## INDICATIONS/ROUTES/DOSAGE

**Psoriatic Arthritis, Plaque Psoriasis**
**PO: ADULTS/ELDERLY:** Initially, titrate dose from day 1–day 5. **Day 1:** 10 mg in AM only. **Day 2:** 10 mg in AM; 10 mg in PM. **Day 3:** 10 mg in AM; 20 mg in PM. **Day 4:** 20 mg in AM; 20 mg in PM. **Day 5:** 20 mg in AM; 30 mg in PM. **Day 6/Maintenance:** 30 mg twice daily.

**Dosage in Renal Impairment (CrCl less than 30 ml/min)**
**Days 1–3:** 10 mg in AM. **Days 4–5:** 20 mg in AM, using only AM schedule. **Day 6/Maintenance:** 30 mg once daily.

**Dosage in Hepatic Impairment**
No dose adjustment.

## SIDE EFFECTS

**Occasional (9%–4%):** Nausea, diarrhea, headache, upper respiratory tract infection. **Rare (3% or less):** Vomiting, nasopharyngitis, upper abdominal pain.

## ADVERSE EFFECTS/TOXIC REACTIONS

Increased risk of depression reported in less than 1% of pts. Weight decrease of 5%–10% of body weight occurred in 10% of pts.

## NURSING CONSIDERATIONS

### BASELINE ASSESSMENT

Obtain baseline weight, vital signs. Question history of depression, severe renal impairment, suicidal ideations. Screen for prior allergic reactions to drug class. Receive full medication history including herbal products. Assess degree of joint pain, range of motion, mobility.

### INTERVENTION/EVALUATION

Be alert for worsening depression, suicidal ideation. Monitor for weight loss. Assess for dehydration if diarrhea occurs. Assess improvement of joint pain, range of motion, mobility.

### PATIENT/FAMILY TEACHING

• Report changes in mood or behavior, thoughts of suicide, self-destructive behavior. Report weight loss of any kind. • Increase fluid intake if dehydration suspected. • Immediately notify physician if pregnancy suspected. • Do not chew, crush, dissolve, or divide tablets.

# aprepitant/ fosaprepitant

a-**prep**-i-tant/fos-a-**prep**-i-tant (Emend)
**Do not confuse fosaprepitant with aprepitant, fosamprenavir, or fospropofol.**

## ◆CLASSIFICATION

**PHARMACOTHERAPEUTIC:** Selective receptor antagonist. **CLINICAL:** Antinausea, antiemetic.

## USES

**PO/IV:** Prevention of nausea, vomiting associated with repeat courses of moderate to high emetogenic cancer chemotherapy. **PO:** Prevention of postop nausea, vomiting.

## PRECAUTIONS

**Contraindications:** Hypersensitivity to aprepitant or fosaprepitant. Concurrent use with pimozide. **Cautions:** Severe hepatic impairment. Concurrent use of medications metabolized through CYP3A4 (**e.g., docetaxol, etoposide, ifosfamide, imatinib, irinotecan, paclitaxel, vinbastine, vincristine, vinorelbine**).

## ACTION

Inhibits substance P receptor, augments antiemetic activity of 5-HT$_3$ receptor antagonists. **Therapeutic Effect:** Prevents acute and delayed phases of chemotherapy-induced emesis.

## PHARMACOKINETICS

Moderately absorbed from GI tract. Crosses blood-brain barrier. Extensively metabolized in liver. Protein binding: greater than 95%. Eliminated primarily by liver metabolism (not excreted renally). **Half-life:** 9–13 hrs.

## ⌛ LIFESPAN CONSIDERATIONS

**Pregnancy/Lactation:** Unknown if drug crosses placenta or is distributed in breast milk. **Children:** Safety and efficacy not established. **Elderly:** No age-related precautions noted.

## INTERACTIONS

**DRUG: Strong CYP3A4 inhibitors (e.g., ketoconazole, clarithromycin)** may increase concentration. **Strong CYP3A4 inducers (e.g., carbamazepine, rifampin)** may decrease concentration. May decrease effectiveness of **hormonal contraceptives, warfarin. HERBAL: St. John's wort** may decrease plasma concentration. **FOOD: Grapefruit products** may increase plasma concentration. **LAB VALUES:** May increase serum BUN, creatinine, glucose, alkaline phosphatase, ALT, AST. May produce proteinuria.

## AVAILABILITY (Rx)

**Capsules (Emend):** 40 mg, 80 mg, 125 mg. **Injection, Powder for Reconstitution (Fosaprepitant):** 150 mg.

## ADMINISTRATION/HANDLING

### PO
• Give without regard to food.

 **IV**

**Reconstitution** • Reconstitute each vial with 5 ml 0.9% NaCl. • Add to 145 ml 0.9% NaCl to provide a final concentration of 1 mg/ml.
**Rate of Administration** • Infuse over 20–30 min 30 min prior to chemotherapy.
**Storage** • Refrigerate unreconstituted vials. • After reconstitution, solution is stable at room temperature for 24 hrs.

## IV INCOMPATIBILITIES

Do not infuse with any solutions containing calcium or magnesium.

## INDICATIONS/ROUTES/DOSAGE

**Prevention of Chemotherapy-Induced Nausea, Vomiting**
**Note:** Administer in combination with a 5-HT$_3$ antagonist and dexamethasone.
**PO: ADULTS, ELDERLY, CHILDREN 12 YRS OR YOUNGER WEIGHING 30 KG OR MORE:** 125 mg 1 hr before chemotherapy on day 1 and 80 mg once daily in the morning on days 2 and 3.
**IV: ADULTS, ELDERLY (SINGLE-DOSE REGIMEN):** 150 mg over 20–30 min 30 min prior to chemotherapy.

**Prevention of Postop Nausea, Vomiting**
**PO: ADULTS, ELDERLY:** 40 mg once within 3 hrs prior to induction of anesthesia.

**Dosage in Renal/Hepatic Impairment**
No dose adjustment. Caution in severe hepatic impairment.

## SIDE EFFECTS

**Frequent (17%–10%):** Fatigue, nausea, hiccups, diarrhea, constipation, anorexia. **Occasional (8%–4%):** Headache, vomiting, dizziness, dehydration, heartburn. **Rare (3% or less):** Abdominal pain, epigastric discomfort, gastritis, tinnitus, insomnia.

## ADVERSE EFFECTS/ TOXIC REACTIONS

Neutropenia, mucous membrane disorders occur rarely.

## NURSING CONSIDERATIONS

### BASELINE ASSESSMENT
Assess for dehydration (poor skin turgor, dry mucous membranes, longitudinal furrows in tongue).

### INTERVENTION/EVALUATION
Monitor hydration, nutritional status, I&O. Assess bowel sounds for peristalsis. Assist with ambulation if dizziness occurs. Provide supportive measures. Monitor daily pattern of bowel activity, stool consistency.

### PATIENT/FAMILY TEACHING
• Relief from nausea/vomiting generally occurs shortly after drug administration. • Report persistent vomiting, headache. • May decrease effectiveness of oral contraceptives.

# argatroban

ar-**gat**-roe-ban
**Do not confuse argatroban with Aggrestat.**

## ◆CLASSIFICATION
**PHARMACOTHERAPEUTIC:** Thrombin inhibitor. **CLINICAL:** Anticoagulant.

## USES

Prophylaxis or treatment of thrombosis in heparin-induced thrombocytopenia (HIT) in pts with HIT or at risk of developing HIT. percutaneous coronary procedures. **OFF-LABEL:** Maintain extracorporeal circuit patency of continuous renal replacement therapy (CRRT) in pts with HIT.

## PRECAUTIONS

**Contraindications:** Hypersensitivity to argatroban, active major bleeding. **Cautions:** Severe hypertension, immediately following lumbar puncture, spinal anesthesia, major surgery, pts with congenital or acquired bleeding disorders, gastrointestinal ulcerations, hepatic impairment, critically ill pts.

## ACTION

Direct thrombin inhibitor that reversibly binds to thrombin-active sites. Inhibits thrombin-catalyzed or thrombin-induced reactions, including fibrin formation, activation of coagulant factors V, VIII, and XIII; inhibits protein C formation, platelet aggregation. **Therapeutic Effect:** Produces anticoagulation.

## PHARMACOKINETICS

Distributed primarily in extracellular fluid. Protein binding: 54%. Metabolized in liver. Primarily excreted in the feces, presumably through biliary secretion. **Half-life:** 39–51 min (prolonged in hepatic failure).

## LIFESPAN CONSIDERATIONS

**Pregnancy/Lactation:** Unknown if excreted in breast milk. **Children:** Safety and efficacy not established in pts younger than 18 yrs. **Elderly:** No age-related precautions noted.

## INTERACTIONS

**DRUG: Antiplatelet agents, other anticoagulants, thrombolytics, NSAIDs** may increase the risk of bleeding. **HERBAL: Dong quai, evening primrose oil, ginkgo, policosanol, willow bark** may increase risk of bleeding. **FOOD:** None known. **LAB VALUES:** Prolongs prothrombin time (PT), activated partial thromboplastin time (aPTT), international normalized ratio (INR). May decrease Hgb, Hct.

## AVAILABILITY (Rx)

**Infusion (Pre-Mix):** 125 mg/125 ml, 250 mg/250 ml. **Injection Solution:** 250 mg/2.5 ml vial.

## ADMINISTRATION/HANDLING

 IV

**Reconstitution** • Dilute each 250-mg vial with 250 ml 0.9% NaCl, D₅W to provide a final concentration of 1 mg/ml.
**Rate of Administration** • Initial rate of administration is based on body weight at 2 mcg/kg/min (e.g., 50-kg pt infuse at 6 ml/hr). Dosage should not exceed 10 mcg/kg/min.
**Storage** • Discard if solution appears cloudy or an insoluble precipitate is noted. • Following reconstitution, stable for 96 hrs at room temperature or refrigerated. • Avoid direct sunlight.

## 🔲 IV INCOMPATIBILITY

Amiodarone (Cardarone).

## 🔲 IV COMPATIBILITIES

Diphenhydramine (Benadryl), dobutamine (Dobutrex), dopamine (Intropin), furosemide (Lasix), midazolam (Versed), morphine, vasopressin (Pitressin). Refer to IV Compatibility Chart in front of book.

## INDICATIONS/ROUTES/DOSAGE

**Heparin-Induced Thrombocytopenia (HIT)**
**IV Infusion: ADULTS, ELDERLY:** Initially, 2 mcg/kg/min administered as a continuous infusion. After initial infusion, dose may be adjusted until steady-state aPTT is 1.5–3 times initial baseline value, not to exceed 100 sec. Dosage should not exceed 10 mcg/kg/min.

**Percutaneous Coronary Intervention**
**IV Infusion: ADULTS, ELDERLY:** Initially, administer bolus of 350 mcg/kg over 3–5 min, then infuse at 25 mcg/kg/min. Check ACT (activated clotting time) 5–10 min following bolus. If ACT is less than 300 sec, give additional bolus 150 mcg/kg, increase infusion to 30 mcg/kg/min.

If ACT is greater than 450 sec, decrease infusion to 15 mcg/kg/min. Once ACT of 300–450 sec achieved, continue dose through duration of procedure.

**Dosage in Renal Impairment**
No dose adjustment.

**Dosage in Hepatic Impairment**
**Moderate to Severe Impairment:**
**ADULTS, ELDERLY:** Initially, 0.5 mcg/kg/min. **CHILDREN:** Initially, 0.2 mcg/kg/min. Adjust dose in increments of 0.05 mcg/kg/min or less.

## SIDE EFFECTS

**Frequent (8%–3%):** Dyspnea, hypotension, fever, diarrhea, nausea, pain, vomiting, infection, cough.

## ADVERSE EFFECTS/ TOXIC REACTIONS

Ventricular tachycardia, atrial fibrillation occur occasionally. Major bleeding, sepsis occur rarely.

## NURSING CONSIDERATIONS

### BASELINE ASSESSMENT

Obtain CBC, PT, aPTT. Determine initial B/P. Minimize need for multiple injection sites, blood draws, catheters.

### INTERVENTION/EVALUATION

Assess for any sign of bleeding: bleeding at surgical site, hematuria, melena, bleeding from gums, petechiae, ecchymoses, bleeding from injection sites. Handle pt carefully and infrequently to prevent bleeding. Assess for decreased B/P, increased pulse rate, complaint of abdominal/back pain, severe headache (may indicate hemorrhage). Monitor ACT, PT, aPTT, platelet count, Hgb, Hct. Question for increase in discharge during menses. Assess for hematuria. Observe skin for any occurring ecchymoses, petechiae, hematoma. Use care in removing any dressing, tape.

### PATIENT/FAMILY TEACHING

• Use electric razor, soft toothbrush to prevent cuts, gingival trauma. • Report any sign of bleeding, including red/dark urine, black/red stool, coffee-ground vomitus, blood-tinged mucus from cough.

---

# *ARIPiprazole    TOP 100

ar-i-**pip**-ra-zole
(Abilify, Abilify Maintena, Aristada)
■ **BLACK BOX ALERT** ■ Increased risk of mortality in elderly pts with dementia-related psychosis, mainly due to pneumonia, HF. Increased risk of suicidal thinking and behavior in children, adolescents, young adults 18–24 yrs with major depressive disorder, other psychiatric disorders.

**Do not confuse Abilify with Ambien, or aripiprazole with esomeprazole, omeprazole, pantoprazole, or rabeprazole (proton pump inhibitors).**

## ◆CLASSIFICATION

**PHARMACOTHERAPEUTIC:** Dopamine agonist. **CLINICAL:** Antipsychotic agent.

## USES

**PO:** Treatment of schizophrenia. Treatment of bipolar disorder. Adjunct treatment in major depressive disorder. Treatment of irritability associated with autistic disorder in children 6–17 yrs of age. Treatment of Tourette disorder. **IM: (Immediate-Release):** Agitation associated with schizophrenia/bipolar disorder. **(Extended-Release):** Treatment of schizophrenia in adults. **Aristada:** Treatment of schizophrenia. **OFF-LABEL:** Schizoaffective disorder, depression with psychotic features, aggression, bipolar disorder (children), conduct disorder (children), psychosis/agitation related to Alzheimer's dementia.

---

## PRECAUTIONS

**Contraindications:** Hypersensitivity to aripiprazole. **Cautions:** Concurrent use of CNS depressants (including alcohol), disorders in which CNS depression is a feature, cardiovascular or cerebrovascular diseases (may induce hypotension), Parkinson's disease (potential for exacerbation), history of seizures or conditions that may lower seizure threshold (Alzheimer's disease), diabetes mellitus. Pts at risk for pneumonia. Elderly with dementia.

## ACTION

Provides partial agonist activity at dopamine and serotonin (5-HT$_{1A}$) receptors and antagonist activity at serotonin (5-HT$_{2A}$) receptors. **Therapeutic Effect:** Improves symptoms associated with schizophrenia, bipolar disorder, autism, depression.

## PHARMACOKINETICS

Well absorbed through GI tract. Protein binding: 99% (primarily albumin). Reaches steady levels in 2 wks. Metabolized in liver. Eliminated in feces (55%), urine (25%). Not removed by hemodialysis. **Half-life:** 75 hrs.

## ⏳ LIFESPAN CONSIDERATIONS

**Pregnancy/Lactation:** Unknown if drug crosses placenta. May be distributed in breast milk. Breastfeeding not recommended. **Children:** Safety and efficacy not established. **Elderly:** May increase serum glucose. May decrease neutrophils, leukocytes.

## INTERACTIONS

**DRUG: Alcohol** may potentiate cognitive and motor effects. **CYP3A4 inducers (e.g., carbamazepine)** may decrease concentration. **CYP3A4 inhibitors (e.g., itraconazole, ketoconazole)** may increase concentration. **HERBAL: St. John's wort** may decrease levels. **Gotu kola, kava kava, St. John's wort, valerian** may increase CNS depression. **FOOD:** None known. **LAB VALUES:** None significant.

## AVAILABILITY (Rx)

**Injection, Prefilled Syringe (Aristada):** 441 mg/1.6 ml, 662 mg/2.4 ml, 882 mg/3.2 ml. **Injection, Solution (Abilify):** 9.75 mg/1.3 ml (7.5 mg/ml). **Solution, Oral:** 1 mg/ml. **Tablets:** 2 mg, 5 mg, 10 mg, 15 mg, 20 mg, 30 mg. **Tablets, Orally Disintegrating:** 10 mg, 15 mg. **Injection, Powder for Reconstitution (Abilify Maintena):** 300 mg, 400 mg.

## ADMINISTRATION/HANDLING

### IM (Abilify)
• For IM use only (inject slowly into deep muscle mass). Do not administer IV or subcutaneous.

### IM (Abilify Maintena)
• Reconstitute 400-mg vial with 1.9 ml Sterile Water for Injection (300-mg vial with 1.5 ml) to provide a concentration of 100 mg/0.5 ml. Once reconstituted, administer in gluteal muscle. Do not administer via IV or subcutaneously.

### PO
• Give without regard to food.

### Orally Disintegrating Tablet
• Remove tablet, place entire tablet on tongue. • Do not break, split tablet. • May give without liquid.

## INDICATIONS/ROUTES/DOSAGE

**Note:** May substitute oral solution/tablet mg per mg up to 25 mg. For 30-mg tablets, give 25 mg oral solution.

**Strong CYP3A4 Inducers:** Aripiprazole dose should be doubled. **Strong CYP3A4 Inhibitors:** Aripiprazole dose should be reduced by 50%.

### Schizophrenia
**PO: ADULTS, ELDERLY:** Initially, 10–15 mg once daily. May increase up to 30 mg/day. Titrate dose at minimum of 2-wk intervals. **CHILDREN 13–17 YRS:** Initially, 2 mg/day for 2 days, then 5 mg/day for 2 days. May further increase to target dose of 10 mg/day. May then increase in

increments of 5 mg up to maximum of 30 mg/day. **IM:** *(Abilify Maintena):* **ADULTS, ELDERLY:** Initially, 400 mg monthly (separate doses by at least 26 days). *(Aristada):* Oral aripiprazole 10 mg/day: initially 441 mg/mos; oral aripiprazole 15 mg/day: initially, 662 mg/mos; oral aripiprazole 20 mg/day, initially, 882 mg q4–6 wks.

### Bipolar Disorder
**PO: ADULTS, ELDERLY: Monotherapy:** Initially, 15 mg once daily. May increase to 30 mg/day. **Adjunct to lithium or valproic acid:** Initially, 10–15 mg. May increase to 30 mg/day based on pt tolerance. **CHILDREN 10–17 YRS:** Initially, 2 mg/day for 2 days, then 5 mg/day for 2 days. May further increase to a target of 10 mg/day. Give subsequent dose increases of 5 mg/day. **Maximum:** 30 mg/day.

### Major Depressive Disorder (Adjunct to Antidepressants)
**PO: ADULTS, ELDERLY:** *(Abilify):* Initially, 2–5 mg/day. May increase up to 15 mg/day. Titrate dose in 5-mg increments of at least 1-wk intervals.

### Agitation with Schizophrenia/Bipolar Disorder
**IM: ADULTS, ELDERLY** *(Abilify):* 5.25–15 mg as a single dose. May repeat after 2 hrs. **Maximum:** 30 mg/day.

### Irritability with Autistic Disorder
**PO: CHILDREN 6–17 YRS:** Initially, 2 mg/day for 7 days followed by increase to 5 mg/day. Subsequent increases made in 5-mg increments at intervals of at least 1 wk. **Maximum:** 15 mg/day.

### Tourette Disorder
**PO: CHILDREN 6–17 YRS WEIGHING 50 KG OR MORE:** 2 mg/day for 2 days; then 5 mg/day for 5 days with target dose of 10 mg on day 8. **Maximum:** 20 mg/day. **LESS THAN 50 KG:** 2 mg/day for 2 days, then 5 mg/day. **Maximum:** 10 mg/day.

### Dosage in Renal/Hepatic Impairment
No dose adjustment.

## SIDE EFFECTS

**Frequent (11%–5%):** Weight gain, headache, insomnia, vomiting. **Occasional (4%–3%):** Light-headedness, nausea, akathisia, drowsiness. **Rare (2% or less):** Blurred vision, constipation, asthenia (loss of strength, energy), anxiety, fever, rash, cough, rhinitis, orthostatic hypotension.

## ADVERSE EFFECTS/TOXIC REACTIONS

Extrapyramidal symptoms, neuroleptic malignant syndrome, tardive dyskinesia, hyperglycemia, ketoacidosis, hyperosmolar coma, CVA, TIA occur rarely. Prolonged QT interval occurs rarely. May cause leukopenia, neutropenia, agranulocytosis.

## NURSING CONSIDERATIONS

### BASELINE ASSESSMENT

Assess behavior, appearance, emotional status, response to environment, speech pattern, thought content. Correct dehydration, hypovolemia. Assess for suicidal tendencies.

### INTERVENTION/EVALUATION

Periodically monitor weight. Monitor for extrapyramidal symptoms (abnormal movement), tardive dyskinesia (protrusion of tongue, puffing of cheeks, chewing/puckering of the mouth). Periodically monitor B/P, pulse (particularly in pts with preexisting cardiovascular disease). Assess for therapeutic response (greater interest in surroundings, improved self-care, increased ability to concentrate, relaxed facial expression).

### PATIENT/FAMILY TEACHING

• Avoid alcohol. • Avoid tasks that require alertness, motor skills until response to drug is established. • Report worsening depression, suicidal ideation, unusual changes in behavior, extrapyramidal effects.

## *armodafinil*

**HIGH ALERT**

ar-moe-**daf**-i-nil
(Nuvigil)
**Do not confuse armodafinil with
modafinil.**

### ◆ CLASSIFICATION

**PHARMACOTHERAPEUTIC:** Alpha₁
agonist. **CLINICAL:** CNS stimulant.

### USES

Treatment of excessive daytime sleepiness associated with obstructive sleep apnea–hypopnea syndrome, narcolepsy, shift-work sleep disorder.

### PRECAUTIONS

**Contraindications:** History of sensitivity to armodafinil or modafinil. **Cautions:** History of mitral valve prolapse, left ventricular hypertrophy, hepatic impairment, recent history of MI, unstable angina, cardiac ischemia, drug abuse, psychosis, depression, mania, renal impairment, elderly.

### ACTION

Exact mechanism unknown. May bind to dopamine reuptake carrier sites in the brain, increasing alpha activity, decreasing delta, theta, and beta activity. **Therapeutic Effect:** Improves wakefulness.

### PHARMACOKINETICS

Well absorbed. Widely distributed. Mainly eliminated by hepatic metabolism with less than 10% excreted by kidneys. Unknown if removed by hemodialysis. **Half-life:** 15 hrs.

### ▧ LIFESPAN CONSIDERATIONS

**Pregnancy/Lactation:** Unknown if distributed in breast milk. Use caution in pregnant women. **Children:** Safety and efficacy not established in pts younger than 17 yrs. **Elderly:** Age-related renal/hepatic impairment may require decreased dosage.

### INTERACTIONS

**DRUG: Carbamazine, erythromycin, ketoconazole, phenobarbital, rifampin** may alter concentration/effect. May reduce effects of **cyclosporine, oral contraceptives.** May increase concentrations of **diazepam, omeprazole, phenytoin, propanolol, tricyclic antidepressants, warfarin. HERBAL:** None significant. **FOOD: Food** slows peak concentration by 2–4 hrs; may affect time of onset, length of drug action. **LAB VALUES:** May increase alkaline phosphatase, GGT. May decrease serum uric acid.

### AVAILABILITY (Rx)

**Tablets:** 50 mg, 150 mg, 200 mg, 250 mg.

### ADMINISTRATION/HANDLING

**PO**
• May give without regard to food.

### INDICATIONS/ROUTES/DOSAGE

**Narcolepsy, Obstructive Sleep Apnea–Hypopnea Syndrome**
**PO: ADULTS, ELDERLY:** 150 or 250 mg/ day given as a single dose in the morning.

**Shift-Work Sleep Disorder**
**PO: ADULTS, ELDERLY:** 150 mg given daily approximately 1 hr prior to the start of work shift.

**Dosage in Renal/Hepatic Impairment**
No dose adjustment. **Severe Hepatic Impairment:** May decrease dose.

### SIDE EFFECTS

**Frequent (17%–7%):** Headache, nausea. **Occasional (5%–4%):** Dizziness, insomnia, dry mouth, diarrhea, anxiety. **Rare (2%):** Depression, fatigue, palpitations, dyspepsia, rash, upper abdominal pain.

### ADVERSE EFFECTS/ TOXIC REACTIONS

Small risk of serious rash, including Stevens-Johnson syndrome.

---

## NURSING CONSIDERATIONS

### BASELINE ASSESSMENT

Obtain baseline evidence of narcolepsy or other sleep disorders, including pattern, environmental situations, lengths of time of sleep episodes. Question for sudden loss of muscle tone (cataplexy) precipitated by strong emotional responses before sleep episode. Assess frequency/severity of sleep episodes prior to drug therapy.

### INTERVENTION/EVALUATION

Monitor sleep pattern, evidence of restlessness during sleep, length of insomnia episodes at night. Assess for dizziness, anxiety; initiate fall precautions.

### PATIENT/FAMILY TEACHING

• Avoid tasks that require alertness, motor skills until response to drug is established. • Avoid or limit alcohol. • Use alternative contraceptives during therapy and 1 mo after discontinuing drug (reduces effectiveness of oral contraceptives). Report rash, depression, diarrhea, insomnia. • Sips of water may relieve dry mouth.

---

## *arsenic trioxide*   **HIGH ALERT**

ar-sen-ik tri-**ox**-ide
(Trisenox)

■ **BLACK BOX ALERT** ■ May prolong QT interval. May lead to multiform ventricular tachycardia (torsade de pointes) or complete AV block. May cause retinoic acid–acute promyelocytic leukemia (RA-APL) syndrome or acute promyelocytic leukemia.

### ◆CLASSIFICATION

**PHARMACOTHERAPEUTIC:** Antineoplastic. **CLINICAL:** Antineoplastic.

### USES

Induction of remission and consolidations in pts with relapsed or refractory acute promyelocytic leukemia (APL).

**OFF-LABEL:** Treatment of myelodysplastic syndrome; initial treatment of APL.

### PRECAUTIONS

**Contraindications:** Hypersensitivity to arsenic. **Cautions:** Renal/hepatic impairment, preexisting QT-interval prolongation, concomitant medications that prolong QT interval. HF, history of torsades de pointes, conditions causing hypokalemia/hypomagnesemia.

### ACTION

Produces morphologic changes and DNA fragmentation in promyelocytic leukemia cells. **Therapeutic Effect:** Induces apoptosis is in APL cells.

### PHARMACOKINETICS

Distributed in liver, kidneys, heart, lungs, hair, and nails. Metabolized in liver. Eliminated by kidneys. **Half-life:** Not available.

### ⌛ LIFESPAN CONSIDERATIONS

**Pregnancy/Lactation:** Distributed in breast milk. May cause fetal harm. **Children:** Safety and efficacy not established in pts younger than 5 yrs. **Elderly:** Age-related renal impairment may require dosage adjustment.

### INTERACTIONS

**DRUG:** May prolong QT interval in pts taking **antiarrhythmics, moxifloxacin, thioridazine. Amphotericin B, cyclosporine, diuretics** may produce electrolyte abnormalities. **HERBAL:** Bilberry, fenugreek, garlic, ginger, ginseng may worsen hypoglycemia. **FOOD:** None known. **LAB VALUES:** May decrease WBC count, Hgb, platelet count, serum magnesium, calcium. May increase serum ALT, AST. Higher risk of hypokalemia than hyperkalemia, hyperglycemia than hypoglycemia.

### AVAILABILITY (Rx)

**Injection Solution:** 1 mg/ml (10 ml).

## ADMINISTRATION/HANDLING

 IV

**◄ALERT►** Central venous line is not required for drug administration.

**Reconstitution** • After withdrawing drug from ampule, dilute with 100–250 ml $D_5W$ or 0.9% NaCl.

**Rate of Administration** • Infuse over 1–2 hrs. • Duration of infusion may be extended up to 4 hrs if acute vasomotor reactions occur.

**Storage** • Store at room temperature. • Diluted solution is stable for 24 hrs at room temperature, 48 hrs if refrigerated.

## ⚙ IV INCOMPATIBILITIES

Do not mix with any other medications.

## INDICATIONS/ROUTES/DOSAGE

**Note:** Obtain baseline 12-lead EKG, electrolytes, creatinine prior to treatment.

**Acute Promyelocytic Leukemia**
**IV: ADULTS, ELDERLY, CHILDREN 5 YRS AND OLDER: Induction:** 0.15 mg/kg/day until bone marrow remission. Do not exceed 60 induction doses. **Consolidation:** Beginning 3–6 wks after completion of induction therapy, 0.15 mg/kg/day for maximum 25 doses over a period of up to 5 wks.

**Dosage in Renal Impairment**
**Mild to Moderate Impairment:** No dose adjustment. **Severe Impairment:** Use caution.

**Dosage in Hepatic Impairment**
Use caution. Monitor for toxicity.

## SIDE EFFECTS

**Expected (75%–50%):** Nausea, cough, fatigue, fever, headache, vomiting, abdominal pain, tachycardia, diarrhea, dyspnea. **Frequent (43%–30%):** Dermatitis, insomnia, edema, rigors, prolonged QT interval, sore throat, pruritus, arthralgia, paresthesia, anxiety. **Occasional (28%–20%):** Constipation, myalgia, hypotension, epistaxis, anorexia, dizziness, sinusitis. **(15%–8%):**

Ecchymosis, nonspecific pain, weight gain, herpes simplex infections, wheezing, flushing, diaphoresis, tremor, hypertension, palpitations, dyspepsia, eye irritation, blurred vision, asthenia (loss of strength, energy), adventitious or diminished breath sounds (crackles). **Rare:** Confusion, petechiae, dry mouth, oral candidiasis, incontinence, pulmonary rhonchi.

## ADVERSE EFFECTS/TOXIC REACTIONS

Seizures, GI hemorrhage, renal impairment or failure, pleural or pericardial effusion, hemoptysis, sepsis occur rarely. Prolonged QT interval, complete AV block, unexplained fever, dyspnea, weight gain, effusion are evidence of arsenic toxicity. Treatment should be halted, steroid therapy instituted.

## NURSING CONSIDERATIONS

### BASELINE ASSESSMENT

Assess CBC, BMP, LFT, coagulation profiles before and frequently during treatment. Ask if pt is breast-feeding.

### INTERVENTION/EVALUATION

Monitor CBC, BMP, LFT. Monitor for arsenic toxicity syndrome (fever, dyspnea, weight gain, confusion, muscle weakness, seizures).

### PATIENT/FAMILY TEACHING

• Avoid crowds, those with known infection. • Avoid tasks that require alertness, motor skills until response to drug is established. • Report high fever, vomiting, difficulty breathing, or rapid heart rate.

---

## asparaginase

as-par-**a**-jin-ace
(Erwinaze, Kidrolase ♣)
**Do not confuse asparaginase with pegaspargase.**

## ◆ CLASSIFICATION

**PHARMACOTHERAPEUTIC:** Enzyme.
**CLINICAL:** Antineoplastic.

 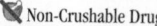

## USES

Treatment of ALL in pts with hypersensitivity to *E. coli*–derived asparaginase. **OFF-LABEL:** Treatment of chronic lymphoblastic leukemia (CLL).

## PRECAUTIONS

**Contraindications:** History of hypersensitivity to asparaginase. History of serious thrombosis, pancreatitis, or hemorrhagic events with prior asparaginase therapy. **Cautions:** Underlying coagulopathy, preexisting hepatic impairment.

## ACTION

Inhibits DNA, RNA, protein synthesis by breaking down asparagine, depriving tumor cells of this essential amino acid. Cell cycle–specific for $G_1$ phase of cell division. **Therapeutic Effect:** Toxic to leukemic cells.

## PHARMACOKINETICS

Metabolized by reticuloendothelial system through slow sequestration. **Half-life: IM:** 39–49 hrs; **IV:** 8–30 hrs.

## ⌛ LIFESPAN CONSIDERATIONS

**Pregnancy/Lactation:** If possible, avoid use during pregnancy, esp. first trimester. Breastfeeding not recommended. **Children/Elderly:** No age-related precautions noted.

## INTERACTIONS

**DRUG:** May increase level of **dexamethasone. HERBAL:** None significant. **FOOD:** None known. **LAB VALUES:** May increase serum ammonia, BUN, uric acid, glucose, partial thromboplastin time (PTT), platelet count, prothrombin time (PT), thrombin time (TT), ALT, AST, alkaline phosphatase, bilirubin. May decrease blood clotting factors (plasma fibrinogen, antithrombin, plasminogen), serum albumin, calcium, cholesterol.

## AVAILABILITY (Rx)

**Injection, Powder for Reconstitution:** 10,000 international units.

## ADMINISTRATION/HANDLING

◄**ALERT►** May be carcinogenic, mutagenic, teratogenic. Handle with extreme care during preparation/administration. Handle voided urine as infectious waste. Powder, solution may irritate skin on contact. Wash area for 15 min if contact occurs.

###  IV

Reconstitute 10,000 international units vial with 5 ml Sterile Water for Injection or 0.9% NaCl to provide a concentration of 2,000 international units/ml. • Shake gently to ensure complete dissolution (vigorous shaking produces foam, some loss of potency). Further dilute in 50–250 ml $D_5W$ or 0.9% NaCl.
**Rate of Administration** • Infuse over at least 30 min.
**Storage** • Refrigerate powder for reconstitution. • Reconstituted solution stable for 8 hrs if refrigerated. • Gelatinous fiber-like particles may develop (remove via 5-micron filter during administration).

### IM

• Add 2 ml 0.9% NaCl injection to 10,000 international units vial to provide a concentration of 5,000 international units/ml. • Administer no more than 2 ml into large muscle mass.

## ▦ IV COMPATIBILITIES

Methotrexate, sodium bicarbonate.

## INDICATIONS/ROUTES/DOSAGE

**Usual Dosage**
**IM: ADULTS, ELDERLY, CHILDREN:** As a substitute for pegaspargase: 25,000 units/m² 3 times/wk for 6 doses. As a substitute for pegaspargase *(E. coli)*: 25,000 units/m² for each planned dose.

**Dosage in Renal/Hepatic Impairment**
No dose adjustment.

## SIDE EFFECTS

**Frequent:** Allergic reaction (rash, urticaria, arthralgia, facial edema, hypotension, respiratory distress), pancreatitis (severe abdominal pain, nausea and vomiting). **Occasional:** CNS effects (confusion, drowsiness, depression, anxiety, fatigue), stomatitis, hypoalbuminemia or uric acid nephropathy (manifested as pedal or lower extremity edema), hyperglycemia. **Rare:** Hyperthermia (including fever or chills), thrombosis, seizures.

## ADVERSE EFFECTS/ TOXIC REACTIONS

Hepatotoxicity usually occurs within 2 wks of initial treatment. Risk of allergic reaction, including anaphylaxis, increases after repeated therapy. Myelosuppression may be severe.

## NURSING CONSIDERATIONS

### BASELINE ASSESSMENT

CBC, BMP, LFT should be performed before therapy begins and when 1 or more wks have elapsed between doses. Before giving medication, agents for adequate airway and allergic reaction (antihistamine, epinephrine, O₂, IV corticosteroid) should be readily available. Assess baseline CNS functions.

### INTERVENTION/EVALUATION

Monitor vital signs, CBC, urinalysis, serum amylase, BMP, LFT, coagulation profile, glucose, uric acid. Discontinue medication at first sign of renal dysfunction (oliguria, anuria), pancreatitis. Monitor for hematologic toxicity (fever, sore throat, signs of local infection, unusual bruising/ bleeding), symptoms of anemia, hypersensitivity reaction.

### PATIENT/FAMILY TEACHING

• Increase fluid intake (protects against renal impairment). • Nausea may decrease during therapy. • Do not have immunizations without physician's approval (drug lowers body's resistance). • Avoid contact with those who have recently received a live virus vaccine. • Notify physician if abdominal pain, rash, nausea, vomiting occurs.

# aspirin (acetylsalicylic acid, ASA)

**TOP 100** **HIGH ALERT**

as-pir-in
(Asaphen E.C. ✤, Ascriptin, Bayer, Bufferin, Durlaza, Ecotrin, Entrophen ✤, Halfprin, Novasen ✤)
**Do not confuse aspirin or Ascriptin with Afrin, Aricept, or Ecotrin with Epogen.**

## FIXED-COMBINATION(S)

**Aggrenox:** aspirin/dipyridamole (an antiplatelet agent): 25 mg/200 mg. **Fiorinal:** aspirin/butalbital/caffeine (a barbiturate): 325 mg/50 mg/40 mg. **Lortab/ASA:** aspirin/hydrocodone (an analgesic): 325 mg/5 mg. **Percodan:** aspirin/oxycodone (an analgesic): 325 mg/2.25 mg, 325 mg/4.5 mg. **Pravigard:** aspirin/ pravastatin (a cholesterol-lowering agent): 81 mg/20 mg, 81 mg/40 mg, 81 mg/80 mg, 325 mg/20 mg, 325 mg/40 mg, 325 mg/80 mg. **Yosprala:** aspirin/omeprazole (a proton pump inhibitor [PPI]) 325 mg/40 mg, 81 mg/40 mg.

## ◆CLASSIFICATION

**PHARMACOTHERAPEUTIC:** Nonsteroidal salicylate. **CLINICAL:** Antiinflammatory, antipyretic, anticoagulant.

## USES

Treatment of mild to moderate pain, fever. Reduces inflammation related to rheumatoid arthritis (RA), juvenile arthritis, osteoarthritis, rheumatic fever. Used as platelet aggregation inhibitor in the prevention of transient ischemic attacks (TIAs), cerebral thromboembolism, MI or reinfarction. **Durlaza:** Reduce risk of MI in pts with CAD or stroke in pts who have had TIA or ischemic stroke. **OFF-LABEL:** Prevention of pre-eclampsia;

alternative therapy for preventing thromboembolism associated with atrial fibrillation when warfarin cannot be used; pericarditis associated with MI; prosthetic valve thromboprophylaxis. Adjunctive treatment of Kawasaki's disease. Complications associated with autoimmune disorders; colorectal cancer.

## PRECAUTIONS

**Contraindications:** Hypersensitivity to salicylates, NSAIDs. Aspirin triad (asthma, rhinitis [with or without nasal polyps], aspirin intolerance). Asthma, rhinitis, nasal polyps; inherited or acquired bleeding disorders; use in children (younger than 16 yrs) for viral infections. Do not use for at least 7 days after tonsillectomy or oral surgery. **Cautions:** Platelet/bleeding disorders, severe renal/hepatic impairment, dehydration, erosive gastritis, peptic ulcer disease, sensitivity to tartrazine dyes, elderly (chronic use of doses 325 mg or greater). Avoid use in pregnancy, especially third trimester.

## ACTION

Inhibits cyclo-oxygenase enzyme via acetylation. Inhibits formation of prostaglandin derivative thromboxane A. **Therapeutic Effect:** Reduces inflammatory response, intensity of pain; decreases fever; inhibits platelet aggregation.

## PHARMACOKINETICS

| Route | Onset | Peak | Duration |
|-------|-------|------|----------|
| PO | 1 hr | 2–4 hrs | 4–6 hrs |

Rapidly and completely absorbed from GI tract; enteric-coated absorption delayed; rectal absorption delayed and incomplete. Protein binding: High. Widely distributed. Rapidly hydrolyzed to salicylate. **Half-life:** 15–20 min (aspirin); 2–3 hrs (salicylate at low dose); more than 20 hrs (salicylate at high dose).

## ⧗ LIFESPAN CONSIDERATIONS

**Pregnancy/Lactation:** Readily crosses placenta; distributed in breast milk. May prolong gestation and labor; decrease fetal birth weight; increase incidence of stillbirths, neonatal mortality, hemorrhage. Avoid use during last trimester (may adversely affect fetal cardiovascular system: premature closure of ductus arteriosus). **Children:** Caution in pts with acute febrile illness (Reye's syndrome). **Elderly:** May be more susceptible to toxicity; lower dosages recommended.

## INTERACTIONS

**DRUG: Alcohol, NSAIDs** may increase risk of GI effects (e.g., ulceration). **Antacids, urinary alkalinizers** increase excretion. **Anticoagulants, heparin, thrombolytics, rivaroxaban, ticagrelor** increase risk of bleeding. **HERBAL:** Avoid **cat's claw, dong quai, evening primrose, feverfew, garlic, ginger, ginkgo, ginseng, green tea, horse chestnut, red clover** (possess antiplatelet activity). **FOOD:** None known. **LAB VALUES:** May alter serum ALT, AST, alkaline phosphatase, uric acid; prolongs prothrombin time (PT), bleeding time. May decrease serum cholesterol, potassium, $T_3$, $T_4$.

## AVAILABILITY (OTC)

**Caplets (Bayer):** 81 mg, 325 mg, 500 mg. **Suppositories:** 300 mg, 600 mg. **Tablets:** 325 mg. **Tablets (Chewable [Bayer, St. Joseph]):** 81 mg.

◤ **Capsule, Extended-Release: (Durlaza)** 162.5 mg. **Tablets (Enteric-Coated [Bayer, Ecotrin, St. Joseph]):** 81 mg, 325 mg, 500 mg, 650 mg.

## ADMINISTRATION/HANDLING

**PO**
• Do not break, crush, dissolve, or divide enteric-coated tablets or extended-release capsule. • May give with water, milk, meals if GI distress occurs.

**Rectal**
• Refrigerate suppositories; do not freeze. • If suppository is too soft, chill for 30 min in refrigerator or run cold water over foil wrapper. • Moisten suppository with cold water before inserting well into rectum.

## INDICATIONS/ROUTES/DOSAGE

### Analgesia, Fever

**PO: ADULTS, ELDERLY, CHILDREN 12 YRS AND OLDER AND 50 KG OR MORE:** 325–650 mg q4–6h or 975 mg q6h prn or 500–1,000 mg q4–6h prn. **Maximum:** 4 g/day. **RECTAL:** 300–600 mg q4h prn. **INFANTS, CHILDREN LESS THAN 50 KG:** 10–15 mg/kg/dose q4–6h. **Maximum:** 4 g/day or 90 mg/kg/day.

### Revascularization

**PO: ADULTS, ELDERLY:** 80–325 mg/day.

### Kawasaki's Disease

**PO: CHILDREN:** 80–100 mg/kg/day in divided doses q6h up to 14 days (until fever resolves for at least 48 hrs). After fever resolves, 1–5 mg/kg once daily for at least 6–8 wks.

### MI, Stroke (Risk Reduction)

**PO: ADULTS, ELDERLY:** *Durlaza:* 162.5 mg once daily.

### Dosage in Renal/Hepatic Impairment

Avoid use in severe impairment.

## SIDE EFFECTS

**Occasional:** GI distress (including abdominal distention, cramping, heartburn, mild nausea); allergic reaction (including bronchospasm, pruritus, urticaria).

## ADVERSE EFFECTS/ TOXIC REACTIONS

High doses of aspirin may produce GI bleeding and/or gastric mucosal lesions. Dehydrated, febrile children may experience aspirin toxicity quickly. Reye's syndrome, characterized by persistent vomiting, signs of brain dysfunction, may occur in children taking aspirin with recent viral infection (chickenpox, common cold, or flu). Low-grade aspirin toxicity characterized by tinnitus, generalized pruritus (may be severe), headache, dizziness, flushing, tachycardia, hyperventilation, diaphoresis, thirst. Marked toxicity characterized by hyperthermia, restlessness, seizures, abnormal breathing patterns, respiratory failure, coma.

## NURSING CONSIDERATIONS

### BASELINE ASSESSMENT

Do not give to children or teenagers who have or recently had viral infections (increases risk of Reye's syndrome). Do not use if vinegar-like odor is noted (indicates chemical breakdown). Assess type, location, duration of pain, inflammation. Inspect appearance of affected joints for immobility, deformities, skin condition. **Therapeutic serum level for antiarthritic effect:** 20–30 mg/dL (toxicity occurs if level is greater than 30 mg/dL).

### INTERVENTION/EVALUATION

Monitor urinary pH (sudden acidification, pH from 6.5 to 5.5, may result in toxicity). Assess skin for evidence of ecchymosis. If given as antipyretic, assess temperature directly before and 1 hr after giving medication. Evaluate for therapeutic response: relief of pain, stiffness, swelling; increased joint mobility; reduced joint tenderness; improved grip strength.

### PATIENT/FAMILY TEACHING

• Do not, chew, crush, dissolve, or divide enteric-coated tablets. • Avoid alcohol. • Report tinnitus or persistent abdominal GI pain, bleeding. • Therapeutic anti-inflammatory effect noted in 1–3 wks. • Behavioral changes, persistent vomiting may be early signs of Reye's syndrome; contact physician.

---

## atazanavir   TOP 100

a-ta-**zan**-a-veer
(Reyataz)
**Do not confuse Reyataz with Retavase.**

### FIXED-COMBINATION(S)

**Evotaz:** atazanavir/cobicistat **(antiretroviral booster):** 300 mg/150 mg.

---

## ◆CLASSIFICATION

**PHARMACOTHERAPEUTIC:** Antiretroviral. **CLINICAL:** Protease inhibitor.

## USES

Treatment of HIV-1 infection in combination with at least two other antiretroviral agents in pts 3 mos and older, weighing 5 kg or more.

## PRECAUTIONS

**Contraindications:** Hypersensitivity to atazanavir. Concurrent use with alfuzosin, ergot derivatives, indinavir, lovastatin, midazolam (oral), pimozide, rifampin, sildenafil (for pulmonary arterial hypertension), St. John's wort, simvastatin, triazolam. **Cautions:** Preexisting conduction system defects (first-, second-, or third-degree AV block), diabetes mellitus, elderly, renal impairment (not recommended in end-stage renal disease or pts on hemodialysis), hemophilia A or B, hepatitis B or C. Do not use in pts younger than 3 mos (potential for kernicterus). Pts with increased transaminase levels prior to use or underlying hepatic disease.

## ACTION

Binds to HIV-1 protease, inhibiting cleavage of viral precursors into functional proteins. **Therapeutic Effect:** Prevents formation of mature HIV viral cells.

## PHARMACOKINETICS

Rapidly absorbed after PO administration. Protein binding: 86%. Extensively metabolized in liver. Eliminated in feces (79%), urine (13%). **Half-life:** 5–8 hrs.

## ⧗ LIFESPAN CONSIDERATIONS

**Pregnancy/Lactation:** Unknown if drug crosses placenta or distributed in breast milk. Lactic acidosis syndrome, hyperbilirubinemia, kernicterus have been reported. **Children:** Safety and efficacy not established in pts younger than 3 mos. **Elderly:** Age-related hepatic impairment may require dose reduction.

## INTERACTIONS

**DRUG:** May increase concentration, toxicity of **amiodarone, atorvastatin, bepridil, clarithromycin, cyclosporine, diltiazem, felodipine, lidocaine, lovastatin, nicardipine, nifedipine, rosuvastatin, sildenafil, simvastatin, sirolimus, tacrolimus, tadalafil, tricyclic antidepressants, vardenafil, verapamil, warfarin.** H$_2$-receptor antagonists, proton pump inhibitors, rifampin may decrease concentration/effects. **Ritonavir, voriconazole** may increase concentration. **HERBAL: St. John's wort** may decrease concentration/effects. **FOOD: High-fat meals** may decrease absorption. **LAB VALUES:** May increase serum bilirubin, ALT, AST, amylase, lipase. May decrease Hgb, neutrophil count, platelets. May alter LDL, triglycerides.

## AVAILABILITY (Rx)

**Capsules:** 150 mg, 200 mg, 300 mg. **Packet, Oral:** 50 mg.

## ADMINISTRATION/HANDLING

**PO**

• Give with food. • Swallow whole; do not break or open capsules. • Administer at least 2 hrs before or 10 hrs after H$_2$ antagonist, 12 hrs after proton pump inhibitor.

## INDICATIONS/ROUTES/DOSAGE

**Note:** Dosage adjustment may be necessary with colchicine, bosentin, H$_2$ antagonists, proton pump inhibitors, PDE5 inhibitors.

**HIV-1 Infection**
**PO: ADULTS, ELDERLY (ANTIRETROVIRAL-NAIVE):** 300 mg and ritonavir 100 mg, or cobicistat 150 mg, once daily, or 400 mg (2 capsules) once daily with food in pts unable to tolerate ritonavir. **CHILDREN 6–17 YRS (NAIVE OR EXPERIENCED) WEIGHING 40 KG OR MORE: Capsules:** 300 mg once daily (with ritonavir 100 mg). **WEIGHING 20–39 KG:** 200 mg once daily (with ritonavir 100 mg). **WEIGHING 15–19 KG:** 150 mg once daily (with ritonavir 100 mg).

**ADULTS, ELDERLY (ANTIRETROVIRAL-EXPERI-ENCED), PREGNANT PTS, CHILDREN WEIGHING 40 KG OR MORE: (Capsule):** 300 mg and ritonavir (Norvir) 100 mg once daily. **WEIGHING 20–39 KG:** 200 mg and ritonavir 100 mg once daily. **WEIGHING 15–19 KG:** 150 mg and ritonavir 100 mg once daily.

*Powder (Naive and Experienced)*
**CHILDREN WEIGHING 25 KG OR MORE:** 300 mg plus ritonavir 100 mg once daily. **WEIGHING 15–24 KG:** 250 mg plus ritonavir 80 mg once daily. **WEIGHING 5–14 KG:** 200 mg plus ritonavir 80 mg once daily.

**HIV-1 Infection (Concurrent Therapy with Efavirenz)**
**PO: ADULTS, ELDERLY:** 400 mg atazanavir, 100 mg ritonavir (as a single dose given with food), and 600 mg efavirenz as a single daily dose on an empty stomach (preferably at bedtime).

**HIV-1 Infection (Concurrent Therapy with Didanosine)**
**PO: ADULTS, ELDERLY:** Give atazanavir with food 2 hrs before or 1 hr after didanosine.

**HIV-1 Infection (Concurrent Therapy with Tenofovir)**
**PO: ADULTS, ELDERLY:** 300 mg atazanavir, 100 mg ritonavir, and 300 mg tenofovir given as a single daily dose with food. **FOR TREATMENT-EXPERIENCED PREGNANT WOMEN DURING SECOND OR THIRD TRIMESTER:** 400 mg with ritonavir 100 mg once daily.

**HIV-1 Infection in Pts with Mild to Moderate Hepatic Impairment**
◄ **ALERT** ► Avoid use in pts with severe hepatic impairment.
**PO: ADULTS, ELDERLY:** 300 mg once daily with food.

**Dosage in Renal Impairment**
**HD** (Naive): 300 mg with ritonavir. (Experienced): Not recommended.

## SIDE EFFECTS

**Frequent (16%–14%):** Nausea, headache. **Occasional (9%–4%):** Rash, vomiting, depression, diarrhea, abdominal pain, fever. **Rare (3% or less):** Dizziness, insomnia, cough, fatigue, back pain.

## ADVERSE EFFECTS/ TOXIC REACTIONS

Severe hypersensitivity reaction (angioedema, chest pain), jaundice may occur.

## NURSING CONSIDERATIONS

### BASELINE ASSESSMENT

Obtain baseline CBC, BMP, LFT before beginning therapy and at periodic intervals during therapy. Offer emotional support.

### INTERVENTION/EVALUATION

Monitor lab results. Assess for nausea, vomiting; assess eating pattern. Monitor daily pattern of bowel activity, stool consistency. Assess skin for rash. Question for evidence of headache. Assess mood for evidence of depression.

### PATIENT/FAMILY TEACHING

• Take with food. • Small, frequent meals may offset nausea, vomiting. • Swallow whole; do not break or open capsules. • Pt must continue practices to prevent HIV transmission. • Atazanavir is not a cure for HIV infection, nor does it reduce risk of transmission to others. • Report dizziness, light-headedness, yellowing of skin or whites of eyes, flank pain or when urinating, blood in urine, skin rash.

---

## *atenolol*     **HIGH ALERT**

a-**ten**-oh-lol
(Apo-Atenol ♣, Tenormin)
■ **BLACK BOX ALERT** ■ Do not abruptly discontinue; taper gradually to avoid acute tachycardia, hypertension, ischemia.
**Do not confuse atenolol with albuterol, timolol, or Tylenol, or Tenormin with Imuran, Norpramin, or thiamine.**

A

◆ CLASSIFICATION

PHARMACOTHERAPEUTIC: Beta$_1$-adrenergic blocker. CLINICAL: Antihypertensive, antianginal, antiarrhythmic.

## USES

Treatment of hypertension, alone or in combination with other agents; management of angina; secondary prevention of post-MI. OFF-LABEL: Arrhythmia (esp. supraventricular and ventricular tachycardia), thyrotoxicosis.

## PRECAUTIONS

Contraindications: Hypersensitivity to atenolol. Cardiogenic shock, uncompensated HF, second- or third-degree heart block (except with functioning pacemaker), sinus bradycardia, sinus node dysfunction, pulmonary edema, pregnancy. Cautions: Renal impairment, peripheral vascular disease, diabetes, thyroid disease, bronchospastic disease, compensated HF, concurrent use with digoxin, verapamil, or diltiazem; myasthenia gravis, psychiatric disease. History of anaphylaxis to allergens, elderly.

## ACTION

Blocks beta$_1$-adrenergic receptors in cardiac tissue. Therapeutic Effect: Slows sinus node heart rate, decreasing cardiac output, B/P. Decreases myocardial oxygen demand.

## PHARMACOKINETICS

| Route | Onset | Peak | Duration |
|-------|-------|--------|----------|
| PO | 1 hr | 2–4 hrs | 24 hrs |

Incompletely absorbed from GI tract. Protein binding: 6%–16%. Minimal liver metabolism. Primarily excreted unchanged in urine. Removed by hemodialysis. Half-life: 6–9 hrs (increased in renal impairment).

## ⧗ LIFESPAN CONSIDERATIONS

Pregnancy/Lactation: Readily crosses placenta; distributed in breast milk. Avoid use during first trimester. May produce bradycardia, apnea, hypoglycemia, hypothermia during delivery; low birth-weight infants. Children: No age-related precautions noted. Elderly: Age-related peripheral vascular disease, renal impairment require caution.

## INTERACTIONS

DRUG: Diuretics, other antihypertensives may increase hypotensive effect. Sympathomimetics, xanthines may mutually inhibit effects. May mask symptoms of hypoglycemia, prolong hypoglycemic effect of insulin, oral antidiabetic medications. NSAIDs may decrease antihypertensive effect. HERBAL: Ephedra, ginseng, yohimbe may worsen hypertension. Garlic may increase antihypertensive effect. FOOD: None known. LAB VALUES: May increase serum ANA titer, serum BUN, creatinine, potassium, uric acid, lipoprotein, triglycerides.

## AVAILABILITY (Rx)

Tablets: 25 mg, 50 mg, 100 mg.

## ADMINISTRATION/HANDLING

PO
• Give without regard to food. • Tablets may be crushed.

## INDICATIONS/ROUTES/DOSAGE

Hypertension
PO: ADULTS: Initially, 25–50 mg once daily. May increase dose up to 100 mg once daily. ELDERLY: Usual initial dose, 25 mg/day. CHILDREN: Initially, 0.5–1 mg/kg/dose given once daily. Range: 0.5–1.5 mg/kg/day. Maximum: 2 mg/kg/day up to 100 mg/day.

Angina Pectoris
PO: ADULTS: Initially, 50 mg once daily. May increase dose up to 200 mg once daily. ELDERLY: Usual initial dose, 25 mg/day.

### Post-MI
**PO: ADULTS:** 100 mg once daily or 50 mg twice daily for 6–9 days post-MI.

### Dosage in Renal Impairment
Dosage interval is modified based on creatinine clearance.

| Creatinine Clearance | Maximum Dosage |
|---|---|
| 15–35 ml/min | 50 mg/day |
| Less than 15 ml/min | 25 mg/day |
| Hemodialysis (HD) | Give dose post-HD or give 25–50 mg supplemental dose |

### Dosage in Hepatic Impairment
No dose adjustment.

## SIDE EFFECTS

Atenolol is generally well tolerated, with mild and transient side effects. **Frequent:** Hypotension manifested as cold extremities, constipation or diarrhea, diaphoresis, dizziness, fatigue, headache, nausea. **Occasional:** Insomnia, flatulence, urinary frequency, impotence or decreased libido, depression. **Rare:** Rash, arthralgia, myalgia, confusion (esp. in the elderly), altered taste.

## ADVERSE EFFECTS/ TOXIC REACTIONS

Overdose may produce profound bradycardia, hypotension. Abrupt withdrawal may result in diaphoresis, palpitations, headache, tremors. May precipitate HF, MI in pts with cardiac disease; thyroid storm in pts with thyrotoxicosis; peripheral ischemia in pts with existing peripheral vascular disease. Hypoglycemia may occur in previously controlled diabetes. Thrombocytopenia (unusual bruising, bleeding) occurs rarely. **Antidote:** Glucagon (see Appendix J for dosage).

## NURSING CONSIDERATIONS

### BASELINE ASSESSMENT

Assess B/P, apical pulse immediately before drug is administered (if pulse is 60/min or less, or systolic B/P is less than 90 mm Hg, withhold medication, contact physician). **Antianginal:** Record onset, quality (sharp, dull, squeezing), radiation, location, intensity, duration of anginal pain, precipitating factors (exertion, emotional stress). Assess baseline renal/hepatic function tests.

### INTERVENTION/EVALUATION

Monitor B/P for hypotension, pulse for bradycardia, respiration for difficulty in breathing, EKG. Monitor daily pattern of bowel activity, stool consistency. Assess for evidence of HF: dyspnea (particularly on exertion or lying down), nocturnal cough, peripheral edema, distended neck veins. Monitor I&O (increased weight, decreased urinary output may indicate HF). Assess extremities for pulse quality, changes in temperature (may indicate worsening peripheral vascular disease). Assist with ambulation if dizziness occurs.

### PATIENT/FAMILY TEACHING

• Do not abruptly discontinue medication. • Compliance with therapy essential to control hypertension, angina. • To reduce hypotensive effect, go from lying to standing slowly. • Avoid tasks that require alertness, motor skills until response to drug is established. • Advise diabetic pts to monitor blood glucose carefully (may mask signs of hypoglycemia). • Report dizziness, depression, confusion, rash, unusual bruising/bleeding. • Outpatients should monitor B/P, pulse before taking medication, following correct technique. • Restrict salt, alcohol intake. • Therapeutic antihypertensive effect noted in 1–2 wks.

# atezolizumab

a-te-zoe-**liz**-ue-mab
(Tecentriq)
**Do not confuse atezolizumab with daclizumab, certolizumab, eculizumab, omalizumab, or tocilizumab.**

## ◆ CLASSIFICATION

**PHARMACOTHERAPEUTIC:** Programmed death-ligand 1 (PD-L1) blocking antibody. Monoclonal antibody. **CLINICAL:** Antineoplastic.

## USES

Treatment of pts with locally advanced or metastatic urothelial carcinoma who have disease progression during or following platinum-containing chemotherapy or have disease progression within 12 mos of neoadjuvant or adjuvant treatment with platinum-containing chemotherapy.

## PRECAUTIONS

**Contraindications:** Hypersensitivity to atezolizumab. **Cautions:** Active infection; baseline anemia, lymphopenia; diabetes; pts at risk for dehydration, electrolyte imbalance; hepatic impairment, peripheral or generalized edema, neuropathy, optic disorders, interstitial lung disease; history of venous thromboembolism, intestinal obstruction, pancreatitis.

## ACTION

Binds to PD-L1 and blocks interaction with both PD-L1 and B7.1 receptors. Releases the PD-1/PD-L1 pathway-mediated inhibition of the immune response (including antitumor immune response). **Therapeutic Effect:** Inhibits T-cell proliferation and cytokine production. Inhibits tumor cell growth and metastasis.

## PHARMACOKINETICS

Metabolization not specified. Steady state reached in 6–9 wks. Elimination not specified. **Half-life:** 27 days.

## ⏳ LIFESPAN CONSIDERATIONS

**Pregnancy/Lactation:** Avoid pregnancy; may cause fetal harm. Unknown if distributed in breast milk; however, human immunoglobulin G is present in break milk. Breastfeeding not recommended during treatment and for at least 5 mos after discontinuation. Females of reproductive potential should use effective contraception during treatment and up to 5 mos after discontinuation. May impair fertility in females. **Children:** Safety and efficacy not established. **Elderly:** No age-related precautions noted.

## INTERACTIONS

**DRUG:** None known. **HERBAL:** None significant. **FOOD:** None known. **LAB VALUES:** May increase serum alkaline phosphatase, ALT, AST, creatinine, glucose. May decrease serum albumin, sodium; lymphocytes, Hgb, Hct, RBCs.

## AVAILABILITY (Rx)

**Injection Solution:** 1,200 mg/20 ml (60 mg/ml).

## ADMINISTRATION/HANDLING

 IV

**Reconstitution** • Visually inspect solution for particulate matter or discoloration. Solution should appear clear to slightly yellow. Discard if solution is cloudy or discolored or if visible particles are present. • Do not shake vial. • Withdraw 20 ml of solution from vial and dilute into a 250-ml polyvinyl chloride, polyethylene, or polyolefin infusion bag containing 0.9% NaCl. Dilute with 0.9% NaCl only. • Mix by gentle inversion. • Do not shake. • Discard partially used or empty vials.
**Rate of Administration** • Infuse over 60 min using sterile, nonpyrogenic, low-protein binding, 0.2–0.22 micron in-line filter. • If first infusion is tolerated, all subsequent infusions may be delivered over 30 mins. • Do not administer as IV bolus.
**Storage** • Refrigerate diluted solution up to 24 hrs or store at room temperature for no more than 6 hrs (includes time of preparation and infusion). • Do not freeze. • Do not shake.

## ▦ IV INCOMPATABILITIES

Do not administer with other medications. Infuse via dedicated line.

---

## INDICATIONS/ROUTES/DOSAGE

### Urothelial Carcinoma

IV: **ADULTS, ELDERLY:** 1,200 mg q3wks until disease progression or unacceptable toxicity occurs. No dose reductions are recommended.

### Dose Modification

Based on Common Terminology Criteria for Adverse Events (CTCAE). **Withhold treatment for any of the following toxic reactions:** Grade 2 or 3 diarrhea or colitis; grade 2 pneumonitis; serum AST or ALT elevation 3–5 times upper limit of normal (ULN) or serum bilirubin elevation 1.5–3 times ULN; symptomatic hypophysitis, adrenal insufficiency, hypothyroidism, hyperthyroidism; grade 3 or 4 hyperglycemia; grade 3 rash; grade 2 ocular inflammatory toxicity, grade 2 or 3 pancreatitis, grade 3 or 4 infection, grade 2 infusion-related reactions. **Restarting treatment after interruption of therapy:** Resume treatment when adverse effects return to grade 0 or 1. **Permanently discontinue for any of the following toxic reactions:** Grade 3 or 4 diarrhea or colitis; grade 3 or 4 pneumonitis; serum AST or ALT elevation greater than 5 times UNL or serum bilirubin elevation 3 times UNL; grade 4 hypophysitis; grade 4 rash; grade 3 or 4 ocular inflammatory toxicity; grade 4 or any grade recurrent pancreatitis; grade 3 or 4 infusion-related reactions; any occurrence of encephalitis, Guillain-Barré, meningitis, meningoencephalitis, myasthenic syndrome/myasthenia gravis.

### Dosage in Renal Impairment

No dose adjustment.

### Dosage in Hepatic Impairment

**Mild impairment:** No dose adjustment. **Moderate to severe impairment:** Not specified; use caution.

## SIDE EFFECTS

**Frequent (52%–18%):** Fatigue, decreased appetite, nausea, pyrexia, constipation, diarrhea, peripheral edema. **Occasional (17%–13%):** Abdominal pain, vomiting, dyspnea, back/neck pain, rash, arthralgia, cough, pruritus.

## ADVERSE EFFECTS/TOXIC REACTIONS

May cause severe immune-mediated events including adrenal insufficiency (0.4% of pts), interstitial lung disease or pneumonitis (3% of pts), colitis or diarrhea (20% of pts), hepatitis (2%–3% of pts), hypophysitis (0.2% of pts), hyperthyroidism (1% of pts), hypothyroidism (4% of pts), rash (up to 37% of pts), new-onset diabetes with ketoacidosis (0.2% of pts), pancreatitis (0.1% of pts); meningoencephalitis, myasthenic syndrome/myasthenia gravis, Guillain-Barré, ocular inflammatory toxicity (less than 1% of pts). Severe, sometimes fatal, infections including sepsis, herpes encephalitis, mycobacterial infection occurred in 38% of pts. Urinary tract infections were there the most common cause of grade 3 or higher infection, occurring in 7% of pts. Severe infusion-related reactions reported in less than 1% of pts. Other adverse events including acute kidney injury, dehydration, dyspnea, encephalitis, hematuria, intestinal obstruction, meningitis, neuropathy, pneumonia, urinary obstruction, venous thromboembolism were reported. Immunogenicity (auto-atezolizumab antibodies) occurred in 42% of pts.

## NURSING CONSIDERATIONS

### BASELINE ASSESSMENT

Obtain baseline CBC, BMP, LFT, thyroid panel, urine pregnancy, urinalysis; vital signs. Screen for history of pituitary/pulmonary/thyroid disease, autoimmune disorders, diabetes, hepatic impairment, venous thromboembolism. Conduct full dermatologic/neurologic/ophthalmologic exam. Verify use of effective contraception in females of reproductive potential. Screen for active infection. Assess hydration status.

## INTERVENTION/EVALUATION

Monitor CBC, BMP, LFT, thyroid panel, vital signs. Diligently monitor for immune-mediated adverse events as listed in Adverse Effects/Toxic Reactions. Notify physician if any CTCAE toxicities occur and initiate proper treatment. Obtain chest X-ray if interstitial lung disease, pneumonitis suspected. Due to high risk for dehydration/diarrhea, strictly monitor I&O. Encourage PO intake. If corticosteroid therapy is initiated for immune-mediated events, monitor capillary blood glucose and screen for corticosteroid side effects. Report any changes in neurologic status including nuchal rigidity with fever, positive Kernig's sign, positive Brudzinski's sign, altered mental status, seizures. Diligently monitor for infection.

## PATIENT/FAMILY TEACHING

• Blood levels will be routinely monitored. • Avoid pregnancy; treatment may cause birth defects. Do not breast-feed. Females of childbearing potential should use effective contraception during treatment and for at least 5 mos after final dose • Treatment may cause serious or life-threatening inflammatory reactions. Report signs and symptoms of treatment-related inflammatory events in the following body systems: colon (severe abdominal pain or diarrhea); eye (blurry vision, double vision, unequal pupil size, sensitivity to light, eyelid drooping); lung (chest pain, cough, shortness of breath); liver (bruising easily, amber-colored urine, clay-colored/tarry stools, yellowing of skin or eyes); pituitary (persistent or unusual headache, dizziness, extreme weakness, fainting, vision changes); thyroid (trouble sleeping, high blood pressure, fast heart rate [overactive thyroid]), (fatigue, goiter, weight gain [underactive thyroid]); neurologic (confusion, headache, seizures, neck rigidity with fever, severe nerve pain or loss of motor function). • Immediately report allergic reactions, bleeding of any kind, signs of infection. • Treatment may cause severe diarrhea. Drink plenty of fluids.

## *atoMOXetine

at-oh-**mox**-e-teen
Apo-Atomoxetine ✤ (Strattera)
■ **BLACK BOX ALERT** ■ Increased risk of suicidal thinking and behavior in children and adolescents with attention-deficit hyperactivity disorder (ADHD).
**Do not confuse atomoxetine with atorvastatin.**

## ◆CLASSIFICATION

**PHARMACOTHERAPEUTIC:** Norepinephrine reuptake inhibitor. **CLINICAL:** Psychotherapeutic agent.

## USES

Treatment of ADHD.

## PRECAUTIONS

**Contraindications:** Hypersensitivity to atomoxetine. Narrow-angle glaucoma, use within 14 days of MAOIs. Pheochromocytoma or history of pheochromocytoma. Severe cardiovascular disease. **Cautions:** Hypertension, tachycardia, cardiovascular disease (e.g., structural abnormalities, cardiomyopathy), urinary retention, moderate or severe hepatic impairment, suicidal ideation, emergent psychotic or manic symptoms, comorbid bipolar disorder, renal impairment, poor metabolizers of CYP2D6 metabolized drugs (e.g., fluoxetine, paroxetine). Pts predisposed to hypotension.

## ACTION

Inhibits reuptake of norepinephrine. **Therapeutic Effect:** Improves symptoms of ADHD.

## PHARMACOKINETICS

Rapidly absorbed after PO administration. Protein binding: 98% (primarily to albumin). Eliminated in urine (80%), feces (17%). Not removed by hemodialysis. **Half-life:** 4–5 hrs (increased in moderate to severe hepatic insufficiency).

## ⏳ LIFESPAN CONSIDERATIONS

**Pregnancy/Lactation:** Unknown if distributed in breast milk. **Children:** Safety and efficacy not established in pts younger than 6 yrs. May produce suicidal thoughts in children and adolescents. **Elderly:** Age-related hepatic/renal impairment, cardiovascular or cerebrovascular disease may increase risk of adverse effects.

## INTERACTIONS

**DRUG:** MAOIs may increase concentration/effect. **Fluoxetine, paroxetine** may increase concentration/effect. Avoid concurrent use of **medications that can increase heart rate or B/P. HERBAL:** None significant. **FOOD:** None known. **LAB VALUES:** May increase hepatic enzymes, serum bilirubin.

## AVAILABILITY (Rx)

**Capsules:** 10 mg, 18 mg, 25 mg, 40 mg, 60 mg, 80 mg, 100 mg.

## ADMINISTRATION/HANDLING

**PO**

• Give without regard to food. • Swallow capsules whole, do not break or open (powder in capsule is ocular irritant). Give as single daily dose in the morning or 2 evenly divided doses in morning and late afternoon/early evening.

## INDICATIONS/ROUTES/DOSAGE

**Attention-Deficit Hyperactivity Disorder (ADHD)**
**PO: ADULTS, CHILDREN 6 YRS AND OLDER WEIGHING 70 KG OR MORE:** 40 mg once daily. May increase after at least 3 days to 80 mg daily. **Maximum:** 100 mg. **Concurrent CYP2D6 Inhibitors:** Initially, 40 mg/day. May increase to 80 mg/day after 4 wks. **CHILDREN 6 YRS AND OLDER WEIGHING LESS THAN 70 KG:** Initially, 0.5 mg/kg/day. May increase after at least 3 days to 1.2 mg/kg/day. **Maximum:** 1.4 mg/kg/day or 100 mg, whichever is less. **Concurrent**

**CYP2D6 Inhibitors:** Initially, 0.5 mg/kg. May increase to 1.2 mg/kg/day after 4 wks.

**Dosage in Hepatic Impairment**
Expect to administer 50% of normal atomoxetine dosage to pts with moderate hepatic impairment and 25% of normal dosage to pts with severe hepatic impairment.

**Dosage in Renal Impairment**
No dose adjustment.

**Dosage with Strong CYP2D6 Inhibitors**
**ADULTS:** Initially, 40 mg/day. May increase to 80 mg/day after minimum of 4 wks. **CHILDREN:** Initially, 0.5 mg/kg/day. May increase to 1.2 mg/kg/day only after minimum 4-wk interval.

## SIDE EFFECTS

**Frequent:** Headache, dyspepsia, nausea, vomiting, fatigue, decreased appetite, dizziness, altered mood. **Occasional:** Tachycardia, hypertension, weight loss, delayed growth in children, irritability. **Rare:** Insomnia, sexual dysfunction in adults, fever.

## ADVERSE EFFECTS/ TOXIC REACTIONS

Urinary retention, urinary hesitancy may occur. In overdose, gastric lavage, activated charcoal may prevent systemic absorption. Severe hepatic injury occurs rarely.

## NURSING CONSIDERATIONS

### BASELINE ASSESSMENT

Assess pulse, B/P before therapy, following dose increases, and periodically during therapy. Assess attention span, interactions with others.

### INTERVENTION/EVALUATION

Monitor urinary output; complaints of urinary retention/hesitancy may be a related adverse reaction. Monitor B/P, pulse periodically and following dose increases. Monitor for growth, attention span, hyperactivity, unusual changes in

---

behavior, suicidal ideation. Assist with ambulation if dizziness occurs. Be alert to mood changes. Monitor fluid and electrolyte status in pts with significant vomiting.

### PATIENT/FAMILY TEACHING

• Avoid tasks that require alertness, motor skills until response to drug is established. • Take last dose early in evening to avoid insomnia. • Report palpitations, fever, vomiting, irritability. • Monitor growth rate, weight. • Report changes in behavior, suicidal ideation, chest pain, palpitations, dyspnea.

---

## *atorvaSTATin    TOP 100

a-**tor**-va-sta-tin
(Apo-Atorvastatin ✦, Lipitor, Novo-Atorvastatin ✦)
**Do not confuse atorvastatin with atomoxetine, lovastatin, nystatin, pitavastatin, pravastatin, or simvastatin, or Lipitor with Levatol, lisinopril, or Zocor.**

### FIXED-COMBINATION(S)

**Caduet:** atorvastatin/amlodipine (calcium channel blocker): 10 mg/2.5 mg, 10 mg/5 mg, 10 mg/10 mg, 20 mg/2.5 mg, 20 mg/5 mg, 20 mg/10 mg, 40 mg/2.5 mg, 40 mg/5 mg, 40 mg/10 mg, 80 mg/5 mg, 80 mg/10 mg.

### ◆CLASSIFICATION

**PHARMACOTHERAPEUTIC:** Hydroxymethylglutaryl CoA (HMG-CoA) reductase inhibitor. **CLINICAL:** Antihyperlipidemic.

### USES

Primary prevention of cardiovascular disease in high-risk pts. Reduces risk of stroke and heart attack in pts with type 2 diabetes with or without evidence of heart disease. Reduces risk of stroke in pts with or without evidence of heart disease with multiple risk factors other than diabetes. Adjunct to diet therapy in management of hyperlipidemias (reduces elevations in total cholesterol, LDL-C, apolipoprotein B triglycerides in pts with primary hypercholesterolemia), homozygous familial hypercholesterolemia, heterozygous familial hypercholesterolemia in pts 10–17 yrs of age, females more than 1 yr postmenarche. **OFF-LABEL:** Secondary prevention in pts who have experienced a noncardioembolic stroke/TIA or following an acute coronary syndrome (ACS) event.

### PRECAUTIONS

**Contraindications:** Hypersensitivity to atorvastatin. Active hepatic disease, breastfeeding, pregnancy, unexplained elevated LFT results. **Cautions:** Anticoagulant therapy; history of hepatic disease; substantial alcohol consumption; pts with prior stroke/TIA; concomitant use of potent CYP3A4 inhibitors; elderly (predisposed to myopathy).

### ACTION

Inhibits HMG-CoA reductase, the enzyme that catalyzes the early step in cholesterol synthesis. **Therapeutic Effect:** Decreases LDL and VLDL, plasma triglyceride levels; increases HDL concentration.

### PHARMACOKINETICS

Poorly absorbed from GI tract. Protein binding: greater than 98%. Metabolized in liver. Primarily eliminated in feces (biliary). **Half-life:** 14 hrs.

### ⊗ LIFESPAN CONSIDERATIONS

**Pregnancy/Lactation:** Distributed in breast milk. Contraindicated during pregnancy. May produce fetal skeletal malformation. **Children:** Safety and efficacy not established. **Elderly:** No age-related precautions noted.

### INTERACTIONS

**DRUG:** Strong CYP3A4 inhibitors (e.g., **clarithromycin, protease inhibitors,**

---

itraconazole) may increase concentration, risk of rhabdomyolysis. **Cyclosporine** may increase concentration. **Gemfibrozil, fibrates, niacin, colchicine** may increase risk of myopathy, rhabdomyolysis. **Strong CYP3A4 inducers (e.g., rifampin, efavirenz)** may decrease concentration. **HERBAL:** St. John's wort may decrease level. **FOOD:** Grapefruit products may increase serum concentrations. **Red yeast rice** may increase serum levels (2.4 mg lovastatin per 600 mg rice). **LAB VALUES:** May increase serum transaminase, creatinine kinase concentrations.

## AVAILABILITY (Rx)

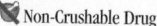 Tablets: 10 mg, 20 mg, 40 mg, 80 mg.

## ADMINISTRATION/HANDLING

### PO
• Give without regard to food or time of day. • Do not break, crush, dissolve, or divide film-coated tablets.

## INDICATIONS/ROUTES/DOSAGE

Do not use in pts with active hepatic disease.
**Note:** Individualize dosage based on baseline LDL/cholesterol, goal of therapy, pt response. **Maximum dose with strong CYP3A4 inhibitors:** 20 mg/day.

### Dyslipidemias
**PO: ADULTS, ELDERLY:** Initially, 10–20 mg/day (40 mg in pts requiring greater than 45% reduction in LDL-C). Range: 10–80 mg/day.

### Heterozygous Hypercholesterolemia
**PO: CHILDREN 10–17 YRS:** Initially, 10 mg/day. **Maximum:** 20 mg/day.

### Dosage in Renal Impairment
No dose adjustment.

### Dosage in Hepatic Impairment
See contraindications.

## SIDE EFFECTS

**Common:** Atorvastatin is generally well tolerated. Side effects are usually mild

and transient. **Frequent (16%):** Headache. **Occasional (5%–2%):** Myalgia, rash, pruritus, allergy. **Rare (less than 2%–1%):** Flatulence, dyspepsia, depression.

## ADVERSE EFFECTS/TOXIC REACTIONS

Potential for cataracts, photosensitivity, myalgia, rhabdomyolysis.

## NURSING CONSIDERATIONS

### BASELINE ASSESSMENT
Obtain baseline cholesterol, triglycerides, LFT. Question for possibility of pregnancy before initiating therapy. Obtain dietary history.

### INTERVENTION/EVALUATION
Monitor for headache. Assess for rash, pruritus, malaise. Monitor cholesterol, triglyceride lab values for therapeutic response. Monitor LFTs, CPK.

### PATIENT/FAMILY TEACHING
• Follow special diet (important part of treatment). • Periodic lab tests are essential part of therapy. • Do not take other medications without consulting physician. • Do not chew, crush, dissolve, or divide tablets. • Report dark urine, muscle fatigue, bone pain. • Avoid excessive alcohol intake, large quantities of grapefruit products.

# atovaquone

a-**toe**-va-kwone
(Mepron)

### ◆CLASSIFICATION
**PHARMACOTHERAPEUTIC:** Systemic anti-infective. **CLINICAL:** Antiprotozoal.

## USES

Treatment or prevention of mild to moderate *Pneumocystis jiroveci* pneumonia (PCP) in pts intolerant to trimethoprim-sulfamethoxazole (TMP-SMZ). **OFF-LABEL:** Treatment of babesiosis.

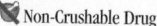

Prophylaxis in HIV pts at high risk for developing *Toxoplasma gondii* encephalitis.

## PRECAUTIONS

**Contraindications:** Development or history of potentially life-threatening allergic reaction to the drug. **Cautions:** Elderly, pts with severe PCP, chronic diarrhea, malabsorption syndromes, severe hepatic impairment.

## ACTION

Inhibits mitochondrial electron transport system at the cytochrome bc1 complex (Complex III) interrupting nucleic acid, adenosine triphosphate synthesis. **Therapeutic Effect:** Antiprotozoal, antipneumocystic activity.

## INTERACTIONS

**DRUG: Rifabutin, rifampin** may decrease concentration. May increase **rifampin** concentration. **HERBAL: Bilberry, fenugreek, garlic, ginger, ginseng** may enhance risk of hypoglycemia. **FOOD: High-fat meals** increase absorption. **LAB VALUES:** May elevate serum ALT, AST, alkaline phosphatase, amylase. May decrease serum sodium.

## AVAILABILITY (Rx)

**Suspension, Oral:** 750 mg/5 ml.

## ADMINISTRATION/HANDLING

**PO**
• Must give with food or high-fat meals. Shake gently prior to using.

## INDICATIONS/ROUTES/DOSAGE

*Pneumocystis Jiroveci* **Pneumonia (PCP)**
**PO: ADULTS, CHILDREN OLDER THAN 12 YRS:** 750 mg twice daily with food for 21 days. **CHILDREN 4–24 MOS:** 45 mg/kg/day in 2 divided doses with food. **Maximum:** 1,500 mg/day. **CHILDREN 1–3 MOS OR OLDER THAN 24 MOS:** 30–40 mg/kg/day in 2 divided doses with food. **Maximum:** 1,500 mg/day. **NEONATES:** 30–40 mg/kg/day in 2 divided doses.

**Prevention of PCP**
**PO: ADULTS, CHILDREN OLDER THAN 12 YRS:** 1,500 mg once daily with food. **CHILDREN 4–24 MOS:** 45 mg/kg/day as single dose. **Maximum:** 1,500 mg/day. **CHILDREN 1–3 MOS OR OLDER THAN 24 MOS:** 30 mg/kg/day as single dose. **Maximum:** 1,500 mg/day.

**Dosage in Renal/Hepatic Impairment**
No dose adjustment.

## SIDE EFFECTS

**Frequent (greater than 10%):** Rash, nausea, diarrhea, headache, vomiting, fever, insomnia, cough. **Occasional (less than 10%):** Abdominal discomfort, thrush, asthenia, anemia, neutropenia.

## ADVERSE EFFECTS/ TOXIC REACTIONS

None known.

## NURSING CONSIDERATIONS

**BASELINE ASSESSMENT**
Obtain baseline lab studies, esp. LFT.

**INTERVENTION/EVALUATION**
Monitor CBC, BMP, LFT, serum amylase. Assess for GI discomfort, nausea, vomiting. Monitor daily pattern of bowel activity, stool consistency. Assess skin for rash. Monitor elderly closely for decreased hepatic, renal, cardiac function. Monitor I&O.

**PATIENT/FAMILY TEACHING**
• Continue therapy for full length of treatment. • Do not take any other medications unless approved by physician. • Report rash, diarrhea, or other new symptoms. • Must be taken with high-fat meal or food.

# atropine

**at**-roe-peen
**Lomotil:** atropine/diphenoxylate
(peristaltic inhibitor): 0.025 mg/
2.5 mg.

## ◆CLASSIFICATION

**PHARMACOTHERAPEUTIC:** Acetylcholine antagonist. **CLINICAL:** Antiarrhythmic, antispasmodic, antidote,
cycloplegic, antisecretory, anticholinergic.

## USES

**Injection:** Preop to inhibit salivation/
secretions; treatment of symptomatic sinus bradycardia; AV block; ventricular
asystole; antidote for organophosphate
pesticide poisoning. Adjuvant to decrease
side effects during reversal of neuromuscular blockage.

## PRECAUTIONS

**Contraindications:** Hypersensitivity to atropine. Narrow-angle glaucoma, pyloric
stenosis, prostatic hypertrophy. **Cautions:** Autonomic neuropathy, paralytic ileus, intestinal atony, severe ulcerative
colitis, toxic megacolon, renal/hepatic impairment, myocardial ischemia, hyperthyroidism, hypertension, tachyarrhythmias,
HF, coronary artery disease, esophageal
reflux or hiatal hernia associated with
reflux esophagitis; infants, children with
spastic paralysis or brain damage; elderly;
biliary tract disease, chronic pulmonary
disease.

## ACTION

Competes with acetylcholine for common
binding sites on muscarinic receptors
located on exocrine glands, cardiac and
smooth muscle ganglia, intramural neurons. **Therapeutic Effect:** Decreases
GI motility, secretory activity, GU muscle
tone (ureter, bladder); abolishes various
types of reflex vagal cardiac slowing or
asystole.

## PHARMACOKINETICS

Rapidly and well absorbed after IM
administration. Widely distributed. Metabolized in liver. Excreted in urine
(30%–50% as unchanged drug). **Half-
life:** 2–3 hrs.

## ⏳ LIFESPAN CONSIDERATIONS

**Pregnancy/Lactation:** Crosses placenta;
distributed in breast milk. **Children/
Elderly:** Increased susceptibility to atropine effects.

## INTERACTIONS

**DRUG: Anticholinergics** may increase
effects. **HERBAL:** None significant.
**FOOD:** None known. **LAB VALUES:** None
significant.

## AVAILABILITY (Rx)

**Injection (AtroPen):** 0.25 mg/0.3 ml,
0.5 mg/0.7 ml, 1 mg/0.7 ml, 2 mg/0.7 ml.
**Injection, Solution:** 0.4 mg/ml, 1 mg/ml.

## ADMINISTRATION/HANDLING

**IV**

• Must be given rapidly (prevents paradoxical slowing of heart rate).

**IM**
• May be given subcutaneously or IM.

## ▦ IV INCOMPATIBILITIES
None known.

## ▦ IV COMPATIBILITIES

Diphenhydramine (Benadryl), droperidol (Inapsine), fentanyl (Sublimaze),
glycopyrrolate (Robinul), heparin, hydromorphone (Dilaudid), midazolam
(Versed), morphine, potassium chloride,
propofol (Diprivan).

## INDICATIONS/ROUTES/DOSAGE
**Preanesthetic**
**IV, IM, Subcutaneous: ADULTS, EL-
DERLY:** 0.4–0.6 mg 30–60 min preop.
**CHILDREN WEIGHING 5 KG OR MORE:** 0.01–
0.02 mg/kg/dose to maximum of 0.4 mg/
dose. Minimum dose: 0.1 mg. **CHILDREN**

---

✤ Canadian trade name       Non-Crushable Drug      🔲 High Alert drug

**WEIGHING LESS THAN 5 KG:** 0.02 mg/kg/dose 30–60 min preop.

**Bradycardia**
**IV: ADULTS, ELDERLY:** 0.5–1 mg q5min, not to exceed total of 3 mg or 0.04 mg/kg. **CHILDREN:** 0.02 mg/kg with a minimum of 0.1 mg to a maximum of 0.5 mg as a single dose. May repeat in 5 min. **Maximum total dose:** 1 mg.

**Dosage in Renal/Hepatic Impairment**
No dose adjustment.

## SIDE EFFECTS

**Frequent:** Dry mouth, nose, throat (may be severe); decreased sweating; constipation; irritation at subcutaneous or IM injection site. **Occasional:** Dysphagia, blurred vision, bloated feeling, impotence, urinary hesitancy. **Ophthalmic:** Mydriasis, blurred vision, photophobia, decreased visual acuity, tearing, dry eyes or dry conjunctiva, eye irritation, crusting of eyelid. **Rare:** Allergic reaction, including rash, urticaria; mental confusion or excitement, particularly in children; fatigue.

## ADVERSE EFFECTS/ TOXIC REACTIONS

Overdose may produce tachycardia, palpitations, hot/dry/flushed skin, absence of bowel sounds, increased respiratory rate, nausea, vomiting, confusion, drowsiness, slurred speech, dizziness, CNS stimulation. Overdose may also produce psychosis as evidenced by agitation, restlessness, rambling speech, visual hallucinations, paranoid behavior, delusions, followed by depression. Ophthalmic form may rarely produce increased IOP.

## NURSING CONSIDERATIONS

**BASELINE ASSESSMENT**
Determine if pt is sensitive to atropine, homatropine, scopolamine.

**INTERVENTION/EVALUATION**
Monitor changes in B/P, pulse, temperature. Observe for tachycardia if pt has cardiac abnormalities. Assess skin turgor, mucous membranes to evaluate hydration status (encourage adequate fluid intake unless NPO for surgery), bowel sounds for peristalsis. Be alert for fever (increased risk of hyperthermia). Monitor I&O, palpate bladder for urinary retention. Monitor daily pattern of bowel activity, stool consistency.

**PATIENT/ FAMILY TEACHING**
• For preop use, explain that warm flushing feeling may occur.

# axitinib

ax-**i**-ti-nib
(Inlyta)
**Do not confuse axitinib with afatinib, ibrutinib, or imatinib.**

## ◆CLASSIFICATION

**PHARMACOTHERAPEUTIC:** Tyrosine kinase inhibitor. **CLINICAL:** Antineoplastic.

## USES

Treatment of advanced renal cell carcinoma after failure of one prior systemic chemotherapy.

## PRECAUTIONS

**Contraindications:** Hypersensitivity to axitinib. **Cautions:** Pts with increased risk or history of thrombotic events, GI perforation or fistula formation, renal/hepatic impairment, hypertension, HF. Do not use in pts with untreated brain metastasis or recent active GI bleeding.

## ACTION

Inhibits vascular endothilial growth factor receptors. **Therapeutic Effect:** Blocks tumor growth, inhibits angiogenesis.

## PHARMACOKINETICS

Undergoes extensive hepatic metabolism. Protein binding: greater than 99%. Eliminated primarily in feces with a lesser amount excreted in urine. **Half-life:** 2.5–6 hrs.

## ⧗ LIFESPAN CONSIDERATIONS

**Pregnancy/Lactation:** May cause fetal harm. Unknown whether distributed in breast milk. **Children:** Safety and efficacy not established in pts younger than 18 yrs. **Elderly:** No age-related precautions noted.

## INTERACTIONS

**DRUG: Strong CYP3A4/5 inhibitors (e.g., erythromycin, itraconazole, ketoconazole, ritonavir)** may significantly increase concentration; do not use concurrently. If used, reduce dose by 50%. Coadministration with **strong CYP3A4/5 inducers (e.g., rifampin, phenytoin, carbamazepine, phenobarbital)** may significantly decrease concentration; do not use concurrently. **HERBAL: St. John's wort** may decrease concentration. **FOOD: Grapefruit products** may increase concentration. **LAB VALUES:** May decrease Hgb, WBC count, platelets, lymphocytes, serum calcium, alkaline phosphatase, albumin, sodium, phosphate, bicarbonate. May increase serum ALT, AST, bilirubin, BUN, creatinine, serum potassium, lipase, amylase; urine protein. May alter serum glucose.

## AVAILABILITY (Rx)

Tablets, film-coated: 1 mg, 5 mg.

## ADMINISTRATION/HANDLING

**PO**

• Give without regard to food. • Swallow tablets whole with full glass of water.

## INDICATIONS/ROUTES/DOSAGE

**Renal Cell Carcinoma**

**PO: ADULTS, ELDERLY:** Initially, 5 mg twice daily, given approximately 12 hrs apart. If tolerated (no adverse events above grade 2, BP normal and no antihypertension use for at least 2 consecutive wks), may increase to 7 mg twice daily, then 10 mg twice daily. For adverse effects, may decrease to 3 mg twice daily,

then 2 mg twice daily if adverse effects persist.

**Dose Modification**
**Dosage with concomitant strong CYP3A4 inhibitors:** Reduce dose by 50%.

**Dosage in Renal Impairment**
No dose adjustment. Use caution in ESRD.

**Dosage in Hepatic Impairment**
**Mild impairment:** No dose adjustment. **Moderate Impairment:** Reduce initial dose by 50%. **Severe Impairment:** Not recommended.

## SIDE EFFECTS

**Frequent (55%–20%):** Diarrhea, hypertension, fatigue, decreased appetite, nausea, dysphonia, palmar-plantar erythrodysesthesia (hand-foot) syndrome, weight loss, vomiting, asthenia, constipation. **Occasional (19%–11%):** Hypothyroidism, cough, stomatitis, arthralgia, dyspnea, abdominal pain, headache, peripheral pain, rash, proteinuria, dysgeusia. **Rare (10%–2%):** Dry skin, dyspepsia, dizziness, myalgia, pruritus, epistaxis, alopecia, hemorrhoids, tinnitus, erythema.

## ADVERSE EFFECTS/ TOXIC REACTIONS

Arterial and venous thrombotic events (MI, CVA), GI perforation, fistula, hemorrhagic events (including cerebral hemorrhage, hematuria, hemoptysis, GI bleeding), hypertensive crisis, cardiac failure have been observed and can be fatal. Hypothyroidism requiring thyroid hormone replacement has been noted. Reversible posterior leukoencephalopathy syndrome (RPLS) has been observed.

## NURSING CONSIDERATIONS

### BASELINE ASSESSMENT

Obtain baseline BMP, LFT, renal function test, urine protein, serum amylase, lipase, phosphate before initiation of, and periodically throughout, treatment. Offer emotional support. Assess medical history, esp. hepatic function abnormalities. B/P should be well controlled prior to initiating treatment. Stop medication at least 24 hrs prior to scheduled surgery. Monitor thyroid function before and periodically throughout treatment.

### INTERVENTION/EVALUATION

Monitor CBC, BMP, LFT, renal function test, urine protein, serum amylase, lipase, phosphate, thyroid tests. Monitor daily pattern of bowel activity, stool consistency. Assess for evidence of bleeding or hemorrhage. Assess for hypertension. For persistent hypertension despite use of antihypertensive medications, dose should be reduced. Permanently discontinue if signs or symptoms of RPLS occur (extreme lethargy, increased B/P from pt baseline, pyuria). Contact physician if changes in voice, redness of skin, or rash is noted.

### PATIENT/FAMILY TEACHING

• Avoid crowds, those with known infection. • Avoid contact with anyone who recently received live virus vaccine; do not receive vaccinations. • Swallow tablet whole; do not chew, crush, dissolve, or divide. • Avoid grapefruit products. • Report persistent diarrhea, extreme fatigue, abdominal pain, yellowing of skin or eyes, bruising easily; bleeding of any kind, esp. bloody stool or urine; confusion, seizure activity, vision loss, trouble speaking, chest pain; difficulty breathing, leg pain or swelling.

---

## *azaTHIOprine

a-za-**thy**-o-preen
(Apo-Azathioprine ✦, Azasan, Imuran)
■ **BLACK BOX ALERT** ■ Chronic immunosuppression increases risk of developing malignancy.
**Do not confuse azathioprine with Azulfidine, azacitidine, or azithromycin, or Imuran with Elmiron, Imdur, or Inderal.**

---

◆ **CLASSIFICATION**

**PHARMACOTHERAPEUTIC:** Immunologic agent. **CLINICAL:** Immunosuppressant.

## USES

Adjunct in prevention of rejection in kidney transplantation. Treatment of rheumatoid arthritis (RA) in pts unresponsive to conventional therapy. **OFF-LABEL:** Treatment of dermatomyositis, polymyositis. Maintenance, remission, or reduction of steroid use in Crohn's disease, lupus nephritis, chronic refractory immune thrombocytopenic purpura.

## PRECAUTIONS

**Contraindications:** Hypersensitivity to azathioprine. Pregnant women with RA, pts previously treated for RA with alkylating agents (cyclophosphamide, chlorambucil, melphalan). **Cautions:** Immunosuppressed pts, pts with hepatic/renal impairment, active infection. Testing for genetic deficiency of thiopurine methyltransferase should be obtained. (Absence or reduced levels increase risk of myelosuppression.)

## PHARMACOKINETICS

Well absorbed from GI tract. Peak levels: 1–2 hrs. Protein binding: 30%. Metabolized in liver. Primarily excreted in urine. **Half-life:** 2 hrs.

## ACTION

Antagonizes purine metabolism, inhibits DNA, protein, and RNA synthesis. **Therapeutic Effect:** Suppresses cell-mediated hypersensitivities; alters antibody production, immune response in transplant recipients. Reduces symptoms of arthritis severity.

## ⧗ LIFESPAN CONSIDERATIONS

**Pregnancy/Lactation:** May depress spermatogenesis, reduction of sperm viability, count. May cause fetal harm. Do not breastfeed. **Children:** Safety and efficacy not established. **Elderly:** No age-related precautions noted.

---

## INTERACTIONS

**DRUG: Allopurinol, sulfamethoxazole/ trimethoprim** may increase activity, toxicity. **Bone marrow depressants** may increase myelosuppression. **Other immunosuppressants** may increase risk of infection or development of neoplasms. May increase effects of **live virus vaccines. HERBAL:** Avoid **cat's claw, echinacea** (immunostimulant properties). **FOOD:** None known. **LAB VALUES:** May decrease Hgb, serum albumin, uric acid, leukocytes, platelet count. May increase serum ALT, AST, alkaline phosphatase, amylase, bilirubin.

## AVAILABILITY (Rx)

**Tablets:** 50 mg (Imuran), 75 mg (Azasan), 100 mg (Azasan).

## ADMINISTRATION/HANDLING

**PO**
• Give with food or in divided doses to reduce potential for GI disturbances.
• Store oral form at room temperature.

## INDICATIONS/ROUTES/DOSAGE

◀**ALERT**▶ Reduce dose to 1/3 or 1/4 usual dose when used with allopurinol or in low/absent thiopurine methyltransfurase genetic deficiency.

**Prevention of Renal Allograft Rejection**
**PO: ADULTS, ELDERLY, CHILDREN:** 3–5 mg/ kg/day on day of transplant (or 1–3 days prior to transplant), then 1–3 mg/kg/day as maintenance dose.

**Rheumatoid Arthritis (RA)**
**PO: ADULTS, ELDERLY:** Initially, 1 mg/kg/ day (50–100 mg) as a single dose or in 2 divided doses for 6–8 wks. May increase by 0.5 mg/kg/day after 6–8 wks at 4-wk intervals. **Maximum:** 2.5 mg/kg/ day. **Maintenance:** Lowest effective dosage. May decrease dose by 0.5 mg/kg or 25 mg/day q4wks (while other therapies, such as rest, physiotherapy, and salicylates, are maintained).

**Dosage in Renal Impairment**
Dosage is modified based on creatinine clearance.

| Creatinine Clearance | Dosage |
|---|---|
| 10–50 ml/min | 75% of normal |
| Less than 10 ml/min | 50% of normal |
| Hemodialysis | 50% of normal (Adults: additional 0.25 mg/kg) |
| Continuous renal replacement therapy (CRRT) | 75% of normal |

**Dosage in Hepatic Impairment**
No dose adjustment.

## SIDE EFFECTS

**Frequent:** Nausea, vomiting, anorexia (particularly during early treatment and with large doses). **Occasional:** Rash. **Rare:** Severe nausea/vomiting with diarrhea, abdominal pain, hypersensitivity reaction.

## ADVERSE EFFECTS/ TOXIC REACTIONS

Increases risk of neoplasia (new abnormal-growth tumors). Significant leukopenia and thrombocytopenia may occur, particularly in pts undergoing renal transplant rejection. Hepatotoxicity occurs rarely.

## NURSING CONSIDERATIONS

### BASELINE ASSESSMENT

**Arthritis:** Assess onset, type, location, and duration of pain, fever, inflammation. Inspect appearance of affected joints for immobility, deformities, skin condition.

### INTERVENTION/EVALUATION

CBC, LFT should be performed weekly during first mo of therapy, twice monthly during second and third mos of treatment, then monthly thereafter. If WBC falls rapidly, dosage should be reduced or discontinued. Assess particularly for delayed myelosuppression. Routinely watch

 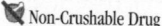

for any change from baseline. **Arthritis:** Assess for therapeutic response: relief of pain, stiffness, swelling; increased joint mobility; reduced joint tenderness; improved grip strength.

### PATIENT/FAMILY TEACHING

• Contact physician if unusual bleeding/bruising, sore throat, mouth sores, abdominal pain, fever occurs. • Therapeutic response in rheumatoid arthritis may take up to 12 wks. • Women of childbearing age must avoid pregnancy.

## azilsartan

a-zil-**sar**-tan
(Edarbi)
■ **BLACK BOX ALERT** ■ May cause fetal injury, mortality. Discontinue as soon as possible once pregnancy is detected.
**Do not confuse azilsartan with losartan, irbesartan, or valsartan.**

### FIXED-COMBINATION(S)

**Edarbyclor:** azilsartan/chlorthalidone, a diuretic: 40 mg/12.5 mg, 40 mg/25 mg.

### ◆CLASSIFICATION

**PHARMACOTHERAPEUTIC:** Angiotensin II receptor blocker (ARB). **CLINICAL:** Antihypertensive.

### USES

Treatment of hypertension alone or in combination with other antihypertensives.

### PRECAUTIONS

**Contraindications:** Hypersensitivity to azilsartan. Concomitant use with aliskiren in pts with diabetes mellitus. **Cautions:** Renal/hepatic impairment, unstented renal artery stenosis, significant aortic/mitral stenosis, severe HF, volume depletion/salt-depleted pts, history of angioedema.

### ACTION

Inhibits vasoconstriction, aldosterone-secreting effects of angiotension II, blocking the binding of angiotension II to $AT_1$ receptors. **Therapeutic Effect:** Produces vasodilation, decreases peripheral resistance, decreases B/P.

### PHARMACOKINETICS

Hydrolyzed to active metabolite in GI tract. Moderately absorbed (60%). Peak plasma concentration: 1.5–3 hrs. Metabolized in liver. Protein binding: greater than 99%. Eliminated in feces (55%), urine (42%). **Half-life:** 11 hrs.

### ☒ LIFESPAN CONSIDERATIONS

**Pregnancy/Lactation:** May cause fetal harm when administered during third trimester. Unknown if distributed in breast milk. Breastfeeding not recommended. **Children:** Safety and efficacy not established. **Elderly:** Elevated creatinine levels may occur in pts older than 75 yrs.

### INTERACTIONS

**DRUG: ACE inhibitors, potassium-sparing diuretics, potassium supplements** may increase risk of hyperkalemia. **NSAIDs, COX-2 inhibitors (e.g., celecoxib)** may decrease effect. **Hypotensive agents** may increase hypotensive effects. **HERBAL: Yohimbe, ephedra, licorice, ginseng** may increase B/P. **Garlic** may enhance antihypertensive effect. **FOOD:** None known. **LAB VALUES:** May increase serum creatinine. May decrease Hgb, Hct.

### AVAILABILITY (Rx)

**Tablets:** 40 mg, 80 mg.

### ADMINISTRATION/HANDLING

**PO**
• May give without regard to food.

### INDICATIONS/ROUTES/DOSAGE

**Hypertension**
**PO: ADULTS, ELDERLY:** 80 mg once daily. Reduce to 40 mg once daily if giving high-dose diuretic concurrently.

---

**Dosage in Renal/Hepatic Impairment**
No dose adjustment.

## SIDE EFFECTS

**Occasional (2%–0.4%):** Diarrhea, orthostatic hypotension. **Rare (0.3%):** Nausea, fatigue, muscle spasm, cough.

## ADVERSE EFFECTS/ TOXIC REACTIONS

Oliguria, acute renal failure may occur in pts with history of renal artery stenosis, severe HF, volume depletion.

## NURSING CONSIDERATIONS

### BASELINE ASSESSMENT

Obtain baseline Hgb, Hct, BMP, LFT. Obtain B/P, apical pulse immediately before each dose, in addition to regular monitoring (be alert to fluctuations). Question for possibility of pregnancy. Assess medication history (esp. diuretics). Question history of hepatic/renal impairment, renal artery stenosis, severe HF.

### INTERVENTION/EVALUATION

Maintain hydration (offer fluids frequently). Monitor serum electrolytes, B/P, pulse, hepatic/renal function. Observe for symptoms of hypotension. If excessive reduction in B/P occurs, place pt in supine position, feet slightly elevated. Correct volume or salt depletion prior to treatment.

### PATIENT/FAMILY TEACHING

• Take measures to avoid pregnancy. If pregnancy occurs, inform physician immediately. • Low blood pressure is more likely to occur if pt takes diuretics or other medications to control hypertension, consumes low-salt diet, experiences vomiting or diarrhea, or becomes dehydrated. • Change positions slowly, particularly from lying to standing position. • Report lightheadedness or dizziness; lie down immediately. • Report swollen extremities or decreased urine output despite fluid intake.

# azithromycin

a-**zith**-roe-**mye**-sin
(Apo-Azithromycin ✦, AzaSite, Novo-Azithromycin ✦, Zithromax, Zithromax TRI-PAK, Zithromax Z-PAK, Zmax)
**Do not confuse azithromycin with azathioprine or erythromycin, or Zithromax with Fosamax or Zovirax.**

## ◆CLASSIFICATION

**PHARMACOTHERAPEUTIC:** Macrolide. **CLINICAL:** Antibiotic.

## USES

**IV/PO:** Treatment of susceptible infections due to *Chlamydia pneumoniae, C. trachomatis, H. influenzae, Legionella, M. catarrhalis, Mycoplasma pneumoniae, N. gonorrhoeae, S. aureus., S. pneumoniae, S. pyogenes,* including mild to moderate infections of upper respiratory tract (pharyngitis, tonsillitis), lower respiratory tract (acute bacterial exacerbations, COPD, pneumonia), uncomplicated skin and skin-structure infections, sexually transmitted diseases (nongonococcal urethritis, cervicitis due to *C. trachomatis*), chancroid. Prevents disseminated *Mycobacterium avium* complex (MAC). Treatment of mycoplasma pneumonia, community-acquired pneumonia, pelvic inflammatory disease (PID). Prevention/treatment of MAC in pts with advanced HIV infection. **OFF-LABEL:** Prophylaxis of endocarditis. Prevention of pulmonary exacerbations in pts with cystic fibrosis. **Ophthalmic:** Treatment of bacterial conjunctivitis caused by susceptible infections due to *H. influenzae, S. aureus, S. mitis, S. pneumoniae.* Prevention of pulmonary exacerbations in pts with cystic fibrosis.

---

✦ Canadian trade name    ⚔ Non-Crushable Drug    🔲 High Alert drug

## PRECAUTIONS

**Contraindications:** Hypersensitivity to azithromycin or other macrolide antibiotics. History of cholestatic jaundice/hepatic impairment associated with prior azithromycin therapy. **Cautions:** Hepatic/renal impairment; myasthenia gravis. Hepatocellular and/or cholestatic hepatitis (with or without jaundice), hepatic necrosis. May prolong QT interval.

## ACTION

Binds to ribosomal receptor sites of susceptible organisms, inhibiting RNA-dependent protein synthesis. **Therapeutic Effect:** Bacteriostatic or bactericidal, depending on drug dosage.

## PHARMACOKINETICS

Rapidly absorbed from GI tract. Protein binding: 7%–50%. Widely distributed. Metabolized in liver. Eliminated primarily by biliary excretion. **Half-life:** 68 hrs.

## ⌛ LIFESPAN CONSIDERATIONS

**Pregnancy/Lactation:** Unknown if distributed in breast milk. **Children:** Safety and efficacy not established in pts younger than 16 yrs for IV use and younger than 6 mos for oral use. **Elderly:** No age-related precautions in those with normal renal function.

## INTERACTIONS

**DRUG:** **Aluminum/magnesium-containing antacids** may decrease concentration (give 1 hr before or 2 hrs after antacid). May increase levels of **amiodarone, cyclosporine, dronedarone, QT-prolonging medications, thioridazine, toremifene, ziprasidone. Quetiapine** may increase concentration. **HERBAL:** None significant. **FOOD:** None known. **LAB VALUES:** May increase serum creatine phosphokinase (CPK), ALT, AST, bilirubin, LDH, potassium.

## AVAILABILITY (Rx)

Injection, Powder for Reconstitution (Zithromax): 500 mg. **Ophthalmic Solution** (AzaSite): 1%. **Suspension, Oral** (Zithromax): 100 mg/5 ml, 200 mg/5 ml. **Suspension, Oral (Extended-Release [Zmax]):** 2-g single-dose packet. **Tablets:** 250 mg, 500 mg, 600 mg.

## ADMINISTRATION/HANDLING

 **IV**

**Reconstitution** • Reconstitute each 500-mg vial with 4.8 ml Sterile Water for Injection to provide concentration of 100 mg/ml. • Shake well to ensure dissolution. • Further dilute with 250 or 500 ml 0.9% NaCl or D₅W to provide final concentration of 2 mg/ml with 250 ml diluent or 1 mg/ml with 500 ml diluent.
**Rate of Administration** • Infuse over 60 min (2 mg/ml). Infuse over 3 hrs (1 mg/ml).
**Storage** • Store vials at room temperature. • Following reconstitution, diluted solution is stable for 24 hrs at room temperature or 7 days if refrigerated.

### PO (Immediate-Release Suspension)

• Give tablets without regard to food.
• May store suspension at room temperature. Stable for 10 days after reconstitution.

### PO (Extended-Release Suspension)

• Do not administer oral suspension with food. Give at least 1 hr before or 2 hrs after meals. • Give Zmax within 12 hrs of reconstitution. • Give tablets with food to decrease GI effects.

### PO

• Tablets: May give with food to decrease GI effects.

### Ophthalmic

• Place gloved finger on lower eyelid and pull out until a pocket is formed between eye and lower lid. • Place prescribed number of drops into pocket. • Instruct pt to close eye gently for 1 to 2 min (so medication will not be squeezed out of sac) and to apply digital pressure to lacrimal sac at inner canthus for 1 min to minimize systemic absorption.

## 🔲 IV INCOMPATIBILITIES

Ceftriaxone (Rocephin), ciprofloxacin (Cipro), famotidine (Pepcid), furosemide (Lasix), ketorolac (Toradol), levofloxacin (Levaquin), morphine, piperacillin/tazobactam (Zosyn), potassium chloride.

## 🔲 IV COMPATIBILITIES

Ceftaroline (Teflaro), doripenem (Doribax), ondansetron (Zofran), tigecycline (Tygacil), diphenhydramine (Benadryl).

## INDICATIONS/ROUTES/DOSAGE

**Usual Dosage Range**
**PO: ADULTS, ELDERLY:** 250–600 mg once daily or 1–2 g as single dose. *(Zmax):* 2 g as a single dose. **CHILDREN 6 MOS AND OLDER:** 5–12 mg/kg (**maximum:** 500 mg) once daily or 30 mg/kg (**maximum:** 1,500 mg) as single dose. *(Zmax):* 60 mg/kg as a single dose. **NEONATES:** 10–20 mg/kg once daily.
**IV: ADULTS, ELDERLY:** 250–500 mg once daily **CHILDREN, NEONATES:** 10 mg/kg once daily.

**Mild to Moderate Respiratory Tract, Skin, Soft Tissue Infections**
**PO: ADULTS, ELDERLY:** 500 mg day 1, then 250 mg days 2–5.

**MAC Prevention**
**PO: ADULTS, ELDERLY:** 1,200 mg once weekly. **CHILDREN:** 20 mg/kg once weekly. **Maximum:** 1,200 mg/dose.

**MAC Treatment**
**PO: ADULTS, ELDERLY:** 600 mg/day with ethambutol. **CHILDREN:** 10–12 mg/kg/day (**maximum:** 500 mg) with ethambutol.

**Otitis Media**
**PO: CHILDREN 6 MOS AND OLDER:** 30 mg/kg as single dose (**maximum:** 1,500 mg) or 10 mg/kg/day for 3 days (**maximum:** 500 mg) or 10 mg/kg on day 1 (**maximum:** 500 mg), then 5 mg/kg on days 2–5 (**maximum:** 250 mg).

**Pharyngitis, Tonsillitis**
**PO: ADULTS, ELDERLY, CHILDREN 16 YRS AND OLDER:** 500 mg on day 1, then 250 mg on days 2–5. **CHILDREN 2–15 YRS:** 12 mg/kg daily for 5 days (**maximum:** 500 mg).

**Pneumonia, Community-Acquired**
**PO *(Zmax):* ADULTS, ELDERLY:** 2 g as single dose.
**PO: ADULTS, ELDERLY, CHILDREN 16 YRS AND OLDER:** 500 mg on day 1, then 250 mg on days 2–5 or 500 mg/day IV for 2 days, then 500 mg/day PO to complete course of therapy. **CHILDREN 6 MOS–15 YRS:** 10 mg/kg on day 1 (**maximum:** 500 mg), then 5 mg/kg (**maximum:** 250 mg) on days 2–5.

**Dosage in Renal/Hepatic Impairment**
Use caution.

**Bacterial Conjunctivitis**
**Ophthalmic: ADULTS, ELDERLY:** 1 drop in affected eye twice daily for 2 days, then 1 drop once daily for 5 days.

## SIDE EFFECTS

**Occasional: Systemic:** Nausea, vomiting, diarrhea, abdominal pain. **Ophthalmic:** Eye irritation. **Rare: Systemic:** Headache, dizziness, allergic reaction.

## ADVERSE EFFECTS/TOXIC REACTIONS

Antibiotic-associated colitis, other superinfections may result from altered bacterial balance in GI tract. Acute interstitial nephritis, hepatotoxicity occur rarely.

## NURSING CONSIDERATIONS

### BASELINE ASSESSMENT

Question for history of hepatitis, allergies to azithromycin, erythromycins. Assess for infection (WBC count, appearance of wound, evidence of fever).

### INTERVENTION/EVALUATION

Check for GI discomfort, nausea, vomiting. Monitor daily pattern of bowel activity and stool consistency. Monitor hepatic function tests, CBC. Assess for hepatotoxicity: malaise, fever, abdominal pain, GI disturbances. Be alert for superinfection: fever, vomiting, diarrhea, anal/genital pruritus, oral mucosal changes (ulceration, pain, erythema).

**PATIENT/FAMILY TEACHING**
• Continue therapy for full length of treatment. • Avoid concurrent administration of aluminum- or magnesium-containing antacids. • Bacterial conjunctivitis: Do not wear contact lenses.

# aztreonam

az-**tree**-o-nam
(Azactam, Cayston)

◆**CLASSIFICATION**
**PHARMACOTHERAPEUTIC:** Monobactam. **CLINICAL:** Antibiotic.

## USES

**Injection:** Treatment of infections caused by susceptible gram-negative microorganisms *P. aeruginosa, E. coli, S. marcescens, K. pneumoniae, P. mirabilis, H. influenzae, Enterobacter, Citrobacter* spp. including lower respiratory tract, skin/skin structure, intraabdominal, gynecologic, complicated/uncomplicated UTIs; septicemia; cystic fibrosis. **Cayston:** Improve respiratory symptoms in cystic fibrosis pts with *P. aeruginosa*. **OFF-LABEL:** Surgical prophylaxis.

## PRECAUTIONS

**Contraindications:** Hypersensitivity to aztreonam. **Cautions:** History of allergy, esp. cephalosporins, penicillins; renal impairment; bone marrow transplant pts with risk factors for toxic epidermal necrolysis (TEN).

## ACTION

Binds to penicillin-binding proteins, which inhibits bacterial cell wall synthesis. **Therapeutic Effect:** Bactericidal.

## PHARMACOKINETICS

Completely absorbed after IM administration. Protein binding: 56%–60%. Partially metabolized by hydrolysis. Primarily excreted unchanged in urine. Removed by hemodialysis. **Half-life:** 1.4–2.2 hrs (increased in renal/hepatic impairment).

## ⧗ LIFESPAN CONSIDERATIONS

**Pregnancy/Lactation:** Crosses placenta, distributed in amniotic fluid; low concentration in breast milk. **Children:** Safety and efficacy not established in pts younger than 9 mos. **Elderly:** Age-related renal impairment may require dosage adjustment.

## INTERACTIONS

**DRUG:** None significant. **HERBAL:** None significant. **FOOD:** None known. **LAB VALUES:** May increase serum alkaline phosphatase, creatinine, LDH, ALT, AST levels. Produces a positive Coombs' test. May prolong partial thromboplastin time (PTT), prothrombin time (PT).

## AVAILABILITY (Rx)

**Injection, Infusion Solution (Azactam):** Premix 1 g/50 ml, 2 g/50 ml. **Injection, Powder for Reconstitution (Azactam):** 1 g, 2 g. **Oral Inhalation, Powder for Reconstitution (Cayston):** 75 mg.

## ADMINISTRATION/HANDLING

 IV

**Reconstitution** • For IV push, dilute each gram with 6–10 ml Sterile Water for Injection. • For intermittent IV infusion, further dilute with 50–100 ml $D_5W$ or 0.9% NaCl. Final concentration not to exceed 20 mg/ml.
**Rate of Administration** • For IV push, give over 3–5 min. • For IV infusion, administer over 20–60 min.
**Storage** • Store vials at room temperature. • Solution appears colorless to light yellow. • Following reconstitution, solution is stable for 48 hrs at room temperature or 7 days if refrigerated.

- Discard if precipitate forms. Discard unused portions.

### IM
- Reconstitute with at least 3 ml diluent per gram of aztreonam. • Shake immediately, vigorously after adding diluent. • Inject deeply into large muscle mass. • Following reconstitution, solution is stable for 48 hrs at room temperature or 7 days if refrigerated.

### Inhalation
- Administer only with an Altera nebulizer system. • Nebulize over 2–3 min. • Give bronchodilator 15 min–4 hrs (short-acting) or 30 min–12 hrs (long-acting) before administration. • Reconstituted solution must be used immediately.

### ▦ IV INCOMPATIBILITIES

Acyclovir (Zovirax), amphotericin (Fungizone), lorazepam (Ativan), metronidazole (Flagyl), vancomycin (Vancocin).

### ▦ IV COMPATIBILITIES

Bumetanide (Bumex), calcium gluconate, cimetidine (Tagamet), diltiazem (Cardizem), diphenhydramine (Benadryl), dobutamine (Dobutrex), dopamine (Intropin), famotidine (Pepcid), furosemide (Lasix), heparin, hydromorphone (Dilaudid), insulin (regular), magnesium sulfate, morphine, potassium chloride, propofol (Diprivan).

## INDICATIONS/ROUTES/DOSAGE

### Severe Infections
IV: **ADULTS, ELDERLY:** 2 g q6–8h. **Maximum:** 8 g/day. **CHILDREN:** 30 mg/kg q6–8h. **Maximum:** 8 g/day.

### Mild to Moderate Infections
IV: **ADULTS, ELDERLY:** 1–2 g q8–12h. **Maximum:** 8 g/day. **CHILDREN:** 30 mg/kg q8h. **Maximum:** 8 g/day.

### Usual Neonatal Dosage
IV: 30 mg/kg/dose q6–12h.

### Cystic Fibrosis
IV: **CHILDREN:** 50 mg/kg/dose q6–8h up to 200 mg/kg/day. **Maximum:** 8 g/day.
Inhalation (Nebulizer): **ADULTS, CHILDREN 7 YRS OR OLDER:** 75 mg 3 times/day (at least 4 hrs apart) for 28 days, then off for 28-day cycle.

### Dosage in Renal Impairment
Dosage and frequency are modified based on creatinine clearance and severity of infection:

| Creatinine Clearance | Dosage |
|---|---|
| 10–30 ml/min | 50% usual dose at usual intervals |
| Less than 10 ml/min | 25% usual dose at usual intervals |
| Hemodialysis | 500 mg–2 g, then 25% of initial dose at usual interval |
| Continuous renal replacement therapy (CRRT) | 2 g, then 1 g q8–12h or 2g q12h |

### Dosage in Hepatic Impairment
Use with caution.

## SIDE EFFECTS

**Frequent (greater than 5%): Cayston:** Cough, nasal congestion, wheezing, pharyngolaryngeal pain, pyrexia, chest discomfort, abdominal pain, vomiting.
**Occasional (less than 3%):** Discomfort and swelling at IM injection site, nausea, vomiting, diarrhea, rash. **Rare (less than 1%):** Phlebitis or thrombophlebitis at IV injection site, abdominal cramps, headache, hypotension.

## ADVERSE EFFECTS/ TOXIC REACTIONS

Antibiotic-associated colitis, other superinfections may result from altered bacterial balance. Severe hypersensitivity reactions, including anaphylaxis, occur rarely.

## NURSING CONSIDERATIONS

### BASELINE ASSESSMENT
Question for history of allergies, esp. to aztreonam, other antibiotics.

### INTERVENTION/EVALUATION
Evaluate for phlebitis, pain at IM injection site. Assess for GI discomfort, nausea, vomiting. Monitor daily pattern of bowel activity, stool consistency. Assess skin for rash. Be alert for superinfection: fever, vomiting, diarrhea, anal/genital pruritus, oral mucosal changes (ulceration, pain, erythema). Monitor renal/hepatic function.

### PATIENT/FAMILY TEACHING
• Report nausea, vomiting, diarrhea, rash.

# baclofen

**bak**-loe-fen
(Apo-Baclofen ✦, Gablofen, Lioresal, Novo-Baclofen ✦)

■ **BLACK BOX ALERT** ■ Abrupt withdrawal of intrathecal form has resulted in severe hyperpyrexia, obtundation, rebound or exaggerated spasticity, muscle rigidity, leading to organ failure, death.
**Do not confuse baclofen with Bactroban or Beclovent, or Lioresal with lisinopril or Lotensin.**

## ◆CLASSIFICATION

**PHARMACOTHERAPEUTIC:** Skeletal muscle relaxant. **CLINICAL:** Antispastic, analgesic in trigeminal neuralgia.

## USES

**Oral:** Management of reversible spasticity associated with multiple sclerosis, spinal cord lesions. **Intrathecal:** Management of severe spasticity of spinal cord or cerebral origin. **OFF-LABEL:** Treatment of bladder spasms, cerebral palsy, intractable hiccups or pain, Huntington's chorea, trigeminal neuralgia.

## PRECAUTIONS

**Contraindications:** Hypersensitivity to baclofen. **Cautions:** Renal impairment, seizure disorder, elderly, autonomic dysreflexia, reduced GI motility, GI or urinary obstruction; respiratory, pulmonary, peptic ulcer disease.

## ACTION

Inhibits transmission of reflexes at spinal cord level. **Therapeutic Effect:** Relieves muscle spasticity.

## PHARMACOKINETICS

Well absorbed from GI tract. Protein binding: 30%. Partially metabolized in liver. Primarily excreted in urine. **Half-life:** 2.5–4 hrs.

## ⧗ LIFESPAN CONSIDERATIONS

**Pregnancy/Lactation:** Unknown if crosses placenta or distributed in breast milk. **Children:** Safety and efficacy not established in pts younger than 12 yrs. Limited published data in children. **Elderly:** Increased risk of CNS toxicity (hallucinations, sedation, confusion, mental depression); age-related renal impairment may require decreased dosage.

## INTERACTIONS

**DRUG:** Potentiated effects when used with other **CNS depressants (e.g., alcohol, alprazolam, lorazepam, morphine, oxycodone, tramadol). HERBAL: Gotu kola, kava kava, St. John's wort, valerian** may increase CNS sedation. **FOOD:** None known. **LAB VALUES:** May increase serum ALT, AST, alkaline phosphatase, glucose.

## AVAILABILITY (Rx)

**Intrathecal Injection Solution:** 50 mcg/ml, 500 mcg/ml, 1,000 mcg/ml, 2,000 mcg/ml. **Tablets:** 10 mg, 20 mg.

## ADMINISTRATION/HANDLING

**PO**
• Give with food or milk. • Tablets may be crushed.

**Intrathecal**
• For screening, a 50 mcg/ml concentration should be used for injection. • For maintenance therapy, solution should be diluted for pts who require concentrations other than 500 mcg/ml or 2,000 mcg/ml.

## INDICATIONS/ROUTES/DOSAGE

◀**ALERT**▶ Avoid abrupt withdrawal.
**Spasticity**
**PO: ADULTS, CHILDREN 12 YRS AND OLDER:** Initially, 5 mg 3 times daily. May increase by 15 mg/day (5 mg/dose) at 3-day intervals. Range: 40–80 mg/day. **Maximum:** 80 mg/day. **ELDERLY:** Initially, 5 mg 2–3 times daily. May gradually increase dosage.

---

✦ Canadian trade name　　　🗑 Non-Crushable Drug　　　🔲 High Alert drug

**3**

**Intrathecal Dose**

**ADULTS, ELDERLY:** Test dose: 50–100 mcg. Dose greater than 50 mcg given in 25-mcg increments, separated by 24 hrs. Following positive response to test dose, maintenance infusion can be given via implanted intrathecal pump. Initial dose is twice the test dose.

**Dosage in Renal Impairment**

Use caution.

**Dosage in Hepatic Impairment**

No dose adjustment.

## SIDE EFFECTS

**Frequent (greater than 10%):** Transient drowsiness, asthenia, dizziness, nausea, vomiting. **Occasional (10%–2%):** Headache, paresthesia, constipation, anorexia, hypotension, confusion, nasal congestion. **Rare (less than 1%):** Paradoxical CNS excitement or restlessness, slurred speech, tremor, dry mouth, diarrhea, nocturia, impotence.

## ADVERSE EFFECTS/ TOXIC REACTIONS

Abrupt discontinuation may produce hallucinations, seizures. Overdose results in blurred vision, seizures, myosis, mydriasis, severe muscle weakness, strabismus, respiratory depression, vomiting.

## NURSING CONSIDERATIONS

### BASELINE ASSESSMENT

Record onset, type, location, duration of muscular spasm, pain. Check for immobility, stiffness, swelling.

### INTERVENTION/EVALUATION

For pts on long-term therapy, BMP, LFT, blood counts should be performed periodically. Assess for paradoxical reaction. Observe for drowsiness, dizziness, ataxia. Assist with ambulation at all times. Evaluate for therapeutic response: decreased intensity of skeletal muscle spasm, pain.

**PATIENT/FAMILY TEACHING**

• Drowsiness usually diminishes with continued therapy. • Avoid tasks that require alertness, motor skills until response to drug is established. • Do not abruptly withdraw medication after long-term therapy (may result in muscle rigidity, rebound spasticity, high fever, altered mental status). • Avoid alcohol, CNS depressants.

# basiliximab

ba-si-**lik**-si-mab
(Simulect)

■ **BLACK BOX ALERT** ■ Must be prescribed by a physician experienced in immunosuppression therapy and organ transplant management.

**Do not confuse basiliximab with daclizumab or brentuximab.**

## ◆CLASSIFICATION

**PHARMACOTHERAPEUTIC:** Monoclonal antibody. **CLINICAL:** Immunosuppressive.

## USES

Adjunct with cyclosporine, corticosteroids in prevention of acute organ rejection in pts receiving renal transplant. **OFF-LABEL:** Treatment of refractory graft-vs-host disease, prevention of liver or cardiac transplant rejection.

## PRECAUTIONS

**Contraindications:** Hypersensitivity to basiliximab. **Cautions:** Re-exposure to subsequent courses of basiliximab.

## ACTION

Binds to and blocks receptor of interleukin-2, a protein that stimulates proliferation of T-lymphocytes, which play a major role in organ transplant rejection. **Therapeutic Effect:** Impairs response of immune system to antigens, prevents acute renal transplant rejection.

## PHARMACOKINETICS

**Half-life:** 4–10 days (adults); 5–17 days (children).

## LIFESPAN CONSIDERATIONS

**Pregnancy/Lactation:** Unknown if crosses placenta or distributed in breast milk. Breastfeeding not recommended. **Children/Elderly:** No age-related precautions noted.

## INTERACTIONS

**DRUG: Tacrolimus** (topical), **trastuzumab** may increase concentration. **HERBAL: Echinacea** may decrease therapeutic effect. **Bilberry, garlic, ginger, ginseng** may increase hypoglycemic effect. **FOOD:** None known. **LAB VALUES:** May alter serum calcium, glucose, potassium; Hgb, Hct. May increase serum cholesterol, BUN, creatinine, uric acid. May decrease serum magnesium, phosphate, platelet count.

## AVAILABILITY (Rx)

**Injection, Powder for Reconstitution:** 10 mg, 20 mg.

## ADMINISTRATION/HANDLING

 IV

**Reconstitution •** Reconstitute 10-mg vial with 2.5 ml or 20-mg vial with 5 ml Sterile Water for Injection. • Shake gently to dissolve. • May further dilute with 25–50 ml 0.9% NaCl or D₅W to a final concentration of 0.4 mg/ml. • Gently invert to avoid foaming. • Do not shake.
**Rate of Administration •** IV bolus over 10 min. • IV infusion over 20–30 min.
**Storage •** Refrigerate unused vials. • After reconstitution, use within 4 hrs (24 hrs if refrigerated). • Discard if precipitate forms.

## IV INCOMPATIBILITIES

Specific information not available. Do not add other medications simultaneously through same IV line.

## INDICATIONS/ROUTES/DOSAGE

**Prophylaxis of Organ Rejection**
**IV: ADULTS, ELDERLY, CHILDREN WEIGHING 35 KG OR MORE:** 20 mg within 2 hrs before transplant surgery and 20 mg 4 days after transplant. **CHILDREN WEIGHING LESS THAN 35 KG:** 10 mg within 2 hrs before transplant surgery and 10 mg 4 days after transplant.

**Dosage in Renal/Hepatic Impairment**
No dose adjustment.

## SIDE EFFECTS

**Frequent (greater than 10%):** GI disturbances (constipation, diarrhea, dyspepsia), CNS effects (dizziness, headache, insomnia, tremor), respiratory tract infection, dysuria, acne, leg or back pain, peripheral edema, hypertension. **Occasional (10%–3%):** Angina, neuropathy, abdominal distention, tachycardia, rash, hypotension, urinary disturbances (urinary frequency, genital edema, hematuria), arthralgia, hirsutism, myalgia.

## ADVERSE EFFECTS/ TOXIC REACTIONS

Severe, acute hypersensitivity reactions including anaphylaxis characterized by hypotension, tachycardia, HF, dyspnea, wheezing, bronchospasm, pulmonary edema, respiratory failure, urticaria, rash, pruritus, sneezing, capillary leak syndrome, cytokine release syndrome have been reported. May increase risk of cytomegalovirus infection.

## NURSING CONSIDERATIONS

### BASELINE ASSESSMENT

Obtain baseline CBC, BMP, serum ionized calcium, phosphate, uric acid; vital signs, particularly B/P, pulse rate. Question current breastfeeding status.

### INTERVENTION/EVALUATION

Diligently monitor CBC, electrolytes, renal function. Assess B/P for hypertension/hypotension; pulse for evidence of tachycardia. Question for GI disturbances, CNS effects, urinary changes. Monitor for presence of wound infection, signs of infection (fever, sore throat, unusual bleeding/bruising), hypersensitivity reaction.

### PATIENT/FAMILY TEACHING

• Report difficulty in breathing or swallowing, palpitations, bruising/bleeding, rash, itching, swelling of lower extremities, weakness. • Female pts should take measures to avoid pregnancy; avoid breastfeeding.

---

## beclomethasone

be-kloe-**meth**-a-sone
(Apo-Beclomethasone ✦, Beconase AQ, QNASL, QVAR, Rivanase AQ ✦)
**Do not confuse beclomethasone with betamethasone or dexamethasone, or Beconase with baclofen.**

### ◆CLASSIFICATION

**PHARMACOTHERAPEUTIC:** Adrenocorticosteroid. **CLINICAL:** Anti-inflammatory, immunosuppressant.

### USES

**Inhalation:** Maintenance and prophylactic treatment of asthma in pts 5 yrs and older. **Intranasal:** Relief of seasonal/perennial rhinitis; prevention of nasal polyp recurrence after surgical removal; treatment of nonallergic rhinitis. **QNASL:** Treatment of seasonal and perennial allergic rhinitis in adults and adolescents 12 yrs and older. **OFF-LABEL:** Prevention of seasonal rhinitis (nasal form).

### PRECAUTIONS

**Contraindications:** Hypersensitivity to beclomethasone. **Oral inhalation:** Acute exacerbation of asthma, status asthmaticus. **Cautions:** Thyroid disease, hepatic impairment, renal impairment, cardiovascular disease, diabetes, glaucoma, cataracts, myasthenia gravis, seizures, risk for osteoporosis, peptic ulcer, ulcerative colitis, elderly; following acute MI. Avoid use in pts with untreated viral, fungal, or bacterial systemic infections.

### ACTION

Controls or prevents inflammation by altering rate of protein synthesis; depresses migration of polymorphonuclear leukocytes, fibroblasts; reverses capillary permeability. **Therapeutic Effect: Inhalation:** Inhibits bronchoconstriction, produces smooth muscle relaxation, decreases mucus secretion. **Intranasal:** Decreases response to seasonal, perennial rhinitis.

### PHARMACOKINETICS

Rapidly absorbed from pulmonary, nasal, GI tissue. Hydrolyzed by pulmonary esterase prior to absorption. Metabolized in liver. Protein binding: 87%. Primarily eliminated in feces (60%), urine (12%). **Half-life:** 2–4.5 hrs.

### ⧗ LIFESPAN CONSIDERATIONS

**Pregnancy/Lactation:** Unknown if crosses placenta or distributed in breast milk. **Children:** Prolonged treatment/high dosages may decrease short-term growth rate, cortisol secretion. **Elderly:** No age-related precautions noted.

### INTERACTIONS

**DRUG:** None significant. **HERBAL: Echinacea** may decrease effects. **FOOD:** None known. **LAB VALUES:** None significant.

## AVAILABILITY (Rx)

Inhalation, Oral (Qvar): 40 mcg/inhalation, 80 mcg/inhalation. **Nasal Inhalation (Beconase AQ):** 42 mcg/inhalation. **QNASL:** 40 mcg/actuation, 80 mcg/actuation.

## ADMINISTRATION/HANDLING

### Inhalation

• Shake container well. • Instruct pt to exhale completely, place mouthpiece between lips, inhale, hold breath as long as possible before exhaling. • Allow at least 1 min between inhalations. • Rinsing mouth after each use (decreases dry mouth, hoarseness, thrush).

### Intranasal

• Instruct pt to clear nasal passages as much as possible before use. • Tilt pt's head slightly forward. • Insert spray tip into nostril, pointing toward nasal passages, away from nasal septum. • Spray into one nostril while pt holds the other nostril closed, concurrently inhaling through nose to permit medication as high into nasal passages as possible.

## INDICATIONS/ROUTES/DOSAGE

### Asthma

**Oral Inhalation** *(QVAR):* **ADULTS, ELDERLY, CHILDREN 12 YRS AND OLDER:** 40–160 mcg twice daily. **Maximum:** 320 mcg twice daily. **CHILDREN 5–11 YRS:** 40 mcg twice daily. **Maximum:** 80 mcg twice daily.

### Rhinitis, Prevention of Recurrence of Nasal Polyps

**Nasal Inhalation** *(Beconase AQ):* **ADULTS, ELDERLY, CHILDREN 12 YRS AND OLDER:** 1–2 sprays in each nostril twice daily. **CHILDREN 6–11 YRS:** 1 spray each nostril twice daily. May increase to 2 sprays 2 times/day. Once adequate control achieved, decrease to 1 spray in each nostril twice daily.

### Allergic Rhinitis

**Nasal Inhalation** *(QNASL):* **ADULTS, ELDERLY, CHILDREN 12 YRS AND OLDER:** 80 mcg/spray: 2 sprays in each nostril daily. **Maximum:** 320 mcg (4 sprays/day). **CHILDREN, 4–11 YRS OF AGE:** 40 mcg/spray: 1 spray each nostril once daily. **Maximum:** 80 mcg/day.

### Dosage in Renal/Hepatic Impairment

No dose adjustment.

## SIDE EFFECTS

**Frequent: Inhalation (14%–4%):** Throat irritation, dry mouth, hoarseness, cough. **Intranasal:** Nasal burning, mucosal dryness. **Occasional: Inhalation (3%–2%):** Localized fungal infection (thrush). **Intranasal:** Nasal-crusting epistaxis, sore throat, ulceration of nasal mucosa. **Rare: Inhalation:** Transient bronchospasm, esophageal candidiasis. **Intranasal:** Nasal and pharyngeal candidiasis, eye pain.

## ADVERSE EFFECTS/ TOXIC REACTIONS

Acute hypersensitivity reaction (urticaria, angioedema, severe bronchospasm) occurs rarely. Change from systemic to local steroid therapy may unmask previously suppressed bronchial asthma condition.

## NURSING CONSIDERATIONS

### BASELINE ASSESSMENT

Establish baseline history for asthma, rhinitis. Question for hypersensitivity to corticosteroids.

### INTERVENTION/EVALUATION

Monitor respiratory status, lung sounds; observe for signs of oral candidiasis. In pts receiving bronchodilators by inhalation concomitantly with inhaled steroid therapy, advise to use bronchodilator several minutes before corticosteroid aerosol (enhances penetration of steroid into bronchial tree).

### PATIENT/FAMILY TEACHING

• Do not change dose schedule or stop taking drug; must taper off gradually under medical supervision. • **Inhalation:** Maintain diligent oral hygiene. • Rinse mouth with water immediately after inhalation (prevents mouth/throat dryness, fungal infection of mouth). • Report sore throat or mouth. • **Intranasal:** Report symptoms that do not improve; or if sneezing, nasal irritation occurs. • Clear nasal passages prior to use. • Improvement may take days to several weeks.

---

# belatacept

bel-**at**-a-sept
(Nulojix)

■ **BLACK BOX ALERT** ■ Must be administered by personnel trained in administration/handling of immunosuppression therapy. Increased risk of malignancies, infection. Increased risk of post-transplant lymphoproliferative disorder (PTLD), mainly in central nervous system. Not recommended for hepatic transplants due to increased risk of graft loss, death.

## ◆ CLASSIFICATION

**PHARMACOTHERAPEUTIC:** Selective T-cell costimulation blocker. **CLINICAL:** Immunosuppressive agent.

## USES

Prevention of acute organ rejection in pts receiving renal transplants (in combination with basiliximab induction, mycophenolate mofetil, corticosteroids). For use in Epstein-Barr virus (EBV) seropositive renal transplant recipients.

## PRECAUTIONS

**Contraindications:** Hypersensitivity to belatacept. Transplant pts who are Epstein-Barr virus (EBV) seronegative or unknown sero-status. **Cautions:** History of opportunistic infections: bacterial, mycobacterial, invasive fungal, viral, protozoal, (histoplasmosis, aspergillosis, candidiasis, coccidioidomycosis, listeriosis, HIV, tuberculosis, pneumocystosis). Recent open wounds, ulcerations. Not recommended in liver transplants. Avoid use of live vaccines.

## ACTION

Inhibits T-lymphocyte proliferation and production of a critical pathway in cellular immune response involved in allograft rejection. **Therapeutic Effect:** Prevents renal transplant rejection.

## PHARMACOKINETICS

**Half-life:** 8–10 days.

## ⧖ LIFESPAN CONSIDERATIONS

**Pregnancy/Lactation:** Unknown if crosses placenta or distributed in breast milk. Must either discontinue breastfeeding or discontinue drug. **Children:** Safety and efficacy not established. **Elderly:** No age-related precautions noted.

## INTERACTIONS

**DRUG:** May increase concentration/effects of **belimumab, mycophenolate. Pimecrolimus, tacrolimus (topical)** may increase concentration/effect. **Live vaccines** not recommended. **HERBAL: Echinacea, cat's claw** may reduce effect. **FOOD:** None known. **LAB VALUES:** May increase serum potassium, cholesterol, uric acid; glucose, urine protein. May decrease serum calcium, magnesium, phosphate, potassium; Hgb, Hct, WBC.

## AVAILABILITY (Rx)

**Lyophilized Powder for Injection:** 250 mg per vial.

## ADMINISTRATION/HANDLING

◄ **ALERT** ► Use only silicone-free disposable syringe provided. Using different syringe may produce translucent particles. Must infuse with sterile, nonpyrogenic, low-protein-binding filter (pore size 0.2–1.2 micron). Administer via dedicated line only.

 **IV**

**Reconstitution** • Calculate number of vials required (solution will equal 25 mg/ml after mixing). • Reconstitute vial with 10.5 ml of suitable diluent (0.9% NaCl,

D$_5$W, or Sterile Water for Injection) using provided syringe, 18- to 20-gauge needle. • Direct stream to glass wall (avoids foaming). • Swirl gently (do not shake). • Discard if opaque particles, discoloration, or foreign particles are present. • Infusion bag must match diluent (0.9% NaCl with 0.9% NaCl, D$_5$W with D$_5$W; may use Sterile Water for Injection with NaCl or D$_5$W). • To mix infusion bag, withdraw and discard volume equal to the volume of reconstituted solution. • Using same silicone-free disposable syringe, gently inject reconstituted solution into 100- to 250-ml bag (based on concentration). • Final concentration of infusion bag should range from 2 mg/ml to 10 mg/ml. • IV infusion stable for 24 hrs at room temperature.

**Rate of Administration** • Infuse over 30 min using infusion set with a 0.2- to 1.2-micron low-protein-binding filter.

**Storage** • Refrigerate vials. • Solution should be clear to slightly opalescent and colorless to slightly yellow. • May refrigerate solution up to 24 hrs. • Discard if reconstituted solution remains at room temperature longer than 24 hrs.

## INDICATIONS/ROUTES/DOSAGE

**Note:** Dosage based on actual body weight at time of transplantation.

**Prophylaxis of Acute Renal Transplant Rejection (in Combination with an Immunosuppressant)**
IV: **ADULTS, ELDERLY:** Initial phase: 10 mg/kg on day 1 (day of transplantation, prior to implantation), day 5, end of wk 2, 4, 8, and 12 after transplantation. Maintenance: 5 mg/kg end of wk 16, then q4wks thereafter (plus or minus 3 days).

**Dosage Modification**
Infusion is based on actual body weight at the time of transplantation; modify dose for weight changes greater than 10% during treatment. Prescribed dose must be evenly divisible by 12.5 to match closest increment (0, 12.5, 25, 37.5, 50, 62.5, 75, 87.5, 100) in mg. For example, the actual dose

for a 64-kg pt is 637.5 mg or 650 mg, not 640 mg.

**Dosage in Renal/Hepatic Impairment**
No dose adjustment.

## SIDE EFFECTS

**Frequent (45%–20%):** Anemia, diarrhea, UTI, peripheral edema, constipation, hypertension, pyrexia, nausea, cough, vomiting, headache. **Occasional (19%–5%):** Abdominal pain, hypotension, arthralgia, hematuria, upper respiratory infection, insomnia, nasopharyngitis, back pain, dyspnea, influenza, dysuria, bronchitis, stomatitis, anxiety, dizziness, abdominal pain, muscle tremor, acne, alopecia, hyperhidrosis.

## ADVERSE EFFECTS/ TOXIC REACTIONS

Serious conditions including malignancies (esp. skin cancer), progressive multifocal leukoencephalopathy (caused by JC virus), cytomegalovirus, polyoma virus nephropathy, viral reactivation (herpes zoster, hepatitis) may occur. Other opportunistic infections (bacterial, fungal, viral, protozoal) may cause tuberculosis, cryptococcal meningitis, Chagas' disease, West Nile encephalitis, Guillain-Barré syndrome, cerebral aspergillosis. Additional complications including chronic allograft nephropathy, renal tubular necrosis, renal artery necrosis, atrial fibrillation, hematoma at incision site, wound dehiscence, lymphocele, arteriovenous fistula thrombosis, hydronephrosis, urinary incontinence, anti-belatacept antibody formation were reported.

## NURSING CONSIDERATIONS

### BASELINE ASSESSMENT

Obtain baseline CBC, serum chemistries, renal function, glomerular filtration rate (GFR), magnesium, ionized calcium, phosphate, lipid panel, urinalysis. Evaluate pt for active tuberculosis or latent infection prior to initiating treatment and periodically during therapy. Induration of

5 mm or greater with tuberculin skin test should be considered a positive result when assessing whether treatment for latent tuberculosis is necessary. Assess baseline mental status to compare any worsening cognitive symptoms. Obtain Epstein-Barr virus (EBV) serology prior to treatment (contraindicated in pts who are EBV seronegative). Note any skin discoloration, ulcers, excoriation, lesions. Question history of hypertension/hypotension, arrhythmia, diabetes, HIV. Receive full medication history. Question possibility of pregnancy.

### INTERVENTION/EVALUATION

Monitor B/P, vital signs, I&O, weight. Diligently monitor CBC, renal function, serum electrolytes (hypokalemia may result in changes in muscle strength, muscle cramps, altered mental status, cardiac arrhythmias). Routinely monitor serum glucose levels for new-onset diabetes after transplantation, corticosteroid use. Monitor for fever, tenderness over transplantation site, skin lesions, changing characteristics of moles, neurologic deterioration related to PTLD or PML.

### PATIENT/FAMILY TEACHING

• Therapy may increase risk of malignancies and life-threatening infections. • Detail concomitant immunosuppressive therapy with basiliximab induction, corticosteroids. • Report history of HIV, opportunistic infections, hepatitis, coughing of blood, or close relatives with active tuberculosis. • Avoid sunlight, sunlamps. • Seek immediate attention if adverse reactions occur. • Do not receive live vaccines. • Report pregnancy or plans of becoming pregnant. • Adhere to strict dosing schedule. • Report chest pain, palpitations, edema, fever, night sweats, weight loss, swollen glands, flu-like symptoms, stomach pain, vomiting, diarrhea, weakness, or urinary changes (color, frequency, odor, concentration, burning, blood).

# belimumab

be-**lim**-oo-mab
(Benlysta)
**Do not confuse belimumab with bevacizumab.**

## ◆CLASSIFICATION

**PHARMACOTHERAPEUTIC:** Monoclonal antibody. **CLINICAL:** Immunosuppressant, anti-lupus agent.

## USES

Treatment for active, autoantibody-positive, systemic lupus erythematosus, in addition to standard therapy.

## PRECAUTIONS

**Contraindications:** Hypersensitivity (anaphylaxis) to belimumab. **Cautions:** Severe, active, chronic infections; depression, pts at risk for suicide, other mood changes. Avoid live vaccines within 30 days before or concurrently with belimumab.

## ACTION

Blocks binding of human B-lymphocyte stimulator protein to receptors on B-lymphocyte. **Therapeutic Effect:** Reduces activity of B-cell–mediated immunity and autoimmune response.

## PHARMACOKINETICS

**Half-life:** 19 days.

## ⏳ LIFESPAN CONSIDERATIONS

**Pregnancy/Lactation:** Unknown if crosses placenta or distributed in breast milk. Contraception recommended during therapy and for at least 4 wks after final treatment. **Children:** Safety and efficacy not established. **Elderly:** No age-related precautions noted.

## INTERACTIONS

**DRUG:** Abatacept, belatacept, etanercept, pimecrolimus, tacrolimus (topical) may increase concentration/effect.

Cyclophosphamide not recommended concomitantly. **HERBAL: Echinacea** may decrease effect. **FOOD:** None known. **LAB VALUES:** May decrease WBC.

## AVAILABILITY (Rx)

**Lyophilized Powder for Injection:** 120 mg, 400 mg.

## ADMINISTRATION/HANDLING

**Reconstitution** • Remove vials from refrigerator and let stand until room temperature (10–15 min). • Reconstitute 120-mg vial with 1.5 ml Sterile Water for Injection or 400-mg vial with 4.8 ml Sterile Water for Injection (both vials will equal final concentration of 80 mg/ml). • Direct stream toward glass wall to avoid foaming. • Gently swirl for 60 sec every 5 min until fully dissolved (usually 10–30 min). • If mechanical reconstitution device used, do not swirl greater than 30 min or exceed 500 rpm. • Small air bubbles expected, acceptable. • Dilute in 250 ml 0.9% NaCl only. • From infusion bag, withdraw and discard volume equal to the volume of reconstituted solution. • Invert bag and gently inject solution to mix. • Infuse within 8 hrs of reconstitution.

**Rate of Administration** • Infuse over 1 hr.

**Storage** • Refrigerate vials/infusion bag until time of use. • Solution should be opalescent and colorless to pale yellow with no particles present. • Discard solution if particulate matter or discoloration observed. • Protect from sunlight.

## ▨ IV INCOMPATIBILITIES

Do not infuse with dextrose-based solution. Use dedicated line only.

## INDICATIONS/ROUTES/DOSAGE

**Active Systemic Lupus Erythematosus**
**IV: ADULTS:** 10 mg/kg at 2-wk intervals for 3 doses, then q4 wks thereafter.

**Dosage in Renal/Hepatic Impairment**
No dose adjustment.

## SIDE EFFECTS

**Frequent (15%–12%):** Nausea, diarrhea. **Occasional (10%–5%):** Pyrexia, nasopharyngitis, bronchitis, insomnia, extremity pain, depression, migraine, pharyngitis. **Rare (less than 4%):** Cystitis, viral gastroenteritis.

## ADVERSE EFFECTS/ TOXIC REACTIONS

May increase risk of mortality. Antibelimumab antibody formation reported in less than 1%. Hypersensitivity reaction including anaphylactic reaction may include urticaria, pruritus, erythema, dyspnea, angioedema, hypotension (13% of pts). Infusion reactions such as nausea, headaches, flushing occur more frequently. Serious infections related to immunosuppression including respiratory tract infection, pneumonia, nasopharyngitis, sinusitis, influenza, UTI, cellulitis, bronchitis, viral reactivation may occur. Mental health issues including psychiatric events (16%) and depression (6%) have been noted. Life-threatening psychiatric events and depression (including suicide) reported in less than 1%. Pts who experienced life-threatening episodes had prior psychiatric history.

## NURSING CONSIDERATIONS

### BASELINE ASSESSMENT

Obtain baseline CBC with differential, BMP, IgG level, vital signs. Assess history of recent immunizations, malignancies, open sores, ulcerations, weight loss, HIV infection, chronic infection. Assess psychiatric history including insomnia, anxiety, depression, impulsiveness, suicidal ideations, mood changes. Question possibility of pregnancy, current breastfeeding.

### INTERVENTION/EVALUATION

Monitor vital signs, CBC. If hypersensitivity reaction occurs, immediately notify physician. Premedication with antihistamines, antipyretics, and/or corticosteroids may prevent subsequent reactions.

---

✦ Canadian trade name     ▨ Non-Crushable Drug     ▨ High Alert drug

Discontinue treatment if anaphylactic reaction occurs; initiate appropriate medical treatment. Routinely inspect skin, paying close attention to areas that are discolored, irregular, or have ill-defined borders (may indicate malignancies). Obtain anti-belimumab antibody titer if immunogenicity suspected. Consider interrupting therapy if acute infection occurs.

### PATIENT/FAMILY TEACHING

• Report any signs of allergic reaction (see Adverse Effects/Toxic Reactions). • If anaphylactic reaction occurs, pt may require rapid sequence intubation. • Allergic reactions include itching, hives, dizziness, or difficulty breathing. • Notify physician if pregnant or plan on becoming pregnant. • Contraception recommended during treatment and at least 4 mos after treatment. • Report suicidal ideation, mood changes, or worsening depression. • Do not receive live vaccines 30 days before or during treatment. • Report any fever, cough, night sweats, flu-like symptoms, skin changes, or painful/burning urination.

# belinostat

beh-**lih**-noh-**stat**
(Beleodaq)

### ◆CLASSIFICATION

**PHARMACOTHERAPEUTIC:** Histone deacetylase inhibitor. **CLINICAL:** Antineoplastic.

## USES

Treatment of relapsed or refractory peripheral T-cell lymphoma (PTCL).

## PRECAUTIONS

**Contraindications:** Hypersensitivity to belinostat. **Cautions:** Pts with high tumor burden, hx of hepatic impairment, thrombocytopenia. Avoid use in pts with active infection.

## ACTION

Inhibits enzymatic activity of histone deacetylases by catalyzing removal of acetyl groups from lysine residues of histones and nonhistone proteins. **Therapeutic Effect:** Inhibits tumor cell growth and metastasis; causes tumor cellular death (apoptosis).

## PHARMACOKINETICS

Limited tissue distribution. Metabolized in liver. Protein binding: 93%–95%. Eliminated primarily in urine as metabolites. **Half-life:** 1.1 hrs.

## ⌛LIFESPAN CONSIDERATIONS

**Pregnancy/Lactation:** Has teratogenic effects; may cause fetal harm/demise. Not recommended in nursing mothers. Unknown if distributed in breast milk. Must either discontinue drug or discontinue breastfeeding. **Children:** Safety and efficacy not established. **Elderly:** No age-related precautions noted.

## INTERACTIONS

**DRUG: Strong UGT1A1 inhibitors (e.g., atazanavir, lopinavir, ritonavir)** may increase concentration/effect. **HERBAL:** None known. **FOOD:** None significant. **LAB VALUES:** May decrease ANC, Hgb/Hct, lymphocytes, platelets, WBC; serum potassium. May increase blood lactic dehydrogenase, serum creatinine.

## AVAILABILITY (Rx)

**Lyophilized Powder for Injection:** 500 mg vial.

## ADMINISTRATION/HANDLING

 **IV**

◄**ALERT**► Use 0.22-micron in-line filter for administration.
**Reconstitution** • Maintain standard chemotherapy preparation and handling precautions. • Reconstitute each vial with 9 ml of Sterile Water for Injection, using suitable syringe for final concentration of 50 mg/ml. • Gently swirl contents

until completely dissolved. • Visually inspect for particulate matter. • Do not use if cloudiness or particulate matter observed. • Withdraw required dosage and mix into infusion bag containing 250 ml of 0.9% NaCl.

**Rate of Administration** • Infuse over 30 min using 0.22-micron in-line filter. • May extend infusion time to 45 min if infusion site pain or other infusion-related symptoms occur.

**Storage** • Reconstituted vial may be stored at room temperature (max 77°F/ 25°C) for up to 12 hrs. • Infusion bag may be stored at room temperature (max 77°F/ 25°C) for up to 36 hrs.

## INDICATIONS/ROUTES/DOSAGE

### Peripheral T-Cell Lymphoma
**IV Infusion: ADULTS/ELDERLY:** 1,000 mg/m$^2$ once daily on days 1–5 of a 21-day cycle. Cycles may be repeated every 21 days until disease progression or unacceptable toxicity.

### Dose Modification
Based on Common Terminology Criteria for Adverse Events (CTCAE). ANC should be greater than or equal to 1,000 cells/ mm$^3$ and platelet count greater than or equal to 50,000 mm$^3$ prior to start of each cycle or prior to resuming treatment following toxicity. Discontinue treatment if ANC nadir less than 500 cells/mm$^3$ or recurrent platelet count nadir less than 25,000 mm$^3$ after two dose reductions. Other toxicities must be CTCAE Grade 2 or less prior to resuming treatment.

### Hematologic Toxicities
**Platelet count greater than 25,000 mm$^3$ or ANC greater than 500 cell/ mm$^3$:** No change. **Platelet count less than 25,000 mm$^3$ or ANC less than 500 cells/mm$^3$:** Decrease dose by 25% (750 mg/m$^2$).

### Nonhematologic Toxicities
**Any CTCAE Grade 3 or 4:** Decrease dose by 25% (750 mg/m$^2$). **Recurrence of CTCAE Grade 3 or 4 Adverse Reaction After Two Dosage Reductions:** Discontinue treatment. **Events for Nausea, Vomiting, Diarrhea:** Only modify dose if duration is greater than 7 days with supportive management. **Pts with Reduced UGT1A1 Activity:** Reduce starting dose to 750 mg/ m$^2$ in pts known to be homozygous for UGT1A1*28 allele.

### Dosage in Renal/Hepatic Impairment
No dose adjustment.

## SIDE EFFECTS

**Frequent (47%–29%):** Nausea, fatigue, pyrexia, vomiting, anemia, vomiting. **Occasional (23%–10%):** Constipation, diarrhea, dyspepsia, rash, peripheral edema, cough, pruritus, chills, decreased appetite, headache, infusion site pain, abdominal pain, hypotension, phlebitis, dizziness.

## ADVERSE EFFECTS/TOXIC REACTIONS

Anemia, lymphopenia, neutropenia, thrombocytopenia are expected responses to therapy. Serious and sometimes fatal infections including pneumonia, sepsis have occurred. May cause hepatotoxicity, LFT abnormalities, tumor lysis syndrome. GI toxicities including severe diarrhea, nausea, vomiting may require use of antiemetic and antidiarrheal medication or result in dosage reduction. Nineteen percent of pts required treatment discontinuation related to toxic anemia, febrile neutropenia, multiorgan failure, ventricular fibrillation (rare).

## NURSING CONSIDERATIONS

### BASELINE ASSESSMENT
Obtain baseline ANC, CBC, BMP, LFT, vital signs; urine pregnancy in women of reproductive potential. Question history of anemia, arrhythmias, hepatic impairment, peripheral edema, or if pt homozygous for UGT1A1 allele (may require reduced starting dose). Question possibility of pregnancy, current

breastfeeding status. Receive full medication history including herbal products.

**INTERVENTION/EVALUATION**

Diligently monitor blood counts (esp. ANC, Hgb/Hct, WBC, platelet count) weekly; hepatic/renal function prior to start of first dose of each cycle, vital signs. Monitor for symptoms of hypokalemia. Screen for tumor lysis syndrome (electrolyte imbalance, uric acid nephropathy, acute renal failure). Obtain EKG if arrhythmia, palpitations occur. Notify physician if any CTCAE toxicities occur (see Appendix M). Offer antiemetics if nausea vomiting occurs.

**PATIENT/FAMILY TEACHING**

• Blood levels will be routinely monitored. • Avoid pregnancy; treatment may cause birth defects or miscarriage. Do not breastfeed. • Report any abdominal pain, black/tarry stools, bruising, yellowing of skin or eyes; dark urine, decreased urine output. • Severe diarrhea may lead to dehydration. • Body aches, burning with urination, chills, cough, difficulty breathing, fever may indicate an acute infection.

---

# benazepril

ben-**ay**-ze-pril
(Lotensin)

■ **BLACK BOX ALERT** ■ May cause fetal injury, mortality. Discontinue as soon as possible once pregnancy is detected.
**Do not confuse benazepril with enalapril, lisinopril, or Benadryl, or Lotensin with Lioresal.**

**FIXED-COMBINATION(S)**

**Lotensin HCT:** benazepril/hydrochlorothiazide (a diuretic): 5 mg/ 625 mg, 10 mg/12.5 mg, 20 mg/ 12.5 mg, 20 mg/25 mg. **Lotrel:** benazepril/amlodipine (a calcium blocker): 2.5 mg/10 mg, 5 mg/ 10 mg, 5 mg/20 mg, 5 mg/40 mg, 10 mg/20 mg, 10 mg/40 mg.

◆ **CLASSIFICATION**

**PHARMACOTHERAPEUTIC:** Angiotensin-converting enzyme (ACE) inhibitor. **CLINICAL:** Antihypertensive.

## USES

Treatment of hypertension. Used alone or in combination with other antihypertensives.

## PRECAUTIONS

**Contraindications:** Hypersensitivity to benazepril. History of angioedema with or without previous treatment with ACE inhibitors. Use with aliskiren in pts with diabetes. **Cautions:** Renal impairment; hypertrophic cardiomyopathy without flow tract obstruction; severe aortic stenosis; before, during, or immediately following major surgery; unstented renal artery stenosis; diabetes mellitus. Concomitant use of potassium-sparing diuretics, potassium supplements.

## ACTION

Decreases rate of conversion of angiotensin I to angiotensin II, a potent vasoconstrictor. Reduces peripheral arterial resistance. **Therapeutic Effect:** Lowers B/P.

## PHARMACOKINETICS

| Route | Onset | Peak | Duration |
|-------|-------|------|----------|
| PO | 1 hr | 2–4 hrs | 24 hrs |

Partially absorbed from GI tract. Protein binding: 97%. Metabolized in liver. Primarily excreted in urine. Minimal removal by hemodialysis. **Half-life:** 35 min; metabolite, 10–11 hrs.

## ⧗ LIFESPAN CONSIDERATIONS

**Pregnancy/Lactation:** Crosses placenta. Unknown if distributed in breast milk. May cause fetal, neonatal mortality or morbidity. **Children:** Safety and efficacy not established. **Elderly:** May be more sensitive to hypotensive effects.

## INTERACTIONS

**DRUG:** **Diuretics (e.g., furosemide),** **antihypertensives** may increase effect. **NSAIDs, sympathomimetics** may decrease effect. **Potassium-sparing diuretics, potassium supplements** may cause hyperkalemia. May increase **cyclosporine, lithium** concentration/ effect. **HERBAL:** **Ephedra, ginseng, licorice** may worsen hypertension. **Black cohosh, periwinkle** may have increased antihypertensive effect. **FOOD:** None known. **LAB VALUES:** May increase serum potassium, ALT, AST, alkaline phosphatase, bilirubin, BUN, creatinine, glucose. May decrease serum sodium, Hgb, Hct. May cause positive ANA titer.

## AVAILABILITY (Rx)

**Tablets:** 5 mg, 10 mg, 20 mg, 40 mg.

## ADMINISTRATION/HANDLING

• Give without regard to food.

## INDICATIONS/ROUTES/DOSAGE

**Hypertension (Monotherapy)**
**PO:** **ADULTS:** Initially, 10 mg/day. **Maintenance:** 10–40 mg/day as single dose or in 2 divided doses. **Maximum:** 80 mg/day. **ELDERLY:** Initially, 5–10 mg/ day. Range: 10–40 mg/day. **CHILDREN 6 YRS AND OLDER:** Initially, 0.2 mg/kg/day (up to 10 mg/day). Range: 0.1–0.6 mg/ kg/day. **Maximum:** 40 mg/day.

**Hypertension (Combination Therapy)**
**PO:** **ADULTS:** Discontinue diuretic 2–3 days prior to initiating benazepril, then dose as noted above. If unable to discontinue diuretic, begin benazepril at 5 mg/day.

**Dosage in Renal Impairment**
**CrCl less than 30 ml/min:** **ADULTS:** Initially, 5 mg/day titrated up to maximum of 40 mg/day. **CHILDREN:** Not recommended. **HD, PD:** 25%–50% of usual dose; supplement dose not necessary.

**Dosage in Hepatic Impairment**
Use caution.

## SIDE EFFECTS

**Frequent (6%–3%):** Cough, headache, dizziness. **Occasional (2%):** Fatigue, drowsiness, nausea. **Rare (less than 1%):** Rash, fever, myalgia, diarrhea, loss of taste.

## ADVERSE EFFECTS/ TOXIC REACTIONS

Excessive hypotension ("first-dose syncope") may occur in pts with HF, severe salt or volume depletion. Angioedema, hyperkalemia occur rarely. Agranulocytosis, neutropenia may be noted in pts with renal impairment, collagen vascular disease (scleroderma, systemic lupus erythematosus). Nephrotic syndrome may occur in pts with history of renal disease.

## NURSING CONSIDERATIONS

### BASELINE ASSESSMENT
Obtain CBC before therapy begins and q2wks for 3 mos, then periodically thereafter. Obtain B/P immediately before each dose, in addition to regular monitoring (be alert to fluctuations).

### INTERVENTION/EVALUATION
Assist with ambulation if dizziness occurs. Monitor B/P, renal function, urinary protein, serum potassium. Monitor CBC with differential if pt has collagen vascular disease or renal impairment. If excessive reduction in B/P occurs, place pt in supine position with legs elevated. Monitor pt with renal impairment, autoimmune disease, or taking drugs that affect leukocytes or immune response.

### PATIENT/FAMILY TEACHING
• To reduce hypotensive effect, go from lying to standing slowly. • Full therapeutic effect may take 2–4 wks. • Skipping doses or noncompliance with drug therapy may produce severe, rebound hypertension. • Report dizziness, persistent cough.

---

# bendamustine

ben-da-**mus**-teen
(Bendeka, Treanda)
**Do not confuse bendamustine
with carmustine or lomustine.**

## ◆ CLASSIFICATION

**PHARMACOTHERAPEUTIC:** Alkylating agent. **CLINICAL:** Antineoplastic.

## USES

Treatment of chronic lymphocytic leukemia (CLL). Treatment of indolent B-cell non-Hodgkin's lymphoma (NHL) that has progressed during or within 6 mos of treatment with rituximab or a rituximab-containing regimen. **OFF-LABEL:** Treatment of mantle cell lymphoma, relapsed multiple myeloma. First-line treatment for follicular lymphoma. Treatment of Waldenström's macroglobulinemia.

## PRECAUTIONS

**Contraindications:** Hypersensitivity to bendamustine, polyethylene glycol 400, or propylene glycol mono-thioglycerol. **Cautions:** Myelosuppression (may increase risk of infection), renal/hepatic impairment, dehydration, HF.

## ACTION

Alkylates and cross-links macromolecules, resulting in DNA, RNA, and protein synthesis inhibition. **Therapeutic Effect:** Inhibits tumor cell growth, causes cell death.

## PHARMACOKINETICS

Metabolized via hydrolysis to metabolites. Protein binding: 64%–95%. Eliminated primarily in feces. **Half-life:** 40 min.

## ⌛ LIFESPAN CONSIDERATIONS

**Pregnancy/Lactation:** May cause fetal harm. Unknown if distributed in breast milk. Impaired spermatogenesis, azoospermia have been reported in male pts. **Children:** Safety and efficacy not established. **Elderly:** No age-related precautions noted.

## INTERACTIONS

**DRUG:** **Ciprofloxacin, fluvoxamine** may increase concentration, decrease plasma concentrations of active metabolites. **CYP1A2 inducers (e.g., omeprazole), nicotine** may decrease concentration. **HERBAL:** None significant. **FOOD:** None known. **LAB VALUES:** May increase serum AST, bilirubin, creatinine, glucose, uric acid. May decrease WBCs, neutrophils, Hgb, platelets; serum potassium, sodium, calcium.

## AVAILABILITY (Rx)

**Injection, Powder for Reconstitution:** *(Treanda):* 25 mg, 100 mg. **Injection, Solution:** *(Treanda):* 90 mg/ml. *(Bendeka):* 100 mg/4 ml.

## ADMINISTRATION/HANDLING

 IV

**Reconstitution** • Reconstitute each 100-mg vial with 20 ml Sterile Water for Injection (25-mg vial with 5 ml) for final concentration of 5 mg/ml. • Powder should completely dissolve in 5 min. • Discard if particulate matter is observed. • Withdraw volume needed for required dose (based on 5 mg/ml concentration) and immediately transfer to 500-ml infusion bag of 0.9% NaCl for final concentration of 0.2–0.6 mg/ml. • Reconstituted solution must be transferred to infusion bag within 30 min of reconstitution. • After transferring, thoroughly mix contents of infusion bag. **Rate of Administration** • Infuse over 30 min for CLL or 60 min for NHL. **Storage** • Reconstituted solution should appear clear and colorless to pale yellow. • Final solution is stable for 24 hrs if refrigerated or 3 hrs at room temperature. • Administration must be completed within these stability time frames.

## INDICATIONS/ROUTES/DOSAGE

**◄ALERT►** Antiemetics are recommended to prevent nausea and vomiting.

### Chronic Lymphocytic Leukemia
**IV Infusion: ADULTS/ELDERLY:** 100 mg/m² given over 30 min daily on days 1 and 2 of a 28-day cycle, up to 6 cycles.

### Non-Hodgkin's Lymphoma
**IV Infusion: ADULTS/ELDERLY:** 120 mg/m² on days 1 and 2 of a 21-day cycle, up to 8 cycles.

### Dose Modification
**Hematologic Toxicity: Grade 4 or greater:** Withhold until ANC 1,000/mm³ or greater, platelet 75,000/mm³ or greater. **CLL: Toxicity Grade 3 or greater:** Reduce dose to 50 mg/m² on days 1 and 2 of each treatment cycle. **Recurrence:** Reduce dose to 25 mg/m² on days 1 and 2 of each cycle. **NHL: Hematologic toxicity Grade 4 or nonhematologic toxicity Grade 3 or greater:** Reduce dose to 90 mg/m² on days 1 and 2 of each cycle; **Recurrence:** Reduce dose to 60 mg/m² on days 1 and 2 of each treatment cycle.

### Dosage in Renal Impairment
Not recommended in pts with CrCl less than 40 ml/min.

### Dosage in Hepatic Impairment
**Mild:** Use caution. **Moderate to Severe:** Not recommended.

## SIDE EFFECTS

**Frequent (24%–16%):** Fever, nausea, vomiting. **Occasional (9%–8%):** Diarrhea, fatigue, asthenia (loss of strength, energy), rash, decreased weight, nasopharyngitis. **Rare (6%–3%):** Chills, pruritus, cough, herpes simplex infections.

## ADVERSE EFFECTS/ TOXIC REACTIONS

Myelosuppression characterized as neutropenia (75% of pts), thrombocytopenia (77% of pts), anemia (89% of pts), leukopenia (61% of pts) is an expected response to therapy. Infection, including pneumonia, sepsis may occur. Tumor lysis syndrome may lead to acute renal failure. Worsening hypertension occurs rarely.

## NURSING CONSIDERATIONS

### BASELINE ASSESSMENT
Question for possibility of pregnancy. Offer emotional support. Obtain baseline CBC, BMP, LFT before treatment begins and routinely thereafter.

### INTERVENTION/EVALUATION
Offer antiemetics to control nausea, vomiting. Monitor daily pattern of bowel activity, stool consistency. Assess skin for evidence of rash. Monitor for signs of infection (fever, chills, cough, flu-like symptoms). Monitor for hypertension. Hematologic nadirs occur in 3rd week of therapy and may require dose delays if recovery to recommended values has not occurred by day 28.

### PATIENT/FAMILY TEACHING
• Avoid crowds, those with known infection. • Avoid contact with anyone who recently received live virus vaccine. • Do not have immunizations without physician's approval (drug lowers body resistance). • Promptly report fever, chills, flu-like symptoms, sore throat, unusual bruising/bleeding from any site. • Male pts should be warned of potential risk to their reproductive capacities.

# benztropine

benz-**trow**-peen
(Cogentin)
**Do not confuse benztropine with bromocriptine or benzonatate.**

## ◆CLASSIFICATION
**PHARMACOTHERAPEUTIC:** Anticholinergic. **CLINICAL:** Antiparkinson agent.

 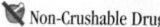

## USES

Treatment of Parkinson's disease, drug-induced extrapyramidal reactions (except tardive dyskinesia).

## PRECAUTIONS

**Contraindications:** Hypersensitivity to benztropine. Children younger than 3 yrs. **Cautions:** Children 3 yrs and older. Glaucoma, heart disease, hypertension, hypotension; pts with tachycardia, arrhythmias, prostatic hypertrophy, hepatic/renal impairment, obstructive diseases of GI/GU tract, urinary retention, elderly, myasthenia gravis, use during hot weather or during exercise.

## ACTION

Possesses anticholinergic effects. **Therapeutic Effect:** Reduces incidence/severity of akinesia, rigidity, tremor.

## PHARMACOKINETICS

Well absorbed following PO and IM administration. Metabolized in liver. PO onset of action: 1–2 hrs, IM onset of action: minutes. Pharmacologic effects may not be apparent until 2–3 days after initiation of therapy and may persist for up to 24 hrs after discontinuation of drug. **Half-life:** Extended (no specific determination).

## ⌛ LIFESPAN CONSIDERATIONS

**Pregnancy/Lactation:** Unknown if drug crosses placenta or is distributed in breast milk. **Children:** Safety and efficacy not established in pts younger than 3 yrs. **Elderly:** Increased risk for adverse reactions.

## INTERACTIONS

**DRUG: CNS depressants** (e.g., **alcohol, alprazolam, lorazepam, morphine, oxycodone, tramadol**) may increase sedation. May increase effects of **anticholinergics. HERBAL:** None significant. **FOOD:** None known. **LAB VALUES:** None significant.

## AVAILABILITY (Rx)

**Injection, Solution:** 1 mg/ml. **Tablets:** 0.5 mg, 1 mg, 2 mg.

## ADMINISTRATION/HANDLING

**IM**
• Inject slow, deep IM.

**PO**
• Give without regard to food. • Give with food if GI upset occurs.

## INDICATIONS/ROUTES/DOSAGE

**Parkinsonism**
**PO: ADULTS, ELDERLY:** Initially, 0.5–1 mg at bedtime or in divided doses. Titrate by 0.5 mg at 5- to 6-day intervals. Usual dose: 1 to 2 mg daily. Range: 0.5–6 mg daily. **Maximum:** 6 mg/day.

**Drug-Induced Extrapyramidal Symptoms**
**PO, IM, IV: ADULTS, ELDERLY:** Initially, 1–2 mg 2–3 times/day. Titrate at 0.5 mg q5–6days. **Usual dose:** 1–4 mg once or twice daily. **Maximum:** 6 mg/day. **CHILDREN OLDER THAN 3 YRS:** 0.02–0.05 mg/kg/dose once or twice daily.

**Acute Dystonic Reactions**
**IV, IM: ADULTS:** Initially, 1–2 mg as a single dose followed by 1–2 mg orally 1–2 times/day for up to 7–28 days to prevent recurrence.

**Dosage in Renal/Hepatic Impairment**
No dose adjustment.

## SIDE EFFECTS

**Frequent:** Drowsiness, dry mouth, blurred vision, constipation, urinary retention, GI upset, photosensitivity. **Occasional:** Headache, memory loss, muscle cramps, anxiety, peripheral paresthesia, orthostatic hypotension, abdominal cramps. **Rare:** Rash, confusion, eye pain.

## ADVERSE EFFECTS/ TOXIC REACTIONS

Overdose may produce severe anticholinergic effects (drowsiness, tachycardia, paralytic ileus, malignant hyperthermia, urinary retention, dyspnea, skin flushing, dryness of mouth/nose/throat). Severe paradoxical reactions (hallucinations, tremor, seizures, toxic psychosis) may occur.

## NURSING CONSIDERATIONS

### BASELINE ASSESSMENT

Assess mental status for confusion, disorientation, agitation, psychotic-like symptoms (medication frequently produces such side effects in pts older than 60 yrs). Note severity of baseline rigidity, tremors.

### INTERVENTION/EVALUATION

Be alert to neurologic effects: headache, drowsiness, mental confusion, agitation. Assess for clinical reversal of symptoms (improvement of tremor of head and hands at rest, mask-like facial expression, shuffling gait, muscular rigidity). Monitor daily pattern of bowel activity, stool consistency, esp. constipation. Monitor I/O. Assess for urinary retention.

### PATIENT/FAMILY TEACHING

• Avoid tasks that require alertness, motor skills until response to drug is established. • Dry mouth, drowsiness, dizziness may be an expected response to drug. • Drowsiness tends to diminish or disappear with continued therapy. • Avoid alcohol. • Report sudden muscle weakness or stiffness. • Report trouble urinating, bladder pain, or distension.

---

# betamethasone

bay-ta-**meth**-a-sone
(Betaderm ✤, Betaject ✤, Betnesol ✤, Betnovate ✤, Celestone, Celestone Soluspan, Diprolene, Diprolene AF, Ectosone ✤, Luxiq, Sernivo)

**Do not confuse betamethasone with dexamethasone or Luxiq with Lasix.**

## FIXED-COMBINATION(S)

**Lotrisone:** betamethasone/clotrimazole (an antifungal): 0.05%/1%.
**Taclonex:** betamethasone/calcipotriene (an antipsoriatic): 0.064%/.005%.

## ◆CLASSIFICATION

**PHARMACOTHERAPEUTIC:** Adrenocorticosteroid. **CLINICAL:** Anti-inflammatory, immunosuppressant.

## USES

**Systemic:** Inflammatory dermatoses (e.g., atopic dermatitis, psoriasis. **Topical:** Relief of inflammatory and pruritic dermatoses. **Foam:** Relief of inflammation, itching associated with dermatosis of the scalp. **Sernivo:** Treatment of mild to moderate plaque psoriasis. **OFF-LABEL:** Accelerate fetal lung maturation in pts with preterm labor.

## PRECAUTIONS

**Contraindications:** Hypersensitivity to betamethasone. Systemic fungal infections; IM administration in idiopathic thrombocytopenia purpura. **Cautions:** Hypothyroidism, hepatic/renal impairment, cardiovascular disease, diabetes, glaucoma, cataracts, myasthenia gravis, pts at risk for osteoporosis/seizures/GI disease, following acute MI, elderly.

## ACTION

Controls rate of protein synthesis, depresses migration of polymorphonuclear leukocytes/fibroblasts, reverses capillary permeability, prevents or controls inflammation. **Therapeutic Effect:** Decreases tissue response to inflammatory process.

## PHARMACOKINETICS

Rapidly absorbed following PO administration. Protein binding: 64%. After topical

---

 ✤ Canadian trade name     Non-Crushable Drug    **HIGH ALERT** High Alert drug application, limited absorption systemically. Metabolized in liver. Excreted in urine. **Half-life:** 6.5 hrs.

## ⧗ LIFESPAN CONSIDERATIONS

**Pregnancy/Lactation:** Crosses placenta, distributed in breast milk. **Children:** Prolonged treatment, high-dose therapy may decrease short-term growth rate, cortisol secretion. **Elderly:** Increased risk for developing hypertension, osteoporosis.

## INTERACTIONS

**DRUG: Amphotericin** may increase risk of hypokalemia. May decrease effects of **insulin, oral hypoglycemics (e.g., glimepiride, metformin, sitagliptin), potassium supplements.** May increase **digoxin** toxicity (due to hypokalemia). **Hepatic enzyme inducers (e.g., carbamazepine, phenobarbital, rifampin)** may decrease effect. **Live virus vaccines** may potentiate virus replication, increase vaccine side effects, decrease pt's antibody response to vaccine. **HERBAL: Cat's claw, echinacea** possess immunostimulant effects. **FOOD:** None known. **LAB VALUES:** May decrease serum calcium, potassium, thyroxine. May increase serum cholesterol, lipids, glucose, sodium, amylase.

## AVAILABILITY (Rx)

**Cream (Diprolene AF):** 0.05%. **Foam (Luxiq):** 0.12%. **Gel:** 0.05%. **Injection, Suspension (Celestone Soluspan):** 3 mg/ml. **Lotion (Diprolene):** 0.05%. **Ointment:** 0.05%, 0.1%. **Topical Spray:** 0.05%.

## ADMINISTRATION/HANDLING

### IM

• Inject slowly, deep IM into large muscle mass.

### Topical

• Gently cleanse area before application. • Apply sparingly and rub into area thoroughly. • Do not apply to face, groin, axillae, or inguinal areas. Not for use on broken skin, areas of infection, or in diaper area. • Do not dispense foam directly into hands; use fingers to apply small amounts.

## INDICATIONS/ROUTES/DOSAGE

**Anti-Inflammation, Immunosuppression, Corticosteroid Replacement Therapy**
**IM: ADULTS, ELDERLY:** 0.25–9 mg/day in 2 divided doses. **CHILDREN:** 0.0175–0.125 mg/kg/day in 3–4 divided doses.

**Relief of Inflamed and Pruritic Dermatoses**
**Topical:** *(Cream/Ointment):* **ADULTS, ELDERLY:** 1–2 times daily. **Foam:** Apply twice daily (morning and night).

**Plaque Psoriasis**
**Topical: ADULTS, ELDERLY:** *(Sernivo):* Apply to affected areas 2 times/day for up to 4 wks.

**Dosage in Hepatic Impairment**
Use caution.

## SIDE EFFECTS

**Frequent: Systemic:** Increased appetite, abdominal distention, nervousness, insomnia, false sense of well-being. **Topical:** Burning, stinging, pruritus. **Occasional: Systemic:** Dizziness, facial flushing, diaphoresis, decreased or blurred vision, mood swings. **Topical:** Allergic contact dermatitis, purpura or blood-containing blisters, thinning of skin with easy bruising, telangiectases, raised dark red spots on skin, angiomas.

## ADVERSE EFFECTS/ TOXIC REACTIONS

Overdose may cause systemic hypercorticism, adrenal suppression.

## NURSING CONSIDERATIONS

### BASELINE ASSESSMENT

Question for hypersensitivity to any corticosteroid, sulfite. Obtain baseline values for height, weight, B/P, serum glucose, electrolytes. Obtain baseline results of initial tests (tuberculosis [TB] skin test, X-rays, EKG).

## INTERVENTION/EVALUATION

Monitor B/P, blood glucose, electrolytes. Apply topical preparation sparingly. Do not use on broken skin or in areas of infection. Do not apply to wet skin, face, inguinal areas.

## PATIENT/FAMILY TEACHING

• Take with food, milk. • Take single daily dose in the morning. • Do not stop abruptly. • Apply topical preparations in a thin layer. • Do not receive smallpox vaccination during or immediately after therapy.

# bethanechol

be-**than**-e-kole

(Duvoid ✤, Urecholine)
**Do not confuse bethanechol with betaxolol.**

## ◆CLASSIFICATION

**PHARMACOTHERAPEUTIC:** Parasympathomimetic choline ester. **CLINICAL:** Cholinergic.

## USES

Treatment of acute postoperative and postpartum nonobstructive urinary retention, retention due to neurogenic bladder. **OFF-LABEL:** Treatment of gastroesophageal reflux.

## PRECAUTIONS

**Contraindications:** Hypersensitivity to bethanechol. Mechanical obstruction of GI/GU tract, GI or bladder wall instability, hyperthyroidism, cardiac disease, bronchial asthma, peptic ulcer. **Cautions:** None known.

## ACTION

Acts directly at cholinergic receptors in smooth muscle of urinary bladder, GI tract. Increases detrusor muscle tone. **Therapeutic Effect:** May initiate urination, bladder emptying. Stimulates gastric, intestinal motility.

## PHARMACOKINETICS

| Route | Onset | Peak | Duration |
|---|---|---|---|
| PO | 30–90 min | 60 min | 6 hrs |

Poorly absorbed following PO administration. Does not cross blood-brain barrier. **Half-life:** Unknown.

## ⧖ LIFESPAN CONSIDERATIONS

**Pregnancy/Lactation:** Unknown if crosses placenta or distributed in breast milk. **Children/Elderly:** No age-related precautions noted.

## INTERACTIONS

**DRUG:** Beta blockers (e.g., labetalol, metoprolol), anticholinesterase inhibitors (donepezil, rivastigmine) may increase effect/toxicity. **HERBAL:** None significant. **FOOD:** None known. **LAB VALUES:** May increase serum amylase, lipase, ALT, AST.

## AVAILABILITY (Rx)

**Tablets:** 5 mg, 10 mg, 25 mg, 50 mg.

## ADMINISTRATION/HANDLING

**PO**
• Administer 1 hr before or 2 hrs after meals.

## INDICATIONS/ROUTES/DOSAGE

**Nonobstructive Urinary Retention, Neurogenic Bladder**
**PO: ADULTS, ELDERLY:** Usual dose: 10–50 mg 3–4 times/day. Minimum effective dose determined by giving 5–10 mg initially, repeating same amount at 1-hr intervals until desired response is achieved. **CHILDREN:** 0.3–0.6 mg/kg/day in 3–4 divided doses.

**Dosage in Renal/Hepatic Impairment**
No dose adjustment.

## SIDE EFFECTS

**Occasional:** Belching, changes in vision, blurred vision, diarrhea, urinary urgency or frequency. **Rare:** Dyspnea, chest tightness, bronchospasm.

---

## ADVERSE EFFECTS/ TOXIC REACTIONS

Overdose produces CNS stimulation (insomnia, anxiety, orthostatic hypotension), cholinergic stimulation (headache, increased salivation/diaphoresis, nausea, vomiting, flushed skin, abdominal pain, seizures).

## NURSING CONSIDERATIONS

### BASELINE ASSESSMENT

Ensure pt has emptied bladder prior to procedure.

### INTERVENTION/EVALUATION

Monitor urine output. Palpate bladder for evidence of urinary retention.

### PATIENT/FAMILY TEACHING

• Report nausea, vomiting, diarrhea, diaphoresis, increased salivary secretions, irregular heartbeat, muscle weakness, severe abdominal pain, difficulty breathing.

## *bevacizumab*

be-va-**siz**-ue-mab
(Avastin)
■ **BLACK BOX ALERT** ■ May result in development of GI perforation, presented as intra-abdominal abscess, fistula, wound dehiscence, wound healing complications. Severe, sometimes fatal, hemorrhagic events including central nervous system/GI/vaginal bleeding, epistaxis, hemoptysis, pulmonary hemorrhage has occurred.
**Do not confuse Avastin with Astelin, or bevacizumab with cetuximab or rituximab.**

## ◆CLASSIFICATION

**PHARMACOTHERAPEUTIC:** Monoclonal antibody. **CLINICAL:** Antineoplastic.

## USES

First- or second-line combination chemotherapy with 5-fluorouracil (5-FU) for treatment of pts with colorectal cancer. Second-line treatment of colorectal cancer after progression of first-line treatment with bevacizumab. Treatment with carboplatin and paclitaxel for nonsquamous, non–small-cell lung cancer (NSCLC). Treatment of renal cell carcinoma (metastatic) with interferon alfa, brain cancer (glioblastoma) that has progressed following prior therapy. Treatment of platinum-resistant recurrent epithelial ovarian, fallopian tube, or primary peritoneal cancer (in combination with paclitaxel, doxorubicin [liposomal] or topotecan). Treatment of platinum-sensitive ovarian cancer. Treatment of persistent, recurrent, or metastatic cervical cancer (in combination with paclitaxel and either cisplatin or topotecan). **OFF-LABEL:** Adjunctive therapy in malignant mesothelioma, ovarian cancer, prostate cancer, age-related macular degeneration. Treatment of metastatic breast cancer.

## PRECAUTIONS

**Contraindications:** Hypersensitivity to bevacizumab. **Cautions:** Cardiovascular disease, acquired coagulopathy, preexisting hypertension, pts at risk of thrombocytopenia. Pts with CNS metastasis. Do not administer within 28 days of major surgery or active bleeding.

## ACTION

Binds to and inhibits vascular endothelial growth factor, a protein that plays a major role in formation of new blood vessels to tumors. **Therapeutic Effect:** Inhibits metastatic disease progression.

## PHARMACOKINETICS

Clearance varies by body weight, gender, tumor burden. **Half-life:** 20 days (range: 11–50 days).

## ⧗ LIFESPAN CONSIDERATIONS

**Pregnancy/Lactation:** May possess teratogenic effects. Potential for fertility impairment. May decrease maternal and fetal body weight; increase risk of skeletal fetal abnormalities. Breastfeeding not recommended. **Children:** Safety and efficacy not established. **Elderly:** Higher incidence of severe adverse reactions in pts older than 65 yrs.

## INTERACTIONS

**DRUG:** Sunitinib may increase concentration/effect. May increase levels of **clozapine, sorafenib, sunitinib. HERBAL:** None significant. **FOOD:** None known. **LAB VALUES:** May decrease Hgb, Hct, platelet count, WBC; serum potassium, sodium. May increase urine protein.

## AVAILABILITY (Rx)

**Injection, Solution:** 25-mg/ml vial. (4 ml, 16 ml)

## ADMINISTRATION/HANDLING

 IV

◀**ALERT**▶ Do not give by IV push or bolus.

**Reconstitution** • Dilute prescribed dose in 100 ml 0.9% NaCl. • Avoid dextrose-containing solutions. • Discard any unused portion.

**Rate of Administration** • Usually given following other chemotherapy. Infuse initial dose over 90 min. • If first infusion is well tolerated, second infusion may be administered over 60 min. • If 60-min infusion is well tolerated, all subsequent infusions may be administered over 30 min. **Storage** • Refrigerate vials. • Diluted solution may be stored for up to 8 hrs if refrigerated.

## ⊗ IV INCOMPATIBILITIES

Do not mix with dextrose solutions.

## INDICATIONS/ROUTES/DOSAGE

**Colorectal Cancer (with fluorouracil-based chemotherapy)**
**IV: ADULTS, ELDERLY:** 5 mg/kg q2wks or 10 mg/kg q2wks in combination with FOLFOX4).

**Colorectal Cancer Progression (following initial bevacizumab/fluorouracil-based chemotherapy)**
**IV: ADULTS, ELDERLY:** 5 mg/kg q2wks or 7.5 mg/kg q3wks (in combination with fluoropyrimidine-irinotecan– or fluoro-pyrimidine-oxaliplatin–based regimen).

**Non–Small-Cell Lung Cancer (NSCLC)**
**IV: ADULTS, ELDERLY:** 15 mg/kg q3wks (in combination with carboplatin and paclitaxel) for 6 cycles.

**Metastatic Renal Cell Carcinoma**
**IV: ADULTS, ELDERLY:** 10 mg/kg once q2wks (with interferon alfa).

**Brain Cancer**
**IV: ADULTS, ELDERLY:** 10 mg/kg q2wks (as monotherapy).

**Ovarian Cancer (Platinum-Resistant)**
**IV: ADULTS, ELDERLY:** 10 mg/kg q2wks with paclitaxel, doxorubicin [liposomal], or wkly topotecan or 15 mg/kg q3wks (with topotecan q3wks).

**Ovarian Cancer (Platinum-Sensitive)**
**IV: ADULTS, ELDERLY:** 15 mg/kg q3wk with carboplatin/paclitaxel for 6–8 cycles then 15 mg/kg q3wks as a single agent or 15 mg/kg with carboplatin/gemcitabine for 6–10 cycles then 15 mg/kg q3wks as a single agent.

**Cervical Cancer**
**IV: ADULTS, ELDERLY:** 15 mg/kg q3wks (in combination with paclitaxel and either cisplatin or topotecan).

**Dose Adjustment for Toxicity**
**Temporary suspension:** Mild to moderate proteinuria, severe hypertension not controlled with medical management. **Permanent discontinuation:** Wound dehiscence requiring intervention, GI perforation, hypertensive crises, serious bleeding, nephrotic syndrome.

**Dosage in Renal/Hepatic Impairment**
No dose adjustment.

## SIDE EFFECTS

**Frequent (73%–25%):** Asthenia, vomiting, anorexia, hypertension, epistaxis, stomatitis, constipation, headache, dyspnea. **Occasional (21%–15%):** Altered taste, dry skin, exfoliative dermatitis, dizziness, flatulence, excessive lacrimation, skin discoloration, weight loss, myalgia. **Rare (8%–6%):** Nail disorder, skin ulcer, alopecia, confusion, abnormal gait, dry mouth.

## ADVERSE EFFECTS/ TOXIC REACTIONS

UTI, manifested as urinary frequency/ urgency, proteinuria, occurs frequently. Most serious adverse effects include HF, deep vein thrombosis, GI perforation, wound dehiscence, hypertensive crisis, nephrotic syndrome, severe hemorrhage. Anemia, neutropenia, thrombocytopenia occur occasionally. Hypersensitivity reactions occur rarely. May increase risk of tracheoesophageal fistula development.

## NURSING CONSIDERATIONS

### BASELINE ASSESSMENT

Obtain baseline CBC, serum potassium, sodium levels and at regular intervals during therapy. Assess for proteinuria with urinalysis. For pts with 2+ or greater urine dipstick reading, a 24-hr urine collection is advised.

### INTERVENTION/EVALUATION

Monitor B/P regularly for hypertension. Assess for asthenia. Assist with ambulation if asthenia occurs. Monitor for fever, chills, abdominal pain, epistaxis. Offer antiemetic if nausea, vomiting occurs. Monitor daily pattern of bowel activity, stool consistency.

### PATIENT/FAMILY TEACHING

• Report abdominal pain, vomiting, constipation, headache. • Do not receive immunizations without physician's approval (lowers body's resistance).
• Avoid contact with anyone who recently received a live virus vaccine.
• Avoid crowds, those with infection.
• Female pts should take measures to avoid pregnancy during treatment.

---

# *bexarotene*

beks-**ar**-oh-teen
(Targretin)
■ **BLACK BOX ALERT** ■ Do not administer to pregnant women (high risk of birth defects).

## ◆CLASSIFICATION

**PHARMACOTHERAPEUTIC:** Retinoid. **CLINICAL:** Antineoplastic.

## USES

**PO:** Treatment of cutaneous T-cell lymphoma (CTCL) in pts refractory to at least one prior systemic therapy. **Topical:** Treatment of cutaneous lesions in pts with refractory CTCL (stage 1A and 1B) or not tolerant of other therapies.

## PRECAUTIONS

**Contraindications:** Hypersensitivity to bexarotene. Pregnancy. **Cautions:** Hepatic impairment, diabetes mellitus, lipid abnormalities, excessive alcohol consumption, biliary tract disease.

## ACTION

Binds to and activates retinoid X receptor subtypes that regulate the genes controlling cellular differentiation and proliferation. **Therapeutic Effect:** Inhibits growth of tumor cell lines of hematopoietic and squamous cell origin, induces tumor regression.

## PHARMACOKINETICS

Moderately absorbed from GI tract. Protein binding: greater than 99%. Metabolized in liver. Primarily eliminated through the hepatobiliary system. **Half-life:** 7 hrs.

---

## ⌛ LIFESPAN CONSIDERATIONS

**Pregnancy/Lactation:** May cause fetal harm. Unknown if distributed in breast milk. **Children:** Safety and efficacy not established. **Elderly:** No age-related precautions noted.

## INTERACTIONS

**DRUG: Bone marrow depressants, medications causing blood dyscrasias** may have adverse additive effects. **CYP3A4 inducers (e.g., phenobarbital, phenytoin, rifampin)** may decrease plasma concentration. **CYP3A4 inhibitors (e.g., erythromycin, gemfibrozil, itraconazole, ketoconazole)** may increase plasma concentration. May reduce **tamoxifen** concentration. **HERBAL: Dong quai, St. John's wort** may decrease plasma concentration/cause photosensitization. **FOOD: Grapefruit products** may increase concentration/toxicity. **LAB VALUES:** May increase serum ALT, AST, bilirubin, cholesterol, glucose, potassium, triglycerides, total cholesterol, LDL. May decrease HDL. CA-125 in ovarian cancer may be increased.

## AVAILABILITY (Rx)

**Capsules (Soft Gelatin [Targretin]):** 75 mg. **Topical Gel (Targretin):** 1%.

## ADMINISTRATION/HANDLING

### PO
• Give following a high-fat meal. • Swallow whole. Do not chew or dissolve.

### Topical
• Generously coat lesions with gel. • Allow to dry before covering. • Avoid applying gel to normal skin surrounding lesions or near mucosal surfaces. • Use of occlusive dressings not recommended.

## INDICATIONS/ROUTES/DOSAGE

**Cutaneous T-Cell Lymphoma Refractory to at Least One Prior Systemic Therapy**
**PO: ADULTS:** 300 mg/m$^2$/day. If no tumor response after 8 wks and initial dose is well tolerated, may increase to 400 mg/m$^2$/day. If not tolerated, may decrease to 200 mg/m$^2$/day, then to 100 mg/m$^2$/day, or temporarily suspended to manage toxicity. **Topical: ADULTS:** Initially, apply once every other day for first wk. May increase at weekly intervals to once daily, then twice daily, then 3 times/day, up to 4 times/day based on tolerance.

**Dosage in Renal/Hepatic Impairment**
No dose adjustment.

## SIDE EFFECTS

**Frequent (79%–20%):** Hyperlipidemia, headache, hypothyroidism, asthenia (loss of strength, energy). **Occasional (17%–7%):** Rash, nausea, peripheral edema, dry skin, abdominal pain, chills, exfoliative dermatitis, diarrhea.

## ADVERSE EFFECTS/TOXIC REACTIONS

Pancreatitis, hepatic failure, pneumonia occur rarely.

## NURSING CONSIDERATIONS

### BASELINE ASSESSMENT
Assess baseline lipid profile, WBC, LFT, thyroid function. Question for possibility of pregnancy.

### INTERVENTION/EVALUATION
Monitor serum cholesterol, triglycerides, CBC, hepatic, thyroid function tests.

### PATIENT/FAMILY TEACHING
• Do not use medicated, drying, abrasive soaps; wash with gentle, bland soap. • Inform physician if pregnant or planning to become pregnant (Pregnancy Category X). • Warn women of childbearing age about potential fetal risk if pregnancy occurs. • Instruct on need for use of 2 reliable forms of contraceptives concurrently during therapy and for 1 mo after discontinuation of therapy, even in infertile, premenopausal women.

---

✦ Canadian trade name     🗲 Non-Crushable Drug     🟥 HIGH ALERT High Alert drug

## *bicalutamide*

bye-ka-**loo**-ta-mide
(Apo-Bicalutamide ✦, Casodex,
Novo-Bicalutamide ✦ )

### ◆CLASSIFICATION

**PHARMACOTHERAPEUTIC:** Antiandrogen hormone. **CLINICAL:** Antineoplastic.

## USES

Treatment of advanced metastatic prostatic carcinoma (in combination with luteinizing hormone-releasing hormone [LHRH] agonist analogues, e.g., leuprolide). Treatment with both drugs must be started at same time. **OFF-LABEL:** Monotherapy for locally advanced prostate cancer.

## PRECAUTIONS

**Contraindications:** Hypersensitivity to bicalutamide. Women, esp. those who are or may become pregnant. **Cautions:** Moderate to severe hepatic impairment, diabetes.

## ACTION

Competitively inhibits androgen action by binding to androgen receptors in target tissue. **Therapeutic Effect:** Prevents testosterone stimulation of cell growth in prostate cancer.

## PHARMACOKINETICS

Well absorbed from GI tract. Protein binding: 96%. Metabolized in liver. Excreted in urine and feces. Not removed by hemodialysis. **Half-life:** 5.8–7 days.

## ⌛ LIFESPAN CONSIDERATIONS

**Pregnancy/Lactation:** May inhibit spermatogenesis in males. Not used in women. **Children:** Safety and efficacy not established. **Elderly:** No age-related precautions noted.

## INTERACTIONS

**DRUG:** May increase effects of **aripiprazole, budesonide, colchicine, fentanyl, salmeterol, saxagliptin.** **HERBAL:** None significant. **FOOD:** None known. **LAB VALUES:** May increase serum ALT, AST, alkaline phosphatase, creatinine, bilirubin, BUN, glucose. May decrease WBC, Hgb.

## AVAILABILITY (Rx)

**Tablets:** 50 mg.

## ADMINISTRATION/HANDLING

**PO**
• Give without regard to food. • Give at same time each day.

## INDICATIONS/ROUTES/DOSAGE

**Prostatic Carcinoma**
**PO: ADULTS, ELDERLY:** 50 mg once daily in morning or evening, given concurrently with an LHRH analogue or after surgical castration.

**Dosage in Renal/Hepatic Impairment**
No dose adjustment.

## SIDE EFFECTS

**Frequent (49%–10%):** Hot flashes, breast pain, muscle pain, constipation, asthenia, diarrhea, nausea. **Occasional (9%–8%):** Nocturia, abdominal pain, peripheral edema. **Rare (7%–3%):** Vomiting, weight loss, dizziness, insomnia, rash, impotence, gynecomastia.

## ADVERSE EFFECTS/ TOXIC REACTIONS

Sepsis, HF, hypertension, iron deficiency anemia, interstitial pneumonitis, pulmonary fibrosis may occur. Severe hepatotoxicity occurs rarely within the first 3–4 mos after treatment initiation.

## NURSING CONSIDERATIONS

### BASELINE ASSESSMENT

Obtain baseline CBC, LFT, PSA, serum testosterone, leuteinizing hormone (LH) levels.

**INTERVENTION/EVALUATION**

Monitor lab studies for changes from baseline. Perform periodic hepatic function tests. If ALT, AST increase over 2 times the upper limit of normal (ULN) or jaundice is noted, discontinue treatment. Monitor for diarrhea, nausea, vomiting.

**PATIENT/FAMILY TEACHING**

• Do not stop taking either medication (both drugs must be continued). • Take medications at same time each day. • Explain possible expectancy of frequent side effects. • Report persistent nausea, vomiting, diarrhea or yellowing of skin or eyes.

---

# bisacodyl

bis-**ak**-oh-dil
Apo-Bisacodyl ♣, Dulcolax

## ◆CLASSIFICATION

**PHARMACOTHERAPEUTIC:** GI stimulant. **CLINICAL:** Laxative.

## USES

Treatment of constipation, colonic evacuation before examinations or procedures.

## PRECAUTIONS

**Contraindications:** Hypersensitivity to bisacodyl. Abdominal pain, appendicitis, intestinal obstruction, nausea, undiagnosed rectal bleeding, vomiting, pregnancy, lactation. **Cautions:** Long-term use may lead to laxative dependence, loss of normal bowel function.

## ACTION

Direct effect on colonic smooth musculature by stimulating intramural nerve plexi. **Therapeutic Effect:** Promotes fluid and electrolyte accumulation in colon, increasing peristalsis, producing laxative effect.

## PHARMACOKINETICS

| Route | Onset | Peak | Duration |
|---|---|---|---|
| PO | 6–12 hrs | N/A | N/A |
| Rectal | 15–60 min | N/A | N/A |

Minimal absorption following PO and rectal administration. Absorbed drug is excreted in urine; remainder is eliminated in feces.

## ⧖ LIFESPAN CONSIDERATIONS

**Pregnancy/Lactation:** Unknown if drug crosses placenta or is distributed in breast milk. **Children:** Use with caution in pts younger than 6 yrs (usually unable to describe symptoms or more severe side effects). **Elderly:** Repeated use may cause weakness, orthostatic hypotension due to fluid, electrolyte imbalance.

## INTERACTIONS

**DRUG: Antacids** may decrease effect, cause premature dissolution of enteric coating and possible gastric irritation. **HERBAL:** None significant. **FOOD: Milk** may cause rapid dissolution of bisacodyl. **LAB VALUES:** May increase serum glucose. May decrease serum potassium (due to fluid loss).

## AVAILABILITY (OTC)

**Suppositories (Dulcolax):** 10 mg.

🔖 **Tablets (Enteric-Coated [Dulcolax]):** 5 mg.

## ADMINISTRATION/HANDLING

**PO**

• Give on empty stomach (faster action). • Offer 6–8 glasses of water a day (aids stool softening). • Administer tablets whole; do not break, crush, dissolve, or divide. • Avoid giving within 1 hr of antacids, milk, other oral medication.

**Rectal, Suppository**

• If suppository is too soft, chill for 30 min in refrigerator or run cold water over foil wrapper. • Moisten suppository with cold water before inserting well into rectum.

---

**Storage** • Store rectal enema, suppositories at room temperature.

# INDICATIONS/ROUTES/DOSAGE

### Treatment of Constipation

**PO: ADULTS, ELDERLY, CHILDREN OLDER THAN 12 YRS:** 5–15 mg as needed. **Maximum:** 30 mg. **CHILDREN 3–12 YRS:** 5–10 mg or 0.3 mg/kg at bedtime or after breakfast.

**Rectal, Suppository: ADULTS, ELDERLY, CHILDREN OLDER THAN 12 YRS:** 10 mg to induce bowel movement. **CHILDREN 2–12 YRS:** 5–10 mg as a single dose. **CHILDREN YOUNGER THAN 2 YRS:** 5 mg.

### Dosage in Renal/Hepatic Impairment
No dose adjustment.

## SIDE EFFECTS

**Frequent:** Some degree of abdominal discomfort, nausea, mild cramps, faintness. **Occasional:** Rectal administration: burning of rectal mucosa, mild proctitis.

## ADVERSE EFFECTS/ TOXIC REACTIONS

Long-term use may result in laxative dependence, chronic constipation, loss of normal bowel function. Overdose may result in electrolyte or metabolic disturbances (hypokalemia, hypocalcemia, metabolic acidosis, alkalosis), persistent diarrhea, vomiting, muscle weakness, malabsorption, weight loss.

## NURSING CONSIDERATIONS

### BASELINE ASSESSMENT

Observe for evidence of constipation. Assess pattern of bowel activity, stool consistency.

### INTERVENTION/EVALUATION

Encourage adequate fluid intake. Assess bowel sounds for peristalsis. Monitor daily pattern of bowel activity, stool consistency; record time of evacuation. Assess for abdominal disturbances. Monitor serum electrolytes in those exposed to prolonged, frequent, or excessive use of medication.

### PATIENT/FAMILY TEACHING

• Institute measures to promote defecation: increase fluid intake, exercise, high-fiber diet. • Do not take antacids, milk, or other medication within 1 hr of taking medication (decreased effectiveness). • Report unrelieved constipation, rectal bleeding, muscle pain or cramps, dizziness, weakness. • Do not chew, crush, dissolve, or divide tablets.

---

# *bisoprolol*

bi-**soe**-proe-lol
(Apo-Bisoprolol ✦, Novo-Bisoprolol ✦, Zebeta)
**Do not confuse Zebeta with DiaBeta or Zetia.**

## FIXED-COMBINATION(S)

**Ziac:** bisoprolol/hydrochlorothiazide (a diuretic): 2.5 mg/6.25 mg, 5 mg/6.25 mg, 10 mg/6.25 mg.

## ◆CLASSIFICATION

**PHARMACOTHERAPEUTIC:** Beta-adrenergic blocker. **CLINICAL:** Antihypertensive.

## USES

Management of hypertension, alone or in combination with other medications. **OFF-LABEL:** Chronic stable angina pectoris, premature ventricular contractions, supraventricular arrhythmias, HF.

## PRECAUTIONS

**Contraindications:** Hypersensitivity to bisoprolol. Cardiogenic shock, marked sinus bradycardia, overt HF, second- or third-degree heart block (except in pts with pacemaker). **Cautions:** Concurrent use of digoxin, verapamil, diltiazem, HF, history of severe anaphylaxis to allergens, renal/ hepatic impairment, hyperthyroidism, diabetes, bronchospastic disease, myasthenia gravis, psychiatric disease, peripheral vascular disease, Raynaud's disease.

## ACTION

Blocks beta$_1$-adrenergic receptors in cardiac tissue. **Therapeutic Effect:** Slows sinus heart rate, decreases B/P.

## PHARMACOKINETICS

Well absorbed from GI tract. Protein binding: 26%–33%. Metabolized in liver. Primarily excreted in urine. Not removed by hemodialysis. **Half-life:** 9–12 hrs (increased in renal impairment).

## ⏳ LIFESPAN CONSIDERATIONS

**Pregnancy/Lactation:** Readily crosses placenta; distributed in breast milk. Avoid use during first trimester. May produce bradycardia, apnea, hypoglycemia, hypothermia during delivery, low birth-weight infants. **Children:** Safety and efficacy not established. **Elderly:** Age-related peripheral vascular disease may increase risk of decreased peripheral circulation.

## INTERACTIONS

**DRUG: Diuretics (e.g., furosemide), other antihypertensives** may increase hypotensive effect. May mask symptoms of hypoglycemia, prolong hypoglycemic effect of **insulin, oral hypoglycemics (e.g., glimepiride, metformin, sitagliptin). NSAIDs** may decrease antihypertensive effect. **Verapamil, diltiazem, digoxin** may increase risk of bradycardia or heart block. **HERBAL: Ephedra, ginseng, yohimbe** may worsen hypertension. **Garlic** may have increased antihypertensive effect. **FOOD:** None known. **LAB VALUES:** May increase ANA titer, serum BUN, creatinine, potassium, uric acid, lipoproteins, triglycerides.

## AVAILABILITY (Rx)

**Tablets:** 5 mg, 10 mg.

## ADMINISTRATION/HANDLING

**PO**
• Give without regard to food.

## INDICATIONS/ROUTES/DOSAGE

**Hypertension**
**PO: ADULTS, ELDERLY:** Initially,    2.5–5 mg/day. May increase to 10 mg, then to 20 mg/day. Usual dose: 5–10 mg once daily.

**Dosage in Renal Impairment**
**ADULTS, ELDERLY: CrCl less than 40 ml/min:** Initially, give 2.5 mg.

**Dosage in Hepatic Impairment**
**Cirrhosis, Hepatitis:** Initially, 2.5 mg.

## SIDE EFFECTS

**Frequent (11%–8%):** Fatigue, headache. **Occasional (4%–2%):** Dizziness, arthralgia, peripheral edema, URI, rhinitis, pharyngitis, diarrhea, nausea, insomnia. **Rare (less than 2%):** Chest pain, asthenia, dyspnea, vomiting, bradycardia, dry mouth, diaphoresis, decreased libido, impotence.

## ADVERSE EFFECTS/TOXIC REACTIONS

Overdose may produce profound bradycardia, hypotension. Abrupt withdrawal may result in diaphoresis, palpitations, headache, tremors. May precipitate HF, MI in pts with cardiac disease, thyroid storm in pts with thyrotoxicosis, peripheral ischemia in those with existing peripheral vascular disease. Hypoglycemia may occur in previously controlled diabetes. Thrombocytopenia, unusual bruising/bleeding occur rarely.

## NURSING CONSIDERATIONS

### BASELINE ASSESSMENT

Assess baseline renal/hepatic function tests. Assess B/P, apical pulse immediately before drug is administered (if pulse is 60/min or less or systolic B/P is less than 90 mm Hg, withhold medication, contact physician).

---

### INTERVENTION/EVALUATION

Monitor B/P, pulse for quality, irregular rate, bradycardia. Assist with ambulation if dizziness occurs. Assess for peripheral edema (usually, first area of lower extremity swelling is behind medial malleolus in ambulatory, sacral area in bedridden). Monitor daily pattern of bowel activity, stool consistency. Assess neurologic status.

### PATIENT/FAMILY TEACHING

• Do not abruptly discontinue medication. • Compliance with therapy regimen is essential to control hypertension. • If dizziness occurs, sit or lie down immediately. • Avoid tasks that require alertness, motor skills until response to drug is established. • Take pulse properly before each dose and report excessively slow pulse rate (less than 60 beats/min). Report numbness of extremities, dizziness. • Do not use nasal decongestants, OTC cold preparations (stimulants) without physician's approval. • Restrict salt, alcohol intake.

---

## *bivalirudin* HIGH ALERT

bye-**val**-i-rue-din
(Angiomax)

### ◆CLASSIFICATION

**PHARMACOTHERAPEUTIC:** Thrombin inhibitor. **CLINICAL:** Anticoagulant.

## USES

Anticoagulant in pts with unstable angina undergoing percutaneous transluminal coronary angioplasty (PTCA) in conjunction with aspirin. Pts with heparin-induced thrombocytopenia (HIT) and thrombosis syndrome (HITTS) while undergoing percutaneous coronary intervention (PCI) (in conjunction with aspirin). **OFF-LABEL:** HIT; ST-segment elevation MI (STEMI) undergoing PCI.

## PRECAUTIONS

**Contraindications:** Hypersensitivity to bivalirudin. Active major bleeding. **Cautions:** Renal impairment, conditions associated with increased risk of bleeding (e.g., bacterial endocarditis, recent major bleeding, CVA, stroke, intracerebral surgery, hemorrhagic diathesis, severe hypertension, severe renal/hepatic impairment, recent major surgery).

## ACTION

Specifically and reversibly inhibits thrombin by binding to its receptor sites. **Therapeutic Effect:** Decreases acute myocardial ischemic complications in pts with unstable angina pectoris.

### PHARMACOKINETICS

| Route | Onset | Peak | Duration |
|-------|-------|------|----------|
| IV | Immediate | N/A | 1 hr |

Primarily eliminated by kidneys. Twenty-five percent removed by hemodialysis. **Half-life:** 25 min (increased in moderate to severe renal impairment).

### ⧖ LIFESPAN CONSIDERATIONS

**Pregnancy/Lactation:** Unknown if drug crosses placenta or is distributed in breast milk. **Pregnancy Category B. Children:** Safety and efficacy not established. **Elderly:** Age-related renal impairment may require dosage adjustment.

## INTERACTIONS

**DRUG: Antiplatelets** (e.g., **aspirin, clopidogrel**), **NSAIDs, thrombolytics** may increase effect. **HERBAL: Ginkgo biloba**, other herbs with anticoagulant/antiplatelet properties may increase risk of bleeding. **FOOD:** None known. **LAB VALUES:** Prolongs activated partial thromboplastin time (aPTT), prothrombin time (PT).

## AVAILABILITY (Rx)

**Injection, Powder for Reconstitution:** 250 mg.

---

## ADMINISTRATION/HANDLING
IV

**Reconstitution** • To each 250-mg vial add 5 ml Sterile Water for Injection. • Gently swirl until fully dissolved. • Dilute each vial in 50 ml D₅W or 0.9% NaCl bag to yield final concentration of 5 mg/ml (1 vial in 50 ml, 2 vials in 100 ml, 5 vials in 250 ml). • If low-rate infusion is used after initial infusion, reconstitute the 250-mg vial with added 5 ml Sterile Water for Injection. • Gently swirl until fully dissolved. • Dilute each vial in 500 ml D₅W or 0.9% NaCl bag to yield final concentration of 0.5 mg/ml. • Produces a clear, colorless solution (do not use if cloudy or contains a precipitate).
**Rate of Administration** • Adjust IV infusion based on aPTT or pt's body weight.
**Storage** • Store unreconstituted vials at room temperature. • Reconstituted solution may be refrigerated for up to 24 hrs. • Final dilution with a concentration of 0.5–5 mg/ml is stable at room temperature for up to 24 hrs.

## IV INCOMPATIBILITIES

Alteplase (Activase), amiodarone (Cordarone), amphotericin B (AmBisome, Abelcet), diazepam (Valium), dobutamine (Dobutrex), reteplase (Retavase), streptokinase (Streptase), vancomycin (Vancocin).

## IV COMPATIBILITIES

Refer to IV compatibility chart in front of book.

## INDICATIONS/ROUTES/DOSAGE

**Anticoagulant in Pts with Unstable Angina, HIT, or HITTS Undergoing PTCA**
**IV: ADULTS, ELDERLY:** 0.75 mg/kg as IV bolus, followed by IV infusion at rate of 1.75 mg/kg/hr for duration of procedure and up to 4 hrs postprocedure. IV infusion may be continued beyond initial 4 hrs at rate of 0.2 mg/kg/hr for up to 20 hrs.

**Dosage in Renal Impairment**
◀**ALERT**▶ Initial bolus dose remains unchanged.

| Creatinine Clearance | Dosage |
|---|---|
| 30 ml/min or greater | 1.75 mg/kg/hr |
| 10–29 ml/min | 1 mg/kg/hr |
| Dialysis | 0.25 mg/kg/hr |

**Dosage in Hepatic Impairment**
No dosage adjustment.

## SIDE EFFECTS

**Frequent (42%):** Back pain. **Occasional (15%–12%):** Nausea, headache, hypotension, generalized pain. **Rare (8%–4%):** Injection site pain, insomnia, hypertension, anxiety, vomiting, pelvic or abdominal pain, bradycardia, nervousness, dyspepsia, fever, urinary retention.

## ADVERSE EFFECTS/ TOXIC REACTIONS

Hemorrhagic events occur rarely, characterized by significant fall in B/P or Hgb/Hct.

## NURSING CONSIDERATIONS

### BASELINE ASSESSMENT

Assess CBC, PT/INR, aPTT, renal function. Determine initial B/P.

### INTERVENTION/EVALUATION

Monitor aPTT, CBC, urine and stool specimen for occult blood, renal function studies. Monitor for evidence of bleeding. Assess for decrease in B/P, increase in pulse rate. Question for increase in vaginal bleeding during menses.

# blinatumomab

**blin**-a-**toom**-oh-mab
(Blincyto)

■ **BLACK BOX ALERT** ■ Cytokine release syndrome (CRS) or neurologic toxicities, which may be life threatening or fatal, have occurred.

Interrupt or discontinue treatment as recommended.

**Do not confuse blinatuxumab with ibritimomab or tositumomab.**

## ◆CLASSIFICATION

**PHARMACOTHERAPEUTIC:** Bispecific CD-19-directed CD3 T-cell engager. **CLINICAL:** Antineoplastic.

## USES

Treatment of Philadelphia chromosome-negative relapsed or refractory B-cell precursor acute lymphoblastic leukemia (ALL).

## PRECAUTIONS

**Contraindications:** Hypersensitivity to blinatumomab. **Cautions:** Baseline anemia, leukopenia, neutropenia, thrombocytopenia; active infection or pts at increased risk of infection (diabetes, indwelling catheters), hepatic/renal impairment, electrolyte imbalance, high tumor burden, history of cognitive or seizure disorders, syncope, elderly.

## ACTION

Activates endogenous T cells by connecting CD3 in the T-cell receptor complex with CD19 on benign and malignant B cells. Mediates proliferation of T cells, release of inflammatory cytokines, production of cytolytic proteins, and upregulation of cell adhesions, resulting in lysis of tumor cells. **Therapeutic Effect:** Inhibits tumor cell growth and metastasis in ALL.

## PHARMACOKINETICS

Widely distributed. Metabolism not specified; degrades into small peptides and amino acids via catabolic pathway. Protein binding: Not specified. Steady state reached within 24 hrs. Elimination not specified; negligible amounts excreted in urine. **Half-life:** 2.1 hrs.

## LIFESPAN CONSIDERATIONS

**Pregnancy/Lactation:** May cause fetal harm. Avoid pregnancy. Unknown if distributed in breast milk. Must either discontinue drug or discontinue breast-feeding. **Children:** Safety and efficacy not established. **Elderly:** May have increased risk of neurologic toxicities including cognitive disorder, encephalopathy, confusion, seizure; serious infections, hepatic impairment.

## INTERACTIONS

**DRUG:** May alter concentration of **medications with a narrow therapeutic index (e.g., cyclosporine, warfarin).** **HERBAL:** None significant. **FOOD:** None known. **LAB VALUES:** May decrease immunoglobulins, Hgb, Hct, neutrophils, leukocytes, platelets; serum albumin, magnesium, phosphate, potassium. May increase serum ALT, AST, bilirubin, GGT, glucose; body weight.

## AVAILABILITY (Rx)

**Injection, Lyophilized Powder for Reconstitution:** 35 mcg/vial.

## ADMINISTRATION/HANDLING

 IV

• Hospitalization is recommended for the first 9 days of the first cycle and the first 2 days of the second cycle. For all subsequent cycle starts and re-initiation (e.g., if treatment is interrupted for 4 or more hrs), supervision by a healthcare professional or hospitalization is recommended. • Do not flush infusion line after administration, esp. when changing infusion bags. Flushing of infusion line can result in excess dosage and complications. • At end of infusion, any used solution in IV bag and IV lines should be disposed of in accordance with local requirements. **Premedication** • Premedicate with dexamethasone 20 mg IV 1 hr prior to the first dose of each cycle, prior to step dose (such as cycle 1 on day 8), or when restarting an infusion after an interruption of 4 or more hrs. **Reconstitution** • Reconstitution guidelines are highly specific. Infusion bags must be prepared by personnel trained in aseptic preparations and admixing of oncologic drugs following strict environmental specifications at a USP <797> compliant facility using ISO Class 5 laminar flow hood or better. • See manufacturer guidelines for details.

**Rate of Administration** • Administer as continuous IV infusion at a constant flow rate using an infusion pump. The pump should be programmable, lockable, nonelastomeric, and have an alarm. • Infusion bags should be infused over 24–48 hrs. Infuse the total 240 ml solution according to the instructions on the pharmacy label of the bag at one of the following constant rates: 10 ml/hr over 24 hrs, or 5 ml/hr over 48 hrs. • Infuse via dedicated line. • Use sterile, nonpyrogenic, low-protein-binding, 0.2-micron in-line filter.

**Storage** • Refrigerate unused vials and IV solution stabilizer until time of use. • Protect from light • Do not freeze. • Reconstituted vials may be stored at room temperature up to 4 hrs or refrigerated up to 24 hrs. • Prepared IV bag solutions may be stored at room temperature up to 48 hrs or refrigerated up to 8 days. • If prepared IV bag solution is not administered with the infusion time frame and temperature indicated, it must be discarded; do not refrigerate again.

# INDICATIONS/ROUTES/DOSAGE

NOTE: See Administration/Handling.

**Acute Lymphoblastic Leukemia (ALL)**
**IV: ADULTS, ELDERLY, CHILDREN:** A single treatment cycle consists of 4 wks of continuous IV infusion followed by a 2-wk treatment-free interval. **PTS WEIGHING 45 KG OR MORE:** (Cycle 1): Administer 9 mcg/day on days 1–7, then at 28 mcg/day on days 8–28 as continuous infusion. (Subsequent Cycles): Administer 28 mcg/day on days 1–28 of a 6-wk treatment cycle. **PTS WEIGHING LESS THAN 45 KG:** (Cycle 1): 5 mcg/m²/day on days 1–7 and 15 mcg/m²/day on days 8–28 as continuous infusion. (Subsequent Cycles): Administer 15 mcg/m²/day on days 1–28 of a 6-wk treatment cycle.

**Dose Modification**
(Based on Common Terminology Criteria for Adverse Events) **Note:** If interruption after an adverse event is no longer than 7 days, continue the same cycle to a total of 28 days of infusion inclusive of the days before and after the interruption in that cycle. If interruption due to an adverse event is longer than 7 days, start new cycle.

*Cytokine Release Syndrome*
**CTCAE Grade 3:** Withhold until resolved, then restart at 9 mcg/day. Increase dose to 28 mcg/day after 7 days if toxicity does not occur. **CTCAE Grade 4:** Permanently discontinue.

*Neurological Toxicity*
**CTCAE Grade 3:** Withhold until no more than Grade 1 for at least 3 days, then restart at 9 mcg/day. Increase dose to 28 mcg/day after 7 days if toxicity does not recur. If toxicity occurred at 9 mcg/day, or if toxicity takes more than 7 days to resolve, permanently discontinue. **CTCAE Grade 4:** Permanently discontinue.

*Seizure*
Permanently discontinue if more than one seizure occurs.

*Other Clinically Relevant Adverse Reactions*
**CTCAE Grade 3:** Withhold no more than Grade 1, then restart at 9 mcg/day. Increase dose to 28 mcg/day after 7 days if toxicity does not recur. If toxicity takes more than 14 days to resolve, permanently discontinue. **CTCAE Grade 4:** Consider permanent discontinuation.

*Elevated Hepatic Enzymes*
Interrupt treatment if ALT/AST rise to greater than 5 times upper limit of normal (UNL) or bilirubin rises to more than 3 times ULN. Consider dose recommendation as listed in other clinically relevant adverse reactions or as ordered by prescriber.

---

### Dosage in Renal Impairment
**CrCl equal to or greater than 30 ml/min:** No dose adjustment. **CrCl less than 30 ml/min or hemodialysis:** Not specified; use caution.

### Dosage in Hepatic Impairment
Not specified; use caution. Hepatic toxicity during treatment: see dose modification.

## SIDE EFFECTS
**Frequent (62%–36%):** Pyrexia, headache. **Occasional (25%–5%):** Peripheral edema, nausea, tremor, constipation, diarrhea, cough, fatigue, dyspnea, insomnia, chills, abdominal pain, dizziness, back pain, extremity pain, vomiting, bone pain, chest pain, decreased appetite, arthralgia, hypotension, hypertension, tachycardia, confusion, paresthesia. **Rare (4%–2%):** Aphasia, memory impairment.

## ADVERSE EFFECTS/TOXIC REACTIONS
Myelosuppression (principally, anemia, leukopenia, neutropenia, thrombocytopenia) is an expected outcome of treatment. Cytokine release syndrome (CRS) may be life threatening or fatal. Symptoms of CRS may include asthenia, hypotension, nausea, pyrexia; elevated ALT/AST, bilirubin; disseminated intravascular coagulation (DIC), capillary leak syndrome, hemophagocytic lymphohistiocytosis/macrophage activation syndrome (HLM/MAS). Infusion reactions have occurred and may be clinically indistinguishable from CRS. Neurologic toxicities such as altered level of consciousness, balance disorders, confusion, disorientation encephalopathy, seizures, speech disorders, syncope occurred in approx. 50% of pts and may affect ability to drive or operate machinery. Median time to onset of neurologic toxicity was 7 days. CTCAE Grade 3 toxicities or higher occurred in 15% of pts. Serious infections such as opportunistic infections, bacterial/viral/fungal infections, sepsis, pneumonia, catheter-site infections occurred in 25% of pts.

Other life-threatening or fatal events may include tumor lysis syndrome, neutropenia/febrile neutropenia, leukoencephalopathy. Medication preparation and administration errors have occurred, resulting in underdose or overdose. Immunogenicity (anti-blinatumomab antibodies) occurred in less than 1% of pts.

## NURSING CONSIDERATIONS

### BASELINE ASSESSMENT
Obtain baseline CBC, BMP, LFTs, serum magnesium, phosphate, ionized calcium, vital signs. Consider electrolyte correction before starting treatment. Screen for home medications requiring narrow therapeutic index. Screen for active infection, history of seizures, hepatic/renal impairment, cognitive disorders. Verify pregnancy status in women of childbearing potential. Assess plans of breastfeeding. Conduct full neurologic assessment.

### INTERVENTION/EVALUATION
Monitor CBC, LFTs, serum electrolytes (correct as indicated), vital signs. Monitor closely for cytokine release syndrome, neurologic toxicities, serious infection, tumor lysis syndrome, hepatic impairment. Keep area around IV site clean to reduce risk of infection. Do adjust setting of infusion pump. Pump changes may result in dosing errors. Do not flush IV line after infusion completion. Initiate fall precautions. Monitor I & O.

### PATIENT/FAMILY TEACHING
• Treatment may cause life-threatening side effects that must be immediately treated by medical personal. • Report symptoms of cytokine release syndrome such as chills, facial swelling, fever, low blood pressure, nausea, vomiting, weakness; any infusion-related reactions such as difficulty breathing or skin rash. • Report any neurologic problems such as confusion, difficulty speaking or slurred speech, loss of consciousness, loss of balance, or seizures. • Treatment may

lower your white blood cell count and increase your risk of infection. Report any signs of infection such as fever, cough, fatigue, or burning with urination. Keep area around IV catheter clean at all times to reduce risk of infection. • Do not change or alter settings on infusion pump, even if the pump alarm sounds. Any changes made to the infusion pump by anyone other than trained medical personal can result in a dose that is too high or too low and may be life threatening. • Report symptoms of liver problems such as bruising, confusion, dark or amber-colored urine, right upper abdominal pain, or yellowing of the skin or eyes. • Avoid tasks that require alertness, motor skills until response to drug is established. Do not drive or operate machinery. • Blood levels will be monitored routinely. • Hospitalization is required when starting therapy.

---

## bortezomib **HIGH ALERT**

bor-**tez**-oh-mib
(Velcade)

### ◆ CLASSIFICATION

**PHARMACOTHERAPEUTIC:** Protease inhibitor. **CLINICAL:** Antineoplastic.

## USES

Treatment of relapsed or refractory mantle cell lymphoma. Initial treatment of multiple myeloma. **OFF-LABEL:** Treatment of Waldenström's macroglobulinemia; peripheral or cutaneous T-cell lymphoma; systemic light-chain amyloidosis.

## PRECAUTIONS

**Contraindications:** Hypersensitivity to bortezomib, boron or mannitol; intrathecal administration. **Cautions:** Concomitant use of CYP3A4 inhibitors, history of syncope, concomitant use of antihypertensives; dehydration, diabetes, hepatic impairment, preexisting cardiac disease, neuropathy.

## ACTION

Inhibits proteasomes (enzyme complexes regulating protein homeostasis within the cell). **Therapeutic Effect:** Produces cell-cycle arrest, apoptosis.

## PHARMACOKINETICS

Widely distributed. Protein binding: 83%. Primarily metabolized by enzymatic action. Significant biliary excretion, with lesser amount excreted in urine. **Half-life:** 9–15 hrs.

## ⧖ LIFESPAN CONSIDERATIONS

**Pregnancy/Lactation:** May induce degenerative effects in ovary, degenerative changes in testes. May affect male/female fertility. Breastfeeding not recommended. Children: Safety and efficacy not established. **Elderly:** Increased incidence of Grade 3 or 4 thrombocytopenia.

## INTERACTIONS

**DRUG: CYP3A4 inhibitors (e.g., itraconazole, ketoconazole)** may increase concentration/toxicity. **CYP3A4 inducers (e.g., rifampin)** may decrease concentration/effect (avoid use). **HERBAL: Green tea, green tea extracts** may diminish effect. **St. John's wort** may decrease level/effect. **FOOD: Grapefruit products** may increase concentration. **LAB VALUES:** May significantly decrease WBC, Hgb, Hct, platelet count, neutrophils.

## AVAILABILITY (Rx)

**Injection, Powder for Reconstitution:** 3.5 mg.

## ADMINISTRATION/HANDLING

🝆 IV

**Reconstitution** • Reconstitute vial with 3.5 ml 0.9% NaCl to provide a concentration of 1 mg/ml.
**Rate of Administration** • Give as bolus IV injection over 3–5 sec.

---

✦ Canadian trade name    🗡 Non-Crushable Drug    **HIGH ALERT** High Alert drug

**3**

**Storage** • Store unopened vials at room temperature. • Once reconstituted, solution may be stored at room temperature for up to 3 days or for 5 days if refrigerated.

**SUBCUTANEOUS**

**Reconstitution** • Reconstitute vial with 1.4 ml 0.9% NaCl to provide a concentration of 2.5 mg/ml.

# INDICATIONS/ROUTES/DOSAGE

**Mantle Cell Lymphoma (Initial Treatment)**
IV: ADULTS, ELDERLY: 1.3 mg/m² days 1, 4, 8, 11 of a 21-day cycle for 6 cycles (in combination with rituximab, cyclophosphamide, doxorubicin, and prednisone).

**Mantle Cell Lymphoma (Relapsed)**
IV: Subcutaneous: ADULTS, ELDERLY: Treatment cycle consists of 1.3 mg/m² twice wkly on days 1, 4, 8, and 11 for 2 wks of a 21-day treatment for 8 cycles.

**Multiple Myeloma (Initial Treatment)**
IV: Subcutaneous: ADULTS, ELDERLY: (with melphalan and prednisone) 1.3 mg/m² on days 1, 4, 8, 11, 22, 25, 29, 32 of a 42-day cycle for 4 cycles, then 1.3 mg/m² on days 1, 8, 22, 29 of a 42-day cycle for 5 cycles.

**Multiple Myeloma (Relapsed)**
IV, Subcutaneous: ADULTS, ELDERLY: 1.3 mg/m² twice wkly for 2 wks on days 1, 4, 8, 11 of a 21-day treatment cycle for 8 cycles.

**Dosage Adjustment Guidelines**
Withhold therapy at onset of Grade 3 nonhematologic or Grade 4 hematologic toxicities, excluding neuropathy. When symptoms resolve, resume therapy at a 25% reduced dosage.

**Dosage Adjustment Guidelines with Neuropathic Pain, Peripheral Sensory Neuropathy**
For Grade 1 toxicity with pain or Grade 2 (interfering with function but not activities of daily living [ADL]), 1 mg/m². For Grade 2 toxicity with pain or Grade 3 (interfering with ADL), withhold drug until toxicity is resolved, then reinitiate with 0.7 mg/m². For Grade 4 toxicity (permanent sensory loss that interferes with function), discontinue bortezomib.

**Dosage in Renal Impairment**
No dose adjustment.

**Dosage in Hepatic Impairment**
**Mild impairment:** No initial adjustment. **Moderate (bilirubin greater than 1.5–3 times ULN) to severe (bilirubin greater than 3 times upper limit of normal/ULN) impairment:** Decrease initial dose to 0.7 mg/m² (based on tolerance may increase to 1 mg/m² or decrease to 0.5 mg/m²).

# SIDE EFFECTS

Expected (65%–36%): Fatigue, malaise, asthenia, nausea, diarrhea, anorexia, constipation, fever, vomiting. Frequent (28%–21%): Headache, insomnia, arthralgia, limb pain, edema, paresthesia, dizziness, rash. Occasional (18%–11%): Dehydration, cough, anxiety, bone pain, muscle cramps, myalgia, back pain, abdominal pain, taste alteration, dyspepsia, pruritus, hypotension (including orthostatic hypotension), rigors, blurred vision.

# ADVERSE EFFECTS/ TOXIC REACTIONS

Thrombocytopenia occurs in 40% of pts. Platelet count peaks at day 11, returns to baseline by day 21. GI, intracerebral hemorrhage are associated with drug-induced thrombocytopenia. Anemia occurs in 32% of pts. New onset or worsening of existing neuropathy occurs in 37% of pts. Symptoms may improve in some pts upon drug discontinuation. Pneumonia occurs occasionally.

## NURSING CONSIDERATIONS

### BASELINE ASSESSMENT

Obtain baseline CBC. Ensure adequate hydration prior to initiation of therapy. Antiemetics, antidiarrheals may be effective in preventing, treating nausea, vomiting, diarrhea.

### INTERVENTION/EVALUATION

Routinely assess B/P; monitor pt for orthostatic hypotension. Maintain strict I&O. Monitor CBC, esp. platelet count, throughout treatment. Monitor renal, hepatic, pulmonary function throughout therapy. Encourage adequate fluid intake to prevent dehydration. Monitor temperature and be alert to high potential for fever. Monitor for peripheral neuropathy (burning sensation, neuropathic pain, paresthesia, hyperesthesia). Avoid IM injections, rectal temperatures, other traumas that may induce bleeding.

### PATIENT/FAMILY TEACHING

• Report new/worsening vomiting, bruising/bleeding, breathing difficulties. • Discuss importance of pregnancy testing, avoidance of pregnancy, measures to prevent pregnancy. • Increase fluid intake. • Avoid tasks that require mental alertness, motor skills until response to drug is established.

---

# bosutinib

boe-**sue**-ti-nib
(Bosulif)

## ◆ CLASSIFICATION

**PHARMACOTHERAPEUTIC:** Tyrosine kinase inhibitor. **CLINICAL:** Antineoplastic.

## USES

Treatment of chronic, accelerated, or blast phase Ph⁺ chronic myelogenous leukemia (CML) with resistance or intolerance to prior therapy.

## PRECAUTIONS

**Contraindications:** Hypersensitivity to bosutinib. **Cautions:** Baseline anemia, thrombocytopenia, neutropenia; hepatic impairment, recent diarrhea, pulmonary edema, HF, fluid retention. Pts with history of pancreatitis, moderate to severe renal impairment. Avoid concurrent use of CYP3A4 inducers/inhibitors.

## ACTION

Inhibits Bcr-Abl tyrosine kinase, a translocation-created enzyme, created by the Philadelphia chromosome (Ph¹) abnormality noted in chronic myelogenous leukemia (CML). Inhibits Src-family kinase including Src, Lyn, and Hck. **Therapeutic Effect:** Inhibits tumor cell growth and proliferation in chronic, accelerated, or blast phase CML.

## PHARMACOKINETICS

Well absorbed following oral administration. Protein binding: 94%. Metabolized in liver. Eliminated in feces (91%), urine (3%). **Half-life:** 22.5 hrs.

## ⌛ LIFESPAN CONSIDERATIONS

**Pregnancy/Lactation:** Potential for embryo/fetal toxicity. Avoid pregnancy. Must use effective contraception during, and for at least 30 days after treatment. Unknown if distributed in breast milk. Avoid breastfeeding. **Children:** Safety and efficacy not established in pts younger than 18 yrs. **Elderly:** No age-related precautions noted.

## INTERACTIONS

**DRUG:** Strong CYP3A inhibitors and/or P-glycoprotein (P-gp) inhibitors (e.g., **clarithromycin, ketoconazole, ritonavir, misoprostol, nafcillin, salmeterol**) and moderate CYP3A4 inhibitors (e.g., **ciprofloxacin, diltiazem, erythromycin, verapamil**) may increase concentration/effect. Strong CYP3A4 inducers (e.g., **rifampin,**

phenytoin, phenobarbital) and **moderate CYP3A4 inducers** (e.g., **bosentan, nafcillin, modafinil**) may decrease concentration/effect. **Proton pump inhibitors** (e.g., **omeprazole, pantoprazole**) may reduce absorption, concentration. **HERBAL: St. John's wort** may decrease effectiveness. **FOOD: Grapefruit products** may decrease bosutinib concentration. **LAB VALUES:** May decrease Hgb, platelets, WBCs, serum phosphorous. May increase ALT, AST, bilirubin, lipase.

## AVAILABILITY (Rx)

Tablets: 100 mg, 500 mg.

## ADMINISTRATION/HANDLING

**PO**
• Give with food. Do not break, crush, dissolve, or divide tablets.

## INDICATIONS/ROUTES/DOSAGE

**Chronic Myelogenous Leukemia (CML)**
**PO: ADULTS, ELDERLY:** 500 mg once daily with food. May increase to 600 mg once daily for poor responders without high-grade adverse reactions.

**CML with Baseline Renal Impairment**
**CrCl less than 30 ml/min:** 300 mg once daily. **CrCl 30–50 ml/min:** 400 mg once daily.

**CML with Baseline Hepatic Impairment**
**PO: ADULTS:** 200 mg once daily with food.

**Dosage Modification**
**Hepatotoxicity:** Withhold treatment until serum ALT, AST less than or equal to 2.5 times ULN. Then, resume at 400 mg once daily with food. Discontinue if recovery lasts longer than 4 wks or hepatotoxicity including elevated serum bilirubin levels are greater than 2 times ULN. **Severe Diarrhea:** Withhold until recovery to low-grade diarrhea. Then, resume at 400 mg once daily with food. **Myelosuppression:** Withhold until absolute neutrophil count greater than 1000 cells/mm$^3$ and platelet count greater than 50,000 cells/mm$^3$. Then, resume at same dose if recovery occurs within 2 wks. May reduce dose to 400 mg for recovery lasting greater than 2 wks.

## SIDE EFFECTS

**Frequent (82%–35%):** Diarrhea, nausea, vomiting, abdominal pain, rash. **Occasional (26%–10%):** Pyrexia, fatigue, headache, cough, peripheral edema, arthralgia, anorexia, upper respiratory infection, asthenia, back pain, nasopharyngitis, dizziness, pruritus.

## ADVERSE EFFECTS/TOXIC REACTIONS

Severe fluid retention may result in pleural effusion, pericardial effusion, pulmonary edema, ascites. Neutropenia, thrombocytopenia, anemia is an expected response of drug therapy. Severe diarrhea may result in fluid loss, electrolyte imbalance, hypotension. Hepatotoxicity occurred in 7%–9% of pts.

## NURSING CONSIDERATIONS

### BASELINE ASSESSMENT
Offer emotional support. Assess baseline weight, BMP, LFT. Confirm negative pregnancy test before initiating treatment. Obtain full medication history including vitamins, herbal products. Screen for peripheral edema, signs/symptoms of HF, anemia.

### INTERVENTION/EVALUATION
Weigh daily and monitor for unexpected rapid weight gain, edema. Monitor for changes in serum electrolytes, LFT during treatment. Offer antiemetics for nausea, vomiting. Monitor daily pattern of bowel activity, stool consistency. Monitor CBC for neutropenia, thrombocytopenia, anemia. Assess for bruising, hematuria, jaundice, right upper abdominal pain, weight loss, or acute infection (fever, diaphoresis, lethargy, productive cough).

## PATIENT/FAMILY TEACHING

• Blood levels will be drawn routinely. • Take medication with meals. • Drink plenty of fluids (diarrhea may result in dehydration). • Swallow whole; do not break, chew, crush, dissolve, or divide tablets. • Strictly avoid pregnancy. • Use contraception during treatment and for at least 30 days after treatment. • Report urine changes, bloody or clay-colored stools, upper abdominal pain, nausea, vomiting, bruising, persistent diarrhea, fever, cough, difficulty breathing, chest pain. • Immediately report any newly prescribed medications. • Avoid alcohol, grapefruit products. • Discuss using antacids for indigestion, heartburn, upset stomach (omeprazole, lansoprazole, pantoprazole may reduce absorption, concentration of bosutinib). • Separate antacid dosing by more than 2 hrs before and after medication.

# brentuximab vedotin

bren-**tux**-i-mab ve-**doe**-tin
(Adcetris)

■ **BLACK BOX ALERT** ■ JC virus infection resulting in progressive multifocal leukoencephalopathy and death can occur.

## ◆CLASSIFICATION

**PHARMACOTHERAPEUTIC:** Monoclonal antibody, antimitotic. **CLINICAL:** Antineoplastic.

## USES

Treatment of Hodgkin's lymphoma after failure of autologous hematopoietic stem cell transplant (HSCT) or after failure of at least two prior multiagent chemotherapy regimens in pts who are not transplant candidates. Treatment of systemic anaplastic large-cell lymphoma (ALCL) after failure of at least one prior multiagent chemotherapy regimen.

## PRECAUTIONS

**Contraindications:** Hypersensitivity to brentuximab. Avoid use with bleomycin (increased risk for pulmonary toxicity). **Cautions:** Renal/hepatic impairment, peripheral neuropathy, infusion reactions, neutropenia, tumor lysis syndrome, Stevens-Johnson syndrome, pregnancy.

## ACTION

Binds to CD30-expressing cells, allowing the antibody to direct the drug to a target on lymphoma cells, disrupting the microtubule network within the cell. **Therapeutic Effect:** Induces cell cycle arrest, cell death.

## PHARMACOKINETICS

Minimally metabolized. Protein binding: 68%–82%. Eliminated primarily in feces (72%). **Half-life:** 4–6 days.

## ⏳ LIFESPAN CONSIDERATIONS

**Pregnancy/Lactation:** May cause fetal harm (embryo-fetal toxicities). Unknown if distributed in breast milk. **Children:** Safety and efficacy not established. **Elderly:** Safety and efficacy not established.

## INTERACTIONS

**DRUG: Strong CYP3A4 inhibitors (e.g., atazanavir, clarithromycin, ketoconazole)** increase concentration/effect. **CYP3A4 inducers (e.g., rifampin)** may reduce concentration/effect. **FOOD:** None known. **HERBAL: Echinacea** may decrease effect. **LAB VALUES:** May decrease Hgb, Hct, WBC, RBC, platelets. May increase serum bicarbonate, lactate dehydrogenase, glucose, albumin, magnesium, sodium.

## AVAILABILITY (Rx)

**Injection, Powder for Reconstitution:** 50-mg single-use vial.

## ADMINISTRATION/HANDLING

**IV**

**Reconstitution** • Reconstitute each 50-mg vial with 10.5 ml Sterile Water for Injection, directing the stream toward wall of vial and not at powder. • Gently swirl (do not shake). • This will yield a concentration of 5 mg/ml. • The dose for pts weighing over 100 kg should be calculated for 100 kg. • Reconstituted solution must be transferred to infusion bag with a minimum 100 ml diluent, yielding a final concentration range of 0.4 mg/ml to 1.8 mg/ml brentuximab. • Gently invert bag to mix solution.
**Rate of Administration** • Infuse over 30 min.
**Storage** • Discard if solution contains particulate or is discolored; solution should appear clear to slightly opalescent, colorless. • May store solution at 36°–46°F. • Use within 24 hrs after reconstitution.

### ▓ IV COMPATIBILITIES
0.9% NaCl, D5W, lactated Ringer's.

## INDICATIONS/ROUTES/DOSAGE
◀ALERT▶ Do not give by IV bolus or IV push.

**Hodgkin's Lymphoma**
**IV Infusion: ADULTS/ELDERLY:** 1.8 mg/kg (maximum: 180 mg) IV infused over 30 min every 3 wks. Continue treatment until a maximum of 16 cycles, disease progression, or unacceptable toxicity occurs.

**Systemic Anaplastic Large-Cell Lymphoma**
**IV Infusion: ADULTS/ELDERLY:** 1.8 mg/kg IV infused over 30 min every 3 wks. Continue treatment until a maximum of 16 cycles, disease progression, or unacceptable toxicity occurs.

**Dosage in Renal Impairment**
**CrCl less than 30 ml/min:** Avoid use.

**Dosage in Hepatic Impairment**
**Mild:** Initial dose 1.2 mg/kg (Maximum: 120 mg) q3wks. **Moderate to Severe:** Avoid use.

## SIDE EFFECTS
◀ALERT▶ Effects present as mild, manageable.
**Frequent (52%–22%):** Peripheral neuropathy, fatigue, respiratory tract infection, nausea, diarrhea, fever, rash, abdominal pain, cough, vomiting. **Occasional (19%–11%):** Headache, dizziness, constipation, chills, bone/muscle pain, insomnia, peripheral edema, alopecia. **Rare (10%–5%):** Anxiety, muscle spasm, decreased appetite, dry skin.

## ADVERSE EFFECTS/ TOXIC REACTIONS
Myelosuppression characterized as neutropenia (54% of pts), peripheral neuropathy (52% of pts), thrombocytopenia (28% of pts), anemia (19% of pts) have occurred. Infusion reactions (including anaphylaxis), Stevens-Johnson syndrome have been reported. Tumor lysis syndrome may lead to acute renal failure. Progressive multifocal leukoencephalopathy (changes in mood, confusion, loss of memory, changes in speech, walking, and vision, decreased strength or weakness on one side of body) has been reported.

## NURSING CONSIDERATIONS

### BASELINE ASSESSMENT
Obtain baseline CBC before treatment begins and as needed to monitor response and toxicity but particularly prior to each dosing cycle. Question for evidence of peripheral neuropathy (hypoesthesia, hyperesthesia, paresthesia, burning sensation, neuropathic pain or weakness). Pts experiencing new or worsening neuropathy may require a delay, dose change, or discontinuation of treatment.

## INTERVENTION/EVALUATION

Offer antiemetics to control nausea, vomiting. Monitor for hematologic toxicity (fever, sore throat, signs of local infection, bruising, unusual bleeding), symptoms of anemia (excessive fatigue, weakness). Assess response to medication. Monitor and report nausea, vomiting, diarrhea. Monitor daily pattern of bowel activity, stool consistency. Assess skin for evidence of rash.

## PATIENT/FAMILY TEACHING

• Avoid crowds, persons with known infections. • Report signs of infection at once (fever, flu-like symptoms). • Avoid contact with those who recently received live virus vaccine. • Do not receive immunizations without physician's approval (drug lowers body resistance). • Promptly report fever, easy bruising or unusual bleeding from any site. • Male pts should be warned of potential risk to their reproductive capacities.

# brexpiprazole

brex-**pip**-ra-zole
(Rexulti)

■ **BLACK BOX ALERT** ■ Elderly pts with dementia-related psychosis are at increased risk of death, mainly due to HF, pneumonia. Increased risk of suicidal thoughts and behaviors in patients aged 24 yrs and younger with major depression, other psychiatric disorders.

**Do not confuse brexpiprazole with aripiprazole, esomeprazole, omeprazole, or pantoprazole, or rabeprazole.**

## ◆CLASSIFICATION

**PHARMACOTHERAPEUTIC:** Dopamine agonist. **CLINICAL:** Antipsychotic agent.

## USES

Adjunctive therapy to antidepressants for the treatment of major depressive disorder. Treatment of schizophrenia.

## PRECAUTIONS

**Contraindications:** Hypersensitivity to brexpiprazole. **Cautions:** Concurrent use of CNS depressants (including alcohol), disorders in which CNS depression is a feature, cardiovascular or cerebrovascular disease (may induce hypotension), Parkinson's disease, history of seizures or conditions that may lower seizure threshold (Alzheimer's disease). Pts at risk for pneumonia, elderly, HF, diabetes. Pts at high risk for suicide. Preexisting low WBC/ANC, history of drug-induced leukopenia/neutropenia, dehydration, concurrent antihypertensive medications.

## ACTION

Exact mechanism of action unknown. Provides partial agonist activity at dopamine and serotonin (5-HT$_{1A}$) receptors and antagonist activity at serotonin (5-HT$_{2A}$) receptors. **Therapeutic Effect:** Diminishes schizophrenic, depressive behavior.

## PHARMACOKINETICS

Widely distributed. Metabolized in liver. Protein binding: greater than 99%. Peak plasma concentration: 4 hrs. Steady state reached in 10–12 days. Eliminated in urine (25%), feces (46%). **Half-life:** 86–91 hrs.

## LIFESPAN CONSIDERATIONS

**Pregnancy/Lactation:** Unknown if distributed in breast milk. May cause extrapyramidal and/or withdrawal symptoms in neonates if given in third trimester. **Children:** Safety and efficacy not established. **Elderly:** May have increased risk for adverse effects due to age-related hepatic, renal, cardiac disease. May increase risk of death in elderly pts with dementia-related psychosis.

---

## INTERACTIONS

**DRUG:** Alcohol may potentiate cognitive and motor effects. **Strong CYP3A4 inducers (e.g., carbamazepine, rifampin)** may decrease concentration/effect. **Strong CYP3A4 inhibitors (e.g., itraconazole, ketoconazole), strong CYP2D6 inhibitors (e.g., fluoxetine, paroxetine)** may increase concentration/effect. **HERBAL:** St John's wort may decrease concentration. **Gotu kola, kava kava, St John's wort, valerian** may increase CNS depression. **FOOD:** None known. **LAB VALUES:** May decrease leukocytes, neutrophils. May increase serum blood glucose, lipid levels.

## AVAILABILITY (Rx)

**Tablets:** 0.25 mg, 0.5 mg, 1 mg, 2 mg, 3 mg, 4 mg.

## ADMINISTRATION/HANDLING

**PO**
• Give without regard to food.

## INDICATIONS/ROUTES/DOSAGE

**Major Depression Disorder (MDD)**
**PO: ADULTS, ELDERLY:** Initially, 0.5–1 mg once daily. May increase at weekly intervals, to 1 mg once daily, then up to target dose of 2 mg once daily. **Maximum:** 3 mg once daily.

**Schizophrenia**
**PO: ADULTS, ELDERLY:** Initially, 1 mg once daily on days 1–4. May increase to 2 mg once daily on days 5–7, then to 4 mg once daily on day 8 based on clinical response and tolerability. **Maximum:** 4 mg once daily.

**Dose Modification**
*Renal Impairment (CrCl less than 60 ml/min)*
**Maximum:** 2 mg once daily for MDD, or 3 mg once daily for schizophrenia.
*Hepatic Impairment*
Maximum recommended dose: 2 mg once daily for MDD, or 3 mg once daily for schizophrenia.

*CYP2D6 Poor Metabolizers or Pts Taking Strong CYP2D6 Inhibitors or Strong CYP3A4 Inhibitors*
Administer half of the usual dose.
*CYP2D6 Poor Metabolizers Taking Strong/Moderate CYP3A4 Inhibitors or Pts Taking Strong/Moderate CYP2D6 Inhibitors with Strong/Moderate CYP3A4 Inhibitors*
Administer a quarter of the usual dose.
*Pts Taking Strong CYP3A4 Inducers*
Double the usual dose over 1–2 wks.

## SIDE EFFECTS

**Occasional (9%–4%):** Headache, nasopharyngitis, dyspepsia, akathisia, somnolence, tremor. **Rare (3%–1%):** Constipation, fatigue, increased appetite, weight gain, anxiety, restlessness, dizziness, diarrhea, blurry vision, dry mouth, salivary hypersecretion, abdominal pain, flatulence, myalgia, abnormal dreams, insomnia, hyperhidrosis.

## ADVERSE EFFECTS/TOXIC REACTIONS

May increase risk of death in elderly pts with dementia-related psychosis. Most deaths appeared to be cardiovascular (e.g., HF, sudden death) or infectious (e.g., pneumonia) in nature. Increased incidence of suicidal thoughts and behaviors in pts 24 yrs and younger was reported. May increase risk of neuroleptic malignant syndrome (NMS). Symptoms of NMS may include hyperpyrexia, muscle rigidity, altered mental status, autonomic instability (irregular pulse or blood pressure, tachycardia, diaphoresis, and cardiac dysrhythmia), elevated creatinine, phosphokinase, myoglobinuria (rhabdomyolysis), acute renal failure. Metabolic changes such as hyperglycemia, ketoacidosis, hyperosmolar coma, diabetes mellitus, dyslipidemia, dystonia, and weight gain may occur. Other adverse effects may include leukopenia, neutropenia, agranulocytosis, orthostatic hypotension, syncope, cerebrovascular events (e.g., CVA, transient ischemic attack), seizures, hyperthermia, dysphagia, cognitive or motor impairment, tardive dyskinesia.

## NURSING CONSIDERATIONS

### BASELINE ASSESSMENT

Obtain baseline BMP, capillary blood glucose, vital signs; CBC in pts with preexisting low WBC or history of leukopenia or neutropenia. Receive full medication history and screen for drug interactions. Assess behavior, appearance, emotional state, response to environment, speech pattern, thought content. Correct dehydration, hypovolemia. Assess for suicidal tendencies, history of dementia-related psychosis, HF, CVA, NMS, diabetes.

### INTERVENTION/EVALUATION

Monitor weight, BMP, capillary blood glucose, vital signs. Diligently monitor for extrapyramidal symptoms, tardive dyskinesia, hypotension, syncope, cerebrovascular or cardiovascular dysfunction, NMS. Assess for therapeutic response (greater interest in surroundings, improved self-care, increased ability to concentrate, relaxed facial expression).

### PATIENT/FAMILY TEACHING

• Avoid alcohol. • Avoid tasks that require alertness, motor skills until response to drug is established. • Report worsening depression, suicidal ideation, usual changes in behavior. • Treatment may cause life-threatening conditions such as involuntary, uncontrollable movements; elevated body temperature, altered mental status, high or low blood pressure, seizures. • Pts with HF or active pneumonia are at increased risk of sudden death. • Immediately report fever, cough, increased sputum production, palpitations, fainting, or signs of HF.

# brivaracetam

briv-a-ra-se-tam
(Briviact)
**Do not confuse brivaracetam with levetiracetam.**

## ◆CLASSIFICATION

**PHARMACOTHERAPEUTIC:** Synaptic vesicle protein 2A ligand. **CLINICAL:** Anticonvulsant.

## USES

Adjunctive therapy in the treatment of partial-onset seizures in pts 16 years and older with epilepsy.

## PRECAUTIONS

**Contraindications:** Hypersensitivity to brivaracetam. **Cautions:** Baseline neutropenia, hepatic impairment; pts at high risk for suicide; history of depression, mood disorder, psychiatric disorder; history of drug abuse.

## ACTION

Exact mechanism unknown. Binds to synaptic proteins that modulate neurotransmitter release in the brain. **Therapeutic Effect:** Prevents seizure activity.

## PHARMACOKINETICS

Rapidly, completely absorbed following PO administration. Metabolized primarily by enzymatic hydrolysis, mediated by hepatic and extrahepatic amidase. Protein binding: less than or equal to 20%. Peak plasma concentration: 1 hr. Primarily eliminated in urine (95%). **Half-life:** 9 hrs.

## ⌛ LIFESPAN CONSIDERATIONS

**Pregnancy/Lactation:** Unknown if distributed in breast milk. Must either discontinue drug or discontinue breastfeeding. **Children:** Safety and efficacy not established pts younger than 16 yrs. **Elderly:** Not specified; use caution.

---

 Canadian trade name     Non-Crushable Drug     **HIGH ALERT** High Alert drug

## INTERACTIONS

**DRUG:** **Rifampin** may decrease concentration/effect. May increase concentration/effect of **phenytoin, carbamazepine. HERBAL: Ginseng, goldenseal, gotu kola, hawthorn, melatonin, valerian** may increase CNS depression. **Ginkgo** may decrease anticonvulsant effect. **FOOD:** None known. **LAB VALUES:** May decrease neutrophils, WBCs. May increase serum phenytoin (free and total) levels.

## AVAILABILITY (Rx)

**Tablets:** 10 mg, 25 mg, 50 mg, 75 mg, 100 mg. **Oral Solution:** 10 mg/ml. **Injection Solution:** 50 mg/5 ml.

## ADMINISTRATION/HANDLING

 **IV**

**Reconstitution** • Visually inspect for particulate matter or discoloration. Do not use if particulate matter or discoloration observed. • May be given without further dilution or may be mixed with 0.9% NaCl, 5% dextrose injection.
**Rate of Administration** • Give over 2–15 min.
**Storage** • Injection solution should appear clear and colorless. • Diluted solution should not be stored more than 4 hrs at room temperature. Do not freeze.

**PO**
• Give without regard to food. • Administer tablets whole; do not crush, cut, dissolve, or divide. • Oral solution should appear slightly viscous, clear, colorless to yellowish in color, and have a raspberry flavor. • Store oral solution at room temperature. • Discard unused oral solution remaining after 5 mos of first opening bottle. • Do not freeze oral solution. Oral solution should be delivered using calibrated measuring device (does not require dilution). May give oral solution via nasogastric tube or gastrostomy tube.

## INDICATIONS/ROUTES/DOSAGE

**Partial-Onset Seizures**
**PO/IV: ADOLESCENTS, ADULTS:** Initially, 50 mg twice daily. **Maintenance:** 25–100 mg twice daily. **Maximum:** 200 mg/day. When initiating treatment, gradual dose escalation is not required. Injection solution should be administered at same dose and same frequency as tablets and oral solution. Gradually taper dose to discontinue treatment.

**Dose Modification**
**Concomitant use with rifampin:** May need to increase brivaracetam dosage by 100% (double dose).

**Dosage in Renal Impairment**
No dosage adjustment. Not recommended in pts with ESRD undergoing dialysis (not studied).

**Dosage in Hepatic Impairment**
**Mild, moderate, severe impairment:** Initially, 25 mg twice daily. **Maintenance:** 25–75 mg twice daily. **Maximum:** 75 mg twice daily.

## SIDE EFFECTS

**Occasional (16%–9%):** Somnolence, sedation, dizziness, fatigue. **Rare (5%–2%):** Nausea, vomiting, ataxia, balance disorder, abnormal coordination, nystagmus, irritability, constipation.

## ADVERSE EFFECTS/TOXIC REACTIONS

Sudden discontinuance may increase risk of seizure frequency and status epilepticus. May increase risk of suicidal thoughts or behavior. Psychiatric events including nonpsychotic behavior (anger, agitation, aggression, anxiety, apathy, depression, hyperactivity, irritability, mood swings, nervousness, restlessness, tearfulness) and psychotic symptoms (psychotic behavior with acute psychosis, delirium, hallucinations, paranoia) occurred in 13% of pts. Hypersensitivity reactions including bronchospasm, angioedema were reported. Clinically significant decreased WBC count (less than 3,000 cells/mm$^3$) and decreased neutrophil count (less than 1000 cells/mm$^3$) occurred in 1.8% and 0.3% of pts, respectively.

## NURSING CONSIDERATIONS

### BASELINE ASSESSMENT

Obtain CBC in pts with baseline neutropenia. Review history of seizure disorder (intensity, frequency, duration, LOC). Initiate seizure precautions, fall precautions. Question history of hypersensitivity reaction, hepatic impairment, psychiatric disorder; history of suicidal thoughts or behavior. Obtain urine pregnancy in female pts of reproductive potential.

### INTERVENTION/EVALUATION

Periodically monitor CBC in pts with neutropenia. Monitor phenytoin levels in pts taking concomitant phenytoin (treatment may increase phenytoin levels). Observe for recurrence of seizure activity. Assess for clinical improvement (decrease in intensity/frequency of seizures). Diligently monitor for depression, changes in behavior, psychosis, suicidal ideation. Assist with ambulation if dizziness occurs.

### PATIENT/FAMILY TEACHING

• Drowsiness usually diminishes with continued therapy. • Avoid tasks that require alertness, motor skills until response to drug is established. • Do not abruptly discontinue medication (may precipitate seizures). • Strict maintenance of drug therapy is essential for seizure control. • Report anxiety, anger, depression, mood swings, hostile behavior, thoughts of suicide, unusual changes in behavior. • Difficulty breathing, swelling of tongue or throat may indicate emergent allergic reaction. • Avoid alcohol.

# budesonide

bue-**des**-oh-nide
(Entocort EC, Pulmicort Flexhaler, Pulmicort Respules, Rhinocort Aqua, Uceris)
**Do not confuse budesonide with Budeprion.**

## FIXED-COMBINATION(S)

**Symbicort:** budesonide/formoterol (bronchodilator): 80 mcg/4.5 mcg, 160 mcg/4.5 mcg.

## ◆CLASSIFICATION

**PHARMACOTHERAPEUTIC:** Glucocorticosteroid. **CLINICAL:** Anti-inflammatory, antiallergy.

## USES

**Nasal:** Management of seasonal or perennial allergic rhinitis, nonallergic rhinitis. **Nebulization:** Maintenance or prophylaxis therapy for asthma. **PO: (Entocort EC):** Treatment of mild to moderate active Crohn's disease. Maintenance of clinical remission of mild to moderate Crohn's disease. **(Uceris):** Induction of remission in active, mild to moderate ulcerative colitis. **Oral Inhalation:** Maintenance and prophylactic treatment of asthma. **OFF-LABEL:** Treatment of vasomotor rhinitis.

## PRECAUTIONS

**Contraindications:** Hypersensitivity to budesonide, primary treatment of status asthmaticus, acute episodes of asthma. Not for relief of acute bronchospasms. **Cautions:** Thyroid disease, hepatic impairment, renal impairment, cardiovascular disease, diabetes, glaucoma, cataracts, myasthenia gravis, pts at risk for osteoporosis, seizures, GI disease, post acute MI, elderly.

## ACTION

Inhibits accumulation of inflammatory cells; controls rate of protein synthesis;

decreases migration of polymorphonuclear leukocytes (reverses capillary permeability and lysosomal stabilization at cellular level). **Therapeutic Effect:** Relieves symptoms of allergic rhinitis, asthma, Crohn's disease.

## PHARMACOKINETICS

| Form | Onset | Peak | Duration |
|------|-------|------|----------|
| Pulmicort Respules | 2–8 days | 4–6 wks | — |
| Rhinocort Aqua | 10 hrs | 2 wks | — |

Minimally absorbed from nasal tissue; moderately absorbed from inhalation. Protein binding: 88%. Primarily metabolized in liver. **Half-life:** 2–3 hrs.

## ⏳ LIFESPAN CONSIDERATIONS

**Pregnancy/Lactation:** Unknown if drug crosses placenta or is distributed in breast milk. **Children:** Prolonged treatment or high dosages may decrease short-term growth rate, cortisol secretion. **Elderly:** No age-related precautions noted.

## INTERACTIONS

**DRUG:** **CYP3A4 inhibitors** (e.g., itraconazole, ketoconazole) may increase concentration. **HERBAL: Echinacea** may decrease effects. **FOOD: Grapefruit products** may increase systemic exposure. **LAB VALUES:** May decrease serum potassium.

## AVAILABILITY (Rx)

**Oral Inhalation Powder (Pulmicort Flexhaler):** 90 mcg per inhalation; 180 mcg per inhalation. **Inhalation Suspension for Nebulization (Pulmicort Respules):** 0.25 mg/2 ml; 0.5 mg/2 ml; 1 mg/2 ml. **Nasal Spray (Rhinocort Aqua):** 32 mcg/spray.

⌛ **Capsules, Enteric-Coated (Entocort EC):** 3 mg. **Tablets, Extended-Release: (Uceris):** 9 mg.

## ADMINISTRATION/HANDLING

**Inhalation**
• Shake container well. Instruct pt to exhale completely, place mouthpiece between lips, inhale, hold breath as long as possible before exhaling. • Allow at least 1 min between inhalations. • Rinsing mouth after each use decreases dry mouth, hoarseness.

**Intranasal**
• Instruct pt to clear nasal passages before use. • Tilt pt's head slightly forward. • Insert spray tip into nostril, pointing toward nasal passages, away from nasal septum. • Spray into one nostril while pt holds other nostril closed and concurrently inspires through nostril to allow medication as high into nasal passages as possible.

**Nebulization**
• Shake well before use. • Administer with mouthpiece or face mask. • Rinse mouth following treatment.

**PO**
• May take with or without food. Swallow whole. Do not break, crush, dissolve, or divide capsule or tablet.

## INDICATIONS/ROUTES/DOSAGE

**Rhinitis**
**Intranasal: ADULTS, ELDERLY, CHILDREN 6 YRS AND OLDER:** 1 spray (32 mcg) in each nostril once daily. **Maximum:** 8 sprays (256 mcg)/day for adults and children 12 yrs and older; 4 sprays (128 mcg)/day for children younger than 12 yrs.

**Bronchial Asthma**
**Nebulization: CHILDREN 12 MOS–8 YRS:** *(Previous therapy with bronchodilators alone):* 0.5 mg/day as single dose or 2 divided doses. **Maximum:** 0.5 mg/day. *(Previous therapy with inhaled corticosteroids):* 0.5 mg/day as single dose or 2 divided doses. **Maximum:** 1 mg/day. *(Previous therapy of oral corticosteroids):* 1 mg/day as single dose in 2 divided doses. **Maximum:** 1 mg/day.
**Oral Inhalation:** *(Pulmicort Flexhaler):* **ADULTS, ELDERLY:** Initially, 360 mcg 2 times/

day. **Maximum:** 720 mcg 2 times/day. **CHILDREN, 6 YRS AND OLDER:** 180 mcg 2 times/day. **Maximum:** 360 mcg 2 times/day.

**Crohn's Disease**
**PO: ADULTS, ELDERLY:** 9 mg once daily for up to 8 wks. Recurring episodes may be treated with a repeat 8-wk course of treatment. Maintenance of remission: 6 mg once daily for 3 mos.

**Ulcerative Colitis**
**PO: ADULTS, ELDERLY:** 9 mg once daily in morning for up to 8 wks.

**Dosage in Renal/Hepatic Impairment**
No dose adjustment.

## SIDE EFFECTS

**Frequent (greater than 3%): Nasal:** Mild nasopharyngeal irritation, burning, stinging, dryness; headache, cough. **Inhalation:** Flu-like symptoms, headache, pharyngitis. **Occasional (3%–1%): Nasal:** Dry mouth, dyspepsia, rebound congestion, rhinorrhea, loss of taste. **Inhalation:** Back pain, vomiting, altered taste, voice changes, abdominal pain, nausea, dyspepsia.

## ADVERSE EFFECTS/ TOXIC REACTIONS

Acute hypersensitivity reaction (urticaria, angioedema, severe bronchospasm) occurs rarely.

## NURSING CONSIDERATIONS

**BASELINE ASSESSMENT**
Question for hypersensitivity to any corticosteroids, components.

**INTERVENTION/EVALUATION**
Monitor for relief of symptoms. Auscultate lung sounds.

**PATIENT/FAMILY TEACHING**
• Improvement noted in 24 hrs, but full effect may take 3–7 days. • Report if no improvement in symptoms, sneezing, nasal irritation occurs.

# bumetanide

bue-**met**-a-nide
(Bumex, Burinex ✦)
■ **BLACK BOX ALERT** ■ Excess dosage can lead to profound diuresis with fluid and electrolyte loss.
**Do not confuse bumetanide with Buminate.**

## ◆CLASSIFICATION

**PHARMACOTHERAPEUTIC:** Loop diuretic. **CLINICAL:** Diuretic.

## USES

Management of edema associated with HF, renal, or hepatic disease.

## PRECAUTIONS

**Contraindications:** Hypersensitivity to bumetanide. Anuria, hepatic coma, severe electrolyte depletion (until condition improves or is corrected). **Cautions:** Severe hypersensitivity to sulfonamides; hypotension.

## ACTION

Enhances excretion of sodium, chloride, and, to lesser degree, potassium, by direct action at ascending limb of loop of Henle and in proximal tubule. **Therapeutic Effect:** Produces diuresis.

## PHARMACOKINETICS

| Route | Onset | Peak | Duration |
|-------|-------|------|----------|
| PO | 30–60 min | 60–120 min | 4–6 hrs |
| IV | Rapid | 15–30 min | 2–3 hrs |

Completely absorbed from GI tract (absorption decreased in HF, nephrotic syndrome). Protein binding: 94%–96%. Partially metabolized in liver. Primarily excreted in urine. Not removed by hemodialysis. **Half-life:** 1–1.5 hrs.

## ⧖ LIFESPAN CONSIDERATIONS

**Pregnancy/Lactation:** Unknown if drug is distributed in breast milk.

---

Children: Safety and efficacy not established. Elderly: May be more sensitive to hypotension/electrolyte effects. Increased risk for circulatory collapse or thrombolytic episode. Age-related renal impairment may require reduced or extended dosage interval.

## INTERACTIONS

DRUG: Agents inducing hypokalemia (e.g., metolazone, hydrochlorothiazide) may increase risk of hypokalemia. May increase risk of lithium toxicity. NSAIDs may increase effect. HERBAL: Ephedra, ginseng, yohimbe may worsen hypertension. Garlic may have increased antihypertensive effect. FOOD: None known. LAB VALUES: May increase serum glucose, BUN, uric acid; urinary phosphate. May decrease serum calcium, chloride, magnesium, potassium, sodium.

## AVAILABILITY (Rx)

Injection Solution: 0.25 mg/ml. Tablets: 0.5 mg, 1 mg, 2 mg.

## ADMINISTRATION/HANDLING

 IV

Rate of Administration • May give undiluted but is compatible with D₅W, 0.9% NaCl, or lactated Ringer's solution. • Administer IV push over 1–2 min. • May give through Y tube or 3-way stopcock. • May give as continuous infusion.
Storage • Store at room temperature. • Stable for 24 hrs if diluted.

### PO
• Give with food to avoid GI upset, preferably with breakfast (may prevent nocturia).

## ▒ IV INCOMPATIBILITY

Midazolam (Versed).

## ▒ IV COMPATIBILITIES

Aztreonam (Azactam), cefepime (Maxipime), dexmedetomidine (Precedex), diltiazem (Cardizem), dobutamine (Dobutrex), furosemide (Lasix), lorazepam (Ativan), milrinone (Primacor), morphine, piperacillin and tazobactam (Zosyn), propofol (Diprivan).

## INDICATIONS/ROUTES/DOSAGE

### Edema
PO: ADULTS, ELDERLY: 0.5–2 mg 1–2 times/day. May repeat in 4–5 hrs for up to 2 doses. Maximum: 10 mg/day.
IV, IM: ADULTS, ELDERLY: 0.5–1 mg/dose; may repeat in 2–3 hrs for up to 2 doses (maximum: 10 mg/day) or 0.5–2 mg/hr by continuous IV infusion.

### Usual Pediatric Dosage
IV, IM, PO: CHILDREN: 0.015–0.1 mg/kg/dose q6–24h. Maximum: 10 mg/day. NEONATES: 0.01–0.05 mg/kg/dose q12–48h.

### Dosage in Renal/Hepatic Impairment
Use caution; contraindicated in anuria, hepatic coma.

## SIDE EFFECTS

Expected: Increased urinary frequency and urine volume. Frequent (5%): Muscle cramps, dizziness, hypotension, headache, nausea. Occasional (3%–1%): Impaired hearing, pruritus, EKG changes, weakness, hives, abdominal pain, dyspepsia, musculoskeletal pain, rash, nausea, vomiting. Rare (less than 1%): Chest pain, ear pain, fatigue, dry mouth, premature ejaculation, impotence, nipple tenderness.

## ADVERSE EFFECTS/TOXIC REACTIONS

Vigorous diuresis may lead to profound water and electrolyte depletion, resulting in hypokalemia, hyponatremia, dehydration, coma, circulatory collapse. Ototoxicity manifested as deafness, vertigo, tinnitus may occur, esp. in pts with severe renal impairment or those taking other ototoxic drugs. Blood dyscrasias, acute hypotensive episodes have been reported.

## NURSING CONSIDERATIONS

### BASELINE ASSESSMENT

Obtain baseline vital signs, esp. B/P for hypotension, before administration. Assess baseline electrolytes, particularly for hypokalemia, hyponatremia. Assess for edema. Observe skin turgor, mucous membranes for hydration status. Initiate I&O, obtain baseline weight.

### INTERVENTION/EVALUATION

Continue to monitor B/P, vital signs, electrolytes, I&O, weight. Note extent of diuresis. Watch for changes from initial assessment (hypokalemia may result in muscle weakness, tremor, muscle cramps, altered mental status, cardiac arrhythmias; hyponatremia may result in confusion, thirst, cold/clammy skin).

### PATIENT/FAMILY TEACHING

• Expect increased urinary frequency/volume. • Report auditory abnormalities (e.g., sense of fullness in ears, tinnitus). • Eat foods high in potassium such as whole grains (cereals), legumes, meat, bananas, apricots, orange juice, potatoes (white, sweet), raisins. • Rise slowly from sitting/lying position.

---

# buprenorphine TOP 100

bue-pre-**nor**-feen
(Belbuca, Buprenex, Butrans, Probuphine, Suboxone, Subutex)

■ **BLACK BOX ALERT** ■ **Transdermal:** Prolonged use during pregnancy may result in neonatal abstinence syndrome. Potential for abuse, misuse, and diversion. Do not exceed dose of one 20 mcg/hr patch due to risk of QT interval prolongation. May cause potentially life-threatening respiratory depression.

**Do not confuse Buprenex with Bumex, or buprenorphine with bupropion.**

## FIXED-COMBINATION(S)

**Brunavail:** buprenorphine/naloxone (narcotic antagonist): 2.1 mg/0.3 mg; 4.2 mg/0.7 mg; 6.3 mg/1 mg. **Suboxone:** buprenorphine/naloxone: 2 mg/0.5 mg, 4 mg/1 mg, 8 mg/2 mg, 12 mg/3 mg. **Zubsolv:** buprenorphine/naloxone: 1.4 mg/0.36 mg; 5.7 mg/1.4 mg.

## ◆CLASSIFICATION

**PHARMACOTHERAPEUTIC:** Opioid agonist, antagonist injection **(Schedule V)**; tablet **(Schedule III)**. **CLINICAL:** Opioid dependence adjunct, analgesic.

## USES

**Sublingual Tablet:** Treatment of opioid dependence. **Implant:** Maintenance treatment of opioid dependence in pts who achieved/sustained prolonged clinical stability on low to moderate doses of a transmucosal buprenorphine product. **Injection:** Relief of moderate to severe pain. **Transdermal, Buccal film:** Moderate to severe chronic pain requiring continuous around-the-clock opioid analgesic for extended period. **OFF-LABEL:** Injection: Heroin/opioid withdrawal in hospitalized pts.

## PRECAUTIONS

**Contraindications:** Hypersensitivity to buprenorphine. **Transdermal patch, Buccal film:** Significant respiratory depression, severe asthma, known or suspected GI obstruction, including paralytic ileus. **Cautions:** Hepatic/renal impairment, elderly, debilitated, pediatric pts, head injury/increased intracranial pressure, pts at risk for respiratory depression, hyperthyroidism, myxedema, adrenal cortical insufficiency (e.g., Addison's disease), urethral stricture, CNS depression, morbid obesity, toxic psychosis, prostatic hypertrophy, delirium tremens, kyphoscoliosis, biliary tract dysfunction, acute pancreatitis, acute abdominal conditions, acute alcoholism,

---

pts with prolonged QT syndrome, concurrent use of antiarrhythmics, hypovolemia, cardiovascular disease, ileus, bowel obstruction, hx of seizure disorder.

## ACTION

Binds to opioid receptors within CNS. **Therapeutic Effect:** Suppresses opioid withdrawal symptoms, cravings. Alters pain perception, emotional response to pain.

## PHARMACOKINETICS

| Route | Onset | Peak | Duration |
|---|---|---|---|
| Sublingual | 15 min | 1 hr | 6 hrs |
| IV | Less than 15 min | Less than 1 hr | 6 hrs |
| IM | 15 min | 1 hr | 6 hrs |

Excreted primarily in feces with lesser amount eliminated in urine. Protein binding: High. **Half-life: Parenteral:** 2–3 hrs; **Sublingual:** 37 hrs (increased in hepatic impairment).

## ⌛ LIFESPAN CONSIDERATIONS

**Pregnancy/Lactation:** Crosses placenta. Distributed in breast milk. Breast-feeding not recommended. Neonatal withdrawal noted in infant if mother was treated with buprenorphine during pregnancy with onset of withdrawal symptoms generally noted on day 1, manifested as hypertonia, tremor, agitation, myoclonus. Apnea, bradycardia, seizures occur rarely. **Children:** Safety and efficacy of injection form not established in those 2–12 yrs. Safety and efficacy of tablet, fixed-combination form not established in pts 16 yrs or younger. **Elderly:** Age-related hepatic impairment may require dosage adjustment.

## INTERACTIONS

**DRUG: CNS depressants, MAOIs** may increase CNS or respiratory depression, hypotension. **CYP3A4 inhibitors (e.g., azole antifungals, macrolide antibiotics, protease inhibitors)** may increase plasma concentration. **CYP3A4 inducers (e.g., carbamazepine, phenytoin, rifampin)** may cause increased clearance of buprenorphine. May decrease effects of **other opioid analgesics. HERBAL: St. John's wort, kava kava, gotu kola, valerian** may increase CNS depression. **FOOD:** None known. **LAB VALUES:** May increase serum amylase, lipase.

## AVAILABILITY (Rx)

**Buccal Film:** 75 mcg, 150 mcg, 300 mcg, 450 mcg, 600 mcg, 750 mcg, 900 mcg. **Implant (Probuphine):** Implant containing 80 mg buprenorphine HCl. **Injection Solution (Buprenex):** 0.3 mg/1 ml. **Tablets, Sublingual:** 2 mg, 8 mg. **Transdermal (Butrans):** 5 mcg/hr, 7.5 mcg/hr, 10 mcg/hr, 15 mcg/hr, 20 mcg/hr.

## ADMINISTRATION/HANDLING

 **IV**

**Reconstitution** • May be diluted with lactated Ringer's solution, D₅W, 0.9% NaCl.
**Rate of Administration** • If given as IV push, administer over at least 2 min.

**IM**
• Give deep IM into large muscle mass.

**Buccal Film**
Moisten inside cheek. Apply with dry finger. Press and hold in place for 5 sec. Keep film in place until dissolved (approx 30 min). Do not chew, swallow, touch, or move film. Do not cut/tear. Avoid areas with open sores/lesions.

**Sublingual**
• Instruct pt to dissolve tablet(s) under tongue; avoid swallowing (reduces drug bioavailability). • For doses greater than 2 tablets, either place all tablets at once or 2 tablets at a time under the tongue.
**Storage** • Store parenteral form at room temperature. • Protect from prolonged exposure to light. • Store tablets at room temperature.

**Transdermal**
- Apply to clean, dry, intact skin of upper outer arm, upper chest, upper back, or side of chest. • Wear for 7 days.
- Wait minimum of 21 days before reapplying to same site. • If patch falls off during 7-day dosing interval, apply new patch to a different skin site.

## ▦ IV INCOMPATIBILITIES

Diazepam (Valium), furosemide (Lasix), lorazepam (Ativan).

## ▦ IV COMPATIBILITIES

Allopurinol (Aloprim, Zyloprim), aztreonam (Azactam), cefepime (Maxipime), diphenhydramine (Benadryl), granisetron (Kytril), haloperidol (Haldol), heparin, linezolid (Zyvox), midazolam (Versed), piperacillin/tazobactam (Zosyn), promethazine (Phenergan), propofol (Diprivan).

## INDICATIONS/ROUTES/DOSAGE

**Opioid Dependence**
**Sublingual: ADULTS, CHILDREN 13 YRS AND OLDER:** 8 mg on day 1, then 16 mg on day 2 and subsequent induction days. Range: 12–16 mg/day of Subutex used as induction with switch to Suboxone for maintenance. **Implant:** Four implants inserted subdermally in upper arm for 6 mos of treatment.

**Moderate to Severe Pain**
**IM/IV: ADULTS, CHILDREN 13 YRS AND OLDER:** 0.3 mg (1 ml) q6–8h prn; may repeat once 30–60 min after initial dose. Range: 0.15–0.6 mg q4–8h prn. **ELDERLY:** 0.15 mg q6h prn. **CHILDREN 2–12 YRS:** 2–6 mcg/kg q4–6h prn.

**Transdermal: ADULTS, ELDERLY: (OPIOID NAIVE):** Initial dose always 5 mcg/hr once q7days. **THOSE ALREADY RECEIVING OPIOIDS:** Refer to conversion chart in package insert. Do not increase dose until pt exposed to previous dose for 72 hrs.

**Buccal: ADULTS, ELDERLY: (OPIOID NAIVE):** Initially, 75 mcg once or q12h for 4 days, then 150 mcg q12h. **(OPIOID EXPERIENCED):** Taper current opioid to no more than 30 mg oral morphine equivalent. Based on opioid dose prior to tapering: 75 mcg once daily or q12h for less than 30 mg; 150 mcg q12h for 30–89 mg; 300 mcg q12h for 90–160 mg.

**Dosage in Renal Impairment**
Use caution.

**Dosage in Hepatic Impairment**
**Injection:** Use caution.
**Transdermal:** No adjustment.

## SIDE EFFECTS

**Frequent (67%–10%):** Sedation, dizziness, nausea. **Butrans (more than 5%):** Nausea, headache, pruritus at application site, dizziness, rash, vomiting, constipation, dry mouth. **Occasional (5%–1%):** Headache, hypotension, vomiting, miosis, diaphoresis. **Rare (less than 1%):** Dry mouth, pallor, visual abnormalities, injection site reaction.

## ADVERSE EFFECTS/ TOXIC REACTIONS

Overdosage results in cold, clammy skin, weakness, confusion, severe respiratory depression, cyanosis, pinpoint pupils, seizures, extreme drowsiness progressing to stupor, coma.

## NURSING CONSIDERATIONS

### BASELINE ASSESSMENT

Obtain baseline B/P, pulse rate. Assess mental status, alertness. Assess type, location, intensity of pain. Obtain history of pt's last opioid use. Assess for early signs of withdrawal symptoms before initiating therapy.

### INTERVENTION/EVALUATION

Monitor for change in respirations, B/P, rate/quality of pulse, mental status. Assess lab results. Initiate deep breathing, coughing exercises, particularly in pts with pulmonary impairment. Assess for clinical improvement; record onset of relief of pain.

Monitor strictly for compliance, signs of abuse or misuse.

### PATIENT/FAMILY TEACHING

• Change positions slowly to avoid dizziness, orthostatic hypotension. • Avoid tasks that require alertness, motor skills until response to drug is established. • Avoid alcohol, sedatives, antidepressants, tranquilizers.

## *buPROPion

bue-**proe**-pee-on
(Aplenzin, Buproban, Forfivo XL, Wellbutrin, Wellbutrin SR, Wellbutrin XL, Zyban)

■ **BLACK BOX ALERT** ■ Increased risk of suicidal thinking and behavior in children, adolescents, young adults 18–24 yrs with major depressive disorder, other psychiatric disorders. Agitation, hostility, depressed mood also reported. Use in smoking cessation may cause serious neuropsychiatric events.

**Do not confuse Aplenzin with Relenza, bupropion with buspirone, Wellbutrin SR with Wellbutrin XL, or Zyban with Diovan or Zagam.**

### ◆CLASSIFICATION

**PHARMACOTHERAPEUTIC:** Aminoketone. **CLINICAL:** Antidepressant, smoking cessation aid.

## USES

Treatment of depression, seasonal affective disorder (SAD). Zyban assists in smoking cessation. **OFF-LABEL:** Treatment of ADHD in adults, children. Depression associated with bipolar disorder.

## PRECAUTIONS

**Contraindications:** Hypersensitivity to buPROPion. Current or prior diagnosis of anorexia nervosa or bulimia, seizure disorder, use within 14 days of MAOIs; concomitant use of other bupropion products; pts undergoing abrupt discontinuation of alcohol or sedatives. Initiation of bupropion in pts receiving linezolid or IV methylene blue. **Aplenzin, Wellbutrin XL (additional):** Conditions increasing seizure risk, severe head injury, stroke, CNS tumor/infection. **Cautions:** History of seizure, cranial or head trauma, cardiovascular disease, history of hypertension or coronary artery disease, elderly, pts at high risk for suicide, renal/hepatic impairment. Concurrent use of antipsychotics, antidepressants, theophylline, steroids, stimulants, hypoglycemic agents, excessive use of alcohol, sedatives/hypnotics, opioids.

## ACTION

Blocks reuptake of neurotransmitters, (dopamine, norepinephrine) at CNS presynaptic membranes. **Therapeutic Effect:** Relieves depression. Eliminates nicotine withdrawal symptoms.

## PHARMACOKINETICS

Rapidly absorbed from GI tract. Protein binding: 84%. Crosses the blood-brain barrier. Metabolized in liver. Primarily excreted in urine. **Half-life:** 14 hrs.

## ⌛ LIFESPAN CONSIDERATIONS

**Pregnancy/Lactation:** Unknown if drug crosses placenta or is distributed in breast milk. **Children:** More sensitive to increased dosage, toxicity; increased risk of suicidal ideation, worsening of depression. Safety and efficacy not established in pts younger than 18 yrs. **Elderly:** More sensitive to anticholinergic, sedative, cardiovascular effects. Age-related renal impairment may require dosage adjustment.

## INTERACTIONS

**DRUG: Ritonavir, efavirenz** may reduce concentration. **Carbamazepine, phenobarbital, phenytoin** may decrease effectiveness. **MAOIs** may increase risk of toxicity. **Levodopa, amantadine** may increase risk of side effects. **HERBAL: Gotu kola, kava kava,**

St. John's wort, valerian may increase CNS depression. **FOOD:** None known. **LAB VALUES:** May decrease WBC.

## AVAILABILITY (Rx)

Tablets (Wellbutrin): 75 mg, 100 mg.

Tablets, Extended-Release (24 hr): 174 mg, 348 mg, 522 mg (Aplenzin); 450 mg (Forfivo XL); 150 mg, 300 mg (Wellbutrin XL). Tablets, Sustained-Release (12 hr): 100 mg, 150 mg, 200 mg (Wellbutrin SR), 150 mg (Zyban).

## ADMINISTRATION/HANDLING

**PO**

• Give without regard to food (give with food if GI irritation occurs). • Give at least 4-hr interval for immediate onset and 8-hr interval for sustained-release tablet to avoid seizures. • Give Aplenzin once daily in the morning. • Avoid bedtime dosage (decreases risk of insomnia). • Do not break, crush, dissolve, or divide sustained-, extended-release preparations.

## INDICATIONS/ROUTES/DOSAGE

**Depression**

**PO** *(Immediate-Release)*: **ADULTS:** Initially, 100 mg twice daily. May increase to 100 mg 3 times/day no sooner than 3 days after beginning therapy. **Maximum:** 150 mg 3 times/day. **ELDERLY:** Initially, 37.5 2 times/day. May increase by 37.5 q3–4days. **Maximum:** 300 mg/day in divided doses.

**PO** *(Sustained-Release)*: **ADULTS:** Initially, 150 mg/day as a single dose in the morning. May increase to 150 mg twice daily as early as day 4 after beginning therapy. **Maximum:** 400 mg/day in 2 divided doses. **ELDERLY:** Initially, 100 mg/day. May increase by 100 mg q3–4days. **Maximum:** 300 mg/day in divided doses.

**PO** *(Extended-Release)*: **ADULTS:** 150 mg once daily. May increase to 300 mg once daily. **Maximum:** 450 mg/day. *(Forfivo XL):* Use only after initial dose titration with other bupropion products.

*(Aplenzin):* Initially, 174 mg once daily in morning; may increase as soon as 4 days to 348 mg/day. **Maximum:** 522 mg/day.

**Smoking Cessation**

**PO:** **ADULTS, ELDERLY:** (Zyban): Initially, 150 mg/day for 3 days, then 150 mg twice daily for 7–12 wks.

**SAD**

**PO:** **ADULTS, ELDERLY:** (Wellbutrin XL): 150 mg/day for 1 wk, then 300 mg/day. Begin in autumn (Sept–Nov). End of treatment begins in spring (Mar–Apr) by decreasing dose to 150 mg/day for 2 wks before discontinuation. **(Aplenzin):** 174 mg once daily. May increase after 1 wk to 348 mg once daily.

**Dosage in Renal Impairment**

Use caution.

**Dosage in Hepatic Impairment**

**Mild to moderate impairment:** Use caution, reduce dosage. **Severe impairment:** Use extreme caution. **Maximum dose:** Aplenzin: 174 mg every other day. Wellbutrin: 75 mg/day. Wellbutrin SR: 100 mg/day or 150 mg every other day. Wellbutrin XL: 150 mg every other day. Zyban: 150 mg every other day.

## SIDE EFFECTS

**Frequent (32%–18%):** Constipation, weight gain or loss, nausea, vomiting, anorexia, dry mouth, headache, diaphoresis, tremor, sedation, insomnia, dizziness, agitation. **Occasional (10%–5%):** Diarrhea, akinesia, blurred vision, tachycardia, confusion, hostility, fatigue.

## ADVERSE EFFECTS/ TOXIC REACTIONS

Risk of seizures increases in pts taking more than 150 mg/dose; in pts with history of bulimia, seizure disorders, discontinuing drugs that may lower seizure threshold.

---

## NURSING CONSIDERATIONS

### BASELINE ASSESSMENT

Assess psychological status, thought content, suicidal tendencies, appearance. For pts on long-term therapy, hepatic/renal function tests should be performed periodically.

### INTERVENTION/EVALUATION

Supervise suicidal-risk pt closely during early therapy and dose changes (as depression lessens, energy level improves, increasing suicide potential). Assess appearance, behavior, speech pattern, level of interest, mood changes.

### PATIENT/FAMILY TEACHING

• Full therapeutic effect may be noted in 4 wks. • Avoid tasks that require alertness, motor skills until response to drug is established. • Report signs/symptoms of seizure, worsening depression, suicidal ideation, unusual behavioral changes. • Avoid alcohol. • Do not chew, crush, dissolve, or divide sustained-, extended-release tablets.

---

# *busPIRone

bue-**spye**-rone
(Apo-Buspirone ✦)
**Do not confuse buspirone with bupropion.**

### ◆ CLASSIFICATION

**PHARMACOTHERAPEUTIC:** Nonbarbiturate. **CLINICAL:** Antianxiety.

## USES

Short-term management (up to 4 wks) of generalized anxiety disorder (GAD). **OFF-LABEL:** Augmenting medication for antidepressants.

## PRECAUTIONS

**Contraindications:** Hypersensitivity to busPIRone. **Cautions:** Concurrent use of MAOIs, severe hepatic/renal impairment (not recommended).

## ACTION

Exact mechanism of action unknown. Binds to serotonin, dopamine at presynaptic neurotransmitter receptors in CNS. **Therapeutic Effect:** Produces anxiolytic effect.

## PHARMACOKINETICS

Rapidly and completely absorbed from GI tract. Protein binding: 95%. Metabolized in liver. Primarily excreted in urine. Not removed by hemodialysis. **Half-life:** 2–3 hrs.

## ⧗ LIFESPAN CONSIDERATIONS

**Pregnancy/Lactation:** Unknown if drug crosses placenta or is distributed in breast milk. **Children:** Safety and efficacy not established. **Elderly:** No age-related precautions noted.

## INTERACTIONS

**DRUG: CNS depressants (e.g., alcohol, alprazolam, lorazepam, morphine, oxycodone, tramadol)** potentiate effect, may increase sedation. **CYP3A4 inhibitors (e.g., erythromycin, ketoconazole)** may increase concentration/effect. **CYP3A4 inducers (e.g., rifampin)** may decrease concentration/effect. May increase effects of **MAOIs. HERBAL: Gotu kola, kava kava, St. John's wort, valerian** may increase CNS depression. **FOOD: Grapefruit products** may increase concentration, risk of toxicity. **LAB VALUES:** May produce false positive urine metanephrine/catecholamine assay test.

## AVAILABILITY (Rx)

**Tablets:** 5 mg, 7.5 mg, 10 mg, 15 mg, 30 mg.

## ADMINISTRATION/HANDLING

### PO

• Give without regard to food.

---

## INDICATIONS/ROUTES/DOSAGE

**Short-Term Management (up to 4 wks) of Anxiety Disorders**
**PO: ADULTS, ELDERLY:** 7.5 mg twice daily. May increase by 5 mg/day every 2–4 days. **Maintenance:** 15–30 mg/day in 2–3 divided doses. **Maximum:** 60 mg/day.

**Dosage in Renal/Hepatic Impairment**
Not recommended in severe impairment.

## SIDE EFFECTS

**Frequent (12%–6%):** Dizziness, drowsiness, nausea, headache. **Occasional (5%–2%):** Nervousness, fatigue, insomnia, dry mouth, light-headedness, mood swings, blurred vision, poor concentration, diarrhea, paresthesia. **Rare:** Muscle pain/stiffness, nightmares, chest pain, involuntary movements.

## ADVERSE EFFECTS/ TOXIC REACTIONS

No evidence of drug tolerance, psychological or physical dependence, withdrawal syndrome. Overdose may produce severe nausea, vomiting, dizziness, drowsiness, abdominal distention, excessive pupil constriction.

## NURSING CONSIDERATIONS

### BASELINE ASSESSMENT

Assess degree/manifestations of anxiety. Offer emotional support. Assess motor responses (agitation, trembling, tension), autonomic responses (cold, clammy hands; diaphoresis).

### INTERVENTION/EVALUATION

For pts on long-term therapy, CBC, LFT, renal function tests should be performed periodically. Assist with ambulation if drowsiness, dizziness occur. Evaluate for therapeutic response: calm facial expression, decreased restlessness, lessened insomnia, mental status.

### PATIENT/FAMILY TEACHING

• Improvement may be noted in 7–10 days, but optimum therapeutic effect generally takes 3–4 wks. • Drowsiness usually disappears during continued therapy. • If dizziness occurs, slowly go from lying to standing. • Avoid tasks that require alertness, motor skills until response to drug is established. • Avoid alcohol, grapefruit products.

# cabazitaxel

ka-**baz**-i-**tax**-el
(Jevtana)

■ **BLACK BOX ALERT** ■ All pts should be premedicated with a corticosteroid, an antihistamine, and an H$_2$ antagonist prior to infusion. Severe hypersensitivity reactions have occurred. Immediately discontinue infusion and give appropriate treatment if hypersensitivity reaction occurs. Neutropenic deaths reported. CBC, particularly ANC, should be obtained prior to and during treatment. Do not administer with neutrophil count 1,500 cells/mm$^3$ or less.

**Do not confuse cabazitaxel with paclitaxel or Paxil, or Jevtana with Januvia, Levitra, or Sentra.**

## ◆CLASSIFICATION

**PHARMACOTHERAPEUTIC:** Microtubule inhibitor. **CLINICAL:** Antineoplastic.

## USES

Used in combination with prednisone for treatment of hormone-refractory metastatic prostate cancer previously treated with a docetaxel-containing regimen.

## PRECAUTIONS

**Contraindications:** Hypersensitivty to cabazitaxel. Severe hepatic impairment (total bilirubin greater than 3 times upper limit of normal [ULN]). Neutrophil count of 1,500/mm$^3$ or less, history of hypersensitivity to polysorbate 80. **Caution:** Mild to moderate hepatic impairment (bilirubin equal to or less than 3 times ULN), elderly, pregnancy, renal impairment (CrCl less than 30 ml/min). Pts at risk for developing GI complications (e.g., GI ulceration, concomitant use of NSAIDs).

## ACTION

Binds to tubulin to promote assembly into microtubules and inhibits disassembly, which inhibits microtubules depolymerization/cell division. **Therapeutic Effect:** Blocks cells in mitotic phase of cell cycle, inhibiting tumor proliferation.

## PHARMACOKINETICS

Widely distributed. Metabolized in liver. Protein binding: 89%–92%. Excreted in feces (76%), urine (3.7%). **Half-life:** 95 hrs.

## ⧗ LIFESPAN CONSIDERATIONS

**Pregnancy/Lactation:** May cause fetal harm. Crosses placental barrier. Breastfeeding not recommended. **Children:** Safety and efficacy not established. **Elderly:** Pts 65 yrs and older have 5% greater risk of developing neutropenia, fatigue, dizziness, fever, urinary tract infection, dehydration.

## INTERACTIONS

**DRUG:** Concurrent use of **strong CYP3A4 inhibitors (e.g., atazanavir, clarithromycin, ketoconazole, ritonavir)** may increase concentration of cabazitaxel and is not recommended. **Strong CYP3A4 inducers (e.g., carbamazepine, phenobarbital, phenytoin, rifabutin, rifampin, rifapentine)** may decrease cabazitaxel concentration effects. **Live virus vaccine** may potentiate virus replication, increase vaccine's side effects, decrease response to vaccine. **HERBAL: St. John's wort, valerian** may increase CNS depression. **St. John's wort** may decrease concentration, effect. **FOOD: Grapefruit products** may increase concentration/effects. **LAB VALUES:** May increase serum bilirubin. May decrease Hgb, Hct, neutrophils, platelets.

## AVAILABILITY (Rx)

**Injection, Single-Use Vials, 2 per Kit:** 60 mg/1.5 ml polysorbate 80 vial and one vial containing 13% ethanol (in diluent).

## ADMINISTRATION/HANDLING

◄**ALERT**► Wear gloves during preparation, handling. Two-step dilution process must be performed under aseptic conditions to prepare second (final) infusion solution. Medication undergoes two dilutions. After second dilution, administration should be initiated within 30 min.

### Reconstitution

**Step 1, First Dilution:** • Each vial of cabazitaxel contains 60 mg/1.5 ml; must first be mixed with entire contents of supplied diluent. • Once reconstituted, resultant solution contains 10 mg/ml of cabazitaxel. • When transferring diluent, direct needle onto inside vial wall and inject slowly to limit foaming. • Remove syringe and needle, then gently mix initial diluted solution by repeated inversions for at least 45 sec to ensure full mixing of drug and diluent. • Do not shake. • Allow any foam to dissipate.

**Step 2, Final Dilution:** • Withdraw recommended dose and further dilute with 250 ml 0.9% NaCl or D5W. • If dose greater than 65 mg is required, use larger volume of 0.9% NaCl or D5W so that concentration of 0.26 mg/ml is not exceeded. • Concentration of final infusion should be between 0.10 and 0.26 mg/ml.

**Rate of Administration** • Infuse over 1 hr using in-line 0.22-micron filter.

**Storage** • Store vials at room temperature. • First dilution solution stable for 30 min. • Final dilution solution stable for 8 hrs at room temperature or 24 hrs if refrigerated.

## INDICATIONS/ROUTES/DOSAGE

◀**ALERT**▶ Antihistamine (dexchlorpheniramine 5 mg, diphenhydramine 25 mg, or equivalent antihistamine), corticosteroid (dexamethasone 8 mg or equivalent steroid), and $H_2$ antagonist (ranitidine 50 mg or equivalent $H_2$ antagonist) should be given at least 30 min prior to each dose to reduce risk/severity of hypersensitivity.

**Hormone-Refractory Metastatic Prostate Cancer**

◀**ALERT**▶ Monitoring of CBC is essential on wkly basis during cycle 1 and before each treatment cycle thereafter so that the dose can be adjusted.

**IV Infusion: ADULTS, ELDERLY:** 25 mg/$m^2$ given as 1-hr infusion every 3 wks in combination with 10 mg prednisone daily throughout treatment.

### Dose Modification

**Grade 3 neutropenia, febrile neutropenia, grade 3 or persistent diarrhea, neuropathy:** Reduce dosage to 20 mg/$m^2$ after treatment interruption.

### Dosage with Strong CYP3A Inhibitors

Consider dose reduction by 25%.

### Dosage in Renal Impairment

**CrCl less than 30 ml/min:** Use with caution.

### Dosage in Hepatic Impairment

**Total bilirubin greater than or equal to ULN or ALT and/or AST greater than or equal to 1.5 times ULN:** Not recommended.

## SIDE EFFECTS

**Frequent (47%–16%):** Diarrhea, fatigue, nausea, vomiting, constipation, esthesia, abdominal pain, anorexia, back pain. **Occasional (13%–5%):** Peripheral neuropathy, fever, dyspnea, cough, arthralgia, dysgeusia, dyspepsia, alopecia, peripheral edema, weight decrease, urinary tract infection, dizziness, headache, muscle spasm, dysuria, hematuria, mucosal inflammation, dehydration.

## ADVERSE EFFECTS/ TOXIC REACTIONS

Hypersensitivity reaction may include generalized rash, erythema, hypotension, bronchospasm. 94% of pts develop grade 1–4 neutropenia and associated complications including anemia, thrombocytopenia, sepsis. GI abnormalities, hypertension, arrhythmias, renal failure may occur.

## NURSING CONSIDERATIONS

### BASELINE ASSESSMENT

Obtain baseline CBC, BMP, LFT, serum testosterone levels prior to initiation of therapy. Offer emotional support.

### INTERVENTION/EVALUATION

Assess CBC, ANC prior to each infusion. Monitor CBC, ANC on wkly basis during cycle 1 and before each treatment cycle thereafter; do not administer if ANC less than 1,500 cells/mm³. Monitor ALT, AST, renal function. Monitor for hypersensitivity reaction (rash, erythema, dyspnea). Encourage adequate fluid intake. Monitor daily pattern of bowel activity, stool consistency. Offer antiemetics if nausea, vomiting occur. Closely monitor for signs/symptoms of neutropenia.

### PATIENT/FAMILY TEACHING

• Report fever, chills, persistent sore throat, unusual bruising/bleeding, pale skin, fatigue. • Avoid tasks that require alertness, motor skills until response to drug is established. • Maintain strict oral hygiene. • Do not have immunizations without physician approval (drug lowers body's resistance). • Avoid those who have received a live virus vaccine. • Avoid crowds, those with cough, sneezing.

---

# cabozantinib

ka-boe-**zan**-ti-nib
(Cabometyx, Cometriq)

■ **BLACK BOX ALERT** ■ Complications including GI perforation and fistula formation have occurred. Severe and sometimes fatal hemorrhaging including hemoptysis, GI bleeding occurred in 3% of pts. Discontinue treatment if visceral perforation, fistula formation (GI, tracheal/esophageal), severe hemorrhaging occurs.

### ◆CLASSIFICATION

**PHARMACOTHERAPEUTIC:** Tyrosine kinase inhibitor. **CLINICAL:** Antineoplastic.

## USES

**Cabometyx:** Treatment of advanced renal cell carcinoma (RCC) in pts who received prior antiangiogenic therapy. **Cometriq:** Treatment of progressive, metastatic medullary thyroid cancer.

## PRECAUTIONS

**Contraindications:** Hypersensitivity to cabozantinib. **Cautions:** Moderate to severe hepatic impairment; baseline thrombocytopenia, anemia, neutropenia; recent surgery or dental procedures, open wounds, chronic electrolyte imbalance, dehydration, hypertension; recent history of hemorrhagic events, hemoptysis.

## ACTION

Inhibits tyrosine kinase activity in tumor cells. Inhibits cell migration, proliferation, survival, and angiogenesis (new blood vessel formation). **Therapeutic Effect:** Inhibits thyroid tumor cell growth and metastasis.

## PHARMOCOKINETICS

Well absorbed after PO administration. Metabolized in liver. Protein binding: 99%. Peak plasma concentration: 2–5 hrs. Excreted in feces (54%), urine (27%). **Half-life:** 55 hrs.

## ⧗ LIFESPAN CONSIDERATIONS

**Pregnancy/Lactation:** May cause fetal harm. Breastfeeding not recommended. Must either discontinue drug or discontinue breastfeeding. Unknown if distributed in breast milk. Female pts of reproductive potential must use effective contraception during treatment and up to 4 mos after discontinuation. **Children:** Safety and efficacy not established. **Elderly:** No age-related precautions noted.

## INTERACTIONS

**DRUG:** Strong CYP3A4 inhibitors (e.g., **clarithromycin, ketoconazole, voriconazole**) may increase concentration/effect. **Strong CYP3A4 inducers** (e.g., **carbamazepine, phenytoin, rifampin**) may decrease concentration/effect. **HERBAL:** St John's wort may decrease effect. **FOOD:** Grapefruit products may increase concentration/effect. **High-fat meals** may increase absorption/exposure. **LAB VALUES:** May decrease lymphocytes, neutrophils, platelets; serum calcium, magnesium, phosphorus, potassium, sodium.

May increase serum ALT, AST, bilirubin, lipase, TSH, urine protein.

## AVAILABILITY (Rx)

Cabometyx (Tablets): 20 mg, 40 mg, 60 mg.

Cometriq (Capsules): 20 mg, 80 mg.

## ADMINISTRATION/HANDLING

### PO

• Give on empty stomach only; do not administer 2 hrs before or 1 hr after meal. Give with water. Administer capsules whole; do not break, cut, dissolve, or divide. Do not crush tablets.

## INDICATIONS/ROUTES/DOSAGES

### Metastatic Medullary Thyroid Cancer

PO: *(Cometriq):* ADULTS, ELDERLY: 140 mg once daily.

### Cometriq

### Dose Modification

*Hematologic/Nonhematologic Reaction, Drug Intolerance*

Interrupt treatment until resolved, then resume at 100 mg once daily (if previously taking 140 mg) or 60 mg once daily (if previously taking 100 mg). If previously taking 60 mg/day, resume 60 mg once daily once toxic effects resolve.

### Renal Cell Carcinoma

PO: *(Cabometyx):* ADULTS, ELDERLY: 60 mg once daily.

### Cabometyx

### Dose Modification

Withhold for Common Terminology Criteria for Adverse Events (CTCAE) grade 4 adverse reactions, and grade 3 or intolerable grade 2 adverse reaction not managed with a dose reduction after resolution/improvement. Previous dose of 60 mg daily: resume at 40 mg daily. Previous dose of 40 mg daily: resume at 20 mg daily. Previous 20 mg daily: resume at 20 mg if tolerated; otherwise discontinue.

### Dosage in Renal Impairment

**Mild to moderate impairment:** No dose adjustment. **Severe impairment:** Use with caution.

### Dosage in Hepatic Impairment

**Mild to moderate impairment:** No dose adjustment. **Severe impairment:** Not recommended.

## SIDE EFFECTS

Frequent (63%–34%): Diarrhea, stomatitis, weight loss, decreased appetite, nausea, fatigue, oral pain, dysgeusia. Occasional (27%–7%): Constipation, abdominal pain, vomiting, asthenia, dysphonia, dry skin, headache, alopecia, dizziness, arthralgia, dysphagia, muscle spasms, erythema, dyspepsia, anxiety, musculoskeletal pain, paresthesia, peripheral neuropathy, hyperkeratosis.

## ADVERSE REACTIONS/TOXIC EFFECTS

May cause GI perforation (3% of pts), GI fistula formation (1% of pts), severe GI hemorrhaging (3% of pts). Malignant hypertension may occur despite continued medical management. Thromboembolic events including venous/arterial thromboembolism, cerebral infarction, MI have been reported. May cause ineffective wound healing or wound dehiscence requiring medical intervention. Osteonecrosis of the jaw may present as mandibular pain, jaw bone erosion, periodontal/gingival infection or ulceration, osteomyelitis, slow healing of the mouth after dental procedures. Palmar-plantar erythrodysesthesia syndrome (PPES), a chemotherapy-induced skin condition that presents as redness, swelling, numbness, skin sloughing of the hands and feet, may occur. Reversible posterior leukoencephalopathy syndrome (RPLS) reported in less than 1% of pts. Proteinuria may indicate nephrotic syndrome.

---

## NURSING CONSIDERATIONS

### BASELINE ASSESSMENT

Obtain CBC with differential, BMP, LFT, serum magnesium, phosphate, ionized calcium; urinalysis; vital signs. Assess for recent surgeries, dental procedures. Obtain negative urine pregnancy before initiating treatment. Receive full medication history including herbal products. Question history of hypertension, hepatic impairment, hemorrhagic events, thromboembolic events such as CVA, DVT, MI. Assess for open wounds, skin lesions. Monitor for osteonecrosis of the jaw.

### INTERVENTION/EVALUATION

Monitor CBC, serum electrolytes, urinalysis. Routinely assess vital signs and report any change in blood pressure. Persistent diastolic hypertension may indicate hypertensive crisis. Obtain EKG for palpitations, chest pain. RPLS should be considered in pt with seizure, headache, visual disturbances, confusion, altered mental status. Assess hydration status. Encourage PO intake. Immediately report any hemorrhaging, bloody stools, abdominal pain, hemoptysis (may indicate GI perforation/fistula formation). Monitor skin for poor healing of chronic wounds, new skin lesions.

### PATIENT/FAMILY TEACHING

• Blood levels will be routinely monitored. Strictly avoid pregnancy. Contraception should be utilized during treatment and up to 4 mos after last dose. • Report any yellowing of skin or eyes, abdominal pain, bruising, black/tarry stools, dark urine, decreased urine output, skin changes. • Neurologic changes including altered mental status, seizures, headache, blurry vision, trouble speaking, one-sided weakness may indicate stroke, high blood pressure crisis, or life-threatening brain swelling. • Do no take herbal products. • Report any jaw pain or oral lesions, skin changes including dermal sloughing, rash, or poor healing of open wounds. • Notify physician before any planned surgeries or dental procedures. • Do not ingest grapefruit products. • Do not take with food. Do not eat at least 2 hrs before or 1 hr after any dose. • Severe diarrhea may lead to dehydration; drink plenty of fluids.

## caffeine citrate

kaf-een **sit**-rate
(Cafcit)

### ◆CLASSIFICATION

**PHARMACOTHERAPEUTIC:** Citrate salt of caffeine. **CLINICAL:** Bronchial smooth muscle relaxant.

### USES

Short-term treatment of apnea in premature infants from 28 wks to younger than 33 wks gestational age.

### PRECAUTIONS

**Contraindications:** Hypersensitivity to caffeine. **Cautions:** Avoid in pts with symptomatic cardiac arrhythmias, agitation, anxiety, tremors.

### ACTION

Stimulates medullary respiratory center. Appears to increase sensitivity of respiratory center to stimulatory effects of $CO_2$. **Therapeutic Effect:** Increases alveolar ventilation, reducing severity, frequency of apneic episodes.

### INTERACTIONS

**DRUG: CNS stimulants** may cause excessive CNS stimulation (e.g., nervousness, insomnia, seizures, arrhythmias). **CYP1A2 inhibitors (e.g., cimetidine, ciprofloxacin)** may increase concentration, risk of side effects. **HERBAL:** None significant. **FOOD:** None known. **LAB VALUES:** May alter serum glucose.

### AVAILABILITY (Rx)

**Injection Solution:** 20 mg/ml. **Oral Solution:** 20 mg/ml.

## ADMINISTRATION/HANDLING

**PO**
- May give without regard to feedings.
- May administer injectable solution orally.

 **IV**
- Infuse loading dose over at least 30 min; maintenance dose over at least 10 min. • May give without further dilution.

### 🔲 IV COMPATIBILITIES

Alprostadil, calcium gluconate, cefotoxime, dexamethasone, dobutamine, dopamine, gentamicin, heparin, vancomycin.

### 🔲 IV INCOMPATIBILITIES

Acyclovir, furosemide.

## INDICATIONS/ROUTES/DOSAGE

**Apnea**
**PO, IV: Loading dose:** 10–20 mg/kg as caffeine citrate (5–10 mg/kg as caffeine base). If theophylline given within previous 72 hrs, a modified dose (50%–75%) may be given. **Maintenance:** 5 mg/kg/day as caffeine citrate (2.5 mg/kg/day as caffeine base) starting 24 hrs after loading dose. Dosage adjusted based on pt response.

## SIDE EFFECTS

**Frequent (10%–5%):** Feeding intolerance, rash.

## ADVERSE EFFECTS/ TOXIC REACTIONS

Sepsis, necrotizing enterocolitis may occur.

## NURSING CONSIDERATIONS

### BASELINE ASSESSMENT

Baseline serum caffeine levels should be measured in infants previously treated with theophylline (preterm infants metabolize theophylline to caffeine).

### INTERVENTION/EVALUATION

Diligently monitor respirations. Assess skin for rash. Monitor heart rate, number/severity of apnea spells, serum caffeine levels.

# calcitonin

kal-si-**toe**-nin
(Calcimar ✦, Fortical, Miacalcin)
**Do not confuse calcitonin with calcitriol, or Miacalcin with Micatin.**

## ◆ CLASSIFICATION

**PHARMACOTHERAPEUTIC:** Synthetic hormone. **CLINICAL:** Calcium regulator, bone resorption inhibitor.

## USES

**Parenteral:** Treatment of Paget's disease, hypercalcemia, postmenopausal osteoporosis in women greater than 5 yrs postmenopause. **Intranasal:** Postmenopausal osteoporosis.

## PRECAUTIONS

**Contraindications:** Hypersensitivity to calcitonin, salmon protein. **Cautions:** None known.

## ACTION

Antagonizes effects of parathyroid hormone. Increases jejunal secretion of water, sodium, potassium, chloride. Inhibits osteoclast bone resorption, increases excretion of calcium, phosphate, sodium, magnesium, potassium. **Therapeutic Effect:** Regulates serum calcium concentrations.

## PHARMACOKINETICS

Nasal form rapidly absorbed. Injection form rapidly metabolized primarily in kidneys. Primarily excreted in urine. **Half-life:** Nasal: 43 min; Injection: 70–90 min.

## ⧗ LIFESPAN CONSIDERATIONS

**Pregnancy/Lactation:** Does not cross placenta; unknown if distributed in breast

---

milk. Safe usage during lactation not established (inhibits lactation in animals). **Children:** Safety and efficacy not established. **Elderly:** No age-related precautions noted.

## INTERACTIONS

**DRUG:** May decrease **lithium** concentration/effects. **HERBAL:** None significant. **FOOD:** None known. **LAB VALUES:** None significant.

## AVAILABILITY (Rx)

**Injection Solution (Miacalcin):** 200 units/ml (calcitonin-salmon). **Nasal Spray (Fortical, Miacalcin Nasal):** 200 units/activation (calcitonin-salmon).

## ADMINISTRATION/HANDLING

**IM, Subcutaneous**
• IM route preferred if injection volume greater than 2 ml. Subcutaneous injection for outpatient self-administration unless volume greater than 2 ml. • Skin test should be performed before therapy in pts suspected of sensitivity to calcitonin. • Bedtime administration may reduce nausea, flushing.

**Intranasal**
• Refrigerate unopened nasal spray. Store at room temperature after initial use. • Instruct pt to clear nasal passages. • Tilt head slightly forward. • Insert spray tip into nostril, pointing toward nasal passages, away from nasal septum. • Spray into one nostril while pt holds other nostril closed and concurrently inspires through nose to deliver medication as high into nasal passage as possible. Spray into one nostril daily. • Discard after 30 doses.

## INDICATIONS/ROUTES/DOSAGE

**Skin Testing before Treatment in Pts with Suspected Sensitivity to Calcitonin-Salmon**
**Note:** A detailed skin testing protocol is available from the manufacturer.

**Paget's Disease**
**IM, Subcutaneous: ADULTS, ELDERLY:** Initially, 100 units/day.

**Postmenopausal Osteoporosis**
**IM, Subcutaneous: ADULTS, ELDERLY:** 100 units every other day with adequate calcium and vitamin D intake.
**Intranasal: ADULTS, ELDERLY:** 200 units/day as a single spray, alternating nostrils daily.

**Hypercalcemia**
**IM, Subcutaneous: ADULTS, ELDERLY:** Initially, 4 units/kg q12h; may increase to 8 units/kg q12h if no response in 2 days; may further increase to 8 units/kg q6h if no response in another 2 days.

**Dosage in Renal/Hepatic Impairment**
No dose adjustment.

## SIDE EFFECTS

**Frequent: IM, Subcutaneous (10%):** Nausea (may occur soon after injection; usually diminishes with continued therapy), inflammation at injection site. **Nasal (12%–10%):** Rhinitis, nasal irritation, redness, mucosal lesions. **Occasional: IM, Subcutaneous (5%–2%):** Flushing of face, hands. **Nasal (5%–3%):** Back pain, arthralgia, epistaxis, headache. **Rare: IM, Subcutaneous:** Epigastric discomfort, dry mouth, diarrhea, flatulence. **Nasal:** Itching of earlobes, pedal edema, rash, diaphoresis.

## ADVERSE EFFECTS/TOXIC REACTIONS

Pts with a protein allergy may develop a hypersensitivity reaction (rash, dyspnea, hypotension, tachycardia).

## NURSING CONSIDERATIONS

**BASELINE ASSESSMENT**
Obtain baseline serum electrolyte levels.

**INTERVENTION/EVALUATION**
Ensure rotation of injection sites; check for inflammation. Assess vertebral bone mass (document stabilization/improvement). Assess for allergic response: rash, urticaria, swelling, dyspnea, tachycardia, hypotension. Monitor serum electrolytes, calcium, alkaline phosphatase.

• Instruct pt/family on aseptic technique, proper injection method of subcutaneous medication, including rotation of sites, proper administration of nasal medication. • Nausea is transient and usually decreases over time. • Immediately report rash, itching, shortness of breath, significant nasal irritation. • Improvement in biochemical abnormalities and bone pain usually occurs in the first few months of treatment. • Improvement of neurologic lesions may take more than a year.

# calcium acetate

(Eliphos, PhosLo)

# calcium carbonate

(Apo-Cal ✸, Caltrate 600 ✸, OsCal ✸, Titralac, Tums)

# calcium chloride

(Cal-Citrate, Citracal, Osteocit ✸)

# calcium glubionate

# calcium gluconate

kal-si-um
**Do not confuse Citracal with Citrucel, OsCal with Asacol, or PhosLo with ProSom.**

## ◆CLASSIFICATION

**PHARMACOTHERAPEUTIC:** Electrolyte replenisher. **CLINICAL:** Antacid, antihypocalcemic, antihyperkalemic, antihypermagnesemic, antihyperphosphatemic.

## USES

**Parenteral (calcium chloride):** Treatment of hypocalcemia, emergency treatment of severe hypermagnesemia. **(calcium gluconate):** Treatment of hypocalcemia, cardiac disturbances secondary to hyperkalemia; adjunctive treatment of rickets, osteomalacia, and magnesium sulfate overdose. **Calcium carbonate:** Antacid, dietary supplement. **Calcium acetate:** Controls hyperphosphatemia in end-stage renal disease. **OFF-LABEL (Calcium chloride):** Calcium channel blocker overdose, severe hyperkalemia, malignant arrhythmias associated with hypermagnesemia.

## PRECAUTIONS

**Contraindications:** Hypersensitivity to calcium formulation. **All preparations:** Calcium-based renal calculi, hypercalcemia, ventricular fibrillation. **Calcium chloride:** Digoxin toxicity. **Calcium gluconate: Neonates:** Concurrent IV use with ceftriaxone. **Cautions:** Chronic renal impairment, hypokalemia, concurrent use with digoxin.

## ACTION

Essential for function, integrity of nervous, muscular, skeletal systems. Plays an important role in normal cardiac/renal function, respiration, blood coagulation, cell membrane and capillary permeability. Assists in regulating release/storage of hormones/neurotransmitters. Neutralizes/reduces gastric acid (increases pH). **Calcium acetate:** Binds with dietary phosphate, forming insoluble calcium phosphate. **Therapeutic Effect:** Replaces calcium in deficiency states; controls hyperphosphatemia in end-stage renal disease; relieves heartburn, indigestion.

## PHARMACOKINETICS

Moderately absorbed from small intestine (absorption depends on presence of vitamin D metabolites, pH). Primarily eliminated in feces.

## ⧗ LIFESPAN CONSIDERATIONS

**Pregnancy/Lactation:** Distributed in breast milk. Unknown whether calcium chloride or calcium gluconate is distributed in breast milk. **Children:** Risk of extreme irritation, possible tissue necrosis or sloughing with IV calcium

---

✸ Canadian trade name        🗞 Non-Crushable Drug        🔲 High Alert drug preparations. Restrict IV use due to small vasculature. **Elderly:** Oral absorption may be decreased.

## INTERACTIONS

**DRUG:** Hypercalcemia may increase **digoxin** toxicity. Oral form may decrease absorption of **biphosphonates (e.g., risedronate), calcium channel blockers, tetracycline derivatives, thyroid products. HERBAL:** None significant. **FOOD:** Food may increase calcium absorption. **LAB VALUES:** May increase serum pH, calcium, gastrin. May decrease serum phosphate, potassium.

## AVAILABILITY

CALCIUM ACETATE (667 mg = 169 mg calcium)
**Gelcap (PhosLo):** 667 mg. **Tablets (Eliphos):** 667 mg.
CALCIUM CARBONATE (1 g = 400 mg calcium)
**Tablets:** 500 mg, 600 mg, 1,250 mg, 1,500 mg. **Tablets (Chewable):** 500 mg, 750 mg, 1,000 mg.
CALCIUM CHLORIDE
**Injection Solution:** 10% (100 mg/ml) equivalent to 27.2 mg elemental calcium per ml.
CALCIUM GLUCONATE (1 g = 93 mg calcium)
**Injection Solution:** 10%.

## ADMINISTRATION/HANDLING

 IV

### Dilution
**Calcium Chloride** • May give undiluted or may dilute with 0.9% NaCl or Sterile Water for Injection.
**Calcium Gluconate** • May give undiluted or may dilute with 100 ml 0.9% NaCl or $D_5W$.

### Rate of Administration
**Calcium Chloride • Note:** Rapid administration may produce bradycardia, metallic/chalky taste, hypotension, sensation of heart, peripheral vasodilation. • **IV push:** Infuse slowly at maximum rate of 50–100 mg/min (in cardiac arrest, may administer over 10–20 sec). • **IV infusion:** Dilute to maximum final concentration of 20 mg/ml and infuse over 1 hr or no faster than 45–90 mg/kg/hr. Give via a central line. Do **NOT** use scalp, small hand or foot veins. Stop infusion if pt complains of pain or discomfort.
**Calcium Gluconate • Note:** Rapid administration may produce vasodilation, hypotension, arrhythmias, syncope, cardiac arrest. • **IV push:** Infuse slowly over 3–5 min or at maximum rate of 50–100 mg/min (in cardiac arrest, may administer over 10–20 sec). • **IV infusion:** Dilute 1–2 g in 100 ml 0.9% NaCl or $D_5W$ and infuse over 1 hr.
**Storage** • Store at room temperature. • Once diluted, stable for 24 hrs at room temperature.

### PO
**Calcium Acetate** • Administer with plenty of fluids during meals to optimize effectiveness.
**Calcium Carbonate** • Administer with or immediately following meals with plenty of water (give with meals if used for phosphate binding). Instruct pt to thoroughly chew chewable tablets before swallowing.

## 🔲 IV INCOMPATIBILITIES

**Calcium chloride:** Amphotericin B complex (Abelcet, AmBisome, Amphotec), pantoprazole (Protonix), phosphate-containing solutions, propofol (Diprivan), sodium bicarbonate. **Calcium gluconate:** Amphotericin B complex (Abelcet, AmBisome, Amphotec), fluconazole (Diflucan).

## 🔲 IV COMPATIBILITIES

**Calcium chloride:** Amikacin (Amikin), dobutamine (Dobutrex), lidocaine, milrinone (Primacor), morphine, norepinephrine (Levophed). **Calcium gluconate:** Ampicillin, aztreonam (Azactam), cefazolin

(Ancef), cefepime (Maxipime), ciprofloxacin (Cipro), dobutamine (Dobutrex), enalapril (Vasotec), famotidine (Pepcid), furosemide (Lasix), heparin, lidocaine, lipids, magnesium sulfate, meropenem (Merrem IV), midazolam (Versed), milrinone (Primacor), norepinephrine (Levophed), piperacillin and tazobactam (Zosyn), potassium chloride, propofol (Diprivan).

## INDICATIONS/ROUTES/DOSAGE

### Hyperphosphatemia

**PO (Calcium Acetate): ADULTS, ELDERLY:** 2 tablets 3 times/day with meals. May increase gradually up to 4 tablets 3 times/day to decrease serum phosphate level to less than 6 mg/dL as long as hypercalcemia does not develop.

### Hypocalcemia

**IV: (Calcium chloride): ADULTS, ELDERLY:** 200–1,000 mg q1–days.

**IV (Calcium Gluconate): ADULTS, ELDERLY:** 1–2 g over 2 hrs. May repeat q60 min until level resolved. **CHILDREN:** 200–500 mg/kg/day in 4 divided doses. **NEONATES:** 200–800 mg/kg/day in 4 divided doses.

### Antacid

**PO (Calcium Carbonate): ADULTS, ELDERLY:** 1–4 tabs as needed. **Maximum:** 8,000 mg/day. **CHILDREN 6–11 YRS:** 750–800 mg. **Maximum:** 3,000 mg/day. **CHILDREN 2–5 YRS:** 375–400 mg. **Maximum:** 1,500 mg/day.

### Cardiac Arrest

**IV (Calcium Chloride): ADULTS, ELDERLY:** 500–1,000 mg over 2–5 min. May repeat as necessary. **CHILDREN, NEONATES:** 20 mg/kg. May repeat in 10 min if necessary. If effective, consider IV infusion of 20–50 mg/kg/hr.

### Supplement

**PO (Calcium carbonate): ADULTS, ELDERLY:** 500 mg–4 g/day in 1–3 divided doses. **CHILDREN OLDER THAN 4 YRS:** 750 mg 3 times/day. **CHILDREN 2–4 YRS:** 750 mg 2 times/day. **(Calcium Citrate): ADULTS, ELDERLY:** 0.5–2 g 2–4 times/day. **CHILDREN:** 45–65 mg/kg/day in 4 divided doses.

### Dosage in Renal/Hepatic Impairment
No dose adjustment.

## SIDE EFFECTS

**Frequent: PO:** Chalky taste. **Parenteral:** Pain, rash, redness, burning at injection site; flushing, nausea, vomiting, diaphoresis, hypotension. **Occasional: PO:** Mild constipation, fecal impaction, peripheral edema, metabolic alkalosis (muscle pain, restlessness, slow respirations, altered taste). **Calcium carbonate:** Milk-alkali syndrome (headache, decreased appetite, nausea, vomiting, unusual fatigue). **Rare:** Urinary urgency, painful urination.

## ADVERSE EFFECTS/ TOXIC REACTIONS

**Hypercalcemia: Early signs:** Constipation, headache, dry mouth, increased thirst, irritability, decreased appetite, metallic taste, fatigue, weakness, depression. **Later signs:** Confusion, drowsiness, hypertension, photosensitivity, arrhythmias, nausea, vomiting, painful urination.

## NURSING CONSIDERATIONS

### BASELINE ASSESSMENT

Assess B/P, EKG and cardiac rhythm, renal function, serum magnesium, phosphate, calcium, ionized calcium.

### INTERVENTION/EVALUATION

Monitor serum BMP, calcium, ionized calcium, magnesium, phosphate; B/P, cardiac rhythm, renal function. Monitor for signs of hypercalcemia.

### PATIENT/FAMILY TEACHING

• Do not take within 1–2 hrs of other oral medications, fiber-containing foods.
• Avoid excessive use of alcohol, tobacco, caffeine.

# canagliflozin

**kan**-a-gli-**floe**-zin
(Invokana)

## CLASSIFICATION

**PHARMACOTHERAPEUTIC:** Sodium-glucose co-transporter 2 (SGLT2) inhibitor. **CLINICAL:** Antidiabetic.

### FIXED-COMBINATION(S)

**Invokamet:** canagliflozin/metformin (an antidiabetic): 50 mg/500 mg, 50 mg/1,000 mg, 150 mg/500 mg, 150 mg/1,000 mg.

## USES

Adjunctive treatment to diet and exercise to improve glycemic controls in pts with type 2 diabetes mellitus.

## PRECAUTIONS

**Contraindications:** History of hypersensitivity to canagliflozin, other SGLT2 inhibitors, severe renal impairment, end-stage renal disease, dialysis. **Cautions:** Not recommended in type 1 diabetes, diabetic ketoacidosis. Concurrent use of diuretics, ACE inhibitors, angiotensin receptor blockers (ARB), other hypoglycemic or nephrotoxic medications; mild to moderate renal impairment, hypovolemia (dehydration/anemia), elderly, episodic hypotension, hyperkalemia, genital mycotic infection.

## ACTION

Increases excretion of urinary glucose by inhibiting reabsorption of filtered glucose in kidney. Inhibits SGLT2 in proximal renal tubule. **Therapeutic Effect:** Lowers serum glucose levels.

## PHARMACOKINETICS

Readily absorbed following PO administration. Metabolized in liver. Peak plasma concentration: 1–2 hrs. Protein binding: 99%. Excreted in feces (42%), urine (33%). **Half-life:** 11–13 hrs.

## LIFESPAN CONSIDERATIONS

**Pregnancy/Lactation:** Unknown if distributed in breast milk. Must either discontinue drug or discontinue breastfeeding. **Children:** Safety and efficacy not established in pts younger than 18 yrs. **Elderly:** May have increased risk for adverse reactions (e.g., hypotension, syncope, dehydration).

## INTERACTIONS

**DRUG:** Phenytoin, **rifampin** may decrease concentration/effect. **Potassium-sparing diuretics** may increase serum potassium level. **Antihypertensives (e.g., amlodipine, lisinopril), beta blockers (e.g., carvedilol, metroprolol), diuretics (e.g., furosemide, HCTZ)** may increase risk of hypotension. **Insulin, oral hypoglycemics** may increase risk of hypoglycemia. May increase concentration/effects of **digoxin.** **HERBAL:** Herbs with hypoglycemic properties **(e.g., fenugreek, garlic, ginger, ginseng, gotu)** may increase risk of hypoglycemia. **FOOD:** None known. **LAB VALUES:** May increase serum low-density lipoprotein-cholesterol (LDL-C), Hgb, creatinine, magnesium, phosphate, potassium. May decrease glomerular filtration rate.

## AVAILABILITY (Rx)

**Tablets:** 100 mg, 300 mg.

## ADMINISTRATION/HANDLING

**PO**
• May give without regard to food. Give before first meal of the day.

## INDICATIONS/ROUTES/DOSAGE

**Type 2 Diabetes Mellitus**
**PO: ADULTS/ELDERLY:** 100 mg daily before first meal. May increase to 300 mg daily if glomerular filtration rate (GFR) greater than 60 ml/min.

**Dosage in Renal Impairment**
**GFR 45–60 ml/min:** 100 mg daily (maximum). **GFR less than 45 ml/min:** Discontinue.

---

**Dosage in Hepatic Impairment**
No dose adjustment.

## SIDE EFFECTS

**Occasional (5%):** Increased urination. **Rare (3%–2%):** Thirst, nausea, constipation.

## ADVERSE EFFECTS/ TOXIC REACTIONS

Symptomatic hypotension (postural dizziness, orthostatic hypotension, syncope) may occur. Genital myocotic (yeast) infections reported in 10% of pts. Hypoglycemic events reported in 1.5% of pts (5% in elderly). Concomitant use of hypoglycemic medications may increase hypoglycemic risk. Hypersensitivity reactions including angioedema, urticaria, rash, pruritus, erythema occurred in 3%–4% of pts. May cause hyperkalemia. May increase risk of ketoacidosis.

## NURSING CONSIDERATIONS

### BASELINE ASSESSMENT

Assess hydration status. Obtain BMP, capillary blood glucose, hemoglobin A1c, LDL-C, digoxin level (if applicable). Assess pt's understanding of diabetes management, routine blood glucose monitoring. Receive full medication history including minerals, herbal products. Question history of co-morbidities, esp. renal or hepatic impairment.

### INTERVENTION/EVALUATION

Monitor serum potassium, cholesterol; capillary blood glucose, hepatic/renal function tests. Assess for hypoglycemia, hypersensitivity reaction. Monitor for signs of hyperkalemia. Screen for glucose-altering conditions: fever, increased activity or stress, surgical procedures. Obtain dietary consult for nutritional education. Encourage PO intake.

### PATIENT/FAMILY TEACHING

• Diabetes mellitus requires lifelong control. • Diet and exercise are principal parts of treatment; do not skip or delay meals. • Test blood sugar regularly. • When taking combination drug therapy or when glucose demands are altered (fever, infection, trauma, stress), have low blood sugar treatment available (glucagon, oral dextrose). • Report suspected pregnancy or plans of breastfeeding. • Monitor daily calorie intake. • Go from lying to standing slowly to prevent dizziness. • Genital itching may indicate yeast infection. • Therapy may increase risk for dehydration/low blood pressure. • Report any palpitations or muscle weakness.

# candesartan

kan-de-**sar**-tan
(Apo-Candesartan ♣, Atacand)
■ **BLACK BOX ALERT** ■ May cause fetal injury, mortality. Discontinue as soon as possible once pregnancy is detected.

## FIXED-COMBINATION(S)

**Atacand HCT:** candesartan/hydrochlorothiazide (a diuretic): 16 mg/12.5 mg, 32 mg/12.5 mg.

## ◆CLASSIFICATION

**PHARMACOTHERAPEUTIC:** Angiotensin II receptor antagonist. **CLINICAL:** Antihypertensive.

## USES

Treatment of hypertension alone or in combination with other antihypertensives, HF: NYHA class II–IV.

## PRECAUTIONS

**Contraindications:** Hypersensitivty to candesartan. Concomitant use with aliskiren in pts with diabetes mellitus. **Cautions:** Significant aortic/mitral stenosis, renal/hepatic impairment, unstented (unilateral/bilateral) renal artery stenosis, HF (may induce hypotension when treatment initiated).

## ACTION

Blocks vasoconstriction, aldosterone-secreting effects of angiotensin II, inhibiting binding of angiotensin II to $AT_1$ receptors. **Therapeutic Effect:** Produces vasodilation; decreases peripheral resistance, B/P.

## PHARMACOKINETICS

| Route | Onset | Peak | Duration |
|-------|-------|------|----------|
| PO | 2–3 hrs | 6–8 hrs | Greater than 24 hrs |

Rapidly, completely absorbed. Protein binding: greater than 99%. Undergoes minor hepatic metabolism to inactive metabolite. Excreted unchanged in urine and in feces through biliary system. Not removed by hemodialysis. **Half-life:** 9 hrs.

## ⌛ LIFESPAN CONSIDERATIONS

**Pregnancy/Lactation:** Unknown if distributed in breast milk. May cause fetal/neonatal morbidity/mortality. **Children:** Safety and efficacy not established in pts younger than 1 yr. **Elderly:** No age-related precautions noted.

## INTERACTIONS

**DRUG:** May increase risk of **lithium** toxicity. **NSAIDs** may decrease effects. **HERBAL: Ephedra, ginseng, yohimbe** may worsen hypertension. **Garlic** may increase antihypertensive effect. **FOOD:** None known. **LAB VALUES:** May increase serum BUN, alkaline phosphatase, bilirubin, creatinine, ALT, AST. May decrease Hgb, Hct.

## AVAILABILITY (Rx)

**Tablets:** 4 mg, 8 mg, 16 mg, 32 mg.

## ADMINISTRATION/HANDLING

**PO**
• Give without regard to food.

## INDICATIONS/ROUTES/DOSAGE

**Hypertension**
**PO: ADULTS, ELDERLY:** Initially, 16 mg once daily. Titrate to response. Range: 8–32 mg/day in 1–2 divided doses. **CHILDREN 6–16 YRS, GREATER THAN 50 KG:** Initially, 8–16 mg/day in 1–2 divided doses. Range: 4–32 mg. **Maximum:** 32 g/day. **50 KG OR LESS:** Initially, 4–8 mg in 1–2 divided doses. Range: 2–16 mg/day. **Maximum:** 32 mg/day. **CHILDREN 1–5 YRS:** Initially, 0.2 mg/kg/day in 1–2 divided doses. Range: 0.05–0.4 mg/kg/day. **Maximum:** 0.4 mg/kg/day.

**HF**
**PO: ADULTS, ELDERLY:** Initially, 4 mg once daily. May double dose at approximately 2-wk intervals up to a target dose of 32 mg/day.

**Dosage in Renal/Hepatic Impairment**
**Mild to moderate impairment:** No dose adjustment. **Severe impairment:** Use caution.

## SIDE EFFECTS

**Occasional (6%–3%):** Upper respiratory tract infection, dizziness, back/leg pain. **Rare (2%–1%):** Pharyngitis, rhinitis, headache, fatigue, diarrhea, nausea, dry cough, peripheral edema.

## ADVERSE EFFECTS/TOXIC REACTIONS

Overdosage may manifest as hypotension, tachycardia. Bradycardia occurs less often. May increase risk of renal failure, hyperkalemia.

## NURSING CONSIDERATIONS

### BASELINE ASSESSMENT

Obtain B/P, apical pulse immediately before each dose, in addition to regular monitoring (be alert to fluctuations). Question for possibility of pregnancy. Assess medication history (esp. diuretic).

Question for history of hepatic/renal impairment, renal artery stenosis. Obtain serum BUN, creatinine, LFT; Hgb, Hct.

### INTERVENTION/EVALUATION

Maintain hydration (offer fluids frequently). Assess for evidence of upper respiratory infection. Assist with ambulation if dizziness occurs. Monitor electrolytes, renal function, urinalysis. Assess B/P for hypertension/hypotension. If excessive reduction in B/P occurs, place pt in supine position, feet slightly elevated.

### PATIENT/FAMILY TEACHING

• Hypertension requires lifelong control. • Inform female pts regarding potential for fetal injury, mortality with second- and third-trimester exposure to candesartan. • Report suspected pregnancy. • Avoid tasks that require alertness, motor skills until response to drug is established. • Report any sign of infection (sore throat, fever). • Do not stop taking medication. • Caution against exercising during hot weather (risk of dehydration, hypotension).

# cangrelor

kan-grel-or
(Kengreal)
**Do not confuse cangrelor with ticagrelor.**

## ◆CLASSIFICATION

**PHARMACOTHERAPEUTIC:** P2Y$_{12}$ platelet inhibitor. **CLINICAL:** Antiplatelet.

## USES

Adjunct to percutaneous coronary intervention (PCI) for reducing risk of periprocedural myocardial infarction, repeat coronary revascularization, and stent thrombosis in pts who have not been treated with a P2Y$_{12}$ platelet inhibitor and are not being given a glycoprotein IIb/IIIa inhibitor.

## PRECAUTIONS

**Contraindications:** Major active bleeding. Hypersensitivity to cangrelor. **Cautions:** Renal impairment; history of intracranial hemorrhage, GI bleeding.

## ACTION

Blocks adenosine diphosphate (ADP)-induced platelet activation and aggregation. Binds selectively and reversibly to P2Y$_{12}$ receptor to prevent further signaling and platelet activation. **Therapeutic Effect:** Reduces platelet aggregation.

## PHARMACOKINETICS

Widely distributed. Metabolized rapidly in circulatory system via dephosphorylation. Protein binding: 97–98%. Peak plasma concentration: 2 min. Platelet function returns to baseline within 1 hr after discontinuing infusion. Eliminated in urine (58%), feces (35%). **Half-Life:** 3–6 min.

## ⧗ LIFESPAN CONSIDERATIONS

**Pregnancy/Lactation:** Unknown if distributed in breastmilk. **Children:** Safety and efficacy not established. **Elderly:** No age-related precautions noted.

## INTERACTIONS

**DRUG:** Clopidogrel, prasugrel have no antiplatelet effect if administered during cangrelor infusion. **HERBAL:** None significant. **FOOD:** None known. **LAB VALUES:** May increase creatinine (in pts with severe renal impairment).

## AVAILABILITY (Rx)

**Injection, Lyophilized Power for Reconstitution:** 50 mg/10 ml vial.

## ADMINISTRATION/HANDLING
 IV

**Reconstitution** • Obtain weight in kg. • For each 50 mg/ml vial, reconstitute with 5 ml of Sterile Water for Injection. • Swirl gently until fully dissolved. Do not shake or agitate. Allow foam to settle. • Visually inspect for particulate

---

matter or discoloration. Solution should appear clear, colorless to pale yellow in color. • Further dilute with 250 ml 0.9% NaCl or 5% Dextrose Injection. • Gently invert bag to mix. • Final concentration of diluted solution: 200 mcg/ml.
**Rate of Administration** • Administer bolus rapidly (less than 1 min), from diluted bag via manual IV push or infusion pump. Ensure bolus dose is completely administered before starting PCI. • Start infusion immediately via dedicated line after administration of bolus.
**Storage** • Diluted solution is stable up to 12 hrs in 5% dextrose or up to 24 hrs in 0.9% NaCl at room temperature.

## INDICATIONS/ROUTES/DOSAGE

**Coronary Revascularization/Cardiac Stent Thrombosis**
**IV Infusion: ADULTS, ELDERLY:** 30 mcg/kg bolus, then 4 mcg/kg/min infusion. Maintenance infusion should be continued for at least 2 hrs or for the duration of PCI (whichever is longer).

**Transition to Oral P2Y12 Therapy**
To maintain platelet inhibition after discontinuation, one oral $P2Y_{12}$ platelet inhibitor should be administered as follows:
• Ticagrelor 180 PO mg at any time during infusion or immediately after discontinuation.
• Prasugrel 60 mg PO immediately after discontinuation (do not administer prasugrel prior to discontinuing infusion).
• Clopidogrel 600 mg PO immediately after discontinuation (do not administer clopidogrel prior to discontinuing infusion).

**Dosage in Renal/Hepatic Impairment**
No dose adjustment.

## SIDE EFFECTS

None known (see Adverse Effects/Toxic Reactions).

## ADVERSE EFFECTS/TOXIC REACTIONS

Bleeding complications including intracranial hemorrhage, other life-threatening/severe/moderate bleeding events occurred in less than 1% of pts. Mild bleeding reported in 15% of pts. Coronary artery dissection, coronary artery perforation, and dyspnea were the most common events leading to discontinuation. Serious hypersensitivity reactions including angioedema, anaphylaxis, anaphylactic shock, bronchospasm, stridor occurred in less than 1% of pts. Worsening renal function was reported in 3% of pts with severe renal impairment. Dyspnea occurred in less than 2% of pts.

## NURSING CONSIDERATIONS

### BASELINE ASSESSMENT
Obtain renal function test in pts with renal impairment. Cross-check dose with co-worker. Question history of renal impairment; colon polyps, gastric/duodenal ulcers, GI bleeding; CVA, head trauma, recent intracranial hemorrhage; hypersensitivity to drug class.

### INTERVENTION/EVALUATION
Report hematuria, epistaxis, coffee ground emesis, black/tarry stools. Assess for headache, altered mental status, stroke-like symptoms, hypertension (may indicate intracranial hemorrhage). Assess peripheral pulses; skin for ecchymosis, petechiae; gums for erythema, gingival bleeding.

### PATIENT/FAMILY TEACHING
• It may take longer to stop bleeding during therapy. • Use soft toothbrush, electric razor to decrease risk of bleeding. • Report any sign of red or dark urine, black or tarry stools, coffee-ground vomitus, blood-tinged mucus, nosebleeds. • Do not vigorously blow nose. • Report any confusion, headache, lethargy, one-sided weakness, trouble speaking.

## capecitabine

kap-e-**sye**-ta-bine
(<u>Xeloda</u>)

■ **BLACK BOX ALERT** ■ May increase anticoagulant effect of warfarin.

**Do not confuse Xeloda with Xenical.**

### ◆CLASSIFICATION

**PHARMACOTHERAPEUTIC:** Antimetabolite. **CLINICAL:** Antineoplastic.

### USES

Treatment of metastatic breast cancer, metastatic colorectal cancer. Adjuvant (postsurgical) treatment of Dukes C colon cancer. **OFF-LABEL:** Gastric cancer, pancreatic cancer, esophageal cancer, ovarian cancer, neuroendocrine tumors, hepatobiliary cancer.

### PRECAUTIONS

**Contraindications:** Severe renal impairment (CrCl less than 30 ml/min), dihydropyrimidine dehydrogenase (DPD) deficiency, hypersensitivity to capecitabine, 5-fluorouracil (5-FU). **Cautions:** Existing bone marrow depression, hepatic impairment, mild to moderate renal impairment, previous cytotoxic therapy/radiation therapy, elderly (60 yrs of age or older).

### ACTION

Enzymatically converted to 5-fluorouracil (5-FU). Inhibits enzymes necessary for synthesis of essential cellular components. **Therapeutic Effect:** Interferes with DNA synthesis, RNA processing, protein synthesis.

### PHARMACOKINETICS

Readily absorbed from GI tract. Protein binding: less than 60%. Metabolized in liver. Primarily excreted in urine. **Half-life:** 45 min.

### ⏳ LIFESPAN CONSIDERATIONS

**Pregnancy/Lactation:** May cause fetal harm. Unknown if distributed in breast milk. **Children:** Safety and efficacy not established in those younger than 18 yrs. **Elderly:** May be more sensitive to GI side effects.

### INTERACTIONS

**DRUG:** May increase concentration, toxicity of **warfarin, phenytoin.** Myelosuppression may be enhanced when given concurrently with **bone marrow depressants. Live virus vaccines** may potentiate virus replication, increase vaccine side effects, decrease pt's antibody response to vaccine. **HERBAL: Echinacea** may decrease level/effects. **FOOD:** None known. **LAB VALUES:** May increase serum alkaline phosphatase, bilirubin, ALT, AST. May decrease Hgb, Hct, WBC count. May increase PT/INR.

### AVAILABILITY (Rx)

**Tablets:** 150 mg, 500 mg.

### ADMINISTRATION/HANDLING

• Give within 30 min after meals with water. • Administer whole; do not cut, crush.

### INDICATIONS/ROUTES/DOSAGE

**Metastatic Breast Cancer, Colorectal Cancer, Adjuvant (Postsurgery) Treatment of Dukes C Colon Cancer**
**PO: ADULTS, ELDERLY:** Initially, 2,500 mg/m²/day in 2 equally divided doses approximately q12h apart for 2 wks. Follow with a 1-wk rest period; given in 3-wk cycles.

**Dosage in Renal Impairment**
**CrCl 51–80 ml/min:** No adjustment. **CrCl 30–50 ml/min:** 75% of normal dose. **CrCl less than 30 ml/min:** Contraindicated.

**Dosage in Hepatic Impairment**
No dose adjustment at start of therapy; interrupt therapy for grade 3 or

4 hyperbilirubinemia until bilirubin is 3 times ULN or less.

## SIDE EFFECTS

**Frequent (55%–25%):** Diarrhea, nausea, vomiting, stomatitis, fatigue, anorexia, dermatitis. **Occasional (24%–10%):** Constipation, dyspepsia, headache, dizziness, insomnia, edema, myalgia, pyrexia, dehydration, dyspnea, back pain. **Rare (less than 10%):** Mood changes, depression, sore throat, epistaxis, cough, visual abnormalities.

## ADVERSE EFFECTS/ TOXIC REACTIONS

Serious reactions include myelosuppression (neutropenia, thrombocytopenia, anemia), cardiovascular toxicity (angina, cardiomyopathy, deep vein thrombosis), respiratory toxicity (dyspnea, epistaxis, pneumonia), lymphedema. Palmar-plantar erythrodysesthesia syndrome (PPES) presenting as redness, swelling, numbness, skin sloughing of hands and feet may occur.

## NURSING CONSIDERATIONS

### BASELINE ASSESSMENT

Assess sensitivity to capecitabine or 5-fluorouracil. Obtain baseline Hgb, Hct, serum chemistries, renal function.

### INTERVENTION/EVALUATION

Monitor for severe diarrhea, nausea, vomiting; if dehydration occurs, fluid and electrolyte replacement therapy should be initiated. Assess hands/feet for PPES. Monitor CBC for evidence of bone marrow depression. Monitor renal/hepatic function. Monitor for blood dyscrasias (fever, sore throat, signs of local infection, unusual bruising/bleeding from any site), symptoms of anemia (excessive fatigue, weakness).

### PATIENT/FAMILY TEACHING

• Report nausea, vomiting, diarrhea, hand-and-foot syndrome, stomatitis. • Do not have immunizations without physician's approval (drug lowers body's resistance). • Avoid contact with those who have recently received live virus vaccine. • Promptly report fever higher than 100.5°F, sore throat, signs of local infection, unusual bruising/bleeding from any site.

# captopril

kap-toe-pril
(Apo-Capto ✳)

■ **BLACK BOX ALERT** ■ May cause injury/death to developing fetus. Discontinue as soon as possible once pregnancy is detected.
**Do not confuse captopril with calcitriol, Capitrol, or carvedilol.**

## FIXED-COMBINATION(S)

**Capozide:** captopril/hydrochlorothiazide (a diuretic): 25 mg/15 mg, 25 mg/25 mg, 50 mg/15 mg, 50 mg/25 mg.

## ◆CLASSIFICATION

**PHARMACOTHERAPEUTIC:** Angiotensin-converting enzyme (ACE) inhibitor. **CLINICAL:** Antihypertensive, vasodilator.

## USES

Treatment of hypertension, HF, diabetic nephropathy, post-MI for prevention of ventricular failure.

## PRECAUTIONS

**Contraindications:** Hypersensitivity to captopril. History of angioedema from previous treatment with ACE inhibitors, concomitant use with aliskiren in pts with diabetes mellitus. **Cautions:** Renal impairment; hypertrophic cardiomyopathy with outflow obstruction, before, during, or immediately after major surgery. Unstented unilateral/bilateral renal artery stenosis. Concomitant use of potassium-sparing diuretics, potassium supplements.

---

## ACTION

Suppresses renin-angiotensin-aldosterone system (prevents conversion of angiotensin I to angiotensin II, a potent vasoconstrictor; may inhibit angiotensin II at local vascular and renal sites). Decreases plasma angiotensin II, increases plasma renin activity, decreases aldosterone secretion. **Therapeutic Effect:** Reduces peripheral arterial resistance, pulmonary capillary wedge pressure; improves cardiac output, exercise tolerance.

## PHARMACOKINETICS

| Route | Onset | Peak | Duration |
|-------|-------|------|----------|
| PO | 0.25 hr | 0.5–1.5 hrs | Dose-related |

Rapidly, well absorbed from GI tract (absorption decreased in presence of food). Protein binding: 25%–30%. Metabolized in liver. Primarily excreted in urine. Removed by hemodialysis. **Half-life:** Less than 3 hrs (increased in renal impairment).

## ⧗ LIFESPAN CONSIDERATIONS

**Pregnancy/Lactation:** Crosses placenta; distributed in breast milk. May cause fetal/neonatal mortality/morbidity. **Children:** Safety and efficacy not established. **Elderly:** May be more sensitive to hypotensive effects.

## INTERACTIONS

**DRUG: Antihypertensives** (e.g., amlodipine, lisinopril), **diuretics** (e.g., furosemide, HCTZ) may increase hypotensive effects. May increase **lithium** concentration, toxicity. **NSAIDs** may decrease antihypertensive effect. **Potassium-sparing diuretics, potassium supplements** may cause hyperkalemia. **HERBAL: Ephedra, ginseng, yohimbe** may worsen hypertension. **Garlic** may increase antihypertensive effect. **FOOD: Licorice** may cause sodium and water retention, hypokalemia. **LAB VALUES:** May increase serum BUN, alkaline phosphatase, bilirubin, creatinine, potassium, ALT, AST. May decrease serum sodium. May cause positive ANA titer.

## AVAILABILITY (Rx)

**Tablets:** 12.5 mg, 25 mg, 50 mg, 100 mg.

## ADMINISTRATION/HANDLING

**PO**

• Administer 1 hr before or 2 hrs after meals for maximum absorption (food may decrease drug absorption). • Tablets may be crushed.

## INDICATIONS/ROUTES/DOSAGE

**Hypertension**

**PO: ADULTS, ELDERLY:** Initially, 12.5–25 mg 2–3 times/day. May increase by 12.5–25 mg/dose at 1–2 wk intervals up to 50 mg 3 times/day. Add diuretic before further increase in dose. **Maximum:** 450 mg/day in 3 divided doses. **CHILDREN:** 0.3–0.5 mg 3 times/day. **Maximum:** 6 mg/kg/day in 2–4 divided doses. **INFANTS:** 0.15–0.3 mg/kg/dose. May titrate up to maximum of 6 mg/kg/day in 1–4 divided doses. Usual range: 2.5–6 mg/kg/day. **NEONATES:** 0.01–0.1 mg/kg/dose q8–24h. **Maximum:** 0.5 mg/kg/dose q6–24h.

**HF**

**PO: ADULTS, ELDERLY:** Initially, 6.25–25 mg 3 times/day. **Target dose:** 50 mg 3 times/day.

**Post-MI**

**PO: ADULTS, ELDERLY:** Initially, 6.25 mg. If tolerated, then 12.5 mg 3 times/day. Increase to 25 mg 3 times/day over several days, up to 50 mg 3 times/day over several wks.

**Diabetic Nephropathy**

**PO: ADULTS, ELDERLY:** 25 mg 3 times/day.

**Dosage in Renal Impairment**

**CrCl 10–50 ml/min:** 75% of normal dosage. **CrCl less than 10 ml/min:** 50% of normal dosage.

**Dosage in Hepatic Impairment**

No dose adjustment.

---

 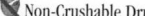

## SIDE EFFECTS

**Frequent (7%–4%):** Rash. **Occasional (4%–2%):** Pruritus, dysgeusia. **Rare (less than 2%):** Headache, cough, insomnia, dizziness, fatigue, paresthesia, malaise, nausea, diarrhea or constipation, dry mouth, tachycardia.

## ADVERSE EFFECTS/TOXIC REACTIONS

Hypotension ("first-dose syncope") may occur in pts with HF and in those who are severely sodium/volume depleted. Angioedema, hyperkalemia occur rarely. Agranulocytosis, neutropenia noted in those with collagen vascular disease (scleroderma, systemic lupus erythematosus), renal impairment. Nephrotic syndrome noted in those with history of renal disease.

## NURSING CONSIDERATIONS

### BASELINE ASSESSMENT

Obtain B/P immediately before each dose, in addition to regular monitoring (be alert to fluctuations). If hypotension occurs, place pt in supine position with legs elevated. In pts with prior renal disease or receiving dosages greater than 150 mg/day, test urine for protein by dipstick method with first urine of day before therapy begins and periodically thereafter. In pts with renal impairment, autoimmune disease, or taking drugs that affect leukocytes or immune response, obtain CBC before beginning therapy, q2wks for 3 mos, then periodically thereafter.

### INTERVENTION/EVALUATION

Assess skin for rash, pruritus. Assist with ambulation if dizziness occurs. Monitor urinalysis for proteinuria. Monitor serum potassium levels in pts on concurrent diuretic therapy. Monitor B/P, serum BUN, creatinine, CBC. Discontinue medication, contact physician if angioedema occurs.

### PATIENT/FAMILY TEACHING

• Full therapeutic effect of B/P reduction may take several wks. • Skipping doses or voluntarily discontinuing drug may produce severe rebound hypertension. • Limit alcohol intake. • Immediately report if swelling of face, lips, or tongue; difficulty breathing, vomiting, diarrhea, excessive perspiration, dehydration, persistent cough, sore throat, fever occur. • Inform physician if pregnant or planning to become pregnant. • Rise slowly from sitting/lying position.

## *carBAMazepine

kar-ba-**maz**-e-peen
(Apo-Carbamazepine ✦, Carbatrol, Carnexiv, Epitol, Equetro, Tegretol, Tegretol XR)

■ **BLACK BOX ALERT** ■ Potentially fatal aplastic anemia, agranulocytosis reported. Potentially fatal, severe dermatologic reactions (e.g., Stevens-Johnson syndrome, toxic epidermal necrolysis) may occur. Risk increased in pts with the variant HLA-β* 1502 allele, almost exclusively in pts of Asian ancestry.
**Do not confuse carbamazepine with oxcarbazepine, or Tegretol with Mebaral, Toprol XL, Toradol, or Trental.**

### ◆CLASSIFICATION

**PHARMACOTHERAPEUTIC:** Iminostilbene derivative. **CLINICAL:** Anticonvulsant, antineuralgic, antimanic, antipsychotic.

## USES

**Carbatrol, Epitol, Tegretol, Tegretol XR:** Treatment of partial seizures with complex symptomatology, generalized tonic-clonic seizures, mixed seizure patterns, pain relief of trigeminal, glossopharyngeal neuralgia. **Carnexiv:** Replacement when oral therapy not feasible in adults with seizures. **Equetro:** Acute manic and mixed episodes associated with bipolar disorder. **OFF-LABEL:** Neuropathic pain in critically ill pts.

## PRECAUTIONS

**Contraindications:** Concomitant use or within 14 days of use of MAOIs, myelosuppression. Concomitant use of delavirdine or other NNRT inhibitors, hypersensitivity to carbamazepine, tricyclic antidepressants. **Cautions:** High risk of suicide, increased IOP, hepatic or renal impairment, history of cardiac impairment, EKG abnormalities, elderly.

## ACTION

Decreases sodium ion influx into neuronal membranes, reducing post-tetanic potentiation at synapses. **Therapeutic Effect:** Produces anticonvulsant effect.

## PHARMACOKINETICS

Slowly, completely absorbed from GI tract. Protein binding: 75%–90%. Metabolized in liver. Primarily excreted in urine. Not removed by hemodialysis. **Half-life:** 25–65 hrs (decreased with chronic use).

## ⧖ LIFESPAN CONSIDERATIONS

**Pregnancy/Lactation:** Crosses placenta; distributed in breast milk. Accumulates in fetal tissue. **Children:** Behavioral changes more likely to occur. **Elderly:** More susceptible to confusion, agitation, AV block, bradycardia, syndrome of inappropriate antidiuretic hormone (SIADH).

## INTERACTIONS

**DRUG: CYP3A4 inhibitors (e.g., cimetidine, clarithromycin, azole antifungals, protease inhibitors)** may increase concentration. **CYP3A4 inducers (e.g., rifampin, phenytoin)** may decrease concentration/effects. May decrease concentration/effects of **hormonal contraceptives, warfarin, trazodone. HERBAL: Evening primrose** may decrease seizure threshold. **Gotu kola, kava kava, St. John's wort, valerian** may increase CNS depression. **FOOD: Grapefruit products** may increase absorption, concentration. **LAB VALUES:** May increase serum BUN, glucose, alkaline phosphatase, bilirubin, ALT, AST, cholesterol, HDL, triglycerides. May decrease serum calcium, thyroid hormone ($T_3$, $T_4$ index) levels. **Therapeutic serum level:** 4–12 mcg/ml; **toxic serum level:** greater than 12 mcg/ml.

## AVAILABILITY (Rx)

**Injection, Soluton (Carnexiv):** 200 mg/20 ml single use vial. **Suspension (Tegretol):** 100 mg/5 ml. **Tablets (Epitol, Tegretol):** 200 mg. **Tablets (Chewable [Tegretol]):** 100 mg.

 **Capsules (Extended-Release [Carbatrol, Equetro]):** 100 mg, 200 mg, 300 mg. **Tablets (Extended-Release [Tegretol XR]):** 100 mg, 200 mg, 400 mg.

## ADMINISTRATION/HANDLING

### PO

• Store oral suspension, tablets at room temperature. • Give with meals to reduce GI distress. • May give extended-release capsules without regard to food. • Extended-release tablets should be given with meals. • Shake oral suspension well. Do not administer simultaneously with other liquid medicine. • Do not crush or open extended-release capsules or tablets. • Extended-release capsules may be opened and sprinkled over food (e.g., applesauce).

### 🜄 IV

Must be diluted with 100 ml 0.9% NaCl or $D_5W$. Solution stable for 4 hrs at room temperature, 24 hrs refrigerated.

## INDICATIONS/ROUTES/DOSAGE

◀**ALERT**▶ Suspension must be given on a 3–4 times/day schedule; tablets on a 2–4 times/day schedule; extended-release capsules 2 times/day. **Carnexiv:** 70% of total oral dose given as four 30 min infusions separated by 6 hrs.

### Seizure Control

**PO: ADULTS, ELDERLY, CHILDREN OLDER THAN 12 YRS:** Initially, 200 mg twice daily (tablet or extended-release or in 4 divided doses as suspension). May increase dosage by 200 mg/day at wkly intervals. Usual dose: 800–1,200 mg/day in 2–4 divided doses. **Maximum:** 1.6–2.4 g/day. **CHILDREN OLDER THAN 15 YRS:** 1,200 mg/day; **CHILDREN 13–15 YRS:** 1,000 mg/day. **CHILDREN 6–12 YRS:** Initially, 100 mg twice daily (tablets) or 4 times/day (oral suspension). May increase by 100 mg/day at wkly intervals. Usual dose: 400–800 mg/day. **Maximum:** 1,000 mg/day. **CHILDREN YOUNGER THAN 6 YRS:** Initially, 10–20 mg/kg/day 2–3 times/day (tablets) or 4 times/day (suspension). May increase at wkly intervals until optimal response and therapeutic levels are achieved. **Maximum:** 35 mg/kg/day.

**Trigeminal, Glossopharyngeal Neuralgia, Diabetic Neuropathy**
**PO: ADULTS, ELDERLY:** Initially, 100 mg twice a day (tablets or extended-release) or 4 times/day (oral suspension). May increase by 100 mg twice daily up to 400–800 mg/day. **Maximum:** 1,200 mg/day.

**Bipolar Disorder**
**PO: ADULTS, ELDERLY (Equetro):** Initially, 400 mg/day in 2 divided doses (tablets) or 4 times/day (oral suspension). May adjust dose in 200-mg increments. **Maximum:** 1,600 mg/day in divided doses.

**Dosage in Renal Impairment**
**CrCl less than 10 ml/min:** 75% of normal dose. **HD:** 75% of normal dose. **CRRT:** 75% of normal dose.

**Dosage in Hepatic Impairment**
Use with caution.

## SIDE EFFECTS

**Frequent (greater than 10%):** Vertigo, somnolence, ataxia, fatigue, leucopenia, rash, urticaria, nausea, vomiting. **Occasional (10%–1%):** Headache, diplopia, blurred vision, thrombocytopenia, dry mouth, edema, fluid retention, increased weight. **Rare (less than 1%):** Tremors, visual disturbances, lymphadenopathy, jaundice, involuntary muscle movements, nystagmus, dermatitis.

## ADVERSE EFFECTS/ TOXIC REACTIONS

Toxic reactions appear as blood dyscrasias (aplastic anemia, agranulocytosis, thrombocytopenia, leukopenia, leukocytosis, eosinophilia), cardiovascular disturbances (HF, hypotension/hypertension, thrombophlebitis, arrhythmias), dermatologic effects (rash, urticaria, pruritus, photosensitivity). Abrupt withdrawal may precipitate status epilepticus.

## NURSING CONSIDERATIONS

### BASELINE ASSESSMENT
CBC, serum iron determination, urinalysis, BUN should be performed before therapy begins and periodically during therapy. **Seizures:** Review history of seizure disorder (intensity, frequency, duration, level of consciousness [LOC]). Initiate seizure precautions. **Neuralgia:** Assess facial pain, stimuli that may cause facial pain. **Bipolar:** Assess mental status, cognitive abilities.

### INTERVENTION/EVALUATION
**Seizures:** Observe frequently for recurrence of seizure activity. Monitor for therapeutic levels. Assess for clinical improvement (decrease in intensity, frequency of seizures). Assess for clinical evidence of early toxicity (fever, sore throat, mouth ulcerations, unusual bruising/bleeding, joint pain). **Neuralgia:** Avoid triggering tic douloureux (draft, talking, washing face, jarring bed, hot/warm/cold food or liquids). **Bipolar:** Monitor for suicidal ideation, behavioral changes. Observe for excessive sedation. **Therapeutic serum level:** 4–12 mcg/ml; **toxic serum level:** greater than 12 mcg/ml.

### PATIENT/FAMILY TEACHING
• Do not abruptly discontinue medication after long-term use (may precipitate seizures). • Strict maintenance of therapy is essential for seizure control. • Avoid tasks that require alertness, motor skills until response to drug is established. • Report visual disturbances. • Blood tests should be repeated frequently during first 3 mos of therapy and at monthly intervals thereafter for 2–3 yrs. • Do not take oral suspension simultaneously with other liquid medicine. • Do not ingest grapefruit products. • Report serious skin reactions.

# carbidopa/levodopa

kar-bi-doe-pa/lee-voe-doe-pa
(Apo-Levocarb ✦, Duopa, Rytary,
Sinemet, Sinemet CR)
**Do not confuse Sinemet with
Serevent.**

## FIXED-COMBINATION(S)

**Stalevo:** carbidopa/levodopa/
entacapone (antiparkinson agent): 12.5
mg/50 mg/200 mg, 18.75 mg/75
mg/200 mg, 25 mg/100 mg/200 mg,
31.25 mg/125 mg/200 mg, 37.5 mg/150
mg/200 mg, 50 mg/200 mg/200 mg.

## ◆CLASSIFICATION

**PHARMACOTHERAPEUTIC:** Dopamine
precursor. **CLINICAL:** Antiparkinson
agent.

## USES

Treatment of Parkinson's disease, post-
encephalitic parkinsonism, symptomatic
parkinsonism following CNS injury by $CO_2$
poisoning, manganese intoxication. **OFF-
LABEL:** Restless legs syndrome.

## PRECAUTIONS

**Contraindications:** Hypersensitivity to car-
bidopa/levodopa. Narrow-angle glaucoma,
use within 14 days of MAOIs. **Cautions:** History of MI, arrhythmias, bronchial asthma,
emphysema, severe cardiac, pulmonary,
renal/hepatic impairment; active peptic ulcer, treated open-angle glaucoma, seizure
disorder, pts at risk for hypotension, elderly.

## ACTION

Converted to dopamine in basal ganglia,
increasing dopamine concentration in
brain, inhibiting hyperactive cholinergic
activity. Carbidopa prevents peripheral
breakdown of levodopa, making more
levodopa available for transport into brain.
**Therapeutic Effect:** Reduces tremor.

## PHARMACOKINETICS

Rapidly and completely absorbed from GI
tract. Widely distributed. Excreted primarily

in urine. Levodopa is converted to dopamine.
Excreted primarily in urine. **Half-life:** 1–2
hrs (carbidopa); 1–3 hrs (levodopa).

## ⧗ LIFESPAN CONSIDERATIONS

**Pregnancy/Lactation:** Unknown if
drug crosses placenta or is distributed in
breast milk. May inhibit lactation. Breastfeeding not recommended. **Children:**
Safety and efficacy not established in
those younger than 18 yrs. **Elderly:** More
sensitive to effects of levodopa. Anxiety,
confusion, nervousness more common
when receiving anticholinergics.

## INTERACTIONS

**DRUG: Isoniazid, antipsychotics,
phenytoin, pyridoxine** may decrease
effects. **MAOIs** may increase concentra-
tion, effects of orthostatic hypotension.
**Selegiline, antihypertensives** may in-
crease risk of orthostatic hypotension.
**HERBAL: Kava kava** may decrease effect.
**FOOD: High-protein** diets may cause de-
creased or erratic response to levodopa.
**LAB VALUES:** May increase serum BUN,
LDH, alkaline phosphatase, bilirubin, ALT,
AST. May decrease Hgb, Hct, WBC.

## AVAILABILITY (Rx)

**Enteral Suspension:** 100 ml cassette containing 4.63 mg carbidopa and 20 mg
levodopa per ml. **Tablets (Immediate-
Release [Sinemet]):** 10 mg carbidopa/100
mg levodopa, 25 mg carbidopa/100 mg levodopa, 25 mg carbidopa/250 mg levodopa.
**Tablets (Orally-Disintegrating Immediate-
Release):** 10 mg carbidopa/100 mg levodopa, 25 mg carbidopa/100 mg levodopa,
25 mg carbidopa/250 mg levodopa.

**⬢ Capsules (Extended-Release [Rytary]):**
carbidopa/levodopa: 23.75 mg/95 mg,
36.25 mg/145 mg, 48.75 mg/195 mg,
61.25 mg/245 mg. **Tablets (Extended-
Release [Sinemet CR]):** 25 mg carbidopa/
100 mg levodopa, 50 mg carbidopa/200
mg levodopa.

## ADMINISTRATION/HANDLING

**Note:** Space doses evenly over waking
hours.

---

✦ Canadian trade name          ⬢ Non-Crushable Drug          🄷🄸 High Alert drug

**Enteral Suspension**

Refrigerate. Remove 20 min prior to administration.

**PO**

• Scored tablets may be crushed. • Give with meals to decrease GI upset. • Do not crush or chew extended-release tablets.

**PO (Parcopa)**

• Place orally-disintegrating tablet on top of tongue. Tablet will dissolve in seconds, pt to swallow with saliva. Not necessary to administer with liquid.

## INDICATIONS/ROUTES/DOSAGE

**Parkinsonism**

**PO: ADULTS, ELDERLY (IMMEDIATE-RELEASE ORALLY DISINTEGRATING TABLET):** Initially, 25/100 mg 3 times/day. May increase every other day by 1 tablet up to 200/2,000 mg daily. **(EXTENDED-RELEASE):** (Sinemet CR) 50/200 mg 2 times/day at least 6 hrs apart. Intervals between doses of Sinemet CR should be 4–8 hrs while awake, with smaller doses at end of day if doses are not equal. May adjust q3 days. **Maximum:** 8 tablets/day. **(RYTARY):** Initially, 23.75/95 mg 3 times/day for 3 days, then to 36.25/145 mg 3 times/day. **Maximum daily dose:** 612.5/2450 mg/day. **(ENTERAL SUSPENSION):** Maximum: 2000 mg (1 container) over 16 hrs through NJ or PEG tube via infusion pump. Also take oral immediate-release in evening after disconnecting pump.

**Dosage in Renal/Hepatic Impairment**

Use with caution.

## SIDE EFFECTS

**Frequent (80%–50%):** Involuntary movements of face, tongue, arms, upper body; nausea/vomiting; anorexia. **Occasional:** Depression, anxiety, confusion, nervousness, urinary retention, palpitations, dizziness, light-headedness, decreased appetite, blurred vision, constipation, dry mouth, flushed skin, headache, insomnia, diarrhea, unusual fatigue, darkening of urine

and sweat. **Rare:** Hypertension, ulcer, hemolytic anemia (marked by fatigue).

## ADVERSE EFFECTS/ TOXIC REACTIONS

High incidence of involuntary choreiform, dystonic, dyskinetic movements in those on long-term therapy. Numerous mild to severe CNS and psychiatric disturbances may occur (reduced attention span, anxiety, nightmares, daytime drowsiness, euphoria, fatigue, paranoia, psychotic episodes, depression, hallucinations).

## NURSING CONSIDERATIONS

### BASELINE ASSESSMENT

Assess symptoms of Parkinson's disease (e.g., rigidity, pill rolling, gait).

### INTERVENTION/EVALUATION

Be alert to neurologic effects (headache, lethargy, mental confusion, agitation). Monitor for evidence of dyskinesia (difficulty with movement). Assess for clinical reversal of symptoms (improvement of tremor of head and hands at rest, mask-like facial expression, shuffling gait, muscular rigidity). Monitor B/P (standing, sitting, supine).

### PATIENT/FAMILY TEACHING

• Avoid tasks that require alertness, motor skills until response to drug is established. • Sugarless gum, sips of water may relieve dry mouth. • Take with food to minimize GI upset. • Effects may be delayed from several wks to mos. • May cause darkening of urine or sweat (not harmful). • Report any uncontrolled movement of face, eyelids, mouth, tongue, arms, hands, legs; mental changes; palpitations; severe or persistent nausea/vomiting; difficulty urinating. • Report exacerbations of asthma, underlying depression, psychosis.

# *CARBOplatin

kar-boe-**plat-in**
(Carboplatin Injection ❦)

■ **BLACK BOX ALERT** ■ Must be administered by personnel trained in administration/handling of chemotherapeutic agents (high potential for severe reactions, including anaphylaxis [may occur within minutes of administration] and sudden death). Profound myelosuppression (anemia, thrombocytopenia) has occurred. Vomiting may occur.
**Do not confuse carboplatin with Cisplatin or oxaliplatin, or with Platinol.**

## ◆CLASSIFICATION

**PHARMACOTHERAPEUTIC:** Platinum coordination complex. **CLINICAL:** Antineoplastic.

## USES

Treatment of ovarian carcinoma. Palliative treatment of recurrent ovarian cancer. **OFF-LABEL:** Brain tumors, Hodgkin's and non-Hodgkin's lymphomas, malignant melanoma, retinoblastoma; treatment of breast, bladder, cervical, endometrial, esophageal, small-cell lung, non–small-cell lung, head and neck, testicular carcinomas; germ cell tumors, osteogenic sarcoma.

## PRECAUTIONS

**Contraindications:** Hypersensitivity to carboplatin. History of severe allergic reaction to cisplatin, platinum compounds, mannitol; severe bleeding, severe myelosuppression. **Cautions:** Moderate bone marrow depression, renal impairment, elderly.

## ACTION

Inhibits DNA synthesis by cross-linking with DNA strands, preventing cell division. **Therapeutic Effect:** Interferes with DNA function.

## PHARMACOKINETICS

Protein binding: Low. Hydrolyzed in solution to active form. Primarily excreted in urine. **Half-life:** 2.6–5.9 hrs.

## ⧗ LIFESPAN CONSIDERATIONS

**Pregnancy/Lactation:** If possible, avoid use during pregnancy, esp. first trimester. May cause fetal harm. Unknown if distributed in breast milk. Breastfeeding not recommended. **Children:** Safety and efficacy not established. **Elderly:** Peripheral neurotoxicity increased, myelotoxicity may be more severe. Age-related renal impairment may require decreased dosage, careful monitoring of blood counts.

## INTERACTIONS

**DRUG: Bone marrow depressants** may increase myelosuppression. **Live virus vaccines** may potentiate virus replication, increase vaccine side effects, decrease pt's antibody response to vaccine. **Nephrotoxic, ototoxic medications** may increase risk of toxicity. **HERBAL:** Avoid **black cohosh, dong quai** in estrogen-dependent tumors. **Echinacea** may decrease level/effects. **FOOD:** None known. **LAB VALUES:** May decrease serum calcium, magnesium, potassium, sodium. May increase serum BUN, alkaline phosphatase, bilirubin, creatinine, AST.

## AVAILABILITY (Rx)

**Injection Solution:** 10 mg/ml.

## ADMINISTRATION/HANDLING

◀**ALERT**▶ May be carcinogenic, mutagenic, teratogenic. Handle with extreme care during preparation/administration.

 **IV**

**Reconstitution •** Dilute with $D_5W$ or 0.9% NaCl to a final concentration as low as 0.5 mg/ml.
**Rate of Administration •** Infuse over 15–60 min. • Rarely, anaphylactic reaction occurs minutes after administration.

Use of epinephrine, corticosteroids alleviates symptoms.

**Storage** • Store vials at room temperature. •After dilution, solution is stable for 8 hrs.

##  IV INCOMPATIBILITY

Amphotericin B complex (Abelcet, AmBisome, Amphotec).

## ⊞ IV COMPATIBILITIES

Etoposide (VePesid), granisetron (Kytril), ondansetron (Zofran), paclitaxel (Taxol), palonosetron (Aloxi).

## INDICATIONS/ROUTES/DOSAGE

**Note:** Doses commonly calculated by target AUC.

**Ovarian Carcinoma (Monotherapy)**
**IV: ADULTS:** 360 mg/m² on day 1, every 4 wks (as single agent), or 300 mg/m² q4 wks (in combination with cyclophosphamide) or target AUC 4–6 (single agent; in previously treated pts). Do not repeat dose until neutrophil and platelet counts are within acceptable levels.

**Dose Modification**
**Platelets less than 50,000 cells/ mm³ or ANC less than 500 cells/ mm³:** Give 75% of dose.

**Dosage in Renal Impairment**
Initial dosage is based on creatinine clearance; subsequent dosages are based on pt's tolerance, degree of myelosuppression.

| Creatinine Clearance | Dosage Day 1 |
| --- | --- |
| 60 ml/min or greater | 360 mg/m² |
| 41–59 ml/min | 250 mg/m² |
| 16–40 ml/min | 200 mg/m² |

**Dosage in Hepatic Impairment**
No dose adjustment.

## SIDE EFFECTS

**Frequent (80%–65%):** Nausea, vomiting. **Occasional (17%–4%):** Generalized pain, diarrhea/constipation, peripheral neuropathy. **Rare (3%–2%):** Alopecia, asthenia, hypersensitivity reaction (erythema, pruritus, rash, urticaria).

## ADVERSE EFFECTS/ TOXIC REACTIONS

Myelosuppression may be severe, resulting in anemia, infection (sepsis, pneumonia), major bleeding. Prolonged treatment may result in peripheral neurotoxicity.

## NURSING CONSIDERATIONS

### BASELINE ASSESSMENT

Obtain EKG, CBC, serum chemistries, renal function test. Offer emotional support. Do not repeat treatment until WBC recovers from previous therapy. Transfusions may be needed in those receiving prolonged therapy (myelosuppression increased in those with previous therapy, renal impairment).

### INTERVENTION/EVALUATION

Monitor pulmonary function studies, hepatic/renal function tests, CBC, serum electrolytes. Monitor for fever, sore throat, signs of local infection, unusual bruising/ bleeding from any site, symptoms of anemia (excessive fatigue, weakness).

### PATIENT/FAMILY TEACHING

• Nausea, vomiting generally abate within 24 hrs. • Do not have immunizations without physician's approval (drug lowers body's resistance). • Avoid contact with those who have recently received live virus vaccine.

# carfilzomib

kar-**fil**-zoh-mib
(Kyprolis)
**Do not confuse carfilzomib with crizotinib, pazopanib.**

## ◆CLASSIFICATION

**PHARMACOTHERAPEUTIC:** Proteasome inhibitor. **CLINICAL:** Antineoplastic.

## USES

Treatment of pts with multiple myeloma who have received at least 2 prior therapies including bortezomib and an immunomodulatory agent and have demonstrated disease progression on or within 60 days of completion of last therapy. In combination with lenalidomide and dexamethasone for treatment of relapsed multiple myeloma who have received 1 to 3 prior therapies.

## PRECAUTIONS

**Contraindications:** Hypersensitivity to carfilzomib. **Cautions:** Preexisting HF, decreased left ventricular ejection fraction, myocardial abnormalities, complications of pulmonary hypertension (e.g., dyspnea), hepatic impairment, thrombocytopenia.

## ACTION

Blocks action of proteasomes, intracellular proteins to induce cell death in rapidly dividing cells. **Therapeutic Effect:** Produces cell cycle arrest and apoptosis.

## PHARMACOKINETICS

Protein Binding: 97%. Rapidly, extensively metabolized. Excreted primarily extrahepatically. Minimal removal by hemodialysis. **Half-life:** Equal to or less than 1 hr on day 1 of cycle 1. Proteasome inhibition was maintained for 48 hrs or longer following first dose of carfilzomib for each week of dosing.

## LIFESPAN CONSIDERATIONS

**Pregnancy/Lactation:** Avoid pregnancy. May cause fetal harm. Unknown if excreted in breast milk. **Children:** Safety and efficacy not established. **Elderly:** No age-related precautions noted.

## INTERACTIONS

**DRUG:** None significant. **HERBAL:** None significant. **FOOD:** None known. **LAB VALUES:** May increase serum creatinine, glucose, creatinine, ALT, AST, bilirubin, calcium. May decrease RBC, Hgb, Hct, absolute neutrophil count (ANC), platelet count; serum magnesium, phosphate, potassium, sodium.

## AVAILABILITY (Rx)

Injection Powder for Reconstitution (Single-Use Vial): 60 mg.

## ADMINISTRATION/HANDLING

 IV

**Reconstitution** • Slowly inject 29 ml Sterile Water for Injection, directing solution to inside wall of vial (minimizes foaming). • Swirl and invert vial slowly for 1 min or until completely dissolved. • Do not shake. • If foaming occurs, rest vial for 2–5 min until subsided. • Withdraw calculated dose from vial and dilute into 50 ml D₅W. • Final concentration of reconstituted solution: 2 mg/ml.
**Rate of administration** • Infuse over 2–10 min. Flush line before and after with NaCl or D₅W. • Do not administer as a bolus.
**Storage** • Refrigerate undiluted vials. • Reconstituted solution may be refrigerated up to 24 hrs. • At room temperature, use diluted solution within 4 hrs.

## ⬛ IV INCOMPATIBILITIES

Do not mix with other IV medications or additives. Infuse via dedicated line. Flush IV administration line with NaCl or D₅W immediately before and after carfilzomib administration.

## INDICATIONS/ROUTES/DOSAGE

**◄ALERT►** Dose is calculated using pts' actual body surface area at baseline. Pts with a body surface area greater than 2.2 m² should receive dose based on a body surface area of 2.2 m². No dose adjustment needed for weight changes of less than or equal to 20%.
**◄ALERT►** Prior to each dose in cycle 1, give 250 ml to 500 ml NaCl bolus. Give an additional 250 ml to 500 ml IV fluid following administration. Continue IV hydration in subsequent cycles (reduces risk of renal toxicity, tumor lysis syndrome). Premedicate with dexamethasone 4 mg PO or IV prior to all doses during cycle 1 and prior to all doses during first cycle of dose escalation to 27 mg/m² (reduces

incidence, severity of infusion reactions). Reinstate dexamethasone premedication (4 mg PO or IV) if symptoms develop or reappear during subsequent cycles.

### Multiple Myeloma

**Note:** Each 28 day cycle consists of carfilzomib on days 1, 2, 8, 9, 15, 16, followed by a 12-day rest period days 17–28.

**IV Infusion: ADULTS, ELDERLY:** Initially, 20 mg/m² given on days 1 and 2. If tolerated, may escalate dose to 27 mg/m² beginning on day 8 of cycle 1 and continue at 27 mg/m² during cycles 2–12. Cycles 13 and beyond: 27 mg/m² on days 1, 2, 15, 16 of a 28-day treatment cycle. Treatment may be continued until disease progression or unacceptable toxicity occurs.

### Dosage Modification for Toxicity

*Hematologic*

**Grade 3 or 4 Neutropenia:** Withhold dose. Continue at same dose if fully recovered prior to next scheduled dose. If recovered to grade 2, reduce dose by one dose level. If dose tolerated, may escalate to previous dose. **Grade 4 Thrombocytopenia:** Withhold dose. Continue at same dose if fully recovered prior to next scheduled dose. If recovered to grade 3, reduce dose by one dose level. If dose tolerated, may escalate to previous dose.

*Cardiac*

**Grade 3 or 4, New Onset or Worsening of HF, Decreased LVF, Myocardial Ischemia:** Withhold dose until resolved or at baseline. After resolution, restart at reduced dose level. If dose tolerated, may escalate to previous dose.

*Hepatic*

**Grade 3 or 4 Elevation of Bilirubin, transaminases:** Withhold dose until resolved or at baseline. After resolution, restart at reduced dose level. If dose tolerated, may escalate to previous dose.

*Peripheral Neuropathy*

**Grade 3 or 4:** Withhold dose until resolved or at baseline. After resolution, restart at reduced dose level. If dose tolerated, may escalate to previous dose.

*Pulmonary Toxicity*

**Pulmonary Hypertension:** Withhold dose until resolved or at baseline. After resolution, restart at reduced dose level. If dose tolerated, may escalate to previous dose. **Grade 3 or 4 Pulmonary Complications:** Withhold dose until resolved or at baseline. After resolution, restart at reduced dose level. If dose tolerated, may escalate to previous dose.

*Renal*

**Serum Creatinine 2 times or Greater from Baseline:** Withhold dose until renal function improves to grade 1 or baseline. Withhold dose until resolved or at baseline. After resolution, restart at reduced dose level. If dose tolerated, may escalate to previous dose.

### Dosage in Renal/Hepatic Impairment

No dose adjustment.

## SIDE EFFECTS

**Frequent (56%–20%):** Fatigue, anemia, nausea, exertional dyspnea, diarrhea, fever, headache, cough, peripheral edema, vomiting, constipation, back pain. **Occasional (18%–14%):** Insomnia, chills, arthralgia, muscle spasms, hypertension, asthenia, extremity pain, dizziness, hypoesthesia (decreased sensitivity to touch), anorexia.

## ADVERSE EFFECTS/ TOXIC REACTIONS

Pneumonia (10% of pts), acute renal failure (4% of pts), pyrexia (3% of pts), and HF (3% of pts) were reported. Adverse reactions leading to discontinuation occurred in 15% of pts. Upper respiratory tract infection reported in 28% of pts. HF, pulmonary edema, decrease in ejection fraction were reported in 7% of pts. Infusion reaction characterized by chills, fever, wheezing, facial flushing, dyspnea, vomiting, chest tightness can occur immediately following or up to 24 hrs after administration. Tumor lysis syndrome occurs rarely.

## NURSING CONSIDERATIONS

### BASELINE ASSESSMENT

Obtain full history of home medications including vitamins, herbal products. Ensure hydration status and maintain throughout treatment. Obtain CBC, serum chemistries. Assess vital signs, $O_2$ saturation. Platelet nadirs occur around day 8 of each 28-day cycle and recover to baseline by start of the next 28-day cycle.

### INTERVENTION/EVALUATION

Monitor for fluid overload. Monitor platelet count frequently; adjust dose according to grade of thrombocytopenia. Obtain serum ALT, AST, bilirubin for evidence of hepatotoxicity. Monitor vital signs, $O_2$ saturation routinely. Monitor cardiac function and manage as needed. Assess for palpitations, tachycardia. Assess for anemia-related dizziness, exertional dyspnea, fatigue, weakness, syncope. Report decreases in Hgb, Hct, platelets, neutrophils. Monitor for acute infection (fever, diaphoresis, lethargy, oral mucosal changes, productive cough), bloody stools, bruising, hematuria, DVT, pulmonary embolism. Encourage nutritional intake and assess anorexia, weight loss. Reinforce birth control compliance. Monitor daily pattern of bowel activity, stool consistency. Offer antiemetics if nausea, vomiting occur. Monitor for symptoms of neutropenia.

### PATIENT/FAMILY TEACHING

• Blood tests will be drawn routinely.
• Immediately report any newly prescribed medications. • May alter taste of food or decrease appetite. • Report bloody stool/ urine, increased bruising, difficulty breathing, weakness, dizziness, palpitations, weight loss. • Maintain strict oral hygiene. • Do not have immunizations without physician approval (drug lowers body's resistance). • Avoid those who have recently taken live virus vaccine. • Avoid crowds, those with symptoms of viral illness.

# cariprazine

kar-**ip**-ra-zeen
(Vraylar)

■ **BLACK BOX ALERT** ■ Elderly pts treated with antipsychotic drugs are at an increased risk of death. Treatment not approved in pts with dementia-related psychosis.

**Do not confuse cariprazine with Compazine or mirtazapine.**

### ◆ CLASSIFICATION

**PHARMACOTHERAPEUTIC:** Serotonin receptor antagonist. **CLINICAL:** Antipsychotic.

## USES

Treatment of schizophrenia. Acute treatment of manic or mixed episodes associated with bipolar I disorder.

## PRECAUTIONS

**Contraindications:** Hypersensitivity to cariprazine. **Cautions:** Baseline leukopenia, neutropenia; hx of drug-induced leukopenia, neutropenia; debilitated, diabetes mellitus, dyslipidemia, elderly, hepatic impairment, Parkinson's disease, pts at risk for hypotension (dehydration, hypovolemia, concomitant use of antihypertensives), pts at risk for aspiration, dysphagia; history of cardiovascular disease (e.g., ischemic heart disease, HF, cardiac arrhythmias); pts at risk for CVA, TIA; hx of seizures. Concomitant use of medications that lower seizure threshold. Avoid concomitant use of CYP3A inducers.

## ACTION

Exact mechanism unknown. Partial agonist of central dopamine $D_2$ and serotonin $5-HT_{1A}$ receptors and antagonist of serotonin $5-HT_{2A}$ receptors. **Therapeutic Effect:** Diminishes symptoms of psychotic behavior.

## PHARMACOKINETICS

Widely distributed. Metabolized in liver. Protein binding: 91–97%. Peak plasma concentration: 3–6 hrs. Mean plasma concentrations decrease approx. 50% after 1 wk from last dose. Excreted primarily in urine (21%). **Half-Life:** 2–4 days.

## ⧗ LIFESPAN CONSIDERATIONS

**Pregnancy/Lactation:** Avoid pregnancy; may cause fetal harm. May increase risk of extrapyramidal symptoms and/or withdraw syndrome in neonates. Unknown if distributed in breast milk. Must either discontinue drug or discontinue breast-feeding. **Children:** Safety and efficacy not established. **Elderly:** May increase risk of adverse effects due to age-related cardiac/hepatic/renal impairment.

## INTERACTIONS

**DRUG:** Strong CYP3A inhibitors (e.g., **clarithromycin, ketoconazole, ritonavir**) may increase concentration/effect. **Strong CYP3A inducers (e.g., carbamazepine, rifampicin), moderate CYP3A inducers (e.g., nafcillin)** may decrease concentration/effect; avoid use. **Alcohol, antidepressants (e.g., sertraline, nortriptyline), benzodiazepines (e.g., diazepam, lorazepam), opioids (e.g., morphine), phenothiazines (e.g., thioridazine), sedative/hypnotics (e.g., zolpidem)** may increase CNS depression. **Antihypertensives (e.g., amlodipine, enalapril, valsartan)** may increase hypotensive effect. **HERBAL:** St. John's wort may decrease concentration/effect. **FOOD:** Grapefruit products may increase concentration/effect. **LAB VALUES:** May increase serum ALT, AST; CPK. May decrease serum sodium.

## AVAILABILITY (Rx)

🛆 **Capsules:** 1.5 mg, 3 mg, 4.5 mg, 6 mg.

## ADMINISTRATION/HANDLING

**PO**
• Give without regard to food. • Administer whole; do not break, crush, cut, or open capsule.

## INDICATIONS/ROUTES/DOSAGE

**Schizophrenia**
**PO: ADULTS, ELDERLY:** Initially, 1.5 mg once daily. May increase to 3 mg on day 2 if tolerated. May further increase in increments of 1.5–3 mg based on clinical response and tolerability. **Range:** 1.5–6 mg once daily.

**Bipolar I Disorder**
**PO: ADULTS, ELDERLY:** 1.5 mg once on day 1, then increase to 3 mg once daily on day 2. May further increase in increments of 1.5–3 mg based on clinical response and tolerability. **Range:** 3–6 mg once daily.
*Concomitant Use of Strong CYP3A Inhibitors*
**Pts starting strong CYP3A inhibitor while on stable dose of cariprazine:** Reduce maintenance cariprazine dose by 50%. Pts taking cariprazine 4.5 mg/day should reduce dosage to 1.5 mg/day or 3 mg/day. Pts taking 1.5 mg/day, adjust dosing to every other day. If the strong CYP3A inhibitor is discontinued, cariprazine may need to be increased. **Pts starting cariprazine while on CYP3A inhibitor:** 1.5 mg once on day 1; no dose on day 2; 1.5 mg once on day 3. After day 3, increase dose to 3 mg once daily as tolerated. If strong CYP3A inhibitor is discontinued, cariprazine may need to be increased.

**Dosage in Renal Impairment**
**Mild to Moderate:** No dose adjustment. **Severe:** Treatment not recommended.

**Dosage in Hepatic Impairment**
**Mild to Moderate:** No dose adjustment. **Severe:** Treatment not recommended.

## SIDE EFFECTS

**Frequent (26%–11%):** Bradykinesia, cogwheel rigidity, drooling, dyskinesia, masked faces, muscle rigidity, dystonia, tremor, salivary hypersecretion, torticollis, trismus, insomnia, akathisia, headache. **Occasional (5%–3%):** Nausea, constipation, restlessness, vomiting, dizziness, agitation, anxiety, dyspepsia, abdominal pain, diarrhea,

---

underlined – top prescribed drug

fatigue, asthenia, back pain, toothache, hypertension, decreased appetite. **Rare (2%–1%):** Dry mouth, weight gain, extremity pain, somnolence, sedation, cough, tachycardia, arthralgia.

## ADVERSE EFFECTS/TOXIC REACTIONS

May increase risk of hypotension, orthostatic hypotension, syncope; diabetes mellitus, DKA, hyperglycemia, hyperglycemic hyperosmolar nonketotic coma; leukopenia, neutropenia, febrile neutropenia; aspiration, dysphagia, gastritis, gastric reflux; extrapyramidal symptoms including akathisia, dystonia, parkinsonism, tardive dyskinesia; suicidal ideation. May cause neuroleptic malignant syndrome (NMS); manifested by alerted mental status, cardiac arrhythmias, diaphoresis, labile blood pressure, malignant hyperthermia, muscle rigidity, rhabdomyolysis, renal failure. May increase risk of death in pts with dementia-related psychosis. Cognitive and motor impairment reported in 7% of pts. May increase seizure-like activity related to decrease in seizure threshold. Infectious processes including nasopharyngitis, urinary tract infection reported in 1% of pts. Hypersensitivity reactions including angioedema, rash, pruritus have occurred.

## NURSING CONSIDERATIONS

### BASELINE ASSESSMENT

Obtain baseline fasting lipid profile, fasting plasma glucose level, vital signs; Hgb A1c in pts with diabetes; ANC, CBC in pts with baseline leukopenia, neutropenia. Receive full medication history including herbal products and screen for interactions. Assess appearance, behavior, speech pattern, levels of interest. Verify pregnancy status. Question history of diabetes, cardiovascular disease, CVA, dysphagia, hepatic impairment, hypersensitivity reaction, TIA, seizures.

### INTERVENTION/EVALUATION

Monitor ANC, CBC, fasting lipid profile, fasting plasma glucose levels periodically. Assess mental status for anxiety, depression, suicidal ideation (esp. at initiation and with change in dosage), social function. Due to long half-life, any change in dosage will not be fully reflected for several wks; monitor closely for adverse effects during the following wks. Monitor for hypersensitivity reaction, dysphagia, tardive dyskinesia, extrapyramidal symptoms, metabolic changes including hyperglycemia. Screen for infection. Monitor for neuroleptic malignant syndrome.

### PATIENT/FAMILY TEACHING

• Immediately report thoughts of suicide or plans to commit suicide. • Avoid tasks that require alertness until response to drug is established. • Therapy may increase blood sugar levels. Monitor for blurry vision, confusion, frequent urination, fruity-smelling breath, thirst, weakness. • Treatment may cause fetal harm. Avoid pregnancy. Do not breastfeed. • Treatment may lower ability to fight infection. • Swallow capsules whole; do not chew, crush, cut, or open capsules. • Do not ingest grapefruit products or herbal products. Report drooling, muscle rigidity, lock jaw, tremors, or inability to control muscle movements. • Treatment may increase risk of seizures. • Report confusion, palpitations, profuse sweating, fluctuating blood pressure, unusually high core body temperature, muscle rigidity, dark-colored urine or decreased urine output; may indicate life-threatening neurologic event called neuroleptic malignant syndrome (NMS).

---

## carmustine

**HIGH ALERT**

kar-**mus**-teen
(BiCNU, Gliadel Wafer)

■ **BLACK BOX ALERT** ■ Profound myelosuppression (leukopenia, thrombocytopenia) is major toxicity. High risk of pulmonary toxicity. Must be administered by personnel trained in administration/handling of chemotherapeutic agents (high potential for severe reactions, including anaphylaxis, sudden death). **Do not confuse carmustine with bendamustine or lomustine.**

### ◆ CLASSIFICATION

**PHARMACOTHERAPEUTIC:** Alkylating agent, nitrosourea. **CLINICAL:** Antineoplastic.

### USES

**BiCNU:** Treatment of brain tumors, Hodgkin's lymphomas, non-Hodgkin's lymphomas, multiple myeloma. **Gliadel Wafer:** Adjunct to surgery to prolong survival in recurrent glioblastoma multiforme. **OFF-LABEL:** Treatment of mycosis fungoides (topical).

### PRECAUTIONS

**Contraindications:** Hypersensitivity to carmustine. **Cautions:** Thrombocytopenia, leukopenia, anemia, renal/hepatic impairment.

### ACTION

Inhibits DNA, RNA synthesis by crosslinking with DNA, RNA strands, preventing cell division. Cell cycle–phase nonspecific. **Therapeutic Effect:** Interferes with DNA, RNA function.

### PHARMACOKINETICS

Crosses blood-brain barrier. Metabolized in liver. Excreted in urine. **Half-life:** 15–30 min.

### ⧖ LIFESPAN CONSIDERATIONS

**Pregnancy/Lactation:** Avoid pregnancy, particularly first trimester; may cause fetal harm. Unknown if distributed in breast milk. Breastfeeding not recommended. **Children:** Safety and efficacy not established. **Elderly:** No age-related precautions noted.

### INTERACTIONS

**DRUG: Bone marrow depressants, cimetidine** may enhance myelosuppressive effect. **Hepatotoxic, nephrotoxic medications** may increase risk of hepatotoxicity, nephrotoxicity. **Live-virus vaccines** may potentiate virus replication, increase vaccine side effects, decrease pt's antibody response to vaccine. **HERBAL: Echinacea** may decrease effects. **FOOD:** None known. **LAB VALUES:** May increase serum BUN, alkaline phosphatase, bilirubin, ALT, AST.

### AVAILABILITY (Rx)

**Injection, Powder for Reconstitution (BiCNU):** 100 mg. **Implant Device (Gliadel Wafer):** 7.7 mg.

### ADMINISTRATION/HANDLING

**◀ALERT▶** May be carcinogenic, mutagenic, teratogenic. Wear protective gloves during preparation of drug; may cause transient burning, brown staining of skin.

 **IV**

**Reconstitution** • Reconstitute 100-mg vial with 3 ml sterile dehydrated (absolute) alcohol, followed by 27 ml Sterile Water for Injection to provide concentration of 3.3 mg/ml. • Further dilute with 50–250 ml D₅W to final concentration of 0.2–1 mg/ml.
**Rate of Administration** • Infuse over 1–2 hrs (shorter duration may produce intense burning pain at injection site, intense flushing of skin, conjunctiva). • Flush IV line with 5–10 ml 0.9% NaCl or D₅W before and after administration to prevent irritation at injection site.
**Storage** • Refrigerate unused vials. • Reconstituted vials are stable for 8 hrs at room temperature or 24 hrs if refrigerated. • Solutions further diluted with D₅W

are stable for 8 hrs at room temperature. • Solutions appear clear, colorless to yellow. • Discard if precipitate forms, color change occurs, or oily film develops on bottom of vial. **Gliadel Wafers:** Store at or below −20°C (−4°F). Unopened pouches may be kept at room temperature for maximum of 6 hrs.

### 🔲 IV INCOMPATIBILITIES

Allopurinol (Aloprim), sodium bicarbonate.

### 🔲 IV COMPATIBILITIES

Granisetron (Kytril), ondansetron (Zofran).

## INDICATIONS/ROUTES/DOSAGE

◀**ALERT**▶ Refer to individual oncology protocols.

**Usual Dosage (Refer to Individual Protocols)**
**IV** *(BiCNU)*: **ADULTS, ELDERLY:** 150–200 mg/m² as a single dose q6wks or 75–100 mg/m² on 2 successive days q6wks.

◀**ALERT**▶ Next dosage is based on clinical and hematologic response to previous dose (platelets greater than 100,000/mm³ and leukocytes greater than 4,000/mm³).
**Implantation** *(Gliadel Wafer)*: **ADULTS, ELDERLY, CHILDREN:** Up to 8 wafers (62.6 mg) may be placed in resection cavity.

**Dosage Modification**
**Leukocytes 2,000–2,999 cells/mm³ or platelets 25,000–74,999 cells/mm³:** Give 70% of dose. **Leukocytes less than 2,000 cells/mm³ or platelets less than 25,000 cells/mm³:** Give 50% of dose.

**Dosage in Renal Impairment**

| Creatinine Clearance (ml/min) | Dosage |
|---|---|
| 46–60 | 80% of dose |
| 31–45 | 75% of dose |
| Less than 31 | Not recommended |

**Dosage in Hepatic Impairment**
Use caution.

## SIDE EFFECTS

**Frequent:** Nausea, vomiting (may last up to 6 hrs). **Occasional:** Diarrhea, esophagitis, anorexia, dysphagia, hyperpigmentation. **Rare:** Thrombophlebitis, burning sensation, pain at injection site.

## ADVERSE EFFECTS/TOXIC REACTIONS

Hematologic toxicity due to myelosuppression occurs frequently. Thrombocytopenia occurs approximately 4 wks after treatment begins and lasts 1–2 wks. Leukopenia is evident 5–6 wks after treatment begins and lasts 1–2 wks. Anemia occurs less frequently. Mild, reversible hepatotoxicity occurs frequently. Prolonged, high-dose therapy may produce impaired renal function, pulmonary toxicity (pulmonary infiltrate/fibrosis).

## NURSING CONSIDERATIONS

### BASELINE ASSESSMENT

Obtain CBC, renal/hepatic function studies before initiation and periodically thereafter.

### INTERVENTION/EVALUATION

Monitor renal/hepatic function tests. Obtain CBC wkly during and for at least 6 wks after therapy ends. Monitor for hematologic toxicity (fever, sore throat, signs of local infection, unusual bruising/bleeding from any site), symptoms of anemia (excessive fatigue, weakness). Monitor for pulmonary toxicity; observe for dyspnea, adventitious breath sounds.

### PATIENT/FAMILY TEACHING

• Maintain adequate hydration (may protect against renal impairment). • Do not have immunizations without physician's approval (drug lowers body's resistance). • Avoid contact with those who have recently received live virus vaccine. • Report nausea, vomiting, fever, sore throat, chills, unusual bleeding/bruising.

---

✢ Canadian trade name     🍸 Non-Crushable Drug     🔳 High Alert drug

## *carvedilol*

TOP 100 | HIGH ALERT

kar-ve-dil-ole
(Apo-Carvedilol ✦, <u>Coreg</u>, Coreg CR, Novo-Carvedilol ✦)
**Do not confuse carvedilol with atenolol or carteolol, or Coreg with Corgard, Cortef, or Cozaar.**

### ◆ CLASSIFICATION

**PHARMACOTHERAPEUTIC:** Beta-adrenergic blocker. **CLINICAL:** Antihypertensive.

### USES

Treatment of mild to severe HF, left ventricular dysfunction following MI, hypertension. **OFF-LABEL:** Treatment of angina pectoris, idiopathic cardiomyopathy.

### PRECAUTIONS

**Contraindications:** Hypersensitivity to carvedilol. Bronchial asthma or related bronchospastic conditions, cardiogenic shock, decompensated HF requiring intravenous inotropic therapy, severe hepatic impairment, second- or third-degree AV block, severe bradycardia, or sick sinus syndrome (except in pts with pacemaker). **Cautions:** Diabetes, myasthenia gravis, mild to moderate hepatic impairment. Withdraw gradually to avoid acute tachycardia, hypertension, and/or ischemia. Pts suspected of having Prinzmetal angina, pheochromocytoma, hx of severe anaphylaxis to allergens.

### ACTION

Possesses nonselective beta-blocking and alpha-adrenergic blocking activity. Causes vasodilation. **Therapeutic Effect:** Hypertension: Reduces cardiac output, exercise-induced tachycardia, reflex orthostatic tachycardia; reduces peripheral vascular resistance. HF: Decreases pulmonary capillary wedge pressure, heart rate, systemic vascular resistance; increases stroke volume index.

### PHARMACOKINETICS

| Route | Onset | Peak | Duration |
|-------|-------|------|----------|
| PO | 30 min | 1–2 hrs | 24 hrs |

Rapidly, extensively absorbed from GI tract. Protein binding: 98%. Metabolized in liver. Excreted primarily via bile into feces. Minimally removed by hemodialysis. **Half-life:** 7–10 hrs. Food delays rate of absorption.

### ⧗ LIFESPAN CONSIDERATIONS

**Pregnancy/Lactation:** Unknown if drug crosses placenta or is distributed in breast milk. May produce bradycardia, apnea, hypoglycemia, hypothermia during delivery; may contribute to low birth-weight infants. **Children:** Safety and efficacy not established. **Elderly:** Incidence of dizziness may be increased.

### INTERACTIONS

**DRUG:** Beta blockers (e.g., **carvedilol, metoprolol**), **calcium channel blockers** (e.g., **diltiazem, verapamil**), **digoxin, CYP2C9 inhibitors** (e.g., **amiodarone, fluconazole**) increase risk of cardiac conduction disturbances. **Diuretics** (e.g., **furosemide, HCTZ**), **other antihypertensives** may potentiate hypotensive effects. **Cimetidine** may increase concentration. May increase concentration of **cyclosporine, digoxin. CYP2D6 inhibitors** (e.g., **fluoxetine, paroxetine**) may increase concentration/side effects; may enhance slowing of HR or cardiac conduction. May increase effects of **insulin, oral hypoglycemics. Rifampin** decreases concentration. **HERBAL:** Ephedra, ginseng, yohimbe may worsen hypertension. Garlic may increase antihypertensive effect. **FOOD:** None known. **LAB VALUE:** May increase serum creatinine, bilirubin, ALT, AST, PT.

### AVAILABILITY (Rx)

**Tablets (Immediate-Release):** 3.125 mg, 6.25 mg, 12.5 mg, 25 mg.
**Capsules (Extended-Release [Coreg CR]):** 10 mg, 20 mg, 40 mg, 80 mg.

## ADMINISTRATION/HANDLING

### PO

• Give with food (slows rate of absorption, reduces risk of orthostatic effects). • Do not crush or cut extended-release capsules. • Capsules may be opened and sprinkled on applesauce for immediate use.

## INDICATIONS/ROUTES/DOSAGE

### Hypertension

PO *(Immediate-Release)*: ADULTS, ELDERLY: Initially, 6.25 mg twice daily. May double at 1–2 wk intervals. **Maximum:** 25 mg twice daily. *(Extended-Release)*: Initially, 20 mg once daily. May increase to 40 mg once daily after 1–2 wks. **Maximum:** 80 mg once daily.

### HF

PO *(Immediate-Release)*: ADULTS, ELDERLY: Initially, 3.125 mg twice daily. May double at 2-wk intervals to highest tolerated dosage. **Maximum: Greater than 85 kg:** 50 mg twice daily; **Less than 85 kg:** 25 mg twice daily. *(Extended-Release)*: Initially, 10 mg once daily for 2 wks. May increase to 20 mg, 40 mg, and 80 mg over successive intervals of at least 2 wks. **Maximum:** 80 mg/day.

### Left Ventricular Dysfunction Following MI

PO *(Immediate-Release)*: ADULTS, ELDERLY: Initially, 3.125–6.25 mg twice daily. May increase at intervals of 3–10 days up to 25 mg twice daily. **Maximum:** 50 mg twice daily. *(Extended-Release)*: Initially, 10–20 mg once daily. May increase incrementally in intervals of 3–10 days. Target dose: 80 mg once daily.

### Dosage in Renal Impairment

No dose adjustment.

### Dosage in Hepatic Impairment

Contraindicated in severe impairment.

## SIDE EFFECTS

**Frequent (6%–4%):** Fatigue, dizziness. **Occasional (2%):** Diarrhea, bradycardia, rhinitis, back pain. **Rare (less than 2%):** Orthostatic hypotension, drowsiness, UTI, viral infection.

## ADVERSE EFFECTS/ TOXIC REACTIONS

Overdose may produce profound bradycardia, hypotension, bronchospasm, cardiac insufficiency, cardiogenic shock, cardiac arrest. Abrupt withdrawal may result in diaphoresis, palpitations, headache, tremors. May precipitate HF, MI in pts with cardiac disease; thyroid storm in pts with thyrotoxicosis; peripheral ischemia in pts with existing peripheral vascular disease. Hypoglycemia may occur in pts with previously controlled diabetes.

## NURSING CONSIDERATIONS

### BASELINE ASSESSMENT

Assess B/P, apical pulse immediately before drug is administered (if pulse is 60 beats/min or less or systolic B/P is less than 90 mm Hg, withhold medication, contact physician).

### INTERVENTION/EVALUATION

Monitor B/P for hypotension, respirations for dyspnea. Take standing systolic B/P 1 hr after dosing as guide for tolerance. Assess pulse for quality, regularity, rate; monitor for bradycardia. Monitor EKG for cardiac arrhythmias. Assist with ambulation if dizziness occurs. Assess for evidence of HF: dyspnea (particularly on exertion or lying down), night cough, peripheral edema, distended neck veins. Monitor I&O (increase in weight, decrease in urine output may indicate HF). Monitor renal/hepatic function tests.

### PATIENT/FAMILY TEACHING

• Full antihypertensive effect noted in 1–2 wks. • Contact lens wearers may experience decreased lacrimation. • Take with food. • Do not abruptly discontinue medication. • Compliance with therapy regimen is essential to control hypertension. • Report excessive fatigue, prolonged dizziness. • Do not use nasal decongestants, OTC cold preparations (stimulants) without physician's approval. • Monitor B/P, pulse before taking medication. • Restrict salt, alcohol intake.

# caspofungin

kas-poe-**fun**-jin
(Cancidas)

♦ **CLASSIFICATION**

**PHARMACOTHERAPEUTIC:** Echinocandin antifungal. **CLINICAL:** Antifungal.

## USES

Treatment of invasive aspergillosis, candidemia, *Candida* infection (intraabdominal abscess, peritonitis, esophageal, pleural space). Empiric therapy for presumed fungal infections in febrile neutropenia.

## PRECAUTIONS

**Contraindications:** Hypersensitivity to caspofungin. **Cautions:** Concurrent use of cyclosporine, hepatic impairment.

## ACTION

Inhibits synthesis of glucan, a vital component of fungal cell wall formation, damaging fungal cell membrane. **Therapeutic Effect:** Fungistatic.

## PHARMACOKINETICS

Distributed in tissue. Protein binding: 97%. Metabolized in liver to active metabolite. Excreted in urine (50%), feces (30%). Not removed by hemodialysis. **Half-life:** 40–50 hrs.

## ⌛ LIFESPAN CONSIDERATIONS

**Pregnancy/Lactation:** May be embryotoxic. Crosses placental barrier. Distributed in breast milk. **Children:** Safety and efficacy not established. **Elderly:** Age-related moderate renal impairment may require dosage adjustment.

## INTERACTIONS

**DRUG: Cyclosporine** may increase concentration. **Rifampin** may decrease concentration. May decrease concentration/effects of **tacrolimus. HERBAL:** None significant. **FOOD:** None known. **LAB VALUES:** May increase serum alkaline phosphatase, bilirubin, creatinine, ALT, AST, urine protein. May decrease serum albumin, bicarbonate, potassium, magnesium; Hgb, Hct.

## AVAILABILITY (Rx)

**Injection, Powder for Reconstitution:** 50-mg, 70-mg vials.

## ADMINISTRATION/HANDLING

 IV

**Reconstitution** • Reconstitute 50-mg or 70-mg vial with 0.9% NaCl, Sterile Water for Injection, or Bacteriostatic Water for Injection. Further dilute in 0.9% NaCl or $D_5W$ to maximum concentration of 0.5 mg/ml.
**Rate of Administration** • Infuse over 60 min.
**Storage** • Refrigerate vials but warm to room temperature before preparing with diluent. • Reconstituted solution, prior to preparation of pt infusion solution, may be stored at room temperature for 1 hr before infusion. • Final infusion solution can be stored at room temperature for 24 hrs or 48 hrs if refrigerated. • Discard if solution contains particulate or is discolored.

## ▦ IV COMPATIBILITIES

Aztreonam (Azactam), daptomycin (Cubicin), fluconazole (Diflucan), linezolid (Zyvox), meropenem (Merrem IV), piperacillin/tazobactam (Zosyn), vancomycin.

## ▦ IV INCOMPATIBILITIES

Cefepime (Maxipime), ceftaroline (Teflaro), ceftazidime (Fortaz), ceftriaxone (Rocephin), furosemide (Lasix).

# INDICATIONS/ROUTES/DOSAGE

### Aspergillosis

**Note:** Continue for minimum 6–12 wks.
**IV: ADULTS, ELDERLY:** Give single 70-mg loading dose on day 1, followed by 50 mg/day thereafter. For pts with moderate hepatic impairment, reduce daily dose to 35 mg. **CHILDREN 3 MOS–17 YRS:** 70 mg/m² on day 1, then 50 mg/m² daily. **Maximum:** 70-mg loading dose, 50-mg daily dose.

### Candidemia

**Note:** Continue for at least 14 days after last positive culture.
**IV: ADULTS, ELDERLY:** Initially, 70 mg followed by 50 mg daily. **CHILDREN 3 MOS–17 YRS:** 70 mg/m² on day 1, then 50 mg/m² daily. **Maximum:** 70-mg loading dose, 50-mg daily dose.

### Esophageal Candidiasis

**Note:** Continue for 7–14 days after symptom resolution.
**IV: ADULTS, ELDERLY:** 50 mg/day. **CHILDREN 3 MOS–17 YRS:** 50 mg/m² daily. **Maximum:** 50 mg.

### Empiric Therapy

**Note:** Continue for minimum 14 days if fungal infection confirmed (continue for 7 days after resolution of neutropenia/clinical symptoms).
**IV: ADULTS, ELDERLY:** Initially 70 mg, then 50 mg/day. May increase to 70 mg/day. **CHILDREN 3 MOS–17 YRS:** 70 mg/m² on day 1, then 50 mg/m² daily. **Maximum:** 70 mg.

### Dosage in Renal Impairment

No dose adjustment.

### Dosage in Hepatic Impairment

**Mild:** No adjustment. **Moderate: Child-Pugh score 7–9:** 35 mg/day. **Severe:** No clinical experience.

## SIDE EFFECTS

**Frequent (26%):** Fever. **Occasional (11%–4%):** Headache, nausea, phlebitis. **Rare (3% or less):** Paresthesia, vomiting, diarrhea, abdominal pain, myalgia, chills, tremor, insomnia.

## ADVERSE EFFECTS/TOXIC REACTIONS

Hypersensitivity reaction (rash, facial edema, pruritus, sensation of warmth) including anaphylaxis may occur. May cause hepatic dysfunction, hepatitis (drug-induced), or hepatic failure.

## NURSING CONSIDERATIONS

### BASELINE ASSESSMENT

Obtain baseline CBC, BMP, LFT, magnesium. Determine baseline temperature. Assess for allergic or hypersensitivity reactions.

### INTERVENTION/EVALUATION

Assess for signs/symptoms of hepatic dysfunction. Monitor LFT in pts with preexisting hepatic impairment. Monitor CBC, serum potassium. Monitor for fever, hypersensitivity reaction.

### PATIENT/FAMILY TEACHING

• Report rash, facial swelling, itching, difficulty breathing, abdominal pain, yellowing of skin or eyes, dark colored urine, nausea.

# cefaclor

**sef**-a-klor
(Apo-Cefaclor ✦, Ceclor ✦, Novo-Cefaclor ✦)
**Do not confuse Cefaclor with cephalexin.**

## ◆CLASSIFICATION

**PHARMACOTHERAPEUTIC:** Second-generation cephalosporin. **CLINICAL:** Antibiotic.

## USES

Treatment of susceptible infections due to *S. pneumoniae, S. pyogenes, S. aureus, H. influenzae, E. coli, M. catarrhalis, Klebsiella* spp., *P. mirabilis,* including acute otitis

---

✦ Canadian trade name      🗡 Non-Crushable Drug      🔲 High Alert drug

media, bronchitis, pharyngitis/tonsillitis, respiratory tract, skin/skin structure, UTIs.

## PRECAUTIONS

**Contraindications:** History of hypersensitivity/anaphylactic reaction to cefaclor, cephalosporins. **Cautions:** Severe renal impairment, history of penicillin allergy. Extended release not approved in children younger than 16 yrs.

## ACTION

Binds to bacterial cell membranes, inhibits cell wall synthesis. **Therapeutic Effect:** Bactericidal.

## PHARMACOKINETICS

Well absorbed from GI tract. Protein binding: 25%. Widely distributed. Partially metabolized in liver. Primarily excreted in urine. Moderately removed by hemodialysis. **Half-life:** 0.6–0.9 hr (increased in renal impairment).

## ⧗ LIFESPAN CONSIDERATIONS

**Pregnancy/Lactation:** Readily crosses placenta. Distributed in breast milk. **Children:** No age-related precautions noted in pts older than 1 mo. **Elderly:** Age-related renal impairment may require dosage adjustment.

## INTERACTIONS

**DRUG: Probenecid** may increase concentration. **HERBAL:** None significant. **FOOD:** None known. **LAB VALUES:** May increase serum BUN, alkaline phosphatase, bilirubin, creatinine, LDH, ALT, AST. May cause positive direct/indirect Coombs' test.

## AVAILABILITY (Rx)

🍶 **Capsules:** 250 mg, 500 mg. **Powder for Oral Suspension:** 125 mg/5 ml, 250 mg/5 ml, 375 mg/5 ml.
**Tablets (Extended-Release):** 500 mg.

## ADMINISTRATION/HANDLING

**PO**
• After reconstitution, oral solution is stable for 14 days if refrigerated.
• Shake oral suspension well before

using. • **Extended-Release:** Swallow whole; do not cut, crush, or divide.
• Give without regard to food; if GI upset occurs, give with food, milk.

## INDICATIONS/ROUTES/DOSAGE

**Usual Dosage**
**PO: ADULTS, ELDERLY:** 250–500 mg q8h or 500 mg q12h (extended-release). **CHILDREN:** 20–40 mg/kg/day divided q8–12h. **Maximum:** 1 g/day.

**Otitis Media**
**PO: CHILDREN:** 40 mg/kg/day divided q12h. **Maximum:** 1 g/day.

**Pharyngitis**
**CHILDREN:** 20 mg/kg/day divided q12h. **Maximum:** 1 g/day.

**Dosage in Renal Impairment**
Use caution.

**Dosage in Hepatic Impairment**
No dose adjustment.

## SIDE EFFECTS

**Frequent:** Oral candidiasis, mild diarrhea, mild abdominal cramping, vaginal candidiasis. **Occasional:** Nausea, serum sickness-like reaction (fever, joint pain; usually occurs after second course of therapy and resolves after drug is discontinued). **Rare:** Allergic reaction (pruritus, rash, urticaria).

## ADVERSE EFFECTS/ TOXIC REACTIONS

Antibiotic-associated colitis, other (abdominal cramps, severe watery diarrhea, fever) superinfections may result from altered bacterial balance in GI tract. Nephrotoxicity may occur, esp. in pts with preexisting renal disease. Pts with history of penicillin allergy are at increased risk for developing a severe hypersensitivity reaction (severe pruritus, angioedema, bronchospasm, anaphylaxis).

---

## NURSING CONSIDERATIONS

### BASELINE ASSESSMENT

Obtain baseline CBC, renal function tests. Question for history of allergies, particularly cephalosporins, penicillins.

### INTERVENTION/EVALUATION

Assess oral cavity for white patches on mucous membranes, tongue (thrush). Monitor daily pattern of bowel activity, stool consistency. Mild GI effects may be tolerable (increasing severity may indicate onset of antibiotic-associated colitis). Monitor I&O, renal function tests for nephrotoxicity. Be alert for superinfection: fever, vomiting, diarrhea, anal/genital pruritus, oral mucosal changes (ulceration, pain, erythema).

### PATIENT/FAMILY TEACHING

• Continue therapy for full length of treatment. • Doses should be evenly spaced. • May cause GI upset (may take with food, milk). • Chewable tablets must be chewed; do not swallow whole. • Refrigerate oral suspension. • Report persistent diarrhea.

## cefadroxil

sef-a-**drox**-il
(Apo-Cefadroxil ✦)

### ◆CLASSIFICATION

**PHARMACOTHERAPEUTIC:** First-generation cephalosporin. **CLINICAL:** Antibiotic.

## USES

Treatment of susceptible infections due to group A streptococci, staphylococci, *S. pneumoniae, H. influenzae, Klebsiella* spp., *E. coli, P. mirabilis,* including impetigo, pharyngitis/tonsillitis, skin/skin structure, UTIs. **OFF-LABEL:** Chronic suppression of prosthetic joint infection.

## PRECAUTIONS

**Contraindications:** History of hypersensitivity/anaphylactic reaction to cefadroxil, cephalosporins. **Cautions:** Severe renal impairment, history of penicillin allergy. History of GI disease (colitis).

## ACTION

Binds to bacterial cell membranes, inhibits cell wall synthesis. **Therapeutic Effect:** Bactericidal.

## PHARMACOKINETICS

Well absorbed from GI tract. Protein binding: 15%–20%. Widely distributed. Primarily excreted unchanged in urine. Removed by hemodialysis. **Half-life:** 1.2–1.5 hrs (increased in renal impairment).

## ⧗ LIFESPAN CONSIDERATIONS

**Pregnancy/Lactation:** Readily crosses placenta. Distributed in breast milk. **Children:** No age-related precautions noted. **Elderly:** Age-related renal impairment may require dosage adjustment.

## INTERACTIONS

**DRUG: Probenecid** may increase concentration. **HERBAL:** None significant. **FOOD:** None known. **LAB VALUES:** May increase serum BUN, alkaline phosphatase, bilirubin, creatinine, LDH, ALT, AST. May cause positive direct/indirect Coombs' test.

## AVAILABILITY (Rx)

▧ **Capsules:** 500 mg. **Powder for Oral Suspension:** 250 mg/5 ml, 500 mg/5 ml. **Tablets:** 1 g.

## ADMINISTRATION/HANDLING

**PO**

• After reconstitution, oral solution is stable for 14 days if refrigerated. • Shake oral suspension well before using. • Give without regard to meals; if GI upset occurs, give with food, milk.

---

✦ Canadian trade name　　　▧ Non-Crushable Drug　　　[HIGH ALERT] High Alert drug

C

## INDICATIONS/ROUTES/DOSAGE

**Usual Dosage**
PO: ADULTS, ELDERLY: 1–2 g/day as single dose or in 2 divided doses. CHILDREN: 30 mg/kg/day in 2 divided doses. **Maximum:** 2 g/day.

**Dosage in Renal Impairment**
After initial 1-g dose, dosage and frequency are modified based on creatinine clearance and severity of infection.

| Creatinine Clearance | Dosage |
|---|---|
| 26–50 ml/min | q12h |
| 10–25 ml/min | q24h |
| Less than 10 ml/min | q36h |

**Dosage in Hepatic Impairment**
No dose adjustment.

## SIDE EFFECTS

**Frequent:** Oral candidiasis, mild diarrhea, mild abdominal cramping, vaginal candidiasis. **Occasional:** Nausea, unusual bruising/bleeding, serum sickness-like reaction (fever, joint pain; usually occurs after second course of therapy and resolves after drug is discontinued). **Rare:** Allergic reaction (rash, pruritus, urticaria), thrombophlebitis (pain, redness, swelling at injection site).

## ADVERSE EFFECTS/TOXIC REACTIONS

Antibiotic-associated colitis, other superinfections (abdominal cramps, severe watery diarrhea, fever) may result from altered bacterial balance in GI tract. Nephrotoxicity may occur, esp. in pts with preexisting renal disease. Pts with history of penicillin allergy are at increased risk for developing a severe hypersensitivity reaction (severe pruritus, angioedema, bronchospasm, anaphylaxis).

## NURSING CONSIDERATIONS

### BASELINE ASSESSMENT

Obtain CBC, renal function tests. Question for history of allergies, particularly cephalosporins, penicillins.

### INTERVENTION/EVALUATION

Assess oral cavity for white patches on mucous membranes, tongue (thrush). Monitor daily pattern of bowel activity, stool consistency. Mild GI effects may be tolerable (increasing severity may indicate onset of antibiotic-associated colitis). Monitor I&O, renal function tests for nephrotoxicity. Be alert for superinfection: fever, vomiting, diarrhea, anal/genital pruritus, oral mucosal changes (ulceration, pain, erythema).

### PATIENT/FAMILY TEACHING

• Continue therapy for full length of treatment. • Doses should be evenly spaced. • May cause GI upset (may take with food, milk). • Refrigerate oral suspension. • Report persistent diarrhea.

## *ceFAZolin

sef-a-**zoe**-lin
**Do not confuse cefazolin with cefoxitin, cefprozil, ceftriaxone, or cephalexin.**

## ◆ CLASSIFICATION

**PHARMACOTHERAPEUTIC:** First-generation cephalosporin. **CLINICAL:** Antibiotic.

## USES

Treatment of susceptible infections due to *S. aureus, S. epidermidis,* group A beta-hemolytic streptococci, *S. pneumoniae, E. coli, P. mirabilis, Klebsiella* spp., *H. influenzae* including biliary tract, bone and joint, genital, respiratory tract, skin/skin structure infections; UTIs, endocarditis, perioperative prophylaxis, septicemia. **OFF-LABEL:** Prophylaxis against infective endocarditis.

## PRECAUTIONS

**Contraindications:** History of hypersensitivity/anaphylactic reaction to cefazolin, cephalosporins. **Cautions:** Severe renal impairment, history of penicillin allergy, history of seizures.

---

*"Tall Man" lettering                    <u>underlined</u> – top prescribed drug

## ACTION

Binds to bacterial cell membranes, inhibits cell wall synthesis. **Therapeutic Effect:** Bactericidal.

## PHARMACOKINETICS

Widely distributed. Protein binding: 85%. Primarily excreted unchanged in urine. Moderately removed by hemodialysis. **Half-life:** 1.4–1.8 hrs (increased in renal impairment).

## ☒ LIFESPAN CONSIDERATIONS

**Pregnancy/Lactation:** Readily crosses placenta; distributed in breast milk. **Children:** No age-related precautions noted. **Elderly:** Age-related renal impairment may require reduced dosage.

## INTERACTIONS

**DRUG: Probenecid** may increase concentration. **HERBAL:** None significant. **FOOD:** None known. **LAB VALUES:** May increase serum BUN, alkaline phosphatase, bilirubin, creatinine, LDH, ALT, AST. May cause positive direct/indirect Coombs' test.

## AVAILABILITY (Rx)

**Injection, Powder for Reconstitution:** 500 mg, 1 g. **Ready-to-Hang Infusion:** 1 g/50 ml, 2 g/100 ml.

## ADMINISTRATION/HANDLING

 IV

**Reconstitution** • Reconstitute each 1 g with at least 10 ml Sterile Water for Injection or 0.9% NaCl. • May further dilute in 50–100 ml $D_5W$ or 0.9% NaCl (decreases incidence of thrombophlebitis). **Rate of Administration** • For IV push, administer over 3–5 min (**maximum concentration:** 100 mg/ml). • For intermittent IV infusion (piggyback), infuse over 30–60 min (**maximum concentration:** 20 mg/ml). **Storage** • Solution appears light yellow to yellow. • Reconstituted solution stable for 24 hrs at room temperature or for 10 days if refrigerated. • IV infusion (piggyback) stable for 48 hrs at room temperature or for 14 days if refrigerated.

**IM**
• To minimize discomfort, inject deep IM slowly. • Less painful if injected into gluteus maximus rather than lateral aspect of thigh.

## ▦ IV INCOMPATIBILITIES

Amikacin (Amikin), amiodarone (Cordarone), hydromorphone (Dilaudid).

## ▦ IV COMPATIBILITIES

Calcium gluconate, dexamethasone (Decadron), diltiazem (Cardizem), famotidine (Pepcid), heparin, insulin (regular), lidocaine, lorazepam (Ativan), magnesium sulfate, meperidine (Demerol), metoclopramide (Reglan), midazolam (Versed), morphine, multivitamins, ondansetron (Zofran), potassium chloride, propofol (Diprivan).

## INDICATIONS/ROUTES/DOSAGE

**Usual Dosage Range**

**IV, IM: ADULTS:** 1–1.5 g q6–12h (usually q8h). **Maximum:** 12 g/day. **CHILDREN OLDER THAN 1 MO:** 25–100 mg/kg/day divided q6–8h. **Maximum:** 6 g/day. **NEONATES OLDER THAN 7 DAYS:** 25 mg/kg/dose q8h. **NEONATES 7 DAYS AND YOUNGER:** 25 mg/kg/dose q12h.

**Dosage in Renal Impairment**
Dosing frequency is modified based on creatinine clearance.

| Creatinine Clearance | Dosage |
| --- | --- |
| 11–34 ml/min | 50% usual dose q12h |
| 10 ml/min or less | 50% usual dose q18–24h |
| HD | 500 mg–1 g q24h |
| PD | 500 mg q12h |
| CRRT | |
| CVVH | Loading dose 2 g, then 1–2 g q12h |
| CVVHD/CVVHDF | Loading dose 2 g, then 1 g q8h or 2 g q12h |

**Dosage in Hepatic Impairment**
No dose adjustment.

## SIDE EFFECTS

**Frequent:** Discomfort with IM administration, oral candidiasis (thrush), mild diarrhea, mild abdominal cramping, vaginal candidiasis. **Occasional:** Nausea, serum sickness-like reaction (fever, joint pain; usually occurs after second course of therapy and resolves after drug is discontinued). **Rare:** Allergic reaction (rash, pruritus, urticaria), thrombophlebitis (pain, redness, swelling at injection site).

## ADVERSE EFFECTS/ TOXIC REACTIONS

Antibiotic-associated colitis, other superinfections (abdominal cramps, severe watery diarrhea, fever) may result from altered bacterial balance in GI tract. Nephrotoxicity may occur, esp. in pts with preexisting renal disease. Pts with history of penicillin allergy are at increased risk for developing severe hypersensitivity reaction (severe pruritus, angioedema, bronchospasm, anaphylaxis).

## NURSING CONSIDERATIONS

### BASELINE ASSESSMENT

Obtain CBC, renal function tests. Question for history of allergies, particularly cephalosporins, penicillins.

### INTERVENTION/EVALUATION

Evaluate IM site for induration and tenderness. Assess oral cavity for white patches on mucous membranes, tongue (thrush). Monitor daily pattern of bowel activity, stool consistency. Mild GI effects may be tolerable (increasing severity may indicate onset of antibiotic-associated colitis). Monitor I&O, renal function tests for nephrotoxicity. Be alert for superinfection: fever, vomiting, diarrhea, anal/genital pruritus, oral mucosal changes (ulceration, pain, erythema).

### PATIENT/FAMILY TEACHING

• Discomfort may occur with IM injection.

# cefdinir

**sef**-di-neer

## ◆CLASSIFICATION

**PHARMACOTHERAPEUTIC:** Third-generation cephalosporin. **CLINICAL:** Antibiotic.

## USES

Treatment of susceptible infections due to *S. pyogenes, S. pneumoniae, H. influenzae, H. parainfluenzae, M. catarrhalis* including community-acquired pneumonia, acute exacerbation of chronic bronchitis, acute maxillary sinusitis, pharyngitis, tonsillitis, uncomplicated skin/skin structure infections, otitis media.

## PRECAUTIONS

**Contraindications:** Hypersensitivity to cefdinir. History of anaphylactic reaction to cephalosporins. **Cautions:** Hypersensitivity to penicillins; renal impairment.

## ACTION

Binds to bacterial cell membranes, inhibits cell wall synthesis. **Therapeutic Effect:** Bactericidal.

## PHARMACOKINETICS

Moderately absorbed from GI tract. Protein binding: 60%–70%. Widely distributed. Not appreciably metabolized. Primarily excreted unchanged in urine. Minimally removed by hemodialysis. **Half-life:** 1–2 hrs (increased in renal impairment).

## ⌛ LIFESPAN CONSIDERATIONS

**Pregnancy/Lactation:** Crosses placenta. Not detected in breast milk. **Children:** Newborns, infants may have lower renal clearance. **Elderly:** Age-related renal impairment may require decreased dosage or increased dosing interval.

---

*"Tall Man" lettering          <u>underlined</u> – top prescribed drug

## INTERACTIONS

**DRUG: Antacids, iron preparations** may interfere with absorption. **Probenecid** increases concentration. **HERBAL:** None significant. **FOOD:** None known. **LAB VALUES:** May produce false-positive reaction for urine ketones. May increase serum alkaline phosphatase, bilirubin, LDH, ALT, AST.

## AVAILABILITY (Rx)

 **Capsules:** 300 mg. **Powder for Oral Suspension:** 125 mg/5 ml, 250 mg/5 ml.

## ADMINISTRATION/HANDLING

**PO**

• Give without regard to food. Give at least 2 hrs before or after antacids or iron supplements. • Twice daily doses should be given 12 hrs apart. • Shake oral suspension well before administering. • Store mixed suspension at room temperature for 10 days.

## INDICATIONS/ROUTES/DOSAGE

**Usual Dosage Range**
**PO: ADULTS, ELDERLY:** 300 mg q12h or 600 mg once daily. **CHILDREN 6 MOS–12 YRS:** 7 mg/kg q12h or 14 mg/kg once daily. **Maximum:** 600 mg/day.

**Dosage in Renal Impairment**
**CrCl less than 30 ml/min:** 300 mg/day or 7 mg/kg as single daily dose. **Maximum:** 300 mg. **Hemodialysis pts:** 300 mg or 7 mg/kg/dose every other day. **Maximum:** 300 mg.

**Dosage in Hepatic Impairment**
No dose adjustment.

## SIDE EFFECTS

**Frequent:** Oral candidiasis, mild diarrhea, mild abdominal cramping, vaginal candidiasis. **Occasional:** Nausea, serum sickness-like reaction (fever, joint pain; usually occurs after second course of therapy and resolves after drug is discontinued). **Rare:** Allergic reaction (rash, pruritus, urticaria).

## ADVERSE EFFECTS/ TOXIC REACTIONS

Antibiotic-associated colitis, other super-infections (abdominal cramps, severe watery diarrhea, fever) may result from altered bacterial balance in GI tract. Nephrotoxicity may occur, esp. in pts with preexisting renal disease. Pts with history of penicillin allergy are at increased risk for developing a severe hypersensitivity reaction (severe pruritus, angioedema, bronchospasm, anaphylaxis).

## NURSING CONSIDERATIONS

### BASELINE ASSESSMENT

Obtain CBC, renal function tests. Question for hypersensitivity to cefdinir or other cephalosporins, penicillins.

### INTERVENTION/EVALUATION

Observe for rash. Monitor daily pattern of bowel activity, stool consistency. Mild GI effects may be tolerable (increasing severity may indicate onset of antibiotic-associated colitis). Be alert for superinfection: fever, vomiting, diarrhea, anal/genital pruritus, oral mucosal changes (ulceration, pain, erythema). Monitor hematology reports.

### PATIENT/FAMILY TEACHING

• Take antacids 2 hrs before or following medication. • Continue medication for full length of treatment; do not skip doses. • Doses should be evenly spaced. • Report persistent severe diarrhea, rash, muscle aches, fever, enlarged lymph nodes, joint pain.

## cefepime

sef-e-**peem**
(Maxipime ✤)
**Do not confuse cefepime with cefixime or ceftazidime.**

## ◆ CLASSIFICATION

**PHARMACOTHERAPEUTIC:** Fourth-generation cephalosporin. **CLINICAL:** Antibiotic.

---

✤ Canadian trade name     Non-Crushable Drug    🔲 High Alert drug

## USES

Susceptible infections due to aerobic gram-negative organisms including *P. aeruginosa*, gram-positive organisms including *S. aureus*. Treatment of empiric febrile neutropenia, intra-abdominal infections, skin/skin structure infections, UTIs, pneumonia. **OFF-LABEL:** Brain abscess, malignant otitis externa, septic lateral/cavernous sinus thrombus.

## PRECAUTIONS

**Contraindications:** History of anaphylactic reaction to penicillins, hypersensitivity to cefepime, cephalosporins. **Cautions:** Renal impairment, history of seizure disorder, GI disease (colitis), elderly.

## ACTION

Binds to bacterial cell wall membranes, inhibits cell wall synthesis. **Therapeutic Effect:** Bactericidal.

## PHARMACOKINETICS

Well absorbed after IM administration. Protein binding: 20%. Widely distributed. Primarily excreted unchanged in urine. Removed by hemodialysis. **Half-life:** 2–2.3 hrs (increased in renal impairment, elderly pts).

## LIFESPAN CONSIDERATIONS

**Pregnancy/Lactation:** Unknown if distributed in breast milk. **Children:** No age-related precautions noted in pts older than 2 mos. **Elderly:** Age-related renal impairment may require reduced dosage or increased dosing interval.

## INTERACTIONS

**DRUG: Probenecid** may increase concentration. May increase **aminoglycoside** concentration. **HERBAL:** None significant. **FOOD:** None known. **LAB VALUES:** May increase serum BUN, alkaline phosphatase, bilirubin, LDH, ALT, AST. May cause positive direct/indirect Coombs' test.

## AVAILABILITY (Rx)

**Injection, Powder for Reconstitution:** 1 g, 2 g. **Injection, Premix:** 1 g (50 ml), 2 g (50 ml).

## ADMINISTRATION/HANDLING

 **IV**

**Reconstitution** • Add 10 ml of diluent for 1-g and 2-g vials. • Further dilute with 50–100 ml 0.9% NaCl or D₅W.
**Rate of Administration** • For intermittent IV infusion (piggyback), infuse over 30 min. For direct IV, administer over 5 min.
**Storage** • Solution is stable for 24 hrs at room temperature, 7 days if refrigerated.

**IM**
• Add 2.4 ml Sterile Water for Injection, 0.9% NaCl, or D₅W to 1-g and 2-g vials. • Inject into a large muscle mass (e.g., upper gluteus maximus).

## IV INCOMPATIBILITIES

Acyclovir (Zovirax), amphotericin (Fungizone), cimetidine (Tagamet), ciprofloxacin (Cipro), cisplatin (Platinol), dacarbazine (DTIC), daunorubicin (Cerubidine), diazepam (Valium), diphenhydramine (Benadryl), dobutamine (Dobutrex), dopamine (Intropin), doxorubicin (Adriamycin), droperidol (Inapsine), famotidine (Pepcid), ganciclovir (Cytovene), haloperidol (Haldol), magnesium, magnesium sulfate, mannitol, metoclopramide (Reglan), morphine, ofloxacin (Floxin), ondansetron (Zofran), vancomycin (Vancocin).

## IV COMPATIBILITIES

Bumetanide (Bumex), calcium gluconate, furosemide (Lasix), hydromorphone (Dilaudid), lorazepam (Ativan), propofol (Diprivan).

## INDICATIONS/ROUTES/DOSAGE

**Usual Dosage Range**
**IV: ADULTS, ELDERLY:** 1–2 g q8–12h.
**CHILDREN:** 50 mg/kg q8–12h not to exceed adult dosing. **NEONATES:** 30 mg/kg/dose q12h.

**IM: ADULTS, ELDERLY:** 0.5–1 g q12h. **CHILDREN:** 50 mg/kg/dose q8–12h not to exceed adult dosing. **NEONATES:** 30 mg/kg/dose q12h.

### Dosage in Renal Impairment

Dosage and frequency are modified based on creatinine clearance and severity of infection.

| Creatinine Clearance | Dosage |
|---|---|
| 30–60 ml/min | 500 mg q24h–2 g q12h |
| 11–29 ml/min | 500 mg–2 g q24h |
| 10 ml/min or less | 250 mg–1 g q24h |
| Hemodialysis | Initially, 1 g, then 0.5–1 g q24h or 1–2 g q48–72h. |
| Peritoneal dialysis | Normal dose q48h |
| Continuous renal replacement therapy | Initially, 2 g, then 1 g q8h or 2 g q12h |

### Dosage in Hepatic Impairment

No dose adjustment.

## SIDE EFFECTS

**Frequent:** Discomfort with IM administration, oral candidiasis (thrush), mild diarrhea, mild abdominal cramping, vaginal candidiasis. **Occasional:** Nausea, serum sickness-like reaction (fever, joint pain; usually occurs after second course of therapy and resolves after drug is discontinued). **Rare:** Allergic reaction (rash, pruritus, urticaria), thrombophlebitis (pain, redness, swelling at injection site).

## ADVERSE EFFECTS/ TOXIC REACTIONS

Antibiotic-associated colitis, other superinfections (abdominal cramps, severe watery diarrhea, fever) may result from altered bacterial balance in GI tract. Nephrotoxicity may occur, esp. in pts with preexisting renal disease. Pts with history of penicillin allergy are at increased risk for developing a severe hypersensitivity reaction (severe pruritus, angioedema, bronchospasm, anaphylaxis).

## NURSING CONSIDERATIONS

### BASELINE ASSESSMENT

Obtain CBC, renal function tests. Question for history of allergies, particularly cephalosporins, penicillins.

### INTERVENTION/EVALUATION

Evaluate IM site for induration and tenderness. Assess oral cavity for white patches on mucous membranes, tongue (thrush). Monitor daily pattern of bowel activity, stool consistency. Mild GI effects may be tolerable (increasing severity may indicate onset of antibiotic-associated colitis). Monitor I&O, CBC, renal function tests for nephrotoxicity. Be alert for superinfection: fever, vomiting, diarrhea, anal/genital pruritus, oral mucosal changes (ulceration, pain, erythema).

### PATIENT/FAMILY TEACHING

• Discomfort may occur with IM injection. • Continue therapy for full length of treatment. • Doses should be evenly spaced. • Report persistent diarrhea.

# cefixime

sef-**ix**-eem
(Suprax)
**Do not confuse cefixime with cefepime, or Suprax with Sporanox or Surbex.**

## ◆CLASSIFICATION

**PHARMACOTHERAPEUTIC:** Third-generation cephalosporin. **CLINICAL:** Antibiotic.

## USES

Treatment of susceptible infections due to *S. pneumoniae, S. pyogenes, M. catarrhalis, H. influenzae, E. coli, P. mirabilis* including otitis media, acute bronchitis, acute exacerbations of chronic bronchitis, pharyngitis, tonsillitis, uncomplicated UTI.

---

## PRECAUTIONS

**Contraindications:** History of hypersensitivity/anaphylactic reaction to cefixime, cephalosporins. **Cautions:** History of penicillin allergy, renal impairment.

## ACTION

Binds to bacterial cell membranes, inhibits cell wall synthesis. **Therapeutic Effect:** Bactericidal.

## PHARMACOKINETICS

Moderately absorbed from GI tract. Protein binding: 65%–70%. Widely distributed. Primarily excreted unchanged in urine. Minimally removed by hemodialysis. **Half-life:** 3–4 hrs (increased in renal impairment).

## ⧗ LIFESPAN CONSIDERATIONS

**Pregnancy/Lactation:** Not recommended during labor and delivery. Unknown if distributed in breast milk. **Children:** Safety and efficacy not established in pts younger than 6 mos. **Elderly:** Age-related renal impairment may require dosage adjustment.

## INTERACTIONS

**DRUG: Probenecid** may increase concentration. May increase **aminoglycoside** concentration. **HERBAL:** None significant. **FOOD:** None known. **LAB VALUES:** May increase serum BUN, alkaline phosphatase, bilirubin, creatinine, LDH, ALT, AST. May cause a positive direct/indirect Coombs' test.

## AVAILABILITY (Rx)

**Oral Suspension:** 100 mg/5 ml, 200 mg/5 ml, 500 mg/5 ml. **Tablets:** 400 mg. **Tablets (Chewable):** 100 mg, 200 mg.

## ADMINISTRATION/HANDLING

**PO**
• Give without regard to food. • After reconstitution, oral suspension is stable for 14 days at room temperature or refrigerated. • Shake oral suspension well before administering. Chewable tablets must be chewed or crushed before swallowing.

## INDICATIONS/ROUTES/DOSAGE

**Usual Dosage**
**PO: ADULTS, ELDERLY, CHILDREN 12 YRS AND OLDER WEIGHING MORE THAN 45 KG:** 400 mg/day as a single dose or in 2 divided doses. **CHILDREN 6 MOS–12 YRS WEIGHING 45 KG OR LESS:** 8 mg/kg/day as a single dose or in 2 divided doses. **Maximum:** 400 mg.

**Dosage in Renal Impairment**
Dosage is modified based on creatinine clearance.

| Creatinine Clearance | Dosage |
|---|---|
| 21–60 ml/min | 260 mg/day |
| 20 ml/min or less | 200 mg/day |
| Hemodialysis | 260 mg/day |

**Dosage in Hepatic Impairment**
No dose adjustment.

## SIDE EFFECTS

**Frequent:** Oral candidiasis (thrush), mild diarrhea, mild abdominal cramping, vaginal candidiasis. **Occasional:** Nausea, serum sickness-like reaction (arthralgia, fever; usually occurs after second course of therapy and resolves after drug is discontinued). **Rare:** Allergic reaction (rash, pruritus, urticaria).

## ADVERSE EFFECTS/ TOXIC REACTIONS

Antibiotic-associated colitis, other superinfections (abdominal cramps, severe watery diarrhea, fever) may result from altered bacterial balance in GI tract. Nephrotoxicity may occur, esp. in pts with preexisting renal disease. Pts with history of penicillin allergy are at increased risk for developing a severe hypersensitivity reaction (severe pruritus, angioedema, bronchospasm, anaphylaxis).

## NURSING CONSIDERATIONS

### BASELINE ASSESSMENT

Obtain CBC, renal function tests. Question for hypersensitivity to cefixime or other cephalosporins, penicillins.

### INTERVENTION/EVALUATION

Assess oral cavity for white patches on mucous membranes, tongue (thrush). Monitor daily pattern of bowel activity, stool consistency. Mild GI effects may be tolerable (increasing severity may indicate onset of antibiotic-associated colitis). Monitor renal function tests for evidence of nephrotoxicity. Be alert for superinfection: fever, vomiting, diarrhea, anal/genital pruritus, oral mucosal changes (ulceration, pain, erythema).

### PATIENT/FAMILY TEACHING

• Continue medication for full length of treatment; do not skip doses. • Doses should be evenly spaced. • May cause GI upset (may take with food or milk). • Report persistent diarrhea.

---

## cefotaxime

sef-oh-**tax**-eem
(Claforan)
**Do not confuse cefotaxime with cefoxitin, ceftizoxime, or cefuroxime, or Claforan with Claritin.**

### ◆CLASSIFICATION

**PHARMACOTHERAPEUTIC:** Third-generation cephalosporin. **CLINICAL:** Antibiotic.

## USES

Treatment of susceptible infections (active vs. most gram-negative [not *Pseudomonas*] and gram-positive cocci [not *Enterococcus*]) including bone, joint, GU, gynecologic, intra-abdominal, lower respiratory tract, skin/skin structure infections; septicemia, meningitis, perioperative prophylaxis. **OFF-LABEL:** Surgical prophylaxis.

## PRECAUTIONS

**Contraindications:** History of hypersensitivity/anaphylactic reaction to cefotaxime, cephalosporins. **Cautions:** History of penicillin allergy, colitis, renal impairment with CrCl less than 30 ml/min.

## ACTION

Binds to bacterial cell membranes, inhibits cell wall synthesis. **Therapeutic Effect:** Bactericidal.

## PHARMACOKINETICS

Widely distributed to CSF. Protein binding: 30%–50%. Partially metabolized in liver to active metabolite. Primarily excreted in urine. Moderately removed by hemodialysis. **Half-life:** 1 hr (increased in renal impairment).

## ⌛ LIFESPAN CONSIDERATIONS

**Pregnancy/Lactation:** Readily crosses placenta. Distributed in breast milk. **Children:** No age-related precautions noted. **Elderly:** Age-related renal impairment may require dosage adjustment.

## INTERACTIONS

**DRUG: Probenecid** may increase concentration. May increase **aminoglycoside** concentration. **HERBAL:** None significant. **FOOD:** None known. **LAB VALUES:** May cause positive direct/indirect Coombs' test. May increase serum BUN, creatinine, ALT, AST, alkaline phosphatase.

## AVAILABILITY (Rx)

**Injection, Powder for Reconstitution:** 500 mg, 1 g, 2 g. **Intravenous Solution (Premix):** 1 g/50 ml, 2 g/50 ml.

## ADMINISTRATION/HANDLING
### 💉 IV

**Reconstitution** • Reconstitute with 10 ml Sterile Water for Injection or 0.9% NaCl to provide a maximum concentration of 100 mg/ml. • May further dilute with 50–100 ml 0.9% NaCl or D₅W.
**Rate of Administration** • For IV push, administer over 3–5 min. • For

intermittent IV infusion (piggyback), infuse over 15–30 min.

**Storage** • Solution appears light yellow to amber. • IV infusion (piggyback) is stable for 24 hrs at room temperature, 5 days if refrigerated. • Discard if precipitate forms.

**IM**

• Reconstitute with Sterile Water for Injection or Bacteriostatic Water for Injection to provide a concentration of 230–330 mg/ml. • To minimize discomfort, inject deep IM slowly. Less painful if injected into gluteus maximus than lateral aspect of thigh. For 2-g IM dose, give at 2 separate sites.

### ▨ IV INCOMPATIBILITIES

Allopurinol (Aloprim), filgrastim (Neupogen), fluconazole (Diflucan), vancomycin (Vancocin).

### ▨ IV COMPATIBILITIES

Diltiazem (Cardizem), famotidine (Pepcid), hydromorphone (Dilaudid), lorazepam (Ativan), magnesium sulfate, midazolam (Versed), morphine, propofol (Diprivan).

### INDICATIONS/ROUTES/DOSAGE

**Usual Dosage Range**

**IV, IM: ADULTS, ELDERLY, CHILDREN WEIGHING 50 KG OR MORE:** 1–2 g q4–12h. **Maximum:** 12 g/day. **CHILDREN 1 MO–12 YRS WEIGHING LESS THAN 50 KG:** 50–180 mg/kg/day in divided doses q4–6h. **Maximum:** 12 g/day. **NEONATES:** 50 mg/kg/dose q8–12h.

**Dosage in Renal Impairment**

| Creatinine Clearance | Dosage Interval |
|---|---|
| 10–50 ml/min | 6–12 hrs |
| Less than 10 ml/min | 24 hrs |
| Hemodialysis | 1–2g q24h |
| Peritoneal dialysis | 1g q24h |
| CVVH | 1–2 g q8–12h |
| CVVHD | 1–2g q8h |
| CVVHDF | 1–2g q6–8h |

**Dosage in Hepatic Impairment**
No dose adjustment.

### SIDE EFFECTS

**Frequent:** Discomfort with IM administration, oral candidiasis (thrush), mild diarrhea, mild abdominal cramping, vaginal candidiasis. **Occasional:** Nausea, serum sickness-like reaction (fever, joint pain; usually occurs after second course of therapy and resolves after drug is discontinued). **Rare:** Allergic reaction (rash, pruritus, urticaria), thrombophlebitis (pain, redness, swelling at injection site).

### ADVERSE EFFECTS/ TOXIC REACTIONS

Antibiotic-associated colitis, other superinfections (abdominal cramps, severe watery diarrhea, fever) may result from altered bacterial balance in GI tract. Nephrotoxicity may occur, esp. in pts with preexisting renal disease. Pts with history of penicillin allergy are at increased risk for developing a severe hypersensitivity reaction (severe pruritus, angioedema, bronchospasm, anaphylaxis).

### NURSING CONSIDERATIONS

**BASELINE ASSESSMENT**

Question for history of allergies, particularly cephalosporins, penicillins.

**INTERVENTION/EVALUATION**

Check IM injection sites for induration, tenderness. Assess oral cavity for white patches on mucous membranes, tongue (thrush). Monitor daily pattern of bowel activity, stool consistency. Mild GI effects may be tolerable (increasing severity may indicate onset of antibiotic-associated colitis). Monitor I&O, renal function tests for nephrotoxicity. Be alert for superinfection: fever, vomiting, diarrhea, anal/genital pruritus, oral mucosal changes (ulceration, pain, erythema).

**PATIENT/FAMILY TEACHING**

• Discomfort may occur with IM injection. • Doses should be evenly spaced. • Continue antibiotic therapy for full length of treatment.

# cefpodoxime

sef-poe-**dox**-eem

## ◆CLASSIFICATION

**PHARMACOTHERAPEUTIC:** Third-generation cephalosporin. **CLINICAL:** Antibiotic.

## USES

Treatment of susceptible infections due to *S. pneumoniae, S. pyogenes, S. aureus, H. influenzae, M. catarrhalis, E. coli, Proteus, Klebsiella* spp., including acute maxillary sinusitis, chronic bronchitis, community-acquired pneumonia, gonorrhea, otitis media, pharyngitis, tonsillitis, skin/skin structure infections, UTIs.

## PRECAUTIONS

**Contraindications:** History of hypersensitivity/anaphylactic reaction to cefpodoxime, cephalosporins. **Cautions:** Renal impairment, history of penicillin allergy.

## ACTION

Binds to bacterial cell membranes, inhibits cell wall synthesis. **Therapeutic Effect:** Bactericidal.

## PHARMACOKINETICS

Well absorbed from GI tract (food increases absorption). Protein binding: 18%–23%. Widely distributed. Primarily excreted unchanged in urine. Partially removed by hemodialysis. **Half-life:** 2.3 hrs (increased in renal impairment, elderly pts).

## ☒ LIFESPAN CONSIDERATIONS

**Pregnancy/Lactation:** Readily crosses placenta. Distributed in breast milk. **Children:** Safety and efficacy not established in pts younger than 6 mos. **Elderly:** Age-related renal impairment may require dosage adjustment.

## INTERACTIONS

**DRUG:** High doses of **antacids containing aluminum, H$_2$ antagonists** may decrease absorption. **Probenecid** may increase concentration. **HERBAL:** None significant. **FOOD:** Food enhances absorption. **LAB VALUES:** May increase serum BUN, alkaline phosphatase, bilirubin, creatinine, LDH, ALT, AST. May cause positive direct/indirect Coombs' test.

## AVAILABILITY (Rx)

**Oral Suspension:** 50 mg/5 ml, 100 mg/5 ml. **Tablets:** 100 mg, 200 mg.

## ADMINISTRATION/HANDLING

**PO**

• Administer tablet with food (enhances absorption). • Administer suspension without regard to food. • After reconstitution, oral suspension is stable for 14 days if refrigerated.

## INDICATIONS/ROUTES/DOSAGE

**Usual Dosage Range**
**PO: ADULTS, ELDERLY, CHILDREN OLDER THAN 12 YRS:** 100–400 mg q12h. **CHILDREN 2 MOS–12 YRS:** 10 mg/kg/day in 2 divided doses. **Maximum:** 200 mg/dose.

**Dosage in Renal Impairment**
For pts with CrCl less than 30 ml/min, usual dose is given q24h. For pts on hemodialysis, usual dose is given 3 times/wk after dialysis.

**Dosage in Hepatic Impairment**
No dose adjustment.

## SIDE EFFECTS

**Frequent:** Oral candidiasis (thrush), mild diarrhea, mild abdominal cramping, vaginal candidiasis. **Occasional:** Nausea, serum sickness-like reaction (fever, joint pain; usually occurs after second course of therapy and resolves after drug is discontinued). **Rare:** Allergic reaction (pruritus, rash, urticaria).

---

## ADVERSE EFFECTS/ TOXIC REACTIONS

Antibiotic-associated colitis, other superinfections (abdominal cramps, severe watery diarrhea, fever) may result from altered bacterial balance in GI tract. Nephrotoxicity may occur, esp. in pts with preexisting renal disease. Pts with history of penicillin allergy are at increased risk for developing a severe hypersensitivity reaction (severe pruritus, angioedema, bronchospasm, anaphylaxis).

## NURSING CONSIDERATIONS

### BASELINE ASSESSMENT

Obtain CBC, renal function tests. Question for history of allergies, particularly cephalosporins, penicillins.

### INTERVENTION/EVALUATION

Assess oral cavity for white patches on mucous membranes, tongue (thrush). Monitor daily pattern of bowel activity, stool consistency. Mild GI effects may be tolerable (increasing severity may indicate onset of antibiotic-associated colitis). Monitor I&O, renal function tests for nephrotoxicity. Be alert for superinfection: fever, vomiting, diarrhea, anal/genital pruritus, oral mucosal changes (ulceration, pain, erythema).

### PATIENT/FAMILY TEACHING

• Doses should be evenly spaced. • Shake oral suspension well before using. • Take tablets with food (enhances absorption). • Continue antibiotic therapy for full length of treatment. • Refrigerate oral suspension. • Report persistent diarrhea.

# cefprozil

**sef**-proe-zil
(Apo-Cefprozil ✱, Cefzil ✱)
**Do not confuse cefprozil with cefazolin, or Cefzil with Cefol, Ceftin, or Kefzol.**

## ◆ CLASSIFICATION

**PHARMACOTHERAPEUTIC:** Second-generation cephalosporin. **CLINICAL:** Antibiotic.

## USES

Treatment of susceptible infections due to *S. pneumoniae, S. pyogenes, S. aureus, H. influenzae, M. catarrhalis* including pharyngitis, tonsillitis, otitis media, secondary bacterial infection of acute bronchitis, acute bacterial exacerbation of chronic bronchitis, uncomplicated skin/skin structure infections, acute sinusitis.

## PRECAUTIONS

**Contraindications:** History of hypersensitivity/anaphylactic reaction to cefprozil, cephalosporins. **Cautions:** Severe renal impairment, history of penicillin allergy.

## ACTION

Binds to bacterial cell membranes, inhibits cell wall synthesis. **Therapeutic Effect:** Bactericidal.

## PHARMACOKINETICS

Well absorbed from GI tract. Protein binding: 36%–45%. Widely distributed. Primarily excreted unchanged in urine. Moderately removed by hemodialysis. **Half-life:** 1.3 hrs (increased in renal impairment).

## ⧗ LIFESPAN CONSIDERATIONS

**Pregnancy/Lactation:** Readily crosses placenta. Distributed in breast milk. **Children:** Safety and efficacy not established in pts younger than 6 mos. **Elderly:** Age-related renal impairment may require dosage adjustment.

## INTERACTIONS

**DRUG: Probenecid** may increase concentration. May increase **aminoglycoside** concentration. **HERBAL:** None significant. **FOOD:** None known. **LAB VALUES:** May cause positive direct/indirect Coombs' test. May increase serum BUN, creatinine, alkaline phosphatase, ALT, AST.

## AVAILABILITY (Rx)

**Oral Suspension:** 125 mg/5 ml, 250 mg/5 ml. **Tablets:** 250 mg, 500 mg.

## ADMINISTRATION/HANDLING

### PO

• Give without regard to food; if GI upset occurs, give with food, milk. • After reconstitution, oral suspension is stable for 14 days if refrigerated. • Shake oral suspension well before using.

## INDICATIONS/ROUTES/DOSAGE

### Usual Dosage Range

**PO: ADULTS, ELDERLY, CHILDREN OLDER THAN 12 YRS:** 250–500 mg q12h or 500 mg q24h. **CHILDREN OLDER THAN 6 MOS-12 YRS:** 7.5–15 mg/kg/day in 2 divided doses. **Maximum:** 500 mg/dose. Do not exceed adult dose.

### Dosage in Renal Impairment

**CrCl less than 30 ml/min:** 50% of usual dose at usual interval. **Hemodialysis:** Administer dose after completion of dialysis.

### Dosage in Hepatic Impairment

No dose adjustment.

## SIDE EFFECTS

**Frequent:** Oral candidiasis (thrush), mild diarrhea, mild abdominal cramping, vaginal candidiasis. **Occasional:** Nausea, serum sickness reaction (fever, joint pain; usually occurs after second course of therapy and resolves after drug is discontinued). **Rare:** Allergic reaction (pruritus, rash, urticaria).

## ADVERSE EFFECTS/ TOXIC REACTIONS

Antibiotic-associated colitis, other superinfections (abdominal cramps, severe watery diarrhea, fever) may result from altered bacterial balance in GI tract. Nephrotoxicity may occur, esp. in pts with preexisting renal disease. Pts with history of penicillin allergy are at increased risk for developing a severe

hypersensitivity reaction (severe pruritus, angioedema, bronchospasm, anaphylaxis).

# NURSING CONSIDERATIONS

## BASELINE ASSESSMENT

Obtain CBC, renal function tests. Question for history of allergies, particularly cephalosporins, penicillins.

## INTERVENTION/EVALUATION

Assess oral cavity for evidence of stomatitis. Monitor daily pattern of bowel activity, stool consistency. Mild GI effects may be tolerable (but increasing severity may indicate onset of antibiotic-associated colitis). Monitor I&O, renal function tests for nephrotoxicity. Be alert for superinfection: fever, vomiting, diarrhea, anal/genital pruritus, oral mucosal changes (ulceration, pain, erythema).

## PATIENT/FAMILY TEACHING

• Doses should be evenly spaced. • Continue antibiotic therapy for full length of treatment. • May cause GI upset (may take with food or milk). • Report persistent diarrhea.

# ceftaroline

sef-**tar**-o-leen
(Teflaro)

## ◆CLASSIFICATION

**PHARMACOTHERAPEUTIC:** Fifth-generation cephalosporin. **CLINICAL:** Antibiotic.

## USES

Treatment of susceptible infections due to gram-positive and gram-negative organisms including *S. pneumoniae*, *S. aureus* (methicillin susceptible only), *H. influenzae*, *Klebsiella pneumoniae*, *E. coli* including acute bacterial skin and skin structure infections, community-acquired bacterial pneumonia.

## PRECAUTIONS

**Contraindications:** History of hypersensitivity/anaphylactic reaction to ceftaroline, cephalosporins. **Cautions:** History of allergy to penicillin, severe renal impairment with CrCl less than 50 ml/min, elderly.

## ACTION

Binds to bacterial cell membranes, inhibits cell wall synthesis. **Therapeutic Effect:** Bactericidal.

## PHARMACOKINETICS

Protein binding: 20%. Widely distributed in plasma. Not metabolized. Primarily excreted unchanged in urine. Hemodialyzable. **Half-life:** 1.6 hrs (increased in renal impairment).

## ⏳ LIFESPAN CONSIDERATIONS

**Pregnancy/Lactation:** Unknown if distributed in breast milk. **Children:** Safety and efficacy not established in pts younger than 18 yrs. **Elderly:** Age-related renal impairment may require dose adjustment.

## INTERACTIONS

**DRUG: Probenecid** may increase concentration. **HERBAL:** None significant. **FOOD:** None known. **LAB VALUES:** May cause positive direct/indirect Coombs' test. May increase serum BUN, creatinine. May decrease serum potassium.

## AVAILABILITY (Rx)

**Injection, Powder for Reconstitution:** 400-mg, 600-mg single-use vial.

## ADMINISTRATION/HANDLING

◀**ALERT**▶ Give by intermittent IV infusion (piggyback). Do not give IV push.
**Reconstitution** • Reconstitute either 400-mg or 600-mg vial with 20 ml Sterile Water for Injection. • Mix gently to dissolve powder. • Further dilute with 50–250 ml D₅W, 0.9% NaCl.
**Rate of Administration** • Infuse over 5–60 min.

**Storage** • Discard if particulate is present. • Following reconstitution, solution should appear clear, light to dark yellow. • Solution is stable for 6 hrs at room temperature or 24 hrs if refrigerated.

## ▦ IV INCOMPATIBILITIES

Fluconazole (Diflucan), vancomycin (Vancocin).

## ▦ IV COMPATIBILITIES

Famotidine (Pepcid), hydromorphone (Dilaudid), lorazepam (Ativan), magnesium sulfate, midazolam (Versed), morphine, propofol (Diprivan).

## INDICATIONS/ROUTES/DOSAGE

**Usual Dosage**
**IV: ADULTS, ELDERLY:** 600 mg q12h.
**CHILDREN 2–18 YRS (WEIGHING MORE THAN 33 KG):** 400 mg q8h or 600 mg q12h.
**(WEIGHING 33 KG OR LESS):** 12 mg/kg q8h.
**CHILDREN 2 MOS TO LESS THAN 2 YRS:** 8 mg/kg q8h.

**Dosage in Renal Impairment**

| Creatinine Clearance | Dosage |
| --- | --- |
| 30–50 ml/min | 400 mg q12h |
| 15–29 ml/min | 300 mg q12h |
| End-stage renal disease, hemodialysis | 200 mg every 12 hrs (give after dialysis) |

**Dosage in Hepatic Impairment**
No dose adjustment.

## SIDE EFFECTS

**Occasional (5%–4%):** Diarrhea, nausea. **Rare (3%–2%):** Allergic reaction (rash, pruritus, urticaria), phlebitis.

## ADVERSE EFFECTS/ TOXIC REACTIONS

Antibiotic-associated colitis, other super infections (abdominal cramps, severe watery diarrhea, fever) may result from altered bacterial balance in GI tract. Nephrotoxicity may occur, esp. with pre-existing renal disease. Pts with history of penicillin allergy are at increased risk for developing a severe hypersensitivity reaction (severe pruritus, angioedema, bronchospasm, anaphylaxis).

## NURSING CONSIDERATIONS

### BASELINE ASSESSMENT

Obtain CBC, renal function tests. Question for hypersensitivity to other cephalosporins, penicillins. For pts on hemodialysis, administer medication after dialysis.

### INTERVENTION/EVALUATION

Assess oral cavity for white patches on mucous membranes, tongue (thrush). Monitor daily pattern of bowel activity, stool consistency. Mild GI effects may be tolerable, but increasing severity may indicate onset of antibiotic-associated colitis. Monitor I&O, renal function tests for evidence of nephrotoxicity. Be alert for superinfection: fever, vomiting, severe genital/anal pruritus, moderate to severe diarrhea, oral mucosal changes (ulceration, pain, erythema).

### PATIENT/FAMILY TEACHING

• Continue medication for full length of treatment. • Doses should be evenly spaced.

## *cefTAZidime/ avibactam

sef-**taz**-i-deem/a-vi-**bak**-tam
(Avycaz)
**Do not confuse ceftazidime with cefazolin or cefepime, or avibactam with sulbactam or tazobactam.**

### ◆CLASSIFICATION

**PHARMACOTHERAPEUTIC:** Cephalosporin/beta-lactamase inhibitor. **CLINICAL:** Antibacterial.

## USES

Used in combination with metronidazole for treatment of complicated intra-abdominal infections caused by the following susceptible microorganisms: *Enterobacter cloacae,* *Escherichia coli, Klebsiella pneumoniae, Klebsiella oxytoca, Proteus mirabilis, Providencia stuartii,* and *Pseudomonas aeruginosa* in pts 18 yrs or older. Treatment of complicated urinary tract infections, including pyelonephritis, caused by the following susceptible microorganisms: *Citrobacter freundii, Citrobacter koseri, Enterobacter aerogenes, Enterobacter cloacae, Escherichia coli, Klebsiella pneumoniae, Proteus spp.,* and *Pseudomonas aeruginosa* in pts 18 yrs or older.

## PRECAUTIONS

**Contraindications:** Hypersensitivity to avibactam-containing products, ceftazidime, cephalosporins. **Cautions:** History of renal impairment, seizure disorder, encephalopathy, recent *Clostridium difficile* (C-diff) infection or antibiotic-associated colitis. Hypersensitivity to penicillins, other beta-lactams.

## ACTION

Inhibits cell wall synthesis by binding to bacterial cell membrane. Bacterial action of ceftazidime is mediated through binding to essential penicillin-binding proteins. Avibactam inactivates some beta-lactamases and protects ceftazidime from degradation by certain beta-lactamases. **Therapeutic Effect:** Bactericidal.

## PHARMACOKINETICS

Widely distributed. Excreted unchanged as parent drug; not significantly metabolized in liver. Protein binding: less than 10%. Removed extensively by hemodialysis (55% of dose). Eliminated in urine (80%–90% unchanged). **Half-life:** 2.7 hrs (dependent on dose and severity of renal impairment).

## ⌛ LIFESPAN CONSIDERATIONS

**Pregnancy/Lactation:** Ceftazidime is excreted in breast milk in low concentrations. Unknown if avibactam is excreted in breast milk. **Children:** Safety and efficacy not established. **Elderly:** May have increased risk of adverse effects (due to renal impairment).

## INTERACTIONS

**DRUG:** None significant. **HERBAL:** None significant. **FOOD:** None known. **LAB VALUES:** May increase serum alkaline phosphatase, ALT, GGT, LDH. May decrease platelets, eosinophils, leukocytes, lymphocytes; serum potassium. May result in positive Coombs' test or false-positive elevated urine glucose.

## AVAILABILITY (Rx)

◀**ALERT**▶ Ceftazidime/avibactam is a combination product.

**Injection, Powder for Reconstitution:** 2 gm ceftazidime/ 0.5 gm avibactam.

## ADMINISTRATION/HANDLING

 IV

**Reconstitution** • Reconstitute vial with 10 ml of one of following solutions with 0.9% NaCl, Sterile Water for Injection or 5% Dextrose injection. • Shake gently until powder completely dissolved. • Visually inspect for particular matter or discoloration. Solution should appear clear to slightly yellow in color. • Final concentration of vial will equal approx. 0.167 g/ml of ceftazidime and 0.042 g/ml of avibactam. • Further dilute with 50 ml to 250 ml 0.9% Nacl or 5% Dextrose injection.

**Rate of Administration** • Infuse over 2 hrs.

**Storage** • Diluted solution may be stored at room temperature up to 12 hrs or refrigerated up to 24 hrs. • Infuse within 12 hrs once removed from refrigerator. • Do not freeze.

## INDICATIONS/ROUTES/DOSAGE

**Complicated Intra-Abdominal Infections**
**IV: ADULTS, ELDERLY:** 2.5 g (ceftazidime 2 g/avibactam 0.5 g) q8h for 5–14 days (in combination with metronidazole).

**Complicated Urinary Tract Infections Including Pyelonephritis**
**IV: ADULTS, ELDERLY:** 2.5 g (2 g ceftazidine/0.5 g avibactam) q8h for 7–14 days.

**Dosage in Renal Impairment**
**Note:** Infuse after hemodialysis on hemodialysis days.
Dosage is modified based on creatinine clearance.

| Creatinine Clearance | Dosage |
|---|---|
| Greater than 50 ml/min: | 2.5 g (2 gm/0.5 g) q8h |
| 31–50 ml/min: | 1.25 g (1 g/0.25 g) q8h |
| 16–30 ml/min: | 0.94 g (0.75 g/0.19 g) q12h |
| 6–15 ml/min: | 0.94 g (0.75 g/0.19 g) q24h |
| Less than or equal to 5 ml/min: | 0.94 g (0.75 g/0.19 g) q48h |

**Dosage in Hepatic Impairment**
No dose adjustment.

## SIDE EFFECTS:

**Occasional (14%–5%):** Vomiting, nausea, abdominal pain, anxiety, rash. **Rare (4%–2%):** Constipation, dizziness.

## ADVERSE EFFECTS/TOXIC REACTIONS

May cause worsening of renal function or acute renal failure in pts with renal impairment. Clinical cure rates were lower in pts with CrCl 30–50 ml/min compared with those with CrCl greater than 50 ml/min, and in pts receiving metronidazole combination therapy. Blood and lymphatic disorders such as agranulocytosis, hemolytic anemia, leukopenia, lymphocytosis, neutropenia, thrombocytopenia were reported. Hypersensitivity reactions, including anaphylaxis or severe skin reactions, have been reported in pts treated with beta-lactam antibacterial drugs. *Clostridium difficile* (C-diff)–associated diarrhea, with severity ranging from mild diarrhea to fatal colitis, was reported. C-diff infection may occur more than 2 mos after treatment completion. Central nervous system reactions including asterixis, coma, encephalopathy, neuromuscular excitability, myoclonus, nonconvulsive status epilepticus, seizures have been reported in pts receiving ceftazidime, esp. in pts with renal impairment. May increase risk of development of drug-resistant bacteria when used in the absence of a proven or strongly suspected bacterial infection. Skin and subcutaneous tissue disorders such as angioedema, erythema multiforme, pruritis, Stevens-Johnson syndrome, toxic epidermal necrolysis were reported in pts receiving ceftazidime. Other reported adverse effects including infusion site inflammation/hematoma/thrombosis, jaundice, candidiasis, dysgeusia, paresthesia, tubulointerstitial nephritis, vaginal inflammation occur rarely.

## NURSING CONSIDERATIONS

### BASELINE ASSESSMENT

Obtain baseline CBC, BUN, serum creatinine, potassium; CrCl, GFR, LFT; bacterial culture and sensitivity; vital signs. Question history of recent C-diff infection, renal impairment, seizure disorder; hypersensitivity reaction to beta-lactams, carbapenem, cephalosporins, PCN. Assess skin for wounds; hydration status. Question pt's usual stool characteristics (color, frequency, consistency).

### INTERVENTION/EVALUATION

Monitor CBC, BMP, renal function periodically. For pts with changing renal function, monitor renal function test daily and adjust dose accordingly. Diligently monitor I&Os. Observe daily pattern of bowel activity, stool consistency (increased severity may indicate antibiotic-associated colitis). If frequent diarrhea occurs, obtain C-diff toxin screen and initiate isolation precautions until test result confirmed; manage proper fluids levels/PO intake, electrolyte levels, protein intake. Antibacterial drugs that are not directed against C-diff infection may need to be discontinued. Report any sign of hypersensitivity reaction.

### PATIENT/FAMILY TEACHING

• It is essential to complete drug therapy despite symptom improvement. Early discontinuation may result in antibacterial resistance or increased risk of recurrent infection. • Report any episodes of diarrhea, esp. the following mos after treatment completion. Frequent diarrhea, fever, abdominal pain, blood-streaked stool may indicate C-diff infection and may be contagious to others. • Report abdominal pain, black/tarry stools, bruising, yellowing of skin or eyes; dark urine, decreased urine output; skin problems such as development of sores, rash, skin bubbling/necrosis. • Drink plenty of fluids. • Report any nervous system changes such as anxiety, confusion, hallucinations, muscle jerking, or seizure-like activity. • Severe allergic reactions such as hives, palpitations, shortness of breath, rash, tongue-swelling may occur.

## *cefTAZidime

sef-**taz**-i-deem
(Fortaz, Tazicef)
**Do not confuse ceftazidime with cefazolin, cefepime, or ceftriaxone.**

### ◆CLASSIFICATION

**PHARMACOTHERAPEUTIC:** Third-generation cephalosporin. **CLINICAL:** Antibiotic.

## USES

Treatment of susceptible infections due to gram-negative organisms (including *Pseudomonas* and *Enterobacteriaceae*) including bone, joint, CNS (including meningitis), gynecologic, intra-abdominal, lower respiratory tract, skin/skin structure infections; UTI, septicemia. Treatment of CNS infections due to *H. influenzae, N. meningitidis,* including meningitis. **OFF-LABEL:** Bacterial endophthalmitis.

## PRECAUTIONS

**Contraindications:** History of hypersensitivity/anaphylactic reaction to ceftazidime, cephalosporins. **Cautions:** Severe renal impairment, history of penicillin allergy, seizure disorder.

## ACTION

Binds to bacterial cell membranes, inhibits cell wall synthesis. **Therapeutic Effect:** Bactericidal.

## PHARMACOKINETICS

Widely distributed including to CSF. Protein binding: 5%–17%. Primarily excreted unchanged in urine. Removed by hemodialysis. **Half-life:** 2 hrs (increased in renal impairment).

## ⧖ LIFESPAN CONSIDERATIONS

**Pregnancy/Lactation:** Readily crosses placenta. Distributed in breast milk. **Children:** No age-related precautions noted. **Elderly:** Age-related renal impairment may require dosage adjustment.

## INTERACTIONS

**DRUG: Probenecid** may increase concentration. May increase **aminoglycoside** concentration. **HERBAL:** None significant. **FOOD:** None known. **LAB VALUES:** May increase serum BUN, alkaline phosphatase, creatinine, LDH, ALT, AST. May cause positive direct/indirect Coombs' test.

## AVAILABILITY (Rx)

**Injection, Powder for Reconstitution (Fortaz, Tazicef):** 500 mg, 1 g, 2 g. **Injection, Premix:** 1 g/50 ml, 2 g/50 ml.

## ADMINISTRATION/HANDLING

◀ **ALERT** ▶ Give by IM injection, direct IV injection (IV push), or intermittent IV infusion (piggyback).

**◨ IV**

**Reconstitution** • Add 10 ml Sterile Water for Injection to each 1 g to provide concentration of 90 mg/ml. • May further dilute with 50–100 ml 0.9% NaCl, $D_5W$, or other compatible diluent.

**Rate of Administration** • For IV push, administer over 3–5 min (**maximum concentration: 180 mg/ml**). • For intermittent IV infusion (piggyback), infuse over 15–30 min.

**Storage** • Solution appears light yellow to amber, tends to darken (color change does not indicate loss of potency). • IV infusion (piggyback) stable for 12 hrs at room temperature or 3 days if refrigerated. • Discard if precipitate forms.

**IM**

• For reconstitution, add 1.5 ml Sterile Water for Injection or lidocaine 1% to 500-mg vial or 3 ml to 1-g vial to provide a concentration of 280 mg/ml. • To minimize discomfort, inject deep IM slowly. Less painful if injected into gluteus maximus than lateral aspect of thigh.

## ▦ IV INCOMPATIBILITIES

Amphotericin B complex (Abelcet, AmBisome, Amphotec), fluconazole (Diflucan), idarubicin, midazolam (Versed), vancomycin (Vancocin).

## ▦ IV COMPATIBILITIES

Diltiazem (Cardizem), famotidine (Pepcid), heparin, hydromorphone (Dilaudid), lipids, morphine, propofol (Diprivan).

## INDICATIONS/ROUTES/DOSAGE

**Usual Dosage Range**

**IV, IM: ADULTS, ELDERLY:** 500 mg–2 g q8–12h.

**IV: CHILDREN 1 MO–12 YRS:** 90–150 mg/kg/day in divided doses q8h. **Maximum:** 6 g/day. **NEONATES 0–4 WKS:** 50 mg/kg/dose q8–12h.

**Dosage in Renal Impairment**

Dosage and frequency are modified based on creatinine clearance and severity of infection.

| Creatinine Clearance | Dosage |
|---|---|
| 31–50 ml/min | 1g q12h |
| 16–30 ml/min | 1g q24h |
| 6–15 ml/min | 500 mg q24h |
| Less than 6 ml/min | 500 mg q48h |
| Hemodialysis | 0.5–1 g q24h or 1–2 g q48–72h (give post hemodialysis on dialysis days) |
| Peritoneal dialysis | Initially, 1 g, then 0.5 g q24h |
| Continuous renal replacement therapy | Initially, 2 g, then 1 g q8h or 2 g q12h |

**Dosage in Hepatic Impairment**
No dose adjustment.

## SIDE EFFECTS

**Frequent:** Discomfort with IM administration, oral candidiasis (thrush), mild diarrhea, mild abdominal cramping, vaginal candidiasis. **Occasional:** Nausea, serum sickness–like reaction (fever, joint pain; usually occurs after second course of therapy and resolves after drug is discontinued). **Rare:** Allergic reaction (pruritus, rash, urticaria), thrombophlebitis (pain, redness, swelling at injection site).

## ADVERSE EFFECTS/ TOXIC REACTIONS

Antibiotic-associated colitis, other superinfections (abdominal cramps, severe watery diarrhea, fever) may result from altered bacterial balance in GI tract. Nephrotoxicity may occur, esp. in pts with preexisting renal disease. Pts with history of penicillin allergy are at increased risk for developing a severe hypersensitivity reaction (severe pruritus, angioedema, bronchospasm, anaphylaxis).

## NURSING CONSIDERATIONS

### BASELINE ASSESSMENT
Obtain CBC, renal function tests. Question for history of allergies, particularly cephalosporins, penicillins.

### INTERVENTION/EVALUATION
Evaluate IV site for phlebitis (heat, pain, red streaking over vein). Assess IM injection sites for induration, tenderness. Check oral cavity for white patches on mucous membranes, tongue (thrush). Monitor daily pattern of bowel activity, stool consistency. Mild GI effects may be tolerable (increasing severity may indicate onset of antibiotic-associated colitis). Monitor I&O, renal function tests for nephrotoxicity. Be alert for superinfection: fever, vomiting, diarrhea, anal/genital pruritus, oral mucosal changes (ulceration, pain, erythema).

### PATIENT/FAMILY TEACHING
• Discomfort may occur with IM injection. • Doses should be evenly spaced. • Continue antibiotic therapy for full length of treatment.

# ceftolozane/ tazobactam

cef-**tol**-oh-zane/tay-zoe-**bak**-tam (Zerbaxa)
**Do not confuse ceftolozane with ceftazidime, or tazobactam with avibactam or sulbactam.**

### ◆CLASSIFICATION

**PHARMACOTHERAPEUTIC:** Cephalosporin/beta-lactamase inhibitor. **CLINICAL:** Antibacterial.

## USES

Used in combination with metronidazole for treatment of complicated intra-abdominal infections caused by the following susceptible gram-negative and gram-positive microorganisms: *Bacteroides fragilis, Enterobacter cloacae, Escherichia coli, Klebsiella oxytoca, Klebsiella pneumoniae, Proteus mirabilis, Pseudomonas aeruginosa, Streptococcus anginosus, Streptococcus constellatus,* and *Streptococcus salivarius* in pts 18 yrs or older. Treatment of complicated urinary tract infections, including pyelonephritis, caused by the following susceptible Gram-negative microorganisms: *Escherichia coli*, *Klebsiella pneumoniae*, *Proteus mirabilis*, and *Pseudomonas aeruginosa* in pts 18 yrs or older.

## PRECAUTIONS

**Contraindications:** Hypersensitivity to ceftolozane/tazobactam, piperacillin/tazobactam, or other beta-lactams. **Cautions:** History of atrial fibrillation, electrolyte imbalance-associated arrhythmias, recent *Clostridium difficile* (C-diff) infection or antibiotic-associated colitis, renal/hepatic impairment, seizure disorder; prior hypersensitivity to penicillins, other cephalosporins.

## ACTION

Inhibits cell wall synthesis by binding to bacterial cell membrane. Bacterial action of ceftolozane is mediated through binding to essential penicillin-binding proteins. Tazobactam inactivates certain beta-lactamases and binds to certain chromosomal and plasmid-mediated bacterial beta-lactamases. **Therapeutic Effect:** Bactericidal.

## PHARMACOKINETICS

Widely distributed. Excreted unchanged as parent drug; not significantly metabolized in liver. Protein binding: 16%–30%. Eliminated in urine (95% unchanged). Removed extensively by hemodialysis. **Half-life:** 2.7 hrs (dependent on dose and severity of renal impairment).

## ⧖ LIFESPAN CONSIDERATIONS

**Pregnancy/Lactation:** Unknown if distributed in breast milk. **Children:** Safety and efficacy not established. **Elderly:** May have increased risk of adverse effects (due to renal impairment).

## INTERACTIONS

**DRUG:** None significant. **FOOD:** None known. **LAB VALUES:** May increase serum alkaline phosphatase, ALT, AST, GGT. May decrease Hgb, Hct, platelets; serum potassium, magnesium, phosphate. May result in positive Coombs' test.

## AVAILABILITY (Rx)

◀**ALERT**▶ Ceftolozane/tazobactam is a combination product.
**Injection, Powder for Reconstitution:** 1 g ceftolozane/0.5 g tazobactam.

## ADMINISTRATION/HANDLING
🜄 IV

**Reconstitution** • Reconstitute vial with 10 ml of Sterile Water for Injection or 0.9% NaCl. • Shake gently until powder is completely dissolved. • Final volume of vial will equal approx. 11.4 ml. • Visually inspect for particular matter or discoloration. Solution should appear clear, colorless to slightly yellow in color. • Withdraw required volume from reconstituted vial and inject into diluent bag containing 100 ml 0.9% NaCl or 5% dextrose injection as follows:

| Ceftolozane/ Tazobactam | Volume to Withdraw from Reconstituted Vial |
|---|---|
| 1.5 g (1 g/0.5 g) | 11.4 ml |
| 750 mg (500 mg/250 mg) | 5.7 ml |
| 375 mg (250 mg/125 mg) | 2.9 ml |
| 150 mg (100 mg/50 mg) | 1.2 ml |

**Rate of Administration** • Infuse over 60 min.
**Storage** • Reconstituted vial may be held for 1 hr prior to transfer to diluent bag. • May refrigerate diluted solution up to 7 days or store at room temperature up to 24 hrs. • Do not freeze.

## INDICATIONS/ROUTES/DOSAGE

**Complicated Intra-abdominal Infections**
**IV: ADULTS, ELDERLY:** 1.5 g (ceftolozane 1 g/tazobactam 0.5 g) q8h for 4–14 days (in combination with metronidazole).

---

**Complicated Urinary Tract Infections Including Pyelonephritis**
IV: **ADULTS, ELDERLY:** 1.5 g (ceftolozane 1 g/tazobactam 0.5 g) q8h for 7 days.

**Dosage in Renal Impairment**
**CrCl 30–50 ml/min:** 750 mg (500 mg/250 mg) q8h. **CrCl 15–29 ml/min:** 375 mg (250 mg/125 mg) q8h.
**End-Stage Renal Disease or on Hemodialysis:** 750 mg (500 mg/250 mg) loading dose, then 150 mg (100 mg/50 mg) maintenance dose q8h for the remainder of the treatment period.
**Note:** Administer after hemodialysis on hemodialysis days.

**Dosage in Hepatic Impairment**
No dose adjustment.

## SIDE EFFECTS

**Occasional (6%–3%):** Nausea, diarrhea, pyrexia, insomnia, headache, vomiting.
**Rare (2%–1%):** Constipation, anxiety, hypotension, rash, abdominal pain, dizziness, tachycardia, dyspnea, urticaria, gastritis, abdominal distension, dyspepsia, flatulence.

## ADVERSE EFFECTS/TOXIC REACTIONS

Clinical cure rates were lower in pts with CrCl 30–50 ml/min compared with those with CrCl greater than 50ml/min, and in pts receiving metronidazole combination therapy. Hypersensitivity reactions including anaphylaxis or severe skin reactions have been reported with use of beta-lactam antibacterial drugs. *Clostridium difficile* (C-diff)–associated diarrhea, with severity ranging from mild diarrhea to fatal colitis, was reported. C-diff infection may occur more than 2 mos after treatment completion. May increase risk of development of drug-resistant bacteria when used in the absence of a proven or strongly suspected bacterial infection. Atrial fibrillation reported in 1.2% of pts. Other reported adverse events such as angina pectoris, infections (candidiasis, oropharyngeal infection,

fungal urinary tract infection), paralytic ileus, venous thrombosis occur rarely.

## NURSING CONSIDERATIONS

### BASELINE ASSESSMENT

Obtain baseline CBC, serum BUN, creatinine; CrCl, GFR, LFT; bacterial culture and sensitivity; vital signs. Question history of atrial fibrillation, recent C-diff infection, hepatic/renal impairment, hypersensitivity reaction to beta-lactams, cephalosporins, penicillins, carbapenem. Assess skin for wounds; hydration status. Question pt's usual stool characteristics (color, frequency, consistency).

### INTERVENTION/EVALUATION

Monitor CBC, BMP, renal function test periodically; serum magnesium, ionized calcium in pts at risk for arrhythmias. For pts with changing renal function, monitor renal function test daily and adjust dose accordingly. Diligently monitor I&Os. Observe daily pattern of bowel activity, stool consistency (increased severity may indicate antibiotic-associated colitis). If frequent diarrhea occurs, obtain C-diff toxin screen and initiate isolation precautions until test result confirmed; manage proper fluids levels/PO intake, electrolyte levels, protein intake. Antibacterial drugs that are not directed against C-diff infection may need to be discontinued. Report any signs of hypersensitivity reaction.

### PATIENT/FAMILY TEACHING

• It is essential to complete drug therapy despite symptom improvement. Early discontinuation may result in antibacterial resistance or increased risk of recurrent infection. • Report any episodes of diarrhea, esp. the following mos after treatment completion. Frequent diarrhea, fever, abdominal pain, blood-streaked stool may indicate C-diff infection and may be contagious to others. • Report abdominal pain, black/tarry stools, bruising, yellowing of skin or eyes; dark urine, decreased urine output. • Drink plenty of fluids. • Severe allergic reactions such as hives palpitations, rash, shortness of breath, tongue swelling may occur.

# *cefTRIAXone

sef-trye-**ax**-own
(Rocephin)
**Do not confuse ceftriaxone with cefazolin, cefoxitin, or ceftazidine.**

## ◆CLASSIFICATION

**PHARMACOTHERAPEUTIC:** Third-generation cephalosporin. **CLINICAL:** Antibiotic.

## USES

Treatment of susceptible infections due to gram-negative aerobic organisms, some gram-positive organisms including respiratory tract, GU tract, skin and skin structure, bone and joint, intra-abdominal, pelvic inflammatory disease (PID), biliary tract/urinary tract infections; bacterial septicemia, meningitis, perioperative prophylaxis, acute bacterial otitis media. **OFF-LABEL:** Complicated gonococcal infections, STDs, Lyme disease, salmonellosis, shigellosis, atypical community-acquired pneumonia.

## PRECAUTIONS

**Contraindications:** History of hypersensitivity/anaphylactic reaction to ceftriaxone, cephalosporins. Hyperbilirubinemic neonates, esp. premature infants, should not be treated with ceftriaxone (can displace bilirubin from its binding to serum albumin, causing bilirubin encephalopathy). Do not administer with calcium-containing IV solutions, including continuous calcium-containing infusion such as parenteral nutrition (in neonates) due to the risk of precipitation of ceftriaxone-calcium salt. **Cautions:** Hepatic impairment, history of GI disease (esp. ulcerative colitis, antibiotic-associated colitis). History of penicillin allergy.

## ACTION

Binds to bacterial cell membranes, inhibits cell wall synthesis. **Therapeutic Effect:** Bactericidal.

## PHARMACOKINETICS

Widely distributed including to CSF. Protein binding: 83%–96%. Primarily excreted unchanged in urine. Not removed by hemodialysis. **Half-life: IV:** 4.3–4.6 hrs; **IM:** 5.8–8.7 hrs (increased in renal impairment).

## ⌛ LIFESPAN CONSIDERATIONS

**Pregnancy/Lactation:** Readily crosses placenta. Distributed in breast milk. **Children:** May displace bilirubin from serum albumin. Contraindicated in hyperbilirubinemic neonates. **Elderly:** Age-related renal impairment may require dosage adjustment.

## INTERACTIONS

**DRUG: Probenecid** may increase excretion. May increase **aminoglycoside** concentration. **HERBAL:** None significant. **FOOD:** None known. **LAB VALUES:** May increase serum BUN, alkaline phosphatase, bilirubin, creatinine, LDH, ALT, AST. May cause positive direct/indirect Coombs' test.

## AVAILABILITY (Rx)

**Injection, Powder for Reconstitution (Rocephin):** 250 mg, 500 mg, 1 g, 2 g. **Intravenous Solution (Rocephin):** 1 g/50 ml, 2 g/50 ml.

## ADMINISTRATION/HANDLING

 IV

**Reconstitution** • Add 2.4 ml Sterile Water for Injection to each 250 mg to provide concentration of 100 mg/ml. • May further dilute with 50–100 ml 0.9% NaCl, D₅W.
**Rate of Administration** • For IV push, administer over 1–4 min (**maximum concentration:** 40 mg/ml). • For intermittent IV infusion (piggyback), infuse over 30 min.

**Storage** • Solution appears light yellow to amber. • IV infusion (piggyback) is stable for 2 days at room temperature, 10 days if refrigerated. • Discard if precipitate forms.

**IM**

• Add 0.9 ml Sterile Water for Injection, 0.9% NaCl, $D_5W$, or lidocaine to each 250 mg to provide concentration of 250 mg/ml. • To minimize discomfort, inject deep IM slowly. Less painful if injected into gluteus maximus than lateral aspect of thigh.

### ▦ IV INCOMPATIBILITIES

Amphotericin B complex (Abelcet, AmBisome, Amphotec), famotidine (Pepcid), fluconazole (Diflucan), labetalol (Normodyne), vancomycin (Vancocin).

### ▦ IV COMPATIBILITIES

Diltiazem (Cardizem), heparin, lidocaine, metronidazole (Flagyl), morphine, propofol (Diprivan).

### INDICATIONS/ROUTES/DOSAGE

**Usual Dosage Range**
**IM/IV: ADULTS, ELDERLY:** 1–2 g q12–24h. **CHILDREN:** 50–100 mg/kg/day in 1–2 divided doses. **Maximum:** 4 g/day (meningitis), 2 g/day (other). **NEONATES:** 50 mg/kg/dose given once daily.

**Dosage in Renal/Hepatic Impairment**
Dosage modification is usually unnecessary but hepatic/renal function test results should be monitored in pts with renal and hepatic impairment or severe renal impairment.

### SIDE EFFECTS

**Frequent:** Discomfort with IM administration, oral candidiasis (thrush), mild diarrhea, mild abdominal cramping, vaginal candidiasis. **Occasional:** Nausea, serum sickness-like reaction (fever; joint pain; usually occurs after second course of therapy and resolves after drug is discontinued). **Rare:** Allergic reaction (rash, pruritus, urticaria), thrombophlebitis (pain, redness, swelling at injection site).

### ADVERSE EFFECTS/TOXIC REACTIONS

Antibiotic-associated colitis, other superinfections (abdominal cramps, severe watery diarrhea, fever) may result from altered bacterial balance in GI tract. Nephrotoxicity may occur, esp. in pts with preexisting renal disease. Pts with history of penicillin allergy are at increased risk for developing a severe hypersensitivity reaction (severe pruritus, angioedema, bronchospasm, anaphylaxis).

### NURSING CONSIDERATIONS

#### BASELINE ASSESSMENT

Obtain CBC, renal function tests. Question for history of allergies, particularly cephalosporins, penicillins.

#### INTERVENTION/EVALUATION

Assess oral cavity for white patches on mucous membranes, tongue (thrush). Monitor daily pattern of bowel activity, stool consistency. Mild GI effects may be tolerable (increasing severity may indicate onset of antibiotic-associated colitis). Monitor I&O, renal function tests for nephrotoxicity, CBC. Be alert for superinfection: fever, vomiting, diarrhea, anal/genital pruritus, oral mucosal changes (ulceration, pain, erythema).

#### PATIENT/FAMILY TEACHING

• Discomfort may occur with IM injection. • Doses should be evenly spaced. • Continue antibiotic therapy for full length of treatment.

### cefuroxime

sef-ue-**rox**-eem
(Apo-Cefuroxime ✸, Ceftin, Zinacef)
**Do not confuse Ceftin with Cefzil or Cipro, cefuroxime with cefotaxime, cefprozil, or deferoxamine, or Zinacef with Zithromax.**

C

## ◆ CLASSIFICATION

**PHARMACOTHERAPEUTIC:** Second-generation cephalosporin. **CLINICAL:** Antibiotic.

## USES

Treatment of susceptible infections due to group B streptococci, pneumococci, staphylococci, *H. influenzae, E. coli, Enterobacter, Klebsiella* including acute/chronic bronchitis, gonorrhea, impetigo, early Lyme disease, otitis media, pharyngitis/tonsillitis, sinusitis, skin/skin structure, UTI, perioperative prophylaxis.

## PRECAUTIONS

**Contraindications:** History of hypersensitivity/anaphylactic reaction to cefuroxime, cephalosporins. **Cautions:** Severe renal impairment, history of penicillin allergy. Pts with hx of colitis, GI malabsorption, seizures.

## ACTION

Binds to bacterial cell membranes, inhibits cell wall synthesis. **Therapeutic Effect:** Bactericidal.

## PHARMACOKINETICS

Rapidly absorbed from GI tract. Protein binding: 33%–50%. Widely distributed including to CSF. Primarily excreted unchanged in urine. Moderately removed by hemodialysis. **Half-life:** 1.3 hrs (increased in renal impairment).

## ⧖ LIFESPAN CONSIDERATIONS

**Pregnancy/Lactation:** Readily crosses placenta. Distributed in breast milk. **Children:** No age-related precautions noted. **Elderly:** Age-related renal impairment may require dosage adjustment.

## INTERACTIONS

**DRUG: Probenecid** may increase concentration. **Antacids, H₂-receptor antagonists (e.g, cimetidine, famotidine)** may decrease absorption. **HERBAL:** None significant. **FOOD:** None known. **LAB VALUES:** May increase serum BUN, creatinine, alkaline phosphatase, bilirubin, LDH, ALT, AST. May cause positive direct/indirect Coombs' test.

## AVAILABILITY (Rx)

**Injection, Powder for Reconstitution:** 750 mg, 1.5 g. **Injection, Solution:** 1.5 g/50 ml. **Oral Suspension (Ceftin):** 125 mg/5 ml, 250 mg/5 ml. **Tablets (Ceftin):** 250 mg, 500 mg.

## ADMINISTRATION/HANDLING

 IV

**Reconstitution** • Reconstitute 750 mg in 8 ml (1.5 g in 14 ml) Sterile Water for Injection to provide a concentration of 100 mg/ml. • For intermittent IV infusion (piggyback), further dilute with 50–100 ml 0.9% NaCl or D₅W.
**Rate of Administration** • For IV push, administer over 3–5 min. • For intermittent IV infusion (piggyback), infuse over 15–30 min.
**Storage** • Solution appears light yellow to amber (may darken, but color change does not indicate loss of potency). • IV infusion (piggyback) is stable for 24 hrs at room temperature, 7 days if refrigerated. • Discard if precipitate forms.

**IM**
• To minimize discomfort, inject deep IM slowly in large muscle mass.

**PO**
• Give tablets without regard to food (give 400-mg dose with food). • If GI upset occurs, give with food, milk. • Avoid crushing tablets due to bitter taste. • Suspension must be given with food. • Suspension stable at room temperature or refrigerated for 10 days.

## ▦ IV INCOMPATIBILITIES

Fluconazole (Diflucan), midazolam (Versed), vancomycin (Vancocin).

## ▦ IV COMPATIBILITIES

Diltiazem (Cardizem), hydromorphone (Dilaudid), morphine, propofol (Diprivan).

## INDICATIONS/ROUTES/DOSAGE

**Usual Dosage**
**IV, IM: ADULTS, ELDERLY, CHILDREN 12 YRS AND OLDER:** 750 mg–1.5 g q8h. **CHILDREN: 3 MOS TO YOUNGER THAN 12 YRS:** 75–150 mg/kg/day divided q8h. **Maximum:** 6 g/day. **NEONATES:** 50 mg/kg/dose q8–12h.
**PO: ADULTS, ELDERLY, CHILDREN 12 YRS AND OLDER:** 250–500 mg twice a day. **CHILDREN 3 MOS TO YOUNGER THAN 12 YRS:** 20–30 mg/kg/day in 2 divided doses. **Maximum:** 1 g/day.

**Dosage in Renal Impairment**
Adult dosage frequency is modified based on creatinine clearance and severity of infection.

| Creatinine Clearance | Dosage |
|---|---|
| **IV** | |
| Greater than 20 ml/min | q8h |
| 10–20 ml/min | q12h |
| Less than 10 ml/min | q24h |
| Peritoneal dialysis | Dose q24h |
| Continuous renal replacement therapy | 1 g q12h |
| **PO** | |
| Greater than 30 ml/min | No adjustment |
| 10–29 ml/min | q24h |
| Less than 10 ml/min | q48h |

**Dosage in Hepatic Impairment**
No dose adjustment.

## SIDE EFFECTS

**Frequent:** Discomfort with IM administration, oral candidiasis (thrush), mild diarrhea, mild abdominal cramping, vaginal candidiasis. **Occasional:** Nausea, serum sickness–like reaction (fever, joint pain; usually occurs after second course of therapy and resolves after drug is discontinued). **Rare:** Allergic reaction (rash, pruritus, urticaria), thrombophlebitis (pain, redness, swelling at injection site).

## ADVERSE EFFECTS/ TOXIC REACTIONS

Antibiotic-associated colitis, other super-infections (abdominal cramps, severe watery diarrhea, fever) may result from altered bacterial balance in GI tract. Nephrotoxicity may occur, esp. in pts with preexisting renal disease. Pts with history of penicillin allergy are at increased risk for developing a severe hypersensitivity reaction (severe pruritus, angioedema, bronchospasm anaphylaxis).

## NURSING CONSIDERATIONS

### BASELINE ASSESSMENT

Obtain CBC, renal function tests. Question for history of allergies, particularly cephalosporins, penicillins.

### INTERVENTION/EVALUATION

Assess oral cavity for white patches on mucous membranes, tongue (thrush). Monitor daily pattern of bowel activity, stool consistency. Mild GI effects may be tolerable (increasing severity may indicate onset of antibiotic-associated colitis). Monitor I&O, renal function tests for nephrotoxicity. Be alert for superinfection: fever, vomiting, diarrhea, anal/genital pruritus, oral mucosal changes (ulceration, pain, erythema).

### PATIENT/FAMILY TEACHING

• Discomfort may occur with IM injection. • Doses should be evenly spaced. • Continue antibiotic therapy for full length of treatment. • May cause GI upset (may take with food, milk).

---

## celecoxib

sel-e-**kox**-ib
(Apo-Celecoxib ✿, Celebrex)
■ **BLACK BOX ALERT** ■ Increased risk of serious cardiovascular thrombotic events, including MI, CVA. Increased risk of severe GI reactions, including ulceration, bleeding, perforation of stomach, intestines.

---

Do not confuse Celebrex with Celexa, Cerebyx, or Clarinex.

## ◆ CLASSIFICATION

**PHARMACOTHERAPEUTIC:** NSAID.
**CLINICAL:** Anti-inflammatory.

## USES

Relief of signs/symptoms of osteoarthritis, rheumatoid arthritis (RA) in adults. Treatment of acute pain, primary dysmenorrhea. Relief of signs/symptoms associated with ankylosing spondylitis. Treatment of juvenile rheumatoid arthritis (JRA).

## PRECAUTIONS

◀ALERT▶ May increase cardiovascular risk when high doses given to prevent colon cancer.
**Contraindications:** Hypersensitivity to celecoxib, sulfonamides. Active GI bleeding. Pts experiencing asthma, urticaria, or allergic reactions to aspirin, other NSAIDs. Treatment of perioperative pain in coronary artery bypass graft (CABG) surgery. **Cautions:** History of GI disease (bleeding/ulcers); concurrent use with aspirin, anticoagulants, smoking; alcohol, elderly, debilitated pts, hypertension, asthma, renal/hepatic impairment. Pts with edema, cerebrovascular disease, ischemic heart disease, HF, known or suspected deficiency of cytochrome P450 isoenzyme 2C9. Pediatric pts with systemic-onset juvenile idiopathic arthritis.

## ACTION

Inhibits cyclooxygenase-2, the enzyme responsible for prostaglandin synthesis. **Therapeutic Effect:** Reduces inflammation, relieves pain.

## PHARMACOKINETICS

Rapidly absorbed from GI tract. Widely distributed. Protein binding: 97%. Metabolized in liver. Primarily eliminated in feces. **Half-life:** 11.2 hrs.

## ⧗ LIFESPAN CONSIDERATIONS

**Pregnancy/Lactation:** Unknown if drug crosses placenta or is distributed in breast milk. Avoid use during third trimester (may adversely affect fetal cardiovascular system: premature closure of ductus arteriosus). **Children:** Safety and efficacy not established in pts younger than 18 yrs. **Elderly:** No age-related precautions noted.

## INTERACTIONS

**DRUG:** May decrease antihypertensive effect of **ACE inhibitors, angiotensin II antagonists. Fluconazole** may significantly increase concentration. May increase **lithium** concentration. **Warfarin** may increase risk of bleeding. **Aspirin** may increase risk of celecoxib-induced GI ulceration, other GI complications. **HERBAL:** Avoid herbs with anticoagulant or antiplatelet activity (e.g., **evening primrose, garlic, ginger, ginseng**). **FOOD:** None known. **LAB VALUES:** May increase serum ALT, AST, alkaline phosphatase, creatinine, BUN. May decrease serum phosphate.

## AVAILABILITY (Rx)

**Capsules:** 50 mg, 100 mg, 200 mg, 400 mg.

## ADMINISTRATION/HANDLING

**PO**
- May give without regard to meals.
- Capsules may be swallowed whole or opened and mixed with applesauce.

## INDICATIONS/ROUTES/DOSAGE

**Note:** Consider reduced initial dose of 50% in poor CYP2C9 metabolizers.
**Osteoarthritis**
**PO: ADULTS, ELDERLY:** 200 mg/day as a single dose or 100 mg twice daily.

**Rheumatoid Arthritis (RA)**
**PO: ADULTS, ELDERLY:** 100–200 mg twice daily.

**Juvenile Rheumatoid Arthritis (JRA)**
**PO: CHILDREN 2 YRS AND OLDER, WEIGHING MORE THAN 25 KG:** 100 mg twice daily. **WEIGHING 10–25 KG:** 50 mg twice daily.

**Acute Pain, Primary Dysmenorrhea**
**PO: ADULTS, ELDERLY:** Initially, 400 mg with additional 200 mg on day 1, if needed. **Maintenance:** 200 mg twice daily as needed.

**Ankylosing Spondylitis**
**PO: ADULTS, ELDERLY:** 200 mg/day as a single dose or in 2 divided doses. May increase to 400 mg/day if no effect is seen after 6 wks.

**Dosage in Renal Impairment**
Not recommended in severe renal impairment.

**Dosage in Hepatic Impairment**
Decrease dose by 50% in pts with moderate hepatic impairment. Not recommended in severe hepatic impairment.

## SIDE EFFECTS

**Frequent (16%–5%):** Diarrhea, dyspepsia, headache, upper respiratory tract infection. **Occasional (less than 5%):** Abdominal pain, flatulence, nausea, back pain, peripheral edema, dizziness, insomnia, rash.

## ADVERSE EFFECTS/ TOXIC REACTIONS

Increased risk of cardiovascular events, (MI, CVA), serious, potentially life-threatening GI bleeding.

### NURSING CONSIDERATIONS

**BASELINE ASSESSMENT**

Assess onset, type, location, duration of pain/inflammation. Inspect appearance of affected joints for immobility, deformity, skin condition. Assess for allergy to sulfa, aspirin, or NSAIDs (contraindicated).

**INTERVENTION/EVALUATION**

Assess for therapeutic response: pain relief; decreased stiffness, swelling; increased joint mobility; reduced joint tenderness; improved grip strength. Observe for bleeding, bruising, weight gain.

**PATIENT/FAMILY TEACHING**
• If GI upset occurs, take with food.
• Avoid aspirin, alcohol (increases risk of GI bleeding). • Immediately report chest pain, jaw pain, sweating, confusion, difficulty speaking, one-sided weakness (may indicate heart attack or stroke).

# cephalexin

sef-a-**lex**-in
(Apo-Cephalex ✿, Keflex)
**Do not confuse cephalexin with cefaclor, cefazolin, or ciprofloxacin.**

## ◆CLASSIFICATION

**PHARMACOTHERAPEUTIC:** First-generation cephalosporin. **CLINICAL:** Antibiotic.

## USES

Treatment of susceptible infections due to staphylococci, group A *streptococcus, K. pneumoniae, E. coli, P. mirabilis, H. influenzae, M. catarrhalis* including respiratory tract, genitourinary tract, skin, soft tissue, bone infections; otitis media; rheumatic fever prophylaxis; follow-up to parenteral therapy. **OFF-LABEL:** Suppression of prosthetic joint infection.

## PRECAUTIONS

**Contraindications:** History of hypersensitivity/anaphylactic reaction to cephalexin, cephalosporins. **Cautions:** Renal impairment, history of GI disease (esp. ulcerative colitis, antibiotic-associated colitis), history of penicillin allergy.

---

C

## ACTION

Binds to bacterial cell membranes, inhibits cell wall synthesis. **Therapeutic Effect:** Bactericidal.

## PHARMACOKINETICS

Rapidly absorbed from GI tract (delayed in young children). Protein binding: 10%–15%. Widely distributed. Primarily excreted unchanged in urine. Moderately removed by hemodialysis. **Half-life:** 0.9–1.2 hrs (increased in renal impairment).

## ⧖ LIFESPAN CONSIDERATIONS

**Pregnancy/Lactation:** Readily crosses placenta. Distributed in breast milk. **Children:** No age-related precautions noted. **Elderly:** Age-related renal impairment may require dosage adjustment.

## INTERACTIONS

**DRUG: Probenecid** may increase concentration. **HERBAL:** None significant. **FOOD:** None known. **LAB VALUES:** May increase serum BUN, creatinine, alkaline phosphatase, bilirubin, LDH, ALT, AST. May cause positive direct/indirect Coombs' test.

## AVAILABILITY (Rx)

🖊 **Capsules:** 250 mg, 500 mg, 750 mg. **Powder for Oral Suspension:** 125 mg/5 ml, 250 mg/5 ml. **Tablets:** 250 mg, 500 mg.

## ADMINISTRATION/HANDLING

**PO**
• After reconstitution, oral suspension is stable for 14 days if refrigerated. • Shake oral suspension well before using. • Give without regard to food. If GI upset occurs, give with food, milk.

## INDICATIONS/ROUTES/DOSAGE

**Usual Dosage Range**
**PO: ADULTS, ELDERLY:** 250–1,000 mg q6h. **Maximum:** 4 g/day. **CHILDREN 1 YR AND OLDER:** 25–100 mg/kg/day in 3–4 divided doses. **Maximum:** 4 g/day.

**Dosage in Renal Impairment**
After usual initial dose, dosing frequency is modified based on creatinine clearance and severity of infection.

| Creatinine Clearance | Dosage |
|---|---|
| 10–50 ml/min | 500 mg q8–12h |
| Less than 10 ml/min | 250–500 mg q12–24h |
| Hemodialysis | 250 mg q12–24h (administer after dialysis session) |

**Dosage in Hepatic Impairment**
No dose adjustment.

## SIDE EFFECTS

**Frequent:** Oral candidiasis, mild diarrhea, mild abdominal cramping, vaginal candidiasis. **Occasional:** Nausea, serum sickness–like reaction (fever, joint pain; usually occurs after second course of therapy and resolves after drug is discontinued). **Rare:** Allergic reaction (rash, pruritus, urticaria).

## ADVERSE EFFECTS/TOXIC REACTIONS

Antibiotic-associated colitis, other superinfections (abdominal cramps, severe watery diarrhea, fever) may result from altered bacterial balance in GI tract. Nephrotoxicity may occur, esp. in pts with preexisting renal disease. Pts with history of penicillin allergy are at increased risk for developing a severe hypersensitivity reaction (severe pruritus, angioedema, bronchospasm, anaphylaxis).

## NURSING CONSIDERATIONS

**BASELINE ASSESSMENT**
Obtain CBC, renal function tests. Question for history of allergies, particularly cephalosporins, penicillins.

**INTERVENTION/EVALUATION**
Assess oral cavity for white patches on mucous membranes, tongue (thrush). Monitor daily pattern of bowel activity, stool consistency. Mild GI effects may be

tolerable (increasing severity may indicate onset of antibiotic-associated colitis). Monitor I&O, renal function tests for nephrotoxicity. Be alert for superinfection: fever, vomiting, diarrhea, anal/genital pruritus, oral mucosal changes (ulceration, pain, erythema). With prolonged therapy, monitor renal/hepatic function tests.

### PATIENT/FAMILY TEACHING

• Doses should be evenly spaced. • Continue therapy for full length of treatment. • May cause GI upset (may take with food, milk). • Refrigerate oral suspension. • Report persistent diarrhea.

# ceritinib

se-**ri**-ti-nib
(Zykadia)
**Do not confuse ceritinib with crizotinib, gefitinib, imatinib, or lapatinib.**

## ◆CLASSIFICATION

**PHARMACOTHERAPEUTIC:** Kinase inhibitor. **CLINICAL:** Antineoplastic.

## USES

Treatment of pts with anaplastic lymphoma kinase (ALK)–positive metastatic non–small cell lung cancer (NSCLC) who have progressed or are intolerant to crizotinib.

## PRECAUTIONS

**Contraindications:** Hypersensitivity to ceritinib. **Cautions:** Bradyarrhythmias/ventricular arrhythmias, diabetes, dehydration, electrolyte imbalance (e.g., hypomagnesemia, hypokalemia), hepatic impairment, HF, ocular disease, pulmonary disease. Medications that prolong QT interval. Not recommended in pts with congenital long QT syndrome. Avoid use of medications that cause bradycardia.

## ACTION

Inhibits tyrosine kinase activity and tumor cell proliferation. Inhibits autophosphorylation of ALK and ALK-dependent signaling proteins. **Therapeutic Effect:** Inhibits lung cancer growth and metastasis.

## PHARMACOKINETICS

Well absorbed after PO administration. Metabolized in liver. Peak plasma concentration: 4–6 hrs. Protein binding: 97%. Eliminated in feces (92%), urine (1.3%). **Half-life:** 41 hrs.

## ⚖ LIFESPAN CONSIDERATIONS

**Pregnancy/Lactation:** Avoid pregnancy; may cause fetal harm. Do not initiate therapy until pregnancy status confirmed. Contraception recommended during treatment and for at least 2 wks after discontinuation. Unknown if distributed in breast milk. Must either discontinue drug or discontinue breastfeeding. **Children:** Safety and efficacy not established. **Elderly:** No age-related precautions noted.

## INTERACTIONS

**DRUG: Strong CYP3A inhibitors (e.g., ketoconazole, ritonavir)** may increase concentration/effect; avoid use. **Strong CYP3A inducers (e.g., carbamazepine, phenobarbital, phenytoin, rifampin)** may decrease concentration/effect; avoid use. **HERBAL: St. John's wort** may decrease effectiveness. **FOOD: All food** may increase absorption/effect. **Grapefruit products** may increase concentration/effect; avoid use. **LAB VALUES:** May decrease Hgb, phosphate. May increase serum ALT, AST, bilirubin, creatinine, glucose, lipase.

## AVAILABILITY (Rx)

🗑 **Capsules:** 150 mg.

## ADMINISTRATION/HANDLING

### PO

• Give on empty stomach only. Do not administer within 2 hrs of meal. • Administer whole; do not break, cut, or open.

## INDICATIONS/ROUTES/DOSAGE

**Non–Small Cell Lung Cancer**
**PO: ADULTS/ELDERLY:** 750 mg once daily until disease progression or unacceptable toxicity.

**Dosage in Renal/Hepatic Impairment**
No dose adjustment.

**Dosage Modification**
*Cardiac*
**QTc interval greater than 500 msec on at least 2 separate EKGs:** Withhold until QTc interval is less than 481 msec, or recovery to baseline (if baseline QTc interval is greater than or equal to 481 msec), then resume with a 150-mg dose reduction.
**QTc prolongation in combination with torsades de pointes or polymorphic ventricular tachycardia or serious arrhythmia:** Permanently discontinue.
**Severe or intolerable diarrhea, nausea, vomiting despite optimal antiemetic or antidiarrheal therapy:** Withhold until improved, then resume with a 150-mg dose reduction.
**Symptomatic, non–life-threatening bradycardia:** Withhold until recovery to asymptomatic bradycardia or heart rate of 60 beats/min or greater. Evaluate concomitant medications known to cause bradycardia and adjust dose as tolerated (reduction not specified).
**Clinically significant, life-threatening bradycardia requiring intervention or life-threatening bradycardia in pts taking concomitant medications known to cause bradycardia or hypotension:** Withhold until recovery to asymptomatic bradycardia or heart rate of 60 beats/min or greater. If concomitant medication can be adjusted or discontinued, then resume with a 150-mg dose reduction.
**Life-threatening bradycardia in pts who are not taking concomitant medications known to cause bradycardia or hypotension:** Permanently discontinue.

**Concomitant use of strong CYP3A inhibitors:** If concomitant use unavoidable, reduce ceritinib dose by one third, rounded to the nearest 150-mg dose strength. After discontinuation of a strong CYP3A inhibitor, resume ceritinib dose that was taken prior to initiating strong CYP3A inhibitor.
*Endocrine*
**Persistent hyperglycemia greater than 250 ml/dL despite optimal antihyperglycemic therapy:** Withhold until hyperglycemia is adequately controlled, then resume with a 150-mg dose reduction. If adequate control cannot be achieved with optimal medical management, then permanently discontinue.
*Hepatic (During Treatment)*
**ALT, AST greater than 5 times upper limit of normal (ULN) with total bilirubin elevation less than or equal to 2 times ULN:** Withhold until recovery to baseline or less than or equal to 2 times ULN, then resume with a 150-mg dose reduction.
**ALT, AST greater than 3 times ULN with total bilirubin elevation greater than or equal to 2 times ULN in the absence of cholestasis or hemolysis:** Permanently discontinue.
*Pulmonary*
**Any grade treatment related to interstitial lung disease/pneumonitis:** Permanently discontinue.
*Intolerability/Toxicity*
**If unable to tolerate 300-mg dose:** Permanently discontinue.

## SIDE EFFECTS

**Frequent (86%–52%):** Diarrhea, nausea, vomiting, abdominal pain, fatigue, asthenia. **Occasional (34%–9%):** Decreased appetite, constipation, paresthesia, muscular weakness, gait disturbance, peripheral motor/sensory neuropathy, hypotonia, polyneuropathy, dyspepsia, gastric reflux disease, dysphagia, rash, maculopapular rash, acneiform dermatitis, vision impairment, blurred vision, photopsia, presbyopia, reduced visual acuity.

---

## ADVERSE EFFECTS/TOXIC REACTIONS

Approximately 60% of pts required at least one dose reduction. Median time to first dose reduction was approximately 7 wks. Decreased Hgb levels reported in 84% of pts. Severe or persistent GI toxicity including nausea, vomiting, diarrhea occurred in 96% of pts; severe cases reported in 14% of pts. Drug-induced hepatotoxicity with elevation of ALT 5 times ULN occurred in 27% of pts. Bradycardia, severe interstitial lung disease (ILD), QT interval prolongation, ILD reported in 3% of pts. Common Terminology Criteria for Adverse Events (CTCAE) grade 3–4 hyperglycemia reported in 13% of pts; diabetics have a sixfold increase in risk; pts receiving corticosteroids have twofold increase in risk. Fatal adverse reactions including pneumonia, respiratory failure, ILD/pneumonitis, pneumothorax, gastric hemorrhage, general physical health deterioration, tuberculosis, cardiac tamponade, sepsis occurred in 5% of pts.

## NURSING CONSIDERATIONS

### BASELINE ASSESSMENT

Obtain baseline CBC, BMP, LFT; serum ionized calcium, magnesium, phosphate; capillary blood glucose, $O_2$ saturation, urine pregnancy, vital signs. Obtain baseline EKG in pts with history of arrhythmias, HF, electrolyte imbalance, or concurrent use of medications known to prolong QTc interval. Question possibility of pregnancy or plans of breastfeeding. Assess hydration status. Screen for history/co-morbidities. Receive full medication history including herbal products; esp. CYP3A inhibitors or inducers, medications that prolong QT interval. Assess visual acuity. Verify ALK-positive NSCLC test prior to initiation.

### INTERVENTION/EVALUATION

Monitor CBC routinely; LFT monthly (or more frequently in pts with elevated hepatic enzymes). Obtain BMP, serum ionized calcium, magnesium if arrhythmia or dehydration occurs. Monitor vital signs (esp. heart rate). Obtain EKG for bradycardia, chest pain, dyspnea; chest X-ray if ILD, pneumonitis, pneumothorax suspected. Worsening cough, fever, or shortness of breath may indicate pneumonitis. Monitor for hepatic dysfunction, hyperglycemia, sepsis, vision changes. Assess hydration status. Encourage PO intake. Offer antidiarrheal medication for loose stool, antiemetic for nausea, vomiting.

### PATIENT/FAMILY TEACHING

• Blood levels, EKGs will be monitored routinely. • Most pts experience diarrhea, nausea, vomiting, which may lead to dehydration; drink plenty of fluids. • Report history of heart problems, including extremity swelling, HF, congenital long QT syndrome, palpitations, syncope. Therapy may decrease your heart rate; report dizziness, chest pain, palpitations, or fainting. • Worsening cough, fever, or shortness of breath may indicate severe lung inflammation. • Avoid pregnancy; contraception recommended during treatment and up to 2 wks after final dose. Do not breastfeed. • Blurry vision, confusion, frequent urination, increased thirst, fruity breath may indicate high blood sugar levels. • Report any yellowing of skin or eyes, upper abdominal pain, bruising, black/tarry stools, dark urine. • Immediately report any newly prescribed medications. • Take on empty stomach only; do not eat 2 hrs before or 2 hrs after any dose. • Avoid alcohol. Do not consume grapefruit products.

---

# certolizumab

ser-toe-**liz**-ue-mab
(Cimzia)

■ **BLACK BOX ALERT** ■ Serious, sometimes fatal, cases of tuberculosis, other fungal infections, or other opportunistic infections including viral and bacterial infection have been reported. Lymphoma reported in children/adolescents receiving other TNF-blocking medications.

◆ **CLASSIFICATION**

**PHARMACOTHERAPEUTIC:** Tumor necrosis factor (TNF) blocker. **CLINICAL:** Crohn's disease agent.

## USES

Treatment of moderate to severe active rheumatoid arthritis, moderate to severe active Crohn's disease, active ankylosing spondylitis, active psoriatic arthritis.

## PRECAUTIONS

**Contraindications:** Hypersensitivity to certolizumab. **Cautions:** Chronic, latent, or localized infection; preexisting or recent-onset CNS demyelinating disorders, moderate to severe HF, underlying hematologic disorders, elderly. Pts who have resided in regions where TB is endemic, pts who are hepatitis B virus carriers. Use of live vaccines.

## ACTION

Binds specifically to TNF-alpha cell, a protein in the immune system that causes inflammation. **Therapeutic Effect:** Reduces signs and symptoms of Crohn's disease and joint destruction associated with rheumatoid arthritis.

## PHARMACOKINETICS

Higher clearance with increasing body weight. Peak plasma concentrations: 54–171 hrs. **Half-life:** 14 days.

## ⧗ LIFESPAN CONSIDERATIONS

**Pregnancy/Lactation:** Unknown if distributed in breast milk. **Children:** Safety and efficacy not established. **Elderly:** Use cautiously due to higher rate of infection.

## INTERACTIONS

**DRUG: Anakinra, other TNF antagonists (e.g., adalimumab, etanercept, infliximab)** may increase risk of infection. **Live virus vaccines** may decrease immune response. **HERBAL: Echinacea** may decrease effect. **FOOD:** None known. **LAB VALUES:** May increase serum alkaline phosphatase, ALT, AST, bilirubin; aPTT.

## AVAILABILITY (Rx)

**Injection, Powder for Reconstitution:** 200 mg. **Injection, Solution:** 200 mg/ml in a single-use prefilled syringe.

## ADMINISTRATION/HANDLING

**Subcutaneous**
**Reconstitution** • Bring to room temperature before reconstitution. • Reconstitute with 1 ml Sterile Water for Injection. • Gently swirl without shaking, using syringe with 20-gauge needle. • Leave undisturbed to fully reconstitute (may take as long as 30 min). • Using a new 20-gauge needle, withdraw reconstituted solution into syringe for final concentration of 1 ml (200 mg). Use separate syringes for multiple vials. • Switch each 20-gauge needle to a 23-gauge needle and inject full contents of each syringe subcutaneously into separate sites on the abdomen or thigh.
**Storage** • Store vial in refrigerator. • Once powder reconstituted, solution should appear clear to opalescent, colorless to pale yellow. • Discard if solution is discolored or contains precipitate. • Reconstituted solution is stable for up to 2 hrs at room temperature or 24 hrs if refrigerated.

## INDICATIONS/ROUTES/DOSAGE

**Note:** Each 400-mg dose is given as two injections of 200 mg each.

---

### Crohn's Disease

**Subcutaneous:** Initially, 400 mg (given as two subcutaneous injections of 200 mg) and at weeks 2 and 4. **Maintenance:** In pts who obtain a therapeutic response, 400 mg every 4 wks.

### Rheumatoid Arthritis, Ankylosing Spondylitis, Psoriatic Arthritis

**Subcutaneous: ADULTS, ELDERLY:** Initially, 400 mg and at weeks 2 and 4. **Maintenance:** 200 mg q2wks or 400 mg q4wks.

### Dosage Modification

Discontinue for hypersensitivity reaction, lupus-like syndrome, serious infection, sepsis, hepatitis B virus reactivation.

### Dosage in Renal/Hepatic Impairment

No dose adjustment.

## SIDE EFFECTS

**Occasional (6%):** Arthralgia. **Rare (less than 1%):** Abdominal pain, diarrhea.

## ADVERSE EFFECTS/ TOXIC REACTIONS

Upper respiratory tract infection occurs in 20% of pts. UTI occurs in 7% of pts. Serious infections such as pneumonia, pyelonephritis occur in 3% of pts. Hypersensitivity reaction (rash, urticaria, hypotension, dyspnea) occurs rarely. May increase risk of malignancies (e.g., lymphoma).

## NURSING CONSIDERATIONS

### BASELINE ASSESSMENT

Obtain baseline CBC, urinalysis, C-reactive protein. Do not initiate treatment in pts with active infections, including chronic or localized infection. TB test should be obtained before initiation.

### INTERVENTION/EVALUATION

Monitor pts for infection during and after treatment. If pt develops an infection, treatment should be discontinued. Monitor lab results, especially WBC count, urinalysis, C-reactive protein for evidence of infection.

### PATIENT/FAMILY TEACHING

• Report cough, fever, flu-like symptoms. • Do not receive live virus vaccine during treatment or within 3 mos after last dose.

## cetirizine

se-**teer**-i-zeen
(Apo-Cetirizine ✦, Reactine ✦, Zyrtec)
**Do not confuse cetirizine with levocetirizine, or Zyrtec with Xanax, Zantac, Zocor, or Zyprexa.**

### FIXED-COMBINATION(S)

**Zyrtec D 12 Hour Tablets:** cetirizine/pseudoephedrine: 5 mg/120 mg.

### ◆CLASSIFICATION

**PHARMACOTHERAPEUTIC:** Second-generation piperazine. **CLINICAL:** Antihistamine.

## USES

Relief of symptoms (sneezing, rhinorrhea, postnasal discharge, nasal pruritus, ocular pruritus, tearing) of upper respiratory allergies, itching due to urticaria.

## PRECAUTIONS

**Contraindications:** Hypersensitivity to cetirizine, hydroxyzine. **Cautions:** Elderly, hepatic/renal impairment.

## ACTION

Competes with histamine for $H_1$-receptor sites on effector cells in GI tract, blood vessels, respiratory tract. **Therapeutic Effect:** Prevents allergic response, produces mild bronchodilation, blocks histamine-induced bronchitis.

## PHARMACOKINETICS

| Route | Onset | Peak | Duration |
|-------|-------|------|----------|
| PO | Less than 1 hr | 4–8 hrs | Less than 24 hrs |

---

✦ Canadian trade name     🔪 Non-Crushable Drug     🅷🅰 High Alert drug

Well absorbed from GI tract. Protein binding: 93%. Undergoes low first-pass metabolism; not extensively metabolized. Primarily excreted in urine (more than 80% as unchanged drug). **Half-life:** 6.5–10 hrs.

## ⧗ LIFESPAN CONSIDERATIONS

**Pregnancy/Lactation:** Not recommended during first trimester of pregnancy. Distributed in breast milk. Breastfeeding not recommended. **Children:** Less likely to cause anticholinergic effects. **Elderly:** More sensitive to anticholinergic effects (e.g., dry mouth, urinary retention). Dizziness, sedation, confusion may occur.

## INTERACTIONS

**DRUG:** Alcohol, other CNS depressants may increase CNS depression. **Anticholinergics (e.g., glycopyrrolate, hyoscyamine, oxybutynin)** may increase anticholinergic effects. **HERBAL:** None significant. **FOOD:** None known. **LAB VALUES:** May suppress wheal and flare reactions to antigen skin testing unless drug is discontinued 4 days before testing.

## AVAILABILITY (Rx)

▧ **Capsule:** 10 mg. **Oral solution:** 5 mg/5 ml. **Syrup:** 5 mg/5 ml. **Tablets:** 5 mg, 10 mg. **Tablets (Chewable):** 5 mg, 10 mg. **Tablet (Dispersible):** 10 mg.

## ADMINISTRATION/HANDLING

**PO**
• Give without regard to food.

## INDICATIONS/ROUTES/DOSAGE

◀ALERT▶ May cause drowsiness at dosage greater than 10 mg/day.

**Upper Respiratory Allergies, Urticaria**
**PO: ADULTS, ELDERLY, CHILDREN OLDER THAN 5 YRS:** Initially, 5–10 mg/day as single dose. **CHILDREN 2–5 YRS:** 2.5 mg/day. May increase up to 5 mg/day as a single dose

or in 2 divided doses. **CHILDREN 12–23 MOS:** Initially, 2.5 mg/day. May increase up to 5 mg/day in 2 divided doses. **CHILDREN 6–11 MOS:** 2.5 mg once daily.

**Dosage in Renal/Hepatic Impairment**
**Adult/elderly pts with renal impairment (CrCl 11–31 ml/min), pts receiving hemodialysis (CrCl less than 7 ml/min), pts with hepatic impairment:** Decrease to 5 mg once daily. **CHILDREN 6–11 YRS:** Less than 2.5 mg once daily. **CHILDREN YOUNGER THAN 6 YRS:** Not recommended.

## SIDE EFFECTS

**Occasional (10%–2%):** Pharyngitis, dry mucous membranes, nausea, vomiting, abdominal pain, headache, dizziness, fatigue, thickening of mucus, drowsiness, photosensitivity, urinary retention.

## ADVERSE EFFECTS/ TOXIC REACTIONS

Children may experience paradoxical reaction (restlessness, insomnia, euphoria, nervousness, tremor). Dizziness, sedation, confusion more likely to occur in elderly.

## NURSING CONSIDERATIONS

### BASELINE ASSESSMENT

Assess lung sounds. Assess severity of rhinitis, urticaria, other symptoms.

### INTERVENTION/EVALUATION

For upper respiratory allergies, increase fluids to maintain thin secretions and offset thirst. Monitor symptoms for therapeutic response.

### PATIENT/FAMILY TEACHING

• Avoid tasks that require alertness, motor skills until response to drug is established. • Avoid alcohol.

# cetuximab

se-**tux**-i-mab
(Erbitux)

■ **BLACK BOX ALERT** ■ Severe infusion reactions (bronchospasm, stridor, urticaria, hypotension, cardiac arrest) have occurred, especially with first infusion in pts with head and neck cancer, cardiopulmonary arrest reported in pts receiving radiation in combination with cetuximab.

**Do not confuse cetuximab with bevacizumab.**

## ◆CLASSIFICATION

**PHARMACOTHERAPEUTIC:** Monoclonal antibody. **CLINICAL:** Antineoplastic.

## USES

As a single agent or in combination with irinotecan for treatment of EGFR-expressing, metastatic colorectal carcinoma in pts who are refractory or intolerant to irinotecan-based chemotherapy. Treatment of advanced squamous cell cancer of head/neck (with radiation). Treatment of recurrent or metastasized squamous cell carcinoma of head/neck progressing after platinum-based therapy. First-line treatment of squamous cell carcinoma of head and neck in combination with platinum-based therapy with 5-FU. **OFF-LABEL:** EGFR-expressing advanced non–small-cell lung cancer (NSCLC). Treatment of unresectable squamous cell skin cancer.

## PRECAUTIONS

**Contraindications:** Hypersensitivty to cetuximab. **Cautions:** Preexisting IgE antibodies to cetuximab, coronary artery disease, HF, arrythmias, pulmonary disease.

## ACTION

Binds to the epidermal growth factor receptor (EGFR), a glycoprotein on normal and tumor cells. **Therapeutic Effect:** Inhibits tumor cell growth, inducing apoptosis (cell death).

## PHARMACOKINETICS

Reaches steady-state levels by the third wkly infusion. Clearance decreases as dose increases. **Half-life:** 114 hrs (range: 75–188 hrs).

## ⧗ LIFESPAN CONSIDERATIONS

**Pregnancy/Lactation:** Crosses placental barrier; may cause fetal harm, abortifactant. Breastfeeding not recommended. **Children:** Safety and efficacy not established. **Elderly:** No age-related precautions noted.

## INTERACTIONS

**DRUG:** None significant. **HERBAL:** None significant. **FOOD:** None known. **LAB VALUES:** May decrease WBCs; serum calcium, magnesium, potassium.

## AVAILABILITY (Rx)

**Injection Solution:** 2 mg/ml (50 ml, 100 ml).

## ADMINISTRATION/HANDLING

 IV

**◀ALERT▶** Do not give by IV push or bolus.

**Reconstitution** • Does not require reconstitution. • Solution should appear clear, colorless; may contain a small amount of visible, white particulates. • Do not shake or dilute. • Infuse with a low protein-binding 0.22-micron in-line filter.

**Rate of Administration** • First dose should be given as a 120-min infusion. • Maintenance infusion should be infused over 60 min. • Maximum infusion rate should not exceed 5 ml/min.

**Storage** • Refrigerate vials. • Infusion containers are stable for up to 12 hrs if refrigerated, up to 8 hrs at room temperature. • Discard unused portions.

## ❖ IV COMPATIBILITY

Irinotecan (Camptosar).

## INDICATIONS/ROUTES/DOSAGE

### Head/Neck Cancer, Metastatic Colorectal Carcinoma

**IV: ADULTS, ELDERLY:** Initially, 400 mg/ $m^2$ as a loading dose. **Maintenance:** 250 mg/ $m^2$ infused over 60 min wkly.

### Dosage in Renal/Hepatic Impairment

No dose adjustment.

## SIDE EFFECTS

**Frequent (90%–25%):** Acneiform rash, malaise, fever, nausea, diarrhea, constipation, headache, abdominal pain, anorexia, vomiting. **Occasional (16%–10%):** Nail disorder, back pain, stomatitis, peripheral edema, pruritus, cough, insomnia. **Rare (9%–5%):** Weight loss, depression, dyspepsia, conjunctivitis, alopecia.

## ADVERSE EFFECTS/ TOXIC REACTIONS

Anemia occurs in 10% of pts. Severe infusion reaction (rapid onset of airway obstruction, hypotension, severe urticaria) occurs rarely. Dermatologic toxicity, pulmonary embolus, leukopenia, renal failure occur rarely.

## NURSING CONSIDERATIONS

### BASELINE ASSESSMENT

Monitor Hgb, Hct, serum potassium, magnesium. Assess for evidence of anemia. Question possibility of pregnancy. Question history of hypersensitivity reaction.

### INTERVENTION/EVALUATION

Monitor for evidence of infusion reaction (rapid onset of bronchospasm, stridor, hoarseness, urticaria, hypotension) during infusion and for at least 1 hr postinfusion. Pts may experience first severe infusion reaction during later infusions. Assess skin for evidence of dermatologic toxicity (development of inflammatory sequelae, dry skin, exfoliative dermatitis, rash). Monitor CBC, serum electrolytes, acute onset or worsening pulmonary symptoms.

### PATIENT/FAMILY TEACHING

• Do not have immunizations without physician's approval (drug lowers resistance). • Avoid contact with anyone who recently received a live virus vaccine. • Avoid crowds, those with infection. • Wear sunscreen, limit sun exposure (sunlight can exacerbate skin reactions). • Avoid pregnancy. • Report cardiac or lung symptoms, severe rash.

---

# *chlorambucil*

klor-**am**-bue-sil
(Leukeran)

**■ BLACK BOX ALERT ■** May cause myelosuppression. Affects fertility; potential for carcinogenic, mutagenic, teratogenic effects. May cause azoospermia.

**Do not confuse Leukeran with Alkeran, Leukine, or Myleran.**

## ◆ CLASSIFICATION

**PHARMACOTHERAPEUTIC:** Alkylating agent, nitrogen mustard. **CLINICAL:** Antineoplastic.

## USES

Treatment of chronic lymphocytic leukemia (CLL), Hodgkin's and non-Hodgkin's lymphomas (NHL). **OFF-LABEL:** Nephrotic syndrome in children, Waldenström's macroglobulinemia.

## PRECAUTIONS

**Contraindications:** Hypersensitivity to chlorambucil. Previous allergic reaction to other alkylating agents, prior resistance to chlorambucil, pregnancy. **Extreme Cautions:** Treatment within 4 wks after full-course radiation therapy or myelosuppressive drug regimen. **Cautions:** History of bone marrow suppression, head trauma, hepatic impairment,

---

nephrotic syndrome, seizure disorder; administration of live vaccines to immunocompromised pts.

## ACTION

Inhibits DNA, RNA synthesis by crosslinking with DNA, RNA strands. **Therapeutic Effect:** Interferes with DNA replication and RNA transcription.

## PHARMACOKINETICS

Rapidly, completely absorbed from GI tract. Protein binding: 99%. Metabolized in liver to active metabolite. Not removed by hemodialysis. **Half-life:** 1.5 hrs; metabolite, 2.5 hrs.

## ⧗ LIFESPAN CONSIDERATIONS

**Pregnancy/Lactation:** If possible, avoid use during pregnancy, esp. first trimester. Breastfeeding not recommended. **Children:** No age-related precautions noted. When taken for nephrotic syndrome, may increase risk of seizures. **Elderly:** No age-related precautions noted.

## INTERACTIONS

**DRUG: Bone marrow depressants** may increase myelosuppression. **Other immunosuppressants (e.g., steroids)** may increase risk of infection or development of neoplasms. **Live virus vaccines** may potentiate virus replication, decrease antibody response to vaccine. **HERBAL: Echinacea** may decrease effects. **FOOD: Acidic foods, spicy foods** may delay absorption. **LAB VALUES:** May increase serum alkaline phosphatase, AST, uric acid.

## AVAILABILITY (Rx)

**Tablets:** 2 mg.

## ADMINISTRATION/HANDLING

**PO**
• Give 30–60 min before food.

## INDICATIONS/ROUTES/DOSAGE

**Chronic Lymphocytic Leukemia (CLL)**
**PO: ADULTS, ELDERLY:** 0.1 mg/kg/day for 3–6 wks or 0.4 mg/kg pulsed doses administered intermittently, biweekly or monthly.

**Hodgkin's Lymphoma (HL)**
**PO: ADULTS, ELDERLY:** 0.2 mg/kg/day for 3–6 wks.

**Non-Hodgkin's Lymphoma (NHL)**
**PO: ADULTS, ELDERLY:** 0.1 mg/kg/day for 3–6 wks.

**Dosage in Renal Impairment**
No dose adjustment.

**Dosage in Hepatic Impairment**
Use caution.

## SIDE EFFECTS

**Expected:** GI effects (nausea, vomiting, anorexia, diarrhea, abdominal distress) generally mild, last less than 24 hrs, occur only if single dose exceeds 20 mg. **Occasional:** Rash, dermatitis, pruritus, oral ulcerations. **Rare:** Alopecia, urticaria, erythema, hyperuricemia.

## ADVERSE EFFECTS/ TOXIC REACTIONS

Hematologic toxicity due to severe myelosuppression occurs frequently, manifested as neutropenia, anemia, thrombocytopenia. After discontinuation of therapy, thrombocytopenia, neutropenia usually last for 1–2 wks, but may persist for 3–4 wks. Neutrophil count may continue to decrease for up to 10 days after last dose. Toxicity appears to be less severe with intermittent drug administration. Overdosage may produce seizures in children. Excessive serum uric acid level, hepatotoxicity occur rarely.

## NURSING CONSIDERATIONS

### BASELINE ASSESSMENT

Obtain CBC before therapy and wkly during therapy, WBC count 3–4 days following each wkly, CBC during first 3–6 wks of therapy (4–6 wks if pt on intermittent dosing schedule).

---

### INTERVENTION/EVALUATION

Monitor CBC, serum uric acid, LFT. Monitor for hematologic toxicity (fever, sore throat, signs of local infection, unusual bruising/bleeding from any site), symptoms of anemia (excessive fatigue, weakness). Assess skin for rash, pruritus, urticaria.

### PATIENT/FAMILY TEACHING

• Increase fluid intake (may protect against hyperuricemia). • Avoid acidic or spicy foods; may delay absorption of medication. • Do not have immunizations without physician's approval (drug lowers resistance). • Avoid contact with those who have recently received live virus vaccine. • Promptly report fever, sore throat, signs of local infection, unusual bruising/bleeding from any site, nausea, vomiting, rash.

# cholestyramine

koe-lee-**stye**-ra-meen
(Novo-Cholamine ✤, Prevalite, Questran, Questran Lite)

### ◆CLASSIFICATION

**PHARMACOTHERAPEUTIC:** Bile acid sequestrant. **CLINICAL:** Antihyperlipoproteinemic.

### USES

Adjunct to diet to decrease elevated serum cholesterol levels in pts with primary hypercholesterolemia. Relief of pruritus associated with elevated levels of bile acids. Regression of arteriosclerosis. **OFF-LABEL:** Treatment of diarrhea (due to bile acids), binding toxicologic agents.

### PRECAUTIONS

**Contraindications:** Hypersensitivity to cholestyramine. Complete biliary obstruction. **Cautions:** GI dysfunction (esp. constipation), recent abdominal surgery, renal impairment, dehydration, concurrent spironolactone therapy.

### ACTION

Binds with bile acids in intestine, forming insoluble complex. Binding results in partial removal of bile acid from enterohepatic circulation. **Therapeutic Effect:** Removes LDL cholesterol from plasma.

### PHARMACOKINETICS

Not absorbed from GI tract. Decreases in serum LDL apparent in 5–7 days and in serum cholesterol in 1 mo. Serum cholesterol returns to baseline about 1 mo after drug discontinuation.

### ⧖ LIFESPAN CONSIDERATIONS

**Pregnancy/Lactation:** Not systemically absorbed. May interfere with maternal absorption of fat-soluble vitamins. **Children:** No age-related precautions noted. Limited experience in pts younger than 10 yrs. **Elderly:** Increased risk of GI side effects, adverse nutritional effects.

### INTERACTIONS

**DRUG:** May increase effects of **anticoagulants (e.g., warfarin)** by decreasing vitamin K level. May decrease **warfarin** absorption. May bind with, decrease absorption of **digoxin, folic acid, penicillins, propranolol, tetracyclines, thiazides, thyroid hormones, oral vancomycin. HERBAL:** None significant. **FOOD:** None known. **LAB VALUES:** May increase serum alkaline phosphatase, magnesium, ALT, AST. May decrease serum calcium, potassium, sodium. May prolong PT.

### AVAILABILITY (Rx)

**Powder for Oral Suspension:** 4 g.

### ADMINISTRATION/HANDLING

**PO**
• Give other drugs at least 1 hr before or 4–6 hrs following cholestyramine (capable of binding drugs in GI tract). • Do not give in dry form (highly irritating). Mix with 3–6 oz water, milk, fruit juice, soup. • Place powder on surface for 1–2 min (prevents lumping), then

mix thoroughly. • Excessive foaming with carbonated beverages reported; use extra large glass, stir slowly. • Administer with meals.

## INDICATIONS/ROUTES/DOSAGE

### Hypercholesterolemia
**PO: ADULTS, ELDERLY:** Initially, 4 g 1–2 times/day. Gradually increase over at least 1-mo intervals. **Maintenance:** 8–16 g/day in divided doses. **Maximum:** 24 g/day, 6 doses/day. **CHILDREN:** 80 mg/kg 3 times/day. **Maximum:** 8 g/day.

### Pruritus
**PO: ADULTS, ELDERLY:** Initially, 4 g 1–2 times/day. **Maintenance:** 4–16 g/day in divided doses. **Maximum:** 24 g/day.

### Dosage in Renal/Hepatic Impairment
No dose adjustment.

## SIDE EFFECTS

**Frequent:** Constipation (may lead to fecal impaction), nausea, vomiting, abdominal pain, indigestion. **Occasional:** Diarrhea, belching, bloating, headache, dizziness. **Rare:** Gallstones, peptic ulcer disease, malabsorption syndrome.

## ADVERSE EFFECTS/ TOXIC REACTIONS

GI tract obstruction, hyperchloremic acidosis, or osteoporosis secondary to calcium excretion may occur. High dosage may interfere with fat absorption, resulting in steatorrhea.

## NURSING CONSIDERATIONS

### BASELINE ASSESSMENT
Question for history of hypersensitivity to cholestyramine, tartrazine, aspirin. Obtain baseline serum cholesterol, triglycerides, electrolytes, LFT.

### INTERVENTION/EVALUATION
Monitor daily pattern of bowel activity, stool consistency. Evaluate food tolerance, abdominal discomfort, flatulence. Monitor cholesterol, triglycerides, PT, LFT, serum electrolytes. Encourage several glasses of water between meals.

### PATIENT/FAMILY TEACHING
• Complete full course of therapy; do not stop or change doses. • Take other drugs at least 1 hr before or 4–6 hrs after cholestyramine. • Never take in dry form; mix with 3–6 oz water, milk, fruit juice, soup (place powder on surface for 1–2 min to prevent lumping, then mix well). • Use extra-large glass, stir slowly when mixing with carbonated beverages due to foaming. • Take with meals, drink several glasses of water between meals. • Eat high-fiber foods (whole-grain cereals, fruits, vegetables) to reduce potential for constipation.

# ciclesonide

sye-**kles**-oh-nide
(Alvesco, Omnaris, Zetonna)

## ◆CLASSIFICATION
**PHARMACOTHERAPEUTIC:** Glucocorticoid. **CLINICAL:** Anti-inflammatory.

## USES

**Intranasal:** Management of seasonal or perennial allergic rhinitis. **Oral Inhalation:** Prophylactic management of bronchial asthma. **OFF-LABEL: Nasal:** Adjunct to antibiotics in empiric treatment of acute bacterial rhinosinusitis.

## PRECAUTIONS

**Contraindications:** Hypersensitivity to ciclesonide. Acute asthma or status asthmaticus, moderate to severe bronchiectasis. **Cautions:** Pts with respiratory TB, untreated systemic infections, ocular herpes simplex.

## ACTION

Inhibits accumulation of inflammatory cells, decreases and prevents tissues from responding to inflammatory process. **Therapeutic Effect:** Relieves symptoms of allergic rhinitis, asthma.

◆ Canadian trade name    🔔 Non-Crushable Drug    📛 High Alert drug

## PHARMACOKINETICS

Minimally absorbed from nasal tissue, moderately absorbed from inhalation. Protein binding: 99%. Metabolized in liver. Excreted in feces (66%), urine (20% or less). **Half-life:** 2–3 hrs.

## ⧗ LIFESPAN CONSIDERATIONS

**Pregnancy/Lactation:** Unknown if drug crosses placenta or distributed in breast milk. **Children:** Safety and efficacy not established in pts younger than 12 yrs. **Elderly:** No age-related precautions noted.

## INTERACTIONS

**DRUG:** Ketoconazole may increase concentration/effect. **HERBAL:** None significant. **FOOD:** None known. **LAB VALUES:** None significant.

## AVAILABILITY (Rx)

**Inhalation (Alvesco):** 80 mcg/spray, 160 mcg/spray. **Nasal Spray (Omnaris):** 50 mcg/spray. **(Zetonna):** 37 mcg/spray.

## ADMINISTRATION/HANDLING

**Inhalation**
• Shaking not necessary. • Wait 2 min before inhaling second dose (allows for deeper bronchial penetration). • Rinse mouth with water immediately after inhalation (prevents mouth/throat dryness).

**Intranasal**
• Instruct pt to clear nasal passages before use. • Tilt head slightly forward. • Insert spray tip into nostril, pointing toward nasal passages, away from nasal septum. • Spray into one nostril while pt holds other nostril closed, concurrently inspires through nose to permit medication as high into nasal passages as possible.

## INDICATIONS/ROUTES/DOSAGE

**Perennial Allergic Rhinitis**
**Intranasal:** ADULTS, ELDERLY, CHILDREN 12 YRS AND OLDER: **(Omnaris):** 2 sprays (100 mcg) in each nostril once a day. **Maximum:** 200 mcg/day. **(Zetonna):** 1 spray (37 mcg) in each nostril daily. **Maximum:** 74 mcg/day.

**Seasonal Allergic Rhinitis**
**Intranasal:** ADULTS, ELDERLY, CHILDREN 6 YRS AND OLDER: **(Omnaris):** 2 sprays (100 mcg) in each nostril once a day. **Maximum:** 200 mcg/day. **(Zetonna):** 1 spray (37 mcg) in each nostril daily. **Maximum:** 74 mcg/day.

**Asthma**
**Inhalation:** ADULTS, ELDERLY, CHILDREN 12 YRS AND OLDER (PREVIOUS THERAPY WITH BRONCHODILATORS ALONE): Initially, 80 mcg 2 times daily. **Maximum:** 320 mcg 2 times daily. (PREVIOUS THERAPY WITH INHALED STEROIDS): Initially, 80 mcg twice daily. **Maximum:** 640 mcg/day. (PREVIOUS THERAPY WITH ORAL STEROIDS): Initially, 320 mcg twice daily. **Maximum:** 640 mcg/day.

**Dosage in Renal/Hepatic Impairment**
No dose adjustment.

## SIDE EFFECTS

**Occasional (6%–4%):** Headache, epistaxis, nasopharyngitis. **Rare (2%):** Ear pain.

## ADVERSE EFFECTS/ TOXIC REACTIONS

Excessive doses over prolonged periods may result in systemic hypercortisolism.

## NURSING CONSIDERATIONS

**BASELINE ASSESSMENT**
Question for hypersensitivity to any corticosteroids. Establish baseline history of asthma, rhinitis.

**INTERVENTION/EVALUATION**
Monitor for relief of symptoms. Monitor rate, depth, rhythm, type of respiration. Assess lung sounds for rhonchi, wheezing, rales. Assess oral mucous membranes for candidiasis.

**PATIENT/FAMILY TEACHING**

• Improvement noted in 24–48 hrs, but full effect may take 1–2 wks for seasonal allergic rhinitis, 5 wks for perennial allergic rhinitis. • Improvement in asthma may take 4 wks or longer. • Oral inhalation not indicated for acute asthma attacks. • Report if no improvement in symptoms, sneezing or nasal irritation occurs.

# cilostazol

sil-**o**-sta-zol
(Pletal)
■ **BLACK BOX ALERT** ■ Contraindicated in pts with HF of any severity, active bleeding.
**Do not confuse Pletal with Plendil.**

## ◆ CLASSIFICATION

**PHARMACOTHERAPEUTIC:** Phosphodiesterase enzyme inhibitor. **CLINICAL:** Antiplatelet.

## USES

Reduces symptoms of intermittent claudication (increases walking distance).

## PRECAUTIONS

**Contraindications:** Hypersensitivity to cilostazol. HF of any severity. **Cautions:** Hemostatic disorders or active bleeding (bleeding peptic ulcer, intracranial bleeding). Severe underlying heart disease, thrombocytopenia, pts receiving other platelet aggregation inhibitors, moderate to severe hepatic impairment, severe renal impairment.

## ACTION

Inhibits phosphodiesterase, increasing cAMP, leading to inhibition of platelet aggregation. **Therapeutic Effect:** Improves walking distance in pts with intermittent claudication.

## PHARMACOKINETICS

Moderately absorbed from GI tract. Protein binding: 95%–98%. Metabolized in liver. Excreted in urine (74%), feces (20%). Not removed by hemodialysis. **Half-life:** 11–13 hrs.

## ⧗ LIFESPAN CONSIDERATIONS

**Pregnancy/Lactation:** Unknown if drug crosses placenta or is distributed in breast milk. **Children:** Safety and efficacy not established. **Elderly:** No age-related precautions noted.

## INTERACTIONS

**DRUG: Aspirin** may potentiate inhibition of platelet aggregation. **CYP3A4 inhibitors (e.g., clarithromycin, diltiazem, fluconazole), CYP2C19 inhibitors (e.g., omeprazole)** may increase concentration/effect. **HERBAL: St. John's wort** may decrease effect. Avoid herbs with antiplatelet activity (**e.g., garlic, ginger, ginkgo**). **FOOD: Grapefruit products** may increase concentration, toxicity. **LAB VALUES:** May increase serum BUN, glucose, uric acid. May decrease platelet count, WBC.

## AVAILABILITY (Rx)

**Tablets:** 50 mg, 100 mg.

## ADMINISTRATION/HANDLING

**PO**
• Give at least 30 min before or 2 hrs after meals. • Do not give with grapefruit products.

## INDICATIONS/ROUTES/DOSAGE

**Intermittent Claudication**
**PO: ADULTS, ELDERLY:** 100 mg twice daily at least 30 min before or 2 hrs after meals. Decrease to 50 mg twice daily during concurrent therapy with CYP3A4 or CYP2C19 inhibitors (e.g., clarithromycin, diltiazem, erythromycin, fluconazole, fluoxetine, omeprazole, sertraline).

**Dosage in Renal/Hepatic Impairment**
No dose adjustment.

## SIDE EFFECTS

**Frequent (34%–10%):** Headache, diarrhea, palpitations, dizziness, pharyngitis.

---

♣ Canadian trade name     🗡 Non-Crushable Drug     📵 High Alert drug

**Occasional (7%–3%):** Nausea, rhinitis, back pain, peripheral edema, dyspepsia, abdominal pain, tachycardia, cough, flatulence, myalgia. **Rare (2%–1%):** Leg cramps, paresthesia, rash, vomiting.

## ADVERSE EFFECTS/TOXIC REACTIONS

Overdose noted as severe headache, diarrhea, hypotension, cardiac arrhythmias. May increase risk of endocardial hemorrhage, fibrosis of left ventricle, intimal thickening of coronary artery.

## NURSING CONSIDERATIONS

### BASELINE ASSESSMENT

Assess CBC (esp. platelet count), BMP, LFT before treatment and periodically during treatment.

### INTERVENTION/EVALUATION

Monitor for improvement of symptoms (e.g., improved walking distance). Monitor lab tests periodically. Monitor for bleeding events, cardiovascular toxicity or lesions.

### PATIENT/FAMILY TEACHING

• Take on an empty stomach (at least 30 min before or 2 hrs after meals). • Do not take with grapefruit products. • Report severe bleeding of any kind.

# cimetidine

sye-**met**-i-deen
(Apo-Cimetidine ✱, Novo-Cimetidine ✱, Tagamet HB 200)
**Do not confuse cimetidine with simethicone.**

## ◆CLASSIFICATION

**PHARMACOTHERAPEUTIC:** H₂-receptor antagonist. **CLINICAL:** Antiulcer, gastric acid secretion inhibitor.

## USES

Short-term treatment of active duodenal ulcer. Prevention of duodenal ulcer recurrence. Treatment of benign gastric ulcer, pathologic GI hypersecretory conditions, gastroesophageal reflux disease (GERD). **OTC use:** Heartburn, acid indigestion. **OFF-LABEL:** *H. pylori* eradication to reduce risk of duodenal ulcer recurrence.

## PRECAUTIONS

**Contraindications:** Hypersensitivity to cimetidine, other H₂ antagonists. **Cautions:** Renal/hepatic impairment, elderly. Concurrent administration of medications utilizing P450 system.

## ACTION

Inhibits histamine action at histamine-2 (H₂)-receptor sites of gastric parietal cells. **Therapeutic Effect:** Reduces gastric acid secretion, gastric volume, hydrogen ion concentration.

## PHARMACOKINETICS

Well absorbed from GI tract. Protein binding: 15%–20%. Widely distributed. Metabolized in liver. Primarily excreted in urine. Not removed by hemodialysis. **Half-life:** 2 hrs (increased in renal impairment).

## ⌛ LIFESPAN CONSIDERATIONS

**Pregnancy/Lactation:** Distributed in breast milk. Possible adverse effects on fetal development. **Children:** Long-term use may induce cerebral toxicity, affect hormonal system. **Elderly:** More likely to experience confusion, esp. pts with renal impairment.

## INTERACTIONS

**DRUG:** May increase concentration, decrease metabolism of **warfarin, phenytoin, propranolol, tricyclic antidepressants.** May decrease concentration/effect of **itraconazole, ketoconazole. HERBAL: St. John's wort** may decrease concentration. **FOOD:** None known. **LAB VALUES:** Interferes with skin tests using allergen extracts. May increase serum prolactin, creatinine, ALT, AST. May decrease parathyroid hormone concentration.

## AVAILABILITY (Rx)

Liquid, Oral: 300 mg/5 ml. Tablets: 200 mg (OTC), 300 mg, 400 mg, 800 mg.

## ADMINISTRATION/HANDLING
### PO
• Give without regard to food. • Best given with meals and at bedtime. • Do not administer within 1 hr of antacids.

## INDICATIONS/ROUTES/DOSAGE

**Active Duodenal Ulcer**
**PO: ADULTS, ELDERLY:** 300 mg 4 times/day or 400 mg twice daily or 800 mg at bedtime for up to 8 wks.

**Prevention of Duodenal Ulcer**
**PO: ADULTS, ELDERLY:** 400 mg at bedtime.

**Gastric Hypersecretory Secretions**
**PO: ADULTS, ELDERLY:** 300–600 mg q6h. **Maximum:** 2,400 mg/day.

**Gastroesophageal Reflux Disease (GERD)**
**PO: ADULTS, ELDERLY:** 800 mg twice daily or 400 mg 4 times/day for 12 wks.

**OTC Use**
**PO: ADULTS, ELDERLY:** 200 mg up to 30 min before meals. **Maximum:** 400 mg/day.

**Usual Pediatric/Neonatal Dosage**
**CHILDREN:** 20–40 mg/kg/day in divided doses q6h. **INFANTS:** 10–20 mg/kg/day in divided doses q6–12h. **NEONATES:** 5–10 mg/kg/day in divided doses q8–12h.

**Dosage in Renal Impairment**
Dosage is modified based on creatinine clearance.

| Creatinine Clearance | Dosage |
|---|---|
| Greater than 50 ml/min | No change |
| 10–50 ml/min | 50% of normal dose |
| Less than 10 ml/min | 300 mg q8–12h |
| Hemodialysis | Dose after dialysis |
| CCRT | 50% of normal dose |
| Peritoneal dialysis | 300 mg q8–12h |

**Dosage in Hepatic Impairment**
Caution in severe impairment.

## SIDE EFFECTS

**Occasional (4%–2%):** Headache. **Elderly, pts with renal impairment, severely ill pts:** Confusion, agitation, psychosis, depression, anxiety, disorientation, hallucinations. Effects reverse 3–4 days after discontinuance. **Rare (less than 2%):** Diarrhea, dizziness, drowsiness, nausea, vomiting, gynecomastia, rash, impotence.

## ADVERSE EFFECTS/TOXIC REACTIONS

None known.

## NURSING CONSIDERATIONS

### BASELINE ASSESSMENT
Obtain baseline renal function test in pts with renal impairment; LFT in pts with hepatic impairment.

### INTERVENTION/EVALUATION
Assess for GI bleeding: hematemesis, blood in stool. Monitor for changes in mental status in elderly, severely ill, those with renal impairment.

### PATIENT/FAMILY TEACHING
• Do not take antacids within 1 hr of cimetidine administration. • Avoid tasks that require alertness, motor skills until response to drug is established. • Avoid smoking, excessive amounts of caffeine. • Report any blood in vomitus/stool, or dark, tarry stool.

## cinacalcet

sin-a-**kal**-set
(Sensipar)

## ◆CLASSIFICATION

**PHARMACOTHERAPEUTIC:** Calcium receptor agonist. **CLINICAL:** Calcimimetic.

 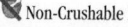

## USES

Treatment of severe hypercalcemia in pts with primary parathyroid carcinoma. Treatment of secondary hyperparathyroidism in pts with chronic renal disease on dialysis. Treatment of severe hypercalcemia in pts with primary hyperparathyroidism unable to undergo parathyroidectomy.

## PRECAUTIONS

**Contraindications:** Hypersensitivity to cinacalcet. Hypocalcemia. **Cautions:** Cardiovascular disease, moderate to severe hepatic impairment, seizure disorder.

## ACTION

Increases sensitivity of calcium-sensing receptor on parathyroid gland to activation by extracellular calcium, thus lowering parathyroid hormone (PTH) levels. **Therapeutic Effect:** Decreases serum calcium, PTH levels.

## PHARMACOKINETICS

Extensively distributed after PO administration. Protein binding: 93%–97%. Metabolized in liver. Excreted in urine (80%), feces (15%). **Half-life:** 30–40 hrs.

## ⧖ LIFESPAN CONSIDERATIONS

**Pregnancy/Lactation:** May cross placental barrier; unknown if distributed in breast milk. Safe usage during lactation not established (potential adverse reaction in infants). **Children:** Safety and efficacy not established. **Elderly:** No age-related precautions noted.

## INTERACTIONS

**DRUG: Strong CYP3A4 inhibitors (e.g., erythromycin, ketoconazole)** increase concentration/effects. Concurrent administration of drugs metabolized by **CYP2D6 enzyme (e.g., flecainide, tricyclic antidepressants, metoprolol, carvedilol)**, may require dosage adjustment. **HERBAL:** None significant. **FOOD: High-fat meals** increase plasma concentration. **LAB VALUES:** May decrease serum calcium, phosphorus.

## AVAILABILITY (Rx)

**Tablets:** 30 mg, 60 mg, 90 mg.

## ADMINISTRATION/HANDLING

**PO**

• Store at room temperature. • Do not break, crush, dissolve, or divide film-coated tablets. • Administer with food or shortly after a meal.

## INDICATIONS/ROUTES/DOSAGE

**Hypercalcemia in Parathyroid Carcinoma; Primary Hyperparathyroidism**
**PO: ADULTS, ELDERLY:** Initially, 30 mg twice daily. Titrate dosage sequentially (60 mg twice daily, 90 mg twice daily, and 90 mg 3–4 times/day) every 2–4 wks as needed to normalize serum calcium level. **Maximum:** 360 mg/day (as 90 mg 4 times/day).

**Secondary Hyperparathyoidism in Pts on Dialysis**
**PO: ADULTS, ELDERLY:** Initially, 30 mg once daily. Titrate dosage sequentially (60, 90, 120, and 180 mg once daily) every 2–4 wks to maintain iPTH level between 150 and 300 pg/ml. **Maximum:** 180 mg/day.

**Dosage in Renal Impairment**
No dose adjustment.

**Dosage in Hepatic Impairment**
**Moderate to Severe:** Use caution.

## SIDE EFFECTS

**Frequent (31%–21%):** Nausea, vomiting, diarrhea. **Occasional (15%–10%):** Myalgia, dizziness. **Rare (7%–5%):** Asthenia, hypertension, anorexia, noncardiac chest pain.

## ADVERSE EFFECTS/ TOXIC REACTIONS

Overdose may lead to hypocalcemia, seizures, worsening of HF.

## NURSING CONSIDERATIONS

### BASELINE ASSESSMENT

Establish baseline serum electrolyte levels (esp. serum calcium, phosphorus, ionized calcium).

### INTERVENTION/EVALUATION

Monitor serum calcium, phosphate, ionized calcium for hyperparathyroidism. Monitor daily pattern of bowel activity, stool consistency. Obtain order for antidiarrheal, antiemetic medication to prevent serum electrolyte imbalance. Assess for evidence of dizziness, institute fall risk precautions.

### PATIENT/FAMILY TEACHING

• Take with food or shortly after a meal. • Do not chew, crush, dissolve, divide film-coated tablets. • Notify physician if vomiting, diarrhea, cramping, muscle pain, numbness occurs.

# ciprofloxacin

sip-roe-**flox**-a-sin
(Apo-Ciproflox ✦, Cetraxal, Ciloxan, Cipro ✦, Cipro XR)

■ **BLACK BOX ALERT** ■ May increase risk of tendonitis, tendon rupture. May exacerbate myasthenia gravis.

**Do not confuse Ciloxan with Cytoxan, or Cipro with Ceftin, or ciprofloxacin with cephalexin.**

### FIXED-COMBINATION(S)

**Cipro HC Otic:** ciprofloxacin/hydrocortisone (a steroid): 0.2%/1%. **CiproDex Otic:** ciprofloxacin/dexamethasone (a corticosteroid): 0.3%/0.1%.

### ◆CLASSIFICATION

**PHARMACOTHERAPEUTIC:** Fluoroquinolone. **CLINICAL:** Antibiotic.

### USES

Treatment of susceptible infections due to *E. coli, K. pneumoniae, E. cloacae, P. mirabilis, P. vulgaris, P. aeruginosa, H. influenzae, M. catarrhalis, S. pneumoniae, S. aureus* (methicillin susceptible), *S. epidermidis, S. pyogenes, C. jejuni, Shigella* spp., *S. typhi* including intra-abdominal, bone, joint, lower respiratory tract, skin/skin structure infections; UTIs, infectious diarrhea, prostatitis, sinusitis, typhoid fever, febrile neutropenia. **Ophthalmic:** Treatment of superficial ocular infections. **OTIC:** Treatment of acute otitis externa due to susceptible strains of *P. aeruginosa* or *S. aureus*. **OFF-LABEL:** Treatment of chancroid. Acute pulmonary exacerbations in cystic fibrosis, disseminated gonococcal infections, prophylaxis to *Neisseria meningitidis* following close contact with infected person. Infectious diarrhea (children); periodontitis.

### PRECAUTIONS

**Contraindications:** Hypersensitivity to ciprofloxacin, other quinolones. Concurrent use of tizanidine. **Cautions:** Renal impairment, CNS disorders, seizures, rheumatoid arthritis, history of QT prolongation, uncorrected hypokalemia, hypomagnesemia, myasthenia gravis. Suspension not used through feeding or gastric tubes. Use in children (due to adverse events to joints/surrounding tissue).

### ACTION

Inhibits enzyme, DNA gyrase, in susceptible bacteria, interfering with bacterial cell replication. **Therapeutic Effect:** Bactericidal.

### PHARMACOKINETICS

Well absorbed from GI tract. Protein binding: 20%–40%. Widely distributed including to CSF. Metabolized in liver. Primarily excreted in urine. Minimal removal by hemodialysis. **Half-life:** 3–5 hrs (increased in renal impairment, elderly).

### ☒ LIFESPAN CONSIDERATIONS

**Pregnancy/Lactation:** Unknown if distributed in breast milk. If possible, do not use during pregnancy/lactation (risk of arthropathy to fetus/infant). **Children:** Arthropathy may occur if given to children younger than 18 yrs. **Elderly:** Age-related renal impairment may require dosage adjustment.

**C**

## INTERACTIONS

**DRUG:** **Antacids, calcium, magnesium, zinc, iron preparations, sucralfate** may decrease absorption. May increase effects of **caffeine, oral anticoagulants (e.g., warfarin).** May decrease concentration of **fosphenytoin, phenytoin.** May increase concentration, toxicity of **theophylline. HERBAL: Dong quai, St. John's wort** may increase photosensitization. **FOOD:** None known. **LAB VALUES:** May increase serum alkaline phosphatase, creatine kinase (CK), LDH, ALT, AST.

## AVAILABILITY (Rx)

**Infusion Solution:** 200 mg/100 ml, 400 mg/200 ml. **Injection, Solution (Cipro):** 10 mg/ml. **Ophthalmic Ointment (Ciloxan):** 0.3%. **Ophthalmic Solution (Ciloxan):** 0.3%. **Otic Solution (Cetraxal):** 0.2% (single-dose container: 0.25 ml). **Suspension, Oral:** 250 mg/5 ml, 500 mg/5 ml. **Tablets (Cipro):** 100 mg, 250 mg, 500 mg, 750 mg.

 **Tablets (Extended-Release):** 500 mg, 1,000 mg.

## ADMINISTRATION/HANDLING

💧 **IV**

**Reconstitution** • Available prediluted in infusion container ready for use. Final concentration not to exceed 2 mg/ml.
**Rate of Administration** • Infuse over 60 min (reduces risk of venous irritation).
**Storage** • Store at room temperature. • Solution appears clear, colorless to slightly yellow.

**PO**

• May be given with food to minimize GI upset. • Give at least 2 hrs before or 6 hrs after antacids, calcium, iron, zinc-containing products. • **Tablets, extended-release:** Administer whole; do not break, crush, cut, or divide. • Do not administer suspension through feeding or gastric tubes. • **NG tube:** Crush immediate-release tablet and mix with water. Flush tube before/after administration.

**Ophthalmic**

• Place gloved finger on lower eyelid and pull out until a pocket is formed between eye and lower lid. • Place ointment or drops into pocket. • Instruct pt to close eye gently for 1–2 min (so medication will not be squeezed out of the sac). • Instruct pt using ointment to roll eyeball to increase contact area of drug to eye. • Instruct pt using solution to apply digital pressure to lacrimal sac at inner canthus for 1 min to minimize systemic absorption. • Do not use ophthalmic solution for injection.

## 🔲 IV INCOMPATIBILITIES

Ampicillin and sulbactam (Unasyn), cefepime (Maxipime), dexamethasone (Decadron), furosemide (Lasix), heparin, hydrocortisone (Solu-Cortef), methylprednisolone (Solu-Medrol), phenytoin (Dilantin), sodium bicarbonate.

## 🔲 IV COMPATIBILITIES

Calcium gluconate, diltiazem (Cardizem), dobutamine (Dobutrex), dopamine (Intropin), lidocaine, lorazepam (Ativan), magnesium, midazolam (Versed), potassium chloride.

## INDICATIONS/ROUTES/DOSAGE

**Note:** Not recommended as first choice in pregnancy/lactation or children younger than 18 yrs due to adverse events related to joints/surrounding tissue.

**Usual Dosage Range**
**PO: ADULTS, ELDERLY:** 250–750 mg q12h.
**CHILDREN:** 20–30 mg/kg/day in 2 divided doses. **Maximum:** 1.5 g/day.
**IV: ADULTS, ELDERLY:** 200–400 mg q12h.
**CHILDREN:** 20–30 mg/kg/day in divided doses q12h. **Maximum:** 800 mg/day.

**Usual Ophthalmic Dosage**
**ADULTS, ELDERLY, CHILDREN:** *(Solution):* 1–2 drops q2h while awake for 2 days, then 1–2 drops q4h while awake for 5 days. *(Ointment):* Apply 3 times/day for 2 days, then 2 times/day for 5 days.

**Usual Otic Dosage**
**ADULTS, ELDERLY, CHILDREN:** 0.25 ml 2 times/day for 7 days.

**Dosage in Renal Impairment**
Dosage and frequency are modified based on creatinine clearance and the severity of the infection.

| Creatinine Clearance | Dosage |
|---|---|
| **Immediate-Release** | |
| 30–50 ml/min | PO: 250–500 mg q12h |
| 5–29 ml/min | 250–500 mg q18h |
| ESRD, HD, PD | 250–500 mg q24h |
| **Extended-Release** | |
| <30 ml/min | 500 mg q24h |
| ESRD, HD, PD | 500 mg q24h |
| IV 5–29 ml/min | 200–400 mg q18–24h |

**Dosage in Hepatic Impairment**
No dose adjustment.

## SIDE EFFECTS

**Frequent (5%–2%):** Nausea, diarrhea, dyspepsia, vomiting, constipation, flatulence, confusion, crystalluria. **Ophthalmic:** Burning, crusting in corner of eye. **Occasional (less than 2%):** Abdominal pain/discomfort, headache, rash. **Ophthalmic:** Altered taste, sensation of foreign body in eye, eyelid redness, itching. **Rare (less than 1%):** Dizziness, confusion, tremors, hallucinations, hypersensitivity reaction, insomnia, dry mouth, paresthesia.

## ADVERSE EFFECTS/ TOXIC REACTIONS

Superinfection (esp. enterococcal, fungal), nephropathy, cardiopulmonary arrest, cerebral thrombosis may occur. Hypersensitivity reaction (rash, pruritus, blisters, edema, burning skin), photosensitivity have occurred. Sensitization to ophthalmic form may contraindicate later systemic use of ciprofloxacin. May exacerbate muscle weakness in pts with myasthenia gravis. Dermatologic conditions such as toxic epidermal necrolyis, Stevens-Johnson syndrome have been reported. Cases of severe hepatotoxicity have occured.

## NURSING CONSIDERATIONS

### BASELINE ASSESSMENT
Question for history of hypersensitivity to ciprofloxacin, quinolones; myasthenia gravis, renal/hepatic impairment.

### INTERVENTION/EVALUATION
Obtain urinalysis for microscopic analysis for crystalluria prior to and during treatment. Evaluate food tolerance. Monitor daily pattern of bowel activity, stool consistency. Encourage hydration (reduces risk of crystalluria). Monitor for dizziness, headache, visual changes, tremors. Assess for chest, joint pain. **Ophthalmic:** Observe therapeutic response.

### PATIENT/FAMILY TEACHING
• Do not skip doses; take full course of therapy. • Maintain adequate hydration to prevent crystalluria. • Do not take antacids within 2 hrs of ciprofloxacin (reduces/destroys effectiveness). • Shake suspension well before using; do not chew microcapsules in suspension. • Sugarless gum, hard candy may relieve bad taste. • Avoid caffeine. • Report tendon pain or swelling. • Avoid exposure to sunlight/artificial light (may cause photosensitivity reaction). • Report persistent diarrhea. • **Ophthalmic:** Crystal precipitate may form, usual resolution in 1–7 days.

## *CISplatin    HIGH ALERT

sis-**pla**-tin

■ **BLACK BOX ALERT** ■ Cumulative renal toxicity may be severe. Dose-related toxicities include myelosuppression, nausea, vomiting. Ototoxicity, especially pronounced in children, noted by tinnitus, loss of high-frequency hearing, deafness. Must be administered by personnel trained in administration/handling of chemotherapeutic agents. Anaphylactic reaction can occur within minutes of administration. Avoid confusion between cisplatin and carboplatin. **Do not confuse cisplatin with carboplatin or oxaliplatin.**

---

 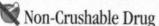

C

## ◆CLASSIFICATION

**PHARMACOTHERAPEUTIC:** Platinum coordination complex. **CLINICAL:** Antineoplastic.

## USES

Treatment of metastatic testicular tumors, metastatic ovarian tumors, advanced bladder carcinoma. **OFF-LABEL:** Breast, cervical, endometrial, esophageal, gastric, head and neck, lung (small-cell, non–small-cell) carcinomas; Hodgkin's and non-Hodgkin's lymphomas; malignant melanoma, neuroblastoma, osteosarcoma, soft tissue sarcoma, Wilms tumor.

## PRECAUTIONS

**Contraindications:** Hypersensitivity to cisplatin. Hearing impairment, myelosuppression, preexisting renal impairment. **Cautions:** Elderly, renal impairment.

## ACTION

Inhibits DNA and, to a lesser extent, RNA protein synthesis by cross-linking with DNA strands. Cell cycle–phase nonspecific. **Therapeutic Effect:** Prevents cellular division.

## PHARMACOKINETICS

Widely distributed. Protein binding: greater than 90%. Undergoes rapid nonenzymatic conversion to inactive metabolite. Excreted in urine. Removed by hemodialysis. **Half-life:** 58–73 hrs (increased in renal impairment).

## ⧖ LIFESPAN CONSIDERATIONS

**Pregnancy/Lactation:** If possible, avoid use during pregnancy, esp. first trimester. Breastfeeding not recommended. **Children:** Ototoxic effects may be more severe. **Elderly:** Age-related renal impairment may require dosage adjustment.

## INTERACTIONS

**DRUG:** May decrease effects of **anticonvulsant medications.** Bone marrow depressants (e.g., **paclitaxel**) may increase myelosuppression. **Live virus vaccines** may potentiate virus replication, increase vaccine side effects, decrease pt's antibody response to vaccine. **Nephrotoxic, ototoxic agents** (e.g., **aminoglycosides**) may increase risk of toxicity. **HERBAL:** Avoid **black cohosh, dong quai** with estrogen-dependent tumors. **Echinacea** may decrease effects. **FOOD:** None known. **LAB VALUES:** May increase serum BUN, creatinine, uric acid, AST. May decrease CrCl, serum calcium, magnesium, phosphate, potassium, sodium. May cause positive Coombs' test.

## AVAILABILITY (Rx)

**Injection Solution:** 1 mg/ml (50 ml, 100 ml, 200 ml).

## ADMINISTRATION/HANDLING

◀**ALERT**▶ Wear protective gloves during handling. May be carcinogenic, mutagenic, teratogenic. Handle with extreme care during preparation/administration.

 **IV**

**Dilution** • Dilute desired dose in 250–1,000 ml 0.9% NaCl, D₅/0.45% NaCl, or D₅/0.9% NaCl to concentration of 0.05–2 mg/ml. Solution should have final NaCl concentration of 0.2% or greater.
**Rate of Administration** • Infuse over 6–8 hrs (per protocol). • Avoid rapid infusion (increases risk of nephrotoxicity, ototoxicity). • Monitor for anaphylactic reaction during first few minutes of infusion.
**Storage** • Protect from sunlight. • Do not refrigerate (may precipitate). Discard if precipitate forms. IV infusion: Stable for 72 hrs at 39°F–77°F.

## ▦ IV INCOMPATIBILITIES

Amphotericin B complex (Abelcet, AmBisome, Amphotec), cefepime (Maxipime), piperacillin and tazobactam (Zosyn), sodium bicarbonate.

## 🏥 IV COMPATIBILITIES

Etoposide (VePesid), granisetron (Kytril), heparin, hydromorphone (Dilaudid), lipids, lorazepam (Ativan), magnesium sulfate, mannitol, morphine, ondansetron (Zofran), palonosetron (Aloxi).

## INDICATIONS/ROUTES/DOSAGE

**Note:** Pretreatment hydration with 1–2 liters of fluid recommended. Adequate hydration, urine output greater than 100 ml/hr should be maintained for 24 hrs after administration. Verify any cisplatin dose exceeding 100 mg/m$^2$/course.

**Bladder Carcinoma**
**IV: ADULTS, ELDERLY:** (Single agent): 50–70 mg/m$^2$ q3–4wks.

**Ovarian Tumors**
**IV: ADULTS, ELDERLY:** 75–100 mg/m$^2$ q3–4wks (combination therapy) or 100 mg/m$^2$ q4wks (single agent).

**Testicular Tumors**
**IV: ADULTS, ELDERLY:** 20 mg/m$^2$ daily for 5 days repeated q3wks (in combination with bleomycin and etoposide).

**Dosage in Renal Impairment**
Dosage is modified based on CrCl, BUN. **◄ALERT►** Repeated courses of cisplatin should not be given until serum creatinine is less than 1.5 mg/100 ml and/or BUN is less than 25 mg/100 ml.

| Creatinine Clearance | Dosage |
|---|---|
| 10–50 ml/min | 75% of normal dose |
| Less than 10 ml/min | 50% of normal dose |
| Hemodialysis | 50% of dose post dialysis |
| Peritoneal dialysis | 50% of dose |
| Continuous renal replacement therapy | 75% of dose |

**Dosage in Hepatic Impairment**
No dose adjustment.

## SIDE EFFECTS

**Frequent:** Nausea, vomiting (occurs in more than 90% of pts, generally beginning 1–4 hrs after administration and lasting up to 24 hrs); myelosuppression (affecting 25%–30% of pts, with recovery generally occurring in 18–23 days). **Occasional:** Peripheral neuropathy (with prolonged therapy [4–7 mos]). Pain/redness at injection site, loss of taste, appetite. **Rare:** Hemolytic anemia, blurred vision, stomatitis.

## ADVERSE EFFECTS/ TOXIC REACTIONS

Anaphylactic reaction (angioedema, wheezing, tachycardia, hypotension) may occur in first few minutes of administration in pt previously exposed to cisplatin. Nephrotoxicity occurs in 28%–36% of pts treated with a single dose, usually during second wk of therapy. Ototoxicity (tinnitus, hearing loss) occurs in 31% of pts treated with a single dose (more severe in children). Symptoms may become more frequent, severe with repeated doses.

## NURSING CONSIDERATIONS

### BASELINE ASSESSMENT

Obtain baseline CBC, BMP, LFT. Pts should be well hydrated before and 24 hrs after medication to ensure adequate urinary output (100 ml/hr), decrease risk of nephrotoxicity.

### INTERVENTION/EVALUATION

Measure all emesis, urine output (general guideline requiring immediate notification of physician: 750 ml/8 hrs, urinary output less than 100 ml/hr). Monitor I&O q1–2h beginning with pretreatment hydration, continue for 48 hrs after dose. Assess vital signs q1–2h during infusion. Monitor urinalysis, serum electrolytes, LFT, renal function tests, CBC, platelet count for changes from baseline.

### PATIENT/FAMILY TEACHING

• Report signs of ototoxicity (tinnitus, hearing loss). • Do not have immunizations without physician's approval (lowers body's resistance). • Avoid contact with those who have recently taken oral polio vaccine. • Report if nausea/vomiting continues at home. • Report signs of peripheral neuropathy.

# citalopram

sye-**tal**-o-pram
(Apo-Citalopram ✦, Celexa)

■ **BLACK BOX ALERT** ■ Increased risk of suicidal thinking and behavior in children, adolescents, young adults 18–24 yrs with major depressive disorder, other psychiatric disorders.

**Do not confuse Celexa with Celebrex, Cerebyx, Ranexa, or Zyprexa.**

## ◆CLASSIFICATION

**PHARMACOTHERAPEUTIC:** Serotonin reuptake inhibitor. **CLINICAL:** Antidepressant.

## USES

Treatment of depression. **OFF-LABEL:** Treatment of alcohol abuse, diabetic neuropathy, obsessive-compulsive disorder, smoking cessation.

## PRECAUTIONS

**Contraindications:** Hypersensitivity to citalopram, use within 14 days of MAOIs, initiation in pts receiving linezolid or methylene blue. Concurrent use with pimozide. **Cautions:** Elderly, hepatic/renal impairment, seizure disorder. Not recommended in pts with congenital long QT syndrome, bradycardia, recent MI, uncompensated HF, hypokalemia, or hypomagnesemia; pts at high risk of suicide.

## ACTION

Blocks uptake of the neurotransmitter serotonin at CNS presynaptic neuronal membranes, increasing its availability at postsynaptic receptor sites. **Therapeutic Effect:** Relieves symptoms of depression.

## PHARMACOKINETICS

Well absorbed after PO administration. Protein binding: 80%. Extensively metabolized in liver. Excreted in urine. **Half-life:** 35 hrs.

## ⧗ LIFESPAN CONSIDERATIONS

**Pregnancy/Lactation:** Distributed in breast milk. **Children:** May cause increased anticholinergic effects, hyperexcitability. **Elderly:** More sensitive to anticholinergic effects (e.g., dry mouth), more likely to experience dizziness, sedation, confusion, hypotension, hyperexcitability.

## INTERACTIONS

**DRUG: CYP2C19 inhibitors (e.g., fluconazole), other medications prolonging QT** interval may increase risk of QT prolongation. **Linezolid, MAOIs, triptans** may cause serotonin syndrome (excitement, diaphoresis, rigidity, hyperthermia, autonomic hyperactivity, coma). **HERBAL: Gotu kola, kava kava, SAMe, St. John's wort, valerian** may increase CNS depression. **St. John's wort** may increase risk of serotonin syndrome. **FOOD:** None known. **LAB VALUES:** May decrease serum sodium.

## AVAILABILITY (Rx)

**Oral Solution:** 10 mg/5 ml. **Tablets:** 10 mg, 20 mg, 40 mg.

## ADMINISTRATION/HANDLING

**PO**
• Give without regard to food.

## INDICATIONS/ROUTES/DOSAGE

**Note:** Doses greater than 40 mg not recommended.

**Depression**
**PO: ADULTS:** Initially, 20 mg once daily in the morning or evening. May increase in 20-mg increments at intervals of no less than 1 wk. **Maximum:** 40 mg/day. **ELDERLY:** 20 mg once daily. **Maximum:** 20 mg/day.

### Dose Modification

**Hepatic impairment; poor metabolizers of CYP2C19; concomitant use of CYP2C19 inhibitors:** 20 mg once daily. **Maximum:** 20 mg/day.

### Dosage in Renal Impairment

**Mild to Moderate:** No dose adjustment. **Severe:** Use caution.

## SIDE EFFECTS

**Frequent (21%–11%):** Nausea, dry mouth, drowsiness, insomnia, diaphoresis. **Occasional (8%–4%):** Tremor, diarrhea, abnormal ejaculation, dyspepsia, fatigue, anxiety, vomiting, anorexia. **Rare (3%–2%):** Sinusitis, sexual dysfunction, menstrual disorder, abdominal pain, agitation, decreased libido.

## ADVERSE EFFECTS/ TOXIC REACTIONS

Overdose manifested as dizziness, drowsiness, tachycardia, confusion, seizures, torsades de pointes, ventricular tachycardia, sudden death. Serotonin syndrome or neuroleptic malignant syndrome (NMS)–like reactions have been reported.

## NURSING CONSIDERATIONS

### BASELINE ASSESSMENT

Hepatic/renal function tests, blood counts should be performed periodically for pts on long-term therapy. Observe, record behavior. Assess psychological status, thought content, sleep pattern, appearance, interest in environment. Screen for bipolar disorder.

### INTERVENTION/EVALUATION

Supervise suicidal-risk pt closely during early therapy (as depression lessens, energy level improves, increasing suicide potential). Assess appearance, behavior, speech pattern, level of interest, mood.

### PATIENT/FAMILY TEACHING

• Do not stop taking medication or increase dosage. • Avoid alcohol. • Avoid tasks that require alertness, motor skills until response to drug is established. • Report worsening depression, suicidal ideation, unusual changes in behavior.

## *cladribine*

klad-ree-bine

■ **BLACK BOX ALERT** ■ Must be administered by personnel trained in administration/handling of chemotherapeutic agents. Myelosuppression, neurologic toxicity, acute nephrotoxicity have been reported. **Do not confuse cladribine with clevidipine, clofarabine, or fludarabine.**

## ◆CLASSIFICATION

**PHARMACOTHERAPEUTIC:** Antimetabolite. **CLINICAL:** Antineoplastic.

## USES

Treatment of active hairy cell leukemia defined by clinically significant anemia, neutropenia, thrombocytopenia. **OFF-LABEL:** Treatment of chronic lymphocytic leukemia, non-Hodgkin's lymphoma, acute myeloid leukemia.

## PRECAUTIONS

**Contraindications:** Hypersensitivity to cladribine. **Cautions:** Renal/hepatic impairment. Preexisting hematologic or immunologic abnormalities; those with high tumor burden. Use of live vaccines.

## ACTION

Disrupts cellular metabolism by incorporating into DNA of dividing cells. Cytotoxic to both actively dividing and quiescent lymphocytes, monocytes. **Therapeutic Effect:** Prevents DNA synthesis.

## PHARMACOKINETICS

Protein binding: 20%. Metabolized in liver. Primarily excreted in urine. **Half-life:** 5.4 hrs.

## ⧖ LIFESPAN CONSIDERATIONS

**Pregnancy/Lactation:** May produce fetal harm; may be embryotoxic, fetotoxic; potential for serious reactions in breastfed infants. **Children:** Safety and efficacy not established. **Elderly:** No age-related precautions noted.

## INTERACTIONS

**DRUG: Bone marrow depressants** may increase myelosuppression. **Live virus vaccines** may potentiate virus replication, increase vaccine side effects, decrease pt's antibody response to vaccine. **HERBAL: Echinacea** may decrease effect. **FOOD:** None known. **LAB VALUES:** May decrease platelets, Hgb, Hct, neutrophils during initial dose of therapy. Resolution of anemia, neutropenia, thrombocytopenia indicates disease progression.

## AVAILABILITY (Rx)

**Injection Solution:** 1 mg/ml (10 ml).

## ADMINISTRATION/HANDLING

 **IV**

**◀ALERT▶** • Wear gloves, protective clothing during handling; if contact with skin, rinse with copious amounts of water.
**Reconstitution** • Must dilute before administration. • Add calculated dose (0.09 mg/kg) to 500 ml 0.9% NaCl.
**Rate of Administration** • Infuse over 0.5–2 hrs.
**Storage** • Refrigerate unopened vials. • May refrigerate diluted solution for no more than 8 hrs. • Diluted solution is stable for at least 24 hrs at room temperature. • Discard unused portion.

## ▓ IV INCOMPATIBILITIES

None known.

## ▓ IV COMPATIBILITIES

Dexamethasone (Decadron), granisetron (Kytril), ondansetron (Zofran).

## INDICATIONS/ROUTES/DOSAGE

**Hairy Cell Leukemia**
**IV Infusion: ADULTS, CHILDREN:** 0.09–0.1 mg/kg/day as continuous infusion for 7 days.

**Dosage in Renal Impairment**

|  | Children | Adults |
| --- | --- | --- |
| CrCl 10–50 | 50% of dose | 75% of dose |
| CrCl less than 10 | 30% of dose | 50% of dose |
| Hemodialysis | 30% of dose | — |
| Peritoneal dialysis | — | 50% of dose |
| Continuous renal replacement therapy | 50% of dose | — |

**Dosage in Hepatic Impairment**
No dose adjustment.

## SIDE EFFECTS

**Frequent (69%–13%):** Fever, fatigue, nausea, rash, headache, injection site reactions, anorexia, vomiting. **Occasional (10%–5%):** Diarrhea, cough, purpura, chills, diaphoresis, constipation, dizziness, petechiae, myalgia, shortness of breath, malaise, pruritus, erythema, insomnia, edema, tachycardia, abdominal/trunk pain, epistaxis, arthralgia.

## ADVERSE EFFECTS/ TOXIC REACTIONS

Myelosuppression characterized as severe neutropenia (WBC less than 500 cells/mm³), severe anemia (Hgb less than 8.5 g/dL), thrombocytopenia occur commonly. High-dose treatment may produce acute nephrotoxicity (increased serum BUN, creatinine levels), neurotoxicity (irreversible motor weakness of upper/lower extremities).

## NURSING CONSIDERATIONS

### BASELINE ASSESSMENT

Obtain baseline CBC, serum chemistries. Offer emotional support. Perform neurologic exam before chemotherapy. Use strict asepsis; protect pt from infection.

## INTERVENTION/EVALUATION

Monitor vital signs during infusion, esp. during first hour. Observe for hypotension, bradycardia (both do not usually occur during same course). Immediately discontinue if severe hypersensitivity reaction occurs. Monitor for and report fever promptly. Assess for signs of infection. Assess skin for evidence of rash, purpura, petechiae. Monitor CBC, serum creatinine, potassium, sodium.

## PATIENT/FAMILY TEACHING

• There is a narrow margin between therapeutic and toxic response. • Avoid crowds, persons with known infections; report signs of infection at once (fever, flu-like symptoms). • Do not have immunizations without physician's approval (drug lowers resistance). • Avoid contact with those who have recently received live virus vaccine. • Avoid pregnancy.

# clarithromycin

kla-**rith**-roe-**mye**-sin
(Apo-Clarithromycin ✦, Biaxin, Biaxin XL, PMS-Clarithromycin ✦)
**Do not confuse clarithromycin with Claritin, clindamycin, or erythromycin.**

## ◆CLASSIFICATION

**PHARMACOTHERAPEUTIC:** Macrolide.
**CLINICAL:** Antibiotic.

## USES

Treatment of susceptible infections due to *C. pneumoniae, H. influenzae, H. parainfluenzae, H. pylori, M. catarrhalis, M. avium, M. pneumoniae, S. aureus, S. pneumoniae, S. pyogenes*, including bacterial exacerbation of bronchitis, otitis media, acute maxillary sinusitis, *Mycobacterium avium* complex (MAC), pharyngitis, tonsillitis, *H. pylori* duodenal ulcer, community acquired pneumonia, skin and soft tissue infections. Prevention of MAC disease. **OFF-LABEL:** Prophylaxis of infective endocarditis, pertussis, Lyme disease.

## PRECAUTIONS

**Contraindications:** Hypersensitivity to clarithromycin, other macrolide antibiotics. History of QT prolongation or ventricular arrhythmias including torsades de pointes. History of cholestatic jaundice or hepatic impairment with prior use of clarithromycin. Concomitant use with colchicine (in pts with renal/hepatic impairment), lovastatin, simvastatin, pimozide, ergotamine, dihydroergotamine. **Cautions:** Hepatic/renal impairment, elderly with severe renal impairment, myasthenia gravis, coronary artery disease. Pts at risk of prolonged cardiac repolarization. Avoid use with uncorrected electrolyes (e.g., hypokalemia, hypomanesemia), clinically significant bradycarida, class IA or III antiarrthmics (see Classification).

## ACTION

Binds to ribosomal receptor sites of susceptible organisms, inhibiting protein synthesis of bacterial cell wall. **Therapeutic Effect:** Bacteriostatic; may be bactericidal with high dosages or very susceptible microorganisms.

## PHARMACOKINETICS

Well absorbed from GI tract. Protein binding: 65%–75%. Widely distributed (except CNS). Metabolized in liver. Primarily excreted in urine. Not removed by hemodialysis. **Half-life:** 3–7 hrs; metabolite, 5–9 hrs (increased in renal impairment).

## ⧗ LIFESPAN CONSIDERATIONS

**Pregnancy/Lactation:** Unknown if distributed in breast milk. **Children:** Safety and efficacy not established in pts younger than 6 mos. **Elderly:** Age-related renal impairment may require dosage adjustment.

## INTERACTIONS

**DRUG:** May increase concentrations, toxicity of **carbamazepine, colchicine, digoxin, ergotamine, theophylline,**

sildenafil, tadalafil, vardenafil. **Rifabutin, rifampin, atorvastatin, efavirenz** may decrease plasma concentration. May increase effect of **warfarin.** May decrease concentration of **zidovudine. Atazanavir, ritonavir** may increase concentration of clarithromycin. **HERBAL: St. John's wort** may decrease plasma concentration. **FOOD:** None known. **LAB VALUES:** May increase serum BUN, ALT, AST, alkaline phosphatase, LDH, creatinine, PT. May decrease WBC.

## AVAILABILITY (Rx)

**Oral Suspension (Biaxin):** 125 mg/5 ml, 250 mg/5 ml. **Tablets (Biaxin):** 250 mg, 500 mg.
**Tablets (Extended-Release [Biaxin XL]):** 500 mg.

## ADMINISTRATION/HANDLING

**PO**

• Give immediate-release tablets, oral suspension without regard to food. • Give q12h (rather than twice daily). • Shake suspension well before each use. • Extended-release tablets should be given with food. • Do not break, crush, dissolve, or divide extended-release tablets.

## INDICATIONS/ROUTES/DOSAGE

**Usual Dosage Range**
**PO: ADULTS, ELDERLY:** 250–500 mg q12h or 1,000 mg once daily (extended-release tablets). **CHILDREN 6 MOS AND OLDER:** *(Immediate-Release):* 7.5 mg/kg q12h. **Maximum:** 500 mg/dose.

**Dosage in Renal Impairment**
**CrCl less than 30 ml/min:** Reduce dose by 50% and administer once or twice daily. **HD:** Administer dose after dialysis complete.

**Combination with atazanavir or ritonavir**

| | |
|---|---|
| CrCl 30–60 ml/min | Decrease dose by 50% |
| CrCl less than 30 ml/min | Decrease dose by 75% |

**Dosage in Hepatic Impairment**
No dose adjustment.

## SIDE EFFECTS

**Occasional (6%–3%):** Diarrhea, nausea, altered taste, abdominal pain. **Rare (2%–1%):** Headache, dyspepsia.

## ADVERSE EFFECTS/TOXIC REACTIONS

Antibiotic-associated colitis, other superinfections (abdominal cramps, severe watery diarrhea, fever) may result from altered bacterial balance in GI tract. Hepatotoxicity, thrombocytopenia occur rarely.

## NURSING CONSIDERATIONS

### BASELINE ASSESSMENT

Question pt for allergies to clarithromycin, erythromycins.

### INTERVENTION/EVALUATION

Monitor daily pattern of bowel activity, stool consistency. Mild GI effects may be tolerable, but increasing severity may indicate onset of antibiotic-associated colitis. Be alert for superinfection: fever, vomiting, diarrhea, anal/genital pruritus, oral mucosal changes (ulceration, pain, erythema).

### PATIENT/FAMILY TEACHING

• Continue therapy for full length of treatment. • Doses should be evenly spaced. • Biaxin may be taken without regard to food. Take Biaxin XL with food. • Report severe diarrhea.

# clindamycin

klin-da-**mye**-sin
(Apo-Clindamycin ♦, Cleocin, Cleocin T, Cleocin Vaginal, Clindagel, Clindamax, Clindesse)

■ **BLACK BOX ALERT** ■ May cause severe, potentially fatal colitis characterized by severe, persistent diarrhea, severe abdominal cramps, passage of blood and mucus.
**Do not confuse Cleocin with Clinoril or Cubicin, or clindamycin with clarithromycin, Claritin, or vancomycin.**

## ◆CLASSIFICATION

**PHARMACOTHERAPEUTIC:** Lincosamide. **CLINICAL:** Antibiotic.

## USES

**Systemic:** Treatment of aerobic gram-positive staphylococci and streptococci (not enterococci), *Fusobacterium*, *Bacteroides* spp., and *Actinomyces* for treatment of respiratory tract infections, skin/soft tissue infections, sepsis, intra-abdominal infections, infections of female pelvis and genital tract, bacterial endocarditis prophylaxis for dental and upper respiratory procedures in penicillin-allergic pts, perioperative prophylaxis. **Topical:** Treatment of acne vulgaris. **Intravaginal:** Treatment of bacterial vaginosis. **OFF-LABEL:** Treatment of actinomycosis, babesiosis, erysipelas, malaria, otitis media, *Pneumocystis jiroveci* pneumonia (PCP), sinusitis, toxoplasmosis. **PO:** Bacterial vaginosis.

## PRECAUTIONS

**Contraindications:** Hypersensitivity to clindamycin. **Cautions:** Severe hepatic dysfunction; history of GI disease (especially colitis).

## ACTION

Inhibits protein synthesis of bacterial cell wall by binding to bacterial ribosomal receptor sites. Topically, decreases fatty acid concentration on skin. **Therapeutic Effect:** Bacteriostatic or bacteriocidal.

## PHARMACOKINETICS

Rapidly absorbed from GI tract. Protein binding: 92%–94%. Widely distributed. Metabolized in liver. Primarily excreted in urine. Not removed by hemodialysis. **Half-life:** 1.6–5.3 hrs (increased in renal/hepatic impairment, premature infants).

## ⊠ LIFESPAN CONSIDERATIONS

**Pregnancy/Lactation:** Readily crosses placenta. Distributed in breast milk. **Topical/vaginal:** Unknown if distributed in breast milk. **Children:** Caution in pts younger than 1 mo. **Elderly:** No age-related precautions noted.

## INTERACTIONS

**DRUG: Adsorbent antidiarrheals** may delay absorption. **Erythromycin** may increase effect. May increase effects of **neuromuscular blockers. HERBAL: St. John's wort** may decrease concentration/effect. **FOOD:** None known. **LAB VALUES:** May increase serum alkaline phosphatase, ALT, AST.

## AVAILABILITY (Rx)

 **Capsules:** 75 mg, 150 mg, 300 mg. **Cream, Vaginal (Cleocin, Clindesse):** 2%. **Gel, Topical (Cleocin T, Clindagel, Clindamax):** 1%. **Infusion, Premix (Cleocin):** 300 mg/50 ml, 600 mg/50 ml, 900 mg/50 ml. **Injection Solution (Cleocin):** 150 mg/ml. **Lotion (Cleocin T, Clindamax):** 1%. **Oral Solution (Cleocin Pediatric):** 75 mg/5 ml. **Suppositories, Vaginal (Cleocin):** 100 mg. **Swabs, Topical (Cleocin T):** 1%.

## ADMINISTRATION/HANDLING

### IV

**Reconstitution** • Dilute 300–600 mg with 50 ml D₅W or 0.9% NaCl (900–1,200 mg with 100 ml).
**Rate of Administration** • Infuse over at least 10–60 min at rate not exceeding 30 mg/min. Severe hypotension, cardiac arrest can occur with rapid administration. • No more than 1.2 g should be given in a single infusion.
**Storage** • Reconstituted IV infusion (piggyback) is stable for 16 days at room temperature, 32 days if refrigerated.

### IM

• Do not exceed 600 mg/dose. • Administer deep IM.

### PO

• Store capsules at room temperature. • After reconstitution, oral solution is stable for 2 wks at room temperature. • Do not refrigerate oral solution (avoids thickening). • Give with at least 8 oz water (minimizes esophageal ulceration). • Give without regard to food.

### Topical
• Wash skin, allow to completely dry before application. • Shake topical lotion well before each use. • Apply liquid, solution, or gel in thin film to affected area. • Avoid contact with eyes or abraded areas.

### Vaginal, Cream or Suppository
• Use one applicatorful or suppository at bedtime. • Fill applicator that comes with cream or suppository to indicated level. • Instruct pt to lie on back with knees drawn upward and spread apart. • Insert applicator into vagina and push plunger to release medication. • Withdraw, wash applicator with soap and warm water. • Wash hands promptly to avoid spreading infection.

### ▥ IV INCOMPATIBILITIES

Allopurinol (Aloprim), fluconazole (Diflucan).

### ▥ IV COMPATIBILITIES

Amiodarone (Cordarone), diltiazem (Cardizem), heparin, hydromorphone (Dilaudid), magnesium sulfate, midazolam (Versed), morphine, multivitamins, propofol (Diprivan).

## INDICATIONS/ROUTES/DOSAGE

### Usual Dosage
**IV, IM: ADULTS, ELDERLY:** 600–2,700 mg/day in 2–4 divided doses. **Maximum:** 4,800 mg/day. **CHILDREN 1 MO–16 YRS:** 20–40 mg/kg/day in 3–4 divided doses. **Maximum:** 2,700 mg/day. **CHILDREN YOUNGER THAN 1 MO:** 5 mg/kg/dose q6–12h. **PO: ADULTS, ELDERLY:** 150–450 mg q6h. **Maximum:** 1,800 mg/day. **CHILDREN 1 MO–16 YRS:** *(Capsule):* 8–40 mg/kg/day in divided doses q6–8h. **Maximum:** 1,800 mg/day. *(Oral Solution):* 8–25 mg/kg/day in 3–4 divided doses. Minimum dose: 37.5 mg 3 times/day. **CHILDREN YOUNGER THAN 1 MO:** 5 mg/kg/dose q6–12h.

### Bacterial Vaginosis
**Intravaginal *(Cream)*: ADULTS:** One applicatorful at bedtime for 3–7 days or 1 suppository at bedtime for 3 days. *(Clindesse)*: **ADULTS:** One applicatorful once daily.

### Acne Vulgaris
**Topical: ADULTS:** Apply thin layer to affected area twice daily.

### Dosage in Renal/Hepatic Impairment
No dose adjustment.

## SIDE EFFECTS

**Frequent: Systemic:** Abdominal pain, nausea, vomiting, diarrhea. **Topical:** Dry, scaly skin. **Vaginal:** Vaginitis, pruritus. **Occasional: Systemic:** Phlebitis; pain, induration at IM injection site, allergic reaction, urticaria, pruritus. **Topical:** Contact dermatitis, abdominal pain, mild diarrhea, burning, stinging. **Vaginal:** Headache, dizziness, nausea, vomiting, abdominal pain. **Rare: Vaginal:** Hypersensitivity reaction.

## ADVERSE EFFECTS/ TOXIC REACTIONS

Antibiotic-associated colitis, other superinfections (abdominal cramps, severe watery diarrhea, fever) may occur during and several wks after clindamycin therapy (including topical form). Blood dyscrasias (leukopenia, thrombocytopenia), nephrotoxicity (proteinuria, azotemia, oliguria) occur rarely. Thrombophlebitis with IV administration.

## NURSING CONSIDERATIONS

### BASELINE ASSESSMENT
Obtain baseline WBC. Question pt for history of allergies. Avoid, if possible, concurrent use of neuromuscular blocking agents.

### INTERVENTION/EVALUATION
Monitor daily pattern of bowel activity, stool consistency. Report diarrhea promptly due to potential for serious colitis (even with topical or vaginal

---

administration). Assess skin for rash (dryness, irritation) with topical application. With all routes of administration, be alert for superinfection: fever, vomiting, diarrhea, anal/genital pruritus, oral mucosal changes (ulceration, pain, erythema).

### PATIENT/FAMILY TEACHING

• Continue therapy for full length of treatment. • Doses should be evenly spaced. • Take oral doses with at least 8 oz water. • Use caution when applying topical clindamycin concurrently with peeling or abrasive acne agents, soaps, alcohol-containing cosmetics to avoid cumulative effect. • Do not apply topical preparations near eyes, abraded areas. • Report severe persistent diarrhea, cramps, bloody stool. • **Vaginal:** In event of accidental contact with eyes, rinse with large amounts of cool tap water. • Do not engage in sexual intercourse during treatment. • Wear sanitary pad to protect clothes against stains. Tampons should not be used.

---

# *cloBAZam

kloe-**ba**-zam
(Apo-Clobazam ✦, Novo-Clobazam ✦, Onfi)
**Do not confuse clobazam with clonazepam or clozapine.**

### ◆CLASSIFICATION

**PHARMACOTHERAPEUTIC:** Benzodiazepine **(Schedule IV). CLINICAL:** Anticonvulsant.

### USES

Adjunctive treatment of seizures associated with Lennox-Gastaut syndrome in pts 2 yrs of age and older. **OFF-LABEL:** Catamenial epilepsy; epilepsy (monotherapy).

### PRECAUTIONS

**Contraindications:** Hypersensitivity to clobazam. **Cautions:** Elderly, debilitated, mild to moderate hepatic impairment, preexisting muscle weakness or ataxia, concomitant CNS depressants, impaired gag reflex, respiratory disease, sleep apnea, concomitant poor CYP2C19 metabolizers, pts at risk for falls, myasthenia gravis, narrow-angle glaucoma.

### ACTION

Potentiates neurotransmission of gamma-aminobutyric acid (GABA) by binding to GABA receptor. Depresses nerve impulse transmission in motor cortex. **Therapeutic Effect:** Decreases seizure activity.

### PHARMOCOKINETICS

Rapidly absorbed after PO administration. Peak plasma concentration: 0.5–4 hrs. Protein binding: 80–90%. Metabolized in liver. Primarily excreted in urine. Unknown if removed by dialysis. **Half-life:** 36–42 hrs.

### ⌛ LIFESPAN CONSIDERATIONS

**Pregnancy/Lactation:** Excreted in breast milk. Hormonal contraceptives may have decreased effectiveness. Nonhormonal contraception recommended. **Children:** Safety and efficacy not established in pts younger than 2 yrs. **Elderly:** May have decreased clearance levels (initial dose 5 mg/day).

### INTERACTIONS

**DRUG: CYP2C19 inhibitors (e.g., fluconazole, fluvoxamine, omeprazole, ticlopidine)** may increase concentration/effects. **Alcohol, other CNS depressants** may increase CNS depression. May decrease effects of **hormonal contraceptives. HERBAL: Gotu kola, kava kava, St. John's wort, valerian** may increase CNS depression. **St. John's wort** may decrease effects. **FOOD:** None known. **LAB VALUES:** None significant.

### AVAILABILITY (Rx)

**Suspension, Oral:** 2.5 mg/ml. **Tablets:** 5 mg, 10 mg, 20 mg.

---

## ADMINISTRATION/HANDLING

- May give without regard to food.
- Tablets may be crushed and mixed with applesauce. • Shake suspension well. Use oral syringe supplied with suspension.

## INDICATIONS/ROUTES/DOSAGE

**Seizure Control (Lennox-Gastaut Syndrome)**
**PO: ADULTS, CHILDREN WEIGHING 30 KG OR LESS:** Initially, 5 mg once daily. Increase to 5 mg twice daily on day 7, then increase to 10 mg twice daily on day 14. **Maximum:** 20 mg/day. **ADULTS, CHILDREN WEIGHING MORE THAN 30 KG:** Initially, 5 mg twice daily. Increase to 10 mg twice daily on day 7, then increase to 20 mg twice daily on day 14. **Maximum:** 40 mg/day.
**ELDERLY WEIGHING MORE THAN 30 KG, HEPATIC IMPAIRMENT, CYP2C19 POOR METABOLIZERS:** Initially, 5 mg once daily for 1 wk, then increase to 5 mg twice daily for 1 wk, then increase to 10 mg twice daily. After 1 wk, may increase to 20 mg twice daily.
**ELDERLY WEIGHING 30 KG OR LESS, HEPATIC IMPAIRMENT, CYP2C19 POOR METABOLIZERS:** Initially, 5 mg once daily for 2 wks, then 5 mg twice daily for 1 wk, then 10 mg twice daily.

**Dosage in Renal Impairment**
No dose adjustment.

## SIDE EFFECTS

**Frequent (26%–10%):** Sleepiness, URI, lethargy. **Occasional (9%–5%):** Drooling, nausea, vomiting, constipation, irritability, ataxia, insomnia, cough, fatigue. **Rare (4%–2%):** Psychomotor hyperactivity, UTI, decreased/increased appetite, dysarthria, pyrexia, dysphagia, bronchitis.

## ADVERSE EFFECTS/TOXIC REACTIONS

May increase risk of suicidal behavior/ideation (less than 1%). Physical dependence can increase with higher doses or concomitant alcohol/drug abuse. Abrupt benzodiazepine withdrawal may present as profuse sweating, cramping, nausea, vomiting, muscle pain, convulsions, psychosis, hallucinations, aggression, tremor, anxiety, insomnia. Overdose may result in confusion, lethargy, diminished reflexes, respiratory depression, coma. **Antidote:** Flumazenil (see Appendix J for dosage). Decreased mobility may potentiate higher risk of pneumonia.

## NURSING CONSIDERATIONS

### BASELINE ASSESSMENT

Offer emotional support. Review history of seizure disorder (frequency, duration, intensity, level of consciousness [LOC]). Question history of alcohol use. Obtain baseline vital signs. Assess history of depression/suicidal ideation.

### INTERVENTION/EVALUATION

Monitor for excess sedation, respiratory depression, suicidal ideation. Implement seizure precautions, observe frequently for seizure activity. Assist with ambulation if drowsiness, dizziness occurs. Evaluate for therapeutic response. Encourage turning, coughing, deep breathing for pts with decreased mobility or who are bedridden.

### PATIENT/FAMILY TEACHING

- Avoid tasks that require alertness, motor skills until response to drug is established. • Do not abruptly discontinue medication. • If tapering, monitor for drug withdrawal symptoms. • Avoid alcohol. • Report depression, aggression, thoughts of suicide/self-harm, excessive drowsiness.

## clofarabine

kloe-**far**-a-bine
(Clolar)
**Do not confuse clofarabine with cladribine or clevidipine.**

### ◆CLASSIFICATION

**PHARMACOTHERAPEUTIC:** Antimetabolite. **CLINICAL:** Antineoplastic.

## USES

Treatment of pediatric pts (1–21 yrs) with relapsed or refractory acute lymphoblastic leukemia (ALL). **OFF-LABEL:** Acute myeloid leukemia (AML) in adults 60 yrs or older. Treatment of relapsed/refractory ALL.

## PRECAUTIONS

**Contraindications:** Hypersensitivity to clofarabine. **Cautions:** Dehydration, hypotension, concomitant nephrotoxic or hepatotoxic medications, renal/hepatic impairment.

## ACTION

Metabolized intracellularly to ribonucleotide reductase. Alters mitochondrial membrane necessary in DNA synthesis. **Therapeutic Effect:** Decreases cell replication, inhibits cell repair. Produces cell death.

## PHARMACOKINETICS

Protein binding: 47%. Metabolized intracellularly. Primarily excreted in urine (40%–60% unchanged). **Half-life:** 5.2 hrs.

## ⧗ LIFESPAN CONSIDERATIONS

**Pregnancy/Lactation:** May cause fetal harm. Breastfeeding not recommended. **Children:** Safety and efficacy not established in pts younger than 1 yr. **Elderly:** No age-related precautions noted.

## INTERACTIONS

**DRUG: Hepatotoxic, nephrotoxic medications** may increase risk of hepatic/renal toxicity. **HERBAL: Echinacea** may decrease effect. **FOOD:** None known. **LAB VALUES:** May increase serum creatinine, uric acid, ALT, AST, bilirubin.

## AVAILABILITY (Rx)

**Injection, Solution:** 1 mg/ml (20-ml vial).

## ADMINISTRATION/HANDLING

 IV

**Reconstitution** • Filter clofarabine through sterile, 0.2-micrometer syringe filter prior to dilution with $D_5W$ or 0.9% NaCl to final concentration of 0.15–0.4 mg/ml.
**Rate of Administration** • Administer over 1–2 hrs. • Continuously infuse IV fluids to decrease risk of tumor lysis syndrome, other adverse events.
**Storage** • Store undiluted or diluted solution at room temperature. • Use diluted solution within 24 hrs.

## ▦ IV INCOMPATIBILITIES

Do not administer any other medication through same IV line.

## INDICATIONS/ROUTES/DOSAGE

**Acute Lymphoblastic Leukemia (ALL)**
**IV: CHILDREN 1–21 YRS:** 52 mg/m² over 2 hrs once daily for 5 consecutive days; repeat q2–6wks following recovery or return to baseline organ function. (Subsequent cycles should begin no sooner than 14 days from day 1 of previous cycle.)

**Dosage in Renal Impairment**
Dosage is modified based on creatinine clearance.

| Creatinine Clearance | Dosage |
|---|---|
| 30–60 ml/min | Decrease dose by 50% |
| Less than 30 ml/min | Use with caution |

**Dosage in Hepatic Impairment**
**Baseline Impairment:** No dose adjustment. **Hepatotoxicity during treatment: Grade 3 or higher increase in bilirubin:** Discontinue. May restart at 25% dose reduction following recovery to baseline.

## SIDE EFFECTS

**Frequent (83%–20%):** Vomiting, nausea, diarrhea, pruritus, headache, fever, dermatitis, rigors, abdominal pain, fatigue, tachycardia, epistaxis, anorexia, petechiae, limb pain, hypotension, anxiety, constipation, edema. **Occasional (19%–11%):** Cough, mucosal inflammation, erythema, flushing, hematuria, dizziness, gingival bleeding, injection site pain, respiratory distress, pharyngitis, back pain, palmar-plantar erythrodysesthesia syndrome, myalgia, oral candidiasis, hypertension, depression, irritability, arthralgia, anorexia. **Rare (10%):** Tremor, weight gain, drowsiness.

## ADVERSE EFFECTS/ TOXIC REACTIONS

Neutropenia occurs in 57% of pts; pericardial effusion in 35%; left ventricular systolic dysfunction in 27%; hepatomegaly, jaundice in 15%; pleural effusion, pneumonia, bacteremia in 10%; capillary leak syndrome in less than 10%.

## NURSING CONSIDERATIONS

### BASELINE ASSESSMENT

Question possibility of pregnancy. Obtain CBC, BMP, LFT, CrCl levels prior to therapy.

### INTERVENTION/EVALUATION

Monitor B/P, LFT, renal function tests, cardiac function, respiratory status, CBC, platelets, uric acid. Monitor daily pattern of bowel activity, stool consistency. Assess for GI disturbances. Assess skin for pruritus, dermatitis, petechiae, erythema on palms of hands and soles of feet. Assess for fever, sore throat; obtain blood cultures to detect evidence of infection. Ensure adequate hydration.

### PATIENT/FAMILY TEACHING

• Do not have immunizations without physician's approval (drug lowers resistance). • Avoid contact with anyone who recently received a live virus vaccine. • Avoid crowds, those with infection. • Avoid pregnancy; pts of childbearing potential should use effective contraception. • Maintain strict oral hygiene and frequent handwashing. • Report fever, respiratory distress, prolonged nausea, vomiting, diarrhea, easy bruising.

# *clomiPRAMINE

kloe-**mip**-rah-meen
(Anafranil, Apo-Clomipramine ✱,
Novo-Clomipramine ✱)

■ **BLACK BOX ALERT** ■ Increased risk of suicidal ideation and behavior in children, adolescents, young adults 18–24 yrs with major depressive disorder, other psychiatric disorders.
**Do not confuse Anafranil with enalapril, or clomipramine with chlorpromazine, clevidipine, clomiphene, or desipramine.**

## ◆CLASSIFICATION

**PHARMACOTHERAPEUTIC:** Tricyclic.
**CLINICAL:** Antidepressant.

## USES

Treatment of obsessive-compulsive disorder. **OFF-LABEL:** Depression, panic attacks.

## PRECAUTIONS

**Contraindications:** Hypersensitivity to clomipramine, other tricyclic agents. Acute recovery period after MI, use within 14 days of MAOIs. Initiation in pts receiving linezolid or methylene blue. **Cautions:** Pts at high risk for suicide, prostatic hypertrophy, history of urinary retention/obstruction, narrow-angle glaucoma, seizures, cardiovascular/hepatic/renal disease, hyperthyroidism, alcoholism, xerostomia, visual problems, elderly, constipation, history of bowel obstruction. Tumors of the adrenal medulla (e.g., pheochromocytoma).

## ACTION

Blocks reuptake of neurotransmitters (norepinephrine, serotonin) at CNS presynaptic membranes, increasing availability at postsynaptic receptor sites. **Therapeutic Effect:** Reduces obsessive-compulsive behavior.

## PHARMACOKINETICS

Rapidly absorbed. Metabolized in liver. Eliminated in urine (51%–60%), feces (24%–32%). **Half-life:** 20–30 hrs.

## ⧗ LIFESPAN CONSIDERATIONS

**Pregnancy/Lactation:** Distributed in breast milk. **Children:** Increased risk of suicidal ideation, behavior noted in children, adolescents. Safety and effectiveness in pts younger than 10 yrs not established. **Elderly:** No age-related precautions noted.

## INTERACTIONS

**DRUG: Alcohol, other CNS depressants** may increase CNS, respiratory depression, hypotensive effect. **Cimetidine, haloperidol** may increase concentration, risk of toxicity. May decrease effects of **clonidine. Phenobarbital** may decrease concentration, antidepressant effect. **MAOIs** may increase risk of neuroleptic malignant syndrome, seizures, hyperpyrexia, hypertensive crisis. **Phenothiazines** may increase anticholinergic, sedative effects. **Sympathomimetics** may increase the risk of cardiac effects. **HERBAL: Gota kola, kava kava, SAMe, St. John's wort, valerian** may increase CNS depression. **FOOD: Grapefruit products** may increase concentration, toxicity. **LAB VALUES:** May alter serum glucose, ECG readings.

## AVAILABILITY (Rx)

🔖 **Capsules:** 25 mg, 50 mg, 75 mg.

## ADMINISTRATION/HANDLING

**PO**
• May give with food to decrease risk of GI disturbance. • Recommend bedtime administration.

## INDICATIONS/ROUTES/DOSAGE

**NOTE:** Following dose titration, may give once-daily dose at bedtime.

**Obsessive-Compulsive Disorder (OCD)**
**PO: ADULTS, ELDERLY:** Initially, 25 mg/day. May gradually increase to 100 mg/day in divided doses in the first 2 wks. **Maximum:** 250 mg/day. **CHILDREN 10 YRS AND OLDER:** Initially, 25 mg/day. May gradually increase up to maximum of 3 mg/kg/day or 100 mg in divided doses (whichever is lowest). **Maintenance:** May further increase to 200 mg/day.

**Dosage in Renal/Hepatic Impairment**
Use caution.

## SIDE EFFECTS

**Frequent (30%–15%):** Ejaculatory failure, dry mouth, somnolence, tremors, dizziness, headache, constipation, fatigue, nausea. **Occasional (14%–5%):** Impotence, diaphoresis, dyspepsia, sexual dysfunction, dysmenorrhea, nervousness, weight gain, pharyngitis. **Rare (less than 5%):** Diarrhea, myalgia, rhinitis, increased appetite, paresthesia, memory impairment, anxiety, rash, pruritus, anorexia, abdominal pain, vomiting, flatulence, flushing, UTI, back pain.

## ADVERSE EFFECTS/ TOXIC REACTIONS

Overdose may produce seizures, cardiovascular effects (severe orthostatic hypotension, dizziness, tachycardia, palpitations, arrhythmias), altered temperature regulation (hyperpyrexia, hypothermia). Abrupt discontinuation after prolonged therapy may produce headache, malaise, nausea, vomiting, vivid dreams. Anemia, agranulocytosis have been noted.

## NURSING CONSIDERATIONS

### BASELINE ASSESSMENT

Assess psychological status, thought content, level of interest, mood, behavior, suicidal ideation.

### INTERVENTION/EVALUATION

Supervise suicidal-risk pt closely during early therapy (as depression lessens, energy level improves, increasing suicide potential). Assess appearance, behavior, speech pattern, level of interest, mood.

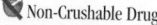

## PATIENT/FAMILY TEACHING

• May cause dry mouth, constipation, blurred vision. Avoid tasks that require alertness, motor skills until response to drug is established. • Tolerance to postural hypotension, sedative, anticholinergic effects usually develop during early therapy. • Maximum therapeutic effect may be noted in 2–4 wks. • Do not abruptly discontinue medication. • Daily dose may be given at bedtime to minimize daytime sedation. • Avoid alcohol. • Report worsening depression, suicidal ideation, change in behavior.

# *clonazePAM

kloe-**naz**-e-pam
(Apo-Clonazepam ✤, Klonopin, Rivotril ✦)
**Do not confuse clonazepam or Klonopin with clobazam, clonidine, clozapine, or lorazepam.**

## ◆CLASSIFICATION

**PHARMACOTHERAPEUTIC:** Benzodiazepine (**Schedule IV**). **CLINICAL:** Anticonvulsant, antianxiety.

## USES

Adjunct in treatment of Lennox-Gastaut syndrome (petit mal variant epilepsy); akinetic, myoclonic seizures; absence seizures (petit mal). Treatment of panic disorder. **OFF-LABEL:** Burning mouth syndrome, REM sleep behavior disorder, essential tremor.

## PRECAUTIONS

**Contraindications:** Hypersensitivity to clonazepam. Active narrow-angle glaucoma, severe hepatic disease, pregnancy. **Cautions:** Renal/hepatic impairment, impaired gag reflex, chronic respiratory disease, elderly, debilitated pts, depression, pts at suicidal risk or drug dependence, comcomitant use of other CNS depressants.

## ACTION

Depresses all levels of CNS; depresses nerve impulse transmission in motor cortex. Suppresses abnormal discharge in petit mal seizures. **Therapeutic Effect:** Produces anxiolytic, anticonvulsant effects.

## PHARMACOKINETICS

| Route | Onset | Peak | Duration |
|-------|-------|------|----------|
| PO | 20–60 min | — | 12 hrs or less |

Well absorbed from GI tract. Protein binding: 85%. Metabolized in liver. Excreted in urine. Not removed by hemodialysis. **Half-life:** 18–50 hrs.

## ⌛ LIFESPAN CONSIDERATIONS

**Pregnancy/Lactation:** Crosses placenta. May be distributed in breast milk. Chronic ingestion during pregnancy may produce withdrawal symptoms, CNS depression in neonates. **Children:** Long-term use may adversely affect physical/mental development. **Elderly:** Usually more sensitive to CNS effects (e.g., ataxia, dizziness, oversedation). Use low dosage, increase gradually.

## INTERACTIONS

**DRUG: Alcohol, other CNS depressants** may increase CNS depressant effect. **CYP3A4 inhibitors (e.g., azole antifungals)** may increase concentration, toxicity. **HERBAL: Gotu kola, kava kava, SAMe, St. John's wort, valerian** may increase CNS depression. **St. John's wort** may decrease concentration/effects. **FOOD:** None known. **LAB VALUES:** None significant.

## AVAILABILITY (Rx)

**Tablets (Klonopin):** 0.5 mg, 1 mg, 2 mg.
**Tablets (Orally Disintegrating):** 0.125 mg, 0.25 mg, 0.5 mg, 1 mg, 2 mg.

## ADMINISTRATION/HANDLING

**PO**
• Give without regard to food. • Swallow whole with water.

---

**Orally Disintegrating Tablet**
• Open pouch, peel back foil; do not push tablet through foil. • Remove tablet with dry hands, place in mouth. • Swallow with or without water. • Use immediately after removing from package.

## INDICATIONS/ROUTES/DOSAGE

**Seizures**
**PO: ADULTS, ELDERLY, CHILDREN 10 YRS AND OLDER:** Initial dose not to exceed 1.5 mg/day in 3 divided doses; may be increased in 0.5- to 1-mg increments every 3 days until seizures are controlled or adverse effects occur. **Maintenance:** 2–8 mg/day in 1–2 divided doses. **Maximum:** 20 mg/day. **INFANTS, CHILDREN YOUNGER THAN 10 YRS OR WEIGHING LESS THAN 30 KG:** 0.01–0.03 mg/kg/day in 2–3 divided doses; may be increased by no more than 0.25–0.5 mg every 3 days until seizures are controlled or adverse effects occur. **Maintenance:** 0.1–0.2 mg/kg/day in 3 divided doses. **Maximum:** 0.2 mg/kg/day.

**Panic Disorder**
**PO: ADULTS, ELDERLY:** Initially, 0.25 mg twice daily. Increase in increments of 0.125–0.25 mg twice daily every 3 days. **Target dose:** 1 mg/day. **Maximum:** 4 mg/day. **Note:** Discontinue gradually by 0.125 mg twice daily q3days until completely withdrawn.

**Dosage in Renal Impairment**
Use caution.

**Dosage in Hepatic Impairment**
**Mild to moderate impairment:** Use with caution. **Severe impairment:** Contraindicated.

## SIDE EFFECTS

**Frequent (37%–11%):** Mild, transient drowsiness; ataxia, behavioral disturbances (aggression, irritability, agitation), esp. in children. **Occasional (10%–5%):** Dizziness, ataxia, URI, fatigue. **Rare (4% or less):** Impaired memory, dysarthria, nervousness, sinusitis, rhinitis, constipation, allergic reaction.

## ADVERSE EFFECTS/ TOXIC REACTIONS

Abrupt withdrawal may result in pronounced restlessness, irritability, insomnia, hand tremors, abdominal/muscle cramps, diaphoresis, vomiting, status epilepticus. Overdose results in drowsiness, confusion, diminished reflexes, coma. **Antidote:** Flumazenil (see Appendix J for dosage).

## NURSING CONSIDERATIONS

### BASELINE ASSESSMENT
Review history of seizure disorder (frequency, duration, intensity, level of consciousness [LOC]). For panic attack, assess motor responses (agitation, trembling, tension), autonomic responses (cold/clammy hands, diaphoresis).

### INTERVENTION/EVALUATION
Observe for excess sedation, respiratory depression, suicidal ideation. Assess children, elderly for paradoxical reaction, particularly during early therapy. Initiate seizure precautions, observe frequently for recurrence of seizure activity. Assist with ambulation if drowsiness, ataxia occur. For pts on long-term therapy, CBC, BMP, LFT should be performed periodically. Evaluate for therapeutic response: decreased intensity and frequency of seizures or, if used in panic attack, calm facial expression, decreased restlessness.

### PATIENT/FAMILY TEACHING
• Avoid tasks that require alertness, motor skills until response to drug is established. • Do not abruptly discontinue medication after long-term therapy. • Strict maintenance of drug therapy is essential for seizure control. • Avoid alcohol. • Report depression, thoughts of suicide/self-harm, excessive drowsiness, GI symptoms, worsening or loss of seizure control.

---

*"Tall Man" lettering ♦ Canadian trade name  Non-Crushable Drug High Alert drug

C

# *cloNIDine

klon-i-deen
(Apo-Clonidine ♣, Catapres,
Catapres-TTS, Dixarit ♣, Duraclon,
Kapvay, Novo-Clonidine ♣)

■ **BLACK BOX ALERT** ■ **Epidural:**
Not to be used for perioperative,
obstetric, or postpartum pain.
**Do not confuse Catapres with
Cataflam, or clonidine with
clomiphene, clorazepam,
Klonopin, or quinidine.**

## ◆CLASSIFICATION

**PHARMACOTHERAPEUTIC:** Antiadrenergic, sympatholytic. **CLINICAL:**
Antihypertensive.

## USES

**Immediate-Release, Transdermal
Patch:** Treatment of hypertension alone
or in combination with other antihypertensive agents. **Kapvay:** Treatment of
attention-deficit hyperactivity disorder
(ADHD). **Epidural:** Combined with opiates for relief of severe pain. **OFF-LABEL:** Opioid or nicotine withdrawal,
prevention of migraine headaches, treatment of diarrhea in diabetes mellitus,
treatment of dysmenorrhea, menopausal
flushing, alcohol dependence, glaucoma,
clozapine-induced sialorrhea, Tourette's
syndrome, insomnia in children.

## PRECAUTIONS

**Contraindications:** Hypersensitivity to
clonidine. **Epidural:** Contraindicated in
pts with bleeding diathesis or infection at
the injection site; pts receiving anticoagulation therapy. **Cautions:** Depression,
elderly. Severe coronary insufficiency,
recent MI, cerebrovascular disease,
chronic renal impairment, pre-existing
bradycardia, sinus node dysfunction,
conduction disturbances; concurrent
use with digoxin, diltiazem, metoprolol,
verapamil.

## ACTION

Stimulates alpha-adrenergic receptors,
reducing sympathetic CNS response. **Epidural:** Prevents pain signal transmission
to brain and produces analgesia at pre-
and post-alpha-adrenergic receptors in
spinal cord. **ADHD:** Mechanism of action
unknown. **Therapeutic Effect:** Reduces
peripheral resistance; decreases B/P,
heart rate. Produces analgesia.

## PHARMACOKINETICS

| Route | Onset | Peak | Duration |
|-------|-------|------|----------|
| PO | 0.5–1 hr | 2–4 hrs | 6–10 hrs |

Well absorbed from GI tract. Transdermal
best absorbed from chest and upper arm;
least absorbed from thigh. Protein binding:
20%–40%. Metabolized in liver. Primarily
excreted in urine. Minimally removed by
hemodialysis. **Half-life:** 6–20 hrs (increased in renal impairment).

## ⊠ LIFESPAN CONSIDERATIONS

**Pregnancy/Lactation:** Crosses placenta.
Distributed in breast milk. **Children:**
More sensitive to effects; use caution.
**Elderly:** May be more sensitive to hypotensive effect. Age-related renal impairment may require dosage adjustment.

## INTERACTIONS

**DRUG:** Discontinuation of concurrent
**beta-blocker (e.g., carvedilol, metoprolol)** therapy may increase risk of clonidine-withdrawal hypertensive crisis. **Tricyclic
antidepressants** may decrease effect
(may require increased dose of clonidine).
**Digoxin, diltiazem, metoprolol, verapamil** may increase risk of serious bradycardia. **HERBAL: Gotu kola, kava kava,
SAMe, St. John's wort, valerian** may
increase CNS depression. **Ephedra, ginseng, yohimbe** may decrease antihypertensive effect. **FOOD:** None known. **LAB
VALUES:** None significant.

## AVAILABILITY (Rx)

**Injection Solution (Duraclon):** 100 mcg/ml,
500 mcg/ml. **Tablets (Catapres):** 0.1 mg,

0.2 mg, 0.3 mg. **Transdermal Patch (Catapres-TTS):** 2.5 mg (release at 0.1 mg/24 hrs), 5 mg (release at 0.2 mg/24 hrs), 7.5 mg (release at 0.3 mg/24 hrs).

**Extended-Release Tablets: (Kapvay):** 0.1 mg. **(Nexiclon XR):** 0.17 mg.

## ADMINISTRATION/HANDLING

### PO
• Give without regard to food. • Tablets may be crushed. • Give last oral dose just before bedtime. • Swallow extended-release tablets whole; do not break, crush, dissolve, or divide.

### Transdermal
• Apply transdermal system to dry, hairless area of intact skin on upper arm or chest. • Rotate sites (prevents skin irritation). • Do not trim patch to adjust dose.

### Epidural
• Must be administered only by medical personnel trained in epidural management.

## ▨ IV INCOMPATIBILITIES
None known.

## ▨ IV COMPATIBILITIES
Bupivacaine (Marcaine, Sensorcaine), fentanyl (Sublimaze), heparin, ketamine (Ketalar), lidocaine, lorazepam (Ativan).

## INDICATIONS/ROUTES/DOSAGE

### Hypertension
**PO: ADULTS:** Initially, 0.1 mg twice a day. Increase by 0.1–0.2 mg q2–4days. **Maintenance:** 0.2–1.2 mg/day in 2–4 divided doses up to maximum of 2.4 mg/day. **ELDERLY:** Initially, 0.1 mg at bedtime. May increase gradually. **CHILDREN 12 YRS AND OLDER:** Initially, 0.2 mg/day in 2 divided doses. May increase gradually at 5- to 7-day intervals in 0.1 mg/day increments. **Maximum:** 2.4 mg/day.
**Transdermal: ADULTS, ELDERLY:** System delivering 0.1 mg/24 hrs up to 0.6 mg/24 hrs q7days. Usual dosage range: 0.1–0.3 mg once wkly.

### Acute Hypertension
**PO: ADULTS:** Initially, 0.1–0.2 mg followed by 0.1 mg every hr if necessary, up to maximum total dose of 0.7 mg.

### Attention-Deficit Hyperactivity Disorder (ADHD)
**PO: CHILDREN 45 KG OR LESS:** Initially 0.05 mg/day at bedtime. May increase in increments of 0.05 mg/day q3–7days up to 0.2 mg/day (27–40.5 kg), 0.3 mg/day (40.5–45 kg). **GREATER THAN 45 KG:** 0.1 mg at bedtime. May increase 0.1 mg/day q3–7 days. **Maximum:** 0.4 mg/day. **Extended-Release Tablet (Kapvay):** **CHILDREN 6 YRS AND OLDER:** Initially, 0.1 mg daily at bedtime. May increase in increments of 0.1 mg/day at wkly intervals (**Maximum:** 0.4 mg/day). Doses should be taken twice daily with higher split dose given at bedtime.

### Severe Pain
**Epidural: ADULTS, ELDERLY:** 30–40 mcg/hr. **CHILDREN:** Range: 0.5–2 mcg/kg/hr, not to exceed adult dose.

### Dosage in Renal/Hepatic Impairment
No dose adjustment.

## SIDE EFFECTS
**Frequent (40%–10%):** Dry mouth, drowsiness, dizziness, sedation, constipation. **Occasional (5%–1%): Tablets, Injection:** Depression, pedal edema, loss of appetite, decreased sexual function, itching eyes, dizziness, nausea, vomiting, nervousness. **Transdermal:** Pruritus, redness or darkening of skin. **Rare (less than 1%):** Nightmares, vivid dreams, feeling of coldness in distal extremities (esp. the digits).

## ADVERSE EFFECTS/ TOXIC REACTIONS
Overdose produces profound hypotension, irritability, bradycardia, respiratory depression, hypothermia, miosis (pupillary constriction), arrhythmias, apnea. Abrupt withdrawal may result in rebound hypertension associated with nervousness, agitation, anxiety, insomnia, paresthesia,

**C**

tremor, flushing, diaphoresis. May produce sedation in pts with acute CVA.

## NURSING CONSIDERATIONS

### BASELINE ASSESSMENT

Obtain B/P immediately before each dose is administered, in addition to regular monitoring (be alert to B/P fluctuations).

### INTERVENTION/EVALUATION

Monitor B/P, pulse, mental status. Monitor daily pattern of bowel activity, stool consistency. If clonidine is to be withdrawn, discontinue concurrent beta-blocker therapy several days before discontinuing clonidine (prevents clonidine withdrawal hypertensive crisis). Slowly reduce clonidine dosage over 2–4 days.

### PATIENT/FAMILY TEACHING

• Sugarless gum, sips of water may relieve dry mouth. • Avoid tasks that require alertness, motor skills until response to drug is established. • To reduce hypotensive effect, rise slowly from lying to standing. • Skipping doses or voluntarily discontinuing drug may produce severe, rebound hypertension. • Avoid alcohol. • If patch loosens during 7-day application period, secure with adhesive cover.

---

## *clopidogrel*

kloe-**pid**-oh-grel
(Apo-Clopidogrel ✸, <u>Plavix</u>)

■ **BLACK BOX ALERT** ■ Diminished effectiveness in CYP2C19 metabolizers increases risk for cardiovascular events. Pts with CYP2C19*2 and/or CYP2C19*3 alleles may have reduced platelet inhibition.
**Do not confuse Plavix with Elavil or Paxil.**

### ◆ CLASSIFICATION

**PHARMACOTHERAPEUTIC:** Thienopyridine derivative. **CLINICAL:** Antiplatelet.

## USES

Unstable angina/non–ST-segment elevation MI. ST-segment elevation, acute MI. Recent MI, stroke, or established peripheral arterial disease. **OFF-LABEL:** Graft patency (saphenous vein), stable coronary artery disease (in combination with aspirin). Initial treatment of acute coronary syndrome in pts allergic to aspirin.

## PRECAUTIONS

**Contraindications:** Hypersensitivity to clopidogrel. Active bleeding (e.g., peptic ulcer, intracranial hemorrhage). **Cautions:** Severe hepatic/renal impairment, pts at risk of increased bleeding (e.g., trauma), concurrent use of anticoagulants. Avoid concurrent use of CYP2C19 inhibitors (e.g., omeprazole).

## ACTION

Inhibits binding of enzyme adenosine phosphate (ADP) to its platelet receptor and subsequent ADP-mediated activation of a glycoprotein complex. **Therapeutic Effect:** Inhibits platelet aggregation.

## PHARMACOKINETICS

| Route | Onset | Peak | Duration |
|-------|-------|------|----------|
| PO | 2 hrs | 5–7 days (with repeated doses of 75 mg/day) | 5 days after last dose |

Rapidly absorbed. Protein binding: 98%. Extensively metabolized by liver. Eliminated equally in the urine and feces. **Half-life:** 8 hrs.

## ⧗ LIFESPAN CONSIDERATIONS

**Pregnancy/Lactation:** Unknown if drug crosses placenta or is distributed in breast milk. **Children:** Safety and efficacy not established. **Elderly:** No age-related precautions noted.

## INTERACTIONS

**DRUG: Aspirin, NSAIDs, warfarin** may increase risk of bleeding. **Proton pump**

---

inhibitors (e.g., omeprazole) may decrease efficacy, increase risk of cardiovascular events. HERBAL: Cat's claw, dong quai, evening primrose, feverfew, garlic, ginger, ginkgo, ginseng, green tea, red clover may have additive antiplatelet effects. FOOD: Grapefruit products may decrease effects. LAB VALUES: May increase serum bilirubin, ALT, AST, cholesterol, uric acid. May decrease neutrophil count, platelet count.

## AVAILABILITY (Rx)

Tablets: 75 mg, 300 mg.

## ADMINISTRATION/HANDLING

PO
• Give without regard to food. • Avoid grapefruit products.

## INDICATIONS/ROUTES/DOSAGE

Reduction of Atherosclerotic Events (Pts with Recent MI, Stroke, PAD)
PO: ADULTS, ELDERLY: 75 mg once daily.

Acute Coronary Syndrome (ACS), Unstable Angina/NSTEMI
PO: ADULTS, ELDERLY: Initially, 300 mg loading dose, then 75 mg once daily (in combination with aspirin).

ACS (STEMI)
PO: ADULTS, ELDERLY 75 YRS OR YOUNGER: Initially 300-mg loading dose, then 75 mg once daily. ELDERLY OLDER THAN 75 YRS: 75 mg once daily.

ACS (PCI)
PO: ADULTS, ELDERLY: Initially, 600 mg, then 75 mg once daily.

Dosage in Renal Impairment
No dose adjustment.

Dosage in Hepatic Impairment
Use caution.

## SIDE EFFECTS

Frequent (15%): Skin disorders. Occasional (8%–6%): Upper respiratory tract infection, chest pain, flu-like symptoms, headache, dizziness, arthralgia. Rare (5%–3%): Fatigue, edema, hypertension, abdominal pain, dyspepsia, diarrhea, nausea, epistaxis, dyspnea, rhinitis.

## ADVERSE EFFECTS/ TOXIC REACTIONS

Agranulocytosis, aplastic anemia/ pancytopenia, thrombotic thrombocytopenic purpura (TTP) occur rarely. Hepatitis, hypersensitivity reaction, anaphylactoid reaction have been reported.

## NURSING CONSIDERATIONS

BASELINE ASSESSMENT
Obtain baseline chemistries, platelet count, PFA level. Perform platelet counts before drug therapy, q2days during first wk of treatment, and wkly thereafter until therapeutic maintenance dose is reached. Abrupt discontinuation of drug therapy produces elevated platelet count within 5 days.

INTERVENTION/EVALUATION
Monitor platelet count for evidence of thrombocytopenia. Assess Hgb, Hct, WBC; serum ALT, AST, bilirubin, BUN, creatinine; signs/symptoms of hepatic insufficiency during therapy.

PATIENT/FAMILY TEACHING
• It may take longer to stop bleeding during drug therapy. • Report any unusual bleeding. • Inform physicians, dentists if clopidogrel is being taken, esp. before surgery is scheduled or before taking any new drug.

C

# *cloZAPine

kloe-za-peen
(Apo-Clozapine ✦, Clozaril, FazaClo, Versacloz)

■ **BLACK BOX ALERT** ■ Significant risk of life-threatening agranulocytosis, increased risk of potentially fatal cardiovascular events, particularly myocarditis, in elderly pts with dementia-related psychosis. May cause severe orthostatic hypotension, bradycardia, syncope, cardiac arrest, dose-dependent seizures.
**Do not confuse clozapine with clonazepam, clonidine, or Klonopin, or Clozaril with Clinoril or Colazal.**

## ◆CLASSIFICATION

**PHARMACOTHERAPEUTIC:** Dibenzodiazepine derivative. **CLINICAL:** Antipsychotic.

## USES

Management of severely ill schizophrenic pts who have failed to respond to other antipsychotic therapy. Treatment of recurrent suicidal behavior in schizophrenia or schizoaffective disorder. **OFF-LABEL:** Schizoaffective disorder, bipolar disorder, childhood psychosis, obsessive-compulsive disorder, agitation related to Alzheimer's dementia.

## PRECAUTIONS

**Contraindications:** Hypersensitivity to clozapine. History of clozapine-induced agranulocytosis or severe granulocytopenia. **Cautions:** History of seizures, cardiovascular disease, myocarditis, respiratory/hepatic/renal impairment, alcohol withdrawal, high risk of suicide, paralytic ileus, myasthenia gravis, pts at risk for aspiration pneumonia, urinary retention, narrow-angle glaucoma, prostatic hypertrophy, xerostomia, visual disturbances, constipation, history of bowel obstruction, diabetes mellitus. History of long QT prolongation/ventricular arrhythmias; concomitant use of medications that prolong QT interval; hypokalemia, hypomagnesemia. **Pregnancy Category B.**

## ACTION

Interferes with binding of dopamine and serotonin receptor sites. **Therapeutic Effect:** Diminishes schizophrenic behavior.

## PHARMACOKINETICS

Readily absorbed from GI tract. Protein binding: 97%. Metabolized in liver. Excreted in urine. **Half-life:** 12 hrs.

## INTERACTIONS

**DRUG:** **Antihypertensive medications** (e.g., amlodipine, lisinopril, valsartan) may increase risk of hypotension. **Alcohol, other CNS depressants** may increase CNS depressant effects. **Bone marrow depressants** may increase myelosuppression. **Cimetidine, citalopram, ciprofloxacin, erythromycin** may increase concentration, risk of adverse effects. **SSRIs (e.g., paroxetine)** may increase concentration. **Lithium** may increase risk of confusion, dyskinesia, seizures. **Medications prolonging QT interval** may increase risk of QT prolongation. **CYP3A4 inducers** (e.g., phenytoin, carbamazepine, rifampin) may decrease concentration/effects. **HERBAL:** St. John's wort may decrease concentration/therapeutic effects. **Kava kava, gotu kola, valerian, St. John's wort** may increase risk of CNS depression. **FOOD:** None known. **LAB VALUES:** May increase serum glucose, cholesterol (rare), triglycerides (rare).

## AVAILABILITY (Rx)

**Suspension, Oral (Versacloz):** 50 mg/ml (100 ml). **Tablets (Clozaril):** 25 mg, 50 mg, 100 mg, 200 mg. **Tablets (Orally Disintegrating [FazaClo]):** 12.5 mg, 25 mg, 100 mg, 150 mg, 200 mg.

---

## ADMINISTRATION/HANDLING

### PO

• Give without regard to food. • **Suspension:** Use oral syringes (provided). Shake well, administer dose immediately after preparing. Suspension stable for 100 days after initial bottle opening.

### Orally Disintegrating Tablets

• Remove from foil blister; do not push tablet through foil. • Remove tablet with dry hands, place in mouth. • Allow to dissolve in mouth, swallow with saliva. • If dose requires splitting tablet, discard unused portion.

## INDICATIONS/ROUTES/DOSAGE

### Schizophrenic Disorders

◀**ALERT**▶ For initiation of therapy, must have WBC equal to or greater than 3,500 cells/mm$^3$ and ANC equal to or greater than 2,000 cells/mm$^3$.
**PO: ADULTS:** Initially, 12.5 mg once or twice daily. May increase by 25–50 mg/day over 2 wks until target dose of 300–450 mg/day is achieved. May further increase by 50–100 mg/day no more than once or twice wkly. Range: 200–600 mg/day. **Maximum:** 900 mg/day. **ELDERLY:** Initially, 12.5 mg/day for 3 days, then 25 mg/day for 3 days. May further increase in increments of 12.5–25 mg daily q3days. **Maximum:** 300 mg/day.

### Suicidal Behavior in Schizophrenia

**PO: ADULTS:** Initially, 12.5 mg 1–2 times/day. May increase in increments of 25–50 mg/day to a target dose of 300–450 mg/day after 2 wks. **Maximum:** 900 mg/day.

### Dose Modification

**Leukopenia/granulocytopenia: Mild: (WBC 3,000–3,500 cells/mm$^3$ and/or ANC 1,500–2,000 cells/mm$^3$):** Continue treatment, monitor WBC and ANC twice wkly until WBC greater than 3,500 cells/mm$^3$ and ANC greater than 2,000 cells/mm$^3$. **Moderate: (WBC 2,000–3,000 cells/mm$^3$ and/or ANC greater than 1,000 cells/mm$^3$–1,500 cells/mm$^3$):** Interrupt therapy, monitor WBC and ANC daily until WBC greater than 3,000 cells/mm$^3$

and ANC greater than 1,500 cells/mm$^3$, then twice wkly until WBC greater than 3,500 cells/mm$^3$ and ANC greater than 2,000 cells/mm$^3$. **Severe: (WBC less than 2,000 cells/mm$^3$ and/or ANC less than 1,500 cells/mm$^3$):** Discontinue treatment. **Discontinue:** QT$_c$ interval greater than 500 msec, cardiomyopathy/myocarditis, hepatotoxicity, or neuroleptic malignant syndrome.

### Dosage in Renal/Hepatic Impairment

No dose adjustment.

## SIDE EFFECTS

**Frequent (39%–14%):** Drowsiness, salivation, tachycardia, dizziness, constipation. **Occasional (9%–4%):** Hypotension, headache, tremor, syncope, diaphoresis, dry mouth, nausea, visual disturbances, nightmares, restlessness, akinesia, agitation, hypertension, abdominal discomfort, heartburn, weight gain. **Rare:** Rigidity, confusion, fatigue, insomnia, diarrhea, rash.

## ADVERSE EFFECTS/ TOXIC REACTIONS

Seizures occur occasionally (3% of pts). Overdose produces CNS depression (sedation, delirium, coma), respiratory depression, hypersalivation. Blood dyscrasias, particularly agranulocytosis, mild leukopenia, may occur.

## NURSING CONSIDERATIONS

### BASELINE ASSESSMENT

Obtain baseline weight, glucose, Hgb A1c, WBC, absolute neutrophil count (ANC) before initiating treatment. Assess behavior, appearance, emotional status, response to environment, speech pattern, thought content.

### INTERVENTION/EVALUATION

Monitor B/P for hypertension/hypotension. Assess pulse for tachycardia (common side effect). Monitor CBC for blood dyscrasias. Monitor WBC, WBC count every wk for first 6 mos, then biweekly for 6 mos. If CBC and ANC are normal after 12 mos, then monthly monitoring of CBC and ANC is recommended. Supervise suicidal-risk pt closely during early therapy (as depression lessens, energy level improves, increasing suicide potential). Assess for therapeutic response (interest in surroundings, improvement in self-care, increased ability to concentrate, relaxed facial expression).

### PATIENT/FAMILY TEACHING

• Do not abruptly discontinue long-term drug therapy. • Avoid tasks that require alertness, motor skills until response to drug is established. • Drowsiness generally subsides during continued therapy. • Avoid alcohol, caffeine. • Report fever, sore throat, flu-like symptoms.

# cobicistat

**koe-bi-sye-**stat
(Tybost)

## FIXED-COMBINATION(S)

**Evotaz:** cobicistat (antiretroviral booster)/atazanavir (antiretroviral): 150 mg/300 mg. **Genvoya:** cobicistat (antiretroviral booster)/emtricitabine/elvitegravir/tenofovir (TAF) (antiretroviral agents): 150 mg/200 mg/150 mg/25 mg. **Prezcobix:** cobicistat (antiretrovial booster)/darunavir (antiretroviral): 150 mg/800 mg. **Stribild:** cobicistat (antiretroviral booster)/emtricitabine/elvitegravir/tenofovir (TDF) (antiretroviral agents): 150 mg/200 mg/150 mg/300 mg.

## ◆CLASSIFICATION

**PHARMACOTHERAPEUTIC:** CYP3A inhibitor. **CLINICAL:** Antiretroviral booster.

## USES

Indicated to increase systemic exposure of atazanavir or darunavir (once daily dosing regimen), in combination with other antiretroviral agents for treatment of HIV-1 infection.

## PRECAUTIONS

**Contraindications:** Concomitant use with alfuzosin, dihydroergotamine, dronedarone, ergotamine, indinavir, irinotecan, lovastatin, methylergonovine, midazolam (oral), nevirapine, rifampin, sildenafil (use in PAH), simvastatin, St. John's wort. **Cautions:** Renal impairment, hypercholesterolemia. Avoid use with nephrotoxic medications. Do not initiate in pts with CrCl less than 70 ml/min. Use with HIV-1 protease inhibitors other than atazanavir or darunavir (once daily) or more than 1 antiretroviral requiring kinetic enhancement is NOT recommended. Co-administration of cobicistat and ritonavir. Cobicistat is not interchangeable with ritonavir.

## ACTION

Inhibits cytochrome P450 3A (CYP3A). **Therapeutic Effect:** Boosts exposure of atazanavir or darunavir. Does not exhibit antiviral activity.

## PHARMACOKINETICS

Readily absorbed after PO administration. Metabolized in liver. Protein binding: 97%–98%. Peak plasma concentration: 3.5 hrs. Eliminated in feces (86%), urine (8%). **Half-life:** 3–4 hrs.

## ⧖ LIFESPAN CONSIDERATIONS

**Pregnancy/Lactation:** Breastfeeding not recommended due to risk of postnatal HIV transmission. Secreted in breast milk. **Children:** Safety and efficacy not established in pts younger than 18 yrs. **Elderly:** Safety and efficacy not established in pts older than 65 yrs. May have increased risk of side effects/adverse reactions, renal failure.

## INTERACTIONS

**DRUG: Note:** See contraindications. **Nephrotoxic medications** may increase risk of acute renal failure. **Efavirenz, etravirine, nevirapine** may decrease cobicistat effectiveness. May increase concentration/effect of **antiarrhythmics (e.g., amiodarone, digoxin), antifungals**

(e.g., ketoconazole), atorvastatin, benzodiazepines, beta blockers (e.g., carvedilol, metoprolol), calcium channel blockers (e.g., amlodipine, diltiazem), clarithromycin, colchicine, cyclosporine, fluticasone, maraviroc, neuroleptics (e.g., risperidone, thioridazine), opioids (e.g., morphine), PDE-5 inhibitors (e.g., sildenafil), SSRIs, tricyclic antidepressants. Antacids, anticonvulsants (e.g., carbamazepine, phenytoin), famotidine, omeprazole may decrease absorption/effect. **HERBAL:** St John's wort contraindicated; may decrease effectiveness. **FOOD:** None known. **LAB VALUES:** May increase serum amylase, ALT, AST, bilirubin, BUN, cholesterol (LDL/HDL), creatine kinase (CK), creatinine, GGT, triglycerides, urine glucose; urine protein, urine RBC. May decrease CrCl.

## AVAILABILITY (Rx)

**Film-Coated Tablets:** 150 mg.

## ADMINISTRATION/HANDLING

**PO**
• Give with food. • Must be administered simultaneously with atazanavir or darunavir. • If pt receiving antacid with cobicistat/atazanavir regimen, do not give aluminum- or magnesium-containing antacids within 2 hrs, H₂-receptor antagonists (e.g., famotidine) within 10 hrs, or proton pump inhibitors (e.g., omeprazole) within 12 hrs of antiretroviral dose.

## INDICATIONS/ROUTES/DOSAGE

**HIV Infection**
**PO: ADULTS/ELDERLY:** 150 mg once daily (see Uses).

**Dosage in Renal Impairment**
No dose adjustment. Not recommended in pts with CrCl less than 70 ml/min when used with tenofovir (TDF).

**Dosage in Hepatic Impairment**
**Mild to Moderate:** No dose adjustment; use caution. **Severe:** Not recommended.

## SIDE EFFECTS

**Occasional (5%):** Jaundice, dermatitis, pruritus, pustular folliculitis, rash, urticaria. **Rare (3%–2%):** Ocular icterus, nausea, diarrhea, headache, depression, abnormal dreams, insomnia.

## ADVERSE REACTIONS/TOXIC EFFECTS

May cause acute renal failure or Fanconi syndrome when administered with tenofovir. Nephrolithiasis reported in 2% of pts. Pts co-infected with hepatitis B or C virus have increased risk for viral reactivation, worsening of hepatic function, or may experience hepatic decompensation and/or failure if therapy is discontinued.

## NURSING CONSIDERATIONS

**BASELINE ASSESSMENT**
Obtain CBC, BMP, CrCl, GFR, lipid panel, LFT, serum phosphate (baseline renal impairment), urine glucose, urine protein, vital signs; CD4+ count, viral load. Screen for hepatitis B or C co-infection, hypercholesterolemia. Receive full medication history including herbal products and screen for contraindications. Question possibility of pregnancy.

**INTERVENTION/EVALUATION**
Diligently monitor hepatic/renal function tests. An increase in serum creatinine greater than 0.4 mg/dL from baseline may indicate renal impairment. Monitor CD4+ count, viral load for treatment effectiveness. Assess skin for urticaria, pruritus, rash. Cough, dyspnea, fever, excess of band cells on CBC may indicate acute infection (WBC test may be unreliable in pts with uncontrolled HIV infection).

**PATIENT/FAMILY TEACHING**
• Offer emotional support. • Take cobicistat with atazanavir or darunavir at the same time each day with food (optimizes absorption). • Antacids may decrease drug effectiveness. • Drug resistance can form if therapy is interrupted; do not run out of supply. • Cobicistat does not cure

C

HIV infection nor reduce risk of transmission. • As immune system strengthens, it may respond to dormant infections hidden within the body. Report body aches, chills, cough, fever, night sweats, shortness of breath. • Treatment may cause kidney failure if used with tenofovir regimen. Report abdominal pain, darkened urine, decreased urine output. • Clay-colored stools, significant weight loss, or yellowing of skin or eyes may indicate liver problem. • Do not take any new medications, including over-the-counter drugs or herbal products, unless approved by your doctor.

# cobimetinib

**koe**-bi-**me**-ti-nib
(Cotellic)
**Do not confuse cobimetinib with cabozantinib, imatinib, or trametinib.**

## ◆CLASSIFICATION

**PHARMACOTHERAPEUTIC:** Kinase inhibitor. **CLINICAL:** Antineoplastic.

## USES

Treatment of pts with unresectable or metastatic melanoma with a BRAF V600E or V600K mutation, in combination with vemurafenib.

## PRECAUTIONS

**Contraindications:** Hypersensitivity to cobimetinib. **Cautions:** Baseline anemia, lymphopenia, thrombocytopenia; cardiomyopathy, hepatic/renal impairment, HF, hypertension, ocular disorders; pts at risk for bleeding (history of gastrointestinal, genitourinary, intracranial, reproductive system bleeding), electrolyte imbalance. Not recommended in pts taking moderate or strong CYP3A inhibitors.

## ACTION

Inhibits mitogen-activated protein kinase/extracellular signal regulated kinase 1 (MEK1) and MEK2. Cobimetinib also prevents vemurafenib-mediated growth enhancement of a wild-type BRAF tumor cell line. **Therapeutic Effect:** Inhibits tumor cell growth and metastasis.

## PHARMACOKINETICS

Widely distributed. Metabolized in liver. Protein binding: 95%. Peak plasma concentration: 2.4 hrs. Steady state reached in 9 days. Eliminated in feces (76%), urine (18%). **Half-life:** 44 hrs.

## ⧖ LIFESPAN CONSIDERATIONS

**Pregnancy/Lactation:** Avoid pregnancy; may cause fetal harm/malformations. Female pts of reproductive potential should use effective contraception during treatment and up to 2 wks after discontinuation. Unknown if distributed in breast milk. Breastfeeding not recommended. May reduce fertility in females and males. **Children:** Safety and efficacy not established. **Elderly:** Safety and efficacy not established.

## INTERACTIONS

**DRUG: Strong CYP3A inhibitors (e.g., clarithromycin, ketoconazole, ritonavir), moderate CYP3A inhibitors (e.g., atazanavir, ciprofloxacin)** may increase concentration/effect. **Strong CYP3A inducers (e.g., carbamazepine, rifampicin), moderate CYP3A inducers (e.g., bosentan, nafcillin)** may decrease concentration/effect. **HERBAL:** St. John's wort may decrease concentration/effect. **FOOD:** None known. **LAB VALUES:** Many increase serum alkaline phosphatase, ALT, AST, creatine phosphokinase, creatinine, GGT. May decrease Hct, Hgb, lymphocytes, platelets, RBCs; serum albumin, calcium, sodium. May increase or decrease serum potassium.

## AVAILABILITY (Rx)

**Tablets:** 20 mg.

## ADMINISTRATION/HANDLING

**PO**
• Give without regard to food. • If dose is missed or vomiting occurs during administration, give next dose at regularly scheduled time.

## INDICATIONS/ROUTES/DOSAGE

**Metastatic Melanoma**
**PO: ADULTS, ELDERLY:** 60 mg (three 20-mg tablets) once daily for first 21 days of 28-day cycle. Continue until disease progression or unacceptable toxicity.

**Concomitant Use of CYP3A Inhibitors**
Reduce dose to 20 mg once daily if short-term (14 days or less) use of moderate CYP3A inhibitors is unavoidable. May resume 60-mg once-daily dose once the short-term CYP3A inhibitor is discontinued. Use an alternative strong or moderate CYP3A inhibitor in pts already taking reduced dose of 20 mg or 40 mg daily.

**Dose Modification**
Based on Common Terminology Criteria for Adverse Events (CTCAE) grading 1–4. See prescribing information for vemurafenib for recommended dose modification.

**Dose Reduction Schedule**
**First dose reduction:** 40 mg once daily. **Second dose reduction:** 20 mg once daily. Permanently discontinue if unable to tolerate 20 mg once daily.

**Cardiomyopathy**
**Asymptomatic decrease in left ventricular ejection fraction (LVEF) greater than 10% from baseline and less than institutional lower limit of normal (LLN):** Withhold treatment for 2 wks, then reassess LVEF. Resume at next lower dose level if LVEF is at or above LLN and the decrease from baseline is 10% or less. Permanently discontinue if LVEF is less than LLN or the decrease from baseline LVEF is more than 10%. **Symptomatic decrease of LVEF from baseline:** Withhold treatment for up to 4 wks, then reassess LVEF. Resume at next lower dose level if symptoms resolve, LVEF is at or above LLN, and the decrease from baseline LVEF is 10% or less. Permanently discontinue if symptoms persist, LVEF is less than LLN, or the decrease from baseline LVEF is more than 10%.

**Dermatologic Reactions**
**Grade 2 (intolerable), grade 3 or 4:** Withhold or reduce dose.

**Hepatotoxicity or Hepatic Laboratory Abnormalities**
**First occurrence, grade 4:** Withhold treatment for up to 4 wks. If improved to grade 0 or 1, resume at next lower dose level. If not improved to grade 0 or 1 within 4 wks, permanently discontinue. **Recurrent grade 4:** Permanently discontinue.

**Hemorrhage**
**Grade 3:** Withhold treatment for up to 4 wks. If not improved to grade 0 or 1, resume at next lower dose level. If not improved within 4 wks, permanently discontinue. **Grade 4:** Permanently discontinue.

**New Primary Malignancies (Cutaneous or Noncutaneous)**
No dose adjustment.

**Nonspecific Adverse Effects**
**Any intolerable grade 2; any grade 3:** Withhold for up to 4 wks. If improved to grade 0 or 1, resume at next lower dose level. If not improved within 4 wks, permanently discontinue. **First occurrence of any grade 4:** Permanently discontinue.

**Ocular Toxicities**
**Serious retinopathy:** Withhold treatment for up to 4 wks. If signs and symptoms improve, resume at next lower dose level. If not improved or symptoms recur at the lower dose within 4 wks, permanently discontinue. **Retinal vein occlusion:** Permanently discontinue.

**Photosensitivity**
**Grade 2 (intolerable); grade 3 or
4:** Withhold treatment for up to 4 wks. If
improved to grade 0 or 1, resume at next
lower dose level. If not improved within
4 wks, permanently discontinue.

**Rhabdomyolysis, CPK Level Elevations**
**Grade 4 CPK elevation or any CPK
elevation with myalgia:** Withhold treatment for up to 4 wks. If improved to
grade 3 or lower, resume at next lower
dose level. If not improved within 4 wks,
permanently discontinue.

**Severe Hypersensitivity Reaction**
Permanently discontinue.

**Renal Impairment**
**Mild to moderate impairment:** No
dose adjustment. **Severe:** Not specified;
use caution.

**Hepatic Impairment**
**Mild impairment:** No dose adjustment.
**Moderate to severe impairment:** Not
specified; use caution.

## SIDE EFFECTS

**Frequent (60%–24%):** Diarrhea, photosensitivity, sunburn, solar dermatitis,
nausea, pyrexia, vomiting. **Occasional
(16%–10%):** Acneiform dermatitis, stomatitis, aphthous stomatitis, mouth ulceration, mucosal inflammation, alopecia, hypertension, vision impairment,
blurred vision, reduced visual acuity,
hyperkeratosis, erythema, chills.

## ADVERSE EFFECTS/TOXIC REACTIONS

Anemia, lymphopenia, thrombocytopenia
is an expected response to therapy. New
primary malignancies including squamous cell carcinoma, keratoacanthoma,
secondary-primary melanomas were reported. Serious, sometimes fatal hemorrhagic events including GI bleeding (4%
of pts), intracranial bleeding (1% of
pts), hematuria (2% of pts), reproductive system hemorrhage (2% of pts) have

occurred. Other hemorrhagic events may
include cerebral/conjunctival/intracranial/
gingival/hemorrhoidal/ovarian/pulmonary/
rectal/uterine/vaginal bleeding; ecchymosis, epistaxis. Grade 3 or 4 cardiomyopathy reported in 26% of pts. Grade 3
or 4 skin reactions including severe rash
occurred in 16% of pts. Ocular toxicities
including retinopathy, chorioretinopathy,
retinal detachment reported in 26% of
pts. Grade 3 or 4 CPK level elevations occurred in 14% of pts and may lead to
rhabdomyolysis. Hepatotoxicity reported
in 7%–11% of pts. Severe photosensitivity
reported in 47% of pts.

## NURSING CONSIDERATIONS

### BASELINE ASSESSMENT

Confirm presence of BRAF V600E or
V600K mutation in tumor specimen pri-
or to initiation. Obtain baseline CBC, BMP,
LFT, CPK; serum albumin, magnesium,
phosphate, ionized calcium; urine pregnancy; vital signs. Obtain ophthalmologic
exam with visual acuity; EKG, echocardiogram for LVEF. Assess skin for moles,
lesions, papillomas. Verify use of effective
contraception in female pts of reproductive potential. Receive full medication
history including herbal products. Question history as listed in Precautions. Assess visual acuity. Assess hydration status.

### INTERVENTION/EVALUATION

Monitor CBC, BMP, LFT, CPK; serum
albumin, magnesium, phosphate, ionized
calcium; vital signs. Assess skin for new
lesions, dermal toxicities at least q2mos
during treatment and for least 6 mos after discontinuation. Assess LVEF by echocardiogram 1 mo after initiation, then
q3mos thereafter until discontinuation. If
treatment interrupted to change in LVEF,
monitor LVEF at 2 wks, 4 wks, 10 wks,
and 16 wks, and then as indicated. Conduct ophthalmologic examinations regularly, esp. with any new or worsening visual
disturbances. Assess for eye pain, visual
changes. Immediately report GI bleeding,
hematuria, unusual reproductive system

hemorrhage; symptoms of intracranial bleeding (aphasia, blindness, confusion, facial droop, hemiplegia, seizures). Monitor for hepatotoxicity; signs of rhabdomyolysis such as dark-colored urine, flank pain, decreased urine output, muscle aches. Due to high risk of diarrhea, strictly monitor I&Os.

### PATIENT/FAMILY TEACHING

• Blood levels monitoring, cardiac function tests, eye exams, skin exams will be conducted frequently. • Treatment may lead to severe anemia, HF, kidney failure, new cancers, severe light sensitivity, liver dysfunction, skin toxicities (such as severe rash, peeling), vision changes. • Report bloody stools, bloody urine, unusual reproductive system bleeding, nose bleeds, coughing up blood; abdominal or flank pain, dark-colored urine, decreased urinary output; stroke-like symptoms; new skin moles or lesions, rash; eye pain, vision changes; heart problems such as shortness of breath, dizziness, fainting, palpitations • Report any newly prescribed medications. • Avoid sunlight, tanning beds. Wear protect clothing, high SPF sunscreen, and lip balm when outdoors. • Treatment may cause fetal harm. Women of childbearing potential should use effective contraception during treatment and up to 2 wks after last dose. Immediately report suspected pregnancy. Do not breastfeed. Treatment may reduce fertility.

## codeine

koe-deen
(Codeine Contin ✤)
**Do not confuse codeine with Cardene or Iodine.**

■ **BLACK BOX ALERT** ■ Respiratory depression, death have occurred in children following tonsillectomy and/or adenoidectomy.

### FIXED-COMBINATION(S)

**Capital with Codeine, Tylenol with Codeine:** acetaminophen/codeine: 120 mg/12 mg per 5 ml. **Tylenol with Codeine:** acetaminophen/codeine: 300 mg/15 mg, 300 mg/30 mg, 300 mg/60 mg.

### ◆CLASSIFICATION

**PHARMACOTHERAPEUTIC:** Opioid agonist. **CLINICAL:** Analgesic: Single entity: **Schedule II:** Fixed-combination form: **Schedule III:** Less than 90 mg, fixed combinations.

### USES

Relief of mild to moderate pain. **OFF-LABEL:** Short-term relief of cough.

### PRECAUTIONS

**Contraindications:** Hypersensitivity to codeine. Respiratory depression in absence of resuscitative equipment, acute or severe bronchial asthma or hypercarbia, paralytic ileus. Postoperative pain management in children following tonsillectomy/adenoidectomy. **Cautions:** Adrenal insufficiency, biliary tract impairment, CNS depression/coma, morbid obesity, prostatic hyperplasia, urinary stricture, thyroid dysfunction, severe renal/hepatic impairment, COPD, respiratory disease, cardiovascular disease, hypovolemia, GI obstruction, head injury, elevated intracranial pressure, history of drug abuse, patients with 2 or more copies of variant CYP2D6*2 allele (may have extensive conversion to morphine), elderly, debilitated pts, seizure disorder, acute alcoholism.

### ACTION

Binds to opioid receptors in CNS. Inhibits ascending pain pathways. **Therapeutic Effect:** Alters perception, emotional response to pain; suppresses cough reflex.

---

✤ Canadian trade name     🗡 Non-Crushable Drug     🔲 High Alert drug

C

## PHARMACOKINETICS

| Route | Onset | Peak | Duration |
|-------|-------|------|----------|
| PO | 30–60 min | 1–1.5 hrs | 4–6 hrs |
| IM | 10–30 min | 0.5–1 hr | 4–6 hrs |

Well absorbed following PO administration. Protein binding: (7–25%.) Metabolized in liver. Excreted in urine. **Half-life:** 2.5–3.5 hrs.

## LIFESPAN CONSIDERATIONS

**Children:** Efficacy not established in pts younger than 2 yrs. **Elderly:** May cause confusion, oversedation; use lower dosing range.

## INTERACTIONS

**DRUG: Alcohol, other CNS depressants** may increase CNS, respiratory depression, hypotension. **Anticholinergics** may increase risk of urinary retention, severe constipation. **MAOIs** may produce a severe, sometimes fatal reaction (reduce dosage to ¼ usual dose). **HERBAL: St. John's wort** may decrease concentration. **Gotu kola, kava kava, SAMe, St. John's wort, valerian** may increase CNS depression. **FOOD:** None known. **LAB VALUES:** May increase serum amylase, lipase.

## AVAILABILITY (Rx)

**Tablets:** 15 mg, 30 mg, 60 mg.

## ADMINISTRATION/HANDLING

**PO**
• May give without regard to food.
• Take with food or milk to decrease adverse GI effects.

## INDICATIONS/ROUTES/DOSAGE

◀ALERT▶ Reduce initial dosage in pts with hypothyroidism, Addison's disease, renal insufficiency, pts using other CNS depressants concurrently. Respiratory depression and death have occurred in children receiving codeine following tonsillectomy and/or adenoidectomy and found to have evidence of being ultrarapid metabolizers of codeine due to a CYP2D6 polymorphism.

**Analgesia**
**PO: ADULTS, ELDERLY:** 15–60 mg q4h as needed. **Maximum total daily dose:** 360 mg. **CHILDREN:** 0.5–1 mg/kg q4–6h. **Maximum:** 60 mg/dose.

**Dosage in Renal Impairment**
Dosage is modified based on creatinine clearance.

| Creatinine Clearance | Dosage |
|----------------------|--------|
| 10–50 ml/min | 75% of usual dose |
| Less than 10 ml/min | 50% of usual dose |

**Dosage in Hepatic Impairment**
Use caution.

## SIDE EFFECTS

◀ALERT▶ Ambulatory pts, pts not in severe pain may experience dizziness, nausea, vomiting, hypotension more frequently than those in supine position or with severe pain. **Frequent:** Constipation, drowsiness, nausea, vomiting. **Occasional:** Paradoxical excitement, confusion, palpitations, facial flushing, decreased urination, blurred vision, dizziness, dry mouth, headache, hypotension (including orthostatic hypotension), decreased appetite, injection site redness, burning, or pain. **Rare:** Hallucinations, depression, abdominal pain, insomnia.

## ADVERSE EFFECTS/ TOXIC REACTIONS

Chronic use may result in paralytic ileus. Overdose may produce cold/clammy skin, confusion, seizures, decreased B/P, restlessness, pinpoint pupils, bradycardia, respiratory depression, decreased LOC, severe weakness. Tolerance to drug's analgesic effect, physical dependence may occur with chronic use.

## NURSING CONSIDERATIONS

### BASELINE ASSESSMENT

**Analgesic:** Assess onset, type, location, duration of pain. Effect of medication is reduced if full pain response recurs before next dose. **Antitussive:** Assess type, severity, frequency of cough, sputum production.

### INTERVENTION/EVALUATION

Monitor daily pattern of bowel activity, stool consistency. Increase fluid intake, environmental humidity to improve viscosity of lung secretions. Initiate deep breathing, coughing exercises. Assess for clinical improvement; record onset of relief of pain, cough.

### PATIENT/FAMILY TEACHING

• Change positions slowly to avoid orthostatic hypotension. • Avoid tasks that require alertness, motor skills until response to drug is established. • Tolerance, dependence may occur with prolonged use of high dosages. • Avoid alcohol.

---

## colchicine

kol-chi-seen
(Colcrys, Mitigare)
**Do not confuse colchicine with Cortrosyn.**

### ◆CLASSIFICATION

**PHARMACOTHERAPEUTIC:** Alkaloid.
**CLINICAL:** Antigout.

## USES

Prevention, treatment of acute gouty arthritis (Colcrys only). Used to reduce frequency of recurrence of familial Mediterranean fever (FMF). **OFF-LABEL:** Treatment of biliary cirrhosis, recurrent pericarditis.

## PRECAUTIONS

**Contraindications:** Hypersensitivity to colchicine. Concomitant use of a P-glycoprotein (e.g., cyclosporine) or strong CYP3A4 inhibitor (e.g., clarithromycin) in presence of renal or hepatic impairment. **Mitigare:** Pts with both renal/hepatic impairment. **Cautions:** Hepatic impairment, elderly, debilitated, renal impairment. Concomitant use of cyclosporine, diltiazem, verapamil, fibrates, statins may increase risk of myopathy.

## ACTION

Decreases leukocyte motility, phagocytosis, lactic acid production. **Therapeutic Effect:** Decreases urate crystal deposits, reduces inflammatory process.

## PHARMACOKINETICS

Rapidly absorbed from GI tract. Oral bioavailability: 45%. Highest concentration is in liver, spleen, kidney. Protein binding: 30%–50%. Reenters intestinal tract by biliary secretion and is reabsorbed from intestines. Partially metabolized in liver via CYP3A4. Eliminated primarily in feces. **Half-life:** 27–31 hrs.

## ⚖ LIFESPAN CONSIDERATIONS

**Pregnancy/Lactation:** Unknown if drug crosses placenta or is distributed in breast milk. **Children:** Safety and efficacy not established. **Elderly:** May be more susceptible to cumulative toxicity. Age-related renal impairment may increase risk of myopathy.

## INTERACTIONS

**DRUG:** May increase concentration of **statins** and increase risk of rhabdomyolysis. **Atazanavir, clarithromycin, cyclosporine, diltiazem, erythromycin, fluconazole, fosamprenavir, indinavir, ketoconazole, ranolazine, ritonavir, saquinavir, verapamil** may increase colchicine concentration, toxicity. **HERBAL:** None significant. **FOOD: Grapefruit products** may increase concentration/toxicity. **LAB VALUES:** May increase serum alkaline phosphatase, AST. May decrease platelet count.

## AVAILABILITY (Rx)

**Tablets (Colcrys):** 0.6 mg. **Capsule (Mitigare):** 0.6 mg.

---

## ADMINISTRATION/HANDLING

### PO

• Give without regard to food. • For FMF, give in 1 or 2 divided doses. • Give with adequate water and maintain fluid intake.

## INDICATIONS/ROUTES/DOSAGE

### Acute Gouty Arthritis

**PO: ADULTS, ELDERLY:** Initially, 1.2 mg at first sign of gout flare, then 0.6 mg 1 hr later. **Coadministration with Strong CYP3A4 Inhibitors:** Initially, 0.6 mg, then 0.3 mg dose 1 hr later. Do not repeat for at least 3 days. **Coadministration with Moderate CYP3A4 Inhibitors:** 1.2 mg once. Do not repeat for at least 3 days. **Coadministration with P-Glycoprotein Inhibitors:** 0.6 mg once. Do not repeat for at least 3 days.

### Gout Prophylaxis

**PO: ADULTS, ELDERLY:** 0.6 mg 1–2 times/day. **Maximum:** 1.2 mg/day. **Coadministration with Strong CYP3A4 Inhibitors:** If dose is 0.6 mg 2 times/day, adjust dose to 0.3 mg once daily; if dose is 0.6 mg once daily, adjust dose to 0.3 mg every other day. **Coadministration with Moderate CYP3A4 Inhibitors:** If dose is 0.6 mg 2 times/day, adjust dose to 0.3 mg twice daily or 0.6 mg once daily; if dose is 0.6 mg once daily, adjust dose to 0.3 mg once daily. **Coadministration with P-Glycoprotein Inhibitors:** If dose is 0.6 mg 2 times/day, adjust dose to 0.3 mg once daily; if dose is 0.6 mg once daily, adjust dose to 0.3 mg every other day.

### FMF

**PO: ADULTS, ELDERLY, CHILDREN OLDER THAN 12 YRS:** 1.2–2.4 mg/day. **Coadministration with strong CYP3A4 inhibitors: Maximum:** 0.6 mg once daily (or 0.3 mg twice daily). **Coadministration with moderate CYP3A4 inhibitors:** 1.2 mg/day (0.6 mg twice daily). **Coadministration with P-glycoprotein inhibitors:** 0.6 mg once daily (or 0.3 mg twice daily). **CHILDREN 6–12 YRS:** 0.9–1.8 mg/day in 1–2 divided doses. **CHILDREN 4–5 YRS:** 0.3–1.8 mg/day in 1–2 divided doses. **Note:** Increase or decrease dose by 0.3 mg/day, not to exceed maximum dose.

### Pericarditis

**PO: ADULTS, ELDERLY:** 0.6 mg 2 times/day.

### Dosage in Renal Impairment

| Creatinine Clearance | Dosage |
| --- | --- |
| Less than 30 ml/min | |
| FMF | 0.3 mg initially |
| Gout prophylaxis | 0.3 mg/day |
| Gout flare | No reduction |
| HD | |
| FMF | 0.3 mg as single dose |
| Gout prophylaxis | 0.3 mg 2–4 times/wk |

### Dosage in Hepatic Impairment

Use caution.

## SIDE EFFECTS

**Frequent:** Nausea, vomiting, abdominal discomfort. **Occasional:** Anorexia. **Rare:** Hypersensitivity reaction, including angioedema.

## ADVERSE EFFECTS/TOXIC REACTIONS

Bone marrow depression (aplastic anemia, agranulocytosis, thrombocytopenia) may occur with long-term therapy. Overdose initially causes burning feeling in skin/throat; severe diarrhea, abdominal pain. Second stage manifests as fever, seizures, delirium, renal impairment (hematuria, oliguria). Third stage causes hair loss, leukocytosis, stomatitis.

## NURSING CONSIDERATIONS

### BASELINE ASSESSMENT

Obtain baseline laboratory studies. **Gout:** Assess involved joints for pain, mobility, edema. **Mediterranean fever:** Assess abdominal pain, fever, chills, erythema, swollen skin lesions.

## INTERVENTION/EVALUATION

Discontinue medication immediately if GI symptoms occur. Encourage high fluid intake (3,000 ml/day). Monitor I&O (output should be at least 2,000 ml/day), CBC, hepatic/renal function tests. Monitor serum uric acid. Assess for therapeutic response: relief of pain, stiffness, swelling; increased joint mobility; reduced joint tenderness; improved grip strength.

## PATIENT/FAMILY TEACHING

• Drink 8–10 glasses (8 oz) of fluid daily while taking medication. • Report skin rash, sore throat, fever, unusual bruising/bleeding, weakness, fatigue, numbness. • Stop medication as soon as gout pain is relieved or at first sign of nausea, vomiting, diarrhea. • Avoid grapefruit products.

# conjugated estrogens

kon-joo-gate-ed ess-troe-jenz
(Cenestin, Enjuvia, Premarin)

■ **BLACK BOX ALERT** ■ Risk of dementia may be increased in postmenopausal women. Do not use to prevent cardiovascular disease. May increase risk of endometrial carcinoma in postmenopausal women.

**Do not confuse Enjuvia with Januvia, or Premarin with Primaxin, Provera, or Remeron.**

## FIXED-COMBINATION(S)

**Duavee:** conjugated estrogen/bazedoxifene (estrogen agonist/antagonist): 0.45 mg/20 mg.

## ◆CLASSIFICATION

**PHARMACOTHERAPEUTIC:** Estrogen.
**CLINICAL:** Hormone.

## USES

**Premarin:** Management of moderate to severe vasomotor symptoms associated with menopause. Treatment of atrophic vaginitis, kraurosis vulvae, female hypogonadism and castration, primary ovarian failure. Retardation of osteoporosis in postmenopausal women. Palliative treatment of inoperable, progressive cancer of the prostate in men and of the breast in postmenopausal women. Abnormal uterine bleeding. Treatment of moderate to severe postmenopausal dyspareunia (painful sexual intercourse). **Cenestin:** Treatment of moderate to severe vasomotor symptoms of menopause, treatment of vulvar/vaginal atrophy. **Enjuvia:** Treatment of moderate to severe vasomotor symptoms, moderate to severe vaginal dryness and pain with intercourse, symptoms of vulvar/vaginal atrophy associated with menopause. **OFF-LABEL:** Prevention of estrogen deficiency–induced premenopausal osteoporosis. **Cream:** Prevention of nosebleeds.

## PRECAUTIONS

**Contraindications:** Hypersensitivity to estrogens. Breast cancer (except in pts being treated for metastatic disease), hepatic disease, history of or current thrombophlebitis, undiagnosed abnormal vaginal bleeding, pregnancy. **Cautions:** Asthma, epilepsy, migraine headaches, diabetes, cardiac/renal dysfunction, history of severe hypocalcemia, lupus erythematosis, porphyria, endometriosis, gallbladder disease, familial defects of lipoprotein metabolism. Hypoparathyroidism, history of cholestatic jaundice.

## ACTION

Responsible for development and maintenance of female reproductive system and secondary sexual characteristics; modulates release of gonadotropin-releasing hormone, reduces follicle-stimulating hormone (FSH), luteinizing hormone (LH). **Therapeutic Effect:** Reduces elevated levels of gonadotropins, LH, and FSH.

**C**

## PHARMACOKINETICS

Well absorbed from GI tract. Widely distributed. Protein binding: 50%–80%. Metabolized in liver. Primarily excreted in urine. **Half-life (total estrone):** 27 hrs.

## ⌛ LIFESPAN CONSIDERATIONS

**Pregnancy/Lactation:** Distributed in breast milk. May cause fetal harm. Breastfeeding not recommended. **Children:** Safety and efficacy not established. **Elderly:** No age-related precautions noted.

## INTERACTIONS

**DRUG:** None significant. **HERBAL: Black cohosh, dong quai** may increase estrogenic activity. **Ginseng, red clover, saw palmetto** may increase hormonal effects. **St. John's wort** may decrease concentration. **FOOD: Grapefruit products** may increase concentration/toxicity. **LAB VALUES:** May increase serum glucose, HDL, calcium, triglycerides. May decrease serum cholesterol, LDH. May affect serum metapyrone testing, thyroid function tests.

## AVAILABILITY (Rx)

**Cream, Vaginal (Premarin):** 0.625 mg/g.
**Injection, Powder for Reconstitution:** 25 mg. **Tablet (Cenestin, Enjuvia, Premarin):** 0.3 mg, 0.45 mg, 0.625 mg, 0.9 mg, 1.25 mg.

## ADMINISTRATION/HANDLING

 **IV**

**Reconstitution** • Reconstitute with Sterile Water for Injection. • Slowly add diluent, shaking gently. • Avoid vigorous shaking.
**Rate of Administration** • Give slowly to prevent flushing reaction.
**Storage** • Refrigerate vials for IV use. • Use immediately following reconstitution.

**PO**
• Administer at same time each day.
• Give with milk, food if nausea occurs.

## 🔲 IV INCOMPATIBILITIES

No information available on Y-site administration.

## INDICATIONS/ROUTES/DOSAGE

**Vasomotor Symptoms Associated with Menopause**
PO: **ADULTS, ELDERLY:** (Premarin): 0.3 mg/day cyclically (21 days on, 7 days off) or continuously. (Enjuvia): 0.3 mg/day. May titrate up to 1.25 mg/day. (Cenestin): 0.45 mg/day. May titrate up to 1.25 mg/day.

**Vulvar and Vaginal Atrophy**
PO: **ADULTS, ELDERLY:** (Cenestin, Enjuvia, Premarin): 0.3 mg/day.
**Intravaginal: ADULTS, ELDERLY:** 0.5–2 g/day cyclically, such as 21 days on and 7 days off.

**Female Hypogonadism**
PO: **ADULTS:** (Premarin): 0.3–0.625 mg/day given either as 3 wks on/1 wk off or 25 days on/5 days off.

**Female Castration, Primary Ovarian Failure**
PO: **ADULTS:** (Premarin): Initially, 1.25 mg/day cyclically given either as 3 wks on/1 wk off or 25 days on/5 days off. Adjust dosage, upward or downward, according to severity of symptoms and pt response. For maintenance, adjust dosage to lowest level that will provide effective control.

**Postmenopausal Osteoporosis Prevention**
PO: **ADULTS, ELDERLY:** (Premarin): 0.3 daily or cyclically, such as 25 days on and 5 days off or 3 wks on and 1 wk off.

**Breast Cancer**
PO: **ADULTS, ELDERLY:** (Premarin): 10 mg 3 times/day for at least 3 mos.

**Prostate Cancer**
PO: **ADULTS, ELDERLY:** (Premarin): 1.25–2.5 mg 3 times/day.

**Abnormal Uterine Bleeding**
IV, IM: **ADULTS:** 25 mg; may repeat once in 6–12 hrs.

**Dyspareunia**
**Intravaginal: ADULTS, ELDERLY:** 0.5 g daily (21 days on, 7 days off).

**Dosage in Renal Impairment**
No dose adjustment.

**Dosage in Hepatic Impairment**
Contraindicated.

## SIDE EFFECTS

**Frequent:** Vaginal bleeding (spotting, breakthrough bleeding), breast pain/tenderness, gynecomastia. **Occasional:** Headache, hypertension, intolerance to contact lenses. **High doses:** Anorexia, nausea. **Rare:** Loss of scalp hair, depression.

## ADVERSE EFFECTS/ TOXIC REACTIONS

Prolonged administration may increase risk of breast, cervical, endometrial, hepatic, vaginal carcinoma; cerebrovascular disease, coronary heart disease, gallbladder disease, hypercalcemia.

### NURSING CONSIDERATIONS

#### BASELINE ASSESSMENT
Question for hypersensitivity to estrogen, hepatic impairment, thromboembolic disorders associated with pregnancy, estrogen therapy. Assess frequency/severity of vasomotor symptoms.

#### INTERVENTION/EVALUATION
Assess B/P periodically. Assess for edema; weigh daily. Monitor for loss of vision, diplopia, migraine, thromboembolic disorder, sudden onset of proptosis.

#### PATIENT/FAMILY TEACHING
• Avoid smoking due to increased risk of heart attack, blood clots. • Avoid grapefruit products. • Diet, exercise important part of therapy when used to retard osteoporosis. • Teach how to perform Homans' test, signs/symptoms of blood clots (report these immediately). • Promptly report signs/symptoms of thromboembolic, thrombotic disorders: sudden severe headache, shortness of breath, vision/speech disturbance, weakness/numbness of an extremity, loss of coordination; pain in chest, groin, leg. • Report abnormal vaginal bleeding, depression. • Teach female pts to perform breast self-exam. • Report weight gain of more than 5 lbs a wk. • Stop taking medication, contact physician if pregnancy is suspected.

# cosyntropin

koe-sin-**troe**-pin
(Cortrosyn)
**Do not confuse Cortrosyn with colchicine, cortisone, or Cotazym.**

## ◆CLASSIFICATION

**PHARMACOTHERAPEUTIC:** Adrenocortical steroid. **CLINICAL:** Glucocorticoid.

## USES

Diagnostic testing of adrenocortical function.

## PRECAUTIONS

**Contraindications:** Hypersensitivity to cosyntropin, corticotropin. **Cautions:** Preexisting allergies, history of allergic reaction to corticotropin.

## ACTION

Stimulates initial reaction in synthesis of adrenal steroids from adrenal cortex. **Therapeutic Effect:** Increases endogenous corticoid synthesis.

## ⚕ LIFESPAN CONSIDERATIONS

**Pregnancy/Lactation:** Unknown if distributed in breast milk. **Children/Elderly:** No age-related precautions noted.

## INTERACTIONS

**DRUG:** None significant. **HERBAL:** None significant. **FOOD:** None known. **LAB VALUES:** None significant.

## AVAILABILITY (Rx)

Powder for Injection: 0.25 mg. Injection, Solution: 0.25 mg/ml.

## ADMINISTRATION/HANDLING

**Reconstitution**

IM: • Reconstitute with 1 ml 0.9% NaCl. • Give as 0.25 mg/ml concentration. IV Push: • Dilute with 2–5 ml 0.9% NaCl over 2 min.

**Storage**

Powder: • Room temperature. Solution: • Refrigerate.

## INDICATIONS/ROUTES/DOSAGE

**Adrenocortical Insufficiency (Diagnostic Use)**

IM, IV: ADULTS, ELDERLY, CHILDREN OLDER THAN 2 YRS: 0.25–0.75 mg. CHILDREN 2 YRS AND YOUNGER: 0.125 mg. NEONATES: 0.015 mg/kg/dose.
IV Infusion: ADULTS, ELDERLY, CHILDREN OLDER THAN 2 YRS: 0.25 mg over 6 hrs at 0.04 mg/hr.

## SIDE EFFECTS

**Occasional:** Nausea, vomiting. **Rare:** Hypersensitivity reaction (fever, pruritus).

## ADVERSE EFFECTS/ TOXIC REACTIONS

None known.

## NURSING CONSIDERATIONS

### BASELINE ASSESSMENT

Hold cortisone, hydrocortisone, spironolactone the day prior to and the day of the test. Ensure that baseline plasma cortisol concentration has been drawn before start of test or 24-hr urine for 17-KS or 17-OHCS is initiated.

### INTERVENTION/EVALUATION

Adhere to time frame for blood draws; monitor urine collection if indicated.

### PATIENT/FAMILY TEACHING

• Explain procedure, purpose of test.

# crizotinib

kriz-o-ti-nib
(Xalkori)

## ◆CLASSIFICATION

**PHARMACOTHERAPEUTIC:** Tyrosine kinase inhibitor. **CLINICAL:** Antineoplastic.

## USES

Treatment of locally advanced or metastatic non–small-cell lung cancer (NSCLC) that is anaplastic lymphoma kinase (ALK) positive. Metastatic NSCLC in pts whose tumors are ROS1 positive.

## PRECAUTIONS

**Contraindications:** Hypersensitivity to crizotinib. **Cautions:** Baseline hepatic impairment, congenital long QT interval syndrome. Pregnancy (avoid use). Concomitant use of CYP3A4 inducers/inhibitors, medications known to cause bradycardia, renal impairment.

## ACTION

Inhibits receptor tyrosine kinases including anaplastic lymphoma kinase (ALK), hepatocyte growth factor receptors (HGFR, c-Met), receptor d'origine nantais (RON). **Therapeutic Effect:** Inhibits tumor cell proliferation and survival.

## PHARMACOKINETICS

Well absorbed after PO administration. Peak plasma concentration: 4–6 hrs. Protein binding: 91%. Metabolized in liver. Excreted in feces (63%) and urine (22%). **Half-life:** 42 hrs.

## ⧗ LIFESPAN CONSIDERATIONS

**Pregnancy/Lactation:** Avoid pregnancy. May cause fetal harm. Contraception should be considered during therapy and for at least 12 wks after discontinuation. Do not initiate therapy until pregnancy status confirmed. Unknown if crosses placenta or distributed in breast milk.

Nursing mothers must discontinue either nursing or drug therapy. **Children:** Safety and efficacy not established. **Elderly:** No age-related precautions noted.

## INTERACTIONS

**DRUG:** **Strong CYP3A inhibitors** including **atazanavir, clarithromycin, itraconazole, ketoconazole, ritonavir, saquinavir, voriconazole** may increase concentration. **Strong CYP3A inducers** including **carbamazepine, phenytoin, rifabutin, rifampin** may decrease concentration. May alter plasma levels of **alfentanil, cyclosporine, dihydroergotamine, ergotamine, fentanyl, pimozide, sirolimus. Proton pump inhibitors, H₂ blockers, antacids** may decrease solubility. May increase plasma levels of **colchicine, dexamethasone, doxorubicin, etoposide, non-nucleoside reverse transcriptase inhibitors, protease inhibitors, quinidine, tacrolimus, vinblastine.** **HERBAL:** **St. John's wort** may decrease effectiveness. **FOOD:** **Grapefruit products** may increase concentration/toxicity (potential for torsades, myelotoxicity). **LAB VALUES:** May increase serum ALT, AST, alkaline phosphatase, bilirubin. May decrease neutrophils, platelets, lymphocytes.

## AVAILABILITY (Rx)

Capsules: 200 mg, 250 mg.

## ADMINISTRATION/HANDLING

• May give without regard to meals.
• Avoid grapefruit products. • Do not break, crush, dissolve, or divide capsules.

## INDICATIONS/ROUTES/DOSAGE

**Non–Small-Cell Lung Cancer**
**(ALK Positive), Metastatic NSCLC, ROS-1 Positive**
**PO: ADULTS:** 250 mg twice daily. **Dosage Modification:** Interrupt and/or reduce to 200 mg twice daily based on graded protocol, including hematologic toxicity (grade 4), elevated LFT with bilirubin

elevation (grade 1), QT prolongation (grade 3). May reduce to 250 mg once daily if indicated. Discontinue treatment for QT prolongation (grade 4), elevated LFT with bilirubin elevation (grades 2, 3, 4), pneumonitis of any grade.

**Dosage in Renal Impairment**
**CrCl Less Than 30 ml/min:** 250 mg once daily.

**Dosage in Hepatic Impairment**
No dose adjustment (see dose for hepatotoxicity during treatment).

**Dosage Modification for Toxicity**
*Hematologic*
**Grade 3 toxicity (WBC 1,000–2,000 cells/mm³, ANC 500–1,000 cells/mm³, platelets 25,000–50,000 cells/mm³), grade 3 anemia:** Withhold treatment until recovery to grade 2 or less, then resume at same dosage. **Grade 4 toxicity (WBC less than 1,000 cells/mm³, ANC less than 500 cells/mm³, platelets less than 25,000 cells/mm³), grade 4 anemia:** Withhold treatment until recovery to grade 2 or less, then resume at 200 mg twice daily. **Grade 4 toxicity on 200 mg twice daily:** Withhold treatment until recovery to grade 2 or less, then resume at 250 mg once daily. **Recurrent grade 4 toxicity on 250 mg once daily:** Permanently discontinue.
*Cardiac*
**Grade 3 QTc prolongation on at least 2 separate EKGs:** Withhold treatment until recovery to baseline or grade 1 or less. Resume at 200 mg twice daily. **Recurrent grade 3 QTc prolongation on 200 mg twice daily:** Withhold treatment until recovery to baseline or grade 1 or less. Resume at 250 mg once daily. **Recurrent Grade 3 QTc prolongation on 250 mg once daily:** Permanently discontinue.
*Bradycardia*
**Grades 2 or 3:** Withhold until recovery to asymptomatic bradycardia or heart rate 60 or more beats/min, evaluate concomitant medications, then resume at 200 mg

twice daily. **Grade 4 due to crizotinib:** Permanently discontinue. **Grade 4 associated with concurrent medications known to cause bradycardia/hypotension:** Withhold until recovery to asymptomatic bradycardia or heart rate 60 or more beats/min, and if concurrent medications can be stopped, resume at 250 mg once daily.

*Pulmonary*

**Pulmonary toxicity:** Permanently discontinue.

## SIDE EFFECTS

**Frequent (62%–27%):** Diplopia, photopsia, photophobia, blurry vision, visual field defect, vitreous floaters, reduced visual acuity, nausea, diarrhea, vomiting, peripheral/localized edema, constipation. **Occasional (20%–4%):** Fatigue, decreased appetite, dizziness, neuropathy, paresthesia, dysgeusia, dyspepsia, dysphagia, esophageal obstruction/pain/spasm/ulcer, odynophagia, reflux esophagitis, rash, abdominal pain/tenderness, stomatitis, glossodynia, glossitis, cheilitis, mucosal inflammation, oropharyngeal pain/discomfort, bradycardia, headache, cough. **Rare (3%–1%):** Musculoskeletal chest pain, insomnia, dyspnea, arthralgia, nasopharyngitis, rhinitis, pharyngitis, URI, back pain, complex renal cysts, chest pain/tightness.

## ADVERSE EFFECTS/ TOXIC REACTIONS

Severe, sometimes fatal treatment-related pneumonitis, pneumonia, dyspnea, pulmonary embolism in less than 2% of pts was noted. Grades 3–4 elevation of hepatic enzymes, increased QT prolongation may require discontinuation. May cause thrombocytopenia, neutropenia, lymphopenia. Severe/worsening vitreous floaters, photopsia may indicate retinal hole, retinal detachment.

## NURSING CONSIDERATIONS

### BASELINE ASSESSMENT

Assess vital signs, $O_2$ saturation. Obtain baseline CBC with differential, serum chemistries, LFT, PT/INR, EKG. Question possibility of pregnancy or plans for breastfeeding. Obtain full medication history including vitamins, herbal products. Detection of ALK-positive NSCLC test needed prior to treatment. Assess history of tuberculosis, HIV, HF, bradyarrhythmias, electrolyte imbalance, medications that prolong QT interval. Assess visual acuity, history of vitreous floaters.

### INTERVENTION/EVALUATION

Assess vital signs, $O_2$ saturation routinely. Monitor CBC with differential monthly, LFT, monthly; increase testing for grades 2, 3, 4 adverse effects. Obtain EKG for bradycardia, electrolyte imbalance, chest pain, difficulty breathing. Monitor for bruising, hematuria, jaundice, right upper abdominal pain, weight loss, or acute infection (fever, diaphoresis, lethargy, oral mucosal changes, productive cough). Report decrease in RBC, Hgb, Hct, platelets, neutrophils, lymphocytes. Worsening cough, fever, or shortness of breath may indicate pneumonitis. Consider ophthalmological evaluation for vision changes. Reinforce birth control compliance.

### PATIENT/FAMILY TEACHING

• Blood levels will be drawn routinely. • Report urine changes, bloody or clay-colored stools, upper abdominal pain, nausea, vomiting, bruising, fever, cough, difficulty breathing. • Report history of liver abnormalities or heart problems including long QT syndrome, syncope, palpitations, extremity swelling. • Immediately report any newly prescribed medications, suspected pregnancy, or vision changes including light flashes, blurred vision, photophobia, or new or increased floaters. • Contraception recommended during treatment and for at least 3 mos after treatment. • Avoid alcohol, grapefruit products.

# cyanocobalamin (vitamin B$_{12}$)

sye-an-oh-koe-**bal**-a-min
(Nascobal)

## ◆ CLASSIFICATION

**PHARMACOTHERAPEUTIC:** Coenzyme.
**CLINICAL:** Vitamin, antianemic.

## USES

Treatment of pernicious anemia, vitamin B$_{12}$ deficiency due to malabsorption diseases, increased B$_{12}$ requirement due to pregnancy, thyrotoxicosis, hemorrhage, malignancy, hepatic/renal disease.

## PRECAUTIONS

**Contraindications:** Hypersensitivity to cyanocobalamin. Hereditary optic nerve atrophy. **Cautions:** Folic acid deficiency, anemia, premature neonates.

## ACTION

Coenzyme for metabolic functions (fat, carbohydrate metabolism, protein synthesis). **Therapeutic Effect:** Necessary for cell growth and replication, hematopoiesis, myelin synthesis.

## PHARMACOKINETICS

In presence of calcium, absorbed systemically in lower half of ileum. Initially, bound to intrinsic factor; this complex passes down intestine, binding to receptor sites on ileal mucosa. Protein binding: High. Metabolized in liver. Primarily eliminated unchanged in urine. Half-life: 6 days.

## ⓧ LIFESPAN CONSIDERATIONS

**Pregnancy/Lactation:** Crosses placenta. Distributed in breast milk. **Children/ Elderly:** No age-related precautions noted.

## INTERACTIONS

**DRUG:** None significant. **HERBAL:** None significant. **FOOD:** None known. **LAB VALUES:** None significant.

## AVAILABILITY (Rx)

**Injection Solution:** 1,000 mcg/ml. **Nasal Spray (Nascobal):** 500 mcg/spray. **Tablets:** 50 mcg, 100 mcg, 250 mcg, 500 mcg, 1,000 mcg. **Tablets (Extended-Release):** 1,000 mcg. **Tablets (Sublingual):** 2,500 mcg.

## ADMINISTRATION/HANDLING

**IM, Subcutaneous**
• Avoid IV route.

**PO**
• May give without regard to food.

**Intranasal**
• Clear both nostrils. • Pull clear cover off top of pump. • Press down firmly and quickly on pump's finger grips until a droplet of gel appears at top. Then press down on finger grips two more times. • Place the tip halfway into nostril, pointing tip toward back of nose. • Press down firmly and quickly on finger grips to release medication into one nostril while pressing other nostril closed. • Massage medicated nostril for a few seconds. • Administer nasal preparation at least 1 hr before or 1 hr after hot foods or liquids are consumed (hot foods can cause nasal secretion, resulting in loss of medication).

## INDICATIONS/ROUTES/DOSAGE

**Pernicious Anemia**
**IM, Subcutaneous: ADULTS, ELDERLY:** 100 mcg/day for 7 days, then every other day for 7 doses, then every 3–4 days for 2–3 wks. **Maintenance:** 100 mcg/mo (PO 1,000–2,000 mcg/day). **CHILDREN:** 30–50 mcg/day for 2 or more wks (to a total dose of 1,000–5,000 mcg). **Maintenance:** 100 mcg/mo. **NEONATES:** 0.2 mcg/kg for 2 days, then 1,000 mcg/day for 2–7 days. **Maintenance:** 100 mcg/mo.

**Vitamin Deficiency**
**IM, Subcutaneous: ADULTS, ELDERLY:** 100 mcg daily for 6–7 days; if improvement, 100 mcg q other day for 7 doses, then q3–4 days for 2–3 wks. **Maintenance:** 100 mcg monthly.

PO: **ADULTS, ELDERLY:** 1,000–2,000 mcg daily for 1–2 wks. **Maintenance:** 1,000 mcg daily.
**Intranasal: ADULTS, ELDERLY:** (NASCOBAL): 500 mcg in one nostril once wkly.

**Dosage in Renal/Hepatic Impairment**
No dose adjustment.

## SIDE EFFECTS

**Occasional:** Diarrhea, pruritus.

## ADVERSE EFFECTS/
## TOXIC REACTIONS

Impurities in preparation may cause rare allergic reaction. Peripheral vascular thrombosis, pulmonary edema, hypokalemia, HF occur rarely.

## NURSING CONSIDERATIONS

### BASELINE ASSESSMENT

Assess for signs, symptoms of vitamin $B_{12}$ deficiency (anorexia, ataxia, fatigue, hyporeflexia, insomnia, irritability, loss of positional sense, pallor, palpitations on exertion).

### INTERVENTION/EVALUATION

Assess for HF, pulmonary edema, hypokalemia in cardiac pts receiving subcutaneous/IM therapy. Monitor serum potassium, serum $B_{12}$, rise in reticulocyte count (peaks in 5–8 days). Assess for reversal of deficiency symptoms (hyporeflexia, loss of positional sense, ataxia, fatigue, irritability, insomnia, anorexia, pallor, palpitations on exertion). Therapeutic response usually dramatic within 48 hrs.

### PATIENT/FAMILY TEACHING

• Lifetime treatment may be necessary with pernicious anemia. • Report symptoms of infection. • Foods rich in vitamin $B_{12}$ include clams, oysters, herring, red snapper, muscle meats, fermented cheese, dairy products, egg yolks. • Use nasal preparation at least 1 hr before or 1 hr after consuming hot foods, liquids.

# cyclobenzaprine

sye-kloe-**ben**-za-preen
(Amrix, Apo-Cyclobenzaprine 🍁, Fexmid, Novo-Cycloprine 🍁)
**Do not confuse cyclobenzaprine with cycloserine or cyproheptadine, or Flexeril with Floxin.**

## ◆CLASSIFICATION

**CLINICAL:** Skeletal muscle relaxant.

## USES

Treatment of muscle spasm associated with acute, painful musculoskeletal conditions. **OFF-LABEL:** Treatment of muscle spasms associated with temporomandibular joint pain (TMJ).

## PRECAUTIONS

**Contraindications:** Hypersensitivity to cyclobenzaprine. Acute recovery phase of MI, arrhythmias, HF, heart block, conduction disturbances, hyperthyroidism, use within 14 days of MAOIs. **Cautions:** Hepatic impairment, history of urinary hesitancy or retention, angle-closure glaucoma, increased intraocular pressure (IOP), elderly.

## ACTION

Centrally acting skeletal muscle relaxant that reduces tonic somatic muscle activity at level of brainstem. **Therapeutic Effect:** Relieves local skeletal muscle spasm.

## PHARMACOKINETICS

| Route | Onset | Peak | Duration |
|-------|-------|------|----------|
| PO | 1 hr | 3–4 hrs | 12–24 hrs |

Well but slowly absorbed from GI tract. Protein binding: 93%. Metabolized in GI tract and liver. Primarily excreted in urine. **Half-life:** 8–37 hrs.

## ⌛ LIFESPAN CONSIDERATIONS

**Pregnancy/Lactation:** Unknown if drug crosses placenta or is distributed in breast milk. **Children:** Safety and efficacy not established. **Elderly:** Increased sensitivity to anticholinergic effects (e.g., confusion, urinary retention).

## INTERACTIONS

**DRUG: Alcohol, other CNS depressant medications** may increase CNS depression. **MAOIs** may increase risk of hypertensive crisis, seizures. **Tramadol** may increase risk of seizures. **HERBAL: Gotu kola, kava kava, SAMe, St. John's wort, valerian** may increase CNS depression. **FOOD:** None known. **LAB VALUES:** None significant.

## AVAILABILITY (Rx)

**Tablets:** 5 mg, 7.5 mg (Flexmid), 10 mg.
**Capsules (Extended-Release [Amrix]):** 15 mg, 30 mg.

## ADMINISTRATION/HANDLING

### PO

• Give without regard to food. • Do not break, crush, dissolve, or divide extended-release capsule. • Give extended-release capsule at same time each day.

## INDICATIONS/ROUTES/DOSAGE

◀ALERT▶ Do not use longer than 2–3 wks.

**Acute, Painful Musculoskeletal Conditions**
**PO: ADULTS, ELDERLY, CHILDREN 15 YRS AND OLDER:** Initially, 5 mg 3 times/day. May increase to 7.5–10 mg 3 times/day. **PO *(Extended-Release)*: ADULTS:** 15–30 mg once daily. Not recommended in elderly.

**Dosage in Renal Impairment**
No dose adjustment.

**Dosage in Hepatic Impairment**
**Note:** Extended-release capsule not recommended in hepatic impairment.
**Mild impairment:** 5 mg 3 times/day.

**Moderate to severe impairment:** Not recommended.

## SIDE EFFECTS

**Frequent (39%–11%):** Drowsiness, dry mouth, dizziness. **Rare (3%–1%):** Fatigue, asthenia, blurred vision, headache, anxiety, confusion, nausea, constipation, dyspepsia, unpleasant taste.

## ADVERSE EFFECTS/ TOXIC REACTIONS

Overdose may result in visual hallucinations, hyperactive reflexes, muscle rigidity, vomiting, hyperpyrexia.

# NURSING CONSIDERATIONS

### BASELINE ASSESSMENT

Record onset, type, location, duration of muscular spasm. Check for immobility, stiffness, swelling.

### INTERVENTION/EVALUATION

Assist with ambulation. Assess for therapeutic response: relief of pain; decreased stiffness, swelling; increased joint mobility; reduced joint tenderness; improved grip strength.

### PATIENT/FAMILY TEACHING

Avoid tasks that require alertness, motor skills until response to drug is established. • Drowsiness usually diminishes with continued therapy. • Avoid alcohol, other depressants while taking medication. • Avoid sudden changes in posture. • Sugarless gum, sips of water may relieve dry mouth.

---

**HIGH ALERT**

# cyclophosphamide

sye-kloe-**foss**-fa-mide
(Procytox ✦)
**Do not confuse cyclophosphamide with cyclosporine or ifosfamide.**

## ◆CLASSIFICATION

**PHARMACOTHERAPEUTIC:** Alkylating agent. **CLINICAL:** Antineoplastic.

✦ Canadian trade name  ⬛ Non-Crushable Drug  ⬛ High Alert drug

## USES

Treatment of acute lymphocytic, acute non-lymphocytic, chronic myelocytic, chronic lymphocytic leukemias; ovarian, breast carcinomas; neuroblastoma; retinoblastoma; Hodgkin's, non-Hodgkin's lymphomas; multiple myeloma; mycosis fungoides; nephrotic syndrome in children. **OFF-LABEL:** Treatment of adrenocortical, bladder, cervical, endometrial, prostatic, testicular carcinomas; Ewing's sarcoma; multiple sclerosis; non–small-cell, small-cell lung cancer; organ transplant rejection; osteosarcoma; ovarian germ cell, primary brain, trophoblastic tumors; rheumatoid arthritis; soft-tissue sarcomas; systemic dermatomyositis; systemic lupus erythematosus; Wilms' tumor.

## PRECAUTIONS

**Contraindications:** Hypersensitivity to cyclophosphamide. Urinary outflow obstruction. **Cautions:** Severe leukopenia, thrombocytopenia, tumor infiltration of bone marrow, previous therapy with other antineoplastic agents, radiation, renal/hepatic/cardiac impairment, active UTI.

## ACTION

Inhibits DNA, RNA protein synthesis by cross-linking with DNA, RNA strands. Cell cycle–phase nonspecific. **Therapeutic Effect:** Prevents cell growth. Potent immunosuppressant.

## PHARMACOKINETICS

Well absorbed from GI tract. Protein binding: 10%–60%. Crosses blood-brain barrier. Metabolized in liver. Primarily excreted in urine. Removed by hemodialysis. **Half-life:** 3–12 hrs.

## ⌛ LIFESPAN CONSIDERATIONS

**Pregnancy/Lactation:** If possible, avoid use during pregnancy. May cause fetal malformations (limb abnormalities, cardiac anomalies, hernias). Distributed in breast milk. Breastfeeding not recommended. **Children:** No age-related precautions noted. **Elderly:** Age-related renal impairment may require dosage adjustment.

## INTERACTIONS

**DRUG: CYP2D6 inducers (e.g., carbamazepine, phenobarbital)** may decrease concentration; **CYP2D6 inhibitors (e.g., paroxetine, amiodarone)** may increase concentration. **Anthracycline agents (e.g., doxorubicin, epirubicin)** may increase risk of cardiomyopathy. **CYP3A4 inhibitors (e.g., ketoconazole)** may increase concentration, risk of adverse effects. **Live virus vaccines** may potentiate virus replication, increase vaccine side effects, decrease pt's antibody response to vaccine. **HERBAL:** Pts with an estrogen-dependent tumor should avoid **black cohosh, dong quai. FOOD:** None known. **LAB VALUES:** May increase serum uric acid.

## AVAILABILITY (Rx)

**Capsules:** 25 mg, 50 mg. **Injection, Powder for Reconstitution:** 500 mg, 1 g, 2 g. **Tablets:** 25 mg, 50 mg.

## ADMINISTRATION/HANDLING

◀ **ALERT** ▶ May be carcinogenic, mutagenic, teratogenic. Handle with extreme care during preparation/administration.

 **IV**

**Reconstitution** • Reconstitute each 100 mg with 5 ml Sterile Water for Injection, 0.9% NaCl, or D₅W to provide concentration of 20 mg/ml. • Shake to dissolve. • Allow to stand until clear.
**Rate of Administration** • Infusion rates vary based on protocol. May give by direct IV injection, IV piggyback, or continuous IV infusion.
**Storage** • Reconstituted solution in 0.9% NaCl is stable for 24 hrs at room temperature or up to 6 days if refrigerated.

**PO**

• Give on an empty stomach. If GI upset occurs, give with food. • Do not cut or crush. • To minimize risk of bladder irritation, do not give at bedtime.

### 🔲 IV INCOMPATIBILITY

Amphotericin B complex (Abelcet, AmBisome, Amphotec).

### 🔲 IV COMPATIBILITIES

Granisetron (Kytril), heparin, hydromorphone (Dilaudid), lorazepam (Ativan), morphine, ondansetron (Zofran), propofol (Diprivan).

### INDICATIONS/ROUTES/DOSAGE

**Note:** Hematologic toxicity may require dose reduction.

**Usual Dosage (Refer to Individual Protocols)**
**IV: ADULTS, ELDERLY, CHILDREN:** (Single agent): 40–50 mg/kg in divided doses over 2–5 days or 10–15 mg/kg q7–10 days or 3–5 mg/kg twice wkly.
**PO: ADULTS, ELDERLY, CHILDREN:** 1–5 mg/kg/day.

**Nephrotic Syndrome**
**PO: ADULTS, CHILDREN:** 2 mg/kg/day for 60–90 days. **Maximum cumulative dose:** 168 mg/kg.

**Dosage in Renal/Hepatic Impairment**
No dose adjustment. Use caution.

### SIDE EFFECTS

**Expected:** Marked leukopenia 8–15 days after initiation. **Frequent:** Nausea, vomiting (beginning about 6 hrs after administration and lasting about 4 hrs); alopecia (33%). **Occasional:** Diarrhea, darkening of skin/fingernails, stomatitis, headache, diaphoresis. **Rare:** Pain/redness at injection site.

### ADVERSE EFFECTS/ TOXIC REACTIONS

Myelosuppression resulting in blood dyscrasias (leukopenia, anemia, thrombocytopenia, hypoprothrombinemia) has been noted. Expect leukopenia to resolve in 17–28 days. Anemia generally occurs after large doses or prolonged therapy. Thrombocytopenia may occur 10–15 days after drug initiation. Hemorrhagic cystitis occurs commonly in long-term therapy (esp. in children). Pulmonary fibrosis, cardiotoxicity noted with high doses. Amenorrhea, azoospermia, hyperkalemia may occur.

### NURSING CONSIDERATIONS

**BASELINE ASSESSMENT**

Obtain CBC wkly during therapy or until maintenance dose is established, then at 2- to 3-wk intervals.

**INTERVENTION/EVALUATION**

Monitor CBC, serum BUN, creatinine, electrolytes; urine output. Monitor WBC counts closely during initial therapy. Monitor for hematologic toxicity (fever, sore throat, signs of local infection, unusual bruising/bleeding from any site), symptoms of anemia (excessive fatigue, weakness). Recovery from marked leukopenia due to myelosuppression can be expected in 17–28 days.

**PATIENT/FAMILY TEACHING**

• Encourage copious fluid intake, frequent voiding (assists in preventing cystitis) at least 24 hrs before, during, after therapy. • Do not have immunizations without physician's approval (drug lowers resistance). • Avoid contact with those who have recently received live virus vaccine. • Promptly report fever, sore throat, signs of local infection, difficulty or pain with urination, unusual bruising/bleeding from any site. • Hair loss is reversible, but new hair growth may have different color, texture.

---

# *cycloSPORINE

sye-kloe-**spor**-in
(Apo-Cyclosporine ♦, Gengraf, Neoral, Restasis, Sandimmune)

■ **BLACK BOX ALERT** ■ Only physicians experienced in management of immunosuppressive therapy and organ transplant pts should prescribe. Renal impairment may occur with high dosage. Increased risk of neoplasia, susceptibility to infections. May cause hypertension, nephrotoxicity. Psoriasis pts: Increased risk of developing skin malignancies.

Do not confuse cyclosporine with cycloserine or cyclophosphamide, Gengraf with ProGraf, Neoral with Neurontin or Nizoral, or Sandimmune with Sandostatin.

## ◆ CLASSIFICATION

**PHARMACOTHERAPEUTIC:** Cyclic polypeptide. **CLINICAL:** Immunosuppressant.

## USES

Prevents organ rejection of kidney, liver, heart in combination with steroid therapy and/or azathioprine. Treatment of chronic allograft rejection in those previously treated with other immunosuppressives. **Capsules/solution:** Treatment of severe, active rheumatoid arthritis, severe recalcitrant plaque psoriasis in nonimmunocompromised adults. **Ophthalmic:** Chronic dry eyes. **OFF-LABEL:** Allogenic stem cell transplants for prevention/treatment of graft-vs-host disease; focal segmental glomerulosclerosis, lupus nephritis, severe ulcerative colitis.

## PRECAUTIONS

**Contraindications:** History of hypersensitivity to cyclosporine, polyoxyethylated castor oil; uncontrolled hypertension, renal impairment, or malignancies in treatment of psoriasis or rheumatoid arthritis.

**Cautions:** Hepatic/renal, impairment. History of seizures. Avoid live vaccines.

## ACTION

Inhibits cellular, humoral immune responses by inhibiting interleukin-2, a proliferative factor needed for T-cell activity. **Therapeutic Effect:** Prevents organ rejection, relieves symptoms of psoriasis, arthritis.

## PHARMACOKINETICS

Variably absorbed from GI tract. Protein binding: 90%. Metabolized in liver. Eliminated primarily by biliary or fecal excretion. Not removed by hemodialysis. **Half-life:** Adults, 10–27 hrs; children, 7–19 hrs.

## 🗵 LIFESPAN CONSIDERATIONS

**Pregnancy/Lactation:** Readily crosses placenta. Distributed in breast milk. Breastfeeding not recommended. **Children:** No age-related precautions noted in transplant pts. **Elderly:** Increased risk of hypertension, increased serum creatinine.

## INTERACTIONS

**DRUG: Allopurinol, bromocriptine, cimetidine, clarithromycin, danazol, diltiazem, oral contraceptives, erythromycin, fluconazole, ketoconazole** may increase concentration, risk of hepatic/renal toxicity. **Rifampin, carbamazepine, phenytoin** may decrease **cyclosporine** concentration. **ACE inhibitors, potassium-sparing diuretics, potassium supplements** may cause hyperkalemia. **Immunosuppressants** may increase risk of infection, lymphoproliferative disorders. **Lovastatin, simvastatin, atorvastatin, pravastatin** may increase risk of rhabdomyolysis. **Live virus vaccines** may potentiate virus replication, increase vaccine side effects, decrease pt's response to vaccine. May increase concentration/toxicity of **digoxin, colchicine. HERBAL:** Avoid **cat's claw, echinacea** (possess immunostimulant properties). **St. John's wort** may decrease plasma concentration. **FOOD: Grapefruit**

**products** may increase absorption/immunosuppression, risk of toxicity. **LAB VALUES:** May increase serum BUN, alkaline phosphatase, amylase, bilirubin, creatinine, potassium, uric acid, ALT, AST. May decrease serum magnesium. **Therapeutic peak serum level:** 50–400 ng/ml; **toxic serum level:** greater than 400 ng/ml.

## AVAILABILITY (Rx)

 Capsules (Gengraf, Neoral [Modified], Sandimmune [Nonmodified]): 25 mg, 50 mg, 100 mg. Injection, Solution (Sandimmune): 50 mg/ml. Ophthalmic Emulsion (Restasis): 0.05%. Oral Solution (Gengraf, Neoral [Modified], Sandimmune [Nonmodified]): 100 mg/ml.

## ADMINISTRATION/HANDLING

◀**ALERT**▶ Oral solution available in bottle form with calibrated liquid measuring device. Oral form should replace IV administration as soon as possible.

### IV

**Reconstitution** • Dilute each ml (50 mg) concentrate with 20–100 ml 0.9% NaCl or D₅W (**maximum concentration:** 2.5 mg/ml).
**Rate of Administration** • Infuse over 2–6 hrs. • Monitor pt continuously for hypersensitivity reaction (facial flushing, dyspnea).
**Storage** • Store parenteral form at room temperature. • Protect IV solution from light. • After diluted, stable for 6 hrs in PVC; 24 hrs in Excel or glass.

### PO

• Administer consistently with relation to time of day and meals. • Oral solution may be mixed in glass container with milk, chocolate milk, orange juice, or apple juice (preferably at room temperature). Stir well. • Drink immediately. • Add more diluent to glass container. Mix with remaining solution to ensure total amount is given. • Dry outside of calibrated liquid measuring device before replacing cover. • Do not rinse

with water. • Avoid refrigeration of oral solution (solution may separate). • Discard oral solution after 2 mos once bottle is opened.

### Ophthalmic

• Invert vial several times to obtain uniform suspension. • Instruct pt to remove contact lenses before administration (may reinsert 15 min after administration). • May use with artificial tears.

## ▦ IV INCOMPATIBILITIES

Acyclovir (Zovirax), amphotericin B complex (Abelcet, AmBisome, Amphotec), magnesium.

## ▦ IV COMPATIBILITY

Propofol (Diprivan).

## INDICATIONS/ROUTES/DOSAGE

### Transplantation, Prevention of Organ Rejection

**NOTE:** Initial dose given 4–12 hrs prior to transplant or postoperatively.
**PO: ADULTS, ELDERLY, CHILDREN: NOT MODIFIED:** Initially, 10–14 mg/kg daily for 1–2 wks, then taper by 5% each wk to maintenance dose of 5–10 mg/kg daily. **MODIFIED:** (dose dependent upon type of transplant): **Renal:** 6–12 mg/kg/day in 2 divided doses. **Hepatic:** 4–12 mg/kg/day in 2 divided doses. **Heart:** 4–10 mg/kg/day in 2 divided doses.
**IV: ADULTS, ELDERLY, CHILDREN:** Initially, 5–6 mg/kg/dose daily. Switch to oral as soon as possible.

### Rheumatoid Arthritis

**PO: ADULTS, ELDERLY: MODIFIED:**Initially, 2.5 mg/kg a day in 2 divided doses. May increase by 0.5–0.75 mg/kg/day after 8 wks with additional increases made at 12 wks. **Maximum:** 4 mg/kg/day.

### Psoriasis

**PO: ADULTS, ELDERLY: MODIFIED:**Initially, 2.5 mg/kg/day in 2 divided doses. May increase by 0.5 mg/kg/day after 4 wks; additional increases may be made q2wks. **Maximum:** 4 mg/kg/day.

**Dry Eye**
**Ophthalmic: ADULTS, ELDERLY:** Instill 1 drop in each affected eye q12h.

**Dosage in Renal Impairment**
Modify dose if serum creatinine levels 25% or above pretreatment levels.

**Dosage in Hepatic Impairment**
**Mild to moderate impairment:** No dose adjustment. **Severe impairment:** Use caution.

## SIDE EFFECTS

**Frequent (26%–12%):** Mild to moderate hypertension, hirsutism, tremor. **Occasional (4%–2%):** Acne, leg cramps, gingival hyperplasia (red, bleeding, tender gums), paresthesia, diarrhea, nausea, vomiting, headache. **Rare (less than 1%):** Hypersensitivity reaction, abdominal discomfort, gynecomastia, sinusitis.

## ADVERSE EFFECTS/
## TOXIC REACTIONS

Mild nephrotoxicity occurs in 25% of renal transplants, 38% of cardiac transplants, 37% of liver transplants, generally 2–3 mos after transplantation (more severe toxicity may occur soon after transplantation). Hepatotoxicity occurs in 4% of renal, 7% of cardiac, and 4% of liver transplants, generally within first mo after transplantation. Both toxicities usually respond to dosage reduction. Severe hyperkalemia, hyperuricemia occur occasionally.

## NURSING CONSIDERATIONS

### BASELINE ASSESSMENT

Obtain baseline serum chemistries, esp. renal function, LFT. If nephrotoxicity occurs, mild toxicity is generally noted 2–3 mos after transplantation; more severe toxicity noted early after transplantation; hepatotoxicity may be noted during first mo after transplantation.

### INTERVENTION/EVALUATION

Diligently monitor serum BUN, creatinine, bilirubin, ALT, AST, LDH levels for evidence of hepatotoxicity/nephrotoxicity (mild toxicity noted by slow rise in serum levels; more overt toxicity noted by rapid rise in levels; hematuria also noted in nephrotoxicity). Monitor serum potassium for evidence of hyperkalemia. Encourage diligent oral hygiene (gingival hyperplasia). Monitor B/P for evidence of hypertension. **Note:** Reference ranges dependent on organ transplanted, organ function, cyclosporine toxicity. Trough levels should be obtained immediately prior to next dose. **Therapeutic serum level:** 50–400 ng/ml; **toxic serum level:** greater than 400 ng/ml.

### PATIENT/FAMILY TEACHING

• Blood levels will be drawn routinely.
• Report severe headache, persistent nausea/vomiting, unusual swelling of extremities, chest pain. • Avoid grapefruit products (increases concentration/effects), St. John's wort (decreases concentration).

---

## *cytarabine*

sye-**tar**-a-bine
(Ara-C, Cytosar-U �, Depo-Cyt)
■ **BLACK BOX ALERT** ■ Must be administered by personnel trained in administration/handling of chemotherapeutic agents. *Conventional:* Potent myelosuppressant. High risk of multiple toxicities (GI, CNS, pulmonary, cardiac). *Liposomal:* Chemical arachnoiditis, manifested by profound nausea, vomiting, fever, may be fatal if untreated. **Do not confuse cytarabine with Cytoxan or vidarabine, or Cytosar with Cytoxan or Neosar.**

◆**CLASSIFICATION**

**PHARMACOTHERAPEUTIC:** Antimetabolite. **CLINICAL:** Antineoplastic.

## USES

**Ara-C:** Remission induction in acute myeloid leukemia (AML), treatment of acute lymphocytic leukemia (ALL) and chronic myelocytic leukemia (CML), prophylaxis and treatment of meningeal leukemia. **Depo-Cyt:** Treatment of lymphomatous meningitis. **OFF-LABEL: Ara-C:** Carcinomatous meningitis, Hodgkin's and non-Hodgkin's lymphomas, myelodysplastic syndrome.

## PRECAUTIONS

**Contraindications:** Hypersensitivity to cytarabine. (Liposomal): Active meningeal infection. **Cautions:** Renal/hepatic impairment, prior drug-induced bone marrow suppression.

## ACTION

Inhibits DNA polymerase. Cell cycle–specific for S phase of cell division. **Therapeutic Effect:** Appears to inhibit DNA synthesis. Potent immunosuppressive activity.

## PHARMACOKINETICS

Widely distributed; moderate amount crosses blood-brain barrier. Protein binding: 15%. Primarily excreted in urine. **Half-life:** 1–3 hrs.

## LIFESPAN CONSIDERATIONS

**Pregnancy/Lactation:** If possible, avoid use during pregnancy. May cause fetal malformations. Unknown if distributed in breast milk. Breastfeeding not recommended. **Children:** No age-related precautions noted. **Elderly:** Age-related renal impairment may require dosage adjustment.

## INTERACTIONS

**DRUG:** May decrease concentration of **digoxin, flucytosine. Live virus vaccines** may potentiate virus replication, increase vaccine side effects, decrease pt's response to vaccine. **HERBAL: Echinacea** may decrease therapeutic effect. **FOOD:** None known. **LAB VALUES:** May increase serum alkaline phosphatase, bilirubin, uric acid, AST.

## AVAILABILITY (Rx)

**Injection, Powder for Reconstitution (Ara-C):** 100 mg, 500 mg, 1 g. **Injection,**

**Solution (Ara-C):** 20 mg/ml, 100 mg/ml. **Injection, Suspension (Depo-Cyt):** 10 mg/ml.

## ADMINISTRATION/HANDLING

**◀ALERT▶** May give by subcutaneous, IV push, IV infusion, intrathecal routes at concentration not to exceed 100 mg/ml. May be carcinogenic, mutagenic, teratogenic (embryonic deformity). Handle with extreme care during preparation/administration. Depo-Cyt for intrathecal use only.

**IV, Subcutaneous, Intrathecal**

 **IV**

**Reconstitution • Ara-C:** Reconstitute with Bacteriostatic Water for Injection. • Dose may be further diluted with 250–1,000 ml D₅W or 0.9% NaCl for IV infusion. • For intrathecal use, reconstitute vial with preservative-free 0.9% NaCl or pt's spinal fluid. Dose usually administered in 5–15 ml of solution, after equivalent volume of CSF removed. • Depo-Cyt: No reconstitution required.
**Rate of Administration • Ara-C:** For IV infusion, give over 1–3 hrs or as continuous infusion.
**Storage • Ara-C:** Store at room temperature. • Reconstituted solution is stable for 48 hrs at room temperature. • Use diluted solution within 24 hrs. • Discard if slight haze develops. • Depo-Cyt: Refrigerate; use within 4 hrs following withdrawal from vial.

## IV INCOMPATIBILITIES

Amphotericin B complex (Abelcet, AmBisome, Amphotec), ganciclovir (Cytovene), heparin, insulin (regular).

## IV COMPATIBILITIES

Dexamethasone (Decadron), diphenhydramine (Benadryl), filgrastim (Neupogen), granisetron (Kytril), hydromorphone (Dilaudid), lorazepam (Ativan), morphine, ondansetron (Zofran), potassium chloride, propofol (Diprivan).

**C**

## INDICATIONS/ROUTES/DOSAGE

Usual Dosage for Induction
(Refer to Individual Protocols)
IV: **ADULTS, ELDERLY, CHILDREN: (Induction):** 100 mg/m$^2$/day continuous infusion for 7 days or 200 mg/m$^2$/day continuous infusion (as 100 mg/m$^2$ over 12 hrs q12h) for 7 days.
Intrathecal: **ADULTS, ELDERLY, CHIDREN:** Usual dose: 30 mg/m$^2$ q4 days. Range: 5–75 mg/m$^2$ daily for 4 days or once q4days until CNS findings normalize, followed by one additional treatment.

Usual Maintenance Dosage
IV: **ADULTS, ELDERLY, CHILDREN:** 70–200 mg/m$^2$/day for 2–5 days q mo.
Subcutaneous: **ADULTS, ELDERLY, CHILDREN:** 1–1.5 mg/m$^2$ as single dose q1–4wks.

Usual Dosage for Depo-Cyt
Intrathecal: **ADULTS, ELDERLY: (Induction):** 50 mg q14 days for 2 doses (wks 1, 3). **(Consolidation):** 50 mg q14 days for 3 doses (wks 5, 7, 9) followed by additional dose at wk 13. **(Maintenance):** 50 mg q28days for 4 doses (wks 17, 21, 25, 29).

Dosage in Renal/Hepatic Impairment
No dose adjustment.

## SIDE EFFECTS

**Frequent: IV, Subcutaneous (33%–16%):** Asthenia, fever, pain, altered taste/smell, nausea, vomiting (risk greater with IV push than with continuous IV infusion). **Intrathecal (28%–11%):** Headache, asthenia, altered taste/smell, confusion, drowsiness, nausea, vomiting. **Occasional: IV, Subcutaneous (11%–7%):** Abnormal gait, drowsiness, constipation, back pain, urinary incontinence, peripheral edema, headache, confusion. **Intrathecal (7%–3%):** Peripheral edema, back pain, constipation, abnormal gait, urinary incontinence.

## ADVERSE EFFECTS/ TOXIC REACTIONS

Myelosuppression resulting in blood dyscrasias (leukopenia, anemia, thrombocytopenia, megaloblastosis, reticulocytopenia) occurring minimally after single IV dose. Leukopenia, anemia, thrombocytopenia should be expected with daily or continuous IV therapy. Cytarabine syndrome (fever, myalgia, rash, conjunctivitis, malaise, chest pain), hyperuricemia may occur. High-dose therapy may produce severe CNS, GI, pulmonary toxicity.

## NURSING CONSIDERATIONS

### BASELINE ASSESSMENT

Obtain baseline CBC, renal function, LFT. Leukocyte count decreases within 24 hrs after initial dose, continues to decrease for 7–9 days followed by brief rise at 12 days, decreases again at 15–24 days, then rises rapidly for next 10 days. Platelet count decreases 5 days after drug initiation to its lowest count at 12–15 days, then rises rapidly for next 10 days.

### INTERVENTION/EVALUATION

Monitor BMP, LFT; serum uric acid. Monitor CBC for evidence of myelosuppression. Monitor for blood dyscrasias (fever, sore throat, signs of local infection, unusual bruising/bleeding from any site), symptoms of anemia (excessive fatigue, weakness). Monitor for signs of neuropathy (gait disturbances, handwriting difficulties, paresthesia).

### PATIENT/FAMILY TEACHING

• Increase fluid intake (may protect against hyperuricemia). • Do not have immunizations without physician's approval (drug lowers resistance). • Avoid contact with those who have recently received live virus vaccine. • Promptly report fever, sore throat, signs of local infection, unusual bruising/bleeding from any site.

# dabigatran

dab-i-**gah**-tran
(Pradaxa)

■ **BLACK BOX ALERT** ■ Risk of thrombotic events (e.g., stroke) increased if dabigatran discontinued for a reason other than pathological bleeding. Spinal or epidural hematoma may occur with neuraxial anesthesia.

## ◆CLASSIFICATION

**PHARMACOTHERAPEUTIC:** Thrombin inhibitor. **CLINICAL:** Anticoagulant.

## USES

Indicated to reduce risk of stroke, systemic embolism in pts with nonvalvular atrial fibrillation. Treatment and reduction of risk of deep vein thrombosis (DVT) and pulmonary embolism (PE). Prophylaxis of DVT and PE in pts who have undergone hip replacement surgery.

## PRECAUTIONS

**Contraindications:** Severe hypersensitivity to dabigatran. Active major bleeding, pts with mechanical prosthetic heart valves. **Cautions:** Renal impairment (CrCl 15–30 ml/min), moderate hepatic impairment, invasive procedures, spinal anesthesia, major surgery, pts with congenital or acquired bleeding disorders, elderly, concurrent use of medication that increases risk of bleeding, valvular heart disease.

## ACTION

Direct thrombin inhibitor that inhibits coagulation by preventing thrombin effects (e.g., inhibition of thrombin-induced platelet aggregation). **Therapeutic Effect:** Produces anticoagulation, preventing development of thrombus.

## PHARMACOKINETICS

Metabolized in liver. Protein binding: 35%. Eliminated primarily in urine. **Half-life:** 12–17 hrs.

## ⌛ LIFESPAN CONSIDERATIONS

**Pregnancy/Lactation:** Unknown if distributed in breast milk. **Children:** Safety and efficacy not established in pts younger than 18 yrs. **Elderly:** Severe renal impairment may require dosage adjustment.

## INTERACTIONS

**DRUG:** Rifampin may decrease concentration. **Antacids, proton pump inhibitors (e.g., omeprazole, pantoprazole)** may decrease level, effect. **Antiplatelet agents (e.g., aspirin, clopidogrel), NSAIDs, other anticoagulants, thrombolytics** may increase risk of bleeding. **HERBAL: Feverfew, ginkgo biloba, green tea, red clover** may increase risk of bleeding. **St. John's wort** may decrease concentration/effect. **FOOD: High-fat meal** delays absorption approximately 2 hrs. **LAB VALUES:** May increase aPTT, PT, INR.

## AVAILABILITY (Rx)

🍶 **Capsules:** 75 mg, 110 mg, 150 mg.

## ADMINISTRATION/HANDLING

**PO**
• May be given without regard to food. Administer with water. • Do not break, cut, open capsules.

## INDICATIONS/ROUTES/ DOSAGE

◀**ALERT**▶ Medication should be discontinued prior to invasive or surgical procedures.

**Treatment/Prevention of DVT/PE**
**PO: ADULTS, ELDERLY:** 150 mg twice daily (after 5–10 days of treatment with parenteral anticoagulants).

**Nonvalvular Atrial Fibrillation**
**PO: ADULTS, ELDERLY:** 150 mg twice daily.

**Prophylaxis following Hip Surgery**
**PO: ADULTS, ELDERLY:** 110 mg on day one (1–4 hr postoperative and established hemostasis), then 220 mg daily up to 35 days' duration.

---

✤ Canadian trade name     🍶 Non-Crushable Drug     🔲 High Alert drug

**Dosage in Renal Impairment (Nonvalvular Atrial Fibrillation)**
**CrCl 15–30 ml/min:** 75 mg twice daily.
**CrCl less than 15, or HD:** Not recommended (removes ~60% over 2–3 hrs).

**Dosage in Hepatic Impairment**
No dosage adjustment.

## SIDE EFFECTS

**Frequent (less than 16%):** Dyspepsia (heartburn, nausea, indigestion), diarrhea, upper abdominal pain.

## ADVERSE EFFECTS/ TOXIC REACTIONS

Severe, sometimes fatal, hemorrhagic events including intracranial hemorrhage, hemorrhagic stroke, GI bleeding may occur. Hypersensitivity reactions, including anaphylaxis, reported in less than 1% of pts.

## NURSING CONSIDERATIONS

### BASELINE ASSESSMENT

Obtain CBC (esp. platelet count), renal function test, PT, aPTT. Question history of mechanical heart valve, recent surgery; hepatic, renal impairment; recent spinal, epidural procedures.

### INTERVENTION/EVALUATION

Assess for any sign of bleeding (hematuria, melena, bleeding from gums, petechiae, bruising). Do not obtain B/P in lower extremities (possible deep vein thrombosis). Assess for decrease in B/P, increase in pulse rate, complaint of abdominal pain, diarrhea. Obtain aPTT, PT, platelet count. Question for increase in discharge during menses. Monitor for hematoma. Use care in removing any dressing, tape.

### PATIENT/FAMILY TEACHING

• Do not chew, crush, open, or divide capsules. • Use electric razor, soft toothbrush to prevent bleeding. • Report any sign of red or dark urine, black or red stool, coffee-ground vomitus, red-speckled mucus from cough. • Keep in original container. • Once bottle is opened, must be used within 60 days. • Open blister pack at time of use.

# dabrafenib

da-**braf**-e-nib
(Tafinlar)
**Do not confuse dabrafenib with dasatinib.**

## ◆CLASSIFICATION

**PHARMACOTHERAPEUTIC:** Kinase inhibitor. **CLINICAL:** Antineoplastic.

## USES

Treatment of unresectable or metastatic melanoma with BRAF V600E mutation as detected by FDA-approved test.
◀**ALERT**▶ Not indicated for treatment of wild-type BRAF melanomas.

## PRECAUTIONS

**Contraindications:** Hypersensitivity to dabrafenib. **Cautions:** Diabetes mellitus, hepatic/renal impairment, dehydration, glucose-6-phosphate dehydrogenase (G6PD) deficiency, pts at increased risk for arrhythmias.

## ACTION

Inhibits BRAF kinase gene mutation, a main cause of tumor cell growth, in the absence of growth factors that are normally required for proliferation. **Therapeutic Effect:** Inhibits tumor cell growth and metastasis.

## PHARMACOKINETICS

Readily absorbed after PO administration. Protein binding: 99.7%. Peak plasma concentration: 2 hrs. Metabolized in liver. Excreted in feces (71%), urine (23%). **Half-life:** 8 hrs.

## ⌛ LIFESPAN CONSIDERATIONS

**Pregnancy/Lactation:** Avoid pregnancy. May cause fetal harm. Must use effective nonhormonal contraception during treatment and for at least 4 wks after treatment (intrauterine device, barrier methods). Unknown if distributed in breast milk. Must either discontinue breastfeeding or discontinue therapy. **Children:** Safety and efficacy not established. **Elderly:** May have increased risk of adverse effects, skin lesions.

## INTERACTIONS

**DRUG: Antacids, H₂-receptors blockers (e.g., famotidine, ranitidine), proton pump inhibitors (e.g., omeprazole, pantoprazole)** may decrease concentration/effect. **CYP3A4 inducers (e.g., carbamazepine, phenytoin, rifampin)** may decrease concentration/effect. **CYP3A4 inhibitors (e.g., clarithromycin, gemfibrozil, ketoconazole)** may increase concentration. May decrease effectiveness of **hormonal contraceptives, warfarin. HERBAL:** St. John's wort may decrease concentration/effect. **FOOD: High-fat meals** may decrease absorption/effect. **LAB VALUES:** May increase serum glucose, alkaline phosphatase. May decrease serum phosphate, sodium.

## AVAILABILITY (Rx)

**Capsules:** 50 mg, 75 mg.

## ADMINISTRATION/HANDLING

**PO**

• Give at least 1 hr before or at least 2 hrs after meal. • Do not break, crush, open, or divide capsule. • Missed dose may be given up to 6 hrs prior to next dose.

## INDICATIONS/ROUTES/DOSAGE

**Metastatic Melanoma**

**PO: ADULTS/ELDERLY:** 150 mg twice daily (about 12 hrs apart) until disease progression or unacceptable toxicity.

**Dose Modification**

Based on Common Terminology Criteria for Adverse Events (CTCAE) grading 1–4.

| Reduction Levels | Dose |
|---|---|
| 1st dose reduction | 100 mg twice daily |
| 2nd dose reduction | 75 mg twice daily |
| 3rd dose reduction | 50 mg twice daily |

**Fever Greater Than 101.3°F or Any Grade 2 or Grade 3 Adverse Event**

Withhold until fever or adverse event resolves to grade 1 or less, then reduce dose by one level. May further decrease each dose level based on tolerability.

**Recurrent Grade 4 Adverse Event or 50-mg Dose Intolerability or Hemodynamic Instability**

Permanently discontinue.

**Dosage in Renal Impairment**

No dosage adjustment.

**Dosage in Hepatic Impairment**

**Mild to moderate impairment:** No dosage adjustment. **Severe impairment:** Use with caution.

## SIDE EFFECTS

**Frequent (37%–17%):** Hyperkeratosis, headache, pyrexia, arthralgia, alopecia, rash. **Occasional (12%–10%):** Back pain, cough, myalgia, constipation, nasopharyngitis, fatigue.

## ADVERSE EFFECTS/ TOXIC REACTIONS

Cutaneous squamous cell carcinoma (cuSCC) and keratocanthomas reported in 11% of pts (esp. elderly, prior skin cancer, chronic sun exposure). Skin reactions including palmar-plantar erythrodysesthesia syndrome (PPES), papilloma have occurred. May increase cell proliferation of wild-type BRAF melanoma or new malignant melanomas. Eye conditions including uveitis, iritis reported. Hyperglycemia reported in 6% of pts. Serious febrile drug reactions including hypotension, rigors, dehydration reported in 4% of pts. Pts with G6PD deficiency have increased risk of hemolytic anemia. Pancreatitis, interstitial nephritis, bullous rash reported in less than 10% of pts.

---

✦ Canadian trade name     Non-Crushable Drug     **HIGH ALERT** High Alert drug

## NURSING CONSIDERATIONS

### BASELINE ASSESSMENT

Obtain BMP, LFT, serum magnesium, phosphate, blood glucose level. Confirm presence of BRAF V600E mutation, negative urine pregnancy before initiating treatment. Assess skin for moles, lesions, papillomas. Baseline ophthalmologic exam, visual acuity. Question current breastfeeding status. Receive full medication history including herbal products.

### INTERVENTION/EVALUATION

Offer emotional support. Monitor serum electrolytes, blood glucose routinely. Obtain CBC if hemolytic anemia suspected. Monitor for signs of hyperglycemia. Assess for skin lesions every 2 mos during treatment and at least 6 mos after discontinuation. Immediately report any vision changes, eye pain/swelling, febrile events, renal impairment.

### PATIENT/FAMILY TEACHING

• Treatment may cause hair loss. • Do not breastfeed. • Avoid pregnancy; nonhormonal contraception should be used during treatment and up to 4 wks after last dose. • Take capsule at least 1 hr before or at least 2 hrs after meal. Swallow whole; do not chew, crush, open, or divide. • Report any increased urination, thirst, confusion, vision changes, eye pain, fever, skin changes including moles or lesions. • Minimize exposure to sunlight. • Males may experience a decreased sperm count. • Report any newly prescribed medications.

## daclatasvir

dak-**lat**-as-vir
(Daklinza)
**Do not confuse daclatasvir with ombitasvir, or Daklinza with Zolinza.**

### ◆CLASSIFICATION

**PHARMACOTHERAPEUTIC:** NS5A inhibitor. **CLINICAL:** Antiviral.

## USES

Treatment of chronic hepatitis C virus (HCV) genotypes 1 or 3 infection, in combination with sofosbuvir with or without riboflavin.

## PRECAUTIONS

**Contraindications:** Hypersensitivity to daclatasvir. Concomitant use of strong CYP3A inducers (e.g., phenytoin, carbamazepine, rifampin, St. John's wort). **Cautions:** Concomitant use of strong or moderate CYP3A inhibitors, moderate CYP3A inducers. Concomitant use of amiodarone is not recommended. History of bradycardia, bradyarrhythmias, cardiovascular disease, severe hepatic disease.

## ACTION

Inhibits NS5A, a nonstructural protein encoded by HCV. Binds to N-terminus of NS5A and inhibits both viral RNA replication and virion assembly. **Therapeutic Effect:** Inhibits viral replication of hepatitis C virus.

## PHARMACOKINETICS

Widely distributed. Metabolized in liver. Protein binding: 99%. Peak plasma concentration: 2 hrs. Eliminated in feces (88%), urine (7%). **Half-life:** 12–15 hrs.

## ⧗ LIFESPAN CONSIDERATIONS

**Pregnancy/Lactation:** Unknown if distributed in breast milk. **Children:** Safety and efficacy not established in pts younger than 18 yrs. **Elderly:** No age-related precautions noted.

## INTERACTIONS

**DRUG: Amiodarone, beta blockers (e.g., metoprolol)** may increase risk of symptomatic bradycardia. **Strong CYP3A inhibitors (e.g., clarithromycin, itraconazole, saquinavir), moderate CYP3A inhibitors (e.g., ciprofloxacin, diltiazem, fosamprenavir)** may increase concentration/effect. **Moderate CYP3A inducers (e.g., dexamethasone, efavirenz, nafcillin)** may decrease concentration/effect. May increase concentration/effect, anticoagulant effect of **dabigatran.** May increase concentration/effect of **digoxin.** May increase risk of myopathy, concentration/effects of **HMG-CoA reductase inhibitors (e.g., atorvastatin, simvastatin). HERBAL: St. John's wort** may decrease concentration/effect; use contraindicated. **FOOD: High-fat, high-caloric meal** may decrease absorption by 28%. **LAB VALUES:** May increase **serum lipase.**

## AVAILABILITY (Rx)

**Tablets:** 30 mg, 60 mg.

## ADMINISTRATION/HANDLING

**PO**
• Give without regard to meals.

## INDICATIONS/ROUTES/DOSAGE

**Note:** Cirrhotic pts with genotype 1a should undergo testing for presence of virus with NSA5A-resistance–associated polymorphisms.

**Chronic HCV Infection (Genotypes 1 and 3)**
**PO: ADULTS, ELDERLY:** 60 mg once daily, in combination with sofosbuvir, for 12 wks.

**Dose Modification**
*Concomitant Use of Strong CYP3A Inhibitors*
30 mg once daily, in combination with sofosbuvir, with or without riboflavin for 12 wks.
*Concomitant Use of Moderate CYP3A Inducers*
90 mg once daily, in combination with sofosbuvir, with or without riboflavin for 12 wks.
*Discontinuation*
If sofosbuvir is permanently discontinued, then daclatasvir should also be discontinued.
*Concomitant Use of Digoxin*
Consider decreasing digoxin dose by 30%–50% or use lowest dose possible to maintain adequate response.

**Dosage in Renal Impairment**
No dose adjustment.

**Dosage in Hepatic Impairment**
No dose adjustment. Safety and efficacy not established in pts with decompensated hepatic cirrhosis or liver transplant pts.

## SIDE EFFECTS

**Occasional (14%–8%):** Headache, fatigue, nausea. **Rare (5%):** Diarrhea.

## ADVERSE EFFECTS/TOXIC REACTIONS

Symptomatic bradycardia and some cases requiring pacemaker intervention have been reported when amiodarone is co-administered with sofosbuvir, in combination with another HCV direct-acting antiviral, including daclatasvir. Bradycardia generally occurred within hrs to days, but may extend up to 2 wks after initiation. Pts taking beta blockers (e.g., metoprolol), those with underlying cardiac disease, or pts with advanced hepatic disease are at increased risk of bradycardia when treated with amiodarone. Transient, asymptomatic elevations of serum lipase levels greater than 3 times upper limit of normal reported in 2% of pts.

## NURSING CONSIDERATIONS

### BASELINE ASSESSMENT
Obtain HCV-RNA level, LFT. Receive full medication history including herbal products and screen for contraindications/interactions, esp. concomitant use of amiodarone or digoxin. Confirm HCV genotype 3. Question history of bradycardia, arrhythmias. Assess hydration status.

### INTERVENTION/EVALUATION
Monitor HCV-RNA level, LFT as indicated. Pts requiring treatment with amiodarone should be monitored with a cardiac monitor in an inpatient setting for the first 48 hrs of initiation. Further outpatient monitoring or self-monitoring of the heart rate should occur on a daily basis for at least the first 2 wks of treatment. Due to the amiodarone's long half-life, pts discontinuing amiodarone just prior to starting sofosbuvir, in combination

with daclatasvir, should have similar cardiac monitoring as listed earlier. Immediately report symptoms of bradycardia.

**PATIENT/FAMILY TEACHING**

• There is an increased risk of drug interactions with other medications. • Do not take any new medications unless approved by physician. • Treatment with amiodarone, an antiarrhythmic drug, may increase the risk of a slow heartbeat and is not recommended during drug therapy. If taking amiodarone, seek immediate medical attention if chest pain, confusion, dizziness, fainting, lethargy, or shortness of breath occur after starting therapy. • Do not take herbal products, esp. St. John's wort. • Daclatasvir must be used in combination with sofosbuvir (an antiviral drug) and should not be used alone.

# daclizumab

dac-**klye**-zue-mab
(Zinbryta)

■ **BLACK BOX ALERT** ■ May cause severe, sometimes life-threatening, hepatic injury including hepatic failure and autoimmune hepatitis. Hepatic injury, including autoimmune hepatitis, may occur at any time during treatment and up to 4 mos after discontinuation. Contraindicated in pts with preexisting hepatic disease or impairment. Immune-mediated disorders including toxic skin reactions, lymphadenopathy, noninfectious colitis were reported. **Do not confuse daclizumab with certolizumab, eculizumab, efalizumab, natalizumab, tocilizumab, vedolizumab.**

## ◆CLASSFICATION

**PHARMACOTHERAPEUTIC:** Interleukin-2 receptor blocking antibody. **CLINICAL:** Multiple sclerosis agent.

## USES

Treatment of adult pts with relapsing forms of multiple sclerosis (MS). Therapy should generally be reserved for pts who have had an inadequate response to 2 or more medications indicated for the treatment of MS.

## PRECAUTIONS

**Contraindications:** Hypersensitivity to daclizumab; preexisting hepatic disease or impairment, including serum ALT or AST at least 2 times upper limit of normal (ULN), history of autoimmune hepatitis or other autoimmune disorders involving the liver. **Cautions:** History of chronic opportunistic infections (esp. fungal infections, viral infections, tuberculosis); history of autoimmune disorders (demyelinating polyneuropathy, Crohn's disease, Guillain-Barré syndrome, Hashimoto's thyroiditis, hyperthyroidism, myasthenia gravis, psoriasis, rheumatoid arthritis, systemic lupus erythematosus, type 1 diabetes, vasculitis); concomitant use of other immunosuppressants; conditions predisposing to infection (e.g., diabetes, kidney failure, open wounds), elderly, HIV infection, hematologic cytopenias; history of depression, suicidal ideation. Concomitant use of live vaccines not recommended during treatment and up to 4 mos after treatment. Avoid use during severe active infection.

## ACTION

Exact mechanism of action unknown. May involve modulation of interleukin-2 mediated activation of lymphocytes, reducing the number of lymphocytes available to CNS. **Therapeutic Effect:** May reduce lymphocyte migration into CNS, which reduces central inflammation.

## PHARMACOKINETICS

Widely distributed. Bioavailability: 90%. Degraded into small peptides and amino acids via catabolic pathway. Peak plasma concentration: 5–7 days. Elimination not specified. **Half-life:** 21 days.

## ⧖ LIFESPAN CONSIDERATIONS

**Pregnancy/Lactation:** Unknown if distributed in breast milk. Monoclonal antibodies are known to cross the placenta. **Children:** Safety and efficacy not established in pts younger than 17 yrs. **Elderly:** Not specified; use caution.

## INTERACTIONS

**DRUG:** None known. **Note:** Use caution with other hepatotoxic medications/supplements. **HERBAL: Echinacea** may decrease effect. **FOOD:** None known. **LAB VALUES:** May increase serum alkaline phosphatase, ALT, AST, bilirubin. May decrease absolute neutrophil count, Hgb, Hct, lymphocytes, RBC.

## AVAILABILITY (Rx)

**Injection Solution:** 150 mg/ml in prefilled syringe.

## ADMINISTRATION/HANDLING

### Subcutaneous

• 30 mins prior to injection, remove syringe from the refrigerator to allow to warm to room temperature. • Do not use external heat sources (e.g., hot water, heating plate). • Visually inspect for particulate matter or discoloration. • Solution should appear colorless to slightly yellow, clear to slightly opalescent in color. Discard if solution is cloudy or discolored or visible particles are observed. • If a dose is missed, inject missed dose as soon as possible if no more than 2 wks have passed. If more than 2 wks have passed, skip missed dose and administer the next dose on schedule.

### Administration

• Insert needle subcutaneously into upper arms, outer thigh, or abdomen and inject solution. • Do not inject into areas of active skin disease or injury such as sunburns, rashes, inflammation, skin infections, or active psoriasis. • Rotate injection sites.

### Storage

• Refrigerate until time of use. • If unable to refrigerate, may store protected from light at room temperature (no more than 30°C [86°F]) up to 30 days. • Do not place syringe back in refrigerator after allowing it to warm to room temperature. • Do not freeze.

## INDICATIONS/ROUTES/DOSAGE

### Multiple Sclerosis, Relapsing

**SQ: ADULTS:** 150 mg once monthly.

### Dose Modification
### Hepatic Impairment

**Serum ALT or AST greater than 5 times ULN; total serum bilirubin greater than 2 times ULN; serum ALT or AST 3 to less than 5 times ULN with total serum bilirubin 1.5 to less than 2 times ULN:** Withhold treatment and investigate for other etiologies of abnormal LFT values. If none are identified, discontinue treatment. If other etiologies are identified, use clinical judgment and consider if it is appropriate to resume treatment when both serum ALT or AST are less than 2 times ULN and total serum bilirubin is less than or equal to ULN. **Suspected autoimmune hepatitis:** Permanently discontinue.

### Immune-Mediated Disorders

**Dermatologic toxicity, serious diffuse or inflammatory rashes; lymphadenopathy, lymphadenitis; noninfectious colitis; other single-organ or multiorgan inflammatory events:** Consider interrupting treatment or permanent discontinuation.

### Other Toxicities

**Allergic reaction, anaphylaxis:** Permanently discontinue. **Severe depression, suicidal ideation:** Consider permanent discontinuation. **Infection:** Withhold treatment until infection fully resolved.

**Dosage in Renal Impairment**
Not specified; use caution.

## SIDE EFFECTS

**Occasional (11%–5%):** Rash, oropharyngeal pain, eczema. **Rare (3%–2%):** Acne, pyrexia, diarrhea, dry skin, erythema.

## ADVERSE EFFECTS/TOXIC REACTIONS

Serious, sometimes life-threatening, hepatic injury including autoimmune hepatitis may occur (less than 1% of pts). Serum ALT or AST elevation reported in 6% of pts. Infections occurred in up to 60% of pts. Respiratory tract infections including nasopharyngitis, upper respiratory tract infection, influenza, bronchitis, pharyngitis, tonsillitis, rhinitis, laryngitis, pneumonia reported in 29%–4% of pts. Dermatitis, folliculitis, skin exfoliation, toxic skin eruption may occur. Lymphadenopathy, lymphadenitis reported in 5%–2% of pts. Other immune-mediated disorders may include immune hemolytic anemia, glomerulonephritis, noninfectious colitis, pancreatitis, rheumatoid arthritis, sarcoidosis, sialadenitis thyroiditis. Depression occurred in 7% of pts. Severe hypersensitivity reactions, including anaphylaxis, angioedema may occur any time during treatment. Immunogenicity (auto-daclizumab antibodies) reported in 8%–19% of pts.

## NURSING CONSIDERATIONS

### BASELINE ASSESSMENT

Obtain baseline LFT, vital signs. Screen for hepatitis B and C virus infection; active infection. Pts should be evaluated for active tuberculosis and tested for latent infection prior to initiating treatment and periodically during therapy. Induration of 5 mm or greater with tuberculin skin testing should be considered a positive test result when assessing for latent tuberculosis infection. Antifungal therapy should be considered for pts who reside in or travel to regions where mycoses are endemic. Question history of autoimmune diseases (as listed in Precautions), depression or suicidal ideation, demyelinating disorders, HIV infection, prior hypersensitivity reactions. Conduct neurologic and dermatologic exam.

### INTERVENTION/EVALUATION

Monitor LFT monthly during treatment and for at least 6 mos after discontinuation. If autoimmune hepatitis is suspected or severe immune-mediated disorder occurs, consider referral to specialist; may require treatment with corticosteroids and other immunosuppressant agents. Monitor for symptoms of tuberculosis, including those who tested negative for latent tuberculosis infection at baseline. Interrupt or discontinue treatment if serious infection, opportunistic infection, or sepsis occurs and initiate appropriate antimicrobial therapy. Diligently monitor for depression or suicidal ideation, hepatotoxicity, hypersensitivity reaction (esp. anaphylaxis, angioedema), lymphadenopathy, noninfectious colitis, other immune-mediated disorders, reactivation of latent infection, toxic skin reactions. Assess neurologic status for symptom improvement. Assess skin for rash, lesions.

### PATIENT/FAMILY TEACHING

• Treatment may depress immune system and reduce ability to fight infection. Report symptoms of infection such as body aches, chills, cough, fatigue, fever. Avoid those with active infection. • Report travel plans to possible endemic areas. • Do not receive live vaccines during treatment and up to 4 mos following last dose. • Expect frequent tuberculosis screening. • Treatment may cause signs of a common cold or flu-like symptoms. • Allergic reactions such as difficulty breathing, hives, rash, swelling of the face or tongue, wheezing can happen at any time. If allergic reaction occurs, seek immediate medical attention. • Treatment may cause worsening of chronic autoimmune disorders; inflammatory disorders such as toxic skin reactions, inflammation of the lymph nodes or colon, or life-threatening inflammation of the liver. • Report abdominal pain, diarrhea, easy bruising, clay-colored stools, dark-amber urine, fatigue, loss of appetite, yellowing of skin or eyes; swelling or pain of lymph nodes. • Immediately report thoughts of suicide or worsening of depression.

# dalbavancin

dal-ba-van-sin
(Dalvance)
**Do not confuse dalbavancin with oritavancin or telavancin.**

## ◆CLASSIFICATION
**PHARMACOTHERAPEUTIC:** Glycopeptide. **CLINICAL:** Antibiotic.

## USES

Treatment of adult pts with acute bacterial skin and skin structure infections (ABSSSI) caused by susceptible strains of gram-positive microorganisms including *Staphylococcus aureus* (methicillin-susceptible and methicillin-resistant strains), *Streptococcus pyogenes*, *Streptococcus agalactiae*, and *Streptococcus anginosus* group (including *S. anginosus*, *S. intermedius*, *S. constellatus*).

## PRECAUTIONS

**Contraindications:** Known hypersensitivity reaction to dalbavancin. **Cautions:** Hepatic/renal impairment, chronic hepatitis, hx alcohol abuse, hx hypersensitivity reaction to glycopeptides (e.g., vancomycin), recent *Clostridium difficile* infection or antibiotic-associated colitis.

## ACTION

Inhibits cell wall synthesis by binding to bacterial cell membrane. **Therapeutic Effect:** Bactericidal.

## PHARMACOKINETICS

Widely distributed. Metabolism not defined. Protein binding: 93%. Primarily eliminated in urine. **Half-life:** 14.4 days.

## ⧖ LIFESPAN CONSIDERATIONS

**Pregnancy/Lactation:** Unknown if distributed in breast milk; use caution. **Children:** Safety and efficacy not established. **Elderly:** No age-related precautions noted.

## INTERACTIONS

**DRUG:** None known. **HERBAL:** None known. **FOOD:** None significant. **LAB VALUES:** May increase serum ALT, AST, bilirubin.

## AVAILABILITY (Rx)

**Injection, Powder for Reconstitution:** 500 mg.

## ADMINISTRATION/HANDLING
 IV

◄**ALERT**► Must be reconstituted with Sterile Water for Injection and subsequently diluted with 5% Dextrose Injection only.
**Reconstitution** • Reconstitute each 500 mg vial with 25 ml of Sterile Water for Injection for final concentration of 20 mg/ml. • To avoid foaming, alternate between gentle swirling and inversion of vial until completely dissolved. Do not shake. • Visually inspect for particulate matter. Solution should appear clear, colorless to yellow. Do not use if particulate matter observed. • Aseptically transfer required dose into 5% dextrose to a final concentration of 1–5 mg/ml.
**Rate of Administration** • Infuse over 30 min.
**Storage** • Store unused vials at room temperature. • Reconstituted vials/diluted bag may be refrigerated or stored at room temperature for up to 48 hrs. • Do not freeze.

---

◆ Canadian trade name     ▼ Non-Crushable Drug     ⬛ High Alert drug

## ▦ IV INCOMPATIBILITIES

Do not infuse with other medications or electrolytes. Saline-based solutions may cause precipitate formation. If using single IV access, flush IV with 5% dextrose before and after each use.

## INDICATIONS/ROUTES/DOSAGE

**Acute Bacterial Skin and Skin Structure Infection**
**IV: ADULTS/ELDERLY:** *(Two-Dose Regimen):* 1,000 mg once, followed by 500 mg once 7 days later. *(Single-Dose Regimen):* 1,500 mg.

**Dosage in Renal Impairment**
**CrCl less than 30 ml/min who are not receiving regularly scheduled hemodialysis:** *(Two-Dose Regimen):* 750 mg once, followed by 375 mg once 7 days later. *(Single-Dose Regimen):* 1,125 mg. **Pts receiving regularly scheduled hemodialysis:** No dose adjustment necessary.

**Dosage in Hepatic Impairment**
**Mild impairment:** No dose adjustment. **Moderate to severe impairment:** Not defined; use caution.

## SIDE EFFECTS

**Occasional (6%–4%):** Nausea, vomiting, diarrhea, headache. **Rare (3%–2%):** Rash, pruritus.

## ADVERSE EFFECTS/TOXIC REACTIONS

Serious hypersensitivity reactions including anaphylaxis or severe skin reactions have been reported with glycopeptide antibacterial agents. Too-rapid infusion may cause "red-man syndrome" reaction, characterizing by flushing of upper body, urticaria, pruritus, rash. *C. difficile–*associated diarrhea with severity ranging from mild diarrhea to fatal colitis has occurred. Drug-induced hepatotoxicity with hepatic enzymes greater than 3 times upper limit normal has been reported. Treatment in the absence of proven or strongly suspected bacterial infection may increase risk of drug-resistant bacteria.

## NURSING CONSIDERATIONS

### BASELINE ASSESSMENT

Obtain baseline CBC, BMP, LFT, wound culture and sensitivity, vital signs. Question history of recent *C. difficile* infection, hepatic/renal impairment, hypersensitivity reaction. Assess skin wound characteristics; hydration status. Question pt's usual stool characteristics (color, frequency, consistency).

### INTERVENTION/EVALUATION

Assess skin infection/wound for improvement. Monitor daily pattern of bowel activity, stool consistency; increasing severity may indicate antibiotic-associated colitis. If frequent diarrhea occurs, obtain *C. difficile* toxin screen and initiate isolation precautions until result confirmed. Encourage PO intake. Monitor I&O. Monitor for "redman syndrome" during infusion; stopping or slowing infusion may decrease reaction.

### PATIENT/FAMILY TEACHING

• It is essential to complete drug therapy despite symptom improvement. Early discontinuation may result in antibacterial resistance or increased risk of recurrent infection. • Report any episodes of diarrhea, esp. following weeks after treatment completion. Frequent diarrhea, fever, abdominal pain, bloodstreaked stool may indicate *C. difficile* infection, which may be contagious to others. • Report abdominal pain, black/tarry stools, bruising, yellowing of skin or eyes, dark urine, decreased urine output. • Do not breastfeed. • Drink plenty of fluids.

# dalfampridine

dal-**fam**-pri-deen
(Ampyra, Fampyra ✦)
**Do not confuse Ampyra with anakinra, or dalfampridine with desipramine.**

## ◆CLASSIFICATION

**PHARMACOTHERAPEUTIC:** Potassium channel blocker. **CLINICAL:** Multiple sclerosis agent.

## USES

Indicated to improve ambulation in pts with MS.

## PRECAUTIONS

**Contraindications:** Hypersensitivity to dalfampridine. History of seizures, moderate to severe renal impairment (CrCl equal to or less than 50 ml/min). **Cautions:** Mild renal impairment (CrCl equal to 51–80 ml/min).

## ACTION

Increases conduction of action potentials in demyelinated axons, inhibiting potassium channels. **Therapeutic Effect:** Improves ambulation in those with multiple sclerosis (MS).

## PHARMACOKINETICS

Rapidly absorbed from GI tract. Minimally metabolized in liver. Primarily excreted in urine. **Half-life:** 5.2–6.5 hrs.

## ⧗ LIFESPAN CONSIDERATIONS

**Pregnancy/Lactation:** Unknown if drug crosses placenta or is distributed in breast milk. **Children:** Safety and efficacy not established in pts younger than 18. **Elderly:** Age-related renal impairment may require dosage adjustment.

## INTERACTIONS

**DRUG:** None significant. **HERBAL:** None significant. **FOOD:** None known. **LAB VALUES:** May increase creatinine clearance.

## AVAILABILITY (Rx)

🌂 **Tablet, Film-Coated, Extended-Release:** 10 mg.

## ADMINISTRATION/HANDLING

**PO**
• May give without regard to food.
• Do not break, crush, dissolve, or divide tablets.

## INDICATIONS/ROUTES/DOSAGE

**Multiple Sclerosis**
**PO: ADULTS 18 YRS AND OLDER, ELDERLY:** 10 mg twice daily.

**Dosage in Renal Impairment**
**CrCl 50 ml/min or less:** Contraindicated.

**Dosage in Hepatic Impairment**
No dose adjustment.

## SIDE EFFECTS

**Frequent (9%–5%):** Insomnia, dizziness, headache, nausea, asthenia, back pain. **Rare (4%–2%):** Paresthesia, nasopharyngitis, constipation, dyspepsia, pharyngolaryngeal pain.

## ADVERSE EFFECTS/ TOXIC REACTIONS

Urinary tract infection occurs in 12% of pts.

## NURSING CONSIDERATIONS

### BASELINE ASSESSMENT

Obtain CBC, BUN, creatinine clearance, serum chemistries prior to treatment and routinely thereafter. Offer emotional support.

### INTERVENTION/EVALUATION

Monitor CBC, serum chemistries, renal function tests, particularly creatinine clearance. Monitor for urinary, respiratory infection. Assess for therapeutic response (improvement in walking as demonstrated by increase in walking speed).

✦ Canadian trade name       🌂 Non-Crushable Drug       🟥 High Alert drug

## PATIENT/FAMILY TEACHING

• Avoid tasks that require alertness, motor skills until response to drug is established. • Report difficulty in sleeping, dizziness, headache, nausea, back pain, loss of strength or energy. • Do not chew, crush, dissolve, or divide tablets.

---

## *dalteparin*

**HIGH ALERT**

**dal**-te-par-in
(Fragmin)
■ **BLACK BOX ALERT** ■ Epidural or spinal anesthesia greatly increases potential for spinal or epidural hematoma, subsequent long-term or permanent paralysis.

### ◆CLASSIFICATION

**PHARMACOTHERAPEUTIC:** Low molecular weight heparin. **CLINICAL:** Anticoagulant.

## USES

Prevention of ischemic complications in pts with unstable angina or non–Q-wave MI. Prevention of deep vein thrombosis (DVT) in pts undergoing hip replacement surgery, or abdominal surgery who are at risk for thromboembolic complications (e.g., pts older than 40 yrs, obese, pts with malignancy, history of DVT or PE, surgery requiring general anesthesia and lasting more than 30 min). Extended treatment of symptomatic venous thromboembolism (VTE) to reduce recurrence of VTE in cancer pts. Prevention of DVT or pulmonary embolism in acutely ill pts with severely restricted mobility.

## PRECAUTIONS

**Contraindications:** Active major bleeding; concurrent heparin therapy; hypersensitivity to dalteparin, heparin, pork products; unstable angina; history of heparin-induced thrombocytopenia; non–Q-wave MI; prolonged venous thromboembolism undergoing epidural/neuraxial anesthesia. **Cautions:** Conditions with increased risk for hemorrhage, bacterial endocarditis, renal/hepatic impairment, uncontrolled hypertension, history of recent GI ulceration/hemorrhage, peptic ulcer disease, pericarditis, preexisting thrombocytopenia, recent childbirth, concurrent use of aspirin.

## ACTION

Antithrombin in presence of low molecular weight heparin inhibits factor Xa, thrombin. Only slightly influences platelet aggregation, PT, aPTT. **Therapeutic Effect:** Produces anticoagulation.

## PHARMACOKINETICS

| Route | Onset | Peak | Duration |
|-------|-------|------|----------|
| Subcutaneous | N/A | 4 hrs | N/A |

Protein binding: less than 10%. **Half-life:** 3–5 hrs.

## ⏳ LIFESPAN CONSIDERATIONS

**Pregnancy/Lactation:** Use with caution, particularly during last trimester, immediate postpartum period (increased risk of maternal hemorrhage). Unknown if distributed in breast milk. **Children:** Safety and efficacy not established. **Elderly:** No age-related precautions noted.

## INTERACTIONS

**DRUG:** Anticoagulants, NSAIDs, platelet inhibitors (e.g., **clopidogrel**), thrombolytic agents may increase risk of bleeding. **HERBAL:** Cat's claw, dong quai, evening primrose, garlic, ginseng, other herbs with anticoagulant/antiplatelet activity may increase antiplatelet activity. **FOOD:** None known. **LAB VALUES:** May increase serum ALT, AST. May decrease serum triglycerides.

## AVAILABILITY (Rx)

**Injection, Solution:** 2,500 units/0.2 ml, 5,000 units/0.2 ml, 7,500 units/0.3 ml, 10,000 units/ml, 25,000 units/ml,

---

12,500 units/0.5 ml, 15,000 units/0.6 ml, 18,000 units/0.72 ml.

## ADMINISTRATION/HANDLING

**Subcutaneous**

• Visually inspect for particulate matter or discoloration. • Subcutaneously insert needle into abdomen, outer thigh, or upper arm region and inject solution. • Do not inject into areas of active skin disease or injury such as sunburns, rashes, inflammation, or infection. Rotate injection sites.

## INDICATIONS/ROUTES/DOSAGE

**Abdominal Surgery, Low to Moderate DVT Risk**

**SQ: ADULTS, ELDERLY:** 2,500 units 1–2 hrs before surgery, then daily for 5–10 days.

**Abdominal Surgery**

**SQ: ADULTS, ELDERLY:** *(Low DVT Risk):* 2,500 units 1–2 hrs before surgery, then daily for 5–10 days. *(High DVT Risk):* 5,000 units evening before surgery or 2,500 units 1–2 hrs before surgery, 2,500 units 12 hrs later, then 5,000 units daily for 5–10 days.

**Total Hip Surgery**

**SQ: ADULTS, ELDERLY:** 2,500 units 1–2 hrs before surgery, then 2,500 units 4–8 hrs after surgery, then 5,000 units/day (starting at least 6 hrs after postsurgical dose) for 7–10 days.

**Unstable Angina, Non–Q-Wave MI**

**SQ: ADULTS, ELDERLY:** 120 units/kg q12h for up to 5–8 days (**maximum:** 10,000 units/dose) given with aspirin. Discontinue dalteparin once clinically stable.

**Venous Thromboembolism (Cancer Pts)**

**SQ: ADULTS, ELDERLY:** Initially (1 mo), 200 units/kg (**maximum:** 18,000 units) daily for 30 days. **Maintenance (2–6 mos):** 150 units/kg once daily (**maximum:** 18,000 units). If platelet count 50,000–100,000/mm³, reduce dose by 2,500 units until platelet count recovers to 100,000/mm³ or more. If platelet count less than 50,000/mm³, discontinue until platelet count recovers to more than 50,000/mm³.

**Prevention of DVT, Acutely Ill Pt, Immobile Pt**

**SQ: ADULTS, ELDERLY:** 5,000 units once daily.

**Dosage in Renal Impairment**

For CrCl less than 30 ml/min, monitor anti-Xa levels to determine appropriate dose.

**Dosage in Hepatic Impairment**

No dose adjustment.

## SIDE EFFECTS

**Occasional (7%–3%):** Hematoma at injection site. **Rare (less than 1%):** Hypersensitivity reaction (chills, fever, pruritus, urticaria, asthma, rhinitis, lacrimation, headache); mild, local skin irritation.

## ADVERSE EFFECTS/ TOXIC REACTIONS

Overdose may lead to bleeding complications ranging from local ecchymoses to major hemorrhage. Thrombocytopenia occurs rarely.

## NURSING CONSIDERATIONS

**BASELINE ASSESSMENT**

Obtain baseline coagulation studies, CBC, esp. platelet count. Determine baseline B/P.

**INTERVENTION/EVALUATION**

Periodically monitor CBC, stool for occult blood (no need for daily monitoring in pts with normal presurgical coagulation parameters). Assess for any sign of bleeding (bleeding at surgical site, hematuria, blood in stool, bleeding from gums, petechiae, bruising/bleeding at injection sites).

• Usual length of therapy is 5–10 days. • Do not take any OTC medication (esp. aspirin) without consulting physician. • Report bleeding, bruising, dizziness, light-headedness, rash, itching, fever, swelling, breathing difficulty. • Rotate injection sites daily. • Teach proper injection technique. • Excessive bruising at injection site may be lessened by ice massage before injection.

# dantrolene

dan-troe-leen
(Dantrium, Revonto, Ryanodex)
■ **BLACK BOX ALERT** ■ Potential for hepatotoxicity.
**Do not confuse Dantrium with danazol or Daraprim, Revontro with Revatio.**

## ◆CLASSIFICATION

**CLINICAL:** Skeletal muscle relaxant.

## USES

**PO:** Relief of symptoms of spasticity due to spinal cord injuries, stroke, cerebral palsy, multiple sclerosis, esp. flexor spasms, concomitant pain, clonus, muscular rigidity. Management of malignant hyperthermia (MH), prevention of MH in susceptible individuals. **Parenteral:** Management of malignant hyperthermia. Prevention of malignant hyperthermia (preoperative/postoperative administration). **Ryanodex:** Treatment of malignant hyperthermia; prevention of malignant hyperthermia in pts at high risk. **OFF-LABEL:** Neuroleptic malignant syndrome.

## PRECAUTIONS

**Contraindications:** Hypersensitivity to dantrolene. **IV:** None known. **PO:** When spasticity used to maintain posture/balance during locomotion or to obtain increased motor function. Active hepatic disease. **Cautions:** Cardiac/pulmonary impairment, history of previous hepatic disease.

## ACTION

Acts directly on skeletal muscle by interfering with release of calcium ion. Reduces calcium ion concentration. **Therapeutic Effect:** Dissociates excitation-contraction coupling. Interferes with catabolic process associated with malignant hyperthermia.

## PHARMACOKINETICS

Poorly absorbed from GI tract. Protein binding: High. Metabolized in liver. Primarily excreted in urine. **Half-life: IV:** 4–8 hrs; **PO:** 8.7 hrs.

## ⧗ LIFESPAN CONSIDERATIONS

**Pregnancy/Lactation:** Readily crosses placenta. Breastfeeding not recommended. **Children:** No age-related precautions noted in pts 5 yrs and older. **Elderly:** No precautions specified.

## INTERACTIONS

**DRUG: CNS depressants** may increase CNS depression with short-term use. **Hepatotoxic medications** may increase risk of hepatic toxicity with chronic use. **CYP3A4 inhibitors (e.g., clarithromycin)** may increase concentration. **HERBAL: Gotu kola, kava kava, St. John's wort, valerian** may increase CNS depression. **FOOD:** None known. **LAB VALUES:** May alter serum ALT, AST.

## AVAILABILITY (Rx)

**Capsules (Dantrium):** 25 mg, 50 mg, 100 mg. **Injection, Powder for Reconstitution (Dantrium, Revonto):** 20-mg vial. **Injection Suspension (Ryanodex):** 250 mg powder.

## ADMINISTRATION/HANDLING

 IV

**Reconstitution** • Reconstitute 20-mg vial with 60 ml Sterile Water for Injection (**not** Bacteriostatic Water for Injection). *(Ryanodex):* 250 mg vial with 5 ml Sterile Water for Injection.

**Rate of Administration** • For therapeutic or emergency dose, give IV over 2–3 min. • For IV infusion, administer over 1 hr. • Diligently monitor for extravasation (high pH of IV preparation). May produce severe complications. *(Ryanodex):* Do not dilute; infuse into IV catheter or indwelling catheter.

**Storage** • Store at room temperature. • Use within 6 hrs after reconstitution. • Solution is clear, colorless. Discard if cloudy, precipitate forms.

**PO**
• Give without regard to food.

## ▨ IV INCOMPATIBILITIES

D₅W, 0.9% NaCl.

## INDICATIONS/ROUTES/ DOSAGE

**Spasticity**
**PO: ADULTS, ELDERLY:** Initially, 25 mg once daily for 7 days; then 25 mg 3 times/day for 7 days; then 50 mg 3 times/day for 7 days; then 100 mg 3 times/day. **Maximum:** 400 mg/day. **CHILDREN:** Initially, 0.5 mg/kg/dose once daily for 7 days; then 0.5 mg/kg/dose 3 times/day for 7 days; then 1 mg/kg/dose 3 times/day for 7 days; then 2 mg/kg/dose 3 times/day. **Maximum:** 400 mg/day.

**Perioperative Prophylaxis for Malignant Hyperthermic Crisis**
**PO: ADULTS, ELDERLY, CHILDREN:** 4–8 mg/kg/day in 3–4 divided doses beginning 1–2 days before surgery; give last dose 3–4 hrs before surgery.
**IV: ADULTS, ELDERLY, CHILDREN:** 2.5 mg/kg about 1.25 hrs before surgery with additional doses as needed.

**Management of Malignant Hyperthermic Crisis**
**IV: ADULTS, ELDERLY, CHILDREN:** Initially, a minimum of 2.5 mg/kg rapid IV; may repeat up to total cumulative dose of 10 mg/kg. May follow with 4–8 mg/kg/day PO in 4 divided doses up to 3 days after crisis. *(Ryanodex):* Minimum dose of 1 mg/kg. **Maximum:** 10 mg/kg (cumulative).

**Dosage in Renal/Hepatic Impairment**
No dose adjustment. Contraindicated with active hepatic disease.

## SIDE EFFECTS

**Frequent:** Drowsiness, dizziness, weakness, general malaise, diarrhea (mild). **Occasional:** Confusion, diarrhea (severe), headache, insomnia, constipation, urinary frequency. **Rare:** Paradoxical CNS excitement or restlessness, paresthesia, tinnitus, slurred speech, tremor, blurred vision, dry mouth, nocturia, impotence, rash, pruritus.

## ADVERSE EFFECTS/ TOXIC REACTIONS

Risk of hepatotoxicity, most notably in females, pts 35 yrs and older, pts taking other hepatotoxic medications concurrently. Overt hepatitis noted most frequently between 3rd and 12th mo of therapy. Overdose results in vomiting, muscular hypotonia, muscle twitching, respiratory depression, seizures.

## NURSING CONSIDERATIONS

### BASELINE ASSESSMENT
Obtain baseline LFT. Record onset, type, location, duration of muscular spasm. Check for immobility, stiffness, swelling.

### INTERVENTION/EVALUATION
Assist with ambulation. For pts on long-term therapy, hepatic/renal function tests, CBC should be performed periodically. Assess for therapeutic response: relief of pain, stiffness, spasm.

### PATIENT/FAMILY TEACHING
• Drowsiness usually diminishes with continued therapy. • Avoid tasks that require alertness, motor skills until response to drug is established. • Avoid alcohol/other depressants. • Report continued weakness, fatigue, nausea, diarrhea, skin rash, itching, bloody/tarry stools.

---

✦ Canadian trade name       🗡 Non-Crushable Drug       ▦ High Alert drug

# dapagliflozin

dap-a-gli-**floe**-zin
(Farxiga)
**Do not confuse dapagliflozin with canagliflozin or empagliflozin.**

## FIXED COMBINATION(S)

**Xigduo XR:** dapagliflozin/metformin (an antidiabetic): 5 mg/500 mg, 5 mg/1,000 mg, 10 mg/500 mg, 10 mg/1,000 mg.

## ◆CLASSIFICATION

**PHARMACOTHERAPEUTIC:** Sodium-glucose co-transporter 2 (SGLT2) inhibitor. **CLINICAL:** Antidiabetic agent.

## USES

Adjunctive treatment to diet and exercise to improve glycemic control in pts with type 2 diabetes mellitus.

## PRECAUTIONS

**Contraindications:** Hypersensitivity to dapagliflozin, other SGLT2 inhibitors; severe renal impairment, dialysis, end-stage renal disease. **Cautions:** Baseline hypotension, mild to moderate renal impairment, elderly, hypovolemia/dehydration (correct before initiating treatment), hx of genital mycotic infection. Not recommended in pts with active bladder cancer, diabetic ketoacidosis, type 1 diabetes mellitus. May be associated with ketoacidosis. Concurrent use of loop diuretics.

## ACTION

Increases excretion of urinary glucose by inhibiting reabsorption of glucose in kidneys by inhibiting SGLT2 in proximal renal tubule. **Therapeutic Effect:** Lowers serum glucose levels, Hgb A1c.

## PHARMACOKINETICS

Rapidly absorbed following PO administration. Metabolized in liver. Protein binding: 91%. Peak plasma concentration: 2 hrs. Eliminated in urine (75%), feces (21%). Unknown if removed by hemodialysis. **Half-life:** 12.9 hrs.

## ⌛ LIFESPAN CONSIDERATIONS

**Pregnancy/Lactation:** Unknown if distributed in breast milk. Must either discontinue drug or discontinue breastfeeding. **Children:** Safety and efficacy not established in pts younger than 18 yrs. **Elderly:** May have increased adverse effects related to renal impairment/volume depletion.

## INTERACTIONS

**DRUG:** None significant. **HERBAL: Fenugreek, garlic, ginkgo, ginger, ginseng** may increase hypoglycemic effect. **FOOD:** None known. **LAB VALUES:** May increase Hct, low-density lipoprotein cholesterol (LDL-C) levels; serum creatinine, phosphate. May decrease eGFR. Expected to decrease Hgb A1c; may yield positive urine glucose test.

## AVAILABILITY (Rx)

▧ **Tablets:** 5 mg, 10 mg.

## ADMINISTRATION/HANDLING

**PO**
• May give without regard to meals.

## INDICATIONS/ROUTES/DOSAGE

**Type 2 Diabetes Mellitus**
**PO: ADULTS/ELDERLY:** Initially, 5 mg once daily in the morning. May increase to 10 mg once daily.

**Dosage in Renal Impairment**
**Mild to moderate impairment (eGFR greater than 60 ml/min):** No dose adjustment necessary; use caution. **Severe impairment (eGFR less than 60 ml/min):** Avoid use. **Development of renal impairment during treatment:** Discontinue if eGFR is persistently less than 60 ml/min.

**Dosage in Hepatic Impairment**
No dose adjustment.

---

**Concomitant Use of Insulin or Insulin Secretagogue**

Consider lowering dose of insulin or insulin secretagogue to reduce risk of hypoglycemia.

### SIDE EFFECTS

**Occasional** (6%–3%): Nasopharyngitis, back pain, increased urination, nausea. **Rare** (2%): Constipation, extremity pain, discomfort with urination.

### ADVERSE REACTIONS/TOXIC EFFECTS

Orthostatic hypotension, postural dizziness, symptomatic hypotension, syncope, volume depletion may occur; pts who are elderly, use loop diuretics, or have baseline renal impairment have increased risk. Genital mycotic (yeast) infections occurred in 6% of pts; most reported cases were vulvovaginal infections in women and balanitis in men. Hypoglycemic events reported in 1.5% of pts (5% in elderly). Hypersensitivity reactions including anaphylaxis, angioedema (tongue/lip swelling), erythema, rash, pruritus, urticaria have occurred. Newly diagnosed bladder cancer occur rarely. Genitourinary infections including cystitis, kidney infection, prostatitis, pyelonephritis, trigonitis, urethritis, UTI occurred in 5.7% of pts.

### NURSING CONSIDERATIONS

#### BASELINE ASSESSMENT

Obtain capillary blood glucose, Hgb A1c, LDL-C, renal function test, urinalysis. Assess hydration status. Correct volume depletion prior to initiating treatment. Assess pt's understanding of diabetes management, routine home glucose monitoring. Receive full medication history including herbal products. Question history of co-morbidities, esp. hypersensitivity reaction, renal impairment, type 1 diabetes. Assess breastfeeding status.

#### INTERVENTION/EVALUATION

Monitor capillary blood glucose, Hgb A1c, renal function tests. Assess for hypoglycemia, hyperglycemia, mycotic infections. Screen for glucose-altering conditions: fever, increased activity or stress, trauma, surgery. Obtain dietary consult for nutritional education. Encourage PO intake. Monitor for hypotension. Monitor for hypersensitivity reaction such as dyspnea, urticaria, angioedema, dizziness.

#### PATIENT/FAMILY TEACHING

• Diabetes mellitus requires lifelong control. Diet and exercise are principal parts of treatment; do not skip or delay meals. • Test blood sugar regularly. • When taking combination drug therapy or when glucose demands are altered (fever, infection, trauma, stress), have low blood sugar treatment available (glucagon, oral dextrose). • Monitor daily calorie intake. • Report suspected pregnancy. Do not breastfeed. • Genital itching or discharge may indicate yeast infection. • Therapy may increase risk for dehydration/low blood pressure, esp. in pts who are elderly, on low-salt diet, have low blood pressure, or take water pills (diuretics). Drink plenty of fluids. • Report any decrease in urine output, dark-colored urine, painful urination, or flank pain. • Therapy may increase risk of bladder cancer; report any blood in urine or painful urination. • May rarely cause allergic reaction; report itching, hives, difficulty breathing, wheezing.

# *DAPTOmycin

**dap**-toe-mye-sin
(Cubicin)
**Do not confuse Cubicin with Cleocin, or daptomycin with dactinomycin.**

## ◆CLASSIFICATION

**PHARMACOTHERAPEUTIC:** Lipopeptide antibacterial agent. **CLINICAL:** Antibiotic.

### USES

Treatment of complicated skin/skin structure infections caused by susceptible strains of gram-positive pathogens, including *Staphylococcus aureus* (methicillin susceptible and methicillin resistant) [MRSA], *Streptococcus pyogenes, Streptococcus agalactiae.* Treatment of *S. aureus* systemic infections caused by methicillin-susceptible and -resistant *S. aureus.* **OFF-LABEL:** Severe infections caused by MRSA or Vancomycin-resistant *Enterococcus* (VRE); treatment of prosthetic joint infection caused by staphylococci or *Enterococcus.*

### PRECAUTIONS

**Contraindications:** Hypersensitivity to daptomycin. **Cautions:** Severe renal impairment (CrCl less than 30 ml/min), concurrent use of other medications associated with myopathy (e.g., statins).

### ACTION

Binds to bacterial membranes and causes rapid depolarization of membrane potential. Inhibits protein, DNA, RNA synthesis. **Therapeutic Effect:** Bactericidal.

### PHARMACOKINETICS

Widely distributed. Protein binding: 90%. Primarily excreted unchanged in urine. Moderately removed by hemodialysis. **Half-life:** 7–8 hrs (increased in renal impairment).

### LIFESPAN CONSIDERATIONS

**Pregnancy/Lactation:** Unknown if drug is distributed in breast milk. **Children:** Safety and efficacy not established in pts younger than 18 yrs. **Elderly:** No age-related precautions noted.

### INTERACTIONS

**DRUG:** Concurrent use with **HMG-CoA reductase inhibitors (e.g., simvastatin)** may cause myopathy. **HERBAL:** None significant. **FOOD:** None known. **LAB VALUES:** May increase CPK, serum potassium. May alter LFT results.

### AVAILABILITY (Rx)

**Injection, Powder for Reconstitution:** 500 mg/vial.

### ADMINISTRATION/HANDLING

 **IV**

**Reconstitution** • Reconstitute 500-mg vial with 10 ml 0.9% NaCl to provide a concentration of 50 mg/ml. May further dilute in 0.9% NaCl. • Do not shake or agitate vial.

**Rate of Administration** • For IV injection, give over 2 min (concentration: 50 mg/ml). • For intermittent IV infusion (piggyback), infuse over 30 min.

**Storage** • Refrigerate. • Appears as pale yellow to light brown lyophilized cake. • Reconstituted solution is stable for 12 hrs at room temperature or up to 48 hrs if refrigerated. • Discard if particulate forms.

### IV INCOMPATIBILITIES

Diluents containing dextrose. If same IV line is used to administer different drugs, flush line with 0.9% NaCl.

### IV COMPATIBILITIES

0.9% NaCl, Lactated Ringer's, aztreonam (Azactam), dopamine, fluconazole (Diflucan), gentamicin, heparin, levofloxacin (Levaquin).

### INDICATIONS/ROUTES/DOSAGE

**Complicated Skin/Skin Structure Infections**
**IV: ADULTS, ELDERLY:** 4 mg/kg every 24 hrs for 7–14 days.

**Systemic Infections**
**IV: ADULTS, ELDERLY:** 6 mg/kg once daily for 2–6 wks.

**Dosage in Renal Impairment**
**CrCl less than 30 ml/min, hemodialysis (HD), peritoneal dialysis (PD):** Dosage is 4 mg/kg q48h for skin and soft tissue infections; 6 mg/kg q48h for staphylococcal bacteremia. **Hemodialysis (HD):** Give dose after dialysis. **Continuous renal replacement therapy:** Continuous

Venovenous Hemodialysis (CVVHD): 8 mg/kg q48h, **Continuous Venovenous Hemofiltration (CVVH)** or Continuous Venovenous Hemodiafiltration **(CVVHDF):** 8 mg/kg q48h or 4–6 mg/kg q24h.

**Dosage in Hepatic Impairment**
No dose adjustment.

## SIDE EFFECTS

**Frequent (6%–5%):** Constipation, nausea, peripheral injection site reactions, headache, diarrhea. **Occasional (4%–3%):** Insomnia, rash, vomiting. **Rare (less than 3%):** Pruritus, dizziness, hypotension.

## ADVERSE EFFECTS/ TOXIC REACTIONS

Skeletal muscle myopathy (muscle pain/ weakness, particularly of distal extremities) occurs rarely. Antibiotic-associated colitis, other superinfections (abdominal cramps, severe diarrhea, fever) may result from altered bacterial balance in GI tract.

## NURSING CONSIDERATIONS

### BASELINE ASSESSMENT

Obtain CPK, blood cultures before first dose (therapy may begin before results are known).

### INTERVENTION/EVALUATION

Assess oral cavity for white patches on mucous membranes, tongue (thrush). Monitor for myopathy (muscle pain, weakness), CPK levels, renal function tests. Monitor daily pattern of bowel activity, stool consistency. Mild GI effects may be tolerable, but increasing severity may indicate onset of antibiotic-associated colitis. Be alert for superinfection: fever, vomiting, diarrhea, anal/genital pruritus, oral mucosal changes (ulceration, pain, erythema). Monitor for dizziness, institute appropriate measures.

### PATIENT/FAMILY TEACHING

* Report rash, headache, nausea, dizziness, constipation, diarrhea, muscle pain, or any other new symptom.

# daratumumab

dar-a-**toom**-ue-mab
(Darzalex)
**Do not confuse daratumumab with adalimumab, ofatumumab, panitumumab, or necitumumab.**

## ◆CLASSIFICATION

**PHARMACOTHERAPEUTIC:** Monoclonal antibody. **CLINICAL:** Antineoplastic.

## USES

Monotherapy for the treatment of pts with multiple myeloma who have received at least three prior lines of therapy including a proteasome inhibitor and an immunomodulatory agent or who are double-refractory to a proteasome inhibitor and an immunomodulatory agent. In combination for treatment of multiple myeloma in pts who have received at least one prior therapy.

## PRECAUTIONS

**Contraindications:** Hypersensitivity to daratumumab. **Cautions:** Obstructive pulmonary disorders (e.g., COPD, emphysema), baseline cytopenias, herpes zoster infection, elderly.

## ACTION

Binds to cell surface glycoprotein CD38 on CD38-expressing tumor cells. Inhibits tumor cell proliferation and induces apoptosis. **Therapeutic Effect:** Inhibits tumor cell growth and metastasis. Promotes tumor cell death.

## PHARMACOKINETICS

Widely distributed. Metabolism not specified. Steady state reached approx. 5 mos into the q4wk dosing period (by 21st infusion). Elimination not specified. **Half-life:** 18 ± 9 days.

## ⌛ LIFESPAN CONSIDERATIONS

**Pregnancy/Lactation:** Avoid pregnancy; may cause fetal harm/malformations.

---

*"Tall Man" lettering ◆ Canadian trade name 🛡 Non-Crushable Drug 🔴 High Alert drug

Monoclonal antibodies are known to cross the placenta. Females of reproductive potential should use effective contraception during treatment and up to 3 mos after discontinuation. Unknown if distributed in breast milk. However, human immunoglobulin G is present in breast milk. **Children:** Safety and efficacy not established. **Elderly:** No age-related precautions noted.

## INTERACTIONS

**DRUG:** None known. **HERBAL:** None significant. **FOOD:** None known. **LAB VALUES:** Drug may be detected on both serum protein electrophoresis and immunofixation assays used to monitor multiple myeloma endogenous M protein. May affect the determination of complete response and disease progression of some pts with immunoglobulin G kappa myeloma protein. May cause positive Coombs' test. Expected to decrease Hgb, Hct, lymphocytes, neutrophils, platelets, RBCs.

## AVAILABILITY (Rx)

**Injection Solution:** 100 mg/5 ml, 400 mg/20 ml.

## ADMINISTRATION/HANDLING

 IV

**Preparation for Administration** • Calculate the dose and number of vials required based on weight in kg. • Solution should appear colorless to pale yellow. Do not use if opaque particles, discoloration, or foreign particles are observed. • Remove a volume from the 0.9% NaCl infusion bag that is equal to the required volume of the dose solution. • Dilute in 1000 ml (first infusion) or 500 ml (subsequent infusions) 0.9% NaCl bag. • Mix by gentle inversion. Do not shake or agitate. • Infusion bags must be made of polyvinylchloride, polypropylene, polyethylene, or polyolefin blend. • Diluted solution may develop very small translucent to white proteinaceous particles; do not use if diluted solution is discolored or if visibly opaque or foreign particles are observed. • Discard used portions of vials.

**Infusion Guidelines** • Prior to administration, premedicate with an IV corticosteroid, acetaminophen, and an IV or oral antihistamine approx. 60 mins before each infusion (see manufacturer guidelines). • Infuse using an inline, sterile, nonpyrogenic, low-protein-binding polyethersulfone filter (0.22 or 0.2 μm). • Infuse via dedicated line using infusion pump. • Do not administer as IV push or bolus. • Infusion should be completed within 15 hrs. • If infusion cannot be completed for any reason, do not save unused portions for reuse. • Postinfusion, administer an oral corticosteroid on the first and second day after each infusion to reduce risk of delayed infusion reactions (see manufacturer guidelines). • In pts with a history of obstructive pulmonary disease, consider short-acting and long-acting bronchodilators and an inhaled corticosteroid postinfusion (may discontinue if no infusion reaction occurs after the first four infusions).

**Rate of Administration** • **First infusion (1000 ml volume):** Infuse at 50 ml/hr for the first 60 mins. Increase in increments of 50 ml/hr q1hr if no infusion reactions occur. **Maximum:** 200 ml/hr. • **Second infusion (500 ml volume):** Infuse at 50 ml/hr for the first 60 mins. Increase in increments of 50 ml/hr q1hr if there were no Grade 1 or greater infusion reactions during the first 3 hrs of first infusion. **Maximum:** 200 ml/hr. • **Subsequent infusions (500 ml volume):** Infuse at 100 ml/hr if there were no Grade 1 or greater infusion reactions during a final infusion rate of greater than or equal to 100 ml/hr in the first two infusions. Increase in increments of 50 ml/hr q1hr if tolerated. **Maximum:** 200 ml/hr.

**Storage** • Refrigerate unused vials. • Do not shake. • May refrigerate diluted solution up to 24 hr. • If diluted solution is refrigerated, allow solution to warm to room temperature before use. • Protect from light.

## ▧ IV INCOMPATIBILITIES

Do not mix with other medications.

## INDICATIONS/ROUTES/DOSAGE

**Multiple Myeloma**
**IV: ADULTS, ELDERLY: (Monotherapy or combination with Lenalidomide/dexamethasone) Wks 1–8:** 16 mg/kg once wkly. **Wks 9–24:** 16 mg/kg once q2wks. **Wk 25 and beyond:** 16 mg/kg once q4wks. **(Combination with bortezomib/dexamethasone) Wks 1–9):** 16 mg/kg once wkly. **Wks 10–24):** 16 mg/kg q3wks. **Wk 25 and beyond:** 16 mg/kg q4wks.

**Dose Modification**
**Infusion Reactions**
Promptly interrupt infusion if any reaction occurs.
**Grade 1 or 2 reaction:** Once symptoms resolve, resume infusion at a decreased rate that is 50% (or less) of previous rate. If no further reactions are observed, may increase infusion rate as appropriate.
**Grade 3 reaction:** If symptoms resolve to grade 2 or less, consider resuming infusion at a decreased rate that is 50% (or less) of previous rate. If no further reactions are observed, may increase rate as appropriate. If a grade 3 reaction recurs, decrease rate as outlined earlier. If grade 3 reaction occurs for a third time, permanently discontinue.
**Grade 4 reaction:** Permanently discontinue.

**Dosage in Renal Impairment**
No dose adjustment.

**Dosage in Hepatic Impairment**
**Mild impairment:** No dose adjustment.
**Moderate to severe impairment:** Not specified; use caution.

## SIDE EFFECTS

**Frequent (37%–14%):** Fatigue, back pain, nausea, pyrexia, cough, nasal congestion, arthralgia, diarrhea, dyspnea, decreased appetite, extremity pain, constipation, vomiting. **Occasional (12%–10%):** Headache, musculoskeletal chest pain, chills, hypertension.

## ADVERSE EFFECTS/TOXIC REACTIONS

Anemia, leukopenia, neutropenia, thrombocytopenia is an expected response to therapy. Infusion reactions occurred in approx. 50% of pts (mostly during first infusion). Infusion reactions can also occur with subsequent infusions (mainly during the infusion or within 4 hrs of completion). Severe infusion reactions may include cough, dyspnea, bronchospasm, hypertension, hypoxia, laryngeal edema, pulmonary edema, wheezing. Less common reactions may include chills, headache, hypotension, rash, nausea pruritus urticaria, vomiting. Infections including pneumonia, upper respiratory tract infection, nasopharyngitis reported in 20%–11% of pts. Herpes zoster reported in 3% of pts. Thrombocytopenia may increase risk of bleeding.

## NURSING CONSIDERATIONS

### BASELINE ASSESSMENT

Obtain CBC, blood type and screen; vital signs. Obtain pregnancy test in female pts of reproductive potential. Question history of COPD, emphysema, herpes infection; prior hypersensitivity reaction to any drug in treatment regimen; prior infusion reaction. Assess nutritional status. Screen for active infection. Offer emotional support.

### INTERVENTION/EVALUATION

Monitor CBC; vital signs periodically. Administer in an environment equipped to monitor for and manage infusion reactions. If infusion reaction of any grade/severity occurs, immediately interrupt infusion and manage symptoms. Accurately record characteristics of infusion reactions (severity, type, time of onset). Reactions may affect future infusion rates. To prevent herpes zoster reactivation in pts with prior history, consider antiviral prophylaxis within 1 wk of starting treatment and continue for 3 mos following discontinuation. Monitor for infection. Monitor daily pattern bowel activity, stool consistency.

**PATIENT/FAMILY TEACHING**

• Blood levels will be monitored periodically. • Treatment may depress your immune system and reduce your ability to fight infection. Report symptoms of infection such as body aches, chills, cough, fatigue, fever. Avoid those with active infection. • Avoid pregnancy. Do not breastfeed. • Severe infusion reactions can occur at any time. Immediately report symptoms of infusion reactions such as chills, cough, difficulty breathing, headache, hives, itching, nausea, rash, stuffy or runny nose, throat tightness, vomiting, wheezing.

---

# darbepoetin alfa  <sup>TOP 100</sup>

**dar**-be-poe-**e**-tin **al**-fa
(Aranesp)

■ **BLACK BOX ALERT** ■ Increased risk of serious cardiovascular events, thromboembolic events, mortality, time-to-tumor progression when administered to a target hemoglobin greater than 11 g/dL. Shortened overall survival and/or increased risk of tumor progression has been reported with breast, cervical, head/neck, NSCL cancers. **Do not confuse Aranesp with Aricept, or darbepoetin with dalteparin or epoetin.**

### ◆CLASSIFICATION

**PHARMACOTHERAPEUTIC:** Glycoprotein. **CLINICAL:** Hematopoietic agent.

## USES

Treatment of anemia associated with chronic renal failure (including pts on dialysis and pts not on dialysis), treatment of anemia caused by concurrent myelosuppressive chemotherapy in pts planned to receive chemotherapy for minimum of 2 additional months. **OFF-LABEL:** Treatment of symptomatic anemia in myelodysplastic syndrome (MDS).

## PRECAUTIONS

**Contraindications:** Hypersensitivity to darbepoetin. Pure red cell aplasia, uncontrolled hypertension. **Cautions:** History of seizures, hypertension. Not recommended in pts with mild to moderate anemia and HF or CAD.

## ACTION

Stimulates formation of RBCs in bone marrow. **Therapeutic Effect:** Induces erythropoiesis, release of reticulocytes from bone marrow into bloodstream.

## PHARMACOKINETICS

Well absorbed after subcutaneous administration. **Half-life:** 48.5 hrs.

## ⧗ LIFESPAN CONSIDERATIONS

**Pregnancy/Lactation:** Unknown if drug crosses placenta or is distributed in breast milk. **Children:** Safety and efficacy not established. **Elderly:** Age-related renal impairment may require dosage adjustment.

## INTERACTIONS

**DRUG:** None significant. **HERBAL:** None significant. **FOOD:** None known. **LAB VALUES:** May decrease serum ferritin, serum transferrin saturation.

## AVAILABILITY (Rx)

**Injection Solution:** 25 mcg/ml, 40 mcg/ml, 60 mcg/ml, 100 mcg/ml, 150 mcg/0.75 ml, 200 mcg/ml, 300 mcg/ml. **Prefilled Syringe:** 25 mcg/0.42 ml, 40 mcg/0.4 ml, 60 mcg/0.3 ml, 100 mcg/0.5 ml, 150 mcg/0.3 ml, 200 mcg/0.4 ml, 300 mcg/0.6 ml, 500 mcg/ml.

## ADMINISTRATION/HANDLING

◄**ALERT**► Avoid excessive agitation of vial; do not shake (will cause foaming).

**IV**

**Reconstitution** • No reconstitution necessary. Do not dilute.

**Rate of Administration** • May be given as IV bolus.

**Storage** • Refrigerate. • Do not shake. Vigorous shaking may denature medication, rendering it inactive.

**Subcutaneous**

• Use 1 dose per vial; do not reenter vial. Discard unused portion.

## ▨ IV INCOMPATIBILITIES

Do not mix with other medications.

## INDICATIONS/ROUTES/DOSAGE

**Anemia in Chronic Renal Failure**

◀ALERT▶ Individualize dosing and use lowest dose to reduce need for RBC transfusions. **ON DIALYSIS:** Initiate when Hgb less than 10 g/dL; reduce or stop dose when Hgb approaches or exceeds 11 g/dL. **NOT ON DIALYSIS:** Initiate when Hgb less than 10 g/dL and Hgb decline would likely result in RBC transfusion; reduce dose or stop if Hgb exceeds 10 g/dL.

**IV, SQ: ADULTS, ELDERLY: ON DIALYSIS:** Initially, 0.45 mcg/kg once wkly or 0.75 mcg/kg once q2wks. **NOT ON DIALYSIS:** 0.45 mcg/kg q4wks.

*Decrease dose by 25%:* If Hgb approaches 12 g/dL or increases greater than 1 g/dL in any 2-wk period.

*Increase dose by 25%:* If Hgb does not increase by 1 g/dL after 4 wks of therapy and Hgb is below target range (with adequate iron stores), do not increase dose more frequently than every 4 wks.

**Note:** If pt does not attain Hgb range of 10–12 g/dL after appropriate dosing over 12 wks, do not increase dose and use minimum effective dose to maintain Hgb level that will avoid red blood cell transfusions. Discontinue treatment if responsiveness does not improve.

**Anemia Associated with Chemotherapy**

◀ALERT▶ Initiate only if Hgb less than 10 g/dL and anticipated duration of myelosuppression is 2 months or longer. Titrate dose to maintain Hgb level and avoid RBC transfusions. Discontinue upon completion of chemotherapy.

**SQ: ADULTS, ELDERLY:** 2.25 mcg/kg once wkly or 500 mcg every 3 wks.

*Increase dose:* If Hgb does not increase by 1 g/dL after 6 wks and Hgb is below target range, increase dose to 4.5 mcg/kg once wkly. No dose adjustment if using q3wk dosing.

*Decrease dose:* Decrease dose by 40% if Hgb increases greater than 1 g/dL in any 2-wk period or Hgb reaches level that will avoid red blood cell transfusions. **Note:** Withhold dose when Hgb exceeds a level needed to avoid RBC transfusions, resume at dose 40% lower when Hgb approaches a level where transfusions may be required.

**Dosage in Renal/Hepatic Impairment**

No dose adjustment.

## SIDE EFFECTS

**Frequent:** Myalgia, hypertension/hypotension, headache, diarrhea. **Occasional:** Fatigue, edema, vomiting, reaction at injection site, asthenia, dizziness.

## ADVERSE EFFECTS/ TOXIC REACTIONS

Vascular access thrombosis, HF, sepsis, arrhythmias, anaphylactic reaction occur rarely.

## NURSING CONSIDERATIONS

### BASELINE ASSESSMENT

Establish baseline CBC (esp. note Hgb, Hct). Assess B/P before drug administration. B/P often rises during early therapy in pts with history of hypertension. Assess serum iron (transferrin saturation should be greater than 20%), serum ferritin (greater than 100 ng/ml) before and during therapy. Consider supplemental iron therapy.

## INTERVENTION/EVALUATION

Monitor serum ferritin, CBC, serum creatinine, BUN, potassium, phosphorus; reticulocyte count. Monitor B/P aggressively for increase (25% of pts taking medication require antihypertension therapy, dietary restrictions).

## PATIENT/FAMILY TEACHING

• Frequent blood tests needed to determine correct dose. • Report swollen extremities, breathing difficulty, extreme fatigue, or severe headache. • Avoid tasks requiring alertness, motor skills until response to drug is established.

# darifenacin

dare-i-**fen**-a-sin
(Enablex)

## ◆CLASSIFICATION

**PHARMACOTHERAPEUTIC:** Muscarinic receptor antagonist. **CLINICAL:** Urinary antispasmodic.

## USES

Management of symptoms of bladder overactivity (urge incontinence, urinary urgency/frequency).

## PRECAUTIONS

**Contraindications:** Hypersensitivity to darifenacin. Uncontrolled narrow-angle glaucoma, paralytic ileus, GI/GU obstruction, urine retention. **Cautions:** Bladder outflow obstruction, hepatic impairment, nonobstructive prostatic hyperplasia, decreased GI motility, constipation, hiatal hernia, reflux esophagitis, ulcerative colitis, controlled narrow-angle glaucoma, myasthenia gravis, concurrent use of strong CYP3A4 inhibitors. Hot weather and/or exercise.

## ACTION

Acts as a direct antagonist at muscarinic receptor sites in cholinergically innervated organs; limits bladder contractions.

**Therapeutic Effect:** Reduces symptoms of bladder irritability/overactivity (urge incontinence, urinary urgency/frequency), improves bladder capacity.

## PHARMACOKINETICS

Well absorbed following PO administration. Protein binding: 98%. Metabolized in liver. Excreted in urine (60%), feces (40%). **Half-life:** 13–19 hrs.

## ⌛ LIFESPAN CONSIDERATIONS

**Pregnancy/Lactation:** Unknown if drug crosses placenta or is distributed in breast milk. **Children:** Safety and efficacy not established. **Elderly:** No age-related precautions noted.

## INTERACTIONS

**DRUG:** CYP3A4 inhibitors (**clarithromycin, erythromycin, protease inhibitors**) may increase concentration/effects. **Anticholinergics** may increase side effects (e.g., dry mouth, constipation). **HERBAL:** St. John's wort may decrease concentration/effects. **FOOD:** None known. **LAB VALUES:** None known.

## AVAILABILITY (Rx)

Tablets (Extended-Release): 7.5 mg, 15 mg.

## ADMINISTRATION/HANDLING

**PO**
• Give without regard to food. • Administer extended-release tablets whole; do not break, crush, dissolve, or divide tablet.

## INDICATIONS/ROUTES/DOSAGE

**Overactive Bladder**
**PO: ADULTS, ELDERLY:** Initially, 7.5 mg once daily. If response is not adequate after at least 2 wks, may increase to 15 mg once daily. Do not exceed 7.5 mg once daily in moderate hepatic impairment or concurrent use with CYP3A4 inhibitors (e.g., clarithromycin, fluconazole, protease inhibitors).

**Dosage in Renal Impairment**
No dose adjustment.

**Dosage Hepatic Impairment**
**Moderate impairment:** Maximum dose: 7.5 mg. **Severe impairment:** Not recommended.

## SIDE EFFECTS

**Frequent (35%–21%):** Dry mouth, constipation. **Occasional (8%–4%):** Dyspepsia, headache, nausea, abdominal pain. **Rare (3%–2%):** Asthenia, diarrhea, dizziness, ocular dryness.

## ADVERSE EFFECTS/ TOXIC REACTIONS

UTI occurs occasionally.

## NURSING CONSIDERATIONS

### BASELINE ASSESSMENT

Monitor voiding pattern, assess signs/symptoms of overactive bladder prior to therapy as baseline.

### INTERVENTION/EVALUATION

Monitor I&O. Palpate bladder for urine retention. Monitor daily pattern of bowel activity, stool consistency for evidence of constipation. Dry mouth may be relieved with sips of water. Assess for relief of symptoms of overactive bladder (urge incontinence, urinary frequency/urgency).

### PATIENT/FAMILY TEACHING

• Swallow tablet whole; do not chew, crush, dissolve, or divide. • Increase fluid intake to reduce risk of constipation. • Avoid tasks that require alertness, motor skills until response to drug is established.

# darunavir TOP 100

dar-**ue**-na-veer
(Prezista)

## FIXED COMBINATION(S)

**Prezcobix:** Darunavir/cobicistat (antiretroviral booster): 800 mg/150 mg.

## ◆CLASSIFICATION

**PHARMACOTHERAPEUTIC:** Protease inhibitor. **CLINICAL:** Antiretroviral.

## USES

Treatment of HIV infection in combination with ritonavir and other antiretroviral agents in adults and children 3 yrs and older.

## PRECAUTIONS

**Contraindications:** Hypersensitivity to darunavir. Concurrent therapy with alfuzosin, colchicine, dihydroergotamine, ergonovine, ergotamine, lovastatin, methylergonovine, oral midazolam, pimozide, ranolazine, rifampin, sildenafil (for treatment of PAH), simvastatin, St. John's wort, triazolam. **Cautions:** Diabetes mellitus, hemophilia, known sulfonamide allergy, hepatic impairment.

## ACTION

Binds to site of HIV-I protease activity, inhibiting cleavage of viral precursors into functional proteins required for infectious HIV. **Therapeutic Effect:** Prevents formation of mature viral cells.

## PHARMACOKINETICS

Readily absorbed following PO administration. Protein binding: 95%. Metabolized in liver. Eliminated in feces (79.5%), urine (13.9%). Not significantly removed by hemodialysis. **Half-life:** 15 hrs.

## ⧗ LIFESPAN CONSIDERATIONS

**Pregnancy/Lactation:** Unknown if drug crosses placenta or is distributed in breast milk. Breastfeeding not recommended. **Children:** Safety and efficacy not established. **Elderly:** No age-related precautions noted.

## INTERACTIONS

**DRUG:** May increase concentration/effects of **amiodarone, bepridil, lidocaine, desipramine, colchicine, beta blockers, midazolam, paroxetine,**

---

sertraline, atorvastatin, clarithromycin, cyclosporine, felodipine, inhaled fluticasone, lovastatin, nicardipine, nifedipine, pravastatin, simvastatin, sirolimus, tacrolimus, trazodone, sildenafil, tadalafil, vardenafil. CYP3A4 inhibitors (e.g., itraconazole, ketoconazole, voriconazole) may increase concentration. May decrease effects of **methadone, oral contraceptives. HERBAL:** St. John's wort may lead to loss of virologic response, potential resistance to darunavir. **FOOD:** Food increases plasma concentration. **LAB VALUES:** May increase aPTT, PT, serum alkaline phosphatase, bilirubin, amylase, lipase, cholesterol, triglycerides, uric acid. May decrease lymphocytes/neutrophil count, platelets, WBC count; serum bicarbonate, albumin, calcium. May alter serum glucose, sodium.

## AVAILABILITY (Rx)

<u>Suspension, oral (Prezista):</u> 100 mg/ml

**🖌 Tablets (Prezista):** 75 mg, 150 mg, 400 mg, 600 mg, 800 mg.

## ADMINISTRATION/HANDLING

**PO**
• Give with food (increases plasma concentration). • Coadministration with ritonavir required. • Do not break, crush, dissolve, or divide film-coated tablets. • Shake suspension prior to each dose. Use provided oral dosing syringe.

## INDICATIONS/ROUTES/DOSAGE

**Note:** Genotypic testing recommended in therapy-experienced pts.

**HIV Infection, Treatment Experienced**
**PO: ADULTS, ELDERLY:** *(With 1 or more darunavir resistance–associated substitution):* 600 mg administered twice daily with 100 mg ritonavir twice daily. *(With no darunavir resistance–associated substitutions):* 800 mg with 100 mg ritonavir or 150 mg cobicistat once daily.

**HIV Infection, Treatment Naive**
**PO: ADULTS, ELDERLY:** 800 mg administered with 100 mg ritonavir or 150 mg cobicistat once daily.

**Usual Dosage During Pregnancy**
**PO: ADULTS:** 600 mg administered twice daily with 100 mg ritonavir twice daily.

**Usual Pediatric Dose**
Treatment naive or treatment experienced with no darunavir resistance–associated substitutions: *(Once daily dosing) (Suspension only):* **14 kg:** 490 mg with 96 mg ritonavir. **13 kg:** 455 mg with 80 mg ritonavir. **12 kg:** 420 mg with 80 mg ritonavir. **11 kg:** 385 mg with 64 mg ritonavir. **10 kg:** 350 mg with 64 mg ritonavir. *(Suspension or Tablets):* **40 kg or greater:** 800 mg with 100 mg ritonavir. **30–39 kg:** 675 mg with 100 mg ritonavir. **15–29 kg:** 600 mg with 100 mg ritonavir.

**Treatment Experienced with 1 or More Darunavir Resistance–Associated Substitution**
Use Tablet or Suspension
**PO: CHILDREN WEIGHING 40 KG OR MORE:** 600 mg twice daily with 100 mg ritonavir. **WEIGHING 30–39 KG:** 450 mg twice daily with 60 mg ritonavir. **WEIGHING 15–29 KG:** 375 mg twice daily with 50 mg ritonavir.

Use Oral Suspension Only
**14 KG TO LESS THAN 15 KG:** 280 mg (48 mg ritonavir) twice daily. **13 KG TO LESS THAN 14 KG:** 260 mg (40 mg ritonavir) twice daily. **12 KG TO LESS THAN 13 KG:** 240 mg (40 mg ritonavir) twice daily. **11 KG TO LESS THAN 12 KG:** 220 mg (32 mg ritonavir) twice daily. **10 KG TO LESS THAN 11 KG:** 200 mg (32 mg ritonavir) twice daily.

**Dosage in Renal Impairment**
No dose adjustment.

**Dosage in Hepatic Impairment**
Not recommended in severe impairment.

## SIDE EFFECTS

**Frequent (19%–13%):** Diarrhea, nausea, headache, nasopharyngitis. **Occasional (3%–2%):** Constipation, abdominal pain, vomiting. **Rare (less than 2%):** Allergic dermatitis, dyspepsia, flatulence, abdominal distention, anorexia, arthralgia, myalgia, paresthesia, memory impairment.

## ADVERSE EFFECTS/ TOXIC REACTIONS

Hypertension, MI, transient ischemic attack occur in less than 2% of pts. Acute renal failure, diabetes mellitus, dyspnea, worsening of hepatic impairment, skin reactions including Stevens-Johnson syndrome, toxic epidermal necrolysis occur rarely.

## NURSING CONSIDERATIONS

### BASELINE ASSESSMENT

Obtain baseline LFT before beginning therapy and at periodic intervals during therapy. Offer emotional support. Obtain full medication history.

### INTERVENTION/EVALUATION

Closely monitor for GI discomfort. Monitor daily pattern of bowel activity, stool consistency. Assess skin for rash, other skin reactions, chemistries, laboratory abnormalities, particularly hepatic profile, glucose, cholesterol, triglycerides. Assess for opportunistic infections (onset of fever, oral mucosa changes, cough, other respiratory symptoms).

### PATIENT/FAMILY TEACHING

• Take medication with food. • Continue therapy for full length of treatment. • Doses should be evenly spaced. • Darunavir is not a cure for HIV infection, nor does it reduce risk of transmission to others. • Pt may continue to experience illnesses, including opportunistic infections. • Diarrhea can be controlled with OTC medication. • Report any skin reactions.

## *dasatinib*

da-**sa**-ti-nib
(Sprycel)
**Do not confuse dasatinib with erlotinib, imatinib, or lapatinib.**

## ◆CLASSIFICATION

**PHARMACOTHERAPEUTIC:** Protein-tyrosine kinase inhibitor. **CLINICAL:** Antineoplastic.

## USES

**Chronic myeloid leukemia (CML):** Treatment of adults with chronic, accelerated, myeloid or lymphoid blast phase of CML with resistance, intolerance to prior therapy, including imatinib. Treatment of Ph+ CML in chronic phase of newly diagnosed pt. **Acute lymphoblastic leukemia:** Treatment of adults with Philadelphia chromosome–positive (Ph+) acute lymphoblastic leukemia (ALL) with resistance or intolerance to prior therapy including imatinib. **OFF-LABEL:** Post–stem cell transplant follow-up treatment of CML. Treatment of GI stromal tumor.

## PRECAUTIONS

**Contraindications:** Hypersensitivity to dasatinib. **Cautions:** Hepatic impairment, myelosuppression (particularly thrombocytopenia), pts prone to fluid retention, those with prolonged QT interval, cardiovascular/pulmonary disease. Concomitant use of anticoagulants, CYP3A4 inducers/inhibitors may increase risk of pulmonary arterial hypertension.

## ACTION

Reduces activity of proteins responsible for uncontrolled growth of leukemia cells by binding to most imatinib-resistant BCR-ABL mutations of pts with CML or ALL. **Therapeutic Effect:** Inhibits proliferation, tumor growth of CML and ALL cancer cell lines.

## PHARMACOKINETICS

Extensively distributed in extravascular space. Protein binding: 96%. Metabolized in liver. Eliminated primarily in feces. **Half-life:** 3–5 hrs.

**D**

## ⧗ LIFESPAN CONSIDERATIONS

**Pregnancy/Lactation:** Has potential for severe teratogenic effects, fertility impairment. Breastfeeding not recommended. **Children:** Safety and efficacy not established in pts younger than 18 yrs. **Elderly:** No age-related precautions noted.

## INTERACTIONS

**DRUG:** **CYP3A4 inhibitors (e.g., atazanavir, clarithromycin, erythromycin, indinavir, ketoconazole, nefazodone, nelfinavir, ritonavir, saquinavir)** may increase concentration. **CYP3A4 inducers (e.g., carbamazepine, phenobarbital, phenytoin, rifampin)** may decrease concentration. **Antacids** alter pH-dependent solubility of dasatinib. **Famotidine, omeprazole** may reduce dasatinib absorption. **HERBAL:** **St. John's wort, echinacea** may decrease concentration. **FOOD:** **Grapefruit products** may increase concentration/toxicity (increased risk of torsades, myelotoxicity). **LAB VALUES:** May decrease WBC, platelets, Hgb, Hct, RBC; serum calcium, phosphates. May increase serum ALT, AST, bilirubin, creatinine.

## AVAILABILITY (Rx)

▨ **Tablets (Film-Coated):** 20 mg, 50 mg, 70 mg, 80 mg, 100 mg, 140 mg.

## ADMINISTRATION/HANDLING

**PO**
• Give without regard to food. • Take with food or large glass of water if GI upset occurs. • Avoid grapefruit products. • Do not break, crush, dissolve, or divide film-coated tablets. • Store at room temperature. • Do not give antacids either 2 hrs prior to or within 2 hrs after dasatinib administration.

## INDICATIONS/ROUTES/DOSAGE

**Note: CYP3A4 Inhibitors:** Consider decreasing dose from 100 mg to 20 mg or 140 mg to 40 mg.

**CYP3A4 Inducers:** Consider increasing dose with monitoring.

**CML (Resistant or Intolerant)**
**PO: ADULTS, ELDERLY: (Chronic phase):** 100 mg once daily. May increase to 140 mg once daily in pts not achieving cytogenetic response. **(Accelerated or blast phase):** 140 mg once daily. May increase to 180 mg once daily in pts not achieving cytogenetic response.

**CML (Newly Diagnosed in Chronic Phase)**
**PO: ADULTS, ELDERLY:** 100 mg once daily. May increase to 140 mg/day in pts not achieving cytogenetic response.

**Ph+ ALL**
**PO: ADULTS, ELDERLY:** 140 mg once daily. May increase to 180 mg once daily in pts not achieving cytogenetic response.

**Dosage in Renal/Hepatic Impairment**
No dose adjustment.

## SIDE EFFECTS

**Frequent (50%–32%):** Fluid retention, diarrhea, headache, fatigue, musculoskeletal pain, fever, rash, nausea, dyspnea. **Occasional (28%–12%):** Cough, abdominal pain, vomiting, anorexia, asthenia, arthralgia, stomatitis, dizziness, constipation, peripheral neuropathy, myalgia. **Rare (less than 12%):** Abdominal distention, chills, weight increase, pruritus.

## ADVERSE EFFECTS/ TOXIC REACTIONS

Pleural effusion occurred in 8% of pts, febrile neutropenia in 7%, GI bleeding, pneumonia in 6%, thrombocytopenia in 5%, dyspnea in 4%; anemia, cardiac failure in 3%.

## NURSING CONSIDERATIONS

### BASELINE ASSESSMENT

Obtain CBC weekly for first mo, biweekly for second mo, and periodically thereafter. Monitor LFT before treatment begins and monthly thereafter.

## INTERVENTION/EVALUATION

Assess lower extremities for pedal edema, early evidence of fluid retention. Weigh daily, monitor for unexpected rapid weight gain. Offer antiemetics to control nausea, vomiting. Monitor daily pattern of bowel activity, stool consistency. Assess oral mucous membranes for evidence of stomatitis. Monitor CBC for neutropenia, thrombocytopenia; monitor hepatic function tests for hepatotoxicity.

## PATIENT/FAMILY TEACHING

• Avoid crowds, those with known infection. • Avoid contact with anyone who recently received live virus vaccine; do not receive vaccinations. • Antacids may be taken up to 2 hrs before or 2 hrs after taking dasatinib. • Avoid grapefruit products. Do not chew, crush, dissolve, or divide tablets.

---

## *DAUNOrubicin    HIGH ALERT

daw-noe-**roo**-bi-sin
(Cerubidine, DaunoXome)

■ **BLACK BOX ALERT** ■ Irreversible cardiotoxicity may occur. Myelosuppresant. Lipid component may cause infusion-related effects (back pain, flushing, chest tightness) within first 5 min of infusion. Must be administered by personnel trained in administration/handling of chemotherapeutic agents. Caution in renal impairment or hepatic dysfunction. Potent vesicant.
**Do not confuse daunorubicin with dactinomycin, doxorubicin, epirubicin, idarubicin, or valrubicin.**

## ◆CLASSIFICATION

**PHARMACOTHERAPEUTIC:** Anthracycline antibiotic. **CLINICAL:** Antineoplastic.

## USES

**Cerubidine:** Treatment of leukemias (acute lymphocytic [ALL], acute myeloid [AML]) in combination with other agents. **DaunoXome:** Advanced HIV-related Kaposi's sarcoma.

## PRECAUTIONS

**Contraindications:** Hypersensitivity to daunorubicin. **Cautions:** Preexisting heart disease or bone marrow suppression, hypertension, concurrent chemotherapeutic agents, elderly, infants, radiation therapy.

## ACTION

Inhibits DNA, DNA-dependent RNA synthesis by binding with DNA strands. Cell cycle–phase nonspecific. **Therapeutic Effect:** Prevents cell division.

## PHARMACOKINETICS

Widely distributed. Protein binding: High. Does not cross blood-brain barrier. Metabolized in liver to active metabolite. Excreted in urine (40%); biliary excretion (40%). **Half-life:** 18.5 hrs; metabolite: 26.7 hrs.

## ⚖ LIFESPAN CONSIDERATIONS

**Pregnancy/Lactation:** If possible, avoid use during pregnancy, esp. first trimester. May cause fetal harm. Breastfeeding not recommended. **Children:** Safety and efficacy not established. **Elderly:** Cardiotoxicity may be more frequent; reduced bone marrow reserves require caution. Age-related renal impairment may require dosage adjustment.

## INTERACTIONS

**DRUG:** Previous use of **doxorubicin**, concurrent use of **cyclophosphamide** increases risk of cardiotoxicity. **Hepatotoxic medications** increase risk of hepatotoxicity. **Bone marrow depressants** may enhance myelosuppression. **Live virus vaccines** may potentiate virus replication, increase vaccine side effects, decrease pt's antibody response to vaccine. **HERBAL:** Echinacea may decrease level/effects. **FOOD:** None known. **LAB VALUES:** May increase serum alkaline phosphatase, bilirubin, uric acid, AST.

## AVAILABILITY (Rx)

**Injection Solution (Cerubidine):** 5 mg/ml. **Injection Solution (DaunoXome):** 2 mg/ml.

## ADMINISTRATION/HANDLING

 IV

◄**ALERT**► **Cerubidine:** Give by IV push or IV infusion. **DaunoXome:** Give by IV infusion. May be carcinogenic, mutagenic, teratogenic. Handle with extreme care during preparation/administration.

**Reconstitution**
**Cerubidine** • May further dilute with 100 ml D₅W or 0.9% NaCl.
**DaunoXome** • Must dilute with equal part D₅W to provide concentration of 1 mg/ml. • Do not use any other diluent.

**Rate of Administration**
**Cerubidine** • For IV push, withdraw desired dose into syringe containing 10–15 ml 0.9% NaCl. Inject over 1–5 min into tubing of rapidly infusing IV solution of D₅W or 0.9% NaCl. • For IV infusion, further dilute with 100 ml D₅W or 0.9% NaCl. Infuse over 15–30 min. • Extravasation produces immediate pain, severe local tissue damage. Aspirate as much infiltrated drug as possible, then infiltrate area with hydrocortisone sodium succinate injection (50–100 mg hydrocortisone) and/or isotonic sodium thiosulfate injection or ascorbic acid injection (1 ml of 5% injection). Apply cold compresses.
**DaunoXome** • Infuse over 60 min. • Do not use in-line filter.

**Storage**
**Cerubidine** • Refrigerate intact vials. Protect from light. Solutions prepared for infusion stable for 24 hrs at room temperature.
**DaunoXome** • Refrigerate unopened vials • Reconstituted solution is stable for 6 hrs if refrigerated. • Do not use if opaque.

## ⚅ IV INCOMPATIBILITIES

Allopurinol (Aloprim), aztreonam (Azactam), cefepime (Maxipime), dexamethasone (Decadron), heparin, piperacillin and tazobactam (Zosyn). **DaunoXome:** Do not mix with any other solution, esp. NaCl or bacteriostatic agents (e.g., benzyl alcohol).

## ⚅ IV COMPATIBILITIES

Granisetron (Kytril), ondansetron (Zofran).

## INDICATIONS/ROUTES/DOSAGE

◄**ALERT**► Refer to individual protocols. **Cerubidine:** Cumulative dose should not exceed 550 mg/m² in adults (increased risk of cardiotoxicity) or 400 mg/m² in those receiving chest irradiation.

**Acute Lymphoblastic Leukemia**
**IV** *(Cerubidine)*: **ADULTS, ELDERLY:** 45 mg/m² on days 1, 2, and 3 (in combination with vincristine, prednisone, asparaginase). **CHILDREN 2 YRS AND OLDER, BODY SURFACE AREA 0.5 m² OR GREATER:** 25 mg/m² on day 1 of every wk for up to 4–6 cycles (in combination with vincristine, prednisone). Cumulative dose not to exceed 300 mg/m². **CHILDREN YOUNGER THAN 2 YRS, BODY SURFACE AREA LESS THAN 0.5 m²:** 1 mg/kg/dose per protocol (in combination with vincristine, prednisone). Cumulative dose not to exceed 10 mg/kg.

**Acute Myeloid Leukemia**
**IV** *(Cerubidine)*: **ADULTS YOUNGER THAN 60 YRS:** 45 mg/m² on days 1, 2, and 3 of induction course, then on days 1 and 2 of subsequent courses (in combination with cytarabine). **ADULTS 60 YRS AND OLDER:** 30 mg/m² on days 1, 2, and 3 of induction course, then on days 1 and 2 of subsequent courses (in combination with cytarabine).

**Kaposi's Sarcoma**
**IV** *(Daunoxome)*: **ADULTS:** 40 mg/m² over 1 hr repeated q2wks until disease progression.

---

**Dosage in Renal Impairment**
**Cerubidine: Serum creatinine greater than 3 mg/dL:** 50% of normal dose.
**Daunoxome: Serum creatinine greater than 3 mg/dL:** 50% of normal dose.

**Dosage in Hepatic Impairment**
**Cerubidine: Bilirubin 1.2–3 mg/dL:** 75% of normal dose. **Bilirubin 3.1–5 mg/dL:** 50% of normal dose. **Bilirubin Greater than 5 mg/dL:** Daunorubicin is not recommended for use in this pt population.
**Daunoxome: Bilirubin 1.2–3 mg/dL:** 75% of normal dose. **Bilirubin greater than 3 mg/dL:** 50% of normal dose.

## SIDE EFFECTS

**Frequent:** Complete alopecia (scalp, axillary, pubic), nausea, vomiting (beginning a few hrs after administration and lasting 24–48 hrs). **DaunoXome:** Mild to moderate nausea, fatigue, fever. **Occasional:** Diarrhea, abdominal pain, esophagitis, stomatitis, transverse pigmentation of fingernails, toenails. **Rare:** Transient fever, chills.

## ADVERSE EFFECTS/ TOXIC REACTIONS

Myelosuppression manifested as hematologic toxicity (severe leukopenia, anemia, thrombocytopenia). Decrease in platelet count, WBC count occurs in 10–14 days, returns to normal level by third week. Cardiotoxicity noted as either acute, transient, abnormal. EKG findings and/or cardiomyopathy manifested as HF (risk increases when cumulative dose exceeds 550 mg/m$^2$ in adults, 300 mg/m$^2$ in children 2 yrs and older, or total dosage greater than 10 mg/kg in children younger than 2 yrs).

## NURSING CONSIDERATIONS

### BASELINE ASSESSMENT

Obtain WBC, platelet, erythrocyte counts before and at frequent intervals during therapy. EKG should be obtained before therapy. Antiemetics may be effective in preventing, treating nausea.

### INTERVENTION/EVALUATION

Monitor for stomatitis. May lead to ulceration within 2–3 days. Assess skin, nailbeds for hyperpigmentation. Monitor hematologic status, renal/hepatic function, serum uric acid. Monitor daily pattern of bowel activity, stool consistency. Monitor for hematologic toxicity (fever, sore throat, signs of local infection, unusual bruising/bleeding from any site), symptoms of anemia (excessive fatigue, weakness).

### PATIENT/FAMILY TEACHING

• Urine may turn reddish color for 1–2 days after beginning therapy. • Hair loss is reversible, but new hair growth may have different color, texture. • New hair growth resumes about 5 wks after last therapy dose. • Maintain strict oral hygiene. • Do not have immunizations without physician's approval (drug lowers resistance). • Avoid contact with those who have recently received live virus vaccine. • Promptly report fever, sore throat, signs of local infection, unusual bruising/bleeding from any site, yellowing of whites of eyes/skin, difficulty breathing. • Increase fluid intake (may protect against hyperuricemia). • Report for persistent nausea, vomiting.

# deferasirox

dee-**fur**-a-sir-ox
(Exjade, Jadenu)
■ **BLACK BOX ALERT** ■ May cause renal/hepatic failure, hepatotoxicity, gastrointestinal hemorrhage.
**Do not confuse deferasirox with deferoxamine.**

## ◆CLASSIFICATION

**PHARMACOTHERAPEUTIC:** Iron-chelating agent. **CLINICAL:** Iron reduction agent.

---

**D**

## USES

Treatment of chronic iron overload due to blood transfusions (transfusional hemosiderosis) or due to non–transfusion-dependent thalassemia syndrome.

## PRECAUTIONS

**Contraindications:** Hypersensitivity to deferasirox. Platelet counts less than 50,000/mm$^3$; poor performance status, high-risk myelodysplastic syndromes or advanced malignancies; CrCl less than 40 ml/min or serum creatinine greater than 2 times the upper limit of normal. **Cautions:** Renal/hepatic impairment, elderly, concurrent medications that may increase GI effects (e.g., NSAIDs).

## ACTION

Selective for iron. Binds iron with high affinity in a 2:1 ratio. **Therapeutic Effect:** Induces iron excretion.

## PHARMACOKINETICS

Well absorbed following PO administration. Protein binding: 99%. Metabolized in liver. Excreted in feces (84%), urine (8%). **Half-life:** 8–16 hrs.

## ⧗ LIFESPAN CONSIDERATIONS

**Pregnancy/Lactation:** Unknown if drug crosses placenta or is distributed in breast milk. **Children:** Not recommended for pts younger than 2 yrs. **Elderly:** No age-related precautions noted.

## INTERACTIONS

**DRUG:** Antacids containing **aluminium, cholestyramine, phenobarbital, phenytoin, rifampin, ritonavir** decrease concentration/effects. May decrease effects of **cyclosporine, simvastatin, oral contraceptives.** May increase concentration of **cyclobenzaprine, olanzapine, tizanidine. HERBAL:** None significant. **FOOD:** Bioavailability is variably increased when given with **food. LAB VALUES:** Decreases serum ferritin. May increase serum ALT, AST, creatinine, urine protein.

## AVAILABILITY (Rx)

**Tablets (Jadenu):** 90 mg, 180 mg, 360 mg.
**Tablets, Soluble (Exjade):** 125 mg, 250 mg, 500 mg.

## ADMINISTRATION/HANDLING

**PO**

• Give on empty stomach 30 min before food. • Do not give simultaneously with aluminum-containing antacids, cholestyramine. • Tablets should not be chewed or swallowed whole. • Disperse tablet by stirring in water, apple juice, orange juice until fine suspension is achieved. • Dosage less than 1 g should be dispersed in 3.5 oz of liquid, dosage more than 1 g should be dispersed in 7 oz of liquid. If any residue remains in glass, resuspend with a small amount of liquid.

## INDICATIONS/ROUTES/DOSAGE

**Iron Overload Due to Transfusions**
**PO: ADULTS, ELDERLY, CHILDREN 2 YRS AND OLDER:** *(Exjade):* Initially, 20 mg/kg once daily. **Maintenance:** (Titrate to individual response and goals.) Adjust dosage by 5 or 10 mg/kg/day every 3–6 mos based on serum ferritin levels. Consider holding for serum ferritin less than 500 mcg/L. **Maximum:** 40 mg/kg once daily. *(Jadenu):* Initially, 14 mg/kg once daily. **Maintenance:** (Titrate to individual response and goals.) Adjust dosage by 3.5 or 7 mg/kg/day based on serum ferritin levels. Consider holding for serum ferritin less than 500 mcg/L. **Maximum:** 28 mcg/kg once daily.

**Thalassemia Syndromes**
**PO: ADULTS, ELDERLY, CHILDREN 10 YRS AND OLDER:** *(Exjade):* Initially, 10 mg/kg once daily. May increase to 20 mg/kg once daily after 4 wks if baseline iron is greater than 15 mg Fe/g dry wgt. *(Jadenu):* Initially, 7 mg/kg once daily. May increase to 14 mg/kg/day after 4 wks if baseline iron greater than 15 mg Fe/g dry wgt. **Maintenance:** *(Exjade/ Jadenu):* Dose adjustments based on

---

serum ferritin and hepatic iron concentrations.

**Dosage in Renal Impairment**
**Note:** See Contraindications.
**ADULTS:** For increase in serum creatinine greater than 33% on 2 consecutive measures, reduce daily dose by 10 mg/kg. **CHILDREN:** For increase in serum creatinine above age-appropriate upper limit of normal on 2 consecutive measures, reduce daily dose by 10 mg/kg. *(Jadenu):* **CrCl 40–60 ml/min:** Reduce starting dose by 50%.

**Dosage in Hepatic Impairment**
For severe or persistent elevations in hepatic function tests, consider dose reduction or discontinuation. **Moderate impairment:** *(Jadenu):* Reduce initial dose by 50%.

## SIDE EFFECTS

**Frequent (19%–10%):** Fever, headache, abdominal pain, cough, nasopharyngitis, diarrhea, nausea, vomiting. **Occasional (9%–4%):** Rash, arthralgia, fatigue, back pain, urticaria. **Rare (1%):** Edema, sleep disorder, dizziness, anxiety.

## ADVERSE EFFECTS/ TOXIC REACTIONS

Bronchitis, pharyngitis, acute tonsillitis, ear infection occur occasionally. Hepatitis, auditory disturbances, ocular abnormalities occur rarely. Acute renal failure, cytopenias (e.g., agranulocytosis, neutropenia, thrombocytopenia) may occur.

## NURSING CONSIDERATIONS

### BASELINE ASSESSMENT

Obtain baseline serum CBC, ferritin, iron, creatinine, ALT, AST, urine protein, then monthly thereafter. Auditory, ophthalmic testing should be obtained before therapy and annually thereafter.

### INTERVENTION/EVALUATION

Treatment should be interrupted if serum ferritin levels are consistently less than 500 mcg/L. Suspend treatment if severe rash occurs.

### PATIENT/FAMILY TEACHING

• Take on empty stomach 30 min before food. • Do not chew or swallow tablet whole; disperse tablet completely in water, apple juice, orange juice; drink resulting suspension immediately. • Do not take aluminum-containing antacids concurrently. • Report severe skin rash, changes in vision/hearing, or yellowing of skin/eyes.

# denosumab

den-**oh**-sue-mab
(Prolia, Xgeva)
**Do not confuse denosumab with daclizumab, or Prolia with Avandia or Zebeta.**

## ◆CLASSIFICATION

**PHARMACOTHERAPEUTIC:** Monoclonal antibody. **CLINICAL:** Bone resorption inhibitor.

## USES

**Prolia:** Treatment of osteoporosis in postmenopausal women at high risk for fracture. Treatment to increase bone mass in men at high risk for fractures; treatment of bone loss in men receiving androgen deprivation therapy for nonmetastatic prostate cancer and in women at high risk for fractures receiving adjuvant aromatase inhibitor therapy for breast cancer. **Xgeva:** Prevention of skeletal-related events (e.g., fracture, spinal cord compression) in pts with bone metastases from solid tumor. Treatment of giant cell tumor of bone in adults and skeletally mature adolescents. Treatment of hypercalcemia of malignancy refractory to biphosphonate therapy. **OFF-LABEL:** Treatment of bone destruction caused by rheumatoid arthritis.

## PRECAUTIONS

**Contraindications:** Hypersensitivity to denosumab. **Prolia:** Preexisting hypocalcemia, pregnancy. **Cautions:** History of hypoparathyroidism, thyroid/parathyroid surgery, malabsorption syndromes, excision of small intestine, immunocompromised pts. Pts with severe renal impairment or receiving dialysis (greater risk for developing hypocalcemia). Pts with impaired immune system or immunosuppressive therapy.

## ACTION

Binds to RANK ligand (transmembrane protein), preventing osteoclast formation. **Therapeutic Effect:** Decreases bone resorption; increases bone mass in osteoporosis; decreases skeletal-related events and tumor-induced bone destruction in solid tumors. Inhibits tumor growth.

## PHARMACOKINETICS

Serum level detected 1 hr after administration. **Half-life:** 32 days.

## ⧗ LIFESPAN CONSIDERATIONS

**Pregnancy/Lactation:** Approved for use only in postmenopausal women. **Children:** Approved for use only in postmenopausal women. **Elderly:** No age-related precautions noted.

## INTERACTIONS

**DRUG:** None significant. **HERBAL:** None significant. **FOOD:** None known. **LAB VALUES:** May decrease serum calcium. May increase serum cholesterol.

## AVAILABILITY (Rx)

**Injection, Solution (Prolia):** 60 mg/ml. **(Xgeva):** 120 mg/1.7 ml.

## ADMINISTRATION/HANDLING

**Subcutaneous**
• Administer in upper arm, upper thigh, or abdomen.
**Storage** • Refrigerate. Use within 14 days once at room temperature. • Solution appears as clear, colorless to pale yellow.

## INDICATIONS/ROUTES/DOSAGE

**Note:** Administer calcium and vitamin D to prevent/treat hypocalcemia.

**Prolia**
Treatment of androgen deprivation–induced bone loss in men with prostate cancer; treatment of aromatase inhibitor–induced bone loss in women with breast cancer; treatment of osteoporosis in men or postmenopausal women.
**SQ: ADULTS, ELDERLY:** 60 mg every 6 mos.

**Xgeva**
**Prevention of Skeletal-Related Events from Solid Tumors**
**SQ: ADULTS, ELDERLY:** 120 mg q4wks.

**Xgeva**
**Giant Cell Tumor of Bone, Hypercalcemia of Malignancy**
**SQ: ADULTS, ELDERLY, MATURE ADOLESCENTS:** 120 mg q4wks with additional doses on days 8 and 15 of first mo of therapy.

**Dosage in Renal/Hepatic Impairment**
No dose adjustment.

## SIDE EFFECTS

**Frequent (35%–12%):** Back pain, extremity pain. **Occasional (8%–5%):** Musculoskeletal pain, vertigo, peripheral edema, sciatica. **Rare (4%–2%):** Bone pain, upper abdominal pain, rash, insomnia, flatulence, pruritus, myalgia, asthenia, GI reflux.

## ADVERSE EFFECTS/ TOXIC REACTIONS

Increases risk of infection, specifically cystitis, upper respiratory tract infection, pneumonia, pharyngitis, herpes zoster (shingles) occur in 2%–6% of pts. Osteonecrosis of the jaw (OJN) was reported. Suppression of bone turnover, pancreatitis have been reported.

**D**

## NURSING CONSIDERATIONS

### BASELINE ASSESSMENT

Hypocalcemia must be corrected prior to treatment. Calcium 1,000 mg/day and vitamin D at least 400 international units/day should be given. Dental exam should be provided prior to treatment.

### INTERVENTION/EVALUATION

Monitor serum magnesium, calcium, ionized calcium, phosphate. In pts predisposed with hypocalcemia and disturbances of mineral metabolism, clinical monitoring of calcium, mineral levels is highly recommended. Adequately supplement all pts with calcium and vitamin D. Monitor for delayed fracture healing.

### PATIENT/FAMILY TEACHING

• Report rash, new-onset eczema. • Seek prompt medical attention if signs, symptoms of severe infection (rash, itching, reddened skin, cellulitis) occur. • Report muscle stiffness, numbness, cramps, spasms (signs of hypocalcemia); swelling or drainage from jaw, mouth, or teeth.

## desloratadine

**des**-lor-a-ta-deen
(Aerius ✸, Clarinex, Clarinex Redi-Tabs)
**Do not confuse Clarinex with Celebrex or Claritin.**

### FIXED-COMBINATION(S)

**Clarinex-D 24 Hour:** desloratadine/pseudoephedrine (a sympathomimetic): 5 mg/240 mg. **Clarinex-D 12 Hour:** desloratadine/pseudoephedrine: 2.5 mg/120 mg.

### ◆CLASSIFICATION

**PHARMACOTHERAPEUTIC:** $H_1$ antagonist. **CLINICAL:** Nonsedating antihistamine.

### USES

Relief of nasal/non-nasal symptoms of seasonal and perennial rhinitis (sneezing, rhinorrhea, itching/tearing of eyes, stuffiness), chronic idiopathic urticaria (hives).

### PRECAUTIONS

**Contraindications:** Hypersensitivity to desloratadine or loratidine. **Cautions:** Renal/hepatic impairment, breastfeeding.

### ACTION

Exhibits selective peripheral histamine $H_1$ receptor blocking action. **Therapeutic Effect:** Prevents allergic response mediated by histamine (rhinitis, urticaria).

### PHARMACOKINETICS

Rapidly absorbed from GI tract. Distributed mainly in liver, lungs, GI tract, bile. Protein binding: 82%. Metabolized in liver. Eliminated in urine, feces. **Half-life:** 27 hrs (increased in elderly, renal/hepatic impairment).

### ⧗ LIFESPAN CONSIDERATIONS

**Pregnancy/Lactation:** Excreted in breast milk. **Children/Elderly:** More sensitive to anticholinergic effects (e.g., dry mouth, nose, throat).

### INTERACTIONS

**DRUG:** Erythromycin, ketoconazole, fluconazole, clarithromycin may increase concentration. **HERBAL:** None significant. **FOOD:** None known. **LAB VALUES:** May suppress wheal, flare reactions to antigen skin testing unless antihistamines are discontinued 4 days before testing.

### AVAILABILITY (Rx)

**Syrup (Clarinex):** 2.5 mg/5 ml. **Tablets (Clarinex):** 5 mg. **Tablet, Oral Dispersable:** 2.5 mg, 5 mg.

---

✸ Canadian trade name  Non-Crushable Drug ▐ High Alert drug

D

## ADMINISTRATION/HANDLING

### PO

• May give with or without food. • **Oral dispersable tablet:** Place directly on tongue (disintegrates immediately). • May take with or without water.

## INDICATIONS/ROUTES/DOSAGE

### Allergic Rhinitis, Urticaria

**PO: ADULTS, ELDERLY, CHILDREN OLDER THAN 12 YRS:** 5 mg once daily. **CHILDREN 6–12 YRS:** 2.5 mg once daily. **CHILDREN 1–5 YRS:** 1.25 mg once daily. **CHILDREN 6–11 MOS:** 1 mg once daily.

### Dosage in Hepatic/Renal Impairment

Dosage is decreased to 5 mg every other day.

## SIDE EFFECTS

**Frequent (12%):** Headache. **Occasional (3%):** Dry mouth, drowsiness. **Rare (less than 3%):** Fatigue, dizziness, diarrhea, nausea.

## ADVERSE EFFECTS/ TOXIC REACTIONS

None known.

## NURSING CONSIDERATIONS

### BASELINE ASSESSMENT

Assess lung sounds for wheezing; skin for urticaria, hives.

### INTERVENTION/EVALUATION

For upper respiratory allergies, increase fluids to decrease viscosity of secretions, offset thirst, replace any loss of fluids. Monitor symptoms for therapeutic response.

### PATIENT/FAMILY TEACHING

• Drink plenty of water (may cause dry mouth). • Avoid tasks that require alertness, motor skills until response to drug is established (may cause drowsiness). • Avoid alcohol.

# desmopressin

des-moe-**press**-in
(Apo-Desmopressin ✦, DDAVP, DDAVP Rhinal Tube, Stimate)

## ◆CLASSIFICATION

**PHARMACOTHERAPEUTIC:** Synthetic pituitary hormone. **CLINICAL:** Antidiuretic.

## USES

**DDAVP Nasal: (DDAVP Rhinal Tube):** Antidiuretic replacement therapy in managing central cranial diabetes insipidus. **Parenteral:** Antidiuretic replacement therapy in managing central cranial diabetes insipidus. Manage polyuria and polydipsia following head trauma or surgery in pituitary region. Maintain hemostasis and control bleeding in hemophilia A, von Willebrand's disease (type I). **Stimate intranasal:** Maintain hemostasis and control bleeding due to spontaneous or trauma-induced injuries in hemophilia A, von Willebrand's disease (type I). **PO:** Antidiuretic replacement therapy in managing central cranial diabetes insipidus, primary management of nocturnal enuresis, management of temporary polyuria, polydipsia following pituitary surgery or head trauma. **OFF-LABEL:** Uremic bleeding occurring with acute/chronic renal failure; prevent surgical bleeding in pts with uremia.

## PRECAUTIONS

**Contraindications:** Hypersensitivity to desmopressin. Hyponatremia, history of hyponatremia, moderate to severe renal impairment. **Cautions:** Predisposition to thrombus formation; conditions with fluid, electrolyte imbalance; coronary artery disease; hypertensive cardiovascular disease, elderly, cystic fibrosis, HF, renal impairment, polydipsia. Avoid use in hemophilia A with factor VIII levels less than 5%; hemophilia B; severe type I, type IIB, platelet-type von Willebrand's disease.

## ACTION

Increases CAMP in renal tubular cells, which increases water permeability, decreasing urine volume. Increases levels of von Willebrand factor, factor VIII, tissue plasminogen activator (tPA). **Therapeutic Effect:** Shortens activated partial thromboplastin time (aPTT), bleeding time. Decreases urinary output.

## PHARMACOKINETICS

| Route | Onset | Peak | Duration |
|---|---|---|---|
| PO | 1 hr | 2–7 hrs | 8–12 hrs |
| IV | 15–30 min | 1.5–3 hrs | 8–12 hrs |
| Intranasal | 15 min–1 hr | 1–5 hrs | 8–12 hrs |

Poorly absorbed after PO, nasal administration. Metabolism: Unknown. **Half-life: PO:** 1.5–2.5 hrs. **Intranasal:** 3.3–3.5 hrs. **IV:** 0.4–4 hrs.

## ☒ LIFESPAN CONSIDERATIONS

**Pregnancy/Lactation:** Unknown if distributed in breast milk. **Children:** Caution in neonates, pts younger than 3 mos (increased risk of fluid balance problems). Careful fluid restrictions recommended in infants. **Elderly:** Increased risk of hyponatremia, water intoxication.

## INTERACTIONS

**DRUG: Carbamazepine, lamotrigine, NSAIDs, SSRIs, tricyclic antidepressants** may increase effect. **Demeclocycline, lithium** may decrease effect. **HERBAL:** None significant. **FOOD:** None known. **LAB VALUES:** May decrease serum sodium.

## AVAILABILITY (Rx)

**Injection Solution (DDAVP):** 4 mcg/ml. **Nasal Solution (DDAVP Rhinal Tube 0.01%):** 100 mcg/ml (10 mcg/spray). **Nasal Spray (Stimate):** 1.5 mg/ml (150 mcg/spray). **Tablets (DDAVP):** 0.1 mg, 0.2 mg.

## ADMINISTRATION/HANDLING

 IV

**Reconstitution** • For IV infusion, dilute in 10–50 ml 0.9% NaCl (10 ml for children 10 kg or less; 50 ml for adults, children greater than 10 kg). **Rate of Administration** • Infuse over 15–30 min. **Storage** • Refrigerate.

**Subcutaneous**
• Withdraw dose from vial. Further dilution not required.

**Intranasal**
• Refrigerate DDAVP Rhinal Tube solution, Stimate nasal spray. • Rhinal Tube solution, Stimate nasal spray are stable for 3 wks at room temperature. • DDAVP nasal spray is stable at room temperature. • Calibrated catheter (rhinyle) is used to draw up measured quantity of desmopressin; with one end inserted in nose, pt blows on other end to deposit solution deep in nasal cavity. • For infants, young children, obtunded pts, air-filled syringe may be attached to catheter to deposit solution.

## INDICATIONS/ROUTES/DOSAGE

**Primary Nocturnal Enuresis**
**PO: CHILDREN 6 YRS AND OLDER:** 0.2–0.6 mg once before bedtime. Limit fluid intake 1 hr prior and at least 8 hrs after dose.

**Central Cranial Diabetes Insipidus**
◄ALERT► Fluid restriction should be observed.
**PO: ADULTS, ELDERLY, CHILDREN 4 YRS AND OLDER:** Initially, 0.05 mg twice daily. Titrate to desired response. Range: 0.1–1.2 mg/day in 2–3 divided doses.
**IV, SQ: ADULTS, ELDERLY, CHILDREN 12 YRS AND OLDER:** 2–4 mcg/day in 2 divided doses or $\frac{1}{10}$ of maintenance intranasal dose.

**Intranasal** *(Use 100 mcg/ml Concentration):* **ADULTS, ELDERLY, CHILDREN OLDER THAN 12 YRS:** 10–40 mcg (0.1–0.4 ml) in 1–3 doses/day. Usual dose: 10 mcg 2 times/day. **CHILDREN 3 MOS–12 YRS:** Initially, 5 mcg (0.05 ml)/day. Range: 5–30 mcg (0.05–0.3 ml)/day as a single or 2 divided doses.

**Hemophilia A, von Willebrand's Disease (Type I)**
**IV Infusion: ADULTS, ELDERLY, CHILDREN:** 0.3 mcg/kg as slow infusion.
**Intranasal** *(Use 1.5 mg/ml Concentration Providing 150 mcg/Spray):* **ADULTS, ELDERLY, CHILDREN WEIGHING MORE THAN 50 KG:** 300 mcg; use 1 spray in each nostril. **ADULTS, ELDERLY, CHILDREN WEIGHING 50 KG OR LESS:** 150 mcg as a single spray. Repeat use based on clinical conditions/laboratory work.

**Dosage in Renal Impairment**
**CrCl less than 50 ml/min:** Not recommended.

**Dosage in Hepatic Impairment**
No dose adjustment.

## SIDE EFFECTS

**Occasional: IV:** Pain, redness, swelling at injection site; headache, abdominal cramps, vulvular pain, flushed skin, mild B/P elevation, nausea with high dosages. **Nasal:** Rhinorrhea, nasal congestion, slight B/P elevation.

## ADVERSE EFFECTS/ TOXIC REACTIONS

Water intoxication, hyponatremia (headache, drowsiness, confusion, decreased urination, rapid weight gain, seizures, coma) may occur in overhydration. Children, elderly pts, infants are esp. at risk.

## NURSING CONSIDERATIONS

### BASELINE ASSESSMENT
Establish baselines for B/P, pulse, weight, serum electrolytes, urine specific gravity. Check lab values for factor VIII coagulant concentration for hemophilia A, von Willebrand's disease; bleeding times.

### INTERVENTION/EVALUATION
Check B/P, pulse with IV infusion. Monitor pt weight, fluid intake; urine volume, urine specific gravity, osmolality, serum electrolytes for diabetes insipidus. Assess factor VIII antigen levels, aPTT, factor VIII activity level for hemophilia.

### PATIENT/FAMILY TEACHING
• Avoid overhydration. • Follow guidelines for proper intranasal administration. • Report headache, shortness of breath, heartburn, nausea, abdominal cramps.

# desvenlafaxine

des-ven-la-**fax**-een
(Khedezia, Pristiq)

■ **BLACK BOX ALERT** ■ Increased risk of suicidal thinking and behavior in children, adolescents, young adults 18–24 yrs with major depressive disorder, other psychiatric disorders.

## ◆CLASSIFICATION

**PHARMACOTHERAPEUTIC:** Phenethylamine derivative. **CLINICAL:** Antidepressant.

## USES
Treatment of major depression disorder (MDD).

## PRECAUTIONS
**Contraindications:** Hypersensitivity to desvenlafaxine or venlafaxine. Use of MAOIs within 14 days or in those currently taking MAOIs (may cause neuroleptic malignant syndrome). Allow at least 7 days after discontinuation before starting an MAOI. Initiation in pts taking linezolid or methylene blue. **Cautions:** Renal impairment, history of seizures, bipolar disorder, pts with suicidal ideation and behavior, increased intraocular

pressure, narrow-angle glaucoma, cardiovascular or cerebrovascular disease, elderly.

## ACTION

Appears to inhibit serotonin and norepinephrine reuptake at CNS neuronal presynaptic membranes (weakly inhibits dopamine reuptake). **Therapeutic Effect:** Produces antidepressant effect.

## PHARMACOKINETICS

Well absorbed from GI tract. Protein binding: 30%. Excreted primarily in urine. Steady-state plasma levels occur in 4–5 days. **Half-life:** 9–11 hrs.

## ⧗ LIFESPAN CONSIDERATIONS

**Pregnancy/Lactation:** Distributed in breast milk. **Children:** Safety and efficacy not established. **Elderly:** No age-related precautions noted.

## INTERACTIONS

**DRUG:** Concurrent use of **MAOIs (e.g., phenelzine, selegiline)** may cause neuroleptic malignant syndrome: hyperthermia, rigidity, myoclonus, autonomic instability (including rapid fluctuations of vital signs), mental status changes, coma, extreme agitation. **Alcohol** may increase CNS depressant effects. May decrease **midazolam** concentration. May increase **desipramine** concentration. **Aspirin, NSAIDs, warfarin** increase risk of bleeding. **Ketoconazole** may increase concentration/effect. **HERBAL: Gotu kola, kava kava, St. John's wort, valerian** may increase CNS depressant effects. **FOOD:** None known. **LAB VALUES:** May increase total serum cholesterol, LDL cholesterol, triglycerides, ALT, AST, prolactin level.

## AVAILABILITY (Rx)

🥄 **Tablets (Extended-Release):** 25 mg, 50 mg, 100 mg.

## ADMINISTRATION/HANDLING

**PO**
• Give without regard to food. • Give with food or milk if GI distress occurs. • Do not break, crush, dissolve, or divide tablets. • Must be swallowed whole, with fluid.

## INDICATIONS/ROUTES/DOSAGE

**Major Depressive Disorder**
**PO: ADULTS:** 50 mg once daily. **Maximum:** 400 mg/day.

**Dosage in Renal Impairment**
**CrCl 30–50 ml/min:** 50 mg once daily (Maximum). **CrCl less than 30 ml/min:** 25 mg once daily or 50 mg every other day (Maximum). **HD:** 25 mg once daily or 50 mg every other day (Maximum).

**Dosage in Hepatic Impairment**
**Mild impairment:** No dosage adjustment. **Moderate to severe impairment:** 50 mg once daily. **Maximum:** 100 mg/day.

## SIDE EFFECTS

**Frequent (22%–20%):** Nausea, headache. **Occasional (13%–7%):** Dizziness, dry mouth, diarrhea, sweating, constipation, insomnia, fatigue. **Rare (5%–2%):** Anorexia, drowsiness, decreased libido, erectile dysfunction in men, anxiety, blurred vision, vomiting, decreased weight, tremor, paresthesia, irritability, abnormal dreams, blurred vision, tinnitus.

## ADVERSE EFFECTS/ TOXIC REACTIONS

Seizures, syncope, extrapyramidal disorder, depersonalization, hypomania, epistaxis occur rarely. Ischemic cardiac events, including myocardial ischemia, MI, coronary occlusion requiring revascularization, may occur. Sustained increase in diastolic B/P (10–15 mm Hg) occurs occasionally.

---

## NURSING CONSIDERATIONS

### BASELINE ASSESSMENT
Obtain initial weight, B/P. Assess appearance, behavior, speech pattern, level of interest, mood, sleep pattern.

### INTERVENTION/EVALUATION
For pts on long-term therapy, LFT should be performed periodically. Assess sleep pattern for evidence of insomnia. Monitor for suicidal ideation (esp. at initiation of therapy or changes in dosage). Assess appearance, behavior, speech pattern, level of interest, mood for therapeutic response.

### PATIENT/FAMILY TEACHING
• Take with food to minimize GI distress. • Do not chew, crush, dissolve, or divide tablets. • Do not increase, decrease, or suddenly discontinue medication. • Therapeutic effect may be noted within 1–4 wks. • Avoid tasks that require alertness, motor skills until response to drug is established. • Avoid alcohol. • Report worsening depression, suicidal ideation, unusual changes in behavior.

---

# dexamethasone

dex-a-**meth**-a-sone
(Apo-Dexamethasone ✦,
Dexamethasone Intensol, DexPak,
Maxidex)
**Do not confuse Decadron with Percodan, or dexamethasone with dextroamphetamine, or Maxidex with Maxzide.**

## FIXED-COMBINATION(S)

**Ciprodex Otic:** dexamethasone/ciprofloxacin (antibiotic): 0.1%/0.3%. **Dexacidin, Maxitrol:** dexamethasone/neomycin/polymyxin (anti-infectives): 0.1%/3.5 mg/10,000 units per g or ml.

## ◆CLASSIFICATION

**PHARMACOTHERAPEUTIC:** Long-acting glucocorticoid. **CLINICAL:** Corticosteroid.

## USES
Used primarily as an anti-inflammatory or immunosuppressant agent in a variety of diseases (e.g., allergic, inflammatory autoimmune). **OFF-LABEL:** Antiemetic, treatment of croup, dexamethasone suppression test (indicator consistent with suicide and/or depression), accelerate fetal lung maturation. Treatment of acute mountain sickness, high-altitude cerebral edema.

## PRECAUTIONS
**Contraindications:** Hypersensitivity to dexamethasone. Systemic fungal infections, cerebral malaria. **Cautions:** Thyroid disease, renal/hepatic impairment, cardiovascular disease, diabetes, glaucoma, cataracts, myasthenia gravis, pts at risk for seizures, osteoporosis, post-MI, elderly.

## ACTION
Suppresses neutrophil migration, decreases production of inflammatory mediators, reverses increased capillary permeability. **Therapeutic Effect:** Decreases inflammation. Suppresses normal immune response.

## PHARMACOKINETICS
Rapidly absorbed from GI tract after PO administration. Widely distributed. Protein binding: High. Metabolized in liver. Primarily excreted in urine. Minimally removed by hemodialysis. **Half-life:** 3–4.5 hrs.

## ⧗ LIFESPAN CONSIDERATIONS
**Pregnancy/Lactation:** Crosses placenta. Distributed in breast milk. **Children:** Prolonged treatment with high-dose therapy may decrease short-term growth rate, cortisol secretion. **Elderly:** Higher risk for developing hypertension, osteoporosis.

---

## INTERACTIONS

**DRUG: Amphotericin** may increase hypokalemia. May increase **digoxin** toxicity caused by hypokalemia. **CYP3A4 inducers (e.g., carbamazepine, phenytoin, rifampin)** may decrease concentration. **CYP3A4 inhibitors (e.g., ketoconazole), macrolide antibiotics** may increase concentration. May decrease effects of **oral antidiabetic agents. Live virus vaccines** may decrease pt's antibody response to vaccine, increase vaccine side effects, potentiate virus replication. **HERBAL: Cat's claw, echinacea** may increase immunosuppressant effect. **FOOD:** Interferes with **calcium** absorption. **LAB VALUES:** May increase serum glucose, lipids, sodium levels. May decrease serum calcium, potassium, thyroxine, WBC.

## AVAILABILITY (Rx)

**Elixir:** 0.5 mg/5 ml. **Injection, Solution:** 4 mg/ml, 10 mg/ml. **Ophthalmic Solution:** 0.1%. **Ophthalmic Suspension (Maxidex):** 0.1%. **Solution, Oral:** 0.5 mg/5 ml. **Solution, Oral Concentrate (Dexamethasone Intensol):** 1 mg/ml. **Tablets:** 0.5 mg, 0.75 mg, 1 mg, 1.5 mg, 2 mg, 4 mg, 6 mg. **Tablets (TaperPak [DexPak]):** 1.5 mg (35 or 51 tablets on taper dose card).

## ADMINISTRATION/HANDLING

 **IV**

◀**ALERT**▶ Dexamethasone sodium phosphate may be given by IV push or IV infusion. Rapid injection may cause genital burning sensation in females.
• For IV push, give over 1–4 min if dose is less than 10 mg. • For IV infusion, mix with 50–100 ml 0.9% NaCl or D₅W and infuse over 15–30 min. • For neonates, solution must be preservative free. • IV solution must be used within 24 hrs.

**IM**
• Give deep IM, preferably in gluteus maximus.

**PO**
• Give with milk, food (to decrease GI effect).

**Ophthalmic Solution, Suspension**
• Place gloved finger on lower eyelid and pull out until a pocket is formed between eye and lower lid. • Place prescribed number of drops or ¼–½ inch ointment into pocket. • Instruct pt to close eye gently for 1–2 min (so medication will not be squeezed out of the sac). • Instruct pt to apply digital pressure to lacrimal sac at inner canthus for 1–2 min to minimize systemic absorption.

## ▩ IV INCOMPATIBILITIES

Ciprofloxacin (Cipro), daunorubicin (Cerubidine), idarubicin (Idamycin), midazolam (Versed).

## ▩ IV COMPATIBILITIES

Cimetidine (Tagamet), cisplatin (Platinol), cyclophosphamide (Cytoxan), cytarabine (Cytosar), docetaxel (Taxotere), doxorubicin (Adriamycin), etoposide (VePesid), furosemide (Lasix), granisetron (Kytril), heparin, hydromorphone (Dilaudid), lorazepam (Ativan), morphine, ondansetron (Zofran), paclitaxel (Taxol), palonosetron (Aloxi), potassium chloride, propofol (Diprivan).

## INDICATIONS/ROUTES/DOSAGE

**Anti-Inflammatory**
**PO, IV, IM: ADULTS, ELDERLY:** 0.75–9 mg/day in divided doses q6–12h. **CHILDREN:** 0.08–0.3 mg/kg/day in divided doses q6–12h.

**Cerebral Edema**
**IV: ADULTS, ELDERLY:** Initially, 10 mg, then 4 mg (IV or IM) q6h. **PO, IV, IM: CHILDREN:** Loading dose of 1–2 mg/kg, then 1–1.5 mg/kg/day in divided doses q4–6h.

**Nausea/Vomiting in Chemotherapy Pts**
**Note:** Refer to individual protocols and emetogenic potential.

**IV: ADULTS, ELDERLY:** 8–20 mg 15–30 min before treatment. **CHILDREN:** 10 mg/m²/dose on days of chemotherapy.

**Physiologic Replacement**
**PO, IV, IM: ADULTS, ELDERLY, CHILDREN:** 0.03–0.15 mg/kg/day in divided doses q6–12h.

**Usual Ophthalmic Dosage, Ocular Inflammatory Conditions**
**ADULTS, ELDERLY, CHILDREN: (Solution):** Initially, 2 drops q1h while awake and q2h at night for 1 day, then reduce to 3–4 times/day. **(Suspension):** 1–2 drops up to 4–6 times/day.

**Dosage in Renal/Hepatic Impairment**
No dose adjustment.

## SIDE EFFECTS

**Frequent: Inhalation:** Cough, dry mouth, hoarseness, throat irritation. **Intranasal:** Burning, mucosal dryness. **Ophthalmic:** Blurred vision. **Systemic:** Insomnia, facial edema (cushingoid appearance ["moon face"]), moderate abdominal distention, indigestion, increased appetite, nervousness, facial flushing, diaphoresis. **Occasional: Inhalation:** Localized fungal infection (thrush). **Intranasal:** Crusting inside nose, epistaxis, sore throat, ulceration of nasal mucosa. **Ophthalmic:** Decreased vision; lacrimation; eye pain; burning, stinging, redness of eyes; nausea; vomiting. **Systemic:** Dizziness, decreased/blurred vision. **Rare: Inhalation:** Increased bronchospasm, esophageal candidiasis. **Intranasal:** Nasal/pharyngeal candidiasis, eye pain. **Systemic:** Generalized allergic reaction (rash, urticaria); pain, redness, swelling at injection site; psychological changes; false sense of well-being; hallucinations; depression.

## ADVERSE EFFECTS/ TOXIC REACTIONS

**Long-term therapy:** Muscle wasting (esp. arms, legs), osteoporosis, spontaneous fractures, amenorrhea, cataracts, glaucoma, peptic ulcer disease, HF. **Ophthalmic:** Glaucoma, ocular hypertension, cataracts. **Abrupt withdrawal following long-term therapy:** Severe joint pain, severe headache, anorexia, nausea, fever, rebound inflammation, fatigue, weakness, lethargy, dizziness, orthostatic hypotension.

## NURSING CONSIDERATIONS

### BASELINE ASSESSMENT
Question for hypersensitivity to any corticosteroids. Obtain baselines for height, weight, B/P, serum glucose, electrolytes.

### INTERVENTION/EVALUATION
Monitor I&O, daily weight, serum glucose. Assess for edema. Evaluate food tolerance. Monitor daily pattern of bowel activity, stool consistency. Report hyperacidity promptly. Check vital signs at least twice daily. Be alert to infection (sore throat, fever, vague symptoms). Monitor serum electrolytes, esp. for hypercalcemia, hypokalemia, paresthesia (esp. lower extremities, nausea/vomiting, irritability), Hgb, occult blood loss. Assess emotional status, ability to sleep.

### PATIENT/FAMILY TEACHING
• Do not change dose/schedule or stop taking drug. • **Must** taper off gradually under medical supervision. • Report fever, sore throat, muscle aches, sudden weight gain, edema, exposure to measles/chickenpox. • Severe stress (serious infection, surgery, trauma) may require increased dosage. • Inform dentist, other physicians of dexamethasone therapy within past 12 mos. • Avoid alcohol, limit caffeine.

**D**

# dexmedetomidine

dex-med-e-**toe**-mye-deen
(Precedex)
**Do not confuse Precedex with
Percocet or Peridex.**

◆**CLASSIFICATION**

**PHARMACOTHERAPEUTIC:** Alpha$_2$
agonist. **CLINICAL:** Nonbarbiturate
sedative, hypnotic.

## USES

Sedation of initially intubated, mechanically ventilated adults in intensive care setting. Use in nonintubated pts requiring sedation before and/or during surgical and other procedures. **OFF-LABEL:** Treatment of shivering, use in children. Awake craniotomy.

## PRECAUTIONS

**Contraindications:** Hypersensitivity to dexmedetomidine. **Cautions:** Heart block, bradycardia, hepatic impairment, hypovolemia, diabetes, hypotension, chronic hypertension, severe ventricular dysfunction, elderly, use of vasodilators or drugs decreasing heart rate.

## ACTION

Selective alpha$_2$-adrenergic agonist. Inhibits norepinephrine release. **Therapeutic Effect:** Produces analgesic, hypnotic, sedative effects.

## PHARMACOKINETICS

Protein binding: 94%. Metabolized in liver. Excreted in urine. **Half-life:** 2 hrs.

## INTERACTIONS

**DRUG:** Sedatives (e.g., **midazolam, lorazepam**), opioids (e.g., **fentanyl, morphine, hydromorphone**), hypnotics (e.g., **zolpidem, temazepam**) may enhance effects. **HERBAL:** None significant. **FOOD:** None known. **LAB VALUES:** May increase serum alkaline phosphatase, potassium, ALT, AST.

## AVAILABILITY (Rx)

**Injection Solution:** 80 mcg/20 ml, 200 mcg/2 ml vials, 4 mcg/ml solutions (50 ml, 100 ml).

## ADMINISTRATION/HANDLING
 **IV**

**Reconstitution** • Dilute 2 ml of dexmedetomidine with 48 ml 0.9% NaCl.
**Rate of Administration** • Individualized, titrated to desired effect. Use controlled infusion pump.
**Storage** • Store at room temperature.

## ▦ IV INCOMPATIBILITIES

Do not mix with any other medications.

## ▦ IV COMPATIBILITIES

Amiodarone (Cordarone), bumetanide (Bumex), calcium gluconate, cisatracurium (Nimbex), dexamethasone, dobutamine, dopamine, magnesium sulfate, norepinephrine (Levophed), propofol (Diprivan).

## INDICATIONS/ROUTES/DOSAGE

**Sedation**

**IV: ADULTS:** Loading dose of 1 mcg/kg over 10 min followed by maintenance infusion of 0.2–0.7 mcg/kg/hr. **ELDERLY:** May require decreased dosage.

**Dosage in Renal Impairment**
No dose adjustment.

**Dosage in Hepatic Impairment**
Use caution.

## SIDE EFFECTS

**Frequent (30%–11%):** Hypotension, nausea. **Occasional (3%–2%):** Pain, fever, oliguria, thirst.

## ADVERSE EFFECTS/ TOXIC REACTIONS

Bradycardia, atrial fibrillation, hypoxia, anemia, pain, pleural effusion may occur with too-rapid IV infusion.

---

## NURSING CONSIDERATIONS

### BASELINE ASSESSMENT

Obtain baseline B/P, heart rate, LOC prior to initiation.

### INTERVENTION/EVALUATION

Assess cardiac monitor for arrhythmia, pulse for bradycardia, B/P for hypotension, level of sedation. Assess respiratory rate, rhythm. Monitor ventilator settings. Discontinue once pt is extubated.

---

# dexmethylphenidate

dex-**meth**-il-**fen**-i-date
(Focalin, <u>Focalin XR</u>)

■ **BLACK BOX ALERT** ■ Chronic use can lead to marked tolerance, psychological dependence. Severe depression may occur during drug withdrawal.

**Do not confuse dexmethylphen-idate with methadone.**

## ◆CLASSIFICATION

**PHARMACOTHERAPEUTIC:** Cerebral cortex stimulator **(Schedule II).** **CLINICAL:** CNS stimulant.

## USES

Treatment of ADHD.

## PRECAUTIONS

**Contraindications:** Hypersensitivity to dexmethylphenidate or methylphenidate. Diagnosis or family history of Tourette's syndrome, glaucoma, history of marked agitation, anxiety, tension, motor tics, use of MAOIs within 14 days. **Cautions:** Cardiovascular disease (HF, recent MI), seizure disorder, psychosis, emotional instability, acute stress reactions, hyperthyroidism. Avoid use in pts with history of alcohol or substance abuse.

## ACTION

Blocks reuptake of norepinephrine, dopamine into presynaptic neurons, increasing release of these neurotransmitters into synaptic cleft. **Therapeutic Effect:** Decreases motor restlessness, fatigue; increases motor activity, mental alertness, attention span; elevates mood.

## PHARMACOKINETICS

Readily absorbed from GI tract. Metabolized in liver. Excreted in urine. **Half-life:** 2.2 hrs.

## ⧗ LIFESPAN CONSIDERATIONS

**Pregnancy/Lactation:** Unknown if excreted in breast milk. **Children:** May be more susceptible to developing anorexia, insomnia, abdominal pain, weight loss. Chronic use may inhibit growth. In psychotic children, may exacerbate symptoms of behavior disturbance, thought disorder. **Elderly:** No age-related precautions noted.

## INTERACTIONS

**DRUG:** May enhance effects of **antihypertensives.** May inhibit metabolism of **phenobarbital, phenytoin, primidone, tricyclic antidepressants;** decreased dosages may be necessary. May alter effects of **warfarin. HERBAL: Ephedra** may cause hypertension, arrhythmias. **Yohimbe** may increase CNS stimulation. **FOOD:** None known. **LAB VALUES:** None known.

## AVAILABILITY (Rx)

**Tablets (Focalin):** 2.5 mg, 5 mg, 10 mg.

**Capsules (Extended-Release [Focalin XR]):** 5 mg, 10 mg, 15 mg, 20 mg, 25 mg, 30 mg, 35 mg, 40 mg.

## ADMINISTRATION/HANDLING

### PO

• Do not give drug in afternoon or evening (causes insomnia). • Tablets may be crushed. • Give without regard to food. • Administer extended-release capsules whole; do not cut or crush. • May sprinkle contents of extended-release capsules on small amount of applesauce. • Give extended-release capsules once each day in the morning, before breakfast.

---

## INDICATIONS/ROUTES/DOSAGE

**NOTE:** If pt taking methylphenidate, initially use one half the dose of methylphenidate for conversion to dexmethylphenidate. Maximum immediate-release dose: 20 mg/day. Maximum extended-release dose: 30 mg/day.

**ADHD**

(Dosage for pts not currently taking methylphenidate)

**Capsules (Extended-Release)**
**PO: ADULTS, ELDERLY:** Initially, 10 mg/day. May increase in increments of 10 mg/day at wkly intervals. **Maximum:** 40 mg/day. **CHILDREN 6 YRS AND OLDER:** Initially, 5 mg/day. May increase in increments of 5 mg/day at wkly intervals. **Maximum:** 30 mg/day.

**Tablets (Immediate-Release)**
**PO: ADULTS, ELDERLY, CHILDREN 6 YRS AND OLDER:** Initially, 2.5 mg 2 times/day. Doses should be given at least 4 hrs apart. May increase in increments of 2.5–5 mg at wkly intervals. **Maximum:** 20 mg/day.

**Dosage in Renal/Hepatic Impairment**
No dose adjustment.

## SIDE EFFECTS

**Frequent:** Abdominal pain, nausea, anorexia, fever. **Occasional:** Tachycardia, arrhythmias, palpitations, insomnia, twitching. **Rare:** Blurred vision, rash, arthralgia.

## ADVERSE EFFECTS/ TOXIC REACTIONS

Withdrawal after prolonged therapy may unmask symptoms of underlying disorder. May lower seizure threshold in pts with history of seizures. Overdose produces excessive sympathomimetic effects (vomiting, tremor, hyperreflexia, seizures, confusion, hallucinations, diaphoresis). Prolonged administration to children may delay growth. Neuroleptic malignant syndrome occurs rarely.

## NURSING CONSIDERATIONS

### BASELINE ASSESSMENT
Evaluate pt for cardiac disease, psychiatric conditions. Obtain baseline vital signs, CBC.

### INTERVENTION/EVALUATION
CBC, B/P, heart rate should be performed routinely during therapy. If paradoxical return of ADHD occurs, dosage should be reduced or discontinued. Weigh, measure pediatric pt regularly to detect delayed growth.

### PATIENT/FAMILY TEACHING
• Report any increase in seizures, chest pain, unexplained syncope. • Avoid caffeine. • Last dose should be given in morning to prevent insomnia. • Report anxiety, fever.

---

**TOP 100**

# dextroamphetamine and amphetamine

dex-troe-am-**fet**-ah-meen/am-**fet**-ah-meen
(Adderall, <u>Adderall-XR</u>)

■ **BLACK BOX ALERT** ■ High potential for abuse. Prolonged administration may lead to drug dependence. Severe cardiovascular events including stroke/MI reported. **Do not confuse Adderall with Inderal.**

## ◆CLASSIFICATION

**PHARMACOTHERAPEUTIC:** Amphetamine **(Schedule II). CLINICAL:** CNS stimulant.

## USES
Treatment of narcolepsy; treatment of ADHD.

## PRECAUTIONS
**Contraindications:** Hypersensitivity to dextroamphetamine, amphetamine, or sympathomimetics. Advanced arteriosclerosis, agitated mental states, glaucoma, history of alcohol or drug abuse, hypersensitivity to sympathomimetic amines, hyperthyroidism, moderate to

---

severe hypertension, symptomatic cardiovascular disease, use of MAOIs within 14 days. **Cautions:** Elderly, debilitated pts, history of seizures, mild hypertension. Preexisting psychotic or bipolar disorder.

## ACTION

Enhances action of dopamine, norepinephrine by blocking reuptake from synapses. Inhibits monoamine oxidase, facilitates release of catecholamines. **Therapeutic Effect:** Increases motor activity, mental alertness; decreases drowsiness, fatigue; suppresses appetite.

## PHARMACOKINETICS

Well absorbed following PO administration. Widely distributed including CNS. Metabolized in liver. Excreted in urine. Removed by hemodialysis. **Half-life:** 10–13 hrs.

## ⧖ LIFESPAN CONSIDERATIONS

**Pregnancy/Lactation:** Distributed in breast milk. **Children:** Safety and efficacy not established in pts younger than 3 yrs. **Elderly:** Age-related cardiovascular, cerebrovascular disease, hepatic/renal impairment may increase risk of side effects.

## INTERACTIONS

**DRUG:** May enhance effects of **tricyclic antidepressants, sympathomimetics. MAOIs** may prolong, intensify effects. May antagonize effects of **hypotensive agents. HERBAL:** None significant. **FOOD:** None known. **LAB VALUES:** May increase plasma corticosteroid.

## AVAILABILITY (Rx)

**Tablets (Adderall):** 5 mg, 7.5 mg, 10 mg, 12.5 mg, 15 mg, 20 mg, 30 mg.

🍃 **Capsules (Extended-Release [Adderall-XR]):** 5 mg, 10 mg, 15 mg, 20 mg, 25 mg, 30 mg.

## ADMINISTRATION/HANDLING

**PO**

• Give tablets at least 6 hrs before bedtime. • Extended-release capsules should be swallowed whole; do not break, crush, or cut. • Avoid afternoon doses to prevent insomnia. • May open capsules and sprinkle on applesauce. Instruct pt not to chew sprinkled beads; take immediately.

## INDICATIONS/ROUTES/DOSAGE

**Narcolepsy**

**PO: ADULTS, CHILDREN OLDER THAN 12 YRS:** Initially, 10 mg/day. Increase by 10 mg/day at wkly intervals until therapeutic response is achieved. **Maximum:** 60 mg/day given in 1–3 divided doses with interval of 4–6 hrs between doses. **CHILDREN 6–12 YRS:** Initially, 5 mg/day. Increase by 5 mg/day at wkly intervals until therapeutic response is achieved. **Maximum:** 60 mg/day given in 1–3 divided doses with interval of 4–6 hrs between doses.

**ADHD**

**ADULTS, ELDERLY: (ADDERALL):** Initially, 5 mg 1–2 times/day. May increase by 5 mg increments at wkly intervals. **Maximum:** 40 mg/day in 1–3 divided doses (usual intervals of 4–6 hrs). **(ADDERALL-XR):** Initially, 20 mg once daily in the morning. May increase up to 60 mg/day. **CHILDREN 13–17 YRS: (ADDERALL):** Initially, 5 mg 1–2 times/day. May increase by 5 mg at wkly intervals. **Maximum:** 40 mg/day in 1–3 divided doses (usual intervals of 4–6 hrs). **(ADDERALL-XR):** Initially, 10 mg once daily in the morning. May increase to 20 mg/day after 1 wk if symptoms are not controlled. May increase up to 60 mg/day. **CHILDREN 6–12 YRS: (ADDERALL):** Initially, 5 mg 1–2 times/day. May increase in 5-mg increments at wkly intervals until optimal response is obtained. **Maximum:** 40 mg/day given in 1–3 divided doses (use intervals of

4–6 hrs between additional doses). (**ADDERALL-XR**): Initially, 5–10 mg once daily in the morning. May increase daily dose in 5- to 10-mg increments at wkly intervals. **Maximum:** 30 mg/day. **CHILDREN 3–5 YRS: (ADDERALL):** Initially, 2.5 mg/day given every morning. May increase daily dose in 2.5-mg increments at wkly intervals until optimal response is obtained. **Maximum:** 40 mg/day given in 1–3 divided doses (use intervals of 4–6 hrs between additional doses). Not recommended in children younger than 3 yrs.

**Dosage in Renal/Hepatic Impairment**
No dose adjustment.

## SIDE EFFECTS

**Frequent:** Increased motor activity, talkativeness, nervousness, mild euphoria, insomnia. **Occasional:** Headache, chills, dry mouth, GI distress, worsening depression in pts who are clinically depressed, tachycardia, palpitations, chest pain, dizziness, decreased appetite.

## ADVERSE EFFECTS/TOXIC REACTIONS

Overdose may produce skin pallor/flushing, arrhythmias, psychosis. Abrupt withdrawal after prolonged use of high doses may produce lethargy (may last for wks). Prolonged administration to children with ADHD may temporarily suppress normal weight/height pattern.

## NURSING CONSIDERATIONS

### BASELINE ASSESSMENT

Assess attention span, impulse control, interaction with others. Screen for drug-seeking behavior, past drug abuse. Obtain baseline B/P.

### INTERVENTION/EVALUATION

Monitor for CNS overstimulation, increase in B/P, growth rate, change in pulse rate, respirations, weight loss.

**Narcolepsy:** Observe/document frequency of narcoleptic episodes. **ADHD:** Observe for improved attention span.

### PATIENT/FAMILY TEACHING

• Normal dosage levels may produce tolerance to drug's anorexic mood-elevating effects within a few wks. • Dry mouth may be relieved with sugarless gum, sips of water. • Take early in day. • Do not break, chew, or crush extended-release capsules. • May mask extreme fatigue. • Report pronounced anxiety, dizziness, decreased appetite, dry mouth, new or worsening behavior, chest pain, palpitations. • Avoid alcohol, caffeine.

## *diazePAM

dye-**az**-e-pam
(Apo-Diazepam ✦, Diastat, Diazepam Intensol, Novo-Dipam ✦, Valium)
**Do not confuse diazepam with diazoxide, diltiazem, Ditropan, or lorazepam, or Valium with Valcyte.**

### ◆ CLASSIFICATION

**PHARMACOTHERAPEUTIC:** Benzodiazepine **(Schedule IV). CLINICAL:** Antianxiety, skeletal muscle relaxant, anticonvulsant.

## USES

Short-term relief of anxiety symptoms, relief of acute alcohol withdrawal. Adjunct for relief of acute musculoskeletal conditions, treatment of seizures (IV route used for termination of status epilepticus). **Gel:** Control of increased seizure activity in refractory epilepsy in pts on stable regimens. **OFF-LABEL:** Treatment of panic disorder. Short-term treatment of spasticity in children with cerebral palsy. Sedation for mechanically vented pts in ICU.

---

## PRECAUTIONS

**Contraindications:** Hypersensitivity to diazepam. Acute narrow-angle glaucoma, untreated open-angle glaucoma, severe respiratory depression, severe hepatic insufficiency, sleep apnea syndrome, myasthenia gravis. Children younger than 6 mos (oral). **Cautions:** Pts receiving other CNS depressants or psychoactive agents, depression, history of drug and alcohol abuse, renal/hepatic impairment, respiratory disease, impaired gag reflex, concurrent use of strong CYP3A4 inhibitors or inducers.

## ACTION

Depresses all levels of CNS by enhancing action of gamma-aminobutyric acid (GABA), a major inhibitory neurotransmitter in the brain. **Therapeutic Effect:** Produces anxiolytic effect, elevates seizure threshold, produces skeletal muscle relaxation.

## PHARMACOKINETICS

Well absorbed from GI tract. Widely distributed. Protein binding: 98%. Excreted in urine. Minimally removed by hemodialysis. **Half-life:** 20–70 hrs (increased in hepatic dysfunction, elderly).

## ⚗ LIFESPAN CONSIDERATIONS

**Pregnancy/Lactation:** Crosses placenta. Distributed in breast milk. May increase risk of fetal abnormalities if administered during first trimester of pregnancy. Chronic ingestion during pregnancy may produce withdrawal symptoms, CNS depression in neonates. **Children/Elderly:** Use small initial doses with gradual increases to avoid ataxia, excessive sedation.

## INTERACTIONS

**DRUG:** Alcohol, CNS depressants may increase CNS depression. **CYP3A4 inducers** (e.g., **carbamazepine, rifampin**) may decrease concentration. **CYP3A4 inhibitors** (e.g., **itraconazole, ketoconazole**) may increase concentration. **HERBAL: Gotu kola, kava kava, St. John's wort, valerian** may increase CNS depression. **St. John's wort** may decrease concentration/effects. **FOOD: Grapefruit products** may increase concentration/effects. **LAB VALUES:** None significant. **Therapeutic serum level:** 0.5–2 mcg/ml; **toxic serum level:** greater than 3 mcg/ml.

## AVAILABILITY (Rx)

**Injection, Solution:** 5 mg/ml. **Oral Concentrate (Diazepam Intensol):** 5 mg/ml. **Oral Solution:** 5 mg/5 ml. **Rectal Gel (Diastat):** 2.5 mg, 10 mg, 20 mg. **Tablet (Valium):** 2 mg, 5 mg, 10 mg.

## ADMINISTRATION/HANDLING

 **IV**

**Rate of Administration** • Give by IV push into tubing of flowing IV solution as close as possible to vein insertion point. • Administer directly into large vein (reduces risk of thrombosis/phlebitis). Do not use small veins (e.g., wrist/dorsum of hand). • Administer IV at rate not exceeding 5 mg/min for adults. For children, give 1–2 mg/min (too-rapid IV may result in hypotension, respiratory depression). • Monitor respirations q5–15min for 2 hrs.

**Storage** • Store at room temperature.

**IM**

• Injection may be painful. Inject deeply into large muscle mass.

**PO**

• Give without regard to meals. • Dilute oral concentrate with water, juice, carbonated beverages; may be mixed in semisolid food (applesauce, pudding). • Tablets may be crushed.

**GEL**

• Insert rectal tip and gently push plunger over 3 sec. Remove tip after 3 additional sec. • Buttocks should be held together for 3 sec after removal.

## ▦ IV INCOMPATIBILITIES

Amphotericin B complex (Abelcet, AmBisome, Amphotec), cefepime (Maxipime), diltiazem (Cardizem), fluconazole (Diflucan), foscarnet (Foscavir), furosemide (Lasix), heparin, hydrocortisone (Solu-Cortef), hydromorphone (Dilaudid), meropenem (Merrem IV), potassium chloride, propofol (Diprivan), vitamins.

## ▦ IV COMPATIBILITIES

Dobutamine (Dobutrex), fentanyl, morphine.

## INDICATIONS/ROUTES/DOSAGE

**Anxiety**
**PO: ADULTS:** 2–10 mg 2–4 times/day. **ELDERLY:** Initially, 1–2 mg 1–2 times/day. **CHILDREN:** 0.12–0.8 mg/kg/day in divided doses q6–8h.
**IV, IM: ADULTS:** 2–10 mg; may repeat in 3–4 hrs if needed. **CHILDREN:** 0.04–0.3 mg/kg/dose q2–4h. **Maximum:** 0.6 mg/kg within 8-hr period.

**Skeletal Muscle Relaxation**
**PO: ADULTS:** 2–10 mg 2–4 times/day. **ELDERLY:** Initially, 1–2 mg 1–2 times/day. **CHILDREN:** 0.12–0.8 mg/kg/day in divided doses q6–8h.

**Alcohol Withdrawal**
**IM, IV: ADULTS, ELDERLY:** Initially, 10 mg, then 5–10 mg 3–4 hrs later. **PO: ADULTS, ELDERLY:** 10 mg 3–4 times during first 24 hrs, then reduce to 5 mg 3–4 times/day as needed.

**Status Epilepticus**
**IV: ADULTS, ELDERLY:** 5–10 mg q5–10 min. **Maximum:** 30 mg. May repeat in 2–4 hrs. **INFANTS, CHILDREN:** 0.1–0.3 mg/kg over 2 min; may repeat after 5–10 min. **Maximum:** 10 mg/dose.

**Control of Increased Seizure Activity (Breakthrough Seizures) in Pts with Refractory Epilepsy Who Are on Stable Regimens of Anticonvulsants**
**PO: ADULTS, ELDERLY:** 2–10 mg 2–4 times/day. **Note:** Do not use gel for more than 5 episodes/mo or more than 1 episode q5days. **Rectal Gel: ADULTS, CHILDREN 12 YRS AND OLDER:** 0.2 mg/kg; may be repeated in 4–12 hrs. **CHILDREN 6–11 YRS:** 0.3 mg/kg; may be repeated in 4–12 hrs. **CHILDREN 2–5 YRS:** 0.5 mg/kg; may be repeated in 4–12 hrs.

**Dosage in Renal Impairment**
Use caution.

**Dosage in Hepatic Impairment**
Use caution. Oral tablets contraindicated in severe hepatic impairment.

## SIDE EFFECTS

**Frequent:** Pain with IM injection, drowsiness, fatigue, ataxia. **Occasional:** Slurred speech, orthostatic hypotension, headache, hypoactivity, constipation, nausea, blurred vision. **Rare:** Paradoxical CNS reactions (hyperactivity/nervousness in children, excitement/restlessness in elderly/debilitated) generally noted during first 2 wks of therapy, particularly in presence of uncontrolled pain.

## ADVERSE EFFECTS/ TOXIC REACTIONS

IV route may produce pain, swelling, thrombophlebitis, carpal tunnel syndrome. Abrupt or too-rapid withdrawal may result in pronounced restlessness, irritability, insomnia, hand tremor, abdominal/muscle cramps, diaphoresis, vomiting, seizures. Abrupt withdrawal in pts with epilepsy may produce increase in frequency/severity of seizures. Overdose results in drowsiness, confusion, diminished reflexes, CNS depression, coma. **Antidote:** Flumazenil (see Appendix J for dosage).

## NURSING CONSIDERATIONS

### BASELINE ASSESSMENT

Assess B/P, pulse, respirations immediately before administration. **Anxiety:** Assess autonomic response (cold, clammy hands, diaphoresis), motor response

 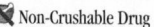

D

(agitation, trembling, tension). **Musculoskeletal spasm:** Record onset, type, location, duration of pain. Check for immobility, stiffness, swelling. **Seizures:** Review history of seizure disorder (length, intensity, frequency, duration, LOC). Observe frequently for recurrence of seizure activity. Initiate seizure precautions.

#### INTERVENTION/EVALUATION

Monitor heart rate, respiratory rate, B/P, mental status. Assess children, elderly for paradoxical reaction, particularly during early therapy. Evaluate for therapeutic response (decrease in intensity/frequency of seizures; calm facial expression, decreased restlessness; decreased intensity of skeletal muscle pain). **Therapeutic serum level:** 0.5–2 mcg/ml; **toxic serum level:** greater than 3 mcg/ml.

#### PATIENT/FAMILY TEACHING

• Avoid alcohol. • Limit caffeine. • May cause drowsiness, avoid tasks that require alertness, motor skills until response to drug is established. • May be habit forming. • Avoid abrupt discontinuation after prolonged use.

## diclofenac

dye-**kloe**-fen-ak
(Apo-Diclo ✦, Cambia, Dyloject, Flector, Pennsaid, Solaraze, Voltaren, Voltaren Gel, Zipsor, Zorvolex)

■ **BLACK BOX ALERT** ■ Increased risk of serious cardiovascular thrombotic events, including myocardial infarction, CVA. Increased risk of severe GI reactions, including ulceration, bleeding, perforation of stomach, intestines. Contraindicated for treatment of perioperative pain in setting of CABG surgery.
**Do not confuse Cataflam with Catapres, diclofenac with Diflucan or Duphalac, or Voltaren with tramadol, Ultram, or Verelan.**

### FIXED-COMBINATION(S)

**Arthrotec:** diclofenac/misoprostol (an antisecretory gastric protectant): 50 mg/200 mcg, 75 mg/200 mcg.

### ◆CLASSIFICATION

**PHARMACOTHERAPEUTIC:** NSAID.
**CLINICAL:** Analgesic, anti-inflammatory.

### USES

**PO: (Immediate-release):** Treatment of rheumatoid arthritis, osteoarthritis, mild to moderate pain, primary dysmenorrhea. **(Zipsor):** Mild to moderate pain. **(Zorvolex):** Mild to moderate pain, osteoarthritic pain. **(Delayed-release):** Treatment of rheumatoid arthritis, osteoarthritis, ankylosing spondylitis. **(Extended-release):** Treatment of rheumatoid arthritis, osteoarthritis. **Oral Solution (Cambia):** Treatment of migraine. **Injection:** Treatment of mild to moderate acute pain and moderate to severe acute pain in adults. **Topical Patch:** Treatment of acute pain due to minor strains, sprains, contusions. **OFF-LABEL:** Treatment of juvenile idiopathic arthritis.

### PRECAUTIONS

**Contraindications:** Hypersensitivity to diclofenac. Pts experiencing asthma, urticaria after taking aspirin, other NSAIDs. Pts with moderate to severe renal impairment in perioperative period who are at risk for volume depletion (injection only); perioperative pain in setting of CABG surgery. **Cautions:** HF, hypertension, renal/hepatic impairment, hepatic porphyria, history of GI disease (e.g., bleeding, ulcers), concomitant use of aspirin or anticoagulants, elderly, debilitated.

### ACTION

Inhibits prostaglandin synthesis, intensity of pain stimulus reaching sensory nerve endings. **Therapeutic Effect:** Produces analgesic, anti-inflammatory effects.

## PHARMACOKINETICS

| Route | Onset | Peak | Duration |
|-------|-------|------|----------|
| PO | 30 min | 2–3 hrs | Up to 8 hrs |

Completely absorbed from GI tract. Protein binding: greater than 99%. Widely distributed. Metabolized in liver. Primarily excreted in urine. Minimally removed by hemodialysis. **Half-life:** 1.2–2 hrs.

## ⧗ LIFESPAN CONSIDERATIONS

**Pregnancy/Lactation:** Crosses placenta. Unknown if distributed in breast milk. Avoid use during third trimester (may adversely affect fetal cardiovascular system: premature closure of ductus arteriosus). **Children:** Safety and efficacy not established. **Elderly:** GI bleeding, ulceration more likely to cause serious adverse effects. Age-related renal impairment may increase risk of hepatic/renal toxicity; reduced dosage recommended.

## INTERACTIONS

**DRUG:** May decrease effects of **acetylcholine, antihypertensives, carbachol, diuretics. Aspirin, other salicylates, warfarin** may increase risk of GI side effects/bleeding. **CYP2C9 inhibitors** (e.g., **voriconazole**) may increase concentration/risk of toxicity. **CYP2C9 inducers** (e.g., **rifampin**) may decrease effect. May increase **cyclosporine** concentration/toxicity. **Ophthalmic:** May decrease antiglaucoma effects of **antiglaucoma agents, epinephrine. HERBAL: Cat's claw, dong quai, evening primrose, garlic, ginseng** may increase antiplatelet activity. **FOOD:** None known. **LAB VALUES:** May increase urine protein, serum BUN, alkaline phosphatase, creatinine, LDH, potassium, ALT, AST. May decrease serum uric acid.

## AVAILABILITY (Rx)

**Adhesive Patch (Flector):** 10×14 cm patch containing 180 mg diclofenac. **Capsules (Zipsor):** 25 mg. **(Zorvolex):** 18 mg, 35 mg. **Intravenous Solution (Dyloject):** 37.5 mg/ml. **Oral Solution (Cambia):** 50-mg packets. **Tablets (Cataflam):** 50 mg.

🍵 **Tablets (Delayed-Release [Voltaren]):** 25 mg, 50 mg, 75 mg. 🍵 **Tablets (Extended-Release [Voltaren XR]):** 100 mg.

## ADMINISTRATION/HANDLING

**PO**
• Do not break, crush, dissolve, or divide enteric-coated tablets. • May give with food, milk, antacids if GI distress occurs. • **Cambia:** Mix one packet in 1–2 oz water, stir well, and instruct pt to drink immediately.

 **IV**

Administer as IV bolus over 15 sec.

**Transdermal Patch**
• Apply to intact skin; avoid contact with eyes. • Do not wear when bathing/showering. • Wash hands after handling.

## INDICATIONS/ROUTES/DOSAGE

**Osteoarthritis**
**PO (Immediate-Release):** ADULTS, ELDERLY: 50 mg 2–3 times/day.
**PO (Extended-Release):** ADULTS, ELDERLY: 100 mg/day as a single dose. May increase to 200 mg/day in 2 divided doses. **(Zorvolex):** 35 mg 3 times/day.

**Rheumatoid Arthritis (RA)**
**PO (Immediate-Release):** ADULTS, ELDERLY: 50 mg 3–4 times/day.
**PO (Extended-Release):** ADULTS, ELDERLY: 100 mg once daily. May increase to 200 mg/day in 2 divided doses.
**PO (Delayed-Release):** ADULTS, ELDERLY: 150–200 mg/day in 2–4 divided doses.

---

**Ankylosing Spondylitis**
**PO** *(Delayed-Release):* **ADULTS, ELDERLY:** 100–125 mg/day in 4–5 divided doses.

**Primary Dysmenorrhea**
**PO** *(Immediate-Release):* **ADULTS, ELDERLY:** 50 mg 3 times/day.

**Pain**
**PO: ADULTS, ELDERLY:** *(Immediate-Release):* 100 mg once, then 50 mg 3 times/day. *(Zipsor):* 25 mg 4 times/day. *(Zorvolex):* 18–35 mg 3 times/day.
**IV:** 37.5 mg q6h prn. **Maximum:** 150 mg/day.
**Topical Patch:** *(Flector):* Apply 2 times/day.

**Migraine (Oral Solution)**
**PO ADULTS, ELDERLY:** 50 mg (one packet) once.

**Dosage in Renal Impairment**
Not recommended in severe impairment.

**Dosage in Hepatic Impairment**
May require dose adjustment. Use caution.

## SIDE EFFECTS

**Frequent (9%–4%): PO:** Headache, abdominal cramps, constipation, diarrhea, nausea, dyspepsia. **Ophthalmic:** Burning, stinging on instillation, ocular discomfort. **Occasional (3%–1%): PO:** Flatulence, dizziness, epigastric pain. **Ophthalmic:** Ocular itching, tearing. **Rare (less than 1%): PO:** Rash, peripheral edema, fluid retention, visual disturbances, vomiting, drowsiness.

## ADVERSE EFFECTS/ TOXIC REACTIONS

Overdose may result in acute renal failure. In pts treated chronically, peptic ulcer, GI bleeding, gastritis, severe hepatic reaction (jaundice), nephrotoxicity (hematuria, dysuria, proteinuria), severe hypersensitivity reaction (bronchospasm, angioedema) occur rarely.

## NURSING CONSIDERATIONS

### BASELINE ASSESSMENT

**Anti-inflammatory:** Assess onset, type, location, duration of pain, inflammation. Inspect appearance of affected joints for immobility, deformities, skin condition.

### INTERVENTION/EVALUATION

Monitor CBC, renal function, LFT, urine output, occult blood test. Monitor for headache, dyspepsia. Monitor daily pattern of bowel activity, stool consistency. Assess for therapeutic response: relief of pain, stiffness, swelling; increased joint mobility; reduced joint tenderness; improved grip strength.

### PATIENT/FAMILY TEACHING

• Swallow tablets whole; do not chew, crush, dissolve, or divide. • Avoid aspirin, alcohol during therapy (increases risk of GI bleeding). • If GI upset occurs, take with food, milk. • Report skin rash, itching, weight gain, changes in vision, black stools, bleeding, jaundice, upper quadrant pain, persistent headache. • **Ophthalmic:** Do not use hydrogel soft contact lenses. • **Topical:** Avoid exposure to sunlight, sunlamps. • Report rash.

## digoxin  `HIGH ALERT`

di-**jox**-in
(Apo-Digoxin ✦, Digitek, Digox, Lanoxin)
**Do not confuse digoxin with Desoxyn or doxepin, or Lanoxin with Lasix, Levoxyl, Levsinex, Lonox, or Mefoxin.**

### ◆CLASSIFICATION

**PHARMACOTHERAPEUTIC:** Cardiac glycoside. **CLINICAL:** Antiarrhythmic, cardiotonic.

## USES

Treatment of mild to moderate HF. Control ventricular response rate in pts with chronic atrial fibrillation. **OFF-LABEL:** Fetal tachycardia with or without hydrops; decrease ventricular rate in supraventricular tachyarrhythmias.

## PRECAUTIONS

**Contraindications:** Hypersensitivity to digoxin. Ventricular fibrillation. **Cautions:** Renal impairment, sinus nodal disease, acute MI (within 6 mos), second- or third-degree heart block (unless functioning pacemaker), concurrent use of strong inducers or inhibitors of P-glycoprotein (e.g., cyclosporine), hyperthyroidism, hypothyroidism, hypokalemia, hypocalcemia.

## ACTION

**HF:** Inhibits sodium/potassium ATPase pump in myocardial cells. Promotes calcium influx. **Supraventricular Arrhythmias:** Suppresses AV node conduction. **Therapeutic Effect: HF:** Increases contractility. **Supraventricular Arrhythmias:** Increases effective refractory period/decreases conduction velocity, decreases heart rate.

## PHARMACOKINETICS

| Route | Onset | Peak | Duration |
|-------|-------|------|----------|
| PO | 0.5–2 hrs | 2–8 hrs | 3–4 days |
| IV | 5–30 min | 1–4 hrs | 3–4 days |

Readily absorbed from GI tract. Widely distributed. Protein binding: 30%. Partially metabolized in liver. Primarily excreted in urine. Minimally removed by hemodialysis. **Half-life:** 36–48 hrs (increased in renal impairment, elderly).

## ⏳ LIFESPAN CONSIDERATIONS

**Pregnancy/Lactation:** Crosses placenta. Distributed in breast milk. **Children:** Premature infants more susceptible to toxicity. **Elderly:** Age-related hepatic/renal impairment may require dosage adjustment. Increased risk of loss of appetite.

## INTERACTIONS

**DRUG: Amiodarone** may increase concentration/toxicity. **Beta blockers (e.g., metoprolol), calcium channel blockers (e.g., diltiazem)** may have additive effect on slowing AV nodal conduction. **Potassium-depleting diuretics (e.g., furosemide)** may increase toxicity due to hypokalemia. **Sympathomimetics (e.g., norepinephrine)** may increase risk of arrhythmias. **HERBAL: Ephedra** may increase risk of arrhythmias. **Licorice** may cause sodium and water retention, loss of potassium. **FOOD: Meals with increased fiber (bran) or high in pectin** may decrease absorption. **LAB VALUES:** None known.

## AVAILABILITY (Rx)

**Oral Solution (Lanoxin):** 50 mcg/ml. **Injection Solution (Lanoxin):** 100 mcg/ml, 250 mcg/ml. **Tablets (Lanoxin):** 62.5 mcg, 125 mcg, 187.5 mcg, 250 mcg.

## ADMINISTRATION/HANDLING

◀**ALERT**▶ IM rarely used (produces severe local irritation, erratic absorption). If no other route possible, give deep into muscle followed by massage. Give no more than 2 ml at any one site.

 **IV**

• May give undiluted or dilute with at least a 4-fold volume of Sterile Water for Injection or D5W (less may cause precipitate). • Use immediately. • Give IV slowly over at least 5 min.

**PO**
• May give without regard to meals.
• Tablets may be crushed.

## ▦ IV INCOMPATIBILITIES

Amphotericin B complex (Abelcet, AmBisome, Amphotec), fluconazole (Diflucan), foscarnet (Foscavir), propofol (Diprivan).

## ✵ IV COMPATIBILITIES

Diltiazem (Cardizem), furosemide (Lasix), heparin, insulin regular, lidocaine, midazolam (Versed), milrinone (Primacor), morphine, potassium chloride.

## INDICATIONS/ROUTES/DOSAGE

**Note:** Loading dose not recommended in HF.

**Loading Dose**

**PO: ADULTS, ELDERLY:** 0.75–1.5 mg. **CHILDREN 10 YRS AND OLDER:** 10–15 mcg/kg. **CHILDREN 5–9 YRS:** 20–35 mcg/kg. **CHILDREN 2–4 YRS:** 30–40 mcg/kg. **CHILDREN 1–23 MOS:** 35–60 mcg/kg. **NEONATE, FULL-TERM:** 25–35 mcg/kg. **NEONATE, PREMATURE:** 20–30 mcg/kg.

**IV: ADULTS, ELDERLY: (Supraventricular tachyarrhythmias):** 0.5–1 mg. **CHILDREN 10 YRS AND OLDER:** 8–12 mcg/kg. **CHILDREN 5–9 YRS:** 15–30 mcg/kg. **CHILDREN 2–4 YRS:** 25–35 mcg/kg. **CHILDREN 1–23 MOS:** 30–50 mcg/kg. **NEONATES, FULL-TERM:** 20–30 mcg/kg. **NEONATES, PREMATURE:** 15–25 mcg/kg.

**Maintenance Dosage**

|  | PO | IV/IM |
|---|---|---|
| Preterm infant | 5–7.5 mcg/kg | 4–6 mcg/kg |
| Full-term infant | 6–10 mcg/kg | 5–8 mcg/kg |
| 1 mo– 2 yrs | 10–15 mcg/kg | 7.5–12 mcg/kg |
| 2–5 yrs | 7.5–10 mcg/kg | 6–9 mcg/kg |
| 5–10 yrs | 5–10 mcg/kg | 4–8 mcg/kg |

**HF**

**PO: ADULTS, ELDERLY:** 0.125–0.25 mg once daily.

**Supraventricular Arrhythmias**

**PO: ADULTS, ELDERLY: Digitalizing dose:** 0.75–1.5 mg. **Maintenance dose:** 0.125–0.5 mg once daily. **IV: Digitalizing dose:** 0.5–1 mg **Maintenance dose:** 0.1–0.4 mg once daily.

**Dosage in Renal Impairment**

Dosage adjustment is based on creatinine clearance. Loading dose: decrease by 50% in end-stage renal disease.

**Maintenance Dose**

| Creatinine Clearance | Dosage |
|---|---|
| 10–50 ml/min | 25%–75% of usual dose or q36h (0.0625 mg q24–36hrs) |
| Less than 10 ml/min (HD, PD, CRRT) | 10%–25% of usual dose or q48h (0.0625 mg q48h) |

**Dosage in Hepatic Impairment**

No dose adjustment.

## SIDE EFFECTS

Dizziness, headache, diarrhea, rash, visual disturbances.

## ADVERSE EFFECTS/ TOXIC REACTIONS

Most common early manifestations of digoxin toxicity are GI disturbances (anorexia, nausea, vomiting), neurologic abnormalities (fatigue, headache, depression, weakness, drowsiness, confusion, nightmares). Facial pain, personality change, ocular disturbances (photophobia, light flashes, halos around bright objects, yellow or green color perception) may occur. Sinus bradycardia, AV block, ventricular arrhythmias noted. **Antidote:** Digoxin immune FAB (see Appendix J for dosage).

## NURSING CONSIDERATIONS

### BASELINE ASSESSMENT

Assess apical pulse. If pulse is 60 or less/min (70 or less/min for children), withhold drug, contact physician. Blood samples are best taken 6–8 hrs after dose or just before next dose.

### INTERVENTION/EVALUATION

Monitor pulse for bradycardia, EKG for arrhythmias for 1–2 hrs after administration (excessive slowing of pulse may be first clinical sign of toxicity). Assess for GI disturbances, neurologic abnormalities (signs of toxicity) q2–4h during loading dose (daily during maintenance). Monitor serum potassium, magnesium, calcium, renal function. **Therapeutic serum level:** 0.8–2 ng/ml; **toxic serum level:** greater than 2 ng/ml.

### PATIENT/FAMILY TEACHING

• Follow-up visits, blood tests are an important part of therapy. • Follow guidelines to take apical pulse and report pulse 60 or less/min (or as indicated by physician). • Wear/carry identification of digoxin therapy and inform dentist, other physician of taking digoxin. • Do not increase or skip doses. • Do not take OTC medications without consulting physician. • Report decreased appetite, nausea/vomiting, diarrhea, visual changes.

# dihydroergotamine

dye-**hye**-droe-er-**got**-a-meen
(D.H.E. 45, Migranal)

■ **BLACK BOX ALERT** ■ Concurrent use with CYP3A4 inhibitors (macrolide antibiotics, azole antifungals, protease inhibitors) increases risk of vasospasm, producing ischemia of brain and peripheral extremities.

### FIXED-COMBINATION(S)

**Cafergot, Wigraine:** ergotamine/caffeine (stimulant): 1 mg/100 mg, 2 mg/100 mg.
**Do not confuse Cafergot with Carafate.**

### ◆CLASSIFICATION

**PHARMACOTHERAPEUTIC:** Ergotamine derivative. **CLINICAL:** Antimigraine.

## USES

Treatment of migraine headache with or without aura. Injection also used to treat cluster headache.

## PRECAUTIONS

**Contraindications:** Hypersensitivity to dihydroergotamine. Uncontrolled hypertension, ischemic heart disease, coronary artery vasospasm (including Prinzmetal's angina), angina pectoris, history of MI following vascular surgery, concurrent use of peripheral and central vasoconstrictors, hemiplegic or basilar migraine, peripheral vascular disease, sepsis, severe renal/hepatic impairment, use of MAOIs within 14 days, use of 5-HT$_B$ agonists within 24 hrs, potent CYP3A4 inhibitors (e.g., azole antifungals, macrolide antibiotics, protease inhibitors), pregnancy, breastfeeding. **Cautions:** Elderly.

## ACTION

Directly stimulates vascular smooth muscle, resulting in peripheral and cerebral vasoconstriction. May have antagonist effects on serotonin. **Therapeutic Effect:** Suppresses vascular headaches, migraine headaches.

## PHARMACOKINETICS

Slowly, incompletely absorbed from GI tract; rapidly and extensively absorbed after rectal administration. Protein binding: greater than 90%. Eliminated in feces by the biliary system. **Half-life:** 21 hrs.

## ⌛ LIFESPAN CONSIDERATIONS

**Pregnancy/Lactation:** Contraindicated in pregnancy (produces uterine stimulant action, resulting in possible fetal death or retarded fetal growth); increases vasoconstriction of placental vascular bed. Drug distributed in breast milk. May produce diarrhea, vomiting in neonate. May prohibit lactation. **Children:** No precautions in pts 6 yrs and older, but use only when unresponsive to other medication. **Elderly:** Age-related occlusive peripheral vascular disease increases risk of peripheral vasoconstriction. Age-related renal impairment may require dosage adjustment.

---

## INTERACTIONS

**DRUG: Beta blockers (e.g., carvedilol, metoprolol), erythromycin** may increase risk of peripheral vasoconstriction. **Ergot alkaloids, 5-HT$_B$ agonists (e.g., sumatriptan), systemic vasoconstrictors** may increase vasopressor effect. **HERBAL:** None significant. **FOOD: Coffee, cola, tea** may increase absorption. **Grapefruit products** may increase concentration, toxicity. **LAB VALUES:** None significant.

## AVAILABILITY (Rx)

**Dihydroergotamine Injection, Solution:** 1 mg/ml. **Intranasal Spray, Solution (Migranal):** 4 mg/ml (0.5 mg/spray).

## INDICATIONS/ROUTES/DOSAGE

**Migraine Headache**
**IM/SQ: ADULTS, ELDERLY:** 1 mg at onset of headache; repeat hourly. **Maximum:** 3 mg/day; 6 mg/wk.
**IV: ADULTS, ELDERLY:** (Give slowly over 2–3 min) 1 mg at onset of headache; repeat hourly. **Maximum:** 2 mg/day; 6 mg/wk.
**Intranasal: ADULTS, ELDERLY:** 1 spray (0.5 mg) into each nostril; repeat in 15 min up to a total of 4 sprays (2 mg). Do not exceed 6 sprays (3 mg) in 24-hr period or 8 sprays (4 mg) in a wk.

**Dosage in Renal/Hepatic Impairment**
Contraindicated in severe impairment.

## SIDE EFFECTS

**Occasional (5%–2%):** Cough, dizziness. **Rare (less than 2%):** Myalgia, fatigue, diarrhea, upper respiratory tract infection, dyspepsia.

## ADVERSE EFFECTS/ TOXIC REACTIONS

Prolonged administration, excessive dosage may produce ergotamine poisoning, manifested as nausea, vomiting, paresthesia of extremities, muscle pain/weakness, precordial pain, significant changes in pulse rate and blood pressure. Vasoconstriction of peripheral arteries/arterioles may result in localized edema, pruritus; feet, hands will become cold, pale. Muscle pain will occur when walking and later, even at rest. Other rare effects include confusion, depression, drowsiness, seizures, gangrene.

## NURSING CONSIDERATIONS

### BASELINE ASSESSMENT

Question for history of peripheral vascular disease, renal/hepatic impairment, possibility of pregnancy. Question onset, location, duration of migraine, possible precipitating symptoms.

### INTERVENTION/EVALUATION

Monitor closely for evidence of ergotamine overdosage as result of prolonged administration or excessive dosage.

### PATIENT/FAMILY TEACHING

• Initiate therapy at first sign of migraine headache. • Report if there is need to progressively increase dose to relieve vascular headaches or if palpitations, nausea, vomiting, paresthesia, pain or weakness of extremities, chest pain. Avoid grapefruit products. • Female pts should avoid pregnancy; if suspected, immediately report.

---

## *dilTIAZem    ᴛᴏᴘ 100

dil-**tye**-a-zem
(Apo-Diltiaz ✦, Cardizem, Cardizem CD, Cardizem LA, Cartia XT, Diltiazem CD, Dilt-XR, Matzim LA, Taztia XT, Tiazac)
**Do not confuse Cardizem with Cardene or Cardene SR, Cartia XT with Procardia XL, diltiazem with Calan, diazepam, or Dilantin, or Tiazac with Ziac.**

## FIXED-COMBINATION(S)

**Teczem:** diltiazem/enalapril (ACE inhibitor): 180 mg/5 mg.

---

## ◆CLASSIFICATION

**PHARMACOTHERAPEUTIC:** Calcium channel blocker. **CLINICAL:** Antianginal, antihypertensive, antiarrhythmic.

## USES

**PO:** Treatment of angina due to coronary artery spasm (Prinzmetal's variant angina), chronic stable angina (effort-associated angina). Treatment of hypertension. **Parenteral:** Temporary control of rapid ventricular rate in atrial fibrillation/flutter. Rapid conversion of paroxysmal supraventricular tachycardia (PSVT) to normal sinus rhythm.

## PRECAUTIONS

**Contraindications: PO:** Acute MI, pulmonary congestion, hypersensitivity to diltiazem, second- or third-degree AV block (except in presence of pacemaker), severe hypotension (less than 90 mm Hg, systolic), sick sinus syndrome (except in presence of pacemaker). **IV:** Hypersensitivity to diltiazem. Sick sinus syndrome or second- or third-degree block (except with functioning pacemaker), cardiogenic shock, administration of IV beta blocker within several hours, atrial fibrillation/flutter associated with accessory bypass tract, severe hypotension, ventricular tachycardia. **Cautions:** Renal/hepatic impairment, HF, concurrent use with beta blocker, hypertrophic obstructive cardiomyopathy.

## ACTION

Inhibits calcium movement across cardiac, vascular smooth-muscle cell membranes (causes dilation of coronary arteries, peripheral arteries, arterioles). **Therapeutic Effect:** Relaxes coronary vascular smooth muscle, increases myocardial oxygen delivery in pts with vasospastic angina, decreases heart rate.

## PHARMACOKINETICS

| Route | Onset | Peak | Duration |
|---|---|---|---|
| PO | 0.5–1 hr | N/A | N/A |
| PO (extended-release) | 2–3 hrs | N/A | N/A |
| IV | 3 min | N/A | N/A |

Well absorbed from GI tract. Protein binding: 70%–80%. Primarily excreted in urine. Not removed by hemodialysis. **Half-life:** 3–8 hrs.

## ⧗ LIFESPAN CONSIDERATIONS

**Pregnancy/Lactation:** Distributed in breast milk. **Children:** No age-related precautions noted. **Elderly:** Age-related renal impairment may require dosage adjustment.

## INTERACTIONS

**DRUG: Beta blockers (e.g., carvedilol, metoprolol), digoxin** may have additive effect on prolonging AV conduction. May increase concentration, risk of toxicity with **carbamazepine, benzodiazepines.** May increase serum **digoxin** concentration. **Rifampin** may decrease concentration/effects. May increase concentration of **statins** and risk of myopathy/rhabdomyolysis. **HERBAL: Ephedra** may worsen arrhythmias, hypertension. **Garlic** may increase antihypertensive effect. **Ginseng, yohimbe** may worsen hypertension. **St. John's wort** may decrease concentration. **FOOD:** None known. **LAB VALUES:** EKG: May increase PR interval.

## AVAILABILITY (Rx)

**Injection, Solution:** 25 mg/5 ml, 50 mg/10 ml, 125 mg/25 ml. **Tablets, Immediate-Release:** 30 mg, 60 mg, 90 mg, 120 mg.

🐾 **Capsules, Extended-Release, 24 Hour:** 120 mg, 180 mg, 240 mg, 300 mg, 360 mg, 420 mg. 🐾 **Capsules, Extended-Release, 12 Hour:** 60 mg, 90 mg, 120 mg. 🐾 **Tablets, Extended-Release, 24 Hour:** 180 mg, 240 mg, 300 mg, 360 mg, 420 mg.

D

---

## ADMINISTRATION/HANDLING

 IV

**Reconstitution** • Add 125 mg to 100 ml D₅W, 0.9% NaCl to provide concentration of 1 mg/ml.
**Rate of Administration** • Infuse per dilution/rate chart provided by manufacturer.
**Storage** • Refrigerate vials. • After dilution, stable for 24 hrs.

### PO
• Give immediate-release tablets before meals and at bedtime. • Tablets may be crushed. • Do not break, crush, dissolve, or divide sustained-release capsules or extended-release capsules or tablets. • Taztia XT capsules may be opened and mixed with applesauce; follow with glass of water. • Cardizem CD, Cardizem LA, Cartia XT, Matzim LA may be given without regard to meals. • Dilacor XR, Dilt-XR to be given on empty stomach.

### ⬛ IV INCOMPATIBILITIES

Acetazolamide (Diamox), acyclovir (Zovirax), ampicillin, ampicillin/sulbactam (Unasyn), diazepam (Valium), furosemide (Lasix), heparin, insulin, nafcillin, phenytoin (Dilantin), rifampin (Rifadin), sodium bicarbonate.

### ⬛ IV COMPATIBILITIES

Albumin, aztreonam (Azactam), bumetanide (Bumex), cefazolin (Ancef), cefotaxime (Claforan), ceftazidime (Fortaz), ceftriaxone (Rocephin), cefuroxime (Zinacef), ciprofloxacin (Cipro), clindamycin (Cleocin), dexmedetomidine (Precedex), digoxin (Lanoxin), dobutamine (Dobutrex), dopamine (Intropin), gentamicin, hydromorphone (Dilaudid), lidocaine, lorazepam (Ativan), metoclopramide (Reglan), metronidazole (Flagyl), midazolam (Versed), morphine, multivitamins, nitroglycerin, norepinephrine (Levophed), potassium chloride, potassium phosphate, tobramycin (Nebcin), vancomycin (Vancocin).

## INDICATIONS/ROUTES/DOSAGE

### Angina
**PO (Immediate-Release)** ADULTS, ELDERLY: Initially, 30 mg 4 times/day. Range: 120–320 mg/day.
**PO (Extended-Release) (Cardizem CD, Cartia XT, DILT-XR):** ADULTS, ELDERLY: Initially, 120–180 mg once daily. May increase at 7–14 day intervals. Range: 120–320 mg. **Maximum:** 480 mg/day.
**(Extended-Release) (Tiazac, Taztia XT):** ADULTS, ELDERLY: Initially, 120–180 mg once daily. May increase at 7–14 day intervals. Range: 120–320 mg/day. **Maximum:** 540 mg/day.
**(Extended-Release) (Cardizem LA, Matzim LA):** Initially, 180 mg/day. May increase at 7–14 day intervals. Range: 120–320 mg. **Maximum:** 360 mg daily.

### Hypertension
**PO Capsule Extended-Release** (once daily dosing) **(Cardizem CD, Cartia XT):** Initially, 180–240 mg/day. May increase after 14 days. Usual dose: 240–360 mg/day. Maximum: 480 mg/day. **(Dilt-XR):** Initially, 180–240 mg/day. May increase after 14 days. Usual dose: 240–360 mg/day. **Maximum:** 540 mg/day. **(Tiazac, Taztia XT):** Initially, 120–240 mg/day. Usual dose: 240–360 mg/day. **Maximum:** 540 mg/day.
**PO Capsule Extended-Release** (twice daily dosing): ADULTS, ELDERLY: Initially, 60–120 mg twice daily. May increase at 14-day intervals. **Maintenance:** 240–360 mg/day.
**PO Tablet Extended-Release** (once daily dosing) **(Cardizem LA, Matzim LA):** ADULTS, ELDERLY: Initially, 180–240 mg/day. May increase at 14-day intervals. Range: 120–540 mg/day. 240–360 mg/day. **Maximum:** 540 mg/day.

**Temporary Control of Rapid Ventricular Rate in Atrial Fibrillation/Flutter; Rapid Conversion of Paroxysmal Supraventricular Tachycardia to Normal Sinus Rhythm**

**IV Push: ADULTS, ELDERLY:** Initially, 0.25 mg/kg (average dose: 20 mg) actual body weight over 2 min. May repeat in 15 min at dose of 0.35 mg/kg (average dose: 25 mg) actual body weight. Subsequent doses individualized.

**IV Infusion: ADULTS, ELDERLY:** After initial bolus injection, may begin infusion at 5–10 mg/hr; may increase by 5 mg/hr up to a maximum of 15 mg/hr. Infusion duration should not exceed 24 hrs. Attempt conversion to PO therapy as soon as possible.

**Dosage in Renal/Hepatic Impairment**
Use with caution.

## SIDE EFFECTS

**Frequent (10%–5%):** Peripheral edema, dizziness, light-headedness, headache, bradycardia, asthenia. **Occasional (5%–2%):** Nausea, constipation, flushing, EKG changes. **Rare (less than 2%):** Rash, micturition disorder (polyuria, nocturia, dysuria, frequency of urination), abdominal discomfort, drowsiness.

## ADVERSE EFFECTS/ TOXIC REACTIONS

Abrupt withdrawal may increase frequency, duration of angina, HF; second- and third-degree AV block occur rarely. Overdose produces nausea, drowsiness, confusion, slurred speech, profound bradycardia. **Antidote:** Glucagon, insulin drip with continuous calcium infusion (see Appendix J for dosage).

## NURSING CONSIDERATIONS

### BASELINE ASSESSMENT

Record onset, type (sharp, dull, squeezing), radiation, location, intensity, duration of anginal pain, precipitating factors (exertion, emotional stress). Assess baseline renal/hepatic function tests. Assess B/P, apical pulse immediately before drug is administered.

### INTERVENTION/EVALUATION

Assist with ambulation if dizziness occurs. Assess for peripheral edema. Monitor pulse rate for bradycardia. Assess B/P, renal function, LFT, EKG with IV therapy. Question for asthenia, headache.

### PATIENT/FAMILY TEACHING

• Do not abruptly discontinue medication. • Compliance with therapy regimen is essential to control anginal pain. • To avoid hypotensive effect, go from lying to standing slowly. • Avoid tasks that require alertness, motor skills until response to drug is established. • Report palpitations, shortness of breath, pronounced dizziness, nausea, constipation. • Avoid alcohol (may increase risk of hypotension or vasodilation).

# dimethyl fumarate

dye-**meth**-il-**fue**-ma-rate
(Tecfidera)

## ◆CLASSIFICATION

**PHARMACOTHERAPEUTIC:** Fumaric acid ester. **CLINICAL:** Multiple sclerosis agent.

## USES

Treatment of relapsing-remitting multiple sclerosis.

## PRECAUTIONS

**Contraindications:** Hypersensitivity to dimethyl fumarate. **Cautions:** Hepatic impairment (may increase hepatic transaminases, lymphopenia (may decrease lymphocyte count).

## ACTION

Exact mechanism of action unknown. May include antiinflammatory action and

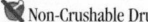

D

cytoprotective properties. **Therapeutic Effect:** Modifies disease progression.

## PHARMACOKINETICS

Undergoes rapid hydrolysis into active metabolite, monomethyl fumarate. Peak concentration: 2–2½ hrs. Protein binding: 27%–45%. Extensively metabolized by esterases. Primarily eliminated as exhaled carbon dioxide (60%). **Half-life:** 1 hr.

## ⧗ LIFESPAN CONSIDERATIONS

**Pregnancy/Lactation:** Unknown if distributed in breast milk. **Children:** Safety and efficacy not established in pts younger than 18 yrs. **Elderly:** No age-related precautions noted.

## INTERACTIONS

**DRUG:** None known. **HERBAL:** None known. **FOOD:** None significant. **LAB VALUES:** May decrease lymphocytes. May increase serum ALT, AST; eosinophils; urine albumin.

## AVAILABILITY (Rx)

**Capsules, Delayed-Release:** 120 mg, 240 mg.

## ADMINISTRATION/HANDLING

**PO**
• Give capsule whole; do not break, crush, dissolve, or divide. • May give without regard to meal. May give with food to decrease flushing reaction and GI effects. • Protect from light.

## INDICATIONS/ROUTES/DOSAGE

**Relapsing-Remitting Multiple Sclerosis**
**PO: ADULTS/ELDERLY:** Initially, 120 mg twice daily for 7 days. Then, increase to 240 mg twice daily.

**Dosage in Renal/Hepatic Impairment**
No dose adjustment.

## SIDE EFFECTS

**Frequent (40%):** Flushing. **Occasional (18%–5%):** Abdominal pain, diarrhea, nausea, vomiting, dyspepsia, pruritus, rash, erythema.

## ADVERSE EFFECTS/ TOXIC REACTIONS

Lymphopenia may increase risk for infection. Severe flushing may lead to noncompliance of therapy.

## NURSING CONSIDERATIONS

### BASELINE ASSESSMENT

Obtain baseline CBC, CMP, urine pregnancy if applicable. Question any plans of breastfeeding. Assess hydration status (urine output, skin turgor). Question history of hepatic impairment, lymphopenia.

### INTERVENTION/EVALUATION

Monitor CBC, LFT. Encourage PO intake. Offer antiemetics for nausea, vomiting. Question any episodes of noncompliance due to flushing, GI symptoms. Monitor for infectious process (fever, malaise, chills, body aches, cough).

### PATIENT/FAMILY TEACHING

• Pts will most likely experience abdominal pain, diarrhea, nausea, and flushing. Side effects may decrease over time. • Take with meals to decrease flushing reaction. • Swallow capsule whole; do not chew, crush, dissolve, or divide. • Two dosage strengths will be provided for starting dose and maintenance dose. • Report any yellowing of skin or eyes, upper abdominal pain, bruising, dark-colored urine, fever, body aches, cough, dehydration.

## dinoprostone

dye-noe-**pros**-tone
(Cervidil, Prepidil, Prostin E$_2$)
■ **BLACK BOX ALERT** ■ To be used only by personnel medically trained in dinoprostone-specific drug effects in a hospital setting.
**Do not confuse Cervidil or Prepidil with bepridil.**

## ◆ CLASSIFICATION

**PHARMACOTHERAPEUTIC:** Prostaglandin. **CLINICAL:** Oxytocic, abortifacient.

## USES

**Vaginal suppository (Prostin E₂):** To induce abortion from wk 12 through wk 20 of pregnancy, to evacuate uterine contents in missed abortion or intrauterine fetal death up to 28 wks gestational age (as calculated from first day of last normal menstrual period), benign hydatidiform mole. **Gel: (Prepidil)** Promote cervical ripening in pregnant women at or near term with medical/obstetric need for labor induction. **Vaginal insert: (Cervidil)** Initiation and/or continuation of cervical ripening in pts at or near term with medical indication for induction of labor.

## PRECAUTIONS

**Contraindications:** Hypersensitivity to dinoprostone. **Gel:** Active cardiac, hepatic, pulmonary, renal disease; acute pelvic inflammatory disease (PID); fetal malpresentation; grand multiparae with 6 or more previous term pregnancy cases with nonvertex presentation; history of cesarean section, major uterine surgery; history of difficult labor, traumatic delivery; hypersensitivity to other prostaglandins; placenta previa, unexplained vaginal bleeding during this pregnancy; pts for whom vaginal delivery is not indicated (vasa previa, active herpes genitalia); significant cephalopelvic disproportion. **Vaginal Suppository:** Active cardiac, hepatic, pulmonary, renal disease; acute PID. **Cautions:** Renal/hepatic impairment, asthma, glaucoma, cardiovascular or pulmonary disease, epilepsy. **Endocervical gel:** With ruptured membrane. **Vaginal gel:** With ruptured membrane, nonvertex or nonsingleton pregnancy, previous uterine pregnancy. **Suppository:** History of hypotension/hypertension, anemia, jaundice, diabetes, compromised uteri, cervicitis, endocervical infections or acute vaginitis.

## ACTION

**Abortifacient:** Stimulates uterine contractions. **Labor Induction:** Relaxes smooth muscle at the cervix .**Therapeutic Effect:** Stimulates myometrial contractions in gravid uterus.

## PHARMACOKINETICS

|  | Onset | Peak | Duration |
|---|---|---|---|
| Uterine stimulation | 10 min (contractions begin) | 1–2 hrs (abortion time) | 2–6 hrs (contractions persist) |

Undergoes rapid enzymatic deactivation primarily in maternal lungs. Protein binding: 73%. Primarily excreted in urine. **Half-life:** Less than 5 min.

## ⧗ LIFESPAN CONSIDERATIONS

**Pregnancy/Lactation: Suppository:** Teratogenic, therefore abortion must be complete. **Gel:** Sustained uterine hyperstimulation may affect fetus (e.g., abnormal heart rate). **Children/Elderly:** Not used in these pt populations.

## INTERACTIONS

**DRUG: Oxytocics** may cause uterine contractions, possibly resulting in uterine rupture, cervical laceration. **HERBAL:** None significant. **FOOD:** None known. **LAB VALUES:** May alter B/P, heart rate. May increase body temperature.

## AVAILABILITY (Rx)

**Endocervical Gel (Prepidil):** 0.5 mg/3 g syringe. **Vaginal Inserts (Cervidil):** 10 mg. **Vaginal Suppositories (Prostin E₂):** 20 mg.

## ADMINISTRATION/HANDLING

**Gel**

• Refrigerate. • Use caution in handling; prevent skin contact. Wash hands thoroughly with soap and water following administration. • Bring to room temperature just before use (avoid forcing the warming process). • Assemble dosing apparatus as described in manufacturer's insert. • Place pt in dorsal position with cervix visualized using a speculum. • Introduce gel into cervical canal just below level of internal os. • Have pt remain in supine position at least 15–30 min (minimizes leakage from cervical canal). • Wait 6–12h after gel administration before initiating oxytocin therapy.

#### Suppository, Vaginal Inserts
• Keep frozen (−4°F); bring to room temperature just before use. • Administer only in hospital setting with emergency equipment available. • Warm suppository to room temperature before removing foil wrapper. • Avoid skin contact (risk of absorption). • Insert high into vagina. • Pt should remain supine for 10 min after administration of suppository, 2 hrs after vaginal insert. • Wait at least 30 min after removing insert before initiating oxytocin therapy.

## INDICATIONS/ROUTES/DOSAGE

#### Abortifacient
**Intravaginal: ADULTS (VAGINAL SUPPOSITORY):** 20 mg (one suppository) high into vagina. May repeat at 3- to 5-hr intervals until abortion occurs. Do not administer for longer than 2 days.

#### Ripening of Unfavorable Cervix
**Intracervical *(Prepidil):* ADULTS (ENDOCERVICAL GEL):** Using catheter supplied, insert 0.5 mg into cervical canal. May repeat 0.5-mg dose q6h prn. **Maximum:** 1.5 mg (7.5 ml) for a 24-hr period.
**Intracervical *(Cervidil):* ADULTS (VAGINAL INSERT):** 10 mg transversely into posterior formix of the vagina (remove upon onset of active labor or 12 hrs after insertion).

## SIDE EFFECTS

**Frequent (66%–33%):** Vomiting, diarrhea, nausea. **Occasional (10%):** Headache, chills/shivering, urticaria, bradycardia, increased uterine pain accompanying abortion, peripheral vasoconstriction. **Rare:** Flushing of skin, vulvar edema.

## ADVERSE EFFECTS/ TOXIC REACTIONS

Overdose may cause uterine contractions with spasm and tetanic contraction, leading to cervical laceration/perforation, uterine rupture/hemorrhage.

## NURSING CONSIDERATIONS

#### BASELINE ASSESSMENT
Offer emotional support. **Suppository:** Obtain orders for antiemetics, antidiarrheals, meperidine, other pain medication for abdominal cramps. Assess any uterine activity, vaginal bleeding. **Gel:** Assess Bishop score. Assess degree of effacement (determines size of shielded endocervical catheter).

#### INTERVENTION/EVALUATION
**Suppository:** Check strength, duration, frequency of contractions. Monitor vital signs q15min until stable, then hourly until abortion complete. Check resting uterine tone. Administer medications for relief of GI effects if indicated or for abdominal cramps. **Gel:** Monitor uterine activity (onset of uterine contractions), fetal status (heart rate), character of cervix (dilation, effacement). Have pt remain recumbent 12 hrs after application with continuous electronic monitoring of fetal heart rate, uterine activity. Record maternal vital signs at least hourly in presence of uterine activity. Reassess Bishop score.

#### PATIENT/FAMILY TEACHING
• **Suppository:** Report promptly fever, chills, foul-smelling/increased vaginal discharge, uterine cramps, pain.

# dinutuximab

din-ue-**tux**-i-mab
(Unituxin)

■ **BLACK BOX ALERT** ■ Life-threatening infusion-related reactions have occurred. Administer required prehydration and premedication, including antihistamines, prior to each infusion. Treatment causes severe neuropathic pain. Administer IV opioids prior to each infusion and for 2 hrs following completion of infusion. Severe peripheral sensory neuropathy occurred in pts with neuroblastoma. Severe motor neuropathy was observed. Discontinue therapy if severe unresponsive pain, severe sensory neuropathy, or moderate to severe peripheral motor neuropathy occurs.

**Do not confuse dinutuximab with brentuximab, cetuximab, rituximab, or siltuximab.**

## ◆CLASSIFICATION

**PHARMACOTHERAPEUTIC:** GD2-binding monoclonal antibody. **CLINICAL:** Antineoplastic.

## USES

Used in combination with granulocyte-macrophage colony-stimulating factor (GM-CSF), interleukin-2 (IL-2), and 13-cis-retinoic acid, for the treatment of pediatric pts with high-risk neuroblastoma who achieve at least a partial response to prior fine-line multiagent, multimodality therapy.

## PRECAUTIONS

**Contraindications:** History of anaphylaxis to dinutuximab. **Cautions:** Active infection; baseline cytopenias; diabetes mellitus, dehydration, electrolyte imbalance, hepatic/renal impairment, peripheral or generalized edema; intolerance of opioids, antipyretics, antihistamines; history of arrhythmias, hypotension, neuropathy, optic disorders.

## ACTION

Binds to glycolipid GD2 expressed on neuroblastoma cells and on normal cells of neuroectodermal origin, including CNS and peripheral nerves. Induces cell lysis of GD2-expressing cells through antibody-dependent cell-mediated cytotoxicity and complement-dependent cytotoxicity. **Therapeutic Effect:** Inhibits tumor cell growth and metastasis.

## PHARMACOKINETICS

Widely distributed. Metabolism not specified. Protein binding: not specified. Elimination not specified. **Half-life:** 10 days.

## ⧗ LIFESPAN CONSIDERATIONS

**Pregnancy/Lactation:** Avoid pregnancy; may cause fetal harm, esp. in third trimester. Unknown if distributed in breast milk. However, human immunoglobulin G is present in human breast milk. Must either discontinue drug or discontinue breastfeeding. Females of reproductive potential must use effective contraception during treatment and for at least 2 mos following discontinuation. **Children:** No age-related precautions noted. **Elderly:** Safety and efficacy not established.

## INTERACTIONS

**DRUG:** None known (not studied). **HERBAL:** None significant. **FOOD:** None known. **LAB VALUES:** May decrease Hgb, Hct, lymphocytes, neutrophils, platelets, RBCs; serum albumin, calcium, magnesium, phosphate, potassium, sodium. May increase serum ALT, AST, bilirubin, creatinine, glucose; urine protein.

## AVAILABILITY (Rx)

**Injection Solution:** 17.5 mg/5 ml (3.5 mg/ml).

## ADMINISTRATION/HANDLING

 IV

*Pretreatment Guidelines*
**IV Hydration** • Administer bolus of 0.9% NaCl 10 ml/kg IV over 1 hr prior to

 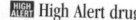

initiation. **Analgesics** • Administer morphine sulfate 50 mcg/kg IV immediately prior to initiation and then continue as morphine sulfate drip at rate of 20–50 mcg/kg/hr during and for 2 hrs following completion of infusion. • Administer additional doses of morphine sulfate 25–50 mcg/kg IV once every 2 hrs as needed for pain, followed by an increase in morphine infusion rate, if clinically stable. • Consider use of fentanyl or hydromorphone if morphine sulfate not tolerated. • If pain is inadequately controlled with opioids, consider use of gabapentin or lidocaine in addition with IV morphine.

**Antihistamines and Antipyretics** • Administer an antihistamine such as diphenhydramine 0.5–1 mg/kg (maximum dose 50 mg) IV over 10–15 min, starting 20 min prior to initiation and as tolerated every 4–6 hrs during infusion. • Administer acetaminophen 10–15 mg/kg (maximum dose 650 mg) 20 minutes prior to each infusion and every 4–6 hrs as needed for fever/pain. • May administer ibuprofen 5–10 mg/kg every 6 hrs as needed for persistent fever/pain.

**Preparation of Infusion** • Visually inspect for particulate matter or discoloration. Do not use if solution is cloudy or contains particulate matter. • Withdraw required volume from vial and inject into 100 ml 0.9% NaCl. • Mix by gently inversion. Do not shake or agitate. • Discard unused portions of vial.

**Rate of Administration** • Initiate infusion rate at 0.875 mg/m2/hr for 30 min via dedicate IV line. May gradually increase rate to maximum rate of 1.75/m2/hr as tolerated. • Do not infuse as IV push or bolus.

**Storage** • Refrigerate vials. • Protect from light by storing in outer carton. • May refrigerate diluted solution up to 4 hrs. • Discard diluted solution 24 hr after preparation.

## ▨ IV INCOMPATABILITIES

Do not mix with other medications.

## INDICATIONS/ROUTES/DOSAGE

**Neuroblastoma**
IV: PEDIATRIC: 17.5 mg/m$^2$/day over 10–20 hrs for 4 consecutive days for maximum of 5 cycles (Tables 1 and 2).

**TABLE 1 SCHEDULE OF DINUTUXIMAB ADMINISTRATION FOR CYCLES 1, 3, AND 5**

| Cycle Day | 1 through 3 | 4 | 5 | 6 | 7 | 8 through 24* |
|---|---|---|---|---|---|---|
| dinutuximab | | X | X | X | X | |

*Cycles 1, 3, and 5 are 24 days in duration.

**TABLE 2 SCHEDULE OF DINUTUXIMAB ADMINISTRATION FOR CYCLES 2 AND 4**

| Cycle Day | 1 through 7 | 8 | 9 | 10 | 11 | 12 through 32* |
|---|---|---|---|---|---|---|
| dinutuximab | | X | X | X | X | |

*Cycles 2 and 4 are 32 days in duration.

**Dose Modification**
*Infusion-Related Reactions*
Mild to moderate adverse reactions such as transient rash, fever, rigors, or localized urticaria that respond promptly to symptomatic treatment: *Onset of Reaction:* Decrease infusion rate to 50% of the previous rate. *After Resolution:* Gradually increase infusion rate up to maximum rate 1.75 mg/m$^2$/hr. Prolonged or severe adverse reactions such as mild bronchospasm without other symptoms, angioedema that does not affect the airway: *Onset of Reaction:* Immediately interrupt infusion. *After Resolution:* If

symptoms resolve rapidly, restart infusion at 50% of the previous rate. *First Recurrence:* Discontinue treatment until the following day. If symptoms resolve and continued treatment is warranted, premedicate with hydrocortisone 1 mg/kg (maximum dose 50 mg) IV and administer dinutuximab infusion at a rate of 0.875 mg/m²/hr in an intensive care unit. *Second Recurrence:* Permanently discontinue.

### Capillary Leak Syndrome
**Moderate to severe, non–life-threatening capillary leak syndrome:** *Onset of Reaction:* Interrupt infusion. After Resolution: Resume infusion rate at 50% of previous rate. **Life-threatening capillary leak syndrome:** *Onset of Reaction:* Discontinue for the current cycle. *After Resolution:* In subsequent cycles, administer at 50% of the previous rate. *First Recurrence:* Permanently discontinue.

### Hypotension Requiring Medical Intervention
*Onset of Reaction:* Interrupt infusion. *After Resolution:* Resume infusion at 50% of the previous rate. If blood pressure remains stable for at least 2 hrs, increase infusion rate as tolerated up to maximum rate of 1.75 mg/m²/hr.

### Severe Systemic Infection or Sepsis
*Onset of Reaction:* Discontinue treatment until resolution of infection, then proceed with subsequent cycles of therapy.

### Neurologic Disorders of the Eye
*Onset of Reaction:* Discontinue infusion until resolution of disorder. *After Resolution:* Reduce dose by 50%. *First Recurrence or if Accompanied by Visual Impairment:* Permanently discontinue.

### Adverse Reactions Requiring Permanent Discontinuation (using CTCAE Grading 1–5)
Grade 3 or 4 anaphylaxis, serum sickness; grade 3 pain unresponsive to maximum supportive measures; grade 4 sensory neuropathy or grade 3 sensory neuropathy that interferes with daily activities for more than 2 wks; grade 2 peripheral motor neuropathy; subtotal or total vision loss; grade 4 hyponatremia despite appropriate fluid management.

**Dosage in Renal/Hepatic Impairment**
Not specified; use caution.

## SIDE EFFECTS
**Frequent (85%–24%):** Pain (abdominal, back, bladder, bone, chest, neck, facial, gingival, musculoskeletal, oropharyngeal, extremity), arthralgia, myalgia, neuralgia, proctalgia, pyrexia, hypotension, vomiting, diarrhea, urticaria, hypoxia. **Occasional (19%–10%):** Tachycardia, edema, hypertension, peripheral neuropathy, weight gain, nausea.

## ADVERSE EFFECTS/TOXIC REACTIONS
Anemia, neutropenia, lymphopenia, thrombocytopenia are expected results of therapy. Severe bone marrow suppression occurred in up to 39% of pts. Serious infusion-related reactions, such as bronchospasm, dyspnea, facial and upper airway edema, hypotension, stridor, and urticaria, may require urgent interventions including bronchodilator therapy, blood pressure support, corticosteroids, infusion interruption, infusion rate reduction, or permanent treatment discontinuation. Severe infusion-related reactions were reported in 26% of pts. Infusion-related reactions usually occurred during or within 24 hrs of infusion completion. Other serious adverse effects may include: severe urticaria (13% of pts); anaphylaxis, cardiac arrest (1% or less of pts); pain despite pretreatment with analgesics including morphine sulfate infusion (85% of pts); grade 3 pain (51% of pts); grade 3 peripheral sensory/motor neuropathy (1% of pts); grade 3–5 capillary leak syndrome (23% of pts); grade 3 hypotension (16% of pts); grade 3 or 4 bacteremia requiring IV antibiotics or other urgent interventions (13% of pts); sepsis (18% of pts); neurologic disorders of the eye including blurred vision, photophobia, mydriasis, fixed or unequal pupils, optic nerve disorder, eyelid ptosis,

papilledema (2%–13% of pts); grade 3 or 4 electrolyte abnormalities including hyponatremia, hypokalemia, hypocalcemia (37%–23% of pts); atypical hemolytic uremic syndrome resulting in anemia, electrolyte imbalance, hypertension, renal insufficiency. Bleeding events including GI/rectal/renal/respiratory/urinary tract/catheter site hemorrhage; disseminated intravascular coagulation, epistaxis, hematemesis, hematochezia, hematuria were reported. Immunogenicity (anti-dinutuximab antibodies) reported in 18% of pts.

## NURSING CONSIDERATIONS

### BASELINE ASSESSMENT

Obtain baseline CBC, BMP, LFT; serum magnesium, ionized calcium, prealbumin, phosphate triglyceride level; capillary blood glucose, urinalysis, urine protein, urine pregnancy test, vital signs. Verify pts have adequate hematologic/hepatic/ophthalmic/respiratory/renal function; proper hydration status prior to start of each infusion. Ensure proper resuscitative equipment/medications are readily available. Obtain baseline visual acuity, pupillary response, neurologic status. Question history of anaphylaxis; intolerance of opioids, antipyretics, antihistamines. Screen for active infection.

### INTERVENTION/EVALUATION

Frequently monitor CBC, BMP, LFT, other serum electrolytes, vital signs. Monitor I&Os. Administer required prehydration and premedication with antihistamine, antipyretics, opioids prior to each infusion and during infusion as indicated. Diligently monitor for infusion-related reactions as listed in Adverse Effects/Toxic Reactions and institute medical support as needed. Monitor for bleeding events of any kind. Consider administration of naloxone if narcotic overdose is suspected. Routinely assess visual acuity, hydration status. Offer emotional support. Initiate fall precautions.

### PATIENT/FAMILY TEACHING

• Serious infusion reactions including anaphylaxis, difficulty breathing, facial swelling, itching, rash, and wheezing may occur during or within 24 hrs of each infusion. • Immediately report any allergic reactions; bleeding of any kind; decreased urine output or dark urine; disorders of the eye including blurry vision, double vision, unequal pupil size, sensitivity to light, eyelid drooping; fever; palpitations; seizures (related to electrolyte imbalance); severe nerve pain or loss of motor function; signs of low blood pressure such as confusion, fainting, pallor; swelling of face, arms, or legs. • Moderate to severe generalized pain is an expected side effect. Medications for pain, fever, and mild allergic reactions will need to be provided before or during each infusion; report any intolerance to such medications. • Therapy is expected to lower blood counts/immune system and may increase risk of bleeding or infection. • Drink plenty of fluids. • Treatment may be harmful to fetuses. Contraception is recommended during therapy and for at least 2 mos after discontinuation in female of childbearing potential.

## *diphenhydrAMINE

dye-fen-**hye**-dra-meen
(Allerdryl ✦, Banophen, Benadryl, Benadryl Children's Allergy, Diphen, Diphenhist, Dytan, Genahist, Nytol ✦)
**Do not confuse Benadryl with benazepril, Bentyl, or Benylin, or diphenhydramine with desipramine, dicyclomine, or dimenhydrinate.**

## FIXED-COMBINATION(S)

**Advil PM:** diphenhydramine/ibuprofen (NSAID): 38 mg/200 mg.

With calamine, an astringent, and camphor, a counterirritant (**Caladryl**).

## ◆ CLASSIFICATION

**PHARMACOTHERAPEUTIC:** Ethanolamine. **CLINICAL:** Antihistamine, anticholinergic, antipruritic, antitussive, antiemetic, antidyskinetic.

## USES

Treatment of allergic reactions including nasal allergies and allergic dermatoses; parkinsonism, including drug-induced extrapyramidal symptoms; prevention/treatment of nausea, vomiting, or vertigo due to motion sickness; antitussive; short-term management of insomnia; adjunct to epinephrine in treatment of anaphylaxis. Topical form used for relief of pruritus from insect bites, skin irritations.

## PRECAUTIONS

**Contraindications:** Hypersensitivity to diphenhydrAMINE. Acute exacerbation of asthma, neonates or premature infants, breastfeeding. **Cautions:** Narrow-angle glaucoma, stenotic peptic ulcer, prostatic hypertrophy, pyloroduodenal/bladder neck obstruction, asthma, COPD, increased IOP, cardiovascular disease, hyperthyroidism, elderly.

## ACTION

Competes with histamine for receptor site on effector cells in GI tract, blood vessels, respiratory tract. **Therapeutic Effect:** Produces anticholinergic, antipruritic, antitussive, antiemetic, antidyskinetic, sedative effects.

## PHARMACOKINETICS

| Route | Onset | Peak | Duration |
|---|---|---|---|
| PO | 15–30 min | 1–4 hrs | 4–6 hrs |
| IV, IM | Less than 15 min | 1–4 hrs | 4–6 hrs |

Well absorbed after PO, parenteral administration. Protein binding: 98%–99%.

Widely distributed. Metabolized in liver. Primarily excreted in urine. **Half-life:** 1–4 hrs. Adults: 7–12 hrs, elderly: 9–18 hrs, children: 4–7 hrs.

## ⏳ LIFESPAN CONSIDERATIONS

**Pregnancy/Lactation:** Crosses placenta. Detected in breast milk (may produce irritability in breastfed infants). Increased risk of seizures in neonates, premature infants if used during third trimester of pregnancy. May prohibit lactation. **Children:** Not recommended in newborns, premature infants (increased risk of paradoxical reaction, seizures). **Elderly:** Increased risk for dizziness, sedation, confusion, hypotension, hyperexcitability.

## INTERACTIONS

**DRUG: Alcohol, other CNS depressants** may increase CNS depressant effects. **Anticholinergics** may increase anticholinergic effects. **HERBAL: Gotu kola, kava kava, St. John's wort, valerian** may increase CNS depression. **FOOD:** None known. **LAB VALUES:** May suppress wheal/flare reactions to antigen skin testing unless drug is discontinued 4 days before testing.

## AVAILABILITY (OTC)

**Capsules:** 25 mg, 50 mg. **Cream:** 1%, 2%. **Injection Solution:** 50 mg/ml. **Syrup:** 12.5 mg/5 ml. **Tablets:** 25 mg, 50 mg. **Tablets, Chewable:** 12.5 mg.

## ADMINISTRATION/HANDLING

 **IV**

• May be given undiluted. • Give IV injection over at least 1 min. **Maximum rate:** 25 mg/min.

**IM**

• Give deep IM into large muscle mass.

**PO**

• Give with food to decrease GI distress. • Scored tablets may be crushed.

---

## ▦ IV INCOMPATIBILITIES

Allopurinol (Aloprim), cefepime (Maxipime), dexamethasone (Decadron), foscarnet (Foscavir).

## ▦ IV COMPATIBILITIES

Atropine, cisplatin (Platinol), cyclophosphamide (Cytoxan), cytarabine (Ara-C), fentanyl, glycopyrrolate (Robinul), heparin, hydrocortisone (Solu-Cortef), hydromorphone (Dilaudid), hydroxyzine (Vistaril), lidocaine, metoclopramide (Reglan), ondansetron (Zofran), potassium chloride, promethazine (Phenergan), propofol (Diprivan).

## INDICATIONS/ROUTES/DOSAGE

**Allergic Reaction**
**PO: ADULTS, ELDERLY:** 25–50 mg q4–8h. **Maximum:** 300 mg/day. **IM, IV:** 10–50 mg/dose. **Maximum:** 400 mg/day. **PO, IV, IM: CHILDREN:** 5 mg/kg/day in divided doses q6–8h. **Maximum:** 300 mg/day.

**Motion Sickness**
**Note:** When used for prophylaxis, give 30 min before motion.
**PO: (Prophylaxis/treatment): ADULTS, ELDERLY:** 25–50 mg q6–8h. **CHILDREN:** 5 mg/kg/day in 3–4 divided doses. **Maximum:** 300 mg/day. **IV/IM: (Treatment): ADULTS, ELDERLY:** 10–50 mg/dose. **Maximum:** 400 mg/day. **CHILDREN:** 5 mg/kg/day in 4 divided doses. **Maximum:** 300 mg/day.

**Antitussive**
**PO: ADULTS, ELDERLY, CHILDREN 12 YRS AND OLDER:** 25 mg q4h. **Maximum:** 150 mg/day.

**Nighttime Sleep Aid**
**PO: ADULTS, ELDERLY, CHILDREN 12 YRS AND OLDER:** 25–50 mg at bedtime. **CHILDREN 2–11 YRS:** 1 mg/kg/dose. **Maximum:** 50 mg.

**Pruritus**
**Topical: ADULTS, ELDERLY, CHILDREN 12 YRS AND OLDER:** Apply 1% or 2% cream or spray 3–4 times/day. **CHILDREN 2–11 YRS:** Apply 1% cream or spray 3–4 times/day.

**Dosage in Renal/Hepatic Impairment**
No dose adjustment.

## SIDE EFFECTS

**Frequent:** Drowsiness, dizziness, muscle weakness, hypotension, urinary retention, thickening of bronchial secretions, dry mouth, nose, throat, lips; in elderly: sedation, dizziness, hypotension. **Occasional:** Epigastric distress, flushing, visual/hearing disturbances, paresthesia, diaphoresis, chills.

## ADVERSE EFFECTS/ TOXIC REACTIONS

Hypersensitivity reactions (eczema, pruritus, rash, cardiac disturbances, photosensitivity) may occur. Overdose symptoms may vary from CNS depression (sedation, apnea, hypotension, cardiovascular collapse, death) to severe paradoxical reactions (hallucinations, tremors, seizures). Children, infants, neonates may experience paradoxical reactions (restlessness, insomnia, euphoria, nervousness, tremors). Overdosage in children may result in hallucinations, seizures, death.

## NURSING CONSIDERATIONS

### BASELINE ASSESSMENT

If pt is having acute allergic reaction, obtain history of recently ingested foods, drugs, environmental exposure, emotional stress. Monitor B/P rate; depth, rhythm, type of respiration; quality, rate of pulse. Assess lung sounds for rhonchi, wheezing, rales.

### INTERVENTION/EVALUATION

Monitor B/P, esp. in elderly (increased risk of hypotension). Monitor children closely for paradoxical reaction.

### PATIENT/FAMILY TEACHING

• Tolerance to antihistaminic effect generally does not occur; tolerance to sedative effect may occur. • Avoid tasks that require alertness, motor skills until response to drug is established. • Dry mouth, drowsiness, dizziness may be an expected response to drug. • Avoid alcohol.

# diphenoxylate with atropine

dye-fen-**ox**-i-late **at**-roe-peen
(Lomotil)
**Do not confuse Lomotil with Lamictal, Lamisil, or Lasix, or Lonox with Lanoxin, Loprox, or Lovenox.**

## FIXED-COMBINATION(S)

**Lomotil:** diphenoxylate/atropine (anticholinergic, antispasmodic): 2.5 mg/0.025 mg.

## ◆CLASSIFICATION

**PHARMACOTHERAPEUTIC:** Meperidine derivative. **CLINICAL:** Antidiarrheal.

## USES

Adjunctive treatment of acute, chronic diarrhea.

## PRECAUTIONS

**Contraindications:** Hypersensitivity to diphenoxylate, atropine. Children younger than 2 yrs, obstructive jaundice, diarrhea associated with pseudomembranous colitis or enterotoxin-producing bacteria. **Cautions:** Children, acute ulcerative colitis, renal/hepatic impairment.

## ACTION

Acts locally and centrally on gastric mucosa. **Therapeutic Effect:** Reduces excessive GI motility and GI propulsion.

## PHARMACOKINETICS

| | Onset | Peak | Duration |
|---|---|---|---|
| Antidiarrheal | 45–60 min | — | 3–4 hrs |

Well absorbed from GI tract. Metabolized in liver. Primarily eliminated in feces. **Half-life:** 2.5 hrs; metabolite: 12–24 hrs.

## ▧ LIFESPAN CONSIDERATIONS

**Pregnancy/Lactation:** Unknown if drug crosses placenta or is distributed in breast milk. **Children:** Not recommended (increased susceptibility to toxicity, including respiratory depression). **Elderly:** More susceptible to anticholinergic effects, confusion, respiratory depression.

## INTERACTIONS

**DRUG: Alcohol, other CNS depressants** may increase CNS depressant effects. **Anticholinergics** may increase effects of atropine. **MAOIs** may precipitate hypertensive crisis. **HERBAL:** None significant. **FOOD:** None known. **LAB VALUES:** May increase serum amylase.

## AVAILABILITY (Rx)

**Liquid (Lomotil):** 2.5 mg diphenoxylate/0.025 mg atropine/5 ml. **Tablets (Lomotil):** 2.5 mg diphenoxylate/0.025 mg atropine.

## ADMINISTRATION/HANDLING

**PO**
• Give without regard to meals. If GI irritation occurs, give with food. • Use liquid for children 2–12 yrs (use graduated dropper for administration of liquid medication).

## INDICATIONS/ROUTES/DOSAGE

**Diarrhea**
**PO: ADULTS, ELDERLY:** Initially, 5 mg (2 tabs or 10 ml) 3–4 times/day. **Maximum:** 20 mg/day. Then reduce dose as needed. **CHILDREN:** 0.3–0.4 mg/kg/day in 4 divided doses (**maximum:** 10 mg/day); then reduce dose as needed.

**D**

**Dosage in Renal/Hepatic Impairment**
No dose adjustment. Use with caution with severe renal/hepatic disease.

## SIDE EFFECTS

**Frequent:** Drowsiness, light-headedness, dizziness, nausea. **Occasional:** Headache, dry mouth. **Rare:** Flushing, tachycardia, urinary retention, constipation, paradoxical reaction (marked by restlessness, agitation), blurred vision.

## ADVERSE EFFECTS/ TOXIC REACTIONS

Dehydration may predispose pt to diphenoxylate toxicity. Paralytic ileus, toxic megacolon (constipation, decreased appetite, abdominal pain with nausea/vomiting) occur rarely. Severe anticholinergic reaction (severe lethargy, hypotonic reflexes, hyperthermia) may result in severe respiratory depression, coma.

## NURSING CONSIDERATIONS

### BASELINE ASSESSMENT
Check baseline hydration status: skin turgor, mucous membranes for dryness, urinary status.

### INTERVENTION/EVALUATION
Encourage adequate fluid intake. Assess bowel sounds for peristalsis. Monitor daily pattern of bowel activity, stool consistency. Record time of evacuation. Assess for abdominal disturbances. Discontinue medication if abdominal distention occurs.

### PATIENT/FAMILY TEACHING
• Avoid tasks that require alertness, motor skills until response to drug is established. • Avoid alcohol. • Report persistent fever, palpitations, diarrhea. • Report abdominal distention.

## *DOBUTamine

doe-**bue**-ta-meen
(Dobutrex ✦)
**Do not confuse dobutamine with dopamine.**

### ◆ CLASSIFICATION
**PHARMACOTHERAPEUTIC:** Sympathomimetic. **CLINICAL:** Cardiac stimulant.

## USES
Short-term management of cardiac decompensation.

## PRECAUTIONS
**Contraindications:** Hypersensitivity to dobutamine. Hypertrophic cardiomyopathy with outflow obstruction. **Cautions:** Atrial fibrillation, hypovolemia, post-MI, concurrent use of MAOIs, elderly.

## ACTION
Direct-action inotropic agent acting primarily on beta₁-adrenergic receptors. **Therapeutic Effect:** Enhances myocardial contractility, increases heart rate.

## PHARMACOKINETICS

| Route | Onset | Peak | Duration |
|-------|-------|------|----------|
| IV | 1–2 min | 10 min | Length of infusion |

Metabolized in liver. Primarily excreted in urine. Not removed by hemodialysis. **Half-life:** 2 min.

## ☒ LIFESPAN CONSIDERATIONS
**Pregnancy/Lactation:** Unknown if drug crosses placenta or is distributed in breast milk. **Children/Elderly:** No age-related precautions noted.

## INTERACTIONS
**DRUG: Sympathomimetics** may increase effects. **HERBAL:** None significant. **FOOD:** None known. **LAB VALUES:** May decrease serum potassium.

## AVAILABILITY (Rx)

**Infusion (Ready-to-Use):** 1 mg/ml (250 ml), 2 mg/ml (250 ml), 4 mg/ml (250 ml). **Injection Solution:** 12.5-mg/ml vial.

## ADMINISTRATION/HANDLING

**◄ALERT►** Correct hypovolemia with volume expanders before dobutamine infusion. Those with atrial fibrillation should be digitalized before infusion. Administer by IV infusion only.

 **IV**

**Reconstitution** • Dilute vial in 0.9% NaCl or D₅W to maximum concentration of 5,000 mcg/ml (5 mg/ml).

**Rate of Administration** • Use infusion pump to control flow rate. • Titrate dosage to individual response. • Infiltration causes local inflammatory changes. • Extravasation may cause dermal necrosis.

**Storage** • Store at room temperature. • Pink discoloration of solution (due to oxidation) does not indicate significant loss of potency if used within recommended time period. • Further diluted solution for infusion is stable for 48 hrs at room temperature, 7 days if refrigerated.

## ⊞ IV INCOMPATIBILITIES

Acyclovir (Zovirax), alteplase (Activase), amphotericin B complex (Abelcet, AmBisome, Amphotec), bumetanide (Bumex), cefepime (Maxipime), foscarnet (Foscavir), furosemide (Lasix), heparin, piperacillin/tazobactam (Zosyn), sodium bicarbonate.

## ⊞ IV COMPATIBILITIES

Amiodarone (Cordarone), calcium chloride, calcium gluconate, diltiazem (Cardizem), dopamine (Intropin), enalapril (Vasotec), epinephrine, famotidine (Pepcid), hydromorphone (Dilaudid), insulin (regular), lidocaine, lorazepam (Ativan), magnesium sulfate, midazolam (Versed), milrinone (Primacor), morphine, nitroglycerin, nitroprusside (Nipride), norepinephrine (Levophed), potassium chloride, propofol (Diprivan).

## INDICATIONS/ROUTES/DOSAGE

**◄ALERT►** Dosage determined by severity of decompensation.

**Cardiac Decompensation**
**IV Infusion: ADULTS, ELDERLY, CHILDREN:** Initially, 0.5–2.5 mcg/kg/min. **Maintenance:** 2–20 mcg/kg/min titrated to desired response. May be infused at a rate of up to 40 mcg/kg/min to increase cardiac output. **NEONATES:** 2–20 mcg/kg/min titrated to desired response.

**Dosage in Renal/Hepatic Impairment**
No dose adjustment.

## SIDE EFFECTS

**Frequent (greater than 5%):** Increased heart rate, B/P. **Occasional (5%–3%):** Pain at injection site. **Rare (3%–1%):** Nausea, headache, anginal pain, shortness of breath, fever.

## ADVERSE EFFECTS/ TOXIC REACTIONS

Overdose may produce marked increase in heart rate (30 beats/min or higher), marked increase in B/P (50 mm Hg or higher), anginal pain, premature ventricular contractions (PVCs).

## NURSING CONSIDERATIONS

**BASELINE ASSESSMENT**

Pt must be on continuous cardiac monitoring. Determine weight (for dosage calculation). Obtain initial B/P, heart rate, respirations. Correct hypovolemia before drug therapy.

**INTERVENTION/EVALUATION**

Continuously monitor for cardiac rate, arrhythmias. Maintain accurate I&O;

D

measure urinary output frequently. Assess serum potassium, plasma dobutamine (therapeutic range: 40–190 ng/ml). Monitor B/P continuously (hypertension risk greater in pts with preexisting hypertension). Check cardiac output, pulmonary wedge pressure/central venous pressure (CVP) frequently. Immediately notify physician of decreased urinary output, cardiac arrhythmias, significant increase in B/P, heart rate, or less commonly, hypotension.

## *DOCEtaxel
`HIGH ALERT`

doe-se-**tax**-el
(Docefrez, Taxotere)

■ **BLACK BOX ALERT** ■ Avoid use with bilirubin more than upper limit of normal (ULN) or serum ALT, AST more than 1.5 times ULN in conjunction with serum alkaline phosphatase more than 2.5 times ULN. Severe hypersensitivity reaction (rash, hypotension, bronchospasm, anaphylaxis) may occur. Fluid retention syndrome (pleural effusions, ascites, edema, dyspnea at rest) has been reported. Pts with abnormal hepatic function, receiving higher doses, and pts with non–small-cell lung carcinoma (NSCLC) and history of prior platinum treatment receiving docetaxel dose of 100 mg/m$^2$ at higher risk for mortality. Avoid use with ANC more than 1,500/mm$^3$.

**Do not confuse docetaxel with paclitaxel or Taxotere with Taxol.**

## ◆CLASSIFICATION

**PHARMACOTHERAPEUTIC:** Antimitotic agent, taxoid. **CLINICAL:** Antineoplastic.

## USES

Treatment of locally advanced or metastatic breast carcinoma after failure of prior chemotherapy. Treatment of metastatic non–small-cell lung cancer. Treatment of metastatic prostate cancer, head and neck cancer (with prednisone). Treatment of advanced gastric adenocarcinoma. **OFF-LABEL:** Bladder, esophageal, ovarian, small-cell lung carcinoma; soft tissue carcinoma, cervical cancer, Ewing's sarcoma, osteosarcoma.

## PRECAUTIONS

**Contraindications:** Hypersensitivity to docetaxel. History of severe hypersensitivity to drugs formulated with polysorbate 80, neutrophil count less than 1,500 cells/mm$^3$. **Cautions:** Hepatic impairment, myelosuppression, concomitant CYP3A4 inhibitors/inducers, fluid retention, pulmonary disease, HF, active infection.

## ACTION

Disrupts microtubular cell network, essential for cellular function. **Therapeutic Effect:** Inhibits cellular mitosis.

## PHARMACOKINETICS

Widely distributed. Protein binding: 94%. Extensively metabolized in liver. Excreted in feces (75%), urine (6%). **Half-life:** 11.1 hrs.

## ⧗ LIFESPAN CONSIDERATIONS

**Pregnancy/Lactation:** May cause fetal harm. Unknown if distributed in breast milk. Breastfeeding not recommended. **Children:** Safety and efficacy not established in pts younger than 16 yrs. **Elderly:** No age-related precautions noted.

## INTERACTIONS

**DRUG: CYP3A4 inhibitors (e.g., erythromycin, ketoconazole)** may increase concentration/toxicity. **CYP3A4 inducers (e.g., rifampin)** may decrease concentration/effects. **Live virus vaccines** may potentiate replication, increase vaccine side effects, decrease pt's antibody response to vaccine. **HERBAL: Echinacea** may decrease concentration. **FOOD:** None known. **LAB VALUES:** May increase serum alkaline phosphatase, bilirubin, ALT, AST. Reduces neutrophil, platelet count, Hgb, Hct.

## AVAILABILITY (Rx)

Injection, Powder for Reconstitution: 20 mg, 80 mg. Injection Solution: 10 mg/ml, 20 mg/ml.

## ADMINISTRATION/HANDLING

 IV

**Reconstitution (Solution)** • Withdraw dose and add to 250–500 ml 0.9% NaCl or D₅W in glass or polyolefin container to provide a final concentration of 0.3–0.74 mg/ml. **(Powder)** Add 1 ml diluent provided to 20-mg vial to provide a concentration of 20 mg/0.8 ml (4 ml to 80-mg vial to provide a concentration of 24 mg/ml). Shake well. Further dilute in 250 ml NaCl or D₅W to a final concentration of 0.3–0.74 mg/ml.

**Rate of Administration** • Administer as a 1-hr infusion. • Monitor closely for hypersensitivity reaction (flushing, localized skin reaction, bronchospasm [may occur within a few min after beginning infusion]).

**Storage** • Store vials between 36°F–77°F. • Protect from bright light. • If refrigerated, stand vial at room temperature for 5 min before administering (do not store in PVC bags). • Diluted solution should be used within 4 hrs (including infusion time).

## ▒ IV INCOMPATIBILITIES

Amphotericin B (Fungizone), methylprednisolone (Solu-Medrol), nalbuphine (Nubain).

## ▒ IV COMPATIBILITIES

Bumetanide (Bumex), calcium gluconate, dexamethasone (Decadron), diphenhydramine (Benadryl), dobutamine (Dobutrex), dopamine (Intropin), furosemide (Lasix), granisetron (Kytril), heparin, hydromorphone (Dilaudid), lorazepam (Ativan), magnesium sulfate, mannitol, morphine, ondansetron (Zofran), palonosetron (Aloxi), potassium chloride.

## INDICATIONS/ROUTES/DOSAGE

◀ **ALERT** ▶ Pt should be premedicated with oral corticosteroids (e.g., dexamethasone 16 mg/day for 5 days beginning day 1 before docetaxel therapy); reduces severity of fluid retention, hypersensitivity reaction.

**Breast Carcinoma**
IV: **ADULTS:** 60–100 mg/m² given over 1 hr q3wks as a single agent. Operable, node positive: 75 mg/m² q3wks for 6 courses (in combination with doxorubicin and cyclophosphamide).

**Non–Small-Cell Lung Carcinoma**
IV: **ADULTS:** 75 mg/m² q3wks (as monotherapy or in combination with cisplatin).

**Prostate Cancer**
IV: **ADULTS, ELDERLY:** 75 mg/m² q3wks with concurrent administration of prednisone.

**Head/Neck Cancer**
IV: **ADULTS, ELDERLY:** 75 mg/m² q3wks (in combination with cisplatin and fluorouracil) for 3–4 cycles, followed by radiation therapy.

**Gastric Adenocarcinoma**
IV: **ADULTS, ELDERLY:** 75 mg/m² q3wks (in combination with cisplatin and fluorouracil).

**Dose Modification for Gastric or Head/Neck Cancer**

| | |
|---|---|
| ALT, AST 2.5 to 5 times ULN and alkaline phosphatase less than or equal to 2.5 times ULN | 80% of dose |
| ALT, AST 1.5 to 5 times ULN and alkaline phosphatase 2.5 to 5 times ULN | 80% of dose |
| ALT, AST greater than 5 times ULN and/or alkaline phosphatase greater than 5 times ULN | Discontinue docetaxel |

**Note:** Toxicity includes febrile neutropenia, neutrophils less than 500/mm³ for longer than 1 wk, severe cutaneous reactions. Also, for NSCLC, platelet nadir less than 25,000/mm³, any CTCAE Grade 3 or 4 nonhematologic toxicity.

**Breast Cancer**
Reduce dose to 75 mg/mm³; if toxicity persists, reduce to 55 mg/mm³.

**Breast Cancer Adjuvant**
Administer when neutrophils are less than 1,500/mm³. If toxicity persists, or grade 3 or 4 stomatitis, reduce dose to 60 mg/mm³.

**Non–Small-Cell Lung Cancer**
*Monotherapy*
Hold dose until toxicity resolves, then reduce dose to 55 mg/mm³. Discontinue if Grade 3 or 4 neuropathy occurs.
*Combination Therapy*
Reduce dose to 65 mg/mm³; may further reduce to 50 mg/mm³ if needed.

**Prostate Cancer**
Reduce dose to 60 mg/mm³; discontinue if toxicity persists.

**Gastric or Head and Neck Cancer**
Reduce dose to 60 mg/mm³; if neutropenic toxicity persists, further reduce to 45 mg/mm³. For Grade 3 or 4 thrombocytopenia, reduce dose from 75 mg/mm³ to 60 mg/mm³; discontinue if toxicity persists.

**Dosage in Renal Impairment**
No dose adjustment.

**Dosage in Hepatic Impairment**
**Total bilirubin more than ULN, or ALT, AST more than 1.5 times ULN with Alkaline Phosphatase more than 2.5 times ULN: Use not recommended.**

## SIDE EFFECTS

**Frequent (80%–19%):** Alopecia, asthenia, hypersensitivity reaction (e.g., dermatitis), which is decreased in pts pretreated with oral corticosteroids; fluid retention, stomatitis, nausea, diarrhea, fever, nail changes, vomiting, myalgia. **Occasional:** Hypotension, edema, anorexia, headache, weight gain, infection (urinary tract, injection site, indwelling catheter tip), dizziness. **Rare:** Dry skin, sensory disorders (vision, speech, taste), arthralgia, weight loss, conjunctivitis, hematuria, proteinuria.

## ADVERSE EFFECTS/ TOXIC REACTIONS

In pts with normal hepatic function, neutropenia (ANC count less than 1,500 cells/mm³), leukopenia (WBC count less than 4,000 cells/mm³) occur in 96% of pts; anemia (hemoglobin level less than 11 g/dL) occurs in 90% of pts; thrombocytopenia (platelet count less than 100,000 cells/mm³) occurs in 8% of pts; infection occurs in 28% of pts. Neurosensory, neuromotor disturbances (distal paresthesia, weakness) occur in 54% and 13% of pts, respectively.

## NURSING CONSIDERATIONS

### BASELINE ASSESSMENT
Obtain baseline ANC, CBC, serum chemistries. Offer emotional support to pt, family. Antiemetics may be effective in preventing, treating nausea/vomiting. Pt should be pretreated with corticosteroids to reduce fluid retention, hypersensitivity reaction.

### INTERVENTION/EVALUATION
Frequently monitor blood counts, particularly ANC count (less than 1,500 cells/mm³ requires discontinuation of therapy). Monitor LFT, serum uric acid levels. Observe for cutaneous reactions (rash with eruptions, mainly on hands, feet). Assess for extravascular fluid accumulation: rales in lungs, dependent edema, dyspnea at rest, pronounced abdominal distention (due to ascites).

### PATIENT/FAMILY TEACHING
• Hair loss is reversible, but new hair growth may have different color or texture. • New hair growth resumes 2–3 mos after last therapy dose. • Maintain

strict oral hygiene. • Do not have immunizations without physician's approval (drug lowers resistance). • Avoid those who have recently taken any live virus vaccine. • Report persistent nausea, diarrhea, respiratory difficulty, chest pain, fever, chills, unusual bleeding, bruising.

# docusate

dok-ue-sate
(Apo-Docusate ✦, Colace, Diocto, Novo-Docusate ✦, Selax ✦, Soflax ✦)
**Do not confuse Colace with Calan or Cozaar, or Surfak with Surbex.**

## FIXED COMBINATION(S)

**Peri-Colace, Senokot-S:** colace/senna (a laxative): 50 mg/8.6 mg.

## ◆CLASSIFICATION

**PHARMACOTHERAPEUTIC:** Bulk-producing laxative. **CLINICAL:** Stool softener.

## USES

Prevention of straining during defecation; constipation associated with hard, dry stools. Relief of occasional constipation.

## PRECAUTIONS

**Contraindications:** Hypersensitivity to docusate. Acute abdominal pain, concomitant use of mineral oil, intestinal obstruction, nausea, vomiting. **Cautions:** Do not use for longer than 1 wk.

## ACTION

Decreases surface film tension by mixing liquid with bowel contents. **Therapeutic Effect:** Increases infiltration of liquid to form softer stool.

## PHARMACOKINETICS

Minimal absorption from GI tract. Acts in small and large intestines. Results usually occur 1–2 days after first dose but may take 3–5 days.

## ⧗ LIFESPAN CONSIDERATIONS

**Pregnancy/Lactation:** Unknown if drug is distributed in breast milk. **Children:** Not recommended in pts younger than 6 yrs. **Elderly:** No age-related precautions noted.

## INTERACTIONS

**DRUG:** None significant. **HERBAL:** None significant. **FOOD:** None known. **LAB VALUES:** None significant.

## AVAILABILITY (OTC)

**Capsules:** 50 mg, 100 mg, 250 mg. **Liquid:** 50 mg/5 ml. **Syrup:** 60 mg/15 ml.

## ADMINISTRATION/HANDLING

• Drink 6–8 glasses of water a day (aids stool softening). • Give each dose with full glass of water, fruit juice. • Administer docusate liquid with milk, fruit juice, infant formula (masks bitter taste).

## INDICATIONS/ROUTES/DOSAGE

**Stool Softener**
**PO: ADULTS, ELDERLY, CHILDREN 12 YRS AND OLDER:** 50–500 mg/day once daily or in divided doses. **CHILDREN 2–11 YRS:** 50–150 mg/day once daily or in divided doses.

## SIDE EFFECTS

**Occasional:** Mild GI cramping, throat irritation (with liquid preparation). **Rare:** Rash.

## ADVERSE EFFECTS/ TOXIC REACTIONS

None known.

## NURSING CONSIDERATIONS

### INTERVENTION/EVALUATION

Encourage adequate fluid intake. Assess bowel sounds for peristalsis. Monitor daily pattern of bowel activity, stool consistency. Record time of evacuation.

D

• Institute measures to promote defecation: increase fluid intake, exercise, high-fiber diet. • Do not use for longer than 1 wk.

# dofetilide

doe-**fet**-i-lide
(Tikosyn)

■ **BLACK BOX ALERT** ■ Pt must be placed in a setting with continuous cardiac monitoring for minimum of 3 days and monitored by staff familiar with treatment of life-threatening arrhythmias.

## ◆CLASSIFICATION

**PHARMACOTHERAPEUTIC:** Potassium channel blocker. **CLINICAL:** Antiarrhythmic: Class III.

## USES

Maintenance of normal sinus rhythm (NSR) in pts with chronic atrial fibrillation/atrial flutter of longer than 1-wk duration who have been converted to NSR. Conversion of atrial fibrillation/flutter to NSR.

## PRECAUTIONS

**Contraindications:** Hypersensitivity to dofetilide. Congenital or acquired prolonged QT syndrome (do not use if baseline QT interval or QTc is greater than 440 msec), severe renal impairment, concurrent use of drugs that may prolong QT interval, hypokalemia, hypomagnesemia, concurrent use with verapamil, dolutegravir, itraconazole, ketoconazole, prochlorperazine, megestrol, cimetidine, hydrochlorothiazide, trimethoprim. Severe renal impairment (CrCl less than 20 ml/min). **Cautions:** Severe hepatic impairment, renal impairment, pts previously taking amiodarone, elderly. Concurrent use of other agents that prolong QT interval. Pts with sick sinus syndrome or second- or third-degree heart block unless functional pacemaker in place.

## ACTION

Prolongs repolarization without affecting conduction velocity by blocking one or more time-dependent potassium currents. No effect on sodium channels, alpha-adrenergic, beta-adrenergic receptors. **Therapeutic Effect:** Terminates reentrant tachyarrhythmias, preventing reinduction.

## PHARMACOKINETICS

Well absorbed following PO administration. 80% eliminated in urine as unchanged drug, 20% excreted as minimally active metabolites. Protein binding: 60%–70%. **Half-life:** 2–3 hrs.

## ⏳ LIFESPAN CONSIDERATIONS

**Pregnancy/Lactation:** Unknown if drug is distributed in breast milk. **Children:** No age-related precautions noted. **Elderly:** Age-related renal impairment may require dosage adjustment.

## INTERACTIONS

**DRUG: Cimetidine, verapamil, itracanazole, ketoconazole, trimethoprim, hydrochlorothiazide** may increase concentration, toxicity. **HERBAL: St. John's wort** may decrease concentration. **Ephedra** may worsen arrhythmias. **FOOD:** None known. **LAB VALUES:** None significant.

## AVAILABILITY (Rx)

**Capsules:** 125 mcg, 250 mcg, 500 mcg.

## ADMINISTRATION/HANDLING

**PO**
• Give without regard to meals. • Do not break, crush, or open capsules.

## INDICATIONS/ROUTES/DOSAGE

◀**ALERT**▶ EKG interval measurements, esp. QTc interval, must be determined prior to first dose.

---

**Antiarrhythmias**

**PO: ADULTS, ELDERLY:** Initially, 500 mcg twice daily. Modify dose in response to QTc interval.

**Dosage in Renal Impairment**

| Creatinine Clearance | Dosage |
|---|---|
| Greater than 60 ml/min | 500 mcg twice daily |
| 40–60 ml/min | 250 mcg twice daily |
| 20–39 ml/min | 125 mcg twice daily |
| Less than 20 ml/min | Contraindicated |

**Dosage in Hepatic Impairment**

No dose adjustment.

## SIDE EFFECTS

**Rare (less than 2%):** Headache, chest pain, dizziness, dyspnea, nausea, insomnia, back/abdominal pain, diarrhea, rash.

## ADVERSE EFFECTS/ TOXIC REACTIONS

Angioedema, bradycardia, cerebral ischemia, facial paralysis, serious arrhythmias (ventricular, various forms of block) have been noted.

## NURSING CONSIDERATIONS

### BASELINE ASSESSMENT

Prior to initiating treatment, QTc intervals must be determined. Do not use if heart rate less than 50 beats/min. Provide continuous EKG monitoring, calculation of creatinine clearance, equipment for resuscitation available for minimum of 3 days. Anticipate proarrhythmic events.

### INTERVENTION/EVALUATION

Assess for conversion of cardiac dysrhythmias and absence of new arrhythmias. Constantly monitor EKG. Provide emotional support. Monitor renal function for electrolyte imbalance (prolonged or excessive diarrhea, sweating, vomiting, thirst).

### PATIENT/FAMILY TEACHING

• Instruct pt on need for compliance and requirement for periodic monitoring of EKG and renal function. • Do not break, crush, or open capsule.

# donepezil

doe-**nep**-e-zil
(Apo-Donepezil ✦, Aricept, Aricept ODT)
**Do not confuse Aricept with Aciphex, Ascriptin, or Azilect.**

## FIXED COMBINATION(S)

**Namzaric:** donepezil/memantine (NMDA receptor antagonist): 10 mg/14 mg, 10 mg/28 mg.

## ◆CLASSIFICATION

**PHARMACOTHERAPEUTIC:** Cholinesterase inhibitor. **CLINICAL:** Cholinergic.

## USES

Treatment of dementia of Alzheimer's disease. **OFF-LABEL:** Treatment of behavioral syndromes in dementia, dementia associated with Parkinson's disease, Lewy body dementia.

## PRECAUTIONS

**Contraindications:** History of hypersensitivity to donepezil, other piperidine derivatives. **Cautions:** Asthma, COPD, bradycardia, bladder outflow obstruction, history of ulcer disease, those taking concurrent NSAIDs, supraventricular cardiac conduction disturbances (e.g., "sick sinus syndrome," Wolff-Parkinson-White syndrome), seizures.

## ACTION

Inhibits enzyme acetylcholinesterase, increasing concentration of acetylcholine at cholinergic synapses, enhancing cholinergic function in CNS. **Therapeutic Effect:** Slows progression of Alzheimer's disease.

## PHARMACOKINETICS

Well absorbed after PO administration. Protein binding: 96%. Extensively metabolized. Eliminated in urine, feces. **Half-life:** 70 hrs.

---

✦ Canadian trade name     Non-Crushable Drug    ⬛ High Alert drug

## ⌛ LIFESPAN CONSIDERATIONS

**Pregnancy/Lactation:** Unknown if drug is distributed in breast milk. **Children:** Safety and efficacy not established. **Elderly:** No age-related precautions noted.

## INTERACTIONS

**DRUG:** May decrease effect of **anticholinergic medications.** May increase synergistic effects of **cholinergic agonists, neuromuscular blockers, succinylcholine. Ketoconazole** may inhibit metabolism. **CYP3A4 inducers (e.g., carbamazepine, rifampin)** may decrease concentration/effects. **HERBAL: St. John's wort** may decrease concentration. **Ginkgo** may increase adverse effects. **FOOD:** None known. **LAB VALUES:** None significant.

## AVAILABILITY (Rx)

**Tablets (Aricept):** 5 mg, 10 mg, 23 mg. **Tablets (Orally Disintegrating [Aricept ODT]):** 5 mg, 10 mg.

## ADMINISTRATION/HANDLING

**PO**
• May be given at bedtime without regard to meals. • Swallow tablets whole; do not break, crush, dissolve, or divide. • **ODT:** Allow to dissolve completely on tongue. • Follow dose with water.

## INDICATIONS/ROUTES/DOSAGE

**Alzheimer's Disease**
**PO: ADULTS, ELDERLY:** Initially 5 mg/day at bedtime. May increase at 4- to 6-wk intervals to 10 mg/day at bedtime. For moderate to severe Alzheimer's, a dose of 23 mg once daily can be administered once pt has been taking 10 mg once daily for at least 3 mos.

**Dosage in Renal/Hepatic Impairment**
No dose adjustment.

## SIDE EFFECTS

**Frequent (11%–8%):** Nausea, diarrhea, headache, insomnia, nonspecific pain, dizziness. **Occasional (6%–3%):** Mild muscle cramps, fatigue, vomiting, anorexia, ecchymosis. **Rare (3%–2%):** Depression, abnormal dreams, weight loss, arthritis, drowsiness, syncope, frequent urination.

## ADVERSE EFFECTS/ TOXIC REACTIONS

Overdose may result in cholinergic crisis (severe nausea, increased salivation, diaphoresis, bradycardia, hypotension, flushed skin, abdominal pain, respiratory depression, seizures, cardiorespiratory collapse). Increasing muscle weakness may occur, resulting in death if muscles of respiration become involved. **Antidote:** Atropine sulfate 1–2 mg IV with subsequent doses based on therapeutic response.

## NURSING CONSIDERATIONS

### BASELINE ASSESSMENT

Assess cognitive function (e.g., memory, attention, reasoning). Obtain baseline vital signs. Assess history for peptic ulcer, urinary obstruction, asthma, COPD, seizure disorder, cardiac conduction disturbances.

### INTERVENTION/EVALUATION

Monitor behavior, mood/cognitive function, activities of daily living. Monitor for cholinergic reaction (GI discomfort/cramping, feeling of facial warmth, excessive salivation/diaphoresis), lacrimation, pallor, urinary urgency, dizziness. Monitor for nausea, diarrhea, headache, insomnia.

### PATIENT/FAMILY TEACHING

• Report nausea, vomiting, diarrhea, diaphoresis, increased salivary secretions, severe abdominal pain, dizziness. • May take without regard to food (best taken at bedtime). • Not a cure for Alzheimer's disease but may slow progression of symptoms.

# *DOPamine

dope-a-meen

■ **BLACK BOX ALERT** ■ If extravasation occurs, infiltrate area with phentolamine (5–10 ml 0.9% NaCl) as soon as possible, no later than 12 hrs after extravasation.
**Do not confuse dopamine with dobutamine or Dopram.**

## ◆CLASSIFICATION

**PHARMACOTHERAPEUTIC:** Sympathomimetic (adrenergic agonist). **CLINICAL:** Cardiac stimulant, vasopressor.

## USES

Adjunct in treatment of shock (e.g., MI, trauma, renal failure, cardiac decompensation, open heart surgery, persisting after adequate fluid volume replacement). **OFF-LABEL:** Symptomatic bradycardia or heart block unresponsive to atropine or cardiac pacing.

## PRECAUTIONS

**Contraindications:** Hypersensitivity to dopamine, sulfites. Pheochromocytoma, ventricular fibrillation. Uncorrected tachyarrhythmias. **Cautions:** Ischemic heart disease, occlusive vascular disease, hypovolemia, recent use of MAOIs (within 2–3 weeks), ventricular arrhythmias, post-MI.

## ACTION

Stimulates adrenergic and dopaminergic receptors. Effects are dose dependent. Lower dosage stimulates dopaminergic receptors, causing renal vasodilation. Higher doses stimulate both dopaminergic and beta$_1$-adrenergic receptors, causing cardiac stimulation and renal vasodilation. **Therapeutic Effect: Low dosage (1–3 mcg/kg/min):** Increases renal blood flow, urinary flow, sodium excretion. **Low to moderate dosage (4–10 mcg/kg/min):** Increases myocardial contractility, stroke volume, cardiac output. **High dosage (greater than 10 mcg/kg/min):** Increases peripheral resistance, vasoconstriction, B/P.

## PHARMACOKINETICS

| Route | Onset | Peak | Duration |
|---|---|---|---|
| IV | 1–2 min | N/A | Less than 10 min |

Widely distributed. Does not cross blood-brain barrier. Metabolized in liver, kidneys, plasma. Primarily excreted in urine. Not removed by hemodialysis. **Half-life:** 2 min.

## ⧗ LIFESPAN CONSIDERATIONS

**Pregnancy/Lactation:** Unknown if drug crosses placenta or is distributed in breast milk. **Children:** Recommended close hemodynamic monitoring (gangrene due to extravasation reported). **Elderly:** No age-related precautions noted.

## INTERACTIONS

**DRUG:** May have increased effects with **vasopressors, vasoconstrictive agents. COMT inhibitors (e.g., entacapone, tolcapone)** may increase level/effects. **HERBAL:** None significant. **FOOD:** None known. **LAB VALUES:** None significant.

## AVAILABILITY (Rx)

**Injection Solution:** 40 mg/ml, 80 mg/ml, 160 mg/ml. **Injection (Premix with Dextrose):** 0.8 mg/ml (250 ml, 500 ml), 1.6 mg/ml (250 ml, 500 ml), 3.2 mg/ml (250 ml).

## ADMINISTRATION/HANDLING

◄**ALERT**► Blood volume depletion must be corrected before administering dopamine (may be used concurrently with fluid replacement).

 **IV**

**Reconstitution •** Available prediluted in 250 or 500 ml D$_5$W or dilute in

250–500 ml 0.9% NaCl or D₅W, to maximum concentration of 3,200 mcg/ml (3.2 mg/ml).

**Rate of Administration** • Administer into large vein (antecubital fossa, central line preferred) to prevent extravasation. • Use infusion pump to control flow rate. • Titrate drug to desired hemodynamic, renal response (optimum urinary flow determines dosage).

**Storage** • Do not use solutions darker than slightly yellow or discolored to yellow, brown, pink to purple (indicates decomposition of drug). • Stable for 24 hrs after dilution.

### ▓ IV INCOMPATIBILITIES

Acyclovir (Zovirax), amphotericin B complex (Abelcet, AmBisome, Amphotec), cefepime (Maxipime), furosemide (Lasix), insulin, sodium bicarbonate.

### ▓ IV COMPATIBILITIES

Amiodarone (Cordarone), calcium chloride, dexmedetomidine (Precedex), diltiazem (Cardizem), dobutamine (Dobutrex), enalapril (Vasotec), epinephrine, heparin, hydromorphone (Dilaudid), labetalol (Trandate), levofloxacin (Levaquin), lidocaine, lorazepam (Ativan), methylprednisolone (Solu-Medrol), midazolam (Versed), milrinone (Primacor), morphine, nicardipine (Cardene), nitroglycerin, norepinephrine (Levophed), piperacillin/tazobactam (Zosyn), potassium chloride, propofol (Diprivan).

### INDICATIONS/ROUTES/DOSAGE

◄ALERT► Effects of dopamine are dose dependent. Titrate to desired response.

**Hemodynamic Support**
**IV Infusion: ADULTS, ELDERLY, CHILDREN:** Range: 2–20 mcg/kg/min. Titrate to desired response. May gradually increase by 5–10 mcg/kg/min increments. **Maximum:** 50 mcg/kg/min. **NEONATES:** 1–20 mcg/kg/min. Titrate to desired response.

### SIDE EFFECTS

**Frequent:** Headache, arrhythmias, tachycardia, anginal pain, palpitations, vasoconstriction, hypotension, nausea, vomiting, dyspnea. **Occasional:** Piloerection (goose bumps), bradycardia, widening of QRS complex.

### ADVERSE EFFECTS/ TOXIC REACTIONS

High doses may produce ventricular arrhythmias. Pts with occlusive vascular disease are at high risk for further compromise of circulation to extremities, which may result in gangrene. Tissue necrosis with sloughing may occur with extravasation of IV solution.

### NURSING CONSIDERATIONS

**BASELINE ASSESSMENT**

Pt must be on continuous cardiac monitoring. Determine weight (for dosage calculation). Obtain initial B/P, heart rate, respirations. Assess potency of IV access.

**INTERVENTION/EVALUATION**

Continuously monitor for cardiac arrhythmias. Measure urinary output frequently. If extravasation occurs, immediately infiltrate affected tissue with 10–15 ml 0.9% NaCl solution containing 5–10 mg phentolamine mesylate. Monitor B/P, heart rate, respirations q15min during administration (more often if indicated). Assess cardiac output, pulmonary wedge pressure, or central venous pressure (CVP) frequently. Assess peripheral circulation (palpate pulses, note color/temperature of extremities). Immediately notify physician of decreased urinary output, cardiac arrhythmias, significant changes in B/P, heart rate, or failure to respond to increase or decrease in infusion rate, decreased peripheral circulation (cold, pale, mottled extremities). Taper dosage before discontinuing (abrupt cessation of therapy may result in marked hypotension). Be alert to excessive vasoconstriction (decreased urine output, increased heart rate, arrhythmias, disproportionate increase in diastolic B/P, decrease in pulse pressure); slow or temporarily stop infusion, notify physician.

# doripenem

dor-i-**pen**-em
(Doribax)
**Do not confuse Doribax with Zovirax, or doripenem with ertapenem, imipenem, or meropenem.**

## ◆CLASSIFICATION

**PHARMACOTHERAPEUTIC:** Carbapenem. **CLINICAL:** Antibiotic.

## USES

Treatment of complicated intra-abdominal infections, complicated UTIs (including pyelonephritis) due to susceptible gram-positive, gram-negative (including *Pseudomonas aeruginosa*), and anaerobic bacteria. **OFF-LABEL:** Treatment of intravascular catheter-related bloodstream infection due to ESBL producing *Escherichia coli* and *Klebsiella* spp. Pneumonia, including ventilator-associated.

## PRECAUTIONS

**Contraindications:** History of serious hypersensitivity to doripenem or other carbapenems (meropenem, imipenem-cilastin, ertapenem). Anaphylactic reactions to beta-lactam antibiotics. **Cautions:** Hypersensitivity to penicillins, cephalosporins. Pts with renal impairment, CNS disorders (e.g., stroke, history of seizures).

## ACTION

Inactivates penicillin-binding proteins, resulting in inhibition of cell wall synthesis. **Therapeutic Effect:** Produces bacterial cell death.

## PHARMACOKINETICS

Penetrates into body fluids, tissues. Widely distributed. Protein binding: 8%.

Primarily excreted in urine. Removed by dialysis. **Half-life:** 1 hr.

##  LIFESPAN CONSIDERATIONS

**Pregnancy/Lactation:** Distributed in breast milk. **Children:** Safety and efficacy not established in pts younger than 18 yrs. **Elderly:** Advanced renal insufficiency, end-stage renal insufficiency may require dosage adjustment.

## INTERACTIONS

**DRUG: Probenecid** reduces renal excretion of doripenem. May decrease **valproic acid** concentration (do not use concurrently). **HERBAL:** None significant. **FOOD:** None known. **LAB VALUES:** May increase serum alkaline phosphatase, ALT, AST. May decrease Hgb, Hct, platelet count; serum potassium.

## AVAILABILITY (Rx)

**Injection, Powder for Reconstitution:** 250 mg, 500 mg.

## ADMINISTRATION/HANDLING

### IV

**Reconstitution** • Reconstitute 250-mg or 500-mg vial with 10 ml Sterile Water for Injection or 0.9% NaCl. • Shake well to dissolve. • Further dilute with 100 ml 0.9% NaCl or D₅W.
**Rate of Administration** • Give by intermittent IV infusion (piggyback). • Do not give IV push. • Infuse over 60 min.
**Storage** • Stable for 12 hrs at room temperature, 72 hrs if refrigerated when diluted in 0.9% NaCl; 4 hrs at room temperature, 24 hrs if refrigerated when diluted in D₅W.

## IV INCOMPATIBILITIES

Diazepam (Valium), potassium phosphate, propofol (Diprivan).

## IV COMPATIBILITIES

Amiodarone, bumetanide (Bumex), calcium gluconate, dexamethasone, diltiazem (Cardizem), diphenhydramine

D

(Benadryl), furosemide (Lasix), heparin, hydrocortisone (Solu-Cortef), hydromorphone (Dilaudid), insulin, labetalol (Trandate), lorazepam (Ativan), magnesium sulfate, methylprednisolone (Solu-Medrol), metoclopramide (Reglan), milrinone, morphine, ondansetron (Zofran), pantoprazole (Protonix), potassium chloride.

## INDICATIONS/ROUTES/DOSAGE

**Intra-Abdominal Infections**
**IV: ADULTS, ELDERLY:** 500 mg q8h for 5–14 days.

**Urinary Tract Infections**
**IV: ADULTS, ELDERLY:** 500 mg q8h for 10–14 days.

**Dosage in Renal Impairment**

| Creatinine Clearance | Dosage |
|---|---|
| Greater than 50 ml/min | No adjustment |
| 30–50 ml/min | 250 mg q8h |
| 11–29 ml/min | 250 mg q12h |
| Hemodialysis | 250 mg q24h, if treating infection caused by *Pseudomonas aeruginosa:* 500 mg q12h on day 1, then 500 g q24h |
| Continuous renal replacement therapy | 250 mg q12h |

**Dosage in Hepatic Impairment**
No dose adjustment.

## SIDE EFFECTS

**Frequent (10%–6%):** Diarrhea, nausea, headache. **Occasional (5%–2%):** Altered mental status, insomnia, rash, abdominal pain, constipation, vomiting, edema, fever. **Rare (less than 2%):** Dizziness, cough, oral candidiasis, anxiety, tachycardia, phlebitis at IV site.

## ADVERSE EFFECTS/ TOXIC REACTIONS

Antibiotic-associated colitis, other superinfections (abdominal cramps, severe watery diarrhea, fever) may occur. Anaphylactic reactions in pts receiving beta-lactams have occurred. Seizures may occur in those with CNS disorders (brain lesions, history of seizures) or with bacterial meningitis or severe impaired renal function.

## NURSING CONSIDERATIONS

### BASELINE ASSESSMENT
Question pt for history of allergies, particularly to beta-lactams, penicillins, cephalosporins. Inquire about history of seizures.

### INTERVENTION/EVALUATION
Monitor for signs of hypersensitivity reaction during first dose. Monitor daily pattern of bowel activity, stool consistency. Monitor for nausea, vomiting. Evaluate hydration status. Evaluate for inflammation at IV injection site. Assess skin for rash. Check mental status; be alert to tremors, possible seizures. Assess sleep pattern for evidence of insomnia.

### PATIENT/FAMILY TEACHING
• Report tremors, seizures, rash, diarrhea, or other new symptoms.

# doxazosin

dox-a-**zoe**-sin
(Apo-Doxazosin ✷, Cardura, Cardura XL)
**Do not confuse Cardura with Cardene, Cordarone, Coumadin, K-Dur, or Ridaura, or doxazosin with doxapram, doxepin, or doxorubicin.**

## ◆CLASSIFICATION

**PHARMACOTHERAPEUTIC:** Alpha-adrenergic blocker. **CLINICAL:** Antihypertensive.

## USES

**Cardura:** Treatment of mild to moderate hypertension. Used alone or in combination with other antihypertensives. Treatment of urinary outflow obstruction and/or obstruction and irritation associated with benign prostatic hyperplasia *(BPH)*: **Cardura XL:** Treatment of urinary outflow obstruction and/or obstruction and irritation associated with benign prostatic hyperplasia. **OFF-LABEL:** Pediatric hypertension. Facilitate distal ureteral stone expulsion. Erectile dysfunction in pts with BPH.

## PRECAUTIONS

**Contraindications:** Hypersensitivity to doxazosin or other quinazolines (prazosin, terazosin). **Cautions:** Constipation, ileus, GI obstruction, hepatic impairment.

## ACTION

**Hypertension:** Selectively blocks alpha$_1$-adrenergic receptors, decreasing peripheral vascular resistance. **BPH:** Inhibits postsynaptic alpha-adrenergic receptors in prostatic stromal and bladder neck tissues. **Therapeutic Effect: Hypertension:** Causes peripheral vasodilation, lowering B/P. **BPH:** Relaxes smooth muscle of bladder, prostate, reducing BPH symptoms.

## PHARMACOKINETICS

| Route | Onset | Peak | Duration |
|---|---|---|---|
| PO (antihypertensive) | 1–2 hrs | 2–6 hrs | 24 hrs |

Well absorbed from GI tract. Protein binding: 98%–99%. Metabolized in liver. Primarily eliminated in feces. Not removed by hemodialysis. **Half-life:** 19–22 hrs.

## ⌛ LIFESPAN CONSIDERATIONS

**Pregnancy/Lactation:** Unknown if drug crosses placenta or is distributed in breast milk. **Children:** Safety and efficacy not established. **Elderly:** May be more sensitive to hypotensive effects.

## INTERACTIONS

**DRUG:** **NSAIDs** may decrease effect. **Hypotension-producing medications (e.g., antihypertensives, diuretics)** may increase effect. **CYP3A4 inhibitors (e.g., atanazavir, ketoconazole)** may increase hypotensive effect. **HERBAL: Ephedra, ginseng, yohimbe** may worsen hypertension. **Garlic** may increase antihypertensive effect. Avoid **saw palmetto** (limited experience with this combination). **FOOD:** None known. **LAB VALUES:** None significant.

## AVAILABILITY (Rx)

**Tablets:** 1 mg, 2 mg, 4 mg, 8 mg.

🔪 **Tablets, Extended-Release:** 4 mg, 8 mg.

## ADMINISTRATION/HANDLING

**PO**
• Give without regard to food. • Do not break, crush, dissolve, or divide extended-release tablet. • Immediate-release tablets given morning or evening; extended-release tablets given with morning meal.

## INDICATIONS/ROUTES/DOSAGE

**Hypertension**
**PO** *(Immediate-Release):* **ADULTS, ELDERLY:** Initially, 0.5–1 mg once daily. May be increased to 2 mg once daily. Thereafter, may increase upward over several weeks to a maximum of 8 mg/day.

**Benign Prostatic Hyperplasia**
**PO** *(Immediate-Release):* **ADULTS, ELDERLY:** Initially, 1 mg/day. May be increased to 2 mg once daily. Thereafter, may increase q1–2wks. **Maximum:** 8 mg/day. *(Extended-Release):* Initially, 4 mg/day. May increase to 8 mg in 3–4 wks. **Note:** When switching to extended-release, omit evening dose prior to starting morning dose.

**Dosage in Renal Impairment**
No dose adjustment.

**Dosage in Hepatic Impairment**
**Mild to moderate impairment:** Use caution. **Severe Impairment:** Avoid use.

## SIDE EFFECTS

**Frequent (20%–10%):** Dizziness, asthenia headache, edema. **Occasional (9%–3%):**

Nausea, pharyngitis, rhinitis, pain in extremities, drowsiness. **Rare (2%–1%):** Palpitations, diarrhea, constipation, dyspnea, myalgia, altered vision, anxiety.

## ADVERSE EFFECTS/ TOXIC REACTIONS

First-dose syncope (hypotension with sudden loss of consciousness) may occur 30–90 min following initial dose of 2 mg or greater, too-rapid increase in dosage, addition of another antihypertensive agent to therapy. First-dose syncope may be preceded by tachycardia (pulse rate 120–160 beats/min).

## NURSING CONSIDERATIONS

### BASELINE ASSESSMENT

Give first dose at bedtime. If initial dose is given during daytime, pt must remain recumbent for 3–4 hrs. Assess B/P, pulse immediately before each dose, and q15–30min until B/P is stabilized (be alert to fluctuations).

### INTERVENTION/EVALUATION

Monitor B/P, I/O. Monitor pulse diligently (first-dose syncope may be preceded by tachycardia). Assess for edema, headache. Assist with ambulation if dizziness, light-headedness occurs.

### PATIENT/FAMILY TEACHING

• Full therapeutic effect may not occur for 3–4 wks. • May cause syncope (fainting); go from lying to standing slowly. • Avoid tasks that require alertness, motor skills until response to drug is established.

# doxepin

dox-e-pin
(Apo-Doxepin ✦, Novo-Doxepin ✦, Prudoxin, Silenor, Sinequan ✦, Zonalon)
■ **BLACK BOX ALERT** ■ Increased risk of suicidal ideation and behavior in children, adolescents, young adults 18–24 yrs with major depressive disorder, other psychiatric disorders.
**Do not confuse doxepin with digoxin, doxapram, doxazosin, Doxidan, or doxycycline, or Sinequan with Seroquel, or Singulair.**

## ◆CLASSIFICATION

**PHARMACOTHERAPEUTIC:** Tricyclic. **CLINICAL:** Antidepressant, antianxiety, antineuralgic, antiulcer, antipruritic.

## USES

Treatment of depression and/or anxiety. **Silenor (only):** Treatment of insomnia in pts with difficulty staying asleep. **Topical:** Treatment of pruritus associated with atopic dermatitis. **OFF-LABEL:** Treatment of neurogenic pain, treatment of anxiety.

## PRECAUTIONS

**Contraindications:** Hypersensitivity to doxepin. Narrow-angle glaucoma, hypersensitivity to other tricyclic antidepressants, urinary retention, use of MAOIs within 14 days. **Cautions:** Cardiac/hepatic/renal disease, pts at risk for suicidal ideation, respiratory compromise, sleep apnea, history of bowel obstruction, increased IOP, glaucoma, history of seizures, history of urinary retention/obstruction, hyperthyroidism, prostatic hypertrophy, hiatal hernia, elderly.

## ACTION

Increases synaptic concentrations of norepinephrine, serotonin. **Therapeutic Effect:** Produces antidepressant, anxiolytic effects.

## PHARMACOKINETICS

**PO:** Rapidly absorbed from GI tract. Protein binding: 80%–85%. Metabolized in liver. Primarily excreted in urine. Not removed by hemodialysis. **Half-life:** 6–8 hrs. **Topical:** Absorbed through skin. Distributed to body tissues.

Metabolized to active metabolite. Excreted in urine.

## ⏳ LIFESPAN CONSIDERATIONS

**Pregnancy/Lactation:** Crosses placenta. Distributed in breast milk. **Children:** Safety and efficacy not established in pts younger than 12 yrs. **Elderly:** Increased risk of toxicity (lower dosages recommended).

## INTERACTIONS

**DRUG: Alcohol, other CNS depressants** may increase CNS, respiratory depression, hypotensive effects. **Cimetidine** may increase concentration, risk of toxicity. **MAOIs** may increase risk of seizures, hyperpyrexia, hypertensive crisis (discontinue at least 2 wks prior to starting doxepin). **Phenothiazines** may increase anticholinergic, sedative effects. **HERBAL: Kava kava, SAMe, St. John's wort, valerian** may increase sedation, risk of serotonin syndrome. **St. John's wort** may decrease concentration/effects. **FOOD:** None known. **LAB VALUES:** May alter serum glucose, EKG readings. **Therapeutic serum level:** 110–250 ng/ml; **toxic serum level:** greater than 300 ng/ml.

## AVAILABILITY (Rx)

**Capsules:** 10 mg, 25 mg, 50 mg, 75 mg, 100 mg, 150 mg. **Cream (Prudoxin, Zonalon):** 5%. **Oral Concentrate:** 10 mg/ml. **Tablets (Silenor):** 3 mg, 6 mg.

## ADMINISTRATION/HANDLING

**PO**
• Give with food, milk if GI distress occurs. • Dilute concentrate in 4-oz glass of water, milk, orange, tomato, prune, pineapple juice. Incompatible with carbonated drinks. • Give larger portion of daily dose at bedtime. • **Silenor:** Give within 30 min of bedtime but not within 3 hrs of a meal.

**Topical**
• Apply thin film of cream on affected areas of skin. • Do not use for more than 8 days. • Do not use occlusive dressing.

## INDICATIONS/ROUTES/DOSAGE

**Depression, Anxiety**
**PO: ADULTS:** Initially, 25–50 mg/day at bedtime or in 2–3 divided doses. May increase gradually to usual dose of 150 mg–300 mg/day (single dose should not exceed 150 mg). **ELDERLY:** Initially, 10–25 mg at bedtime. May increase by 10–25 mg/day every 3–7 days.

**Insomnia (Silenor only)**
**PO: ADULTS:** 3–6 mg. **ELDERLY:** 3 mg (give within 30 min of bedtime). May increase to 6 mg once daily.

**Pruritus Associated with Atopic Dermatitis**
**Topical: ADULTS, ELDERLY:** Apply thin film 4 times/day at 3- to 4-hr intervals. Not recommended for more than 8 days.

**Dosage in Renal Impairment**
No dose adjustment.

**Dosage in Hepatic Impairment**
Use lower initial dose; adjust gradually. **Silenor:** Initially, 3 mg once daily.

## SIDE EFFECTS

**Frequent: PO:** Orthostatic hypotension, drowsiness, dry mouth, headache, increased appetite, weight gain, nausea, unusual fatigue, unpleasant taste. **Topical:** Edema, increased pruritus, eczema, burning, tingling, stinging at application site, altered taste, dizziness, drowsiness, dry skin, dry mouth, fatigue, headache, thirst. **Occasional: PO:** Blurred vision, confusion, constipation, hallucinations, difficult urination, eye pain, irregular heartbeat, fine muscle tremors, nervousness, impaired sexual function, diarrhea, diaphoresis, heartburn, insomnia. **Silenor:** Nausea, upper respiratory infection. **Topical:** Anxiety, skin irritation/cracking, nausea. **Rare: PO:** Allergic reaction, alopecia, tinnitus, breast enlargement. **Topical:** Fever, photosensitivity.

---

✦ Canadian trade name   🜂 Non-Crushable Drug   [HIGH ALERT] High Alert drug

## ADVERSE EFFECTS/ TOXIC REACTIONS

Abrupt or too-rapid withdrawal may result in headache, malaise, nausea, vomiting, vivid dreams. Overdose may produce confusion, severe drowsiness, agitation, tachycardia, arrhythmias, shortness of breath, vomiting.

## NURSING CONSIDERATIONS

### BASELINE ASSESSMENT

Assess B/P, pulse, EKG (those with history of cardiovascular disease). Perform CBC, serum electrolyte tests before long-term therapy. Assess pt's appearance, behavior, level of interest, mood, suicidal ideation, sleep pattern.

### INTERVENTION/EVALUATION

Monitor B/P, pulse, weight. Perform CBC, serum electrolyte tests periodically to assess renal/hepatic function. Monitor mental status, suicidal ideation. Supervise suicidal-risk pt closely during early therapy (as depression lessens, energy level improves, increasing suicide potential). Assess appearance, behavior, speech pattern, level of interest, mood. **Therapeutic serum level:** 110–250 ng/ml; **toxic serum level:** greater than 300 ng/ml.

### PATIENT/FAMILY TEACHING

• Do not discontinue abruptly. • Change positions slowly to avoid dizziness. • Avoid tasks that require alertness, motor skills until response to drug is established. • Do not cover affected area with occlusive dressing after applying cream. • May cause dry mouth. • Avoid alcohol, limit caffeine. • May increase appetite. • Avoid exposure to sunlight/artificial light source. • Therapeutic effect may be noted within 2–5 days, maximum effect within 2–3 wks. • Report worsening depression, suicidal ideation, unusual changes in behavior (esp. at initiation of therapy or with changes in dosage).

---

# *DOXOrubicin    HIGH ALERT

dox-o-**rue**-bi-sin
(Adriamycin, Caelyx ✦, Doxil, Lipodox)

■ **BLACK BOX ALERT** ■ May cause concurrent or cumulative myocardial toxicity. Acute allergic or anaphylaxis-like infusion reaction may be life-threatening. Severe myelosuppresion may occur. Must be administered by personnel trained in administration/handling of chemotherapeutic agents. Secondary acute myelogenous leukemia and myelodysplastic syndrome have been reported. Potent vesicant.
**Do not confuse doxorubicin with dactinoycin, daunorubicin, doxazosin, epirubicin, idarubicin, or valrubicin, or Adriamycin with Aredia or idamycin.**

## ◆ CLASSIFICATION

**PHARMACOTHERAPEUTIC:** Anthracycline antibiotic. **CLINICAL:** Antineoplastic.

## USES

**Adriamycin:** Treatment of acute lymphocytic leukemia (ALL), acute myeloid leukemia (AML), Hodgkin's lymphoma, malignant lymphoma; breast, gastric, small-cell lung, ovarian, epithelial, thyroid, bladder carcinomas; neuroblastoma, Wilms tumor, osteosarcoma, soft tissue sarcoma. **Doxil, Lipodox:** Treatment of AIDS-related Kaposi's sarcoma, advanced ovarian cancer. Used with bortezomib to treat multiple myeloma in pts who have not previously received bortezomib and have received at least one previous treatment. **OFF-LABEL: Adriamycin:** Multiple myeloma, endometrial carcinoma, uterine sarcoma; head and neck cancer, liver, kidney cancer. **Doxil:** Metastatic breast cancer, Hodgkin's lymphoma, cutaneous T-cell lymphomas, advanced soft tissue sarcomas, recurrent or metastatic cervical cancer, advanced or metastatic uterine sarcoma.

## PRECAUTIONS

**Contraindications:** Hypersensitivity to doxorubicin. **Adriamycin:** Severe hepatic impairment, severe myocardial insufficiency, recent MI (within 4–6 wks), severe arrhythmias. Previous or concomitant treatment with high accumulative doses of doxorubicin, daunorubicin, idarubicin, or other anthracyclines or anthracenediones; severe, persistent drug-induced myelosuppression or baseline ANC count less than 1,500/mm³. **Doxil:** Breastfeeding (Canada). **Cautions:** Hepatic impairment. Cardiomyopathy, preexisting myelosuppression, severe HF. Pts who received radiation therapy.

## ACTION

Inhibits DNA, DNA-dependent RNA synthesis by binding with DNA strands. Liposomal encapsulation increases uptake by tumors, prolongs drug action, may decrease toxicity. **Therapeutic Effect:** Prevents cell division.

## PHARMACOKINETICS

Widely distributed. Protein binding: 74%–76%. Does not cross blood-brain barrier. Metabolized in liver. Primarily eliminated by biliary system. Not removed by hemodialysis. **Half-life:** 20–48 hrs.

## LIFESPAN CONSIDERATIONS

**Pregnancy/Lactation:** If possible, avoid use during pregnancy, esp. first trimester. Breastfeeding not recommended. **Children/Elderly:** Cardiotoxicity may be more frequent in pts younger than 2 yrs or older than 70 yrs.

## INTERACTIONS

**DRUG: Cyclosporine** may increase risk of hematologic toxicity. **Bone marrow depressants** may increase myelosuppression. **Daunorubicin** may increase risk of cardiotoxicity. **Live virus vaccines** may potentiate virus replication, increase vaccine side effects, decrease pt's antibody response to vaccine. **HERBAL: St. John's wort** may decrease concentration. Avoid **black cohosh, dong quai** in estrogen-dependent tumors. **FOOD:** None known. **LAB VALUES:** May cause EKG changes, increase serum uric acid. May reduce neutrophil, RBC counts.

## AVAILABILITY (Rx)

**Injection, Powder for Reconstitution:** 10 mg, 20 mg, 50 mg. **Injection Solution (Adriamycin):** 2 mg/ml (5-ml, 10-ml, 25-ml, 100-ml vial). **Lipid Complex (Doxil, Lipodox):** 2 mg/ml (10 ml, 25 ml).

## ADMINISTRATION/HANDLING

◄**ALERT**► Wear gloves. If powder or solution comes in contact with skin, wash thoroughly. Avoid small veins; swollen/edematous extremities; areas overlying joints, tendons. **Doxil:** Do not use with in-line filter or mix with any diluent except D₅W. May be carcinogenic, mutagenic, teratogenic. Handle with extreme care during preparation/administration.

 **IV**

**Reconstitution** • Reconstitute vials of powder with 0.9% NaCl to provide concentration of 2 mg/ml. • Shake vial; allow contents to dissolve. • Withdraw appropriate volume of air from vial during reconstitution (avoids excessive pressure buildup). • May be further diluted with 50–1,000 ml D₅W or 0.9% NaCl and given as continuous infusion. **Doxil:** Dilute each dose in 250 ml D₅W (doses greater than 90 mg in 500 ml D₅W).
**Rate of Administration (Adriamycin):**
• For IV push, administer into tubing of freely running IV infusion of D₅W or 0.9% NaCl, preferably via butterfly needle over 3–5 min (avoids local erythematous streaking along vein and facial flushing). • Must test for flashback q30sec to be certain needle remains in vein during injection. IV piggyback over 15–60 min or

**D**

continuous infusion. • Extravasation produces immediate pain, severe local tissue damage. Terminate administration immediately; withdraw as much medication as possible, obtain extravasation kit, follow protocol. **Doxil:** Give as infusion over 60 min. Do not use in-line filter.

**Storage** • **Adriamycin powder:** Store at room temperature. • Reconstituted vials stable for 7 days at room temperature, 15 days if refrigerated. Infusions stable for 48 hrs at room temperature. • Protect from prolonged exposure to sunlight; discard unused solution. • **Adriamycin solution:** Refrigerate vials. Solutions diluted in $D_5W$ or 0.9% NaCl stable for 48 hrs at room temperature. • **Doxil:** Refrigerate unopened vials. After solution is diluted, use within 24 hrs.

## ▦ IV INCOMPATIBILITIES

**Doxorubicin:** Allopurinol (Aloprim), amphotericin B complex (Abelcet, AmBisome, Amphotec), cefepime (Maxipime), furosemide (Lasix), ganciclovir (Cytovene), heparin, piperacillin/tazobactam (Zosyn), propofol (Diprivan). **Doxil:** Do not mix with any other medications.

## ▦ IV COMPATIBILITIES

Dexamethasone (Decadron), diphenhydramine (Benadryl), granisetron (Kytril), hydromorphone (Dilaudid), lorazepam (Ativan), morphine, ondansetron (Zofran).

## INDICATIONS/ROUTES/DOSAGE

◀ALERT▶ Refer to individual protocols.

**Usual Dosage**
**IV** *(Adriamycin):* **ADULTS:** **(Single-agent Therapy)** 60–75 mg/m² as a single dose every 21 days, 20 mg/m² once wkly. **(Combination Therapy):** 40–75 mg/m² q21–28 days. Because of risk of cardiotoxicity, do not exceed cumulative dose of 550 mg/m² (400–450 mg/m² for

those previously treated with related compounds or irradiation of cardiac region). **CHILDREN:** 35–75 mg/m² as a single dose q3wks or 20–30 mg/m² wkly, or 60–90 mg/m² as continuous infusion over 96 hrs q3–4wks.

**Kaposi's Sarcoma**
**IV** *(Doxil, Lipodox):* **ADULTS:** 20 mg/m² q3wks infused over 30 min.

**Ovarian Cancer**
**IV** *(Doxil, Lipodox):* **ADULTS:** 50 mg/m² q4wks.

**Multiple Myeloma**
**IV** *(Doxil, Lipodox):* **ADULTS:** 30 mg/m²/dose on day 4 q3wks (in combination with bortezomib).

**Dosage in Renal Impairment**
No dose adjustment.

**Dose Modifications**
*Adriamycin*
**Neutropenic Fever/Infection:** Reduce dose to 75%. **ANC less than 1,000/mm³:** Delay treatment until ANC 1,000/mm³ or more. **Platelets less than 100,000/mm³:** Delay treatment until platelets 100,000/mm³ or more.
*Doxil*
**Adjustments for Hand-Foot Syndrome, Stomatitis, Hematologic Toxicities:** Refer to manufacturer's guidelines.

**Dosage in Hepatic Impairment**
**ADRIAMYCIN**

| Hepatic Function | Dosage |
| --- | --- |
| ALT, AST 2–3 times ULN | 75% of normal dose |
| ALT, AST greater than 3 times ULN or bilirubin 1.2–3 mg/dL | 50% of normal dose |
| Bilirubin 3.1–5 mg/dL | 25% of normal dose |
| Bilirubin greater than 5 mg/dL | Not recommended |

ULN = upper limit of normal.

**DOXIL**

| Hepatic Function | Dosage |
|---|---|
| Bilirubin 1.2–3 mg/dL | 50% of normal dose |
| Bilirubin greater than 3 mg/dL | 25% of normal dose |

## SIDE EFFECTS

**Frequent:** Complete alopecia (scalp, axillary, pubic hair), nausea, vomiting, stomatitis, esophagitis (esp. if drug is given on several successive days), reddish urine. **Doxil:** Nausea. **Occasional:** Anorexia, diarrhea; hyperpigmentation of nailbeds, phalangeal, dermal creases. **Rare:** Fever, chills, conjunctivitis, lacrimation.

## ADVERSE EFFECTS/ TOXIC REACTIONS

Myelosuppression manifested as hematologic toxicity (principally leukopenia and, to lesser extent, anemia, thrombocytopenia) generally occurs within 10–15 days, returns to normal levels by third wk. Cardiotoxicity (either acute, manifested as transient EKG abnormalities, or chronic, manifested as HF) may occur.

## NURSING CONSIDERATIONS

### BASELINE ASSESSMENT

Obtain ANC, CBC, erythrocyte counts before and at frequent intervals during therapy. Obtain EKG before therapy, LFT before each dose. Antiemetics may be effective in preventing, treating nausea.

### INTERVENTION/EVALUATION

Monitor for stomatitis (burning or erythema of oral mucosa at inner margin of lips, difficulty swallowing). Observe IV injection site for infiltration, vein irritation. May lead to ulceration of mucous membranes within 2–3 days. Assess dermal creases, nailbeds for hyperpigmentation. Monitor hematologic status, renal/hepatic function studies, serum uric acid levels. Monitor daily pattern of bowel activity, stool consistency. Monitor for hematologic toxicity (fever, sore throat, signs of local infection, unusual bruising/bleeding from any site), symptoms of anemia (excessive fatigue, weakness).

### PATIENT/FAMILY TEACHING

• Hair loss is reversible, but new hair growth may have different color, texture. New hair growth resumes 2–3 mos after last therapy dose. • Maintain strict oral hygiene. • Do not have immunizations without physician's approval (drug lowers resistance). • Avoid contact with those who have recently received live virus vaccine. • Promptly report fever, sore throat, signs of local infection, unusual bruising/bleeding from any site. • Report persistent nausea/vomiting. • Avoid alcohol (may cause GI irritation, a common side effect with liposomal doxorubicin).

---

## doxycycline [TOP 100]

dox-i-**sye**-kleen
(Actilate, Adoxa, Apo-Doxy ,
Avidoxy, Doryx, Doxy-100,
Monodox, Oracea, Vibramycin,
Vibra-Tabs ✦).
**Do not confuse doxycycline with dicyclomine or doxepin, Monodox with Maalox, Oracea with Orencia, Vibramycin with Vancomycin or Vibativ, or Vibra-Tabs with Vibativ.**

## ◆CLASSIFICATION

**PHARMACOTHERAPEUTIC:** Tetracycline. **CLINICAL:** Antibiotic.

## USES

Treatment of susceptible infections due to *H. ducreyi, Pasteurella pestis, P. tularensis, Bacteroides* spp., *V. cholerae, Brucella* spp., *Rickettsiae, Y. pestis, Francisella tularensis, M. pneumoniae* including brucellosis, chlamydia, cholera, granuloma inguinale, lymphogranuloma venereum, malaria prophylaxis, nongonococcal urethritis, pelvic inflammatory disease (PID), plague, psittacosis, relapsing fever, rickettsia infections, primary and secondary syphilis, tularemia. **(Oracea):** Treatment of inflammatory lesions in adults with rosacea. **OFF-LABEL:** Sclerosing agent for pleural effusion; vancomycin-resistant enterococci (VRE); alternative for MRSA, treatment of refractory periodontitis, juvenile periodontitis.

## PRECAUTIONS

**Contraindications:** Hypersensitivity to doxycycline, other tetracyclines. **Cautions:** History or predisposition to oral candidiasis (Oracea). Avoid use during pregnancy, during tooth development in children. Avoid prolonged exposure to sunlight.

## ACTION

Inhibits bacterial protein synthesis by binding to ribosomes. **Therapeutic Effect:** Bacteriostatic.

## PHARMACOKINETICS

Rapidly absorbed after PO administration. Protein binding: 90%. Partially excreted in urine; partially eliminated in bile. **Half-life:** 15–24 hrs.

## ⏳ LIFESPAN CONSIDERATIONS

**Pregnancy/Lactation:** Crosses placenta; distributed in breast milk. **Children:** May cause permanent discoloration of teeth, enamel hypoplasia. **Elderly:** No age-related precautions noted.

## INTERACTIONS

**DRUG: Antacids containing aluminum, calcium, magnesium; laxatives containing magnesium, oral iron preparations** decrease absorption. **Barbiturates, carbamazepine, phenytoin** may decrease concentration. **Cholestyramine, colestipol** may decrease absorption. May decrease effects of **oral contraceptives. HERBAL: Dong quai, St. John's wort** may increase photosensitization. **St. John's wort** may

decrease concentration/effects. **FOOD:** None known. **LAB VALUES:** May increase serum alkaline phosphatase, amylase, bilirubin, ALT, AST. May alter CBC.

## AVAILABILITY (Rx)

**Capsules:** 40 mg, 50 mg, 75 mg, 100 mg, 150 mg. **Injection, Powder for Reconstitution:** 100 mg. **Oral Suspension:** 25 mg/5 ml. **Syrup:** 50 mg/5 ml. **Tablets:** 20 mg, 50 mg, 75 mg, 100 mg, 150 mg.

## ADMINISTRATION/HANDLING

◀**ALERT**▶ Do not administer IM or subcutaneous. Space doses evenly around clock.

 **IV**

**Reconstitution** • Reconstitute each 100-mg vial with 10 ml Sterile Water for Injection for concentration of 10 mg/ml. • Further dilute each 100 mg with at least 100 ml D₅W, 0.9% NaCl, lactated Ringer's.
**Rate of Administration** • Give by intermittent IV infusion (piggyback). • Infuse over 1–4 hrs.
**Storage** • After reconstitution, IV infusion (piggyback) is stable for 12 hrs at room temperature or 72 hrs if refrigerated. • Protect from direct sunlight. Discard if precipitate forms.

### PO

• Store capsules, tablets at room temperature. • Oral suspension is stable for 2 wks at room temperature. • Give with full glass of fluid. • Instruct pt to sit up for 30 min after taking to reduce risk of esophageal irritation and ulceration. • Give without regard to food. Oracea should be given 1 hr before or 2 hrs after meals. • Avoid concurrent use of antacids, milk; separate by 2 hrs.

## ▦ IV INCOMPATIBILITIES

Allopurinol (Aloprim), heparin, piperacillin/tazobactam (Zosyn).

## ▓ IV COMPATIBILITIES

Acyclovir (Zovirax), amiodarone (Cordarone), dexmedetomidine (Precedex), diltiazem (Cardizem), granisetron (Kytril), hydromorphone (Dilaudid), magnesium sulfate, meperidine (Demerol), morphine, ondansetron (Zofran), propofol (Diprivan).

## INDICATIONS/ROUTES/DOSAGE

**Usual Dosage**
**IV/PO: ADULTS, ELDERLY, CHILDREN OLDER THAN 8 YRS; WEIGHING MORE THAN 45 KG**: 100–200 mg/day in 1–2 divided doses. **CHILDREN OLDER THAN 8 YRS; WEIGHING 45 KG OR LESS**: 2–5 mg/kg/day (**maximum**: 200 mg/day) in 1–2 divided doses.

**Dosage in Renal/Hepatic Impairment**
No dose adjustment.

## SIDE EFFECTS

**Frequent:** Anorexia, nausea, vomiting, diarrhea, dysphagia, photosensitivity (may be severe). **Occasional:** Rash, urticaria.

## ADVERSE EFFECTS/ TOXIC REACTIONS

Superinfection (esp. fungal), benign intracranial hypertension (headache, visual changes) may occur. Hepatotoxicity, fatty degeneration of liver, pancreatitis occur rarely.

## NURSING CONSIDERATIONS

**BASELINE ASSESSMENT**

Question for history of allergies, esp. to tetracyclines, sulfites.

**INTERVENTION/EVALUATION**

Monitor daily pattern of bowel activity, stool consistency. Assess skin for rash. Monitor LOC due to potential for increased intracranial pressure (ICP). Be alert for superinfection: fever, vomiting, diarrhea, anal/genital pruritus, oral mucosal changes (ulceration, pain, erythema). Monitor CBC, renal/hepatic function tests.

**PATIENT/FAMILY TEACHING**

• Avoid unnecessary exposure to sunlight. • Do not take with antacids, iron products. • Complete full course of therapy. • After application of dental gel, avoid brushing teeth, flossing the treated areas for 7 days. • Report severe diarrhea.

D

# dronabinol

droe-**nab**-i-nol
(Marinol, Syndros)
**Do not confuse dronabinol with droperidol.**

## ◆CLASSIFICATION

**PHARMACOTHERAPEUTIC:** Controlled substance (**Schedule III**).
**CLINICAL:** Antinausea, antiemetic, appetite stimulant.

## USES

Prevention, treatment of nausea/vomiting due to cancer chemotherapy; appetite stimulant in AIDS. **OFF-LABEL:** Cancer-related anorexia.

## PRECAUTIONS

**Contraindications:** Hypersensitivity to dronabinol, sesame oil, tetrahydrocannabinol products, marijuana. **Cautions:** History of psychiatric illness, schizophrenia, history of substance abuse, mania, depression, seizure disorder, hepatic impairment, elderly.

## ACTION

Exact mechanism unknown. May inhibit endorphins in brain's emetic center, suppress prostaglandins synthesis or effect on cannabinoid receptor in CNS. **Therapeutic Effect:** Inhibits nausea/vomiting, stimulates appetite.

## PHARMACOKINETICS

Well absorbed after PO administration, only 10%–20% reaches systemic circulation. Protein binding: 97%. Undergoes first-pass

---

metabolism. Highly lipid soluble. Primarily excreted in feces. **Half-life:** 25–36 hrs.

## ⧖ LIFESPAN CONSIDERATIONS

**Pregnancy/Lactation:** Unknown if drug crosses placenta. Distributed in breast milk. **Children:** Not recommended. **Elderly:** Monitor carefully during therapy.

## INTERACTIONS

**DRUG: Alcohol, other CNS suppressants** may increase CNS depression. **Sympathomimetics, tricyclic antidepressants** may increase risk of hypertension, tachycardia. **Anticholinergics** may increase drowsiness, tachycardia. **HERBAL: St. John's wort** may decrease concentration. **FOOD:** None known. **LAB VALUES:** None significant.

## AVAILABILITY (Rx)

**Capsules (Gelatin [Marinol]):** 2.5 mg, 5 mg, 10 mg. **Oral Solution (Syndros):** 5 mg/ml.

## ADMINISTRATION/HANDLING

**PO**
• Store in cool environment. May refrigerate capsules. • May administer without regard to meals. Give before meals if used for appetite stimulant. **Oral solution:** Always use enclosed calibrated syringe. Take each dose with a full glass of water.

## INDICATIONS/ROUTES/DOSAGE

**Prevention of Chemotherapy-Induced Nausea and Vomiting**
**PO: ADULTS, ELDERLY, CHILDREN:** *(Marinol):* Initially, 5 mg/m$^2$ 1–3 hrs before chemotherapy, then q2–4h after chemotherapy for total of 4–6 doses/day. May increase by 2.5 mg/m$^2$ up to 15 mg/m$^2$ per dose. *(Syndros):* Initially, 2.1–4.2 mg/m$^2$ 1–2 hrs prior to chemotherapy, then q2–4 hrs after chemotherapy for total of 4–6 doses/day. May increase in increments of 2.1 mg/m$^2$. **Maximum:** 12.6 mg/m$^2$/dose.

**Appetite Stimulant**
**PO: ADULTS, ELDERLY:** *(Marinol):* Initially, 2.5 mg twice daily (before lunch and dinner). Range: 2.5–20 mg/day. *(Syndros):* Initially, 2.1 mg twice daily. May gradually increase dose in 2.1-mg increments. **Maximum:** 8.4 mg twice daily.

**Dosage in Renal/Hepatic Impairment**
No dose adjustment.

## SIDE EFFECTS

**Frequent (24%–3%):** Euphoria, dizziness, paranoid reaction, drowsiness. **Occasional (less than 3%–1%):** Asthenia, ataxia, confusion, abnormal thinking, depersonalization. **Rare (less than 1%):** Diarrhea, depression, nightmares, speech difficulties, headache, anxiety, tinnitus, flushed skin.

## ADVERSE EFFECTS/ TOXIC REACTIONS

Mild intoxication may produce increased sensory awareness (taste, smell, sound), altered time perception, reddened conjunctiva, dry mouth, tachycardia. Moderate intoxication may produce memory impairment, urinary retention. Severe intoxication may produce lethargy, decreased motor coordination, slurred speech, orthostatic hypotension.

## NURSING CONSIDERATIONS

**BASELINE ASSESSMENT**
Assess dehydration status if excessive vomiting occurs (skin turgor, mucous membranes, urinary output).

**INTERVENTION/EVALUATION**
Supervise closely for serious mood, behavior responses, esp. in pts with history of psychiatric illness. Monitor B/P, heart rate.

**PATIENT/FAMILY TEACHING**
• Change positions slowly to avoid dizziness. • Relief from nausea/vomiting generally occurs within 15 min of drug administration. • Do not take any other

medications, including OTC, without physician approval. • Avoid alcohol, barbiturates. • Avoid tasks that require alertness, motor skills until response to drug is established. • For appetite stimulation, take before lunch and dinner.

# dulaglutide

**doo**-la-**gloo**-tide
(Trulicity)

■ **BLACK BOX ALERT** ■ Contraindicated in pts with a personal/family history of medullary thyroid carcinoma (MTC) or in pts with multiple endocrine neoplasia syndrome type 2 (MEN2). Unknown if dulaglutide causes thyroid cell tumors in humans. **Do not confuse dulaglutide with albiglutide or liraglutide.**

## ◆CLASSIFICATION

**PHARMACOTHERAPEUTIC:** GLP-1 receptor agonist. **CLINICAL:** Antidiabetic.

## USES

Adjunct to diet and exercise to improve glycemic controls in pts with type 2 diabetes mellitus.

## PRECAUTIONS

**Contraindications:** Hypersensitivity to dulaglutide, other GLP-1 receptor agonists. Personal/family history of medullary thyroid carcinoma or multiple endocrine neoplasia syndrome type 2. **Cautions:** Pts with increased serum calcitonin, thyroid nodules, hx pancreatitis, renal/hepatic impairment. Not recommended in pts with severe GI disease, diabetic ketoacidosis, or type 1 diabetes.

## ACTION

Activates GLP-1 receptors in pancreatic beta cells increasing intracellular cyclic AMP. **Therapeutic Effect:** Augments glucose-dependent insulin release, slows gastric emptying. Improves glycemic control.

## PHARMACOKINETICS

Readily absorbed following subcutaneous administration. Degraded into amino acids by general protein catabolism. Peak plasma concentration: 24–72 hrs. Steady state reached in 2–4 wks. Elimination not specified. **Half-life:** 5 days.

## ☒ LIFESPAN CONSIDERATIONS

**Pregnancy/Lactation:** Unknown if distributed in breast milk. Must either discontinue drug or discontinue breastfeeding. **Children:** Safety and efficacy not established in pts younger than 18 yrs. **Elderly:** No age-related precautions noted.

## INTERACTIONS

**DRUG: Insulin, insulin secretagogues (e.g., glyburide)** may increase risk of hypoglycemia. May reduce rate of absorption of oral medications. **HERBAL: Garlic,** other herbs with hypooglycemic activity may increase risk of hypoglycemia. **FOOD:** None known. **LAB VALUES:** Expected to decrease serum glucose, Hgb A1c. May increase amylase, lipase.

## AVAILABILITY (Rx)

**Prefilled Injector Pen or Syringe:** 0.75 mg/0.5 ml, 1.5 mg/0.5 ml.

## ADMINISTRATION/HANDLING

**Subcutaneous**
• Administer any time of day, without regard to meals, on same day each week. • May change administration day if last dose was given more than 3 days prior. If dose missed, administer within 3 days of missed dose. If more than 3 days have passed after missed dose, wait until next regularly scheduled dose to administer. **Administration** • Subcutaneously insert needle into abdomen, thigh, or upper arm region and inject solution. • Do not reuse needle. • Rotate injection sites each week. **Storage** • Refrigerate unused pens/syringes; do not freeze. • May store at

D

room temperature for up to 14 days.
• Protect from light.

## INDICATIONS/ROUTES/DOSAGE

### Type 2 Diabetes Mellitus

**SQ: ADULTS/ELDERLY:** 0.75 mg once wkly. May increase to 1.5 mg once wkly if glycemic response inadequate. **Maximum:** 1.5 mg wkly.

### Dose Modification

**Concomitant Use with Insulin Secretagogue (e.g., Sulfonylurea) or Insulin:** Consider reduced dose of insulin secretagogue or insulin based on glycemic goal.

### Dosage in Renal Impairment

No dose adjustment.

### Dosage in Hepatic Impairment

Use caution.

## SIDE EFFECTS

**Occasional (12%–6%):** Nausea, diarrhea, vomiting, abdominal pain. **Rare (4% or less):** Decreased appetite, dyspepsia, fatigue, asthenia.

## ADVERSE EFFECTS/TOXIC REACTIONS

May increase risk of acute renal failure or worsening of chronic renal impairment (esp. with dehydration), severe gastroparesis, pancreatitis, thyroid C-cell tumors. May increase risk of hypoglycemia when used with other hypoglycemic agents or insulin. Dyspnea, pruritus, rash may indicate hypersensitivity reaction. May prolong PR interval by 2–3 msec or may rarely cause first-degree AV block, tachycardia. Immunogenicity (antidulaglutide antibody formation) reported. Some pts with antibody formation also tested positive for antibodies to GLP-1 and human albumin.

## NURSING CONSIDERATIONS

### BASELINE ASSESSMENT

Obtain baseline fasting glucose level, Hgb A1c, BMP. Question history of medullary thyroid carcinoma, multiple endocrine neoplasia syndrome type 2, pancreatitis, renal impairment; first-degree AV block, PR interval prolongation. Receive full medication history and screen for use of other hypoglycemic agents or insulin. Assess pt's understanding of diabetes management, routine home glucose monitoring, medication self-administration. Assess hydration status.

### INTERVENTION/EVALUATION

Monitor capillary blood glucose levels, Hgb A1c; renal function test in pts with renal impairment reporting severe GI reactions including diarrhea, gastroparesis, vomiting. Screen for thyroid tumors (dysphagia, dyspnea, persistent hoarseness, neck mass). If tumor suspected, consider endocrinologist consultation. Clinical significance of serum calcitonin level or thyroid ultrasound with GLP-1–associated thyroid tumors is debated/unknown. Assess for hypoglycemia, hyperglycemia, hypersensitivity/allergic reaction. Screen for glucose-altering conditions: fever, stress, surgical procedures, trauma. Obtain dietary consult for nutritional education. Encourage PO intake.

### PATIENT/FAMILY TEACHING

• Diabetes mellitus requires lifelong control. Diet and exercise are principal parts of treatment; do not skip or delay meals. Test blood sugar regularly. Monitor daily calorie intake. • When taking additional medications to lower blood sugar or when glucose demands are altered (fever, infection, stress trauma), have low blood sugar treatment available (glucagon, oral dextrose). • Report suspected pregnancy or plans for breastfeeding. • Therapy may increase risk of thyroid cancer; report lumps or swelling of the neck; hoarseness, shortness of breath, trouble swallowing. • Persistent, severe abdominal pain that radiates to the back (with or without vomiting) may indicate acute pancreatitis. • Rash, itching, hives may indicate allergic reaction.

# *DULoxetine

du-**lox**-e-teen
(Cymbalta, Irenka)

■ **BLACK BOX ALERT** ■ Increased risk of suicidal thinking and behavior in children, adolescents, young adults 18–24 yrs with major depressive disorder, other psychiatric disorders.

**Do not confuse duloxetine with fluoxetine or paroxetine.**

## ◆CLASSIFICATION

**PHARMACOTHERAPEUTIC:** Serotonin norepinephrine reuptake inhibitor (SNRI). **CLINICAL:** Antidepressant.

## USES

Treatment of major depression. Management of pain associated with diabetic neuropathy, or chronic musculoskeletal pain. Treatment of generalized anxiety disorder. **Cymbalta only:** Treatment of fibromyalgia. **OFF-LABEL:** Treatment of stress incontinence.

## PRECAUTIONS

**Contraindications:** Hypersensitivity to duloxetine. Uncontrolled narrow-angle glaucoma. Use of MAOI intended to treat psychiatric disorder (concurrent or within 14 days of discontinuing MAOI). Initiation of MAOI intended to treat psychiatric disorder within 5 days of discontinuing duloxetine. Initiation of duloxetine in pt receiving linezolid or IV methylene blue. **Cautions:** Renal impairment, history of alcoholism, chronic hepatic disease, history of mania, pts with suicidal ideation or behavior. Concurrent use with inhibitors of CYP1A2 or thioridazine, CNS depressants. Hypertension, controlled narrow-angle glaucoma, pts with impaired GI motility. Concomitant use of NSAIDs (may increase risk of bleeding), history of seizures. Use of medications that lower seizure threshold; elderly; pts at high risk for suicide.

## ACTION

Appears to inhibit serotonin and norepinephrine reuptake at CNS neuronal presynaptic membranes; is a less potent inhibitor of dopamine reuptake. **Therapeutic Effect:** Produces antidepressant effect.

## PHARMACOKINETICS

Well absorbed from GI tract. Protein binding: greater than 90%. Metabolized in liver. Excreted in urine (70%), feces (20%). **Half-life:** 8–17 hrs.

## ⧗ LIFESPAN CONSIDERATIONS

**Pregnancy/Lactation:** May produce neonatal adverse reactions (constant crying, feeding difficulty, hyperreflexia, irritability). Unknown if distributed in breast milk. Breastfeeding not recommended. **Children:** Safety and efficacy not established. **Elderly:** Caution required when increasing dosage.

## INTERACTIONS

**DRUG: Alcohol** increases risk of hepatic injury. **CYP1A2** and **CYP2D6 inhibitors (e.g., fluoxetine, fluvoxamine, paroxetine, quinidine, quinolone antimicrobials)** may increase plasma concentration. **MAOIs** may cause serotonin syndrome (autonomic hyperactivity, coma, diaphoresis, excitement, hyperthermia, rigidity). **Aspirin, NSAIDs** may increase risk of bleeding. May increase concentration, potential toxicity of **tricyclic antidepressants. Serotonergic drugs (e.g., triptans, lithium, tramadol)** may increase risk of serotonin syndrome. **HERBAL: Gotu kola, kava kava, St. John's wort, valerian** may increase CNS depression. **St. John's wort** may increase risk of serotonin syndrome. **FOOD:** None known. **LAB VALUES:** May increase serum bilirubin, ALT, AST, alkaline phosphatase.

## AVAILABILITY (Rx)

🖋 **Capsules (Delayed-Release, Enteric-Coated Pellets) (Cymbalta):** 20 mg, 30 mg, 60 mg. **(Irenka):** 40 mg.

## ADMINISTRATION/HANDLING

◄ALERT► Allow at least 14 days to elapse between use of MAOIs and duloxetine.

**PO**
- Give without regard to meals. Give with food, milk if GI distress occurs.
- Do not break, crush, cut delayed-release capsules. • Contents of capsule may be sprinkled on applesauce or mixed in apple juice and swallowed (without chewing) immediately.

## INDICATIONS/ROUTES/DOSAGE

**Fibromyalgia**
**PO: ADULTS ELDERLY:** Initially, 30 mg/day for 1 wk. Increase to 60 mg/day.

**Major Depressive Disorder**
**PO: ADULTS, ELDERLY:** Initially, 40–60 mg/day in 1 or 2 divided doses. For doses greater than 60 mg/day, titrate in increments of 30 mg/day over 1 wk. **Maximum:** 120 mg/day.

**Diabetic Neuropathy Pain**
**PO: ADULTS, ELDERLY:** 60 mg once daily. **Maximum:** 60 mg/day.

**Generalized Anxiety Disorder**
**PO: ADULTS, ELDERLY:** Initially, 30–60 mg once daily. May increase up to 120 mg/day in 30-mg increments wkly. **CHILDREN 7–17 YRS:** Initially, 30 mg once daily. After 2 wks, may increase to 60 mg once daily. May further increase in increments of 30 mg/day at wkly intervals. **Maximum:** 120 mg/day.

**Chronic Musculoskeletal Pain**
**PO: ADULTS, ELDERLY:** 30 mg once daily for 1 wk, then increase to 60 mg once daily. **Maximum:** 60 mg/day.

**Dosage in Renal/Hepatic Impairment**
**Renal:** Not recommended with CrCl less than 30 ml/min or ESRD. **Hepatic:** Not recommended.

## SIDE EFFECTS

**Frequent (20%–11%):** Nausea, dry mouth, constipation, insomnia. **Occasional (9%–5%):** Dizziness, fatigue, diarrhea, drowsiness, anorexia, diaphoresis, vomiting. **Rare (4%–2%):** Blurred vision, erectile dysfunction, delayed or failed ejaculation, anorgasmia, anxiety, decreased libido, hot flashes.

## ADVERSE EFFECTS/TOXIC REACTIONS

May slightly increase heart rate. Colitis, dysphagia, gastritis, irritable bowel syndrome occur rarely.

## NURSING CONSIDERATIONS

### BASELINE ASSESSMENT

Assess appearance, behavior, speech pattern, level of interest, mood, sleep pattern, suicidal tendencies. Question pain level, intensity, location of pain.

### INTERVENTION/EVALUATION

For pts on long-term therapy, serum chemistry profile to assess hepatic/renal function should be performed periodically. Supervise suicidal-risk pt closely during early therapy (as depression lessens, energy level improves, increasing suicide potential). Monitor B/P, mental status, anxiety, social functioning, serum glucose levels.

### PATIENT/FAMILY TEACHING

- Therapeutic effect may be noted within 1–4 wks. • Do not abruptly discontinue medication. • Avoid tasks that require alertness, motor skills until response to drug is established. • Inform physician of intention of pregnancy or if pregnancy occurs. • Report anxiety, agitation, panic attacks, worsening of depression. • Avoid heavy alcohol intake (associated with severe hepatic injury).

# edoxaban

e-**dox**-a-ban
(Savaysa)

■ **BLACK BOX ALERT** ■ Avoid use in pts with creatinine clearance (CrCl) greater than 95 ml/min (increased risk of ischemic stroke). Premature discontinuation of oral anticoagulant in the absence of alternative anticoagulation may increase risk of ischemic events. If treatment is discontinued for any reason other than pathologic bleeding or completion of course of therapy, consider coverage with another anticoagulant as described in transition guideline. Epidural or spinal hematomas may occur in pts who are receiving neuraxial anesthesia or undergoing spinal puncture, which may result in long-term or permanent paralysis.

**Do not confuse edoxaban with apixaban or rivaroxaban.**

## ◆CLASSIFICATION

**PHARMACOTHERAPEUTIC:** Factor Xa inhibitor. **CLINICAL:** Anticoagulant.

## USES

To reduce risk of stroke and systemic embolism (SE) in pts with nonvalvular atrial fibrillation (NVAF). Treatment of deep vein thrombosis (DVT) and pulmonary embolism (PE) following 5–10 days of initial therapy with a parenteral anticoagulant.

## PRECAUTIONS

**Contraindications:** Hypersensitivity to edoxaban. Major active bleeding. **Cautions:** Elderly, pts at increased risk of bleeding (e.g., prior CVA, thrombocytopenia, severe uncontrolled hypertension; history of bleeding ulcers, upper or lower GI bleeding), recent surgery, renal/hepatic impairment. Avoid concomitant use with aspirin, heparin, low molecular weight heparin (LMWH), NSAIDs, P-gp Inducers (e.g., rifampin). Not recommended in pts with CrCl greater than 95 ml/min (increased risk of ischemic stroke); mechanical heart valves; moderate to severe mitral stenosis.

## ACTION

Selectively blocks active site of factor Xa, a key factor in the intrinsic and extrinsic pathway of blood coagulation cascade. Inhibits platelet activation and fibrin clot formation. **Therapeutic Effect:** Inhibits blood coagulation.

## PHARMACOKINETICS

Readily absorbed after PO administration. Peak plasma concentration: 1–2 hrs. Steady state reached within 3 days. Protein binding: 55%. Primarily eliminated in urine (50%), biliary/intestinal excretion (remaining %). Not removed by hemodialysis. **Half-life:** 10–14 hrs.

## ⚕ LIFESPAN CONSIDERATIONS

**Pregnancy/Lactation:** Unknown if excreted in breast milk. **Children:** Safety and efficacy not established. **Elderly:** May have increased risk of bleeding due to age-related renal impairment.

## INTERACTIONS

**DRUG: Anticoagulants** (e.g., **warfarin**), **antiplatelets** (e.g., **clopidogrel**), **NSAIDs** (e.g., **ibuprofen**), **fibrinolytic therapy** (e.g., **TPA**) may increase concentration/effect; may increase risk of bleeding. **HERBAL:** None significant. **FOOD:** None known. **LAB VALUES:** May increase AST, ALT. May prolong aPTT, PT/INR.

## AVAILABILITY (Rx)

🔹 **Tablets:** 15 mg, 30 mg, 60 mg.

## ADMINISTRATION/HANDLING

### PO
• Give without regard to meals. • Do not administer within 2 hrs of removal of epidural or intrathecal catheters.

## INDICATIONS/ROUTES/DOSAGE

**Nonvalvular Atrial Fibrillation**
**PO: ADULTS, ELDERLY:** 60 mg once daily.

 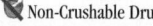

E

### DVT/PE

**PO: ADULTS, ELDERLY:** 60 mg once daily following 5–10 days of initial therapy with a parenteral anticoagulant.

### Dose Modification

**Body weight less than or equal to 60 kg or concomitant use of certain P-gp inhibitors:** 30 mg once daily.

### Dosage in Renal Impairment
#### DVT/PE

**CrCl 15–50 ml/min:** 30 mg once daily. **CrCl less than 15 ml/min:** Not recommended.

#### NVAF

**CrCl greater than 95 ml/min:** Not recommended. **CrCl 51–95 ml/min:** No dose adjustment. **CrCl 15–50 ml/min:** 30 mg once daily. **CrCl less than 15 ml/min:** Not recommended.

### Dosage in Hepatic Impairment

**Mild impairment:** No dose adjustment. **Moderate to severe impairment:** Not recommended.

### Discontinuation for Surgery or Other Interventions

Discontinue at least 24 hrs before invasive surgical procedures. May restart as soon as adequate hemostasis is achieved, noting that the time of onset of pharmacodynamic effect is 1–2 hrs.

### Transition Guideline to Edoxaban

**From warfarin or other vitamin K antagonists:** Discontinue warfarin and start edoxaban when INR is less than or equal to 2.5. **From oral anticoagulants other than warfarin or other vitamin K antagonists:** Discontinue current oral anticoagulant and start edoxaban at the time of the next scheduled dose of the other oral anticoagulant. **From LMWH:** Discontinue LMWH and start edoxaban at the time of the next scheduled dose of LMWH. **From low unfractionated heparin:** Discontinue infusion and start edoxaban 4 hrs later.

### Transition Guideline from Edoxaban to Other Anticoagulant

**To Warfarin:** **Oral option:** For pts taking edoxaban 60 mg, reduce to 30 mg and begin warfarin concomitantly. For pts taking edoxaban 30 mg, reduce dose to 15 mg and begin warfarin concomitantly. Once stable INR greater than or equal to 2, discontinue edoxaban and continue warfarin. **Parenteral option:** Discontinue edoxaban and administer parenteral anticoagulant and warfarin at the time of next scheduled edoxaban dose. Once stable INR greater than or equal to 2, discontinue parenteral anticoagulant and continue warfarin. **To non–vitamin K-dependent oral anticoagulant or parenteral anticoagulant:** Discontinue edoxaban and start other oral anticoagulant at the time of the next scheduled dose.

### SIDE EFFECTS

**Rare (4%):** Rash.

## ADVERSE EFFECTS/TOXIC REACTIONS

Hemorrhagic events including intracranial hemorrhage, hemorrhagic stroke, cutaneous/GI/GU/oral/pharyngeal/urethral/vaginal bleeding, epistaxis, epidural/spinal hematoma (esp. with epidural catheters, spinal trauma) were reported. Discontinuation in the absence of other adequate anticoagulants may increase the risk of ischemic events, stroke. May increase risk of epidural or spinal hematomas, which can lead to long-term or permanent paralysis. Protamine sulfate, vitamin K, tranexamic acid are not expected to reverse anticoagulant effect. Interstitial lung disease was reported in less than 1% of pts.

## NURSING CONSIDERATIONS

### BASELINE ASSESSMENT

Obtain baseline renal function test, esp. creatinine clearance; PT/INR in pts transitioning on or off warfarin therapy. Do not initiate if CrCl greater than 95 ml/min. Question history of bleeding disorders, recent surgery, spinal procedures,

---

intracranial hemorrhage, bleeding ulcers, open wounds, anemia, renal/hepatic impairment. Receive full medication history including herbal products.

### INTERVENTION/EVALUATION

Monitor renal function test; occult urine/stool, urine output. Monitor for symptoms of hemorrhage: abdominal/back pain, headache, altered mental status, weakness, paresthesia, aphasia, vision changes, GI bleeding. Question for increase in menstrual bleeding/discharge. Assess peripheral pulses; skin for ecchymosis, petechiae. Assess urine output for hematuria.

### PATIENT/FAMILY TEACHING

• Do not discontinue current blood thinning regimen or take any newly prescribed medication unless approved by physician who started anticoagulant therapy. • Suddenly stopping therapy may increase risk of stroke or blood clots. Refill prescriptions so next scheduled dose is not missed. • Immediately report bleeding of any kind. • Avoid alcohol, aspirin, NSAIDs. • Consult physician before surgery/dental work. • Use electric razor, soft toothbrush to prevent bleeding. • Report any numbness, muscular weakness, signs of stroke (confusion, headache, one-sided weakness, trouble speaking), bloody stool or urine, nosebleeds. • Monitor changes in urine output.

---

# efavirenz

e-**fav**-ir-enz
(Sustiva)

## FIXED COMBINATION(S)

**Atripla:** efavirenz/emtricitabine (an antiretroviral)/tenofovir (an antiretroviral): 600 mg/200 mg/300 mg.

## ◆CLASSIFICATION

**PHARMACOTHERAPEUTIC:** Nonnucleoside reverse transcriptase inhibitor. **CLINICAL:** Antiretroviral.

## USES

Treatment of HIV infection, in combination with at least two other appropriate antiretroviral agents, in adults and children 3 mos and older weighing at least 3.5 kg.

## PRECAUTIONS

**Contraindications:** Hypersensitivity to efavirenz. Concurrent use with bepridil, ergot derivatives, midazolam, St. John's wort, triazolam. **Cautions:** History of mental illness, seizures, suspected hepatitis B or C infection, history of substance abuse, hepatic impairment (class A). Avoid pregnancy.

## ACTION

Binds to reverse transcriptase, blocking RNA and DNA-dependent DNA polymerase activity including HIV-1 replication. **Therapeutic Effect:** Interrupts HIV replication, slowing progression of HIV infection.

## PHARMACOKINETICS

Rapidly absorbed after PO administration. Protein binding: 99%. Metabolized in liver. Eliminated in feces (16%–61%), urine (14%–34%). **Half-life:** 40–55 hrs.

## ⬛ LIFESPAN CONSIDERATIONS

**Pregnancy/Lactation:** Breastfeeding not recommended. **Children:** Safety and efficacy not established in pts younger than 3 yrs; may have increased incidence of rash. **Elderly:** No age-related precautions noted.

## INTERACTIONS

**DRUG: Ergot derivatives, midazolam, triazolam** may cause serious or life-threatening reactions (cardiac arrhythmias, prolonged sedation, respiratory depression). Decreases plasma concentrations of **amprenavir, atazanavir, boceprevir, telaprevir, indinavir, saquinavir.** Increases plasma concentrations of **ritonavir. CYP3A4 inducers (e.g., phenobarbital, rifabutin, rifampin)** decrease concentration/effects.

---

May alter **warfarin** plasma concentration. **HERBAL: St. John's wort** may decrease concentration/effects. **FOOD: High-fat meals** may increase drug absorption. **LAB VALUES:** May produce false-positive urine test results for cannabinoid. May increase serum ALT, AST, GGT, amylase, glucose, triglycerides, cholesterol. May decrease neutrophils.

## AVAILABILITY (Rx)

**Capsules:** 50 mg, 200 mg.

**Tablets:** 600 mg.

## ADMINISTRATION/HANDLING

### PO

• Give with water at bedtime (decreases CNS adverse effects). • Avoid high-fat meals (may increase absorption) • Capsules may be opened and added to small amount of food/liquid. Administer within 30 min. • Do not break, crush, dissolve, or divide tablets.

## INDICATIONS/ROUTES/DOSAGE

### HIV Infection

**PO: ADULTS, ELDERLY, CHILDREN WEIGHING 40 KG OR MORE:** 600 mg once daily at bedtime. **CHILDREN WEIGHING 32.5 KG–LESS THAN 40 KG:** 400 mg once daily. **CHILDREN WEIGHING 25 KG–LESS THAN 32.5 KG:** 350 mg once daily. **CHILDREN WEIGHING 20 KG–LESS THAN 25 KG:** 300 mg once daily. **CHILDREN WEIGHING 15 KG–LESS THAN 20 KG:** 250 mg once daily. **CHILDREN WEIGHING 7.5 KG–LESS THAN 15 KG:** 200 mg once daily. **CHILDREN WEIGHING 5 KG–LESS THAN 7.5 KG:** 150 mg once daily. **CHILDREN WEIGHING 3.5 KG–LESS THAN 5 KG:** 100 mg once daily.

### Dosage: Concurrent Rifampin

**PO: ONLY IF PT WEIGHS 50 KG OR GREATER:** 800 mg once daily.

### Dosage: Concurrent Voriconazole

**PO:** Reduce efavirenz to 300 mg once daily; increase voriconazole to 400 mg q12h.

### Dosage in Renal Impairment

No dose adjustment.

### Dosage in Hepatic Impairment

**Mild impairment:** Use caution. **Moderate to severe impairment:** Not recommended.

## SIDE EFFECTS

**Frequent (52%): Mild to severe:** Dizziness, vivid dreams, insomnia, confusion, impaired concentration, amnesia, agitation, depersonalization, hallucinations, euphoria. **Occasional: Mild to moderate:** Maculopapular rash (27%); nausea, fatigue, headache, diarrhea, fever, cough (less than 26%).

## ADVERSE EFFECTS/ TOXIC REACTIONS

Serious adverse psychiatric experiences (aggressive reactions, agitation, delusions, emotional lability, mania, neurosis, paranoia, psychosis, suicide) have been reported. Grade 4 rash, Stevens-Johnson syndrome, erythema multiforme occurs rarely. Hepatotoxicity with serum ALT, AST elevation greater than 5 times upper limit of normal reported in 5% of pts. May induce immune reconstitution syndrome (inflammatory response to dormant opportunistic infections or acceleration of autoimmune disorders).

## NURSING CONSIDERATIONS

### BASELINE ASSESSMENT

Offer emotional support. Obtain baseline ALT, AST in pts with history of hepatitis B or C virus infection; serum cholesterol or triglycerides before initiating therapy and at intervals during therapy. Receive full medication history including herbal products (high risk of drug interaction).

### INTERVENTION/EVALUATION

Monitor for CNS, psychological symptoms: severe acute depression (including suicidal ideation or attempts), dizziness, impaired concentration, drowsiness, abnormal dreams, insomnia (begins during first or second day of therapy, generally resolves in 2–4 wks). Assess for evidence of rash (common side effect). Monitor LFT for abnormalities. Assess for headache, nausea, diarrhea.

### PATIENT/FAMILY TEACHING

• Avoid high-fat meals during therapy. • Report appearance of skin rash immediately. • CNS, psychological symptoms occur in more than half of pts (dizziness, impaired concentration, delusions, depression). • Take medication every day as prescribed. • Do not alter dose or discontinue medication without informing physician. • Do not chew, crush, dissolve, or divide tablets. • Avoid tasks that require alertness, motor skills until response to drug is established. • Avoid alcohol. • Efavirenz is not a cure for HIV infection, nor does it reduce risk of transmission to others.

---

# elbasvir/grazoprevir

el-bas-vir/graz-oh-pre-vir
(Zepatier)
**Do not confuse elbasvir with daclatasvir, ombitasvir or grazoprevir with boceprevir or simeprevir.**

### ◆CLASSIFICATION

**PHARMACOTHERAPEUTIC:** NS5A inhibitor/protease inhibitor. **CLINICAL:** Antiviral.

## USES

Treatment of chronic hepatitis C virus genotypes 1 or 4 infection in adults, with or without ribavirin.

## PRECAUTIONS

**Contraindications:** Hypersensitivity to elbasvir or grazoprevir, decompensated hepatic cirrhosis, moderate or severe hepatic impairment; concomitant use of organic anion transporting polypeptides 1B1/3 (OATP1B1/3) inhibitors, strong CYP3A inducers. Concomitant use of atazanavir, carbamazepine, cyclosporine, darunavir, efavirenz, lopinavir, phenytoin, rifampin, saquinavir, St. John's wort, tipranavir. Any contraindications or hypersensitivity to ribavirin (if used with treatment regimen). **Cautions:** HIV infection, mild hepatic impairment. Safety and efficacy not established in pts with hepatitis B virus coinfection, liver transplant recipients.

## ACTION

Elbasvir inhibits hepatitis C virus (HCV) NS5A protein, which is essential for viral RNA replication and virion assembly. Grazoprevir inhibits HCV NS3/4A protease needed for processing HCV-encoded polyproteins, which is essential for viral replication. **Therapeutic Effect:** Inhibits viral replication of hepatitis C virus.

## PHARMACOKINETICS

Widely distributed. Metabolized in liver. Protein binding: elbasvir (99.9%), grazoprevir (98.8%). Peak plasma concentration: 3 hrs. Steady state reached in approx. 6 days. Eliminated in feces (greater than 90%), urine (less than 1%). **Half-life:** elbasvir: 24 hrs; grazoprevir: 31 hrs.

## ⧗ LIFESPAN CONSIDERATIONS

**Pregnancy/Lactation:** Use caution in pregnancy. Unknown if distributed in breast milk. When used with ribavirin, breastfeeding and pregnancy are contraindicated during treatment and up to 6 mos after discontinuation. **Children:** Safety and efficacy not established in pts younger than 18 yrs. **Elderly:** May have increased risk of hepatotoxicity.

## INTERACTIONS

**DRUG: Anticonvulsants (e.g., carbamazepine, phenytoin), antimycobacterials (e.g., rifabutin, rifampin), efavirenz** may significantly decrease concentration/effect; use contraindicated. **Atazanavir, darunavir, lopinavir, tipranavir, cyclosporine**

---

**E**

may significantly increase risk of hepatotoxicity; use contraindicated. **Moderate CYP3A inducers (e.g., etravirine, modafinil, nafcillin)** may decrease concentration/effect. **Elvitegravir/ cobicistat/emtricitabine/tenofovir (disoproxil or alafenamide)**, ketoconazole may increase concentration/ effect. May increase concentration/effect of **atorvastatin, fluvastatin, hydrocodone, lovastatin, nimodipine, rosuvastatin, simvastatin, tacrolimus. Acetaminophen** may increase risk of hepatotoxicity. **HERBAL: St. John's wort** may decrease concentration/effect; use contraindicated. **FOOD: Grapefruit products** may increase grazoprevir concentration/effect. **LAB VALUES:** May decrease Hgb. May increase serum ALT, bilirubin.

## AVAILABILITY (Rx)

**Fixed-Dose Combination Tablets:** elbasvir 50 mg/grazoprevir 100 mg.

## ADMINISTRATION/HANDLING

**PO**
• Give without regard to meals.

## INDICATIONS/ROUTES/DOSAGE

**Note:** NS5A resistance testing recommended in HCV genotype 1a infected pts prior to initiating treatment with Zepatier.

**Chronic Hepatitis C Virus Infection**
**PO: ADULTS, ELDERLY:** 1 tablet once daily (with or without ribavirin).

**Treatment Regimen and Duration**
**PO: ADULTS, ELDERLY: Genotype 1a:** Treatment-naïve or peginterferon alfa **(PegIFN)/ribavirin (RBV)–experienced without baseline NS5A polymorphisms:** 1 tablet once daily for 12 wks. **Genotype 1a:** Treatment-naïve or PegIFN/RBV–experienced **with baseline NS5A polymorphisms:** 1 tablet once daily with ribavirin for 16 wks. **Genotype 1b:** Treatment-naïve or PegIFV/RBV–experienced: 1 tablet once daily for 12 wks. **Genotype 1a**

or 1b: PegIFV/RBV/protease inhibitor–experienced: 1 tablet once daily with ribavirin for 12 wks. **Genotype 4: Treatment-naïve:** 1 tablet once daily for 12 wks. **Genotype 4: PegIFN/RBV–experienced:** 1 tablet once daily with ribavirin for 16 wks.

**Treatment-Induced Hepatotoxicity**
Consider discontinuation in pts with persistent serum ALT elevation greater than 10 times upper limit of normal (ULN). Permanently discontinue if serum ALT elevation is accompanied with elevated alkaline phosphatase, conjugated bilirubin, prolonged INR, or signs of acute hepatic inflammation.

**Dosage in Renal Impairment**
No dose adjustment.

**Dosage in Hepatic Impairment**
**Mild impairment:** No dose adjustment. **Moderate to severe impairment:** Contraindicated.

## SIDE EFFECTS

**Occasional (11%–3%):** Fatigue, headache, diarrhea, nausea, insomnia, dyspnea, rash, pruritus, irritability. **Rare (2%):** Abdominal pain, arthralgia.

## ADVERSE EFFECTS/TOXIC REACTIONS

Serum ALT elevation up to 5 times ULN reported in 1% of pts. Serum bilirubin elevation greater than 2.5 times ULN occurred in 6% of pts. Serum ALT elevation occurred more frequently in the elderly, female pts, and pts of Asian ancestry.

## NURSING CONSIDERATIONS

**BASELINE ASSESSMENT**
Obtain CBC, LFT, HCV-RNA level; pregnancy test in female pts of reproductive potential. Confirm hepatitis C genotype. In pts with HCV genotype 1a, recommend testing for the presence of NS5A resistance-associated polymorphisms prior to

initiation. Receive full medication history including herbal products; screen for contraindications. Question history of chronic anemia, hepatitis B virus infection, HIV infection, liver transplantation.

**INTERVENTION/EVALUATION**

Obtain LFT at wk 8, then as clinically indicated. For pts receiving 16 wks of therapy, obtain additional LFT at wk 12. Monitor CBC periodically; HCV-RNA levels at wks 4, 8, 12, 16 and as clinically indicated. Monitor for hepatotoxicity. Assess for anemia-related dizziness, exertional dyspnea, fatigue, weakness, syncope. Encourage nutritional intake. Assess for decreased appetite, weight loss. Obtain monthly pregnancy tests in females of reproductive potential if treated with ribavirin.

**PATIENT/FAMILY TEACHING**

• Blood levels will be drawn routinely. • Treatment may be used in combination with ribavirin (inform pt of side effects/toxic reactions). If therapy includes ribavirin, female pts of reproductive potential should avoid pregnancy during treatment and up to 6 mos after last dose. • Do not take newly prescribed medication unless approved by the doctor who originally started treatment. • Do not take herbal products, esp. St. John's wort. • Avoid alcohol, grapefruit products. • Report signs of treatment-induced liver injury such as abdominal pain, clay-colored stool, dark amber urine, decreased appetite, fatigue, weakness, yellowing of the skin or eyes. • Maintain proper nutritional intake.

# eletriptan

el-e-**trip**-tan
(Relpax)

◆**CLASSIFICATION**

**PHARMACOTHERAPEUTIC:** Serotonin receptor agonist. **CLINICAL:** Antimigraine.

# USES

Treatment of acute migraine headache with or without aura.

# PRECAUTIONS

**Contraindications:** Hypersensitivity to eletriptan. Arrhythmias associated with conduction disorders, cerebrovascular syndrome including strokes and transient ischemic attacks (TIAs), coronary artery disease, hemiplegic or basilar migraine, ischemic heart disease, peripheral vascular disease including ischemic bowel disease, severe hepatic impairment, uncontrolled hypertension; use within 24 hrs of treatment with another 5-HT$_1$ agonist, an ergotamine-containing or ergot-type medication such as dihydroergotamine (DHE) or methysergide. Recent use (within 72 hrs) of strong CYP3A4 inhibitors (e.g., clarithromycin, ketoconazole, itraconazole, ritonavir). **Cautions:** Mild to moderate renal/hepatic impairment, controlled hypertension, history of CVA.

# ACTION

Binds selectively to serotonin receptors, producing vasoconstrictive effect on cranial blood vessels. **Therapeutic Effect:** Relieves migraine headache.

# PHARMACOKINETICS

Well absorbed after PO administration. Metabolized by liver. Eliminated in urine. **Half-life:** 4.4 hrs (increased in hepatic impairment, elderly [older than 65 yrs]).

# ⧗ LIFESPAN CONSIDERATIONS

**Pregnancy/Lactation:** May decrease possibility of ovulation. Distributed in breast milk. **Children:** Safety and efficacy not established in pts younger than 18 yrs. **Elderly:** Increased risk of hypertension in those older than 65 yrs.

# INTERACTIONS

**DRUG: CYP3A4 inhibitors (e.g., clarithromycin, itraconazole, ketoconazole, nefazodone, nelfinavir, ritonavir)** may decrease metabolism.

Ergotamine-containing medications may produce vasospastic reaction. **HERBAL:** None significant. **FOOD:** None known. **LAB VALUES:** None significant.

## AVAILABILITY (Rx)

**Tablets:** 20 mg, 40 mg.

## ADMINISTRATION/HANDLING

**PO**

• May take without regard to food. Do not break, crush, dissolve, or divide film-coated tablets.

## INDICATIONS/ROUTES/DOSAGE

**Acute Migraine Headache**
**PO: ADULTS, ELDERLY:** 20–40 mg. **Maximum:** 40 mg. If headache improves but then returns, dose may be repeated after 2 hrs. **Maximum:** 80 mg/day.

**Dosage in Renal/Hepatic Impairment**
No dose adjustment. Not recommended in severe hepatic impairment.

## SIDE EFFECTS

**Occasional (6%–5%):** Dizziness, drowsiness, asthenia, nausea. **Rare (3%–2%):** Paresthesia, headache, dry mouth, warm or hot sensation, dyspepsia, dysphagia.

## ADVERSE EFFECTS/ TOXIC REACTIONS

Cardiac reactions (ischemia, coronary artery vasospasm, MI), noncardiac vasospasm-related reactions (hemorrhage, CVA) occur rarely, particularly in pts with hypertension, obesity, diabetes, strong family history of coronary artery disease; smokers; males older than 40 yrs; postmenopausal women.

## NURSING CONSIDERATIONS

### BASELINE ASSESSMENT

Question pt regarding onset, location, duration of migraine, possible precipitating symptoms. Obtain baseline B/P for evidence of uncontrolled hypertension (contraindication).

### INTERVENTION/EVALUATION

Assess for relief of migraine headache, potential for photophobia, phonophobia (sound sensitivity), nausea, vomiting.

### PATIENT/FAMILY TEACHING

• Take a single dose as soon as symptoms of an actual migraine attack appear. • Medication is intended to relieve migraine headaches, not to prevent or reduce number of attacks. • Avoid tasks that require alertness, motor skills until response to drug is established. • Immediately report palpitations, pain/tightness in chest/ throat, sudden or severe abdominal pain, pain/weakness of extremities.

# elotuzumab

el-oh-**tooz**-ue-mab
(Empliciti)
**Do not confuse elotuzumab with alemtuzumab, eculizumab, evolocumab, pertuzumab, gemtuzumab, trastuzumab.**

◆**CLASSIFICATION**

**PHARMACOTHERAPEUTIC:** Monoclonal antibody. **CLINICAL:** Antineoplastic.

## USES

Treatment of multiple myeloma (in combination with lenalidomide and dexamethasone) in pts who have received one to three prior therapies.

## PRECAUTIONS

**Contraindications:** Hypersensitivity to elotuzumab. **Cautions:** Diabetes, baseline cytopenias, hypertension; history of chronic opportunistic infections (esp. viral infections, fungal infections), conditions predisposing to infection (e.g., diabetes, kidney failure, open wounds). Concomitant use of medications known to cause bradycardia (e.g., antiarrhythmics, beta blockers, calcium channel blockers). Concomitant use of live vaccines not recommended during treatment and up to 3 mos after discontinuation. Avoid use during severe active infection.

## ACTION

Binds to and specifically targets signaling lymphocytic activation molecule family member 7 (SLAMF7), a protein that is expressed on most myeloma and natural killer cells. Directly activates natural killer cells and facilitates cellular death. **Therapeutic Effect:** Inhibits tumor cell growth and metastasis.

## PHARMACOKINETICS

Widely distributed. Metabolism not specified. Elimination not specified. **Half-life:** Not specified; 97% of steady-state concentration is expected to be eliminated within 82 days.

## ⚖ LIFESPAN CONSIDERATIONS

**Pregnancy/Lactation:** Avoid pregnancy; may cause fetal harm/malformations when used with lenalidomide. Unknown if distributed in breast milk. However, immunoglobulin G (IgG) is present in breast milk. Breastfeeding contraindicated when used with concomitant lenalidomide treatment. **Men:** Lenalidomide is present in semen. Recommend use of barrier methods during sexual activity. **Children:** Safety and efficacy not established. **Elderly:** No age-related precautions noted.

## INTERACTIONS

**DRUG:** None known (not studied). **HERBAL:** Echinacea may decrease effect. **FOOD:** None known. **LAB VALUES:** May be detected on both serum protein electrophoresis and immunofixation assays used to monitor multiple myeloma endogenous M protein. May affect the determination of complete response and disease progression of some pts with IgG kappa myeloma protein. Expected to decrease lymphocytes, leukocytes, platelets. May decrease serum albumin, bicarbonate, calcium. May increase serum alkaline phosphatase, ALT, AST, glucose, potassium.

## AVAILABILITY (Rx)

**Injection, Powder for Reconstitution:** 300 mg, 400 mg.

## ADMINISTRATION/HANDLING
🔧 IV

**Reconstitution** • Calculate the dose and number of vials required based on weight in kg. • Reconstitute the 300-mg vial with 13 ml of Sterile Water for Injection or the 400-mg vial with 17 ml of Sterile Water for Injection using an 18-g or lower (e.g., 17, 16, or 15) needle. • Gently roll vial upright to mix. To dissolve any powder left on top of vial or stopper, gently invert vial several times. • Do not shake or agitate. • The powder should dissolve in less than 10 mins. • After dissolution, allow vials to stand for 5–10 mins. • Visually inspect solution for particulate matter of discoloration. Solution should appear clear, colorless to slightly yellow. Discard if solution is cloudy or discolored or if foreign particles are observed. Each vial contains an overfill volume to allow for a specific withdraw of 12 ml (300-mg vial) or 16 ml (400-mg vial). • Final concentration of withdrawn volume (without overfill) will equal 25 mg/ml. • Dilute in 230 ml of 0.9% NaCl or 5% Dextrose injection in polyvinyl chloride or polyolefin infusion bag. • Mix by gentle inversion; do not shake or agitate. • The volume may be adjusted in order to not exceed 5 ml/kg of pt weight at any given dose.
**Infusion Guidelines** • Prior to administration, premedicate with dexamethasone, acetaminophen, antihistamine (H1 blocker, plus H2 blocker) approx. 45–90 mins before each infusion (see manufacturer guidelines). • Use an inline, sterile, nonpyrogenic, low-protein-binding filter (0.2–1.2 mm). • Infuse via dedicated line using an infusion pump.

**E**

**Rate of Administration • First Infusion (Cycle 1, Dose 1):** Infuse at 0.5 ml/min for the first 30 mins. If no infusion reactions occur, may increase to 1 ml/min for next 30 mins. If tolerated, may increase to 2 ml/min. **Maximum rate:** 2 ml/min. • **Second Infusion (Cycle 1, Dose 2):** Initiate at 1 ml/min for first 30 mins if no infusion reactions occurred during first infusion. If tolerated, may increase to 2 ml/min until infusion completed. **Maximum rate:** 2 ml/min. • **Subsequent Infusions (Cycle 1, Dose 3 and 4, All Subsequent Infusions):** Initiate at 2 ml/min until completion if no infusion reactions occurred during prior infusion. **Maximum rate:** 2 ml/min. In pts who have received four cycles of treatment, infusion rate may be increased to maximum rate of 5 ml/min. **Storage** • Refrigerate intact vials until time of use. • Do not freeze or shake. • Refrigerate diluted solution up to 24 hrs • May store at room temperature up to 8 hrs (of the total 24 hrs). • Diluted solution must be administered within 24 hrs of reconstitution. • Protect from light.

## ▨ IV INCOMPATABILITIES

Do not mix with other medications.

## INDICATIONS/ROUTES/DOSAGE

**Multiple Myeloma**
**IV: ADULTS, ELDERLY: Cycles 1 and 2:** 10 mg/kg once wkly on days 1, 8, 15, 22 of 28-day cycle (in combination with lenalidomide and dexamethasone).
**Cycles 3 and beyond:** 10 mg/kg once q2wks on days 1 and 15 of 28-day cycle (in combination with lenalidomide and dexamethasone). Continue until disease progression or unacceptable toxicity.

**Dose Modification**
**Infusion Reactions**
**Grade 2 or higher reaction:** Interrupt infusion until symptoms improve. Once resolved to Grade 1 or 0, resume infusion at 0.5 ml/min. If tolerated, increase in increments of 0.5 ml/min q30mins

back to previous rate. May further increase rate as indicated if no reaction recurs. If infusion reaction recurs, stop infusion and do not restart for that day.

**Dosage in Renal/Hepatic Impairment**
Not specified; use caution.

## SIDE EFFECTS

**Frequent (61%–20%):** Fatigue, diarrhea, pyrexia, constipation, cough, peripheral neuropathy, decreased appetite. **Occasional (16%–10%):** Extremity pain, headache, vomiting, decreased weight, oropharyngeal pain, hypoesthesia, mood change, night sweats.

## ADVERSE EFFECTS/TOXIC REACTIONS

All cases were reported in combination with lenalidomide and dexamethasone. Infusion reactions reported in 10% of pts. Most infusion reactions were Grade 3 and lower. Lymphopenia, leukopenia, thrombocytopenia are expected responses to therapy. Infections were reported in 81% of pts. Grade 3 or 4 infections occurred in 28% of pts. Nasopharyngitis (25% of pts), upper respiratory tract infection (23% of pts), opportunistic infection (22% of pts), herpes zoster (14% of pts), fungal infection (10% of pts), influenza; second primary malignancies, skin malignancies, solid tumors, malignant neoplasms; tachycardia, bradycardia, systolic or diastolic hypertension, hypotension; pulmonary embolism may occur. Hepatotoxicity with elevation of serum alkaline phosphatase greater than 2 times upper limit of normal (ULN), serum ALT/AST greater than 3 times ULN, total bilirubin greater than 2 times ULN reported in 3% of pts. Other adverse effects may include cataracts (12% of pts), hyperglycemia (89% of pts), hypersensitivity reaction (greater than 5% of pts). Immunogenicity (auto-elotuzumab antibodies) occurred in 19% of pts. Thrombocytopenia may increase risk of bleeding.

---

## NURSING CONSIDERATIONS

### BASELINE ASSESSMENT

Obtain CBC, BMP, LFT; serum ionized calcium; capillary blood glucose, vital signs; pregnancy test in female pts of reproductive potential. Obtain baseline EKG in pts concurrently using of medications known to cause bradycardia. Question history of chronic opportunistic infections, diabetes, hepatic impairment, pulmonary embolism; prior infusion or hypersensitivity reactions. Screen for medications known to cause bradycardia, hyperglycemia. Screen for active infection. Offer emotional support.

### INTERVENTION/EVALUATION

Obtain CBC, BMP, LFT, ionized calcium periodically. Administer in an environment equipped to monitor for and manage infusion reactions. If infusion reaction of any grade/severity occurs, immediately interrupt infusion and manage symptoms. Accurately record characteristics of infusion reactions (severity, type, time of onset). Infusion reactions may affect future infusion rates. Monitor HR, BP q30mins during infusion and for at least 2 hrs after completion in pts with prior hemodynamic reactions. Cough, dyspnea, hypoxia, tachycardia may indicate pulmonary embolism. Monitor for bradycardia, cataracts, hyperglycemia, hyperkalemia, hypersensitivity reaction, hepatotoxicity, neuropathy, tachycardia. Assess for new primary malignancies (solid tumors, skin cancers); skin for new lesions, moles. Monitor daily pattern bowel activity, stool consistency.

### PATIENT/FAMILY TEACHING

• Blood levels, EKGs will be monitored routinely. • Treatment may depress your immune system and reduce your ability to fight infection. Report symptoms of infection such as body aches, chills, cough, fatigue, fever. Avoid those with active infection. • Therapy may decrease your heart rate, esp. in those taking medications that lower heart rate; report dizziness, chest pain, palpitations, or fainting. • Avoid pregnancy. Do not breastfeed. • Male pts should use condoms during sexual activity. • Treatment includes a steroid that may raise blood sugar levels; report dehydration, blurry vision, confusion, frequent urination, increased thirst, fruity breath. • Report allergic reactions of any kind. • Abdominal pain, easy bruising, clay-colored stools, dark-amber urine, fatigue, loss of appetite, yellowing of skin or eyes may indicate liver problem.

# eltrombopag

el-**trom**-boe-pag
(Promacta, Revolade ♣)

■ **BLACK BOX ALERT** ■ May cause hepatotoxicity. Measure serum ALT, AST, and bilirubin prior to initiation of eltrombopag, every 2 wks during dose adjustment phase, and monthly following establishment of a stable dose. If bilirubin is elevated, perform fractionation. Discontinue eltrombopag if ALT levels increase to 3 times or greater upper limit of normal and are progressive, persistent for 4 or more wks, accompanied by increased direct bilirubin, clinical symptoms of hepatic injury, or evidence of hepatic decompensation.

## ◆CLASSIFICATION

**PHARMACOTHERAPEUTIC:** Thrombopoietin receptor agonist. **CLINICAL:** Prevents thrombocytopenia.

## USES

Treatment of thrombocytopenia in pts with chronic immune (idiopathic) thrombocytopenic purpura (ITP) with insufficient response with corticosteroids, immunoglobulins, or splenectomy. Use only in pts who are at increased risk for bleeding; should not be used to normalize platelet counts. Treatment of thrombocytopenia in pts with chronic hepatitis C infection to allow the initiation and maintenance of

**E**

interferon-based therapy. Treatment of severe aplastic anemia in pts having an insufficient response to immunosuppressive therapy.

## PRECAUTIONS

**Contraindications:** Hypersensitivity to eltrombopag. **Cautions:** Preexisting hepatic impairment, renal impairment (any degree), myelodysplastic syndrome (may increase risk for hematologic malignancies). Pts with known risk for thromboembolism, risk for cataracts.

## ACTION

Interacts with the human thrombopoietin receptor and initiates signaling cascades. **Therapeutic Effect:** Induces proliferation and differentiation of megakaryocytes from bone marrow progenitor cells.

## PHARMACOKINETICS

Readily absorbed from gastrointestinal tract. Primarily distributed in blood cells. Protein binding: 99%. Extensively metabolized including oxidation, conjugation with glucuronic acid or cysteine. Excreted primarily in feces. **Half-life:** 26–35 hrs.

## ⧗ LIFESPAN CONSIDERATIONS

**Pregnancy/Lactation:** Unknown if distributed in breast milk. **Children:** Safety and efficacy not established. **Elderly:** Use caution due to increased frequency of hepatic, renal, cardiac dysfunction.

## INTERACTIONS

**DRUG:** May increase concentration/ toxicity of **atorvastatin, fluvastatin, methotrexate, nateglinide, pravastatin, repaglinide, rifampin, rosuvastatin. Aluminum, antacids, calcium, iron, magnesium** may decrease concentration/effects. **HERBAL:** None significant. **FOOD: Dairy products** may decrease concentration/effects. **LAB VALUES:** May increase serum ALT, AST.

## AVAILABILITY (Rx)

**Tablets:** 12.5 mg, 25 mg, 50 mg, 75 mg, 100 mg. **Oral Suspension:** 25 mg.

## ADMINISTRATION/HANDLING

### PO

• Give on an empty stomach, either 1 hr before or 2 hrs after meal. • Give at least 4 hrs before or 4 hrs after ingestion of antacids, food high in calcium or minerals, or calcium-fortified juices.

## INDICATIONS/ROUTES/DOSAGE

**Aplastic Anemia**
**PO: ADULTS, ELDERLY:** 50 mg once daily (25 mg for pts of East Asian ancestry or hepatic impairment). Titrate dose based on platelet response. Adjust dose to maintain platelets more than 50,000/ mm$^3$. **Maximum:** 150 mg/day.

**ITP**
**PO: ADULTS, ELDERLY, CHILDREN 6 YRS AND OLDER:** Initially, 50 mg once daily (25 mg for pts of East Asian ancestry or moderate to severe hepatic insufficiency or children 1 to 5 yrs of age). Then, adjust dose (25 mg to 75 mg once daily) to achieve and maintain platelet count of 50,000 mm$^3$ or greater as necessary to reduce risk of bleeding. **Maximum:** 75 mg once daily.

**Chronic Hepatitis C–associated Thrombocytopenia**
**PO: ADULTS, ELDERLY:** Initially, 25 mg once daily. Titrate dose based on platelet response. **Maximum:** 100 mg once daily.

**Dosage Adjustment Based on Platelet Response**

| | |
|---|---|
| Less than 50,000/mm$^3$ (after at least 2 wks) | Increase by 25 mg q2 wks up to 100 mg/day |
| 200,000/mm$^3$ or more and 400,000/mm$^3$ or less | Decrease by 25 mg |
| More than 400,000/mm$^3$ | Withhold; when less than 150,000/mm$^3$, resume with dose reduced by 25 mg |
| More than 400,000/mm$^3$ after 2 wks at lowest dose | Discontinue |

**Dosage in Renal Impairment**
No dose adjustment.

**Dosage in Hepatic Impairment**
**ITP**

| | |
|---|---|
| Mild to severe | Initial: 25 mg/day |
| East Asian ancestry | Initial: 12.5 mg/day |

**Chronic Hepatitis C**
No dose adjustment.

**Aplastic Anemia**
Initial dose 25 mg once daily.

## SIDE EFFECTS

**Frequent (6%–4%):** Nausea, vomiting, menorrhagia. **Occasional (3%–2%):** Myalgia, paresthesia, dyspepsia, ecchymosis, cataract, conjunctival hemorrhage.

## ADVERSE EFFECTS/ TOXIC REACTIONS

May cause hepatotoxicity. Increases risk of reticulin fiber deposits within bone marrow (may lead to bone marrow fibrosis). May produce hematologic malignancies. May cause excessive increase in platelets, leading to thrombotic complications.

## NURSING CONSIDERATIONS

### BASELINE ASSESSMENT

Assess CBC and peripheral blood smears, LFT. Examine peripheral blood smear to establish extent of RBC and WBC abnormalities. Conduct ocular examination.

### INTERVENTION/EVALUATION

Monitor CBC, platelet counts, peripheral blood smears, LFT throughout and following discontinuation. Monitor for cataracts during therapy.

### PATIENT/FAMILY TEACHING

• Lab values will be closely monitored throughout therapy and for at least 4 wks after last dose. • Report any yellowing of the skin or eyes, unusual darkening of the urine, unusual tiredness, pain in right upper stomach area. • Report changes in vision.

# eluxadoline

**el**-ux-**ad**-oh-leen
(Viberzi)

## ◆CLASSIFICATION

**PHARMACOTHERAPEUTIC:** Mu-opioid receptor agonist. **CLINICAL:** Antidiarrheal.

E

## USES

Treatment of irritable bowel syndrome with diarrhea in adults.

## PRECAUTIONS

**Contraindications:** Hypersensitivity to eluxadoline. Known or suspected biliary duct obstruction, sphincter of Oddi disease or dysfunction; severe hepatic impairment; severe constipation or sequelae from constipation, or known or suspected mechanical GI obstruction. History of alcoholism, alcohol abuse, alcohol addiction, or consumption of more than 3 alcoholic beverages/day. History of pancreatitis; structural disease of the pancreas, including known or suspected ancreatic duct obstruction. **Cautions:** Pts without a gallbladder, mild to moderate hepatic impairment, respiratory disease.

## ACTION

Affects mu-opioid receptors involved with gut motility, pain sensations, and secretion of liquids within the digestive tract. **Therapeutic Effect:** Reduces abdominal pain and diarrhea (without causing constipation).

## PHARMACOKINETICS

Metabolism not specified. Protein binding: 81%. Peak plasma concentration: 1.5 hrs. Primarily eliminated in feces (82%), urine (less than 1%). **Half-life:** 3.7–6 hrs.

## ☒ LIFESPAN CONSIDERATIONS

**Pregnancy/Lactation:** Unknown if distributed in breast milk. **Children:** Safety

---

 ◆ Canadian trade name    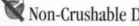 Non-Crushable Drug    High Alert drug

E

and efficacy not established. **Elderly:** No age-related precautions noted.

## INTERACTIONS

**DRUG:** **OATP1B1 inhibitors** (e.g., cyclosporine, atazanavir, ritonavir, rifampin), **strong CYP inhibitors** (e.g., **ciprofloxacin, gemfibrozil, fluconazole, clarithromycin**) may increase concentration/effect. **Drugs that cause constipation** (e.g., alosetron, anticholinergics [e.g., **diphenhydramine**], loperamide, opioids [e.g., **morphine**] may increase risk of serious constipation-associated adverse effects. May increase concentration of **rosuvastatin**, increasing risk of myopathy/rhabdomyolysis. May increase effects of **CYP3A substrates with narrow therapeutic index** (e.g., cyclosporine, sirolimus, tacrolimus). **HERBAL:** None significant. **FOOD:** High-fat meals may decrease absorption. **LAB VALUES:** May increase serum ALT, AST, lipase.

## AVAILABILITY (Rx)

Tablets: 75 mg, 100 mg.

## ADMINISTRATION/HANDLING

**PO**

• Administer with food. • If scheduled dose is missed, give next dose at the regular time; do not give 2 doses at once.

## INDICATIONS/ROUTES/DOSAGE

**Irritable Bowel Syndrome–Associated Diarrhea**

**PO: ADULTS, ELDERLY:** 100 mg twice daily. May decrease to 75 mg twice daily if unable to tolerate 100 mg dose.

**Dose Modification**

**Pts without a gallbladder, or are unable to tolerate 100-mg dose, or are receiving concomitant OATP1B1 inhibitors:** 75 mg twice daily.

**Pts who develop severe constipation for more than 4 days:** Permanently discontinue.

**Dosage in Renal Impairment**

Not specified; use caution.

**Dosage in Hepatic Impairment**

**Mild to moderate impairment:** 75 mg twice daily. **Severe impairment:** Contraindicated.

## SIDE EFFECTS

**Occasional (8%–4%):** Constipation, nausea, abdominal pain (upper or lower), upper respiratory tract infection, vomiting. **Rare (3%–1%):** Abdominal distention, dizziness, flatulence, rash, urticaria, fatigue, sedation, somnolence, euphoric mood.

## ADVERSE EFFECTS/TOXIC REACTIONS

May increase risk of sphincter of Oddi spasm (esp. in pts without a gallbladder), resulting in pancreatitis or hepatic enzyme elevation that may be associated with or without acute abdominal pain, or nausea/vomiting; 80% of pts reported sphincter of Oddi spasm within the first week of treatment. May also increase risk of pancreatitis that is not associated with sphincter of Oddi spasm. Infectious processes including upper respiratory tract infection, bronchitis, nasopharyngitis, viral gastroenteritis were reported. May cause hypersensitivity reaction including asthma, bronchospasm, respiratory failure, wheezing.

## NURSING CONSIDERATIONS

### BASELINE ASSESSMENT

Obtain baseline LFT in pts with baseline hepatic impairment. Receive full medication history and screen for interactions requiring lower dosage. Question pt's usual stool characteristics (color, frequency, consistency). Question history of alcoholism, biliary duct obstruction, mechanical GI obstruction, hepatic impairment, hypersensitivity reaction, pancreatic disease, respiratory disease, sphincter of Oddi disease or spasm. Assess hydration status.

**INTERVENTION/EVALUATION**

Monitor for abdominal pain that radiates to the back or shoulder, with or without nausea or vomiting (esp. during first few weeks of treatment). Obtain LFT, serum lipase level if acute pancreatitis, sphincter of Oddi spasm, biliary tract obstruction suspected. Monitor for hypersensitivity reaction including dyspnea, rash, wheezing. Observe and record daily pattern of bowel activity, stool consistency. Encourage PO intake. If an acute overdose occurs, a narcotic mu-opioid antagonist such as naloxone may be considered if reversal of overdose-related adverse effects is needed.

**PATIENT/FAMILY TEACHING**

• Therapy may cause inflammation of the pancreas (pancreatitis) or elevated liver-associated abdominal pain, esp. during the first few weeks of treatment. Report any new or worsening abdominal pain that radiates to the back or shoulder, with or without nausea/vomiting. • Avoid chronic or acute excessive use of alcohol; may increase risk of liver or pancreas injury. • If a dose is missed, take the next dose at the regular time; do not take 2 doses at once. • Report constipation lasting longer than 4 days. • Avoid medications that cause constipation (e.g., antidiarrheals, narcotics). • Report signs of allergic reaction; respiratory problems such as worsening of asthma, bronchitis, wheezing. • Drink plenty of fluids.

# elvitegravir

el-vi-**teg**-ra-vir
(Vitekta)
**Do not confuse elvitegravir with dolutegravir or raltegravir.**

## FIXED COMBINATION(S)

**Genvoya, Stribild:** elvitegravir (an integrase inhibitor)/cobicistat (an antiretroviral booster)/emtricitabine/ tenofovir (antiretroviral agents): 150 mg/150 mg/200 mg/300 mg.

## ◆CLASSIFICATION

**PHARMACOTHERAPEUTIC:** Integrase strand transfer inhibitor. **CLINICAL:** Antiretroviral agent.

## USES

Used in combination with an HIV protease inhibitor, co-administered with ritonavir and other antiretroviral medications for the treatment of HIV-1 infection in antiretroviral treatment–experienced adults.

## PRECAUTIONS

**Contraindications:** Hypersensitivity to elvitegravir. **Cautions:** Diabetes, hepatic impairment, hypercholesterolemia. Not recommended with a HIV protease inhibitor and cobicistat combination; co-administration of HIV-1 protease inhibitors other than atazanavir, darunavir, fosamprenavir, lopinavir, and tipranavir.

## ACTION

Inhibits HIV integrase by preventing integration of HIV-1 DNA into host DNA, blocking formation of HIV-1 provirus. **Therapeutic Effect:** Interferes with HIV replication, slowing progression of HIV infection.

## PHARMACOKINETICS

Readily absorbed after PO administration. Metabolized in liver. Protein binding: 98%–99%. Peak plasma concentration: 4 hrs. Eliminated in feces (95%), urine (7%). **Half-life:** 8.7 hrs.

## ⏳ LIFESPAN CONSIDERATIONS

**Pregnancy/Lactation:** Breastfeeding not recommend due to risk of postnatal HIV transmission. Unknown if distributed in human breast milk. **Children:** Safety and efficacy not established in pts younger than 18 yrs. **Elderly:** Safety and efficacy not established in pts older than

E

65 yrs. May have increased risk of adverse reactions, hepatic impairment.

## INTERACTIONS

**DRUG:** Antacids, aluminum/calcium/magnesium/iron supplements, antiretrovirals (e.g., efavirenz, nevirapine), corticosteroids (e.g., dexamethasone), anticonvulsants (e.g., carbamazepine, phenytoin), rifampin may decrease concentration/effect. May increase concentrations/effects of **ketoconazole, rifampin. Antifungals** (e.g., ketoconazole), **atazanavir, lopinavir** may increase concentration/effect. May decrease concentration/effect of **hormonal contraceptives. HERBAL:** St John's wort may decrease effectiveness. **FOOD:** None known. **LAB VALUES:** May increase serum ALT, AST, amylase bilirubin, cholesterol, creatine kinase (CK), GGT, glucose, lipase, triglycerides, urine glucose, urine RBC. May decrease neutrophils.

## AVAILABILITY (Rx)

Tablets: 85 mg, 150 mg.

## ADMINISTRATION/HANDLING

**PO**
• Must be taken with food. • Must be administered with a protease inhibitor, in combination with ritonavir and another antiretroviral drug. • If pt receiving antacid, do not give aluminum- or magnesium-containing antacids within 2 hrs of dose.

## INDICATIONS/ROUTES/DOSAGE

**HIV Infection**
**ADULTS, ELDERLY:** 150 mg once daily. *(Co-administered with atazanavir/ritonavir or lopinavir/ritonavir):* **PO:** **ADULTS, ELDERLY:** 85 mg once daily.

**Dosage in Renal Impairment**
No dose adjustment.

**Dosage in Hepatic Impairment**
**Mild to moderate impairment:** No dose adjustment. **Severe impairment:** Not recommended.

## SIDE EFFECTS

**Occasional (7%–4%):** Diarrhea, nausea.
**Rare (3%):** Headache.

## ADVERSE REACTIONS/TOXIC EFFECTS

May induce immune recovery syndrome (inflammatory response to dormant opportunistic infections such as *Mycobacterium avium,* cytomegalovirus, *Pneumocystis carinii* pneumonia [PCP], tuberculosis, or acceleration of autoimmune disorders such as Graves' disease, polymyositis, Guillain-Barré). Pts coinfected with hepatitis B or C virus have increased risk for viral reactivation and worsening of hepatic function and may experience hepatic decompensation and/or failure if therapy is discontinued. Elevation of hepatic enzymes greater than 5 times upper limit of normal reported in 2% of pts.

## NURSING CONSIDERATIONS

**BASELINE ASSESSMENT**
Obtain BMP, CBC, lipid panel, LFT, urine glucose, vital signs; CD4+ count, viral load level. Screen for hepatitis B or C co-infection, hypercholesterolemia. Receive full medication history including herbal products. Question possibility of pregnancy; history of diabetes, hypercholesterolemia.

**INTERVENTION/EVALUATION**
Monitor CBC, hepatic function, lipid levels. Monitor CD4+ count, viral load for treatment effectiveness. Cough, dyspnea, fever, excess of band cells on CBC may indicate acute infection (WBC count may be unreliable in pts with uncontrolled HIV infection). Screen for immune reconstitution syndrome.

**PATIENT/FAMILY TEACHING**
• Offer emotional support. • Take elvitegravir with a HIV protease inhibitor, combined with ritonavir at the same time each day with food (optimizes absorption). • Antacids may decrease drug

underlined – top prescribed drug

effectiveness; do not take within 2 hrs of dose • Treatment regimen does not cure HIV infection, nor reduce risk of transmission. • Drug resistance can form if therapy is interrupted; do not run out of supply. • As immune system strengthens, it may respond to dormant infections hidden within the body. Report body aches, chills, cough, fever, night sweats, shortness of breath. • Treatment may cause liver dysfunction; report abdominal pain, darkened urine, clay-colored stools, significant weight loss, or yellowing of skin or eyes.• Do not take any new medications, including over-the-counter drugs or herbal products, unless approved by your doctor.

# empagliflozin

em-pa-gli-**floe**-zin
(Jardiance)
**Do not confuse empagliflozin with canagliflozin or dapagliflozin.**

## FIXED COMBINATION(S)

**Glyxambi:** empagliflozin/linagliptin (an antidiabetic): 10 mg/5 mg, 25 mg/5 mg. **Synjardy:** Empagliflozin/metformin (an antidiabetic): 5 mg/500 mg, 5 mg/1000 mg, 12.5 mg/500 mg, 12.5 mg/1000 mg.

## ◆CLASSIFICATION

**PHARMACOTHERAPEUTIC:** Sodium-glucose co-transporter 2 (SGLT2) inhibitor. **CLINICAL:** Antidiabetic.

## USES

Adjunctive treatment to diet and exercise to improve glycemic controls in pts with type 2 diabetes mellitus. Reduce risk of cardiovascular death in pts with type 2 diabetes and cardiovascular disease.

## PRECAUTIONS

**Contraindications:** History of hypersensitivity to empagliflozin, other SGLT2 inhibitors, severe renal impairment, end-stage renal disease, dialysis. **Cautions:** Not recommended in type 1 diabetes, diabetic ketoacidosis. Concurrent use of diuretics, other hypoglycemic medications, mild to moderate renal impairment, hypovolemia (dehydration/anemia), elderly, those with low systolic B/P, hyperlipidemia, pts with history of genital mycotic infection. May cause ketoacidosis.

## ACTION

Increases excretion of urinary glucose by inhibiting reabsorption of filtered glucose in kidney. Inhibits SGLT2 in proximal renal tubule. **Therapeutic Effect:** Lowers serum glucose levels.

## PHARMACOKINETICS

Readily absorbed following PO administration. Metabolized in liver by glucuronidation. Peak plasma concentration: 1.5 hrs. Protein binding: 86%. Excreted in urine (54%) and feces (41%). **Half-life:** 12.4 hrs.

## ⧗ LIFESPAN CONSIDERATIONS

**Pregnancy/Lactation:** Unknown if distributed in breast milk. Must either discontinue drug or discontinue breastfeeding. **Children:** Safety and efficacy not established in pts younger than 18 yrs. **Elderly:** May have increased risk for adverse reactions (e.g., hypotension, syncope, dehydration).

## INTERACTIONS

**DRUG: Diuretics (e.g., HCTZ, furosemide)** may increase risk of hypotension/volume depletion. **Insulin, insulin secretagogues (e.g., glyburide)** may increase risk of hypoglycemia. May increase concentration/effect of **digoxin. HERBAL:** Herbs with hypoglycemic properties **(e.g., fenugreek, garlic, ginger, ginseng, gotu)** may increase risk of hypoglycemia. **FOOD:** None known. **LAB VALUES:** May increase low-density lipoprotein cholesterol (LDL-C), serum creatinine. May decrease glomerular filtration rate.

## AVAILABILITY (Rx)

▼ **Tablets:** 10 mg, 25 mg.

 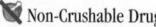

## ADMINISTRATION/HANDLING

### PO

May give without regard to food in the morning.

## INDICATIONS/ROUTES/DOSAGE

### Type 2 Diabetes Mellitus, Reduce Risk of Cardiovascular Death

**PO: ADULTS/ELDERLY:** Initially, 10 mg once daily in the morning. May increase to 25 mg once daily.

### Dosage in Renal impairment

**GFR 45 ml/min or greater:** No dose adjustment. **GFR less than 45 ml/min:** Discontinue. Do not initiate.

### Dosage in Hepatic Impairment

No dose adjustment.

## SIDE EFFECTS

**Occasional (9.3%–5.4%):** UTI, female genital mycotic infection. **Rare (4 %–1.1%):** Upper respiratory tract infection, increased urination, dyslipidemia, arthralgia, male genital mycotic infections, nausea.

## ADVERSE REACTIONS/ TOXIC EFFECTS

Symptomatic hypotension (postural dizziness, orthostatic hypotension, syncope) may occur. Genital myocotic (yeast) infections reported in 6.5% of pts. Hypoglycemic events reported (concomitant use of hypoglycemic medications may increase hypoglycemic risk).

## NURSING CONSIDERATIONS

### BASELINE ASSESSMENT

Assess hydration status. Obtain serum chemistries, capillary blood glucose, hemoglobin A1c, LDL-C. Assess pt's understanding of diabetes management, routine home glucose monitoring. Receive full medication history including minerals, herbal products. Question history of co-morbidities, esp. renal or hepatic impairment.

### INTERVENTION/EVALUATION

Monitor serum cholesterol, blood glucose, renal function, LFT. Assess for hypoglycemia (diaphoresis, tremors, dizziness, anxiety, headache, tachycardia, perioral numbness, hunger, diplopia, difficulty concentrating), hyperglycemia (polyuria, polyphagia, polydipsia, nausea, vomiting, fatigue, Kussmaul respirations), hypersensitivity reaction. Screen for glucose-altering conditions: fever, increased activity or stress, surgical procedures. Obtain dietary consult for nutritional education. Encourage PO intake.

### PATIENT/FAMILY TEACHING

• Diabetes mellitus requires lifelong control. • Diet and exercise are principal parts of treatment; do not skip or delay meals. • Test blood sugar regularly. When taking combination drug therapy or when glucose demands are altered (fever, infection, trauma, stress), have low blood sugar treatment available (glucagon, oral dextrose). • Report suspected pregnancy or plans of breastfeeding. • Monitor daily calorie intake. • Slowly go from lying to standing to prevent dizziness. • Therapy may increase risk for dehydration/low blood pressure. • Genital itching may indicate yeast infection. Report any signs of UTI (e.g., burning while urinating, cloudy urine, pelvic pain, back pain).

## emtricitabine   TOP 100

em-tri-**sye**-ta-bine
(Emtriva)

■ **BLACK BOX ALERT** ■ Serious, sometimes fatal, hypersensitivity reaction, lactic acidosis, severe hepatomegaly with steatosis (fatty liver) have occurred. May exacerbate hepatitis B virus infection after completing treatment.

## FIXED-COMBINATION(S)

**Descovy:** emtricitabine/tenofovir alafenamide (TAF) (a nucleotide reverse transcriptase inhibitor): 200 mg/25 mg.

**Atripla:** emtricitabine/efavirenz (an antiretroviral)/tenofovir disoproxil fumarate (TDF) (an antiretroviral): 200 mg/600 mg/300 mg. **Complera:** emtricitabine/rilpivirine (an antiretroviral)/tenofovir disoproxil fumarate (TDF) (an antiretroviral): 200 mg/25 mg/300 mg. **Genvoya:** emtricitabine/elvitegravir (an integrase inhibitor)/cobicistat (a pharmacokinetic enhancer)/tenofovir alafenamide (TAF) (a nucleotide reverse transcriptase inhibitor): 200 mg/150 mg/150 mg/10 mg. **Truvada:** emtricitabine/tenofovir disoproxil fumarate (TDF) (an antiretroviral): 200 mg/300 mg. **Stribild:** emtricitabine/elvitegravir (an integrase inhibitor)/cobicistat (a pharmacokinetic enhancer)/tenofovir disoproxil fumarate (TDF) (a nucleotide reverse transcriptase inhibitor): 200 mg/150 mg/150 mg/300 mg.
**Odefsey:** emtricitabine/rilpivirine (non-nucleoside reverse transcriptase inhibitor [NNRTI])/tenofovir alafenamide (TAF) (a nucleotide reverse transcriptase inhibitor): 200 mg/25 mg/25 mg.

### ◆CLASSIFICATION

**PHARMACOTHERAPEUTIC:** Nucleoside reverse transcriptase inhibitor. **CLINICAL:** Antiretroviral agent.

## USES

Used in combination with at least two other antiretroviral agents for treatment of HIV-1 infection.

## PRECAUTIONS

**Contraindications:** Hypersensitivity to emtricitabine. **Cautions:** Renal impairment, history of hepatitis, diabetes.

## ACTION

Inhibits HIV-1 reverse transcriptase by incorporating itself into viral DNA, resulting in chain termination. **Therapeutic Effect:** Impairs HIV replication, slowing progression of HIV infection.

## PHARMACOKINETICS

Rapidly, extensively absorbed from GI tract. Protein binding: less than 4%. Excreted primarily in urine. **Half-life:** 10 hrs.

## ⌛ LIFESPAN CONSIDERATIONS

**Pregnancy/Lactation:** Breastfeeding not recommended. **Children:** Safety and efficacy not established. **Elderly:** Age-related renal impairment may require dosage adjustment.

## INTERACTIONS

**DRUG:** None significant. **HERBAL:** None significant. **FOOD:** None known. **LAB VALUES:** May increase serum amylase, lipase, ALT, AST, triglycerides. May alter serum glucose.

## AVAILABILITY (Rx)

**Capsules:** 200 mg. **Oral Solution:** 10 mg/ml.

## ADMINISTRATION/HANDLING

**PO**
• Give without regard to food.

## INDICATIONS/ROUTES/DOSAGE

**HIV**
*Capsules*
**PO: ADULTS, ELDERLY, CHILDREN 3 MOS–17 YRS, WEIGHING MORE THAN 33 KG:** 200 mg once daily.
*Oral Solution*
**PO: ADULTS, ELDERLY:** 240 mg once daily. **CHILDREN 3 MOS–17 YRS WEIGHING MORE THAN 33 KG:** 6 mg/kg once daily. **Maximum:** 240 mg once daily. **CHILDREN 0–3 MOS:** 3 mg/kg/day.

**Dosage in Renal Impairment**

| Creatinine Clearance | Capsule | Oral Solution |
|---|---|---|
| 30–49 ml/min | 200 mg q48h | 120 mg q24h |
| 15–29 ml/min | 200 mg q72h | 80 mg q24h |
| Less than 15 ml/min; hemodialysis pts | 200 mg q96h | 60 mg q24h (administer after dialysis) |

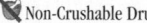

Administer after dialysis on dialysis days.

**Dosage in Hepatic Impairment**
No dose adjustment.

## SIDE EFFECTS

**Frequent (23%–13%):** Headache, rhinitis, rash, diarrhea, nausea. **Occasional (14%–4%):** Cough, vomiting, abdominal pain, insomnia, depression, paresthesia, dizziness, peripheral neuropathy, dyspepsia, myalgia. **Rare (3%–2%):** Arthralgia, abnormal dreams.

## ADVERSE EFFECTS/ TOXIC REACTIONS

Lactic acidosis, hepatomegaly with steatosis (excess fat in liver) occur rarely; may be severe.

## NURSING CONSIDERATIONS

### BASELINE ASSESSMENT
Obtain LFT, serum triglycerides before beginning and at periodic intervals during therapy. Offer emotional support.

### INTERVENTION/EVALUATION
Monitor daily pattern of bowel activity, stool consistency. Question for evidence of nausea, pruritus. Assess skin for rash, urticaria. Monitor serum chemistry tests, LFT for marked abnormalities; signs/ symptoms of lactic acidosis.

### PATIENT/FAMILY TEACHING
• May cause redistribution of body fat. • Continue therapy for full length of treatment. • Emtricitabine is not a cure for HIV infection, nor does it reduce risk of transmission to others. • Pts may continue to acquire illnesses associated with advanced HIV infection. • Avoid tasks that require alertness, motor skills until response to drug is established. • Report persistent or severe abdominal pain, nausea, vomiting, numbness.

# enalapril

en-**al**-a-pril
(Apo-Enalapril ✹, Epaned, Novo-Enalapril ✹, Vasotec)

■ **BLACK BOX ALERT** ■ May cause fetal injury. Discontinue as soon as possible once pregnancy is detected.

**Do not confuse enalapril with Anafranil, Elavil, Eldepryl, or ramipril.**

## FIXED-COMBINATION(S)

**Lexxel:** enalapril/felodipine (calcium channel blocker): 5 mg/2.5 mg, 5 mg/5 mg. **Teczem:** enalapril/diltiazem (calcium channel blocker): 5 mg/180 mg. **Vaseretic:** enalapril/hydrochlorothiazide (diuretic): 5 mg/12.5 mg, 10 mg/25 mg.

## ◆CLASSIFICATION

**PHARMACOTHERAPEUTIC:** Angiotensin-converting enzyme (ACE) inhibitor. **CLINICAL:** Antihypertensive, vasodilator.

## USES

Treatment of hypertension alone or in combination with other antihypertensives. Adjunctive therapy for symptomatic HF. Treatment of asymptomatic left ventricular dysfunction. **(Epaned):** Treatment of hypertension in adults and children older than 1 mo. **OFF-LABEL:** Proteinuria in steroid-resistant nephrotic syndrome.

## PRECAUTIONS

**Contraindications:** Hypersensitivity to enalapril. History of angioedema from previous treatment with ACE inhibitors. Idiopathic/hereditary angioedema. Concomitant use of aliskiren in pts with diabetes. **Cautions:** Renal impairment, hypertrophic cardiomyopathy with outflow tract obstruction; severe aortic stenosis; before, during, or immediately after major surgery. Concomitant use of potassium supplement; unstented unilateral or bilateral renal artery stenosis.

## ACTION

Suppresses renin-angiotensin-aldosterone system (prevents conversion of angiotensin I to angiotensin II, a potent vasoconstrictor; may inhibit angiotensin II at local vascular, renal sites). Decreases plasma angiotensin II, increases plasma renin activity, decreases aldosterone secretion. **Therapeutic Effect:** In hypertension, reduces peripheral arterial resistance. In HF, increases cardiac output; decreases peripheral vascular resistance, B/P, pulmonary capillary wedge pressure, heart size.

## PHARMACOKINETICS

| Route | Onset | Peak | Duration |
|-------|-------|------|----------|
| PO | 1 hr | 4–6 hrs | 24 hrs |
| IV | 15 min | 1–4 hrs | 6 hrs |

Readily absorbed from GI tract. Protein binding: 50%–60%. Primarily excreted in urine. Removed by hemodialysis. **Half-life:** 11 hrs (increased in renal impairment).

## ⌛ LIFESPAN CONSIDERATIONS

**Pregnancy/Lactation:** Crosses placenta. Distributed in breast milk. May cause fetal/neonatal mortality, morbidity. **Children:** Safety and efficacy not established. **Elderly:** May be more susceptible to hypotensive effects.

## INTERACTIONS

**DRUG:** Alcohol, **antihypertensive agents (e.g., amlodipine, clonidine, valsartan), diuretics (e.g., furosemide, torsemide)** may increase effects. **NSAIDs** may decrease antihypertensive effect, increase risk of possible acute renal failure. **Potassium-sparing diuretics (e.g., spironolactone, triamterene), potassium supplements** may cause hyperkalemia. May increase **lithium** concentration, toxicity. **HERBAL:** **Ephedra, ginseng, yohimbe** may worsen hypertension. **Garlic** may increase

antihypertensive effect. **Licorice** may cause sodium/water retention, loss of potassium. **FOOD:** None known. **LAB VALUES:** May increase serum BUN, alkaline phosphatase, bilirubin, creatinine, potassium, ALT, AST. May decrease serum sodium. May cause positive ANA titer.

## AVAILABILITY (Rx)

**Injection Solution:** 1.25 mg/ml. **Powder for Oral Solution *(Epaned):*** 1 mg/ml (after reconstitution). **Tablets:** 2.5 mg, 5 mg, 10 mg, 20 mg.

## ADMINISTRATION/HANDLING

 **IV**

**Reconstitution •** May give undiluted or dilute with D₅W or 0.9% NaCl.
**Rate of Administration •** For IV push, give undiluted over 5 min. • For IV piggyback, infuse over 10–15 min.
**Storage •** Store parenteral form at room temperature. • Use only clear, colorless solution. • Diluted IV solution is stable for 24 hrs at room temperature.

**PO**
• Give without regard to food. • Tablets may be crushed.

**Epaned**
• Reconstitute with 150 ml Ora-Sweet SF (provided) to produce a 1 mg/ml concentration. Stable for 60 days after reconstitution.

## ▥ IV INCOMPATIBILITIES

Amphotericin B (Fungizone), amphotericin B complex (Abelcet, AmBisome, Amphotec), cefepime (Maxipime), phenytoin (Dilantin).

## ▥ IV COMPATIBILITIES

Calcium gluconate, dexmedetomidine (Precedex), dobutamine (Dobutrex), dopamine (Intropin), fentanyl (Sublimaze), heparin, lidocaine, magnesium sulfate, morphine, nitroglycerin, potassium chloride, potassium phosphate, propofol (Diprivan).

## INDICATIONS/ROUTES/DOSAGE

### Hypertension

**PO: ADULTS, ELDERLY:** Initially, 2.5–5 mg/day (2.5 mg if pt taking a diuretic). May increase at 1–2 wk intervals. Range: 10–40 mg/day in 1–2 divided doses. **CHILDREN 1 MO–16 YRS:** Initially, 0.08 mg/kg/day in 1–2 divided doses. **Maximum:** 5 mg/day. **NEONATES:** 0.04–0.1 mg/kg/day given q24h. **Epaned: ADULTS, ELDERLY:** Initially, 5 mg once daily. **CHILDREN:** Initially, 0.08 mg/kg once daily. **Maximum:** 5 mg.

**IV: ADULTS, ELDERLY:** 0.625–1.25 mg q6h up to 5 mg q6h.

### Adjunctive Therapy for HF

**PO: ADULTS, ELDERLY:** Initially, 2.5 mg twice daily. Titrate slowly at 1–2 wk intervals. Range: 5–40 mg/day in 2 divided doses. Target: 10–20 mg twice daily.

### Asymptomatic Left Ventricular Dysfunction

**PO: ADULTS, ELDERLY:** 2.5 mg twice daily. Titrate up to 20 mg/day.

### Dosage in Renal Impairment

**CrCl greater than 30 ml/min:** No dosage adjustment. **CrCl 30 ml/min or less: (HTN):** Initially, 2.5 mg/day. Titrate until B/P controlled. **(HF):** Initially, 2.5 mg twice daily. May increase by 2.5 mg/dose at greater than 4-day intervals. **Maximum:** 40 mg/day.
**Hemodialysis:** Initially, 2.5 mg on dialysis days, adjust dose on non-dialysis days depending on B/P.

### Dosage in Hepatic Impairment

No dose adjustment.

## SIDE EFFECTS

**Frequent (7%–5%):** Headache, dizziness. **Occasional (3%–2%):** Orthostatic hypotension, fatigue, diarrhea, cough, syncope. **Rare (less than 2%):** Angina, abdominal pain, vomiting, nausea, rash, asthenia.

## ADVERSE EFFECTS/ TOXIC REACTIONS

Excessive hypotension ("first-dose syncope") may occur in pts with HF, severe salt or volume depletion. Angioedema (facial, lip swelling), hyperkalemia occur rarely. Agranulocytosis, neutropenia may be noted in pts with renal impairment, collagen vascular diseases (scleroderma, systemic lupus erythematosus). Nephrotic syndrome may be noted in those with history of renal disease.

## NURSING CONSIDERATIONS

### BASELINE ASSESSMENT

Obtain B/P immediately before each dose (be alert to fluctuations). In pts with renal impairment, autoimmune disease, or taking drugs that affect leukocytes/immune response, CBC should be performed before beginning therapy, q2wks for 3 mos, then periodically thereafter.

### INTERVENTION/EVALUATION

Assist with ambulation if dizziness occurs. Monitor CBC, serum BUN, potassium, creatinine, B/P. Monitor daily pattern of bowel activity, stool consistency.

### PATIENT/FAMILY TEACHING

• To reduce hypotensive effect, go from lying to standing slowly. • Several wks may be needed for full therapeutic effect of B/P reduction. • Skipping doses or voluntarily discontinuing drug may produce severe, rebound hypertension. • Limit alcohol intake. • Report vomiting, diarrhea, diaphoresis, persistent cough, difficulty in breathing; swelling of face, lips, tongue.

---

## *enoxaparin*    TOP 100   HIGH ALERT

en-**ox**-a-par-in
(Lovenox)

■ **BLACK BOX ALERT** ■ Epidural or spinal anesthesia greatly increases potential for spinal or epidural hematoma, subsequent long-term or permanent paralysis.

---

Do not confuse Lovenox with Lasix, Levaquin, Lotronex, or Protonix.

### ◆CLASSIFICATION

**PHARMACOTHERAPEUTIC:** Low molecular weight heparin. **CLINICAL:** Anticoagulant.

## USES

DVT prophylaxis following hip or knee replacement surgery, abdominal surgery, or pts with severely restricted mobility during acute illness. Treatment of acute coronary syndrome (ACS): unstable angina, non–Q-wave MI, acute ST-segment elevation MI (STEMI). Treatment of DVT with or without pulmonary embolism (PE) (inpatient); without PE (outpatient). **OFF-LABEL:** DVT prophylaxis following moderate-risk general surgery, gynecologic surgery; management of venous thromboembolism (VTE) during pregnancy. Bariatric surgery, mechanical heart valve to bridge anticoagulation, percutaneous coronary intervention (PCI) adjunctive therapy.

## PRECAUTIONS

**Contraindications:** Hypersensitivity to enoxaparin. Active major bleeding, concurrent heparin therapy, hypersensitivity to heparin, pork products, thrombocytopenia associated with positive in vitro test for antiplatelet antibodies. Not for IM use. **Cautions:** Conditions with increased risk of hemorrhage, platelet defects, renal impairment (renal failure), elderly, uncontrolled arterial hypertension, history of recent GI ulceration or hemorrhage. When neuraxial anesthesia (epidural or spinal anesthesia) or spinal puncture is used, pts anticoagulated or scheduled to be anticoagulated with enoxaparin for prevention of thromboembolic complications are at risk for developing an epidural or spinal hematoma that can result in long-term or permanent paralysis. Bacterial endocarditis, hemorrhagic stroke, history HIT, severe hepatic disease.

## ACTION

Potentiates action of antithrombin III, inactivates coagulation factor Xa. **Therapeutic Effect:** Produces anticoagulation. Does not significantly influence PT, aPTT.

## PHARMACOKINETICS

| Route | Onset | Peak | Duration |
|---|---|---|---|
| Subcutaneous | N/A | 3–5 hrs | 12 hrs |

Well absorbed after subcutaneous administration. Eliminated primarily in urine. Not removed by hemodialysis. **Half-life:** 4.5–7 hrs.

## ⧖ LIFESPAN CONSIDERATIONS

**Pregnancy/Lactation:** Use with caution, particularly during third trimester, immediate postpartum period (increased risk of maternal hemorrhage). Unknown if distributed in breast milk. **Children:** Safety and efficacy not established. **Elderly:** May be more susceptible to bleeding.

## INTERACTIONS

**DRUG: Antiplatelet agents, aspirin, NSAIDs, thrombolytics** may increase risk of bleeding. **HERBAL: Cat's claw, dong quai, evening primrose, feverfew, garlic, ginger, ginkgo, ginseng** may increase antiplatelet action. **FOOD:** None known. **LAB VALUES:** Increases serum alkaline phosphatase, ALT, AST. May decrease Hgb, Hct, RBCs.

## AVAILABILITY (Rx)

**Injection Solution:** 30 mg/0.3 ml, 40 mg/0.4 ml, 60 mg/0.6 ml, 80 mg/0.8 ml, 100 mg/ml, 120 mg/0.8 ml, 150 mg/ml in prefilled syringes.

## ADMINISTRATION/HANDLING

◀**ALERT**▶ Do not mix with other injections, infusions. Do not give IM.

**Subcutaneous**
• Parenteral form appears clear, colorless to pale yellow. • Store at room

E

temperature. • Instruct pt to lie down before administering by deep subcutaneous injection. • Inject between left and right anterolateral and left and right posterolateral abdominal wall. • Introduce entire length of needle (½ inch) into skin fold held between thumb and forefinger, holding skin fold during injection.

## INDICATIONS/ROUTES/ DOSAGE

### Prevention of Deep Vein Thrombosis (DVT) After Hip and Knee Surgery

**SQ: ADULTS, ELDERLY:** 30 mg twice daily, generally for 7–10 days, with initial dose given within 12–24 hrs following surgery. Once-daily dosing following hip surgery: 40 mg with initial dose within 9–15 hrs before surgery.

### Prevention of DVT After Abdominal Surgery

**SQ: ADULTS, ELDERLY:** 40 mg/day for 7–10 days, with initial dose given 2 hrs prior to surgery.

### Prevention of DVT After Bariatric Surgery

**BMI 50 or less (kg/m²):** 40 mg q12h. **BMI greater than 50 kg/m²:** 60 mg q12h.

### Prevention of Long-Term DVT in Nonsurgical Acute Illness

**SQ: ADULTS, ELDERLY:** 40 mg once daily; continue until risk of DVT has diminished (usually 6–11 days).

### Prevention of Ischemic Complications of Unstable Angina, Non–Q-Wave MI (with Oral Aspirin Therapy)

**SQ: ADULTS, ELDERLY:** 1 mg/kg q12h (with oral aspirin).

### STEMI

**SQ: ADULTS YOUNGER THAN 75 YRS:** 30 mg IV once plus 1 mg/kg q12h (**maximum:** 100 mg first 2 doses only). **ADULTS 75 YRS OR OLDER:** 0.75 mg/kg (**maximum:** 75 mg first 2 doses only) q12h.

### Acute DVT

**SQ: ADULTS, ELDERLY: (Inpatient):** 1 mg/kg q12h or 1.5 mg/kg once daily. **(Outpatient):** 1 mg/kg q12h.

### Usual Pediatric Dosage

**SQ: CHILDREN 2 MOS AND OLDER:** 0.5 mg/kg q12h (prophylaxis); 1 mg/kg q12h (treatment). **NEONATES, INFANTS YOUNGER THAN 2 MOS:** 0.75/mg/kg/dose q12h (prophylaxis); 1.5 mg/kg/dose q12h (treatment).

### Dosage in Renal Impairment

Clearance is decreased when CrCl is less than 30 ml/min. Monitor and adjust dosage as necessary.

| Use | Dosage |
|---|---|
| Abdominal surgery, pts with acute illness | 30 mg once/day |
| Hip, knee surgery | 30 mg once/day |
| DVT, angina, MI | 1 mg/kg once/day |
| STEMI: (<75 yrs) | 30 mg IV once plus 1 mg/kg q24h |
| STEMI (75 yrs or greater) | 1 mg/kg q24h |
| NSTEMI | 1 mg/kg q24h |

### Dosage in Hepatic Impairment

Use caution.

## SIDE EFFECTS

**Occasional (4%–1%):** Injection site hematoma, nausea, peripheral edema.

## ADVERSE EFFECTS/ TOXIC REACTIONS

May lead to bleeding complications ranging from local ecchymoses to major hemorrhage. May cause heparin-induced thrombocytopenia (HIT). **Antidote:** IV injection of protamine sulfate (1% solution) equal to dose of enoxaparin injected. One mg protamine sulfate neutralizes 1 mg enoxaparin. One additional dose of 0.5 mg protamine sulfate per 1 mg enoxaparin may be given if aPTT tested 2–4 hrs after first injection remains prolonged.

## NURSING CONSIDERATIONS

### BASELINE ASSESSMENT

Obtain baseline CBC. Note platelet count. Assess potential risk of bleeding.

### INTERVENTION/EVALUATION

Periodically monitor CBC, platelet count, stool for occult blood (no need for daily monitoring in pts with normal presurgical coagulation parameters). Assess for any sign of bleeding (bleeding at surgical site, hematuria, blood in stool, bleeding from gums, petechiae, bruising, bleeding from injection sites).

### PATIENT/FAMILY TEACHING

• Usual length of therapy is 7–10 days.
• Do not take any OTC medication (esp. aspirin) without consulting physician.
• Report unusual bleeding or bruising.

# entecavir

en-**tek**-a-veer
(Baraclude, Apo-Entecavir ✦)
■ **BLACK BOX ALERT** ■ Serious, sometimes fatal, hypersensitivity reaction, lactic acidosis, severe hepatomegaly with steatosis (fatty liver) have occurred. May cause HIV resistance in chronic hepatitis B pts. Severe acute exacerbations of hepatitis B virus infection may occur upon discontinuation of entecavir.

## ◆CLASSIFICATION

**PHARMACOTHERAPEUTIC:** Reverse transcriptase inhibitor. **CLINICAL:** Antiretroviral agent.

## USES

Treatment of chronic hepatitis B virus (HBV) infection with evidence of active viral replication and evidence of either persistent transaminase elevations or histologically active disease or evidence of decompensated hepatic disease. **OFF-LABEL:** HBV reinfection prophylaxis, post–liver transplant, HIV/HBV coinfection.

## PRECAUTIONS

**Contraindications:** Hypersensitivity to entecavir. **Cautions:** Renal impairment, pts receiving concurrent therapy that may reduce renal function. Pts at risk for hepatic disease.

## ACTION

Inhibits hepatitis B viral polymerase, an enzyme blocking reverse transcriptase activity. **Therapeutic Effect:** Interferes with viral DNA synthesis.

## PHARMACOKINETICS

Poorly absorbed from GI tract. Protein binding: 13%. Extensively distributed into tissues. Partially metabolized in liver. Eliminated primarily in urine. **Half-life:** 5–6 days (increased in renal impairment).

## ⧗ LIFESPAN CONSIDERATIONS

**Pregnancy/Lactation:** Unknown if drug crosses placenta or is distributed in breast milk. **Children:** Safety and efficacy not established in pts younger than 16 yrs. **Elderly:** Age-related renal impairment may require dosage adjustment.

## INTERACTIONS

**DRUG: Ganciclovir, ribavirin, valganciclovir** may increase concentration. **HERBAL:** None significant. **FOOD: Food** delays absorption, decreases concentration. **LAB VALUES:** May increase serum amylase, lipase, bilirubin, ALT, AST, creatinine, glucose. May decrease serum albumin; platelets.

## AVAILABILITY (Rx)

**Oral Solution:** 0.05 mg/ml. **Tablets:** 0.5 mg, 1 mg.

## ADMINISTRATION/HANDLING

### PO

• Administer tablets on an empty stomach (at least 2 hrs after a meal and 2 hrs

 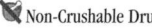

before the next meal). • Do not dilute, mix oral solution with water or any other liquid. • Each bottle of oral solution is accompanied by a dosing spoon. Before administering, hold spoon in vertical position, fill it gradually to mark corresponding to prescribed dose.

**Storage** • Store tablets, oral solution at room temperature.

## INDICATIONS/ROUTES/DOSAGE

**Chronic Hepatitis B (No Previous Nucleoside Treatment)**
**PO: ADULTS, ELDERLY, CHILDREN 16 YRS AND OLDER:** 0.5 mg once daily. **CHILDREN 2 YRS AND OLDER: (Weighing more than 30 kg):** 0.5 mg once daily (tablet or solution). **(27–30 kg):** 0.45 mg once daily (solution). **(24–26 kg):** 0.4 mg once daily (solution). **(21-23 kg):** 0.35 mg once daily (solution). **(18–20 kg):** 0.3 mg once daily (solution). **(15–17 kg):** 0.25 mg once daily (solution). **(12–14 kg):** 0.2 mg once daily (solution). **(10–11 kg):** 0.15 mg once daily (solution).

**Chronic Hepatitis B (Receiving Lamivudine, Known Lamivudine Resistance, Decompensated Liver Disease)**
**PO: ADULTS, ELDERLY, CHILDREN 16 YRS AND OLDER:** 1 mg once daily. **CHILDREN 2 YRS AND OLDER: (Weighing more than 30 kg):** 1 mg once daily (tablet or solution). **(27–30 kg):** 0.9 mg once daily (solution). **(24–26 kg):** 0.8 mg once daily (solution). **(21–23 kg):** 0.7 mg once daily (solution). **(18–20 kg):** 0.6 mg once daily (solution). **(15–17 kg):** 0.5 mg once daily (solution). **(12–14 kg):** 0.4 mg once daily (solution). **(10–11 kg):** 0.3 mg once daily (solution).

**Dosage in Renal Impairment**

| Creatinine Clearance | Dosage |
| --- | --- |
| 50 ml/min and greater | 0.5 mg once daily |
| 30–49 ml/min | 0.25 mg once daily |
| 10–29 ml/min | 0.15 mg once daily |
| 9 ml/min and less | 0.05 mg once daily |

**Dosage in Hepatic Impairment**
No dose adjustment.

## SIDE EFFECTS

**Occasional (4%–3%):** Headache, fatigue. **Rare (less than 1%):** Diarrhea, dyspepsia, nausea, vomiting, dizziness, insomnia.

## ADVERSE EFFECTS/ TOXIC REACTIONS

Lactic acidosis, severe hepatomegaly with steatosis have been reported. Severe, acute exacerbations of hepatitis B have been reported in pts who have discontinued therapy; reinitiation of antihepatitis B therapy may be required. Hematuria occurs occasionally. May cause development of HIV resistance if HIV untreated.

## NURSING CONSIDERATIONS

### BASELINE ASSESSMENT

Obtain baseline laboratory tests, esp. LFT before beginning therapy and at periodic intervals during therapy. Offer emotional support. Obtain full medication history.

### INTERVENTION/EVALUATION

Hepatic function should be monitored closely with both clinical and laboratory follow-up for at least several mos in pts who discontinue antihepatitis B therapy. For pts on therapy, closely monitor serum amylase, lipase, bilirubin, ALT, AST, creatinine, glucose, albumin; platelet count. Assess for evidence of GI discomfort.

### PATIENT/FAMILY TEACHING

• Take medication at least 2 hrs after a meal and 2 hrs before the next meal. • Avoid transmission of hepatitis B infection to others through sexual contact, blood contamination. • Immediately report unusual muscle pain, abdominal pain with nausea/vomiting, cold feeling in extremities, dizziness (signs and symptoms signaling onset of lactic acidosis).

# enzalutamide

en-za-**loo**-ta-mide
(XTANDI)
**Do not confuse enzalutamide
with bicalutamide, flutamide, or
nilutamide.**

## ◆CLASSIFICATION

**PHARMACOTHERAPEUTIC:** Antiandrogen renal inhibitor. **CLINICAL:** Antineoplastic.

## USES

Treatment of metastatic castration-resistant prostate cancer.

## PRECAUTIONS

**Contraindications:** Hypersensitivity to enzalutamide. Women who are pregnant or may become pregnant (not indicated in female population). **Cautions:** History of seizure, underlying brain injury with loss of consciousness, transient ischemic attack within past 12 mos, CVA, brain metastases, brain arteriovenous abnormality, use of concurrent medications that may lower seizure threshold.

## ACTION

Inhibits androgen binding to androgen receptors in target tissue, and inhibits interaction with DNA. **Therapeutic Effect:** Decreases proliferation, induces cell death of prostate cancer cells.

## PHARMACOKINETICS

Readily absorbed in GI tract. Maximum plasma concentration achieved in 0.5–3 hrs. Metabolized in liver. Protein binding: (97%–98%). Primarily excreted in urine. **Half-life:** 5.8 days (Range: 2.8–10.2 days).

## ⏳ LIFESPAN CONSIDERATIONS

**Pregnancy/Lactation:** Not used in female population. **Children:** Safety and efficacy not established. **Elderly:** No age-related precautions noted.

## INTERACTIONS

**DRUG: Strong CYP2C8, CYP3A4 inhibitors (e.g., gemfibrozil, itraconazole)** may increase concentration. **Moderate or strong CYP3A4 inducers** may decrease concentration. **HERBAL:** None significant. **FOOD: All foods** may increase absorption. **LAB VALUES:** May increase serum ALT, AST, bilirubin. May decrease Hgb, Hct, platelets, WBC count.

## AVAILABILITY (Rx)

🖫 **Capsules:** 40 mg.

## ADMINISTRATION/HANDLING

**PO •** May give with or without food. Take at same time each day. Swallow whole. • Do not break, crush, dissolve, or open capsules.

## INDICATIONS/ROUTES/DOSAGE

**Metastatic Castration-Resistant Prostate Cancer**
**PO: ADULTS, ELDERLY:** 160 mg (4 × 40 mg capsules) given once daily.

**Dose Modification**
If a Grade 3 or greater toxicity or an intolerable side effect occurs, withhold dosing for 1 week or until symptoms improve to Grade 2 or less, then resume at same dose or a reduced dose (120 mg or 80 mg). **Concurrent use of strong CYP2C8 inhibitors:** Avoid use (if possible). If concurrent use is necessary, reduce the enzalutamide dose to 80 mg once daily. **Concurrent use of strong CYP3A4 inducers:** Increase dose to 240 mg once daily.

**Dosage in Renal/Hepatic Impairment**
No dose adjustment.

## SIDE EFFECTS

**Common (51%):** Asthenia. **Frequent (26%–15%):** Back pain, diarrhea, arthralgia, hot flashes, peripheral edema, musculoskeletal pain. **Occasional (12%–6%):** Headache, dizziness, insomnia, hematuria, paresthesia, anxiety, hypertension. **Rare (4%–2%):**

E

---

✦ Canadian trade name    🖫 Non-Crushable Drug    🚨 High Alert drug

Mental impairment disorders (includes amnesia, memory impairment, cognitive disorder, attention deficit), hematuria (includes pollakiuria, pruritus, dry skin).

## ADVERSE EFFECTS/ TOXIC REACTIONS

Upper respiratory tract infection occurs in 11% of pts; lower respiratory tract and lung infection (includes pneumonia, bronchitis) occur in slightly less (9% of pts). Spinal cord compression and cauda equina syndrome occurs in 7% of pts.

## NURSING CONSIDERATIONS

### BASELINE ASSESSMENT

Offer emotional support. Obtain baseline CBC, ALT, AST, bilirubin periodically throughout therapy. Assess bowel activity, stool consistency. If coadministered with warfarin (CYP2C9 substrate), perform additional INR monitoring.

### INTERVENTION/EVALUATION

Assess for peripheral edema. Question level of fatigue, weakness. Question presence of back pain, arthralgia, or headache. Assess level of anxiety. Monitor B/P for hypertension. Assess for hematuria. Question pt regarding sleeping pattern.

### PATIENT/FAMILY TEACHING

• Sexually active men must wear condom during treatment and for 1 wk after treatment due to potential risks to fetus. • Women who are pregnant or are planning pregnancy may not touch medication without gloves. • Dizziness, headache, muscle weakness, leg swelling/discomfort should be reported. • Immediately report fever or cough. • Routine lab testing will occur during treatment.

---

## *EPINEPHrine     `HIGH ALERT`

ep-i-**nef**-rin
(Adrenalin, EpiPen, EpiPen Jr., Twinject)

**Do not confuse epinephrine with ephedrine.**

### FIXED-COMBINATION(S)

**LidoSite:** epinephrine/lidocaine (anesthetic): 0.1%/10%.

## ◆CLASSIFICATION

**PHARMACOTHERAPEUTIC:** Sympathomimetic (adrenergic agonist). **CLINICAL:** Antiglaucoma, bronchodilator, cardiac stimulant, antiallergic, antihemorrhagic, priapism reversal agent.

## USES

Treatment of allergic reactions (including anaphylactic reactions). Treatment of hypotension associated with septic shock. Added to local anesthetics to decrease systemic absorption and increase duration of activity of local anesthetic. Decreases superficial hemorrhage. **OFF-LABEL:** Ventricular fibrillation or pulseless ventricular tachycardia unresponsive to initial defibrillatory shocks; pulseless electrical activity, asystole, hypotension unresponsive to volume resuscitation; bradycardia/hypotension unresponsive to atropine or pacing; inotropic support.

## PRECAUTIONS

**Contraindications:** Hypersensitivity to epinephrine. **Note:** There are no absolute contraindications with injectable epinephrine in a life-threatening situation. **IV:** Narrow-angle glaucoma, thyrotoxicosis, diabetes, hypertension, other cardiovascular disorders. **Inhalation:** Concurrent use or within 2 wks of MAOIs. **Cautions:** Elderly, diabetes mellitus, hypertension, Parkinson's disease, thyroid disease, cerebrovascular or cardiovascular disease, concurrent use of tricyclic antidepressants. History of prostate enlargement, urinary retention.

## ACTION

Stimulates alpha-adrenergic receptors (vasoconstriction, pressor effects),

---

beta₁-adrenergic receptors (cardiac stimulation), beta₂-adrenergic receptors (bronchial dilation, vasodilation). **Therapeutic Effect:** Relaxes smooth muscle of bronchial tree, produces cardiac stimulation, dilates skeletal muscle vasculature.

## PHARMACOKINETICS

| Route | Onset | Peak | Duration |
|---|---|---|---|
| IM | 5–10 min | 20 min | 1–4 hrs |
| Subcutaneous | 5–10 min | 20 min | 1–4 hrs |
| Inhalation | 3–5 min | 20 min | 1–3 hrs |

Well absorbed after parenteral administration; minimally absorbed after inhalation. Metabolized in liver, other tissues, sympathetic nerve endings. Excreted in urine. Ophthalmic form may be systemically absorbed as a result of drainage into nasal pharyngeal passages. Mydriasis occurs within several min and persists several hrs; vasoconstriction occurs within 5 min and lasts less than 1 hr.

## ⚥ LIFESPAN CONSIDERATIONS

**Pregnancy/Lactation:** Crosses placenta. Distributed in breast milk. **Children/Elderly:** No age-related precautions noted.

## INTERACTIONS

**DRUG:** May decrease effects of **beta blockers** (e.g., **carvedilol, metoprolol**). **Digoxin, sympathomimetics** may increase risk of arrhythmias. **Ergonovine, methergine, oxytocin** may increase vasoconstriction. **MAOIs, tricyclic antidepressants** may increase cardiovascular effects. **HERBAL: Ephedra, yohimbe** may increase CNS stimulation. **FOOD:** None known. **LAB VALUES:** May decrease serum potassium.

## AVAILABILITY (Rx)

**Injection, Solution (Prefilled Syringes): (EpiPen):** 0.3 mg/0.3 ml, **(EpiPen Jr.):** 0.15 mg/0.3 ml, **(Twinject):** 0.15 mg/0.15 ml. **Injection, Solution:** 0.1 mg/ml (1:10,000), 1 mg/ml (1:1,000).

**Solution for Oral Inhalation (Adrenalin):** 2.25% (0.5 ml).

## ADMINISTRATION/HANDLING

 **IV**

**Reconstitution** • For injection, dilute each 1 mg of 1:1,000 solution with 10 ml 0.9% NaCl to provide 1:10,000 solution and inject each 1 mg or fraction thereof over 1 min or more (except in cardiac arrest). • For infusion, further dilute with 250–500 ml D₅W. Maximum concentration 64 mcg/ml.
**Rate of Administration** • For IV infusion, give at 1–10 mcg/min (titrate to desired response).
**Storage** • Store parenteral forms at room temperature. • Do not use if solution appears discolored or contains a precipitate.

**Subcutaneous**
• Shake ampule thoroughly. • Use tuberculin syringe for injection into lateral deltoid region. • Massage injection site (minimizes vasoconstriction effect). Use only 1:1,000 solution.

**Nebulizer**
• No more than 10 drops Adrenalin Chloride solution 1:100 should be placed in reservoir of nebulizer. • Place nozzle just inside pt's partially opened mouth. • As bulb is squeezed once or twice, instruct pt to inhale deeply, drawing vaporized solution into lungs. • Rinse mouth with water immediately after inhalation (prevents mouth/throat dryness). • When nebulizer is not in use, replace stopper, keep in upright position.

## ▦ IV INCOMPATIBILITIES

Ampicillin, pantoprazole (Protonix), sodium bicarbonate.

## ▦ IV COMPATIBILITIES

Calcium chloride, calcium gluconate, dexmedetomidine (Precedex), diltiazem (Cardizem), dobutamine (Dobutrex), dopamine (Intropin), fentanyl (Sublimaze), heparin, hydromorphone (Dilaudid), lorazepam (Ativan), midazolam (Versed), milrinone (Primacor), morphine, nitroglycerin, norepinephrine (Levophed), potassium chloride, propofol (Diprivan).

## INDICATIONS/ROUTES/ DOSAGE

**Anaphylaxis**
**IM, SQ: ADULTS, ELDERLY:** 0.2–0.5 mg (0.2–0.5 ml of 1:1,000 solution). May repeat q5–15 min if anaphylaxis persists. **CHILDREN:** 0.01 mg/kg (0.01 ml/kg of a 1:1,000 solution) q5–15 min. **Maximum single dose:** 0.3 mg.

**Hypotension (Shock)**
**IV INFUSION: ADULTS, ELDERLY:** 0.05–2 mcg/kg/min. Titrate to desired mean arterial pressure (MAP). May adjust dose by 0.05–0.2 mcg/kg/min.

**Cardiac Arrest**
**IV: ADULTS, ELDERLY:** Initially, 1 mg. May repeat q3–5min as needed. **CHILDREN:** Initially, 0.01 mg/kg (0.1 ml/kg of a 1:10,000 solution). May repeat q3–5min as needed.
**Endotracheal: ADULTS, ELDERLY:** 2–2.5 mg q3–5 min as needed. **CHILDREN:** 0.1 mg/kg (0.1 ml/kg of a 1:1,000 solution). May repeat q3–5min as needed.

**Dosage in Renal/Hepatic Impairment**
No dose adjustment.

## SIDE EFFECTS

**Frequent: Systemic:** Tachycardia, palpitations, anxiety. **Ophthalmic:** Headache, eye irritation, watering of eyes. **Occasional: Systemic:** Dizziness, light-headedness, facial flushing, headache, diaphoresis, increased B/P, nausea, trembling, insomnia, vomiting, fatigue. **Ophthalmic:** Blurred/decreased vision, eye pain. **Rare: Systemic:** Chest discomfort/pain, arrhythmias, bronchospasm, dry mouth/throat.

## ADVERSE EFFECTS/ TOXIC REACTIONS

Excessive doses may cause acute hypertension, arrhythmias. Prolonged/excessive use may result in metabolic acidosis due to increased serum lactic acid. Metabolic acidosis may cause disorientation, fatigue, hyperventilation, headache, nausea, vomiting, diarrhea.

## NURSING CONSIDERATIONS

**INTERVENTION/EVALUATION**

Monitor changes of B/P, HR. Assess lung sounds for rhonchi, wheezing, rales. Monitor ABGs. In cardiac arrest, adhere to ACLS protocols.

**PATIENT/FAMILY TEACHING**

• Avoid excessive use of caffeine. • Report any new symptoms (tachycardia, shortness of breath, dizziness) immediately: may be systemic effects.

# eplerenone

ep-**ler**-e-none
(Inspra)
**Do not confuse Inspra with Spiriva.**

## ◆CLASSIFICATION

**PHARMACOTHERAPEUTIC:** Aldosterone receptor antagonist. **CLINICAL:** Antihypertensive.

## USES

Treatment of hypertension alone or in combination with other antihypertensive agents. Treatment of HF following acute myocardial infarction (AMI).

## PRECAUTIONS

**Contraindications:** Hypersensitivity to eplerenone. Concurrent use with strong CYP3A4 inhibitors (e.g., ketoconazole, itraconazole), CrCl less than 30 ml/min, serum potassium level greater than

5.5 mEq/L. **Hypertension (Additional):** Type 2 diabetes with microalbuminuria; CrCl less than 50 ml/min; serum creatinine greater than 2 mg/dL in men, greater than 1.8 mg/dL in women; concomitant use of potassium supplements or potassium-sparing diuretics. **Cautions:** Hyperkalemia, HF, post-MI, diabetes, mild renal impairment.

## ACTION

Binds to mineralocorticoid receptors in kidney, heart, blood vessels, brain, blocking binding of aldosterone. **Therapeutic Effect:** Reduces B/P.

## PHARMACOKINETICS

Absorption unaffected by food. Protein binding: 50%. Metabolized in liver. Excreted in urine (67%), feces (32%). Not removed by hemodialysis. **Half-life:** 4–6 hrs.

## ⏳ LIFESPAN CONSIDERATIONS

**Pregnancy/Lactation:** Unknown if drug crosses placenta or is distributed in breast milk. **Children:** Safety and efficacy not established. **Elderly:** No age-related precautions noted.

## INTERACTIONS

**DRUG: ACE inhibitors (e.g., enalapril, lisinopril), angiotensin II antagonists (e.g., losartan, valsartan), potassium-sparing diuretics (e.g., spironolactone), potassium supplements** increase risk of hyperkalemia. **CYP3A4 inhibitors (e.g., itraconazole, ketoconazole)** increase concentration five-fold (use is contraindicated). **NSAIDs** may decrease antihypertensive effect. **HERBAL: St. John's wort** decreases effectiveness. **FOOD: Grapefruit products** may increase potential for hyperkalemia, arrhythmias. **LAB VALUES:** May increase serum potassium, ALT, AST, cholesterol, triglycerides, serum creatinine, uric acid. May decrease serum sodium.

## AVAILABILITY (Rx)

🔖 **Tablets:** 25 mg, 50 mg.

## ADMINISTRATION/HANDLING

• Do not break, crush, dissolve, or divide film-coated tablets. • May give without regard to food.

## INDICATIONS/ROUTES/DOSAGE

**Hypertension**
**PO: ADULTS, ELDERLY:** Initially, 50 mg once daily. If 50 mg once daily produces an inadequate B/P response, may increase dosage to 50 mg twice daily. If pt is concurrently receiving CYP3A4 inhibitors (e.g., erythromycin, saquinavir, verapamil, or fluconazole), reduce initial dose to 25 mg once daily.

**HF Following MI**
**PO: ADULTS, ELDERLY:** Initially, 25 mg once daily. If tolerated, titrate up to 50 mg once daily within 4 wks.

**Dosage Adjustment for Serum Potassium Concentrations in HF**
**Less than 5 mEq/L:** Increase dose from 25 mg daily to 50 mg daily or increase dose from 25 mg every other day to 25 mg daily.
**5–5.4 mEq/L:** No adjustment needed.
**5.5–5.9 mEq/L:** Decrease dose from 50 mg daily to 25 mg daily. Decrease dose from 25 mg daily to 25 mg every other day. Decrease dose from 25 mg every other day to withhold medication.
**6 mEq/L or Greater:** Withhold medication until potassium is less than 5.5 mEq/L, then restart at 25 mg every other day.

**Dosage in Renal Impairment**
Use is contraindicated in pts with hypertension with CrCl less than 50 ml/min or serum creatinine greater than 2 mg/dL in males or greater than 1.8 mg/dL in females. All other indications, CrCl less than 30 ml/min, use is contraindicated.

E

---

**Dosage in Hepatic Impairment**
No dose adjustment.

## SIDE EFFECTS

**Rare (3%–1%):** Dizziness, diarrhea, cough, fatigue, flu-like symptoms, abdominal pain.

## ADVERSE EFFECTS/ TOXIC REACTIONS

Hyperkalemia may occur, particularly in pts with type 2 diabetes mellitus and microalbuminuria.

## NURSING CONSIDERATIONS

### BASELINE ASSESSMENT

Obtain B/P, apical pulse immediately before each dose, in addition to regular monitoring (be alert to fluctuations). If excessive reduction in B/P occurs, place pt in supine position, feet slightly elevated.

### INTERVENTION/EVALUATION

Assist with ambulation if dizziness occurs. Monitor serum potassium levels. Assess B/P for hypertension/hypotension. Monitor daily pattern of bowel activity, stool consistency. Assess for evidence of flu-like symptoms.

### PATIENT/FAMILY TEACHING

• Avoid tasks that require alertness, motor skills until response to drug is established (possible dizziness effect). • Hypertension requires lifelong control. • Avoid exercising during hot weather (risk of dehydration, hypotension). • Do not use salt substitutes containing potassium.

## epoetin alfa    TOP 100

e-**poe**-e-tin **al**-fa
(Epogen, Eprex ✦, Procrit)
■ **BLACK BOX ALERT** ■ Increased risk of serious cardiovascular events, thromboembolic events, mortality, time-to-tumor progression in pts with head and neck cancer, metastatic breast cancer, non–small-cell lung cancer when administered to a target hemoglobin of more than 11 g/dL. Increases rate of deep vein thrombosis in perioperative pts not receiving anticoagulant therapy.
**Do not confuse epoetin with darbepoetin, or Epogen with Neupogen.**

## ◆CLASSIFICATION

**PHARMACOTHERAPEUTIC:** Glycoprotein. **CLINICAL:** Erythropoietin.

## USES

Treatment of anemia in pts receiving or who have received myelosuppressive chemotherapy for a planned minimum of 2 mos of chemotherapy pts with chronic renal failure to decrease need for RBC transfusion; HIV-infected pts on zidovudine (AZT) therapy when endogenous erythropoietin levels are 500 mUnits/ml or less; pts scheduled for elective noncardiac, nonvascular surgery, reducing need for allogenic blood transfusions when perioperative Hgb is greater than 10 or less than or equal to 13 g/dl and high risk for blood loss. **OFF-LABEL:** Anemia in myelodysplastic syndromes.

## PRECAUTIONS

**Contraindications:** Hypersensitivity to epoetin. Pure red cell aplasia, uncontrolled hypertension. **Cautions:** History of seizures or controlled hypertension. **Cancer pts:** Tumor growth, shortened survival may occur when Hgb levels of 11 g/dL or greater are achieved with epoetin alfa. **Chronic renal failure pts:** Increased risk for serious cardiovascular reactions (e.g., stroke, MI) when Hgb levels greater than 11 g/dL are achieved with epoetin alfa.

## ACTION

Stimulates division, differentiation of erythroid progenitor cells in bone marrow. **Therapeutic Effect:** Induces erythropoiesis, releases reticulocytes from bone marrow.

## PHARMACOKINETICS

Well absorbed after subcutaneous administration. Following administration, an increase in reticulocyte count occurs within 10 days, and increases in Hgb, Hct, and RBC count are seen within 2–6 wks. **Half-life:** 4–13 hrs.

##  LIFESPAN CONSIDERATIONS

**Pregnancy/Lactation:** Unknown if drug crosses placenta or is distributed in breast milk. **Children:** Safety and efficacy not established in pts 12 yrs and younger. **Elderly:** No age-related precautions noted.

## INTERACTIONS

**DRUG:** None significant. **HERBAL:** None significant. **FOOD:** None known. **LAB VALUES:** May increase serum BUN, phosphorus, potassium, creatinine, uric acid, sodium. May decrease bleeding time, iron concentration, serum ferritin.

## AVAILABILITY (Rx)

**Injection Solution (Epogen, Procrit):** 2,000 units/ml, 3,000 units/ml, 4,000 units/ml, 10,000 units/ml, 20,000 units/ml, 40,000 units/ml.

## ADMINISTRATION/HANDLING

◄ALERT► Avoid excessive agitation of vial; do not shake (foaming).

### IV

**Reconstitution** • No reconstitution necessary.
**Rate of Administration** • May be given as an IV bolus.
**Storage** • Refrigerate. • Vigorous shaking may denature medication, rendering it inactive.

#### Subcutaneous

• Mix in syringe with bacteriostatic 0.9% NaCl with benzyl alcohol 0.9% (bacteriostatic saline) at a 1:1 ratio (benzyl alcohol acts as local anesthetic; may reduce injection site discomfort). • Use 1 dose per vial; do not reenter vial. Discard unused portion.

## IV INCOMPATIBILITIES

Do not mix injection form with other medications.

## INDICATIONS/ROUTES/DOSAGE

### Anemia Associated with Chemotherapy

◄ALERT► Begin therapy only if Hgb less than 10 g/dL and anticipated duration of myelosuppressive chemotherapy is greater than 2 mos. Use minimum effective dose to maintain Hgb level that will avoid red blood cell transfusions. Discontinue upon completion of chemotherapy.

**SQ: ADULTS, ELDERLY:** Initially, 150 units/kg 3 times/wk (commonly used dose of 10,000 units 3 times/wk) or 40,000 units once wkly. **IV: CHILDREN 5 YRS AND OLDER:** 600 units/kg once wkly. **Maximum:** 40,000 units.

*Increase dose:* **ADULTS, ELDERLY:** If Hgb does not increase by greater than 1 g/dL and remains below 10 g/dL after initial 4 wks, may increase to 300 units/kg 3 times/wk or 60,000 units once wkly. **CHILDREN:** If Hgb does not increase by greater than 1 g/dL and remains less than 10 g/dL after initial 4 wks of once-wkly dosing, may increase dose to 900 units/kg/wk. **Maximum:** 60,000 units once wkly.

*Decrease dose:* Decrease dose by 25% if Hgb increases greater than 1 g/dL in any 2-wk period or Hgb levels reaches level that will avoid red blood cell transfusions.

### Reduction of Allogenic Blood Transfusions in Elective Surgery

**SQ: ADULTS, ELDERLY:** 300 units/kg/day for 10 days before and 4 days after surgery.

### Anemia in Chronic Renal Failure

◄ALERT► Individualize dose, using lowest dose to reduce need for RBC transfusions. **ON DIALYSIS:** Initiate when Hgb less than 10 g/dL; reduce dose or discontinue if Hgb approaches or exceeds 11 g/dL. **NOT ON DIALYSIS:** Initiate

 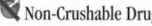

when Hgb less than 10 g/dL; reduce dose or stop if Hgb exceeds 10 g/dL.

**IV, SQ: ADULTS, ELDERLY:** 50–100 units/kg 3 times/wk. **CHILDREN:** 50 units/kg 3 times/wk.

**Maintenance: *Decrease dose by 25%:*** If Hgb increases greater than 1 g/dL in any 2-wk period. ***Increase dose by 25%:*** If Hgb does not increase by greater than 1 g/dL after 4 wks of therapy. Do not increase dose more frequently than every 4 wks.

**Note:** If pt does not attain adequate response after appropriate dosing over 12 wks, do not continue to increase dose and use minimum effective dose to maintain Hgb level that will avoid red blood cell transfusions.

**HIV Infection in Pts Treated with Zidovudine (AZT)**
**IV, SQ: ADULTS:** Initially, 100 units/kg 3 times/wk for 8 wks; may increase by 50–100 units/kg 3 times/wk. Evaluate response q4–8wks thereafter. Adjust dosage by 50–100 units/kg 3 times/wk. If dosages larger than 300 units/kg 3 times/wk are not eliciting response, it is unlikely pt will respond. **Maintenance:** Titrate to maintain desired Hgb level. Hgb levels should not exceed 12 g/dL. If Hgb greater than 12 g/dL, resume treatment with 25% dose reduction when Hgb drops below 11 g/dL. Discontinue if Hgb increase not attained with 300 units/kg for 8 wks.

**Dosage in Renal/Hepatic Impairment**
No dose adjustment.

## SIDE EFFECTS

**Pts Receiving Chemotherapy**
**Frequent (20%–17%):** Fever, diarrhea, nausea, vomiting, edema. **Occasional (13%–11%):** Asthenia, shortness of breath, paresthesia. **Rare (5%–3%):** Dizziness, trunk pain.

**Pts with Chronic Renal Failure**
**Frequent (24%–11%):** Hypertension, headache, nausea, arthralgia. **Occasional (9%–7%):** Fatigue, edema, diarrhea, vomiting, chest pain, skin reactions at administration site, asthenia, dizziness.

**Pts with HIV Infection Treated with AZT**
**Frequent (38%–15%):** Fever, fatigue, headache, cough, diarrhea, rash, nausea. **Occasional (14%–9%):** Shortness of breath, asthenia, skin reaction at injection site, dizziness.

## ADVERSE EFFECTS/ TOXIC REACTIONS

Hypertensive encephalopathy, thrombosis, cerebrovascular accident, MI, seizures occur rarely. Hyperkalemia occurs occasionally in pts with chronic renal failure, usually in those who do not comply with medication regimen, dietary guidelines, frequency of dialysis regimen.

## NURSING CONSIDERATIONS

### BASELINE ASSESSMENT

Assess B/P before drug initiation (80% of pts with chronic renal failure have history of hypertension). B/P often rises during early therapy in pts with history of hypertension. Consider that all pts eventually need supplemental iron therapy. Assess serum iron (should be greater than 20%), serum ferritin (should be greater than 100 ng/ml) before and during therapy. Establish baseline CBC (esp. note Hct).

### INTERVENTION/EVALUATION

Assess CBC routinely (esp. Hgb, Hct). Monitor aggressively for increased B/P (25% of pts require antihypertensive therapy, dietary restrictions). Monitor temperature, esp. in cancer pts on chemotherapy and zidovudine-treated HIV pts. Monitor serum BUN, uric acid, creatinine, phosphorus, potassium, esp. in chronic renal failure pts.

### PATIENT/FAMILY TEACHING

• Frequent laboratory assessments needed to determine correct dosage.

**E**

• Immediately report any severe headache. • Avoid potentially hazardous activity during first 90 days of therapy (increased risk of seizures in pts with chronic renal failure during first 90 days). • Specific dietary regimen must be maintained.

# eprosartan

ep-roe-**sar**-tan
(Teveten)

■ **BLACK BOX ALERT** ■ May cause fetal injury, mortality. Discontinue as soon as possible once pregnancy is detected.

## FIXED COMBINATION(S)

**Teveten HCT:** eprosartan/hydrochlorothiazide (a diuretic): 400 mg/12.5 mg.

## ◆CLASSIFICATION

**PHARMACOTHERAPEUTIC:** Angiotensin II receptor antagonist. **CLINICAL:** Antihypertensive.

## USES

Treatment of hypertension (alone or in combination with other medications).

## PRECAUTIONS

**Contraindications:** Hypersensitivity to eprosartan. Concomitant use with aliskiren in pts with diabetes. **Cautions:** Unstented unilateral/bilateral renal artery stenosis, preexisting renal insufficiency. Concomitant use of potassium-sparing medications (e.g., spironolactone), potassium supplements, pts who are volume depleted.

## ACTION

Potent vasodilator. Blocks vasoconstrictor, aldosterone-secreting effects of angiotensin II, inhibiting binding of angiotensin II to $AT_1$ receptors. **Therapeutic Effect:** Causes vasodilation, decreases peripheral resistance, decreases B/P.

## PHARMACOKINETICS

Rapidly absorbed after PO administration. Protein binding: 98%. Minimally metabolized in liver. Primarily excreted via urine, biliary system. Minimally removed by hemodialysis. **Half-life:** 5–9 hrs.

## ⏳ LIFESPAN CONSIDERATIONS

**Pregnancy/Lactation:** Has caused fetal and neonatal morbidity and mortality. Potential for adverse effects on breastfeeding infant. Breastfeeding not recommended. **Children:** Safety and efficacy not established. **Elderly:** No age-related precautions noted.

## INTERACTIONS

**DRUG: Potassium-sparing diuretics (e.g., spironolactone, triamterene), potassium supplements** may increase risk of hyperkalemia. May produce additive effect with **antihypertensive agents. HERBAL: Ephedra, ginseng, yohimbe** may worsen hypertension. **Garlic** may increase antihypertensive effect. **FOOD:** None known. **LAB VALUES:** May increase serum BUN, alkaline phosphatase, bilirubin, creatinine, ALT, AST. May decrease Hgb, Hct.

## AVAILABILITY (Rx)

🔖 **Tablets:** 400 mg, 600 mg.

## ADMINISTRATION/HANDLING

**PO**
• Give without regard to food. • Do not break, crush, dissolve, or divide tablets.

## INDICATIONS/ROUTES/DOSAGE

**Hypertension**
**PO: ADULTS, ELDERLY:** Initially, 600 mg/day. Range: 400–800 mg/day as single dose or 2 divided doses.

**Dosage in Renal Impairment**
**Mild impairment:** No dose adjustment. **Moderate to severe impairment: Maximum:** 600 mg/day.

---

**Dosage in Hepatic Impairment**
No dose adjustment. **Severe impairment: Maximum:** 600 mg/day.

## SIDE EFFECTS

**Occasional (5%–2%):** Headache, cough, dizziness. **Rare (less than 2%):** Muscle pain, fatigue, diarrhea, upper respiratory tract infection, dyspepsia.

## ADVERSE EFFECTS/ TOXIC REACTIONS

Overdosage may manifest as hypotension, tachycardia. Bradycardia occurs less often.

## NURSING CONSIDERATIONS

### BASELINE ASSESSMENT

Obtain B/P, apical pulse immediately before each dose, in addition to regular monitoring (be alert to fluctuations). Question for possibility of pregnancy, history of hepatic/renal impairment, renal artery stenosis. Assess medication history (esp. diuretics).

### INTERVENTION/EVALUATION

Monitor B/P, pulse, serum BUN, creatinine, electrolytes, urinalysis.

### PATIENT/FAMILY TEACHING

• Inform female pt regarding consequences of second- and third-trimester exposure to medication. • Avoid tasks that require alertness, motor skills until response to drug is established. • Restrict sodium, alcohol intake. • Follow diet, control weight. • Do not stop taking medication; hypertension requires lifelong control. • Check B/P regularly. • Do not chew, crush, dissolve, or divide tablets; take whole.

## eptifibatide
**HIGH ALERT**

ep-ti-**fye**-ba-tide
(Integrilin)

◆**CLASSIFICATION**

**PHARMACOTHERAPEUTIC:** Glycoprotein IIb/IIIa inhibitor. **CLINICAL:** Antiplatelet, antithrombotic.

## USES

Treatment of pts with acute coronary syndrome (ACS), including those managed medically and those undergoing percutaneous coronary intervention (PCI). **OFF-LABEL:** Support PCI during ST-elevation myocardial infarction (STEMI).

## PRECAUTIONS

**Contraindications:** Hypersensitivity to eptifibatide. Active abnormal bleeding within previous 30 days; history of bleeding diathesis; history of stroke within 30 days or history of hemorrhagic stroke; severe hypertension (systolic B/P greater than 200 mmHg or diastolic B/P greater than 110 mmHg); major surgery within previous 6 wks, dependency on hemodialysis. **Cautions:** Renal impairment, hemorrhagic retinopathy, platelet count less than 100,000/mm$^3$, elderly, history of bleeding disorder. Medications that increase risk of bleeding (e.g., oral anticoagulants, NSAIDs). **Pregnancy Category B.**

## ACTION

Blocks platelet glycoprotein IIb/IIIa receptor (binding site for fibrinogen, von Willebrand factor). **Therapeutic Effect:** Prevents thrombus formation within coronary arteries. Prevents platelet aggregation.

## PHARMACOKINETICS

Protein binding: 25%. Excreted in urine. **Half-life:** 2.5 hrs.

## INTERACTIONS

**DRUG: Anticoagulants, heparin, NSAIDs, antiplatelets (e.g., clopidogrel), thrombolytic agents** may increase risk of bleeding. **HERBAL: Cat's claw, dong quai, evening primrose, feverfew, garlic, ginger, ginkgo, ginseng** may increase antiplatelet effects. **FOOD:** None known. **LAB VALUES:** Increases PT, aPTT. Decreases platelet count. Prolongs clotting time.

## AVAILABILITY (Rx)

**Injection Solution:** 0.75 mg/ml, 2 mg/ml.

## ADMINISTRATION/HANDLING

 IV

**Reconstitution** • Withdraw bolus dose from 10-ml vial (2 mg/ml); for IV infusion, withdraw from 100-ml vial (0.75 mg/ml). • IV push and infusion administration may be given undiluted.
**Rate of Administration** • Give bolus dose IV push over 1–2 min.
**Storage** • Store vials in refrigerator. • Solution appears clear, colorless. • Do not shake. • Discard any unused portion left in vial or if preparation contains *any* opaque particles.

### ▦ IV INCOMPATIBILITIES

Administer via dedicated line; do not add other medications to infusion solution.

### ▦ IV COMPATIBILITIES

Amiodarone (Cordarone), argatroban, bivalirudin, metoprolol (Lopressor).

## INDICATIONS/ROUTES/DOSAGE

**Adjunct to Percutaneous Coronary Intervention (PCI)**
**IV Bolus, IV Infusion: ADULTS, ELDERLY:** 180 mcg/kg (**maximum:** 22.6 mg) before PCI initiation; then continuous drip of 2 mcg/kg/min and a second 180 mcg/kg (**maximum:** 22.6 mg) bolus 10 min after the first. **Maximum:** 15 mg/hr. Continue until hospital discharge or for up to 18–24 hrs. Minimum 12 hrs is recommended. Concurrent aspirin and heparin therapy is recommended.

**Acute Coronary Syndrome (ACS)**
**IV Bolus, IV Infusion: ADULTS, ELDERLY:** 180 mcg/kg over 1–2 min (**maximum:** 22.6 mg) bolus then 2 mcg/kg/min until discharge or coronary artery bypass graft, up to 72 hrs. **Maximum:** 15 mg/hr. Concurrent aspirin and heparin therapy is recommended.

**Dosage in Renal Impairment**
**CrCl Less than 50 ml/min:** Use 180 mcg/kg bolus (**maximum:** 22.6 mg) and 1 mcg/kg/min infusion (**maximum:** 7.5 mg/hr). **End-Stage Renal Disease (Dialysis):** Contraindicated.

**Dosage in Hepatic Impairment**
No dose adjustment.

## SIDE EFFECTS

**Occasional (7%):** Hypotension.

## ADVERSE EFFECTS/ TOXIC REACTIONS

Minor to major bleeding complications may occur, most commonly at arterial access site for cardiac catheterization.

## NURSING CONSIDERATIONS

### BASELINE ASSESSMENT

Assess platelet count, Hgb, Hct before treatment and during therapy. If platelet count less than 90,000/mm$^3$, additional platelet counts should be obtained routinely to avoid thrombocytopenia.

### INTERVENTION/EVALUATION

Diligently monitor for potential bleeding, particularly at other arterial, venous puncture sites. If possible, urinary catheters, nasogastric tubes should be avoided.

## *eriBULin

er-i-**bue**-lin
(Halaven)
**Do not confuse eribulin with epirubicin or erlotinib.**

## ◆CLASSIFICATION

**PHARMACOTHERAPEUTIC:** Microtubule inhibitor. **CLINICAL:** Antineoplastic.

## USES

Treatment of metastatic breast cancer in pts who previously received at least 2 chemotherapeutic regimens for treatment. Treatment of metastatic liposarcoma in pts who received a prior anthracycline-containing regimen.

## PRECAUTIONS

**Contraindications:** Hypersensitivity to eribulin. **Cautions:** Prolonged QTc (congenital, other medications that prolong QT interval), hypokalemia, hypomagnesium, hepatic/renal impairment, moderate to severe neuropathy, HF.

## ACTION

Binds directly on microtubules during active stage of $G_2$ and M phases of cell cycle, preventing formation of microtubules, an essential part of process of separation of chromosomes. **Therapeutic Effect:** Blocks cells in mitotic phase of cell division, leading to cell death.

## PHARMACOKINETICS

Extensively metabolized in liver. Protein binding: 49%–65%. Excreted in feces (82%), urine (9%). **Half-life:** 40 hrs.

## ⌛ LIFESPAN CONSIDERATIONS

**Pregnancy/Lactation:** May cause embryo-fetal toxicity. Unknown if distributed in breast milk. **Children:** Safety and efficacy not established in pts younger than 18 yrs. **Elderly:** No age-related precautions noted.

## INTERACTIONS

**DRUG:** None significant. **FOOD:** None known. **HERBAL:** None significant. **LAB VALUES:** May decrease WBC, Hgb, Hct, platelet count, potassium. May increase ALT.

## AVAILABILITY (Rx)

**Injection, Solution:** 1 mg/2 ml (0.5-mg/ml).

## ADMINISTRATION/HANDLING

 IV

**Reconstitution** • May administer undiluted or dilute in 100 ml 0.9% NaCl.
**Rate of Administration** • Administer over 2–5 min.
**Storage** • Store at room temperature. • Once diluted, syringe or diluted

solution may be stored for up to 4 hrs at room temperature or up to 24 hrs if refrigerated.

## ▨ IV INCOMPATIBILITIES

Do not dilute with D$_5$W or administer through IV line containing solutions with dextrose or in same IV line with other medications.

## INDICATIONS/ROUTES/DOSAGE

**Metastatic Breast Cancer, Liposarcoma**
**IV: ADULTS, ELDERLY:** 1.4 mg/m$^2$ over 2–5 min on days 1 and 8 of 21-day cycle.

**Dosage in Renal Impairment**
**Mild:** No dose adjustment. **Moderate to severe impairment (CrCl 15–49 ml/min):** 1.1 mg/m$^2$/dose.

**Dosage in Hepatic Impairment**
**Mild:** 1.1 mg/m$^2$/dose. **Moderate impairment:** 0.7 mg/m$^2$/dose. **Severe impairment:** Use not recommended.

**Recommended Dose Delays**
Do not administer day 1 or day 8 of treatment for any of the following: ANC less than 1,000/mm$^3$, platelets less than 75,000/mm$^3$, Grade 3 or 4 nonhematologic toxicities. Day 8 dose may be delayed for maximum of 1 wk. If toxicities do not resolve or improve to Grade 2 severity by day 15, omit dose. If toxicities resolve or improve to Grade 2 severity by day 15, continue treatment at reduced dose and initiate next cycle no sooner than 2 wks later. Do not re-escalate dose after it has been reduced.

## SIDE EFFECTS

**Common (54%–35%):** Fatigue, asthenia, alopecia, peripheral sensory neuropathy, nausea. **Frequent (25%–18%):** Constipation, arthralgia/myalgia, decreased weight, anorexia, pyrexia, headache, diarrhea, vomiting. **Occasional (16%–9%):** Back pain, dyspnea, cough, bone pain, extremity pain, urinary tract infection, oral mucosal inflammation.

## ADVERSE EFFECTS/ TOXIC REACTIONS

Neutropenia occurs in 82% of pts, with 57% developing grade 3 neutropenia. Severe neutropenia (ANC less than 500/mm³) lasting more than 1 wk occurred in 12%. Anemia occurs in 58% of pts. Peripheral neuropathy occurs in 8% of pts but is the most common adverse reaction requiring discontinuation of therapy. Prolonged QTc may be noted on or after day 8 of treatment.

## NURSING CONSIDERATIONS

### BASELINE ASSESSMENT

Question for possibility of pregnancy. Obtain baseline CBC, serum chemistries before treatment begins. Obtain CBC prior to each dose.

### INTERVENTION/EVALUATION

Diligently monitor for neutropenia, peripheral neuropathy (most frequent cause of drug discontinuation). Monitor for symptoms of neuropathy (burning sensation, hyperesthesia, hypoesthesia, paresthesia, discomfort, neuropathic pain). Assess hands, feet for erythema. Monitor CBC for evidence of neutropenia, thrombocytopenia. Assess mouth for stomatitis (erythema, ulceration, mucosal burning).

### PATIENT/FAMILY TEACHING

• Avoid crowds, those with known infection. • Avoid contact with anyone who recently received live virus vaccine. • Do not have immunizations without physician's approval (drug lowers body resistance). • Promptly report fever over 100.5°F, chills, cough, burning or pain urinating, numbness, tingling, burning sensation, erythema of hands/feet.

---

## *erlotinib*

**HIGH ALERT**

er-**loe**-ti-nib
(Tarceva)
**Do not confuse erlotinib with dasatinib, eribulin, geftinib, imatinib, or lapatinib.**

---

## ◆CLASSIFICATION

**PHARMACOTHERAPEUTIC:** Human epidermal growth factor. **CLINICAL:** Antineoplastic.

## USES

Treatment of locally advanced or metastatic non–small-cell lung cancer (NSCLC) after failure of at least one prior chemotherapy regimen (as monotherapy). Treatment of locally advanced, unresectable, or metastatic pancreatic cancer (in combination with gemcitabine). Maintenance treatment of locally advanced or metastatic NSCLC that has not progressed after 4–6 cycles of first-line platinum-based chemotherapy.

## PRECAUTIONS

**Contraindications:** Hypersensitivity to erlotinib. **Cautions:** Severe hepatic/renal impairment cardiovascular disease. Concurrent use of strong CYP3A4 inhibitors and inducers, pts at risk for GI perforation (e.g., peptic ulcer disease, diverticular disease). Total serum bilirubin greater than 3 times upper limit of normal.

## ACTION

Reversibly inhibits overall epidermal growth factor receptor (EGFR)–tyrosine kinase activity. **Therapeutic Effect:** Produces tumor cell death.

## PHARMACOKINETICS

About 60% is absorbed after PO administration; bioavailability is increased by food to almost 100%. Protein binding: 93%. Extensively metabolized in liver. Primarily eliminated in feces (83%), urine (8%). **Half-life:** 24–36 hrs.

## ▨ LIFESPAN CONSIDERATIONS

**Pregnancy/Lactation:** Unknown if drug crosses placenta or is distributed in breast milk. **Children:** Safety and efficacy not established. **Elderly:** No age-related precautions noted.

---

E

## INTERACTIONS

**DRUG:** **CYP3A4 inhibitors (e.g., atanzavir, clarithromycin, indinavir, itraconazole, ketoconazole, nefazodone, nelfinavir, ritonavir, saquinavir)** may increase concentration/effects. **CYP3A4 inducers (e.g., carbamazepine, phenobarbital, phenytoin, rifampin)** may decrease concentration/effects. **Proton pump inhibitors (e.g., omeprazole), H₂antagonists (e.g., ranitidine)** may decrease absorption/effects (avoid use of **proton pump inhibitors.** Give ertapenem 10 hrs after or 2 hrs prior to **H₂ antagonists).** **HERBAL:** **St. John's wort** may decrease concentration/effects. **FOOD:** **Grapefruit** products may increase potential for myelotoxicity. **LAB VALUES:** May increase serum bilirubin, ALT, AST.

## AVAILABILITY (Rx)

**Tablets:** 25 mg, 100 mg, 150 mg.

## ADMINISTRATION/HANDLING

**PO**
• Give at least 1 hr before or 2 hrs after ingestion of food. • Avoid grapefruit products. • May dissolve in 3–4 oz water and give orally or via feeding tube.

## INDICATIONS/ROUTES/DOSAGE

**◄ALERT►** Dosage adjustment for toxicity: Reduce dose in 50-mg increments.

**Lung Cancer**
**PO: ADULTS, ELDERLY:** 150 mg/day until disease progression or unacceptable toxicity occurs.

**Pancreatic Cancer**
**PO: ADULTS, ELDERLY:** 100 mg/day, in combination with gemcitabine, until disease progression or unacceptable toxicity occurs.

**Dosage in Renal Impairment**
Interrupt dosing for Grade 3 or 4 renal toxicity during treatment.

**Dosage in Hepatic Impairment**
Use extreme caution. Reduce starting dose to 75 mg and individualize dose escalation if tolerated.

## SIDE EFFECTS

**Frequent (greater than 10%):** Fatigue, anxiety, headache, depression, insomnia, rash, pruritus, dry skin, erythema, diarrhea, anorexia, nausea, vomiting, mucositis, constipation, dyspepsia, weight loss, dysphagia, abdominal pain, arthralgia, dyspnea, cough. **Occasional (10%–1%):** Keratitis. **Rare (less than 1%):** Corneal ulceration.

## ADVERSE EFFECTS/ TOXIC REACTIONS

UTI occurs occasionally. Pneumonitis, GI bleeding occur rarely.

## NURSING CONSIDERATIONS

### BASELINE ASSESSMENT
Obtain CBC, serum electrolytes, hepatic enzyme levels before beginning therapy.

### INTERVENTION/EVALUATION
Assess LFT and CBC, renal function, serum electrolytes, hydration status periodically.

### PATIENT/FAMILY TEACHING
• Take drug on empty stomach. • Report rash, blood in stool, diarrhea, irritated eyes, fever. • Avoid grapefruit products.

---

# ertapenem

er-ta-**pen**-em
(Invanz)
**Do not confuse ertapenem with doripenem, imipenem, or meropenem, or Invanz with Avinza.**

◆**CLASSIFICATION**
**PHARMACOTHERAPEUTIC:** Carbapenem. **CLINICAL:** Antibiotic.

---

## USES

Treatment of susceptible infections due to *S. aureus* (methicillin-susceptible only), *S. agalactiae, S. pneumoniae* (penicillin-susceptible only), *S. pyogenes, E. coli, H. influenzae* (beta-lactamase negative strains only), *K. pneumoniae, M. catarrhalis, Bacteroides* spp., *C. clostridioforme, Peptostreptococcus* spp., including moderate to severe intra-abdominal, skin/skin structure infections; community-acquired pneumonia; complicated UTI; acute pelvic infection; adult diabetic foot infections without osteomyelitis. Prevention of surgical site infection. OFF-LABEL: Treatment of IV catheter–related bloodstream infection; prosthetic joint infection.

## PRECAUTIONS

**Contraindications:** Hypersensitivity to ertapenem. History of anaphylactic hypersensitivity to beta-lactams (e.g., imipenem and cilastin, meropenem), hypersensitivity to amide-type local anesthetics (IM). **Cautions:** Hypersensitivity to penicillins, cephalosporins, renal impairment, CNS disorders, esp. brain lesions or history of seizures, elderly.

## ACTION

Penetrates bacterial cell wall of microorganisms, binds to penicillin-binding proteins, inhibiting cell wall synthesis. **Therapeutic Effect:** Produces bacterial cell death.

## PHARMACOKINETICS

Almost completely absorbed after IM administration. Protein binding: 85%–95%. Widely distributed. Primarily excreted in urine (80%), feces (10%). Removed by hemodialysis. **Half-life:** 4 hrs.

## ⧖ LIFESPAN CONSIDERATIONS

**Pregnancy/Lactation:** Distributed in breast milk. **Children:** Safety and efficacy not established in pts younger than 18 yrs. **Elderly:** Advanced or end-stage renal insufficiency may require dosage adjustment.

## INTERACTIONS

**DRUG: Probenecid** may increase concentration/effect. May decrease concentration/effect of **valproic acid.** **HERBAL:** None significant. **FOOD:** None known. **LAB VALUES:** May increase serum alkaline phosphatase, ALT, AST, bilirubin, BUN, creatinine, glucose, PT, aPTT, sodium. May decrease platelet count, Hgb, Hct, WBC.

## AVAILABILITY (Rx)

**Injection, Powder for Reconstitution:** 1 g.

## ADMINISTRATION/HANDLING
 IV

**Reconstitution** • Dilute 1-g vial with 10 ml 0.9% NaCl or Bacteriostatic Water for Injection. • Shake well to dissolve. • Further dilute with 50 ml 0.9% NaCl (**maximum concentration: 20 mg/ml**).
**Rate of Administration** • Give by intermittent IV infusion (piggyback). Do not give IV push. • Infuse over 30 min.
**Storage** • Solution appears colorless to yellow (variation in color does not affect potency). • Discard if solution contains precipitate. • Reconstituted solution is stable for 6 hrs at room temperature or 24 hrs if refrigerated.

**IM**
• Reconstitute with 3.2 ml 1% lidocaine HCl injection (without epinephrine). • Shake vial thoroughly. • Inject deep in large muscle mass (gluteal or lateral part of thigh). • Administer suspension within 1 hr after preparation.

## ▒ IV INCOMPATIBILITIES

Do not mix or infuse with any other medications. Do not use diluents or IV solutions containing dextrose.

## ▒ IV COMPATIBILITIES

Heparin, potassium chloride, tigecycline (Tygacil), Sterile Water for Injection, 0.9% NaCl.

E

---

## INDICATIONS/ROUTES/DOSAGE

**Usual Dosage Range**
**IM, IV: ADULTS, ELDERLY, CHILDREN 13 YRS AND OLDER:** 1 g/day. **CHILDREN 3 MOS–12 YRS:** 15 mg/kg 2 times/day. **Maximum:** 1 g/day.

**Dosage in Renal Impairment**

| | |
|---|---|
| CrCl 30 ml/min or less | 500 mg once daily |
| Hemodialysis | If daily dose given within 6h prior to HD, give 150 mg dose after HD. |
| Peritoneal dialysis | 500 mg once daily |

**Dosage in Hepatic Impairment**
No dose adjustment.

## SIDE EFFECTS

**Frequent (10%–6%):** Diarrhea, nausea, headache. **Occasional (5%–2%):** Altered mental status, insomnia, rash, abdominal pain, constipation, chest pain, vomiting, edema, fever. **Rare (less than 2%):** Dizziness, cough, oral candidiasis, anxiety, tachycardia, phlebitis at IV site.

## ADVERSE EFFECTS/ TOXIC REACTIONS

Antibiotic-associated colitis, other superinfections (abdominal cramps, severe watery diarrhea, fever) may result from altered bacterial balance in GI tract. Anaphylactic reactions have been reported. Seizures may occur in those with CNS disorders (brain lesions, history of seizures), bacterial meningitis, severe renal impairment.

## NURSING CONSIDERATIONS

### BASELINE ASSESSMENT

Question for history of allergies, particularly to beta-lactams, penicillins, cephalosporins. Inquire about history of seizures. Monitor WBC count.

### INTERVENTION/EVALUATION

Monitor renal/hepatic function. Monitor daily pattern of bowel activity, stool consistency. Monitor for nausea, vomiting.

Evaluate hydration status. Evaluate for inflammation at IV injection site. Assess skin for rash. Observe mental status; be alert to tremors, possible seizures. Assess sleep pattern for evidence of insomnia.

### PATIENT/FAMILY TEACHING

• Report tremors, seizures, rash, prolonged diarrhea, chest pain, other new symptoms.

# erythromycin

er-**ith**-roe-**mye**-sin
(Akne-Mycin, Apo-Erythro Base ✦, EES, Erybid ✦, Eryc, EryDerm, EryPed, Ery-Tab, Erythrocin, PCE Dispertab)
**Do not confuse Eryc with Emcyt, or erythromycin with azithromycin or clarithromycin.**

## FIXED-COMBINATION(S)

**Eryzole, Pediazole:** erythromycin/ sulfisoxazole (sulfonamide): 200 mg/ 600 mg per 5 ml.

## ◆CLASSIFICATION

**PHARMACOTHERAPEUTIC:** Macrolide. **CLINICAL:** Antibiotic, antiacne.

## USES

Treatment of susceptible infections due to *S. pyogenes, S. pneumoniae, S. aureus, M. pneumoniae, Legionella, Chlamydia, N. gonorrheae, E. histolytica,* including syphilis, nongonococcal urethritis, diphtheria, pertussis, chancroid, *Campylobacter* gastroenteritis. **Topical:** Treatment of acne vulgaris. **Ophthalmic:** Prevention of gonococcal ophthalmia neonatorum, superficial ocular infections. **OFF-LABEL: Systemic:** Treatment of acne vulgaris, chancroid, *Campylobacter* enteritis, gastroparesis, Lyme disease, preoperative gut sterilization. **Topical:** Treatment of minor bacterial skin infections. **Ophthalmic:** Treatment of blepharitis, conjunctivitis, keratitis, chlamydial trachoma.

## PRECAUTIONS

**Contraindications:** Hypersensitivity to erythromycin. Concomitant administration with ergot derivatives, lovastatin, simvastatin. **Cautions:** Elderly, myasthenia gravis, strong CYP3A4 inhibitor, hepatic impairment, pts with prolonged QT intervals, uncorrected hypokalemia or hypomagnesemia, concurrent use of class IA or III antiarrhythmics.

## ACTION

Penetrates bacterial cell membranes, reversibly binds to bacterial ribosomes, inhibiting protein synthesis. **Therapeutic Effect:** Bacteriostatic.

## PHARMACOKINETICS

Variably absorbed from GI tract (depending on dosage form used). Protein binding: 70%–90%. Widely distributed. Metabolized in liver. Primarily eliminated in feces by bile. Not removed by hemodialysis. **Half-life:** 1.4–2 hrs (increased in renal impairment).

## ⧖ LIFESPAN CONSIDERATIONS

**Pregnancy/Lactation:** Crosses placenta. Distributed in breast milk. Erythromycin estolate may increase hepatic enzymes in pregnant women. **Children/ Elderly:** No age-related precautions noted. High dosage in pts with decreased hepatic/renal function increases risk of hearing loss.

## INTERACTIONS

**DRUG:** May increase concentration of **buspirone, cyclosporine, calcium channel blockers (e.g., diltiazem, verapamil), statins (e.g., atorvastatin, simvastatin).** May inhibit metabolism of **carbamazepine. Hepatotoxic medications** may increase risk of hepatotoxicity. May increase risk of **theophylline** toxicity. May increase effects of **warfarin. HERBAL:** St. John's wort

may decrease concentration. **FOOD: Grapefruit** may increase potential for torsades. **LAB VALUES:** May increase serum alkaline phosphatase, bilirubin, ALT, AST.

## AVAILABILITY (Rx)

**Gel, Topical:** 2%. **Injection, Powder for Reconstitution:** 500 mg, 1 g. **Ointment, Ophthalmic:** 0.5%. **Ointment, Topical (Akne-Mycin):** 2%. **Oral Suspension (EES, EryPed):** 100 mg/2.5 ml, 200 mg/5 ml, 400 mg/5 ml. **Tablet as Base:** 250 mg, 333 mg, 500 mg. **Tablet as Ethylsuccinate (EES):** 400 mg.

 **Capsules, Delayed-Release (Eryc):** 250 mg. **Tablets, Delayed-Release (Ery-Tab):** 250 mg, 333 mg, 500 mg.

## ADMINISTRATION/HANDLING

### IV

**Reconstitution** • Reconstitute each 500 mg with 10 ml Sterile Water for Injection without preservative to provide a concentration of 50 mg/ml. • Further dilute with 100–250 ml D₅W or 0.9% NaCl to maximum concentration of 5 mg/ml.

**Rate of Administration** • For intermittent IV infusion (piggyback), infuse over 20–60 min.

**Storage** • Store parenteral form at room temperature. • Initial reconstituted solution in vial is stable for 2 wks refrigerated or 24 hrs at room temperature. • Diluted IV solution stable for 8 hrs at room temperature or 24 hrs if refrigerated. • Discard if precipitate forms.

### PO

• May give with food to decrease GI upset. Do not give with milk or acidic beverages. • Oral suspension is stable for 35 days at room temperature. • Do not crush delayed-release capsules, tablets.

### Ophthalmic

• Place gloved finger on lower eyelid and pull out until a pocket is formed between eye and lower lid. • Place ¼–½ inch of ointment into pocket. • Instruct pt to close eye gently for 1–2 min (so medication will not be squeezed out of the sac) and to roll eyeball to increase contact area of drug to eye.

### 🔳 IV INCOMPATIBILITIES

Fluconazole (Diflucan), furosemide (Lasix), heparin, metoclopramide (Reglan).

### 🔳 IV COMPATIBILITIES

Amiodarone (Cordarone), diltiazem (Cardizem), hydromorphone (Dilaudid), lidocaine, lorazepam (Ativan), magnesium sulfate, midazolam (Versed), morphine, multivitamins, potassium chloride.

## INDICATIONS/ROUTES/DOSAGE

**Usual Dosage Range**
**PO: ADULTS, ELDERLY: BASE:** 250–500 mg q6–12h. **CHILDREN:** 30–50 mg/kg/day in 2–4 divided doses. **Maximum:** 2 g/day. **ETHYLSUCCINATE: ADULTS, ELDERLY:** 400–800 mg q6–12h. **Maximum:** 4 g/day. **CHILDREN:** 30–50 mg/kg/day in divided doses. **Maximum:** 3.2 g/day. **NEONATES:** 10 mg/kg/dose q8–12h. **IV: ADULTS, ELDERLY:** 15–20 mg/kg/day divided q6h. **Maximum:** 4 g/day. **CHILDREN, INFANTS:** 15–20 mg/kg/day divided q6h. **Maximum:** 4 g /day. **NEONATES:** 10 mg/ks/dose q8–12h.

**Dosage in Renal/Hepatic Impairment**
No dose adjustment.

## SIDE EFFECTS

**Frequent: IV:** Abdominal cramping/discomfort, phlebitis/thrombophlebitis. **Topical:** Dry skin (50%). **Occasional:** Nausea, vomiting, diarrhea, rash, urticaria. **Rare: Ophthalmic:** Sensitivity reaction with increased irritation, burning, itching, inflammation. **Topical:** Urticaria.

## ADVERSE EFFECTS/ TOXIC REACTIONS

Antibiotic-associated colitis, other super infections (abdominal cramps, severe watery diarrhea, fever), reversible cholestatic hepatitis may occur. High dosage in pts with renal impairment may lead to reversible hearing loss. Anaphylaxis occurs rarely. Ventricular arrhythmias, prolonged QT interval occur rarely with IV form.

## NURSING CONSIDERATIONS

### BASELINE ASSESSMENT
Question for history of allergies (particularly erythromycins), hepatitis.

### INTERVENTION/EVALUATION
Monitor daily pattern of bowel activity, stool consistency. Assess skin for rash. Assess for hepatotoxicity (malaise, fever, abdominal pain, GI disturbances). Be alert for superinfection: fever, vomiting, diarrhea, anal/genital pruritus, oral mucosal changes (ulceration, pain, erythema). Check for phlebitis (heat, pain, red streaking over vein). Monitor for high-dose hearing loss.

### PATIENT/FAMILY TEACHING
• Continue therapy for full length of treatment. • Doses should be evenly spaced. • Take medication with 8 oz water 1 hr before or 2 hrs following food or beverage. • **Ophthalmic:** Report burning, itching, inflammation. • **Topical:** Report excessive skin dryness, itching, burning. • Improvement of acne may not occur for 1–2 mos; maximum benefit may take 3 mos; therapy may last mos or yrs. • Use caution if using other topical acne preparations containing peeling or abrasive agents, medicated or abrasive soaps, cosmetics containing alcohol (e.g., astringents, aftershave lotion).

# escitalopram

es-sye-**tal**-o-pram
(Apo-Escitalopram✦, Cipralex ✦, Lexapro)

■ **BLACK BOX ALERT** ■ Increased risk of suicidal ideation and behavior in children, adolescents, young adults 18–24 yrs with major depressive disorder, other psychiatric disorders.

## ◆CLASSIFICATION

**PHARMACOTHERAPEUTIC:** Serotonin reuptake inhibitor. **CLINICAL:** Antidepressant.

## USES

Treatment of major depressive disorder. Treatment of generalized anxiety disorder (GAD). **OFF-LABEL:** Seasonal affective disorder (SAD) in children and adolescents, pervasive developmental disorders (e.g., autism), vasomotor symptoms associated with menopause.

## PRECAUTIONS

**Contraindications:** Hypersensitivity to escitalopram. Use of MAOI intended to treat psychiatric disorders (concurrent or within 14 days of discontinuing either escitalopram or MAOI). Initiation in pts receiving linezolid or IV methylene blue. Concurrent use with pimozide. **Cautions:** Hepatic/renal impairment, history of seizures, concurrent use of CNS depressants, pts at high risk of suicide, concomitant aspirin, NSAIDs, warfarin (may potentiate bleeding risk), elderly, metabolic disease; recent history of MI, cardiovascular disease.

## ACTION

Blocks uptake of neurotransmitter serotonin at neuronal presynaptic membranes, increasing its availability at postsynaptic receptor sites. **Therapeutic Effect:** Antidepressant effect.

## PHARMACOKINETICS

Well absorbed after PO administration. Protein binding: 56%. Primarily metabolized in liver. Primarily excreted in feces, with a lesser amount eliminated in urine. **Half-life:** 35 hrs.

## ⌛ LIFESPAN CONSIDERATIONS

**Pregnancy/Lactation:** Distributed in breast milk. **Children:** May cause increased anticholinergic effects or hyperexcitability. **Elderly:** More sensitive to anticholinergic effects (e.g., dry mouth), more likely to experience dizziness, sedation, confusion, hypotension, hyperexcitability.

## INTERACTIONS

**DRUG: Alcohol, other CNS suppressants** may increase CNS depression. **Linezolid, aspirin, NSAIDs, warfarin** may increase risk of bleeding. **MAOIs** may cause serotonin syndrome (autonomic hyperactivity, diaphoresis, excitement, hyperthermia, rigidity, neuroleptic malignant syndrome, coma). **Sumatriptan** may cause weakness, hyperreflexia, poor coordination. **HERBAL: Gotu kola, kava kava, SAMe, St. John's wort, valerian** may increase CNS depression. **Ginkgo biloba, St. John's wort** may increase risk of serotonin syndrome. **FOOD:** None known. **LAB VALUES:** May decrease serum sodium.

## AVAILABILITY (Rx)

**Oral Solution:** 5 mg/5 ml.

**Tablets:** 5 mg, 10 mg, 20 mg.

## ADMINISTRATION/HANDLING

**PO**

• Give without regard to food. • Do not break, crush, dissolve, or divide tablets.

## INDICATIONS/ROUTES/DOSAGE

**Depression**

**PO: ADULTS:** Initially, 10 mg once daily in the morning or evening. May increase to 20 mg after a minimum of 1 wk. **ELDERLY:** 10 mg/day. **CHILDREN 12–17 YRS:**

Initially, 10 mg once daily. May increase to 20 mg/day after at least 3 wks. **Maximum:** 20 mg once daily. Recommended: 10 mg once daily.

**Generalized Anxiety Disorder**

PO: **ADULTS:** Initially, 10 mg once daily in morning or evening. May increase to 20 mg after minimum of 1 wk. **ELDERLY:** 10 mg/day.

**Dosage in Renal Impairment**

**Mild to moderate impairment:** No dose adjustment. **Severe impairment:** Use caution in pts with CrCl less than 20 ml/min.

**Dosage in Hepatic Impairment**

10 mg/day.

## SIDE EFFECTS

**Frequent (21%–11%):** Nausea, dry mouth, drowsiness, insomnia, diaphoresis. **Occasional (8%–4%):** Tremor, diarrhea, abnormal ejaculation, dyspepsia, fatigue, anxiety, vomiting, anorexia. **Rare (3%–2%):** Sinusitis, sexual dysfunction, menstrual disorder, abdominal pain, agitation, decreased libido.

## ADVERSE EFFECTS/ TOXIC REACTIONS

Overdose manifested as dizziness, drowsiness, tachycardia, confusion, seizures.

## NURSING CONSIDERATIONS

**BASELINE ASSESSMENT**

For pts on long-term therapy, LFT, renal function tests, blood counts should be performed periodically. Observe, record behavior. Assess psychological status, thought content, sleep pattern, appearance, interest in environment.

**INTERVENTION/EVALUATION**

Supervise suicidal-risk pt closely during early therapy (as depression lessens, energy level improves, suicide potential increases). Assess appearance, behavior, speech pattern, level of interest, mood.

Monitor for suicidal ideation (esp. at beginning of therapy or when doses are increased or decreased), social interaction, mania, panic attacks.

**PATIENT/FAMILY TEACHING**

• Do not stop taking medication or increase dosage. • Avoid alcohol. • Avoid tasks that require alertness, motor skills until response to drug is established. • Report worsening depression, suicidal ideation, unusual changes in behavior.

# esmolol

es-moe-lol
(Brevibloc)
**Do not confuse Brevibloc with Bumex or Buprenex, or esmolol with Osmitrol.**

## ◆CLASSIFICATION

**PHARMACOTHERAPEUTIC:** Beta$_1$-adrenergic blocker. **CLINICAL:** Antiarrhythmic.

## USES

Rapid, short-term control of ventricular rate in supraventricular tachycardia (SVT), atrial fibrillation or flutter; treatment of tachycardia and/or hypertension (esp. intraop or postop). Treatment of noncompensatory sinus tachycardia. **OFF-LABEL:** Postoperative hypertension or SVT in children. Arrhythmia and/or rate control in ACS, intubation, thyroid storm, pheochromocytoma, electroconvulsive therapy.

## PRECAUTIONS

**Contraindications:** Hypersensitivity to esmolol. Cardiogenic shock, uncompensated cardiac failure, second- or third-degree heart block (except in pts with pacemaker), severe sinus bradycardia, sick sinus syndrome in close proximity to esmolol, IV administration of calcium blockers, pulmonary hypertension. **Cautions:** Compensated HF; concurrent use of digoxin, verapamil, diltiazem. Diabetes, myasthenia gravis, renal impairment, history of anaphylaxis to allergens. Hypovolemia, hypertension, bronchospastic disease, peripheral vascular disease, Raynaud's disease.

## ACTION

Selectively blocks beta$_1$-adrenergic receptors. **Therapeutic Effect:** Slows sinus heart rate, decreases cardiac output, reducing B/P.

## PHARMACOKINETICS

Rapidly metabolized primarily by esterase in cytosol of red blood cells. Protein binding: 55%. Less than 1%–2% excreted in urine. **Half-life:** 9 min.

## ⧖ LIFESPAN CONSIDERATIONS

**Pregnancy/Lactation:** Crosses placenta; distributed in breast milk. **Children:** Safety and efficacy not established. **Elderly:** No age-related precautions noted.

## INTERACTIONS

**DRUG: Opioids (e.g., fentanyl, morphine), calcium channel blockers (e.g., diltiazem, verapamil),** MAOIs may increase level/effects. **HERBAL: Yohimbe** may decrease effects. **FOOD:** None known. **LAB VALUES:** None significant.

## AVAILABILITY (Rx)

**Injection Solution:** 10 mg/ml (250 ml), 20 mg/ml (100 ml).

## ADMINISTRATION/HANDLING

◀**ALERT**▶ Give by IV infusion. Avoid butterfly needles, very small veins (can cause thrombophlebitis).

 **IV**

**Rate of Administration** • Administer by controlled infusion device; titrate to tolerance and response. • Infuse IV loading dose over 1–2 min. • Hypotension (systolic B/P less than 90 mm Hg)

is greatest during first 30 min of IV infusion.

**Storage** • Use only clear and colorless to light yellow solution. • Discard solution if discolored or precipitate forms.

## ▩ IV INCOMPATIBILITIES

Amphotericin B complex (Abelcet, AmBisome, Amphotec), furosemide (Lasix).

## ▩ IV COMPATIBILITIES

Amiodarone (Cordarone), dexmedetomidine (Precedex), diltiazem (Cardizem), dopamine (Intropin), heparin, magnesium, midazolam (Versed), potassium chloride, propofol (Diprivan).

## INDICATIONS/ROUTES/DOSAGE

**Rate Control in Supraventricular Arrhythmias**

**IV: ADULTS, ELDERLY:** Initially, loading dose of 500 mcg/kg/min for 1 min, followed by 50 mcg/kg/min for 4 min. If optimum response is not attained in 5 min, give second loading dose of 500 mcg/kg/min for 1 min, followed by infusion of 100 mcg/kg/min for 4 min. A third (and final) loading dose can be given and infusion increased by 50 mcg/kg/min, up to 200 mcg/kg/min, for 4 min. Once desired response is attained, increase infusion by no more than 25 mcg/kg/min. Infusion usually administered over 24–48 hrs in most pts. Range: 50–200 mcg/kg/min (average dose 100 mcg/kg/min).

**Intraop/Postop Tachycardia Hypertension (Immediate Control)**

**IV: ADULTS, ELDERLY:** Initially, 1 mg/kg over 30 sec, then 150 mcg/kg/min infusion up to 300 mcg/kg/min.

**Dosage in Renal/Hepatic Impairment**
No dose adjustment.

## SIDE EFFECTS

Generally well tolerated, with transient, mild side effects. **Frequent:** Hypotension (systolic B/P less than 90 mm Hg) manifested as dizziness, nausea, diaphoresis, headache, cold extremities, fatigue. **Occasional:** Anxiety, drowsiness, flushed skin, vomiting, confusion, inflammation at injection site, fever.

## ADVERSE EFFECTS/ TOXIC REACTIONS

Overdose may produce profound hypotension, bradycardia, dizziness, syncope, drowsiness, breathing difficulty, bluish fingernails or palms of hands, seizures. May potentiate insulin-induced hypoglycemia in diabetic pts.

## NURSING CONSIDERATIONS

### BASELINE ASSESSMENT

Assess B/P, apical pulse immediately before drug is administered (if pulse is 60 or less/min or systolic B/P is 90 mm Hg or less, withhold medication, contact physician).

### INTERVENTION/EVALUATION

Monitor B/P for hypotension, EKG, heart rate, respiratory rate, development of diaphoresis, dizziness (usually first sign of impending hypotension). Assess pulse for quality, irregular rate, bradycardia, extremities for coldness. Assist with ambulation if dizziness occurs. Assess for nausea, diaphoresis, headache, fatigue.

# esomeprazole

es-o-**mep**-ra-zole
(Apo-Esomeprazole ♦, Nexium, Nexium 24 HR)
**Do not confuse esomeprazole with aripiprazole or omeprazole, or Nexium with Nexavar.**

## FIXED-COMBINATION(S)

**Vimovo:** esomeprazole/naproxen (NSAID): 20 mg/375 mg, 20 mg/500 mg.

## ◆CLASSIFICATION

**PHARMACOTHERAPEUTIC:** Proton pump inhibitor. **CLINICAL:** Gastric acid inhibitor.

## USES

**PO:** Short-term treatment (4–8 wks) of erosive esophagitis; maintenance treatment of healing of erosive esophagitis; symptomatic gastroesophageal reflux disease (GERD). Treatment of pathologic hypersecretory conditions, including Zollinger-Ellison syndrome. Used in triple therapy with amoxicillin and clarithromycin for treatment of *H. pylori* infection in pts with duodenal ulcer. Reduces risk of NSAID-induced gastric ulcer. (OTC) Treatment of frequent heartburn (2 or more days/wk). **IV:** Treatment of GERD with erosive esophagitis. Reduce risk of ulcer re-bleeding postprocedures.

## PRECAUTIONS

**Contraindications:** Hypersensitivity to esomeprazole, other proton pump inhibitors. **Cautions:** May increase risk of hip, wrist, spine fractures; hepatic impairment; elderly; Asian populations. Concurrent use of CYP3A4 inducers (e.g., rifampin).

## ACTION

Converted to active metabolites that irreversibly bind to, inhibit enzymes on surface of gastric parietal cells. Inhibits hydrogen ion transport into gastric lumen. **Therapeutic Effect:** Increases gastric pH; reduces gastric acid production.

## PHARMACOKINETICS

Well absorbed after PO administration. Protein binding: 97%. Extensively metabolized in liver. Primarily excreted in urine. **Half-life:** 1–1.5 hrs.

## ☒ LIFESPAN CONSIDERATIONS

**Pregnancy/Lactation:** Unknown if drug crosses placenta or is distributed in breast milk. **Children:** Safety and efficacy not established. **Elderly:** No age-related precautions noted.

## INTERACTIONS

**DRUG:** May decrease concentration/ effects of **atazanavir, digoxin, iron, ketoconazole.** May increase effect of **warfarin.** May decrease effect of **clopidogrel. CYP3A4 inducers (e.g., rifampin)** may decrease concentration/effects. **HERBAL:** St. John's wort may decrease concentration/effects. **FOOD:** None known. **LAB VALUES:** None significant.

## AVAILABILITY (Rx)

**Injection, Powder for Reconstitution:** 20 mg, 40 mg. **Oral Suspension, Delayed-Release Packets:** 2.5 mg, 5 mg, 10 mg, 20 mg, 40 mg.

 **Capsules (Delayed-Release [Nexium]):** 20 mg, 40 mg. **[Nexium 24 HR]:** 20 mg.

## ADMINISTRATION/HANDLING

🔲 IV

**Reconstitution** • For IV push, add 5 ml of 0.9% NaCl to esomeprazole vial. **Infusion** • For IV infusion, dissolve content of one vial in 50 ml 0.9% NaCl, or D₅W. **Rate of Administration** • For IV push, administer over not less than 3 min. For intermittent infusion (piggyback) infuse over 10–30 min. • Flush line with 0.9% NaCl, or D₅W, both before and after administration. **Storage** • Use only clear and colorless to very slightly yellow solution. • Discard solution if particulate forms. • IV infusion stable for 12 hrs in 0.9% NaCl or lactated Ringer's; 6 hrs in D₅W.

**PO (Capsules)**
• Give 1 hr or more before eating (best before breakfast). • Do not crush, cut capsule; administer whole. • For pts with difficulty swallowing capsules, open capsule and mix pellets with 1 tbsp applesauce. Swallow immediately without chewing.

**PO (Oral Suspension)**
• Empty contents into 5 ml water for 2.5 mg, 5 mg; 15 ml for 10 mg, 20 mg, 40

mg and stir. • Let stand 2–3 min to thicken. • Stir and drink within 30 min.

## 🔲 IV INCOMPATIBILITIES

Do not mix esomeprazole with any other medications through the same IV line or tubing.

## 🔲 IV COMPATIBILITIES

Ceftaroline (Teflaro), doripenem (Doribax).

## INDICATIONS/ROUTES/DOSAGE

**Erosive Esophagitis**
**PO: ADULTS, ELDERLY, CHILDREN 12 YRS AND OLDER:** 20–40 mg once daily for 4–8 wks. May continue for additional 4–8 wks. **CHILDREN 1–11 YRS, WEIGHING 20 KG OR MORE:** 10–20 mg/day for up to 8 wks. **WEIGHING LESS THAN 20 KG:** 10 mg/ day for up to 8 wks.

**Maintenance Therapy for Erosive Esophagitis**
**PO: ADULTS, ELDERLY:** 20 mg/day.

**Treatment of NSAID-Induced Gastric Ulcers**
**PO: ADULTS, ELDERLY:** 20 mg/day for 4–8 wks.

**Prevention of NSAID-Induced Gastric Ulcer**
**PO: ADULTS, ELDERLY:** 20–40 mg once daily for up to 6 mos.

**Gastroesophageal Reflux Disease (GERD)**
**IV: ADULTS, ELDERLY:** 20 or 40 mg once daily for up to 10 days. **CHILDREN 1–17 YRS, WEIGHING 55 KG OR MORE:** 20 mg once daily; **1–17 YRS, WEIGHING LESS THAN 55 KG:** 10 mg once daily; **1 MO TO LESS THAN 1 YR:** 0.5 mg/kg once daily. **PO: ADULTS, ELDERLY, CHILDREN, 12–17 YRS:** 20 mg once daily for up to 8 wks. **CHILDREN 1–11 YRS:** 10 mg/day for up to 8 wks.

**Zollinger-Ellison Syndrome**
**PO: ADULTS, ELDERLY:** 40 mg 2 times/day. Doses up to 240 mg/day have been used.

---

E

### Duodenal Ulcer Caused by *Helicobacter Pylori*

**PO: ADULTS, ELDERLY:** 40 mg (esomeprazole) once daily, with amoxicillin 1,000 mg and clarithromycin 500 mg twice daily for 10 days.

### Heartburn (OTC)

**PO: ADULTS, ELDERLY:** 20 mg/day for 14 days. May repeat after 4 mos if needed.

### Dosage in Renal Impairment

No dose adjustment.

### Dosage in Hepatic Impairment

**Mild to moderate impairment:** No dose adjustment. **Severe impairment:** Doses should not exceed 20 mg/day.

## SIDE EFFECTS

**Frequent     (7%):** Headache. **Occasional (3%–2%):** Diarrhea, abdominal pain, nausea. **Rare (less than 2%):** Dizziness, asthenia, vomiting, constipation, rash, cough.

## ADVERSE EFFECTS/ TOXIC REACTIONS

Pancreatitis, hepatotoxicity, interstitial nephritis occur rarely.

## NURSING CONSIDERATIONS

### BASELINE ASSESSMENT

Assess epigastric/abdominal pain. Question history of hepatic impairment, pathologic bone fractures.

### INTERVENTION/EVALUATION

Evaluate for therapeutic response (relief of GI symptoms). Question if GI discomfort, nausea, diarrhea occur. Monitor for occult blood, observe for hemorrhage in pts with peptic ulcer.

### PATIENT/FAMILY TEACHING

• Report headache. • Take at least 1 hr before eating. • If swallowing capsules is difficult, open capsule and mix pellets with 1 tbsp applesauce. Swallow immediately without chewing.

# estradiol

es-tra-**dye**-ole
(Alora, Climara, Delestrogen, Depo-Estradiol, Divigel, Elestrin, Estrace, Estraderm, Estrasorb, Estring, Estrogel, Evamist, Femring, Femtrace, Menostar, Minivelle, Vagifem, Vivelle-Dot)

■ **BLACK BOX ALERT** ■ Increased risk of dementia when given to women 65 yrs and older. Use of estrogen without progestin increases risk of endometrial cancer in postmenopausal women with intact uterus. Increased risk of invasive breast cancer in postmenopausal women using conjugated estrogens with medroxyprogesterone. Do not use to prevent cardiovascular disease or dementia.

**Do not confuse Alora with Aldara, or Estraderm with Testoderm.**

## FIXED-COMBINATION(S)

**Activella:** estradiol/norethindrone (hormone): 1 mg/0.5 mg. **Climara PRO:** estradiol/levonorgestrel (progestin): 0.045 mg/24 hr, 0.015 mg/24 hr. **Combi-patch:** estradiol/norethindrone (hormone): 0.05 mg/0.14 mg, 0.05 mg/0.25 mg. **Femhrt:** estradiol/norethindrone (hormone): 5 mcg/1 mg. **Lunelle:** estradiol/medroxy-progesterone (progestin): 5 mg/25 mg per 0.5 ml.

## ◆CLASSIFICATION

**PHARMACOTHERAPEUTIC:** Estrogen. **CLINICAL:** Estrogen, antineoplastic.

## USES

Treatment of moderate to severe vasomotor symptoms associated with menopause, vulvar and vaginal atrophy associated with menopause, hypoestrogenism (due to hypogonadism, primary ovarian failure), metastatic breast cancer (palliation) in men and postmenopausal women, advanced prostate cancer (palliation), prevention of osteoporosis in menopausal women.

## PRECAUTIONS

**Contraindications:** Hypersensitivity to estradiol, angioedema, hepatic dysfunction or disease, undiagnosed abnormal vaginal bleeding, active or history of arterial thrombosis, estrogen-dependent cancer, known or suspected breast cancer (except for pts being treated for metastatic disease), pregnancy, thrombophlebitis or thromboembolic disorders. **Cautions:** Renal insufficiency, diabetes mellitus, endometriosis, severe hypocalcemia, hyperlipidemias, asthma, epilepsy, migraines, SLE, hypertension, hypocalcemia, hypothyroidism, history of jaundice due to past estrogen use or pregnancy, cardiovascular disease, obesity, porphyria, severe hypocalcemia.

## ACTION

Modulates pituitary secretion of gonadotropins; follicle-stimulating hormone (FSH), luteinizing hormone (LH). **Therapeutic Effect:** Promotes normal growth/development of female sex organs.

## PHARMACOKINETICS

Well absorbed from GI tract. Widely distributed. Protein binding: 50%–80%. Metabolized in liver. Primarily excreted in urine. **Half-life:** Unknown.

## ⏳ LIFESPAN CONSIDERATIONS

**Pregnancy/Lactation:** Distributed in breast milk. May be harmful to infant. Breastfeeding not recommended. **Children:** Caution in pts for whom bone growth is not complete (may accelerate epiphyseal closure). **Elderly:** No age-related precautions noted.

## INTERACTIONS

**DRUG: CYP3A4 inducers (e.g., carbamazepine, rifampin)** may decrease concentration/effects. **CYP3A4 inhibitors (e.g., ketoconazole, ritonavir)** may increase concentration/effect. **HERBAL:** Avoid **black cohosh, dong quai, saw palmetto;** may enhance toxic/adverse effects. **St. John's wort** may decrease concentration/effects of estrogens. **FOOD:** None known. **LAB VALUES:** May increase serum glucose, calcium, HDL, triglycerides. May decrease serum cholesterol, LDL. May affect metapyrone testing, thyroid function tests.

## AVAILABILITY (Rx)

**Emulsion, Topical (Estrasorb):** 4.35 mg estradiol/1.74 g pouch (contents of 2 pouches deliver estradiol 0.05 mg/day). **Gel, Topical: (Divigel):** 0.1% (0.25-g packet delivers estradiol 0.25 mg, 0.5 g-packet delivers estradiol 0.5 mg, 1-g packet delivers 1 mg). **(Elestrin):** 0.06% delivers 0.52 mg estradiol/actuation. **(Estrogel):** 0.06% delivers 0.75 mg/actuation. **Injection (Cypionate): Depo-Estradiol:** 5 mg/ml. **(Valerate): Delestrogen:** 10 mg/ml, 20 mg/ml, 40 mg/ml. **Tablets: (Estrace):** 0.5 mg, 1 mg, 2 mg. **(Femtrace):** 0.9 mg. **Topical Spray (Evamist):** 1.53 mg/spray. **Transdermal System (Alora):** twice wkly: 0.025 mg/24 hrs, 0.05 mg/24 hrs, 0.075 mg/24 hrs, 0.1 mg/24 hrs. **Transdermal System (Climara):** once wkly: 0.025 mg/24 hrs, 0.0375 mg/24 hrs, 0.05 mg/24 hrs, 0.06 mg/24 hrs, 0.075 mg/24 hrs, 0.1 mg/24 hrs. **Transdermal System (Menostar):** once wkly: 0.014 mg/24 hrs. **Transdermal System (Minivelle, Vivelle-Dot):** twice wkly: 0.025 mg/24 hrs, 0.0375 mg/24 hrs, 0.05 mg/24 hrs, 0.075 mg/24 hrs, 0.1 mg/24 hrs. **Vaginal Cream (Estrace):** 0.1 mg/g. **Vaginal Ring (Estring):** 2 mg (releases 7.5 mcg/day over 90 days). **Vaginal Ring (Femring):** 0.05 mg/day (total estradiol 12.4 mg-release 0.05 mg/day over 3 mos); 0.1 mg/day (total estradiol 24.8 mg-release 0.1 mg/day over 3 mos). **Vaginal Tablet (Vagifem):** 10 mcg.

---

## ADMINISTRATION/HANDLING

### IM
- Rotate vial to disperse drug in solution.
- Inject deep IM in large muscle mass.

### PO
- Administer at same time each day.
- Administer with food.

### Transdermal
- Remove old patch; select new site (buttocks are alternative application site).
- Peel off protective strip to expose adhesive surface. • Apply to clean, dry, intact skin on trunk of body (area with as little hair as possible). • Press in place for at least 10 sec (do not apply to breasts or waistline).

### Vaginal
- Apply at bedtime for best absorption. • Insert end of filled applicator into vagina, directed slightly toward sacrum; push plunger down completely. • Avoid skin contact with cream (prevents skin absorption).

## INDICATIONS/ROUTES/DOSAGE

### Prostate Cancer
**IM** *(Delestrogen):* **ADULTS, ELDERLY:** 30 mg or more q1–2wks.
**PO: ADULTS, ELDERLY:** 1–2 mg tid for at least 3 mos.

### Breast Cancer
**PO: ADULTS, ELDERLY:** 10 mg 3 times/day for at least 3 mos.

### Osteoporosis Prophylaxis in Postmenopausal Females
**PO: ADULTS, ELDERLY:** 0.45–0.5 mg/day cyclically (3 wks on, 1 wk off).
**Transdermal** *(Climara):* **ADULTS, ELDERLY:** Initially, 0.025 mg/24 hrs wkly, adjust dose as needed.
**Transdermal** *(Alora, Minivelle, Vivelle-Dot):* **ADULTS, ELDERLY:** Initially, 0.025 mg/24 hrs patch twice wkly, adjust dose as needed.
**Transdermal** *(Menostar):* **ADULTS, ELDERLY:** 0.014 mg/24 hrs patch wkly.

### Female Hypoestrogenism
**PO: ADULTS, ELDERLY:** 1–2 mg/day, adjust dose as needed.
**IM** *(Depo-Estradiol):* **ADULTS, ELDERLY:** 1.5–2 mg monthly.
**IM** *(Delestrogen):* **ADULTS, ELDERLY:** 10–20 mg q4wks.

### Vasomotor Symptoms Associated with Menopause
**PO: ADULTS, ELDERLY:** 1–2 mg/day cyclically (3 wks on, 1 wk off), adjust dose as needed.
**IM** *(Depo-Estradiol):* **ADULTS, ELDERLY:** 1–5 mg q3–4wks.
**IM** *(Delestrogen):* **ADULTS, ELDERLY:** 10–20 mg q4wks.
**Topical Emulsion** *(Estrasorb):* **ADULTS, ELDERLY:** 3.48 g (contents of 2 pouches) once daily in the morning.
**Topical Gel** *(Estrogel):* **ADULTS, ELDERLY:** 1.25 g/day.
**Transdermal Spray** *(Evamist):* Initially, 1 spray daily. May increase to 2–3 sprays daily.
**Transdermal** *(Climara):* **ADULTS, ELDERLY:** 0.025 mg/24 hrs wkly. Adjust dose as needed.
**Transdermal ADULTS, ELDERLY:** *(Alora):* 0.05 mg/24 hrs twice wkly. *(Vivelle-Dot):* 0.0375 mg/24 hrs twice wkly.
**Vaginal Ring** *(Femring):* **ADULTS, ELDERLY:** 0.05 mg. May increase to 0.1 mg if needed.

### Vaginal Atrophy
**Vaginal Ring** *(Estring):* **ADULTS, ELDERLY:** 2 mg.
**Vaginal Cream** *(Estrace):* Insert 2–4 g/day intravaginally for 2 wks, then reduce dose by ½ initial dose for 2 wks, then maintenance dose of 1 g 1–3 times/wk.

### Atrophic Vaginitis
**Vaginal Tablet** *(Vagifem):* **ADULTS, ELDERLY:** Initially, 1 tablet/day for 2 wks. **Maintenance:** 1 tablet twice wkly.

### Dosage in Renal Impairment
No dose adjustment.

---

**Dosage in Hepatic Impairment**
Contraindicated.

## SIDE EFFECTS

**Frequent:** Anorexia, nausea, swelling of breasts, peripheral edema marked by swollen ankles and feet. **Transdermal:** Skin irritation, redness. **Occasional:** Vomiting (esp. with high doses), headache (may be severe), intolerance to contact lenses, hypertension, glucose intolerance, brown spots on exposed skin. **Vaginal:** Local irritation, vaginal discharge, changes in vaginal bleeding (spotting, breakthrough, prolonged bleeding). **Rare:** Chorea (involuntary movements), hirsutism (abnormal hairiness), loss of scalp hair, depression.

## ADVERSE EFFECTS/ TOXIC REACTIONS

Prolonged administration increases risk of gallbladder disease, thromboembolic disease, breast/cervical/vaginal/endometrial/hepatic carcinoma. Cholestatic jaundice occurs rarely.

## NURSING CONSIDERATIONS

### BASELINE ASSESSMENT

Assess frequency/severity of vasomotor symptoms. Question for hypersensitivity to estrogen, previous jaundice, thromboembolic disorders associated with pregnancy, estrogen therapy. Question for possibility of pregnancy.

### INTERVENTION/EVALUATION

Monitor B/P, weight, serum calcium, glucose, LFT. Monitor for loss of vision, sudden onset of proptosis, diplopia, migraine, thromboembolic disorders.

### PATIENT/FAMILY TEACHING

• Limit alcohol, caffeine. • Avoid grapefruit products. • Immediately report sudden headache, vomiting, disturbance of vision/speech, numbness/weakness of extremities, chest pain, calf pain, shortness of breath, severe abdominal pain, mental depression, unusual bleeding. • Avoid smoking. • Report abnormal vaginal bleeding. • Never place patch on breast or waistline.

# eszopiclone

e-**zop**-i-klone
(Lunesta)
**Do not confuse Lunesta with Neulasta.**

## ◆ CLASSIFICATION

**PHARMACOTHERAPEUTIC:** Nonbenzodiazepine **(Schedule IV). CLINICAL:** Hypnotic.

## USES

Treatment of insomnia.

## PRECAUTIONS

**Contraindications:** Hypersensitivity to eszopiclone. **Cautions:** Hepatic impairment, compromised respiratory function, COPD, sleep apnea, clinical depression, suicidal ideation, history of drug dependence; concomitant CNS depressants, strong CYP3A4 inhibitors (e.g., ketoconazole); elderly.

## ACTION

May interact with GABA-receptor complexes at binding domains located close to or allosterically coupled to benzodiazepine receptors. **Therapeutic Effect:** Prevents insomnia, difficulty maintaining normal sleep.

## PHARMACOKINETICS

Rapidly absorbed following PO administration. Protein binding: 52%–59%. Metabolized in liver. Excreted in urine. **Half-life:** 5–6 hrs.

## ⌛ LIFESPAN CONSIDERATIONS

**Pregnancy/Lactation:** Unknown if drug crosses placenta or is distributed in breast milk. **Children:** Safety and efficacy not established. **Elderly:** Pts with

---

 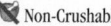

impaired motor or cognitive performance may require dosage adjustment.

## INTERACTIONS

**DRUG:** Alcohol, anticonvulsants (e.g., carbamazepine, phenytoin), antihistamines (e.g., diphenhydramine), other CNS depressants may increase CNS depression. CYP3A4 inhibitors (e.g., clarithromycin, itraconazole, ketoconazole, nelfinavir, ritonavir) may increase concentration/toxicity. **HERBAL:** Gotu kola, kava kava, St. John's wort, valerian may increase CNS depression. **FOOD:** Onset of action may be reduced if taken with or immediately after a **high-fat meal. LAB VALUES:** None known.

## AVAILABILITY (Rx)

Tablets, Film-Coated: 1 mg, 2 mg, 3 mg.

## ADMINISTRATION/HANDLING

**PO**
- Should be administered immediately before bedtime. • Do not give with or immediately following a high-fat or heavy meal. • Do not break, crush, dissolve, or divide tablet.

## INDICATIONS/ROUTES/DOSAGE

**Insomnia**
**PO: ADULTS:** 1 mg before bedtime. **Maximum:** 3 mg. **Concurrent use with CYP3A4 inhibitors (e.g., clarithromycin, erythromycin, azole antifungals):** 1 mg before bedtime; if needed, dose may be increased to 2 mg. **ELDERLY, DEBILITATED PTS:** Initially, 1 mg before bedtime. **Maximum:** 2 mg.

**Sleep Maintenance Difficulty**
**PO: ADULTS:** 2 mg before bedtime.

**Dosage in Renal Impairment**
No dose adjustment.

**Dosage in Hepatic Impairment**
Use caution. Initially, 1 mg immediately before bedtime. **Maximum:** 2 mg.

## SIDE EFFECTS

**Frequent (34%–21%):** Unpleasant taste, headache. **Occasional (10%–4%):** Drowsiness, dry mouth, dyspepsia, dizziness, nervousness, nausea, rash, pruritus, depression, diarrhea. **Rare (3%–2%):** Hallucinations, anxiety, confusion, abnormal dreams, decreased libido, neuralgia.

## ADVERSE EFFECTS/TOXIC REACTIONS

Chest pain, peripheral edema occur occasionally.

## NURSING CONSIDERATIONS

### BASELINE ASSESSMENT

Assess B/P, pulse, respirations. Raise bed rails, provide call light. Provide environment conducive to sleep (quiet environment, low or no lighting).

### INTERVENTION/EVALUATION

Assess sleep pattern of pt. Evaluate for therapeutic response (decrease in number of nocturnal awakenings, increase in length of sleep).

### PATIENT/FAMILY TEACHING

- Take only when experiencing insomnia. Do not take when insomnia is not present. • Do not break, chew, crush, dissolve, or divide tablet. Take whole. • Avoid alcohol. • At least 8 hrs must be devoted for sleep time before daily activity begins. • Take immediately before bedtime. • Report insomnia that worsens or persists longer than 7–10 days, abnormal thoughts or behavior, memory loss, anxiety.

---

## etanercept    TOP 100

e-**tan**-er-sept
(Enbrel)
■ **BLACK BOX ALERT** ■ Serious, potentially fatal, infections, including bacterial sepsis, tuberculosis, have occurred. Lymphomas, other malignancies may occur (reported in children/adolescents).

**Do not confuse Enbrel with Levbid.**

## ◆CLASSIFICATION

**PHARMACOTHERAPEUTIC:** Protein, TNF inhibitor. **CLINICAL:** Antiarthritic.

## USES

Treatment of moderate to severely active rheumatoid arthritis (RA). Treatment of moderately to severely active polyarticular juvenile idiopathic arthritis (JIA), ankylosing spondylitis, psoriatic arthritis. Treatment of chronic, moderate to severe plaque psoriasis. **OFF-LABEL:** Treatment of acute graft-versus-host disease.

## PRECAUTIONS

**Contraindications:** Hypersensitivity to etanercept. Serious active infection or sepsis. **Cautions:** History of recurrent infections, illnesses that predispose to infection (e.g., diabetes, travel from areas of endemic mycosis). History of HF, decreased left ventricular function, significant hematologic abnormalities; moderate to severe alcoholic hepatitis, elderly, preexisting or recent-onset CNS demyelinating disorder.

## ACTION

Binds to tumor necrosis factor (TNF), blocking its interaction with cell surface receptors. Elevated levels of TNF, involved in inflammatory and immune responses, are found in synovial fluid of rheumatoid arthritis pts. **Therapeutic Effect:** Relieves symptoms of arthritis, psoriasis, spondylitis.

## PHARMACOKINETICS

Well absorbed after subcutaneous administration. **Half-life:** 72–132 hrs.

## ⌛ LIFESPAN CONSIDERATIONS

**Pregnancy/Lactation:** Unknown if distributed in breast milk. **Children:** No age-related precautions noted in pts 4 yrs and older. **Elderly:** No age-related precautions noted.

## INTERACTIONS

**DRUG: Anakinra** may increase risk of infection. Use of **live virus vaccines** may potentiate virus replication, increase vaccine side effect, decrease pt's antibody response to vaccine. **HERBAL: Echinacea** may decrease effects. **FOOD:** None known. **LAB VALUES:** May increase serum alkaline phosphatase, ALT, AST, bilirubin.

## AVAILABILITY (Rx)

**Injection, Solution (Prefilled Syringe):** 25 mg/0.5 ml, 50 mg/ml. **Injection, Solution (Autoinjector):** 50 mg/ml.

## ADMINISTRATION/HANDLING

**◄ALERT►** Do not add other medications to solution. Do not use filter during reconstitution or administration.

**Subcutaneous**
• Refrigerate prefilled syringes. • Inject into thigh, abdomen, upper arm. Rotate injection sites. • Give new injection at least 1 inch from an old site and never into area where skin is tender, bruised, red, hard. • Once reconstituted, may be stored in vial for up to 14 days refrigerated.

## INDICATIONS/ROUTES/DOSAGE

**Rheumatoid Arthritis (RA), Psoriatic Arthritis, Ankylosing Spondylitis**
**SQ: ADULTS, ELDERLY:** 25 mg twice wkly given 72–96 hrs apart or 50 mg once wkly. **Maximum:** 50 mg/wk.

**Juvenile Rheumatoid Arthritis (JIA)**
**SQ: CHILDREN 2–17 YRS:** Twice wkly: 0.4 mg/kg 2 times/wk given 72–96 hrs apart. **Maximum dose:** 25 mg. Once wkly: 0.8 mg/kg/dose. **Maximum dose:** 50 mg/wk.

**Plaque Psoriasis**
**SQ: ADULTS, ELDERLY:** 50 mg twice wkly (give 3–4 days apart) for 3 mos. (25 mg or 50 mg once wkly have also been used) **Maintenance:** 50 mg once wkly. **CHILDREN 4 YRS AND OLDER:** 0.8 mg/kg once wkly. **Maximum Dose:** 50 mg/wk.

E

Dosage in Renal/Hepatic Impairment
No dose adjustment.

## SIDE EFFECTS

**Frequent (37%):** Injection site erythema, pruritus, pain, swelling; abdominal pain, vomiting (more common in children than adults). **Occasional (16%–4%):** Headache, rhinitis, dizziness, pharyngitis, cough, asthenia, abdominal pain, dyspepsia. **Rare (less than 3%):** Sinusitis, allergic reaction.

## ADVERSE EFFECTS/ TOXIC REACTIONS

Infection (pyelonephritis, cellulitis, osteomyelitis, wound infection, leg ulcer, septic arthritis, diarrhea, bronchitis, pneumonia) occurs in 29%–38% of pts. Rare adverse effects include heart failure, hypertension, hypotension, pancreatitis, GI hemorrhage.

## NURSING CONSIDERATIONS

### BASELINE ASSESSMENT

Assess onset, type, location, duration of pain, inflammation. If significant exposure to varicella virus has occurred during treatment, therapy should be temporarily discontinued and treatment with varicella-zoster immune globulin should be considered.

### INTERVENTION/EVALUATION

Assess for improvement of joint swelling, pain, tenderness. Monitor erythrocyte sedimentation rate (ESR), C-reactive protein level, CBC with differential, platelet count. Observe for signs of infection.

### PATIENT/FAMILY TEACHING

• Instruct pt in subcutaneous injection technique, including areas of body acceptable as injection sites. • Injection site reaction generally occurs in first mo of treatment and decreases in frequency during continued therapy. • Do not receive live vaccines during treatment. • Report persistent fever, bruising, bleeding, pallor.

# ethambutol

eth-**am**-bue-tol
(Etibi ✦, Myambutol)

◆**CLASSIFICATION**

**PHARMACOTHERAPEUTIC:** Isonicotinic acid derivative. **CLINICAL:** Antitubercular.

## USES

In conjunction with other antitubercular agents for treatment of pulmonary tuberculosis. **OFF-LABEL:** Treatment of atypical mycobacterial infections (e.g., *Mycobacterium avium* complex [MAC]).

## PRECAUTIONS

**Contraindications:** Hypersensitivity to ethambutol. Optic neuritis. Use in young children, unconscious pts, or anyone unable to report visual changes. **Cautions:** Renal/hepatic dysfunction, ocular defects (diabetic retinopathy, cataracts), recurrent ocular inflammatory conditions. Not recommended for children 13 yrs and younger (unless benefit outweighs risk).

## ACTION

Inhibits arabinosyl transferase causing impaired mycobacterial cell wall synthesis. **Therapeutic Effect:** Suppresses multiplication of mycobacteria.

## PHARMACOKINETICS

Rapidly, well absorbed from GI tract. Protein binding: 20%–30%. Widely distributed. Metabolized in liver. Primarily excreted in urine. Removed by hemodialysis. **Half-life:** 3–4 hrs (increased in renal impairment).

## ⧗ LIFESPAN CONSIDERATIONS

**Pregnancy/Lactation:** Crosses placenta. Distributed in breast milk. **Children:** Safety and efficacy not established in pts younger than 13 yrs.

**Elderly:** Age-related renal impairment may require dosage adjustment.

## INTERACTIONS

**DRUG: Aluminum hydroxide** may decrease concentration/effect. **HERBAL:** None significant. **FOOD:** None known. **LAB VALUES:** May increase serum uric acid.

## AVAILABILITY (Rx)

**Tablets:** 100 mg, 400 mg.

## ADMINISTRATION/HANDLING

**PO**

• May be crushed and mixed with apple juice or applesauce. • Administer at least 4 hrs before giving aluminum hydroxide. • Give with food (decreases GI upset).

## INDICATIONS/ROUTES/DOSAGE

**Tuberculosis**
**PO: ADULTS, ELDERLY:** 15–25 mg/kg once daily (**maximum:** 1.5–2.5 g/day). **CHILDREN: (HIV negative):** 15–20 mg/kg/day (**maximum:** 1 g/day) or 50 mg/kg twice wkly (**maximum:** 2.5 g/dose). **(HIV exposed/infected):** 15–25 mg/kg/day. **Maximum:** 2.5 g/day.

**Dosage in Renal Impairment**
Dosage interval is modified based on creatinine clearance.

| Creatinine Clearance | Dosage |
|---|---|
| 10–50 ml/min | q24–36h |
| Less than 10 ml/min | q48h |
| Hemodialysis | Administer post HD |
| Peritoneal dialysis | Administer q48h |
| Continuous renal replacement therapy | Administer q24–36h |

**Dosage in Hepatic Impairment**
Use caution.

## SIDE EFFECTS

**Occasional:** Acute gouty arthritis (chills, pain, swelling of joints with hot skin), confusion, abdominal pain, nausea, vomiting, anorexia, headache. **Rare:** Rash, fever, blurred vision, red-green color blindness.

## ADVERSE EFFECTS/ TOXIC REACTIONS

Optic neuritis (more common with high-dosage, long-term therapy), peripheral neuritis, thrombocytopenia, anaphylactoid reaction occur rarely.

## NURSING CONSIDERATIONS

### BASELINE ASSESSMENT

Evaluate baseline CBC, renal function, LFT, and monitor periodically.

### INTERVENTION/EVALUATION

Assess for vision changes (altered color perception, decreased visual acuity may be first signs). Give with food if GI distress occurs. Monitor serum uric acid. Assess for hot, painful, swollen joints, esp. great toe, ankle, knee (gout). Report numbness, tingling, burning of extremities (peripheral neuritis).

### PATIENT/FAMILY TEACHING

• Do not skip doses; take for full length of therapy (may take mos or yrs). • Immediately report any visual changes (visual effects generally reversible with discontinuation of ethambutol but in rare cases may take up to 1 yr to disappear or may be permanent). • Promptly report swelling or pain of joints, numbness or tingling/burning of extremities, fever, chills.

---

# *etoposide, VP-16*  **HIGH ALERT**

e-**toe**-poe-side
(Etopophos, Toposar, VePesid ✦)
■ **BLACK BOX ALERT** ■ Severe myelosuppression with resulting infection, bleeding may occur. Must be administered by personnel trained in administration/handling of chemotherapeutic agents.
**Do not confuse etoposide with etidronate, or VePesid with Pepcid or Versed.**

---

## ◆CLASSIFICATION

**PHARMACOTHERAPEUTIC:** Epipodo-phyllotoxin. **CLINICAL:** Antineoplastic.

## USES

Treatment of refractory testicular tumors, small-cell lung carcinoma. **OFF-LABEL:** Acute lymphocytic, acute nonlymphocytic leukemias; Ewing's and Kaposi's sarcoma; Hodgkin's and non-Hodgkin's lymphomas; endometrial, gastric, non–small-cell lung carcinomas; multiple myeloma; myelodys-plastic syndromes; neuroblastoma; osteo-sarcoma; ovarian germ cell tumors; pri-mary brain, gestational trophoblastic tumors; soft tissue sarcomas; Wilms tumor.

## PRECAUTIONS

**Contraindications:** Hypersensitivity to et-oposide. **Cautions:** Hepatic/renal im-pairment, myelosuppression, elderly, pts with low serum albumin.

## ACTION

Induces single- and double-stranded breaks in DNA. Cell cycle-dependent and phase-specific; most effective in S and $G_2$ phases of cell division. **Therapeutic Effect:** Inhibits, alters DNA synthesis.

## PHARMACOKINETICS

Variably absorbed from GI tract. Rapidly distributed, low concentrations in CSF. Protein binding: 97%. Metabolized in liver. Primarily excreted in urine. Not removed by hemodialysis. **Half-life:** 3–12 hrs.

## ⧗ LIFESPAN CONSIDERATIONS

**Pregnancy/Lactation:** If possible, avoid use during pregnancy, esp. first trimester. May cause fetal harm. Breastfeeding not recom-mended. **Children:** Safety and efficacy not established. **Elderly:** Age-related renal im-pairment may require dosage adjustment.

## INTERACTIONS

**DRUG: Bone marrow depressants** may increase myelosuppression. **Live-virus vaccines** may potentiate virus replication, increase vaccine side effects, decrease pt's antibody response to vaccine. **HERBAL: Echinacea, St. John's wort** may decrease concentration. **FOOD:** None known. **LAB VALUES:** Expected decrease of leukocytes, platelets, RBC, Hgb, Hct.

## AVAILABILITY (Rx)

**Capsules:** 50 mg. **Injection, Powder for Reconstitution (Water-Soluble [Etopophos]):** 100 mg. **Injection Solution (Toposar):** 20 mg/ml (5 ml, 25 ml, 50 ml).

## ADMINISTRATION/HANDLING

**◀ALERT▶** Administer by slow IV infu-sion. Wear gloves when preparing solution. If powder or solution comes in contact with skin, wash immediately and thoroughly with soap, water. May be carcinogenic, muta-genic, teratogenic. Handle with extreme care during preparation, administration.

 **IV**

**Reconstitution**
**Vepesid** • Dilute each 100 mg (5 ml) with at least 250 ml $D_5W$ or 0.9% NaCl to provide concentration of 0.4 mg/ml (500 ml for concentration of 0.2 mg/ml). May dilute to a concentration as low as 0.1 mg/ml.
**Etopophos** • Reconstitute each 100 mg with 5–10 ml Sterile Water for Injection, $D_5W$, or 0.9% NaCl to provide concentra-tion of 20 mg/ml or 10 mg/ml, respec-tively. • May give without further dilution or further dilute to concentration as low as 0.1 mg/ml with 0.9% NaCl or $D_5W$.
**Rate of administration**
**Vepesid** • Infuse slowly, at least 30–60 min (rapid IV may produce marked hypotension) at a rate not to exceed 100 mg/m²/hr. • Monitor for anaphylactic reaction during infusion (chills, fever, dyspnea, diaphoresis, lacrimation, sneez-ing, throat, back, chest pain).
**Etopophos** • May give over as little as 5 min up to 210 min.
**Storage**
**Vepesid** • Store injection at room tem-perature before dilution. • Concentrate

---

for injection is clear, yellow. • Diluted solution is stable at room temperature for 96 hrs at 0.2 mg/ml, 24 hrs at 0.4 mg/ml. • Discard if crystallization occurs. **Etopophos** • Refrigerate vials. • Stable at room temperature for 24 hrs or for 7 days if refrigerated after reconstitution.

**PO**
**Storage** • Refrigerate gelatin capsules.

### ▦ IV INCOMPATIBILITIES

**VePesid:** Cefepime (Maxipime), filgrastim (Neupogen). **Etopophos:** Amphotericin B (Fungizone), cefepime (Maxipime), chlorpromazine (Thorazine), methylprednisolone (Solu-Medrol), prochlorperazine (Compazine).

### ▦ IV COMPATIBILITIES

**VePesid:** Carboplatin (Paraplatin), cisplatin (Platinol), cytarabine (Cytosar), daunorubicin (Cerubidine), doxorubicin (Adriamycin), granisetron (Kytril), mitoxantrone (Novantrone), ondansetron (Zofran). **Etopophos:** Carboplatin (Paraplatin), cisplatin (Platinol), cytarabine (Cytosar), dacarbazine (DTIC-Dome), daunorubicin (Cerubidine), dexamethasone (Decadron), diphenhydramine (Benadryl), doxorubicin (Adriamycin), granisetron (Kytril), magnesium sulfate, mannitol, mitoxantrone (Novantrone), ondansetron (Zofran), potassium chloride.

## INDICATIONS/ROUTES/DOSAGE

◀ALERT▶ Dosage individualized based on clinical response, tolerance to adverse effects. Treatment repeated at 3- to 4-wk intervals. Refer to individual protocols.

**Refractory Testicular Tumors**
**IV: ADULTS:** 50–100 mg/m$^2$/day on days 1–5, or 100 mg/m$^2$/day on days 1, 3, 5 (as combination therapy). Give q3–4wks for 3–4 courses.

**Small-Cell Lung Carcinoma**
**PO: ADULTS:** Twice the IV dose rounded to nearest 50 mg. Give once daily for doses 200 mg or less, in divided doses for dosages greater than 200 mg.

**IV: ADULTS:** 35 mg/m$^2$/day for 4 consecutive days up to 50 mg/m$^2$/day for 5 consecutive days q3–4wks (as combination therapy).

**Dosage in Renal Impairment**

| Creatinine Clearance | Dosage |
|---|---|
| 15–50 ml/min | 75% of normal dose |
| Less than 15 ml/min | Consider further dose reduction. |

**Dosage in Hepatic Impairment**
No dose adjustment.

## SIDE EFFECTS

**Frequent (66%–43%):** Mild to moderate nausea/vomiting, alopecia. **Occasional (13%–6%):** Diarrhea, anorexia, stomatitis. **Rare (2% or less):** Hypotension, peripheral neuropathy.

## ADVERSE EFFECTS/ TOXIC REACTIONS

Myelosuppression manifested as hematologic toxicity, principally anemia, leukopenia (occurring 7–14 days after drug administration), thrombocytopenia (occurring 9–16 days after administration), and, to lesser extent, pancytopenia. Bone marrow recovery occurs by day 20. Hepatotoxicity occurs occasionally.

## NURSING CONSIDERATIONS

### BASELINE ASSESSMENT

Obtain CBC before and at frequent intervals during therapy. Antiemetics readily control nausea, vomiting.

### INTERVENTION/EVALUATION

Monitor Hgb, Hct, WBC, platelet count, B/P, hepatic/renal function tests. Monitor daily pattern of bowel activity, stool consistency. Monitor for hematologic toxicity (fever, sore throat, signs of local infection, unusual bruising/bleeding from any site), symptoms of anemia (excessive fatigue, weakness). Assess for paresthesia (peripheral neuropathy). Monitor for stomatitis.

E

• Hair loss is reversible, but new hair growth may have different color, texture. • Do not have immunizations without physician's approval (drug lowers resistance). • Avoid contact with those who have recently received live virus vaccine. • Promptly report fever, sore throat, signs of local infection, unusual bruising or bleeding from any site, burning or pain with urination, numbness in extremities, yellowing of skin or eyes.

# everolimus　

e-veer-oh-li-mus
(Afinitor, Afinitor Disperz, Zortress)
**Do not confuse Afinitor with Lipitor, or everolimus with sirolimus, tacrolimus, or temsirolimus.**

■ **BLACK BOX ALERT** ■ Immunosuppressant (may result in infection, malignancy including lymphoma or skin cancer); increased risk of nephrotoxicity in renal transplants (avoid standard doses of cyclosporine); increased risk of renal arterial or venous thrombosis in renal transplants.

## ◆CLASSIFICATION

**PHARMACOTHERAPEUTIC:** Enzyme inhibitor. **CLINICAL:** Antineoplastic, immunosuppressant.

## USES

**Afinitor:** Treatment of advanced renal cell carcinoma after failure of treatment with sunitinib or sorafenib. Treatment of subependymal giant cell astrocytoma (SEGA) associated with tuberous sclerosis. Treatment of progressive neuroendocrine tumors of pancreatic origin and progressive, well-differentiated, non-functional neuroendocrine tumors of GI or lung origin. Treatment of advanced hormone receptor–positive, HER2-negative breast cancer in postmenopausal women. Treatment of tuberous sclerosis complex (TSC) not requiring immediate surgery. **Afinitor Disperz:** Treatment of SEGA associated with TSC requiring intervention but that cannot be curatively resected. **Zortress:** Prophylaxis of organ rejection after kidney/liver transplant at low to moderate immunologic risk. **OFF-LABEL:** Relapsed or refractory Waldenström's macroglobulinemia. Treatment of progressive advanced carcinoid tumors.

## PRECAUTIONS

**Contraindications:** Hypersensitivity to everolimus, sirolimus, other rapamycin derivatives. **Cautions:** Noninfectious pneumonitis; viral, fungal, or bacterial infection; oral ulceration; mucositis; current immunosuppression; hereditary galactose intolerance; renal/hepatic impairment; hyperlipidemia; concurrent use of CYP3A4 inducers and inhibitors (see Interactions). Medications known to cause angioedema.

## ACTION

Binds to the FK binding protein, reducing protein synthesis and cell proliferation. Also reduces lipoma volume. **Therapeutic Effect:** Reduces cell proliferation, produces cell death.

## PHARMACOKINETICS

Peak concentration occurs in 1–2 hrs following administration, with steady-state levels achieved in 2 wks. Undergoes extensive hepatic metabolism. Protein binding: 74%. Eliminated in feces (80%), urine (5%). **Half-life:** 30 hrs.

## ⧖ LIFESPAN CONSIDERATIONS

**Pregnancy/Lactation:** May cause fetal harm. Unknown if distributed in breast milk. **Children:** Safety and efficacy not established. **Elderly:** No age-related precautions noted.

## INTERACTIONS

**DRUG: CYP3A4 inhibitors (e.g., atazanavir, clarithromycin, indinavir, itraconazole, ketoconazole, nefazodone, nelfinavir, ritonavir, saquinavir, voriconazole)** may increase concentration. **CYP3A4 inducers (e.g.,**

carbamazepine, dexamethasone, phenobarbital, phenytoin, rifabutin, rifampin, rifapentine) may decrease concentration. **P-gp inhibitors (e.g., cyclosporine)** may increase everolimus concentration, toxicity. **Statins** may increase risk of rhabdomyolysis. **FOOD: High-fat meals** may reduce plasma concentration. **Grapefruit products** may increase concentration (potential for myelotoxicity, nephrotoxicity). **HERBAL:** St. John's wort may decrease plasma concentration. **LAB VALUES:** May increase serum BUN, creatinine, glucose, triglycerides, lipids. May decrease WBCs, neutrophils, Hgb, platelets.

## AVAILABILITY (Rx)

**Tablets (Zortress):** 0.25 mg, 0.5 mg, 0.75 mg. **Tablets (Afinitor):** 2.5 mg, 5 mg, 7.5 mg, 10 mg. **Tablets for Oral Suspension (Afinitor Disperz):** 2 mg, 3 mg, 5 mg.

## ADMINISTRATION/HANDLING

• Give without regard to food. • Swallow whole. Do not crush/cut Afinitor or Zortress. • Avoid direct contact of crushed tablets with skin or mucous membranes. If unable to swallow, disperse Afinitor Disperz in water with gentle stirring, give immediately.

## INDICATIONS/ROUTES/DOSAGE

**◀ALERT▶** If pt requires coadministration of a strong CYP3A4 inducers (e.g., carbamazepine, dexamethasone, phenobarbital, phenytoin, rifabutin, rifampin), consider doubling the dose. If strong inducer is discontinued, reduce everolimus to dose used prior to initiation. If moderate CYP3A4 inhibitors are required, reduce dose by 50%.

**Renal Carcinoma, Neuroendocrine Tumors, Breast Cancer, TSC**
**PO: ADULTS, ELDERLY: (Afinitor):** 10 mg once daily at same time every day. Coadministration with CYP3A4 inhibitors or P-gp inhibitors: 2.5 mg once daily. May increase to 5 mg/day. Coadministration

with CYP3A4 inducers: Increase by 5-mg increments up to 20 mg/day.

**SEGA with TSC**
**PO: ADULTS, CHILDREN:** 4.5 mg/m² once daily. **Coadministration with CYP3A4 inhibitors or P-gb inhibitors:** 2.5 mg/m²/day. **Coadministration with CYP3A4 inducers:** 9 mg/m²/day.

**Renal Transplant Prophylaxis**
**PO: ADULTS, ELDERLY: (Zortress):** Initially, 0.75 mg 2 times/day. Give in combination with basiliximab and concurrently with reduced doses of cyclosporine and corticosteroids.

**Liver Transplant Prophylaxis**
**PO: ADULTS, ELDERLY: (Zortress):** Initially, 1 mg 2 times/day. Adjust dose at 4–5-day intervals based on serum concentration, tolerability, and response.

**Astrocytoma**
**PO: ADULTS, ELDERLY:** Initially, 4.5 mg/m2 once daily, titrated to attain trough concentration of 5–15 ng/ml. **If trough greater than 15 ng/ml:** reduce dose by 2.5 mg/day (tablets) or 2 mg/day (tablets for oral suspension). **If trough less than 15 ng/ml:** increase dose by 2.5 mg/day (tablets) or 2 mg/day (tablets for oral suspension).

**Dosage in Renal Impairment**
No dose adjustment.

**Dosage in Hepatic Impairment**

| | Mild | Moderate | Severe |
|---|---|---|---|
| Breast Cancer PNET, RCC, renal angiomyolipoma | 7.5 mg/day or 5 mg/day | 5 mg/day or 2.5 mg/day | 2.5 mg/day |
| Liver/Renal transplant | Reduce dose by 33% | Reduce dose by 50% | Reduce dose by 50% |
| SEGA | No change | No change | Initial dose 2.5 mg/m²/day |

---

✦ Canadian trade name      **Non-Crushable Drug**      **High Alert drug**

## SIDE EFFECTS

**Common (44%–26%):** Stomatitis, asthenia. Diarrhea, cough, rash, nausea. **Frequent (25%–20%):** Peripheral edema, anorexia, dyspnea, vomiting, pyrexia. **Occasional (19%–10%):** Mucosal inflammation, headache, epistaxis, pruritus, dry skin, epigastric distress, extremity pain. **Rare (less than 10%):** Abdominal pain, insomnia, dry mouth, dizziness, paresthesia, eyelid edema, hypertension, nail disorder, chills.

## ADVERSE EFFECTS/ TOXIC REACTIONS

Noninfectious pneumonitis characterized as hypoxia, pleural effusion, cough, or dyspnea was reported in 14% of pts; Grade 3 noninfectious pneumonitis reported in 4%. Localized and systemic infections, including pneumonia, other bacterial infections, and invasive fungal infections, have occurred due to everolimus immunosuppressive properties. Renal failure occurs in 3% of pts.

## NURSING CONSIDERATIONS

### BASELINE ASSESSMENT

Assess medical history, esp. renal function, use of other immunosuppressants. Obtain CBC, BMP, LFT before treatment begins and routinely thereafter.

### INTERVENTION/EVALUATION

Offer antiemetics to control nausea, vomiting. Monitor daily pattern of bowel activity, stool consistency. Assess skin for evidence of rash, edema. Monitor CBC, particularly Hgb, platelet, neutrophil count; BUN, creatinine, LFT. Monitor for shortness of breath, fatigue, hypertension. Assess mouth for stomatitis, mucositis.

### PATIENT/FAMILY TEACHING

• Take dose at same time each day. • Avoid crowds, those with known infection. • Avoid contact with anyone who recently received live virus vaccine. • Do not have immunizations without physician's approval (drug lowers body resistance). • Promptly report fever, unusual bruising/bleeding from any site. • Avoid direct contact of crushed tablets with skin or mucous membrane (wash thoroughly if contact occurs). • Avoid grapefruit products.

# evolocumab

e-voe-**lok**-ue-mab
(Repatha)
■ **BLACK BOX ALERT** ■ Do not confuse evolocumab with alirocumab or raxibacumab.

## ◆CLASSIFICATION

**PHARMACOTHERAPEUTIC:** Proprotein convertase subtilison kexin 9 (PCSK9) inhibitor. **CLINICAL:** Antihyperlipidemic, monoclonal antibody.

## USES

Adjunct to diet and maximally tolerated statin therapy for the treatment of adults with heterozygous familial hypercholesterolemia or clinical atherosclerotic cardiovascular disease, who require additional lowering of low-density lipoprotein cholesterol (LDL-C). Adjunct to diet and other LDL-lowering therapies (e.g., statins, ezetimibe, LDL apheresis) in pts with homozygous familial hypercholesterolemia who requires additional lowering of LDL-C.

## PRECAUTIONS

**Contraindications:** Hypersensitivity to evolocumab. **Cautions:** Active infection.

## ACTION

Binds to and inhibits circulating PCSK9 from binding to LDL receptor (LDLR), preventing LDLR degradation and allowing LDLR to recycle back to the liver surface. Increases number of LDLR available to clear LDL from the blood. **Therapeutic Effect:** Lowers LDL-C levels.

## PHARMACOKINETICS

Distributed primarily in circulatory system. Metabolized and eliminated by protein degradation into small peptides, amino acids. Peak plasma concentration: 3–4 days. Steady state reached in 12 wks. **Half-life:** 11–17 days.

## ⏳ LIFESPAN CONSIDERATIONS

**Pregnancy/Lactation:** May cross placental barrier, esp. during second and third trimester. Unknown if distributed in breast milk; however, human immunoglobulin G is present breast milk. Must either discontinue drug or discontinue breastfeeding. **Children:** Safety and efficacy not established in pts with homozygous familial hypercholesterolemia who are younger than 13 yrs. Safety and efficacy not established pts with heterozygous familial hypercholesterolemia or primary hypercholesterolemia. **Elderly:** No age-related precautions noted.

## INTERACTIONS

**DRUG:** None known. **HERBAL:** None significant. **FOOD:** None known. **LAB VALUES:** Expected to decrease serum LDL-C levels.

## AVAILABILITY (Rx)

**Injection Solution:** 140 mg/mL in single-use prefilled syringe, auto-injector. 420 mg/3.5 mL single use Pushtronex system (on body infusor with prefilled cartridge).

## ADMINISTRATION/HANDLING

**Subcutaneous** • Remove auto-injector/prefilled syringe from refrigerator and allow to passively warm to room temperature. • Visually inspect for particulate matter or discoloration. Solution should appear clear to opalescent, colorless to pale yellow in color. Do not use if solution is cloudy, discolored, contains particles; if the auto-injector/prefilled syringe has been dropped, or if the cap is missing or not securely attached. • Once cap is removed, subcutaneously insert needle into abdomen, outer thigh, or upper arm region and inject solution. • Do not inject into areas of active skin disease or injury such as sunburns, skin rashes, inflammation, or skin infections. • If using auto-injector, depress gray button until a click is heard and allow 15 sec to pass to ensure solution is fully injected. • Rotate injection sites.

**Storage** • Refrigerate auto-injector/prefilled syringe in original carton. • May store at room temperature for no more than 30 days. • Protect from direct light. • Do not freeze.

## INDICATIONS/ROUTES/DOSAGE

**Heterozygous Familial Hypercholesterolemia**
**SQ: ADULTS, ELDERLY:** 140 mg q2wks or 420 mg once monthly. Give 420 mg dose as 3 separate injections within 30 min. If switching between regimens, give the first dose of the new regimen on the next scheduled date of the prior regimen. If a q2wk or once monthly dose is missed, either administer as soon as possible if there are more than 7 days until the next scheduled dose or skip the missed dose and administer the next dose according to the original schedule.

**Homozygous Familial Hypercholesterolemia**
**SQ: ADULTS, ELDERLY:** 420 mg once monthly as 3 separate injections within 30 min. If a once monthly dose is missed, administer as soon as possible if there are more than 7 days until the next scheduled dose or skip the missed dose according to the original schedule.

**Dosage in Renal/Hepatic Impairment**
**Mild to moderate impairment:** No dose adjustment. **Severe impairment:** Not studied; use caution.

## SIDE EFFECTS

**Occasional (6%–3%):** Back pain, injection site reactions (bruising, erythema, localized pain), cough, headache, myalgia, dizziness, musculoskeletal pain, hypertension, diarrhea.

## ADVERSE EFFECTS/TOXIC REACTIONS

Serious hypersensitivity reactions (e.g., pruritus, rash, urticaria) reported in (5.1% of pts). Infectious processes such as gastroenteritis (3% of pts), influenza (7.5% of pts), nasopharyngitis (10.5% of pts), sinusitis (4.2% of pts), upper respiratory tract infection (9.3% of pts), UTI (4.5% of pts) have occurred. Musculoskeletal events including arthralgia, back pain, myalgia reported in 14% of pts. Immunogenicity (auto-evolocumab antibodies) occurred in less than 1% of pts.

## NURSING CONSIDERATIONS

### BASELINE ASSESSMENT

Obtain baseline LDL-C level. Verify whether pt is positive for heterozygous or homozygous familial hypercholesterolemia. Question history of hypersensitivity reaction. Assess potential injection sites for sunburns, skin rashes, inflammation, skin infections. Verify pregnancy status.

### INTERVENTION/EVALUATION

Obtain LDL-C level within 4–8 wks after initiation or with any change in dosage. Monitor for hypersensitivity reaction. If hypersensitivity reaction occurs, discontinue therapy and treat symptoms accordingly; monitor until symptoms resolve. Monitor for respiratory infections, musculoskeletal events.

### PATIENT/FAMILY TEACHING

• A health care provider will show you how to properly mix and inject your medication. You must demonstrate correct preparation and injection techniques before using medication at home. • Inject dose under the skin (SQ) of your outer thigh, abdomen, or upper arm; do not inject into muscle or vein. • Rotate injection sites. • Discard used needles using regulated sharps containers. • Treatment may cause serious allergic reactions such as difficulty breathing, itching, hives, rash. If allergic reaction occurs, seek immediate medical attention. • Do not reuse auto-injector/prefilled syringes. • Report symptoms of infection.

# exemestane

ex-e-**mes**-tane
(Aromasin)
**Do not confuse Aromasin with Arimidex, or exemestane with estramustine.**

## ◆CLASSIFICATION

**PHARMACOTHERAPEUTIC:** Hormone.
**CLINICAL:** Antineoplastic.

## USES

Treatment of advanced breast cancer in postmenopausal women whose disease has progressed following tamoxifen therapy. Adjuvant treatment of postmenopausal women with estrogen-receptor positive early breast cancer after 2–3 yrs of tamoxifen therapy for completion of 5 consecutive yrs of adjuvant hormonal therapy. **OFF-LABEL:** Reduces risk of invasive breast cancer in postmenopausal women; treatment of endometrial cancer, uterine sarcoma.

## PRECAUTIONS

**Contraindications:** Hypersensitivity to exemestane. Women who are pregnant or may become pregnant; use in premenopausal women. **Cautions:** Concomitant use of estrogen-containing agents, strong CYP3A4 inducers (e.g., phenobarbital, rifampin).

## ACTION

Inactivates aromatase, the principal enzyme that converts androgens to estrogens in both premenopausal and postmenopausal women, lowering circulating estrogen level. **Therapeutic Effect:** Inhibits

---

growth of breast cancers stimulated by estrogens.

## PHARMACOKINETICS

Rapidly absorbed after PO administration. Protein binding: 90%. Distributed extensively into tissues. Metabolized in liver; eliminated in urine and feces. **Half-life:** 24 hrs.

## ⌛ LIFESPAN CONSIDERATIONS

**Pregnancy/Lactation:** Indicated for postmenopausal women. **Children:** Not indicated for use in this pt population. **Elderly:** No age-related precautions noted.

## INTERACTIONS

**DRUG: CYP3A4 inducers (e.g., phenobarbital, rifampin)** may decrease concentration/effect. **HERBAL: St. John's wort** may decrease concentration. Avoid **black cohosh, dong quai** in estrogen-dependent tumors. **FOOD:** None known. **LAB VALUES:** May increase serum alkaline phosphatase, ALT, AST.

## AVAILABILITY (Rx)

**Tablets:** 25 mg.

## ADMINISTRATION/HANDLING

**PO**
• Give after meals.

## INDICATIONS/ROUTES/DOSAGE

**Breast Cancer (Early)**
**PO: ADULTS, ELDERLY:** 25 mg once daily after a meal (following 2–3 yrs tamoxifen therapy) for total duration of 5 yrs.

**Breast Cancer (Advanced)**
**PO: ADULTS, ELDERLY:** 25 mg once daily after a meal. 50 mg/day when used concurrently with potent CYP3A4 inducers (e.g., rifampin, phenytoin).

**Dosage in Renal/Hepatic Impairment**
No dose adjustment.

## SIDE EFFECTS

**Frequent (22%–10%):** Fatigue, nausea, depression, hot flashes, pain, insomnia, anxiety, dyspnea. **Occasional (8%–5%):** Headache, dizziness, vomiting, peripheral edema, abdominal pain, anorexia, flu-like symptoms, diaphoresis, constipation, hypertension. **Rare (4%):** Diarrhea.

## ADVERSE EFFECTS/ TOXIC REACTIONS

MI has been noted.

## NURSING CONSIDERATIONS

### INTERVENTION/EVALUATION

Monitor for onset of depression. Assess sleep pattern. Monitor for and assist with ambulation if dizziness occurs. Assess for headache. Offer antiemetic for nausea/vomiting.

### PATIENT/FAMILY TEACHING

• Report if nausea, hot flashes become unmanageable. • Avoid tasks that require alertness, motor skills until response to drug is established. • Best taken after meals and at same time each day.

---

## *exenatide*    `HIGH ALERT`

ex-**en**-a-tide
(Bydureon, Byetta)
■ **BLACK BOX ALERT** ■ (Bydureon): Risk of thyroid C-cell tumors.

## ◆CLASSIFICATION

**PHARMACOTHERAPEUTIC:** Incretin mimetic. **CLINICAL:** Antidiabetic.

## USES

Adjunct to diet, exercise to improve glycemic control in pts with type 2 diabetes mellitus.

## PRECAUTIONS

**Contraindications:** Hypersensitivity to exenatide. Bydureon only: History of

---

medullary thyroid carcinoma. Pts with multiple endocrine neoplasia syndrome type 2 (MEN2). **Cautions:** Diabetic keto-acidosis, type 1 diabetes mellitus. Pts with renal transplantation or moderate renal impairment. Not recommended in severe renal impairment, severe GI disease, pancreatitis.

## ACTION

Stimulates release of insulin from beta cells of pancreas, mimics enhancement of glucose-dependent insulin secretion, suppresses elevated glucagon secretion, slows gastric emptying (central action increases satiety). **Therapeutic Effect:** Improves glycemic control by increasing postmeal insulin secretion, decreasing postmeal glucagon levels, delaying gastric emptying, and increasing satiety.

## PHARMACOKINETICS

Minimal systemic metabolism. Eliminated by glomerular filtration with subsequent proteolytic degradation. **Half-life:** 2.4 hrs.

## ⧖ LIFESPAN CONSIDERATIONS

**Pregnancy/Lactation:** Unknown if distributed in breast milk. **Children:** Safety and efficacy not established. **Elderly:** No age-related precautions noted.

## INTERACTIONS

**DRUG:** May decrease effects of **digoxin, lovastatin.** May increase bleeding time, risk of bleeding when used with **warfarin. HERBAL:** None significant. **FOOD:** None known. **LAB VALUES:** None known.

## AVAILABILITY (Rx)

**Injection, Solution (Prefilled Pen):** (Byetta) 10 mcg/0.04 ml (2.4 ml); 5 mcg/0.02 ml (1.2 ml). **Injection, Suspension (Bydureon):** 2 mg.

## ADMINISTRATION/HANDLING

**Subcutaneous**
• May be given in thigh, abdomen, upper arm. • Rotation of injection sites is

essential; maintain careful injection site record. • Give within 60 min before morning and evening meals. Give suspension immediately after powder is suspended. **Storage** • Refrigerate prefilled pens. • Discard if freezing occurs. • May be stored at room temperature after first use. • Discard pen 30 days after initial use.

## INDICATIONS/ROUTE/DOSAGE

**Diabetes Mellitus**
**SQ: ADULTS, ELDERLY:** (Byetta) 5 mcg per dose given twice daily at any time within the 60-min period before the morning and evening meals. Dose may be increased to 10 mcg twice daily after 1 mo of therapy. (Bydureon): 2 mg once q7days.

**Dosage in Renal Impairment**
**Mild impairment:** No dose adjustment. **Moderate impairment:** Use caution. **Severe impairment (CrCl less than 30 ml/min or ESRD):** Not recommended.

**Dosage in Hepatic Impairment**
No dose adjustment.

## SIDE EFFECTS

**(Byetta) Frequent (44%):** Nausea. **Occasional (13%–6%):** Diarrhea, vomiting, dizziness, anxiety, dyspepsia. **Rare (less than 6%):** Weakness. **(Bydureon) 5% or greater:** Nausea, diarrhea, headache, constipation, vomiting, dyspepsia, injection site pruritus or nodule.

## ADVERSE EFFECTS/ TOXIC REACTIONS

With concurrent sulfonylurea, hypoglycemia occurs in 36% when given a 10-mcg dose of exenatide, 16% when given a 5-mcg dose. May cause acute pancreatitis.

## NURSING CONSIDERATIONS

### BASELINE ASSESSMENT

Check serum glucose before administration. Discuss lifestyle to determine extent of learning, emotional needs. Ensure follow-up instruction if pt or family does not thoroughly understand diabetes management, glucose-testing technique. At least 1 mo should elapse to assess response to drug before new dose adjustment is made.

**INTERVENTION/EVALUATION**

Monitor serum glucose, food intake, renal function. Assess for hypoglycemia (cool wet skin, tremors, dizziness, anxiety, headache, tachycardia, numbness in mouth, hunger, diplopia), hyperglycemia (polyuria, polyphagia, polydipsia, nausea, vomiting, dim vision, fatigue, deep rapid breathing). Be alert to conditions that alter glucose requirements (fever, increased activity or stress, surgical procedure).

**PATIENT/FAMILY TEACHING**

• Diabetes mellitus requires lifelong control. • Prescribed diet and exercise are principal parts of treatment. Do not skip, delay meals. • Continue to adhere to dietary instructions, regular exercise program, regular testing of serum glucose. • When taking combination therapy with a sulfonylurea, have source of glucose available to treat symptoms of hypoglycemia. • Report any unexplained severe abdominal pain with or without nausea or vomiting.

# ezetimibe

**TOP 100**

e-zet-i-mib
(Apo-Ezetimibe✤, Ezetrol ✤, <u>Zetia</u>)
**Do not confuse Zetia with Zebeta or Zestril.**

## FIXED-COMBINATION(S)

**Liptruzet:** ezetimibe/atorvastatin (statin): 10 mg/10 mg, 10 mg/20 mg, 10 mg/40 mg, 10 mg/80 mg. **Vytorin:** ezetimibe/simvastatin (statin): 10 mg/10 mg, 10 mg/20 mg, 10 mg/40 mg, 10 mg/80 mg.

## ◆CLASSIFICATION

**PHARMACOTHERAPEUTIC:** Antihyperlipidemic. **CLINICAL:** Anticholesterol agent.

## USES

Adjunct to diet for treatment of primary hypercholesterolemia (monotherapy or in combination with HMG-CoA reductase inhibitors [statins]), homozygous sitosterolemia, homozygous familial hypercholesterolemia (combined with atorvastatin or simvastatin). Mixed hyperlipidemia (in combination with fenofibrate).

## PRECAUTIONS

**Contraindications:** Hypersensitivity to ezetimibe. Concurrent use of an HMG-CoA reductase inhibitor (atorvastatin, fluvastatin, lovastatin, pravastatin, simvastatin) in pts with active hepatic disease or unexplained persistent elevations in serum transaminase; pregnancy and breastfeeding (when used with a statin). **Cautions:** Severe renal or mild hepatic impairment. Not recommended in those with moderate or severe hepatic impairment.

## ACTION

Inhibits cholesterol absorption in brush border of small intestine, leading to decrease in delivery of intestinal cholesterol to liver. **Therapeutic Effect:** Reduces total serum cholesterol, LDL, triglyceride; increases HDL.

## PHARMACOKINETICS

Well absorbed following PO administration. Protein binding: greater than 90%. Metabolized in small intestine and liver. Excreted in feces (78%), urine (11%). **Half-life:** 22 hrs.

## ⏳ LIFESPAN CONSIDERATIONS

**Pregnancy/Lactation:** Unknown if drug crosses placenta or is distributed in breast milk. **Children:** Safety and efficacy not established in pts 10 yrs or younger. **Elderly:** Age-related mild hepatic impairment may require dosage adjustment.

## INTERACTIONS

**DRUG: Antacids containing aluminum or magnesium, cyclosporine, fenofibrate, gemfibrozil** increase concentration. **Cholestyramine resin** decreases effectiveness. **HERBAL:** None significant. **FOOD:** None known. **LAB VALUES:** May increase serum alkaline phosphatase, bilirubin, ALT, AST.

## AVAILABILITY (Rx)

**Tablets:** 10 mg.

## ADMINISTRATION/HANDLING

• Give without regard to food. • May give at same time as statins. Give at least 2 hrs before or 4 hrs after bile acid sequestrants.

## INDICATIONS/ROUTES/DOSAGE

**Hypercholesterolemia**
**PO: ADULTS, ELDERLY, CHILDREN, 10 YRS AND OLDER:** Initially, 10 mg once daily, given with or without food. If pt is also receiving a bile acid sequestrant, give ezetimibe at least 2 hrs before or at least 4 hrs after bile acid sequestrant.

**Dosage in Renal Impairment**
No dose adjustment.

**Dosage in Hepatic Impairment**
**Mild impairment:** No dose adjustment. **Moderate to severe impairment:** Not recommended.

## SIDE EFFECTS

**Occasional (4%–3%):** Back pain, diarrhea, arthralgia, sinusitis, abdominal pain. **Rare (2%):** Cough, pharyngitis, fatigue, depression.

## ADVERSE EFFECTS/ TOXIC REACTIONS

Hepatitis, hypersensitivity reaction, myopathy, rhabdomyolysis occur rarely.

## NURSING CONSIDERATIONS

### BASELINE ASSESSMENT
Obtain diet history, esp. fat consumption. Obtain serum cholesterol, triglycerides, hepatic function tests, blood counts during initial therapy and periodically during treatment. Treatment should be discontinued if hepatic enzyme levels persist more than 3 times normal limit.

### INTERVENTION/EVALUATION
Monitor daily pattern of bowel activity, stool consistency. Question pt for signs/symptoms of back pain, abdominal disturbances. Monitor serum cholesterol, triglycerides for therapeutic response.

### PATIENT/FAMILY TEACHING
• Periodic laboratory tests are essential part of therapy. • Do not stop medication without consulting physician. • Report muscular or bone pain. • May take at same time as statins. Take at least 2 hrs before or 4 hrs after cholestyramine, colestipol, colesevelam.

## ezogabine

e-**zog**-a-bine
(Potiga)
■ **BLACK BOX ALERT** ■ Retinal abnormalities may progress to vision loss.

## ◆CLASSIFICATION

**PHARMACOTHERAPEUTIC:** Potassium channel opener **(Schedule V).**
**CLINICAL:** Anticonvulsant.

## USES

Adjunctive therapy for treatment of partial-onset seizures in pts 18 yrs of age and older.

## PRECAUTIONS

**Contraindications:** Hypersensitivity to ezogabine. **Cautions:** Hepatic/renal impairment, BPH, urinary retention, chronic cognitive impairment, prolonged QT interval, psychiatric history, pts at risk for suicide. Hypokalemia, hypomagnesemia, familial long-QT syndrome, medications that prolong QT interval, hypothyroidism, HF, ventricular arrhythmias, elderly.

## ACTION

Binds to voltage-gated potassium channels, stabilizing the channels in open formation and enhancing the M current. **Therapeutic Effect:** Regulates neuronal excitability, suppressing seizure activity.

## PHARMACOKINETICS

Rapidly absorbed after PO administration. Peak concentration: 0.5–2 hrs. Protein binding: 80%. Metabolized by glucuronidation and acetylation. Primarily excreted in urine (85%), feces (14%). **Half-life:** 7–11 hrs.

## ☒ LIFESPAN CONSIDERATIONS

**Pregnancy/Lactation:** Unknown if drug crosses placenta or is distributed in breast milk. Must either discontinue breastfeeding or discontinue drug regimen. **Children:** Safety and efficacy not established in pts under 18 yrs of age. **Elderly:** Dosage adjustment recommended for pts older than 65 yrs.

## INTERACTIONS

**DRUG: Phenytoin, carbamazepine** may decrease plasma concentration/effects. **Alcohol** may increase concentration/adverse effects. May inhibit clearance of **digoxin. HERBAL:** None known. **FOOD:** None significant. **LAB VALUES:** May create falsely elevated urine bilirubin level.

## AVAILABILITY (Rx)

**Tablets:** 50 mg, 200 mg, 300 mg, 400 mg.

## ADMINISTRATION/HANDLING

• May give without regard to food. Swallow tablets whole.

## INDICATIONS/ROUTES/DOSAGE

### Partial Seizures

**◀ALERT▶** Increase at wkly intervals by no more than 50 mg 3 times daily (150 mg/day).

**PO: ADULTS:** Initially, 100 mg 3 times daily. May increase to maintenance dose of 200–400 mg 3 times daily (600–1,200 mg daily). **Maximum:** 1,200 mg/day. **ELDERLY:** Initially, 50 mg 3 times/day. May increase wkly to therapeutic level. **Maximum:** 250 mg 3 times/day (750 mg/day).

### Dosage Modification

**Renal Impairment (CrCl less than 50 ml/min or ESRD):** 50 mg 3 times/day for 7 days. Then increase to therapeutic level. **Maximum:** 200 mg 3 times/day (600 mg/day). **Mild Hepatic Impairment (Child-Pugh score less than 9):** Initially, 50 mg 3 times/day for 7 days. Then increase to therapeutic level. **Maximum:** 250 mg 3 times/day (750 mg/day). **Severe Hepatic Impairment (Child-Pugh score greater than 9):** Initially, 50 mg 3 times/day for 7 days. Then increase to therapeutic level. **Maximum:** 200 mg 3 times/day (600 mg/day). **Discontinuation:** Reduce gradually over period of at least 3 wks.

## SIDE EFFECTS

**Frequent (23%–15%):** Dizziness, somnolence, fatigue. **Occasional (8%–4%):** Tremor, vertigo, abnormal coordination, nausea, diplopia, attention disturbance, memory impairment, asthenia, blurred vision, gait disturbance, aphasia, dysarthria, balance disorder. **Rare (3%–1%):** Constipation, anxiety, weight gain, dyspepsia, amnesia, dysphasia, disorientation, dysuria, urinary hesitation, hematuria, urine discoloration, psychotic behavior.

## ADVERSE EFFECTS/ TOXIC REACTIONS

Urinary retention requiring catheterization, prolonged QT interval, myoclonus, peripheral edema, hypokinesia, dysphasia, hyperhydrosis, malaise reported in less than 2% of pts. Hydronephrosis associated with baseline renal impairment, increased risk of psychosis, hallucinations, suicidal ideation, depression, aggression, mania noted.

## NURSING CONSIDERATIONS

### BASELINE ASSESSMENT

Review history of seizure disorder (intensity, frequency, duration, LOC). Question history of BPH, urinary retention, cognitive impairment, psychiatric disorder, hepatic/renal impairment, alcoholism, prolonged QT syndrome. Obtain full medication history including digoxin, antiarrhythmics, adjunct anticonvulsant therapy. Obtain baseline EKG, digoxin level if applicable. Question possibility of pregnancy or current breastfeeding.

### INTERVENTION/EVALUATION

Initiate seizure precautions and observe for seizure activity. Assist with ambulation if dizziness occurs. Monitor for depression, suicidal ideation, unusual behavior, mania, anxiety. Routinely monitor digoxin levels. Monitor QT interval for pts with HF, ventricular hypertrophy, hypokalemia, hypomagnesemia.

### PATIENT/FAMILY TEACHING

• Monitor closely for seizure activity.
• Immediately report any new medications, trouble urinating, palpitations, pregnancy, or plans to breastfeed. • Avoid alcohol.
• Report any thoughts of suicide, aggressive behavior, depression, anxiety, trouble sleeping, impulsiveness, unusual behavior.
• Noncompliance may lead to increased risk of seizures.

# famciclovir

fam-**sye**-klo-veer
(Apo-Famciclovir ✦, Famvir)
**Do not confuse famciclovir
with acyclovir, ganciclovir, or
valganciclovir; or Famvir with
Femara.**

## ◆CLASSIFICATION

**PHARMACOTHERAPEUTIC:** Synthetic
nucleoside. **CLINICAL:** Antiviral.

## USES

Treatment of acute herpes zoster (shingles) in immunocompetent pts, treatment and suppression of recurrent genital herpes in immunocompetent pts, treatment of recurrent mucocutaneous herpes simplex in HIV-infected pts. Treatment of recurrent herpes labialis (cold sores) in immunocompetent pts.

## PRECAUTIONS

**Contraindications:** Hypersensitivity to famciclovir, penciclovir. **Cautions:** Renal impairment. Avoid use in galactose intolerance, severe lactose deficiency, or glucose-galactose malabsorption syndromes.

## ACTION

Inhibits HSV-2 polymerase, inhibiting herpes viral DNA synthesis and replication. **Therapeutic Effect:** Suppresses replication of herpes simplex virus, varicella-zoster virus.

## PHARMACOKINETICS

Rapidly absorbed. Protein binding: 20%–25%. Rapidly metabolized to penciclovir by enzymes in GI tract, liver, plasma. Eliminated unchanged in urine. Removed by hemodialysis. **Half-life:** 2–3 hrs (increased in severe renal failure).

## ⧗ LIFESPAN CONSIDERATIONS

**Pregnancy/Lactation:** Unknown if excreted in breast milk. **Children:** Safety and efficacy not established. **Elderly:** Age-related renal impairment may require dosage adjustment.

## INTERACTIONS

**DRUG: Probenecid, methotrexate** may increase adverse effects. **HERBAL:** None significant. **FOOD:** None known. **LAB VALUES:** May increase ALT, AST, amylase, bilirubin, lipase. May decrease neutrophils, platelets.

## AVAILABILITY (Rx)

**Tablets:** 125 mg, 250 mg, 500 mg.

## ADMINISTRATION/HANDLING

**PO**
• Give without regard to meals. • Give with food to decrease GI distress.

## INDICATIONS/ROUTES/DOSAGE

**Herpes Zoster (Shingles)**
**PO: ADULTS:** 500 mg q8h for 7 days. Begin as soon as possible after diagnosis and within 72 hrs of rash onset. (**HIV pts**): 500 mg 3 times/day for 7–10 days.

**Genital Herpes Simplex (Initial)**
**PO: ADULTS:** 250 mg 3 times/day for 7–10 days.

**Genital Herpes Simplex (Recurrence)**
**PO: ADULTS:** 1,000 mg twice daily for 1 day; or 125 mg 2 times/day for 5 days; or 500 mg once, then 250 mg 2 times/day for 2 days.

**Genital Herpes Simplex (Suppression)**
**PO: ADULTS:** 250 mg twice daily for up to 1 yr.

**Genital Herpes Simplex in HIV Pts**
**PO: ADULTS:** 500 mg twice daily for 7 days or 5–10 days.

**F**

---

✦ Canadian trade name     🪓 Non-Crushable Drug     🄷🄸🄶🄷 High Alert drug

**Herpes Labialis (Cold Sores)**
**PO: ADULTS, ELDERLY: (Immunocompetent):** 1,500 mg as a single dose. Initiate at first sign or symptoms. **(HIV pts):** 500 mg 2 times/day for 5–10 days.

**Dosage in Renal Impairment**
Dosage and frequency are modified based on creatinine clearance and disease process.

| Creatinine Clearance | Herpes Zoster | Recurrent Genital Herpes (single-day regimen) | Recurrent Genital Herpes (suppression) | Recurrent Herpes Labialis Treatment (single-day regimen) | Recurrent Orolabial or Genital Herpes in HIV Pts |
|---|---|---|---|---|---|
| 40–59 ml/min | 500 mg q12h | 500 mg q12h | — | 750 mg | — |
| 20–39 ml/min | 500 mg q24h | 500 mg | 125 mg q12h | 500 mg | 500 mg q24h |
| Less than 20 ml/min | 250 mg q24h | 250 mg | 125 mg q24h | 250 mg | 250 mg q24h |
| Hemodialysis | 250 mg after each hemodialysis session | 250 mg after each hemodialysis session | 125 mg after each hemodialysis session | 250 mg after each hemodialysis session | 250 mg after each hemodialysis session |

**Dosage in Hemodialysis Pts**
**Herpes zoster:** 250 mg after each dialysis treatment. **Genital herpes:** 125 mg after each dialysis treatment.

**Dosage in Hepatic Impairment**
No dose adjustment.

## SIDE EFFECTS

**Frequent (23%–12%):** Headache, nausea. **Occasional (10%–2%):** Dizziness, drowsiness, paresthesia (esp. feet), diarrhea, vomiting, constipation, decreased appetite, fatigue, fever, pharyngitis, sinusitis, pruritus. **Rare (less than 2%):** Insomnia, abdominal pain, dyspepsia, flatulence, back pain, arthralgia.

## ADVERSE EFFECTS/ TOXIC REACTIONS

Urticaria, severe skin rash, hallucinations, confusion (delirium, disorientation occur predominantly in elderly) has been reported.

## NURSING CONSIDERATIONS

### BASELINE ASSESSMENT

Obtain baseline chemistry tests, esp. renal function. Question history of galactose intolerance, severe lactose deficiency, glucose-galactose malabsorption, renal impairment. Assess herpetic lesions.

### INTERVENTION/EVALUATION

Evaluate cutaneous lesions. Be alert to neurologic effects: headache, dizziness. Provide analgesics, comfort measures. Monitor renal function, hepatic enzymes, CBC.

### PATIENT/FAMILY TEACHING

• Drink adequate fluids. • Fingernails should be kept short, hands clean. • Do not touch lesions with fingers to avoid spreading infection to new site. • **Genital herpes:** Continue therapy for full length of treatment. • Avoid contact with lesions during duration of outbreak to prevent cross-contamination. • Use condoms during sexual activity. • Report if lesions recur or do not improve. • Slowly go from lying to standing to avoid dizziness. • Avoid tasks that require alertness, motor skills until response to drug is established.

# famotidine

fa-**moe**-ta-deen
(Acid Reducer Maximum Strength,
Apo-Famotidine ✦, Pepcid,
Ulcidine ✦)
**Do not confuse famotidine,
cimetidine, ranitidine, with
fluoxetine or furosemide.**

## FIXED-COMBINATION(S)

**Duexis:** famotidine/ibuprofen (an
NSAID): 26.6 mg/800 mg. **Pepcid
Complete:** famotidine/calcium chloride/magnesium hydroxide (antacids): 10 mg/800 mg/165 mg.

## ◆CLASSIFICATION

**PHARMACOTHERAPEUTIC:** H$_2$ receptor antagonist. **CLINICAL:** Antiulcer, gastric acid secretion inhibitor.

## USES

Short-term treatment of active duodenal ulcer. Prevention, maintenance of duodenal ulcer recurrence. Treatment of active benign gastric ulcer, pathologic GI hypersecretory conditions. Short-term treatment of gastroesophageal reflux disease (GERD). OTC formulation for relief of heartburn, acid indigestion, sour stomach. **OFF-LABEL:** *H. pylori* eradication, risk reduction of duodenal ulcer recurrence (part of multidrug regimen), stress ulcer prophylaxis in critically ill pts, relief of gastritis.

## PRECAUTIONS

**Contraindications:** Hypersensitivity to famotidine, other H$_2$ antagonists. **Cautions:** Renal/hepatic impairment, elderly, thrombocytopenia.

## ACTION

Inhibits histamine action of H$_2$ receptors of parietal cells. **Therapeutic Effect:** Inhibits gastric acid secretion (fasting, nocturnal, or stimulated by food, caffeine, insulin).

## PHARMACOKINETICS

| Route | Onset | Peak | Duration |
|---|---|---|---|
| PO | 1 hr | 1–4 hrs | 10–12 hrs |
| IV | 0.5 hr | 0.5–3 hrs | 10–12 hrs |

Rapidly, incompletely absorbed from GI tract. Protein binding: 15%–20%. Partially metabolized in liver. Primarily excreted in urine. Not removed by hemodialysis. **Half-life:** 2.5–3.5 hrs (increased in renal impairment).

## ⧗ LIFESPAN CONSIDERATIONS

**Pregnancy/Lactation:** Unknown if drug crosses placenta or is distributed in breast milk. **Children:** No age-related precautions noted. **Elderly:** Confusion more likely to occur, esp. in pts with renal/hepatic impairment.

## INTERACTIONS

**DRUG:** May decrease absorption of **atazanavir, itraconazole, ketoconazole.** **HERBAL:** None significant. **FOOD:** None known. **LAB VALUES:** Interferes with skin tests using allergen extracts. May increase serum alkaline phosphatase, ALT, AST. May decrease platelet count.

## AVAILABILITY (Rx)

**Infusion, Premix:** 20 mg in 50 ml 0.9% NaCl. **Injection, Solution:** 10 mg/ml (2 ml vial). **Powder for Oral Suspension (Pepcid):** 40 mg/5 ml. **Tablets:** 10 mg. **(Pepcid):** 20 mg, 40 mg. **Tablets, Chewable:** 20 mg.

## ADMINISTRATION/HANDLING
 IV

**Reconstitution •** For IV push, dilute 20 mg with 5–10 ml 0.9% NaCl. • For intermittent IV infusion (piggyback), dilute with 50–100 ml D$_5$W, or 0.9% NaCl. **Rate of Administration •** Give IV push over at least 2 min. • Infuse piggyback over 15–30 min.
**Storage •** Refrigerate unused vials. • IV solution appears clear, colorless. • After dilution, IV solution is stable for 48 hrs if refrigerated.

F

**PO**

• Store tablets, suspension at room temperature. • Following reconstitution, oral suspension is stable for 30 days at room temperature. • Give without regard to meals. • Shake suspension well before use.

## ▣ IV INCOMPATIBILITIES

Amphotericin B complex (Abelcet, AmBisome, Amphotec), piperacillin/tazobactam (Zosyn).

## ▣ IV COMPATIBILITIES

Calcium gluconate, dexamethasone (Decadron), dexmedetomidine (Precedex), dobutamine (Dobutrex), dopamine (Intropin), doxorubicin (Adriamycin), furosemide (Lasix), heparin, hydromorphone (Dilaudid), insulin (regular), lidocaine, lorazepam (Ativan), magnesium sulfate, midazolam (Versed), morphine, nitroglycerin, norepinephrine (Levophed), ondansetron (Zofran), potassium chloride, potassium phosphate, propofol (Diprivan).

## INDICATIONS/ROUTES/DOSAGE

**Duodenal Ulcer**
**PO: ADULTS, ELDERLY: Acute therapy:** 40 mg/day at bedtime or 20 mg twice daily for 4–8 wks. **Maintenance:** 20 mg/day at bedtime.

**Peptic Ulcer**
**PO: CHILDREN 1–16 YRS:** 0.5 mg/kg/day at bedtime or 2 divided doses. **Maximum:** 40 mg/day.

**Gastric Ulcer**
**PO: ADULTS, ELDERLY: (Acute therapy):** 40 mg/day at bedtime.

**Gastroesophageal Reflux Disease (GERD)**
**PO: ADULTS, ELDERLY:** 20 mg twice daily for 6 wks. **CHILDREN 1–16 YRS:** 1 mg/kg/day in 2 divided doses. **Maximum:** 40 mg 2 times/day. **CHILDREN 3 MOS–11 MOS:** 0.5 mg/kg/dose twice daily. **CHILDREN YOUNGER THAN 3 MOS, NEONATES:** 0.5 mg/kg/dose once daily.

**Esophagitis**
**PO: ADULTS, ELDERLY, CHILDREN 12 YRS AND OLDER:** 20–40 mg twice daily for up to 12 wks.

**Hypersecretory Conditions**
**PO: ADULTS, ELDERLY, CHILDREN 12 YRS AND OLDER:** Initially, 20 mg q6h. May increase up to 160 mg q6h.

**Acid Indigestion, Heartburn (OTC Use)**
**PO: ADULTS, ELDERLY, CHILDREN 12 YRS AND OLDER:** 10–20 mg q12h. May take 15–60 min before eating. **Maximum:** 2 doses/day.

**Usual Parenteral Dosage**
**IV: ADULTS, ELDERLY, CHILDREN OLDER THAN 12 YRS:** 20 mg q12h. **CHILDREN 1–12 YRS:** 0.25–0.5 mg/kg q12h. **Maximum:** 40 mg/day.

**Dosage in Renal Impairment**

| Creatinine Clearance | Dosage |
|---|---|
| Less than 50 ml/min | 50% normal dose or increase dosing interval to 48 hrs |

**Dosage in Hepatic Impairment**
No dose adjustment.

## SIDE EFFECTS

**Occasional (5%):** Headache. **Rare (2% or less):** Confusion, constipation, diarrhea, dizziness.

## ADVERSE EFFECTS/ TOXIC REACTIONS

Agranulocytosis, pancytopenia, thrombocytopenia occur rarely.

## NURSING CONSIDERATIONS

### BASELINE ASSESSMENT

Assess epigastric/abdominal pain. Verify platelet count in critically ill pts.

### INTERVENTION/EVALUATION

Monitor daily pattern of bowel activity, stool consistency. Monitor for headache.

Assess for confusion in elderly. Consider interrupting treatment in pts who develop thrombocytopenia.

**PATIENT/FAMILY TEACHING**
• May take without regard to meals, antacids. • Report headache. • Avoid excessive amounts of coffee, aspirin. • Report persistent symptoms of heartburn, acid indigestion, sour stomach.

# febuxostat

fe-**bux**-oh-stat
(Uloric)
**Do not confuse febuxostat with panobinostat or Femstat.**

## ◆ CLASSIFICATION

**PHARMACOTHERAPEUTIC:** Xanthine oxidase inhibitor. **CLINICAL:** Antigout agent.

## USES

Management of hyperuricemia in pts with gout. Not recommended for treatment of asymptomatic hyperuricemia.

## PRECAUTIONS

**Contraindications:** Hypersensitivity to febuxostat. Concomitant use with azathioprine, mercaptopurine. **Cautions:** Severe renal/hepatic impairment, history of heart disease or stroke. Hypersensitivity to allopurinol. Pts at risk for urate formation.

## ACTION

Decreases uric acid production by inhibiting the enzyme xanthine oxidase. **Therapeutic Effect:** Reduces uric acid concentrations in serum and urine.

## PHARMACOKINETICS

Well absorbed from GI tract. Widely distributed. Protein binding: 99%. Metabolized in liver. Eliminated in urine (49%), feces (45%). Removed by hemodialysis. **Half-life:** 5–8 hrs.

## ⧗ LIFESPAN CONSIDERATIONS

**Pregnancy/Lactation:** Unknown if drug crosses placenta or is distributed in breast milk. **Children:** Safety and efficacy not established. **Elderly:** No age-related precautions noted.

## INTERACTIONS

**DRUG:** May increase concentration, toxicity of **azathioprine, mercaptopurine, theophylline.** **HERBAL:** None significant. **FOOD:** None known. **LAB VALUES:** May increase serum alkaline phosphatase, ALT, AST, LDH, amylase, sodium, potassium, cholesterol, triglycerides, BUN, creatinine. May decrease platelets, Hgb, Hct, neutrophils. May prolong prothrombin time.

## AVAILABILITY (Rx)

**Tablets:** 40 mg, 80 mg.

## ADMINISTRATION/HANDLING

**PO**
• Give without regard to meals or antacids.

## INDICATIONS/ROUTES/DOSAGE

**◄ALERT►** Recommended concomitant NSAID or colchicine with initiation of therapy and continue for up to 6 mos to prevent exacerbations of gout.

**Hyperuricemia**
**PO:** **ADULTS, ELDERLY:** Initially, 40 mg once daily. If pt does not achieve serum uric acid level less than 6 mg/dL after 2 wks with 40 mg, may give 80 mg once daily. **Maximum:** 120 mg/day.

**Dosage in Renal/Hepatic Impairment**
**Mild to moderate impairment:** No dose adjustment. **Severe impairment:** Use caution.

## SIDE EFFECTS

**Rare (1%):** Nausea, arthralgia, rash, dizziness.

---

## ADVERSE EFFECTS/ TOXIC REACTIONS

Hepatic function abnormalities occur in 6% of pts. May increase risk of thromboembolic events including CVA, MI.

## NURSING CONSIDERATIONS

### BASELINE ASSESSMENT

Assess baseline renal function, LFT; concomitant use with azathioprine, mercaptopurine, theophylline (contraindicated).

### INTERVENTION/EVALUATION

Discontinue medication immediately if rash appears. Encourage high fluid intake (3,000 ml/day). Monitor I&O (output should be at least 2,000 ml/day). Monitor CBC, serum uric acid, renal function, LFT. Assess urine for cloudiness, unusual color, odor. Assess for therapeutic response (reduced joint tenderness, swelling, redness, limitation of motion). Monitor for symptoms of CVA, MI.

### PATIENT/FAMILY TEACHING

• Encourage drinking 8–10 glasses (8 oz) of fluid daily while taking medication. • Report rash, chest pain, shortness of breath, symptoms suggestive of stroke. • Gout attacks may occur for several months after starting treatment (medication is not a pain reliever). • Continue taking even if gout attack occurs.

---

# felodipine

fe-**loe**-di-peen
(Plendil ✦)
**Do not confuse Plendil with Isordil, Pletal, Prilosec, or Prinivil, or Renedil with Prinivil.**

## FIXED-COMBINATION(S)

**Lexxel:** felodipine/enalapril (ACE inhibitor): 2.5 mg/5 mg, 5 mg/5 mg.

## ◆CLASSIFICATION

**PHARMACOTHERAPEUTIC:** Calcium channel blocker. **CLINICAL:** Antihypertensive, antianginal.

## USES

Management of hypertension. May be used alone or with other antihypertensives. **OFF-LABEL:** Management of pediatric hypertension.

## PRECAUTIONS

**Contraindications:** Hypersensitivity to felodipine or other calcium channel blocker. **Cautions:** Severe left ventricular dysfunction, HF, hepatic impairment, hypertrophic cardiomyopathy with outflow tract obstruction, peripheral edema, severe aortic stenosis, elderly. Concomitant CYP3A4 inhibitors (see Appendix I).

## ACTION

Inhibits calcium movement across cardiac, vascular smooth muscle cell membranes. **Therapeutic Effect:** Relaxes coronary vascular smooth muscle and causes vasodilation. Increases myocardial oxygen delivery.

## PHARMACOKINETICS

| Route | Onset | Peak | Duration |
|-------|-------|------|----------|
| PO | 2–5 hrs | N/A | 24 hrs |

Rapidly, completely absorbed from GI tract. Protein binding: greater than 99%. Metabolized in liver. Primarily excreted in urine. Not removed by hemodialysis. **Half-life:** 11–16 hrs.

## ⧗ LIFESPAN CONSIDERATIONS

**Pregnancy/Lactation:** Unknown if drug crosses placenta or is distributed in breast milk. **Children:** Safety and efficacy not established. **Elderly:** May experience greater hypotensive response. Constipation may be more problematic.

## INTERACTIONS

**DRUG:** CYP3A4 inhibitors (e.g., **ketoconazole, erythromycin, cimetidine**) may increase concentration. **HERBAL:** **St. John's wort** may decrease concentration. **Ephedra, ginseng, yohimbe** may worsen hypertension. **Garlic** may increase antihypertensive effect. **FOOD:** Grapefruit

---

**products** may increase absorption, concentration. **LAB VALUES:** None significant.

## AVAILABILITY (Rx)

Tablets (Extended-Release): 2.5 mg, 5 mg, 10 mg.

## ADMINISTRATION/HANDLING

### PO

• Give with or without food. • Do not break, crush, dissolve, or divide extended-release tablets. Swallow whole.

## INDICATIONS/ROUTES/DOSAGE

### Hypertension

**PO: ADULTS:** Initially, 5 mg/day as single dose. Increase by 5 mg at 2-wk intervals. Usual dose: 5–10 mg once daily. **ELDERLY:** Initially, 2.5 mg/day. Adjust dosage at no less than 2-wk intervals. Usual dose: 2.5–10 mg once daily. **CHILDREN 6 YRS AND OLDER:** Initially, 2.5 mg once daily. May increase at 2-wk intervals. **Maximum:** 10 mg/day.

### Dosage in Renal Impairment
No dose adjustment.

### Dosage in Hepatic Impairment
Initially, 2.5 mg once daily. Titrate carefully.

## SIDE EFFECTS

**Frequent (22%–18%):** Headache, peripheral edema. **Occasional (6%–4%):** Flushing, respiratory infection, dizziness, light-headedness, asthenia. **Rare (less than 3%):** Angina, gingival hyperplasia, paresthesia, abdominal discomfort, anxiety, muscle cramping, cough, diarrhea, constipation.

## ADVERSE EFFECTS/ TOXIC REACTIONS

Overdose produces nausea, drowsiness, confusion, slurred speech, hypotension, bradycardia.

## NURSING CONSIDERATIONS

### BASELINE ASSESSMENT

Assess B/P, apical pulse immediately before drug administration (if pulse is 60 or less/

min or systolic B/P is less than 90 mm Hg, withhold medication, contact physician).

### INTERVENTION/EVALUATION

Assist with ambulation if dizziness occurs. Assess for peripheral edema. Monitor pulse rate for bradycardia. Assess skin for flushing. Monitor hepatic function. Question for headache, asthenia.

### PATIENT/FAMILY TEACHING

• Do not abruptly discontinue medication. • Compliance with therapy regimen is essential to control hypertension. • To avoid hypotensive effect, go from lying to standing slowly. • Avoid tasks that require alertness, motor skills until response to drug is established. • Report palpitations, shortness of breath, pronounced dizziness, nausea. • Swallow tablet whole; do not chew, crush, dissolve, or divide. • Avoid grapefruit products, alcohol. • Report exacerbation of angina.

---

# fenofibrate  `TOP 100`

fen-o-**fye**-brate
(Antara, Apo-Fenofibrate ✦, Fenoglide, Fibricor, Lipofen, Lofibra, Novo-Fenofibrate ✦, Tricor, Triglide, Trilipix)
**Do not confuse Tricor with Fibricor or Tracleer.**

## ◆CLASSIFICATION

**PHARMACOTHERAPEUTIC:** Fibric acid derivative. **CLINICAL:** Antihyperlipidemic.

## USES

Adjunct to diet for reduction of low-density lipoprotein cholesterol (LDL-C), total cholesterol, triglycerides (types IV and V hyperlipidemia), apo-lipoprotein B, and to increase high-density lipoprotein cholesterol (HDL-C) in pts with primary hypercholesterolemia, mixed dyslipidemia.

---

✦ Canadian trade name    Non-Crushable Drug    `HIGH ALERT` High Alert drug

## PRECAUTIONS

**Contraindications:** Hypersensivity to fenofibrate. Active hepatic disease, preexisting gallbladder disease, severe renal/hepatic dysfunction (including primary biliary cirrhosis, unexplained persistent hepatic function abnormality), breastfeeding. **Cautions:** Anticoagulant therapy (e.g., warfarin), history of hepatic disease, venous thromboembolism, mild to moderate renal impairment, substantial alcohol consumption, statin or colchicine therapy (increased risk of myopathy, rhabdomyolysis), elderly.

## ACTION

Downregulates apoprotein C-III and upregulates apoprotein A-I, increasing VLDL catabolism. **Therapeutic Effect:** Decreases triglycerides, increases HDL.

## PHARMACOKINETICS

Well absorbed from GI tract. Absorption increased when given with food. Protein binding: 99%. Metabolized in liver. Excreted in urine (60%), feces (25%). Not removed by hemodialysis. **Half-life:** 10–35 hrs.

## ⧗ LIFESPAN CONSIDERATIONS

**Pregnancy/Lactation:** Safety in pregnancy not established. Breastfeeding not recommended. **Children:** Safety and efficacy not established. **Elderly:** No age-related precautions noted.

## INTERACTIONS

**DRUG:** Potentiates effects of **anticoagulants (e.g., warfarin). Bile acid sequestrants** may impede absorption. **Cyclosporine** may increase concentration, risk of nephrotoxicity. **Colchicine, HMG-CoA reductase inhibitors (statins)** may increase risk of severe myopathy, rhabdomyolysis, acute renal failure. **HERBAL:** None significant. **FOOD: All foods** increase absorption. **LAB VALUES:** May increase serum creatine kinase (CK), ALT, AST. May decrease Hgb, Hct, WBC; serum uric acid.

## AVAILABILITY (Rx)

**Capsules:** *(Antara):* 30 mg, 90 mg. *(Lipofen):* 50 mg, 150 mg. *(Lofibra):* 67 mg, 134 mg, 200 mg. *(Trilipix):* 45 mg, 135 mg. **Tablets:** *(Fenoglide):* 40 mg, 120 mg. *(Fibricor):* 35 mg, 105 mg. *(Lofibra):* 54 mg, 160 mg. *(Tricor):* 48 mg, 145 mg. *(Triglide):* 160 mg.

## ADMINISTRATION/HANDLING

### PO

• Give Fenoglide, Lipofen, Lofibra with meals. • Antara, Fibricor, Tricor, Triglide, and Trilipix may be given without regard to food. Antara, Fenoglide, Lipafen: Swallow whole; do not open (capsules), crush, dissolve, or cut.

## INDICATIONS/ROUTES/DOSAGE

**Hypertriglyceridemia**
PO *(Antara):* ADULTS, ELDERLY: 30–90 mg/day.
PO *(Fenoglide):* ADULTS, ELDERLY: 40–120 mg/day with meals.
PO *(Fibricor):* ADULTS, ELDERLY: 35–105 mg/day.
PO *(Lipofen):* ADULTS, ELDERLY: 50–150 mg/day with meals.
PO *(Lofibra):* ADULTS, ELDERLY: 67–200 mg/day with meals.
PO *(Tricor):* ADULTS, ELDERLY: 48–145 mg/day.
PO *(Triglide):* ADULTS, ELDERLY: 160 mg/day.
PO *(Trilipix):* ADULTS, ELDERLY: 45–135 mg/day.

**Hypercholesterolemia, Mixed Hyperlipidemia**
PO *(Antara):* ADULTS, ELDERLY: 90 mg/day.
PO *(Fenoglide):* ADULTS, ELDERLY: 120 mg/day with meals.
PO *(Fibricor):* ADULTS, ELDERLY: 105 mg/day.
PO *(Lipofen):* ADULTS, ELDERLY: 150 mg/day with meals.
PO *(Lofibra):* ADULTS, ELDERLY: 200 mg/day with meals.
PO *(Tricor):* ADULTS, ELDERLY: 145 mg/day.

**PO** *(Triglide):* **ADULTS, ELDERLY:** 160 mg/day.
**PO** *(Trilipix):* **ADULTS, ELDERLY:** 135 mg/day.

**Dosage in Renal Impairment**
Monitor renal function before adjusting dose. Decrease dose or increase dosing interval for pts with renal failure.

| Initial doses: | Antara: 30 mg/day Fenoglide: 40 mg/day Lipofen: 50 mg/day | Lofibra: 67 mg/day Tricor: 48 mg/day Triglide: 50 mg/day |
|---|---|---|

**Dosage in Hepatic Impairment**
Contraindicated.

## SIDE EFFECTS

**Frequent (8%–4%):** Pain, rash, headache, asthenia, fatigue, flu-like symptoms, dyspepsia, nausea/vomiting, rhinitis. **Occasional (3%–2%):** Diarrhea, abdominal pain, constipation, flatulence, arthralgia, decreased libido, dizziness, pruritus. **Rare (less than 2%):** Increased appetite, insomnia, polyuria, cough, blurred vision, eye floaters, earache.

## ADVERSE EFFECTS/ TOXIC REACTIONS

May increase cholesterol excretion into bile, leading to cholelithiasis. Pancreatitis, hepatitis, thrombocytopenia, agranulocytosis occur rarely.

## NURSING CONSIDERATIONS

**BASELINE ASSESSMENT**
Obtain diet history, esp. fat consumption. Obtain serum cholesterol, triglycerides, LFT, CBC during initial therapy and periodically during treatment. Treatment should be discontinued if hepatic enzyme levels persist greater than 3 times normal limit.

**INTERVENTION/EVALUATION**
For pts on concurrent therapy with HMG-CoA reductase inhibitors, monitor for complaints of myopathy (muscle pain,

weakness). Monitor serum creatine kinase (CK). Monitor serum cholesterol, triglyceride for therapeutic response.

**PATIENT/FAMILY TEACHING**
• Report severe diarrhea, constipation, nausea. • Report skin rash/irritation, insomnia, muscle pain, tremors, dizziness.

## *fentaNYL

**fen**-ta-nil
(Abstral, <u>Actiq</u>, Apo-Fentanyl ✦ <u>Duragesic</u>, Fentora, Ionsys, Lazanda, Onsolis, Subsys)

■ **BLACK BOX ALERT** ■ Physical and psychological dependence may occur with prolonged use. Must be alert to abuse, misuse, or diversion. May cause life-threatening hypoventilation, respiratory depression, or death. Use with strong or moderate CYP3A4 inhibitors may result in potentially fatal respiratory depression. **Buccal:** Tablet and lozenge contain enough medication that may be fatal to children. **Transdermal patch:** Serious or life-threatening hypoventilation has occurred. Limit use to children 2 yrs of age and older. Exposure to direct heat source increases drug release, resulting in overdose/death.
**Do not confuse fentanyl with alfentanil or sufentanil.**

## ◆ CLASSIFICATION

**PHARMACOTHERAPEUTIC:** Opioid, narcotic agonist **(Schedule II).** **CLINICAL:** Analgesic.

## USES

**Injection: (Fentanyl):** Pain relief, preop medication; adjunct to general or regional anesthesia. **Abstral:** Treatment of breakthrough pain in cancer pts 18 yrs of age and older. **Actiq:** Treatment of breakthrough pain in chronic cancer or AIDS-related pain. **Duragesic:** Management of chronic pain *(transdermal).* **Fentora:** Breakthrough pain in pts on chronic opioids. **Ionsys:** Short-term management of acute postoperative pain in adults. **Lazanda:** Management of breakthrough pain in cancer. **Onsolis:** Breakthrough pain in pts with cancer currently receiving opioids and tolerant to opioid therapy. **Subsys:** Treatment of breakthrough cancer pain.

## PRECAUTIONS

**Contraindications:** Hypersensitivity to fentanyl. **Transdermal:** Severe respiratory disease depression, paralytic ileus, intermittent pain. **Transmucosal, transmucosal, lozenges, buccal films:** Management of acute or postoperative pain, pts not opioid tolerant. **Cautions:** Bradycardia; renal, hepatic, respiratory disease; head injuries; altered LOC; biliary tract disease; acute pancreatitis; cor pulmonale; significant COPD; increased ICP; use of MAOIs within 14 days; elderly; morbid obesity.

## ACTION

Binds to opioid receptors in CNS, reducing stimuli from sensory nerve endings, inhibits ascending pain pathways. **Therapeutic Effect:** Alters pain reception, increases pain threshold.

## PHARMACOKINETICS

| Route | Onset | Peak | Duration |
|---|---|---|---|
| IV | 1–2 min | 3–5 min | 0.5–1 hr |
| IM | 7–15 min | 20–30 min | 1–2 hrs |
| Transdermal | 6–8 hrs | 24 hrs | 72 hrs |
| Transmucosal | 5–15 min | 20–30 min | 1–2 hrs |

Well absorbed after IM or topical administration. Transmucosal form absorbed through buccal mucosa and GI tract. Protein binding: 80%–85%. Metabolized in liver. Primarily eliminated by biliary system. **Half-life:** 2–4 hrs IV; 17 hrs transdermal; 6.6 hrs transmucosal.

## ⏳ LIFESPAN CONSIDERATIONS

**Pregnancy/Lactation:** Readily crosses placenta. Unknown if distributed in breast milk. May prolong labor if administered in latent phase of first stage of labor or before cervical dilation of 4–5 cm has occurred. Respiratory depression may occur in neonate if mother received opiates during labor. **Children:** Neonates more susceptible to respiratory depressant effects. Patch: Safety and efficacy not established in pts younger than 12 yrs. **Elderly:** May be more susceptible to respiratory depressant effects. Age-related renal impairment may require dosage adjustment.

## INTERACTIONS

**DRUG: CYP3A4 inducers (e.g., rifampin, modafinil)** may decrease concentration, effects. **Alcohol, CNS depressant medications** may increase CNS depression. **CYP3A4 inhibitors (e.g., erythromycin, itraconazole, ketoconazole, protease inhibitors [e.g., ritonavir])** may increase effects and potential for respiratory depression. **HERBAL: Gotu kola, kava kava, St. John's wort, valerian** may increase CNS depression. **St. John's wort** may decrease concentration, effects. **FOOD: Grapefruit products** may increase potential for respiratory depression with oral, transmucosal forms. **LAB VALUES:** May increase serum amylase, lipase.

## AVAILABILITY (Rx)

**Buccal Tablet (Fentora):** 100 mcg, 200 mcg, 400 mcg, 600 mcg, 800 mcg. **Buccal Soluble Film (Onsolis):** 200 mcg, 400 mcg, 600 mcg, 800 mcg, 1,200 mcg. **Injection Solution:** 50 mcg/ml. **Nasal Spray (Lazanda):** 100 mcg/spray, 400 mcg/spray. **Sublingual Tablets (Abstral):** 100 mcg, 200 mcg, 300 mcg, 400 mcg, 600 mcg, 800 mcg. **Sublingual Spray (Subsys):** 100 mcg, 200 mcg, 400 mcg, 600 mcg, 800 mcg. **Transdermal Patch (Duragesic):** 12 mcg/hr, 25 mcg/hr, 50 mcg/hr, 75 mcg/hr, 100 mcg/hr. **Transmucosal Lozenges (Actiq):** 200 mcg, 400 mcg, 600 mcg, 800 mcg, 1,200 mcg, 1,600 mcg.

## ADMINISTRATION/HANDLING

 IV

**Rate of Administration** • Give by slow IV injection (over 1–2 min). • Too-rapid injection increases risk of severe adverse reactions (skeletal/thoracic muscle rigidity resulting in apnea, laryngospasm, bronchospasm, peripheral circulatory collapse, anaphylactoid effects, cardiac arrest).

**Storage** • Store parenteral form at room temperature. • Opiate antagonist (naloxone) should be readily available.

**Transdermal**
• Apply to hairless area of intact skin of upper torso. • Use flat, nonirritated site. • Firmly press evenly and hold for 30 sec, ensuring adhesion is in full contact with skin and edges are completely sealed. • Use only water to cleanse site before application (soaps, oils may irritate skin). • Rotate sites of application. • Carefully fold used patches so that system adheres to itself; discard in toilet.

**Buccal Film**
• Wet inside of cheek. • Place film inside mouth with pink side of unit against cheek. • Press film against cheek and hold for 5 sec. • Leave in place until dissolved (15–30 min). • Do not chew, swallow, cut film. • Liquids may be given after 5 min of application; food after film dissolves.

**Buccal Tablets**
• Place tablet above a rear molar between upper cheek and gum. • Dissolve over 30 min. • Swallow remaining pieces with water. • Do not split tablet.

**Sublingual Spray**
• Open blister pack with scissors immediately prior to use. • Spray contents underneath tongue.

**Sublingual Tablets**
• Place under tongue. • Dissolves rapidly. • Do not suck, chew, or swallow tablet.

**Nasal**
• Prime device before use by spraying into pouch. • Insert nozzle about ½ inch into nose, pointing toward bridge of nose, tilting bottle slightly. • Press down firmly until hearing a "click" and number on counting window advances by one. Do not blow nose for at least 30 min following administration.

**Transmucosal**
• Suck lozenge vigorously. • Allow to dissolve over 15 min. • Do not chew.

### ❖ IV INCOMPATIBILITIES

Azithromycin (Zithromax), pantoprazole (Protonix), phenytoin (Dilantin).

### ❖ IV COMPATIBILITIES

Atropine, bupivacaine (Marcaine, Sensorcaine), clonidine (Duraclon), dexmedetomidine (Precedex), diltiazem (Cardizem), diphenhydramine (Benadryl), dobutamine (Dobutrex), dopamine (Intropin), droperidol (Inapsine), heparin, hydromorphone (Dilaudid), ketorolac (Toradol), lorazepam (Ativan), metoclopramide (Reglan), midazolam (Versed), milrinone (Primacor), morphine, nitroglycerin, norepinephrine (Levophed), ondansetron (Zofran), potassium chloride, propofol (Diprivan).

## INDICATIONS/ROUTES/DOSAGE

**Note:** Doses titrated to desired effect dependent upon degree of analgesia, pt status.

**Acute Pain Management (Fentanyl)**
**IM/IV: ADULTS, ELDERLY:** 25–100 mcg/dose q1–2h as needed. **CHILDREN:** 0.5–2 mcg/kg/dose q1–2h as needed. **INFANTS (IV push):** 1–4 mcg/kg/dose q2–4h.

**Continuous IV Infusion (Fentanyl)**
**ADULTS, ELDERLY:** 1–2 mcg/kg/hr. **CHILDREN:** 0.5–3 mcg/kg/hr.

**Usual Buccal Dose (Fentora)**
**ADULTS, ELDERLY:** Initially, 100 mcg. Titrate dose, providing adequate analgesia with tolerable side effects.

**Usual Buccal Soluble Film Dose (Onsolis)**
**Note:** All pts must initiate with 200 mcg.

**ADULTS, ELDERLY:** Initially, 200 mcg up to 1,200 mcg. **Maximum:** No more than 4 doses/day, separate by at least 2 hrs.

**Usual Nasal Dose (Lazanda)**
**Nasal: ADULTS, ELDERLY:** Initially, 100 mcg. Titrate from 100 mcg to 200 mcg to 400 mcg to 800 mcg **(maximum).** Wait at least 2 hrs between doses; no more than 4 doses in 24 hrs.

**Usual Sublingual Tablet Dose (Abstral)**
**ADULTS, ELDERLY:** Initially, 100 mcg, then titrate to desired dose/effect. Wait at least 2 hrs between doses; no more than 4 doses in 24 hrs.

**Usual Sublingual Spray Dose (Subsys)**
**ADULTS, ELDERLY:** Initially, 100 mcg. May repeat in 30 min if pain not relieved. Must wait at least 4 hours before treating another episode of pain.

**Usual Transdermal Dose (Duragesic)**
**ADULTS, ELDERLY, CHILDREN 12 YRS AND OLDER:** Initially, 12–25 mcg/hr. May increase after 3 days.

**Usual Transmucosal Dose (Actiq)**
**ADULTS, CHILDREN:** 200–1200 mcg for breakthrough pain. Limit to 4 applications/day.

**Dosage in Renal/Hepatic Impairment**
**Injection:** No dose adjustment.
**Transdermal patch: Mild to moderate impairment:** Reduce dose by 50%.
**Severe impairment:** Not recommended.

## SIDE EFFECTS

**Frequent: IV:** Postop drowsiness, nausea, vomiting. **Transdermal (10%–3%):** Headache, pruritus, nausea, vomiting, diaphoresis, dyspnea, confusion, dizziness, drowsiness, diarrhea, constipation, decreased appetite. **Occasional: IV:** Postop confusion, blurred vision, chills, orthostatic hypotension, constipation, difficulty urinating. **Transdermal (3%–1%):** Chest pain, arrhythmias, erythema, pruritus, syncope, agitation, skin irritations.

## ADVERSE EFFECTS/ TOXIC REACTIONS

Overdose or too-rapid IV administration may produce severe respiratory depression, skeletal/thoracic muscle rigidity (may lead to apnea, laryngospasm, bronchospasm, cold/clammy skin, cyanosis, coma). Tolerance to analgesic effect may occur with repeated use. **Antidote:** Naloxone (see Appendix J for dosage).

## NURSING CONSIDERATIONS

### BASELINE ASSESSMENT

Resuscitative equipment, opiate antagonist (naloxone 0.5 mcg/kg) should be available for initial use. Establish baseline B/P, respirations. Assess type, location, intensity, duration of pain.

### INTERVENTION/EVALUATION

Assist with ambulation. Encourage post-op pt to turn, cough, deep breathe q2h. Monitor respiratory rate, B/P, heart rate, oxygen saturation. Assess for relief of pain.

### PATIENT/FAMILY TEACHING

• Avoid alcohol; do not take other medications without consulting physician. • Avoid tasks that require alertness, motor skills until response to drug is established. • Teach pt proper transdermal, buccal, lozenge administration. **Transdermal:** Avoid saunas (increases drug release time). • Use as directed to avoid overdosage; potential for physical dependence with prolonged use. • Report constipation, absence of pain relief. • Taper slowly after long-term use.

# ferric gluconate

fer-ick **gloo**-koe-nate
(Ferrlecit)

# ferrous fumarate

fer-us **fue**-ma-rate
(Ferrocite, Palafer ✦)

# ferrous gluconate

**fer**-us **gloo**-koe-nate
(Apo-Ferrous Gluconate ✦, Fergon)

# ferrous sulfate

**fer**-us **sul**-fate
(Apo-Ferrous Sulfate ✦, Fer-In-Sol,
Fer-Iron, Slow-Fe)

## ◆CLASSIFICATION

**PHARMACOTHERAPEUTIC:** Enzymatic
mineral. **CLINICAL:** Iron preparation.

## USES

Prevention, treatment of iron deficiency
anemia.

## PRECAUTIONS

**Contraindications:** Hypersensitivity to iron
salts. Hemochromatosis, hemolytic anemias. **Cautions:** Peptic ulcer, regional
enteritis, ulcerative colitis, pts receiving
frequent blood transfusions.

## ACTION

Essential component in formation of
Hgb, myoglobin, enzymes. Promotes effective erythropoiesis and transport, utilization of oxygen. **Therapeutic Effect:**
Prevents iron deficiency.

## PHARMACOKINETICS

Absorbed in duodenum and upper jejunum. Ten percent absorbed in pts with
normal iron stores; increased to 20%–
30% in pts with inadequate iron stores.
Primarily bound to serum transferrin.
Excreted in urine, sweat, sloughing of
intestinal mucosa, menses. **Half-life:**
6 hrs.

## ⧗ LIFESPAN CONSIDERATIONS

**Pregnancy/Lactation:** Crosses placenta;
distributed in breast milk. **Children/
Elderly:** No age-related precautions
noted.

## INTERACTIONS

**DRUG: Antacids, calcium supple-
ments, pancreatin, pancrelipase** may
decrease absorption of ferrous compounds. May decrease absorption of
**etidronate, quinolones, tetracyclines.**
**HERBAL:** None significant. **FOOD: Cereal,
coffee, dietary fiber, eggs, milk, tea**
decrease absorption. **LAB VALUES:**
May increase serum bilirubin, iron. May
decrease serum calcium.

## AVAILABILITY (OTC)

**Ferric Gluconate**
**Injection, solution:** 12.5 mg/ml.

**Ferrous Fumarate**
**Tablets (Ferrocite):** 324 mg (106 mg elemental iron).

**Ferrous Gluconate**
**Tablets:** 240 mg (27 mg elemental iron)
(Fergon), 325 mg (36 mg elemental iron).

**Ferrous Sulfate**
**Oral Solution (Fer-In-Sol, Fer-Iron):** 75
mg/ml (15 mg/ml elemental iron).
**Tablets:** 325 mg (65 mg elemental iron).
**Syrup:** 300 mg/5 ml.
✇ **Tablets (Timed-Release [Slow-Fe]):**
160 mg (50 mg elemental iron).

## ADMINISTRATION/HANDLING

**PO**
• Store all forms (tablets, capsules,
suspension, drops) at room temperature. • Ideally, give between meals
with water or juice but may give with
meals if GI discomfort occurs. • Transient staining of mucous membranes,
teeth occurs with liquid iron preparation. To avoid staining, place liquid on
back of tongue with dropper or
straw. • Do not give with milk or milk
products. • Do not break, crush, dissolve, or divide timed-release tablets.

## INDICATIONS/ROUTES/DOSAGE

**Iron Deficiency Anemia**
Dosage is expressed in terms of milligrams of elemental iron. Assess degree

---

 ✦ Canadian trade name    ✇ Non-Crushable Drug    🔺HIGH ALERT High Alert drug

of anemia, pt weight, presence of any bleeding. Expect to use periodic hematologic determinations as guide to therapy. **IV:** *(Ferric Gluconate):* **ADULTS, ELDERLY:** 125 mg/dose. Usual dose: 1,000 mg given over 8 sessions.
**PO** *(Ferrous Fumarate):* **ADULTS, ELDERLY:** 100–200 mg/day in 2–3 divided doses. **CHILDREN:** 3–6 mg/kg/day in 2–3 divided doses.
**PO** *(Ferrous Gluconate):* **ADULTS, ELDERLY:** 100–200 mg/day in 2–3 divided doses. **CHILDREN:** 3–6 mg/kg/day in 2–3 divided doses.
**PO** *(Ferrous Sulfate):* **ADULTS, ELDERLY:** 100–200 mg/day in 2–3 divided doses. **CHILDREN:** 3–6 mg/kg/day in 2–3 divided doses.

**Prevention of Iron Deficiency**
**PO** *(Ferrous Fumarate):* **ADULTS, ELDERLY:** 60 mg/day. **CHILDREN:** 30 mg/day with folic acid.
**PO** *(Ferrous Gluconate):* **ADULTS, ELDERLY:** 60 mg/day. **CHILDREN:** 30 mg/day with folic acid.
**PO** *(Ferrous Sulfate):* **ADULTS, ELDERLY:** 60 mg/day. **CHILDREN:** 30 mg/day with folic acid.

## SIDE EFFECTS

**Occasional:** Mild, transient nausea. **Rare:** Heartburn, anorexia, constipation, diarrhea.

## ADVERSE EFFECTS/ TOXIC REACTIONS

Large doses may aggravate existing GI tract disease (peptic ulcer, regional enteritis, ulcerative colitis). Severe iron poisoning occurs most often in children, manifested as vomiting, severe abdominal pain, diarrhea, dehydration, followed by hyperventilation, pallor, cyanosis, cardiovascular collapse.

### NURSING CONSIDERATIONS

#### BASELINE ASSESSMENT

Assess nutritional status, dietary history. Question history of hemachromatosis, hemolytic anemia, ulcerative colitis.

#### INTERVENTION/EVALUATION

Monitor serum iron, total iron-binding capacity, reticulocyte count, Hgb, ferritin. Monitor daily pattern of bowel activity, stool consistency. Assess for clinical improvement, record relief of iron deficiency symptoms (fatigue, irritability, pallor, paresthesia of extremities, headache).

#### PATIENT/FAMILY TEACHING

• Expect stool color to darken. • Oral liquid may stain teeth. • To prevent mucous membrane and teeth staining with liquid preparation, use dropper or straw and allow solution to drop on back of tongue. • If GI discomfort occurs, take after meals or with food. • Do not take within 2 hrs of other medication or eggs, milk, tea, coffee, cereal.

# fesoterodine

fes-oh-**ter**-oh-deen
(Toviaz)
**Do not confuse fesoterodine with fexofenadine or tolteradine.**

## ♦CLASSIFICATION

**PHARMACOTHERAPEUTIC:** Muscarinic receptor antagonist. **CLINICAL:** Antispasmodic.

## USES

Treatment of overactive bladder with symptoms including urinary incontinence, urgency, frequency.

## PRECAUTIONS

**Contraindications:** Hypersensitivity to fesoterodine. Gastric retention, uncontrolled narrow-angle glaucoma, urinary retention. **Cautions:** Severe renal impairment, severe hepatic impairment, clinically significant bladder outflow obstruction (risk of urinary retention), GI obstructive disorders (e.g., pyloric stenosis [risk of gastric retention], treated narrow-angle glaucoma, myasthenia gravis, concurrent therapy with strong CYP3A4 inhibitors, elderly, use in hot weather.

## ACTION

Exhibits antimuscarinic activity by interceding via cholinergic muscarinic receptors, thereby mediating urinary bladder contraction. **Therapeutic Effect:** Decreases urinary frequency, urgency.

## PHARMACOKINETICS

Well absorbed following PO administration. Protein binding: 50%. Rapidly and extensively hydrolyzed to its active metabolite. Primarily excreted in urine. **Half-life:** 7 hours.

## ⌛ LIFESPAN CONSIDERATIONS

**Pregnancy/Lactation:** Unknown if distributed in breast milk. **Children:** Safety and efficacy not established. **Elderly:** Increased incidence of antimuscarinic adverse events including dry mouth, constipation, dyspepsia, increase in residual urine, dizziness, urinary tract infections higher in pts 75 yrs of age and older.

## INTERACTIONS

**DRUG:** CYP3A4 inhibitors (e.g., clarithromycin, erythromycin, itraconazole, ketoconazole, miconazole) may increase concentration. **HERBAL:** None significant. **FOOD:** Grapefruit products may increase potential for urinary retention, constipation. **LAB VALUES:** May increase serum ALT, GGT.

## AVAILABILITY (Rx)

🔰 Tablets, Extended-Release: 4 mg, 8 mg.

## ADMINISTRATION/HANDLING

**PO**
• May be administered with or without food. • Swallow whole; do not break, crush, dissolve, or divide tablet.

## INDICATIONS/ROUTES/DOSAGE

**Overactive Bladder**
**PO: ADULTS, ELDERLY:** Initially, 4 mg once daily. May increase to 8 mg once

daily. Maximum dose for pts with concurrent use of strong CYP3A4 inhibitors (e.g., erythromycin, ketoconazole) is 4 mg once daily.

**Dosage in Renal Impairment**
**PO: ADULTS, ELDERLY: Maximum dose:** 4 mg with CrCl less than 30 ml/min.

**Dosage in Hepatic Impairment**
**Mild to moderate impairment:** No dose adjustment. **Severe impairment:** Not recommended.

## SIDE EFFECTS

**Frequent (34%–18%):** Dry mouth. **Occasional (6%–3%):** Constipation, urinary tract infection dry eyes. **Rare (2% or less):** Nausea, dysuria, back pain, rash, insomnia, peripheral edema.

## ADVERSE EFFECTS/ TOXIC REACTIONS

Severe anticholinergic effects including abdominal cramps, facial warmth, excessive salivation/lacrimation, diaphoresis, pallor, urinary urgency, blurred vision.

## NURSING CONSIDERATIONS

### BASELINE ASSESSMENT

Assess urinary pattern (e.g., urinary frequency, urgency). Obtain baseline chemistries. Question history as listed in Precautions. Receive full medication history.

### INTERVENTION/EVALUATION

Assist with ambulation if dizziness occurs. Question for visual changes. Monitor incontinence, postvoid residuals. Monitor daily pattern of bowel activity, stool consistency.

### PATIENT/FAMILY TEACHING

• May produce constipation and urinary retention. • Blurred vision may occur; use caution until drug effects have been determined. • Heat prostration (due to decreased sweating) can occur if used in a hot environment. • Do not ingest grapefruit products.

# fexofenadine

**fex**-oh-**fen**-a-deen
(Allegra, Allegra Children's)
**Do not confuse Allegra with Viagra, or fexofenadine with fesoterodine.**

## FIXED-COMBINATION(S)

**Allegra-D 12 Hour:** fexofenadine/pseudoephedrine (sympathomimetic): 60 mg/120 mg. **Allegra-D 24 Hour:** fexofenadine/pseudoephedrine (sympathomimetic): 180 mg/240 mg.

## ◆CLASSIFICATION

**PHARMACOTHERAPEUTIC:** Piperidine. **CLINICAL:** Antihistamine.

## USES

Relief of symptoms associated with allergic rhinitis. Treatment of chronic idiopathic urticaria.

## PRECAUTIONS

**Contraindications:** Hypersensitivity to fexofenadine. **Cautions:** Renal impairment. Orally disintegrating tablet not recommended in children younger than 6 yrs.

## ACTION

Competes with histamine in GI tract, blood vessels, and respiratory tract. **Therapeutic Effect:** Relieves allergic rhinitis symptoms.

## PHARMACOKINETICS

|    | Onset  | Peak | Duration          |
|----|--------|------|-------------------|
| PO | 60 min | —    | 12 hrs or greater |

Rapidly absorbed after PO administration. Protein binding: 60%–70%. Does not cross blood-brain barrier. Minimally metabolized. Eliminated in feces (80%), urine (11%). Not removed by hemodialysis. **Half-life:** 14.4 hrs (increased in renal impairment).

## ⧖ LIFESPAN CONSIDERATIONS

**Pregnancy/Lactation:** Unknown if drug crosses placenta or is distributed in breast milk. **Children:** Safety and efficacy not established in pts younger than 12 yrs. **Elderly:** No age-related precautions noted.

## INTERACTIONS

**DRUG: Aluminum-** and **magnesium-containing antacids** may decrease absorption if given within 15 min of fexofenadine. May increase concentrations of **erythromycin, ketoconazole. HERBAL: St. John's wort** may decrease concentration. **FOOD: Fruit juices** may decrease bioavailability. **LAB VALUES:** May suppress wheal, flare reactions to antigen skin testing unless drug is discontinued at least 4 days before testing.

## AVAILABILITY (Rx)

**Oral Suspension:** 30 mg/5 ml. **Tablets:** 30 mg, 60 mg, 180 mg. **Tablets (Orally Disintegrating):** 30 mg.

## ADMINISTRATION/HANDLING

**PO**
• Give without regard to food. • Avoid giving with fruit juices (apple, grapefruit, orange). Administer with water only. • Shake suspension well before use.

**PO (Orally Disintegrating Tablet)**
• Take on empty stomach. • Remove from blister pack; immediately place on tongue. • May take with or without liquid. • Do not split or cut.

## INDICATIONS/ROUTES/DOSAGE

**Allergic Rhinitis**
**PO: ADULTS, ELDERLY, CHILDREN 12 YRS AND OLDER:** 60 mg twice daily or 180 mg once daily. **CHILDREN 2–11 YRS:** 30 mg twice daily.

**Urticaria**
**PO: ADULTS, ELDERLY, CHILDREN 12 YRS AND OLDER:** 60 mg twice daily or 180 mg once daily. **CHILDREN 2–11 YRS:** 30 mg twice daily. **CHILDREN 6 MOS–LESS THAN 2 YRS:** 15 mg twice daily.

**Dosage in Renal Impairment (CrCl Less Than 80 ml/min)**
PO: **ADULTS, ELDERLY, CHILDREN 12 YRS AND OLDER:** 60 mg once daily. **CHILDREN 2–11 YRS:** 30 mg once daily. **CHILDREN 6 MOS–LESS THAN 2 YRS:** 15 mg once daily.

**Dosage in Hepatic Impairment**
No dose adjustment.

## SIDE EFFECTS

**Rare (less than 2%):** Drowsiness, headache, fatigue, nausea, vomiting, abdominal distress, dysmenorrhea.

## ADVERSE EFFECTS/ TOXIC REACTIONS

Hypersensitivity reaction occurs rarely.

## NURSING CONSIDERATIONS

### BASELINE ASSESSMENT

If pt is having an allergic reaction, obtain history of recently ingested foods, drugs, environmental exposure, emotional stress. Monitor rate, depth, rhythm, type of respiration; quality, rate of pulse. Assess lung sounds for rhonchi, wheezing, rales.

### INTERVENTION/EVALUATION

Assess for therapeutic response; relief from allergy: itching, red, watery eyes, rhinorrhea, sneezing.

### PATIENT/FAMILY TEACHING

• Avoid tasks that require alertness, motor skills until response to drug is established. • Avoid alcohol during antihistamine therapy. • Coffee, tea may help reduce drowsiness. • Do not take with any fruit juices.

# fidaxomicin

fye-**dax**-oh-**mye**-sin
(Dificid)

## ◆CLASSIFICATION

**PHARMACOTHERAPEUTIC:** Macrolide. **CLINICAL:** Antibiotic.

## USES

Treatment of *C. difficile*–associated diarrhea.

## PRECAUTIONS

**Contraindications:** Hypersensitivity to fidaxomicin. **Cautions:** History of anemia, neutropenia, macrolide allergy.

## ACTION

Binds to ribosomal sites of susceptible organisms, inhibiting RNA-dependent protein synthesis by RNA polymerase. **Therapeutic Effect:** Bactericidal against *Clostridium difficile*.

## PHARMACOKINETICS

Minimal systemic absorption following PO administration. Mainly confined to GI tract. Excreted primarily in feces (92%). **Half-life:** 9 hrs.

## ☒ LIFESPAN CONSIDERATIONS

**Pregnancy/Lactation:** Unknown if distributed in breast milk. **Children:** Safety and efficacy not established. **Elderly:** No age-related precautions noted.

## INTERACTIONS

**DRUG: Cyclosporine** may increase serum concentration, effects. **HERBAL:** None known. **FOOD:** None significant. **LAB VALUES:** May increase serum ALT, AST, bilirubin, alkaline phosphatase.

## AVAILABILITY (Rx)

**Tablets:** 200 mg.

## ADMINISTRATION/HANDLING

• Give without regard to food.

## INDICATIONS/ROUTES/DOSAGE

*Clostridium Difficile*–Associated Diarrhea
PO: **ADULTS:** 200 mg twice daily for 10 days.

**Dosage in Renal/Hepatic Impairment**
No dose adjustment.

## SIDE EFFECTS

**Frequent (62%–33%):** Nausea, vomiting, abdominal pain. **Rare (less than 2%):** Pruritus, rash.

## ADVERSE EFFECTS/ TOXIC REACTIONS

Less than 2% reported events most likely related to diarrhea-associated illness including volume loss, dehydration, GI bleeding, bloating, megacolon, abdominal distention/tenderness, flatulence, dyspepsia, dysphasia, intestinal obstruction, bicarbonate loss, hyperglycemia, metabolic acidosis, and increased hepatic function tests. GI tract infection may cause bleeding, decreased platelets, decreased RBC count.

## NURSING CONSIDERATIONS

### BASELINE ASSESSMENT

Verify positive *C. difficile* toxin test before initiating treatment. Implement infection control measures. Obtain baseline CBC, electrolytes, renal function, fecal occult blood test. Assess abdominal pain, bowel sounds, and stool characteristics (color, frequency, consistency). Assess hydration status.

### INTERVENTION/EVALUATION

Monitor for volume loss, dehydration, hypotension. Encourage nutrition/fluid intake. Monitor daily pattern of bowel activity, stool consistency. Routinely assess bowel sounds. Screen for intestinal obstruction (increased nausea, abdominal pain, hyperactive bowel sounds) and consider abdominal X-ray if suspected.

### PATIENT/FAMILY TEACHING

• Complete drug therapy, despite symptom improvement. Early discontinuation may result in antibacterial resistance and increased risk of recurrent infection. • Report weakness, fatigue, pale skin, dizziness, or red/dark, tarry stools relating to GI bleeding.

## filgrastim              TOP 100

fil-**gras**-tim
(Granix, <u>Neupogen</u>, Zarxio)
**filgrastim-sndz**
(Zarxio)
**Do not confuse Neupogen with Epogen, Neulasta, Neumega, or Nutramigen.**

### ◆CLASSIFICATION

**PHARMACOTHERAPEUTIC:** Biologic modifier. **CLINICAL:** Granulocyte colony-stimulating factor (G-CSF).

## USES

**Granix:** Decreases duration of severe neutropenia in pts with malignancies receiving chemotherapy associated with severe neutropenia, fever. **Neupogen, Zarxio:** Reduces neutropenia duration, sequelae in pts with nonmyeloid malignancies having myeloablative therapy followed by bone marrow transplant (BMT). Mobilization of hematopoietic progenitor cells into peripheral blood for collection by apheresis. Treatment of chronic, severe neutropenia. Decreases incidence of infection in pts with malignancies receiving chemotherapy associated with increased incidence of severe neutropenia with fever. Reduces time to neutrophil recovery/duration of fever after induction/consolidation chemotherapy in AML pts. **Neupogen:** Increases survival in pts acutely exposed to myelosuppressive doses of radiation. **OFF-LABEL:** Treatment of AIDS-related neutropenia in pts receiving zidovudine; drug-induced neutropenia; anemia in myelodysplastic syndrome; hepatitis C treatment-associated neutropenia.

## PRECAUTIONS

**Contraindications:** Hypersensitivity to filgrastim. (Neupogen) Hypersensitivity to *Escherichia coli*–derived proteins. **Cautions:** Malignancy with myeloid characteristics (due to G-CSF's potential to act as growth factor), gout, psoriasis, neutrophil count greater than 50,000 cells/mm³, sickle cell disease, concomitant use of other drugs that may result in thrombocytopenia. Do not use 24 hrs before or after cytotoxic chemotherapy.

## ACTION

Stimulates production, maturation, activation of neutrophils. **Therapeutic Effect:** Increases migration and cytotoxicity of neutrophils.

## PHARMACOKINETICS

Readily absorbed. Onset of action: 24 hrs (plateaus in 3–5 days). WBC return to normal in 4–7 days. Not removed by hemodialysis. **Half-life:** 3.5 hrs.

## ⏳ LIFESPAN CONSIDERATIONS

**Pregnancy/Lactation:** Unknown if drug crosses placenta or is distributed in breast milk. **Children/Elderly:** No age-related precautions noted.

## INTERACTIONS

**DRUG:** None significant. **HERBAL:** None significant. **FOOD:** None known. **LAB VALUES:** May increase LDH, leukocyte alkaline phosphatase (LAP) scores, serum alkaline phosphatase, uric acid.

## AVAILABILITY (Rx)

**Injection Solution: (Neupogen):** 300 mcg/ml, 480 mcg/1.6 ml **Neupogen):** 300 mcg/0.5 ml; 480 mcg/0.8 ml. **Injection, Prefilled Syringe: (Granix, Zarxio):** 300 mcg/0.5 ml, 480 mcg/0.8 ml.

## ADMINISTRATION/HANDLING

◀**ALERT**▶ May be given by subcutaneous injection, short IV infusion (15–30 min), or continuous IV infusion. Do not dilute with normal saline.

 **IV**

**Reconstitution** • Allow vial to warm to room temperature (approx. 30 mins). • Visually inspect for particulate matter or discoloration. • Dilute in D₅W from

concentration of 300 mcg/ml to 5 mcg/ml (do not dilute to a final concentration less than 5 mcg/ml). Diluted solutions of 5–15 mcg/ml should have addition of albumin to a final concentration of 2 mg/ml. • Do not dilute with saline.

**Rate of Administration** • For intermittent infusion (piggyback), infuse over 15–30 min. • For continuous infusion, give single dose over 4–24 hrs. • In all situations, flush IV line with D₅W before and after administration.

**Storage** • Refrigerate vials and syringes. • Stable for up to 24 hrs at room temperature (provided vial contents are clear and contain no particulate matter).

**Subcutaneous**

• Aspirate syringe before injection (avoid intra-arterial administration).

**Storage** • Store in refrigerator, but remove before use and allow to warm to room temperature.

## ▓ IV INCOMPATIBILITIES

Amphotericin (Fungizone), cefepime (Maxipime), cefotaxime (Claforan), cefoxitin (Mefoxin), ceftizoxime (Cefizox), ceftriaxone (Rocephin), clindamycin (Cleocin), dactinomycin (Cosmegen), etoposide (VePesid), fluorouracil, furosemide (Lasix), heparin, mannitol, methylprednisolone (Solu-Medrol), mitomycin (Mutamycin), prochlorperazine (Compazine).

## ▓ IV COMPATIBILITIES

Bumetanide (Bumex), calcium gluconate, hydromorphone (Dilaudid), lorazepam (Ativan), morphine, potassium chloride.

## INDICATIONS/ROUTES/DOSAGE

◀**ALERT**▶ Begin therapy at least 24 hrs after last dose of chemotherapy and at least 24 hrs after bone marrow infusion. Dosing based on actual body weight.

**Chemotherapy-Induced Neutropenia**
*Neupogen, Zarxio*
**IV or SQ Infusion, SQ Injection:** **ADULTS, ELDERLY, CHILDREN:** Initially, 5 mcg/kg/day. May increase by 5 mcg/kg

for each chemotherapy cycle based on duration/severity of neutropenia; continue for up to 14 days or until absolute neutrophil count (ANC) reaches 10,000/mm³.
**Granix**
**SQ: ADULTS, ELDERLY:** 5 mcg/kg/day. Continue until nadir has passed and neutrophil count recovered to normal range.

**Bone Marrow Transplant**
**IV or SQ Infusion:** *(Neupogen, Zarxio)* **ADULTS, ELDERLY, CHILDREN:** 10 mcg/kg/day. Adjust dosage daily during period of neutrophil recovery based on neutrophil response.

**Mobilization of Progenitor Cells**
**IV or SQ Infusion:** *(Neupogen, Zarxio)* **ADULTS:** 10 mcg/kg/day in donors beginning at least 4 days before first leukapheresis and continuing until last leukapheresis (usually for 6–7 days).

**Chronic Neutropenia,**
**Congenital Neutropenia**
**SQ:** *(Neupogen, Zarxio)* **ADULTS, CHILDREN:** 6 mcg/kg/dose twice daily. Adjust dose based on ANC/clinical response.

**Idiopathic or Cyclic Neutropenia**
**SQ:** *(Neupogen, Zarxio)* **ADULTS, CHILDREN:** 5 mcg/kg/dose once daily. Adjust dose based on ANC/clinical response.

**Dosage in Renal/Hepatic Impairment**
No dose adjustment.

## SIDE EFFECTS

**Frequent (57%–11%):** Nausea/vomiting, mild to severe bone pain (more frequent with high-dose IV form, less frequent with low-dose subcutaneous form), alopecia, diarrhea, fever, fatigue. **Occasional (9%–5%):** Anorexia, dyspnea, headache, cough, rash. **Rare (less than 5%):** Psoriasis, hematuria, proteinuria, osteoporosis.

## ADVERSE EFFECTS/ TOXIC REACTIONS

Long-term administration occasionally produces chronic neutropenia, splenomegaly. Acute respiratory distress syndrome, alveolar hemorrhage and hemoptysis (pts undergoing peripheral blood progenitor cell collection mobilization), capillary leak syndrome, cutaneous vasculitis, glomerulonephritis, leukocytosis, MI, thrombocytopenia, sickle cell crisis, splenic rupture may occur.

## NURSING CONSIDERATIONS

### BASELINE ASSESSMENT
CBC, platelet count should be obtained before therapy initiation and twice wkly thereafter.

### INTERVENTION/EVALUATION
In septic pts, be alert for adult respiratory distress syndrome. Closely monitor those with preexisting cardiac conditions. Monitor B/P (transient decrease in B/P may occur), temperature, CBC with differential, platelet count, serum uric acid, hepatic function tests.

### PATIENT/FAMILY TEACHING
• Report fever, chills, severe bone pain, chest pain, palpitations.

# finasteride

fin-**as**-ter-ide
(Apo-Finasteride ✿, Propecia, Proscar)
**Do not confuse finasteride with furosemide, or Proscar with ProSom, Provera, or Prozac.**

## ◆CLASSIFICATION
**PHARMACOTHERAPEUTIC:** Androgen hormone inhibitor. **CLINICAL:** Benign prostatic hyperplasia agent.

## USES
**Proscar:** Reduces risk of acute urinary retention, need for surgery in symptomatic benign prostatic hyperplasia (BPH) alone or in combination with doxazosin (Cardura). **Propecia:** Treatment of male

pattern hair loss. **OFF-LABEL:** Treatment of female hirsutism.

## PRECAUTIONS

**Contraindications:** Hypersensitivity to finasteride, pregnancy or women of childbearing potential. **Cautions:** Hepatic impairment, urinary outflow obstruction, urinary retention. Women who are attempting to conceive should avoid exposure to crushed or broken tablets.

## ACTION

Inhibits 5-alpha reductase, an intracellular enzyme that converts testosterone into dihydrotestosterone (DHT) in prostate gland, resulting in decreased serum DHT. **Therapeutic Effect:** Reduces size of prostate gland.

## PHARMACOKINETICS

| Route | Onset | Peak | Duration |
|---|---|---|---|
| PO (reduction of DHT) | 8 hrs | — | 24 hrs |

Rapidly absorbed from GI tract. Protein binding: 90%. Widely distributed. Metabolized in liver. **Half-life:** 6–8 hrs. Onset of clinical effect: 3–6 mos of continued therapy.

## ⧖ LIFESPAN CONSIDERATIONS

**Pregnancy/Lactation:** Physical handling of tablet by those who are or may become pregnant may produce abnormalities of external genitalia of male fetus. **Children:** Not indicated for use in children. **Elderly:** No age-related precautions noted.

## INTERACTIONS

**DRUG:** None significant. **HERBAL: St. John's wort** may decrease concentration. Avoid concurrent use with **saw palmetto** (not adequately studied). **FOOD:** None known. **LAB VALUES:** Decreases serum prostate-specific antigen (PSA) level, even in presence of prostate cancer. Decreases dihydrotestosterone (DHT). Increases follicle-stimulating hormone (FSH), luteinizing hormone (LH), testosterone.

## AVAILABILITY (Rx)

🔖 **Tablets:** 1 mg (Propecia), 5 mg (Proscar).

## ADMINISTRATION/HANDLING

**PO**
• Do not break, crush, dissolve, or divide film-coated tablets. • Give without regard to meals.

## INDICATIONS/ROUTES/DOSAGE

**Benign Prostatic Hyperplasia (BPH)**
**PO: ADULTS, ELDERLY:** *(Proscar):* 5 mg once daily (as single agent or in combination with doxazosin).

**Hair Loss**
**PO: ADULTS:** *(Propecia):* 1 mg/day.

**Dosage in Renal Impairment**
No dose adjustment.

**Dosage in Hepatic Impairment**
Use caution.

## SIDE EFFECTS

**Rare (4%–2%):** Gynecomastia, sexual dysfunction (impotence, decreased libido, decreased volume of ejaculate).

## ADVERSE EFFECTS/ TOXIC REACTIONS

Hypersensitivity reaction, circumoral swelling, testicular pain occur rarely.

### NURSING CONSIDERATIONS

#### BASELINE ASSESSMENT

Digital rectal exam, serum prostate-specific antigen (PSA) determination should be performed in pts with benign prostatic hyperplasia (BPH) before initiating therapy and periodically thereafter.

#### INTERVENTION/EVALUATION

Diligently monitor I&O, esp. in pts with large residual urinary volume, severely diminished urinary flow, or obstructive uropathy.

F

• Treatment may cause impotence, decreased volume of ejaculate. • May not notice improved urinary flow even if prostate gland shrinks. • Must take medication longer than 6 mos, and it is unknown if medication decreases need for surgery. • Because of potential risk to male fetus, women who are or may become pregnant should not handle tablets or be exposed to pt's semen.

# fingolimod
TOP 100

fin-**goe**-li-mod
(Gilenya)

## ◆CLASSIFICATION
**PHARMACOTHERAPEUTIC:** Immuno-modulator. **CLINICAL:** Multiple sclerosis agent.

## USES
Treatment of pts with relapsing forms of multiple sclerosis (MS) to reduce frequency of clinical exacerbations, delay accumulation of physical disability.

## PRECAUTIONS
**Contraindications:** Hypersensitivity to fingolimod. Sick sinus syndrome, second-degree or higher conduction block (unless pt has functioning pacemaker). Baseline QT interval 500 msec or greater. Concurrent use of class I or III antiarrhythmic. Recent (within 6 mos) MI, unstable angina, stroke, TIA, decompensated requiring hospitalization or NYHA class III/IV HF. **Cautions:** Concomitant use of antiarrhythmics, beta blockers, calcium channel blockers, immunosuppresants, immune modulators, antineoplastics, QT interval–prolonging medications (e.g., amiodarone, ciprofloxacin); bradycardia, severe hepatic impairment, ischemic heart disease, diabetes, hypokalemia, hypomagnesemia; history of syncope, uveitis; pts at risk for developing bradycardia or heart block.

## ACTION
Blocks capacity of lymphocytes to move out from lymph nodes, reducing number of lymphocytes available to the CNS. **Therapeutic Effect:** May involve reduction of lymphocyte migration into central nervous system, which reduces central inflammation.

## PHARMACOKINETICS
Metabolized by the enzyme sphingosine kinase to active metabolite. Highly distributed in red blood cells (85%). Minimally metabolized in liver. Protein binding: 99.7%. Primarily excreted in urine. **Half-life:** 6–9 days.

## ⧖ LIFESPAN CONSIDERATIONS
**Pregnancy/Lactation:** May cause fetal harm. Unknown if distributed in breast milk. **Children:** Safety and efficacy not established in pts younger than 18 yrs. **Elderly:** Age-related severe hepatic impairment may increase risk of adverse reactions.

## INTERACTIONS
**DRUG: Antineoplastics, immunosuppressives, immunomodulators** may increase risk of immunosuppression. **Ketoconazole** may increase concentration/adverse effects. May decrease effect of **vaccines.** May increase effects of **QT-prolonging medications. HERBAL: Echinacea** may decrease concentration. **FOOD:** None known. **LAB VALUES:** Expect decrease in neutrophil count. May increase serum alkaline phosphatase, ALT, AST, bilirubin, triglycerides.

## AVAILABILITY (Rx)
**Capsules:** 0.5 mg.

## ADMINISTRATION/HANDLING
**PO**
• May give without regard to food.

## INDICATIONS/ROUTES/DOSAGE
**Multiple Sclerosis**
**PO: ADULTS 18 YRS AND OLDER, ELDERLY:** 0.5 mg once daily.

**Dosage in Renal/Hepatic Impairment**
**Mild to moderate impairment:** No dose adjustment. **Severe impairment:** Use caution.

## SIDE EFFECTS

**Frequent (25%–10%):** Headache, diarrhea, back pain, cough. **Occasional (8%–5%):** Dyspnea, clinical depression, dizziness, hypertension, migraine, paresthesia, decreased weight. **Rare (4%–2%):** Blurred vision, alopecia, eye pain, asthenia, eczema, pruritus.

## ADVERSE EFFECTS/ TOXIC REACTIONS

May increase risk of infections (influenza, herpes viral infection, bronchitis, sinusitis, gastroenteritis, ear infection) in 13%–4% of pts. Pts with diabetes or history of uveitis are at increased risk for developing macular edema.

## NURSING CONSIDERATIONS

### BASELINE ASSESSMENT

Obtain baseline CBC, serum chemistries prior to initial treatment. At initial treatment (within first 4–6 hrs after dose), medication reduces heart rate, AV conduction, followed by progressive increase after first day of treatment. Obtain baseline vitals, with particular attention to pulse rate. Perform ophthalmologic evaluation prior to treatment and 3–4 mos after initiation of treatment.

### INTERVENTION/EVALUATION

Monitor for bradycardia for 6 hrs after first dose, then as appropriate. Periodically monitor CBC, serum chemistries, particularly lymphocyte count (expected to decrease approximately 80% from baseline with continued treatment). Monitor for signs of systemic or local infection.

### PATIENT/FAMILY TEACHING

• Obtain regular eye examinations during and for 2 mos following treatment. • Use effective methods of contraception during and for 3 mos following treatment. • Report fever, chills, aches, weakness, cough, nausea, symptoms of infection, visual changes, yellowing of skin, eyes, dark urine.

# fluconazole

flu-**kon**-a-zole
(Apo-Fluconazole ✦, Diflucan, Novo-Fluconazole ✦)
**Do not confuse Diflucan with diclofenac, Diprivan, or disulfiram, or fluconazole with fluoxetine, furosemide, or itraconazole.**

## ◆CLASSIFICATION

**PHARMACOTHERAPEUTIC:** Synthetic azole. **CLINICAL:** Systemic antifungal.

## USES

Antifungal prophylaxis in pts undergoing bone marrow transplant; candidiasis (esophageal, oropharyngeal, urinary tract, vaginal); systemic Candida infections (e.g., candidemia); treatment of cryptococcal meningitis. **OFF-LABEL:** Cryptococcal pneumonia, candidal intertrigo.

## PRECAUTIONS

**Contraindications:** Hypersensitivity to fluconazole. Concomitant administration of QT-prolonging medications (e.g., erythromycin, pimozide). **Cautions:** Hepatic/renal impairment, hypersensitivity to other triazoles (e.g., itraconazole, terconazole), imidazoles (e.g., butoconazole, ketoconazole). Medications or conditions known to cause arrhythmias.

## ACTION

Interferes with cytochrome P-450 activity, an enzyme necessary for ergosterol formation. **Therapeutic Effect:** Directly damages fungal membrane, altering its function. Fungistatic.

## PHARMACOKINETICS

Well absorbed from GI tract. Widely distributed, including to CSF. Protein binding: 11%. Partially metabolized in liver. Excreted unchanged primarily in urine. Partially removed by hemodialysis. **Half-life:** 20–30 hrs (increased in renal impairment).

## LIFESPAN CONSIDERATIONS

**Pregnancy/Lactation:** Unknown if distributed in breast milk. **Children:** No age-related precautions noted. **Elderly:** Age-related renal impairment may require dosage adjustment.

## INTERACTIONS

**DRUG:** May increase concentration/effect of **cyclosporine, sirolimus, tacrolimus. Isoniazid, rifampin** may increase drug metabolism. May increase concentration/effects of **oral antidiabetic medication.** May decrease metabolism of **phenytoin, warfarin. HERBAL:** None significant. **FOOD:** None known. **LAB VALUES:** May increase serum alkaline phosphatase, bilirubin, ALT, AST.

## AVAILABILITY (Rx)

**Injection, Solution, Pre-Mix:** 100 mg (50 ml), 200 mg (100 ml), 400 mg (200 ml). **Powder for Oral Suspension:** 10 mg/ml, 40 mg/ml. **Tablets:** 50 mg, 100 mg, 150 mg, 200 mg.

## ADMINISTRATION/HANDLING
 **IV**

**Rate of Administration** • Do not exceed maximum flow rate of 200 mg/hr.
**Storage** • Store at room temperature. • Do not remove from outer wrap until ready to use. • Squeeze inner bag to check for leaks. • Do not use parenteral form if solution is cloudy, precipitate forms, seal is not intact, or it is discolored. • Do not add supplementary medication.

**PO**
• Give without regard to meals.

## IV INCOMPATIBILITIES

Amphotericin B (Fungizone), amphotericin B complex (Abelcet, AmBisome, Amphotec), ampicillin (Polycillin), calcium gluconate, cefotaxime (Claforan), ceftriaxone (Rocephin), cefuroxime (Zinacef), chloramphenicol (Chloromycetin), clindamycin (Cleocin), co-trimoxazole (Bactrim), diazepam (Valium), digoxin (Lanoxin), erythromycin (Erythrocin), furosemide (Lasix), haloperidol (Haldol), hydroxyzine (Vistaril), imipenem and cilastatin (Primaxin).

## IV COMPATIBILITIES

Dexmedetomidine (Precedex), diltiazem (Cardizem), dobutamine (Dobutrex), dopamine (Intropin), heparin, lipids, lorazepam (Ativan), midazolam (Versed), propofol (Diprivan).

## INDICATIONS/ROUTES/DOSAGE

◄**ALERT**► PO and IV therapy equally effective; IV therapy for pt intolerant of drug or unable to take orally. Oral suspension stable for 14 days at room temperature or refrigerated.

**Usual Dosage**
**Note:** Duration and dose dependent on location/severity of infection.
**PO/IV: ADULTS, ELDERLY:** 150 mg once or **loading dose:** 200–800 mg. **Maintenance dose:** 200–800 mg once daily. **CHILDREN AND NEONATES: Loading dose:** 6–12 mg/kg. **Maintenance dose:** 3–12 mg/kg once daily. **Maximum:** 600 mg/day.

**Dosage in Renal Impairment**
After a loading dose of 400 mg, daily dosage is based on creatinine clearance.

| Creatinine Clearance | Dosage |
| --- | --- |
| Greater than 50 ml/min | 100% |
| 50 ml/min or less | 50% |
| Dialysis | 50% |
| CCRT | 400–800 mg as loading dose |
| CVVH | then 200–800 mg/day |
| CVVHDF | 400–800 mg as loading dose, then 400–800 mg/day |

**Dosage in Hepatic Impairment**
Use caution.

## SIDE EFFECTS

**Occasional (4%–1%):** Hypersensitivity reaction (chills, fever, pruritus, rash), dizziness, drowsiness, headache, constipation, diarrhea, nausea, vomiting, abdominal pain.

## ADVERSE EFFECTS/ TOXIC REACTIONS

Exfoliative skin disorders, serious hepatic injury, blood dyscrasias (eosinophilia, thrombocytopenia, anemia, leukopenia) have been reported rarely.

## NURSING CONSIDERATIONS

### BASELINE ASSESSMENT

Obtain LFT; serum potassium in critically ill pts. Receive full medication history and screen for interactions. Assess areas of infection. Assess infected area. Establish baselines for CBC, serum potassium, hepatic function.

### INTERVENTION/EVALUATION

Assess for hypersensitivity reaction (chills, fever). Monitor CBC, BMP, LFT. Report rash, itching promptly. Monitor temperature at least daily. Monitor daily pattern of bowel activity, stool consistency. Assess for dizziness; provide assistance as needed.

### PATIENT/FAMILY TEACHING

• Report dark urine, pale stool, jaundiced skin or sclera of eyes, rash, pruritus. • Pts with oropharyngeal infections should maintain fastidious oral hygiene. • Consult physician before taking any other medication.

---

## fludarabine

floo-**dar**-a-been
(Fludara)

**■ BLACK BOX ALERT ■** Must be administered by certified chemotherapy personnel. Severe neurologic

toxicity reported. Life-threatening hemolytic anemia, autoimmune thrombocytopenic purpura, hemophilia have occurred. Risk of severe myelosuppression (anemia, thrombocytopenia, neutropenia). Concurrent use with pentostatin may produce severe/fatal pulmonary toxicity.
**Do not confuse Fludara with FUDR, or fludarabine with cladribine or Flumadine.**

## ◆CLASSIFICATION

**PHARMACOTHERAPEUTIC:** Antimetabolite. **CLINICAL:** Antineoplastic.

## USES

Treatment of progressive or refractory B-cell chronic lymphocytic leukemia (CLL) in pts who have not responded to or have not progressed with another standard alkylating agent. **OFF-LABEL:** Treatment of non-Hodgkin's lymphoma, relapsed acute lymphocytic leukemia (ALL) or acute myeloid leukemia (AML) in children, Waldenström's macroglobulinemia, reduced-intensity conditioning regimens prior to allogeneic hematopoietic stem-cell transplantation.

## PRECAUTIONS

**Contraindications:** Hypersensitivity to fludarabine. **Cautions:** Renal insufficiency, pre-existing hematological disorders (e.g., granulocytopenia), seizure disorder, spasticity, peripheral neuropathy, infection, fever, immunodeficiency.

## ACTION

Inhibits DNA synthesis by interfering with DNA polymerase alpha, ribonucleotide reductase, DNA primase. **Therapeutic Effect:** Induces cell death.

## PHARMACOKINETICS

Rapidly dephosphorylated in serum, then phosphorylated intracellularly to active triphosphate. Primarily excreted in urine. **Half-life:** 7–20 hrs.

---

## ⧖ LIFESPAN CONSIDERATIONS

**Pregnancy/Lactation:** If possible, avoid use during pregnancy, esp. first trimester. May cause fetal harm. Not known whether distributed in breast milk. Breastfeeding not recommended. **Children:** Safety and efficacy not established. **Elderly:** Age-related renal impairment may require dosage adjustment.

## INTERACTIONS

**DRUG: Pentostatin** may increase risk of pulmonary toxicity. **Bone marrow depressants** may increase risk of myelo-suppression. **Live virus vaccines** may potentiate virus replication, increase vaccine side effects, decrease pt's antibody response to vaccine. **HERBAL:** None significant. **FOOD:** None known. **LAB VALUES:** May increase serum alkaline phosphatase, AST, uric acid.

## AVAILABILITY (Rx)

**Injection, Powder for Reconstitution (Fludara):** 50 mg. **Injection, Solution:** 25 mg/ml.

## ADMINISTRATION/HANDLING

◄**ALERT**► Give by IV infusion. Do not add to other IV infusions. Avoid small veins; swollen, edematous extremities; areas overlying joints, tendons.

 **IV**

**Reconstitution** • Handle with extreme care during preparation/administration. If contact with skin or mucous membranes occurs, wash thoroughly with soap and water; rinse eyes profusely with plain water. • Reconstitute 50-mg vial with 2 ml Sterile Water for Injection to provide concentration of 25 mg/ml. • Further dilute with 100–125 ml 0.9% NaCl or D₅W.
**Rate of Administration** • Infuse over 30 min.
**Storage** • Store in refrigerator. • Reconstituted vials stable for 16 days at room temperature or refrigerated. • Diluted solutions stable for 48 hrs at room temperature or refrigerated.

## ▦ IV INCOMPATIBILITIES

Acyclovir (Zovirax), amphotericin B (Fungizone), daunorubicin, hydroxyzine (Vistaril), prochlorperazine (Compazine).

## ▦ IV COMPATIBILITIES

Heparin, hydromorphone (Dilaudid), lorazepam (Ativan), magnesium sulfate, morphine, multivitamins, potassium chloride.

## INDICATIONS/ROUTES/DOSAGE

**Chronic Lymphocytic Leukemia**
**IV: ADULTS:** 25 mg/m² daily for 5 consecutive days. Continue for up to 3 additional cycles. Begin each course of treatment every 28 days.

**Dosage in Renal Impairment**

| Creatinine Clearance | Dosage |
|---|---|
| **IV** | |
| 50–79 ml/min | 20 mg/m² |
| 30–49 ml/min | 15 mg/m² |
| Less than 30 ml/min | Not recommended |

**Dosage in Hepatic Impairment**
No dose adjustment.

## SIDE EFFECTS

**Frequent (60%–11%):** Fever, nausea/vomiting, chills. **Occasional (20%–10%):** Fatigue, generalized pain, rash, diarrhea, cough, asthenia, stomatitis, dyspnea, peripheral edema. **Rare (7%–3%):** Anorexia, sinusitis, dysuria, myalgia, paresthesia, headache, visual disturbances.

## ADVERSE EFFECTS/ TOXIC REACTIONS

Pneumonia occurs frequently. Severe hematologic toxicity (anemia, thrombocytopenia, neutropenia), GI bleeding may occur. Tumor lysis syndrome may begin with flank pain, hematuria; may also include hypercalcemia, hyperphosphatemia, hyperuricemia, resulting in renal failure. High-dosage therapy may produce acute leukemia, blindness, coma. Neurotoxicity (progressive demyelinating encephalopathy, mental status deterioration) occurs rarely.

## NURSING CONSIDERATIONS

### BASELINE ASSESSMENT

Assess baseline CBC, BMP, LFT, uric acid and monitor during treatment. Drug should be discontinued if intractable vomiting, diarrhea, stomatitis, GI bleeding occurs.

### INTERVENTION/EVALUATION

Assess for fatigue, visual disturbances, peripheral edema. Assess for onset of pneumonia. Monitor for dyspnea, cough, rapid decrease in WBC count, intractable vomiting, diarrhea, GI bleeding (bright red or tarry stool). Assess oral mucosa for stomatitis. Assess skin for rash. Be alert to possible tumor lysis syndrome (onset of flank pain, hematuria), signs of neurotoxicity.

### PATIENT/FAMILY TEACHING

• Avoid crowds, exposure to infection. • Maintain strict oral hygiene. • Promptly report fever, sore throat, signs of local infection, unusual bruising/bleeding from any site. • Report persistent nausea/vomiting.

---

## fluorouracil, 5-FU  [HIGH ALERT]

flure-oh-ue-ra-sil
(Adrucil, Carac, Efudex, Fluoroplex, Tolak)

■ **BLACK BOX ALERT** ■ Must be administered by personnel trained in administration/handling of chemotherapeutic agents.
**Do not confuse Efudex with Efidac.**

◆**CLASSIFICATION**

**PHARMACOTHERAPEUTIC:** Antimetabolite. **CLINICAL:** Antineoplastic.

## USES

**Parenteral:** Treatment of carcinoma of colon, rectum, breast, stomach, pancreas. **Topical:** Treatment of multiple actinic or solar keratoses, superficial basal cell carcinomas. **OFF-LABEL: Parenteral:** Treatment of carcinoma of: bladder, cervical, endometrial, head/neck, anal, esophageal, renal cell, unknown primary cancer.

## PRECAUTIONS

**Contraindications:** Hypersensitivity to fluorouracil. Myelosuppression, poor nutritional status, potentially serious infections. **Cautions:** History of high-dose pelvic irradiation, hepatic/renal impairment, palmar-plantar erythrodysesthia syndrome (hand and foot syndrome), previous use of alkylating agents. Pts with widespread metastatic marrow involvement.

## ACTION

Blocks formation of thymidylic acid. Cell cycle–specific for S phase of cell division. **Therapeutic Effect:** Inhibits DNA, RNA synthesis. **Topical:** Destroys rapidly proliferating cells.

## PHARMACOKINETICS

Widely distributed. Crosses blood-brain barrier. Metabolized in liver. Primarily excreted by lungs as carbon dioxide. Removed by hemodialysis. **Half-life:** 16 min.

## ⌛ LIFESPAN CONSIDERATIONS

**Pregnancy/Lactation:** If possible, avoid use during pregnancy, esp. first trimester. May cause fetal harm. Unknown if distributed in breast milk. Breastfeeding not recommended. **Children:** No age-related precautions noted. **Elderly:** Age-related renal impairment may require dosage adjustment.

## INTERACTIONS

**DRUG: Bone marrow depressants** may increase risk of myelosuppression. **Live virus vaccines** may potentiate virus

---

F

replication, increase vaccine side effects, decrease pt's antibody response to vaccine. **HERBAL: Echinacea** may decrease effects. Avoid use of **black cohosh, dong quai** in pts with estrogen-dependent tumors. **FOOD:** None known. **LAB VALUES:** May decrease serum albumin. **Topical:** May cause eosinophilia, leukocytosis, thrombocytopenia, toxic granulation.

## AVAILABILITY (Rx)

**Cream, Topical (Carac):** 0.5%. **(Tolak):** 4%, **(Efudex):** 5%. **(Fluoroplex):** 1%. **Injection Solution (Adrucil):** 50 mg/ml. **Solution, Topical (Efudex):** 2%, 5%.

## ADMINISTRATION/HANDLING

**◄ALERT►** Give by IV injection or IV infusion. Do not add to other IV infusions. Avoid small veins, swollen/edematous extremities, areas overlying joints, tendons. May be carcinogenic, mutagenic, teratogenic. Handle with extreme care during preparation/administration.

 **IV**

**Reconstitution** • IV push does not need to be diluted or reconstituted. • Inject through Y-tube or 3-way stopcock of free-flowing solution. • For IV infusion, further dilute with 50–1,000 ml D₅W or 0.9% NaCl. **Rate of Administration** • Give IV push slowly over 1–2 min. • IV infusion is administered over 30 min–24 hrs (refer to individual protocols). • Extravasation produces immediate pain, severe local tissue damage. **Storage** • Store at room temperature. • Solution appears colorless to faint yellow. Slight discoloration does not adversely affect potency or safety. • If precipitate forms, redissolve by heating, shaking vigorously; allow to cool to body temperature. • Diluted solutions stable for 72 hrs at room temperature.

## IV INCOMPATIBILITIES

Amphotericin B complex (Abelcet, AmBisome, Amphotec), filgrastim (Neupogen), ondansetron (Zofran), vinorelbine (Navelbine).

## IV COMPATIBILITIES

Granisetron (Kytril), heparin, hydromorphone (Dilaudid), leucovorin, morphine, potassium chloride, propofol (Diprivan).

## INDICATIONS/ROUTES/DOSAGE

**Note:** Refer to individual protocols.

**Usual Therapy**
**IV Bolus: ADULTS, ELDERLY:** 400–500 mg/m²/day for 4–5 days or 500–600 mg/m²/dose q3–4wks.
**IV Infusion: ADULTS, ELDERLY:** 15 mg/kg/day or 500 mg/m²/day over 4 hrs for 5 days or 800–1200 mg/m² over 24–120 hrs.

**Multiple Actinic or Solar Keratoses**
**Topical (Carac): ADULTS, ELDERLY:** Apply once daily for up to 4 wks.
**Topical (Efudex): ADULTS, ELDERLY:** Apply twice daily for 2–4 wks.
**Topical (Fluoroplex):** Apply twice daily for 2–6 wks.
**Topical (Tolak):** Apply once daily for 4 wks.

**Basal Cell Carcinoma**
**Topical (Efudex 5%): ADULTS, ELDERLY:** Apply twice daily for 3–6 wks up to 10–12 wks.

**Dosage in Renal Impairment**
No dose adjustment.

**Dosage in Hepatic Impairment**
Use extreme caution.

## SIDE EFFECTS

**Parenteral: Frequent (greater than 10%):** Alopecia, dermatitis, anorexia, diarrhea, esophagitis, dyspepsia, stomatitis. **Occasional (10%–1%):** Cardiotoxicity (angina, EKG changes), skin dryness, epithelial fissuring, nausea, vomiting, excessive lacrimation, blurred vision. **Rare (less than 1%):** Headache, photosensitivity, somnolence, allergic reaction, dyspnea, hypotension, MI, pulmonary edema. **Topical: Occasional:**

Erythema, skin ulceration, pruritus, hyperpigmentation, dermatitis, insomnia, stomatitis, irritability, photosensitivity, excessive lacrimation, blurred vision.

## ADVERSE EFFECTS/TOXIC REACTIONS

Earliest sign of toxicity (4–8 days after beginning therapy) is stomatitis (dry mouth, burning sensation, mucosal erythema, ulceration at inner margin of lips). Most common dermatologic toxicity is pruritic rash (generally on extremities, less frequently on trunk). Leukopenia (WBC less than 3500/mm$^3$) generally occurs within 9–14 days after drug administration but may occur as late as 25th day. Thrombocytopenia (platelets less than 100,000/mm$^3$) occasionally occurs within 7–17 days after administration. Pancytopenia, agranulocytosis occur rarely.

## NURSING CONSIDERATIONS

### BASELINE ASSESSMENT

Obtain baseline CBC with differential, serum renal function, LFT and monitor during therapy.

### INTERVENTION/EVALUATION

Monitor for rapidly falling WBC, platelet count; intractable diarrhea, GI bleeding (bright red or tarry stool). Assess oral mucosa for stomatitis. Drug should be discontinued if intractable diarrhea, stomatitis, GI bleeding occurs. Assess skin for rash.

### PATIENT/FAMILY TEACHING

• Maintain strict oral hygiene. • Report signs/symptoms of infection, unusual bruising/bleeding, visual changes, nausea, vomiting, diarrhea, chest pain, palpitations. • Avoid sunlight, artificial light sources; wear protective clothing, sunglasses, sunscreen. • **Topical:** Apply only to affected area. • Do not use occlusive coverings. • Be careful near eyes, nose, mouth. • Wash hands thoroughly after application. • Treated areas may be unsightly for several weeks after therapy.

# *FLUoxetine

floo-**ox**-e-teen
(Apo-Fluoxetine ♣, Novo-Fluoxetine ♣, Prozac, Prozac Weekly, Sarafem)

■ **BLACK BOX ALERT** ■ Increased risk of suicidal thinking and behavior in children, adolescents, young adults 18–24 yrs of age with major depressive disorder, other psychiatric disorders.

**Do not confuse fluoxetine with duloxetine, famotidine, fluconazole, fluvastatin, fluvoxamine, fosinopril, furosemide, or paroxetine, or Prozac with Paxil, Prilosec, Prograf, Proscar, or ProSom, or Sarafem with Serophene.**

## FIXED-COMBINATION(S)

**Symbyax:** fluoxetine/olanzapine (an antipsychotic): 25 mg/6 mg, 25 mg/12 mg, 50 mg/6 mg, 50 mg/12 mg.

## ◆CLASSIFICATION

**PHARMACOTHERAPEUTIC:** Selective serotonin reuptake inhibitor (SSRI). **CLINICAL:** Antidepressant, antiobsessional agent, antibulimic.

## USES

Treatment of major depressive disorder (MDD), obsessive-compulsive disorder (OCD), binge-eating and vomiting in moderate to severe bulimia nervosa, premenstrual dysphoric disorder (PMDD), panic disorder with or without agoraphobia. Treatment of resistant or bipolar 1 depression (with olanzapine). OFF-LABEL: Treatment of fibromyalgia, post-traumatic stress disorder (PTSD), Raynaud's phenomena, social anxiety disorder, selective mutism.

## PRECAUTIONS

**Contraindications:** Hypersensitivity to fluoxetine. Use of MAOIs within 5 wks of discontinuing fluoxetine or within 14 days

F

of discontinuing MAOIs. Initiation in pts receiving linezolid or methylene blue. Use with thioridazine. **Cautions:** Seizure disorder, cardiac dysfunction (e.g., history of MI), diabetes, pts with risk factors for QT prolongation, concurrent use of medication that increase QT interval, renal/hepatic impairment, pts at high risk for suicide, in pts where weight loss is undesirable, elderly. Pts at risk of acute narrow-angle glaucoma or with increased intraocular pressure.

## ACTION

Selectively inhibits serotonin uptake in CNS, enhancing serotonergic function. **Therapeutic Effect:** Relieves depression; reduces obsessive-compulsive, bulimic behavior.

## PHARMACOKINETICS

Well absorbed from GI tract. Crosses blood-brain barrier. Protein binding: 94%. Metabolized in liver. Primarily excreted in urine. Not removed by hemodialysis. **Half-life:** 2–3 days; metabolite, 7–9 days.

## ⧗ LIFESPAN CONSIDERATIONS

**Pregnancy/Lactation:** Unknown whether drug crosses placenta or is distributed in breast milk. **Children:** May be more sensitive to behavioral side effects (e.g., insomnia, restlessness). **Elderly:** No age-related precautions noted.

## INTERACTIONS

**DRUG: NSAIDs, antiplatelets** (e.g., **clopidogrel**), **anticoagulants** (e.g., **warfarin**) may increase risk of bleeding. **Alcohol, other CNS depressants** may increase CNS depression. **MAOIs** may produce serotonin syndrome and neuroleptic malignant syndrome. May increase concentration/toxicity of **phenytoin, tricyclic antidepressants. HERBAL: Gotu kola, kava kava, St. John's wort, valerian** may increase CNS depression. **St. John's wort** may increase effects, risk of serotonin syndrome.

**FOOD:** None known. **LAB VALUES:** May decrease serum sodium. May increase serum ALT, AST.

## AVAILABILITY (Rx)

**Capsules:** 10 mg, 20 mg, 40 mg. **Oral Solution:** 20 mg/5 ml. **Tablets:** 10 mg, 20 mg, 60 mg.

🖉 **Capsules (Delayed-Release [Prozac Weekly]):** 90 mg.

## ADMINISTRATION/HANDLING

### PO
• Give without regard to food, but give with food, milk if GI distress occurs. • **Bipolar disorder:** Give once daily in evening. • **Depression OCD:** Give once daily in morning or twice daily (morning and noon). • **Bulimia:** Give once daily in morning.

## INDICATIONS/ROUTES/DOSAGE

◀**ALERT**▶ Use lower or less frequent doses in pts with renal/hepatic impairment, pts with concurrent disease or multiple medications, the elderly.

**Depression**
**PO: ADULTS, ELDERLY:** Initially, 5–20 mg each morning. May increase after several wks by 20 mg/day. **Maximum:** 80 mg/day as single or 2 divided doses. **Prozac Weekly:** 90 mg/wk, begin 7 days after last dose of 20 mg in pts maintained on 20 mg/day. **CHILDREN 8–18 YRS:** Initially, 5–10 mg/day. Titrate upward as needed. Usual dosage: 20 mg/day.

**Panic Disorder**
**PO: ADULTS, ELDERLY:** Initially, 10 mg/day. May increase to 20 mg/day after 1 wk. **Maximum:** 60 mg/day.

**Bulimia Nervosa**
**PO: ADULTS:** 60 mg each morning. May titrate to 60 mg over several days.

**Obsessive-Compulsive Disorder (OCD)**
**PO: ADULTS, ELDERLY:** Initially, 20 mg/day. May increase after several wks. Usual dose: 20–60 mg/day. **Maximum:** 80 mg/

day. **CHILDREN 7–18 YRS:** Initially, 10 mg/day. May increase to 20 mg/day after 2 wks. Range: 20–60 mg/day.

**Depression Associated with Bipolar Disorder**
**PO: ADULTS, ELDERLY CHILDREN 10–17 YRS:** *(with olanzapine):* Initially, 20 mg/day. May increase after several wks. Range: 20–50 mg/day.

**Premenstrual Dysphoric Disorder (PMDD) (Sarafem)**
**PO: ADULTS:** 20 mg/day continuously **or** 20 mg/day beginning 14 days prior to menstruation and continuing through first full day of menses (repeated with each cycle).

**Dosage in Renal/Hepatic Impairment**
Use caution.

## SIDE EFFECTS
**Frequent (greater than 10%):** Headache, asthenia, insomnia, anxiety, drowsiness, nausea, diarrhea, decreased appetite. **Occasional (9%–2%):** Dizziness, tremor, fatigue, vomiting, constipation, dry mouth, abdominal pain, nasal congestion, diaphoresis, rash. **Rare (less than 2%):** Flushed skin, light-headedness, impaired concentration.

## ADVERSE EFFECTS/ TOXIC REACTIONS
May increase risk of suicide. Agitation, coma, diarrhea, delerium, hallucinations, hyperreflexia, hyperthermia, tachycardia, seizures may indicate life-threatening serotonin syndrome.

## NURSING CONSIDERATIONS
### BASELINE ASSESSMENT
Assess appearance, behavior, mood, suicidal tendencies. For pts on long-term therapy, baseline renal function, LFT, blood counts should be performed at baseline and periodically thereafter.

### INTERVENTION/EVALUATION
Supervise suicidal-risk pt closely during early therapy (as depression lessens, energy level improves, increasing suicide potential). Monitor mental status, anxiety, social functioning, appetite, nutritional intake. Monitor daily pattern of bowel activity, stool consistency. Assess skin for rash. Monitor serum LFT, glucose, sodium; weight.

### PATIENT/FAMILY TEACHING
• Maximum therapeutic response may require 4 or more wks of therapy. • Do not abruptly discontinue medication. • Avoid tasks that require alertness, motor skills until response to drug is established. • Avoid alcohol. • To avoid insomnia, take last dose of drug before 4 PM.

# fluticasone

floo-**tik**-a-sone
(Apo-Fluticasone ❖, Arnuity Ellipta, Cutivate, <u>Flonase</u>, Flonase Allergy Relief, Flovent Diskus, Flovent HFA, Veramyst)
**Do not confuse Cutivate with Ultravate, or Flonase with Flovent.**

## FIXED-COMBINATION(S)
**Advair, Advair Diskus, Advair HFA:** fluticasone/salmeterol (bronchodilator): 100 mcg/50 mcg, 250 mcg/50 mcg, 500 mcg/50 mcg. **Breo Ellipta:** Fluticasone/vilanterol (bronchodilator): 100 mcg/25 mcg. **Dymista:** Fluticasone/azelastine (an antihistamine): 50 mcg/137 mcg per spray.

## ◆CLASSIFICATION
**PHARMACOTHERAPEUTIC:** Corticosteroid. **CLINICAL:** Anti-inflammatory, antipruritic.

**F**

## USES

**Nasal: (Flonase):** Management of nasal symptoms of perennial nonallergic rhinitis in adults and children 4 yrs and older. **(Veramyst):** Management of seasonal and perennial allergic rhinitis in adults, children 2 yrs and older. **Topical:** Relief of inflammation/pruritus associated with steroid-responsive disorders (e.g., contact dermatitis, eczema), atopic dermatitis. **Inhalation:** Maintenance treatment of bronchial asthma. Assists in reducing, discontinuing oral corticosteroid therapy.

## PRECAUTIONS

**Contraindications:** Hypersensitivity to fluticasone. (Arnuity Ellipta, Flovent Diskus): Severe hypersensitivity to milk proteins or lactose. **Inhalation:** Primary treatment of status asthmaticus, acute exacerbation of asthma, other acute asthmatic conditions. **Cautions:** Untreated systemic ocular herpes simplex; untreated fungal, bacterial infection; active or quiescent tuberculosis. Thyroid disease, cardiovascular disease, diabetes, glaucoma, hepatic/renal impairment, cataracts, myasthenia gravis, seizures, GI disease, risk for osteoporosis, untreated localized infection of nasal mucosa. Following acute MI; concurrent use with strong CYP3A4 inhibitors.

## ACTION

Controls rate of protein synthesis, depresses migration of polymorphonuclear leukocytes, reverses capillary permeability, stabilizes lysosomal membranes. **Therapeutic Effect:** Prevents, controls inflammation.

## PHARMACOKINETICS

**Inhalation/intranasal:** Protein binding: 91%. Metabolized in liver. Excreted in urine. **Half-life:** 3–7.8 hrs. **Topical:** Amount absorbed depends on affected area and skin condition (absorption increased with fever, hydration, inflamed or denuded skin).

## ⧗ LIFESPAN CONSIDERATIONS

**Pregnancy/Lactation:** Unknown if drug crosses placenta or is distributed in breast milk. **Children:** Safety and efficacy not established in pts younger than 4 yrs. Children 4 yrs and older may experience growth suppression with prolonged or high doses. **Elderly:** No age-related precautions noted.

## INTERACTIONS

**DRUG:** CYP3A4 inhibitors (**ritonavir, nelfinavir, clarithromycin, itraconazole, ketoconazole**) may increase concentration. **Ritonavir** may reduce serum cortisol concentration. **HERBAL: Echinacea, St. John's wort** may decrease concentration/effects. **FOOD:** None known. **LAB VALUES:** None significant.

## AVAILABILITY (Rx)

**Aerosol for Oral Inhalation (Flovent HFA):** 44 mcg/inhalation, 110 mcg/inhalation, 220 mcg/inhalation. **Cream (Cutivate):** 0.05%. **Ointment (Cutivate):** 0.005%. **Powder for Oral Inhalation (Flovent Diskus):** 50 mcg/blister, 100 mcg/blister, 250 mcg/blister. **(Arnuity Ellipta):** 100 mcg/actuation, 200 mcg/actuation. **Suspension Intranasal Spray: (Flonase, Flonase Allergy Relief):** 50 mcg/inhalation. **(Veramyst):** 27.5 mcg/spray.

## ADMINISTRATION/HANDLING

**Inhalation**

• Shake container well. Instruct pt to exhale completely. Place mouthpiece fully into mouth, inhale, hold breath as long as possible before exhaling. • Allow at least 1 min between inhalations. • Rinsing mouth after each use decreases dry mouth, hoarseness.

**Intranasal**

• Instruct pt to clear nasal passages as much as possible before use (topical nasal decongestants may be needed 5–15 min before use). • Tilt head slightly forward. • Insert spray tip into 1 nostril, pointing toward inflamed nasal turbinates, away from nasal septum. • Pump medication into 1 nostril while pt holds other nostril closed, concurrently inspires through nose.

## INDICATIONS/ROUTES/DOSAGE

### Allergic Rhinitis
**Intranasal:** *(Flonase):* **ADULTS, ELDERLY:** Initially, 200 mcg (2 sprays in each nostril once daily or 1 spray in each nostril q12h). **Maintenance:** 1 spray in each nostril once daily. May increase to 100 mcg (2 sprays) in each nostril. **Maximum:** 200 mcg/day. **CHILDREN 4 YRS AND OLDER:** Initially, 100 mcg (1 spray in each nostril once daily). **Maximum:** 200 mcg/day (2 sprays each nostril).
*(Veramyst):* **ADULTS, ELDERLY, CHILDREN 12 YRS AND OLDER:** 110 mcg (2 sprays in each nostril) once daily. **Maintenance:** 55 mcg (1 spray in each nostril) once daily. **CHILDREN 2–11 YRS:** 55 mcg (1 spray in each nostril) once daily. May increase to 110 mcg (2 sprays each nostril) once daily.

### Usual Topical Dosage
**Note:** Ointment for adults only.
**Topical: ADULTS, ELDERLY, CHILDREN 3 MOS AND OLDER:** Apply sparingly to affected area once or twice daily.

### Maintenance Treatment of Asthma
**Inhalation Powder** *(Arnuity Ellipta):* **ADULTS, ELDERLY, CHILDREN 12 YRS AND OLDER:** 100–200 mcg once daily. **Maximum:** 200 mcg/day.

### Maintenance Treatment for Asthma (Previously Treated with Bronchodilators)
**Inhalation Powder** *(Flovent Diskus):* **ADULTS, ELDERLY, CHILDREN 12 YRS AND OLDER:** Initially, 100 mcg twice daily. **Maximum:** 500 mcg/twice daily.
**Inhalation ADULTS, ELDERLY, CHILDREN 12 YRS AND OLDER:** *(Flovent HFA):* 88 mcg twice daily. **Maximum:** 440 mcg twice daily.

### Maintenance Treatment for Asthma (Previously Treated with Inhaled Steroids)
**Inhalation Powder** *(Flovent Diskus):* **ADULTS, ELDERLY, CHILDREN 12 YRS AND OLDER:** Initially, 100–250 mcg twice daily. **Maximum:** 500 mcg twice daily.
**Inhalation ADULTS, ELDERLY, CHILDREN 12 YRS AND OLDER:** *(Flovent HFA):* 88–220 mcg twice daily. **Maximum:** 440 mcg twice daily.

### Maintenance Treatment for Asthma (Previously Treated with Oral Steroids)
**Inhalation Powder** *(Flovent Diskus):* **ADULTS, ELDERLY, CHILDREN 12 YRS AND OLDER:** 500–1,000 mcg twice daily.
**Inhalation ADULTS, ELDERLY, CHILDREN 12 YRS AND OLDER:** *(Flovent HFA):* 440–880 mcg twice daily.

### Usual Pediatric Dose (4–11 Yrs)
**Flovent Diskus:** Initially, 50 mcg twice daily. May increase to 100 mcg twice daily. **Flovent HFA:** 88 mcg twice daily.

### Dosage in Renal/Hepatic Impairment
No dose adjustment. *(Arnuity Ellipta):* Use caution in hepatic impairment.

## SIDE EFFECTS

**Frequent: Inhalation:** Throat irritation, hoarseness, dry mouth, cough, temporary wheezing, oropharyngeal candidiasis (particularly if mouth is not rinsed with water after each administration). **Intranasal:** Mild nasopharyngeal irritation, nasal burning, stinging, dryness, rebound congestion, rhinorrhea, altered sense of taste. **Occasional: Inhalation:** Oral candidiasis. **Intranasal:** Nasal/pharyngeal candidiasis, headache. **Topical:** Stinging, burning of skin.

## ADVERSE EFFECTS/ TOXIC REACTIONS

None known.

## NURSING CONSIDERATIONS

### BASELINE ASSESSMENT
Establish baseline history of skin disorder, asthma, rhinitis.

### INTERVENTION/EVALUATION
Monitor rate, depth, rhythm, type of respiration; quality/rate of pulse. Assess lung sounds for rhonchi, wheezing, rales. Assess oral mucous membranes for evidence of candidiasis. Monitor growth in pediatric pts. **Topical:** Assess involved area for therapeutic response to irritation.

### PATIENT/FAMILY TEACHING
• Pts receiving bronchodilators by inhalation concomitantly with steroid inhalation therapy should use bronchodilator several min before corticosteroid aerosol (enhances penetration of steroid into bronchial tree). • Do not change dose/schedule or stop taking drug; must taper off gradually under medical supervision. • Maintain strict oral hygiene. • Rinse mouth with water immediately after inhalation (prevents mouth/throat dryness, oral fungal infection). • Increase fluid intake (decreases lung secretion viscosity). • **Intranasal:** Clear nasal passages before use. • Report if no improvement in symptoms or sneezing/nasal irritation occurs. • Improvement noted in several days. • **Topical:** Rub thin film gently into affected area. • Use only for prescribed area and no longer than ordered. • Avoid contact with eyes.

## *fluvoxaMINE

floo-**vox**-a-meen
(Apo-Fluvoxumine ✤, Luvox CR, Novo-Fluvoxamine ✦)

■ **BLACK BOX ALERT** ■ Increased risk of suicidal ideation and behavior in children, adolescents, young adults 18–24 yrs with major depressive disorder, other psychiatric disorders.

**Do not confuse fluvoxamine with flavoxate or fluoxetine, or Luvox with Lasix, Levoxyl, or Lovenox.**

## ◆CLASSIFICATION

**PHARMACOTHERAPEUTIC:** Serotonin reuptake inhibitor. **CLINICAL:** Antidepressant, antiobsessive.

## USES

**Immediate-Release:** Treatment of obsessive-compulsive disorder (OCD) in adults and children 8–17 yrs of age. **Extended-Release:** Treatment of OCD in adults. **OFF-LABEL:** Treatment of social anxiety disorder (SAD), post-traumatic stress disorder (PTSD).

## PRECAUTIONS

**Contraindications:** Hypersensitivity to fluvoxamine. Use of MAOIs concurrently or within 14 days of discontinuing MAOIs or fluvoxamine. Concomitant use with alosetron, pimozide, ramelteon, thioridazine, or tizanidine. Initiation of fluvoxamine in pts receiving linezolid or methylene blue. **Cautions:** Renal/hepatic impairment; elderly; impaired platelet aggregation; concurrent use of NSAIDs, aspirin; seizure disorder; pts that are volume depleted; third trimester of pregnancy; pts with high suicide risk; risk of bleeding or receiving concurrent anticoagulant therapy.

## ACTION

Selectively inhibits neuronal reuptake of serotonin. **Therapeutic Effect:** Relieves depression, symptoms of obsessive-compulsive disorder (OCD).

## PHARMACOKINETICS

Well absorbed following PO administration. Protein binding: 77%. Metabolized in liver. Excreted in urine. **Half-life:** 15–20 hrs.

## ⧗ LIFESPAN CONSIDERATIONS

**Pregnancy/Lactation:** Unknown if drug crosses the placenta; distributed in breast milk. **Children:** Safety and efficacy not established in pts younger than 8 yrs. **Elderly:** Potential for reduced serum clearance; maintain caution.

---

## INTERACTIONS

**DRUG:** May increase concentration, risk of toxicity of **benzodiazepines (e.g., alprazolam, lorazepam), carbamazepine, clozapine, theophylline. Lithium, tryptophan** may enhance fluvoxamine's serotonergic effects. **MAOIs** may increase risk of serotonin syndrome (hyperthermia, rigidity, myoclonus). **Tricyclic antidepressants (e.g., amitriptyline)** may increase concentration. May increase effects of **warfarin. HERBAL: Valerian, St. John's wort, SAMe, kava kava** may increase risk of serotonin syndrome or CNS depression. Avoid **herbs with antiplatelet activity (e.g., cat's claw, feverfew, ginger). FOOD:** None known. **LAB VALUES:** May decrease serum sodium.

## AVAILABILITY (Rx)

**Tablets:** 25 mg, 50 mg, 100 mg.

**Capsules (Extended-Release):** 100 mg, 150 mg.

## ADMINISTRATION/HANDLING

• Do not break, crush, dissolve, or divide extended-release capsules. • May give with or without food.

## INDICATIONS/ROUTES/DOSAGE

**Obsessive-Compulsive Disorder (OCD)**
**PO** *(Immediate-Release):* **ADULTS:** Initially, 50 mg at bedtime; may increase by 50 mg every 4–7 days. Dosages greater than 100 mg/day should be given in 2 divided doses with larger dose given at bedtime. Usual dose: 100–300 mg/day. **Maximum:** 300 mg/day. *(Extended-Release)* Initially, 100 mg once daily at bedtime. May increase by 50 mg at no less than 1-wk intervals. Range: 100–300 mg/day. **Maximum:** 300 mg/day. **CHILDREN 8–17 YRS** *(Immediate-Release):* Initially, 25 mg at bedtime; may increase by 25 mg every 4–7 days. Dosages greater than 50 mg/day should be given in 2 divided doses with larger dose given at bedtime. **Maximum: (CHILDREN 8–11 YRS):** 200 mg/day. **(CHILDREN 12–17 YRS):** 300 mg/day.

**Dosage in Renal/Hepatic Impairment**
No dose adjustment.

## SIDE EFFECTS

**Frequent (40%–21%):** Nausea, headache, drowsiness, insomnia. **Occasional (14%–8%):** Dizziness, diarrhea, dry mouth, asthenia, dyspepsia, constipation, abnormal ejaculation. **Rare (6%–3%):** Anorexia, anxiety, tremor, vomiting, flatulence, urinary frequency, sexual dysfunction, altered taste.

## ADVERSE EFFECTS/ TOXIC REACTIONS

Agitation, coma, diarrhea, delerium, hallucinations, hyperreflexia, hyperthermia, tachycardia, seizures may indicate life-threatening serotonin syndrome.

## NURSING CONSIDERATIONS

### BASELINE ASSESSMENT
Obtain baseline chemistries, esp. renal function, LFT.

### INTERVENTION/EVALUATION
Supervise suicidal-risk pt closely during early therapy (as depression lessens, energy level improves, increasing suicide potential). Assess appearance, behavior, speech pattern, level of interest, mood. Assist with ambulation if dizziness, drowsiness occurs. Monitor daily pattern of bowel activity, stool consistency.

### PATIENT/FAMILY TEACHING
• Maximum therapeutic response may require 4 wks or more of therapy. • Dry mouth may be relieved by sugarless gum, sips of water. • Do not abruptly discontinue medication. • Avoid tasks that require alertness, motor skills until response to drug is established.

# folic acid

foe-lik **as**-id
(Apo-Folic ✦)
**Do not confuse folic acid with folinic acid.**

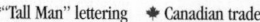

F

## ◆CLASSIFICATION

**PHARMACOTHERAPEUTIC:** Coenzyme.
**CLINICAL:** Nutritional supplement.

## USES

Treatment of megaloblastic and macrocytic anemias due to folate deficiency.

## PRECAUTIONS

**Contraindications:** Hypersensitivity to folic acid. **Cautions:** Anemias (aplastic, normocytic, pernicious, refractory) when anemia present with vitamin $B_{12}$ deficiency.

## ACTION

Stimulates production of platelets, RBCs, WBCs in folate deficiency anemia. **Therapeutic Effect:** Essential for nucleoprotein synthesis, maintenance of normal erythropoiesis.

## PHARMACOKINETICS

PO form almost completely absorbed from GI tract (upper duodenum). Protein binding: High. Metabolized in liver. Excreted in urine. Removed by hemodialysis.

## ⌛ LIFESPAN CONSIDERATIONS

**Pregnancy/Lactation:** Distributed in breast milk. **Children/Elderly:** No age-related precautions noted.

## INTERACTIONS

**DRUG:** May decrease effects of **phenobarbital, phenytoin, primidone, raltitrexed. HERBAL: Green tea** may increase concentration. **FOOD:** None known. **LAB VALUES:** May decrease vitamin $B_{12}$ concentration.

## AVAILABILITY (Rx)

**Capsules:** 0.8 mg, 5 mg, 20 mg. **Injection Solution:** 5 mg/ml. **Tablets:** 0.4 mg (OTC), 0.8 mg (OTC), 1 mg.

## ADMINISTRATION/HANDLING

**PO**
• May give without regard to food.

**IV**
May give 5 mg or less undiluted over at least 1 min, or dilute with 50 ml 0.9% NaCl or $D_5W$ and infuse over 30 min.

## INDICATIONS/ROUTES/DOSAGE

**Anemia**
**IM/IV/SQ/PO: ADULTS, ELDERLY, CHILDREN 4 YRS AND OLDER:** 0.4 mg/day. **CHILDREN YOUNGER THAN 4 YRS:** Up to 0.3 mg/day. **INFANTS:** 0.1 mg/day. **PREGNANT/LACTATING WOMEN:** 0.8 mg/day.

**Prevention of Neural Tube Defects**
**PO: WOMEN OF CHILDBEARING AGE:** 400–800 mcg/day. **WOMEN AT HIGH RISK OR FAMILY HISTORY OF NEURAL TUBE DEFECTS:** 4 mg/day.

## SIDE EFFECTS

None known.

## ADVERSE EFFECTS/ TOXIC REACTIONS

Allergic hypersensitivity occurs rarely with parenteral form. Oral folic acid is nontoxic.

## NURSING CONSIDERATIONS

### BASELINE ASSESSMENT

Pernicious anemia should be ruled out with Schilling test and vitamin $B_{12}$ blood level before initiating therapy (may produce irreversible neurologic damage). Resistance to treatment may occur if decreased hematopoiesis, alcoholism, antimetabolite drugs, deficiency of vitamin $B_6$, $B_{12}$, C, E is evident.

### INTERVENTION/EVALUATION

Assess for therapeutic improvement: improved sense of well-being, relief from iron deficiency symptoms (fatigue, shortness of breath, sore tongue, headache, pallor).

### PATIENT/FAMILY TEACHING

• Eat foods rich in folic acid, including fruits, vegetables, organ meats.

# fondaparinux

fon-**dap**-a-rin-ux
(Arixtra)

■ **BLACK BOX ALERT** ■ Epidural or spinal anesthesia greatly increases potential for spinal or epidural hematoma, subsequent long-term or permanent paralysis.

## ◆CLASSIFICATION

**PHARMACOTHERAPEUTIC:** Factor Xa inhibitor. **CLINICAL:** Antithrombotic.

## USES

Prevention of venous thromboembolism in pts undergoing total hip replacement, hip fracture surgery, knee replacement surgery, abdominal surgery. Treatment of acute deep vein thrombosis (DVT), acute pulmonary embolism. **OFF-LABEL:** Prophylaxis of DVT in pts with history of heparin-induced thrombocytopenia (HIT), acute symptomatic superficial vein thrombosis of the legs.

## PRECAUTIONS

**Contraindications:** Hypersensitivity to fondaparinux, active major bleeding, bacterial endocarditis, prophylaxis treatment in pts with body weight less than 50 kg, severe renal impairment (CrCl less than 30 ml/min), thrombocytopenia associated with antiplatelet antibody formation in presence of fondaparinux. **Cautions:** Conditions with increased risk of bleeding, bacterial endocarditis, active ulcerative GI disease, hemorrhagic stroke; shortly after brain, spinal, or ophthalmologic surgery; concurrent platelet inhibitors, severe uncontrolled hypertension, history of CVA, history of heparin-induced thrombocytopenia, renal/hepatic impairment, elderly, indwelling epidural catheter use.

## ACTION

Factor Xa inhibitor that selectively binds to antithrombin and increases its affinity for factor Xa, inhibiting factor Xa, stopping blood coagulation cascade. **Therapeutic Effect:** Indirectly prevents formation of thrombin and subsequently fibrin clot.

## PHARMACOKINETICS

Well absorbed after subcutaneous administration. Undergoes minimal, if any, metabolism. Highly bound to antithrombin III. Distributed mainly in blood and to a minor extent in extravascular fluid. Excreted unchanged in urine. Removed by hemodialysis. **Half-life:** 17–21 hrs (increased in renal impairment).

## ☒ LIFESPAN CONSIDERATIONS

**Pregnancy/Lactation:** Use with caution, particularly during third trimester, immediate postpartum period (increased risk of maternal hemorrhage). Unknown if excreted in breast milk. **Children:** Safety and efficacy not established. **Elderly:** Age-related renal impairment may increase risk of bleeding.

## INTERACTIONS

**DRUG:** Anticoagulants, antiplatelet medications, aspirin, drotrecogin alfa, NSAIDs, thrombolytics may increase risk of bleeding. **HERBAL:** Cat's claw, dong quai, evening primrose, feverfew, garlic, ginger, ginkgo, ginseng, horse chestnut, red clover, Omega-3 may increase antiplatelet activity. **FOOD:** None known. **LAB VALUES:** May cause reversible increases in serum creatinine, ALT, AST. May decrease Hgb, Hct, platelet count.

## AVAILABILITY (Rx)

**Injection, Solution:** 2.5 mg/0.5 ml, 5 mg/0.4 ml, 7.5 mg/0.6 ml, 10 mg/0.8 ml.

## ADMINISTRATION/HANDLING

Subcutaneous
• Parenteral form appears clear, colorless. Discard if discoloration or particulate matter is noted. • Store at room temperature. • Do not expel air bubble from prefilled syringe before injection. • Insert needle subcutaneously into

upper arms, outer thigh, or abdomen and inject solution. • Do not inject into areas of active skin disease or injury such as sunburns, rashes, inflammation, skin infections, or active psoriasis. • Rotate injection sites.

## INDICATIONS/ROUTES/DOSAGE

◄**ALERT**► For subcutaneous administration only.

**Prevention of Venous Thromboembolism**

SQ: **ADULTS WEIGHING 50 KG OR MORE:** 2.5 mg once daily for 5–9 days after surgery (up to 10 days following abdominal surgery; 11 days following hip or knee replacement). Initial dose should be given no earlier than 6–8h after surgery. Initiate dose once hemeostasis established. **WEIGHING LESS THAN 50 KG:** Contraindicated.

**Treatment of Venous Thromboembolism, Pulmonary Embolism**

**Note:** Start warfarin on first treatment day and continue fondaparinux until INR reaches 2 to 3 for at least 24 hr. Usual duration of fondaparinux: 5–9 days.

SQ: **ADULTS, ELDERLY WEIGHING MORE THAN 100 KG:** 10 mg once daily. **ADULTS, ELDERLY WEIGHING 50–100 KG:** 7.5 mg once daily. **ADULTS, ELDERLY WEIGHING LESS THAN 50 KG:** 5 mg once daily.

**Dosage in Renal Impairment**

**CrCl greater than 50 ml/min:** No dose adjustment. **CrCl 30–50 ml/min:** Use caution (50% dose reduction or use of low-dose heparin). **CrCl less than 30 ml/min:** Contraindicated.

**Dosage in Hepatic Impairment**

**Mild to moderate impairment:** No dose adjustment. **Severe impairment:** Use caution.

## SIDE EFFECTS

**Frequent (19%–11%):** Anemia, fever, nausea. **Occasional (10%–4%):** Edema, constipation, rash, vomiting, insomnia, increased wound drainage, hypokalemia. **Rare (less than 4%):** Dizziness, hypotension, confusion, urinary retention, injection site hematoma, diarrhea, dyspepsia, headache.

## ADVERSE EFFECTS/ TOXIC REACTIONS

Accidental overdose may lead to bleeding complications ranging from local ecchymoses to major hemorrhage. Thrombocytopenia occurs rarely.

## NURSING CONSIDERATIONS

**BASELINE ASSESSMENT**

Assess CBC, renal function test. Evaluate potential risk for bleeding. Question history of recent surgery, trauma, intracranial hemorrhage, GI bleeding.

**INTERVENTION/EVALUATION**

Periodically monitor CBC, esp. platelet count, stool for occult blood (no need for daily monitoring in pts with normal presurgical coagulation parameters). Assess for any signs of bleeding: bleeding at surgical site, hematuria, blood in stool, bleeding from gums, petechiae, ecchymosis, bleeding from injection sites. Monitor B/P, pulse; hypotension, tachycardia may indicate bleeding, hypovolemia.

**PATIENT/FAMILY TEACHING**

• Usual length of therapy is 5–9 days. • Do not take any OTC medication (esp. aspirin, NSAIDs). • Report swelling of hands/feet, unusual back pain, unusual bleeding/bruising, weakness, sudden or severe headache.

# foscarnet

foss-**kar**-net
(Foscavir)

■ **BLACK BOX ALERT** ■ Renal toxicity occurs to some degree in majority of pts. For use only in immunocompromised pts with cytomegalovirus (CMV) retinitis and mucocutaneous acyclovir-resistant herpes simplex virus (HSV) infection. Seizures due to electrolyte/mineral imbalance may occur.

## ◆CLASSIFICATION

**PHARMACOTHERAPEUTIC:** Phosphonic acid derivative. **CLINICAL:** Antiviral.

## USES

Treatment of acyclovir-resistant mucocutaneous HSV in immunocompromised pts; treatment of CMV retinitis in HIV pts. **OFF-LABEL:** Other CMV infections (e.g., colitis, esophagitis); CMV prophylaxis for cancer pts receiving alemtuzumab or allogenic stem cell transplant.

## PRECAUTIONS

**Contraindications:** Hypersensitivity to foscarnet. **Cautions:** Neurologic/cardiac abnormalities, history of hepatic/renal impairment, altered calcium, other electrolyte imbalances.

## ACTION

Selectively inhibits binding sites on virus-specific DNA polymerase, HIV reverse transcriptase. **Therapeutic Effect:** Inhibits replication of herpes virus. Virustatic.

## PHARMACOKINETICS

Sequestered into bone, cartilage. Protein binding: 14%–17%. Primarily excreted unchanged in urine. Removed by hemodialysis. **Half-life:** 3.3–6.8 hrs (increased in renal impairment).

## ⊠ LIFESPAN CONSIDERATIONS

**Pregnancy/Lactation:** Unknown if distributed in breast milk. **Children:** Safety and efficacy not established. **Elderly:** Age-related renal impairment may require dosage adjustment.

## INTERACTIONS

**DRUG: Nephrotoxic medications (e.g., lisinopril, IV contrast dye,** **vancomycin)** may increase risk of renal toxicity. **Pentamidine (IV)** may cause reversible hypocalcemia, hypomagnesemia, nephrotoxicity. **HERBAL:** None significant. **FOOD:** None known. **LAB VALUES:** May increase serum alkaline phosphatase, bilirubin, creatinine, ALT, AST. May decrease serum magnesium, potassium. May alter serum calcium, phosphate.

## AVAILABILITY (Rx)

**Injection Solution:** 24 mg/ml (250 ml).

## ADMINISTRATION/HANDLING

 IV

**Reconstitution •** Standard 24 mg/ml solution may be used without dilution when central venous catheter is used for infusion; 24 mg/ml solution *must* be diluted to maximum concentration of 12 mg/ml when peripheral vein catheter is being used. • Dilute only with D₅W or 0.9% NaCl solution.

**Rate of Administration •** Because dosage is calculated on body weight, unneeded quantity should be removed before start of infusion to avoid overdosage. Aseptic technique must be used and solution administered within 24 hrs of first entry into sealed bottle. • Do not give by IV injection or rapid infusion (increases toxicity). • Administer at rate not exceeding 1 mg/kg/min. • To minimize toxicity and phlebitis, use central venous lines or veins with adequate blood flow to permit rapid dilution, dissemination. • Use IV infusion pump to prevent accidental overdose.

**Storage •** Store parenteral vials at room temperature. • After dilution, stable for 24 hrs at room temperature. • Do not use if solution is discolored or particulate forms.

## ▦ IV INCOMPATIBILITIES

Acyclovir (Zovirax), amphotericin B (Fungizone), calcium, co-trimoxazole (Bactrim), diazepam (Valium), digoxin (Lanoxin), diphenhydramine (Benadryl), dobutamine (Dobutrex), ganciclovir (Cytovene),

---

haloperidol (Haldol), leucovorin, magnesium, midazolam (Versed), pentamidine (Pentam IV), prochlorperazine (Compazine), vancomycin (Vancocin).

### 🏵 IV COMPATIBILITIES

Dopamine (Intropin), heparin, hydromorphone (Dilaudid), lorazepam (Ativan), morphine, potassium chloride.

## INDICATIONS/ROUTES/DOSAGE

**Cytomegalovirus (CMV) Retinitis**
**IV: ADULTS, ELDERLY, ADOLESCENTS:** Initially, 60 mg/kg q8h or 90 mg/kg q12h for 2–3 wks. **Maintenance:** 90–120 mg/kg/day as a single IV infusion.

**Herpes Simplex Infection**
**IV: ADULTS, ELDERLY, ADOLESCENTS:** 40 mg/kg q8–12h for 2–3 wks or until healed.

**Dosage in Renal Impairment**
Dosages are individualized based on creatinine clearance. Refer to dosing guide provided by manufacturer.

**Dosage in Hepatic Impairment**
No dose adjustment.

## SIDE EFFECTS

**Frequent (65%–30%):** Fever, nausea, vomiting, diarrhea. **Occasional (29%–5%):** Anorexia, pain/inflammation at injection site, rigors, malaise, altered B/P, headache, paresthesia, dizziness, rash, diaphoresis, abdominal pain. **Rare (4%–1%):** Back/chest pain, edema, flushing, pruritus, constipation, dry mouth.

## ADVERSE EFFECTS/ TOXIC REACTIONS

Nephrotoxicity occurs to some extent in most pts. Seizures, serum mineral/electrolyte imbalances may be life-threatening.

### NURSING CONSIDERATIONS

**BASELINE ASSESSMENT**
Obtain baseline CBC, serum electrolyte levels, renal function test, vital signs. Risk of renal impairment can be reduced by

sufficient fluid intake to ensure diuresis prior to and during therapy.

**INTERVENTION/EVALUATION**
Monitor serum chemistries, renal function tests. Assess for signs of hypocalcemia (perioral paresthesia, paresthesia of extremities), hypokalemia (weakness, muscle cramps, paresthesia of extremities, irritability). Assess for tremors; provide safety measures for potential seizures. Assess for bleeding, anemia, developing superinfections. Obtain periodic ophthalmologic exams.

**PATIENT/FAMILY TEACHING**
• Report perioral tingling, numbness in extremities, paresthesia during or following infusion (may indicate electrolyte abnormalities). • Tremors should be reported promptly due to potential for seizures.

## fosinopril

foe-**sin**-oh-pril
(Apo-Fosinopril 🍁)

**■ BLACK BOX ALERT ■** May cause fetal injury, mortality. Discontinue as soon as possible once pregnancy is detected.
**Do not confuse fosinopril with Fosamax, or lisinopril, or Monopril with Accupril, minoxidil, moexipril, or ramipril.**

### ◆ CLASSIFICATION

**PHARMACOTHERAPEUTIC:** ACE inhibitor. **CLINICAL:** Antihypertensive.

## USES

Treatment of hypertension, used alone or in combination with other antihypertensives. Treatment of HF.

## PRECAUTIONS

**Contraindications:** Hypersensitivity to fosinopril. History of angioedema from previous treatment with ACE inhibitors. Concomitant use with aliskiren in pts with diabetes. **Cautions:** Renal/hepatic impairment, pts with sodium depletion or on diuretic therapy, dialysis, hypovolemia, hypertrophic cardiomyopathy with outflow tract obstruction, hyperkalemia, concomitant use of potassium supplements, unstented unilateral/bilateral renal stenosis, diabetes, severe aortic stenosis. Before, during, or immediately after major surgery.

## ACTION

Suppresses renin-angiotensin-aldosterone system (prevents conversion of angiotensin I to angiotensin II, a potent vasoconstrictor; may inhibit angiotensin II at local vascular, renal sites). Decreases plasma angiotensin II, increases plasma renin activity, decreases aldosterone secretion. **Therapeutic Effect:** Reduces B/P.

## PHARMACOKINETICS

| Route | Onset | Peak | Duration |
|-------|-------|------|----------|
| PO | 1 hr | 2–6 hrs | 24 hrs |

Slowly absorbed from GI tract. Protein binding: 97%–98%. Metabolized in liver and GI mucosa. Primarily excreted in urine. Minimal removal by hemodialysis. **Half-life:** 11.5 hrs.

## ⏳ LIFESPAN CONSIDERATIONS

**Pregnancy/Lactation:** Crosses placenta. Distributed in breast milk. May cause fetal or neonatal mortality or morbidity. **Children:** Safety and efficacy not established. Neonates, infants may be at increased risk for oliguria, neurologic abnormalities. **Elderly:** May be more sensitive to hypotensive effects.

## INTERACTIONS

**DRUG: Alcohol, antihypertensive agents** (e.g., **amlodipine, valsartan**), **diuretics** (e.g., **furosemide, HCTZ**), **NSAIDs** may increase effects. **Potassium-sparing diuretics** (e.g., **spironolactone**), **potassium supplements** may cause hyperkalemia. May increase **lithium** concentration/toxicity. **Antacids** may decrease absorption. **HERBAL: Ephedra,**

**ginseng, yohimbe** may worsen hypertension. **Garlic** may increase antihypertensive effect. **Licorice** may cause sodium/water retention, loss of potassium. **FOOD:** None known. **LAB VALUES:** May increase serum BUN, alkaline phosphatase, bilirubin, creatinine, potassium, ALT, AST. May decrease serum sodium. May cause positive antinuclear antibody titer (ANA).

## AVAILABILITY (Rx)

**Tablets:** 10 mg, 20 mg, 40 mg.

## ADMINISTRATION/HANDLING

**PO**
• Give without regard to food. • Tablets may be crushed.

## INDICATIONS/ROUTES/DOSAGE

**Hypertension**
**PO: ADULTS, ELDERLY:** Initially, 10 mg/day. **Maintenance:** 20–40 mg/day as a single dose or 2 divided doses. **Maximum:** 80 mg/day. **CHILDREN 6–16 YRS WEIGHING MORE THAN 50 KG:** Initially, 5–10 mg/day. **Maximum:** 40 mg/day.

**HF**
**PO: ADULTS, ELDERLY:** Initially, 5–10 mg/day. May increase dose over several wks. **Maintenance:** 20–40 mg/day. **Maximum:** 40 mg/day.

**Dosage in Renal Impairment**
Reduce initial dose to 5 mg in pts with HF.

**Dosage in Hepatic Impairment**
No dose adjustment.

## SIDE EFFECTS

**Frequent (12%–9%):** Dizziness, cough. **Occasional (4%–2%):** Hypotension, nausea, vomiting, upper respiratory tract infection.

## ADVERSE EFFECTS/ TOXIC REACTIONS

Excessive hypotension ("first-dose syncope") may occur in pts with HF, severely

---

salt/volume depleted. Angioedema (swelling of face/lips), hyperkalemia occur rarely. Agranulocytosis, neutropenia may be noted in pts with renal impairment, collagen vascular disease (scleroderma, systemic lupus erythematosus). Nephrotic syndrome may be noted in those with history of renal disease.

## NURSING CONSIDERATIONS

### BASELINE ASSESSMENT

Obtain B/P immediately before each dose, in addition to regular monitoring (be alert to fluctuations). Renal function tests should be performed before beginning therapy. In pts with renal impairment, autoimmune disease, or taking drugs that affect leukocytes or immune response, CBC, differential count should be performed before therapy begins and q2wks for 3 mos, then periodically thereafter.

### INTERVENTION/EVALUATION

If excessive reduction in B/P occurs, place pt in supine position with legs elevated. Assist with ambulation if dizziness occurs. Assess for urinary frequency. Auscultate lung sounds for rales, wheezing in pts with HF. Monitor renal function tests, CBC, urinalysis for proteinuria. Observe for angioedema (swelling of face, lips, tongue). Monitor serum potassium in those on concurrent diuretic therapy.

### PATIENT/FAMILY TEACHING

• Report any sign of infection (sore throat, fever). • Several wks may be needed for full therapeutic effect of B/P reduction. • Skipping doses or voluntarily discontinuing drug may produce severe, rebound hypertension. • To reduce hypotensive effect, go from lying to standing slowly. • Immediately report swelling of face, lips, tongue, difficulty breathing, vomiting, excessive perspiration, persistent cough. • Avoid potassium salt substitutes.

# fosphenytoin

fos-**fen**-i-toyn
(Cerebyx)
**Do not confuse Cerebyx with Celebrex or Celexa, or fosphenytoin with fospropofol.**

## ◆CLASSIFICATION

**PHARMACOTHERAPEUTIC:** Hydantoin. **CLINICAL:** Anticonvulsant.

## USES

Acute treatment, control of generalized convulsive status epilepticus; prevention, treatment of seizures occurring during neurosurgery; short-term substitution for oral phenytoin.

## PRECAUTIONS

**Contraindications:** Hypersensitivity to fosphenytoin, phenytoin, other hydantoins. Adams-Stokes syndrome; second- or third-degree AV block; sinus bradycardia; SA block; concurrent use of delavirdine. **Cautions:** Porphyria, diabetes, hypothyroidism, hypotension, severe myocardial insufficiency, renal/hepatic disease, hypoalbuminemia.

## ACTION

Stabilizes neuronal membranes, limits spread of seizure activity. Decreases sodium, calcium ion influx into neurons. Decreases post-tetanic potentiation, repetitive discharge. **Therapeutic Effect:** Decreases seizure activity.

## PHARMACOKINETICS

Completely absorbed after IM administration. Protein binding: 95%–99%. Rapidly and completely hydrolyzed to phenytoin after IM or IV administration. Time of complete conversion to phenytoin: 4 hrs after IM injection; 2 hrs after IV infusion. **Half-life:** 8–15 min (for conversion to phenytoin). (Phenytoin: 12–29 hrs.)

## ⚗ LIFESPAN CONSIDERATIONS

**Pregnancy/Lactation:** May increase frequency of seizures during pregnancy. Increased risk of congenital malformations. Unknown if excreted in breast milk. **Children:** Safety and efficacy not established. **Elderly:** Lower dosage recommended.

## INTERACTIONS

**DRUG: Alcohol, other CNS depressants** may increase CNS depression. **Amiodarone, anticoagulants, cimetidine, disulfiram, fluoxetine, isoniazid, sulfonamides** may increase concentration/effects, risk of toxicity. **CYP3A4 inhibitors (e.g., fluconazole, ketoconazole, miconazole)** may increase concentration. **HERBAL:** None significant. **FOOD:** None known. **LAB VALUES:** May increase serum glucose, GGT, alkaline phosphatase.

## AVAILABILITY (Rx)

**Injection Solution:** 75 mg/ml (equivalent to 50 mg phenytoin equivalents (PE)/ml phenytoin).

## ADMINISTRATION/HANDLING

 IV

**Reconstitution** • Dilute in D₅W or 0.9% NaCl to a concentration ranging from 1.5–25 mg PE/ml.
**Rate of Administration** • Administer at rate less than 150 mg PE/min (decreases risk of hypotension, arrhythmias). Children: 1–3 mg PE/kg/min. **Maximum:** 150 mg PE/min.
**Storage** • Refrigerate. • Do not store at room temperature for longer than 48 hrs. • After dilution, solution is stable for 8 hrs at room temperature or 24 hrs if refrigerated.

## ▨ IV INCOMPATIBILITY

Midazolam (Versed).

## ▨ IV COMPATIBILITIES

Lorazepam (Ativan), phenobarbital, potassium chloride.

## INDICATIONS/ROUTES/DOSAGE

◄**ALERT**► 150 mg fosphenytoin yields 100 mg phenytoin. Dosage, concentration solution, infusion rate of fosphenytoin are expressed in terms of phenytoin equivalents (PE).

**Status Epilepticus**
**IV: ADULTS: Loading dose:** 15–20 mg PE/kg infused at rate of 100–150 mg PE/min. Follow with maintenance dose of either fosphenytoin or phenytoin.

**Nonemergent Seizures**
**IV, IM: ADULTS: Loading dose:** 10–20 mg PE/kg. **Maintenance:** 4–6 mg PE/kg/day in divided doses.

**Short-Term Substitution for Oral Phenytoin**
**IV, IM: ADULTS:** May substitute for oral phenytoin at same total daily dose.

**Dosage in Renal/Hepatic Impairment**
No dose adjustment.

## SIDE EFFECTS

**Frequent:** Dizziness, paresthesia, tinnitus, pruritus, headache, drowsiness. **Occasional:** Morbilliform rash.

## ADVERSE EFFECTS/ TOXIC REACTIONS

Toxic fosphenytoin serum concentration may produce ataxia (muscular incoordination), nystagmus (rhythmic oscillation of eyes), diplopia, lethargy, slurred speech, nausea, vomiting, hypotension. As drug level increases, extreme lethargy may progress to coma.

## NURSING CONSIDERATIONS

### BASELINE ASSESSMENT

Review history of seizure disorder (intensity, frequency, duration, LOC). Initiate seizure precautions. Obtain vital signs, medication history (esp. use of phenytoin, other anticonvulsants). Observe clinically.

## INTERVENTION/EVALUATION

Monitor EKG, measure cardiac function, respiratory function, B/P during and immediately following infusion (10–20 min). Discontinue if skin rash appears. Interrupt or decrease rate if hypotension, arrhythmias are detected. Assess pt postinfusion (may feel dizzy, ataxic, drowsy). Monitor free and total dilatin levels (2 hrs after IV infusion or 4 hrs after IM injection).

## PATIENT/FAMILY TEACHING

• If noncompliance is cause of acute seizures, discuss and address reasons for noncompliance. • Avoid tasks that require alertness, motor skills until response to drug is established.

# frovatriptan

froe-va-**trip**-tan
(Frova)

◆CLASSIFICATION

**PHARMACOTHERAPEUTIC:** Serotonin receptor agonist. **CLINICAL:** Antimigraine.

## USES

Treatment of acute migraine headache with or without aura in adults.

## PRECAUTIONS

**Contraindications:** Hypersensitivity to frovatriptan. Management of basilar or hemiplegic migraine, cerebrovascular or peripheral vascular disease, coronary artery disease, ischemic heart disease (angina pectoris, history of MI, silent ischemia, Prinzmetal's angina), severe hepatic impairment (Child-Pugh grade C), uncontrolled hypertension, use within 24 hrs of ergotamine-containing preparations or another serotonin receptor agonist. **Cautions:** Mild to moderate hepatic impairment, pt profile suggesting cardiovascular risks. History of seizures or structural brain lesions.

## ACTION

Agonist for serotonin in cranial arteries causing vasoconstriction and reduction of inflammation. **Therapeutic Effect:** Relieves migraine headache.

## PHARMACOKINETICS

Well absorbed after PO administration. Protein binding: 15%. Metabolized in liver. Primarily eliminated in feces (62%), urine (32%). **Half-life:** 26 hrs (increased in hepatic impairment).

## ⧖ LIFESPAN CONSIDERATIONS

**Pregnancy/Lactation:** Unknown if drug is excreted in breast milk. **Children:** Safety and efficacy not established. **Elderly:** Not recommended for use in this pt population.

## INTERACTIONS

**DRUG: Ergotamine-containing medications** may produce vasospastic reaction. **SSRI, SNRI (e.g., duloxetine, fluoxetine, fluvoxamine, paroxetine, sertraline, venlafaxine)** may produce weakness, hyperreflexia, uncoordination. **HERBAL:** None significant. **FOOD:** None known. **LAB VALUES:** None significant.

## AVAILABILITY (Rx)

▧ **Tablets:** 2.5 mg.

## ADMINISTRATION/HANDLING

**PO**

• Give with fluids as soon as symptoms appear. • Do not break, crush, dissolve, or divide film-coated tablets.

## INDICATIONS/ROUTES/DOSAGE

**Acute Migraine Headache**
**PO: ADULTS, ELDERLY:** Initially, 2.5 mg. If headache improves but then returns, dose may be repeated after at least 2 hrs. **Maximum:** 7.5 mg/day.

**Dosage in Renal Impairment**
No dose adjustment.

Dosage in Hepatic Impairment
**Mild to moderate impairment:** No dose adjustment. **Severe impairment:** Use caution.

## SIDE EFFECTS

**Occasional (8%–4%):** Dizziness, paresthesia, fatigue, flushing. **Rare (3%–2%):** Hot/cold sensation, dry mouth, dyspepsia.

## ADVERSE EFFECTS/ TOXIC REACTIONS

Cardiac reactions (ischemia, coronary artery vasospasm, MI), noncardiac vasospasm-related reactions (cerebral hemorrhage, CVA) occur rarely, particularly in pts with hypertension, obesity, smokers, diabetes, strong family history of coronary artery disease; males older than 40 yrs; postmenopausal women.

## NURSING CONSIDERATIONS

### BASELINE ASSESSMENT

Question for history of peripheral vascular disease, renal/hepatic impairment, possibility of pregnancy. Question regarding onset, location, duration of migraine, possible precipitating factors.

### INTERVENTION/EVALUATION

Assess for relief of migraine headache, potential for photophobia, phonophobia (sound sensitivity), nausea, vomiting.

### PATIENT/FAMILY TEACHING

• Take a single dose as soon as symptoms of an actual migraine attack appear. • Medication is intended to relieve migraine headaches, not to prevent or reduce number of attacks. • Avoid tasks that require alertness, motor skills until response to drug is established. • Immediately report palpitations, pain, tightness in chest or throat, sudden or severe abdominal pain, pain or weakness of extremities.

# *fulvestrant*

ful-**vest**-rant
(Faslodex)
**Do not confuse Faslodex with Fosamax.**

## ◆CLASSIFICATION

**PHARMACOTHERAPEUTIC:** Estrogen antagonist. **CLINICAL:** Antineoplastic.

## USES

Treatment of hormone receptor–positive metastatic breast cancer in postmenopausal women with disease progression following antiestrogen therapy.

## PRECAUTIONS

**Contraindications:** Hypersensitivity to fulvestrant. **Cautions:** Thrombocytopenia, bleeding diathesis, anticoagulant therapy, hepatic impairment, reduced hepatic blood flow, pregnancy.

## ACTION

Competes with endogenous estrogen at estrogen receptor binding sites. **Therapeutic Effect:** Inhibits tumor growth.

## PHARMACOKINETICS

Extensively, rapidly distributed after IM administration. Protein binding: 99%. Metabolized in liver. Eliminated by hepatobiliary route; excreted in feces. **Half-life:** 40 days in postmenopausal women. Peak serum levels occur in 7–9 days.

## LIFESPAN CONSIDERATIONS

**Pregnancy/Lactation:** Do not administer to pregnant women. Unknown if excreted in breast milk. May cause fetal harm. **Children:** Not used in this pt population. **Elderly:** No age-related precautions noted.

## INTERACTIONS

**DRUG:** None significant. **HERBAL:** None significant. **FOOD:** None known. **LAB VALUES:** May increase ALT, AST.

F

---

F

## AVAILABILITY (Rx)
**Injection, Solution:** 50 mg/ml.

## ADMINISTRATION/HANDLING
**IM**
• Administer slowly into upper, outer quadrant or ventrogluteal area of buttock as two injections, one in each buttock over 1–2 min.

## INDICATIONS/ROUTES/DOSAGE
**Breast Cancer**
**IM: ADULTS, ELDERLY:** Initially, 500 mg (two 250-mg injections) on days 1, 15, and 29. **Maintenance:** 500 mg once monthly thereafter.

**Dosage in Renal Impairment**
No dose adjustment.

**Dosage in Hepatic Impairment**
**Mild impairment:** No dose adjustment. **Moderate impairment:** Reduce initial and maintenance dose to 250 mg. **Severe impairment:** Use caution (not studied).

## SIDE EFFECTS
**Frequent (26%–13%):** Nausea, hot flashes, pharyngitis, asthenia, vomiting, vasodilation, headache. **Occasional (12%–5%):** Injection site pain, constipation, diarrhea, abdominal pain, anorexia, dizziness, insomnia, paresthesia, bone/back pain, depression, anxiety, peripheral edema, rash, diaphoresis, fever. **Rare (2%–1%):** Vertigo, weight gain.

## ADVERSE EFFECTS/ TOXIC REACTIONS
UTI occurs occasionally. Vaginitis, anemia, thromboembolic phenomena, leukopenia occur rarely.

## NURSING CONSIDERATIONS
**BASELINE ASSESSMENT**
Estrogen receptor assay should be done before beginning therapy. Baseline radiologic testing should be performed initially and periodically thereafter for evidence of tumor regression.

**INTERVENTION/EVALUATION**
Monitor serum chemistries, plasma lipids. Be alert to increased bone pain, ensure adequate pain relief. Check for edema, esp. of dependent areas. Monitor for and assist with ambulation if asthenia or dizziness occurs. Assess for headache. Offer antiemetic for nausea/ vomiting.

**PATIENT/FAMILY TEACHING**
• Notify physician if nausea/vomiting, asthenia (loss of strength, energy), hot flashes become unmanageable.

---

# furosemide    TOP 100

fur-**oh**-se-myde
(Apo-Furosemide ✣, Lasix, Novo-Semide ✣)

■ **BLACK BOX ALERT** ■ Large amounts can lead to profound diuresis with water and electrolyte depletion.
**Do not confuse furosemide with famotidine, finasteride, fluconazole, fluoxetine, loperamide, or torsemide, or Lasix with Lidex, Lovenox, Luvox, or Luxiq.**

## ◆CLASSIFICATION
**PHARMACOTHERAPEUTIC:** Loop diuretic. **CLINICAL:** Diuretic.

## USES
Treatment of edema associated with HF and renal/hepatic disease; acute pulmonary edema. Treatment of hypertension, either alone or in combination with other antihypertensives.

## PRECAUTIONS
**Contraindications:** Hypersensitivity to furosemide. Anuria. **Cautions:** Hepatic cirrhosis, hepatic coma, severe electrolyte depletion, prediabetes, diabetes, systemic

lupus erythematosus. Pts with prostatic hyperplasia/urinary stricture.

## ACTION

Enhances excretion of sodium, chloride, potassium by direct action at ascending limb of loop of Henle. **Therapeutic Effect:** Produces diuresis, lowers B/P.

## PHARMACOKINETICS

| Route | Onset | Peak | Duration |
|---|---|---|---|
| PO | 30–60 min | 1–2 hrs | 6–8 hrs |
| IV | 5 min | 20–60 min | 2 hrs |
| IM | 30 min | N/A | N/A |

Moderately absorbed from GI tract. Protein binding: greater than 98%. Partially metabolized in liver. Primarily excreted in urine (nonrenal clearance increases in severe renal impairment). Not removed by hemodialysis. **Half-life:** 30–90 min (increased in renal/hepatic impairment, neonates).

## ⧗ LIFESPAN CONSIDERATIONS

**Pregnancy/Lactation:** Crosses placenta. Distributed in breast milk. **Children:** Half-life increased in neonates; may require increased dosage interval. **Elderly:** May be more sensitive to hypotensive, electrolyte effects, developing circulatory collapse, thromboembolic effect. Age-related renal impairment may require dosage adjustment.

## INTERACTIONS

**DRUG: Amphotericin B, nephrotoxic ototoxic medications (e.g., lisinopril, IV contrast dye, vancomycin)** may increase risk of nephrotoxicity, ototoxicity. May increase risk of **lithium** toxicity. **Other medications causing hypokalemia (e.g., HCTZ, laxatives)** may increase risk of hypokalemia. **HERBAL: Ephedra, ginseng, yohimbe** may worsen hypertension. **Garlic** may increase antihypertensive effect. **FOOD:** None known. **LAB VALUES:** May increase serum glucose, BUN, uric acid. May decrease serum calcium, chloride, magnesium, potassium, sodium.

## AVAILABILITY (Rx)

**Injection Solution:** 10 mg/ml. **Oral Solution:** 10 mg/ml, 40 mg/5 ml. **Tablets:** 20 mg, 40 mg, 80 mg.

## ADMINISTRATION/HANDLING

 **IV**

**Rate of Administration** • May give undiluted but is compatible with D₅W or 0.9% NaCl. • May be diluted for infusion to 1–2 mg/ml (**maximum:** 10 mg/ml). • Administer each 40 mg or fraction by IV push over 1–2 min. Do not exceed administration rate of 4 mg/min for short-term intermittent infusion.

**Storage** • Solution appears clear, colorless. • Discard yellow solutions. • Stable for 24 hrs at room temperature when mixed with 0.9% NaCl or D₅W.

**IM**

• Temporary pain at injection site may be noted.

**PO**

• Administer on empty stomach. • Give with food to avoid GI upset, preferably with breakfast (may prevent nocturia). • Food may decrease diuretic effect.

## ▦ IV INCOMPATIBILITIES

Ciprofloxacin (Cipro), diltiazem (Cardizem), dobutamine (Dobutrex), dopamine (Intropin), doxorubicin (Adriamycin), droperidol (Inapsine), esmolol (Brevibloc), famotidine (Pepcid), filgrastim (Neupogen), fluconazole (Diflucan), gemcitabine (Gemzar), gentamicin (Garamycin), idarubicin (Idamycin), labetalol (Trandate), metoclopramide (Reglan), midazolam (Versed), milrinone (Primacor), nicardipine (Cardene), ondansetron (Zofran), quinidine, thiopental (Pentothal), vinblastine (Velban), vincristine (Oncovin), vinorelbine (Navelbine).

## ▦ IV COMPATIBILITIES

Amiodarone (Cordarone), bumetanide (Bumex), calcium gluconate, cimetidine

---

◆ Canadian trade name     🗡 Non-Crushable Drug     🔲 High Alert drug

F

(Tagamet), dexmedetomidine (Precedex), heparin, hydromorphone (Dilaudid), lidocaine, lipids, morphine, nitroglycerin, norepinephrine (Levophed), potassium chloride, propofol (Diprivan).

## INDICATIONS/ROUTES/DOSAGE

### Edema, HF
**PO: ADULTS, ELDERLY:** Initially, 20–80 mg/dose; may increase by 20–40 mg/dose q6–8h. May titrate up to 600 mg/day in severe edematous states. **CHILDREN:** Initially, 2 mg/kg/dose. May increase by 1–2 mg/kg/dose at 6–8 hr intervals. **Maximum:** 6 mg/kg/dose. **NEONATES:** 1 mg/kg/dose 1–2 times/day.

**IV, IM: ADULTS, ELDERLY:** 20–40 mg/dose; may increase by 20 mg/dose q1–2h. **Maximum single dose:** 160–200 mg. **CHILDREN:** Initially, 1 mg/kg/dose. May increase by 1 mg/kg/dose no sooner than 2 hrs after previous dose. **Maximum:** 6 mg/kg/dose. **NEONATES:** 1–2 mg/kg/dose q12–24h.

**IV Infusion: ADULTS, ELDERLY:** Bolus of 40–100 mg over 1–2 min, followed by infusion of 10–40 mg/hr; may double q2h. **Maximum:** 80–160 mg/hr. **CHILDREN:** 0.05 mg/kg/hr; titrate to desired effect. **NEONATES:** Initially, 0.2 mg/kg/hr. May increase by 0.1 mg/kg/hr q12–24h. **Maximum:** 0.4 mg/kg/hr.

### Dosage in Renal Impairment
Avoid use in oliguric states.

### Dosage in Hepatic Impairment
No dose adjustment. Decreased effect, increased sensitivity to hypokalemia/volume depletion in cirrhosis.

## SIDE EFFECTS

**Expected:** Increased urinary frequency/volume. **Frequent:** Nausea, dyspepsia, abdominal cramps, diarrhea or constipation, electrolyte disturbances. **Occasional:** Dizziness, light-headedness, headache, blurred vision, paresthesia, photosensitivity, rash, fatigue, bladder spasm, restlessness, diaphoresis. **Rare:** Flank pain.

## ADVERSE EFFECTS/TOXIC REACTIONS

Vigorous diuresis may lead to profound water loss/electrolyte depletion, resulting in hypokalemia, hyponatremia, dehydration. Sudden volume depletion may result in increased risk of thrombosis, circulatory collapse, sudden death. Acute hypotensive episodes may occur, sometimes several days after beginning therapy. Ototoxicity (deafness, vertigo, tinnitus) may occur, esp. in pts with severe renal impairment. Can exacerbate diabetes mellitus, systemic lupus erythematosus, gout, pancreatitis. Blood dyscrasias have been reported.

## NURSING CONSIDERATIONS

### BASELINE ASSESSMENT
Check vital signs, esp. B/P, pulse, for hypotension before administration. Assess baseline renal function, serum electrolytes, esp. serum sodium, potassium. Assess skin turgor, mucous membranes for hydration status; observe for edema. Assess muscle strength, mental status. Note skin temperature, moisture. Obtain baseline weight. Initiate I&O monitoring.

### INTERVENTION/EVALUATION
Monitor B/P, vital signs, serum electrolytes, I&O, weight. Note extent of diuresis. Watch for symptoms of electrolyte imbalance: Hypokalemia may result in changes in muscle strength, tremor, muscle cramps, altered mental status, cardiac arrhythmias; hyponatremia may result in confusion, thirst, cold/clammy skin.

### PATIENT/FAMILY TEACHING
• Expect increased frequency, volume of urination. • Report palpitations, signs of electrolyte imbalances (noted previously), hearing abnormalities (sense of fullness in ears, tinnitus). • Eat foods high in potassium such as whole grains (cereals), legumes, meat, bananas, apricots, orange juice, potatoes (white, sweet), raisins. • Avoid sunlight, sunlamps.

---

# gabapentin

ga-ba-**pen**-tin
(Apo-Gabapentin ✦, Fanatrex
FusePaq, Gralise, Horizant, Neurontin)
**Do not confuse Neurontin with
Motrin, Neoral, nitrofurantoin,
Noroxin, or Zarontin.**

## ◆ CLASSIFICATION

**PHARMACOTHERAPEUTIC:** Gamma-aminobutyric acid analogue. **CLINICAL:** Anticonvulsant, antineuralgic.

## USES

**Neurontin:** Adjunct in treatment of partial seizures (with or without secondary generalized seizures) in children 13 yrs and older and adults. Adjunct to treatment of partial seizures in children 3–12 yrs; management of postherpetic neuralgia (PHN). **Horizant:** Treatment of moderate to severe primary restless legs syndrome (RLS), PHN. **Gralise:** Management of PHN. **OFF-LABEL:** Treatment of neuropathic pain, diabetic peripheral neuropathy, vasomotor symptoms, fibromyalgia, postoperative pain adjunct.

## PRECAUTIONS

**Contraindications:** Hypersensitivity to gabapentin. **Cautions:** Severe renal impairment, elderly, history of suicidal behavior; substance abuse.

## ACTION

Binds to gabapentin binding sites in brain and may modulate release of excitatory neurotransmitters. **Therapeutic Effect:** Reduces seizure activity, neuropathic pain.

## PHARMACOKINETICS

Well absorbed from GI tract (not affected by food). Protein binding: less than 5%. Widely distributed. Crosses blood-brain barrier. Primarily excreted unchanged in urine. Removed by hemodialysis. **Half-life:** 5–7 hrs (increased in renal impairment, elderly).

## ⧗ LIFESPAN CONSIDERATIONS

**Pregnancy/Lactation:** Unknown if distributed in breast milk. **Children:** Safety and efficacy not established in pts 3 yrs and younger. **Elderly:** Age-related renal impairment may require dosage adjustment.

## INTERACTIONS

**DRUG: Antacids** decrease absorption. **Benzodiazepines (e.g., lorazepam), opiates (e.g., morphine, fentanyl), other CNS depressants** may increase CNS depression. **HERBAL: Evening primrose** may decrease seizure threshold. **Gotu kola, kava kava, St. John's wort, valerian** may increase CNS depression. **FOOD:** None known. **LAB VALUES:** May alter serum glucose; WBC count. May increase serum alkaline phosphatase, ALT, AST, bilirubin.

## AVAILABILITY (Rx)

**Capsules (Neurontin):** 100 mg, 300 mg, 400 mg. **Oral Solution (Neurontin):** 250 mg/5 ml. **Oral Suspension (Fanatrex FusePaq):** 25 mg/ml. **Tablets (Neurontin):** 600 mg, 800 mg. **Tablets (Gralise):** 300 mg, 600 mg.

🗲 **Tablets, Extended-Release:** (Horizant) 300 mg, 600 mg.

## ADMINISTRATION/HANDLING

**PO**
**Immediate-Release/Solution** • Give without regard to meals; may give with food to avoid, reduce GI upset. • Swallow extended-release tablets whole; do not break, crush, dissolve, or divide. Take with evening meal.

## INDICATIONS/ROUTES/DOSAGE

**Note:** When given 3 times/day, maximum time between doses should not exceed 12 hrs. If treatment is discontinued or anticonvulsant therapy is added, do so gradually over at least 1 wk (reduces risk of loss of seizure control).

**Adjunctive Therapy for Seizure Control**
**PO: ADULTS, ELDERLY, CHILDREN 13 YRS AND OLDER:** Initially, 300 mg 3 times/day. May titrate dosage. **Range:** 900–1,800 mg/day

G

---

in 3 divided doses. **Maximum:** 3,600 mg/day. **CHILDREN 3–12 YRS:** Initially, 10–15 mg/kg/day in 3 divided doses. May titrate up to 25–35 mg/kg/day (for children 5–12 yrs) and 40 mg/kg/day (for children 3–4 yrs). **Maximum:** 50 mg/kg/day.

**Adjunctive Therapy for Neuropathic Pain**
**PO: ADULTS, ELDERLY:** Initially, 100 mg 3 times/day; may increase by 300 mg/day at wkly intervals. **Maximum:** 3,600 mg/day in 3 divided doses. **CHILDREN:** Initially, 5 mg/kg/dose at bedtime, followed by 5 mg/kg/dose for 2 doses on day 2, then 5 mg/kg/dose for 3 doses on day 3. **Maximum:** 300 mg. Range: 8–35 mg/kg/day in 3 divided doses.

**Postherpetic Neuralgia**
**PO: ADULTS, ELDERLY:** *(Neurontin):* 300 mg once on day 1, 300 mg twice daily on day 2, and 300 mg 3 times/day on day 3 as needed. Range: 1,800–3,600 mg/day. *(Gralise):* 300 mg once on day 1; 600 mg once on day 2; 900 mg once daily on days 3–6; 1,200 mg once daily on days 7–10; 1,500 mg once daily on days 11–14; then 1,800 mg once daily.

**RLS**
**PO: ADULTS, ELDERLY (HORIZANT):** 600 mg once daily at about 5 PM.

**Dosage in Renal Impairment**
Dosage and frequency are modified based on creatinine clearance:

**Dosage in Hepatic Impairment**
No dose adjustment.

## SIDE EFFECTS

**Frequent (19%–10%):** Fatigue, drowsiness, dizziness, ataxia. **Occasional (8%–3%):** Nystagmus, tremor, diplopia, rhinitis, weight gain, peripheral edema. **Rare (less than 2%):** Anxiety, dysarthria, memory loss, dyspepsia, pharyngitis, myalgia.

## ADVERSE EFFECTS/ TOXIC REACTIONS

Abrupt withdrawal may increase seizure frequency, increased risk of suicidal behavior/thoughts. Overdosage may result in slurred speech, drowsiness, lethargy, diarrhea. Drug reaction with eosinophilia and systemic symptoms (multiorgan hypersensitivity) was reported. Hypersensitivity reaction, including anaphylaxis and angioedema, can occur at any time.

## NURSING CONSIDERATIONS

### BASELINE ASSESSMENT
Review history of seizure disorder (type, onset, intensity, frequency, duration, LOC). Assess location, intensity of neuralgia/neuropathic pain.

### INTERVENTION/EVALUATION
Provide safety measures as needed. Monitor seizure frequency/duration, renal function, weight, behavior in children. Monitor for signs/symptoms of depression, suicidal tendencies, other unusual behavior; hypersensitivity reaction.

| Creatinine Clearance | Neurontin Dosage (Immediate-release) | Gralise Dosage (Extended-release) | Horizant Dosage | |
| --- | --- | --- | --- | --- |
| | | | **RLS** | **PHN** |
| 30–59 ml/min | 200–700 mg q12h | 600–1,800 mg once/day | 300–600 mg/day | Same |
| 16–29 ml/min | 200–700 mg once daily | Not recommended | 300 mg/day | Same |
| Less than 16 ml/min | 100–300 mg once daily | Not recommended | 300 mg q48 h | Same |
| Hemodialysis | 125–350 mg following HD | Not recommended | Not recommended | 300–600 mg following HD |

underlined – top prescribed drug

**PATIENT/FAMILY TEACHING**
• Use only as prescribed; do not abruptly stop taking drug (may increase seizure frequency). • Avoid tasks that require alertness, motor skills until response to drug is established. • Avoid alcohol. • Carry identification card/bracelet to note seizure disorder/anticonvulsant therapy. • Report suicidal ideation, depression, unusual behavioral changes (esp. with changes in dosage), worsening of seizure activity or loss of seizure control. Seek medical attention for allergic reactions including difficulty breathing, coughing, wheezing, throat tightness, swelling of face or tongue.

# galantamine

gal-**an**-ta-meen
(Razadyne, Razadyne ER,
Reminyl ER ✦)
**Do not confuse Razadyne with
Rozerem, or Reminyl with
Amaryl.**

## ◆CLASSIFICATION

**PHARMACOTHERAPEUTIC:** Cholinesterase inhibitor. **CLINICAL:** Antidementia.

## USES

Treatment of mild to moderate dementia of Alzheimer's type. **OFF-LABEL:** Diabetic neuropathy, neuropathic pain, postoperative pain (adjunct), hot flashes.

## PRECAUTIONS

**Contraindications:** Hypersensitivity to galantamine. **Cautions:** Moderate renal/hepatic impairment (not recommended in severe impairment), history of ulcer disease, asthma, COPD, bladder outflow obstruction, supraventricular cardiac conduction conditions (except with pacemaker), seizure disorder, concurrent medications that slow cardiac conduction through SA or AV node. Elderly with low body weight and/or serious co-morbidities.

## ACTION

Elevates acetylcholine concentrations by slowing degeneration of acetylcholine released by still intact cholinergic neurons. May increase serotonin levels. **Therapeutic Effect:** Slows progression of Alzheimer's disease.

## PHARMACOKINETICS

Rapidly, completely absorbed from GI tract. Protein binding: 18%. Distributed to blood cells; binds to plasma proteins, mainly albumin. Metabolized in liver. Excreted in urine. **Half-life:** 7 hrs.

## ⧗ LIFESPAN CONSIDERATIONS

**Pregnancy/Lactation:** Unknown if drug crosses placenta or is distributed in breast milk. **Children:** Not prescribed for this pt population. **Elderly:** No age-related precautions noted, but use is not recommended in those with severe hepatic/renal impairment (CrCl less than 9 ml/min).

## INTERACTIONS

**DRUG:** May interfere with the effects of **bethanechol, succinylcholine. Cimetidine, ketoconazole, paroxetine** may increase concentration/effect. **HERBAL: St. John's wort** may decrease concentration. **FOOD:** None known. **LAB VALUES:** None significant.

## AVAILABILITY (Rx)

**Oral Solution (Razadyne):** 4 mg/ml. **Tablets (Razadyne):** 4 mg, 8 mg, 12 mg.

🦺 **Capsules (Extended-Release [Razadyne ER]):** 8 mg, 16 mg, 24 mg.

## ADMINISTRATION/HANDLING

**PO**
• Give tablet or solution with morning and evening meals. • Mix oral solution with nonalcoholic beverage, take immediately. • Extended-release capsule should be given with breakfast. Swallow whole. Do not break, crush, cut, or divide.

**G**

## INDICATIONS/ROUTES/DOSAGE

**Note:** If therapy interrupted for 3 or more days, restart at lowest dose; then increase gradually.

**Alzheimer's Disease**
**PO** *(Immediate-Release Tablets, Oral Solution):* **ADULTS, ELDERLY:** Initially, 4 mg twice daily (8 mg/day). After a minimum of 4 wks (if well tolerated), may increase to 8 mg twice daily (16 mg/day). After another 4 wks, may increase to 12 mg twice daily (24 mg/day). Range: 16–24 mg/day in 2 divided doses.
**PO** *(Extended-Release):* **ADULTS, ELDERLY:** Initially, 8 mg once daily for 4 wks; then increase to 16 mg once daily for 4 wks or longer. If tolerated, may increase to 24 mg once daily. Range: 16–24 mg once daily.

**Dosage in Renal/Hepatic Impairment**
**Moderate impairment:** Maximum dosage is 16 mg/day. **Severe impairment:** Not recommended.

## SIDE EFFECTS

**Frequent (17%–7%):** Nausea, vomiting, diarrhea, anorexia, weight loss. **Occasional (5%–4%):** Abdominal pain, insomnia, depression, headache, dizziness, fatigue, rhinitis. **Rare (less than 3%):** Tremors, constipation, confusion, cough, anxiety, urinary incontinence.

## ADVERSE EFFECTS/ TOXIC REACTIONS

Overdose may cause cholinergic crisis (increased salivation, lacrimation, urination, defecation, bradycardia, hypotension, muscle weakness). Treatment aimed at generally supportive measures, use of anticholinergics (e.g., atropine).

## NURSING CONSIDERATIONS

### BASELINE ASSESSMENT

Assess cognitive, behavioral, functional deficits of pt. Obtain baseline serum renal function, LFT.

### INTERVENTION/EVALUATION

Monitor cognitive, behavioral, functional status of pt. Evaluate EKG, periodic rhythm strips in pts with underlying arrhythmias. Assess for evidence of GI disturbances (nausea, vomiting, diarrhea, anorexia, weight loss).

### PATIENT/FAMILY TEACHING

• Take with meals (reduces risk of nausea). • Avoid tasks that require alertness, motor skills until response to drug is established. • Report persistent GI disturbances, excessive salivation, diaphoresis, excessive tearing, excessive fatigue, insomnia, depression, dizziness, increased muscle weakness.

# ganciclovir

gan-**sye**-kloe-veer
(Cytovene)

■ **BLACK BOX ALERT** ■ Toxicity presents as neutropenia, thrombocytopenia, anemia. Studies suggest carcinogenic and teratogenic effects, inhibition of spermatogenesis.
**Do not confuse Cytovene with Cytosar, or ganciclovir with famciclovir or acyclovir.**

### ◆CLASSIFICATION

**PHARMACOTHERAPEUTIC:** Synthetic nucleoside. **CLINICAL:** Antiviral.

## USES

Treatment of cytomegalovirus (CMV) retinitis in immunocompromised pts (e.g., HIV), prophylaxis of CMV infection in transplant pts. **OFF-LABEL:** CMV retinitis.

## PRECAUTIONS

**Contraindications:** Hypersensitivity to acyclovir, ganciclovir. **Cautions:** Neutropenia, thrombocytopenia, renal impairment, children (long-term safety not determined due to potential for long-term carcinogenic, adverse reproductive effects), pregnancy. Absolute neutrophil count less than 500/mm³, platelet count less than 25,000/mm³.

## ACTION

Competes with viral DNA polymerase and incorporation into growing viral DNA chains. **Therapeutic Effect:** Interferes with DNA synthesis, viral replication.

## PHARMACOKINETICS

Widely distributed (including CSF and ocular tissue). Protein binding: 1%–2%. Excreted primarily in urine. Removed by hemodialysis. **Half-life:** 1.7–5.8 hrs (increased in renal impairment).

## 🔟 LIFESPAN CONSIDERATIONS

**Pregnancy/Lactation:** Avoid pregnancy. Female pts of reproductive potential should use effective contraception during treatment. Do not breastfeed. May be resumed no sooner than 72 hrs after the last dose. **Children:** Safety and efficacy not established in pts younger than 12 yrs. **Elderly:** Age-related renal impairment may require dosage adjustment.

## INTERACTIONS

**DRUG: Bone marrow depressants** may increase myelosuppression. **Imipenem** may increase risk for seizures. **HERBAL:** None significant. **FOOD:** None known. **LAB VALUES:** May increase serum alkaline phosphatase, ALT, AST, bilirubin, BUN, creatinine.

## AVAILABILITY (Rx)

**Injection, Powder for Reconstitution (Cytovene):** 500 mg.

## ADMINISTRATION/HANDLING

 IV

**Reconstitution** • Reconstitute 500-mg vial with 10 ml Sterile Water for Injection to provide concentration of 50 mg/ml; do **not** use Bacteriostatic Water (contains parabens, which is incompatible with ganciclovir). • Further dilute with 100 ml D₅W, 0.9% NaCl to provide a concentration of 10 mg/ml or less for infusion.
**Rate of Administration** • Administer only by IV infusion over at least 1 hr. • Do not give by IV push or rapid IV infusion

(increases risk of toxicity). Flush line with 0.9% NaCl before and after administration. **Storage** • Store vials at room temperature. Do not refrigerate. • Reconstituted solution in vial is stable for 12 hrs at room temperature. • After dilution, use within 24 hrs. • Discard if precipitate forms, discoloration occurs. • Avoid exposure to skin, eyes, mucous membranes. • Use latex gloves, safety glasses during preparation/handling of solution. • Avoid inhalation. • If solution contacts skin or mucous membranes, wash thoroughly with soap and water; rinse eyes thoroughly with plain water.

## 🔲 IV INCOMPATIBILITIES

Aldesleukin (Proleukin), amifostine (Ethyol), aztreonam (Azactam), cefepime (Maxipime), cytarabine (ARA-C), doxorubicin (Adriamycin), fludarabine (Fludara), foscarnet (Foscavir), gemcitabine (Gemzar), ondansetron (Zofran), piperacillin and tazobactam (Zosyn), sargramostim (Leukine), vinorelbine (Navelbine).

## 🔲 IV COMPATIBILITIES

Amphotericin B, enalapril (Vasotec), filgrastim (Neupogen), fluconazole (Diflucan), granisetron (Kytril), propofol (Diprivan).

## INDICATIONS/ROUTES/DOSAGE

**Cytomegalovirus (CMV) Retinitis**
IV: **ADULTS, CHILDREN 3 MOS AND OLDER:** 5 mg/kg/dose q12h for 14–21 days, then 5 mg/kg/day as a single daily dose or 6 mg/kg 5 days/wk.

**Prevention of CMV in Transplant Pts**
IV: **ADULTS, CHILDREN:** 5 mg/kg/dose q12h for 7–14 days, then 5 mg/kg/day as a single daily dose. Duration dependent on clinical condition and degree of immunosuppression.

**Congenital CMV**
IV: **NEONATES:** 6 mg/kg/dose q12h for 6 wks (if HIV positive, longer duration may be considered).

**Dosage in Renal Impairment**
Dosage and frequency are modified based on creatinine clearance (see table).

| Creatinine Clearance | Dosage | |
| | IV Induction | IV Maintenance |
| --- | --- | --- |
| 50–69 ml/min | 2.5 mg/kg q12h | 2.5 mg/kg q24h |
| 25–49 ml/min | 2.5 mg/kg q24h | 1.25 mg/kg q24h |
| 10–24 ml/min | 1.25 mg/kg q24h | 0.625 mg/kg q24h |
| Less than 10 ml/min | 1.25 mg/kg 3 times/wk | 0.625 mg/kg 3 times/wk |
| Hemodialysis (give after HD on HD days) | 1.25 mg/kg q48–72h | 0.625 mg/kg q48–72h |
| Peritoneal dialysis | 1.25 mg/kg 3 times/wk | 0.625 mg/kg 3 times/wk |
| Continuous renal replacement therapy | | |
| Continuous venovenous hemofiltration | 2.5 mg/kg q24h | 1.25 mg/kg q24h |
| Continuous venovenous hemodialysis/ continuous venovenous hemodiafiltration | 2.5 mg/kg q12h | 2.5 mg/kg q24h |

**Dosage in Hepatic Impairment**
No dose adjustment.

## SIDE EFFECTS

**Frequent (41%–13%):** Diarrhea, fever, nausea, abdominal pain, vomiting. **Occasional (11%–6%):** Diaphoresis, infection, paresthesia, flatulence, pruritus. **Rare (4%–2%):** Headache, stomatitis, dyspepsia, phlebitis.

## ADVERSE EFFECTS/ TOXIC REACTIONS

Hematologic toxicity occurs commonly: leukopenia (41%–29% of pts), anemia (25%–19% of pts). Intraocular implant occasionally results in visual acuity loss, vitreous hemorrhage, retinal detachment. GI hemorrhage occurs rarely.

## NURSING CONSIDERATIONS

### BASELINE ASSESSMENT
Obtain baseline CBC, BMP, LFT. Perform baseline ophthalmic exam. Obtain specimens for support of differential diagnosis (urine, feces, blood, throat) since retinal infection is usually due to hematogenous dissemination.

### INTERVENTION/EVALUATION
Monitor I&O, ensure adequate hydration (minimum 1,500 ml/24 hrs). Diligently evaluate hematology reports for neutropenia, thrombocytopenia, leukopenia. Obtain periodic ophthalmic examinations. Question pt regarding visual acuity, therapeutic improvement, complications. Assess for rash, pruritus.

### PATIENT/FAMILY TEACHING
• Ganciclovir provides suppression, not cure, of cytomegalovirus (CMV) retinitis. • Frequent blood tests, eye exams are necessary during therapy due to toxic nature of drug. • Report any new symptom promptly. • May temporarily or permanently inhibit sperm production in men, suppress fertility in women. • Barrier contraception should be used during and for 90 days after therapy due to mutagenic potential.

# gefitinib

ge-fi-ti-nib
(Iressa)
**Do not confuse gefitinib with erlotinib, dasatinib, imatinib, or lapatinib.**

## ◆CLASSIFICATION

**PHARMACOTHERAPEUTIC:** Tyrosine kinase inhibitor. **CLINICAL:** Antineoplastic.

## USES

First-line treatment of metastatic non-small-cell lung cancer (NSCLC) whose tumors have epidermal growth factor receptor (EGFR) exon 19 deletions or exon 21 substitution mutations.

## PRECAUTIONS

**Contraindications:** Hypersensitivity to gefitinib. **Cautions:** Hepatic impairment, lung disease, ocular disease, concurrent administration of CYP3A4 inducers and inhibitors.

## ACTION

Inhibits epidermal growth factor receptor–tyrosine kinase (EGFR-TK), a key driver in tumor cell growth. Interrupts angiogenesis and metastasis. **Therapeutic Effect:** Inhibits tumor cell proliferation and survival.

## PHARMACOKINETICS

Slowly absorbed following PO administration. Peak plasma levels in 3–7 hrs. Protein binding: 90%. Metabolized in liver. Excreted primarily in feces (86%). **Half-life:** 48 hrs.

## ⏳ LIFESPAN CONSIDERATINS

**Pregnancy/Lactation:** Avoid pregnancy. Unknown if crosses placenta or distributed in breast milk. Nursing mothers must either discontinue breastfeeding or discontinue therapy. **Children:** Safety and efficacy not established in those younger than 18 yrs. **Elderly:** No age-related precautions noted.

## INTERACTIONS

**DRUG: CYP3A4 inhibitors (e.g., clarithromycin, ketoconazole)** may increase concentration. **CYP3A4 inducers (e.g., phenytoin, rifampin)** may decrease concentration. **H2 antagonists (e.g., famotidine), proton pump inhibitors (e.g., pantoprazole)** may decrease concentration. May increase bleeding risk with **warfarin.** **HERBAL:** St. John's wort may decrease effectiveness. **FOOD:** Avoid grapefruit products. **LAB VALUES:** May increase serum AST, ALT, bilirubin, urine protein.

## AVAILABILITY (RX)

**Tablets:** 250 mg.

## ADMINISTRATION/HANDLING

• May give without regard to meals. • Avoid grapefruit products. • Do not crush or cut. Swallow whole or administer as dispersion in water. Gently swirl glass for up to 20 min and immediately ingest once dispersed.

## INDICATIONS/ROUTES/DOSAGE

**NSCLC**
**PO: ADULTS, ELDERLY:** 250 mg once daily, with or without food. (Concurrent CYP3A4 inducers: consider increasing dose to 500 mg once daily.)

**Dosage in Renal Impairment**
No dose adjustment.

**Dosage in Hepatic Impairment**
**Mild impairment:** No dose adjustment. **Moderate to severe impairment:** Use with caution.

## SIDE EFFECTS

**Frequent (47%–15%):** Skin reactions (e.g., acne, pruritus, rash, xeroderma), diarrhea, decreased appetite, vomiting. **Occasional (7%–5%):** Stomatitis, conjunctivitis, blepharitis, dry eye, nail disorders (e.g., infection).

## ADVERSE EFFECTS/TOXIC REACTIONS

Hepatotoxicity, interstitial lung disease, gastrointestinal perforation, severe or persistent diarrhea, ocular disorders including keratitis, bullous and exfoliative skin disorders.

## NURSING CONSIDERATIONS

### BASELINE ASSESSMENT

Obtain baseline CBC with differential, serum chemistries, hepatic function test, thyroid function test, PT/INT (if taking warfarin), EGFR mutation serostatus. Question possibility of pregnancy or plans of breastfeeding. Receive full medication history including vitamins, minerals, herbal products. Assess visual acuity.

**INTERVENTION/EVALUATON**

Assess vital signs, oxygen saturation routinely. Routinely monitor CBC with differential, hepatic function tests. Worsening cough, fever, or shortness of breath may indicate interstitial lung disease. Consider ophthalmologic evaluation for vision changes. Monitor for bruising, hematuria, jaundice, right upper abdominal pain, weight loss, or acute infection (fever, diaphoresis, lethargy, productive cough). Monitor for skin lesions.

**PATIENT/FAMILY TEACHING**

Blood levels will be drawn routinely. Report urine changes, bloody or clay-colored stools, upper abdominal pain, nausea, vomiting, bruising, fever, cough, difficulty breathing. Immediately report any newly prescribed medications, suspected pregnancy, vision changes (eye pain, bleeding, sensitivity to light), or persistent diarrhea, dehydration. Avoid alcohol. Avoid grapefruit products.

---

## *gemcitabine*

jem-**sye**-ta-been
(Gemzar)
**Do not confuse gemcitabine with gemtuzumab, Gemzar with Zinecard.**

### ◆CLASSIFICATION

**PHARMACOTHERAPEUTIC:** Antimetabolite. **CLINICAL:** Antineoplastic.

## USES

Metastatic breast cancer in combination with paclitaxel. Treatment of locally advanced (stage II, III) or metastatic (stage IV) adenocarcinoma of pancreas. In combination with cisplatin for treatment of locally advanced or metastatic non–small-cell lung cancer (NSCLC). Treatment of advanced ovarian cancer (in combination with carboplatin) that has relapsed. **OFF-LABEL:** Treatment of biliary tract carcinoma, bladder carcinoma, germ cell tumors (e.g., testicular), Hodgkin's lymphoma, non-Hodgkin's lymphoma, cervical cancer.

## PRECAUTIONS

**Contraindications:** Hypersensitivity to gemcitabine. **Cautions:** Renal/hepatic impairment, pregnancy, elderly, concurrent radiation therapy, impaired pulmonary function.

## ACTION

Inhibits ribonucleotide reductase, the enzyme necessary for catalyzing DNA synthesis. **Therapeutic Effect:** Produces death of cells undergoing DNA synthesis.

## PHARMACOKINETICS

Not extensively distributed after IV infusion (increased with length of infusion). Protein binding: less than 10%. Metabolized intracellularly by nucleoside kinases. Excreted primarily in urine. **Half-life:** Influenced by duration of infusion. Infusion 1 hr or less: 42–94 min; infusion 3–4 hrs: 4–10.5 hrs.

## ⧗ LIFESPAN CONSIDERATIONS

**Pregnancy/Lactation:** If possible, avoid use during pregnancy, esp. first trimester. May cause fetal harm. Unknown if distributed in breast milk. Breastfeeding not recommended. **Children:** Safety and efficacy not established. **Elderly:** Increased risk of hematologic toxicity.

## INTERACTIONS

**DRUG: Bone marrow depressants** may increase risk of myelosuppression. **Live virus vaccines** may potentiate virus replication, increase vaccine side effects, decrease pt's antibody response to vaccine. **HERBAL:** Echinacea may decrease effects. **FOOD:** None known.

**LAB VALUES:** May increase serum BUN, alkaline phosphatase, bilirubin, creatinine, ALT, AST. May decrease Hgb, Hct, leukocyte count, platelet count.

## AVAILABILITY (Rx)

**Injection, Powder for Reconstitution:** 200-mg, 1-g, 2-g vials. **Injection, Solution:** 38 mg/ml.

## ADMINISTRATION/HANDLING
 IV

**Reconstitution** • Use gloves when handling/preparing gemcitabine. • Reconstitute with 0.9% NaCl injection without preservative to provide concentration of 38 mg/ml. • Shake to dissolve. Further diluted with 50–500 ml 0.9% NaCl to a concentration as low as 0.1 mg/ml.
**Rate of Administration** • Infuse over 30 min. • Infusion time greater than 60 min increases toxicity.
**Storage** • Store at room temperature (refrigeration may cause crystallization). • Reconstituted vials or diluted solutions are stable for 24 hrs at room temperature. Do not refrigerate.

## 🌀 IV INCOMPATIBILITIES

Acyclovir (Zovirax), amphotericin B (Fungizone), cefotaxime (Claforan), furosemide (Lasix), ganciclovir (Cytovene), imipenem/cilastatin (Primaxin), irinotecan (Camptosar), methotrexate, methylprednisolone (Solu-Medrol), mitomycin (Mutamycin), piperacillin/tazobactam (Zosyn), prochlorperazine (Compazine).

## 🌀 IV COMPATIBILITIES

Bumetanide (Bumex), calcium gluconate, dexamethasone (Decadron), diphenhydramine (Benadryl), dobutamine (Dobutrex), dopamine (Intropin), granisetron (Kytril), heparin, hydrocortisone (Solu-Cortef), lorazepam (Ativan), ondansetron (Zofran), potassium chloride.

## INDICATIONS/ROUTES/DOSAGE
**◄ALERT►** Dosage is individualized based on clinical response, tolerance to adverse effects. When used in combination therapy, consult specific protocols for optimum dosage, sequence of drug administration.

**Breast Cancer**
**IV: ADULTS, ELDERLY:** (in combination with paclitaxel): 1,250 mg/m² over 30 min on days 1 and 8 of each 21-day cycle.

**Non–Small-Cell Lung Cancer (NSCLC)**
**IV: ADULTS, ELDERLY, CHILDREN:** (in combination with cisplatin): 1,000 mg/m² on days 1, 8, and 15, repeated every 28 days; or 1,250 mg/m² on days 1 and 8. Repeat every 21 days.

**Ovarian Cancer**
**IV: ADULTS, ELDERLY:** (in combination with carboplatin): 1,000 mg/m² on days 1 and 8 of each 21-day cycle.

**Pancreatic Cancer**
**IV: ADULTS:** 1,000 mg/m² once wkly for up to 7 wks or until toxicity necessitates decreasing dosage or withholding the dose, followed by 1 wk of rest. Subsequent cycles should consist of once-wkly dose for 3 consecutive wks out of every 4 wks.

**Dosage in Renal/Hepatic Impairment**
No dose adjustment.

**Dosage Reduction Guidelines**
**Pancreatic Cancer, Non–Small-Cell Lung Cancer (NSCLC)**
Dosage adjustments should be based on granulocyte count and platelet count, as follows:

| Absolute Granulocyte Counts (cells/mm³) | Platelet Count (cells/mm³) | % of Full Dose |
|---|---|---|
| 1,000 | 100,000 | 100 |
| 500–999 | 50,000–99,000 | 75 |
| Less than 500 or | Less than 50,000 | Hold |

**G**

---

**Breast Cancer**

| Absolute Granulocyte Counts (cells/mm³) | Platelet Count (cells/mm³) | % of Full Dose |
|---|---|---|
| Equal to or greater than 1,200 and | Greater than 75,000 | 100 |
| 1,000–1,199 or | 50,000–75,000 | 75 |
| 700–999 and | Equal to or greater than 50,000 | 50 |
| Less than 700 or | Less than 50,000 | Hold |

**Ovarian Cancer**

| Absolute Granulocyte Counts (cells/mm³) | Platelet Count (cells/mm³) | % of Full Dose |
|---|---|---|
| 1,500 or greater and | 100,000 or greater | 100 |
| 1,000–1,499 and/or | 75,000–99,999 | 50 |
| Less than 1,000 and/or | Less than 75,000 | Hold |

## SIDE EFFECTS

**Frequent (69%–20%):** Nausea, vomiting, generalized pain, fever, mild to moderate pruritic rash, mild to moderate dyspnea, constipation, peripheral edema. **Occasional (19%–10%):** Diarrhea, petechiae, alopecia, stomatitis, infection, drowsiness, paresthesia. **Rare:** Diaphoresis, rhinitis, insomnia, malaise.

## ADVERSE EFFECTS/ TOXIC REACTIONS

Severe myelosuppression (anemia, thrombocytopenia, leukopenia) occurs commonly.

## NURSING CONSIDERATIONS

### BASELINE ASSESSMENT

Obtain baseline CBC, renal function, LFT, and periodically thereafter (CBC, platelets before each dose). Drug should be suspended or dosage modified if myelosuppression is detected.

### INTERVENTION/EVALUATION

Assess all lab results prior to each dose. Monitor for dyspnea, fever, pruritic rash, dehydration. Assess oral mucosa for erythema, ulceration at inner margin of lips, sore throat, difficulty swallowing (stomatitis). Assess skin for rash. Monitor daily pattern of bowel activity, stool consistency. Provide antiemetics as needed.

### PATIENT/FAMILY TEACHING

• Avoid crowds, exposure to infection. • Maintain strict oral hygiene. • Promptly report fever, sore throat, signs of local infection, easy bruising, rash, yellowing of skin or eyes. • Report nausea or vomiting that continues at home.

# gemfibrozil

jem-**fye**-broe-zil
(Apo-Gemfibrozil ✦, Lopid, Novo-Gemfibrozil ✦)
**Do not confuse Lopid with Levbid, Lipitor, Lodine, or Slo-Bid.**

## ◆CLASSIFICATION

**PHARMACOTHERAPEUTIC:** Fibric acid derivative. **CLINICAL:** Antihyperlipidemic.

## USES

Treatment of hypertriglyceridemia in types IV and V hyperlipidemia in pts who are at greater risk for pancreatitis and those who have not responded to dietary intervention. Reduce risk of coronary heart disease (CHD) development in pts without symptoms who have decreased HDL, increased LDL, increased triglycerides.

## PRECAUTIONS

**Contraindications:** Hypersensitivity to gemfibrozil. Hepatic impairment (including primary biliary cirrhosis), preexisting gallbladder disease, severe renal impairment, concurrent use with repaglinide or simvastatin. **Cautions:** Concurrent use with statins, mild to moderate renal impairment. anticoagulant therapy (e.g., warfarin).

## ACTION

Exact mechanism of action unknown. Can inhibit lipolysis of fat in adipose tissue; decrease hepatic uptake of free fatty acids (reduces hepatic triglyceride production) or inhibit hepatic secretion of very low density lipoprotein (VLDL). **Therapeutic Effect:** Lowers serum cholesterol, triglycerides (decreases VLDL, LDL; increases HDL).

## PHARMACOKINETICS

Well absorbed from GI tract. Protein binding: 99%. Metabolized in liver. Primarily excreted in urine. Not removed by hemodialysis. **Half-life:** 1.5 hrs.

## ⧗ LIFESPAN CONSIDERATIONS

**Pregnancy/Lactation:** Unknown if drug crosses placenta or is distributed in breast milk. Decision to discontinue breastfeeding or drug should be based on potential for serious adverse effects. **Children:** Not recommended in pts younger than 2 yrs (cholesterol necessary for normal development). **Elderly:** Age-related renal impairment may require dosage adjustment.

## INTERACTIONS

**DRUG: Statins (e.g., atorvastatin, simvastatin)** may increase risk for myopathy/rhabdomyolysis. May increase effects of **repaglinide, warfarin.** Bile acid–binding resins (e.g., colestipol) may decrease concentration. **HERBAL:** None significant. **FOOD:** None known. **LAB VALUES:** May increase serum alkaline phosphatase, bilirubin, creatine kinase, LDH, ALT, AST. May decrease Hgb, Hct, leukocyte counts, serum potassium.

## AVAILABILITY (Rx)

**Tablets:** 600 mg.

## ADMINISTRATION/HANDLING

**PO**
• Give 30 min before morning and evening meals.

## INDICATIONS/ROUTES/DOSAGE

**Hyperlipidemia**
**PO: ADULTS, ELDERLY:** 600 mg twice daily 30 min before breakfast and dinner.

**Dosage in Renal Impairment**
Use caution. Contraindicated in severe impairment.

**Dosage in Hepatic Impairment**
Contraindicated.

## SIDE EFFECTS

**Frequent (20%):** Dyspepsia. **Occasional (10%–2%):** Abdominal pain, diarrhea, nausea, vomiting, fatigue. **Rare (less than 2%):** Constipation, acute appendicitis, vertigo, headache, rash, pruritus, altered taste.

## ADVERSE EFFECTS/ TOXIC REACTIONS

Cholelithiasis, cholecystitis, acute appendicitis, pancreatitis, malignancy occur rarely.

## NURSING CONSIDERATIONS

### BASELINE ASSESSMENT

Obtain diet history, esp. fat/alcohol consumption. Obtain serum glucose, triglyceride, cholesterol, LFT.

### INTERVENTION/EVALUATION

Monitor LDL, VLDL, serum triglycerides, cholesterol lab results for therapeutic response. Monitor daily pattern of bowel activity, stool consistency. Assess for rash, pruritus. Question for headache, dizziness. Monitor LFT, hematology tests. Assess for abdominal pain, esp. right upper quadrant or epigastric pain suggestive of adverse gallbladder effects. Monitor serum glucose in pts receiving insulin, oral antihyperglycemics.

### PATIENT/FAMILY TEACHING

• Follow special diet (important part of treatment). • Take before meals. • Periodic lab tests are essential part of therapy. • Report pronounced dizziness, blurred vision, abdominal pain, diarrhea, nausea, vomiting.

# gentamicin

jen-ta-**mye**-sin
(Gentak)

■ **BLACK BOX ALERT** ■ Aminoglycoside antibiotics may cause neurotoxicity, nephrotoxicity. Risk of ototoxicity directly proportional to dosage, duration of treatment; ototoxicity usually is irreversible, precipitated by tinnitus, vertigo. May cause fetal harm if given during pregnancy.

**Do not confuse gentamicin with vancomycin.**

## ◆CLASSIFICATION

**PHARMACOTHERAPEUTIC:** Aminoglycoside. **CLINICAL:** Antibiotic.

## USES

**Parenteral:** Treatment of infections susceptible to *Pseudomonas, Proteus, Serratia,* and other gram-negative organisms and gram-positive *Staphylococcus* including skin/skin structure, bone, joint, respiratory tract, intra-abdominal, complicated urinary tract, acute pelvic infections; burns; septicemia; meningitis. **Ophthalmic:** Ophthalmic infections caused by susceptible bacteria. **OFF-LABEL:** Surgical (preoperative) prophylaxis.

## PRECAUTIONS

**Contraindications:** Hypersensitivity to gentamicin, other aminoglycosides (cross-sensitivity) or their components. **Cautions:** Elderly, neonates due to renal insufficiency or immaturity, neuromuscular disorders (potential for respiratory depression), vestibular or cochlear impairment, renal impairment, hypocalcemia, myasthenia gravis. Pediatric pts on extracorporeal membrane oxygenation.

## ACTION

Irreversibly binds to protein of bacterial ribosomes. **Therapeutic Effect:** Interferes with protein synthesis of susceptible microorganisms. Bactericidal.

## PHARMACOKINETICS

Rapid, complete absorption after IM administration. Protein binding: less than 30%. Widely distributed (does not cross blood-brain barrier, low concentrations in CSF). Excreted unchanged in urine. Removed by hemodialysis. **Half-life:** 2–4 hrs (increased in renal impairment, neonates; decreased in cystic fibrosis, burn, or febrile pts).

## ⌛ LIFESPAN CONSIDERATIONS

**Pregnancy/Lactation:** Readily crosses placenta; unknown if distributed in breast milk. **Children:** Caution in neonates: Immature renal function increases half-life and toxicity. **Elderly:** Age-related renal impairment may require dosage adjustment.

## INTERACTIONS

**DRUG:** **Nephrotoxic** (e.g., **lisinopril, IV contrast dye), ototoxic medications** (e.g., **cisplatin, furosemide)** may increase risk of nephrotoxicity, ototoxicity. May increase neuromuscular blockade with concurrent use of **neuromuscular blockers** (e.g., **succinylcholine).** **HERBAL:** None significant. **FOOD:** None known. **LAB VALUES:** May increase serum BUN, creatinine, bilirubin, LDH, ALT, AST. May decrease serum calcium, magnesium, potassium, sodium. **Therapeutic serum level:** peak: 4–10 mcg/ml; trough: 0.5–2 mcg/ml. **Toxic serum level:** peak: greater than 10 mcg/ml; trough: greater than 2 mcg/ml.

## AVAILABILITY (Rx)

**Injection, Infusion:** 60 mg/50 ml, 80 mg/50 ml, 80 mg/100 ml, 100 mg/50 ml, 100 mg/100 ml, 120 mg/100 ml. **Injection, Solution:** 10 mg/ml, 40 mg/ml. **Ointment, Ophthalmic:** 0.3%. **Solution, Ophthalmic (Gentak):** 0.3%.

## ADMINISTRATION/HANDLING

 **IV**

**Reconstitution •** Dilute with 50–100 ml D₅W or 0.9% NaCl. Amount of diluent for infants, children depends on individual needs.

**Rate of Administration** • Infuse over 30–60 min for adults, older children; over 60–120 min for infants, young children.

**Storage** • Store vials at room temperature. • Solution appears clear or slightly yellow. • Intermittent IV infusion (piggyback) is stable for 48 hrs at room temperature or refrigerated. • Discard if precipitate forms.

**IM**

• To minimize discomfort, give deep IM slowly. • Less painful if injected into gluteus maximus than lateral aspect of thigh.

**Ophthalmic**

• Place gloved finger on lower eyelid and pull out until a pocket is formed between eye and lower lid. • Place prescribed number of drops or ¼–½ inch ointment into pocket. Instruct pt to close eye gently for 1–2 min (so medication will not be squeezed out of the sac). • **Solution:** Instruct pt to apply digital pressure to lacrimal sac at inner canthus for 1 min to minimize systemic absorption. • **Ointment:** Instruct pt to roll eyeball to increase contact area of drug to eye. • Remove excess solution or ointment around eye with tissue.

### ▨ IV INCOMPATIBILITIES

Allopurinol (Aloprim), amphotericin B complex (Abelcet, AmBisome, Amphotec), furosemide (Lasix), heparin, heta-starch (Hespan), idarubicin (Idamycin), indomethacin (Indocin), propofol (Diprivan).

### ▨ IV COMPATIBILITIES

Amiodarone (Cordarone), dexmedetomidine (Precedex), diltiazem (Cardizem), enalapril (Vasotec), filgrastim (Neupogen), hydromorphone (Dilaudid), insulin, lorazepam (Ativan), magnesium sulfate, midazolam (Versed), morphine, multivitamins.

### INDICATIONS/ROUTES/DOSAGE

◀**ALERT**▶ Space parenteral doses evenly around the clock. Dosage based on ideal body weight. Peak, trough levels are determined periodically to maintain desired serum concentrations and minimize risk of toxicity.

**Usual Parenteral Dosage**

**IM, IV: ADULTS, ELDERLY: (Conventional):** 1–2.5 mg/kg/dose q8–12h. **(Once Daily):** 4–7 mg/kg/dose q24h. **CHILDREN 5 YRS AND OLDER:** 2–2.5 mg/kg/dose q8h. **INFANTS, CHILDREN YOUNGER THAN 5 YRS:** 2.5 mg/kg/dose q8h. **NEONATES (GREATER THAN 2 KG) PNA 8–28 days:** 4 mg/kg/dose q12–24h; **PNA 7 days or less:** 4 mg/kg/dose q24h. **(1–2 KG) PNA 8–28 days:** 4–5 mg/kg/dose q24–48h; **PNA 7 days or less:** 5 mg/kg/dose q48h. **(LESS THAN 1 KG) PNA 15–28 days:** 4–5 mg/kg/dose q24–48h; **PNA 14 days or less:** 5 mg/kg/dose q48h.

**Hemodialysis (HD)**

**Note:** Administer after HD on dialysis days.

**Loading dose:** 2–3 mg/kg, then 1 mg/kg q48–72h for mild UTI or synergy (consider redose for pre- or post-HD concentrations less than 1 mg/L); 1–1.5 mg/kg q48–72h for moderate to severe UTI (consider redose for pre-HD concentration less than 1.5–2 mg/L or post-HD concentrations less than 1 mg/L); 1.5–2 mg/kg q48–72h for systemic gram-negative rod infection (consider redose for pre-HD concentration less than 3–5 mg/L or post-HD concentrations less than 2 mg/L).

**Continuous Renal Replacement Therapy (CRRT)**

**Loading dose:** 2–3 mg/kg, then 1 mg/kg q24–36h for mild UTI or synergy (redose when concentration less than 1 mg/L); 1–1.5 mg/kg q24–36h for moderate to severe UTI (redose when concentration less than 1.5–2 mg/L; 1.5–2 mg/kg q24–48h for systemic gram-negative infection (redose when concentration less than 3–5 mg/L).

G

**Usual Ophthalmic Dosage**
**Ophthalmic Ointment:** ADULTS, ELDERLY:
Apply ½-inch strip to conjunctival sac
2–4 times/day.
**Ophthalmic Solution:** ADULTS, ELDERLY,
CHILDREN: 1–2 drops q2–4h up to
2 drops/hr.

**Dosage in Renal Impairment**
**Conventional Dosing:**

| Creatinine Clearance | Dosage |
|---|---|
| Greater than 60 ml/mil | q8h |
| 41–60 ml/min | q12h |
| 20–40 ml/min | q24h |
| Less than 20 ml/min | Loading dose, then monitor levels to determine dosage interval |

**Dosage in Hepatic Impairment**
Monitor plasma concentrations.

## SIDE EFFECTS

**Occasional: IM:** Pain, induration at
injection site. **IV:** Phlebitis, thrombophlebitis, hypersensitivity reactions (fever,
pruritus, rash, urticaria). **Ophthalmic:**
Burning, tearing, itching, blurred vision.
**Rare:** Alopecia, hypertension, fatigue.

## ADVERSE EFFECTS/ TOXIC REACTIONS

Nephrotoxicity (increased serum
BUN, creatinine; decreased creatinine
clearance) may be reversible if drug is
stopped at first sign of symptoms.
Irreversible ototoxicity (tinnitus, dizziness, diminished hearing), neurotoxicity (headache, dizziness, lethargy,
tremor, visual disturbances) occur occasionally. Risk increases with higher
dosages, prolonged therapy, or if solution is applied directly to mucosa.
Superinfections, particularly with
fungi, may result from bacterial imbalance via any route of administration.
Ophthalmic application may cause
paresthesia of conjunctiva, mydriasis.

## NURSING CONSIDERATIONS

### BASELINE ASSESSMENT
Dehydration must be treated before beginning parenteral therapy. Establish baseline
hearing acuity. Question for history of allergies, esp. aminoglycosides, sulfites (parabens for topical/ophthalmic routes).

### INTERVENTION/EVALUATION
Monitor I&O (maintain hydration), urinalysis (casts, RBCs, WBCs, decrease in
specific gravity). Be alert to ototoxic,
neurotoxic symptoms (see Adverse
Effects/Toxic Reactions). Check IM injection site for induration. Evaluate IV site
for phlebitis (heat, pain, red streaking
over vein). Assess for rash (**Ophthalmic:** redness, burning, itching, tearing).
Be alert for superinfection (genital/anal
pruritus, changes in oral mucosa, diarrhea). When treating pts with neuromuscular disorders, assess respiratory response
carefully. **Therapeutic serum level:**
peak: 4–10 mcg/ml; peak levels are 2–
3 times greater with once-daily dosing
trough: 0.5–2 mcg/ml. **Toxic serum
level:** peak: greater than 10 mcg/ml;
trough: greater than 2 mcg/ml.

### PATIENT/FAMILY TEACHING
• Discomfort may occur with IM injection. • Blurred vision, tearing may occur briefly after each ophthalmic dose.
• Report any hearing, visual, balance,
urinary problems, even after therapy is
completed. • **Ophthalmic:** Report if
tearing, redness, irritation continues.

# glatiramer    TOP 100

gla-**tir**-a-mer
(Copaxone, Glatopa)
**Do not confuse Copaxone with
Compazine.**

## ◆CLASSIFICATION
**PHARMACOTHERAPEUTIC:** Immunosuppressive. **CLINICAL:** Neurologic
agent for multiple sclerosis.

## USES

Treatment of relapsing, remitting multiple sclerosis.

## PRECAUTIONS

**Contraindications:** Hypersensitivity to glatiramer, mannitol. **Cautions:** Pts exhibiting immediate postinjection reaction (flushing, chest pain, palpitations, anxiety, dyspnea, urticaria).

## ACTION

Induces/activates T-lymphocyte suppressor cells specific to myelin antigens. May also interfere with the antigen-presenting function of immune cells. **Therapeutic Effect:** Slows progression of multiple sclerosis.

## PHARMACOKINETICS

Substantial fraction of glatiramer is hydrolyzed locally. Some fraction of injected material enters lymphatic circulation, reaching regional lymph nodes; some may enter systemic circulation intact.

## ⧗ LIFESPAN CONSIDERATIONS

**Pregnancy/Lactation:** Unknown if distributed in breast milk. **Children:** Safety and efficacy not established. **Elderly:** Safety and efficacy not established.

## INTERACTIONS

**DRUG:** None significant. **HERBAL: Echinacea** may decrease effects. **FOOD:** None known. **LAB VALUES:** None significant.

## AVAILABILITY (Rx)

**Injection Solution:** (Copaxone, Glatopa) 20 mg/ml in prefilled syringes, (Copaxone) 40 mg/ml in prefilled syringes.

## ADMINISTRATION/HANDLING

**Subcutaneous**
• Refrigerate syringes (bring to room temperature before use). • May be stored at room temperature for up to 1 mo. • Avoid heat, intense light. • Inject into deltoid region, abdomen, gluteus maximus, or lateral aspect of thigh. • Prefilled syringe suitable for single use only; discard unused portions.

## INDICATIONS/ROUTES/DOSAGE

**Multiple Sclerosis**
**SQ: ADULTS, ELDERLY:** 20 mg once daily or 40 mg 3 times/wk.

**Dosage in Renal/Hepatic Impairment**
No dose adjustment.

## SIDE EFFECTS

**Expected (73%–40%):** Pain, erythema, inflammation, pruritus at injection site, asthenia. **Frequent (27%–18%):** Arthralgia, vasodilation, anxiety, hypertonia, nausea, transient chest pain, dyspnea, flu-like symptoms, rash, pruritus. **Occasional (17%–10%):** Palpitations, back pain, diaphoresis, rhinitis, diarrhea, urinary urgency. **Rare (less than 9%):** Anorexia, fever, neck pain, peripheral edema, ear pain, facial edema, vertigo, vomiting.

## ADVERSE EFFECTS/ TOXIC REACTIONS

Infection occurs commonly. Lymphadenopathy occurs occasionally.

## NURSING CONSIDERATIONS

### BASELINE ASSESSMENT
Establish baseline neurologic function.

### INTERVENTION/EVALUATION
Observe injection site for reaction. Monitor for fever, chills (evidence of infection). Observe for improvement in neurologic function.

### PATIENT/FAMILY TEACHING
• Report difficulty in breathing/swallowing, rash, itching, swelling of lower extremities, fatigue. • Avoid pregnancy.

## *glimepiride* `HIGH ALERT`

glye-**mep**-ir-ide
(Amaryl, Apo-Glimepiride ✦, Novo-Glimepiride ✦)

---

**Do not confuse Amaryl with Altace, Amerge, or Reminyl, Avandaryl with Benadryl, or glimepiride with glipizide or glyburide.**

### FIXED-COMBINATION(S)

**Avandaryl:** glimepiride/rosiglitazone (an antidiabetic): 1 mg/4 mg, 2 mg/4 mg, 4 mg/4 mg.
**Duetact:** glimepiride/pioglitazone (an antidiabetic): 2 mg/30 mg, 4 mg/30 mg.

### ◆CLASSIFICATION

**PHARMACOTHERAPEUTIC:** Third-generation sulfonylurea. **CLINICAL:** Antidiabetic agent.

### USES

Adjunct to diet, exercise in management of non–insulin-dependent diabetes mellitus (type 2, NIDDM).

### PRECAUTIONS

**Contraindications:** Hypersensitivity to glimepiride. Diabetic ketoacidosis (with or without coma). **Cautions:** Renal/hepatic impairment, glucose-altering conditions (fever, trauma, infection), G6PD deficiency, elderly, malnourished. Allergy to sulfa.

### ACTION

Promotes release of insulin from beta cells of pancreas, decreases glucose output from liver, increases insulin sensitivity at peripheral sites. **Therapeutic Effect:** Lowers serum glucose.

### PHARMACOKINETICS

| Route | Onset | Peak | Duration |
|-------|-------|------|----------|
| PO | N/A | 2–3 hrs | 24 hrs |

Completely absorbed from GI tract. Protein binding: greater than 99%. Metabolized in liver. Excreted in urine (60%), feces (40%). **Half-life:** 5–9.2 hrs.

### ⧗ LIFESPAN CONSIDERATIONS

**Pregnancy/Lactation:** Avoid pregnancy. Unknown if distributed in breast milk. **Children:** Safety and efficacy not established. **Elderly:** Hypoglycemia may be difficult to recognize. Age-related renal impairment may increase sensitivity to glucose-lowering effect.

### INTERACTIONS

**DRUG: Beta blockers (e.g., carvedilol, metoprolol)** may increase hypoglycemic effect, mask signs of hypoglycemia. **Cimetidine, ciprofloxacin, fluconazole, ranitidine, large doses of salicylates** may increase effect. **Corticosteroids (e.g., dexamethasone, prednisone), thiazide diuretics (e.g., HCTZ)** may decrease effect. **HERBAL: Garlic** may worsen hypoglycemia. **FOOD:** None known. **LAB VALUES:** May increase LDH concentrations, serum alkaline phosphatase, ALT, AST, bilirubin, C-peptide.

### AVAILABILITY (Rx)

**Tablets:** 1 mg, 2 mg, 4 mg.

### ADMINISTRATION/HANDLING

**PO**
* Give with breakfast or first main meal.

### INDICATIONS/ROUTES/DOSAGE

**Diabetes Mellitus**
**PO: ADULTS:** Initially, 1–2 mg once daily with breakfast or first main meal. May increase by 1–2 mg q1–2wks, based on serum glucose response. **Maximum:** 8 mg/day. **ELDERLY:** Initially, 1 mg/day. Titrate dose to avoid hypoglycemia.

**Dosage in Renal Impairment**
Initially, 1 mg/day, then titrate dose based on fasting serum glucose levels.

**Dosage in Hepatic Impairment**
No dose adjustment (not studied).

## SIDE EFFECTS

**Rare (less than 3%):** Altered taste, dizziness, drowsiness, weight gain, constipation, diarrhea, heartburn, nausea, vomiting, stomach fullness, headache, photosensitivity, peeling of skin, pruritus, rash.

## ADVERSE EFFECTS/ TOXIC REACTIONS

Overdose or insufficient food intake may produce hypoglycemia (esp. with increased glucose demands). GI hemorrhage, cholestatic hepatic jaundice, leukopenia, thrombocytopenia, pancytopenia, agranulocytosis, aplastic or hemolytic anemia occur rarely.

## NURSING CONSIDERATIONS

### BASELINE ASSESSMENT

Check serum glucose level. Discuss lifestyle to determine extent of learning, emotional needs. Ensure follow-up instruction if pt or family does not thoroughly understand diabetes management or serum glucose testing technique.

### INTERVENTION/EVALUATION

Monitor serum glucose level, food intake. Assess for hypoglycemia (cool/wet skin, tremors, dizziness, anxiety, headache, tachycardia, perioral numbness, hunger, diplopia), hyperglycemia (polyuria, polyphagia, polydipsia, nausea, vomiting, dim vision, fatigue, deep or rapid breathing). Be alert to conditions that alter glucose requirements (fever, increased activity or stress, trauma, surgical procedure).

### PATIENT/ FAMILY TEACHING

• Prescribed diet is principal part of treatment; do not skip or delay meals. • Avoid alcohol. • Carry candy, sugar packets, other quick-acting sugar supplements for immediate response to hypoglycemia. • Wear medical alert identification. • Check with physician when glucose demands are altered (fever, infection, trauma, stress, heavy physical activity). • Avoid direct exposure to sunlight.

# *glipiZIDE

**glip**-i-zide
(Glucotrol, Glucotrol XL)
**Do not confuse glipizide with glimepiride or glyburide, or Glucotrol with Glucophage or Glucotrol XL.**

## FIXED-COMBINATION(S)

Glipizide/metformin (an antidiabetic): 2.5 mg/250 mg, 2.5 mg/500 mg, 5 mg/500 mg.

## ◆CLASSIFICATION

**PHARMACOTHERAPEUTIC:** Second-generation sulfonylurea. **CLINICAL:** Antidiabetic agent.

## USES

Adjunct to diet, exercise in management of non–insulin-dependent diabetes mellitus (type 2, NIDDM).

## PRECAUTIONS

**Contraindications:** Hypersensitivity to glipizide. Diabetic ketoacidosis with or without coma, type 1 diabetes mellitus. **Cautions:** Elderly, malnourished, concomitant use of beta blockers, pts with G6PD deficiency, hepatic/renal impairment. Avoid use of extended-release tablets in pts with stricture/narrowing of GI tract.

## ACTION

Promotes release of insulin from beta cells of pancreas, decreases glucose output from liver, increases insulin sensitivity at peripheral sites. **Therapeutic Effect:** Lowers serum glucose.

## PHARMACOKINETICS

| Route | Onset | Peak | Duration |
|---|---|---|---|
| PO | 15–30 min | 2–3 hrs | 12–24 hrs |
| Extended-release | 2–3 hrs | 6–12 hrs | 24 hrs |

Well absorbed from GI tract. Protein binding: 92%–99%. Metabolized in liver. Excreted in urine. **Half-life:** 2–4 hrs.

## ⏳ LIFESPAN CONSIDERATIONS

**Pregnancy/Lactation:** Insulin is drug of choice during pregnancy; glipizide given within 1 mo of delivery may produce neonatal hypoglycemia. Drug crosses placenta. Distributed in breast milk. **Children:** Safety and efficacy not established. **Elderly:** Hypoglycemia may be difficult to recognize. Age-related renal impairment may increase sensitivity to glucose-lowering effect.

## INTERACTIONS

**DRUG: Beta blockers (e.g., carvedilol, metoprolol)** may increase hypoglycemic effect, mask signs of hypoglycemia. **Corticosteroids (e.g., dexamethasone, prednisone), thiazide diuretics (e.g., HCTZ)** may decrease effect. **HERBAL: Garlic** may worsen hypoglycemia. **FOOD:** None known. **LAB VALUES:** May increase serum alkaline phosphatase, LDH, ALT, AST, bilirubin, C-peptide.

## AVAILABILITY (Rx)

**Tablets (Glucotrol):** 5 mg, 10 mg.

🔖 **Tablets (Extended-Release [Glucotrol XL]):** 2.5 mg, 5 mg, 10 mg.

## ADMINISTRATION/HANDLING

**PO**
• Give immediate-release tablets 30 min before meals. Give extended-release tablets with breakfast. • Do not crush, cut, dissolve, or divide extended-release tablets.

## INDICATIONS/ROUTES/DOSAGE

**Diabetes Mellitus**
**PO: ADULTS: (Immediate-Release):** Initially, 5 mg/day. Adjust dosage in 2.5- to 5-mg increments at intervals of several days. Immediate-release tablet: **Maximum once-daily dose:** 15 mg. **Maximum dose/day:** 40 mg. **(Extended-Release):** Initially, 5 mg/day. May increase dose no more frequently than q7days. **Maximum dose:** 20 mg/day. **ELDERLY: (Immediate-Release):** Initially,

2.5–5 mg/day. May increase by 2.5–5 mg/day q1–2wks. **(Extended-Release):** Initially, 2.5 mg/day. Dosing should be on lower end of adult dosing.

**Dosage in Renal Impairment**
For CrCl of 50 ml/min or less, reduce dose by 50%.

**Dosage in Hepatic Impairment**
**(Immediate-Release):** Initial dose: 2.5 mg/day.

## SIDE EFFECTS

**Rare (less than 3%):** Altered taste, dizziness, drowsiness, weight gain, constipation, diarrhea, heartburn, nausea, vomiting, headache, photosensitivity, peeling of skin, pruritus, rash.

## ADVERSE EFFECTS/ TOXIC REACTIONS

Overdose or insufficient food intake may produce hypoglycemia (esp. with increased glucose demands). GI hemorrhage, cholestatic hepatic jaundice, leukopenia, thrombocytopenia, pancytopenia, agranulocytosis, aplastic or hemolytic anemia occur rarely.

## NURSING CONSIDERATIONS

### BASELINE ASSESSMENT

Check serum glucose level. Discuss lifestyle to determine extent of learning, emotional needs. Ensure follow-up instruction if pt or family does not thoroughly understand diabetes management or serum glucose testing technique.

### INTERVENTION/EVALUATION

Monitor serum glucose level, food intake. Assess for hypoglycemia (cool/wet skin, tremors, dizziness, anxiety, headache, tachycardia, perioral numbness, hunger, diplopia), hyperglycemia (polyuria, polyphagia, polydipsia, nausea, vomiting, dim vision, fatigue, deep or rapid breathing). Be alert to conditions that alter glucose requirements (fever, increased activity or stress, trauma, surgical procedure).

### PATIENT/ FAMILY TEACHING

• Prescribed diet is principal part of treatment; do not skip or delay meals. • Avoid alcohol. • Carry candy, sugar packets, other quick-acting sugar supplements for immediate response to hypoglycemia. • Wear medical alert identification. • Check with physician when glucose demands are altered (fever, infection, trauma, stress, heavy physical activity). • Avoid direct exposure to sunlight.

# glucagon

**gloo**-ka-gon
(GlucaGen, GlucaGen Diagnostic Kit, Glucagon Emergency Kit)

### ◆ CLASSIFICATION

**PHARMACOTHERAPEUTIC:** Glucose elevating agent. **CLINICAL:** Antihypoglycemic, antispasmodic, antidote.

### USES

Treatment of severe hypoglycemia in diabetic pts. Diagnostic aid in radiographic examination to temporarily inhibit GI tract movement. **OFF-LABEL:** Hypoglycemia secondary to insulin or oral hypoglycemic therapy. Toxicity associated with beta blockers, calcium channel blockers.

### PRECAUTIONS

**Contraindications:** Hypersensitivity to glucagon. Known insulinoma, pheochromocytoma, glucagonoma (except GlucaGen). **Cautions:** History of insulinoma, pheochromocytoma, prolonged fasting, starvation, adrenal insufficiency, chronic hypoglycemia. Avoid use in pts with hereditary galactose intolerance.

### ACTION

Promotes hepatic glycogenolysis, gluconeogenesis. Stimulates cAMP, an enzyme, resulting in increased serum glucose concentration. **Therapeutic Effect:** Increases serum glucose level.

### PHARMACOKINETICS

| Route | Onset | Peak | Duration |
|-------|-------|------|----------|
| IV | 5–20 min | — | 60–90 min |
| IM | 30 min | — | 60–90 min |
| SQ | 30–45 min | — | 60–90 min |

Metabolized in liver. **Half-life:** 3–10 min.

### ⧖ LIFESPAN CONSIDERATIONS

**Pregnancy/Lactation:** Unknown if drug crosses placenta or is distributed in breast milk. **Children/Elderly:** No age-related precautions noted.

### INTERACTIONS

**DRUG:** May increase effects of **anticoagulants.** **HERBAL:** None significant. **FOOD:** None known. **LAB VALUES:** May decrease serum potassium.

### AVAILABILITY (Rx)

Injection Powder (GlucaGen, GlucaGen Diagnostic Kit, Glucagon Emergency Kit): 1 mg.

### ADMINISTRATION/HANDLING

◀**ALERT**▶ Place pt in side-lying position to prevent aspiration (glucagon, hypoglycemia may produce nausea/vomiting).

**IV, IM, SQ**
**Reconstitution** • Reconstitute with 1 ml sterile diluent to provide concentration of 1 mg/ml.
**Rate of Administration** • Pt usually awakens in 5–20 min. Although 1–2 additional doses may be administered, concern for effects of continuing cerebral hypoglycemia requires consideration of parenteral glucose. • When pt awakens, give supplemental carbohydrate to restore hepatic glycogen and prevent secondary hypoglycemia. If pt fails to respond to glucagon, IV dextrose is necessary.
**Storage** • Store vial at room temperature. • After reconstitution, is stable for 48 hrs if refrigerated. If reconstituted with Sterile Water for Injection, use immediately. Do not use glucagon solution unless clear.

 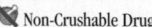

### ▨ IV INCOMPATIBILITIES

Do not mix glucagon with any other medications.

### INDICATIONS/ROUTES/DOSAGE

**Hypoglycemia**

◀**ALERT**▶ Administer IV dextrose if pt fails to respond to glucagon.

**IV, IM, SQ: ADULTS, ELDERLY, CHILDREN WEIGHING MORE THAN 20 KG:** 1 mg. May repeat in 15 min. **CHILDREN WEIGHING 20 KG OR LESS:** 0.5 mg. May repeat in 15 min. **NEONATES:** 0.02–0.2 mg/kg/dose. **Maximum:** 1 mg. May repeat in 20 min if needed.

**Diagnostic Aid**

**IV: ADULTS, ELDERLY:** 0.25–2 mg 10 min prior to procedure. **IM:** 1–2 mg 10 minutes prior to procedure.

**Dosage in Renal/Hepatic Impairment**

No dose adjustment.

### SIDE EFFECTS

**Occasional:** Nausea, vomiting. **Rare:** Allergic reaction (urticaria, respiratory distress, hypotension).

### ADVERSE EFFECTS/ TOXIC REACTIONS

Overdose may produce persistent nausea/vomiting, hypokalemia (severe fatigue, decreased appetite, palpitations, muscle cramps).

### NURSING CONSIDERATIONS

**BASELINE ASSESSMENT**

Obtain immediate assessment, including history, clinical signs/symptoms. If presence of hypoglycemic coma is established, give glucagon promptly.

**INTERVENTION/EVALUATION**

Monitor serum glucose, B/P, pulse, mental status. Monitor response time carefully. Have IV dextrose readily available in event pt does not respond. Assess for possible allergic reaction (urticaria, respiratory difficulty, hypotension). When pt is conscious, give oral carbohydrate.

**PATIENT/FAMILY TEACHING**

• Recognize significance of identifying symptoms of hypoglycemia: pale, cool skin, anxiety, difficulty concentrating, headache, hunger, nausea, shakiness, diaphoresis, unusual fatigue, unusual weakness, unconsciousness. • If symptoms of hypoglycemia develop, give sugar form first (orange juice, honey, hard candy, sugar cubes, table sugar dissolved in water or juice) followed by cheese and crackers, half a sandwich, glass of milk.

---

## *glyBURIDE

**glye**-bue-ride
(Apo-Glyburide ✦, DiaBeta, Euglucon ✦, Glynase)
**Do not confuse DiaBeta with Zebeta, glyburide with glimepiride, glipizide, or Glucotrol.**

### FIXED-COMBINATION(S)

**Glucovance:** glyburide/metformin (an antidiabetic): 1.25 mg/250 mg, 2.5 mg/500 mg, 5 mg/500 mg.

### ◆CLASSIFICATION

**PHARMACOTHERAPEUTIC:** Second-generation sulfonylurea. **CLINICAL:** Antidiabetic agent.

### USES

Adjunct to diet, exercise in management of stable, mild to moderately severe non–insulin-dependent diabetes mellitus (type 2, NIDDM).

### PRECAUTIONS

**Contraindications:** Hypersensitivity to glyburide. Diabetic ketoacidosis with or without coma, type 1 diabetes mellitus, concurrent use with bosentan. **Cautions:** Stress, elderly, debilitated, malnourished, severe hepatic/renal impairment, G6PD deficiency, adrenal and/or pituitary insufficiency.

## ACTION

Promotes release of insulin from beta cells of pancreas, decreases glucose output from liver, increases insulin sensitivity at peripheral sites. **Therapeutic Effect:** Lowers serum glucose level.

## PHARMACOKINETICS

| Route | Onset | Peak | Duration |
|---|---|---|---|
| PO | 0.25–1 hr | 1–2 hrs | 12–24 hrs |

Well absorbed from GI tract. Protein binding: 99%. Metabolized in liver. Primarily excreted in urine. Not removed by hemodialysis. **Half-life:** 5–16 hrs.

## ⧖ LIFESPAN CONSIDERATIONS

**Pregnancy/Lactation:** Crosses placenta. Distributed in breast milk. May produce neonatal hypoglycemia if given within 2 wks of delivery. **Children:** Safety and efficacy not established. **Elderly:** Hypoglycemia may be difficult to recognize. Age-related renal impairment may increase sensitivity to glucose-lowering effect.

## INTERACTIONS

**DRUG:** **Beta blockers (e.g., carvedilol, metoprolol)** may increase hypoglycemic effect, mask signs of hypoglycemia. **Corticosteroids (e.g., dexamethasone, prednisone), thiazide diuretics (e.g., HCTZ)** may decrease effect. **HERBAL:** **Garlic,** other herbs with hypoglycemic properties may enhance effect. **FOOD:** None known. **LAB VALUES:** May increase serum alkaline phosphatase, LDH, ALT, AST, bilirubin, C-peptide.

## AVAILABILITY (Rx)

**Tablets (DiaBeta):** 1.25 mg, 2.5 mg, 5 mg. **Tablets, Micronized (Glynase):** 1.5 mg, 3 mg, 6 mg.

## ADMINISTRATION/HANDLING

**PO**
• May give with food at same time each day.

## INDICATIONS/ROUTES/DOSAGE

**Diabetes Mellitus**
**PO** *(Diabeta):* **ADULTS:** Initially, 1.25–5 mg. May increase by 2.5 mg/day at wkly intervals. **Maintenance:** 1.25–20 mg/day. **Maximum:** 20 mg/day. **ELDERLY:** Initially, 1.25–2.5 mg/day. May increase by 1.25–2.5 mg/day at 1- to 3-wk intervals.
**PO** *(Glynase):* **ADULTS, ELDERLY:** Initially 0.75–3 mg/day. May increase by 1.5 mg/day at wkly intervals. **Maintenance:** 0.75–12 mg/day as a single dose or in divided doses. **Maximum:** 12 mg/day.

**Dosage in Renal Impairment**
Not recommended for pts with CrCl less than 50 ml/min.

**Dosage in Hepatic Impairment**
No dose adjustment.

## SIDE EFFECTS

**Rare (less than 3%):** Altered taste, dizziness, drowsiness, weight gain, constipation, diarrhea, heartburn, nausea, vomiting, headache, photosensitivity, peeling of skin, pruritis, rash.

## ADVERSE EFFECTS/ TOXIC REACTIONS

Overdose or insufficient food intake may produce hypoglycemia (esp. in pts with increased glucose demands). Cholestatic jaundice, leukopenia, thrombocytopenia, pancytopenia, agranulocytosis, aplastic or hemolytic anemia occur rarely.

## NURSING CONSIDERATIONS

**BASELINE ASSESSMENT**
Check serum glucose level. Discuss lifestyle to determine extent of learning, emotional needs. Ensure follow-up instruction if pt or family does not thoroughly understand diabetes management or glucose testing technique.

**INTERVENTION/EVALUATION**
Monitor serum glucose level, food intake. Assess for hypoglycemia (cool/wet skin,

G

tremors, dizziness, anxiety, headache, tachycardia, perioral numbness, hunger, diplopia); hyperglycemia (polyuria, polyphagia, polydipsia, nausea, vomiting, dim vision, fatigue, deep or rapid breathing). Be alert to conditions that alter glucose requirements (fever, increased activity or stress, trauma, surgical procedure).

**PATIENT/ FAMILY TEACHING**

• Prescribed diet is principal part of treatment; do not skip or delay meals. • Avoid alcohol. • Carry candy, sugar packets, other quick-acting sugar supplements for immediate response to hypoglycemia. • Wear medical alert identification. • Check with physician when glucose demands are altered (fever, infection, trauma, stress, heavy physical activity). • Avoid direct exposure to sunlight.

---

# golimumab

goe-**lim**-ue-mab
(Simponi, Simponi Aria)
**Do not confuse Simponi (subcutaneous) with Simponi Aria (intravenous).**

■ **BLACK BOX ALERT** ■ Tuberculosis (TB), invasive fungal infections, other opportunistic infections reported. Discontinue treatment if active infection or sepsis occurs. Test for TB prior to and during treatment, regardless of initial result; if positive, start treatment for TB prior to initiating therapy. Lymphoma, other malignancies reported in pts treated with tumor necrosis factor blockers.

## ◆CLASSIFICATION

**PHARMACOTHERAPEUTIC:** Monoclonal antibody. **CLINICAL:** Immune modulator, antirheumatic, tumor necrosis factor (TNF) blocking agent.

## USES

**Simponi:** Used alone or in combination with methotrexate for the treatment of adult pts with active psoriatic arthritis. Used in combination with methotrexate for the treatment of adult pts with moderately to severely active rheumatoid arthritis. Used alone for the treatment of adult pts with active ankylosing spondylitis. Treatment of moderate to severe ulcerative colitis.
**Simponi Aria:** Used in combination with methotrexate for treatment of adult pts with moderately to severely active rheumatoid arthritis.

## PRECAUTIONS

**Contraindications:** Hypersensitivity to golimumab. **Cautions:** Elderly, concomitant immunosuppressants, comorbid conditions predisposing to infections (e.g., diabetes). Do not start during an active infection. Residence or travel from areas of endemic mycosis; tuberculosis, underlying hematologic disorders, preexisting or recent-onset demyelinating disorders (e.g., multiple sclerosis, polyneuropathy), pts with HF or decreased left ventricular function. Avoid concomitant use with live vaccines, abatacept, or anakinra (increased incidence of serious infections).

## ACTION

Binds specifically to tumor necrosis factor (TNF) alpha, blocking its interaction with cell surface TNF receptors. **Therapeutic Effect:** Alters biologic activity of TNF alpha, reduces inflammation, may alter pathophysiology of rheumatoid arthritis.

## PHARMACOKINETICS

Serum concentration reaches steady state by wk 12. Elimination pathway not specified. **Half-life:** 12–14 days.

## ⧖ LIFESPAN CONSIDERATIONS

**Pregnancy/Lactation:** Unknown if distributed in breast milk. Must either discontinue drug or discontinue breastfeeding. **Children:** Safety and efficacy not established in pts younger than 18 yrs. **Elderly:** May have increased risk of serious infections, malignancy.

## INTERACTIONS

**DRUG: Anakinra, abatacept, rituximab, natalizumab, immunosuppressive therapy** may increase risk of infections. May decrease efficacy of immune response of **vaccines. HERBAL: Echinacea** may decrease effects. **FOOD:** None known. **LAB VALUES:** May increase ALT, AST. May decrease Hgb, leukocytes, neutrophils, platelets.

## AVAILABILITY (Rx)

Injection Solution (Simponi): 50 mg/ 0.5 ml, 100 mg/ml in single-dose prefilled autoinjector or prefilled syringe. Injection Solution (Simponi Aria): 50 mg/ 4 ml per single-use vial (12.5 mg/ml).

## ADMINISTRATION/HANDLING

**Simponi Subcutaneous**

• Remove prefilled syringe or autoinjector from refrigerator. Allow to sit at room temperature for 30 min; do not warm in any other way. • Avoid areas where skin is scarred, tender, bruised, red, scaly, hard. Recommended injection site is front of middle thighs, although lower abdomen 2 in below naval or outer, upper arms are acceptable. • Inject within 5 min after cap has been removed.

**Autoinjector** • Push open end of autoinjector firmly against skin at 90-degree angle. • Do not pull autoinjector away from skin until a first "click" sound is heard and then a second "click" sound (injection is finished and needle is pulled back). This usually takes 3 to 6 sec but may take up to 15 sec for the second "click" to be heard. If autoinjector is pulled away from skin before injection is completed, full dose may not be administered.

**Prefilled Syringe** • Gently pinch skin and hold firmly. Use a quick, dart-like motion to insert needle into pinched skin at a 45-degree angle.

**Storage** • Refrigerate; do not freeze. Do not shake. • Solution appears slightly opalescent, colorless to light yellow. Discard if cloudy or contains particulate.

**Simponi Aria**
◄ALERT► Use in-line 0.22 micron filter.

 **IV**

**Reconstitution** • Calculate dosage and number of vials needed based on pt weight. • Visually inspect for particulate matter. • Dilute in 100 ml 0.9% NaCl. • Prior to mixing, withdraw and discard volume of 0.9% NaCl equal to the volume of patient-dosed solution. • Slowly inject solution into bag and gently mix. • Do not shake.

**Rate of Administration** • Infuse over 30 min using an in-line low-protein–binding 0.22-micron filter.

**Storage** • Refrigerate vials, prefilled syringes • Vial solution should be colorless to light yellow and opalescent. • It is normal for solution to develop fine translucent particles since drug is a protein. • Do not use if opaque particles, discoloration, or other foreign particles present. • May store diluted solution at room temperature up to 4 hrs.

## IV INCOMPATIBILITIES

Do not infuse concomitantly with other drugs.

## INDICATIONS/ROUTES/DOSAGE

**Active Psoriatic Arthritis**

**SQ:** *(Simponi):* **ADULTS, ELDERLY:** 50 mg once monthly. Use alone or in combination with methotrexate or other nonbiologic DMARD.

**Moderate to Severe Active Rheumatoid Arthritis (with methotrexate)**

**SQ:** *(Simponi):* **ADULTS, ELDERLY:** 50 mg once monthly.

**IV Infusion:** *(Simponi Aria):* **ADULTS, ELDERLY:** 2 mg/kg at wk 0 and wk 4. Then decrease frequency to every 8 wks.

**Active Ankylosing Spondylitis**

**SQ:** *(Simponi):* **ADULTS, ELDERLY:** 50 mg once monthly. Use alone or in combination

 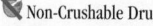
**G**

with methotrexate or other nonbiologic DMARD.

**Ulcerative Colitis**
**SQ:** *(Simponi):* **ADULTS, ELDERLY:** Initially, 200 mg; then 100 mg 2 wks later, and then 100 mg q4wks thereafter.

**Dosage in Renal/Hepatic Impairment**
No dose adjustment.

## SIDE EFFECTS

**Frequent (13%):** Laryngitis, nasopharyngitis, pharyngitis, rhinitis, upper respiratory tract infection. **Occasional (3%–2%):** Bronchitis, hypertension, rash, pyrexia. **Rare (less than 1%):** Dizziness, paresthesia, constipation.

## ADVERSE EFFECTS/ TOXIC REACTIONS

Neutropenia, lymphopenia may increase risk of infection. New-onset psoriasis, exacerbation of preexisting psoriasis have been reported. Serious infections including sepsis, pneumonia, cellulitis, TB, invasive fungal infections reported. May increase risk of lymphoma, melanoma, new malignancies. New onset or exacerbation of CNS demyelinating disorders, including multiple sclerosis, or worsening of HF have occurred. Viral reactivation of herpes zoster, HIV, hepatitis B may occur. Pts who receive TNF blockers have risk of autoantibody formation (immunogenicity). Hypersensitivity reactions including anaphylaxis reported. May induce lupus-like symptoms (butterfly rash, new joint pain, peripheral edema, UV sensitivity).

## NURSING CONSIDERATIONS

### BASELINE ASSESSMENT

Obtain baseline LFT, CBC, vital signs, urine pregnancy. Obtain B-type natriuretic peptide (BNP) level and review echocardiogram for pts with history of HF. Do not initiate therapy if active infection suspected. Evaluate for active TB and test for latent infection prior to and during treatment. Induration of 5 mm or greater with tuberculin skin test should be considered a positive result when assessing for latent TB. Antifungal therapy should be considered for those who reside or travel to regions where mycoses are endemic. Question history of anemia, HF, CNS disorders, hepatic impairment, HIV, malignancies. Assess skin for moles, lesions. Receive full medication history including vitamins, herbal products.

### INTERVENTION/EVALUATION

Monitor CBC, LFT every 4–8 wks, then periodically. Screen pts for TB (night sweats, hemoptysis, weight loss, fever) regardless of baseline tuberculin skin test result. Monitor hepatitis B carriers during treatment and several mos after treatment. If any viral reactivation occurs, interrupt treatment and consider antiviral therapy. Discontinue treatment if acute infection, opportunistic infection, sepsis occur and initiate appropriate antimicrobial therapy. Routinely assess skin for new lesions. Peripheral edema, difficulty breathing, course crackles on lung auscultation, elevated BNP may indicate worsening HF. Monitor for hypersensitivity reactions.

### PATIENT/FAMILY TEACHING

• Therapy may lower immune system response. Do not receive live vaccines. • Report history of HIV, fungal infections, HF, hepatitis B, multiple sclerosis, TB, or close relatives who have active TB. Report travel plans to possible endemic areas. Blood levels, TB screening will be routinely monitored. • Hives, swelling of face, difficulty breathing may indicate allergic reaction. • Do not breastfeed. • Abdominal pain, yellowing of skin or eyes, dark-amber urine, clay-colored stools, fatigue, loss of appetite may indicate liver problems. • Decreased platelet count may increase risk of bleeding. • Swelling of hands or feet, difficulty breathing may indicate HF.

# *goserelin*

**HIGH ALERT**

**goe**-se-**rel**-in
(Zoladex, Zoladex LA ✦)

## ◆CLASSIFICATION

**PHARMACOTHERAPEUTIC:** Gonadotropin-releasing hormone analogue. **CLINICAL:** Antineoplastic.

## USES

Treatment of locally confined prostate cancer. Palliative treatment of advanced carcinoma of prostate as alternative when orchiectomy, estrogen therapy is either not indicated or unacceptable. In combination with an antiestrogen before and during radiation therapy for early stages of prostate cancer. Management of endometriosis. Treatment of advanced breast cancer in premenopausal and perimenopausal women. Endometrial thinning before ablation for dysfunctional uterine bleeding.

## PRECAUTIONS

**Contraindications:** Hypersensitivity to goserelin. Pregnancy (except when used for palliative treatment of advanced breast cancer). **Cautions:** Women of childbearing potential until pregnancy has been excluded. Pts at risk for decreased bone density; diabetes.

## ACTION

Stimulates release of luteinizing hormone (LH) and follicle-stimulating hormone (FSH) from anterior pituitary. **Therapeutic Effect:** In females, reduces ovarian, uterine, mammary gland size; regresses hormone-responsive tumors. In males, decreases testosterone level, reduces growth of abnormal prostate tissue.

## PHARMACOKINETICS

Protein binding: 27%. Metabolized in liver. Excreted in urine. **Half-life:** 4.2 hrs (male); 2.3 hrs (female).

## ⌛ LIFESPAN CONSIDERATIONS

**Pregnancy/Lactation:** Crosses placenta; unknown if distributed in breast milk. **Children:** Safety and efficacy not established. **Elderly:** No age-related precautions noted.

## INTERACTIONS

**DRUG:** None significant. **HERBAL:** None significant. **FOOD:** None known. **LAB VALUES:** May increase serum prostatic acid phosphatase, testosterone, calcium.

## AVAILABILITY (Rx)

**Injection, Solution (Zoladex):** 3.6 mg, 10.8 mg.

## ADMINISTRATION/HANDLING

**Subcutaneous**
• Insert needle subcutaneously into upper arms, outer thigh, or abdomen and inject solution. • Do not inject into areas of active skin disease or injury such as sunburns, rashes, inflammation, skin infections, or active psoriasis. • Rotate injection sites.

## INDICATIONS/ROUTES/DOSAGE

**Prostatic Carcinoma, Advanced**
**SQ: ADULTS OLDER THAN 18 YRS, ELDERLY:** 3.6 mg every 28 days or 10.8 mg q12wks subcutaneously into upper abdominal wall.

**Prostate Carcinoma, Locally Confined**
**SQ: ADULTS, ELDERLY:** (in combination with an antiestrogen and radiotherapy, begin 8 wks prior to radiotherapy): 3.6 mg once. Report in 28 days with 10.8 mg or 3.6 mg q28days for 4 doses.

**Breast Carcinoma, Endometriosis**
**SQ: ADULTS:** 3.6 mg every 28 days subcutaneously into upper abdominal wall.

**Endometrial Thinning**
**SQ: ADULTS:** 3.6 mg subcutaneously into upper abdominal wall as a single dose or in 2 doses 4 wks apart.

G

---

**Endometriosis**
**SQ: ADULTS:** 3.6 mg every 28 days for 6 mos.

**Dosage in Renal/Hepatic Impairment**
No dose adjustment.

## SIDE EFFECTS

**Frequent (60%–13%):** Headache, hot flashes, depression, diaphoresis, sexual dysfunction, impotence, lower urinary tract symptoms. **Occasional (10%–5%):** Pain, lethargy, dizziness, insomnia, anorexia, nausea, rash, upper respiratory tract infection, hirsutism, abdominal pain. **Rare:** Pruritus.

## ADVERSE EFFECTS/ TOXIC REACTIONS

Arrhythmias, HF, hypertension occur rarely. Ureteral obstruction, spinal cord compression has been observed (immediate orchiectomy may be necessary).

## NURSING CONSIDERATIONS

### INTERVENTION/EVALUATION

Monitor pt closely for worsening signs/symptoms of prostatic cancer, esp. during first mo of therapy.

### PATIENT/FAMILY TEACHING

• Use nonhormonal methods of contraception during therapy. • Report suspected pregnancy or regular menstruation persists. • Breakthrough menstrual bleeding may occur if dose is missed.

---

# granisetron

gra-**nis**-e-tron
(Kytril ✤, Sancuso, Sustol)
**Do not confuse granisetron with dolasetron, ondansetron, or palonosetron.**

## ◆CLASSIFICATION

**PHARMACOTHERAPEUTIC:** Serotonin receptor antagonist (5-HT₃). **CLINICAL:** Antiemetic.

## USES

Prevention of nausea/vomiting associated with emetogenic cancer therapy and cancer radiation therapy. **OFF-LABEL:** Prevention, treatment of postop nausea, vomiting. Breakthrough treatment of chemotherapy-associated nausea/vomiting.

## PRECAUTIONS

**Contraindications:** Hypersensitivity to granisetron. **Cautions:** Hypersensitivity to other 5-HT₃ receptor antagonists, congenital QT prolongation, concomitant administration of medications that prolong QT interval, electrolyte abnormalities, cumulative high-dose anthracycline therapy. Following abdominal surgery or in chemotherapy-induced nausea, vomiting (may mask progressive ileus or gastric distention), hepatic disease.

## ACTION

Selectively blocks serotonin stimulation at receptor sites at chemoreceptor trigger zone, vagal nerve terminals. **Therapeutic Effect:** Prevents nausea/vomiting.

## PHARMACOKINETICS

| Route | Onset | Peak | Duration |
|-------|-------|------|----------|
| IV | 1–3 min | N/A | 24 hrs |

Rapidly, widely distributed to tissues. Protein binding: 65%. Metabolized in liver. Eliminated in urine (48%), feces (38%). **Half-life:** 10–12 hrs (increased in elderly).

## ⧗ LIFESPAN CONSIDERATIONS

**Pregnancy/Lactation:** Unknown if distributed in breast milk. **Children:** Safety and efficacy not established in pts younger than 2 yrs. **Elderly:** No age-related precautions noted.

## INTERACTIONS

**DRUG:** None significant. **HERBAL:** None significant. **FOOD:** None known. **LAB VALUES:** May increase serum ALT, AST.

---

## AVAILABILITY (Rx)

**Injection, Extended Release (Sustol):** 10 mg/0.4 ml single dose syringe. **Injection Solution:** 0.1 mg/ml, 1 mg/ml. **Oral Solution:** 2 mg/10 ml. **Tablets:** 1 mg. **Transdermal Patch (Sancuso):** 52-cm² patch containing 34.3 mg granisetron delivering 3.1 mg/24 hrs.

## ADMINISTRATION/HANDLING

 **IV**

**Reconstitution** • May be given undiluted or dilute with 20–50 ml 0.9% NaCl or D₅W. Do not mix with other medications. **Rate of Administration** • May give undiluted as IV push over 30 sec. • For IV piggyback, infuse over 5–10 min depending on volume of diluent used. **Storage** • Appears as a clear, colorless solution. • Store at room temperature. • After dilution, stable for 3 days at room temperature or 7 days if refrigerated. • Inspect for particulates, discoloration.

**PO**

• Give 30 min to 1 hr prior to initiating chemotherapy.

**Subcutaneous**

Administer in skin of back of upper arm, abdomen (at least 1 in away from umbilicus). Avoid areas of compromised skin. Administer over 20–30 sec.

**Transdermal**

• Apply to clean, dry, intact skin on upper outer arm. • Remove immediately from pouch before application. • Do not cut patch.

## ▨ IV INCOMPATIBILITY

Amphotericin B (Fungizone).

## ▨ IV COMPATIBILITIES

Allopurinol (Aloprim), bumetanide (Bumex), calcium gluconate, carboplatin (Paraplatin), cisplatin (Platinol), cyclophosphamide (Cytoxan), cytarabine (Ara-C), dacarbazine (DTIC-Dome), dexamethasone (Decadron), dexmedetomidine (Precedex), diphenhydramine (Benadryl), docetaxel (Taxotere), doxorubicin (Adriamycin), etoposide (VePesid), gemcitabine (Gemzar), magnesium, mitoxantrone (Novantrone), paclitaxel (Taxol), potassium.

## INDICATIONS/ROUTES/DOSAGE

**Prevention of Chemotherapy-Induced Nausea/Vomiting**
**PO: ADULTS, ELDERLY:** 2 mg up to 1 hr before chemotherapy or 1 mg up to 1 hr before, with a second dose 12 hrs later.
**IV: ADULTS, ELDERLY, CHILDREN 2 YRS AND OLDER:** 10 mcg/kg/dose (**maximum:** 1 mg/dose) within 30 min of chemotherapy. **Maximum:** 1 mg.
**Subcutaneous: ADULTS, ELDERLY:** 10 mg at least 30 min before chemotherapy. Do not repeat more frequently than 7 days.
**Transdermal: ADULTS, ELDERLY:** Apply 24–48 hrs prior to chemotherapy. Remove minimum 24 hrs after completion of chemotherapy. May be worn up to 7 days, depending on chemotherapy duration.

**Prevention of Radiation-Induced Nausea/Vomiting**
**PO: ADULTS, ELDERLY:** 2 mg once daily, given 1 hr before radiation therapy.

**Postop Nausea/Vomiting**
**IV: ADULTS, ELDERLY:** 1 mg as a single postop dose. **CHILDREN OLDER THAN 4 YRS:** 20–40 mcg/kg. **Maximum:** 1 mg.

**Dosage in Renal/Hepatic Impairment**
No dose adjustment. **(Sustol) Moderate:** No more frequently than 14 days. **Severe:** Not recommended.

## SIDE EFFECTS

**Frequent (21%–14%):** Headache, constipation, asthenia. **Occasional (8%–6%):** Diarrhea, abdominal pain. **Rare (less than 2%):** Altered taste, fever.

## ADVERSE EFFECTS/ TOXIC REACTIONS

Hypersensitivity reaction, hypertension, hypotension, arrhythmias (sinus bradycardia, atrial fibrillation, AV block, ventricular ectopy), EKG abnormalities occur rarely.

## NURSING CONSIDERATIONS

### BASELINE ASSESSMENT

Assess hydration status. Ensure that granisetron is given within 30 min of starting chemotherapy.

### INTERVENTION/EVALUATION

Monitor for therapeutic effect. Assess for headache. Monitor for dehydration due to recurrent vomiting. Monitor daily pattern of bowel activity, stool consistency.

### PATIENT/FAMILY TEACHING

• Granisetron is effective shortly following administration; prevents nausea/vomiting.
• Transitory taste disorder may occur.

## *guaiFENesin

gwye-**fen**-e-sin
(Mucinex, Robitussin ✦)
**Do not confuse guaifenesin with guanfacine, or Mucinex with Mucomyst.**

### FIXED-COMBINATION(S)

**Mucinex D:** guaifenesin/pseudoephedrine (a sympathomimetic): 600 mg/60 mg, 1,200 mg/120 mg. **Mucinex DM:** guaifenesin/dextromethorphan (a cough suppressant): 600 mg/30 mg, 1,200 mg/60 mg. **Robitussin AC:** guaifenesin/codeine (a narcotic analgesic): 100 mg/10 mg, 75 mg/2.5 mg per 5 ml. **Robitussin DM:** guaifenesin/dextromethorphan (a cough suppressant): 100 mg/10 mg per 5 ml.

### ◆CLASSIFICATION

**PHARMACOTHERAPEUTIC:** Respiratory expectorant. **CLINICAL:** Expectorant.

### USES

Helps loosen phlegm and thin bronchial secretions, making cough more productive.

### PRECAUTIONS

**Contraindications:** Hypersensitivity to guaifenesin. **Cautions:** Avoid OTC use in children younger than 2 yrs.

### ACTION

Stimulates respiratory tract secretions by decreasing adhesiveness, viscosity of mucus. **Therapeutic Effect:** Promotes removal of viscous mucus.

### PHARMACOKINETICS

Well absorbed from GI tract. Metabolized in liver. Excreted in urine. **Half-life:** 1 hr.

### ⌛ LIFESPAN CONSIDERATIONS

**Pregnancy/Lactation:** Unknown if drug crosses placenta or is distributed in breast milk. **Children:** Caution advised in pts younger than 2 yrs with persistent cough. **Elderly:** No age-related precautions noted.

### INTERACTIONS

**DRUG:** None significant. **HERBAL:** None significant. **FOOD:** None known. **LAB VALUES:** None significant.

### AVAILABILITY (OTC)

**Liquid:** 100 mg/5 ml. **Syrup:** 100 mg/5 ml. **Tablets:** 200 mg, 400 mg.

💊 **Tablets, Extended-Release: (Mucinex):** 600 mg, 1,200 mg.

### ADMINISTRATION/HANDLING

**PO**
• Store syrup, liquid, tablets at room temperature. • Give without regard to meals. • Do not break, crush, dissolve, or divide extended-release tablet.

### INDICATIONS/ROUTES/DOSAGE

**Expectorant**
**PO: ADULTS, ELDERLY, CHILDREN OLDER THAN 12 YRS:** 200–400 mg q4h. **Maximum:** 2.4 g/day. **CHILDREN 6–12 YRS:** 100–200 mg q4h. **Maximum:** 1.2 g/day. **CHILDREN 2–5 YRS:** 50–100 mg q4h. **Maximum:** 600 mg/day. **CHILDREN 6 MOS–2 YRS:** 25–50 mg q4h. **Maximum:** 300 mg/day.

PO *(Extended-Release):* **ADULTS, ELDERLY, CHILDREN OLDER THAN 12 YRS:** 600–1,200 mg q12h. **Maximum:** 2.4 g/day.

## SIDE EFFECTS

**Rare:** Dizziness, headache, rash, diarrhea, nausea, vomiting, abdominal pain.

## ADVERSE EFFECTS/ TOXIC REACTIONS

Overdose may produce nausea, vomiting.

## NURSING CONSIDERATIONS

### BASELINE ASSESSMENT

Assess type, severity, frequency of cough.

### INTERVENTION/EVALUATION

Initiate deep breathing, coughing exercises, particularly in pts with pulmonary impairment. Assess for clinical improvement; record onset of relief of cough. Increase fluid intake, environmental humidity to lower viscosity of lung secretions.

### PATIENT/FAMILY TEACHING

• Avoid tasks that require alertness, motor skills until response to drug is established. • Do not take for chronic cough. • Report persistent cough if fever, rash, headache, sore throat is present with cough. • Maintain adequate hydration.

---

# *guanFACINE

gwan-fah-seen
(Intuniv)
**Do not confuse guanfacine with guaifenesin or guanidine.**

## ◆CLASSIFICATION

**PHARMACOTHERAPEUTIC:** Alpha$_{2A}$-adrenergic agonist. **CLINICAL:** Psychotherapeutic agent.

## USES

Treatment of attention-deficit/hyperactivity disorder (ADHD). **OFF-LABEL:** Tic disorder, aggression, Tourette's syndrome.

## PRECAUTIONS

**Contraindications:** Hypersensitivity to guanfacine. **Cautions:** Renal/hepatic impairment.

## ACTION

Interacts with alpha$_{2A}$-adrenergic receptors in prefrontal cortex of brain. Reduces sympathetic outflow. Behaviors (inattention, hyperactivity, impulsiveness) related to ADHD may be controlled in this part of the brain. **Therapeutic Effect:** Improves symptoms of ADHD.

## PHARMACOKINETICS

Readily absorbed from GI tract. Protein binding: 70%. Metabolized in liver. Excreted in urine. **Half-life:** 14–22 hrs.

## ⌛ LIFESPAN CONSIDERATIONS

**Pregnancy/Lactation:** Unknown if distributed in breast milk. **Children:** Safety and efficacy not established in pts younger than 6 yrs. Efficacy beyond 9 wks and safety beyond 2 yrs of treatment not established for children and adolescents older than 6 yrs. **Elderly:** Safety and efficacy not established. Not used in this pt population.

## INTERACTIONS

**DRUG: CYP3A4 inhibitors (e.g., atazanavir, clarithromycin, ketoconazole, saquinavir)** may increase risk of hypotension, bradycardia, sedation. **Rifampin** may decrease concentration. May increase **valproic acid** concentration. Increased risk of cardiovascular effects with **antihypertensives. Alcohol, antipsychotics, barbiturates (e.g., phenobarbital), benzodiazepines (e.g, lorazepam), sedative/hypnotics (e.g., zolpidem)** may produce additive sedative effects. **HERBAL:** None significant. **FOOD: High-fat meals** may increase concentration. **LAB VALUES:** None significant.

## AVAILABILITY (Rx)

💊 **Tablets:** 1 mg, 2 mg. **Tablets, Extended-Release:** 1 mg, 2 mg, 3 mg, 4 mg.

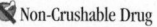

## ADMINISTRATION/HANDLING

### PO

• Do not give with high-fat meal. • Do not break, crush, dissolve or divide extended-release tablets.

## INDICATIONS/ROUTES/DOSAGE

◄ALERT► Dosing should be considered on a mg/kg basis.

### ADHD

**PO: CHILDREN 6 YRS AND OLDER, (IMMEDIATE-RELEASE) GREATER THAN 45 KG:** Initially, 1 mg once daily at bedtime. May increase by 1 mg/day q3–4 days. **Maximum:** 4 mg/day. **45 KG OR LESS:** Initially, 0.5 mg once daily at bedtime. May increase by 0.5 mg/day q3–4 days. **Maximum:** 27–40.5 kg: 2 mg/day; 40.6–45 kg: 3 mg/day. **(EXTENDED-RELEASE):** Begin at dose of 1 mg/day and adjust in increments of no more than 1 mg/wk until clinical response and tolerability are observed. Maintain dose within range of 1–4 mg once daily. If switching from immediate-release guanfacine, discontinue that treatment and titrate with extended-release guanfacine. When discontinuing, taper dose in decrements of no more than 1 mg every 3–7 days.

**Dosage in Renal/Hepatic Impairment**
Use caution.

## SIDE EFFECTS

**Frequent (38%–10%):** Lethargy, headache, fatigue, upper abdominal pain. **Occasional (6%–3%):** Nausea, lethargy, dizziness, irritability, hypotension or decreased B/P, decreased appetite, dry mouth, constipation. **Rare (2%–1%):** Dyspepsia, asthenia increased B/P, increased weight, orthostatic hypotension, increased urinary frequency.

## ADVERSE EFFECTS/ TOXIC REACTIONS

Abrupt discontinuation may produce infrequent, transient elevations in B/P above original baseline (taper dose in decrements of no more than 1 mg every 3–7 days). Abrupt withdrawal following prolonged administration of high dosage may produce extreme fatigue (may last for wks). Prolonged administration to children may produce suppression of weight and/or height patterns. AV block, bradycardia, arrhythmias occur rarely.

## NURSING CONSIDERATIONS

### BASELINE ASSESSMENT

Obtain baseline vital signs, serum chemistries. Measure pulse, B/P prior to initiation of therapy, following dose increases, and periodically during therapy.

### INTERVENTION/EVALUATION

Assist with ambulation if sedation, dizziness, fatigue, lethargy occur. Be alert to mood changes. Assess for nausea, headache. Monitor B/P, serum chemistries, particularly renal/hepatic function for change from baseline. Monitor daily pattern of bowel activity, stool consistency.

### PATIENT/FAMILY TEACHING

• Avoid tasks that require alertness, motor skills until response to drug is established. • Avoid alcohol. • Dry mouth may be relieved with sugarless gum, sips of water. • Advise pts to avoid becoming dehydrated, overheated. • Do not substitute for immediate-release guanfacine tablets. • Swallow extended-release tablets whole; do not chew, crush, dissolve, or divide. • Do not take with high-fat meal.

# haloperidol

hal-o-**per**-i-dol
(Apo-Haloperidol ✦, Haldol, Haldol Decanoate, Novo-Peridol ✦)

■ **BLACK BOX ALERT** ■ Increased risk of mortality in elderly pts with dementia-related psychosis with use of injections.
**Do not confuse Haldol with Halcion or Stadol.**

## ◆CLASSIFICATION

**PHARMACOTHERAPEUTIC:** Butyrophenone antipsychotic. **CLINICAL:** Antipsychotic, antiemetic, antidyskinetic.

## USES

Treatment of schizophrenia, Tourette's disorder (controls tics and vocal utterances), severe behavioral problems in children with combative explosive hyperexcitability without immediate provocation. Management of psychotic disorder, short-term treatment of hyperactive children. **OFF-LABEL:** Treatment of nonschizophrenic psychosis, alcohol dependence, psychosis/agitation related to Alzheimer's dementia, emergency sedation of severely agitated/psychotic pts.

## PRECAUTIONS

**Contraindications:** Hypersensitivity to haloperidol, CNS depression, coma, myelosuppression, Parkinson's disease, severe cardiac/hepatic disease. **Cautions:** Renal/hepatic impairment, cardiovascular disease, history of seizures, prolonged QT syndrome, medications that prolong QT interval, hypothyroidism, thyrotoxicosis, electrolyte imbalance (e.g., hypokalemia, hypomagnesemia), EEG abnormalities, narrow–angle glaucoma, elderly, pts at risk for pneumonia, decreased GI motility, urinary retention, BPH, visual disturbances. Pts at risk for orthostatic hypotension (e.g., cerebrovascular disease).

## ACTION

Competitively blocks postsynaptic dopamine receptors in brain. **Therapeutic Effect:** Produces tranquilizing effect. Strong extrapyramidal, antiemetic effects; weak anticholinergic, sedative effects.

## PHARMACOKINETICS

Readily absorbed from GI tract. Protein binding: 92%. Metabolized in liver. Excreted in urine. Not removed by hemodialysis. **Half-life:** 20 hrs.

## ⌛ LIFESPAN CONSIDERATIONS

**Pregnancy/Lactation:** Crosses placenta. Distributed in breast milk. **Children:** More susceptible to dystonias; not recommended in pts younger than 3 yrs. **Elderly:** More susceptible to orthostatic hypotension, anticholinergic effects, sedation; increased risk for extrapyramidal effects. Decreased dosage recommended.

## INTERACTIONS

**DRUG: Alcohol, other CNS depressants (e.g., diphenhydramine, gabapentin, lorazepam, morphine)** may increase CNS depression. **CYP3A4 inducers (e.g., carbamazepine)** may decrease concentration. **Medications prolonging QT interval (e.g., amiodarone, ciprofloxacin, ondansetron)** may increase risk of QT prolongation. **Medications producing extrapyramidal symptoms (EPS) (e.g., diphenhydramine, benztropine)** may increase EPS. **HERBAL: Gotu kola, kava kava, St. John's wort, valerian** may increase CNS depression. **FOOD:** None known. **LAB VALUES:** None significant. **Therapeutic serum level:** 0.2–1 mcg/ml; **toxic serum level:** Greater than 1 mcg/ml.

## AVAILABILITY (Rx)

**Injection, Oil (Decanoate [Haldol Decanoate]):** 50 mg/ml, 100 mg/ml. **Injection, Solution (Lactate [Haldol]):** 5 mg/ml. **Oral Concentrate:** 2 mg/ml. **Tablets (Haldol):** 0.5 mg, 1 mg, 2 mg, 5 mg, 10 mg, 20 mg.

H

## ADMINISTRATION/HANDLING

**IV**

**◄ALERT►** Only haloperidol lactate is given IV.

**Reconstitution** • May give undiluted. • May add to 50–100 ml of $D_5W$.

**Rate of Administration** • Give IV push at rate of 5 mg/min. • Infuse IV piggyback over 30 min. • For IV infusion, up to 25 mg/hr has been used (titrated to pt response).

**Storage** • Discard if precipitate forms, discoloration occurs. • Store at room temperature; do not freeze. • Protect from light.

**IM**

**Parenteral Administration** • Pt should remain recumbent for 30–60 min to minimize hypotensive effect. • Prepare Decanoate IM injection using 21-gauge needle. • Do not exceed maximum volume of 3 ml per IM injection site. • Inject slow, deep IM into upper outer quadrant of gluteus maximus.

**PO**

• Give without regard to meals. • Scored tablets may be crushed. • Dilute oral concentrate with water or juice. • Avoid skin contact with oral concentrate; may cause contact dermatitis.

### ▓ IV INCOMPATIBILITIES

Allopurinol (Aloprim), amphotericin B complex (Abelcet, AmBisome, Amphotec), cefepime (Maxipime), fluconazole (Diflucan), foscarnet (Foscavir), heparin, nitroprusside (Nipride), piperacillin/tazobactam (Zosyn).

### ▓ IV COMPATIBILITIES

Dobutamine (Dobutrex), dopamine (Intropin), fentanyl (Sublimaze), hydromorphone (Dilaudid), lidocaine, lorazepam (Ativan), midazolam (Versed), morphine, nitroglycerin, norepinephrine (Levophed), propofol (Diprivan).

## INDICATIONS/ROUTES/DOSAGE

**Usual Dosage**

**IM _(Lactate):_ ADULTS, ELDERLY:** 2–5 mg q4–8h as needed. **CHILDREN 6–12 YRS:** 1–3 mg/dose q4–8h as needed. **Maximum:** 0.15 mg/kg/day. Change to PO as soon as possible. _(Decanoate):_ **ADULTS, ELDERLY:** Initially, 10–20 times stabilized oral dose. **Maximum:** 100 mg. **Maintenance:** 10–15 times daily oral dose or 50–200 mg q4wks.

**PO: ADULTS:** 0.5–5 mg 2–3 times/day. **Usual dose:** 5–20 mg/day. **Maximum:** 100 mg/day. **ELDERLY:** 0.2–2 mg/day. **Usual dose:** 5–20 mg/day. **Maximum:** 100 mg/day. **CHILDREN WEIGHING MORE THAN 40 KG, ADOLESCENTS:** 0.5–15 mg/day in 2–3 divided doses. May increase at no less than 5–7 days. **Maximum:** 15 mg/day. **CHILDREN 3–12 YRS (15–40 KG):** 0.25–0.5 mg/day. May increase by 0.25–0.5 mg q5–7days. Range: 0.05–0.15 mg/kg/day in 2–3 divided doses. **Maximum:** 15 mg/day.

**Tourette's Disorder**

**PO: CHILDREN 3–12 YRS:** 0.05–0.075 mg/kg/day in 2–3 divided doses.

**Dosage in Renal/Hepatic Impairment**

No dose adjustment.

## SIDE EFFECTS

**Frequent:** Blurred vision, constipation, orthostatic hypotension, dry mouth, swelling or soreness of female breasts, peripheral edema. **Occasional:** Allergic reaction, difficulty urinating, decreased thirst, dizziness, diminished sexual function, drowsiness, nausea, vomiting, photosensitivity, lethargy.

## ADVERSE EFFECTS/ TOXIC REACTIONS

Extrapyramidal symptoms (EPS) appear to be dose related and typically occur in first few days of therapy. Marked drowsiness/lethargy, excessive salivation, fixed stare may be mild to severe in intensity. Less frequently noted are severe akathisia (motor restlessness), acute dystonias: torticollis (neck muscle spasm), opisthotonos (rigidity of back muscles), oculogyric crisis (rolling back of eyes). Tardive dyskinesia (tongue protrusion, puffing of cheeks, chewing/puckering of the mouth) may occur during long-term therapy or after drug discontinuance and may be irreversible. Elderly female pts have greater risk of developing this reaction.

## NURSING CONSIDERATIONS

### BASELINE ASSESSMENT

Assess behavior, appearance, emotional status, response to environment, speech pattern, thought content. Assess LOC. Screen for co-morbidities as listed in Precautions (esp. seizure disorder, long QT syndrome).

### INTERVENTION/EVALUATION

Monitor B/P, heart rate/rhythm. Supervise suicidal-risk pt closely during early therapy (as depression lessens, energy level improves, increasing suicide potential). Monitor for rigidity, tremor, mask-like facial expression, fine tongue movement. Assess for therapeutic response (interest in surroundings, improvement in self-care, increased ability to concentrate, relaxed facial expression). Monitor EKG and QT interval. **Therapeutic serum level:** 0.2–1 mcg/ml; **toxic serum level:** greater than 1 mcg/ml.

### PATIENT/FAMILY TEACHING

• Full therapeutic effect may take up to 6 wks. • Do not abruptly withdraw from long-term drug therapy. • Sugarless gum, sips of water may relieve dry mouth. • Drowsiness generally subsides during continued therapy. • Avoid tasks that require alertness, motor skills until response to drug is established. • Avoid alcohol. • Report muscle stiffness. • Avoid exposure to sunlight, overheating, dehydration (increased risk of heatstroke).

# heparin

hep-a-rin
(Hepalean Leo ♦, Hep-Lock)
**Do not confuse heparin with Hepspan.**

## ◆CLASSIFICATION

**PHARMACOTHERAPEUTIC:** Sulfated polysaccharide; blood modifier. **CLINICAL:** Anticoagulant.

## USES

Prophylaxis and treatment of thromboembolic disorders; anticoagulant for extracorporeal and dialysis procedures; maintain patency of IV devices. **OFF-LABEL:** STEMI, non-STEMI, unstable angina, anticoagulant used during percutaneous coronary intervention.

## PRECAUTIONS

**Contraindications:** Hypersensitivity to heparin. Severe thrombocytopenia, uncontrolled active bleeding (unless secondary to disseminated intravascular coagulation [DIC]), history of heparin-induced thrombocytopenia (HIT), heparin-induced thrombocytopenia with thrombosis (HITT), or pts who test positive for HIT antibody. **Cautions:** Allergy to pork. Pts at risk for bleeding (e.g., congenital/acquired bleeding disorders, active GI ulcerative disease, hemophilia, concomitant platelet inhibitors, severe hypertension, menses, recent lumbar puncture or spinal anesthesia; recent major surgery, trauma). Use of preservative-free heparin recommended in neonates, infants, pregnant or nursing mothers.

## ACTION

Interferes with blood coagulation by blocking conversion of prothrombin to thrombin and fibrinogen to fibrin. **Therapeutic Effect:** Prevents further extension of existing thrombi or new clot formation. No effect on existing clots.

## PHARMACOKINETICS

Well absorbed following subcutaneous administration. Protein binding: Very high. Metabolized in liver. Removed from circulation via uptake by reticuloendothelial system. Primarily excreted in urine. Not removed by hemodialysis. **Half-life:** 1–6 hrs.

## ⧗ LIFESPAN CONSIDERATIONS

**Pregnancy/Lactation:** Use with caution, particularly during last trimester, immediate postpartum period (increased risk of maternal hemorrhage). Does not cross placenta. Not distributed in breast milk. **Children:** No age-related precautions noted. Benzyl alcohol preservative may cause gasping syndrome in infants. **Elderly:** More susceptible to hemorrhage. Age-related renal impairment may increase risk of bleeding.

## INTERACTIONS

**DRUG: Other anticoagulants (e.g., dabigatran, warfarin), platelet aggregation inhibitors (e.g., aspirin, clopidogrel), thrombolytics (e.g., tissue plasminogen activator [TPA])** may increase risk of bleeding. **HERBAL: Cat's claw, dong quai, evening primrose, feverfew, garlic, ginkgo, ginseng, horse chestnut, red clover** have additional antiplatelet activity. **FOOD:** None known. **LAB VALUES:** May increase free fatty acids, serum ALT, AST, aPTT. May decrease serum cholesterol.

## AVAILABILITY (Rx)

**Injection Solution:** 10 units/ml (Hep-Lock), 100 units/ml, 1,000 units/ml, 5,000 units/ml, 10,000 units/ml, 20,000 units/ml. **Premix Solution for Infusion:** 25,000 units/250 ml infusion, 25,000 units/500 ml infusion.

## ADMINISTRATION/HANDLING

◄**ALERT►** Do not give by IM injection (pain, hematoma, ulceration, erythema).

 **IV**

◄**ALERT►** Used in full-dose therapy. Intermittent IV dosage produces higher incidence of bleeding abnormalities. Continuous IV route preferred.
**Reconstitution • ** Premix solution requires no reconstitution.
**Rate of Administration • ** Infuse and titrate per protocol using infusion pump.
**Storage • ** Store at room temperature.

**Subcutaneous**
◄**ALERT►** Used in low-dose therapy. • After withdrawal of heparin from vial, change needle before injection (prevents leakage along needle track). • Inject above iliac crest or in abdominal fat layer. Do not inject within 2 inches of umbilicus or any scar tissue. • Withdraw needle rapidly, apply prolonged pressure at injection site. Do not massage or apply heat/cold to injection site. • Rotate injection sites.

## ▦ IV INCOMPATIBILITIES

Amiodarone (Cordarone), amphotericin B complex (Abelcet, AmBisome, Amphotec), ciprofloxacin (Cipro), dacarbazine (DTIC), diazepam (Valium), dobutamine (Dobutrex), doxorubicin (Adriamycin), filgrastim (Neupogen), gentamicin (Garamycin), haloperidol (Haldol), idarubicin (Idamycin), labetalol (Trandate), nicardipine (Cardene), phenytoin (Dilantin), quinidine, tobramycin (Nebcin), vancomycin (Vancocin).

## ▦ IV COMPATIBILITIES

Ampicillin/sulbactam (Unasyn), aztreonam (Azactam), calcium gluconate, cefazolin (Ancef), ceftazidime (Fortaz), ceftriaxone (Rocephin), dexmedetomidine (Precedex), digoxin (Lanoxin), diltiazem (Cardizem), dopamine (Intropin), enalapril (Vasotec), famotidine (Pepcid), fentanyl (Sublimaze), furosemide (Lasix), hydromorphone (Dilaudid), insulin, lidocaine, lorazepam (Ativan), magnesium sulfate, methylprednisolone (Solu-Medrol), midazolam (Versed), milrinone (Primacor), morphine, nitroglycerin, norepinephrine (Levophed), oxytocin (Pitocin), piperacillin/tazobactam (Zosyn), procainamide (Pronestyl), propofol (Diprivan).

## INDICATIONS/ROUTES/DOSAGE

**Line Flushing**
**IV: ADULTS, ELDERLY, CHILDREN:** 100 units q6–8h. **INFANTS WEIGHING LESS THAN 10 KG:** 10 units q6–8h.

**Acute Coronary Syndrome**
**IV Infusion: ADULTS, ELDERLY:** 60 units/kg bolus (**maximum: 4,000 units**), then 12 units/kg/hr (**maximum: 1,000 units/hr**).

**Treatment of DVT/PE**
**IV Infusion: ADULTS, ELDERLY:** 80 units/kg bolus (**maximum: 5,000 units**), then 18 units/kg/hr adjusted according to aPTT.

**Usual Pediatric/Neonatal Dose**
**IV Infusion:** 75 units/kg bolus over 10 min, then initial maintenance dose of 20 units/kg/hr. Adjust to maintain aPTT of 60–85 sec.

**Thromboembolic Prophylaxis**
**SQ: ADULTS, ELDERLY:** 5,000 units q8–12h.

**Dosage in Renal/Hepatic Impairment**
No dose adjustment.

## SIDE EFFECTS

**Occasional:** Pruritus, burning (particularly on soles of feet) caused by vasospastic reaction. **Rare:** Pain, cyanosis of extremity 6–10 days after initial therapy lasting 4–6 hrs, hypersensitivity reaction (chills, fever, pruritus, urticaria, asthma, rhinitis, lacrimation, headache).

## ADVERSE EFFECTS/ TOXIC REACTIONS

Bleeding complications ranging from local ecchymoses to major hemorrhage (cutaneous/GI/genitourinary/intracranial/nasal/oral/pharyngeal/urethral/vaginal bleeding) occur more frequently in high-dose therapy, intermittent IV infusion, women 60 yrs and older. HIT can cause life-threatening thromboembolism such as CVA, MI, DVT, pulmonary embolism, renal artery thrombosis, mesenteric thrombosis. **Antidote:** Protamine sulfate 1–1.5 mg IV for every 100 units heparin subcutaneous within 30 min of overdose, 0.5–0.75 mg for every 100 units heparin subcutaneous if within 30–60 min of overdose, 0.25–0.375 mg for every 100 units heparin subcutaneous if 2 hrs have elapsed since overdose, 25–50 mg if heparin was given by IV infusion.

## NURSING CONSIDERATIONS

**BASELINE ASSESSMENT**

Cross-check dose with co-worker. Determine aPTT before administration and 24 hrs following initiation of therapy, then q24–48hrs for first wk of therapy or until maintenance dose is established. Follow with aPTT determinations 1–2 times wkly for 3–4 wks. In long-term therapy, monitor 1–2 times/mo.

**INTERVENTION/EVALUATION**

Monitor aPTT (therapeutic range at 1.5–2.5 times normal) diligently. Assess CBC, platelet count, ALT, AST. If platelet count decreases more than 50% from baseline, obtain stat HIT antibody test. If HIT antibody positive, discontinue heparin and consider treatment with direct thrombin inhibitor (e.g., argatroban); avoid all heparin products and place heparin allergy on chart. Monitor urine and stool for occult blood. Assess for decrease in B/P, increase in pulse rate, complaint of abdominal/back pain, severe headache (may be evidence of hemorrhage). Question for increase in amount of discharge during menses. Assess peripheral pulses; skin for ecchymosis, petechiae. Check for

H

excessive bleeding from minor cuts, scratches. Assess gums for erythema, gingival bleeding. Assess urine output for hematuria. Avoid IM injections due to potential for hematomas. When converting to warfarin (Coumadin) therapy, monitor PT/INR results (will be 10%–20% higher while heparin is given concurrently).

### PATIENT/FAMILY TEACHING

• Use electric razor, soft toothbrush to prevent bleeding. • Report red or dark urine, black or red stool, coffee-ground vomitus, blood-tinged mucus from cough, signs of stroke, nosebleeds, or increase in menstruation. • Do not use any OTC medication without physician approval (may interfere with platelet aggregation). • Wear or carry identification that notes anticoagulant therapy. • Inform dentist, other physicians of heparin therapy. • Limit alcohol.

# *hydrALAZINE

hye-**dral**-a-zeen
(Apo-Hydralazine ✹, Apresoline ✹, Novo-Hylazin ✹)
**Do not confuse hydralazine with hydroxyzine.**

## FIXED-COMBINATION(S)

**Apresazide:** hydralazine/hydrochlorothiazide (a diuretic): 25 mg/25 mg, 50 mg/50 mg, 100 mg/50 mg. **BiDil:** hydralazine/isosorbide (a nitrate): 37.5 mg/20 mg.

## ◆CLASSIFICATION

**PHARMACOTHERAPEUTIC:** Vasodilator. **CLINICAL:** Antihypertensive.

## USES

Management of moderate to severe hypertension. **OFF-LABEL:** Hypertension secondary to eclampsia, preeclampsia. Treatment of HF with reduced ejection fraction, postoperative hypertension.

## PRECAUTIONS

**Contraindications:** Hypersensitivity to hydralazine. Coronary artery disease, mitral valvular rheumatic heart disease, dissecting aortic aneurysm. **Cautions:** Renal impairment, cerebrovascular disease, positive ANA titer, pulmonary hypertension.

## ACTION

Direct vasodilating effects on arterioles. **Therapeutic Effect:** Decreases B/P, systemic vascular resistance.

## PHARMACOKINETICS

| Route | Onset | Peak | Duration |
|-------|-------|------|----------|
| PO | 20–30 min | N/A | Up to 8 hrs |
| IV | 5–20 min | N/A | 1–4 hrs |

Well absorbed from GI tract. Widely distributed. Protein binding: 85%–90%. Metabolized in liver. Primarily excreted in urine. Not removed by hemodialysis. **Half-life:** 3–7 hrs (increased in renal impairment).

## ⧗ LIFESPAN CONSIDERATIONS

**Pregnancy/Lactation:** Drug crosses placenta. Unknown if distributed in breast milk. Thrombocytopenia, leukopenia, petechial bleeding, hematomas have occurred in newborns (resolved within 1–3 wks). **Children:** No age-related precautions noted. **Elderly:** More sensitive to hypotensive effects. Age-related renal impairment may require dosage adjustment.

## INTERACTIONS

**DRUG: Diuretics (e.g., furosemide, HCTZ), other antihypertensives (e.g., amlodipine, clonidine, lisinopril, valsartan)** may increase hypotensive effect. **HERBAL: Ephedra, ginseng, yohimbe** may worsen hypertension. **Garlic** may increase antihypertensive effect. **FOOD: Any foods** may increase absorption. **LAB VALUES:** May produce positive direct Coombs' test.

## AVAILABILITY (Rx)

**Injection Solution:** 20 mg/ml. **Tablets:** 10 mg, 25 mg, 50 mg, 100 mg.

## ADMINISTRATION/HANDLING

 IV

**Rate of Administration** • May give undiluted. • Administer slowly: maximum rate 5 mg/min (0.2 mg/kg/min for children). **Storage** • Store at room temperature.

**PO**
• Best given with food at regularly spaced meals. • Tablets may be crushed.

## ▦ IV INCOMPATIBILITIES

Ampicillin (Polycillin), furosemide (Lasix).

## ▦ IV COMPATIBILITIES

Dobutamine (Dobutrex), heparin, hydrocortisone (Solu-Cortef), nitroglycerin, potassium chloride.

## INDICATIONS/ROUTES/DOSAGE

**Hypertension**
**PO: ADULTS, ELDERLY:** Initially, 10 mg 4 times/day for first 2–4 days. May increase to 25 mg 4 times/day balance of first wk. May increase by 10–25 mg/dose gradually q2–5 days to 50 mg 4 times/day. Usual range: 25–100 mg in 2–3 divided doses. **Maximum:** 300 mg/day in divided doses. **CHILDREN:** Initially, 0.75–1 mg/kg/day in 2–4 divided doses. May increase over 3–4 wks. **Maximum:** 7.5 mg/kg/day (5 mg/kg/day in infants). **Maximum daily dose:** 200 mg/day in divided doses. **IV, IM: ADULTS, ELDERLY:** Initially, 10–20 mg/dose q4–6h. May increase to 40 mg/dose. **CHILDREN:** Initially, 0.1–0.2 mg/kg/dose (**maximum:** 20 mg) q4–6h, as needed, up to 1.7–3.5 mg/kg/day in 4–6 divided doses.

**Dosage in Renal Impairment**
Dosage interval is based on creatinine clearance.

| Creatinine Clearance | Dosage |
| --- | --- |
| 10–50 ml/min | q8h |
| Less than 10 ml/min | q8–24h |

**Dosage in Hepatic Impairment**
No dose adjustment.

## SIDE EFFECTS

**Occasional:** Headache, anorexia, nausea, vomiting, diarrhea, palpitations, tachycardia, angina pectoris. **Rare:** Constipation, ileus, edema, peripheral neuritis (paresthesia), dizziness, muscle cramps, anxiety, hypersensitivity reactions (rash, urticaria, pruritus, fever, chills, arthralgia), nasal congestion, flushing, conjunctivitis.

## ADVERSE EFFECTS/ TOXIC REACTIONS

High dosage may produce lupus erythematosus–like reaction (fever, facial rash, muscle/joint aches, glomerulonephritis, splenomegaly). Severe orthostatic hypotension, skin flushing, severe headache, myocardial ischemia, cardiac arrhythmias may develop. Profound shock may occur with severe overdosage.

## NURSING CONSIDERATIONS

**BASELINE ASSESSMENT**
Obtain B/P, pulse immediately before each dose, in addition to regular monitoring (be alert to fluctuations).

**INTERVENTION/EVALUATION**
Monitor B/P, pulse, ANA titer. Monitor for headache, palpitations, tachycardia. Assess for peripheral edema of hands, feet.

**PATIENT/FAMILY TEACHING**
• To reduce hypotensive effect, go from lying to standing slowly. • Report muscle/joint aches, fever (lupus-like reaction), flu-like symptoms. • Limit alcohol use.

## *hydroCHLOROthiazide

**hye**-dro-**klor**-oh-**thy**-ah-zide
(Apo-Hydro ✦, Microzide)
**Do not confuse Microzide with Maxzide.**

## FIXED-COMBINATION(S)

**Accuretic:** hydrochlorothiazide/ quinapril (an angiotensin-converting enzyme [ACE] inhibitor): 12.5 mg/

10 mg, 12.5 mg/20 mg, 25 mg/20 mg. **Aldactazide:** hydrochlorothiazide/spironolactone (a potassium-sparing diuretic): 25 mg/25 mg, 50 mg/50 mg. **Aldoril:** hydrochlorothiazide/methyldopa (an antihypertensive): 15 mg/250 mg, 25 mg/250 mg, 30 mg/500 mg, 50 mg/500 mg. **Amturnide:** hydrochlorothiazide/aliskiren (renin inhibitor)/amlodipine (calcium channel blocker): 12.5 mg/150 mg/5 mg, 12.5 mg/300 mg/5 mg, 25 mg/300 mg/5 mg, 12.5 mg/300 mg/10 mg, 25 mg/300 mg/10 mg. **Apresazide:** hydrochlorothiazide/hydralazine (a vasodilator): 25 mg/25 mg, 50 mg/50 mg, 50 mg/100 mg. **Atacand HCT:** hydrochlorothiazide/candesartan (an angiotensin II receptor antagonist): 12.5 mg/16 mg, 12.5 mg/32 mg. **Avalide:** hydrochlorothiazide/irbesartan (an angiotensin II receptor antagonist): 12.5 mg/150 mg, 12.5 mg/300 mg, 25 mg/300 mg. **Benicar HCT:** hydrochlorothiazide/olmesartan (an angiotensin II receptor antagonist): 12.5 mg/20 mg, 12.5 mg/40 mg, 25 mg/40 mg. **Capozide:** hydrochlorothiazide/captopril (an ACE inhibitor): 15 mg/25 mg, 15 mg/50 mg, 25 mg/25 mg, 25 mg/50 mg. **Diovan HCT:** hydrochlorothiazide/valsartan (an angiotensin II receptor antagonist): 12.5 mg/80 mg, 12.5 mg/160 mg. **Dutoprol:** hydrochlorothiazide/metoprolol (a beta blocker): 12.5 mg/25 mg, 12.5 mg/50 mg, 12.5 mg/100 mg. **Dyazide/Maxide:** hydrochlorothiazide/triamterene (a potassium-sparing diuretic): 25 mg/37.5 mg, 25 mg/50 mg, 50 mg/75 mg. **Exforge HCT:** hydrochlorothiazide/amlodipine (a calcium channel blocker)/valsartan (an angiotensin II receptor blocker): 12.5 mg/5 mg/160 mg, 25 mg/5 mg/160 mg, 12.5 mg/10 mg/160 mg, 25 mg/10 mg/160 mg, 25 mg/10 mg/320 mg. **Hyzaar:** hydrochlorothiazide/losartan (an angiotensin II receptor antagonist): 12.5 mg/50 mg, 12.5 mg/100 mg, 25 mg/100 mg. **Inderide:** hydrochlorothiazide/propranolol (a beta blocker): 25 mg/40 mg, 25 mg/80 mg, 50 mg/80 mg, 50 mg/120 mg, 50 mg/160 mg. **Lopressor HCT:** hydrochlorothiazide/metoprolol (a beta blocker): 25 mg/50 mg, 25 mg/100 mg, 50 mg/100 mg. **Lotensin HCT:** hydrochlorothiazide/bepridil (a calcium channel blocker): 6.25 mg/5 mg, 12.5 mg/10 mg, 12.5 mg/20 mg, 25 mg/20 mg. **Micardis HCT:** hydrochlorothiazide/telmisartan (an angiotensin II receptor antagonist): 12.5 mg/40 mg, 12.5 mg/80 mg. **Moduretic:** hydrochlorothiazide/amiloride (a potassium-sparing diuretic): 50 mg/5 mg. **Normozide:** hydrochlorothiazide/labetalol (a beta blocker): 25 mg/100 mg, 25 mg/300 mg. **Prinzide/Zestoretic:** hydrochlorothiazide/lisinopril (an ACE inhibitor): 12.5 mg/10 mg, 12.5 mg/20 mg, 25 mg/20 mg. **Tekturna HCT:** hydrochlorothiazide/aliskiren (a renin inhibitor): 12.5 mg/150 mg, 25 mg/300 mg. **Teveten HCT:** hydrochlorothiazide/eprosartan (an angiotensin II receptor antagonist): 12.5 mg/600 mg, 25 mg/600 mg. **Timolide:** hydrochlorothiazide/timolol (a beta blocker): 25 mg/10 mg. **Tribenzor:** hydrochlorothiazide/olmesartan/amlodipine: 12.5 mg/20 mg/5 mg, 12.5 mg/40 mg/5 mg, 25 mg/40 mg/5 mg, 12.5 mg/40 mg/10 mg, 25 mg/40 mg/10 mg. **Uniretic:** hydrochlorothiazide/moexipril (an ACE inhibitor): 12.5 mg/7.5 mg, 25 mg/15 mg. **Vaseretic:** hydrochlorothiazide/enalapril (an ACE inhibitor): 12.5 mg/5 mg, 25 mg/10 mg. **Ziac:** hydrochlorothiazide/bisoprolol (a beta blocker): 6.25 mg/5 mg, 6.25 mg/10 mg.

## ◆CLASSIFICATION

**PHARMACOTHERAPEUTIC:** Sulfonamide derivative. **CLINICAL:** Thiazide diuretic, antihypertensive.

## USES

Treatment of mild to moderate hypertension, edema in HF, hepatic cirrhosis, renal dysfunction (e.g., nephrotic syndrome). **OFF-LABEL:** Treatment of calcium nephrolithiasis.

## PRECAUTIONS

**Contraindications:** Hypersensitivity to hydrochlorothiazide. Anuria, history of hypersensitivity to sulfonamides or thiazide diuretics. **Cautions:** Severe renal/hepatic impairment, prediabetes or diabetes mellitus, elderly or debilitated, history of gout, moderate to high serum cholesterol, hypercalcemia, hypokalemia.

## ACTION

Inhibits sodium reabsorption in distal renal tubules, causing excretion of sodium, potassium, hydrogen ions, water. **Therapeutic Effect:** Promotes diuresis; reduces B/P.

## PHARMACOKINETICS

| Route | Onset | Peak | Duration |
|---|---|---|---|
| PO (diuretic) | 2 hrs | 4–6 hrs | 6–12 hrs |

Variably absorbed from GI tract. Primarily excreted unchanged in urine. Not removed by hemodialysis. **Half-life:** 5.6–14.8 hrs.

## ▒ LIFESPAN CONSIDERATIONS

**Pregnancy/Lactation:** Crosses placenta. Small amount distributed in breast milk. Breastfeeding not recommended. **Children:** No age-related precautions noted, except jaundiced infants may be at risk for hyperbilirubinemia. **Elderly:** May be more sensitive to hypotensive, electrolyte effects. Age-related renal impairment may require dosage adjustment.

## INTERACTIONS

**DRUG: Cholestyramine, colestipol** may decrease absorption, effects. **Antihypertensives (e.g., amlodipine, clonidine, lisinopril, valsartan)** may increase hypotensive effect. May increase risk of **digoxin** toxicity associated with hydrochlorothiazide-induced hypokalemia. May increase risk of **lithium** toxicity. **HERBAL: Ephedra, ginseng, yohimbe** may diminish effect. **Black cohosh, periwinkle** may increase antihypertensive effect. **FOOD:** None known. **LAB VALUES:** May increase serum glucose, cholesterol, LDL, bilirubin, calcium, creatinine, uric acid, triglycerides. May decrease urinary calcium, serum magnesium, potassium, sodium.

## AVAILABILITY (Rx)

**Capsules (Microzide):** 12.5 mg. **Tablets:** 12.5 mg, 25 mg, 50 mg.

## ADMINISTRATION/HANDLING

**PO**
• May take with or without food. If GI upset occurs, give with food or milk, preferably with breakfast (may prevent nocturia). • Give last dose no later than 6 PM unless instructed otherwise.

## INDICATIONS/ROUTES/DOSAGE

**Edema**
**PO: ADULTS:** 25–100 mg/day in 1–2 divided doses. May give on alternate days or on 3–5 days/wk.

**Hypertension**
**PO: ADULTS:** Initially, 12.5–25 mg once daily. May increase up to 50 mg/day in 1–2 divided doses.

**Usual Elderly Dosage**
**PO:** 12.5–25 mg once daily. Titrate in 12.5-mg increments.

**Usual Pediatric Dosage (Edema/HTN)**
**PO: CHILDREN 2–17 YRS:** 1–2 mg/kg/day. **Maximum:** 50 mg/day. **CHILDREN 6 MOS–2 YRS:** 1–2 mg/kg/day in 1–2 divided doses. **Maximum:** 37.5 mg/day.

H

**CHILDREN YOUNGER THAN 6 MOS:** 1–3 mg/kg/day in 2 divided doses. **Maximum: 37.5 mg/day.**

**Dosage in Renal Impairment**
**CrCl less than 30 ml/min:** Generally not effective. Avoid use with CrCl less than 10 ml/min.

**Dosage in Hepatic Impairment**
Use caution.

## SIDE EFFECTS

**Expected:** Increased urinary frequency, urine volume. **Frequent:** Potassium depletion. **Occasional:** Orthostatic hypotension, headache, GI disturbances, photosensitivity.

## ADVERSE EFFECTS/ TOXIC REACTIONS

Vigorous diuresis may lead to profound water loss/electrolyte depletion, resulting in hypokalemia, hyponatremia, dehydration. Acute hypotensive episodes may occur. Hyperglycemia may occur during prolonged therapy. Pancreatitis, blood dyscrasias, pulmonary edema, allergic pneumonitis, dermatologic reactions occur rarely. Overdose can lead to lethargy, coma without changes in electrolytes or hydration.

## NURSING CONSIDERATIONS

### BASELINE ASSESSMENT

Check vital signs, esp. B/P for hypotension before administration. Assess baseline electrolytes, esp. for hypokalemia. Evaluate skin turgor, mucous membranes for hydration status. Evaluate for peripheral edema. Assess muscle strength, mental status. Note skin temperature, moisture. Obtain baseline weight. Monitor I&O.

### INTERVENTION/EVALUATION

Continue to monitor B/P, vital signs, electrolytes, I&O, daily weight. Note extent of diuresis. Watch for changes from initial assessment (hypokalemia may result in weakness, tremor, muscle cramps, nausea, vomiting, altered mental status, tachycardia; hyponatremia may result in confusion, thirst, cold/clammy skin). Be esp. alert for potassium depletion in pts taking digoxin (cardiac arrhythmias). Potassium supplements are frequently ordered. Check for constipation (may occur with exercise diuresis).

### PATIENT/FAMILY TEACHING

• Expect increased frequency, volume of urination. • To reduce hypotensive effect, go from lying to standing slowly. • Eat foods high in potassium, such as whole grains (cereals), legumes, meat, bananas, apricots, orange juice, potatoes (white, sweet), raisins. • Protect skin from sun, ultraviolet light (photosensitivity may occur).

---

## *HYDROcodone  [TOP 100] [HIGH ALERT]

hye-droe-**koe**-done
(Hycodan ✹, Hysingla ER, Robidone ✹, Zohydro ER)
**Do not confuse Hycodan with Vicodin.**

### FIXED-COMBINATION(S)

**Hycet:** hydrocodone/acetaminophen: 7.5 mg/325 mg per 15 ml. **Hycodan:** hydrocodone/homatropine (an anticholinergic): 5 mg/1.5 mg. **Hycotuss, Vituss in:** hydrocodone/guaifenesin (an expectorant): 5 mg/100 mg. **Norco:** hydrocodone/acetaminophen: 5 mg/325 mg, 7.5 mg/325 mg, 10 mg/325 mg. **Reprexain CIII:** hydrocodone/ibuprofen (an NSAID): 5 mg/200 mg. **Rezira:** hydrocodone/pseudoephedrine (a nasal decongestant): 5 mg/60 mg per 5 ml. **Tussend:** hydrocodone/pseudoephedrine (a sympathomimetic)/guaifenesin (an expectorant): 2.5 mg/30 mg/100 mg per 5 ml. **Vicodin:** hydrocodone/acetaminophen: 5 mg/300 mg. **Vicodin ES:** hydrocodone/acetaminophen: 7.5 mg/300 mg. **Vicodin HP:** hydrocodone/acetaminophen:

---

10 mg/300 mg. **Vicoprofen:** hydrocodone/ibuprofen (an NSAID): 7.5 mg/200 mg. **Xodol:** hydrocodone/acetaminophen: 5 mg/300 mg, 7.5 mg/300 mg, 10 mg/300 mg. **Zutripto:** hydrocodone/chlorpheniramine (an antihistamine)/pseudoephedrine (a nasal decongestant): 5 mg/4 mg/60 mg.

◆**CLASSIFICATION**

**PHARMACOTHERAPEUTIC:** Opioid agonist **(Schedule III). CLINICAL:** Narcotic analgesic, antitussive.

## USES

Relief of moderate to moderately severe pain, nonproductive cough. **Hysingla ER, Zohydro ER:** Around-the-clock management of moderate to severe chronic pain.

## PRECAUTIONS

**Contraindications:** Hypersensitivity to hydrocodone. Significant respiratory depression, acute or severe bronchial asthma or hypercarbia, paralytic ileus. **Cautions:** Adrenal insufficiency, biliary tract disease, pancreatitis, CNS depression/coma, acute alcoholism, hypothyroidism; severe renal, hepatic, or pulmonary impairment; urinary stricture, prostatic hypertrophy, seizures, elderly, debilitated, other CNS depressants, history of substance abuse.

## ACTION

Binds with opioid receptors in CNS. **Therapeutic Effect:** Reduces intensity of incoming pain stimuli from sensory nerve endings, altering pain perception, emotional response to pain; suppresses cough reflex.

## PHARMACOKINETICS

| Route | Onset | Peak | Duration |
|---|---|---|---|
| PO (analgesic) | 10–20 min | 30–60 min | 4–6 hrs |
| PO (antitussive) | N/A | N/A | 4–6 hrs |

Well absorbed from GI tract. Metabolized in liver. Primarily excreted in urine. **Half-life:** 3.8 hrs (increased in elderly).

## ⏳ LIFESPAN CONSIDERATIONS

**Pregnancy/Lactation:** Readily crosses placenta. Distributed in breast milk. May prolong labor if administered in latent phase of first stage of labor or before cervical dilation of 4–5 cm has occurred. Respiratory depression may occur in neonate if mother received opiates during labor. Regular use of opiates during pregnancy may produce withdrawal symptoms (irritability, excessive crying, tremors, hyperactive reflexes, fever, vomiting, diarrhea, yawning, sneezing, seizures) in the neonate. **Children:** Pts younger than 2 yrs may be more susceptible to respiratory depression. **Elderly:** May be more susceptible to respiratory depression, may cause paradoxical excitement. Age-related renal impairment, prostatic hypertrophy or obstruction may increase risk of urinary retention; dosage adjustment recommended.

## INTERACTIONS

**DRUG: Alcohol, other CNS depressants** (e.g., diphenhydramine, gabapentin, haloperidol lorazepam, morphine) may increase CNS or respiratory depression, hypotension. **MAOIs, tricyclic antidepressants** (e.g., amitriptyline, doxepin) may alter effect of hydrocodone. **CYP3A4 inhibitors** (e.g., clarithromycin, ketoconazole) may increase or prolong opioid effects. **HERBAL: Gotu kola, kava kava, St. John's wort, valerian** may increase CNS depression. **FOOD:** None known. **LAB VALUES:** May increase serum amylase, lipase.

## AVAILABILITY (Rx)

🖾 **Capsules, Extended-Release (Zohydro ER):** 10 mg, 15 mg, 20 mg, 30 mg, 40 mg, 50 mg. **Tablets, Extended-Release (Hysingla ER):** 20 mg, 30 mg, 40 mg, 60 mg, 80 mg, 100 mg, 120 mg.

## ADMINISTRATION/HANDLING

### PO
• Give without regard to meals.
• Extended-release capsules/tablets must be swallowed whole. Do not cut, crush, or dissolve.

## INDICATIONS/ROUTES/DOSAGE

### Analgesia (Combination Products)
**PO: ADULTS, CHILDREN WEIGHING 50 KG OR MORE:** Initially, 5–10 mg q3–4h as needed. **ADULTS, CHILDREN WEIGHING LESS THAN 50 KG:** Initially, 0.1–0.2 mg/kg q3–4h as needed. **ELDERLY:** 2.5–5 mg q4–6h.

### Analgesia (Extended-Release)
**PO: ADULTS, ELDERLY: (Zohydro ER):** Initially, 10 mg q12h. May increase by 10 mg q12h q3–7 days to achieve adequate analgesia. **(Hysingla ER):** Initially, 20 mg q24h. May titrate q3-5 days.

### Cough (Combination Products)
**PO: ADULTS, ELDERLY:** 5–10 mg q4–6h as needed. **Maximum:** 15 mg/dose. **CHILDREN:** 0.6 mg/kg/day in 3–4 divided doses at intervals of at least 4 hrs. **Maximum single dose:** 10 mg (children older than 12 yrs), 5 mg (children 2–12 yrs), 1.25 mg (children younger than 2 yrs).

### Dosage in Renal Impairment
No dose adjustment.

### Dosage in Hepatic Impairment
Use caution.

## SIDE EFFECTS

**Frequent:** Lethargy, hypotension, diaphoresis, facial flushing, dizziness, drowsiness. **Occasional:** Urine retention, blurred vision, constipation, dry mouth, headache, nausea, vomiting, difficult/painful urination, euphoria, dysphoria.

## ADVERSE EFFECTS/ TOXIC REACTIONS

Overdose results in respiratory depression, skeletal muscle flaccidity, cold/ clammy skin, cyanosis, extreme drowsiness progressing to seizures, stupor, coma. Tolerance to analgesic effect, physical dependence may occur with repeated use. Prolonged duration of action, cumulative effect may occur in those with hepatic/renal impairment. **Antidote:** Naloxone (see Appendix J).

## NURSING CONSIDERATIONS

### BASELINE ASSESSMENT
Obtain vital signs. If respirations are 12/ min or less (20/min or less in children), withhold medication, contact physician. **Analgesic:** Assess onset, type, location, duration of pain. Effect of medication is reduced if full pain recurs before next dose. **Antitussive:** Assess type, severity, frequency of cough.

### INTERVENTION/EVALUATION
Palpate bladder for urinary retention. Monitor daily pattern of bowel activity, stool consistency. Initiate deep breathing and coughing exercises, particularly in pts with pulmonary impairment. Assess for clinical improvement; record onset of relief of pain, cough. Monitor LOC.

### PATIENT/FAMILY TEACHING
• Go from lying to standing slowly to avoid orthostatic hypotension. • Avoid tasks that require alertness, motor skills until response to drug is established. • Avoid alcohol. • Tolerance or dependence may occur with prolonged use at high dosages. • Report nausea, vomiting, constipation, shortness of breath, difficulty breathing.

# hydrocortisone

hye-droe-**kor**-ti-sone
(Anusol HC, Caldecort, Colocort, Cortaid, Cortef, Cortenema, Cortizone-10, Preparation H Hydrocortisone, Proctocort, Solu-Cortef, Westcort).

**Do not confuse hydrocortisone with hydrochlorothiazide, hydrocodone, or hydroxychloroquine, Cortef with Coreg, or Solu-Cortef with Solu-Medrol.**

## FIXED-COMBINATION(S)

**Cortisporin:** hydrocortisone/neomycin/polymyxin (an anti-infective): 5 mg/10,000 units/5 mg, 10 mg/10,000 units/5 mg. **Liposivir:** hydrocortisone/acyclovir (an antiviral): 1%/5%.

## ◆CLASSIFICATION

**PHARMACOTHERAPEUTIC:** Adrenal corticosteroid. **CLINICAL:** Glucocorticoid.

## USES

**Systemic:** Management of adrenocortical insufficiency, anti-inflammatory, immunosuppressive. **Topical:** Inflammatory dermatoses, adjunctive treatment of ulcerative colitis, atopic dermatitis, inflamed hemorrhoids. **OFF-LABEL:** Management of septic shock. Treatment of thyroid storm.

## PRECAUTIONS

**Contraindications:** Hypersensitivity to hydrocortisone. Fungal, tuberculosis, viral skin lesions; serious infections, IM administration in idiopathic thrombocytopenia purpura. **Cautions:** Thyroid dysfunction, cirrhosis, hypertension, osteoporosis, thromboembolic tendencies or thrombophlebitis, HF, seizure disorders, diabetes, respiratory tuberculosis, untreated systemic infections, renal/hepatic impairment, acute MI, myasthenia gravis, glaucoma, cataracts, increased intraocular pressure, elderly.

## ACTION

Inhibits accumulation of inflammatory cells at inflammation sites, phagocytosis, lysosomal enzyme release, synthesis and/or release of mediators of inflammation. Reverses increased capillary permeability. **Therapeutic Effect:** Prevents/suppresses cell-mediated immune reactions. Decreases/prevents tissue response to inflammatory process.

## PHARMACOKINETICS

| Route | Onset | Peak | Duration |
|-------|-------|------|----------|
| IV | N/A | 4–6 hrs | 8–12 hrs |

Well absorbed after IM administration. Widely distributed. Metabolized in liver. **Half-life:** Plasma, 1.5–2 hrs; biologic, 8–12 hrs.

## ⧖ LIFESPAN CONSIDERATIONS

**Pregnancy/Lactation:** Crosses placenta; distributed in breast milk. May produce cleft palate if used chronically during first trimester. Breastfeeding not recommended. **Children:** Prolonged treatment or high dosages may decrease short-term growth rate, cortisol secretion. **Elderly:** May be more susceptible to developing hypertension or osteoporosis.

## INTERACTIONS

**DRUG:** May decrease effects of **diuretics (e.g., furosemide), insulin, oral hypoglycemics (e.g., glimepiride, metformin, sitagliptin), potassium supplements.** Hepatic enzyme inducers **(e.g., carbamazepine, phenytoin, rifampin)** may decrease effects. **Live virus vaccines** may decrease pt's antibody response to vaccine, increase vaccine side effects, potentiate virus replication. **HERBAL: St. John's wort** may decrease concentration. **Cat's claw, echinacea** may increase immunostimulant properties. **FOOD:** None known. **LAB VALUES:** May increase serum glucose, lipids, sodium. May decrease serum calcium, potassium, thyroxine; WBC count.

## AVAILABILITY (Rx)

**Cream, Rectal (Cortizone-10, Preparation H Hydrocortisone):** 1%, 2.5%. **Cream, Topical:** 0.5%, 1%, 2.5%. **Injection, Powder for Reconstitution (Solu-Cortef):** 100 mg, 250 mg, 500 mg, 1 g. **Ointment, Topical:** 0.5%, 1%, 2.5%. **Suppository (Anusol HC):** 25 mg. **Suspension, Rectal**

H

(**Colocort, Cortenema**): 100 mg/60 ml.
**Tablets (Cortef):** 5 mg, 10 mg, 20 mg.

## ADMINISTRATION/HANDLING

 IV

**Hydrocortisone Sodium Succinate**
**Reconstitution •** Initially, reconstitute vial per manufacturer's instructions. • May further dilute with $D_5W$ or 0.9% NaCl. For IV push, dilute to 50 mg/ml; for intermittent infusion, dilute to 1 mg/ml. **Note:** 100–3,000 mg may be added to 50 ml $D_5W$ or 0.9% NaCl.
**Rate of Administration •** Administer IV push over 3–5 min (over 10 min for doses 500 mg or greater). Give intermittent infusion over 20–30 min.
**Storage •** Store at room temperature. • Once reconstituted, stable for 3 days at room temperature. Once further diluted with 0.9% NaCl or $D_5W$ stability concentration dependent: 1 mg/ml (24 hrs) 2 mg/ml to 60 mg/ml (4 hrs).

**PO**
• Give with food or milk if GI distress occurs.

**Rectal**
• Shake homogeneous suspension well. • Instruct pt to lie on left side with left leg extended, right leg flexed. • Gently insert applicator tip into rectum, pointed slightly toward navel (umbilicus). Slowly instill medication.

**Topical**
• Gently cleanse area before application. • Use occlusive dressings only as ordered. • Apply sparingly; rub into area thoroughly.

## ▓ IV INCOMPATIBILITIES

Ciprofloxacin (Cipro), diazepam (Valium), midazolam (Versed), phenytoin (Dilantin).

## ▓ IV COMPATIBILITIES

Amphotericin, calcium gluconate, cefepime (Maxipime), digoxin (Lanoxin),

diltiazem (Cardizem), diphenhydramine (Benadryl), dopamine (Intropin), insulin, lidocaine, lorazepam (Ativan), magnesium sulfate, morphine, norepinephrine (Levophed), procainamide (Pronestyl), potassium chloride, propofol (Diprivan).

## INDICATIONS/ROUTES/DOSAGE

**Acute Adrenal Insufficiency**
**IV: ADULTS, ELDERLY:** 100 mg IV bolus, then 50–75 mg q6h for 24 hrs, then taper slowly. **CHILDREN:** 1–2 mg/kg IV bolus, then 150–250 mg/day in divided doses q6–8h. **INFANTS:** 1–2 mg/kg/dose IV bolus, then 25–150 mg/day in divided doses q6–8h.

**Anti-Inflammation, Immunosuppression**
**IV, IM: ADULTS, ELDERLY:** 15–240 mg q12h. **CHILDREN:** 1–5 mg/kg/day in divided doses q12h.
**PO: ADULTS, ELDERLY:** 15–240 mg q12h. **CHILDREN:** 2.5–10 mg/kg/day in divided doses q6–8h.

**Physiologic Replacement**
**PO: CHILDREN:** 8–10 mg/m²/day in 3 divided doses.

**Status Asthmaticus**
**IV: ADULTS, ELDERLY, CHILDREN:** 1–2 mg/kg/dose q6h for 24 hrs. **Maintenance:** 0.5–1 mg/kg q6h.

**Adjunctive Treatment of Ulcerative Colitis**
**Rectal (Enema): ADULTS, ELDERLY:** 100 mg at bedtime for 21 nights or until clinical and proctologic remission occurs (may require 2–3 mos of therapy).
**Rectal Foam: ADULTS, ELDERLY:** 1 applicator 1–2 times/day for 2–3 wks, then every second day until therapy ends.
**Usual Topical Dosage: ADULTS, ELDERLY:** Apply sparingly 2–4 times/day.

**Dosage in Renal/Hepatic Impairment**
No dose adjustment.

## SIDE EFFECTS

**Frequent:** Insomnia, heartburn, anxiety, abdominal distention, diaphoresis, acne, mood swings, increased appetite, facial flushing, delayed wound healing, increased susceptibility to infection, diarrhea or constipation. **Occasional:** Headache, edema, change in skin color, frequent urination. **Topical:** Pruritus, redness, irritation. **Rare:** Tachycardia, allergic reaction (rash, hives), psychological changes, hallucinations, depression. **Topical:** Allergic contact dermatitis, purpura. **Systemic:** Absorption more likely with use of occlusive dressings or extensive application in young children.

## ADVERSE EFFECTS/ TOXIC REACTIONS

**Long-term therapy:** Hypocalcemia, hypokalemia, muscle wasting (esp. arms, legs), osteoporosis, spontaneous fractures, amenorrhea, cataracts, glaucoma, peptic ulcer, HF. **Abrupt withdrawal after long-term therapy:** Nausea, fever, headache, sudden severe joint pain, rebound inflammation, fatigue, weakness, lethargy, dizziness, orthostatic hypotension.

## NURSING CONSIDERATIONS

### BASELINE ASSESSMENT

Obtain baseline weight, B/P, serum glucose, cholesterol, electrolytes. Review results of initial tests (tuberculosis [TB] skin test, X-rays, EKG).

### INTERVENTION/EVALUATION

Assess for edema. Be alert to infection (reduced immune response): sore throat, fever, vague symptoms. Monitor daily pattern of bowel activity, stool consistency. Monitor electrolytes, B/P, weight, serum glucose. Monitor for hypocalcemia (muscle twitching, cramps), hypokalemia (weakness, paresthesia [esp. lower extremities], nausea/vomiting, irritability, EKG changes). Assess emotional status, ability to sleep.

### PATIENT/FAMILY TEACHING

• Report fever, sore throat, muscle aches, sudden weight gain, swelling, visual disturbances, behavioral changes. • Do not take aspirin or any other medication without consulting physician. • Limit caffeine, avoid alcohol. • Inform dentist, other physicians of cortisone therapy now or within past 12 mos. • Caution against overusing joints injected for symptomatic relief. • **Topical:** Apply after shower or bath for best absorption. • Do not cover or use occlusive dressings unless ordered by physician; do not use tight diapers, plastic pants, coverings. • Avoid contact with eyes.

---

## *HYDROmorphone HIGH ALERT

H

hye-droe-**mor**-fone
(Apo-Hydromorphone ✦, Dilaudid, Dilaudid HP, Exalgo, Hydromorph Contin ✦)

■ **BLACK BOX ALERT** ■ High abuse potential, respiratory depression risk. Other opioids, alcohol, CNS depressants increase risk of potentially fatal respiratory depression. Highly concentrated (Dilaudid HP, 10 mg/ml) form not to be interchanged with less concentrated (Dilaudid) form; overdose, death may result. Exalgo: For use in opioid-tolerant pts. Do not crush, break, chew, or dissolve. Swallow whole.

**Do not confuse Dilaudid with demerol or Dilantin, or hydromorphone with hydrocodone or morphine.**

## ◆CLASSIFICATION

**PHARMACOTHERAPEUTIC:** Opioid agonist **(Schedule II). CLINICAL:** Narcotic analgesic, antitussive.

## USES

Relief of moderate to severe pain. Extended-release tablet (Exalgo): Around the clock, continuous analgesia for extended period.

## PRECAUTIONS

**Contraindications:** Hypersensitivity to hydromorphone. Acute or severe asthma, severe respiratory depression. **Additional**

---

**Product-Specific Contraindications: Dilaudid liquids and tablets:** Obstetric analgesia. **Dilaudid injection:** Opioid-intolerant pts, pts at risk of developing GI obstruction. **Exalgo:** Opioid-intolerant pts, preexisting GI surgery/diseases causing GI narrowing, GI obstruction, paralytic ileus. **Cautions:** Severe hepatic, renal, respiratory disease; hypothyroidism, adrenal cortical insufficiency, seizures, acute alcoholism, head injury, intracranial lesions, increased intracranial pressure, prostatic hypertrophy, Addison's disease, urethral stricture, pancreatitis, biliary tract disease, cardiovascular disease, morbid obesity, delirium tremens, toxic psychosis, pts with CNS depression or coma, pts with depleted blood volume, obstructive bowel disorder.

## ACTION

Binds to opioid receptors in CNS, reducing intensity of pain stimuli from sensory nerve endings. **Therapeutic Effect:** Alters perception, emotional response to pain; suppresses cough reflex.

## PHARMACOKINETICS

| Route | Onset | Peak | Duration |
|---|---|---|---|
| PO | 30 min | 90–120 min | 4 hrs |
| IV | 10–15 min | 15–30 min | 2–3 hrs |
| IM | 15 min | 30–60 min | 4–5 hrs |
| SQ | 15 min | 30–90 min | 4 hrs |
| Rectal | 15–30 min | N/A | N/A |

Well absorbed from GI tract after IM administration. Widely distributed. Metabolized in liver. Excreted in urine. **Half-life:** 2.6–4 hrs.

## ⏳ LIFESPAN CONSIDERATIONS

**Pregnancy/Lactation:** Readily crosses placenta. Unknown if distributed in breast milk. May prolong labor if administered in latent phase of first stage of labor or before cervical dilation of 4–5 cm has occurred. Respiratory depression may occur in neonate if mother receives opiates during labor. Regular use of opiates during pregnancy may produce withdrawal symptoms in the neonate (irritability, excessive crying, tremors, hyperactive reflexes, fever, vomiting, diarrhea, yawning, sneezing, seizures). **Children:** Pts younger than 2 yrs may be more susceptible to respiratory depression. **Elderly:** May be more susceptible to respiratory depression, may cause paradoxical excitement. Age-related renal impairment, prostatic hypertrophy or obstruction may increase risk of urinary retention; dosage adjustment recommended.

## INTERACTIONS

**DRUG: Alcohol, other CNS depressants (e.g., diphenhydramine, gabapentin, lorazepam, morphine)** may increase CNS, respiratory depression, hypotension. **HERBAL: Gotu kola, kava kava, St. John's wort, valerian** may increase CNS depression. **FOOD:** None known. **LAB VALUES:** May increase serum amylase, lipase.

## AVAILABILITY (Rx)

**Injection, Solution (Dilaudid):** 1 mg/ml, 2 mg/ml, 4 mg/ml, 10 mg/ml. **Liquid, Oral:** 1 mg/ml. **Suppository (Dilaudid):** 3 mg. **Tablets (Dilaudid):** 2 mg, 4 mg, 8 mg.

 **Tablets, Extended-Release (Exalgo):** 8 mg, 12 mg, 16 mg, 32 mg.

## ADMINISTRATION/HANDLING

### 💉 IV

◀**ALERT**▶ High concentration injection (10 mg/ml) should be used only in pts tolerant to opiate agonists, currently receiving high doses of another opiate agonist for severe, chronic pain due to cancer.

**Reconstitution** • May give undiluted. • May further dilute with 5 ml Sterile Water for Injection or 0.9% NaCl.

**Rate of Administration** • Administer IV push very slowly (over 2–3 min). • Rapid IV increases risk of severe adverse reactions (chest wall rigidity, apnea, peripheral circulatory collapse, anaphylactoid effects, cardiac arrest).

**Storage** • Store at room temperature; protect from light. • Slight yellow discoloration of parenteral form does not indicate loss of potency.

**IM, SQ**
• Use short 25- to 30-gauge needle for subcutaneous injection. • Administer slowly; rotate injection sites. • Pts with circulatory impairment experience higher risk of overdosage due to delayed absorption of repeated administration.

**PO**
• Give without regard to meals. • Tablets may be crushed. • Extended-release tablets must be swallowed whole; do not break, crush, dissolve, or divide.

**Rectal**
• Refrigerate suppositories. • Moisten suppository with cold water before inserting well up into rectum.

## 🕸 IV INCOMPATIBILITIES

Amphotericin B complex (Abelcet, AmBisome, Amphotec), cefazolin (Ancef, Kefzol), diazepam (Valium), phenobarbital, phenytoin (Dilantin).

## 🕸 IV COMPATIBILITIES

Dexmedetomidine (Precedex), diltiazem (Cardizem), diphenhydramine (Benadryl), dobutamine (Dobutrex), dopamine (Intropin), fentanyl (Sublimaze), furosemide (Lasix), heparin, lorazepam (Ativan), magnesium sulfate, metoclopramide (Reglan), midazolam (Versed), milrinone (Primacor), morphine, propofol (Diprivan).

## INDICATIONS/ROUTES/DOSAGE

**Analgesia**
**PO: ADULTS, ELDERLY:** *(Immediate-Release):* Initially 2–4 mg q4–6h prn (tablets) or 2.5–10 mg q3–6h prn (liquid). Range: 2–8 mg/dose. **CHILDREN, ADOLESCENTS WEIGHING MORE THAN 50 KG:** 1–2 mg q3–4h. **CHILDREN OLDER THAN 6 MOS AND WEIGHING LESS THAN 50 KG:** 0.03–0.08 mg/kg/dose q3–4h.

*(Extended-Release):* **(For use in opioid-tolerant pts) ADULTS, ELDERLY:** Range: 8–64 mg once daily.
**IV: ADULTS, ELDERLY, CHILDREN WEIGHING MORE THAN 50 KG: (For use in opiate-naive pts)** 1 mg q2–3h (pts with prior opioid exposure may require higher doses.) **CHILDREN WEIGHING 50 KG OR LESS:** 0.03–0.06 mg/kg q4h prn.
**Rectal: ADULTS, ELDERLY:** 3 mg q6–8h.

**Patient-Controlled Analgesia (PCA)**
**IV: ADULTS, ELDERLY:** (Usual concentration: 0.2 mg/ml). Initially, 0.1–0.2 mg. Range: 0.05–0.4 mg. Lockout interval: 6 min. Range: 5–10 min.
**Epidural: ADULTS, ELDERLY:** Bolus dose of 0.4–1 mg; infusion rate: 0.03–0.3 mg/hr; demand dose: 0.02–0.05 mg. Lockout interval: 10–15 min.

**Dosage in Renal/Hepatic Impairment**
Decrease initial dose; use with caution.

## SIDE EFFECTS

**Frequent:** Drowsiness, dizziness, hypotension (including orthostatic hypotension), decreased appetite. **Occasional:** Confusion, diaphoresis, facial flushing, urinary retention, constipation, dry mouth, nausea, vomiting, headache, pain at injection site. **Rare:** Allergic reaction, depression.

## ADVERSE EFFECTS/ TOXIC REACTIONS

Overdose results in respiratory depression, skeletal muscle flaccidity, cold/clammy skin, cyanosis, extreme drowsiness progressing to seizures, stupor, coma. Tolerance to analgesic effect, physical dependence may occur with repeated use. Prolonged duration of action, cumulative effect may occur in those with hepatic/renal impairment. **Antidote:** Naloxone (see Appendix J).

## NURSING CONSIDERATIONS

### BASELINE ASSESSMENT
Obtain vital signs. If respirations are 12/min or less (20/min or less in children),

withhold medication, contact physician. **Analgesic:** Assess onset, type, location, duration of pain. Effect of medication is reduced if full pain recurs before next dose. **Antitussive:** Assess type, severity, frequency of cough.

### INTERVENTION/EVALUATION

Monitor vital signs; assess for pain relief, cough. To prevent pain cycles, instruct pt to request pain medication as soon as discomfort begins. Monitor daily pattern of bowel activity, stool consistency (esp. in long-term use). Initiate deep breathing and coughing exercises, particularly in pts with pulmonary impairment. Assess for clinical improvement; record onset of relief of pain, cough.

### PATIENT/FAMILY TEACHING

• Avoid alcohol. • Avoid tasks that require alertness/motor skills until response to drug is established. • Tolerance or dependence may occur with prolonged use at high dosages. • Change positions slowly to avoid orthostatic hypotension. • Do not chew, crush, dissolve, or divide extended-release tablets.

---

# hydroxychloroquine

hye-drox-ee-**klor**-oh-kwin
(Apo-Hydroxyquine ✤, Plaquenil)
■ **BLACK BOX ALERT** ■ Should be given by physicians familiar with prescribing information before use. **Do not confuse hydroxychloroquine with hydrocortisone or hydroxyzine, or Plaquenil with Platinol.**

### ◆CLASSIFICATION

**PHARMACOTHERAPEUTIC:** Aminoquinoline antimalarial. **CLINICAL:** Antimalarial, antirheumatic.

### USES

Suppression and treatment of acute attacks of malaria. Treatment of systematic lupus erythematosus, rheumatoid arthritis (RA). **OFF-LABEL:** Porphyria, treatment of Q fever.

### PRECAUTIONS

**Contraindications:** Hypersensitivity to hydroxychloroquine. Porphyria, psoriasis, retinal or visual field changes. **Cautions:** Alcoholism, hepatic disease, G6PD deficiency. Concomitant use of hepatotoxic medications. Children are esp. susceptible to hydroxychloroquine fatalities.

### ACTION

Concentrates in parasite acid vesicles, interfering with parasite protein (DNA/RNA) synthesis. Inhibits movement of neutrophils, and chemotaxis of eosinophils. **Therapeutic Effect:** Inhibits parasite growth.

### PHARMACOKINETICS

Variable rate of absorption. Widely distributed in body tissues (eyes, kidneys, liver, lungs). Protein binding: 45%. Partially metabolized in liver. Partially excreted in urine. **Half-life:** 32 days (in plasma), 50 days (in blood).

### ⧗ LIFESPAN CONSIDERATIONS

**Pregnancy/Lactation:** Crosses placenta; distributed in breast milk. **Children:** Long-term therapy not recommended. **Elderly:** No age-related precautions noted.

### INTERACTIONS

**DRUG:** May increase concentration of **dapsone. HERBAL: Echinacea** may decrease concentration. **FOOD:** None known. **LAB VALUES:** None significant.

### AVAILABILITY (Rx)

**Tablets:** 200 mg (155 mg base).

### ADMINISTRATION/HANDLING

**PO**
• Give with food or milk.

---

## INDICATIONS/ROUTES/DOSAGE

**Treatment of Acute Malaria**
**PO:**

| Dose | Times | Adults/Elderly | Children |
|------|-------|---------|----------|
| Initial | Day 1 | 800 mg | 13 mg/kg |
| Second | 6 hrs later | 400 mg | 6.5 mg/kg |
| Third | Day 2 | 400 mg | 6.5 mg/kg |
| Fourth | Day 3 | 400 mg | 6.5 mg/kg |

**Suppression of Malaria**
**PO: ADULTS, ELDERLY:** 400 mg base wkly on same day each wk, beginning 2 wks before entering an endemic area and continuing for 4–6 wks after leaving the area. **CHILDREN:** 6.5 mg/kg/wk, beginning 2 wks before entering an endemic area and continuing for 4–6 wks after leaving the area. If therapy is not begun before exposure, administer a loading dose of 13 mg/kg in 2 equally divided doses 6 hrs apart and continue treatment for 8 wks.

**Rheumatoid Arthritis (RA)**
**PO: ADULTS, ELDERLY:** Initially, 400–600 mg (310–465 mg base) daily, gradually increase to optimum response level. **Maintenance (usually within 4–12 wks):** Decrease dose by 50% and then continue at maintenance dose of 200–400 mg (155–310 mg base) daily. Maximum effect may not be seen for several mos.

**Lupus Erythematosus**
**PO: ADULTS, ELDERLY:** Initially, 400 mg (310 mg base) once or twice daily for several wks or mos. **Maintenance:** 200–400 mg/day (155–310 mg base).

**Dosage in Renal/Hepatic Impairment**
Use caution.

## SIDE EFFECTS

**Frequent:** Transient headache, anorexia, nausea, vomiting. **Occasional:** Visual disturbances, anxiety, fatigue, pruritus (esp. palms, soles, scalp), irritability, personality changes, diarrhea, photosensitivity.

**Rare:** Stomatitis, dermatitis, impaired hearing.

## ADVERSE EFFECTS/TOXIC REACTIONS

Ocular toxicity (esp. retinopathy) may progress even after drug is discontinued. **Prolonged therapy:** Peripheral neuritis, neuromyopathy, hypotension, EKG changes, agranulocytosis, aplastic anemia, thrombocytopenia, seizures, psychosis. **Overdosage:** Headache, vomiting, visual disturbances, drowsiness, seizures, hypokalemia followed by cardiovascular collapse, death.

## NURSING CONSIDERATIONS

### BASELINE ASSESSMENT
Evaluate CBC, LFT vision.

### INTERVENTION/EVALUATION
Monitor CBC, LFT. Observe for muscular weakness. Evaluate for GI distress. Assess skin/buccal mucosa; inquire about pruritus. Report impaired vision/hearing immediately.

### PATIENT/FAMILY TEACHING
• Avoid exposure to direct sunlight. • Avoid alcohol. • Explain need for eye exams q3mos with prolonged therapy. • Immediately report **any** new visual difficulties, muscular weakness, impaired hearing, tinnitus, numbness, tremors, rash, persistent diarrhea, emotional changes.

# hydroxyurea HIGH ALERT

hye-**drox**-ee-yoo-**ree**-ah
(Apo-Hydroxyurea ♣, Droxia, Hydrea)

■ **BLACK BOX ALERT** ■ Must be administered by personnel trained in administration/handling of chemotherapeutic agents or in treatment of sickle cell anemia. Carcinogenic risk; secondary leukemias reported with long-term treatment.
**Do not confuse hydroxyurea with hydroxyzine.**

H

## ◆CLASSIFICATION

**PHARMACOTHERAPEUTIC:** Synthetic urea analogue. **CLINICAL:** Antineoplastic.

## USES

Treatment of melanoma, resistant chronic myelocytic leukemia, recurrent, metastatic, inoperable ovarian carcinoma. Used in combination with radiation therapy for local control of primary squamous cell carcinoma of head/neck, excluding lip. Treatment of sickle cell anemia with at least 3 painful crises in previous 12 mos. **OFF-LABEL:** Treatment of hematologic conditions (e.g., polycythemia vera), cervical cancer, essential thrombocythemia, hyperleukocytosis due to AML, treatment of meningiomas.

## PRECAUTIONS

**Contraindications:** Hypersensitivity to hydroxyurea. **Cautions:** WBC count less than 2,500/mm³ or platelet count less than 100,000/mm³, severe anemia. Previous irradiation therapy, concurrent use with other cytoxic drugs, renal/hepatic impairment, elderly; pts with sickle cell anemia if neutrophils less than 2,000/mm³, platelets less than 80,000/mm³, Hgb less than 4.5 g/dL, or reticulocytes less than 80,000/mm³ when Hgb less than 9 g/dL.

## ACTION

Inhibits DNA synthesis without interfering with RNA synthesis or protein. In sickle cell anemia, increases RBC hemoglobin levels, thereby decreasing concentration of sickled cells; alters adhesion of RBCs to endothelium. **Therapeutic Effect:** Interferes with normal repair process of cancer cells damaged by irradiation.

## PHARMACOKINETICS

Well absorbed from GI tract. Protein binding: 75%–80%. Metabolized in liver. Excreted in urine as urea and unchanged drug. **Half-life:** 3–4 hrs.

## ⧗ LIFESPAN CONSIDERATIONS

**Pregnancy/Lactation:** Crosses placenta; distributed in breast milk. May cause fetal harm. **Children:** Safety and efficacy not established. **Elderly:** More sensitive to hydroxyurea effects; may require lower dosage.

## INTERACTIONS

**DRUG: Bone marrow depressants (e.g., alemtuzumab, methotrexate)** may increase myelosuppression. **Live virus vaccines** may potentiate virus replication, increase vaccine side effects, decrease the pt's antibody response to vaccine. **HERBAL: Echinacea** may decrease effect. **FOOD:** None known. **LAB VALUES:** May increase serum BUN, creatinine, uric acid.

## AVAILABILITY (Rx)

**Capsules:** 200 mg (Droxia), 300 mg (Droxia), 400 mg (Droxia), 500 mg (Hydrea).

## ADMINISTRATION/HANDLING

Do not open capsules.

## INDICATIONS/ROUTES/DOSAGE

◀**ALERT**▶ Antineoplastic therapy interrupted when platelet count less than 100,000/mm³ or WBC count less than 2,500/mm³. Resume when counts return to normal.

Sickle cell anemia therapy interrupted when neutrophils less than 2,000/mm³, platelets less than 80,000/mm³, Hgb less than 4.5 g/dL, or reticulocytes less than 80,000/mm³ with Hgb less than 9 g/dL. Reduce dose by 2.5 mg/kg/day following recovery.

**Antineoplastic Uses**
**PO: ADULTS, ELDERLY:** 15 mg/kg/day. Adjust dose based on tumor type, disease state, response, pt risk factors. May give alone or in combination with other agents.

**Sickle Cell Anemia**
**PO: ADULTS, ELDERLY:** Initially, 15 mg/kg once daily. May increase by 5 mg/kg/day

every 12 wks. **Maximum:** 35 mg/kg/day. **CHILDREN 6 MOS AND OLDER:** 20 mg/kg/dose once daily; increase by 5 mg/kg/day q8wk until mild myelosuppression is achieved. **Maximum:** 35 mg/kg/day.

**Dosage in Renal Impairment**
Reduce dose to 7.5 mg/kg/day for CrCl 60 ml/min or less.

**Dosage in Hepatic Impairment**
No dose adjustment.

## SIDE EFFECTS

**Frequent:** Nausea, vomiting, anorexia, constipation or diarrhea. **Occasional:** Mild, reversible rash; facial flushing, pruritus, fever, chills, malaise. **Rare:** Alopecia, headache, drowsiness, dizziness, disorientation.

## ADVERSE EFFECTS/ TOXIC REACTIONS

Myelosuppression manifested as hematologic toxicity (leukopenia and, to a lesser extent, thrombocytopenia, anemia).

## NURSING CONSIDERATIONS

### BASELINE ASSESSMENT

Obtain bone marrow studies, renal function, LFT before therapy begins, periodically thereafter. Obtain Hgb, WBC, platelet count, serum uric acid at baseline and wkly during therapy. Pts with marked renal impairment may develop visual or auditory hallucinations, marked hematologic toxicity.

### INTERVENTION/EVALUATION

Monitor daily pattern of bowel activity, stool consistency. Monitor for hematologic toxicity (fever, sore throat, signs of local infection, unusual bleeding/bruising at any site), symptoms of anemia (excessive fatigue, weakness). Assess skin for rash, erythema. Monitor CBC with differential, renal/hepatic function, uric acid.

### PATIENT/FAMILY TEACHING

• Promptly report fever, sore throat, signs of local infection, unusual bleeding/bruising at any site.

# *hydrOXYzine

hye-**drox**-ee-zeen
(Apo-Hydroxyzine ✸, Atarax ✸, Novo-Hydroxyzin ✸, Vistaril)
**Do not confuse hydroxyzine with hydralazine or hydroxyurea, or Vistaril with Restoril, Versed, or Zestril.**

## ◆CLASSIFICATION

**PHARMACOTHERAPEUTIC:** Piperazine derivative. **CLINICAL:** Antihistamine, antianxiety, antispasmodic, antiemetic, antipruritic.

## USES

Antiemetic, treatment of anxiety/agitation, antipruritic.

## PRECAUTIONS

**Contraindications:** Hypersensitivity to hydroxyzine. Early pregnancy; subcutaneous, intravenous administration. **Cautions:** Narrow-angle glaucoma, prostatic hypertrophy, bladder neck obstruction, asthma, COPD, elderly.

## ACTION

Competes with histamine for receptor sites in GI tract, blood vessels, respiratory tract. **Therapeutic Effect:** Produces anxiolytic, anticholinergic, antihistaminic, analgesic effects; relaxes skeletal muscle; controls nausea, vomiting.

## PHARMACOKINETICS

| Route | Onset | Peak | Duration |
|-------|----------|------|----------|
| PO | 15–30 min | N/A | 4–6 hrs |

Well absorbed from GI tract and after parenteral administration. Metabolized in liver to active metabolite cetirizine. Primarily excreted in urine. Not removed by hemodialysis. **Half-life:** 3–7 hrs (increased in elderly, hepatic impairment). (Cetirizine half-life: 8–20 hrs.)

---

*"Tall Man" lettering  ✦ Canadian trade name  ⬛ Non-Crushable Drug  ⬛ High Alert drug

H

## ⧗ LIFESPAN CONSIDERATIONS

**Pregnancy/Lactation:** Unknown if drug crosses placenta or is distributed in breast milk. **Children:** Not recommended in newborns or premature infants (increased risk of anticholinergic effects). Paradoxical excitement may occur. **Elderly:** Increased risk of dizziness, sedation, confusion. Hypotension, hyperexcitability may occur.

## INTERACTIONS

**DRUG: Alcohol, other CNS depressants (e.g., diphenhydramine, gabapentin, lorazepam, morphine)** may increase CNS depressant effects. **HERBAL: Gotu kola, kava kava, St. John's wort, valerian** may increase CNS depression. **FOOD:** None known. **LAB VALUES:** May cause false-positive urine 17-hydroxycorticosteroid determinations.

## AVAILABILITY (Rx)

**Oral Solution:** 10 mg/5 ml. **Syrup:** 10 mg/5 ml. **Tablets:** 10 mg, 25 mg, 50 mg. 🖋 **Capsules:** 25 mg, 50 mg, 100 mg.

## ADMINISTRATION/HANDLING

**PO**
- May give without regard to food.
- Shake oral suspension well.
- Scored tablets may be crushed; do not break, crush, or open capsule.

## INDICATIONS/ROUTES/DOSAGE

**Anxiety**
**PO: ADULTS, ELDERLY:** 50–100 mg 4 times/day or 37.5–75 mg/day in divided doses.

**Pruritus**
**PO: ADULTS, ELDERLY:** 25 mg 3–4 times/day. **CHILDREN 6 YRS AND OLDER:** 50–100 mg/day in divided doses. **CHILDREN YOUNGER THAN 6 YRS:** 50 mg/day in divided doses.

**Dosage in Renal/Hepatic Impairment**
No dose adjustment. Change dosing interval to q24h in pts with primary biliary cirrhosis.

## SIDE EFFECTS

Side effects are generally mild, transient. **Frequent:** Drowsiness, dry mouth, marked discomfort with IM injection. **Occasional:** Dizziness, ataxia, asthenia, slurred speech, headache, agitation, increased anxiety. **Rare:** Paradoxical reactions (hyperactivity, anxiety in children; excitement, restlessness in elderly or debilitated pts) generally noted during first 2 wks of therapy, particularly in presence of uncontrolled pain.

## ADVERSE EFFECTS/TOXIC REACTIONS

Hypersensitivity reaction (wheezing, dyspnea, chest tightness) may occur.

## NURSING CONSIDERATIONS

### BASELINE ASSESSMENT

**Anxiety:** Offer emotional support. Assess motor responses (agitation, trembling, tension), autonomic responses (cold/clammy hands, diaphoresis). **Antiemetic:** Assess for dehydration (poor skin turgor, dry mucous membranes, longitudinal furrows in tongue).

### INTERVENTION/EVALUATION

For pts on long-term therapy, CBC, BMP, LFT should be performed periodically. Monitor lung sounds for signs of hypersensitivity reaction. Monitor serum electrolytes in pts with severe vomiting. Assess for paradoxical reaction, particularly during early therapy. Assist with ambulation if drowsiness, light-headedness occur.

### PATIENT/FAMILY TEACHING

- Marked discomfort may occur with IM injection. • Sugarless gum, sips of water may relieve dry mouth. • Drowsiness usually diminishes with continued therapy. • Avoid tasks that require alertness, motor skills until response to drug is established.

---

# hyoscyamine

hye-oh-**sye**-a-meen
(Anaspaz, Hyosyne, Levbid, Levsin,
Levsin S/L, Nu-Lev, Symax SL, Symax SR)
**Do not confuse Anaspaz with
Anaprox, or Levbid with
Lithobid or Lopid.**

## FIXED COMBINATIONS

**Donnatal:** hyoscyamine/atropine (anticholinergic)/phenobarbital (sedative)/
scopolamine (anticholinergic): 0.1037
mg/0.0194 mg/16.2 mg/0.0065 mg.

## ◆CLASSIFICATION

**PHARMACOTHERAPEUTIC:** Anticholinergic. **CLINICAL:** Antimuscarinic,
antispasmodic.

## USES

Adjunctive therapy for relief of biliary/renal
colic; control of acute episodes of gastric
secretion, hypermotility in spastic colitis,
pylorospasm, and abdominal cramps; relieve symptoms of infant colic; control hypermotility in spastic bladder and cystitis;
adjunctive therapy in treatment of neurogenic bladder.

## PRECAUTIONS

**Contraindications:** Hypersensitivity   to
hyoscyamine. GI/GU obstruction, myasthenia gravis, narrow-angle glaucoma,
paralytic ileus, severe ulcerative colitis.
**Cautions:** Hyperthyroidism, HF, cardiac
arrhythmias, prostatic hypertrophy, neuropathy, chronic lung disease, biliary
tract disease, children with spastic
paralysis.

## ACTION

Inhibits action of acetylcholine at postganglionic (muscarinic) receptor sites. **Therapeutic Effect:** Decreases secretions
(bronchial, salivary, sweat gland, gastric
juices). Reduces motility of GI, urinary
tracts.

## PHARMACOKINETICS

| Route | Onset | Peak | Duration |
|---|---|---|---|
| PO | 15–30 min | — | 4–6 hrs |

Well absorbed following PO administration. Protein binding: 50%. Metabolized in liver. Excreted in urine. Removed by hemodialysis. **Half-life:**
3.5 hrs (immediate-release); 7 hrs
(sustained-release).

## ⌛ LIFESPAN CONSIDERATIONS

**Pregnancy/Lactation:** Crosses   placenta; distributed in breast milk. **Children:** Safety and efficacy not established.
**Elderly:** No   age-related   precautions
noted.

## INTERACTIONS

**DRUG: Antacids** may decrease absorption. **Other   anticholinergics   (e.g.,
atropine,   glycopyrrolate)** may
increase effects. **HERBAL:** None significant. **FOOD:** None known. **LAB VALUES:** None significant.

## AVAILABILITY (Rx)

**Capsules,   Timed-Release:** 0.375   mg.
**Elixir (Hyosyne, Levsin):** 0.125 mg/5 ml.
**Injection, Solution:** 0.5   mg/ml. **Solution, Oral Drops:** 0.125 mg/ml. **Tablets:**
0.125   mg. **Tablets,   Orally Disintegrating:** 0.125   mg. **Tablets,   Sublingual:**
0.125 mg.

🔪 **Tablets, Extended-Release:** 0.375 mg.

## ADMINISTRATION/HANDLING

**PO**
• Give   before   meals. • Immediaterelease tablets may be crushed, chewed.
• Extended-release tablet should be administered whole. • Allow orally disintegrating tablet placed on tongue to dissolve before swallowing; may give with
or without water. • Sublingual: Place
under tongue.

**Parenteral**
• May give undiluted.

---

**H**

## INDICATIONS/ROUTES/DOSAGE

**GI Tract Disorders**

**PO** *(Immediate-Release):* **ADULTS, ELDERLY, CHILDREN 12 YRS AND OLDER:** 0.125–0.25 mg q4h as needed. **Maximum:** 1.5 mg/day. **CHILDREN 2–11 YRS:** 0.0625–0.125 mg q4h as needed. **Maximum:** 0.75 mg/day. **ADULTS, ELDERLY:** *(Extended-Release):* 0.375–0.75 mg q12h. **Maximum:** 1.5 mg/day.

**IV, IM: ADULTS, ELDERLY, CHILDREN 12 YRS AND OLDER:** 0.25–0.5 mg. May repeat as needed up to 4 times/day at 4-hr intervals.

**Hypermotility of Lower Urinary Tract**

**PO** *(Sublingual):* **ADULTS, ELDERLY:** 0.15–0.3 mg 4 times/day. *(Extended-Release):* 0.375 mg q12h.

**Infant Colic**

**PO:** **INFANTS:** Drops dosed q4h as needed (based on weight): 2.3 kg: 3 drops; 3.4 kg: 4 drops; 5 kg: 5 drops; 7 kg: 6 drops; 10 kg: 8 drops; 15 kg: 11 drops.

**Dosage in Renal/Hepatic Impairment**
No dose adjustment.

## SIDE EFFECTS

**Frequent:** Dry mouth, decreased diaphoresis, constipation. **Occasional:** Blurred vision, bloated feeling, urinary hesitancy, drowsiness (with high dosage), headache, intolerance to light, loss of taste, anxiety, flushing, insomnia, impotence, mental confusion or excitement (particularly in elderly, children), temporary light-headedness (with parenteral form), local irritation (with parenteral form). **Rare:** Dizziness, faintness.

## ADVERSE EFFECTS/ TOXIC REACTIONS

Overdose may produce temporary paralysis of ciliary muscle, pupillary dilation, tachycardia, palpitations, hot/dry/flushed skin, absence of bowel sounds, hyperthermia, increased respiratory rate, EKG abnormalities, nausea, vomiting, rash over face/upper trunk, CNS stimulation, psychosis (agitation, restlessness, rambling speech, visual hallucinations, paranoid behavior, delusions) followed by depression.

## NURSING CONSIDERATIONS

### BASELINE ASSESSMENT

Before giving medication, instruct pt to void (reduces risk of urinary retention). Question history of myasthenia gravis, narrow-angle glaucoma, BPH, ulcerative colitis.

### INTERVENTION/EVALUATION

Monitor daily pattern of bowel activity, stool consistency. Palpate bladder for urinary retention. Monitor changes in B/P, temperature. Assess skin turgor, mucous membranes to evaluate hydration status (encourage adequate fluid intake), bowel sounds for peristalsis. Be alert for fever (increased risk of hyperthermia).

### PATIENT/FAMILY TEACHING

• May cause dry mouth; maintain proper oral hygiene (lack of saliva may increase risk of cavities). • Report rash, eye pain, difficulty in urinating, constipation. • Avoid tasks that require alertness, motor skills until response to drug is established. • Avoid hot baths, saunas.

# ibandronate

eye-**ban**-droe-nate
(Boniva)

## ◆CLASSIFICATION

**PHARMACOTHERAPEUTIC:** Bisphosphonate. **CLINICAL:** Calcium regulator.

## USES

Treatment/prevention of osteoporosis in postmenopausal women. **OFF-LABEL:** Hypercalcemia of malignancy; reduces bone pain and skeletal complications from metastatic bone disease due to breast cancer.

## PRECAUTIONS

**Contraindications:** Hypersensitivity to ibandronate, other bisphosphonates; oral tablets in pts unable to stand or sit upright for at least 60 min; pts with abnormalities of the esophagus that would delay emptying, hypocalcemia. **Cautions:** GI diseases (duodenitis, dysphagia, esophagitis, gastritis, ulcers [drug may exacerbate these conditions]), renal impairment with CrCl less than 30 ml/min.

## ACTION

Inhibits bone resorption via activity on osteoclasts. **Therapeutic Effect:** Reduces rate of bone resorption, resulting in increased bone mineral density.

## PHARMACOKINETICS

Absorbed in upper GI tract. Extent of absorption impaired by food, beverages (other than plain water). Protein binding: 85%–99%. Rapidly binds to bone. Unabsorbed portion eliminated in urine. **Half-life: PO:** 37–157 hrs; **IV:** 5–25 hrs.

## ⧖ LIFESPAN CONSIDERATIONS

**Pregnancy/Lactation:** Potential for teratogenic effects. Unknown if distributed in breast milk. Breastfeeding not recommended. **Children:** Safety and efficacy not established. **Elderly:** No age-related precautions noted.

## INTERACTIONS

**DRUG: Antacids containing aluminum, calcium, magnesium; vitamin D** decrease absorption. **Aspirin, NSAIDs** may increase GI irritation. **HERBAL:** None significant. **FOOD: Beverages (other than plain water), dietary supplements, food** interfere with absorption. **LAB VALUES:** May decrease serum alkaline phosphatase. May increase serum cholesterol.

## AVAILABILITY (Rx)

**Injection Solution:** 3 mg/3 ml syringe.
**Tablets:** 150 mg.

## ADMINISTRATION/HANDLING

**PO**

• Give 60 min before first food or beverage of the day, on an empty stomach with 6–8 oz plain water (not mineral water) while pt is standing or sitting in upright position. • Pt cannot lie down for 60 min following drug administration. • Instruct pt to swallow whole; do not break, crush, dissolve, or divide tablet (potential for oropharyngeal ulceration).

 **IV**

• Give over 15–30 sec. • Give over 1 hr for metastatic bone disease; over 1–2 hrs for hypercalcemia of malignancy.

## INDICATIONS/ROUTES/DOSAGE

**Osteoporosis**

**PO** *(Prevention/Treatment):* **ADULTS, ELDERLY:** 150 mg once monthly.
**IV** *(Treatment):* **ADULTS, ELDERLY:** 3 mg q3mos.

**Dosage in Renal Impairment**
Not recommended for pts with CrCl less than 30 ml/min.

**Dosage in Hepatic Impairment**
No dose adjustment.

## SIDE EFFECTS

**Frequent (13%–6%):** Back pain, dyspepsia, peripheral discomfort, diarrhea, headache, myalgia. **IV:** Abdominal pain, dyspepsia, constipation, nausea, diarrhea. **Occasional (4%–3%):** Dizziness, arthralgia, asthenia. **Rare (2% or less):** Vomiting, hypersensitivity reaction.

## ADVERSE EFFECTS/ TOXIC REACTIONS

Upper respiratory infection occurs occasionally. Overdose results in hypocalcemia, hypophosphatemia, significant GI disturbances.

## NURSING CONSIDERATIONS

### BASELINE ASSESSMENT

Hypocalcemia, vitamin D deficiency must be corrected before beginning therapy. Obtain laboratory baselines, esp. serum chemistries, renal function. Obtain results of bone density study.

### INTERVENTION/EVALUATION

Monitor electrolytes, esp. serum calcium, phosphate. Monitor renal function tests.

### PATIENT/FAMILY TEACHING

• Expected benefits occur only when medication is taken with full glass (6–8 oz) of plain water, first thing in the morning and at least 60 min before first food, beverage, medication of the day. Any other beverage (mineral water, orange juice, coffee) significantly reduces absorption of medication. • Do not chew, crush, dissolve, or divide tablets; swallow whole. • Do not lie down for at least 60 min after taking medication (potentiates delivery to stomach, reduces risk of esophageal irritation). • Report swallowing difficulties, pain when swallowing, chest pain, new/ worsening heartburn. • Consider weight-bearing exercises; modify behavioral factors (e.g., cigarette smoking, alcohol consumption). • Calcium and vitamin D supplements should be taken if dietary intake inadequate.

# ibrutinib

eye-**broo**-ti-nib
(Imbruvica)
**Do not confuse ibrutinib with axitinib, dasatinib, erlotinib, gefitinib, imatinib, nilotinib, ponatinib, sorafenib, sunitinib, or vandetanib.**

## ◆CLASSIFICATION

**PHARMACOTHERAPEUTIC:** Kinase inhibitor. **CLINICAL:** Antineoplastic.

## USES

Treatment of pts with mantle cell lymphoma (MCL) who have received at least one prior therapy, chronic lymphocytic leukemia (CLL) with at least one prior therapy or with 17p deletion, first-line treatment of CLL. Waldenstrom's macroglobulemia (WM).

## PRECAUTIONS

**Contraindications:** Hypersensitivity to ibrutinib. **Cautions:** Hepatic/renal impairment, elderly, pregnancy, history of GI disease (e.g., bleeding, ulcers).

## ACTION

Inhibits enzymatic activity of Bruton's tyrosine kinase (BTK), a signaling molecule that promotes malignant B-cell proliferation and survival. **Therapeutic Effect:** Inhibits tumor cell growth and metastasis.

## PHARMACOKINETICS

Readily absorbed following PO. Metabolized in liver. Peak plasma concentration: 1–2 hrs. Protein binding: 97%. Excreted in feces (80%), urine (10%). **Half-life:** 4–6 hrs.

## ⧗ LIFESPAN CONSIDERATIONS

**Pregnancy/Lactation:** May cause fetal harm. Avoid pregnancy. Unknown if distributed in breast milk. Must either discontinue drug or discontinue breastfeeding. **Children:** Safety and efficacy not established.

**Elderly:** Increased risk of cardiac events (atrial fibrillation, hypertension), infections (pneumonia, cellulitis), GI events (diarrhea, dehydration, bleeding).

## INTERACTIONS

**DRUG: Strong CYP3A4 inhibitors (e.g., ketoconazole, clarithromycin)** may increase plasma concentration/effect; avoid use. **Strong CYP3A4 inducers (e.g., rifampin, phenytoin)** may decrease plasma concentration/effect; avoid use. **Anticoagulants (e.g., warfarin), antiplatelets (e.g., aspirin, clopidogrel), NSAIDs** may increase risk of bleeding. **HERBAL: St. John's wort** may decrease concentration/effect. **FOOD: Grapefruit products, Seville oranges** may increase concentration/effect. **All foods** may increase absorption/concentration. **LAB VALUES:** May decrease Hgb, Hct, neutrophils, platelets.

## AVAILABILITY (Rx)

Capsules: 140 mg.

## ADMINISTRATION/HANDLING

**PO**

• Give with water. • Do not break, crush, or open capsule.

## INDICATIONS/ROUTES/DOSAGE

**Mantle Cell Lymphoma**
**PO: ADULTS/ELDERLY:** 560 mg (4 × 140-mg capsules) once daily.

**CLL, WM**
**PO: ADULTS, ELDERLY:** 420 mg (3 × 140 mg) once daily.

**Dose Modification**
Based on Common Terminology Criteria for Adverse Events (CTCAE).

**Any Grade 3 or Greater Nonhematologic Event, Grade 3 or Greater Neutropenia with Infection or Fever, or Any Grade 4 Hematologic Toxicities**
Interrupt treatment until resolution to grade 1 or baseline, then restart at initial dose. If toxicity reoccurs, interrupt treatment until resolution to grade 1 or baseline, then reduce dose to 420 mg daily (one capsule less). If toxicity reoccurs, interrupt treatment until resolution to grade 1 or baseline, then reduce dose to 280 mg once daily (one capsule less). If toxicity still occurs at 280 mg dose, discontinue treatment.

**Concomitant Use of Moderate CYP3A4 Inhibitors (e.g., Fluconazole, Diltiazem, Verapamil)**
Start at reduced dose of 140 mg daily. If toxicity occurs, either discontinue treatment or find alternate agent with less CYP3A inhibition.

**Concomitant Short-Term Use of Strong CYP3A4 Inhibitors (7 days or less) (e.g., Antifungals, Antibiotics)**
Interrupt treatment until strong CYP3A medications no longer needed.

**Concomitant Chronic Use of Strong CYP3A4 Inhibitors or Inducers**
Treatment not recommended.

**Dosage in Renal Impairment**
No dose adjustment.

**Dosage in Hepatic Impairment**
**Mild impairment:** Decrease dose to 140 mg. **Moderate to severe impairment:** Avoid use.

## SIDE EFFECTS

**Frequent (51%–23%):** Diarrhea, fatigue, musculoskeletal pain, peripheral edema, nausea, bruising, dyspnea, constipation, rash, abdominal pain, vomiting. **Occasional (21%–11%):** Decreased appetite, cough, pyrexia, stomatitis, asthenia, dizziness, muscle spasms, dehydration, headache, dyspepsia, petechiae, arthralgia.

## ADVERSE EFFECTS/ TOXIC REACTIONS

Anemia, lymphopenia, neutropenia, thrombocytopenia is expected response to therapy. Treatment-emergent myelosuppression (grade 3–4 CTCAE) reported in 41%

of pts: neutropenia (29%), thrombocytopenia (17%), anemia (9%). Infections including upper respiratory tract infection, UTI, pneumonia, skin infection, sinusitis were reported. Hemorrhagic events including epistaxis, GI bleeding, hematuria, intracranial hemorrhage, subdural hematoma reported in 5% of pts. Serious and fatal cases of renal toxicity reported: increased serum creatinine 1.5 times upper limit of normal (ULN) (67% of pts), increased serum creatinine 1.53 times UNL (9% of pts). Second primary malignancies including skin cancer (4%), other carcinomas (1%) occurred.

## NURSING CONSIDERATIONS

### BASELINE ASSESSMENT

Obtain baseline vital signs, CBC, serum chemistries, LFT, PT/INR if on anticoagulants. Question history of arrhythmias, HF, GI bleed, hepatic/renal impairment, peripheral edema, pulmonary disease. Obtain negative urine pregnancy before initiating treatment. Assess hydration status. Receive full medication history including herbal products. Assess skin for open/unhealed wounds, lesions, moles. Conduct baseline neurologic exam.

### INTERVENTION/EVALUATION

Monitor CBC monthly; LFT, serum chemistries, renal function routinely. Monitor stool frequency, consistency, characteristics. Immediately report hemorrhagic events: epistaxis, hematuria, hemoptysis, melena. Encourage PO intake. Obtain EKG for arrhythmias, dyspnea, palpitations. Screen for possible intracranial hemorrhage: altered mental status, aphasia, hemiparesis, unequal pupils, homonymous hemianopsia (blindness of one half of vision on same side of both eyes). Monitor for renal toxicity (anuria, hypertension, generalized edema, flank pain). Assess skin for new lesions.

### PATIENT/FAMILY TEACHING

• Blood levels will be monitored routinely. • Difficulty breathing, fever, cough, burning with urination, body aches, chills may indicate acute infection. • Avoid pregnancy. • Report any black/tarry stools, bruising, nausea, RUQ abdominal pain, yellowing of skin or eyes, palpitations, nose bleeds, blood in urine or stool, decreased urine output. • Avoid alcohol. • Do not take herbal products. • Do not ingest grapefruit products. • Severe diarrhea may lead to dehydration. • Contact physician before any planned surgical/dental procedures. • Immediately report neurological changes: confusion, one-sided paralysis, difficulty speaking, partial blindness. • Do not receive live vaccines. • Do not break, crush, or open capsule.

# ibuprofen

eye-bue-**pro**-fen
(Advil, Apo-Ibuprofen ✦, Caldolor, Motrin, NeoProfen, Novo-Profen ✦)

■ **BLACK BOX ALERT** ■ Increased risk of serious cardiovascular thrombotic events, including myocardial infarction, CVA. Increased risk of severe GI reactions, including ulceration, bleeding, perforation.
**Do not confuse Motrin with Neurontin.**

## FIXED-COMBINATION(S)

**Children's Advil Cold:** ibuprofen/pseudoephedrine (a nasal decongestant): 100 mg/15 mg per 5 ml. **Combunox:** ibuprofen/oxycodone (a narcotic analgesic): 400 mg/5 mg. **Duexis:** ibuprofen/famotidine (an $H_2$ antagonist): 800 mg/26.6 mg. **Reprexain CIII:** ibuprofen/hydrocodone (a narcotic analgesic): 200 mg/5 mg. **Vicoprofen:** ibuprofen/hydrocodone (a narcotic analgesic): 200 mg/7.5 mg.

## ◆CLASSIFICATION

**PHARMACOTHERAPEUTIC:** NSAID. **CLINICAL:** Antirheumatic, analgesic, antipyretic, antidysmenorrheal, vascular headache suppressant.

## USES

**Oral:** Treatment of fever, rheumatoid disorders, osteoarthritis, mild to moderate pain, primary dysmenorrhea. **Caldolor:** Mild to moderate pain; severe pain in combination with an opioid analgesic; fever. **NeoProfen:** Induces closure in clinically significant patent ductus arteriosus (PDA) in premature infants weighing between 500 and 1,500 g who are no more than 32 wks gestational age when usual medical management is ineffective. **OFF-LABEL:** Treatment of cystic fibrosis, pericarditis. Juvenile idiopathic arthritis.

## PRECAUTIONS

**Contraindications:** History of hypersensitivity to ibuprofen, aspirin, other NSAIDs. Treatment of perioperative pain in coronary artery bypass graft (CABG) surgery. Aspirin triad (bronchial asthma, aspirin intolerance, rhinitis). **NeoProfen:** Infants with proven or suspected untreated infection, elevated total bilirubin, congenital heart disease in whom patency of the patent ductus arteriosus is necessary for satisfactory pulmonary or systemic blood flow (e.g., pulmonary atresia), bleeding, thrombocytopenia, coagulation defects, suspected necrotizing enterocolitis, significant renal impairment. **Cautions:** Pts with fluid retention, HF, dehydration, coagulation disorders, concurrent use with aspirin, anticoagulants, steroids; history of GI disease (e.g., bleeding, ulcers), smoking, use of alcohol, elderly, debilitated, hepatic/renal impairment, asthma.

## ACTION

Inhibits prostaglandin synthesis. **Therapeutic Effect:** Produces analgesic, antiinflammatory effects; decreases fever.

## PHARMACOKINETICS

| Route | Onset | Peak | Duration |
|---|---|---|---|
| PO (analgesic) | 0.5 hr | N/A | 4–6 hrs |
| PO (antirheumatic) | 2 days | 1–2 wks | N/A |

Rapidly absorbed from GI tract. Protein binding: 90%–99%. Metabolized in liver. Primarily excreted in urine. Not removed by hemodialysis. **Half-life:** 2–4 hrs.

##  LIFESPAN CONSIDERATIONS

**Pregnancy/Lactation:** Unknown if drug crosses placenta or is distributed in breast milk. Avoid use during third trimester (may adversely affect fetal cardiovascular system: premature closure of ductus arteriosus). **Children:** Safety and efficacy not established in pts younger than 6 mos. **Elderly:** GI bleeding, ulceration more likely to cause serious adverse effects. Age-related renal impairment may increase risk of hepatic/renal toxicity; reduced dosage recommended.

## INTERACTIONS

**DRUG:** May decrease effects of **antihypertensives (e.g., amlodipine, lisinopril, valsartan), diuretics (e.g., furosemide). Aspirin, other salicylates** may increase risk of GI side effects, bleeding. May increase effects of **oral anticoagulants (e.g., warfarin).** May increase concentration, risk of toxicity of **lithium, methotrexate. HERBAL: Cat's claw, dong quai, evening primrose, feverfew, garlic, ginkgo, ginseng, horse chestnut, red clover** may increase antiplatelet activity. **FOOD:** None known. **LAB VALUES:** May prolong bleeding time. May alter serum glucose level. May increase serum BUN, creatinine, potassium, ALT, AST. May decrease serum calcium, glucose; Hgb, Hct, platelets.

## AVAILABILITY (Rx)

**Capsules:** 200 mg. **Injection, Solution (NeoProfen):** 10 mg/ml. **(Caldolor):** 100 mg/ml. **Suspension, Oral:** 100 mg/5 ml. **Suspension, Oral Drops:** 40 mg/ml. **Tablets:** 200 mg, 400 mg, 600 mg, 800 mg. **Tablets, Chewable:** 50 mg, 100 mg.

## ADMINISTRATION/HANDLING

IV (Caldolor)

**Reconstitution** • Dilute with $D_5W$ or 0.9% NaCl to final concentration of 4 mg/ml or less.

---

**Rate of Administration** • Infuse over at least 30 min.
**Storage** • Store at room temperature.
• Stable for 24 hrs after dilution.

 **IV (NeoProfen)**

**Reconstitution** • Dilute to appropriate volume with $D_5W$ or 0.9% NaCl.
• Discard any remaining medication after first withdrawal from vial.
**Rate of Administration** • Administer via IV port nearest the insertion site.
• Infuse continuously over 15 min.
**Storage** • Store at room temperature.
• Stable for 30 min after dilution.

**PO**
• Give with food, milk, antacids if GI distress occurs.

## INDICATIONS/ROUTES/DOSAGE

**Fever**
**PO: ADULTS, ELDERLY:** 200–400 mg q4–6h prn. **CHILDREN 6 MOS AND OLDER:** 5–10 mg/kg q6–8h. **Maximum:** 400 mg/dose; 1,200 mg/day.
**IV: ADULTS, ELDERLY:** 400 mg q4–6h or 100–200 mg q4h prn. **Maximum:** 3.2 g/day.
**CHILDREN 12–17 YRS:** 400 mg q4–6h prn. **Maximum:** 2,400 mg/day. **CHILDREN 6 MOS–11 YRS:** 10 mg/kg q4–6h prn. **Maximum/dose:** 400 mg. **Maximum:** 40 mg/kg up to 2,400 mg/day.

**Osteoarthritis, Rheumatoid Disorders**
**PO: ADULTS, ELDERLY:** 400–800 mg 3–4 times/day. **Maximum:** 3.2 g/day.

**Pain**
**PO: ADULTS, ELDERLY, CHILDREN 12 YRS AND OLDER:** 200–400 mg q4–6h prn. **CHILDREN 6 MOS–11 YRS:** 4–10 mg/kg q6–8h prn. **Maximum:** 40 mg/kg/day. **IV: ADULTS, ELDERLY:** 400–800 mg q6h prn. **Maximum:** 3.2 g/day.

**Primary Dysmenorrhea**
**PO: ADULTS:** 200–400 mg q4–6h prn. **Maximum:** 1,200 mg/day.

**Patent Ductus Arteriosus (PDA)**
**IV: INFANTS:** Initially, 10 mg/kg then 2 doses of 5 mg/kg, after 24 hrs and 48 hrs. All doses based on birth weight.

**Dosage in Renal Impairment**
Hold if anuria or oliguria evident. Avoid use in severe impairment.

**Dosage in Hepatic Impairment**
Avoid use in severe impairment.

## SIDE EFFECTS

**Occasional (9%–3%):** Nausea, vomiting, dyspepsia, dizziness, rash. **Rare (less than 3%):** Diarrhea or constipation, flatulence, abdominal cramps or pain, pruritus, increased B/P.

## ADVERSE EFFECTS/ TOXIC REACTIONS

Overdose may result in metabolic acidosis. Rare reactions with long-term use include peptic ulcer, GI bleeding, gastritis, severe hepatic reaction (cholestasis, jaundice), nephrotoxicity (dysuria, hematuria, proteinuria, nephrotic syndrome), severe hypersensitivity reaction (particularly in pts with systemic lupus erythematosus or other collagen diseases). **NeoProfen:** Hypoglycemia, hypocalcemia, respiratory failure, UTI, edema, atelectasis may occur. **Caldolor:** Abdominal pain, anemia, cough, dizziness, dyspnea, edema, hypertension, nausea, vomiting have been reported.

## NURSING CONSIDERATIONS

### BASELINE ASSESSMENT

Assess onset, type, location, duration of pain, inflammation. Inspect appearance of affected joints for immobility, deformities, skin condition. Assess temperature.

### INTERVENTION/EVALUATION

Monitor for evidence of nausea, dyspepsia. Monitor CBC, renal function, LFT. Assess skin for rash. Observe for bleeding, bruising, occult blood loss. Evaluate for therapeutic response: relief of pain, stiffness, swelling; increased joint mobility; reduced joint tenderness; improved grip strength. Monitor for fever.

### PATIENT/FAMILY TEACHING

• Avoid aspirin, alcohol during therapy (increases risk of GI bleeding). • If GI upset occurs, take with food, milk, antacids. • May cause dizziness. • Report ringing in ears, persistent stomach pain, respiratory difficulty, unusual bruising/bleeding, swelling of extremities, chest pain/palpitations.

---

## *IDArubicin    HIGH ALERT

eye-da-**rue**-bi-sin
(Idamycin PFS)

■ **BLACK BOX ALERT** ■ Cardiotoxicity may occur (HF, arrhythmias, cardiomyopathy). Severe myelosuppressant. Must be administered by personnel trained in administration/handling of chemotherapeutic agents. Severe local tissue damage, necrosis if extravasation occurs. Dosage reduction recommended with renal/hepatic impairment.
**Do not confuse Idamycin with Adriamycin, or idarubicin with daunorubicin, doxorubicin, or epirubicin.**

### ◆CLASSIFICATION

**PHARMACOTHERAPEUTIC:** Anthracycline antibiotic. **CLINICAL:** Antineoplastic.

### USES

Treatment of acute myeloid leukemia (AML). **OFF-LABEL:** Acute lymphocytic leukemia (ALL).

### PRECAUTIONS

**Contraindications:** Hypersensitivity to idarubicin. **Cautions:** Renal/hepatic impairment, concurrent radiation therapy, anemia, bone marrow depression, active infections, arrhythmias, cardiomyopathy, severe HF.

### ACTION

Inhibits DNA/RNA synthesis by intercalating between DNA base pairs. **Therapeutic Effect:** Produces apoptosis of rapidly dividing cells.

### PHARMACOKINETICS

Widely distributed. Protein binding: 97%. Rapidly metabolized in liver. Primarily eliminated by biliary excretion. Not removed by hemodialysis. **Half-life:** 12–27 hrs.

### ⌛ LIFESPAN CONSIDERATIONS

**Pregnancy/Lactation:** If possible, avoid use during pregnancy (may be embryotoxic). Unknown if drug is distributed in breast milk (advise to discontinue breastfeeding before drug initiation). **Children:** Safety and efficacy not established. **Elderly:** Cardiotoxicity may be more prevalent. Caution in pts with inadequate bone marrow reserves. Age-related renal impairment may require dosage adjustment.

### INTERACTIONS

**DRUG:** May decrease effects of **antigout medications (e.g., allopurinol, probenecid). Bone marrow depressants (e.g., alemtuzumab, methotrexate)** may increase myelosuppression. **Live virus vaccines** may potentiate virus replication, increase vaccine side effects, decrease pt's antibody response to vaccine. **HERBAL:** None significant. **FOOD:** None known. **LAB VALUES:** May increase serum alkaline phosphatase, bilirubin, uric acid, ALT, AST. May cause EKG changes.

### AVAILABILITY (Rx)

**Injection Solution:** 1 mg/ml in 5-ml, 10-ml, 20-ml vials.

### ADMINISTRATION/HANDLING

◄**ALERT**► Give by free-flowing IV infusion (**never** subcutaneous or IM). Gloves, gowns, eye goggles recommended during preparation/administration of medication. If powder/solution comes in contact with skin, wash thoroughly. Avoid small veins, swollen/edematous extremities, areas overlying joints/tendons.

---

**IV**

**Reconstitution** • May give undiluted or dilute with 0.9% NaCl or D₅W.

**Rate of Administration** • Administer IV push into tubing of freely running IV infusion of D₅W or 0.9% NaCl, preferably via butterfly needle, **slowly** over 3–5 min. • May give intermittent infusion over 10–15 min. • Extravasation produces immediate pain, severe local tissue damage. Terminate infusion immediately. Apply cold compresses for 30 min immediately, then q30min 4 times/day for 3 days. Keep extremity elevated.

**Storage** • Refrigerate vials. • Diluted solutions in 0.9% NaCl or D₅W are stable for 72 hrs at room temperature or 7 days if refrigerated.

### ⊞ IV INCOMPATIBILITIES

Acyclovir (Zovirax), allopurinol (Aloprim), ampicillin and sulbactam (Unasyn), cefazolin (Ancef, Kefzol), cefepime (Maxipime), ceftazidime (Fortaz), clindamycin (Cleocin), dexamethasone (Decadron), furosemide (Lasix), hydrocortisone (Solu-Cortef), lorazepam (Ativan), methotrexate, piperacillin and tazobactam (Zosyn), sodium bicarbonate, teniposide (Vumon), vancomycin (Vancocin), vincristine (Oncovin).

### ⊞ IV COMPATIBILITIES

Diphenhydramine (Benadryl), granisetron (Kytril), magnesium, potassium.

## INDICATIONS/ ROUTES/DOSAGE

◀**ALERT**▶ Refer to individual protocols.

#### AML

**IV: ADULTS, ELDERLY: (Induction):** 12 mg/m²/day for 3 days (in combination with cytarabine). A second induction cycle may be administered if necessary.

**Dosage in Renal Impairment**
**ADULTS:** CrCl 10–50 ml/min: Give 75% of dose. CrCl less than 10 ml/min: Give 50% of dose. **CHILDREN:** CrCl less than 50 ml/min: Give 75% of dose.

**Hemodialysis, Peritoneal Dialysis, Continuous Renal Replacement Therapy:** Administer 75% of dose.

**Dosage in Hepatic Impairment**
**Bilirubin 2.6–5 mg/dL:** Give 50% of dose. **Bilirubin greater than 5 mg/dL:** Avoid use.

## SIDE EFFECTS

**Frequent (82%–50%):** Nausea, vomiting, complete alopecia (scalp, axillary, pubic hair), abdominal cramping, diarrhea, mucositis. **Occasional (46%–20%):** Hyperpigmentation of nailbeds, phalangeal, dermal creases; fever, headache. **Rare:** Conjunctivitis, neuropathy.

## ADVERSE EFFECTS/ TOXIC REACTIONS

Myelosuppression (principally leukopenia and, to lesser extent, anemia, thrombocytopenia) generally occurs within 10–15 days after starting therapy, returns to normal levels by third wk. Cardiotoxicity (either acute, manifested as transient EKG abnormalities, or chronic, manifested as HF) may occur.

## NURSING CONSIDERATIONS

### BASELINE ASSESSMENT

Obtain CBC, BMP, LFT. Obtain EKG before therapy. Antiemetic medication before and during therapy may prevent or relieve nausea, vomiting. Inform pt of high potential for alopecia.

### INTERVENTION/EVALUATION

Monitor CBC, serum electrolytes, EKG, renal function, LFT. Monitor for hematologic toxicity (fever, sore throat, signs of local infection, unusual bruising/bleeding from any site), symptoms of anemia (excessive fatigue, weakness). Avoid IM injections, rectal temperatures, other trauma that may precipitate bleeding. Check infusion site frequently for extravasation (causes severe local necrosis). Assess for potentially fatal HF (dyspnea, rales, pulmonary edema), life-threatening arrhythmias.

### PATIENT/FAMILY TEACHING

• Total body hair loss is frequent but reversible. • New hair growth resumes 2–3 mos after last therapy dose and may have different color, texture. • Maintain strict oral hygiene. • Avoid crowds, those with infections. • Report fever, sore throat, bruising/ bleeding. • Urine may turn pink or red. • Frequent lab testing is a normal part of therapy. • Use contraceptive measures.

# idelalisib

eye-**del**-a-**lis**-ib
(Zydelig)

■ **BLACK BOX ALERT** ■ Fatal and/or serious hepatotoxicity may occur. Monitor hepatic function prior to and during treatment. Fatal and/or serious and severe diarrhea or colitis may occur. Monitor for GI symptoms. Fatal and serious pneumonitis may occur. Monitor for pulmonary symptoms and bilateral interstitial infiltrates. Interrupt, then reduce or discontinue treatment if hepatotoxicity, severe diarrhea, or pneumonitis occurs. Fatal and serious intestinal perforation may occur. Discontinue if perforation suspected.

## ◆CLASSIFICATION

**PHARMACOTHERAPEUTIC:** Kinase inhibitor. **CLINICAL:** Antineoplastic.

## USES

Treatment of relapsed chronic lymphocytic leukemia (CLL), in combination with rituximab, in pts for whom rituximab alone would not be considered appropriate therapy due to other co-morbidities. Treatment of relapsed follicular B-cell non-Hodgkin's lymphoma (FL) or relapsed small lymphocytic lymphoma (SLL) in pts who have received at least two prior systemic therapies.

## PRECAUTIONS

**Contraindications:** History of serious allergic reactions to idelalisib (e.g., anaphylaxis, toxic epidermal necrolysis). **Cautions:** Baseline anemia, leukopenia, neutropenia, thrombocytopenia; GI bleeding, hepatic impairment. Pts with active infection, high tumor burden. Avoid concomitant use of hepatotoxic or promotility medications.

## ACTION

Inhibits several cell signaling pathways including B-cell receptor signaling and CXCR4 and CXCR5 signaling, which are involved in trafficking B cells to lymph nodes and bone marrow. **Therapeutic Effect:** Induces apoptosis and inhibits proliferation in cell lines derived from malignant B cells and primary tumor cells.

## PHARMACOKINETICS

Well absorbed following PO administration. Metabolized in liver. Protein binding: 84%. Peak plasma concentration: 1.5 hrs. Eliminated in feces (78%), urine (14%). **Half-life:** 8.3 hrs.

## ⌛ LIFESPAN CONSIDERATIONS

**Pregnancy/Lactation:** May cause fetal harm; avoid pregnancy. Use effective contraception during treatment and for at least 1 mo after discontinuation. Unknown if distributed in breast milk. Must either discontinue drug or discontinue breastfeeding. **Children:** Safety and efficacy not established in pts younger than 18 yrs. **Elderly:** May have increased risk of side effects/adverse reactions.

## INTERACTIONS

**DRUG:** **Strong CYP3A4 inducers (e.g., rifampin, phenytoin)** may decrease concentration/effect. **Strong CYP3A4 inhibitors (ketoconazole, ritonavir)** may increase concentration/ effect. **HERBAL:** **St. John's wort** may decrease concentration/effect. **FOOD:** None known. **LAB VALUES:** May increase serum ALT, AST, bilirubin, GGT; triglycerides.

May decrease Hgb, neutrophils, platelets, serum sodium. May increase or decrease lymphocytes, serum glucose.

## AVAILABILITY (Rx)

Tablets: 100 mg, 150 mg.

## ADMINISTRATION/HANDLING

### PO

• Give without regard to meals. • Swallow tablets whole.

## INDICATIONS/ROUTES/DOSAGE

**Chronic Lymphocytic Leukemia (in Combination with Rituximab), Follicular B-cell Non-Hodgkin's Lymphoma, Small Lymphocytic Lymphoma**
PO: ADULTS/ELDERLY: 150 mg twice daily. Continue until disease progression or unacceptable toxicity.

**Dose Modification**
*Elevated ALT, AST*
3–5 Times Upper Limit of Normal (ULN): Maintain dose. 5–20 Times ULN: Monitor serum ALT, AST wkly. Withhold until ALT, AST less than 1 times ULN, then resume at 100 mg twice daily. Greater Than 20 Times ULN: Permanently discontinue.
*Elevated Bilirubin*
1.5–3 Times ULN: Monitor serum bilirubin wkly. Maintain dose.
3–10 Times ULN: Monitor serum bilirubin wkly. Withhold until bilirubin less than 1 times ULN, then resume at 100-mg dose.
Greater Than 10 Times ULN: Permanently discontinue.
*Diarrhea*
Moderate Diarrhea: Maintain dose. Severe Diarrhea or Hospitalization: Withhold until resolved, then resume at 100-mg dose. Life-Threatening Diarrhea: Permanently discontinue.
*Neutropenia*
ANC 1,000–1,500 cells/mm³: Maintain dose. ANC 500–1,000 cells/mm³: Monitor ANC wkly and maintain dose. ANC Less Than 500 cells/mm³: Permanently discontinue.

*Thrombocytopenia*
Platelets 50,000–75,000/mm³: Maintain dose. Platelets 25,000–50,000/mm³: Monitor platelet count wkly and maintain dose. Platelets Less Than 25,000/mm³: Monitor platelet count wkly. Withhold until platelets greater than 25,000 mm³, then resume at 100-mg dose.
*Pneumonitis*
Any Symptoms: Permanently discontinue.

**Dosage in Renal Impairment**
No dose adjustment.

**Dosage in Hepatic Impairment**
Use caution. See dose modification.

## SIDE EFFECTS

### CLL
Frequent (35%–21%): Pyrexia, nausea, diarrhea, chills. Occasional (10%–5%): Headache, vomiting, generalized pain, arthralgia, stomatitis, gastric reflux, nasal congestion.

### Non-Hodgkin's Lymphoma
Frequent (47%–21%): Diarrhea, fatigue, nausea, cough, pyrexia, abdominal pain, rash. Occasional (17%–10%): Dyspnea, decreased appetite, vomiting, asthenia, night sweats, insomnia, headache, peripheral edema.

## ADVERSE EFFECTS/TOXIC REACTIONS

Thrombocytopenia, neutropenia, leukopenia, lymphopenia are expected responses to therapy, but more severe reactions, including bone marrow failure, febrile neutropenia, may occur. Fatal and/or serious events including hepatotoxicity (14% of pts), severe diarrhea or colitis (14% of pts), hypersensitivity reactions (including anaphylaxis), pneumonitis, intestinal perforation were reported. Neutropenia occurred in 31% of pts, which may greatly increase risk of infection. Severe skin reactions including toxic epidermal necrolysis, generalized rash, exfoliative rash were reported. Other infections processes may include bronchitis, *Clostridium difficile* colitis, pneumonia, sepsis, UTI. Fatal and/ or serious intestinal perforation may occur.

## NURSING CONSIDERATIONS

### BASELINE ASSESSMENT

Obtain ANC, CBC, BMP, LFT, PT/INR, vital signs, urine pregnancy. Receive full medication history including herbal products. Question possibility of pregnancy, current breastfeeding status, use of contraceptive measures in female pts of reproductive potential. Questions history of hypersensitivity reaction or acute skin reactions to drug class. Perform full dermatologic exam with routine assessment.

### INTERVENTION/EVALUATION

Diligently monitor blood counts (esp. ANC, CBC, platelet count) frequently. Any interruption of therapy or dosage change may require wkly lab monitoring until symptoms resolve. Obtain *C. difficile* toxin PCR if severe diarrhea occurs. Screen for acute cutaneous reactions, allergic reactions, other acute infections (sepsis, UTI), hepatic impairment, pulmonary events (dyspnea, pneumonitis, pneumonia), or tumor lysis syndrome (electrolyte imbalance, uric acid nephropathy, acute renal failure). Monitor strict I&Os, hydration status, stool frequency and consistency.

### PATIENT/FAMILY TEACHING

• Blood levels will be routinely monitored. Any change in dose or interruption of therapy may require blood draws every week • Avoid pregnancy; do not breastfeed. • Report abdominal pain, amber or bloody urine, bruising, black/tarry stools, persistent diarrhea, yellowing of skin or eyes. • Fever, cough, burning with urination, body aches, chills may indicate acute infection. • Avoid alcohol. • Immediately report difficult breathing, severe coughing, chest tightness. • Therapy may cause severe allergic reactions, intestinal tearing, or skin rashes or severe diarrhea related to an infected colon. • Do not take any over-the-counter medications including herbal products unless approved by your doctor.

# ifosfamide    HIGH ALERT

eye-**fos**-fa-mide
(Ifex)

■ **BLACK BOX ALERT** ■ Hemorrhagic cystitis may occur. Severe myelosuppressant. May cause CNS toxicity, including confusion, coma. Must be administered by personnel trained in administration/handling of chemotherapeutic agents. May cause severe nephrotoxicity, resulting in renal failure.
**Do not confuse ifosfamide with cyclophosphamide.**

## ◆CLASSIFICATION

**PHARMACOTHERAPEUTIC:** Alkylating agent. **CLINICAL:** Antineoplastic.

## USES

Treatment of germ cell testicular carcinoma (used in combination with other chemotherapy agents and with concurrent mesna). **OFF-LABEL:** Small cell lung, non–small-cell lung, ovarian, cervical, bladder cancer; soft tissue sarcomas, Hodgkin's, non-Hodgkin's lymphomas; osteosarcoma; head and neck, Ewing's sarcoma.

## PRECAUTIONS

**Contraindications:** Hypersensitivity to ifosfamide. Urinary outflow obstruction. **Cautions:** Renal/hepatic impairment, compromised bone marrow reserve, active urinary tract infection, preexisting cardiac disease, prior radiation therapy. Avoid use in pts with WBCs less than 2,000/mm³ and platelets less than 50,000/mm³.

## ACTION

Inhibits DNA, RNA protein synthesis by cross-linking with DNA, RNA strands, preventing cell growth. Cell cycle–phase nonspecific. **Therapeutic Effect:** Interferes with DNA, RNA function.

## PHARMACOKINETICS

Metabolized in liver. Protein binding: Negligible. Crosses blood-brain barrier (to a limited extent). Primarily excreted in urine. Removed by hemodialysis. **Half-life:** 11–15 hrs (high dose); 4–7 hrs (low dose).

## ⌛ LIFESPAN CONSIDERATIONS

**Pregnancy/Lactation:** If possible, avoid use during pregnancy, esp. first trimester. May cause fetal harm. Distributed in breast milk. Breastfeeding not recommended. **Children:** Not intended for this pt population. **Elderly:** Age-related renal impairment may require dosage adjustment.

## INTERACTIONS

**DRUG: Bone marrow depressants (e.g., alemtuzumab, methotrexate)** may increase myelosuppression. **Live virus vaccines** may potentiate virus replication, increase vaccine side effects, decrease pt's antibody response to vaccine. **HERBAL: St. John's wort** may decrease concentration. **FOOD:** None known. **LAB VALUES:** May increase serum BUN, bilirubin, creatinine, uric acid, ALT, AST.

## AVAILABILITY (Rx)

**Injection, Powder for Reconstitution (Ifex):** 1 g, 3 g. **Injection, Solution:** 50 mg/ml.

## ADMINISTRATION/HANDLING

◀**ALERT**▶ Hemorrhagic cystitis occurs if mesna is not given concurrently. Mesna should always be given with ifosfamide.

 **IV**

**Reconstitution** • Reconstitute vial with Sterile Water for Injection or Bacteriostatic Water for Injection to provide concentration of 50 mg/ml. Shake to dissolve. • Further dilute with 50–1,000 ml D₅W or 0.9% NaCl to provide concentration of 0.6–20 mg/ml. **Rate of Administration** • Infuse over minimum of 30 min. • Give with at least 2,000 ml PO or IV fluid (prevents bladder toxicity). • Give with protectant against hemorrhagic cystitis (i.e., mesna). **Storage** • Store vials of powder at room temperature. • Refrigerate vials

of solution. • After reconstitution with Bacteriostatic Water for Injection, vials and diluted solutions stable for 24 hrs if refrigerated.

## ▦ IV INCOMPATIBILITIES

Cefepime (Maxipime), methotrexate.

## ▦ IV COMPATIBILITIES

Granisetron (Kytril), ondansetron (Zofran).

## INDICATIONS/ROUTES/DOSAGE

◀**ALERT**▶ Dosage individualized based on clinical response, tolerance to adverse effects. When used in combination therapy, consult specific protocols for optimum dosage, sequence of drug administration.

**Germ Cell Testicular Carcinoma**
**IV: ADULTS:** 1,200 mg/m²/day for 5 consecutive days. Repeat q3wks or after recovery from hematologic toxicity. Administer with mesna (to prevent bladder toxicity).

**Dosage in Renal/Hepatic Impairment**
Use caution.

## SIDE EFFECTS

**Frequent (83%–58%):** Alopecia, nausea, vomiting. **Occasional (15%–5%):** Confusion, drowsiness, hallucinations, infection. **Rare (less than 5%):** Dizziness, seizures, disorientation, fever, malaise, stomatitis (mucosal irritation, glossitis, gingivitis).

## ADVERSE EFFECTS/ TOXIC REACTIONS

Hemorrhagic cystitis with hematuria, dysuria occurs frequently if protective agent (mesna) is not used. Myelosuppression (leukopenia, thrombocytopenia) occurs frequently. Pulmonary toxicity, hepatotoxicity, nephrotoxicity, cardiotoxicity, CNS toxicity (confusion, hallucinations, drowsiness, coma) may require discontinuation of therapy.

## NURSING CONSIDERATIONS

### BASELINE ASSESSMENT

Obtain urinalysis before each dose. If hematuria occurs (greater than 10 RBCs per field), therapy should be withheld until resolution occurs. Obtain WBC, platelet count, Hgb before each dose.

### INTERVENTION/EVALUATION

Monitor hematologic studies, urinalysis, renal function, LFT. Assess for fever, sore throat, signs of local infection, unusual bruising/bleeding from any site, symptoms of anemia (excessive fatigue, weakness).

### PATIENT/FAMILY TEACHING

• Alopecia is reversible, but new hair growth may have a different color or texture. • Drink plenty of fluids (protects against cystitis). • Do not have immunizations without physician's approval (drug lowers resistance). • Avoid contact with those who have recently received live virus vaccine. • Avoid crowds, those with infections. • Report unusual bleeding/bruising, fever, chills, sore throat, joint pain, sores in mouth or on lips, yellowing skin or eyes.

# iloperidone

eye-loe-**per**-i-doan
(Fanapt)

■ **BLACK BOX ALERT** ■ Elderly pts with dementia-related psychosis are at increased risk for mortality due to cerebrovascular events.
**Do not confuse iloperidone with amiodarone or dronedarone.**

## ◆CLASSIFICATION

**PHARMACOTHERAPEUTIC:** Piperidinyl-benzisoxazole derivative. **CLINICAL:** Antipsychotic.

## USES

Acute treatment of schizophrenia in adults.

## PRECAUTIONS

**Contraindications:** Hypersensitivity to iloperidone. **Cautions:** Cardiovascular disease (HF, history of MI, ischemia, cardiac conduction abnormalities), cerebrovascular disease (increases risk of CVA in pts with dementia, seizure disorders). Pts at risk for orthostatic hypotension. Pts with bradycardia, hypokalemia, hypomagnesemia may be at greater risk for torsades de pointes. History of seizures, conditions lowering seizure threshold, high risk of suicide, risk of aspiration pneumonia, congenital QT syndrome, concurrent use of medications that prolong QT interval, decreased GI motility, urinary retention, BPH, xerostomia, visual problems, hepatic impairment, narrow-angle glaucoma, diabetes, elderly.

## ACTION

Exact mechanism mediated through combination of dopamine type 2 ($D_2$) and serotonin type 2 ($5-HT_2$) antagonisms. **Therapeutic Effect:** Diminishes symptoms of schizophrenia and reduces incidence of extrapyramidal side effects.

## PHARMACOKINETICS

Steady-state concentration occurs in 3–4 days. Well absorbed from GI tract (unaffected by food). Protein binding: 95%. Metabolized in liver. Primarily excreted in urine, with a lesser amount eliminated in feces. **Half-life:** 18–33 hrs.

## ☒ LIFESPAN CONSIDERATIONS

**Pregnancy/Lactation:** Unknown if drug crosses placenta or is excreted in breast milk. Breastfeeding not recommended. **Children:** Safety and efficacy not established. **Elderly:** More susceptible to postural hypotension. Increased risk of cerebrovascular events, mortality, including stroke in elderly pts with psychosis.

## INTERACTIONS

**DRUG:** Alcohol, CNS depressants (e.g., **diphenhydramine, lorazepam,**

**morphine**) may increase CNS depression. **Strong CYP3A4 inhibitors (e.g., clarithromycin, ketoconazole)** or **strong CYP2D6 inhibitors (e.g., fluoxetine, paroxetine)** may increase concentration. **Medications causing prolongation of QT interval (e.g., amiodarone, dofetilide, sotalol)** may increase effects on cardiac conduction, leading to malignant arrhythmias (torsades de pointes). **HERBAL:** Gotu kola, kava kava, St. John's wort, valerian may increase CNS depression. **St. John's wort** may decrease concentration. **FOOD:** None known. **LAB VALUES:** May increase serum prolactin levels.

## AVAILABILITY (Rx)

**Tablets:** 1 mg, 2 mg, 4 mg, 6 mg, 8 mg, 10 mg, 12 mg.

## ADMINISTRATION/HANDLING

**PO**
• Give without regard to food. • Tablets may be crushed.

## INDICATIONS/ROUTES/DOSAGE

**Note:** Titrate to the proper dose range with dosage adjustments not to exceed 2 mg twice daily q24h.

**Schizophrenia**
**PO: ADULTS:** To avoid orthostatic hypotension, begin with 1 mg twice daily, then adjust dosage to 2 mg twice daily, 4 mg twice daily, 6 mg twice daily, 8 mg twice daily, 10 mg twice daily, and 12 mg twice daily on days 2, 3, 4, 5, 6, and 7, respectively, to reach target daily dose of 12–24 mg/day in 2 divided doses. **Note:** Reduce dose by 50% when receiving strong CYP2D6 or CYP3A4 inhibitors or poor metabolizers of CYP2D6 (see Interactions).

**Dosage in Renal Impairment**
No dose adjustment.

**Dosage in Hepatic Impairment**
**Mild impairment:** No adjustment. **Moderate impairment:** Use caution. **Severe impairment:** Not recommended.

## SIDE EFFECTS

**Frequent (20%–12%):** Dizziness, drowsiness, tachycardia. **Occasional (10%–4%):** Nausea, dry mouth, nasal congestion, weight increase, diarrhea, fatigue, orthostatic hypotension. **Rare (3%–1%):** Arthralgia, musculoskeletal stiffness, abdominal discomfort, nasopharyngitis, tremor, hypotension, rash, ejaculatory failure, dyspnea, blurred vision, lethargy.

## ADVERSE EFFECTS/ TOXIC REACTIONS

Extrapyramidal disorders, including tardive dyskinesia (protrusion of tongue, puffing of cheeks, chewing/puckering of the mouth), occur in 4% of pts. Upper respiratory infection occurs in 3% of pts. QT interval prolongation may produce torsades de pointes, a form of ventricular tachycardia. Neuroleptic malignant syndrome (e.g., hyperpyrexia, muscle rigidity, altered mental status, irregular pulse or B/P) has been noted.

## NURSING CONSIDERATIONS

**BASELINE ASSESSMENT**
Assess pt's behavior, appearance, emotional status, response to environment, speech pattern, thought content. EKG should be obtained to assess for QT prolongation before instituting medication.

**INTERVENTION/EVALUATION**
Monitor for orthostatic hypotension; assist with ambulation. Monitor for fine tongue movement (may be first sign of tardive dyskinesia, possibly irreversible). Monitor serum potassium, magnesium in pts at risk for electrolyte disturbances. Assess for therapeutic response (greater interest in surroundings, improved self-care, increased ability to concentrate, relaxed facial expression).

**PATIENT/FAMILY TEACHING**
• Avoid tasks that require alertness, motor skills until response to drug is established. • Be alert to symptoms of orthostatic hypotension; slowly go from lying to standing. • Report if feeling faint,

experience heart palpitations or if fever or muscle rigidity occurs. • Report extrapyramidal symptoms (e.g., involuntary muscle movements, tics) immediately.

## imatinib

im-**at**-in-ib
(Gleevec)
**Do not confuse imatinib with dasatininb, erlotinib, lapatinib, nilotinib, sorafenib, or sunitinib.**

### ◆CLASSIFICATION

**PHARMACOTHERAPEUTIC:** Protein tyrosine kinase inhibitor. **CLINICAL:** Antineoplastic.

## USES

Newly diagnosed chronic-phase Philadelphia chromosome positive chronic myeloid leukemia (Ph+ CML) in children and adults. Pts in blast crisis, accelerated phase, or chronic phase Ph+ CML who have already failed interferon therapy. Adults with relapsed or refractory Ph+ acute lymphoblastic leukemia (ALL). Treatment in children with Ph+ ALL. Adults with myelodysplastic/myeloproliferative disease (MDS/MPD) associated with platelet-derived growth factor receptor (PDGFR) gene rearrangements. Adults with aggressive systemic mastocytosis (ASM) without mutation of the D816V c-Kit or unknown mutation status of the c-Kit. Adults with hypereosinophilic syndrome (HES) and/or chronic eosinophilic leukemia (CEL) with positive, negative, or unknown FIP1L1-PDGFR fusion kinase. Adults with dermatofibrosarcoma protuberans (DFSP) that is unresectable, recurrent, and/or metastatic. Pts with malignant gastrointestinal stromal tumors (GIST) that are unresectable and/or metastatic. Prevention of cancer recurrence in pts following surgical removal of GIST. **OFF-LABEL:** Treatment of desmoid tumors (soft tissue sarcoma). Post–stem cell transplant

(allogenic), follow-up treatment in recurrent CML. Treatment of advanced or metastatic melanoma.

## PRECAUTIONS

**Contraindications:** Hypersensitivity to imatinib. **Cautions:** Hepatic/renal impairment, thyroidectomy pts, hypothyroidism, gastric surgery pts. Pts in whom fluid accumulation is poorly tolerated (e.g., HF, hypertension, pulmonary disease).

## ACTION

Inhibits Bcr-Abl tyrosine kinase, an enzyme created by Philadelphia chromosome abnormality found in pts with chronic myeloid leukemia. **Therapeutic Effect:** Suppresses tumor growth during the three stages of CML: blast crisis, accelerated phase, chronic phase. Induces apoptosis.

## PHARMACOKINETICS

Well absorbed after PO administration. Protein binding: 95%. Metabolized in liver. Eliminated in feces (68%), urine (13%). **Half-life:** 18 hrs; metabolite, 40 hrs.

## 🔲 LIFESPAN CONSIDERATIONS

**Pregnancy/Lactation:** May cause fetal harm. Breastfeeding not recommended. **Children:** Safety and efficacy not established. **Elderly:** Increased frequency of fluid retention.

## INTERACTIONS

**DRUG: CYP3A4 inducers (e.g., carbamazepine, phenytoin, rifampin)** may decrease concentration. **CYP3A4 inhibitors (e.g., clarithromycin, erythromycin, ketoconazole)** may increase concentration. **Bone marrow depressants (e.g., alemtuzumab, methotrexate)** may increase myelosuppression. **Live virus vaccines** may potentiate virus replication, increase vaccine side effects, decrease pt's antibody response to vaccine. May reduce effect of **warfarin. HERBAL: St. John's wort** decreases concentration. **FOOD: Grapefruit products** may increase concentration. **LAB VALUES:** May increase serum bilirubin, ALT, AST, creatinine. May decrease platelet count, RBC, WBC count; serum potassium, albumin, calcium.

## AVAILABILITY (Rx)

Tablets: 100 mg, 400 mg.

## ADMINISTRATION/HANDLING

### PO

• Give with a meal and large glass of water. • Tablets may be dispersed in water or apple juice (stir until dissolved; give immediately). Do not crush or chew tablets.

## INDICATIONS/ROUTES/DOSAGE

**Ph+ Chronic Myeloid Leukemia (CML) (Chronic Phase)**
PO: ADULTS, ELDERLY: 400 mg once daily; may increase to 600 mg/day. CHILDREN: 340 mg/m²/day. **Maximum:** 600 mg.

**Ph+ CML (Accelerated Phase)**
PO: ADULTS, ELDERLY: 600 mg once daily. May increase to 800 mg/day in 2 divided doses (400 mg twice daily). CHILDREN: 340 mg/m²/day. **Maximum:** 600 mg.

**Ph+ Acute Lymphoblastic Leukemia (ALL)**
PO: ADULTS, ELDERLY: 600 mg once daily.

**Gastrointestinal Stromal Tumors (GIST) (Following Complete Resection)**
PO: ADULTS, ELDERLY: 400–600 mg/day.

**GIST (Unresectable)**
PO: ADULTS, ELDERLY: 400–800 mg/day.

**Aggressive Systemic Mastocytosis (ASM) with Eosinophilia**
PO: ADULTS, ELDERLY: Initially, 100 mg/day. May increase up to 400 mg/day.

**ASM without Mutation of the D816V C-Kit or Unknown Mutation Status of C-Kit**
PO: ADULTS, ELDERLY: 400 mg once daily.

**Dermatofibrosarcoma Protuberans (DFSP)**
PO: ADULTS, ELDERLY: 400 mg twice daily.

**Hypereosinophilic Syndrome (HES)/ Chronic Eosinophilic Leukemia (CEL)**
PO: ADULTS, ELDERLY: 400 mg once daily.

**HES/CEL with Positive or Unknown FIP1L1-PDGFR Fusion Kinase**
PO: ADULTS, ELDERLY: Initially, 100 mg/day. May increase up to 400 mg/day.

**Myelodysplastic/Myeloproliferative Disease (MDS/MPD)**
PO: ADULTS, ELDERLY: 400 mg once daily.

**Usual Dosage for Children (2 Yrs and Older)**
Ph+ CML (Chronic Phase, Recurrent or Resistant): 340 mg/m²/day. **Maximum:** 600 mg/day.
Ph+ CML (Chronic Phase, Newly Diagnosed, Ph+ ALL): 340 mg/m²/day. **Maximum:** 600 mg/day.

**Dosage with Strong CYP3A4 Inducers**
Increase dose by 50% with careful monitoring.

**Dosage in Renal Impairment**

| Creatinine Clearance | Maximum Dose |
| --- | --- |
| 40–59 ml/min | 600 mg |
| 20–39 ml/min | 400 mg |
| Less than 20 ml/min | 100 mg |

**Dosage in Hepatic Impairment**
**Mild to moderate impairment:** No adjustment. **Severe impairment:** Reduce dosage by 25%.

## SIDE EFFECTS

Frequent (68%–24%): Nausea, diarrhea, vomiting, headache, fluid retention, rash, musculoskeletal pain, muscle cramps, arthralgia. Occasional (23%–10%): Abdominal pain, cough, myalgia, fatigue, fever, anorexia, dyspepsia, constipation, night sweats, pruritus, dizziness, blurred vision, somnolence. Rare (less than 10%): Nasopharyngitis, petechiae, asthenia, epistaxis.

## ADVERSE EFFECTS/ TOXIC REACTIONS

Severe fluid retention (pleural effusion, pericardial effusion, pulmonary edema, ascites), hepatotoxicity occur rarely. Neutropenia, thrombocytopenia are expected responses to the therapy. Respiratory toxicity is manifested as dyspnea, pneumonia. Heart damage (left ventricular dysfunction, HF) may occur.

## NURSING CONSIDERATIONS

### BASELINE ASSESSMENT

Obtain baseline CBC, serum chemistries, renal function test. Monitor LFT before beginning treatment, monthly thereafter.

### INTERVENTION/EVALUATION

Assess periorbital area, lower extremities for early evidence of fluid retention. Monitor for unexpected, rapid weight gain. Offer antiemetics to control nausea, vomiting. Monitor daily pattern of bowel activity, stool consistency. Monitor CBC wkly for first mo, biweekly for second mo, periodically thereafter for evidence of neutropenia, thrombocytopenia; assess hepatic function tests for hepatotoxicity. Monitor renal function, serum electrolytes. Duration of neutropenia or thrombocytopenia ranges from 2–4 wks.

### PATIENT/FAMILY TEACHING

• Avoid crowds, those with known infection. • Avoid contact with anyone who recently received live virus vaccine; do not receive vaccinations. • Take with food and a full glass of water. • Avoid grapefruit products. • Report chest pain, swelling of extremities, weight gain greater than 5 lb, easy bruising/bleeding. • Avoid tasks that require alertness, motor skills until response to drug is established.

## imipenem/cilastatin

im-i-**pen**-em/sye-la-**stat**-in
(Primaxin)
**Do not confuse imipenem with doripenem, ertapenem, or meropenem, or Primaxin with Premarin or Primacor.**

## ◆CLASSIFICATION

**PHARMACOTHERAPEUTIC:** Fixed-combination carbapenem. **CLINICAL:** Antibiotic.

## USES

Treatment of susceptible infections due to gram-negative (ESBL *Escherichia coli* and *Klebsiella, Enterobacter* spp. PsAs), gram-positive (MSSA, *Streptococcus* spp.), anaerobic organisms including respiratory tract, skin/skin structure, gynecologic, bone, joint, intra-abdominal, complicated or uncomplicated UTIs; endocarditis (caused by *S. aureus*); polymicrobic infections; septicemia; serious nosocomial infections. **OFF-LABEL:** Hepatic abscess, neutropenic fever, melioidosis.

## PRECAUTIONS

**Contraindications:** Hypersensitivity to imipenem/cilastatin. **Cautions:** CNS disorders (e.g., brain lesions and history of seizures), sensitivity to beta-lactams (e.g., penicillins, cephalosporins), renal impairment, elderly.

## ACTION

**Imipenem:** Penetrates bacterial cell membrane, inhibiting cell wall synthesis. **Cilastatin:** Competitively inhibits the enzyme dehydropeptidase, preventing renal metabolism of imipenem. **Therapeutic Effect:** Produces bacterial cell death.

## PHARMACOKINETICS

Readily absorbed after IM administration. Protein binding: **Imipenem:** 20%; **Cilastatin:** 40%. Widely distributed. Metabolized in kidneys. Primarily excreted in urine. Removed by hemodialysis. **Half-life:** 1 hr (increased in renal impairment).

## ☒ LIFESPAN CONSIDERATIONS

**Pregnancy/Lactation:** Crosses placenta. Distributed in cord blood, amniotic fluid, breast milk. **Children:** No precautions noted. **Elderly:** Age-related renal impairment may require dosage adjustment.

---

## INTERACTIONS

**DRUG:** May decrease concentration of **valproic acid. HERBAL:** None significant. **FOOD:** None known. **LAB VALUES:** May increase serum alkaline phosphatase, BUN, bilirubin, creatinine, LDH, ALT, AST. May decrease Hgb, Hct.

## AVAILABILITY (Rx)

**Injection, Powder for Reconstitution (Primaxin):** 250 mg, 500 mg.

## ADMINISTRATION/HANDLING

 IV

**Reconstitution** • Dilute each 250- or 500-mg vial with 100–250 ml D₅W or 0.9% NaCl. Final concentration not to exceed 5 mg/ml.
**Rate of Administration** • Give by intermittent IV infusion (piggyback). • Do not give IV push. • Infuse over 20–30 min (doses greater than 500 mg over 40–60 min). • Observe pt during initial 30 min of first-time infusion for possible hypersensitivity reaction.
**Storage** • Solution appears colorless to yellow; discard if solution turns brown. • IV infusion (piggyback) is stable for 4 hrs at room temperature, 24 hrs if refrigerated. • Discard if precipitate forms.

## IV INCOMPATIBILITIES

Allopurinol (Aloprim), amphotericin B complex (Abelcet, AmBisome, Amphotec), fluconazole (Diflucan).

## IV COMPATIBILITIES

Diltiazem (Cardizem), insulin, propofol (Diprivan).

## INDICATIONS/ROUTES/DOSAGE

**Usual Dosage Ranges**
**IV: ADULTS, ELDERLY, WEIGHING 70 KG OR MORE:** 250 mg q6h up to 1,000 mg q6h.
**60–69 KG:** 250 mg q8h up to 1 g q8h.
**50–59 KG:** 125 mg q6h up to 750 mg q8h.
**40–49 KG:** 125 mg q6h up to 500 mg q8h.
**30–39 KG:** 125 mg q8h up to 500 mg q8h.
**CHILDREN OLDER THAN 3 MOS–12 YRS:** 15–25 mg/kg q6h. **Maximum:** 4 g/day.
**CHILDREN 1–3 MOS:** 25 mg/kg q6h. **CHILDREN 1–4 WKS:** 20–25 mg/kg q8h. **CHILDREN YOUNGER THAN 1 WK:** 20–25 mg/kg q12h.

**Dosage in Renal Impairment**
Dosage and frequency are modified based on creatinine clearance and severity of infection. (See table.)

**Dosage in Hepatic Impairment**
Consider reducing dose frequency.

| Creatinine Clearance (ml/min) | 70 kg or greater | 60–69 kg | 50–59 kg | 40–49 kg | 30–39 kg |
|---|---|---|---|---|---|
| 41–70 | 250 mg q8h– 750 mg q8h | 125 mg q6h– 750 mg q8h | 125 mg q6h– 500 mg q6h | 125 mg q6h– 500 mg q8h | 125 mg q8h– 250 mg q6h |
| 21–40 | 250 mg q12h– 500 mg q6h | 250 mg q12h– 500 mg q8h | 125 mg q8h– 500 mg q8h | 125 mg q12h– 250 mg q6h | 125 mg q12h– 250 mg q8h |
| 6–20 | 250 mg q12h– 500 mg q12h | 125 mg q12h– 500 mg q12h | 125 mg q12h– 500 mg q12h | 125 mg q12h– 250 mg q12h | 125 mg q12h– 250 mg q12h |

## SIDE EFFECTS

**Occasional (3%):** Diarrhea, nausea, vomiting. **Rare (1%):** Rash.

## ADVERSE EFFECTS/ TOXIC REACTIONS

Antibiotic-associated colitis, other superinfections (abdominal cramps, severe watery diarrhea, fever) may result from altered bacterial balance in GI tract. Anaphylactic reactions have been reported.

## NURSING CONSIDERATIONS

### BASELINE ASSESSMENT

Question for history of allergies, particularly to beta-lactams, penicillins, cephalosporins. Inquire about history of seizures.

## INTERVENTION/EVALUATION

Monitor renal, hepatic, hematologic function tests. Evaluate for phlebitis (heat, pain, red streaking over vein), pain at IV injection site. Assess for GI discomfort, nausea, vomiting. Monitor daily pattern of bowel activity, stool consistency. Assess skin for rash. Be alert to tremors, possible seizures.

# imipramine

i-**mip**-ra-meen
Novo-Pramine ✤, Tofranil, Tofranil-PM)

■ **BLACK BOX ALERT** ■ Increased risk of suicidal ideation and behavior in children, adolescents, young adults 18–24 yrs with major depressive disorder, other psychiatric disorders. **Do not confuse imipramine with amitriptyline, desipramine, or Norpramin.**

◆**CLASSIFICATION**

**PHARMACOTHERAPEUTIC:** Tricyclic antidepressant. **CLINICAL:** Antidepressant, antineuritic, antipanic, antineuralgic, antinarcoleptic adjunct, anticataplectic, antibulimic.

## USES

Treatment of depression. Treatment of nocturnal enuresis in children older than 6 yrs. **OFF-LABEL:** Treatment of attention-deficit/hyperactivity disorder (ADHD), post-traumatic stress disorder (PTSD), neurogenic pain, panic disorder.

## PRECAUTIONS

**Contraindications:** Hypersensitivity to imipramine. Acute recovery period after MI, use within 14 days of MAOIs; initiation of imipramine in pts with concurrent use with linezolid or IV methylene blue. **Cautions:** Prostatic hypertrophy; history of urinary retention, history of bowel obstruction; glaucoma, diabetes mellitus, history of seizures, hyperthyroidism; cardiac, hepatic, renal disease; increased intraocular pressure, pts with high risk for suicide. Decreased GI motility, paralytic ileus, visual problems, respiratory disease, elderly.

## ACTION

Blocks reuptake of neurotransmitters (norepinephrine, serotonin) at presynaptic membranes, increasing concentration at postsynaptic receptor sites. **Therapeutic Effect:** Relieves depression, controls nocturnal enuresis.

## INTERACTIONS

**DRUG: Alcohol, other CNS depressants (e.g., diphenhydramine, lorazepam, morphine)** may increase hypotensive effects, CNS, respiratory depression. **Cimetidine, fluoxetine** may increase concentration, risk of toxicity. **Phenytoin, barbiturates** may decrease concentration. **HERBAL: Kava kava, SAMe, St. John's wort, valerian** may increase risk of serotonin syndrome, CNS depression. **St. John's wort** may decrease concentration. **FOOD: Grapefruit products** may increase concentration/toxicity. **LAB VALUES:** May alter serum glucose, EKG readings. **Therapeutic serum level:** 225–300 ng/ml; **toxic serum level:** greater than 500 ng/ml.

## AVAILABILITY (Rx)

**Capsules (Tofranil-PM):** 75 mg, 100 mg, 125 mg, 150 mg. **Tablets (Tofranil):** 10 mg, 25 mg, 50 mg.

## ADMINISTRATION/HANDLING

**PO**
• Give with food, milk if GI distress occurs.

## INDICATIONS/ROUTES/DOSAGE

**Depression**
**PO: ADULTS: (Outpatient):** Initially, 75 mg/day. May gradually increase to 150 mg/day as single dose at bedtime or in divided doses. **Maintenance:** 50–150 mg/day. **Maximum:** 200 mg/day. **(Inpatient):** Initially, 100–150 mg/day. May increase to 200 mg/day. May further increase to 250–300 mg/day after 2 wks. May give as single dose at bedtime or

in divided doses. **Maximum:** 300 mg/day. Initially, 75–100 mg/day in 3–4 divided doses. May gradually increase to maximum of 200 mg/day (outpatient) or 300 mg/day (inpatient). **ELDERLY, ADOLESCENTS:** Initially, 25–50 mg/day at bedtime. May increase by 10–25 mg every 3–7 days. **Maximum:** 100 mg/day. **CHILDREN:** 1.5 mg/kg/day. May increase by 1 mg/kg every 3–4 days. **Maximum:** 5 mg/kg/day in 1–4 divided doses.

**Enuresis**
**PO: CHILDREN, 6 YRS AND OLDER:** Initially, 25 mg 1 hr before bedtime. May increase by 25 mg if inadequate response seen after 1 wk. **Maximum:** 2.5 mg/kg/day or 50 mg at bedtime for ages 6–12 yrs; 75 mg at bedtime for ages over 12 yrs.

**Dosage in Renal/Hepatic Impairment**
No dose adjustment.

## SIDE EFFECTS

**Frequent:** Drowsiness, fatigue, dry mouth, blurred vision, constipation, delayed micturition, orthostatic hypotension, diaphoresis, impaired concentration, increased appetite, urinary retention, photosensitivity. **Occasional:** GI disturbances (nausea, metallic taste). **Rare:** Paradoxical reactions (agitation, restlessness, nightmares, insomnia), extrapyramidal symptoms (EPS) (particularly fine hand tremor).

## ADVERSE EFFECTS/ TOXIC REACTIONS

Overdose may produce seizures, cardiovascular effects (severe orthostatic hypotension, dizziness, tachycardia, palpitations, arrhythmias). May result in altered temperature regulation (hyperpyrexia, hypothermia). Abrupt withdrawal from prolonged therapy may produce headache, malaise, nausea, vomiting, vivid dreams.

## NURSING CONSIDERATIONS

### BASELINE ASSESSMENT

Assess appearance, behavior, speech pattern, level of interest, mood. Obtain renal function, LFT.

### INTERVENTION/EVALUATION

Supervise suicidal-risk pt closely during early therapy (as depression lessens, energy level improves, increasing suicide potential). Monitor appearance, behavior, speech pattern, level of interest, mood. For pts on long-term therapy, hepatic/renal function tests, blood counts should be performed periodically. Monitor daily pattern of bowel activity, stool consistency. Monitor B/P, pulse for hypotension, arrhythmias. Assess for urinary retention by bladder palpation. **Therapeutic serum level:** 225–300 ng/ml; **toxic serum level:** greater than 500 ng/ml.

### PATIENT/FAMILY TEACHING

• Report worsening depression, thoughts of suicide, agitation, irritability. • Slowly go from lying to standing to avoid hypotensive effect. • Tolerance to postural hypotension, sedative, anticholinergic effects usually develops during early therapy. • Avoid tasks that require alertness, motor skills until response to drug is established. • Therapeutic effect may be noted within 2–5 days, maximum effect within 2–3 wks. • Sugarless gum, sips of water may relieve dry mouth. • Do not abruptly discontinue medication. • Limit caffeine; avoid alcohol.

## immune globulin IV (IGIV)

im-**mune glob**-u-lin
(Bivigam, Carimune NF, Flebogamma DIF, Gammagard Liquid, Gammagard S/D, Gammaplex, Gamunex-C, Hizentra, Octagam 5%, Privigen)
■ **BLACK BOX ALERT** ■ Acute renal impairment characterized by increased serum creatinine, oliguria, acute renal failure, osmotic nephrosis, particularly pts with any degree of renal insufficiency, diabetes mellitus, volume depletion, sepsis, and those older than age 65 yrs. Thrombosis may occur.

## ◆CLASSIFICATION

**PHARMACOTHERAPEUTIC:** Immune globulin, blood product. **CLINICAL:** Immunizing agent.

## USES

Treatment of pts with primary humoral immunodeficiency syndromes, acute/chronic immune idiopathic thrombocytopenic purpura (ITP), prevention of coronary artery aneurysms associated with Kawasaki disease, prevention of recurrent bacterial infections in pts with hypogammaglobulinemia associated with B-cell chronic lymphocytic leukemia (CLL). Treatment of chronic inflammatory demyelinating polyneuropathies. Provide passive immunity in pts with hepatitis A, measles, rubella, varicella. **OFF-LABEL:** Guillain-Barré syndrome; myasthenia gravis; prevention of acute infections in immunosuppressed pts; prevention, treatment of infection in high-risk, preterm, low-birth-weight neonates; treatment of multiple sclerosis, HIV-associated thrombocytopenia.

## PRECAUTIONS

**Contraindications:** Hypersensitivity to immune globulin. Selective IgA deficiency, hyperprolinemia (Hizentra, Privigen), severe thrombocytopenia, coagulation disorders where IM injections contraindicated. **Cautions:** Cardiovascular disease, history of thrombosis, renal impairment.

## ACTION

Replacement therapy for primary/secondary immunodeficiencies and IgG antibodies against bacteria, viral antigens; interferes with receptors on cells of reticuloendothelial system for autoimmune cytopenias/idiopathic thrombocytopenia purpura (ITP); increases antibody titer and antigen-antibody reaction potential. **Therapeutic Effect:** Provides passive immunity replacement for immunodeficiencies, increases antibody titer.

## PHARMACOKINETICS

Evenly distributed between intravascular and extravascular space. **Half-life:** 21–23 days.

## ⏳ LIFESPAN CONSIDERATIONS

**Pregnancy/Lactation:** Unknown if drug crosses placenta or is distributed in breast milk. **Children/Elderly:** No age-related precautions noted.

## INTERACTIONS

**DRUG: Live virus vaccines** may increase vaccine side effects, potentiate virus replication, decrease pt's antibody response to vaccine. **HERBAL:** None significant. **FOOD:** None known. **LAB VALUES:** None significant.

## AVAILABILITY (Rx)

Injection, Powder for Reconstitution (Carimune NF): 3 g, 6 g, 12 g. (Gammagard S/D): 5 g, 10 g. Injection, Solution (Bivigam 10%, Flebogamma DIF 5%, 10%, Gammagard Liquid 10%, Gammaplex 5%, Gamunex-C 10%, Octagam 5%, Privigen 10%).

## ADMINISTRATION/HANDLING

 IV

◀**ALERT**▶ Monitor vital signs, B/P diligently during and immediately after IV administration (precipitous fall in B/P may indicate anaphylactic reaction). Stop infusion immediately. Epinephrine should be readily available.

**Reconstitution •** Reconstitute only with diluent provided by manufacturer. • Discard partially used or turbid preparations.

**Rate of Administration •** Give by infusion only. • After reconstitution, administer via separate tubing. • Rate of infusion varies with product used.

**Storage •** Refer to individual IV preparations for storage requirements, stability after reconstitution.

## 🔲 IV INCOMPATIBILITIES

Do not mix with any other medications.

---

## INDICATIONS/ROUTES/DOSAGE

### Primary Immunodeficiency Syndrome
**IV: ADULTS, ELDERLY, CHILDREN:** *(Privigen):* 200–800 mg/kg q3–4wks. *(Carimune NF):* 400–800 mg/kg q3–4 wks. *(Flebogamma DIF, Gammagard, Gamunex-C, Octagam):* 300–600 mg/kg/q3–4wks. *(Bivigam, Gammaplex):* 300–800 mg/kg q3–4wks.

### Idiopathic Thrombocytopenic Purpura (ITP)
**IV: ADULTS, ELDERLY, CHILDREN:** *(Carimune NF):* 400 mg/kg/day for 2–5 days. **Maintenance:** 400–1,000 mg/kg/dose to maintain platelet count or control bleeding. *(Gammagard):* **1,000 MG/KG:** up to 3 additional doses may be given on alternate days.

### Kawasaki Disease
**Note:** Must be used with aspirin.
**IV: ADULTS, ELDERLY, CHILDREN:** *(Gammagard):* 1,000 mg/kg as single dose or 400 mg/kg/day for 4 consecutive days. Begin within 7 days of onset of fever. **American Heart Association Guidelines:** 2,000 mg/kg as a single dose given over 10–12 hrs within 10 days of disease onset.

### Chronic Leukocytic Leukemia (CLL)
**IV: ADULTS, ELDERLY, CHILDREN:** *(Gammagard):* 400 mg/kg/dose q3–4wks.

### Chronic Inflammatory Demyelinating Polyneuropathy
**IV: ADULTS, ELDERLY, CHILDREN:** *(Gamunex-C):* 2,000 mg/kg divided over 2–4 days (consecutive). **Maintenance:** 1,000 mg/kg/day q3wks or 500 mg/kg for 2 consecutive days q3wks.

### Dosage in Renal Impairment
Caution when giving IV.

### Dosage in Hepatic Impairment
No dose adjustment.

## SIDE EFFECTS

**Frequent:** Tachycardia, backache, headache, arthralgia, myalgia. **Occasional:** Fatigue, wheezing, injection site rash/pain, leg cramps, urticaria, bluish color of lips/nailbeds, light-headedness.

## ADVERSE EFFECTS/ TOXIC REACTIONS

Anaphylactic reactions occur rarely but incidence increases with repeated injections. Epinephrine should be readily available. Overdose may produce chest tightness, chills, diaphoresis, dizziness, facial flushing, nausea, vomiting, fever, hypotension. Hypersensitivity reaction (anxiety, arthralgia, dizziness, flushing, myalgia, palpitations, pruritus) occurs rarely.

## NURSING CONSIDERATIONS

### BASELINE ASSESSMENT
Inquire about exposure history to disease for pt/family as appropriate. Have epinephrine readily available. Pt should be well hydrated prior to administration.

### INTERVENTION/EVALUATION
Control rate of IV infusion carefully; too-rapid infusion increases risk of precipitous fall in B/P, signs of anaphylaxis (facial flushing, chest tightness, chills, fever, nausea, vomiting, diaphoresis). Assess pt closely during infusion, esp. first hr; monitor vital signs continuously. Stop infusion if aforementioned signs noted. For treatment of idiopathic thrombocytopenic purpura (ITP), monitor platelet count.

### PATIENT/FAMILY TEACHING
• Explain rationale for therapy. • Report sudden weight gain, fluid retention, edema, decreased urine output, shortness of breath.

# indacaterol

in-da-ka-ter-ol
(Arcapta Neohaler, Onbrez Breezhaler ✦)

■ **BLACK BOX ALERT** ■ Long-acting beta₂-adrenergic agonists (LABAs) have an increased risk of asthma-related deaths. Not indicated for treatment of asthma.

## ◆CLASSIFICATION

**PHARMACOTHERAPEUTIC:** Long-acting beta₂-adrenergic agonist. **CLINICAL:** Bronchodilator.

## USES

Long-term maintenance treatment of airflow obstruction in pts with chronic obstructive pulmonary disease (COPD), including chronic bronchitis and emphysema.

## PRECAUTIONS

◀ALERT▶ Not indicated for the treatment of asthma, acute exacerbations of COPD.
**Contraindications:** Hypersensitivity to indacaterol. Monotherapy in treatment of asthma. **Cautions:** Cardiovascular disease (coronary insufficiency, arrhythmias, hypertension, history of hypersensitivity to sympathomimetics), seizure disorders, hyperthyroidism, hypokalemia, diabetes mellitus. May cause paradoxical bronchospasm, severe asthma.

## ACTION

Stimulates beta₂-adrenergic receptors in lungs, resulting in relaxation of bronchial smooth muscle. **Therapeutic Effect:** Relieves bronchospasm, reduces airway resistance, improves bronchodilation.

## PHARMACOKINETICS

Extensive activation of systemic beta-adrenergic receptors; acts primarily in lungs. Protein binding: 94%–95%. Metabolized in liver. Steady-state level: 12–15 days. Primarily excreted in feces. **Half-life:** 45–126 hrs.

## ⧖ LIFESPAN CONSIDERATIONS

**Pregnancy/Lactation:** Unknown if drug crosses placenta or is distributed in breast milk. **Children:** Safety and efficacy not established. **Elderly:** May be more sensitive to tremor, tachycardia due to age-related increased sympathetic sensitivity.

## INTERACTIONS

**DRUG:** May decrease effectiveness of **beta blockers** (e.g., **carvedilol, metoprolol**). Diuretics (e.g., furosemide, HCTZ), corticosteroids (e.g., dexamethasone, prednisone), xanthine derivatives may increase risk of hypokalemia. **Drugs that can prolong QT interval** (e.g., erythromycin, quinidine, thioridazine), antiarrhythmics (e.g., amiodarone), **MAOIs, tricyclic antidepressants** (e.g., **amitriptyline, doxepin**) may potentiate cardiovascular effects (increased risk of ventricular arrhythmias). **Erythromycin, ketoconazole, ritonavir, verapamil** may increase serum concentration. **HERBAL:** None significant. **FOOD:** None known. **LAB VALUES:** May decrease serum potassium. May increase serum glucose.

## AVAILABILITY (Rx)

**Powder for Inhalation:** 75 mcg (in blister packs).

## ADMINISTRATION/HANDLING

**Inhalation**
• Open cap of Neohaler by pulling upward, then open mouthpiece. • Remove capsule from blister package and place in center of chamber. Firmly close until click is heard. • Hold inhaler upright and pierce capsule by pressing side buttons once only. • Instruct pt to exhale completely. Place mouthpiece into mouth, close lips, and inhale quickly and deeply through mouth (this causes capsule to spin, dispensing the drug). A slight whirring noise should occur. If not, this may indicate capsule is stuck. Gently tap inhaler to loosen and reattempt. • Pt should hold breath as long as possible before exhaling. • Check capsule to ensure all the powder is gone. Instruct pt to reinhale if powder remains.
**Storage** • Store at room temperature. • Maintain capsules within individual blister pack until time of use. • Do not store capsules in Neohaler device.

## INDICATIONS/ROUTES/DOSAGE

**Maintenance Therapy and Prevention of COPD**
**Inhalation: ADULTS, ELDERLY:** 75 mcg (1 capsule) once daily via Neohaler inhalation device.

**Dosage in Renal/Hepatic Impairment**
No dose adjustment.

## SIDE EFFECTS

**Occasional (7%–5%):** Cough, nasopharyngitis, headache. **Rare (2%):** Oropharyngeal pain, nausea.

## ADVERSE EFFECTS/ TOXIC REACTIONS

Peripheral edema, diabetes mellitus, hyperglycemia, sinusitis, URI reported in greater than 2% of pts. Excessive sympathomimetic stimulation, hypokalemia may produce palpitations, arrhythmias, angina pectoris, tachycardia, muscle cramps, weakness. Hyperglycemia symptoms present with increased thirst, polyuria, dry mouth, drowsiness/confusion, blurred vision. Severe shortness of breath may indicate paradoxical bronchospasm, deteriorating COPD. Serious asthma-related events including death reported.

## NURSING CONSIDERATIONS

### BASELINE ASSESSMENT

Assess rate, depth, rhythm, type of respirations. Monitor EKG, serum potassium, ABG determinations, $O_2$ saturation, pulmonary function test. Assess lung sounds for wheezing (bronchoconstriction), rales. Obtain baseline electrolytes, blood glucose. Receive full medication history and screen for possible drug interactions. Question for history of asthma, angina pectoris, diabetes mellitus, peripheral edema.

### INTERVENTION/EVALUATION

Routinely monitor serum electrolytes, blood glucose, $O_2$ saturation. Recommend

discontinuation of short-acting beta$_2$-agonists (use only for symptomatic relief of acute respiratory symptoms). Monitor for palpitations, tachycardia, serum hypokalemia. Inspect oropharyngeal cavity for irritation.

### PATIENT/FAMILY TEACHING

• Follow manufacturer guidelines for proper use of inhaler. • Increase fluid intake (decreases lung secretion viscosity). • Rinse mouth with water after inhalation to decrease mouth/throat irritation. • Avoid excessive use of caffeine derivatives (chocolate, coffee, tea, cola). • An immediate cough lasting 15 sec may occur after inhaler use. • Report any fever, productive cough, body aches, difficulty breathing.

# indapamide

in-**dap**-a-mide
(Apo-Indapamide ✤, Lozide ✤, Novo-Indapamide ✤)
**Do not confuse indapamide with lopidine.**

## ◆CLASSIFICATION

**PHARMACOTHERAPEUTIC:** Thiazide.
**CLINICAL:** Diuretic, antihypertensive.

## USES

Management of mild to moderate hypertension. Treatment of edema associated with HF. **OFF-LABEL:** Calcium nephrolithiasis.

## PRECAUTIONS

**Contraindications:** Hypersensitivity to indapamide. Anuria, sulfonamide-derived drugs. **Cautions:** History of hypersensitivity to sulfonamides or thiazide diuretics. Severe renal disease, hepatic impairment, prediabetes, diabetes mellitus, elderly, severe hyponatremia, elevated serum cholesterol.

## ACTION

**Diuretic:** Blocks reabsorption of water, sodium, potassium at cortical diluting segment of distal renal tubule. **Antihypertensive:** Reduces plasma, extracellular fluid volume, and peripheral vascular resistance by direct effect on blood vessels. **Therapeutic Effect:** Promotes diuresis, reduces B/P.

## PHARMACOKINETICS

Almost completely absorbed following PO administration. Protein binding: 71%–79%. Metabolized in liver. Eliminated in urine. **Half-life:** 14–18 hrs.

## ⌛ LIFESPAN CONSIDERATIONS

**Pregnancy/Lactation:** Unknown if drug crosses placenta or is distributed in breast milk. **Children:** Safety and efficacy not established. **Elderly:** May be more sensitive to hypotensive, electrolyte effects.

## INTERACTIONS

**DRUG:** May increase risk of **lithium** toxicity. **HERBAL: Ephedra, ginseng, licorice, yohimbe** may worsen hypertension. **Black cohosh** may increase antihypertensive effect. **FOOD:** None known. **LAB VALUES:** May increase plasma renin activity. May decrease protein-bound iodine; serum calcium, potassium, sodium.

## AVAILABILITY (Rx)

**Tablets:** 1.25 mg, 2.5 mg.

## ADMINISTRATION/HANDLING

### PO

• Give with food, milk if GI upset occurs, preferably with breakfast (may prevent nocturia).

## INDICATIONS/ROUTES/DOSAGE

**Edema**
**PO: ADULTS:** Initially, 2.5 mg/day, may increase to 5 mg/day after 1 wk.

**Hypertension**
**PO: ADULTS, ELDERLY:** Initially, 1.25 mg. May increase to 2.5 mg/day after 4 wks or 5 mg/day after additional 4 wks. Usual dose: 1.25–2.5 mg/day.

**Dosage in Renal/Hepatic Impairment**
Use caution.

## SIDE EFFECTS

**Frequent (5% and greater):** Fatigue, paresthesia of extremities, tension, irritability, agitation, headache, dizziness, lightheadedness, insomnia, muscle cramps. **Occasional (less than 5%):** Urinary frequency, urticaria, rhinorrhea, flushing, weight loss, orthostatic hypotension, depression, blurred vision, nausea, vomiting, diarrhea, constipation, dry mouth, impotence, rash, pruritus.

## ADVERSE EFFECTS/ TOXIC REACTIONS

Vigorous diuresis may lead to profound water and electrolyte depletion, resulting in hypokalemia, hyponatremia, dehydration. Acute hypotensive episodes may occur. Hyperglycemia may be noted during prolonged therapy. Pancreatitis, blood dyscrasias, pulmonary edema, allergic pneumonitis, dermatologic reactions occur rarely. Overdose can lead to lethargy, coma without changes in electrolytes or hydration.

## NURSING CONSIDERATIONS

### BASELINE ASSESSMENT

Check vital signs, esp. B/P for hypotension, before administration. Assess baseline electrolytes, particularly hypokalemia. Observe for edema; assess skin turgor, mucous membranes for hydration status. Assess muscle strength, mental status. Note skin temperature, moisture. Obtain baseline weight. Initiate I&O.

### INTERVENTION/EVALUATION

Continue to monitor B/P, vital signs, electrolytes, I&O, weight. Note extent of diuresis. Watch for electrolyte disturbances (hypokalemia may result in weakness, tremor, muscle cramps, nausea, vomiting, altered mental status, tachycardia; hyponatremia may result in confusion, thirst, cold/clammy skin).

---

✦ Canadian trade name    🐄 Non-Crushable Drug    🔲 High Alert drug

## PATIENT/FAMILY TEACHING

• Expect increased frequency, volume of urination. • To reduce hypotensive effect, go from lying to standing slowly. • Eat foods high in potassium such as whole grains (cereals), legumes, meat, bananas, apricots, orange juice, potatoes (white, sweet), raisins. • Take early in the day to avoid nocturia.

# indomethacin

in-doe-**meth**-a-sin
(Indocin, Novo-Methacin ✦,
Tivorbex)

■ **BLACK BOX ALERT** ■ Increased risk of serious cardiovascular thrombotic events, including myocardial infarction, CVA. Increased risk of severe GI reactions, including ulceration, bleeding, perforation.
**Do not confuse Indocin with Imodium, Minocin, or Vicodin.**

## ◆CLASSIFICATION

**PHARMACOTHERAPEUTIC:** NSAID.
**CLINICAL:** Anti-inflammatory, analgesic.

## USES

Treatment of active stages of rheumatoid arthritis, osteoarthritis, ankylosing spondylitis, acute gouty arthritis. Relieves acute bursitis, tendonitis. **(Tivorbex):** Treatment of mild to moderate acute pain in adults. **(IV Form):** For closure of hemodynamically significant patent ductus arteriosus of premature infants. **OFF-LABEL:** Management of preterm labor.

## PRECAUTIONS

**Contraindications:** Hypersensitivity to aspirin, indomethacin, other NSAIDs. Perioperative pain in setting of CABG surgery. History of asthma, urticaria, allergic reactions after taking aspirin, other NSAIDs. **Suppositories:** History of proctitis, recent rectal bleeding. **Injection:** In preterm infants with untreated/systemic infection or congenital heart disease where patency of PDA

necessary for pulmonary or systemic blood flow; bleeding, thrombocytopenia, coagulation defects, necrotizing enterocolitis, significant renal dysfunction. **Cautions:** Cardiac dysfunction, fluid retention, HF, hypertension, renal/hepatic impairment, epilepsy; concurrent aspirin, steroids, anticoagulant therapy. Treatment of juvenile rheumatoid arthritis in children. History of GI disease (bleeding or ulcers), elderly, debilitated, asthma, depression, Parkinson's disease.

## ACTION

Produces antipyretic, analgesic, anti-inflammatory effects by inhibiting prostaglandin synthesis. **Therapeutic Effect:** Reduces inflammatory response, fever, intensity of pain. Closure of patent ductus arteriosus.

## PHARMACOKINETICS

| Route | Onset | Peak | Duration |
|-------|-------|------|----------|
| PO | 30 min | — | 4–6 hrs |

Well absorbed from GI tract. Protein binding: 99%. Metabolized in liver. Excreted in urine. **Half-life:** 4.5 hrs.

## ⌛ LIFESPAN CONSIDERATIONS

**Pregnancy/Lactation:** Crosses placenta; distributed in breast milk. **Children:** Safety and efficacy not established in those younger than 14 yrs. **Elderly:** GI bleeding, ulceration increase risk of serious adverse effects.

## INTERACTIONS

**DRUG:** May decrease effects of **antihypertensives (e.g., amlodipine, lisinopril, valsartan), diuretics (e.g., furosemide). Aspirin, other salicylates** may increase risk of GI side effects, bleeding. **Bone marrow depressants (e.g., alemtuzumab, methotrexate)** may increase risk of hematologic reactions. May increase risk of bleeding with **heparin, anticoagulants, thrombolytics.** May increase concentration, risk of toxicity of **lithium.** May increase risk of cyclosporine, methotrexate toxicity. **HERBAL:** Cat's claw, dong quai, evening primrose, feverfew, garlic, ginkgo, ginseng, horse chestnut, red clover may increase antiplatelet activity. **FOOD:** None known. **LAB VALUES:** May prolong bleeding time. May alter serum glucose. May increase serum BUN, creatinine, potassium, ALT, AST. May decrease serum sodium, platelet count, leukocytes.

## AVAILABILITY (Rx)

**Capsules:** 25 mg, 50 mg. **(Tivorbex):** 20 mg, 40 mg. **Injection, Powder for Reconstitution (Indocin IV):** 1 mg. **Oral Suspension (Indocin):** 25 mg/5 ml. **Suppository:** 50 mg.

🖤 **Capsules, Extended-Release:** 75 mg.

## ADMINISTRATION/HANDLING
🖤 IV

**Reconstitution •** To 1-mg vial, add 1–2 ml preservative-free Sterile Water for Injection or 0.9% NaCl to provide concentration of 1 mg/ml or 0.5 mg/ml, respectively. • Do not further dilute.
**Rate of Administration •** Administer over 20–30 min.
**Storage •** Use IV solution immediately following reconstitution. • IV solution appears clear; discard if cloudy or precipitate forms. • Discard unused portion.

### PO
• Give after meals or with food, antacids. • Do not break, crush, or open extended-release capsule. Swallow whole.

## 🖤 IV INCOMPATIBILITIES
Amino acid injection, calcium gluconate, dobutamine (Dobutrex), dopamine (Intropin), gentamicin (Garamycin), tobramycin (Nebcin).

## 🖤 IV COMPATIBILITIES
Insulin, potassium.

## INDICATIONS/ROUTES/DOSAGE
**Moderate to Severe Rheumatoid Arthritis (RA), Osteoarthritis, Ankylosing Spondylitis**
**PO: RECTAL: ADULTS, ELDERLY (Immediate-Release):** Initially, 25–50 mg 2–3 times/day; increased by 25–50 mg/wk up to 200 mg/day. **(Extended-Release):** Initially, 75 mg once daily. May increase to 75 mg twice daily. **Maximum:** 150 mg/day. **CHILDREN 2 YRS AND OLDER (Immediate-Release):** 1–2 mg/kg/day in 2–4 divided doses. **Maximum:** 4 mg/kg/day not to exceed 150–200 mg/day.

**Acute Gouty Arthritis**
**PO: ADULTS, ELDERLY (Immediate-Release):** 50 mg 3 times/day for 3–5 days.

**Acute Bursitis, Tendonitis**
**PO: RECTAL: ADULTS, ELDERLY: (Immediate-Release):** 75–150 mg/day in 3–4 divided doses for 7–14 days. **(Extended-Release):** 75–150 mg/day in 1–2 doses/day.

**Acute Pain**
**PO: ADULTS, ELDERLY: (Tivorbex):** 20 mg 3 times/day or 40 mg 2–3 times/day.

**Patent Ductus Arteriosus**
**IV: NEONATES:** Initially, 0.2 mg/kg. Subsequent doses are based on age, as follows: **NEONATES OLDER THAN 7 DAYS:** 0.25 mg/kg for 2nd and 3rd doses. **NEONATES 2–7 DAYS:** 0.2 mg/kg for 2nd and 3rd doses. **NEONATES LESS THAN 48 HRS:** 0.1 mg/kg for 2nd and 3rd doses. In general, dosing interval is 12 hrs if urine output is greater than 1 ml/kg/hr after prior dose, 24 hrs if urine output is less than 1 ml/kg/hr but greater than 0.6 ml/kg/hr. Dose is held if urine output is less than 0.6. ml/kg/hr or if neonate is anuric.

**Dosage in Renal Impairment**
**Mild to moderate impairment:** No dose adjustment. **Severe impairment:** Not recommended.

I

---

**Dosage in Hepatic Impairment**
Use caution.

## SIDE EFFECTS

**Frequent (11%–3%):** Headache, nausea, vomiting, dyspepsia, dizziness. **Occasional (less than 3%):** Depression, tinnitus, diaphoresis, drowsiness, constipation, diarrhea. **Patent ductus arteriosus:** Bleeding abnormalities. **Rare:** Hypertension, confusion, urticaria, pruritus, rash, blurred vision.

## ADVERSE EFFECTS/ TOXIC REACTIONS

Paralytic ileus, ulceration of esophagus, stomach, duodenum, small intestine may occur. Pts with renal impairment may develop hyperkalemia with worsening of renal impairment. May aggravate depression or other psychiatric disturbances, epilepsy, parkinsonism. Nephrotoxicity (dysuria, hematuria, proteinuria, nephrotic syndrome) occurs rarely. Metabolic acidosis/alkalosis, bradycardia occur rarely in neonates with patent ductus arteriosus.

## NURSING CONSIDERATIONS

### BASELINE ASSESSMENT

Assess onset, type, location, duration of pain, fever, inflammation. Inspect appearance of affected joints for immobility, deformities, skin condition.

### INTERVENTION/EVALUATION

Monitor serum BUN, creatinine, potassium, LFT. Monitor for evidence of nausea, dyspepsia. Assist with ambulation if dizziness occurs. Evaluate for therapeutic response: relief of pain, stiffness, swelling; increased joint mobility; reduced joint tenderness; improved grip strength. Observe for weight gain, edema, bleeding, bruising. In neonates, also monitor heart rate, heart sounds for murmur, B/P, urine output, EKG, serum sodium, glucose, platelets.

### PATIENT/FAMILY TEACHING

• Avoid aspirin, alcohol during therapy (increases risk of GI bleeding). • If GI upset occurs, take with food, milk.

• Avoid tasks that require alertness, motor skills until response to drug is established. • Report ringing in ears, persistent stomach pain, unusual bruising/bleeding.

---

## *inFLIXimab

in-**flix**-i-mab
(Remicade)

■ **BLACK BOX ALERT** ■ Risk of severe/fatal opportunistic infections (tuberculosis, sepsis, fungal), reactivation of latent infections. Rare cases of very aggressive, usually fatal hepatosplenic T-cell lymphoma reported in adolescents, young adults with Crohn's disease.
**Do not confuse infliximab with rituximab, or Remicade with Reminyl.**

## ◆CLASSIFICATION

**PHARMACOTHERAPEUTIC:** Monoclonal antibody. **CLINICAL:** GI anti-inflammatory.

## USES

In combination with methotrexate, reduces signs/symptoms, inhibits progression of structural damage, improves physical function in moderate to severe active rheumatoid arthritis (RA), psoriatic arthritis. Reduces signs/symptoms, induces and maintains remission in moderate to severe active Crohn's disease. Reduces number of draining enterocutaneous/rectovaginal fistulas, maintains fistula closure in fistulizing Crohn's disease. Reduces sign/symptoms of active ankylosing spondylitis. Treatment of chronic severe plaque psoriasis in pts who are candidates for systemic therapy. Reduces sign/symptoms, induces and maintains clinical remission and mucosal healing, eliminates corticosteroid use in moderate to severe active ulcerative colitis.

## PRECAUTIONS

**Contraindications:** Hypersensitivity to infliximab. Moderate to severe HF (doses greater than 5 mg/kg should be avoided).

---

Sensitivity to murine proteins, sepsis, serious active infection. **Cautions:** Hematologic abnormalities, history of COPD, pre-existing or recent onset CNS demyelinating disorders, seizures, mild HF, history of recurrent infections, conditions predisposing pt to infections (e.g., diabetes), pts exposed to tuberculosis, elderly, chronic hepatitis B virus infection.

## ACTION

Binds to tumor necrosis factor (TNF), inhibiting functional activity of TNF (induction of proinflammatory cytokines, enhanced leukocytic migration, activation of neutrophils/eosinophils). **Therapeutic Effect:** Prevents disease and allows diseased joints to heal.

## PHARMACOKINETICS

Absorbed into GI tissue; primarily distributed in vascular compartment. **Half-life:** 8–9.5 days.

## LIFESPAN CONSIDERATIONS

**Pregnancy/Lactation:** Unknown if distributed in breast milk. **Children:** Safety and efficacy not established. **Elderly:** Use cautiously due to higher rate of infection.

## INTERACTIONS

**DRUG:** Anakinra, abatacept may increase risk of infection. **Immunosuppressants** may reduce frequency of infusion reactions, antibodies to infliximab. **Live virus vaccines** may decrease immune response (do not give concurrently). **HERBAL:** Echinacea may decrease effects. **FOOD:** None known. **LAB VALUES:** May increase serum alkaline phosphatase, ALT, AST, bilirubin.

## AVAILABILITY (Rx)

**Injection, Powder for Reconstitution:** 100 mg.

## ADMINISTRATION/HANDLING

IV

**Reconstitution** • Reconstitute each vial with 10 ml Sterile Water for Injection, using 21-gauge or smaller needle. Direct stream of Sterile Water for Injection to glass wall of vial. • Swirl vial gently to dissolve contents (do not shake). • Allow solution to stand for 5 min and inject into 250-ml bag 0.9% NaCl; gently mix. Concentration should range between 0.4 and 4 mg/ml. • Begin infusion within 3 hrs after reconstitution.

**Rate of Administration** • Administer IV infusion over at least 2 hrs using a low protein-binding filter.

**Storage** • Refrigerate vials. • Solution should appear colorless to light yellow and opalescent; do not use if discolored or particulate forms.

## ▨ IV INCOMPATIBILITIES

Do not infuse in same IV line with other agents.

## INDICATIONS/ROUTES/ DOSAGE

◀ **ALERT** ▶ Premedicate with antihistamines, acetaminophen, steroids to prevent/manage infusion reactions.

**Rheumatoid Arthritis (RA)**
**IV Infusion: ADULTS, ELDERLY: (in combination with methotrexate):** 3 mg/kg followed by additional doses at 2 and 6 wks after first infusion, then q8wks thereafter. Range: 3–10 mg/kg at 4- to 8-wk intervals.

**Crohn's Disease**
**IV Infusion: ADULTS, ELDERLY, CHILDREN 6 YRS AND OLDER:** 5 mg/kg followed by additional doses at 2 and 6 wks after first infusion, then q8wks thereafter. For adults who respond then lose response, consideration may be given to treatment with 10 mg/kg.

**Ankylosing Spondylitis**
**IV Infusion: ADULTS, ELDERLY:** 5 mg/kg followed by additional doses at 2 and 6 wks after first infusion, then q6wks thereafter.

**Psoriatric Arthritis**
**IV Infusion: ADULTS, ELDERLY:** 5 mg/kg followed by additional doses at 2 and

6 wks after first infusion, then q8wks thereafter. May be used with or without methotrexate.

**Plaque Psoriasis**
**IV Infusion: ADULTS, ELDERLY:** 5 mg/kg followed by additional doses at 2 and 6 wks after first infusion, then q8wks thereafter.

**Ulcerative Colitis**
**IV Infusion: ADULTS, ELDERLY, CHILDREN 6 YRS AND OLDER:** 5 mg/kg followed by additional doses at 2 and 6 wks after first infusion, then q8wks thereafter.

**Dosage in Renal/Hepatic Impairment**
No dose adjustment.

## SIDE EFFECTS

**Frequent (22%–10%):** Headache, nausea, fatigue, fever. **Occasional (9%–5%):** Fever/chills during infusion, pharyngitis, vomiting, pain, dizziness, bronchitis, rash, rhinitis, cough, pruritus, sinusitis, myalgia, back pain. **Rare (4%–1%):** Hypotension or hypertension, paresthesia, anxiety, depression, insomnia, diarrhea, UTI.

## ADVERSE EFFECTS/ TOXIC REACTIONS

Serious infections, including sepsis, occur rarely. Potential for hypersensitivity reaction, lupus-like syndrome, severe hepatic reaction, HF.

## NURSING CONSIDERATIONS

**BASELINE ASSESSMENT**
Evaluate baseline hydration status (skin turgor urinary status).

**INTERVENTION/EVALUATION**
Monitor urinalysis, erythrocyte sedimentation rate (ESR), B/P. Monitor for signs of infection. Monitor daily pattern of bowel activity, stool consistency. **Crohn's disease:** Monitor C-reactive protein, frequency of stools. Assess for abdominal pain. **Rheumatoid arthritis (RA):** Monitor C-reactive protein.

Assess for decreased pain, swollen joints, stiffness.

**PATIENT/FAMILY TEACHING**
• Report persistent fever, cough, abdominal pain, swelling of ankles/feet.

## *insulin*

in-su-lin
**Rapid-acting:** (Afrezza):
**INHALATION POWDER, INSULIN ASPART:** (Novolog), **INSULIN GLULISINE:** (Apidra), **INSULIN LISPRO:** (Humalog)
**Short-acting: REGULAR INSULIN:** (Humulin R, Novolin R)
**Intermediate-acting: NPH:** (Humulin N, Novolin N)
**Long-acting: INSULIN DEGLUDEC:** (Tresiba), **INSULIN DETEMIR:** (Levemir), **INSULIN GLARGINE:** (Basaglar, Lantus, Toujeo)

■ **BLACK BOX ALERT** ■ (Afrezza): Acute bronchospasms reported in pts with asthma and COPD.
**Do not confuse Novolog with Humalog or Novolin.**

## FIXED-COMBINATION(S)

**Humalog Mix 75/25:** lispro suspension 75% and lispro solution 25%. **Humulin Mix 50/50:** NPH 50% and regular 50%. **Humulin 70/30, Novolin 70/30:** NPH 70% and rapid-acting regular 30%. **Novolog Mix 70/30:** aspart suspension 70% and aspart solution 30%. **Ryzodeg 70/30:** degludec suspension 70% and aspart solution 30%. **Soliqua 100/33:** glargine 100 units/ml and lixisenatide (a GLP-1 receptor agonist) 33 mcg/ml. **Xultophy 100/3.6:** degludec 100 units/ml and liraglutide (a GLP-1 receptor agonist) 3.6 mg/ml.

## ◆CLASSIFICATION

**PHARMACOTHERAPEUTIC:** Exogenous insulin. **CLINICAL:** Antidiabetic.

## USES

Treatment of insulin-dependent type 1 diabetes mellitus; non–insulin-dependent type 2 diabetes mellitus (NIDDM) to improve glycemic control. **OFF-LABEL: Insulin aspart, insulin lispro, insulin regular:** Gestational diabetes, mild to moderate diabetic ketoacidosis, mild to moderate hyperosmolar hyperglycemic state. **Insulin NPH:** Gestational diabetes.

## PRECAUTIONS

**Contraindications:** Hypersensitivity to insulin, use during episodes of hypoglycemia. **Afrezza:** Chronic lung disease. **Cautions:** Pts at risk for hypokalemia; renal/hepatic impairment, elderly. Afrezza: Must be used with a long-acting insulin in type 1 diabetes. Not recommended for use in diabetic ketoacidosis or in smokers. **Afrezza:** Pts with active lung cancer, history of lung cancer or at risk for lung cancer.

## ACTION

Acts via specific receptor to regulate metabolism of carbohydrates, protein, and fats. Acts on liver, skeletal muscle, and adipose tissue. **Liver:** Stimulates hepatic glycogen synthesis, synthesis of fatty acids. **Muscle:** Increases protein, glycogen synthesis. **Adipose tissue:** Stimulates lipoproteins to provide free fatty acids, triglyceride synthesis. **Therapeutic Effect:** Controls serum glucose levels.

## PHARMACOKINETICS

**Rapid-Acting**

|  | Onset (min) | Peak (hrs) | Duration (hrs) |
|---|---|---|---|
| Aspart (Novolog) | 10–20 | 1–3 | 3–5 |
| Glulisine (Apidra) | 5–15 | 0.75–1.25 | 2–4 |
| Insulin Human (Afrezza) | 15–30 | 1 | 2 |
| Lispro (Humalog) | 15–30 | 0.5–2.5 | 3–6.5 |

**Short-Acting**

|  | Onset (min) | Peak (hrs) | Duration (hrs) |
|---|---|---|---|
| Regular (Humulin R) | 30–60 | 1–5 | 6–10 |
| Regular (Novolin R) | 30–60 | 1–5 | 6–10 |

**Intermediate-Acting**

|  | Onset (hrs) | Peak (hrs) | Duration (hrs) |
|---|---|---|---|
| NPH (Humulin N) | 1–2 | 6–14 | 16–24+ |
| NPH (Novolin N) | 1–2 | 6–14 | 16–24+ |

**Long-Acting**

|  | Onset (hrs) | Peak (hrs) | Duration (hrs) |
|---|---|---|---|
| Degludec (Tresiba) | 0.5–1.5 | 12 | 42 |
| Detemir (Levemir) | 3–4 | 3–9 | 6–23 |
| Glargine (Lantus) | 3–4 | No peak | 24 |
| Glargine (Toujeo) | Over 6 | No peak | Over 24 |

## LIFESPAN CONSIDERATIONS

**Pregnancy/Lactation:** Insulin is drug of choice for diabetes in pregnancy; close medical supervision is needed. Following delivery, insulin needs may drop for 24–72 hrs, then rise to pre-pregnancy levels. Not distributed in breast milk; lactation may decrease insulin requirements. **Children:** No age-related precautions noted. **Elderly:** Decreased vision, fine motor tremors may lead to inaccurate self-dosing.

## INTERACTIONS

**DRUG: Alcohol** may increase risk of hypoglycemia. **Beta blockers (e.g., carvedilol, metoprolol)** may alter effects; may mask signs, prolong periods of hypoglycemia. **Glucocorticoids, thiazide diuretics** may increase serum glucose. **HERBAL: Garlic, ginger, ginseng** may increase risk of hypoglycemia. **FOOD:** None known. **LAB VALUES:** May decrease serum magnesium, phosphate, potassium.

## AVAILABILITY

### Rapid-Acting
(Afrezza) Inhalation Powder: 4 units, 8 units, 12 units as single-use inhalation cartridges. Aspart (Novolog): 100 units/ml vial, 3 ml cartridge, 3 ml Flex-Pen. Glulisine (Apidra): 100 units/ml vial, 3 ml cartridge. Lispro (Humalog): 100 units/ml vial, 3 ml cartridge, 3 ml pen.

### Short-Acting
Regular (Humulin R): 100 units/ml vial, U-500 Kwik Pen. Regular (Novolin R): 100 units/ml vial, 3 ml cartridge, 3 ml Innolet prefilled syringe.

### Intermediate-Acting
NPH (Humulin N): 100 units/ml vial, 3 ml pen. NPH (Novolin N): 100 units/ml vial, 3 ml cartridge, 3 ml Innolet prefilled syringe.

### Long-Acting
Detemir (Levemir): 100 units/ml vial, 3 ml Flex-Pen. Glargine (Lantus): 100 units/ml vial, 3 ml cartridge.

### Intermediate- and Short-Acting Mixtures
Humulin 50/50, Humulin 70/30, Humalog Mix 75/25, Humalog Mix 50/50, Novolin 70/30, Novolog Mix 70/30.

## ADMINISTRATION/HANDLING

### IV (Regular and Insulin Glulisine [Apidra])
• Use only if solution is clear. • May give undiluted.

### Rapid-Acting
Afrezza • Administer using a single inhalation/cartridge. Give at beginning of a meal.
Aspart (Novolog) • May give subcutaneous, IV infusion. • Can mix with NPH (draw aspart into syringe first; inject immediately after mixing). • After first use, stable at room temperature for 28 days. • Administer 5–10 min before meals.

Glulisine (Apidra) • May mix with NPH (draw glulisine into syringe first; inject immediately after mixing). • After first use, stable at room temperature for 28 days. • Administer 15 min before or within 20 min after starting a meal.
Lispro (Humalog) • For subcutaneous use only. • May mix with NPH. Stable for 28 days at room temperature; syringe is stable for 14 days if refrigerated. • After first use, stable at room temperature for 28 days. • Administer 15 min before or immediately after meals.

### Short-Acting
Regular (Humulin R, Novolin R) • May give subcutaneous, IM, IV. • May mix with NPH for immediate use or for storage for future use. Stable for 1 mo at room temperature, 3 mos if refrigerated. • Can mix with Sterile Water for Injection or 0.9% NaCl. • After first use, stable at room temperature for 28 days. • Administer 30 min before meals.

### Intermediate-Acting
NPH (Humulin N, Novolin N) • For subcutaneous use only. • May mix with aspart (Novolog) or lispro (Humalog). Draw aspart or lispro first and use immediately. • May mix with regular (Humulin R, Novolin R) insulin. Draw regular insulin first, use immediately or may store for future use (up to 28 days). • After first use, stable at room temperature for 28 days. • Administer 15 min before meals when mixed with aspart or lispro; 30 min before meals when mixed with regular insulin.

### Long-Acting
Degludec (Tresiba) • For subcutaneous use only. • Do not mix with other insulins. • After first use, stable at room temperature for 56 days. • May take once daily any time of day.
Detemir (Levemir) • For subcutaneous use only. • Do not mix with other insulins. • After first use, stable at room temperature for 42 days. • Evening

dose given at dinner or at bedtime. Twice-daily regimens can be given 12 hrs after morning dose.

**Glargine (Lantus, Toujeo)** • For subcutaneous use only. • Do not mix with other insulins. • After first use, stable at room temperature for 28 days. • Administer once daily at same time. Meal timing is not applicable.

**Subcutaneous**

• Check serum glucose concentration before administration; dosage highly individualized. • Subcutaneous injections may be given in thigh, abdomen, upper arm, buttocks, upper back if there is adequate adipose tissue. • Rotation of injection sites is essential; maintain careful record. • Prefilled syringes should be stored in vertical or oblique position to avoid plugging; plunger should be pulled back slightly and syringe rocked to remix solution before injection.

### ▦ IV INCOMPATIBILITIES

Diltiazem (Cardizem), dopamine (Intropin), nafcillin (Nafcil).

### ▦ IV COMPATIBILITIES

Amiodarone (Cordarone), ampicillin/sulbactam (Unasyn), cefazolin (Ancef), digoxin (Lanoxin), dobutamine (Dobutrex), famotidine (Pepcid), gentamicin, heparin, magnesium sulfate, metoclopramide (Reglan), midazolam (Versed), milrinone (Primacor), morphine, nitroglycerin, potassium chloride, propofol (Diprivan), vancomycin (Vancocin).

## INDICATIONS/ROUTES/DOSAGE

**Note:** Insulin requirments vary dramatically between pts requiring dosage adjustment.

**Type 1 Diabetes:** Multiple daily injections, guided by glucose monitoring or continuous subcutaneous insulin infusions, is standard of care.

**Initial dose:** 0.5–1 unit/kg/day in divided doses. **Maintenance:** 0.5–1.2 units/day in divided doses.

**Type 2 Diabetes:** General goal is to achieve HbA$_{1c}$ less than 7% using safe medication titration.

**Afrezza:** Dosage based on metabolic needs, blood glucose results, glycemic goal control.

**Dosage in Renal Impairment**

| Creatinine Clearance | Dose |
|---|---|
| 10–50 ml/min | 75% normal dose |
| Less than 10 ml/min | 25–50% normal dose |

**Dosage in Hepatic Impairment**
Insulin requirement may be reduced.

## SIDE EFFECTS

**Occasional:** Localized redness, swelling, itching (due to improper insulin injection technique), allergy to insulin cleansing solution. **Infrequent:** Somogyi effect (rebound hyperglycemia) with chronically excessive insulin dosages. Systemic allergic reaction (rash, angioedema, anaphylaxis), lipodystrophy (depression at injection site due to breakdown of adipose tissue), lipohypertrophy (accumulation of subcutaneous tissue at injection site due to inadequate site rotation). **Rare:** Insulin resistance.

## ADVERSE EFFECTS/TOXIC REACTIONS

Severe hypoglycemia (due to hyperinsulinism) may occur with insulin overdose, decrease/delay of food intake, excessive exercise, pts with brittle diabetes. Diabetic ketoacidosis may result from stress, illness, omission of insulin dose, long-term poor insulin control.

## NURSING CONSIDERATIONS

### BASELINE ASSESSMENT

Check blood glucose level. Discuss lifestyle to determine extent of learning, emotional needs. If given IV, obtain serum chemistries (esp. serum potassium).

### INTERVENTION/EVALUATION

Assess for hypoglycemia (refer to pharmacokinetics table for peak times and duration): cool, wet skin, tremors, dizziness, headache, anxiety, tachycardia, numbness in mouth, hunger, diplopia. Assess sleeping pt for restlessness, diaphoresis. Check for hyperglycemia: polyuria (excessive urine output), polyphagia (excessive food intake), polydipsia (excessive thirst), nausea/vomiting, dim vision, fatigue, deep and rapid breathing (Kussmaul respirations). Be alert to conditions altering glucose requirements: fever, trauma, increased activity/stress, surgical procedure.

### PATIENT/FAMILY TEACHING

• Instruct on proper technique for drug administration, testing of glucose, signs/symptoms of hypoglycemia and hyperglycemia. • Prescribed diet is an essential part of treatment; do not skip/delay meals. • Carry candy, sugar packets, other sugar supplements for immediate response to hypoglycemia. • Wear or carry medical alert identification. • Check with physician when insulin demands are altered (e.g., fever, infection, trauma, stress, heavy physical activity). • Do not take other medication without consulting physician. • Weight control, exercise, hygiene (including foot care), not smoking are integral parts of therapy. • Protect skin, limit sun exposure. • Inform dentist, physician, surgeon of medication before any treatment is given.

---

## interferon alfa-2b   HIGH ALERT

in-ter-feer-on
(Intron-A)

■ **BLACK BOX ALERT** ■ May cause or aggravate fatal or life-threatening autoimmune disorders, ischemia, neuropsychiatric symptoms (profound depression, suicidal thoughts/behaviors), infectious disorders.

**Do not confuse interferon alfa-2b with interferon alfa-2a, interferon alfa-n3, or peginterferon alfa-2b, or Intron with Peg-Intron.**

### FIXED-COMBINATION(S)

**Rebetron:** interferon alfa-2b/ribavirin (an antiviral): 3 million units/200 mg.

## ◆CLASSIFICATION

**PHARMACOTHERAPEUTIC:** Biologic response modifier. **CLINICAL:** Antineoplastic.

## USES

Treatment of hairy cell leukemia, condylomata acuminata (genital, venereal warts), malignant melanoma, AIDS-related Kaposi's sarcoma, chronic hepatitis C virus infection (including children 3 yrs of age and older), chronic hepatitis B (including children 1 yr and older), follicular non-Hodgkin's lymphoma. **OFF-LABEL:** Treatment of bladder, cervical, renal carcinoma; chronic myelocytic leukemia; laryngeal papillomatosis; multiple myeloma; cutaneous T-cell lymphoma; mycosis fungoides; West Nile virus.

## PRECAUTIONS

**Contraindications:** Hypersensitivity to interferon alfa-2b. Decompensated hepatic disease, autoimmune hepatitis. **In combination with ribavirin:** Women who are pregnant, males with pregnant partners, pts with hemoglobinemias (e.g., sickle cell anemia, CrCl less than 50 ml/min). **Cautions:** Renal/hepatic impairment, seizure disorder, compromised CNS function, cardiac diseases, myelosuppression, concurrent use of medications causing myelosuppression, pulmonary impairment, multiple sclerosis, diabetes, thyroid disease, coagulopathy, hypertension, preexisting eye disorders, history of psychiatric disorders. History of autoimmune disorders, MI, arrhythmias, cardiac abnormalities.

## ACTION

Inhibits viral replication in virus-infected cells, suppresses cell proliferation, augments specific cytotoxicity of lymphocytes. **Therapeutic Effect:** Prevents rapid growth of malignant cells; inhibits hepatitis virus.

## PHARMACOKINETICS

Well absorbed after IM, subcutaneous administration. Undergoes proteolytic

---

degradation during reabsorption in kidneys. **Half-life:** 2–3 hrs.

## ⏳ LIFESPAN CONSIDERATIONS

**Pregnancy/Lactation:** If possible, avoid use during pregnancy. Breastfeeding not recommended. **Children:** Safety and efficacy not established. **Elderly:** Neurotoxicity, cardiotoxicity may occur more frequently. Age-related renal impairment may require dosage adjustment.

## INTERACTIONS

**DRUG: Bone marrow depressants (e.g., alemtuzumab, methotrexate)** may increase myelosuppression. **HERBAL:** None significant. **FOOD:** None known. **LAB VALUES:** May increase PT, aPTT, LDH, serum alkaline phosphatase, ALT, AST. May decrease Hgb, Hct, leukocyte, platelet counts.

## AVAILABILITY (Rx)

**Injection, Powder for Reconstitution:** 10 million units, 18 million units, 50 million units.

## ADMINISTRATION/HANDLING

 IV

**Reconstitution •** Prepare immediately before use. • Reconstitute with diluent provided by manufacturer. • Withdraw desired dose and further dilute with 100 ml 0.9% NaCl to provide final concentration of at least 10 million international units/100 ml.
**Rate of Administration •** Administer over 20 min.
**Storage •** Refrigerate unopened vials. • Following reconstitution, stable for 24 hrs if refrigerated.

**IM, Subcutaneous**
**IM •** Administer in evening (if possible).
**SQ •** Reconstitute with recommended amount of Sterile Water for Injection. Agitate gently; do not shake.

## 🔳 IV INCOMPATIBILITIES

$D_5W$. Do not mix with other medications via Y-site administration.

## 🔳 IV COMPATIBILITIES

0.9% NaCl, lactated Ringer's.

## INDICATIONS/ROUTES/DOSAGE

**Hairy Cell Leukemia**
**IM, SQ: ADULTS:** 2 million units/$m^2$ 3 times/wk for 2–6 mos. If severe adverse reactions occur, modify dose or temporarily discontinue drug.

**Condylomata Acuminata**
**Intralesional: ADULTS:** 1 million units/lesion 3 times/wk for 3 wks. May administer a second course at 12–16 wks. Use only 10-million-unit vial, and reconstitute with no more than 1 ml diluent. **Maximum:** 5 lesions per treatment.

**AIDS-Related Kaposi's Sarcoma**
**IM, SQ: ADULTS:** 30 million units/$m^2$ 3 times/wk. Use only 50-million-unit vials. Continue until disease progression or maximal response achieved after 16 wks. If severe adverse reactions occur, modify dose or temporarily discontinue drug.

**Chronic Hepatitis C**
**IM, SQ: ADULTS:** 3 million units 3 times/wk for up to 6 mos. For pts who tolerate therapy and whose ALT level normalizes within 16 wks, therapy may be extended for up to 18–24 mos. May be used in combination with ribavirin. **CHILDREN, 3–17 YRS (WITH HIV CO-INFECTION):** 3–5 million units/$m^2$ 3 times/wk with ribavirin for 48 wks.

**Chronic Hepatitis B**
**IM, SQ: ADULTS:** 30–35 million units wkly, either as 5 million units/day or 10 million units 3 times/wk for 16 wks.
**SQ: CHILDREN 1–17 YRS:** 3 million units/$m^2$ 3 times/wk for 1 wk, then 6 million units/$m^2$ 3 times/wk for 16–24 wks. **Maximum:** 10 million units 3 times/wk.

**Malignant Melanoma**
**IV: ADULTS:** Initially, 20 million units/m$^2$ 5 times/wk for 4 wks. **Maintenance:** 10 million units subcutaneously 3 times/wk for 48 wks.

**Follicular Non-Hodgkin's Lymphoma**
**SQ: ADULTS:** 5 million units 3 times/wk for up to 18 mos.

**Dosage in Renal Impairment**
Do not use when combined with ribavirin.

**Dosage in Hepatic Impairment**
No dose adjustment (see Contraindications).

## SIDE EFFECTS

**Frequent:** Flu-like symptoms (fever, fatigue, headache, myalgia, anorexia, chills), rash (hairy cell leukemia, Kaposi's sarcoma only). **Pts with Kaposi's sarcoma:** All previously mentioned side effects plus depression, dyspepsia, dry mouth or thirst, alopecia, rigors. **Occasional:** Dizziness, pruritus, dry skin, dermatitis, altered taste. **Rare:** Confusion, leg cramps, back pain, gingivitis, flushing, tremor, anxiety, eye pain.

## ADVERSE EFFECTS/ TOXIC REACTIONS

Hypersensitivity reactions occur rarely. Severe flu-like symptoms appear dose-related.

## NURSING CONSIDERATIONS

### BASELINE ASSESSMENT

CBC, blood chemistries, urinalysis, renal function, LFT should be performed before initial therapy and routinely thereafter.

### INTERVENTION/EVALUATION

Offer emotional support. Monitor all levels of clinical function (numerous side effects). Encourage PO intake, particularly during early therapy. Monitor for worsening depression, suicidal ideation, associated behaviors.

### PATIENT/FAMILY TEACHING

• Clinical response occurs in 1–3 mos.
• Flu-like symptoms tend to diminish with continued therapy. • Some symptoms may be alleviated or minimized by bedtime doses. • Do not have immunizations without physician's approval (drug lowers resistance). • Avoid contact with those who have recently received live virus vaccine. • Avoid tasks that require alertness, motor skills until response to drug is established. • Sips of tepid water may relieve dry mouth. • Report depression, thoughts of suicide, unusual behavior.

---

**TOP 100**

# interferon beta-1a

in-ter-**feer**-on
(Avonex, Rebif)
**Do not confuse Avonex with Avelox, or interferon beta-1a with interferon beta-1b.**

## ◆ CLASSIFICATION

**PHARMACOTHERAPEUTIC:** Biologic response modifier. **CLINICAL:** Multiple sclerosis agent.

## USES

Treatment of relapsing multiple sclerosis to slow progression of physical disability, decrease frequency of clinical exacerbations.

## PRECAUTIONS

**Contraindications:** Hypersensitivity to natural or recombinant interferon, human albumin (only for albumin-containing products). **Cautions:** Depression, severe psychiatric disorders, hepatic impairment, increased serum ALT at baseline, alcohol abuse, cardiovascular disease, seizure disorders, myelosuppression.

## ACTION

Alters expression and response to surface antigens and may enhance immune cell activity. **Therapeutic Effect:** Slows progression of multiple sclerosis.

## PHARMACOKINETICS

Peak serum levels attained 3–15 hrs after IM administration. Biologic markers increase within 12 hrs and remain elevated for 4 days. **Half-life:** 10 hrs (Avonex); 69 hrs (Rebif).

## ⌛ LIFESPAN CONSIDERATIONS

**Pregnancy/Lactation:** Has abortifacient potential. Unknown if distributed in breast milk. **Children:** Safety and efficacy not established. **Elderly:** No information available.

## INTERACTIONS

**DRUG: Alcohol, hepatotoxic drugs (e.g., acetaminophen, simvastatin)** may increase risk of hepatic injury. **HERBAL:** None significant. **FOOD:** None known. **LAB VALUES:** May increase serum glucose, BUN, alkaline phosphatase, bilirubin, calcium, ALT, AST. May decrease Hgb, neutrophil, platelet, WBC counts.

## AVAILABILITY (Rx)

**Injection, Powder for Reconstitution (Avonex):** 30 mcg. **Injection Solution (Prefilled Syringe):** 22 mcg/0.5 ml (Rebif), 30 mcg/0.5 ml (Avonex Prefilled Syringe), 44 mcg/0.5 ml (Rebif). **Titration Pack (Prefilled Syringe [Rebif]):** 8.8 mcg/0.2 ml, 22 mcg/0.5 ml.

## ADMINISTRATION/HANDLING

**IM (Avonex) Syringe**
• Refrigerate syringe. • Allow to warm to room temperature before use. • May store up to 7 days at room temperature.

**IM (Avonex) Vial**
• Refrigerate vials (may store at room temperature up to 30 days). • Following reconstitution, may refrigerate again but use within 6 hrs if refrigerated. • Reconstitute 30-mcg *MicroPin* (6.6 million international units) vial with 1.1 ml diluent (supplied by manufacturer). • Gently swirl to dissolve medication; do not shake. • Discard if discolored or particulate forms. • Discard unused portion (contains no preservative).

**Subcutaneous (Rebif)**
• Refrigerate. May store at room temperature up to 30 days. Avoid heat, light.

• Administer at same time of day 3 days each wk. Separate doses by at least 48 hrs.

## INDICATIONS/ROUTES/DOSAGE

**Relapsing Multiple Sclerosis**
**IM *(Avonex):* ADULTS:** 30 mcg once wkly.
**SQ *(Rebif):* ADULTS: (Target dose 44 mcg 3 times/wk):** Initially, 8.8 mcg 3 times/wk for 2 wks, then 22 mcg 3 times/wk for 2 wks, then 44 mcg 3 times/wk thereafter. **(Target dose 22 mcg 3 times/wk):** Initially, 4.4 mcg 3 times/wk for 2 wks, then 11 mcg 3 times/wk for 2 wks, then 22 mcg 3 times/wk thereafter.

**Dosage in Renal Impairment**
No dose adjustment.

**Dosage in Hepatic Impairment (Rebif)**
Use with caution in pts with history of active hepatic disease or ALT more than 2.5 times upper limit of normal (ULN).

## SIDE EFFECTS

**Frequent (67%–11%):** Headache, flu-like symptoms, myalgia, upper respiratory tract infection, depression with suicidal ideation, generalized pain, asthenia, chills, sinusitis, infection. **Occasional (9%–4%):** Abdominal pain, arthralgia, chest pain, dyspnea, malaise, syncope. **Rare (3%):** Injection site reaction, hypersensitivity reaction.

## ADVERSE EFFECTS/ TOXIC REACTIONS

Anemia occurs in 8% of pts. Hepatic failure has been reported.

## NURSING CONSIDERATIONS

### BASELINE ASSESSMENT
Obtain CBC, BMP, LFT. Assess home situation for support of therapy.

### INTERVENTION/EVALUATION
Assess for headache, flu-like symptoms, myalgia. Periodically monitor lab results, re-evaluate injection technique. Assess for depression, suicidal ideation.

### PATIENT/FAMILY TEACHING

• Do not change schedule, dosage without consulting physician. • Follow guidelines for reconstitution of product and administration, including aseptic technique. • Use puncture-resistant container for used needles, syringes; dispose of used needles, syringes properly. • Injection site reactions may occur. These do not require discontinuation of therapy, but type and extent should be carefully noted. Report flu-like symptoms (fever, chills, fatigue, muscle aches).

---

**TOP 100**

# interferon beta-1b

in-ter-**feer**-on
(Betaseron, Extavia)
**Do not confuse interferon beta-1b with interferon beta-1a.**

### ◆CLASSIFICATION

**PHARMACOTHERAPEUTIC:** Biologic response modifier. **CLINICAL:** Multiple sclerosis agent.

## USES

Reduces frequency of clinical exacerbations in pts with relapsing-remitting multiple sclerosis (recurrent attacks of neurologic dysfunction). Treatment of early stages of multiple sclerosis.

## PRECAUTIONS

**Contraindications:** Hypersensitivity to albumin, interferon. **Cautions:** Depression, severe psychiatric disorders, hepatic/renal impairment, alcohol abuse, cardiovascular disease, seizure disorders, myelosuppression, pulmonary disease.

## ACTION

Exact mechanism unknown. Participates in immunoregulation by enhancing oxidative metabolism of macrophages, antibody dependent cellular cytotoxicity and activating natural killer cells. **Therapeutic Effect:** Improves MRI lesions, decreases relapse rate and disease severity in multiple sclerosis.

## PHARMACOKINETICS

Slowly absorbed following subcutaneous administration. **Half-life:** 8 min–4.3 hrs.

## ⧗ LIFESPAN CONSIDERATIONS

**Pregnancy/Lactation:** Unknown if distributed in breast milk. **Children:** Safety and efficacy not established. **Elderly:** No information available.

## INTERACTIONS

**DRUG:** None significant. **HERBAL:** None significant. **FOOD:** None known. **LAB VALUES:** May increase bilirubin, ALT, AST. May decrease neutrophil, lymphocyte, WBC counts.

## AVAILABILITY (Rx)

**Injection, Powder for Reconstitution:** 0.3 mg.

## ADMINISTRATION/HANDLING

**Subcutaneous**

• Store vials at room temperature. • After reconstitution, stable for 3 hrs if refrigerated. • Use within 3 hrs of reconstitution. • Discard if discolored or precipitate forms. • Reconstitute 0.3-mg (9.6 million international units) vial with 1.2 ml diluent (supplied by manufacturer) to provide concentration of 0.25 mg/ml (8 million units/ml). • Gently swirl to dissolve medication; do not shake. • Withdraw 1 ml solution and inject subcutaneous into arms, abdomen, hips, thighs using 27-gauge needle. • Discard unused portion (contains no preservative).

## INDICATIONS/ROUTES/DOSAGE

**Relapsing-Remitting Multiple Sclerosis**
**SQ: ADULTS:** Initially, 0.0625 mg every other day; gradually increase by 0.0625 mg every 2 wks. Target dose: 0.25 mg every other day.

**Dosage in Renal/Hepatic Impairment**
No dose adjustment.

---

## SIDE EFFECTS

**Frequent (85%–21%):** Injection site reaction, headache, flu-like symptoms, fever, asthenia, myalgia, sinusitis, diarrhea, dizziness, altered mental status, constipation, diaphoresis, vomiting. **Occasional (15%–4%):** Malaise, drowsiness, alopecia.

## ADVERSE EFFECTS/ TOXIC REACTIONS

Seizures occur rarely.

## NURSING CONSIDERATIONS

### BASELINE ASSESSMENT

Obtain CBC, BMP, LFT. Assess home situation for support of therapy.

### INTERVENTION/EVALUATION

Periodically monitor lab results, reevaluate injection technique. Assess for nausea (high incidence). Monitor sleep pattern. Monitor daily pattern of bowel activity, stool consistency. Assist with ambulation if dizziness occurs. Monitor food intake.

### PATIENT/FAMILY TEACHING

• Report flu-like symptoms (fever, chills, fatigue, muscle aches); occur commonly but decrease over time. • Wear sunscreen, protective clothing if exposed to sunlight, ultraviolet light until tolerance known.

# interferon gamma-1b

in-ter-**feer**-on
(Actimmune)

## ◆CLASSIFICATION

**PHARMACOTHERAPEUTIC:** Biologic response modifier. **CLINICAL:** Immunologic agent.

## USES

Reduces frequency, severity of serious infections due to chronic granulomatous disease. Delays time to disease progression in pts with severe, malignant osteopetrosis.

## PRECAUTIONS

**Contraindications:** Hypersensitivity to interferon gamma-1b, *Escherichia coli*–derived products. **Cautions:** Seizure disorders, compromised CNS function, preexisting cardiac disease (e.g., ischemia, HF, arrhythmias), hepatic disease, myelosuppression.

## ACTION

Exact mechanism unknown. Enhances oxidative metabolism of macrophages, antibody-dependent cellular cytotoxicity; activates natural killer cells. **Therapeutic Effect:** Decreases signs/symptoms of serious infections in chronic granulomatous disease.

## PHARMACOKINETICS

Slowly absorbed after subcutaneous administration. **Half-life:** 3–6 hrs.

## ⏳ LIFESPAN CONSIDERATIONS

**Pregnancy/Lactation:** Unknown if drug crosses placenta or is distributed in breast milk. **Children:** Safety and efficacy not established in pts younger than 1 yr. Flu-like symptoms may occur more frequently. **Elderly:** No information available.

## INTERACTIONS

**DRUG: Bone marrow depressants (e.g., alemtuzumab, methotrexate)** may increase myelosuppression. **HERBAL:** None significant. **FOOD:** None known. **LAB VALUES:** May increase serum ALT, AST, alkaline phosphatase, LDH, triglycerides, cortisol concentrations. May decrease leukocytes, neutrophils, platelets.

## AVAILABILITY (Rx)

**Injection Solution:** 100 mcg/0.5 ml (2 million units).

## ADMINISTRATION/HANDLING

**◄ALERT►** Avoid excessive agitation of vial; do not shake.

**Subcutaneous**

• Refrigerate vials. Do not freeze. • Do not keep at room temperature for more than 12 hrs; discard after 12 hrs. • Vials are single dose; discard unused portion. • Solution is clear, colorless. Do not use if discolored or precipitate forms. • When given 3 times/wk, rotate injection sites.

## INDICATIONS/ROUTES/DOSAGE

**Chronic Granulomatous Disease; Severe, Malignant Osteopetrosis**

**SQ: ADULTS, ELDERLY, CHILDREN OLDER THAN 1 YR:** 50 mcg/m$^2$ (1 million units/m$^2$) 3 times/wk in pts with body surface area (BSA) greater than 0.5 m$^2$; 1.5 mcg/kg/dose 3 times/wk in pts with BSA 0.5 m$^2$ or less.

**Dosage in Renal/Hepatic Impairment**
No dose adjustment.

## SIDE EFFECTS

**Frequent (52%–14%):** Fever, headache, rash, chills, fatigue, diarrhea. **Occasional (13%–10%):** Vomiting, nausea. **Rare (6%–3%):** Weight loss, myalgia, anorexia.

## ADVERSE EFFECTS/ TOXIC REACTIONS

May exacerbate preexisting CNS dysfunction (manifested as decreased mental status, gait disturbance, dizziness), cardiac abnormalities.

## NURSING CONSIDERATIONS

### BASELINE ASSESSMENT

CBC, serum electrolytes, urinalysis, renal function, LFT should be performed before initial therapy and at 3-mo intervals during course of treatment.

### INTERVENTION/EVALUATION

Monitor for flu-like symptoms. Assess skin for evidence of rash.

### PATIENT/FAMILY TEACHING

• Flu-like symptoms (fever, chills, fatigue, muscle aches) are generally mild and tend to disappear as treatment continues. Symptoms may be minimized with bedtime administration. • Avoid tasks that require alertness, motor skills until response to drug is established. • If home use prescribed, follow guidelines for proper technique of administration; care in proper disposal of needles, syringes. • Vials should remain refrigerated.

# interleukin-2 (aldesleukin)

in-ter-**loo**-kin
(Proleukin)

■ **BLACK BOX ALERT** ■ High-dose therapy is associated with capillary leak syndrome resulting in significant hypotension and reduced organ perfusion. Use restricted to pts with normal cardiac/pulmonary function. Increased risk of disseminated infection (sepsis, bacterial endocarditis). Withhold treatment for pts developing moderate-to-severe lethargy or drowsiness (continued treatment may result in coma). Must be administered by personnel trained in administration/handling of chemotherapeutic agents.
**Do not confuse aldesleukin with oprelvekin.**

## ◆CLASSIFICATION

**PHARMACOTHERAPEUTIC:** Biologic response modifier. **CLINICAL:** Antineoplastic.

## USES

Treatment of metastatic renal cell carcinoma, metastatic melanoma. **OFF-LABEL:** Treatment of acute myeloid leukemia (AML).

## PRECAUTIONS

**Contraindications:** Hypersensitivity to aldesleukin. Abnormal pulmonary function or thallium stress test results, bowel ischemia or perforation, coma or toxic psychosis lasting longer than 48 hrs, GI bleeding requiring surgery, intubation lasting more than 72 hrs, organ allografts, pericardial tamponade, renal dysfunction requiring dialysis for longer than 72 hrs, repetitive or difficult-to-control seizures; retreatment in pts who experience any of the following toxicities: angina, MI, recurrent chest pain with EKG changes, sustained ventricular tachycardia, uncontrolled or unresponsive cardiac rhythm disturbances. **Extreme Caution:** Pts with normal thallium stress tests and pulmonary function tests who have history of cardiac or pulmonary disease. **Cautions:** Pts with fixed requirements for large volumes of fluid (e.g., those with hypercalcemia), history of seizures, renal/hepatic impairment, autoimmune disease, inflammatory disorders.

## ACTION

Promotes proliferation, differentiation, recruitment of T and B cells, lymphokine-activated and natural killer cells, thymocytes. **Therapeutic Effect:** Enhances cytolytic activity in lymphocytes.

## PHARMACOKINETICS

Primarily distributed into plasma, lymphocytes, lungs, liver, kidney, spleen. Metabolized to amino acids in cells lining the kidneys. **Half-life:** 80–120 min.

## LIFESPAN CONSIDERATIONS

**Pregnancy/Lactation:** Avoid use in those of either sex not practicing effective contraception. **Children:** Safety and efficacy not established. **Elderly:** Age-related renal impairment may require dosage adjustment; will not tolerate toxicity.

## INTERACTIONS

**DRUG: Antihypertensives** may increase hypotensive effect. **Cardiotoxic, hepatotoxic, myelotoxic, nephrotoxic medications** may increase risk of toxicity. **Glucocorticoids** may decrease effects. **HERBAL:** None significant. **FOOD:** None

known. **LAB VALUES:** May increase serum BUN, alkaline phosphatase, bilirubin, creatinine, ALT, AST. May decrease serum calcium, magnesium, phosphorus, potassium, sodium.

## AVAILABILITY (Rx)

**Injection, Powder for Reconstitution (Proleukin):** 22 million units (1.3 mg) (18 million units/ml = 1.1 mg/ml when reconstituted).

## ADMINISTRATION/HANDLING

◄ALERT► Hold administration in pts who develop moderate to severe lethargy or drowsiness (continued administration may result in coma).

 **IV**

**Reconstitution** • Reconstitute 22 million units vial with 1.2 ml Sterile Water for Injection to provide concentration of 18 million units/ml (1.1 mg/ml). • Bacteriostatic Water for Injection or NaCl should not be used to reconstitute because of increased aggregation. • During reconstitution, direct Sterile Water for Injection at the side of vial. Swirl contents gently to avoid foaming. Do not shake.
**Rate of Administration** • Further dilute dose in 50 ml $D_5W$ to a final concentration between 0.49 and 1.1 million international units/ml (30–70 mcg/ml) and infuse over 15 min. Do not use an in-line filter. • Solution should be warmed to room temperature before infusion. • Monitor diligently for drop in mean arterial B/P (sign of capillary leak syndrome [CLS]). Continued treatment may result in significant hypotension (less than 90 mm Hg or a 20 mm Hg drop from baseline systolic pressure), edema, pleural effusion, altered mental status.
**Storage** • Refrigerate vials; do not freeze. • Reconstituted solution is stable for 48 hrs refrigerated or at room temperature (refrigeration preferred).

## IV INCOMPATIBILITIES

Ganciclovir (Cytovene), pentamidine (Pentam), prochlorperazine (Compazine), promethazine (Phenergan).

## IV COMPATIBILITIES

Calcium gluconate, dopamine (Intropin), heparin, lorazepam (Ativan), magnesium, potassium.

## INDICATIONS/ROUTES/DOSAGE

**Metastatic Melanoma, Metastatic Renal Cell Carcinoma**
**IV: ADULTS 18 YRS AND OLDER:** 600,000 units/kg q8h for 14 doses; followed by 9 days of rest, then another 14 doses for a total of 28 doses per course. Course may be repeated if tumor shrinkage observed after rest period of at least 7 wks from date of hospital discharge.

**Dosage in Renal/Hepatic Impairment**
No dose adjustment. Do not initiate if serum creatinine greater than 1.5 mg/dl.

**Dosage Modification for Toxicity**
Withhold or interrupt therapy; do not reduce dose. Retreatment contraindicated with the following toxicities: Sustained ventricular tachycardia, uncontrolled arrhythmias; chest pain/EKG changes consistent with angina or MI; cardiac tamponade, repetitive/refractory seizures; GI bleeding; bowel ischemia/perforation; renal failure requiring dialysis; coma lasting more than 48 hrs.

## SIDE EFFECTS

Side effects are generally self-limited and resolve within 2–3 days after discontinuing therapy. **Frequent (89%–48%):** Fever, chills, nausea, vomiting, hypotension, diarrhea, oliguria/anuria, altered mental status, irritability, confusion, depression, sinus tachycardia, pain (abdominal, chest, back), fatigue, dyspnea, pruritus. **Occasional (47%–17%):** Edema, erythema, rash, stomatitis, anorexia, weight gain, infection (UTI, injection site, catheter tip), dizziness. **Rare (15%–4%):** Dry skin, sensory

disorders (vision, speech, taste), dermatitis, headache, arthralgia, myalgia, weight loss, hematuria, conjunctivitis, proteinuria.

## ADVERSE EFFECTS/ TOXIC REACTIONS

Anemia, thrombocytopenia, leukopenia occur commonly. GI bleeding, pulmonary edema occur occasionally. Capillary leak syndrome (CLS) results in hypotension (systolic pressure less than 90 mm Hg or a 20 mm Hg drop from baseline systolic pressure), extravasation of plasma proteins and fluid into extravascular space, loss of vascular tone. May result in cardiac arrhythmias, angina, MI, respiratory insufficiency. Fatal malignant hyperthermia, cardiac arrest, CVA, pulmonary emboli, bowel perforation/gangrene, severe depression leading to suicide occur in less than 1% of pts.

## NURSING CONSIDERATIONS

**BASELINE ASSESSMENT**

Pts with bacterial infection and with indwelling central lines should be treated with antibiotic therapy before treatment begins. All pts should be neurologically stable with a negative CT scan before treatment begins. CBC, BMP, LFT, chest X-ray should be performed before therapy begins and daily thereafter.

**INTERVENTION/EVALUATION**

Monitor CBC with differential, amylase, electrolytes, renal function, LFT, weight, pulse oximetry. Discontinue medication at first sign of hypotension and hold for moderate to severe lethargy (physician must decide whether therapy should continue). Assess for altered mental status (irritability, confusion, depression), weight gain/loss. Maintain strict I&O. Assess for extravascular fluid accumulation (rales in lungs, edema in dependent areas).

**PATIENT/FAMILY TEACHING**

• Nausea may decrease during therapy.
• At home, increase fluid intake (protects against renal impairment). • Do not

have immunizations without physician's approval (drug lowers resistance). • Avoid exposure to persons with infection. • Report fever, chills, lower back pain, difficulty with urination, unusual bleeding/bruising, black tarry stools, blood in urine, petechial rash (pinpoint red spots on skin). • Report symptoms of depression or suicidal ideation immediately.

# ipilimumab

ip-i-**lim**-ue-mab
(Yervoy)

■ **BLACK BOX ALERT** ■ Severe and fatal immune-mediated adverse reactions due to T-cell activation and proliferation are capable of involving any organ system. Specific reactions include enterocolitis, hepatitis, dermatitis, neuropathy, endocrinopathy. Majority of immune-mediated reactions may initially manifest during treatment or weeks to months after treatment. Permanently discontinue treatment and initiate high-dose corticosteroid therapy for severe immune-mediated adverse reactions. Assess all pts for signs/symptoms of enterocolitis, hepatitis, dermatitis (including toxic epidermal necrolysis), neuropathy, endocrinopathy and evaluate clinical chemistries including hepatic function tests and thyroid tests at baseline and before each treatment.

## ◆CLASSIFICATION

**PHARMACOTHERAPEUTIC:** Human cytotoxic T-lymphocyte antigen 4 (CTLA-4)-blocking antibody. **CLINICAL:** Antineoplastic.

## USES

Treatment of unresectable or metastatic melanoma. Adjuvant treatment of pts with cutaneous melanoma with pathologic involvement of regional lymph nodes and have undergone complete resection, including total lymphadenectomy.

## PRECAUTIONS

**Contraindications:** Hypersensitivity to ipilimumab. **Cautions:** Hepatic impairment, chronic peripheral neuropathy, thyroid/adrenal/pituitary dysfunction, autoimmune disorders (ulcerative colitis, Crohn's disease, lupus, sarcoidosis).

## ACTION

Augments T-cell activation and proliferation. Binds to cytotoxic T-lymphocyte-associated antigen 4 (CTLA-4) and blocks interaction of CTLA-4 with its ligands. **Therapeutic Effect:** Inhibits tumor cell growth.

## PHARMACOKINETICS

Metabolized in liver. Steady state reached by third dose. **Half-life:** 14.7 days.

## ⌛ LIFESPAN CONSIDERATIONS

**Pregnancy/Lactation:** May cause fetal harm. Unknown if distributed in breast milk. Discontinue drug or discontinue breastfeeding. **Children:** Safety and efficacy not established. **Elderly:** No age-related precautions noted.

## INTERACTIONS

**DRUG:** None significant. **HERBAL:** None significant. **FOOD:** None known. **LAB VALUES:** May increase serum ALT, AST, bilirubin; eosinophils.

## AVAILABILITY (Rx)

**Injection, Solution:** 5 mg/ml (10 ml, 40 ml vials).

## ADMINISTRATION/HANDLING
🖐 IV

**◀ALERT▶** Use sterile, nonpyrogenic, low protein-binding in-line filter. Use dedicated line only.
**Reconstitution** • Calculate number of vials needed for injection. • Inspect for particulate matter or discoloration. • Allow vials to stand at room temperature for approximately 5 min. • Withdraw proper volume and transfer to infusion

---

bag. Dilute in NaCl or $D_5W$ with final concentration ranging from 1–2 mg/ml. • Mix diluted solution by gentle inversion. Do not shake or agitate.

**Rate of Administration** • Infuse over 90 min. Flush with 0.9% NaCl or $D_5W$ at end of infusion.

**Storage** • Solution should be translucent to white or pale yellow with amorphous particles. • Discard vial if cloudy or discolored. • Refrigerate vials until time of use. • May store diluted solution either under refrigeration or at room temperature for no more than 24 hrs.

# INDICATIONS/ROUTES/DOSAGE

### Metastatic Melanoma

**IV: ADULTS:** 3 mg/kg q3wks for 4 doses. Doses may be delayed due to toxicity, but all doses must be given within 16 wks of initial dose.

◄ALERT► Pts who are presenting with severe immune-mediated adverse reactions must immediately discontinue drug therapy and start prednisone 1 mg/kg/day.

### Cutaneous Melanoma

**IV: ADULTS:** 10 mg/kg q3wks for 4 doses, then 10 mg/kg q12wks for up to 3 yrs. If toxicity occurs, doses are omitted (not delayed).

### Dosage Modification

Hold scheduled dose for moderate immune-mediated adverse reactions. Pts with complete or partial resolution of adverse reactions and who are receiving less than 7.5 mg/day of prednisone may resume scheduled doses. Permanently discontinue for persistent moderate adverse reactions or inability to reduce corticosteroid dose to 7.5 mg/day, failure to complete full treatment course in 16 wks, any severe or life-threatening adverse reactions.

### Dosage in Renal/Hepatic Impairment

No dose adjustment.

### Hepatotoxicity during Treatment

**ALT/AST greater than 2.5 times upper limit of normal (ULN) or bilirubin greater than 1.5–3 times ULN:** Withhold treatment. **ALT/AST greater than 5 times ULN or bilirubin greater than 3 times ULN:** Permanently discontinue.

# SIDE EFFECTS

**Frequent (42%):** Fatigue. **Occasional (32%–29%):** Diarrhea, pruritus, rash, colitis.

# ADVERSE EFFECTS/ TOXIC REACTIONS

Severe and fatal immune-mediated adverse reactions have occurred. Enterocolitis (7% of pts) may present with fever, ileus, abdominal pain, GI bleeding, intestinal perforation, severe dehydrating diarrhea. Endocrinopathies (4% of pts), including hypopituitarism, adrenal insufficiency, hypogonadism, hypothyroidism may present with fatigue, headache, mental status change, unusual bowel habits, hypotension and may require emergent hormone replacement therapy. Dermatitis including toxic epidermal necrolysis (2% of pts) may present with full-thickness ulceration or necrotic, bullous, hemorrhagic manifestations. Hepatotoxicity (1% of pts), defined as LFT greater than 2.5–5 times ULN, may present with right upper abdominal pain, jaundice, black/tarry stools, bruising, dark-colored urine, nausea, vomiting. Neuropathy (1% of pts), including Guillain-Barré syndrome or myasthenia gravis, may present with weakness, sensory alterations, paresthesia, paralysis. Other serious adverse reactions such as pneumonitis, meningitis, nephritis, eosinophilia, pericarditis, myocarditis, angiopathy, temporal arteritis, vasculitis, polymyalgia rheumatica, conjunctivitis, blepharitis, episcleritis, scleritis, leukocytoclastic vasculitis, erythema multiforme, psoriasis, pancreatitis, arthritis, autoimmune thyroiditis reported. Anti-ipilimumab antibodies reported in 1.1% of pts. All severe immune-mediated adverse reactions require immediate high-dose corticosteroid therapy.

## NURSING CONSIDERATIONS

### BASELINE ASSESSMENT

Obtain baseline CBC, complete metabolic profile, LFT, TSH, free T4, urine pregnancy. Screen for history of hepatic impairment, chronic neuropathy, thyroid/adrenal/pituitary dysfunction, autoimmune disorders. Focused assessment relating to possible adverse reactions includes abdominal area (inspection, auscultation, percussion, palpation, bowel pattern, symmetry), skin (color, lesions, mucosal inspection, edema), neurologic (mental status, gait, numbness, tingling, pain, strength, visual acuity), hormonal glands (lymph node inspection/palpation, pyrexia, goiter, palpitations). Question possibility of pregnancy or plans of breastfeeding. Receive full medication history including vitamins, minerals, herbal products.

### INTERVENTION/EVALUATION

Monitor vital signs, hepatic function, thyroid panel before each dose. Continue focused assessment and screen for life-threatening immune-mediated adverse reactions. If adverse reactions occur, immediately notify physician and initiate proper treatment. Report suspected pregnancy. Obtain CBC, blood cultures for fever, suspected infection. EKG for palpitations, chest pain, difficulty breathing, dizziness. If prednisone therapy initiated, monitor capillary blood glucose and screen for side effects.

### PATIENT/FAMILY TEACHING

• Inform pt that serious and fatal adverse reactions indicate inflammation to certain systems: intestines (diarrhea, dark/tarry stools, abdominal pain), liver (yellowing of the skin, dark-colored urine, right upper quadrant pain, bruising), skin (rash, mouth sores, blisters, ulcers), nerves (weakness, numbness, tingling, difficulty breathing, paralysis), hormonal glands (headaches, weight gain, palpitations, changes in mood or behavior, dizziness), eyes (blurry vision, double vision, eye pain/redness).

• Prednisone therapy may be started if adverse reactions occur. • May cause fetal harm, stillbirth, premature delivery. • Blood levels will be drawn before each dose. • Report any chest pain, palpitations, fever, swollen glands, stomach pain, vomiting, or any sign of adverse reactions.

---

# ipratropium

ip-ra-**troe**-pee-um
(Atrovent, Atrovent HFA, Novo-Ipramide ✦, Nu-Ipratropium ✦, PMS-Ipratropium ✦)
**Do not confuse Atrovent with Alupent or Serevent, or ipratropium with tiotropium.**

### FIXED-COMBINATION(S)

**Combivent, DuoNeb:** ipratropium/albuterol (a bronchodilator): *Aerosol:* 18 mcg/90 mcg per actuation. *Solution:* 0.5 mg/2.5 mg per 3 ml.

### ◆CLASSIFICATION

**PHARMACOTHERAPEUTIC:** Anticholinergic. **CLINICAL:** Bronchodilator.

## USES

**Inhalation, Nebulization:** Maintenance treatment of bronchospasm due to COPD, bronchitis, emphysema, asthma. Not indicated for immediate bronchospasm relief. **Nasal Spray:** Symptomatic relief of rhinorrhea associated with the common cold and allergic/nonallergic rhinitis.

## PRECAUTIONS

**Contraindications:** History of hypersensitivity to ipratropium, atropine. **Cautions:** Narrow-angle glaucoma, prostatic hypertrophy, bladder neck obstruction, myasthenia gravis.

## ACTION

Blocks action of acetylcholine at parasympathetic sites in bronchial smooth

---

 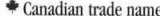

muscle. **Therapeutic Effect:** Causes bronchodilation, inhibits nasal secretions.

## PHARMACOKINETICS

| Route | Onset | Peak | Duration |
|---|---|---|---|
| Inhalation | 1–3 min | 1.5–2 hrs | Up to 4 hrs |
| Nasal | 5 min | 1–4 hrs | 4–8 hrs |

Minimal systemic absorption after inhalation. Metabolized in liver (systemic absorption). Primarily eliminated in feces. **Half-life:** 1.5–4 hrs (nasal).

## ⧗ LIFESPAN CONSIDERATIONS

**Pregnancy/Lactation:** Unknown if distributed in breast milk. **Children/Elderly:** No age-related precautions noted.

## INTERACTIONS

**DRUG:** Anticholinergics (e.g., glycopyrolate, scopolamine), medications with anticholinergic properties may increase toxicity. **HERBAL:** None significant. **FOOD:** None known. **LAB VALUES:** None significant.

## AVAILABILITY (Rx)

**Aerosol for Oral Inhalation (Atrovent HFA):** 17 mcg/actuation. **Solution, Intranasal Spray:** 0.03%; 0.06%. **Solution for Nebulization:** 0.02% (500 mcg).

## ADMINISTRATION/HANDLING

**Inhalation**
• Shake container well. • Instruct pt to exhale completely, place mouthpiece between lips, inhale deeply through mouth while fully depressing top of canister. Hold breath as long as possible before exhaling slowly. • Allow at least 1 minute between inhalations. • Rinse mouth with water immediately after inhalation (prevents mouth/throat dryness).

**Nebulization**
• May be administered with or without dilution in 0.9% NaCl. • Stable for 1 hr when mixed with albuterol. • Give over 5–15 min.

**Nasal**
• Store at room temperature. • Initial pump priming requires 7 actuations of pump. • If used regularly as recommended, no further priming is required. If not used for more than 4 hrs, pump will require 2 actuations, or if not used for more than 7 days, the pump will require 7 actuations to reprime.

## INDICATIONS/ROUTES/DOSAGE

**Bronchodilator for COPD**
**Inhalation: ADULTS, ELDERLY, CHILDREN OLDER THAN 12 YRS:** 2 inhalations 4 times/day. **Maximum:** 12 inhalations/day.
**Nebulization: ADULTS, ELDERLY, CHILDREN OLDER THAN 12 YRS:** 500 mcg (1 unit dose vial) 3–4 times/day (doses 6–8 hrs apart).

**Asthma Exacerbation**
**Note:** Should be given in combination with a short-acting beta-adrenergic agonist.
**Inhalation: ADULTS, ELDERLY, CHILDREN OLDER THAN 12 YRS:** 8 inhalations q20min as needed for up to 3 hrs. **CHILDREN 6–12 YRS:** 4–8 inhalations q20min as needed for up to 3 hrs. **CHILDREN 5 YRS OR YOUNGER:** 2 inhalations q20 min for 1 hr.
**Nebulization: ADULTS, ELDERLY, CHILDREN OLDER THAN 12 YRS:** 500 mcg q20min for 3 doses, then as needed. **CHILDREN 6–12 YRS:** 250–500 mcg q20min for 3 doses, then as needed. **CHILDREN 5 YRS OR YOUNGER:** 250 mcg q20 min for 1 hr.

**Rhinorrhea (Perennial Allergic/Nonallergic Rhinitis)**
**Intranasal *(0.03%):* ADULTS, ELDERLY, CHILDREN 6 YRS AND OLDER:** 2 sprays per nostril 2–3 times/day.

**Rhinorrhea (Common Cold)**
**Intranasal *(0.06%):* ADULTS, ELDERLY, CHILDREN 12 YRS AND OLDER:** 2 sprays per nostril 3–4 times/day for up to 4 days. **CHILDREN 5–11 YRS:** 2 sprays per nostril 3 times/day for up to 4 days.

Rhinorrhea (Seasonal Allergy)
**Intranasal** *(0.06%):* **ADULTS, ELDERLY, CHILDREN 5 YRS AND OLDER:** 2 sprays per nostril 4 times/day for up to 3 wks.

**Dosage in Renal/Hepatic Impairment**
No dose adjustment.

## SIDE EFFECTS
**Frequent: Inhalation (6%–3%):** Cough, dry mouth, headache, nausea. **Nasal:** Dry nose/mouth, headache, nasal irritation. **Occasional: Inhalation (2%):** Dizziness, transient increased bronchospasm. **Rare (less than 1%): Inhalation:** Hypotension, insomnia, metallic/unpleasant taste, palpitations, urinary retention. **Nasal:** Diarrhea, constipation, dry throat, abdominal pain, nasal congestion.

## ADVERSE EFFECTS/ TOXIC REACTIONS
Worsening of angle-closure glaucoma, acute eye pain, hypotension occur rarely.

## NURSING CONSIDERATIONS

### BASELINE ASSESSMENT
Offer emotional support (high incidence of anxiety due to difficulty in breathing, sympathomimetic response to drug).

### INTERVENTION/EVALUATION
Monitor rate, depth, rhythm, type of respiration; quality, rate of pulse. Assess lung sounds for rhonchi, wheezing, rales. Monitor ABGs. Observe lips, fingernails for cyanosis (blue or dusky color in light-skinned pts; gray in dark-skinned pts). Observe for retractions (clavicular, sternal, intercostal), hand tremor. Evaluate for clinical improvement (quieter, slower respirations, relaxed facial expression, cessation of retractions). Monitor for improvement of rhinorrhea.

### PATIENT/ FAMILY TEACHING
• Increase fluid intake (decreases lung secretion viscosity). • Do not take more than 2 inhalations at any one time (excessive use may produce paradoxical

bronchoconstriction, decreased bronchodilating effect). • Rinsing mouth with water immediately after inhalation may prevent mouth and throat dryness. • Avoid excessive use of caffeine derivatives (chocolate, coffee, tea, cola, cocoa).

# irbesartan
ir-be-**sar**-tan
(Apo-lrbesartan*, Avapro)
■ **BLACK BOX ALERT** ■ May cause fetal injury, mortality if used during second or third trimester of pregnancy.
**Do not confuse Avapro with Anaprox.**

### FIXED-COMBINATION(S)
**Avalide:** irbesartan/hydrochlorothiazide (a diuretic): 150 mg/12.5 mg, 300 mg/12.5 mg, 300 mg/25 mg.

## ◆CLASSIFICATION
**PHARMACOTHERAPEUTIC:** Angiotensin II receptor antagonist. **CLINICAL:** Antihypertensive.

## USES
Treatment of hypertension alone or in combination with other antihypertensives. Treatment of diabetic nephropathy in pts with type 2 diabetes. **OFF-LABEL:** Reduce proteinuria in children with chronic kidney disease.

## PRECAUTIONS
**Contraindications:** Hypersensitivity to irbesartan. Concomitant use with aliskiren in pts with diabetes. **Cautions:** Renal impairment, unstented unilateral or bilateral renal artery stenosis, dehydration, HF, idiopathic or hereditary angioedema or angioedema associated with ACE inhibitor therapy.

## ACTION
Blocks vasoconstriction, aldosterone-secreting effects of angiotensin II, inhibiting

binding of angiotensin II to $AT_1$ receptors. **Therapeutic Effect:** Produces vasodilation, decreases peripheral resistance, decreases B/P.

## PHARMACOKINETICS

| Route | Onset | Peak | Duration |
|-------|-------|------|----------|
| PO | — | 1–2 hrs | Greater than 24 hrs |

Rapidly, completely absorbed after PO administration. Protein binding: 90%. Metabolized in liver. Eliminated in feces (80%), urine (20%). Not removed by hemodialysis. **Half-life:** 11–15 hrs.

## ⌛ LIFESPAN CONSIDERATIONS

**Pregnancy/Lactation:** Unknown if distributed in breast milk. May cause fetal or neonatal morbidity or mortality. **Children:** Safety and efficacy not established. **Elderly:** No age-related precautions noted.

## INTERACTIONS

**DRUG: Diuretics (e.g., furosemide, HCTZ)** produce additive hypotensive effects. **Potassium-sparing diuretics (e.g., spironolactone, triamterene), potassium supplements** may increase risk of hyperkalemia. **NSAIDs** may decrease antihypertensive effect. **HERBAL: Ephedra, ginseng, yohimbe** may worsen hypertension. **Garlic** may increase antihypertensive effect. **FOOD:** None known. **LAB VALUES:** May slightly increase serum BUN, creatinine. May decrease Hgb.

## AVAILABILITY (Rx)

**Tablets:** 75 mg, 150 mg, 300 mg.

## ADMINISTRATION/HANDLING

**PO**
• Give without regard to meals.

## INDICATIONS/ROUTES/DOSAGE

**Hypertension**
**PO: ADULTS, ELDERLY, CHILDREN 13 YRS AND OLDER:** Initially, 75–150 mg/day. May increase to 300 mg/day. **CHILDREN**

**6–12 YRS:** Initially, 75 mg/day. May increase to 150 mg/day.

**Nephropathy**
**PO: ADULTS, ELDERLY:** Target dose of 300 mg once daily.

**Dosage in Renal/Hepatic Impairment**
No dose adjustment.

## SIDE EFFECTS

**Occasional (9%–3%):** Upper respiratory tract infection, fatigue, diarrhea, cough. **Rare (2%–1%):** Heartburn, dizziness, headache, nausea, rash.

## ADVERSE EFFECTS/ TOXIC REACTIONS

Overdose may manifest as hypotension, syncope, tachycardia. Bradycardia occurs less often.

## NURSING CONSIDERATIONS

### BASELINE ASSESSMENT

Obtain B/P, apical pulse immediately before each dose, in addition to regular monitoring (be alert to fluctuations). If excessive reduction in B/P occurs, place pt in supine position, feet slightly elevated. Question possibility of pregnancy. Assess medication history (esp. diuretic therapy).

### INTERVENTION/EVALUATION

Maintain hydration (offer fluids frequently). Assess for evidence of upper respiratory infection. Assist with ambulation if dizziness occurs. Monitor electrolytes, renal function, urinalysis, B/P, pulse. Assess for hypotension.

### PATIENT/ FAMILY TEACHING

• May cause fetal or neonatal morbidity or mortality. • Avoid tasks that require alertness, motor skills until response to drug is established (possible dizziness effect); ensure appropriate birth control measures are in place. • Report any sign of infection (sore throat, fever). • Avoid exercising during hot weather (risk of dehydration, hypotension).

# irinotecan

**eye**-ri-noe-**tee**-kan
(Camptosar, Onivyde)

■ **BLACK BOX ALERT** ■ Can induce both early and late forms of severe diarrhea. Early diarrhea (during or shortly after administration) accompanied by salivation, rhinitis, lacrimation, diaphoresis, flushing. Late diarrhea (occurring more than 24 hrs after administration) can be prolonged and life-threatening. May produce severe, profound myelosuppression. Administer under supervision of experienced cancer chemotherapy physician.

## ◆CLASSIFICATION

**PHARMACOTHERAPEUTIC:** DNA topoisomerase inhibitor. **CLINICAL:** Antineoplastic.

## USES

**Camptosar:** Treatment of metastatic carcinoma of colon or rectum. **Onivyde:** Treatment of metastatic adenocarcinoma of the pancreas (in combination with 5-fluorouracil and leucovorin). **OFF-LABEL:** Non–small-cell lung cancer; small-cell lung cancer; CNS tumor; cervical, gastric, pancreatic, ovarian, esophageal cancer; Ewing's sarcoma; brain tumor.

## PRECAUTIONS

**Contraindications:** Hypersensitivity to irinotecan. **Cautions:** Pt previously receiving pelvic, abdominal irradiation (increased risk of myelosuppression), pts older than 65 yrs, hepatic dysfunction, hyperbilirubinemia, renal impairment, preexisting pulmonary disease.

## ACTION

Interacts with topoisomerase I, an enzyme that relieves torsional strain in DNA by inducing reversible single-strand breaks. Prevents religation of these single-stranded breaks resulting in damage to double-strand DNA, cell death. **Therapeutic Effect:** Produces cytotoxic effect on cancer cells.

## PHARMACOKINETICS

Metabolized in liver. Protein binding: 95% (metabolite). Excreted in urine and eliminated by biliary route. **Half-life:** 6–12 hrs; metabolite, 10–20 hrs.

##  LIFESPAN CONSIDERATIONS

**Pregnancy/Lactation:** May cause fetal harm. Unknown if distributed in breast milk. Breastfeeding not recommended. **Children:** Safety and efficacy not established. **Elderly:** Risk of diarrhea significantly increased.

## INTERACTIONS

**DRUG: CYP3A4 inducers (e.g., phenytoin, phenobarbital, carbamazepine)** may decrease concentration/effects. **CYP3A4 inhibitors (e.g., ketoconazole)** increase concentration. Avoid **live vaccines** during treatment. **HERBAL: St. John's wort** may decrease irinotecan effectiveness. **FOOD:** None known. **LAB VALUES:** May increase serum alkaline phosphatase, AST. May decrease Hgb, leukocytes, platelets.

## AVAILABILITY (Rx)

**Injection Solution:** 20 mg/ml (2 ml, 5 ml, 15 ml, 25 ml).

## ADMINISTRATION/HANDLING
💧 IV

**Camptosar**
**Reconstitution** • Dilute in D₅W (preferred) or 0.9% NaCl to concentration of 0.12–2.8 mg/ml.
**Rate of Administration** • Administer all doses as IV infusion over 30–90 min. • Assess for extravasation (flush site with Sterile Water for Injection, apply ice if extravasation occurs).
**Storage** • Store vials at room temperature, protect from light. • Solution diluted with D₅W is stable for 24 hrs at room

temperature or 48 hrs if refrigerated.
• Solution diluted with 0.9% NaCl is stable for 24 hrs at room temperature.
• Do not refrigerate solution if diluted with 0.9% NaCl.

**Onivyde**
**Reconstitution** • Withdraw dose from vial and dilute with 500 ml D$_5$W or 0.9% NaCl. Mix gently.
**Rate of Administration** • Infuse over 90 min.
**Storage** • Refrigerate vials; do not freeze. • Protect from light. • Stable for 4 hrs at room temperature or 24 hrs refrigerated.

### 🞖 IV INCOMPATIBILITY
Gemcitabine (Gemzar).

## INDICATIONS/ROUTES/DOSAGE
**Note:** Genotyping of UGT1A1 available. Pts who are homozygous for the UGT1A1*28 allele are at increased risk for neutropenia. Decreased dose is recommended.

**Carcinoma of the Colon, Rectum**
**IV** *(Single-Agent Therapy):* **ADULTS, ELDERLY:** **(WEEKLY REGIMEN):** Initially, 125 mg/m$^2$ once wkly for 4 wks, followed by a rest period of 2 wks. Additional courses may be repeated q6wks. Dosage may be adjusted in 25–50 mg/m$^2$ increments to as high as 150 mg/m$^2$ or as low as 50 mg/m$^2$. **(THREE-WEEK REGIMEN):** 350 mg/m$^2$ q3wks. Dosage may be adjusted to as low as 200 mg/m$^2$.
*(In Combination with Leucovorin and 5-Fluorouracil):* **REGIMEN ONE:** 125 mg/m$^2$ on days 1, 8, 15, 22. **REGIMEN TWO:** 180 mg/m$^2$ on days 1, 15, 29.

**Pancreatic Cancer**
**IV Infusion: ADULTS, ELDERLY:** 70 mg/m$^2$ once q2wks (in combination with leucovorin and 5-fluorouracil).

**Dosage in Renal Impairment**
No dose adjustment.

**Dosage in Hepatic Impairment**

| Bilirubin | Dose |
|---|---|
| More than upper limit of normal to 2 mg/dL or less: | Reduce dose one level |
| More than 2 mg/dL: | Not recommended |

## SIDE EFFECTS
**Expected (64%–32%):** Nausea, alopecia, vomiting, diarrhea. **Frequent (29%–22%):** Constipation, fatigue, fever, asthenia, skeletal pain, abdominal pain, dyspnea. **Occasional (19%–16%):** Anorexia, headache, stomatitis, rash.

## ADVERSE EFFECTS/ TOXIC REACTIONS
Hematologic toxicity characterized by anemia, leukopenia, thrombocytopenia, and neutropenia, sepsis occur frequently.

## NURSING CONSIDERATIONS
### BASELINE ASSESSMENT
Offer emotional support. Assess hydration status, electrolytes, CBC before each dose. Premedicate with antiemetics on day of treatment, starting at least 30 min before administration. Inform pt of possibility of alopecia.

### INTERVENTION/EVALUATION
Monitor daily pattern of bowel activity, stool consistency. Monitor hydration status, I&O, electrolytes, CBC, renal function, LFT. Monitor infusion site for signs of inflammation. Assess skin for rash.

### PATIENT/ FAMILY TEACHING
• Report diarrhea, vomiting, fever, lightheadedness, dizziness. • Do not have immunizations without physician's approval (drug lowers resistance). • Avoid contact with those who have recently received live virus vaccine. • Avoid crowds, those with infections.

# iron dextran

iron **dex**-tran
(Dexiron ✽, Infed, Infufer ✽)
■ **BLACK BOX ALERT** ■ Potentially fatal anaphylactic-type reaction has been associated with parenteral administration.
**Do not confuse DexFerrum with Desferal, or iron dextran with iron sucrose.**

## ◆CLASSIFICATION

**PHARMACOTHERAPEUTIC:** Trace element. **CLINICAL:** Hematinic iron preparation.

## USES

Treatment of anemia, iron deficiency. Use only when PO administration is not feasible or when rapid replenishment of iron is warranted.

## PRECAUTIONS

**Contraindications:** Hypersensitivity to iron formulation. All anemias not associated with iron deficiency anemia (pernicious, aplastic, normocytic, refractory). **Caution:** Serious hepatic impairment. History of allergies, bronchial asthma, rheumatoid arthritis, preexisting cardiac disease. Avoid use during acute kidney infection.

## ACTION

Essential component in formation of Hgb. Necessary for effective erythropoiesis, transport and utilization of oxygen. Serves as cofactor of several essential enzymes. **Therapeutic Effect:** Replenishes Hgb, depleted iron stores.

## PHARMACOKINETICS

Readily absorbed after IM administration. Most absorption occurs within 72 hrs; remainder within 3–4 wks. Bound to protein to form hemosiderin, ferritin, or transferrin. No physiologic system of elimination. Small amounts lost daily in shedding of skin, hair, nails and in feces, urine, perspiration. **Half-life:** 5–20 hrs.

## ⌛ LIFESPAN CONSIDERATIONS

**Pregnancy/Lactation:** May cross placenta in some form (unknown). Trace distributed in breast milk. **Children/Elderly:** No age-related precautions noted.

## INTERACTIONS

**DRUG:** None significant. **HERBAL:** None significant. **FOOD:** None known. **LAB VALUES:** None significant.

## AVAILABILITY (Rx)

**Injection Solution (Infed):** 50 mg/ml.

## ADMINISTRATION/HANDLING

◀**ALERT**▶ Test dose is generally given before full dosage; monitor pt for several min after injection due to potential for anaphylactic reaction.

 **IV**

**Reconstitution** • May give undiluted or dilute in 250–1,000 ml 0.9% NaCl for infusion. • Avoid dilution in dextrose (increased pain/phlebitis).
**Rate of Administration** • Do not exceed IV bolus administration rate of 50 mg/min (1 ml/min). Too-rapid IV rate may produce flushing, chest pain, hypotension, tachycardia, shock. • Infuse diluted solution over 1–6 hrs. • Pt must remain recumbent 30–45 min after IV administration (minimizes postural hypotension).
**Storage** • Store at room temperature.

**IM**
• Draw up medication with one needle; use new needle for injection (minimizes skin staining). • Administer deep IM in upper outer quadrant of buttock only. • Use Z-tract technique (displacement of subcutaneous tissue lateral to injection site before inserting needle) to minimize skin staining.

## ▨ IV INCOMPATIBILITIES

Do not mix with other medications.

## INDICATIONS/ROUTES/DOSAGE

0.5-ml test dose (0.25 ml in infants). Give prior to initiating iron dextran therapy.
◄ALERT► Discontinue oral iron preparations before administering iron dextran. Dosage expressed in terms of milligrams of elemental iron. Dosage individualized based on degree of anemia, pt weight, presence of any bleeding. Use periodic hematologic determinations as guide to therapy.
◄ALERT► Not normally given in first 4 mos of life.

**Iron Deficiency Anemia**
**IV, IM: ADULTS, ELDERLY, CHILDREN WEIGHING MORE THAN 15 KG:** Dose in ml (50 mg elemental iron/ml) = 0.0442 (desired Hgb less observed Hgb) $\times$ lean body weight (in kg) + (0.26 $\times$ lean body weight). Give 2 ml or less once daily until total dose reached.
**CHILDREN WEIGHING 5–15 KG:** Dose in ml (50 mg elemental iron/ml) = 0.0442 (desired Hgb less observed Hgb) $\times$ body weight (in kg) + (0.26 $\times$ body weight). Give 2 ml or less once daily until total dose reached.

**Maximum Daily Dosages**
**ADULTS WEIGHING MORE THAN 50 KG:** 100 mg. **CHILDREN WEIGHING MORE THAN 10 KG:** 100 mg. **CHILDREN WEIGHING 5–10 KG:** 50 mg. **CHILDREN WEIGHING LESS THAN 5 KG:** 25 mg.

**Dosage in Renal/Hepatic Impairment**
No dose adjustment.

## SIDE EFFECTS

**Frequent:** Allergic reaction (rash, pruritus), backache, myalgia, chills, dizziness, headache, fever, nausea, vomiting, flushed skin, pain/redness at injection site, brown discoloration of skin, metallic taste.

## ADVERSE EFFECTS/ TOXIC REACTIONS

Anaphylaxis occurs rarely in first few min following injection. Leukocytosis, lymphadenopathy occur rarely.

## NURSING CONSIDERATIONS

### BASELINE ASSESSMENT

Do not give concurrently with oral iron form (excessive iron may produce excessive iron storage [hemosiderosis]). Be alert to pts with rheumatoid arthritis (RA), iron deficiency anemia (acute exacerbation of joint pain, swelling may occur). Inguinal lymphadenopathy may occur with IM injection. Assess for adequate muscle mass before injecting medication.

### INTERVENTION/EVALUATION

Question pt regarding soreness, pain, inflammation at/near IM injection site. Monitor IM site for abscess formation, necrosis, atrophy, swelling, brownish color of skin. Check IV site for phlebitis. Monitor serum ferritin. Monitor daily pattern of bowel activity, stool consistency.

### PATIENT/FAMILY TEACHING

• Pain, brown staining may occur at injection site. • Oral iron should not be taken when receiving iron injections. • Stools often become black with iron therapy but is harmless unless accompanied by red streaking, sticky consistency of stool, abdominal pain/cramping, which should be reported to physician. • Oral hygiene, hard candy, gum may reduce metallic taste. • Immediately report fever, back pain, headache.

# iron sucrose

iron **soo**-krose
(Venofer)
**Do not confuse iron sucrose with iron dextran.**

## ◆CLASSIFICATION

**PHARMACOTHERAPEUTIC:** Trace element. **CLINICAL:** Hematinic iron preparation.

## USES

Treatment of iron deficiency anemia in chronic kidney disease. **OFF-LABEL:** Chemotherapy-associated anemia.

## PRECAUTIONS

**Contraindications:** Hypersensitivity to iron sucrose. **Cautions:** History of allergies, bronchial asthma; hepatic impairment, rheumatoid arthritis, preexisting cardiac disease. Pts at risk for significant hypotension.

## ACTION

Essential component in formation of Hgb. Necessary for effective erythropoiesis, transport and utilization of oxygen. Serves as cofactor of several essential enzymes. **Therapeutic Effect:** Replenishes body iron stores in pts on chronic hemodialysis who have iron deficiency anemia and are receiving erythropoietin.

## PHARMACOKINETICS

Distributed mainly in blood and to some extent in extravascular fluid. Iron sucrose is dissociated into iron and sucrose by reticuloendothelial system. Sucrose component is eliminated mainly by urinary excretion. **Half-life:** 6 hrs.

## ⌛ LIFESPAN CONSIDERATIONS

**Pregnancy/Lactation:** Unknown if drug crosses placenta or is distributed in breast milk. **Children:** Safety and efficacy not established. **Elderly:** Age-related renal impairment may require dosage adjustment.

## INTERACTIONS

**DRUG:** None significant. **HERBAL:** None significant. **FOOD:** None known. **LAB VALUES:** Increases Hgb, Hct; serum ferritin, transferrin.

## AVAILABILITY (Rx)

**Injection Solution:** 20 mg of elemental iron/ml in 2.5-ml, 5-ml, 10-ml vials.

## ADMINISTRATION/HANDLING

◀**ALERT**▶ Administer directly into dialysis line during hemodialysis.

 **IV**

**Reconstitution** • May give undiluted as slow IV injection or IV infusion. For IV infusion, dilute 100-mg (5-ml) vial in maximum of 100 ml 0.9% NaCl immediately before infusion. (Do not dilute to concentration less than 1 mg/ml in children.) • Dilute large doses in maximum of 250 ml 0.9% NaCl.

**Rate of Administration** • For IV injection, administer 100–200 mg (5–10 ml) over 2–5 min. • For IV infusion, administer 100 mg over at least 15 min; 300 mg over 1.5 hrs; 400 mg over 2.5 hrs; 500 mg over 3.5–4 hrs.

**Storage** • Store at room temperature. • Following dilution, stable for 7 days at room temperature or if refrigerated.

## ▨ IV INCOMPATIBILITIES

Do not mix with other medications or add to parenteral nutrition solution for IV infusion.

## INDICATIONS/ROUTES/DOSAGE

**Iron Deficiency Anemia**
Dosage is expressed in terms of milligrams of elemental iron.
**IV: ADULTS, ELDERLY (HEMODIALYSIS-DEPENDENT PTS):** 5 ml iron sucrose (100 mg elemental iron) delivered during dialysis; administer 1–3 times/wk to total dose of 1,000 mg in 10 doses. Give no more than 3 times/wk. **CHILDREN 2 YRS AND OLDER:** 0.5 mg/kg/dose (**Maximum:** 100 mg) q4wks for 3 doses. **(PERITONEAL DIALYSIS-DEPENDENT PTS):** Two infusions of 300 mg over 90 min 14 days apart followed by a single 400-mg dose over 2½ hrs 14 days later. **CHILDREN 2 YRS AND OLDER:** 0.5 mg/kg/dose (**Maximum:** 100 mg) q4wks for 3 doses. **(NON–DIALYSIS-DEPENDENT PTS):** 200 mg over 2–5 min on 5 different occasions within 14 days.

I

**CHILDREN 2 YRS AND OLDER:** 0.5 mg/kg/dose (**Maximum:** 100 mg) q4wks for 3 doses.

**Dosage in Renal/Hepatic Impairment**
No dose adjustment.

## SIDE EFFECTS

**Frequent (36%–23%):** Hypotension, leg cramps, diarrhea.

## ADVERSE EFFECTS/ TOXIC REACTIONS

Too-rapid IV administration may produce severe hypotension, headache, vomiting, nausea, dizziness, paresthesia, abdominal/muscle pain, edema, cardiovascular collapse. Hypersensitivity reaction occurs rarely.

## NURSING CONSIDERATIONS

### INTERVENTION/EVALUATION

Initially, monitor Hgb, Hct, serum ferritin, transferrin monthly, then q2–3mos thereafter. Reliable serum iron values can be obtained 48 hrs following administration.

# isavuconazonium

eye-sa-vue-**kon**-a-**zoe**-nee-um
(Cresemba)

## ◆ CLASSIFICATION

**PHARMACOTHERAPEUTIC:** Azole antifungal derivative. **CLINICAL:** Antifungal.

## USES

Treatment of invasive aspergillosis and invasive mucormycosis in pts 18 yrs and older.

## PRECAUTIONS

**Contraindications:** Hypersensitivity to isavuconazonium or isavuconazole, concomitant use of strong CYP3A inhibitors (e.g., ketoconazole, ritonavir), strong CYP3A inducers (e.g., carbamazepine, rifampin, St. John's wort), history of short QT syndrome. **Cautions:** Renal/hepatic impairment, hypersensitivity to other azoles. Pts at risk for acute pancreatitis; concomitant use of nephrotoxic medications; pts at risk for hypokalemia, hypomagnesemia. Concomitant use of medications that prolong QT interval.

## ACTION

Isavuconazonium is the prodrug of isavuconazole. Interferes with fungal cytochrome activity, decreasing ergosterol synthesis, inhibiting fungal cell membrane formation. **Therapeutic Effect:** Damages fungal cell wall membrane.

## PHARMACOKINETICS

Widely distributed. Metabolized in liver. Protein binding: greater than 99%. Peak plasma concentration: 2–3 hrs. Eliminated in feces (46%), urine (46%). **Half-life:** 130 hrs.

## ⧗ LIFESPAN CONSIDERATIONS

**Pregnancy/Lactation:** May cause fetal harm. Avoid pregnancy. Avoid breastfeeding while taking Cresemba. **Children:** Safety and efficacy not established in pts younger than 18 yrs. **Elderly:** No age-related precautions noted.

## INTERACTIONS

**DRUG:** Strong **CYP3A4 inhibitors (e.g., ketoconazole, ritonavir)** may increase concentration/effect. **Strong CYP3A4 inducers (e.g., carbamazepine, rifampin)** may decrease concentration/effect. May increase concentration/effects of **atorvastatin, bupropion, cyclosporine, digoxin, midazolam, mycophenolate mofetil/sirolimus, tacrolimus.** **HERBAL:** St. John's wort may decrease concentration/effect. **FOOD:** None known. **LAB VALUES:** May increase serum alkaline phosphatase, ALT, AST, bilirubin. May decrease serum potassium, magnesium.

## AVAILABILITY (Rx)

**Injection Powder:** 372 mg/vial (equivalent to 200 mg isavuconazole).

**Capsules:** 186 mg (equivalent to 100 mg isavuconazole).

## ADMINISTRATION/HANDLING
 IV

**Reconstitution** • Reconstitute vial with 5 ml Sterile Water for Injection. • Gently shake until completely dissolved. • Visually inspect for particulate matter or discoloration. Solution may contain visible translucent to white particles. • Inject reconstituted solution into 250 ml 0.9% NaCl or 5% Dextrose injection. • Gently invert bag to mix. Do not shake or agitate. Do not use pneumatic transport system. • Diluted solution may also contain visible translucent to white particles (which will be removed by in-line filter).
**Administration** • Do not give as IV push or bolus. Flush IV line with 0.9% NaCl or 5% Dextrose injection prior to and after infusion.
**Rate of Administration** • Infuse over 60 min (minimum) using 0.2- to 1.2-micron in-line filter.
**Storage** • Diluted solution may be stored at room temperature up to 6 hrs or refrigerated up to 24 hrs. • Do not freeze.

**PO**
• Give without regard to meals. • Do not cut, crush, divide, or open capsules.

## INDICATIONS/ROUTES/DOSAGE
**Note:** 372 mg is equivalent to 200 mg isavuconazole.

**Invasive Aspergillosis, Invasive Mucormycosis**
**IV: ADULTS, ELDERLY: Loading dose:** 372 mg q8h for 6 doses (48 hrs). **Maintenance:** 372 mg once daily. **PO: ADULTS, ELDERLY: Loading dose:** 372 mg (2 capsules) q8h for 6 doses (48 hrs). **Maintenance:** 372 mg (2 capsules) once daily.

**Dosage in Renal Impairment**
No dose adjustment.

**Dosage in Hepatic Impairment**
**Mild to moderate impairment:** No dose adjustment. **Severe impairment:** Not specified; use caution.

## SIDE EFFECTS
**Frequent (28%–17%):** Nausea, vomiting, diarrhea, abdominal pain, headache, dyspnea. **Occasional (15%–6%):** Peripheral edema, constipation, fatigue, insomnia, back pain, delirium, agitation, confusion, disorientation, chest pain, rash, pruritus, hypotension, anxiety, dyspepsia, injection site reaction, decreased appetite.

## ADVERSE EFFECTS/TOXIC REACTIONS
Severe hepatic injury including cholestasis, hepatitis, hepatic failure reported in pts with underlying medical conditions (e.g., hematologic malignancies). Infusion-related reactions including chills, dizziness, dyspnea, hypoesthesia, hypotension, paresthesia may occur. Acute respiratory failure, renal failure, Stevens-Johnson syndrome; serious hypersensitivity reaction including anaphylaxis were reported.

## NURSING CONSIDERATIONS

### BASELINE ASSESSMENT
Obtain baseline LFT. Confirm negative pregnancy test before initiating treatment. Specimens for fungal culture, histopathology should be obtained prior to initiating therapy. Receive full medication history and screen for interactions/contraindications. Question history of hypersensitivity reaction, hepatic impairment.

### INTERVENTION/EVALUATION
Monitor BMP, LFT periodically. Monitor for infusion-related reactions, hypersensitivity reactions, anaphylaxis. Monitor I&O. Report worsening of hepatic/renal function.

### PATIENT/FAMILY TEACHING
• Swallow capsule whole; do not chew, crush, cut, or open capsules. • Treatment may cause fetal harm. Females of

reproductive potential should use effective contraception. Immediately report suspected pregnancy. • Do not take herbal products such as St. John's wort. • Report liver problems such as upper abdominal pain, bleeding, dark or amber-colored urine, nausea, vomiting, or yellowing of the skin or eyes. • Report decreased urinary out, extremity swelling, dark-colored urine; skin changes such as rash, skin bubbling, or sloughing.

## isoniazid

eye-soe-**nye**-a-zid
(Isotamine ✦)

■ **BLACK BOX ALERT** ■ Severe, potentially fatal hepatitis may occur.

### FIXED-COMBINATION(S)

**Rifamate:** isoniazid/rifampin (antitubercular): 150 mg/300 mg.
**Rifater:** isoniazid/pyrazinamide/rifampin (antitubercular): 50 mg/300 mg/120 mg.

### ◆CLASSIFICATION

**PHARMACOTHERAPEUTIC:** Isonicotinic acid derivative. **CLINICAL:** Antitubercular.

## USES

Treatment of susceptible mycobacterial infection due to *Mycobacterium tuberculosis*. Treatment of latent tuberculosis.

## PRECAUTIONS

**Contraindications:** Hypersensitivity to isoniazid (including drug-induced hepatitis) hepatic disease, hepatic injury or severe adverse reactions with previous isoniazid therapy. **Cautions:** Chronic hepatic disease, alcoholism, severe renal impairment. Pregnancy, pts at risk for peripheral neuropathy, HIV infection, history of hypersensitivity reactions to latent TB infection medications.

## ACTION

Inhibits mycolic acid synthesis. Causes disruption of bacterial cell wall, loss of acid-fast properties in susceptible mycobacteria. **Therapeutic Effect:** Bactericidal against actively growing intracellular, extracellular susceptible mycobacteria.

## PHARMACOKINETICS

Readily absorbed from GI tract. Protein binding: 10%–15%. Widely distributed (including to CSF). Metabolized in liver. Primarily excreted in urine. Removed by hemodialysis. **Half-life:** 0.5–5 hrs.

## ⌛ LIFESPAN CONSIDERATIONS

**Pregnancy/Lactation:** Prophylaxis usually postponed until after delivery. Crosses placenta. Distributed in breast milk. **Children:** No age-related precautions noted. **Elderly:** More susceptible to developing hepatitis.

## INTERACTIONS

**DRUG: Alcohol may** increase isoniazid metabolism, risk of hepatotoxicity. May increase toxicity of **carbamazepine, phenytoin. Hepatotoxic medications (e.g., acetaminophen, simvastatin)** may increase risk of hepatotoxicity. May decrease **ketoconazole** concentration. **HERBAL:** None significant. **FOOD: Foods containing tyramine** may cause hypertensive crisis. **LAB VALUES:** May increase serum bilirubin, ALT, AST.

## AVAILABILITY (Rx)

**Oral Solution:** 50 mg/5 ml. **Solution, Injection:** 100 mg/ml. **Tablets:** 100 mg, 300 mg.

## ADMINISTRATION/HANDLING

**PO**
• Give 1 hr before or 2 hrs following meals (may give with food to decrease GI upset, but will delay absorption).
• Administer at least 1 hr before antacids, esp. those containing aluminum.

## INDICATIONS/ROUTES/DOSAGE

### Active Tuberculosis (in Combination with One or More Antituberculars)

**IM/PO: ADULTS, ELDERLY:** 5 mg/kg once daily. **Usual dose:** 300 mg. **CHILDREN:** 10–15 mg/kg once daily. **Maximum:** 300 mg. **Note:** Give isoniazid with rifampin, pyrazinamide, and with or without ethambutol for 8 wks, then give with rifampin for 18 wks.

### Latent Tuberculosis

**Note:** Give for 9 mos.
**IM/PO: ADULTS, ELDERLY:** 5 mg/kg/day (**maximum:** 300 mg) or 15 mg/kg twice wkly (**maximum:** 900 mg). **CHILDREN:** 10–20 mg/kg/day as a single daily dose. **Maximum:** 300 mg/day or 20–40 mg/kg 2 times/wk. **Maximum:** 900 mg/dose.

### Dosage in Renal Impairment

No dose adjustment.

### Dosage in Hepatic Impairment

Use caution. Contraindicated with acute hepatic disease.

## SIDE EFFECTS

**Frequent:** Nausea, vomiting, diarrhea, abdominal pain. **Rare:** Pain at injection site, hypersensitivity reaction.

## ADVERSE EFFECTS/ TOXIC REACTIONS

Neurotoxicity (ataxia, paresthesia), optic neuritis, hepatotoxicity occur rarely.

## NURSING CONSIDERATIONS

### BASELINE ASSESSMENT

Question for history of hypersensitivity reactions, hepatic injury or disease, sensitivity to nicotinic acid or chemically related medications. Ensure collection of specimens for culture, sensitivity. Evaluate initial LFT.

### INTERVENTION/EVALUATION

Monitor LFT, assess for hepatitis: anorexia, nausea, vomiting, weakness, fatigue, dark urine, jaundice (withhold concurrent INH therapy and inform physician promptly). Assess for paresthesia of extremities (pts esp. at risk for neuropathy may be given pyridoxine prophylactically: malnourished, elderly, diabetics, pts with chronic hepatic disease [including alcoholics]). Be alert for fever, skin eruptions (hypersensitivity reaction).

### PATIENT/FAMILY TEACHING

• Do not skip doses; continue taking isoniazid for full length of therapy (6–24 mos). • Take preferably 1 hr before or 2 hrs following meals (with food if GI upset). • Avoid alcohol during treatment. • Do not take any other medications, including antacids, without consulting physician. • Must take isoniazid at least 1 hr before antacid. • Avoid tuna, sauerkraut, aged cheeses, smoked fish (consult list of tyramine-containing foods) that may cause hypertensive reaction (red/itching skin, palpitations, light-headedness, hot or clammy feeling, headache). • Report any new symptom, immediately for vision difficulties, nausea/vomiting, dark urine, yellowing of skin/eyes (jaundice), fatigue, paresthesia of extremities.

# isosorbide dinitrate

eye-soe-**sor**-bide
(ISDN ✦, IsoDitrate ER, Dilatrate-SR, Isordil)

# isosorbide mononitrate

(Apo-ISMN ✦)
**Do not confuse Imdur with Imuran, Inderal, or K-Dur, Isordil with Inderal, Isuprel, or Plendil.**

## FIXED-COMBINATION(S)

**BiDil:** isosorbide dinitrate/hydralazine (a vasodilator): 20 mg/37.5 mg.

## ◆CLASSIFICATION

**PHARMACOTHERAPEUTIC:** Nitrate.
**CLINICAL:** Antianginal.

## USES

**Dinitrate:** Prevention and treatment of angina pectoris. **Mononitrate:** Prevention of angina pectoris.

## PRECAUTIONS

**Contraindications:** Hypersensitivity to nitrates, concurrent use of sildenafil, tadalafil, vardenafil. **Cautions:** Inferior wall MI, head trauma, increased intracranial pressure (ICP), orthostatic hypotension, blood volume depletion from diuretic therapy, systolic B/P less than 90 mm Hg, hypertrophic cardiomyopathy, alcohol consumption.

## ACTION

Stimulates intracellular cyclic guanosine monophosphate. **Therapeutic Effect:** Relaxes vascular smooth muscle of arterial, venous vasculature. Decreases preload, afterload, cardiac oxygen demand.

## PHARMACOKINETICS

| Route | Onset | Peak | Duration |
|---|---|---|---|
| **Dinitrate** | | | |
| Sublingual | 3 min | N/A | 1–2 hrs |
| PO | 45–60 min | N/A | up to 8 hrs |
| **Mononitrate** | | | |
| PO (extended-release) | 30–60 min | N/A | 12–24 hrs |

Dinitrate poorly absorbed and metabolized in liver to its active metabolite isosorbide mononitrate. Mononitrate well absorbed after PO administration. Primarily excreted in urine. **Half-life:** Dinitrate, 1–4 hrs; mononitrate, 4 hrs.

## ⌛ LIFESPAN CONSIDERATIONS

**Pregnancy/Lactation:** Unknown if drug crosses placenta or is distributed in breast milk. **Children:** Safety and efficacy not established. **Elderly:** May be more sensitive to hypotensive effects. Age-related renal impairment may require dosage adjustment.

## INTERACTIONS

**DRUG:** Alcohol, **antihypertensives** (e.g., **amlodipine, lisinopril, valsartan**) may increase risk of orthostatic hypotension. **Sildenafil, tadalafil, vardenafil** may potentiate hypotensive effects (concurrent use of these agents is contraindicated). **HERBAL:** None significant. **FOOD:** None known. **LAB VALUES:** May increase urine catecholamine, urine vanillylmandelic acid levels.

## AVAILABILITY (Rx)

*Dinitrate*
**Tablets:** 5 mg, 10 mg, 20 mg, 30 mg, 40 mg.

**Capsules, Extended-Release:** 40 mg.
**Tablets, Extended-Release:** 40 mg.

*Mononitrate*
**Tablets:** 10 mg, 20 mg.

**Tablets, Extended-Release:** 30 mg, 60 mg, 120 mg.

## ADMINISTRATION/HANDLING

**PO**
• Best if taken on an empty stomach.
• Do not administer around the clock.
• Oral tablets may be crushed. • Do not crush/break sustained-, extended-release form.

## INDICATIONS/ROUTES/DOSAGE

**Angina**
**PO** *(Isosorbide Dinitrate) (Immediate-Release):* **ADULTS, ELDERLY:** Initially, 5–20 mg 2–3 times/day. **Maintenance:** 10–40 mg 2–3 times/day.

*(Sustained-Release):* **ADULTS, ELDERLY:** 40 mg 1–2 times/day. **Maximum:** 160 mg/day.

**PO** *(Isosorbide Mononitrate) (Immediate-Release)*: **ADULTS, ELDERLY:** 5–20 mg twice daily given 7 hrs apart.
*(Sustained-Release):* Initially, 30–60 mg/day in morning as a single dose. May increase dose at 3-day intervals. **Maximum daily single dose:** 240 mg.

**Dosage in Renal/Hepatic Impairment**
No dose adjustment.

## SIDE EFFECTS

**Frequent:** Headache (may be severe) occurs mostly in early therapy, diminishes rapidly in intensity, usually disappears during continued treatment. **Occasional:** Transient flushing of face/neck, dizziness, weakness, orthostatic hypotension, nausea, vomiting, restlessness. GI upset, blurred vision, dry mouth. **Sublingual:** **Frequent:** Burning, tingling at oral point of dissolution.

## ADVERSE EFFECTS/ TOXIC REACTIONS

Discontinue if blurred vision occurs. Severe orthostatic hypotension manifested by syncope, pulselessness, cold/clammy skin, diaphoresis has been reported. Tolerance may occur with repeated, prolonged therapy, but may not occur with extended-release form. Minor tolerance with intermittent use of sublingual tablets. High dosage tends to produce severe headache.

## NURSING CONSIDERATIONS

### BASELINE ASSESSMENT

Record onset, type (sharp, dull, squeezing), radiation, location, intensity, duration of anginal pain; precipitating factors (exertion, emotional stress). If headache occurs during management therapy, administer medication with meals.

### INTERVENTION/EVALUATION

Assist with ambulation if light-headedness, dizziness occurs. Assess for facial/neck flushing. Monitor number of anginal episodes, orthostatic B/P.

### PATIENT/FAMILY TEACHING

• Do not chew, crush, dissolve, or divide sublingual, extended-release, sustained-release forms. • Take sublingual tablets while sitting down. • Go from lying to standing slowly (prevents dizziness effect). • Take oral form on empty stomach (however, if headache occurs during management therapy, take medication with meals). • Dissolve sublingual tablet under tongue; do not swallow. • Avoid alcohol (intensifies hypotensive effect). • If alcohol is ingested soon after taking nitrates, possible acute hypotensive episode (marked drop in B/P, vertigo, pallor) may occur. • Report signs/symptoms of hypotension, angina.

# itraconazole

it-ra-**kon**-a-zole
(Onmel, Sporanox)

■ **BLACK BOX ALERT** ■ Serious cardiovascular events, including HF, ventricular tachycardia, torsade de pointes, death, have occurred due to concurrent use with pimozide, quinidine, dofetilide, ergot alkaloids, felodipine, lovastatin, methadone, midazolam (oral), simvastatin, triazolam, or levomethadyl. Negative inotropic effects observed following IV administration. Contraindicated for treatment of onychomycosis in pts with HF, ventricular dysfunction.
**Do not confuse itraconazole with fluconazole, or Sporanox with Suprax or Topamax.**

## ◆CLASSIFICATION

**PHARMACOTHERAPEUTIC:** Imidazole/triazole type antifungal. **CLINICAL:** Antifungal.

## USES

**Oral capsules:** Treatment of aspergillosis, blastomycosis, esophageal and oropharyngeal candidiasis, empiric treatment in febrile neutropenia, histoplasmosis, onychomycosis. **Oral solution:** Treatment of oral and esophageal candidiasis. **Oral tablet:** Treatment of onychomycosis of toenail.

## PRECAUTIONS

**Contraindications:** Hypersensitivity to itraconazole, other azoles. Treatment of onychomycosis in pts with evidence of ventricular dysfunction (e.g., HF or history of HF); concurrent use of dofetilide, dronedarone, eplerenone, ergot derivatives, felodipine, irinotecan, lovastatin, lurasidone, methadone, midazolam (oral), pimozide, ranolazine, simvastatin, ticagrelor, triazolam, quinidine; concurrent use with colchicine, fesoterodine, solifenacin in pts with renal/hepatic impairment; treatment of onychomycosis in women who are pregnant or are intending to become pregnant. **Cautions:** Preexisting hepatic impairment (not recommended in pts with active hepatic disease, elevated LFTs), renal impairment, pts with risk factors for HF (e.g., COPD, myocardial ischemia).

## ACTION

Inhibits synthesis of ergosterol (vital component of fungal cell formation). **Therapeutic Effect:** Damages fungal cell membrane, altering its function. Fungistatic.

## PHARMACOKINETICS

Moderately absorbed from GI tract. Absorption is increased when taken with food. Protein binding: 99%. Widely distributed, primarily in fatty tissue, liver, kidneys. Metabolized in liver. Primarily excreted in urine. Not removed by hemodialysis. **Half-life:** 16–26 hrs.

## ⌛ LIFESPAN CONSIDERATIONS

**Pregnancy/Lactation:** Distributed in breast milk. **Children:** Safety and efficacy not established. **Elderly:** Age-related renal impairment may require dosage adjustment.

## INTERACTIONS

**DRUG:** May increase concentration/toxicity of **calcium channel–blocking agents** (e.g., felodipine, nifedipine), **carbamazepine, cyclosporine, digoxin, ergot alkaloids, HMG-CoA reductase inhibitors** (e.g., lovastatin, simvastatin), **midazolam, oral antidiabetic agents** (e.g., glyburide, glipizide), **protease inhibitors** (e.g., indinavir, ritonavir, saquinavir), **sirolimus, tacrolimus, triazolam, warfarin. CYP3A4 inducers** (e.g., carbamazepine, isoniazid, phenobarbital, phenytoin, rifampin) may decrease concentration/effects. May inhibit metabolism of **busulfan, docetaxel, vinca alkaloids. Erythromycin** may increase risk of cardiac toxicity. **Antacids, $H_2$ antagonists, proton pump inhibitors** may decrease absorption. **HERBAL:** St. John's wort may decrease concentration. **FOOD: Grapefruit products** may alter absorption. **LAB VALUES:** May increase serum alkaline phosphatase, bilirubin, ALT, AST, LDH. May decrease serum potassium.

## AVAILABILITY (Rx)

**Capsules:** 100 mg. **Oral Solution:** 10 mg/ml. **Tablet:** 200 mg.

## ADMINISTRATION/HANDLING

**PO**
• Give capsules and tablets with food (increases absorption). • Give solution on empty stomach. Swish vigorously in mouth, then swallow.

## INDICATIONS/ROUTES/DOSAGE

**Note:** Capsules/tablets are not bioequivalent with oral solution.

**Blastomycosis, Histoplasmosis**
**PO: ADULTS, ELDERLY:** Initially, 200 mg once daily. May increase in increments of 100 mg/day up to 400 mg/day. **Life-threatening infections:** 200 mg 3 times/day for first 3 days of therapy. Continue for at least 3 mos.

**Aspergillosis**
**PO: ADULTS, ELDERLY:** 200–400 mg daily for 3 mos. **Life-threatening**

**infections:** 200 mg 3 times/day for first 3 days of therapy. Continue 200–400 mg/day for at least 3 mos.

**Esophageal Candidiasis**
**PO: ADULTS, ELDERLY:** Swish 100–200 mg (10–20 ml) in mouth for several seconds, then swallow once daily for a minimum of 3 wks. Continue for 2 wks after resolution of symptoms. **Maximum:** 200 mg/day.

**Oropharyngeal Candidiasis**
**PO: ADULTS, ELDERLY:** 200 mg (10 ml) oral solution, swish and swallow once daily for 7–14 days.

**Onychomycosis (Fingernail)**
**PO: ADULTS, ELDERLY:** 200 mg twice daily for 7 days, off for 21 days, repeat 200 mg twice daily for 7 days.

**Onychomycosis (Toenail)**
**PO: ADULTS, ELDERLY:** 200 mg once daily for 12 wks.

**Dosage in Renal/Hepatic Impairment**
Use caution.

## SIDE EFFECTS

**Frequent (11%–9%):** Nausea, rash. **Occasional (5%–3%):** Vomiting, headache, diarrhea, hypertension, peripheral edema, fatigue, fever. **Rare (2% or less):** Abdominal pain, dizziness, anorexia, pruritus.

## ADVERSE EFFECTS/ TOXIC REACTIONS

Hepatitis (anorexia, abdominal pain, unusual fatigue/weakness, jaundiced skin/sclera, dark urine) occurs rarely.

## NURSING CONSIDERATIONS

### BASELINE ASSESSMENT
Determine baseline temperature, LFT. Assess allergies. Receive full medication history (numerous contrainidications/cautions).

### INTERVENTION/EVALUATION
Assess for signs, symptoms of hepatic dysfunction. Monitor LFT in pts with pre-existing hepatic impairment.

### PATIENT/ FAMILY TEACHING
• Take capsules with food, liquids if GI distress occurs. • Therapy will continue for at least 3 mos, until lab tests, clinical presentation indicate infection is controlled. • Immediately report unusual fatigue, yellow skin, dark urine, pale stool, anorexia, nausea, vomiting. • Avoid grapefruit products.

# ivabradine

eye-**vab**-ra-deen
(Corlanor)

## ◆CLASSIFICATION
**PHARMACOTHERAPEUTIC:** Hyperpolarization-activated cyclic nucleotide-gated (HCN) channel blocker. **CLINICAL:** Reduces risk of worsening HF.

## USES
To reduce the risk of hospitalization for worsening HF in pts with stable, symptomatic chronic HF with left ventricular ejection fraction less than or equal to 35%, who are in sinus rhythm with a resting heart rate greater than or equal to 70 bpm, and either are on maximally tolerated dose of beta blockers or have a contraindication to beta blocker use.

## PRECAUTIONS
**Contraindications:** Hypersensitivity to ivabradine. Acute decompensated HF, B/P less than 90/50 mm Hg, sick sinus syndrome; sinoatrial block or third-degree AV block (unless a functional pacemaker is present), resting heart rate less than 60 bpm prior to initiation, severe hepatic impairment, pacemaker dependence (heart rate maintained exclusively by a pacemaker), concomitant use of strong

CYP3A4 inhibitors. **Cautions:** History of atrial fibrillation, hypertension. Avoid concomitant use of diltiazem or verapamil. Avoid use in pts with second-degree heart block (unless a functioning pacemaker is present). Pts at risk for bradycardia. Not recommended with pacemakers set to rate of 60 bpm or greater.

## ACTION

Reduces spontaneous pacemaker activity of the cardiac sinus node by blocking HCN channels that are responsible for cardiac current, which regulates heart rate. Does not affect ventricular repolarization or myocardial contractility. Also inhibits retinal current involved in reducing bright light in retina. **Therapeutic Effect:** Reduces heart rate.

## PHARMACOKINETICS

Widely distributed. Metabolized in liver and intestines. Protein binding: 70%. Peak plasma concentration: 1 hr. Eliminated in feces, urine (% not specified). **Half-life:** 6 hrs.

## ☒ LIFESPAN CONSIDERATIONS

**Pregnancy/Lactation:** May cause fetal harm. Females of reproductive potential should use effective contraception. Unknown if distributed in breast milk. Must either discontinue drug or discontinue breastfeeding. If treatment is decided to be absolutely necessary, pregnant pts should be closely monitored for destabilizing HF, esp. during the first trimester. Pregnant women with chronic HF in the third trimester should be closely monitored for preterm birth. **Children:** Safety and efficacy not established. **Elderly:** No age-related precautions noted.

## INTERACTIONS

**DRUG: Beta blockers (e.g., labetolol, metoprolol), negative chronotropes (e.g., amiodarone, digoxin, diltiazem, verapamil)** may increase risk of bradycardia. **Diltiazem, verapamil** may increase concentration/effect; may

further increase risk of bradycardia. **Strong CYP3A4 inhibitors (e.g., clarithromycin, itraconazole)** may increase concentration/effect. **CYP3A4 inducers (e.g., phenytoin, rifampin)** may decrease concentration/effect. **HERBAL: St. John's wort** may decrease concentration/effect. **FOOD: Grapefruit products** may increase concentration/effect. **LAB VALUES:** None significant.

## AVAILABILITY (Rx)

**Tablets:** 5 mg, 7.5 mg.

## ADMINISTRATION/HANDLING

**PO**
• Give with meals. May divide 5-mg tablet, providing 2.5-mg dose.

## INDICATIONS/ROUTES/DOSAGE

**HF**
**PO: ADULTS, ELDERLY:** Initially, 5 mg twice daily for 14 days, then adjust dose to resting heart rate of 50–60 bpm. Further adjustments based on resting heart rate and tolerability. **Maximum dose:** 7.5 mg twice daily. **Pts with history of conduction defects, pts in whom bradycardia could lead to hemodynamic compromise:** Initiate therapy at 2.5 mg twice daily.

### Dose Modification
Adjust dose to maintain a resting heart between 50–60 bpm as follows:

| Heart rate | Dose Adjustment |
|---|---|
| Greater than 60 bpm | Increase by 2.5 mg (given twice daily) up to maximum dose of 7.5 mg daily. |
| 50–60 bpm | Maintain dose. |
| Less than 50 bpm or symptomatic bradycardia | Decrease by 2.5 mg (given twice daily); if current dose is 2.5 mg twice daily, permanently discontinue. |

### Dosage in Renal Impairment
**Mild to moderate impairment:** No dose adjustment. **Severe impairment:** Use caution.

**Dosage in Hepatic Impairment**
**Mild to moderate impairment:** No
dose adjustment. **Severe impairment:**
Contraindicated.

## SIDE EFFECTS

**Occasional (10%–3%):** Bradycardia, hypertension, phosphenes (visual disturbances, luminous phenomena), visual brightness.

## ADVERSE EFFECTS/TOXIC REACTIONS

May increase risk of atrial fibrillation (8.3% of pts). Bradycardia, sinus arrest, or heart block may occur. Bradycardia occurred in 10% of pts. Risk factors for bradycardia may include sinus node dysfunction, conduction defects (e.g., first- or second-degree AV block, bundle branch block), ventricular dyssynchrony, or use of negative chronotropic drugs. Phosphenes, a transient enhanced brightness in the visual field (which may include halos, stroboscopic or kaleidoscopic effect, colored bright lights, or multiple images) may occur. Phosphenes are usually triggered by sudden variations in light intensity and generally occur within the first 2 mos of treatment. Other adverse reactions such as angioedema, diplopia, erythema, hypotension, pruritus, rash, syncope, urticaria, vertigo, visual impairment occur rarely. Overdose may lead to severe and prolonged bradycardia requiring temporary cardiac pacing or infusion of IV beta-stimulating agents.

## NURSING CONSIDERATIONS

### BASELINE ASSESSMENT

Obtain baseline HR, B/P. Confirm negative pregnancy test before initiating therapy. Receive full medication history and screen for interactions. Screen for contraindications as listed in Precautions. Question history of atrial fibrillation, bradycardia, hypertension.

### INTERVENTION/EVALUATION

Frequently monitor HR, B/P. Diligently monitor for atrial fibrillation, bradycardia, syncope. If symptomatic bradycardia occurs, temporary cardiac pacing or infusion of beta-stimulating agents may be warranted. Immediately report suspected pregnancy. Monitor for hypersensitivity reaction. Monitor for visual changes. Initiate fall precautions.

### PATIENT/FAMILY TEACHING

• Take medication with meals. • Avoid grapefruit products, herbal supplements such as St. John's wort. • Treatment may cause fetal harm. Female pts of reproductive potential should use effective contraception during treatment. • Report symptoms of low heart rate such as confusion, dizziness, fatigue, fainting, low blood pressure, pallor. • Report symptoms of atrial fibrillation such as chest pressure, palpitations, shortness of breath. • Treatment may cause luminous phenomena (phosphenes), a transient visual brightness that may include halos, light sensitivity, or colored bright lights. • Avoid tasks that require alertness, motor skills until response to drug is established. • Report allergic reactions such as hives, itching, rash, tongue swelling.

# ivacaftor

**eye**-va-**kaf**-tor
(Kalydeco)

## FIXED COMBINATION(S)

**Orkambi:** ivacaftor/lumacaftor (cystic fibrosis transmembrane conductance regulator): 125 mg/200 mg.

## ◆CLASSIFICATION

**PHARMACOTHERAPEUTIC:** Cystic fibrosis transmembrane conductance regulator potentiator. **CLINICAL:** Cystic fibrosis agent.

## USES

Treatment of cystic fibrosis in pts age 2 yrs and older who have a G551D mutation in the cystic fibrosis transmembrane conductance regulator *(CFTR)* gene.

## PRECAUTIONS

**Contraindications:** Hypersensitivity to ivacaftor. **Cautions:** Moderate to severe hepatic/renal impairment.

## ACTION

Potentiates a specific protein to facilitate, regulate chloride ions, water transport. In cystic fibrosis pts with a specific gene mutation (G551D), a defect in chloride and water transport results in formation of thick mucus in lungs. **Therapeutic Effect:** Improves lung function, fewer respiratory exacerbations.

## PHARMACOKINETICS

Readily absorbed. Peak concentration occurs in 4 hrs. Metabolized in liver. Protein binding: 99%. Primarily excreted in feces. **Half-life:** 12 hrs.

## ⧖ LIFESPAN CONSIDERATIONS

**Pregnancy/Lactation:** Distributed in breast milk. **Children:** Safety and efficacy in children younger than 6 yrs not established. **Elderly:** No age-related precautions noted.

## INTERACTIONS

**DRUG:** Strong CYP3A4 inducers (e.g., **carbamazepine, rifampin**) substantially decreases concentration/effects. Concurrent use not recommended. **Strong CYP3A4 inhibitors (e.g., clarithromycin, ketoconazole)** significantly increases concentration. **Moderate CYP3A4 inhibitors (e.g., erythromycin, fluconazole)** may increase concentration and should not be given concurrently. **HERBAL:** St. John's wort decreases concentration/effects. **FOOD:** Grapefruit products, Seville oranges should be avoided (increases concentration). **High-fat meals** increase absorption. **LAB VALUES:** May increase serum ALT, AST.

## AVAILABILITY (Rx)

**Oral Granules:** 50 mg, 75 mg. **Tablets, Film-Coated:** 150 mg.

## ADMINISTRATION/HANDLING

**PO**
• Give with a high-fat meal (e.g., eggs, butter, peanut butter, cheese pizza).

## INDICATIONS/ROUTES/DOSAGE

**Cystic Fibrosis**
**PO: ADULTS, CHILDREN 6 YRS AND OLDER:** One 150-mg tablet q12h with fat-containing food. **Total daily dose:** 300 mg. **CHILDREN 2–6 YRS, WEIGHING 14 KG OR MORE:** 75-mg packet q12hr. **CHILDREN 2–6 YRS, WEIGHING LESS THAN 14 KG:** 50-mg packet q12hr.

**Concurrent Use with Moderate CYP3A4 Inhibitors (e.g., fluconazole)**
**PO: ADULTS, CHILDREN 6 YRS AND OLDER:** 150 mg once daily.

**Concurrent Use with Strong CYP3A4 Inhibitors (e.g., clarithromycin, ketoconazole)**
**PO: ADULTS, CHILDREN 6 YRS AND OLDER:** 150 mg twice wkly.

**Dosage in Renal Impairment**
**Mild to moderate impairment:** No dose adjustment. **Severe impairment, ESRD:** Use caution.

**Dosage in Hepatic Impairment**
**Mild impairment:** No dose adjustment. **Moderate impairment: ADULTS, ELDERLY:** 150 mg once daily. **CHILDREN WEIGHING 14 KG OR MORE:** 75 mg once daily. **CHILDREN WEIGHING LESS THAN 14 KG:** 50 mg once daily. **Severe impairment:** 150 mg once daily or q48h. Use caution.

## SIDE EFFECTS

**Frequent (24%–10%):** Headache, nasal congestion, abdominal discomfort, diarrhea, nausea, rash. **Occasional (6%–5%):** Rhinitis, dizziness, arthralgia, bacteria in sputum. **Rare (4% and Less):** Myalgia, wheezing, acne.

## ADVERSE EFFECTS/ TOXIC REACTIONS

Upper respiratory infections occurs in 22% of pts, nasopharyngitis in 15%. Increase in ALT, AST occurs in 6% of pts.

## NURSING CONSIDERATIONS

### BASELINE ASSESSMENT

If the pt's genotype is unknown, an FDA-cleared CF mutation test should be used to detect presence of the G551D mutation. Assess hepatic function prior to and periodically during therapy.

### INTERVENTION/EVALUATION

Patients who develop increased ALT, AST levels should be closely monitored until the abnormalities resolve. Dosing should be interrupted if transaminases (ALT or AST) are greater than 5 times upper limit of normal. Transaminases should be obtained every 3 mos during the first year of treatment, and annually thereafter.

### PATIENT/FAMILY TEACHING

• Always take medication with fatty food. • Avoid grapefruit products and Seville oranges. • Adhere to routine laboratory testing as a part of treatment regimen. • Report headache, diarrhea, rash, signs and symptoms of respiratory infection.

# ixabepilone

**ix**-ab-**ep**-i-lone
(Ixempra)

■ **BLACK BOX ALERT** ■ Combination therapy with capecitabine is contraindicated in pts with ALT or AST greater than 2.5 times upper limit of normal (ULN) or bilirubin greater than 1 times ULN. Increased risk of toxicity, neutropenia-related mortality.

## ◆CLASSIFICATION

**PHARMACOTHERAPEUTIC:** Epothilone microtubule inhibitor, antimitotic agent. **CLINICAL:** Antineoplastic.

## USES

Combination therapy with capecitabine for treatment of metastatic or locally advanced breast cancer in pts after failure of anthracycline, taxane therapy. As monotherapy, treatment of metastatic or locally advanced breast cancer in pts after failure of anthracycline, taxane, and capecitabine therapy. **OFF-LABEL:** Treatment of endometrial cancer.

## PRECAUTIONS

**Contraindications:** Hypersensitivity to ixabepilone. Severe hypersensitivity reaction (grade 3 or 4) to Cremophor, baseline neutrophil count less than 1,500/mm³ or platelet count less than 100,000 cells/mm³. **Combination Capecitabine Therapy:** ALT or AST greater than 2.5 times normal range, bilirubin greater than 1 times normal range. **Cautions:** Diabetes mellitus, existing moderate to severe neuropathy, history of cardiovascular disease. **Monotherapy:** ALT or AST greater than 5 times normal range, bilirubin greater than 3 times normal range.

## ACTION

Binds directly on microtubules during active stage of G2 and M phases of cell cycle, preventing formation of microtubules, an essential part of the process of separation of chromosomes. **Therapeutic Effect:** Blocks cells in mitotic phase of cell division, leading to cell death.

## PHARMACOKINETICS

Metabolized in liver. Protein binding: 77%. Excreted in feces (65%), urine (21%). **Half-life:** 52 hrs.

## ⌛ LIFESPAN CONSIDERATIONS

**Pregnancy/Lactation:** May cause fetal harm. Unknown if distributed in breast milk. **Children:** Safety and efficacy not established. **Elderly:** Higher incidence of severe adverse reactions in those older than 65 yrs.

## INTERACTIONS

**DRUG:** CYP3A4 inhibitors (e.g., **atazanavir, clarithromycin, indinavir, itraconazole, ketoconazole, nefazodone, ritonavir, voriconazole**) may increase concentration. CYP3A4 inducers (e.g., **carbamazepine, dexamethasone, phenobarbital, phenytoin, rifabutin, rifampin, rifapentin**) may decrease concentration. **HERBAL: St. John's wort** may decrease plasma concentration. **FOOD: Grapefruit products** may increase plasma concentration. **LAB VALUES:** May increase serum ALT, AST, bilirubin. May decrease WBCs, Hgb, platelets.

## AVAILABILITY (Rx)

**Injection, Solution: Kit:** 15 mg kit supplied with diluent for Ixempra, 8 ml; 45 mg supplied with diluent for Ixempra, 23.5 ml.

## ADMINISTRATION/HANDLING

 **IV**

**Reconstitution** • Withdraw diluent and slowly inject into vial. • Gently swirl and invert until powder is completely dissolved. • Further dilute with 250 ml lactated Ringer's. • Solution may be stored in vial for a maximum of 1 hr at room temperature. • Final concentration for infusion must be between 0.2 mg/ml and 0.6 mg/ml. • Mix infusion bag by manual rotation.
**Rate of Administration** • Administer through an in-line filter of 0.2 to 1.2 microns. • Infuse over 3 hrs. Administration must be completed within 6 hrs of reconstitution.
**Storage** • Refrigerate kit. • Prior to reconstitution, kit should be removed from refrigerator and allowed to stand at room temperature for approximately 30 min. • When vials are initially removed from refrigerator, a white precipitate may be observed in the diluent vial. • This precipitate will dissolve to form a clear solution once diluent warms to room temperature. • Once diluted with lactated Ringer's, solution is stable at room temperature and room light for a maximum of 6 hrs.

## INDICATIONS/ROUTES/DOSAGE

**◄ALERT►** An $H_1$ antagonist (diphenhydramine 50 mg PO or equivalent) and an $H_2$ antagonist (ranitidine 150–300 mg PO or equivalent) must be given prior to beginning treatment with ixabepilone. Pts who experienced a previous hypersensitivity reaction to ixabepilone require pretreatment with corticosteroids (e.g., dexamethasone 20 mg IV, 30 min before infusion or PO, 1 hr before infusion) in addition to pretreatment with $H_1$ and $H_2$ antagonists.

**Breast Cancer**
**IV: ADULTS, ELDERLY:** 40 mg/m² infused over 3 hrs q3 wks. **Maximum:** 88 mg.

**Monotherapy Dosage Adjustments for Hepatic Impairment**
**Mild Hepatic Impairment (ALT and AST Less Than 2.5 Times Upper Limit of Normal (ULN) and Bilirubin Less Than 1 Time ULN)**
**IV: ADULTS, ELDERLY:** 40 mg/m² infused over 3 hrs q3 wks.
**Mild Hepatic Impairment (ALT and AST Greater Than 2.5 Times ULN and Less Than 10 Times ULN and Bilirubin Greater Than 1 Time ULN and Less Than 1.5 Times ULN)**
**IV: ADULTS, ELDERLY:** 32 mg/m² infused over 3 hrs q3 wks.

**Moderate Hepatic Impairment (ALT and AST Less Than 10 Times ULN and Bilirubin Greater Than 1.5 Times ULN and Less Than 3 Times ULN)**
**IV Infusion: ADULTS, ELDERLY:** 20–30 mg/m² infused over 3 hrs q3 wks.

### Dosage with Strong CYP3A4 Inhibitors/Inducers

**Inhibitors:** Consider dose reduction to 20 mg/m².

**Inducers:** Consider dose increase to 60 mg/m².

### Dosage in Renal Impairment

No dose adjustment.

### Dose Modification

Dosage adjustment based on grade of neuropathy, hematologic conditions.

#### Hematologic

**Neutrophils Less Than 500/mm³ for 7 Days or Longer:** Reduce dose by 20%. **Neutropenic Fever:** Reduce dose by 20%. **Platelets Less Than 25,000/mm³ (Less Than 50,000/mm³ with Bleeding):** Reduce dose by 20%.

#### Neuropathy

**Grade 2 for 7 Days or Longer or Grade 3 for Less Than 7 Days:** Reduce dose by 20%. **Grade 3 for 7 Days or Longer:** Discontinue treatment. **Grade 3 (Other Than Neuropathy):** Reduce dose by 20%. **Grade 4:** Discontinue treatment.

## SIDE EFFECTS

**Common (62%):** Peripheral sensory neuropathy. **Frequent (56%–46%):** Fatigue, asthenia, myalgia, arthralgia, alopecia, nausea. **Occasional (29%–11%):** Vomiting, stomatitis, mucositis, diarrhea, musculoskeletal pain, anorexia, constipation, abdominal pain, headache. **Rare (9%–5%):** Skin rash, nail disorder, edema, hand-foot syndrome (blistering/rash/peeling of skin on palms of hands, soles of feet), pyrexia, dizziness, pruritus, gastroesophageal reflux disease (GERD), hot flashes, taste disorder, insomnia.

## ADVERSE EFFECTS/TOXIC REACTIONS

Neuropathy occurs early during treatment; 75% of new onset or worsening neuropathy occurred during first 3 cycles. Diabetics may be at increased risk for severe neuropathy manifested as grade 4 neutropenia. Neutropenia, leukopenia occurs commonly; anemia, thrombocytopenia occur rarely.

## NURSING CONSIDERATIONS

### BASELINE ASSESSMENT

Question possibility of pregnancy. Obtain baseline CBC, serum chemistries, LFT before treatment begins as baseline and monitor for hepatotoxicity, peripheral neuropathy (most frequent cause of drug discontinuation).

### INTERVENTION/EVALUATION

Monitor for symptoms of neuropathy (burning sensation, hyperesthesia, hypoesthesia, paresthesia, discomfort, neuropathic pain). Assess hands and feet for erythema. Monitor CBC for evidence of neutropenia, thrombocytopenia; LFT for hepatotoxicity. Assess mouth for stomatitis, mucositis.

### PATIENT/FAMILY TEACHING

• Avoid crowds, those with known infection. • Avoid contact with those who have recently received live virus vaccine. • Do not have immunizations without physician's approval (drug lowers resistance). • Promptly report fever over 100.5°F, chills, numbness, tingling, burning sensation, erythema of hands/feet.

# ixazomib

ix-**az**-oh-mib
(Ninlaro)
**Do not confuse ixazomib with bortezomib, carfilzomib, idelalisib, or ixekizumab.**

## ◆CLASSIFICATION

**PHARMACOTHERAPEUTIC:** Proteasome inhibitor. **CLINICAL:** Antineoplastic.

## USES

Treatment of multiple myeloma (in combination with lenalidomide and dexamethasone)

 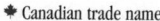

in pts who have received at least 1 prior therapy.

## PRECAUTIONS

**Contraindications:** Severe hypersensitivity to ixazomib. **Cautions:** Baseline neutropenia, thrombocytopenia; hepatic/renal impairment, chronic peripheral edema, predisposing factors to infection (e.g., diabetes, renal failure, open wounds). Concomitant use of strong CYP3A inducers not recommended.

## ACTION

Inhibits activity of beta 5 subunit of the 20S proteasome, leading to cell cycle arrest and tumor cell death (apoptosis). **Therapeutic Effect:** Inhibits tumor cells growth and metastasis.

## PHARMACOKINETICS

Well absorbed following oral administration. Widely distributed. Metabolized in liver. Protein binding: 99%. Peak plasma concentration: 1 hr. Eliminated in urine (62%), feces (22%). Not removed by hemodialysis. **Half-life:** 9.5 days.

## ⏳ LIFESPAN CONSIDERATIONS

**Pregnancy/Lactation:** Avoid pregnancy; may cause fetal harm/malformations. Female and male pts of reproductive potential should use effective contraception during treatment and up to 3 mos after discontinuation. Unknown if distributed in breast milk. Breastfeeding not recommended. **Children:** Safety and efficacy not established. **Elderly:** No age-related precautions noted.

## INTERACTIONS

**DRUG: Strong CYP3A inducers (e.g., carbamazepine, phenytoin, rifampin)** may decrease concentration/effect; avoid use. **HERBAL: St. John's wort** may decrease concentration/effect. **FOOD: High-fat meals** may decrease absorption/concentration. **LAB VALUES:** Expected to decrease neutrophils, platelets.

## AVAILABILITY (Rx)

**Capsules:** 2.3 mg, 3 mg, 4 mg.

## ADMINISTRATION/HANDLING

### PO
• Capsule contents are hazardous; use cytotoxic precautions during handling and disposal. • Administer capsule whole; do not break, cut, crush, or open. • Give at least 1 hr before or 2 hrs after food. • Give on the same day each wk and at the same time that day. If a dose is missed, do not administer within 72 hrs of next scheduled dose. • If vomiting occurs after dosing, do not readminister; give dose at next scheduled time.

## INDICATIONS/ROUTES/DOSAGE

### Multiple Myeloma
**PO: ADULTS, ELDERLY:** 4 mg once wkly on days 1, 8, and 15 of 28-day cycle, in combination with lenalidomide 25 mg daily (on days 1–21 of 28-day cycle) and dexamethasone 40 mg (on days 1, 8, 15, and 22 of 28-day cycle). Continue until disease progression or unacceptable toxicity.

### Dose Reduction Schedule
**Initial dose:** 4 mg. **First dose reduction:** 3 mg. **Second dose reduction:** 2.3 mg. **Unable to tolerate 2.3-mg dose:** Permanently discontinue.

### Dose Modification
Based on Common Terminology Criteria for Adverse Events (CTCAE).

### Thrombocytopenia
**Platelet count less than 30,000 cells/mm³:** Withhold ixazomib and lenalidomide until platelet count is 30,000 cells/mm³ or greater, then resume ixazomib at the same dose and resume lenalidomide at reduced dose level (see manufacturer guidelines).
**Recurrence of platelet count less than 30,000 cells/mm³:** Withhold ixazomib and lenalidomide until platelet

count is 30,000 cells/mm³ or greater, then resume ixazomib at reduced dose level and resume lenalidomide at the same dose.

**Additional occurrences:** Alternate dose modification of ixazomib and lenalidomide.

**Neutropenia**

**Absolute neutrophil count (ANC) less than 500 cells/mm³:** Withhold ixazomib and lenalidomide until ANC is 500 cells/mm³ or greater, then resume ixazomib at the same dose and resume lenalidomide at reduced dose level (see manufacturer guidelines).

**Recurrence of ANC less than 500 cells/mm³:** Withhold ixazomib and lenalidomide until ANC is 500 cells/mm³ or greater, then resume ixazomib at reduced dose level and resume lenalidomide at the same dose.

**Additional occurrences:** Alternate dose modification of ixazomib and lenalidomide.

**Rash**

**Grade 2 or 3 rash:** Withhold lenalidomide until resolved to grade 1 or 0, then resume lenalidomide at next lower dose level (see manufacturer guidelines) and resume ixazomib at the same dose.

**Recurrence of grade 2 or 3 rash:** Withhold ixazomib and lenalidomide until recovery to grade 1 or 0, then resume ixazomib at reduced dose level and resume lenalidomide at the same dose.

**Grade 4 rash:** Permanently discontinue.

**Additional occurrences:** Alternate dose modification of ixazomib and lenalidomide.

**Peripheral Neuropathy**

**Grade 1 (with pain) or grade 2:** Withhold ixazomib until resolved to baseline or improved to grade 1 or 0 without pain (at prescriber's discretion), then resume ixazomib at the same dose.

**Grade 2 (with pain) or grade 3:** Withhold ixazomib until resolved to baseline or improved to grade 1 or 0 without pain (at prescriber's discretion), then resume ixazomib at reduced dose level.

**Grade 4:** Permanently discontinue.

**Any Other Nonhematologic Toxicity**

**Grade 3 or 4:** Withhold ixazomib until resolved to baseline or improved to grade 1 or 0 (at physician's discretion), then resume ixazomib at reduced dose level.

**Dosage in Renal Impairment**

**Mild to moderate impairment:** Not specified; use caution. **Severe impairment, end-stage renal disease:** Reduce starting dose to 3 mg.

**Dosage in Hepatic Impairment**

**Mild impairment:** No dose adjustment. **Moderate to severe impairment:** Reduce starting dose to 3 mg.

## SIDE EFFECTS

**Frequent (42%–26%):** Diarrhea, constipation, nausea. **Occasional (22%–5%):** Vomiting, back pain, blurry vision, dry eye.

## ADVERSE EFFECTS/TOXIC REACTIONS

Neutropenia, thrombocytopenia are expected responses to therapy. Thrombocytopenia reported in 78% of pts; neutropenia in 67% of pts. Severe diarrhea may lead to discontinuation of treatment. Peripheral neuropathy reported in 28% of pts (sensory neuropathies were the most common type). Peripheral edema occurred in 28% of pts. Dermatologic toxicities including maculopapular and macular rash may occur. Infectious processes including upper respiratory tract infection (19% of pts), conjunctivitis (6% of pts) may occur. Other toxic reactions including neutrophilic dermatosis, posterior reversible encephalopathy, Stevens-Johnson syndrome, thrombotic thrombocytopenic purpura, transverse myelitis, treatment-induced hepatotoxicity, tumor lysis syndrome, occur rarely.

## NURSING CONSIDERATIONS

### BASELINE ASSESSMENT

Obtain ANC, CBC (esp. platelet count), renal function test (in pts with renal impairment), LFT; pregnancy test in female pts of reproductive potential. Screen for active infection. Question history of peripheral neuropathy, peripheral edema, hepatic/renal impairment, current hemodialysis status. Receive full medication history including herbal supplements. Offer emotional support. Assess hydration status. Obtain baseline visual acuity. Obtain dietary consult for nutritional support.

### INTERVENTION/EVALUATION

Monitor ANC, platelet count at least monthly; more frequently during first 3 cycles; LFT in pts with hepatic impairment. Consider concomitant granulocyte colony-stimulating factor (e.g., filgrastim, pegfilgrastim) in pts with neutropenia. Monitor for dehydration, electrolyte imbalance if diarrhea occurs. Offer antiemetics for nausea; antidiarrheals for diarrhea. Monitor for infection (esp. in pts with neutropenia); dermal toxicity, skin rashes, petechiae; peripheral neuropathy (with or without pain); peripheral edema. Monitor daily pattern bowel activity, stool consistency. Monitor for side effects of dexamethasone (e.g., hyperglycemia, weight loss, decreased appetite), lenalidomide (see prescribing information). Reversible posterior leukoencephalopathy syndrome should be considered in pts with altered mental status, confusion, headache, seizures, visual disturbances. Obtain visual acuity if vision becomes blurry.

### PATIENT/FAMILY TEACHING

• Treatment may depress your immune system and reduce your ability to fight infection. Report symptoms of infection such as body aches, chills, cough, fatigue, fever. Avoid those with active infection. • Female and male pts of reproductive potential should use effective contraception during treatment and up to 3 mos after last dose. Do not breastfeed. Immediately report suspected pregnancy. • Do not take ixazomib and dexamethasone at the same time. Take dexamethasone with food to minimize GI upset. • Swallow capsules whole; do not chew, crush, or open. Take dose at least 1 hr before or 2 hrs after any food. • Do not expose the capsule contents to the skin or eyes. If eyes are exposed to the capsule powder, thoroughly flush eyes with water. If skin is exposed to the capsule powder, thoroughly wash skin with soap and water. • Treatment may cause nerve pain; extreme sensitivity to touch; muscle weakness; or prickling, tingling, numbness in your hands and feet. • Report swelling of the legs, ankles, feet. • Report neurologic changes such as blurry vision, confusion, headache, seizures; may indicate life-threatening brain swelling. • Treatment may increase risk of bleeding. • Do not take herbal supplements, esp. St. John's wort.

# ixekizumab

ix-ee-**kiz**-ue-mab
(Taltz)
**Do not confuse ixekizumab with daclizumab, eculizumab, gevokizumab, secukinumab, or ustekinumab.**

## ◆CLASSIFICATION

**PHARMACOTHERAPEUTIC:** Human interleukin-17A antagonist. Monoclonal antibody. **CLINICAL:** Antipsoriasis agent.

## USES

Treatment of moderate to severe plaque psoriasis in adults who are candidates for systemic therapy or phototherapy.

## PRECAUTIONS

**Contraindications:** Hypersensitivity to ixekizumab. **Cautions:** Baseline neutropenia, thrombocytopenia; inflammatory bowel disease (Crohn's disease, ulcerative colitis), HIV infection, concomitant immunosuppressant therapy, conditions predisposing to infection (e.g., diabetes, renal failure, open wounds), pts who have been exposed to tuberculosis. Concomitant use of live vaccines not recommended.

## ACTION

Binds to and inhibits interaction of interleukin-17A receptor, a cytokine that is involved in inflammatory and immune response. May reduce epidermal neutrophils in psoriatic plaques. **Therapeutic Effect:** Alters biologic immune response; reduces inflammation.

## PHARMACOKINETICS

Widely distributed. Degraded into small peptides and amino acids via catabolic pathway. Peak plasma concentration: 4 days. Steady state reached in 8–10 wks. Elimination not specified. **Half-life:** 13 days.

## ⧖ LIFESPAN CONSIDERATIONS

**Pregnancy/Lactation:** Unknown if distributed in breast milk. However, human immunoglobulin G is present in breastmilk and is known to cross placenta. **Children:** Safety and efficacy not established in pts younger than 18 yrs. **Elderly:** No age-related precautions noted.

## INTERACTIONS

**DRUG:** Avoid use of **live vaccines.** May decrease therapeutic response. **HERBAL:** **Echinacea** may decrease effect. **FOOD:** None known. **LAB VALUES:** May decrease neutrophil, platelets. May decrease diagnostic effect of *Coccidioides immitis* skin test.

## AVAILABILITY (Rx)

**Auto-injector Pen:** 80 mg/ml. **Prefilled Syringe:** 80 mg/ml.

## ADMINISTRATION/HANDLING

**Subcutaneous**
• Follow instructions for preparation according to manufacturer guidelines.

• Remove autoinjector or prefilled syringe from refrigerator and allow to warm to room temperature (approx. 30 mins) with needle cap intact. • Visually inspect for particulate matter or discoloration. Solution should appear clear, colorless to slightly yellow in color. Do not use if solution is cloudy, discolored, or if visible particles are observed.

**Administration** • Insert needle subcutaneously into upper arms, outer thigh, or abdomen and inject solution. • Do not inject into areas of active skin disease or injury such as sunburns, skin rashes, inflammation, skin infections, or active psoriasis. • Rotate injection sites.

**Storage** • Refrigerate until time of use. • Do not freeze. • Do not shake. • Protect from light.

## INDICATIONS/ROUTES/DOSAGE

**Plaque Psoriasis**
**SQ: ADULTS, ELDERLY:** Initially, 160 mg (two injections of 80 mg) once, then 80 mg at wks 2, 4, 6, 8, 10, 12, then 80 mg once q4wks.

**Dosage in Renal Impairment**
Not specified; use caution.

**Dosage in Hepatic Impairment**
Not specified; use caution.

## SIDE EFFECTS

**Occasional (17%):** Injections site reactions (pain, erythema). **Rare (2%):** Nausea.

## ADVERSE EFFECTS/TOXIC REACTIONS

May increase risk of infection including tuberculosis. Infections including upper respiratory tract infection (14% of pts), nasopharyngitis (14% of pts), tinea infections (2% of pts) have occurred. Cytopenias including neutropenia (11% of pts), thrombocytopenia (3% of pts) were reported. May cause exacerbation of Crohn's disease and ulcerative colitis. Hypersensitivity reactions, including angioedema, occur rarely. Immunogenicity (auto-ixekizumab antibodies) occurred in less than 9% of pts.

## NURSING CONSIDERATIONS

### BASELINE ASSESSMENT

Obtain CBC in pts with known history of neutropenia, thrombocytopenia. Screen for active infection. Pts should be evaluated for active tuberculosis and tested for latent infection prior to initiating treatment and periodically during therapy. Induration of 5 mm or greater with tuberculin skin testing should be considered a positive test result when assessing if treatment for latent tuberculosis is necessary. Consider administration of age-appropriate immunizations (if applicable) before initiation. Question history of Crohn's disease, ulcerative colitis, hypersensitivity reaction. Conduct dermatologic exam; record characteristics of psoriatic lesions.

### INTERVENTION/EVALUATION

Monitor for symptoms of tuberculosis, including pts who tested negative for latent tuberculosis infection prior to initiating therapy. Interrupt or discontinue treatment if serious infection, opportunistic infection, or sepsis occurs and initiate appropriate antimicrobial therapy. Assess skin for improvement of lesions. Monitor for hypersensitivity reaction, symptoms of inflammatory bowel disease.

### PATIENT/FAMILY TEACHING

• A healthcare provider will show you how to properly prepare and inject your medication. You must demonstrate correct preparation and injection techniques before using medication at home. • Treatment may depress your immune system response and reduce your ability to fight infection. Report symptoms of infection such as body aches, chills, cough, fatigue, fever. Avoid people with active infection. • Do not receive live vaccines. • Expect frequent tuberculosis screening. • Report travel plans to possible endemic areas. • Immediately report difficulty breathing, itching, hives, rash, swelling of the face or tongue; may indicate allergic reaction. • Treatment may cause worsening of Crohn's disease or cause inflammatory bowel disease. Report abdominal pain, diarrhea, weight loss.

# ketoconazole

kee-toe-kon-a-zole
(Apo-Ketoconazole ✦, Extina,
Nizoral, Nizoral AD, Xolegel)
■ **BLACK BOX ALERT** ■ Potentially
fatal hepatotoxicity has occurred;
serious cardiovascular events
(QT prolongation, torsades de
pointes, ventricular tachycardia,
ventricular fibrillation, fatalities)
have occurred.
**Do not confuse Nizoral with
Nasarel, Neoral, or Nitrol.**

## ◆ CLASSIFICATION

**PHARMACOTHERAPEUTIC:** Imidazole derivative. **CLINICAL:** Antifungal.

## USES

**PO:** Treatment of susceptible fungal infections including histoplasmosis, blastomycosis, coccidioidomycosis, paracoccidioi-
domycosis, chromomycosis. **Shampoo:**
Treatment of dandruff. Treatment of tinea
versicolor. **Topical:** Treatment of tineas,
pityriasis versicolor, cutaneous candidiasis, seborrhea dermatitis, dandruff. **Xolegel:** Treatment of seborrheic dermatitis.
**OFF-LABEL: Systemic:** Treatment of advanced prostate cancer.

## PRECAUTIONS

**Contraindications:** Hypersensitivity to ketoconazole. Acute or chronic liver disease; concurrent use with alprazolam,
colchicine, dofetilide, eplerenone, ergot
derivatives, methadone, midazolam, quinidine irinotecan, ranolazine, statins, triazolam. **Cautions:** Hepatic impairment,
concomitant use of drugs decreasing gastric acidity (e.g., antacids, H₂ antagonists,
proton pump inhibitors).

## ACTION

Alters cell wall permeability, inhibits phos-
pholipids/enzymes of fungi. **Therapeutic
Effect:** Damages fungal cell membrane,
altering its function. Fungistatic.

## PHARMACOKINETICS

Well absorbed from GI tract following PO
administration (absorption decreases as
pH of gastric contents increases). Protein
binding: 93%–96%. Metabolized in liver.
Primarily excreted in bile. Negligible systemic absorption following topical absorption. Ketoconazole is not detected in
plasma after shampooing, topical administration. **Half-life:** 8 hrs.

## ⧗ LIFESPAN CONSIDERATIONS

**Pregnancy/Lactation:** Oral form distributed in breast milk. Unknown if topical form crosses placenta or is distributed in breast milk. **Children: Cream,
shampoo:** Safety and efficacy not established. **Oral form:** Safety and efficacy not established in pts younger than
2 yrs. **Elderly:** No age-related precautions noted.

## INTERACTIONS

**DRUG:** May increase concentration/tox-
icity of **cyclosporine, digoxin, ergot
alkaloids, midazolam, protease inhibitors (e.g., indinavir, ritonavir,
saquinavir), sirolimus, tacrolimus,
triazolam, warfarin. Isoniazid, rifampin** may decrease concentration/
effects. **Antacids, H₂ antagonists (e.g.,
cimetidine, famotidine), proton pump
inhibitors (e.g., omeprazole)** may
decrease absorption. **HERBAL: St. John's
wort** may decrease concentration. **FOOD:**
None known. **LAB VALUES:** May increase
serum alkaline phosphatase, bilirubin,
ALT, AST. May decrease serum corticosteroid, testosterone.

## AVAILABILITY (Rx)

**Foam (Extina):** 2%. **Gel (Xolegel):** 2%.
**Shampoo (Nizoral AD [OTC]):** 1%. **Tablets (Nizoral):** 200 mg.

## ADMINISTRATION/HANDLING

**PO**
• Give with food to minimize GI irritation. • Tablets may be crushed. • Ketoconazole requires acidity; give antacids,

K

anticholinergics, $H_2$ blockers at least 2 hrs following dosing.

**Shampoo**
• Apply to wet hair, massage for 1 min, rinse thoroughly, reapply for 3 min, rinse.

**Topical**
• Apply, rub gently into affected/surrounding area.

## INDICATIONS/ROUTES/DOSAGE

**Usual Dosage**
**PO: ADULTS, ELDERLY:** 200–400 mg once daily. **CHILDREN 2 YRS AND OLDER:** 3.3–6.6 mg/kg once daily.
**Topical: ADULTS, ELDERLY:** Apply to affected area 1–2 times/day for 2–4 wks.
**Shampoo: ADULTS, ELDERLY:** Use twice wkly for 4 wks, allowing at least 3 days between shampooing. Use intermittently to maintain control.

**Dosage in Renal Impairment**
No dose adjustment.

**Dosage in Hepatic Impairment**
Use caution.

## SIDE EFFECTS

**Occasional (10%–3%):** Nausea, vomiting. **Rare (less than 2%):** Abdominal pain, diarrhea, headache, dizziness, photophobia. **Topical:** Burning, irritation, pruritus.

## ADVERSE EFFECTS/TOXIC REACTIONS

Hematologic toxicity (thrombocytopenia, hemolytic anemia, leukopenia) occurs occasionally. Hepatotoxicity may occur within first wk to several mos after starting therapy. Anaphylaxis occurs rarely.

## NURSING CONSIDERATIONS

### BASELINE ASSESSMENT
Confirm culture or histologic test for accurate diagnosis; therapy may begin before results known. Receive full medication history and screen for contraindications.

### INTERVENTION/EVALUATION
Monitor LFT; be alert for hepatotoxicity: dark urine, pale stools, jaundice, fatigue, anorexia, nausea, or vomiting (unrelieved by giving medication with food). Monitor CBC for hematologic toxicity. Monitor daily pattern of bowel activity, stool consistency. Assess for dizziness, provide assistance as needed. Evaluate skin for rash, urticaria, pruritus. **Topical:** Check for localized burning, pruritus, irritation.

### PATIENT/FAMILY TEACHING
• Prolonged therapy (wks or mos) is usually necessary. • Avoid alcohol. • May cause dizziness; avoid tasks that require alertness, motor skills until response to drug is established. • Take antacids, antiulcer medications at least 2 hrs after ketoconazole. • Report dark urine, pale stool, yellow skin or eyes, vomiting, increased irritation in topical use, onset of other new symptoms. • **Topical:** Rub well into affected areas. • Avoid contact with eyes. • Keep skin clean, dry; wear light clothing for ventilation. • Separate personal items in direct contact with affected area. • **Shampoo:** Initially, use 2 times/wk for 4 wks with at least 3 days between shampooing; frequency then determined by response to medication.

# ketorolac

kee-**toe**-role-ak
(Acular, Acular LS, Acuvail, Apo-Ketorolac ✦, Novo-Ketorolac ✦, Sprix, Toradol ✦)

■ **BLACK BOX ALERT** ■ Increased risk of serious cardiovascular thrombotic events, including myocardial infarction, CVA. Increased risk of severe GI reactions, including ulceration, bleeding, perforation.
**Do not confuse Acular with Acthar or Ocular, ketorolac with Ketalar, or Toradol with Foradil, Inderal, Tegretol, or tramadol.**

## ◆CLASSIFICATION

**PHARMACOTHERAPEUTIC:** NSAID. **CLINICAL:** Analgesic, intraocular anti-inflammatory.

## USES

**PO, injection, nasal:** Short-term (5 days or less) relief of mild to moderate pain. **Ophthalmic:** Relief of ocular itching due to seasonal allergic conjunctivitis. Treatment postop for inflammation following cataract extraction, pain following incisional refractive surgery. **OFF-LABEL:** Prevention, treatment of ocular inflammation (ophthalmic form).

## PRECAUTIONS

**Contraindications:** Hypersensitivity to ketorolac, aspirin or other NSAIDs. Intracranial bleeding, hemorrhagic diathesis, high risk of bleeding; concomitant use of aspirin, NSAIDs, probenecid or pentoxifylline; labor and delivery, advanced renal impairment or risk of renal failure, active or history of peptic ulcer disease, chronic inflammation of GI tract, recent or history of GI bleeding/ulceration. Perioperative pain in setting of CABG surgery. Prophylaxis before major surgery. **Cautions:** Hepatic impairment, history of GI tract disease, asthma, coagulation disorders, receiving anticoagulants, fluid retention, HF, renal impairment, inflammatory bowel disease, smoking, use of alcohol, elderly, debilitated.

## ACTION

Inhibits prostaglandin synthesis, reduces prostaglandin levels in aqueous humor. **Therapeutic Effect:** Reduces intensity of pain stimulus, reduces intraocular inflammation.

## PHARMACOKINETICS

Readily absorbed from GI tract after IM administration. Protein binding: 99%. Metabolized in liver. Primarily excreted in urine. Not removed by hemodialysis. **Half-life:** 5–9 hrs (increased in renal impairment, in elderly).

## ⌛ LIFESPAN CONSIDERATIONS

**Pregnancy/Lactation:** Unknown if distributed in breast milk. Avoid use during third trimester (may adversely affect fetal cardiovascular system: premature closure of ductus arteriosus). **Children:** Safety and efficacy not established, but doses of 0.5 mg/kg have been used. **Elderly:** GI bleeding, ulceration more likely to cause serious adverse effects. Age-related renal impairment may increase risk of hepatic/renal toxicity; decreased dosage recommended.

## INTERACTIONS

**DRUG:** May decrease effects of **antihypertensives (e.g., amlodipine, lisinopril), diuretics (e.g., furosemide, HCTZ). Aspirin, NSAIDs, other salicylates** may increase risk of GI side effects, bleeding. May increase risk of bleeding with **heparin, oral anticoagulants (e.g., warfarin), thrombolytics.** May increase concentration, risk of toxicity of **lithium.** May increase risk of **methotrexate** toxicity. **Probenecid** may increase concentration. **HERBAL: Cat's claw, dong quai, evening primrose, feverfew, garlic, ginkgo, ginseng, horse chestnut, red clover** may decrease antiplatelet activity, risk of bleeding. **FOOD:** None known. **LAB VALUES:** May prolong bleeding time. May increase serum ALT, AST, BUN, potassium, creatinine.

## AVAILABILITY (Rx)

**Injection Solution (Toradol):** 15 mg/ml, 30 mg/ml. **Nasal Spray (Sprix):** 1.7-g bottle provides 8 sprays (15.75 mg/spray). **Ophthalmic Solution:** 0.4% (Acular LS), 0.45% (Acuvail), 0.5% (Acular). **Tablets (Toradol):** 10 mg.

K

---

## ADMINISTRATION/HANDLING

 **IV**

• Give undiluted as IV push. • Give over at least 15 sec.

**IM**

• Give deep IM slowly into large muscle mass.

**PO**

• Give with food, milk, antacids if GI distress occurs.

**Ophthalmic**

• Place gloved finger on lower eyelid and pull out until pocket is formed between eye and lower lid. Place prescribed number of drops into pocket. • Instruct pt to close eye gently for 1–2 min (so medication will not be squeezed out of the sac) and to apply digital pressure to lacrimal sac at inner canthus for 1 min to minimize system absorption.

## ▨ IV INCOMPATIBILITY

Promethazine (Phenergan).

## ▨ IV COMPATIBILITIES

Fentanyl (Sublimaze), hydromorphone (Dilaudid), morphine, nalbuphine (Nubain).

## INDICATIONS/ROUTES/DOSAGE

**Pain Management**

**PO: ADULTS, ELDERLY:** Initially, 20 mg (10 mg for elderly), then 10 mg q4–6h. **Maximum:** 40 mg/24 hrs.
**IM: ADULTS YOUNGER THAN 65 YRS:** 60 mg once or 30 mg q6h. **Maximum:** 120 mg/24 hrs. **ADULTS 65 YRS AND OLDER, PTS WITH RENAL IMPAIRMENT, PTS WEIGHING LESS THAN 50 KG:** 30 mg once or 15 mg q6h. **Maximum:** 60 mg/24 hrs.
**IV: ADULTS YOUNGER THAN 65 YRS:** 30 mg once or 30 mg q6h. **Maximum:** 120 mg/24 hrs. **ADULTS 65 YRS AND OLDER, PTS WITH RENAL IMPAIRMENT, PTS WEIGHING LESS THAN 50 KG:** 15 mg once or 15 mg q6h. **Maximum:** 60 mg/24 hrs.

**Nasal Spray: ADULTS, ELDERLY YOUNGER THAN 65 YRS:** 31.5 mg (1 spray each nostril) q6–8h. **Maximum daily dose:** 126 mg. **ADULTS 65 YRS AND OLDER, PTS WEIGHING LESS THAN 50 KG:** 15.75 (1 spray in one nostril) mg q6–8h. **Maximum daily dose:** 63 mg.

**Allergic Conjunctivitis**
**Ophthalmic: ADULTS, ELDERLY, CHILDREN 3 YRS AND OLDER:** 1 drop 4 times/day.

**Cataract Extraction**
**Ophthalmic: ADULTS, ELDERLY:** 1 drop 4 times/day. Begin 24 hrs after surgery and continue for 2 wks.

**Refractive Surgery**
**Ophthalmic: ADULTS, ELDERLY:** 1 drop 4 times/day for 3 days.

**Dosage in Renal Impairment**
See dosage section.

**Dosage in Hepatic Impairment**
Use caution.

## SIDE EFFECTS

**Frequent (17%–12%):** Headache, nausea, abdominal cramps/pain, dyspepsia. **Occasional (9%–3%):** Diarrhea. **Nasal:** Nasal discomfort, rhinalgia, increased lacrimation, throat irritation, rhinitis. **Ophthalmic:** Transient stinging, burning. **Rare (3%–1%):** Constipation, vomiting, flatulence, stomatitis. **Ophthalmic:** Ocular irritation, allergic reactions (manifested by pruritus, stinging), superficial ocular infection, keratitis.

## ADVERSE EFFECTS/TOXIC REACTIONS

Peptic ulcer, GI bleeding, gastritis, severe hepatic reaction (cholestasis, jaundice) occur rarely. Nephrotoxicity (glomerular nephritis, interstitial nephritis, nephrotic syndrome) may occur in pts with preexisting renal impairment. Acute hypersensitivity reaction (fever, chills, joint pain) occurs rarely.

**K**

## NURSING CONSIDERATIONS

### BASELINE ASSESSMENT

Assess onset, type, location, duration of pain. Obtain baseline renal/hepatic function tests.

### INTERVENTION/EVALUATION

Monitor renal function, LFT, urinary output. Monitor daily pattern of bowel activity, stool consistency. Observe for occult blood loss. Assess for therapeutic response: relief of pain, stiffness, swelling; increased joint mobility; reduced joint tenderness; improved grip strength. Monitor for bleeding (may also occur with ophthalmic route due to systemic absorption).

### PATIENT/ FAMILY TEACHING

• Avoid aspirin, alcohol. • Report abdominal pain, bloody stools, or vomiting blood. • If GI upset occurs, take with food, milk. • **Ophthalmic:** Transient stinging, burning may occur upon instillation. • Do not administer while wearing soft contact lenses.

**K**

# labetalol

la-**bayt**-a-lol
(Apo-Labetalol ❖, Normodyne ❖, Trandate ❖)
**Do not confuse labetalol with betaxolol, metoprolol or propranolol, or Trandate with tramadol or Trental.**

## FIXED-COMBINATION(S)

**Normozide:** labetalol/hydrochlorothiazide (a diuretic): 100 mg/25 mg, 200 mg/25 mg, 300 mg/25 mg.

## ◆CLASSIFICATION

**PHARMACOTHERAPEUTIC:** Alpha-, beta-adrenergic blocker. **CLINICAL:** Antihypertensive.

## USES

Management of mild to severe hypertension. IV for severe hypertension. **OFF-LABEL:** Management of preeclampsia, severe hypertension in pregnancy, hypertension during acute ischemic stroke, pediatric hypertension.

## PRECAUTIONS

**Contraindications:** Hypersensitivity to labetalol. Bronchial asthma, cardiogenic shock, uncompensated HF, second- or third-degree heart block (except in pts with functioning pacemaker), severe bradycardia, conditions associated with severe, prolonged hypotension. **Cautions:** Compensated HF, severe anaphylaxis to allergens, myasthenia gravis, psychiatric disease, hepatic impairment, pheochromocytoma, diabetes mellitus; concurrent use with digoxin, verapamil, or diltiazem; arterial obstruction, elderly. Pts with peripheral vascular disease, Raynaud's disease.

## ACTION

Blocks alpha$_1$-, beta$_1$-, beta$_2$- (large doses) adrenergic receptor sites. **Therapeutic Effect:** Slows sinus heart rate; decreases peripheral vascular resistance, B/P.

## PHARMACOKINETICS

| Route | Onset | Peak | Duration |
|---|---|---|---|
| PO | 0.5–2 hrs | 2–4 hrs | 8–12 hrs |
| IV | 2–5 min | 5–15 min | 2–4 hrs |

Incompletely absorbed from GI tract. Bioavailability: 25%. Protein binding: 50%. Metabolized in liver. Primarily excreted in urine. Not removed by hemodialysis. **Half-life:** 6–8 hrs.

## ⧖ LIFESPAN CONSIDERATIONS

**Pregnancy/Lactation:** Drug crosses placenta. Small amount distributed in breast milk. **Children:** Safety and efficacy not established. **Elderly:** Age-related peripheral vascular disease may increase susceptibility to decreased peripheral circulation.

## INTERACTIONS

**DRUG:** May decrease effects of **beta$_2$-adrenergic agonists (e.g., arformoterol, salmeterol), theophylline. Beta blockers (e.g., carvedilol, metoprolol), digoxin** may increase risk of bradycardia. **HERBAL: Ephedra, ginseng, yohimbe** may worsen hypertension. **Garlic** may increase antihypertensive effect. **Licorice** may cause water retention, increased serum sodium, decreased serum potassium. **FOOD:** None known. **LAB VALUES:** May increase serum antinuclear antibody titer (ANA), BUN, LDH, alkaline phosphatase, bilirubin, creatinine, potassium, triglycerides, lipoprotein, uric acid, ALT, AST.

## AVAILABILITY (Rx)

**Injection Solution:** 5 mg/ml. **Tablets (Trandate):** 100 mg, 200 mg, 300 mg.

## ADMINISTRATION/HANDLING

 **IV**

◀**ALERT**▶ Prolonged duration of action: Monitor several hrs after administration. Excessive administration may result in prolonged hypotension and/or bradycardia.
**Reconstitution •** For IV infusion, dilute in D$_5$W to provide concentration of 1–2 mg/ml.

**Rate of Administration** • For IV push, administer at a rate of 10 mg/min. • For IV infusion, administer at rate of 2 mg/min initially. Rate is adjusted according to B/P. • Monitor B/P immediately before and q5–10min during IV administration (maximum effect occurs within 5 min).

**Storage** • Store at room temperature. • After dilution, IV solution is stable for 72 hrs. • Solution appears clear, colorless to light yellow. • Discard if discolored or precipitate forms.

**PO**
• Give without regard to food. • Tablets may be crushed.

### ▨ IV INCOMPATIBILITIES

Amphotericin B complex (Abelcet, AmBisome, Amphotec), ceftaroline (Teflaro), ceftriaxone (Rocephin), furosemide (Lasix), heparin, nafcillin (Nafcil).

### ▨ IV COMPATIBILITIES

Amiodarone (Cordarone), calcium gluconate, dexmedetomidine (Precedex), diltiazem (Cardizem), dobutamine (Dobutrex), dopamine (Intropin), enalapril (Vasotec), fentanyl (Sublimaze), hydromorphone (Dilaudid), lidocaine, lorazepam (Ativan), magnesium sulfate, midazolam (Versed), milrinone (Primacor), morphine, nitroglycerin, norepinephrine (Levophed), potassium chloride, potassium phosphate, propofol (Diprivan).

### INDICATIONS/ROUTES/DOSAGE

**Hypertension**
**PO: ADULTS, ELDERLY:** Initially, 100 mg twice daily. Adjust in increments of 100 mg twice daily q2–3days. Usual dose: 100–300 mg twice daily. **Maximum:** 2.4 g/day. **CHILDREN:** 1–3 mg/kg/day in 2 divided doses. **Maximum:** 10–12 mg/kg/day up to 1,200 mg/day.

**Severe Hypertension, Hypertensive Crisis**
**IV: ADULTS:** Initially, 20 mg (bolus over 2 min). Additional doses of 40–80 mg may be given at 10-min intervals, up to total dose of 300 mg.

**IV Infusion: ADULTS:** Initially, 2 mg/min up to total dose of 300 mg. **CHILDREN:** 0.4–1 mg/kg/hr. **Maximum:** 3 mg/kg/hr.

**Dosage in Renal Impairment**
No dose adjustment.

**Dosage in Hepatic Impairment**
Use caution.

### SIDE EFFECTS

**Frequent (20%–11%):** Drowsiness, dizziness, excessive fatigue. **Occasional (10% or less):** Dyspnea, peripheral edema, depression, anxiety, constipation, diarrhea, nasal congestion, weakness, diminished sexual function, transient scalp tingling, insomnia, nausea, vomiting, abdominal discomfort. **Rare:** Altered taste, dry eyes, increased urination, paresthesia.

### ADVERSE EFFECTS/ TOXIC REACTIONS

May precipitate, aggravate HF due to decreased myocardial stimulation. Abrupt withdrawal may precipitate myocardial ischemia, producing chest pain, diaphoresis, palpitations, headache, tremor. May mask signs, symptoms of acute hypoglycemia (tachycardia, B/P changes) in diabetic pts.

### NURSING CONSIDERATIONS

**BASELINE ASSESSMENT**
Assess baseline renal function, LFT. Assess B/P, apical pulse immediately before drug administration (if pulse is 60/min or less or systolic B/P is lower than 90 mm Hg, withhold medication, contact physician).

**INTERVENTION/EVALUATION**
Monitor B/P for hypotension. Assess pulse for quality, irregular rate, bradycardia. Monitor EKG for cardiac arrhythmias. Assist with ambulation if dizziness occurs. Assess for evidence of HF: dyspnea (particularly on exertion or lying down), night cough, peripheral edema, distended neck veins. Monitor I&O (increase in weight, decrease in urine output may indicate HF).

• Do not discontinue drug except upon advice of physician (abrupt discontinuation may precipitate heart failure). • Slowly go from lying to standing. • Compliance with therapy regimen is essential to control hypertension, arrhythmias. • Avoid tasks that require alertness, motor skills until response to drug is established. • Report shortness of breath, excessive fatigue, weight gain, prolonged dizziness, headache. • Do not use nasal decongestants, OTC cold preparations (stimulants) without physician approval. • Limit alcohol.

# lacosamide

la-**koe**-sa-myde
(Vimpat)
**Do not confuse lacosamide with zonisamide.**

## ◆CLASSIFICATION

**PHARMACOTHERAPEUTIC:** Succinimide **(Schedule V). CLINICAL:** Anticonvulsant.

## USES

Monotherapy or adjunctive therapy for treatment of partial-onset seizures in pts 17 yrs and older.

## PRECAUTIONS

**Contraindications:** Hypersensitivity to lacosamide. **Cautions:** Renal/hepatic impairment, cardiac conduction problems (e.g., marked first-degree AV block, second-degree or higher AV block, sick sinus syndrome without pacemaker), myocardial ischemia, HF, pts at risk of suicide.

## ACTION

Selectively enhances slow inactivation of sodium channels, stabilizing hyperexcitable neuronal membranes and inhibits neuronal firing. **Therapeutic Effect:** Produces anticonvulsant effect.

## PHARMACOKINETICS

Completely absorbed following PO administration. Protein binding: 15%. Peak plasma concentration: 1–4 hrs after oral dosing and is reached at the end of IV infusion. Primarily excreted in urine. Steady-state levels achieved in 3 days. Removed by hemodialysis. **Half-life:** 13 hrs.

## ⧗ LIFESPAN CONSIDERATIONS

**Pregnancy/Lactation:** Unknown if distributed in breast milk. **Children:** Safety and efficacy not established in pts younger than 17 yrs. **Elderly:** No age-related precautions noted.

## INTERACTIONS

**DRUG: Strong CYP2C9 inhibitors (e.g., fluconazole), strong CYP3A4 inhibitors (e.g., clarithromycin, ketoconazole)** may increase concentration/effects. **HERBAL:** None significant. **FOOD:** None known. **LAB VALUES:** May increase serum ALT; proteinuria.

## AVAILABILITY (Rx)

**Injection Solution:** 10 mg/ml (20 ml).
**Oral Solution:** 10 mg/ml.

**Tablets:** 50 mg, 100 mg, 150 mg, 200 mg.

## ADMINISTRATION/HANDLING

**PO**
• Give without regard to meals. • Do not break, crush, dissolve, or divide film-coated tablets. • Oral solution should be administered with a calibrated measuring device. • Discard any unused portion after 7 wks.

**IV**
• Appears as a clear, colorless solution. • Discard unused portion or if precipitate or discoloration is present. May give without further dilution. • If mixing with diluent, may be stored for 24 hrs at room temperature. Infuse over 30–60 min.

##  IV COMPATIBILITIES

0.9% NaCl, $D_5$W, lactated Ringer's.

## INDICATIONS/ROUTES/DOSAGE

**Note:** IV dose is same as oral dose. May give undiluted or mixed in compatible diluent and infused over 30–60 min.

#### Partial-Onset Seizures
*Monotherapy*
**PO/IV: ADULTS, CHILDREN 17 YRS AND OLDER:** Initially, 100 mg twice daily. May increase by 50 mg twice daily at wkly intervals. **Maintenance:** 150–200 mg twice daily.
*Adjunctive Therapy*
**PO/IV: ADULTS, CHILDREN 17 YRS AND OLDER:** Initially, 50 mg twice daily. May increase by 50 mg twice daily at wkly intervals. **Maintenance:** 100–200 mg twice daily.

#### Switch from IV to PO
When switching from IV to PO form, use same equivalent daily dosage and frequency as IV administration.

#### Switch from PO to IV
When switching from PO to IV form, initial total daily IV dosage should be equivalent to total daily dosage and frequency of PO form and should be infused IV over 30–60 min.

#### Dosage in Renal Impairment
Use caution when titrating. **Mild to moderate impairment:** No dose adjustment. **Severe impairment, end-stage renal disease:** Maxiumum: 300 mg/day.

#### Dosage in Hepatic Impairment
Use caution when titrating. **Mild to moderate impairment: Maximum:** 300 mg/day. **Severe impairment:** Not recommended.

## SIDE EFFECTS

**Frequent (31%–13%):** Dizziness, headache. **Occasional (11%–5%):** Nausea, double vision, vomiting, fatigue, blurred vision, ataxia, tremor, nystagmus. **Rare (4%–2%):** Vertigo, diarrhea, gait disturbances, memory impairment, depression, pruritus, injection site discomfort.

## ADVERSE EFFECTS/ TOXIC REACTIONS

Increased risk of suicidal ideation, behavior. Dose-dependent prolongations in PR interval noted. Leukopenia, anemia, thrombocytopenia occur rarely.

## NURSING CONSIDERATIONS

### BASELINE ASSESSMENT
Review history of seizure disorder (intensity, frequency, duration, level of consciousness). Initiate seizure precautions. Renal function, LFT, CBC should be performed before therapy begins and periodically during therapy.

### INTERVENTION/EVALUATION
Observe for recurrence of seizure activity. Assess for clinical improvement (decrease in intensity/frequency of seizures). Assist with ambulation if dizziness occurs. Assess for suicidal ideation, depression, behavioral changes. Drug should be withdrawn gradually (over a minimum of 1 wk) to minimize potential for increased seizure frequency.

### PATIENT/FAMILY TEACHING
• Strict maintenance of drug therapy is essential for seizure control. • Avoid tasks that require alertness, motor skills until response to drug is established. • Avoid alcohol. • Report depression, suicidal ideation, unusual behavioral changes.

# lactulose

**lak**-tyoo-lose
(Apo-Lactulose ✦, Constulose, Enulose, Generlac, Kristalose)
**Do not confuse lactulose with lactose.**

### ◆CLASSIFICATION
**PHARMACOTHERAPEUTIC:** Lactose derivative. **CLINICAL:** Hyperosmotic laxative, ammonia detoxicant.

---

## USES

Prevention, treatment of portal-systemic encephalopathy (including hepatic pre-coma, coma); treatment of constipation.

## PRECAUTIONS

**Contraindications:** Hypersensitivity to lactulose. Pts requiring a low-galactose diet. **Cautions:** Diabetes mellitus, hepatic impairment, dehydration.

## ACTION

Inhibits diffusion of $NH_3$ into blood by converting $NH_3$ to $NH_4^+$; enhances diffusion of $NH_3$ from blood to gut, where it is converted to $NH_4^+$; produces osmotic effect in colon. **Therapeutic Effect:** Promotes increased peristalsis, bowel evacuation; decreases serum ammonia concentration.

## PHARMACOKINETICS

Poorly absorbed from GI tract. Extensively metabolized in colon. Primarily excreted in feces.

## ⧖ LIFESPAN CONSIDERATIONS

**Pregnancy/Lactation:** Unknown if drug crosses placenta or is distributed in breast milk. **Children:** Avoid use in pts younger than 6 yrs (usually unable to describe symptoms). **Elderly:** No age-related precautions noted.

## INTERACTIONS

**DRUG:** None significant. **HERBAL:** None significant. **FOOD:** None known. **LAB VALUES:** May decrease serum potassium (GI loss).

## AVAILABILITY (Rx)

**Packets (Kristalose):** 10 g, 20 g. **Solution, Oral:** 10 g/15 ml.

## ADMINISTRATION/HANDLING

### PO
• Store solution at room temperature. • Solution appears pale yellow to yellow, viscous liquid. Cloudiness, darkened solution does not indicate potency loss. • Drink water, juice, milk with each dose (aids stool softening, increases palatability). • Mix packets with 4 oz water.

### Rectal
• Lubricate anus with petroleum jelly before enema insertion. • Insert carefully (prevents damage to rectal wall) with nozzle toward navel. • Squeeze container until entire dose expelled. • Instruct pt to retain 30–60 min in divided doses. **Maximum:** 60 ml/day (40 g/day).

## INDICATIONS/ROUTES/DOSAGE

### Constipation
**PO: ADULTS, ELDERLY:** 15–30 ml (10–20 g)/day, up to 60 ml (40 g)/day. **CHILDREN:** 1–3 ml/kg/day (0.7–2 g/kg/day). **Maximum:** 40 g/day (60 ml/day).

### Prevention of Portal-Systemic Encephalopathy
**ADULTS, ELDERLY:** 30–45 ml (20–30 g) 3–4 times/day. Adjust dose q1–2 days to produce 2–3 soft stools/day. **CHILDREN:** 40–90 ml/day in divided doses 3–4 times/day. **INFANTS:** 2.5–10 ml/day in 3–4 divided doses. Adjust dose q1–2 days to produce 2–3 soft stools/day.

### Treatment of Portal-Systemic Encephalopathy
**PO: ADULTS, ELDERLY:** Initially, 30–45 ml (20–30 g) every hr to induce rapid laxation. Then, 30–45 ml 3–4 times/day. Adjust dose q1–2days to produce 2–3 soft stools/day.

### Rectal Administration (as Retention Enema)
200 g (300 ml) diluted with 700 ml water or NaCl via rectal balloon catheter. Retain 30–60 min q4–6h. (Transition to oral prior to stopping rectal administration.)

### Dosage in Renal/Hepatic Impairment
No dose adjustment.

## SIDE EFFECTS

**Occasional:** Abdominal cramping, flatulence, increased thirst, abdominal discomfort. **Rare:** Nausea, vomiting.

## ADVERSE EFFECTS/ TOXIC REACTIONS

Severe diarrhea indicates overdose. Long-term use may result in laxative dependence, chronic constipation, loss of normal bowel function.

### NURSING CONSIDERATIONS

#### INTERVENTION/EVALUATION

Encourage adequate fluid intake. Assess bowel sounds for peristalsis. Monitor daily pattern of bowel activity, stool consistency; record time of evacuation. Assess for abdominal disturbances. Monitor serum electrolytes in pts with prolonged, frequent, excessive use of medication.

#### PATIENT/FAMILY TEACHING

• Evacuation occurs in 24–48 hrs of initial dose. • Institute measures to promote defecation: increase fluid intake, exercise, high-fiber diet.

## *lamiVUDine

la-**miv**-yoo-deen
(Apo-Lamivudine ✦ , Epivir, Epivir-HBV, Heptovir ✦)

■ **BLACK BOX ALERT** ■ Serious, sometimes fatal lactic acidosis, severe hepatomegaly with steatosis (fatty liver) have occurred. Pts must be monitored for chronic hepatitis B infection for several months following therapy. Do not use Epivir-HBV for treatment of HIV infection.
**Do not confuse Epivir with Combivir, or lamivudine with lamotrigine.**

### FIXED-COMBINATION(S)

**Combivir:** lamivudine/zidovudine (an antiviral): 150 mg/300 mg.
**Epzicom:** lamivudine/abacavir (an antiviral): 300 mg/600 mg. **Triumeq:** lamivudine/abacavir (antiretroviral)/dolutegravir (integrase inhibitor): 300 mg/600 mg/50 mg.
**Trizivir:** lamivudine/zidovudine/abacavir (an antiviral): 150 mg/300 mg/300 mg.

## ◆CLASSIFICATION

**PHARMACOTHERAPEUTIC:** Nucleoside reverse transcriptase inhibitor. **CLINICAL:** Antiviral.

## USES

**Epivir:** Treatment of HIV infection in combination with at least two other antiretroviral agents. **Epivir-HBV:** Treatment of chronic hepatitis B infection associated with evidence of hepatitis B viral replication and active hepatic inflammation. **OFF-LABEL:** Prophylaxis in health care workers at risk of acquiring HIV after occupational exposure to virus. Use as part of multidrug regimen.

## PRECAUTIONS

**Contraindications:** Hypersensitivity to lamivudine. **Cautions:** Use in children with history of pancreatitis or risk factors for developing pancreatitis. Use in combination with interferon alfa with or without ribavirin in HIV/HBV coinfected pts; renal/hepatic impairment.

## ACTION

Inhibits HIV reverse transcriptase by viral DNA chain termination. Inhibits RNA-, DNA-dependent DNA polymerase, an enzyme necessary for HIV, hepatitis B replication. **Therapeutic Effect:** Slows HIV replication, reduces progression of HIV infection, chronic hepatitis B.

## PHARMACOKINETICS

Rapidly, completely absorbed from GI tract. Protein binding: less than 36%. Widely distributed (crosses blood-brain barrier). Primarily excreted unchanged in urine. Not removed by hemodialysis

L

or peritoneal dialysis. **Half-life: Children:** 2 hrs. **Adults:** 5–7 hrs.

## ⌛ LIFESPAN CONSIDERATIONS

**Pregnancy/Lactation:** Drug crosses placenta. Unknown if distributed in breast milk. Breastfeeding not recommended (possibility of HIV transmission). **Children:** Safety and efficacy not established in pts younger than 3 mos. **Elderly:** Age-related renal impairment may require dosage adjustment.

## INTERACTIONS

**DRUG: Zalcitabine** may inhibit absorption of both drugs; avoid concurrent administration. **HERBAL:** None significant. **FOOD:** None known. **LAB VALUES:** May increase Hgb, neutrophil count; serum amylase, ALT, AST, bilirubin.

## AVAILABILITY (Rx)

**Oral Solution:** 5 mg/ml (Epivir-HBV), 10 mg/ml (Epivir). **Tablets:** 100 mg (Epivir-HBV), 150 mg (Epivir), 300 mg (Epivir).

## ADMINISTRATION/HANDLING

**PO**
• Give without regard to meals.

## INDICATIONS/ROUTES/DOSAGE

**HIV Infection**
**PO: ADULTS, ELDERLY:** 150 mg twice daily or 300 mg once daily. **CHILDREN 4 MOS–16 YRS:** *(Oral Solution):* 4 mg/kg twice daily (up to 150 mg/dose). **INFANTS 1–3 MOS:** 4 mg/kg twice daily. **NEONATES YOUNGER THAN 30 DAYS:** 2 mg/kg twice daily. *(Tablets):* **25 KG OR MORE:** 150 mg 2 times/day or 300 mg once daily. **20–24 KG:** 75 mg in AM and 150 mg in PM or 225 mg once daily. **14–19 KG:** 75 mg 2 times/day or 150 mg once daily.

**Chronic Hepatitis B**
**PO: ADULTS:** 100 mg/day. **CHILDREN 2–17 YRS:** 3 mg/kg/day. **Maximum:** 100 mg/day.

### Dosage in Renal Impairment
Dosage and frequency are modified based on creatinine clearance.

| Creatinine Clearance | Dosage HIV | Dosage Hepatitis B |
|---|---|---|
| 30–49 ml/min | 150 mg once/daily | 100 mg first dose, then 50 mg once/daily |
| 15–29 ml/min | 150 mg first dose, then 100 mg once/daily | 100 mg first dose, then 25 mg once/daily |
| 5–14 ml/min | 150 mg first dose, then 50 mg once/daily | 35 mg first dose, then 15 mg once/daily |
| Less than 5 ml/min | 50 mg first dose, then 25 mg once/daily | 35 mg first dose, then 10 mg once/daily |

**Hemodialysis:** Dosing post-HD recommended.

### Dosage in Hepatic Impairment
No dose adjustment.

## SIDE EFFECTS

**Frequent (35%–10%):** Headache, nausea, malaise, fatigue, nasal disturbances, diarrhea, cough, musculoskeletal pain, neuropathy, insomnia, dizziness, fever, chills. **Occasional (9%–5%):** Depression, myalgia, abdominal cramps, dyspepsia, arthralgia.

## ADVERSE EFFECTS/ TOXIC REACTIONS

Pancreatitis occurs in 13% of pediatric pts. Anemia, neutropenia, thrombocytopenia occur rarely. Lactic acidosis, severe hepatomegaly with steatosis have been reported.

## NURSING CONSIDERATIONS

### BASELINE ASSESSMENT
Obtain baseline renal function test, LFT. Screen HIV pts for hepatitis B infection before initiating therapy.

## INTERVENTION/EVALUATION

Monitor serum BUN, creatinine, amylase, lipase, ALT, AST, bilirubin. Assess for headache, nausea, cough. Monitor daily pattern of bowel activity, stool consistency. Modify diet or administer laxative as needed. Assess for dizziness, sleep pattern. If pancreatitis in children occurs, movement aggravates abdominal pain; sitting up, flexing at the waist may relieve the pain.

## PATIENT/FAMILY TEACHING

• Continue therapy for full length of treatment. • Doses should be evenly spaced. • Lamivudine is not a cure for HIV infection, nor does it reduce risk of transmission to others. • Avoid tasks requiring alertness, motor skills until response to drug is established. • Avoid alcohol. • Closely monitor for symptoms of pancreatitis (severe, steady abdominal pain often radiating to the back, clammy skin, hypotension; nausea/vomiting may accompany abdominal pain).

---

# *lamoTRIgine

la-**moe**-tri-jeen
(Apo-Lamotrigine ✦, Lamictal, Lamictal ODT, Lamictal XR)

■ **BLACK BOX ALERT** ■ Severe, potentially life-threatening skin rashes have been reported, including Stevens-Johnson syndrome. Risk increased with coadministration with valproic acid and rapid-dose titration.

**Do not confuse Lamictal with Lamisil or Lomotil, or lamotrigine with labetalol or lamivudine.**

## ◆CLASSIFICATION

**PHARMACOTHERAPEUTIC:** Phenyltriazine. **CLINICAL:** Anticonvulsant.

## USES

**Immediate-Release:** Adjunctive therapy in adults and children with generalized tonic-clonic seizures and partial seizures, treatment of adults and children with generalized seizures of Lennox-Gastaut syndrome. Conversion to monotherapy in adults treated with another enzyme-inducing antiepileptic drug (EIAED) (e.g., valproic acid, carbamazepine, phenytoin, phenobarbital, primidone). Long-term maintenance treatment of bipolar disorder. Treatment of pts 2 yrs and older with primary generalized tonic-clonic seizures. **Extended-release:** Adjunctive therapy for primary generalized tonic-clonic and partial-onset seizures in pts 13 yrs and older. Conversion to monotherapy in pt 13 yrs and older with partial seizures receiving treatment with a single antiepileptic drug (AED).

## PRECAUTIONS

**Contraindications:** Hypersensitivity to lamotrigine. **Cautions:** Renal/hepatic impairment, pts at high risk of suicide, pts taking estrogen-containing oral contraceptives, history of adverse hematologic reaction.

## ACTION

May block voltage-sensitive sodium channels, stabilizing neuronal membranes, regulating presynaptic transmitter release of excitatory amino acids. **Therapeutic Effect:** Produces anticonvulsant activity. Delays time to occurrence of acute mood episodes (mania, depression, hypomania).

## ⏳ LIFESPAN CONSIDERATIONS

**Pregnancy/Lactation:** Distributed in breast milk. Breastfeeding not recommended. Increased fetal risk of oral cleft formation has been noted with use during pregnancy. **Children:** Safety and efficacy in pts 18 yrs and younger with bipolar disorder, younger than 13 yrs with epilepsy not established. **Elderly:** Age-related renal impairment may require dosage adjustment.

---

## INTERACTIONS

**DRUG: Carbamazepine, phenobarbital, primidone, phenytoin, rifampin** may decrease concentration. **Valproic acid** may increase concentration/effects. May decrease effects of **oral contraceptives**. **HERBAL: Evening primrose** may decrease seizure threshold. **FOOD:** None known. **LAB VALUES:** None significant.

## AVAILABILITY (Rx)

**Tablets:** 25 mg, 100 mg, 150 mg, 200 mg. **Tablets (Chewable):** 5 mg, 25 mg. **Tablets (Orally Disintegrating):** 25 mg, 50 mg, 100 mg, 200 mg.

**Tablets (Extended-Release):** 25 mg, 50 mg, 100 mg, 200 mg, 250 mg, 300 mg.

## ADMINISTRATION/HANDLING

### PO

• Give without regard to food. • Chewable tablets may be dispensed in water or diluted fruit juice, or swallowed whole. • Extended-release tablets must be swallowed whole; do not break, crush, dissolve, or divide. • Place orally disintegrating tablet on tongue, allow to dissolve. Pt must not break, cut, or chew. Can be swallowed without regard to food or water.

## INDICATIONS/ROUTES/DOSAGE

**Lennox-Gastaut, Primary Generalized Tonic-Clonic Seizures, Partial Seizures**
**PO: ADULTS, ELDERLY, CHILDREN OLDER THAN 12 YRS:** Initially, 25 mg/day for 2 wks, then increase to 50 mg/day for 2 wks. After 4 wks, may increase by 50 mg/day at 1- to 2-wk intervals. **Maintenance:** 225–375 mg/day in 2 divided doses. **CHILDREN 2–12 YRS:** Initially, 0.3 mg/kg/day in 1–2 divided doses for 2 wks, then increase to 0.6 mg/kg/day in 1–2 divided doses for 2 wks. After 4 wks, may increase by 0.6 mg/kg/day at 1- to 2-wk intervals. **Maintenance:** 4.5–7.5 mg/kg/day in 2 divided doses. **Maximum:** 300 mg/day in 2 divided doses.

**Adjusted Dosage with Antiepileptic Drugs Containing Valproic Acid**
**PO: ADULTS, ELDERLY, CHILDREN OLDER THAN 12 YRS:** Initially, 25 mg every other day for 2 wks, then increase to 25 mg/day for 2 wks. After 4 wks, may increase by 25–50 mg/day at 1- to 2-wk intervals. **Maintenance:** 100–400 mg/day in 2 divided doses (100–200 mg/day when taking lamotrigine with valproic acid alone). **CHILDREN 2–12 YRS:** Initially, 0.15 mg/kg/day in 1–2 divided doses for 2 wks, then increase to 0.3 mg/kg/day in 1–2 divided doses for 2 wks. After 4 wks, may increase by 0.3 mg/kg/day at 1- to 2-wk intervals. **Maintenance:** 1–5 mg/kg/day in 2 divided doses. **Maximum:** 200 mg/day in 2 divided doses.

**Adjusted Dosage with EIAED without Valproic Acid**
**PO: ADULTS, ELDERLY, CHILDREN OLDER THAN 12 YRS:** Initially, 50 mg/day for 2 wks, then increase to 100 mg/day in 2 divided doses for 2 wks. After 4 wks, may increase by 100 mg/day at 1- to 2-wk intervals. **Maintenance:** 300–500 mg/day in 2 divided doses. **CHILDREN 2–12 YRS:** Initially, 0.6 mg/kg/day in 1–2 divided doses for 2 wks, then increase to 1.2 mg/kg/day in 1–2 divided doses for 2 wks. After 4 wks, may increase by 1.2 mg/kg/day at 1- to 2-wk intervals. **Maintenance:** 5–15 mg/kg/day in 2 divided doses. **Maximum:** 400 mg/day in 2 divided doses.

**Usual Maintenance Range for Extended-Release Tablets**
**PT TAKING VALPROIC ACID:** 200–250 mg once daily. **PT TAKING EIAED WITHOUT VALPROIC ADIC:** 400–600 mg once daily. **PT NOT TAKING EIAED:** 300–400 mg once daily.

**Conversion to Monotherapy for Pts Receiving EIAEDs**
**PO: ADULTS, ELDERLY, CHILDREN 16 YRS AND OLDER:** 500 mg/day in 2 divided doses. Titrate to desired dose while maintaining EIAED at fixed level, then withdraw EIAED by 20% each wk over a 4-wk period.

---

**Conversion to Monotherapy for Pts Receiving Valproic Acid**

**PO: ADULTS, ELDERLY, CHILDREN 16 YRS AND OLDER:** Titrate lamotrigine to 200 mg/day, maintaining valproic acid dose. Maintain lamotrigine dose and decrease valproic acid to 500 mg/day, no greater than 500 mg/day/wk, then maintain 500 mg/day for 1 wk. Increase lamotrigine to 300 mg/day and decrease valproic acid to 250 mg/day. Maintain for 1 wk, then discontinue valproic acid and increase lamotrigine by 100 mg/day each wk until maintenance dose of 500 mg/day reached.

**Bipolar Disorder**

**PO: ADULTS, ELDERLY:** Initially, 25 mg/day for 2 wks, then 50 mg/day for 2 wks, then 100 mg/day for 1 wk, then 200 mg/day beginning with wk 6.

**Bipolar Disorder in Pts Receiving EIAEDs**

**PO: ADULTS, ELDERLY:** 50 mg/day for 2 wks, then 100 mg/day for 2 wks, then 200 mg/day for 1 wk, then 300 mg/day for 1 wk, then up to usual maintenance dose 400 mg/day in divided doses.

**Bipolar Disorder in Pts Receiving Valproic Acid**

**PO: ADULTS, ELDERLY:** 25 mg/day every other day for 2 wks, then 25 mg/day for 2 wks, then 50 mg/day for 1 wk, then 100 mg/day. **Usual maintenance dose with valproic acid:** 100 mg/day.

**Usual Dosage for Lamictal XR**

**Adjunct Therapy:** Range: 200–600 mg/day.

**Conversion to Monotherapy:** Range: 250–500 mg/day.

**Discontinuation Therapy**

◄**ALERT**► A dosage reduction of approximately 50%/wk over at least 2 wks is recommended.

**Dosage in Renal Impairment**

◄**ALERT**► Decreased dosage may be effective in pts with significant renal impairment.

**Dosage in Hepatic Impairment**

**Mild impairment:** No dose adjustment. **Moderate to severe impairment without ascites:** Reduce dose by 25%. **Severe impairment with ascites:** Reduce dose by 50%.

## SIDE EFFECTS

**Frequent (38%–14%):** Dizziness, headache, diplopia, ataxia, nausea, blurred vision, drowsiness, rhinitis. **Occasional (10%–5%):** Rash, pharyngitis, vomiting, cough, flu-like symptoms, diarrhea, dysmenorrhea, fever, insomnia, dyspepsia. **Rare:** Constipation, tremor, anxiety, pruritus, vaginitis, hypersensitivity reaction.

## ADVERSE EFFECTS/ TOXIC REACTIONS

Abrupt withdrawal may increase seizure frequency. Serious rashes, including Stevens-Johnson syndrome, have been reported.

## NURSING CONSIDERATIONS

### BASELINE ASSESSMENT

Review history of seizure disorder (type, onset, intensity, frequency, duration, LOC), medication history (esp. other anticonvulsants), other medical conditions (e.g., renal impairment). Initiate seizure precautions. Assess baseline mood, behavior.

### INTERVENTION/EVALUATION

Report occurrence of rash (drug discontinuation may be necessary). Assist with ambulation if dizziness, ataxia occurs. Assess for clinical improvement (decreased intensity/frequency of seizures). Assess for visual abnormalities, headache. Monitor for suicidal ideation, depression, behavioral changes.

### PATIENT/ FAMILY TEACHING

• Take medication only as prescribed; do not abruptly discontinue medication after long-term therapy. • Avoid alcohol. • Avoid tasks that require alertness,

 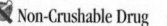

motor skills until response to drug is established. • Carry identification card/bracelet to note anticonvulsant therapy. • Strict maintenance of drug therapy is essential for seizure control. • Report any rash, fever, swelling of glands, worsening depression, suicidal ideation, unusual changes in behavior, worsening of seizure control. • May cause photosensitivity reaction; avoid exposure to sunlight, ultraviolet light.

# lansoprazole

lan-**soe**-pra-zole
(Apo-Lansoprazole ✸, First Lansoprazole, Prevacid, Prevacid Solu-Tab, Prevacid 24HR)
**Do not confuse lansoprazole with aripiprazole or dexlansoprazole, or Prevacid with Pravachol, Prilosec, or Prinivil.**

### FIXED-COMBINATION(S)

**Prevacid NapraPac:** lansoprazole/naproxen (an NSAID): 15 mg/375 mg, 15 mg/500 mg. **Prevpac:** Combination card containing amoxicillin 500 mg (4 capsules), lansoprazole 30 mg (2 capsules), clarithromycin 500 mg (2 tablets).

### ◆CLASSIFICATION

**CLINICAL:** Proton pump inhibitor.

### USES

Short-term treatment (4 wks and less) of healing, symptomatic relief of active duodenal ulcer; short-term treatment (8 wks and less) for healing, symptomatic relief of erosive esophagitis. Long-term treatment of pathologic hypersecretory conditions, including Zollinger-Ellison syndrome. Short-term treatment (8 wks and less) of active benign gastric ulcer, *H. pylori*–associated duodenal ulcer (part of multidrug regimen), maintenance treatment for healed duodenal ulcer. Treatment of gastroesophageal reflux disease (GERD), NSAID-associated gastric ulcer. Reduce risk of NSAID-associated gastric ulcer in pts with history of gastric ulcer requiring NSAIDs. **OTC:** Relief of frequent heartburn (2 or more days/wk). **IV:** Short-term treatment of erosive esophagitis. **OFF-LABEL:** Stress ulcer prophylaxis in critically ill.

### PRECAUTIONS

**Contraindications:** Hypersensitivity to lansoprazole, other proton pump inhibitors. **Cautions:** Hepatic impairment. May increase risk of hip, wrist, spine fractures; GI infections.

### ACTION

Inhibits the $(H^+, K^+)$–ATPase enzyme system, blocking the final step in gastric acid secretion. **Therapeutic Effect:** Suppresses gastric acid secretion.

### PHARMACOKINETICS

Rapid, complete absorption (food may decrease absorption) once drug has left stomach. Protein binding: 97%. Distributed primarily to gastric parietal cells. Metabolized in liver. Eliminated in bile and urine. Not removed by hemodialysis. **Half-life:** 1.5 hrs (increased in hepatic impairment, elderly).

### ⌛ LIFESPAN CONSIDERATIONS

**Pregnancy/Lactation:** Unknown if distributed in breast milk. **Children:** Safety and efficacy not established. **Elderly:** No age-related precautions noted but doses greater than 30 mg not recommended.

### INTERACTIONS

**DRUG:** May decrease concentration of **atazanavir.** May interfere with absorption of **ampicillin, digoxin, iron salts, ketoconazole.** Sucralfate may delay absorption. May increase effect of **warfarin.** May decrease effect of **clopidogrel. HERBAL: St. John's wort** may decrease concentration/effect. **FOOD: Food** may decrease absorption. **LAB VALUES:** May increase serum LDH, alkaline phosphatase, bilirubin, cholesterol, creatinine, ALT, AST, triglycerides, uric acid; Hgb, Hct. May produce abnormal albumin/globulin ratio, electrolyte balance, platelet, RBC, WBC count.

## AVAILABILITY (Rx)

**Tablets, Orally Disintegrating (Prevacid Solu-Tab):** 15 mg, 30 mg. **Powder for Oral Suspension (First Lansoprazole):** 3 mg/ml.

**Capsules (Delayed-Release): (Prevacid):** 15 mg, 30 mg. **(Prevacid 24HR):** 15 mg.

## ADMINISTRATION/HANDLING

**PO**
• Best if taken before breakfast • Do not cut/crush delayed-release capsules. • If pt has difficulty swallowing capsules, open capsules, sprinkle granules on 1 tbsp of applesauce, give immediately. Do not crush or allow pt to chew granules.

**PO (Solu-Tab)**
• Place tablet on tongue; allow to dissolve, then swallow. • May give via oral syringe or nasogastric tube. • May dissolve in 4 ml (15 mg) or 10 ml (30 mg) water.

## INDICATIONS/ROUTES/DOSAGE

**Duodenal Ulcer**
**PO: ADULTS, ELDERLY:** 15 mg/day, before morning meal for up to 4 wks. **Maintenance:** 15 mg/day.

**Erosive Esophagitis**
**PO: ADULTS, ELDERLY:** 30 mg/day, before morning meal for up to 8 wks. If healing does not occur within 8 wks (in 5%–10% of cases), may give for additional 8 wks. **Maintenance:** 15 mg/day. **CHILDREN 1–11 YRS, WEIGHING GREATER THAN 30 KG:** 30 mg/day; **WEIGHING 30 KG OR LESS:** 15 mg/day.

**Gastric Ulcer**
**PO: ADULTS:** 30 mg/day for up to 8 wks.

**NSAID Gastric Ulcer**
**PO: ADULTS, ELDERLY:** (Healing): 30 mg/day for up to 8 wks. (Prevention): 15 mg/day for up to 12 wks.

**Gastroesophageal Reflux Disease (GERD)**
**PO: ADULTS:** 15 mg/day for up to 8 wks. **CHILDREN 12–17 YRS:** 30 mg/day up to 8 wks. **CHILDREN 1–11 YRS, WEIGHING GREATER THAN 30 KG:** 30 mg/day; **WEIGHING 30 KG OR LESS:** 15 mg/day.

*H. Pylori* **Infection**
**PO: ADULTS, ELDERLY:** (triple drug therapy including amoxicillin, clarithromycin) 30 mg q12h for 10–14 days or (with amoxicillin) 30 mg 3 times/day for 14 days.

**Pathologic Hypersecretory Conditions (Including Zollinger-Ellison Syndrome)**
**PO: ADULTS, ELDERLY:** Initially, 60 mg/day. Individualize dosage according to pt needs and for as long as clinically indicated. Administer doses greater than 120 mg/day in divided doses.

**Heartburn (OTC)**
**PO: ADULTS, ELDERLY:** 15 mg once daily for 14 days. May repeat q4mos.

**Dosage in Renal Impairment**
No dose adjustment.

**Dosage in Hepatic Impairment**
Consider dose reduction in severe impairment.

## SIDE EFFECTS

**Occasional (3%–2%):** Diarrhea, abdominal pain, rash, pruritus, altered appetite. **Rare (1%):** Nausea, headache.

## ADVERSE EFFECTS/ TOXIC REACTIONS

Bilirubinemia, eosinophilia, hyperlipemia occur rarely. May increase risk of *C. difficile* infection.

---

## NURSING CONSIDERATIONS

### BASELINE ASSESSMENT

Obtain baseline lab values. Assess for epigastric/abdominal pain, evidence of GI bleeding, ecchymosis.

### INTERVENTION/EVALUATION

Monitor CBC, hepatic/renal function tests. Assess for therapeutic response (relief of GI symptoms). Question if diarrhea, abdominal pain, nausea occurs. Obtain *C. difficile* PCR test in pts with persistent diarrhea, fever, abdominal pain.

### PATIENT/ FAMILY TEACHING

• Do not chew, crush delayed-release capsules. • For pts who have difficulty swallowing capsules, open capsules, sprinkle granules on 1 tbsp of applesauce, swallow immediately.

# lapatinib

la-pa-tin-ib
(Tykerb)
■ **BLACK BOX ALERT** ■ Hepatotoxicity (serum ALT or AST more than 3 times upper limit of normal [ULN] and total bilirubin more than 2 times ULN), possibly severe, has occurred. **Do not confuse lapatinib with dasatinib, erlotinib, or imatinib.**

## ◆CLASSIFICATION

**PHARMACOTHERAPEUTIC:** Tyrosine kinase inhibitor. **CLINICAL:** Antineoplastic.

## USES

Combination treatment with capecitabine for treatment of human epidermal growth receptor type 2 (HER2) overexpressing advanced or metastatic breast cancer in pts who have received prior therapy including an anthracycline, a taxane, and trastuzumab. Combination treatment with letrozole for treatment of postmenopausal women with *HER2* overexpressing hormone receptor-positive metastatic breast cancer for whom hormonal therapy is indicated. **OFF-LABEL:** Treatment (in combination with trastuzumab) of *HER2*-overexpressing metastatic breast cancer that progressed on prior trastuzumab-containing therapy. Treatment of *HER2*-overexpressing metastatic breast cancer with brain metastasis.

## PRECAUTIONS

**Contraindications:** Hypersensitivity to lapatinib. **Cautions:** Left ventricular function abnormalities, prolonged QT interval or medications known to prolong QT interval, hepatic impairment. History of treatment with anthracyclines, chest wall irradiation. Avoid concurrent use with strong CYP3A4 inhibitors or inducers.

## ACTION

Inhibitory action against kinases targeting intracellular components of epidermal growth factor receptor ErbB1 and a second receptor, human epidermal receptor (HER2 [ErbB2]). **Therapeutic Effect:** Inhibits ErbB-driven tumor cell growth, produces tumor regression, inhibits metastasis.

## PHARMACOKINETICS

| Route | Onset | Peak | Duration |
|-------|-------|------|----------|
| PO | 30 min | 4 hrs | — |

Steady-state level occurs within 6–7 days. Incomplete and variable oral absorption. Undergoes extensive metabolism. Protein binding: 99%. Minimally excreted in feces and plasma. **Half-life:** 24 hrs.

## ⏳ LIFESPAN CONSIDERATIONS

**Pregnancy/Lactation:** May cause fetal harm. Unknown if distributed in breast milk. **Children:** Safety and efficacy not established. **Elderly:** No age-related precautions noted.

## INTERACTIONS

**DRUG:** May increase **digoxin** levels. **CYP3A4 inhibitors (e.g., clarithromycin, ketoconazole, ritonavir)** may increase plasma concentration. **CYP3A4**

inducers (**e.g., carbamazepine, phenytoin, rifampin**) may decrease plasma concentration. **HERBAL: St. John's wort** decreases plasma concentration. **FOOD: Grapefruit products** may increase plasma concentration (potential for torsades, myelotoxicity). **LAB VALUES:** May increase serum ALT, AST, bilirubin. May decrease neutrophils, Hgb, platelets.

## AVAILABILITY (Rx)

Tablets: 250 mg.

## ADMINISTRATION/HANDLING

**PO**
• Do not break, crush, dissolve, or divide film-coated tablets. • Give at least 1 hr before or 1 hr after food. Take full dose at same time each day.

## INDICATIONS/ROUTES/DOSAGE

**Breast Cancer**
**PO: ADULTS, ELDERLY: (With capecitabine):** 1,250 mg (5 tablets) once daily. **(With letrozole):** 1,500 mg once daily continuously with letrozole. Continue until disease progresses or unacceptable toxicity.

**Dose Modification**
**Cardiac Toxicity**
Discontinue with decreased left ventricular ejection fraction grade 2 or higher, or in pts with an ejection fraction that drops to lower limit of normal. May be started at a reduced dose (1,000 mg/day) at a minimum of 2 wks when ejection fraction returns to normal and pt is asymptomatic.

**Pulmonary Toxicity**
Discontinue with symptoms indicative of interstitial lung disease or pneumonitis grade 3 or higher.

**Severe Hepatic Impairment**
**With capecitabine:** 750 mg/day. **With letrozole:** 1,000 mg/day.

**CYP3A4 Inhibitors/Inducers**
Concomitant use of CYP3A4 inhibitors may require dose reduction of lapatinib (e.g., decrease to 500 mg/day with careful monitoring); CYP3A4 inducers may require dose increase of lapatinib (e.g., increase to 4,500 mg with capecitabine or 5,500 mg with letrozole).

**Dosage in Renal Impairment**
No dose adjustment.

**Dosage in Hepatic Impairment**
**Mild to moderate impairment:** No dose adjustment. **Severe impairment:** See dose modification.

## SIDE EFFECTS

**Common (65%–44%):** Diarrhea, hand-foot syndrome (blistering/rash/peeling of skin on palms of hands, soles of feet), nausea. **Frequent (28%–26%):** Rash, vomiting. **Occasional (15%–10%):** Mucosal inflammation, stomatitis, extremity pain, back pain, dry skin, insomnia.

## ADVERSE EFFECTS/ TOXIC REACTIONS

Decreases in left ventricular ejection grade 3 or higher have been observed; 20% decrease relative to baseline is considered toxic.

## NURSING CONSIDERATIONS

**BASELINE ASSESSMENT**
Question for possibility of pregnancy. Obtain baseline CBC, serum chemistries before treatment begins and monthly thereafter.

**INTERVENTION/EVALUATION**
Offer antiemetics to control nausea, vomiting. Monitor daily pattern of bowel activity, stool consistency. Monitor CBC (particularly Hgb, platelets, neutrophil count), LFT. Assess hands and feet for erythema/blistering/peeling. Monitor for shortness of breath, palpitations, fatigue (decreased cardiac ejection fraction).

**PATIENT/FAMILY TEACHING**
• Avoid crowds, those with known infection. • Avoid contact with those who recently received live virus vaccine.

L

---

✦ Canadian trade name    Non-Crushable Drug    **HIGH ALERT** High Alert drug

• Do not have immunizations without physician's approval (drug lowers resistance). • Promptly report fever, unusual bruising/bleeding from any site. • Ensure use of appropriate birth control measures in women.

# leflunomide

lee-**floo**-noe-myde
(Apo-Leflunomide ✹, Arava)

■ **BLACK BOX ALERT** ■ Do not use during pregnancy. Women of childbearing potential must be counseled regarding fetal risk, use of reliable contraceptives confirmed, possibility of pregnancy excluded. Severe hepatic injury may occur.

## ◆CLASSIFICATION

**PHARMACOTHERAPEUTIC:** Immunomodulatory agent. **CLINICAL:** Antiinflammatory, antirheumatic.

## USES

Treatment of active rheumatoid arthritis (RA). Improve physical function in pts with rheumatoid arthritis. **OFF-LABEL:** Treatment of cytomegalovirus (CMV) disease. Prevention of acute/chronic rejection in recipients of solid organ transplants.

## PRECAUTIONS

**Contraindications:** Hypersensitivity to leflunomide. Pregnancy or plans for pregnancy. Severe hepatic impairment. **Cautions:** Hepatic/renal impairment, hepatitis B or C infection, pts with immunodeficiency or bone marrow dysplasias, breastfeeding mothers, history of new/recurrent infections, significant hematologic abnormalities, diabetes, concomitant use of neurotoxic medications, elderly.

## ACTION

Inhibits pyrimidine synthesis, resulting in antiproliferative and anti-inflammatory effects. **Therapeutic Effect:** Reduces signs/symptoms of RA, retards structural damage.

## PHARMACOKINETICS

Well absorbed after PO administration. Protein binding: greater than 99%. Metabolized in GI wall, liver. Excreted through renal, biliary systems. Not removed by hemodialysis. **Half-life:** 16 days.

## ⧗ LIFESPAN CONSIDERATIONS

**Pregnancy/Lactation:** Can cause fetal harm. Unknown if distributed in breast milk. Breastfeeding not recommended. **Children:** Safety and efficacy not established in pts younger than 18 yrs. **Elderly:** No age-related precautions noted.

## INTERACTIONS

**DRUG:** Rifampin may increase concentration/effects. **Hepatotoxic medications (e.g., acetaminophen, ketoconazole, simvastatin)** may increase risk of side effects, hepatotoxicity. Use of **live virus vaccine** not recommended. **HERBAL:** Echinacea may decrease effects. **FOOD:** None known. **LAB VALUES:** May increase serum ALT, AST, alkaline phosphatase, bilirubin.

## AVAILABILITY (Rx)

**Tablets:** 10 mg, 20 mg.

## ADMINISTRATION/HANDLING

### PO
• Give without regard to food.

## INDICATIONS/ROUTES/DOSAGE

**Rheumatoid Arthritis (RA)**
**PO: ADULTS, ELDERLY:** Initially, 100 mg/day for 3 days, then 10–20 mg/day. (Loading dose may be omitted in pts at increased risk of hepatitis or toxicity.)

**Dosage in Renal Impairment**
No dose adjustment.

**Dosage in Hepatic Impairment**
**ALT 2–3 Times Upper Limit of Normal (ULN):** Not recommended. **Persistent ALT Level Greater Than 3 Times ULN:** Discontinue and initiate accelerated drug elimination.

## SIDE EFFECTS

**Frequent (20%–10%):** Diarrhea, respiratory tract infection, alopecia, rash, nausea.

## ADVERSE EFFECTS/ TOXIC REACTIONS

May cause immunosuppression. Transient thrombocytopenia, leukopenia, hepatotoxicity occur rarely.

## NURSING CONSIDERATIONS

### BASELINE ASSESSMENT

Question for possibility of pregnancy. Obtain baseline CBC, LFT. Assess limitations in activities of daily living due to rheumatoid arthritis (RA).

### INTERVENTION/EVALUATION

Monitor tolerance to medication. Assess symptomatic relief of RA (relief of pain; improved range of motion, grip strength, mobility). Monitor LFT.

### PATIENT/FAMILY TEACHING

• May take without regard to food.
• Improvement may take longer than 8 wks. • Avoid pregnancy.

# lenalidomide

len-a-**lid**-o-myde
(Revlimid)

■ **BLACK BOX ALERT** ■ Analogue to thalidomide. High potential for significant birth defects. Hematologic toxicity (thrombocytopenia, neutropenia) occurs in 80% of pts. Greatly increases risk for DVT, pulmonary embolism in multiple myeloma pts.

**Do not confuse lenalidomide with thalidomide.**

## ◆ CLASSIFICATION

**PHARMACOTHERAPEUTIC:** Isoxazole immunomodulator. **CLINICAL:** Immunosuppressive agent.

## USES

Treatment of low- to intermediate-risk myelodysplastic syndrome (MDS) in pts with deletion 5q cytogenetic abnormality with transfusion-dependent anemia. Treatment of multiple myeloma (in combination with dexamethasone). Treatment of relapsed or refractory mantle cell lymphoma. **OFF-LABEL:** Systemic amyloidosis, lower-risk myelodysplastic syndrome, non-Hodgkin's lymphoma, maintenance treatment for multiple myeloma (following autologous stem cell transplant). Relapsed or refractory chronic lymphocytic leukemia (CLL).

## PRECAUTIONS

**Contraindications:** Hypersensitivity to lenalidomide. Pregnancy, women capable of becoming pregnant. **Cautions:** Renal/hepatic impairment. History of arterial thromboembolic events, hypertension, hyperlipidemia. Avoid use in pts with glucose intolerance, lactase deficiency.

## ACTION

Inhibits secretion of pro-inflammatory cytokines, increases secretion of anti-inflammatory cytokines. Enhances cell-mediated immunity by stimulation of T-cells. **Therapeutic Effect:** Inhibits myeloma cell growth; induces cell cycle arrest and cell death.

## PHARMACOKINETICS

Well absorbed following PO administration. Protein binding: 30%. Eliminated in urine. **Half-life:** 3 hrs (increased in renal impairment).

## ☒ LIFESPAN CONSIDERATIONS

**Pregnancy/Lactation:** Contraindicated in women who are or may become pregnant, who are not using two reliable forms of contraception, or who are not abstinent.

L

---

✦ Canadian trade name     🦺 Non-Crushable Drug     HIGH ALERT High Alert drug

Can cause severe birth defects, fetal death. Unknown if distributed in breast milk; breastfeeding not recommended. **Children:** Safety and efficacy not established in pts younger than 18 yrs. **Elderly:** Age-related renal impairment may require caution in dosage selection. Risk of toxic reactions greater in those with renal insufficiency.

## INTERACTIONS

**DRUG: Erythropoietin, dexamethasone, oral contraceptives** may increase risk of deep vein thrombosis, pulmonary embolism. May increase concentration of digoxin. **HERBAL:** Avoid **echinacea** (has immunostimulant properties). **FOOD:** None known. **LAB VALUES:** May decrease WBC count, Hgb, Hct platelets, troponin I, serum creatinine, sodium, $T_3$, $T_4$. May decrease serum bilirubin, glucose, potassium, magnesium.

## AVAILABILITY (Rx)

💊 Capsules: 2.5 mg, 5 mg, 10 mg, 15 mg, 25 mg.

## ADMINISTRATION/HANDLING

• Store at room temperature. • Do not break, crush, dissolve, or divide capsules. • Swallow whole with water.

## INDICATIONS/ROUTES/DOSAGE

**Myelodysplastic Syndrome**
**PO: ADULTS, ELDERLY:** 10 mg once daily.

**Dosage Adjustments for Myelodysplastic Syndrome**
*Platelets:*
**Thrombocytopenia within 4 wks with 10 mg/day**
**Baseline platelets 100,000/mm³ or greater:** If platelets less than 50,000/mm³, hold treatment. Resume at 5 mg/day when platelets return to 50,000/mm³ or greater. **Baseline platelets less than 100,000/mm³:** If platelets fall to 50% of baseline, hold treatment. Resume at 5 mg/day if baseline is 60,000/mm³ or greater and platelets return to 50,000/mm³ or greater. Resume at 5 mg/day if baseline is less than 60,000/mm³ and platelets return to 30,000/mm³ or greater.

**Thrombocytopenia after 4 wks with 10 mg/day:** If platelets less than 30,000/mm³ OR less than 50,000/mm³ with platelet transfusion, hold treatment. Resume at 5 mg/day when platelets return to 30,000/mm³ or greater.

**Thrombocytopenia developing with 5 mg/day:** If platelets less than 30,000/mm³ OR less than 50,000/mm³ with platelet transfusion, hold treatment. Resume at 5 mg every other day when platelets return to 30,000/mm³ or greater.

*Neutrophils:*
**Neutropenia within 4 wks with 10 mg/day**
**Baseline absolute neutrophil count (ANC) 1,000/mcl or greater:** If ANC less than 750/mm³, hold treatment. Resume at 5 mg/day when ANC 1,000/mm³ or greater. **Baseline ANC less than 1,000/mm³:** If ANC less than 500/mm³, hold treatment. Resume at 5 mg/day when ANC 500/mm³ or greater.

**Neutropenia after 4 wks with 10 mg/day:** If ANC less than 500/mm³ for 7 days or longer or associated with fever, hold treatment. Resume at 5 mg/day when ANC 500/mm³ or greater.

**Neutropenia developing with 5 mg/day:** If ANC less than 500/mm³ for 7 days or longer or associated with fever, hold treatment. Resume at 5 mg every other day when ANC 500/mm³ or greater.

**Mantle Cell Lymphoma**
**PO: ADULTS, ELDERLY:** 25 mg once daily on days 1–21 of repeated 28-day cycle.

**Multiple Myeloma**
**PO: ADULTS, ELDERLY:** 25 mg/day on days 1–21 of repeated 28-day cycle (in combination with dexamethasone).

**Dosage Adjustments for Multiple Myeloma**
*Platelets:*
**Thrombocytopenia:** If platelets fall to less than 30,000/mm³, hold treatment,

monitor CBC. Resume at 15 mg/day when platelets 30,000/mm³ or greater. For each subsequent fall to less than 30,000/mm³, hold treatment and resume at 5 mg/day less than previous dose when platelets return to 30,000/mm³ or greater. Do not dose to less than 5 mg/day.

**Neutrophils:**
**Neutropenia:** If neutrophils fall to less than 1,000/mm³, hold treatment, add G-CSF, follow CBC wkly. Resume at 25 mg/day when neutrophils return to 1,000/mm³ and neutropenia is the only toxicity. Resume at 15 mg/day if other toxicity is present. For each subsequent fall to less than 1,000/mm³, hold treatment and resume at 5 mg/day less than previous dose when neutrophils return to 1,000/mm³ or greater. Do not dose to less than 5 mg/day.

**Dosage in Renal Impairment**

| | Creatinine Clearance 30–59 ml/min | Creatinine Clearance Less Than 30 ml/min (Nondialysis Dependent) | Creatinine Clearance Less Than 30 ml/min (Dialysis Dependent) |
|---|---|---|---|
| Myelodysplastic syndrome | 5 mg once daily | 2.5 mg once daily | 2.5 mg once daily (give after dialysis) |
| Multiple myeloma | 10 mg once daily | 15 mg q48h | 5 mg once daily (give after dialysis) |

**Dosage in Hepatic Impairment**
No dose adjustment.

## SIDE EFFECTS

**Frequent (49%–31%):** Diarrhea, pruritus, rash, fatigue. **Occasional (24%–12%):** Constipation, nausea, arthralgia, fever, back pain, peripheral edema, cough, dizziness, headache, muscle cramps, epistaxis, asthenia, dry skin, abdominal pain. **Rare (10%–5%):** Extremity pain, vomiting, generalized edema, anorexia, insomnia, night sweats, myalgia, dry mouth, ecchymosis, rigors, depression, dysgeusia, palpitations.

## ADVERSE EFFECTS/ TOXIC REACTIONS

Significant increased risk of deep vein thrombosis (DVT), pulmonary embolism. Thrombocytopenia occurs in 62% of pts, neutropenia in 59% of pts, and anemia in 12% of pts. Upper respiratory infection (nasopharyngitis, pneumonia, sinusitis, bronchitis, rhinitis), UTI occur occasionally. Cellulitis, peripheral neuropathy, hypertension, hypothyroidism occur in approximately 6% of pts.

## NURSING CONSIDERATIONS

### BASELINE ASSESSMENT
Obtain baseline CBC. Due to high potential for human birth defects/fetal death, female pts must avoid pregnancy 4 wks before therapy, during therapy, during dose interruptions, and 4 wks following therapy. Two reliable forms of contraception must be used even if pt has history of infertility unless it is due to hysterectomy or menopause that has occurred for at least 24 consecutive mos. Confirm two negative pregnancy tests before therapy initiation.

### INTERVENTION/EVALUATION
Monitor CBC, BMP, serum magnesium as appropriate. Perform pregnancy tests on women of childbearing potential: wkly during the first 4 wks, then at 4-wk intervals in pts with regular menstrual cycles or q2wks in pts with irregular menstrual cycles. Monitor for hematologic toxicity; obtain CBC wkly during first 8 wks of therapy and at least monthly thereafter. Observe for signs, symptoms of thromboembolism (shortness of breath, chest pain, extremity pain, swelling, stroke-like symptoms).

**L**

---

✦ Canadian trade name          🗡 Non-Crushable Drug          **HIGH ALERT** High Alert drug

## PATIENT/FAMILY TEACHING

• Two reliable forms of birth control must be used before, during, and after therapy for female pts. • A pregnancy test must be performed within 10–14 days and 24 hrs before therapy begins. • Males must always use a latex condom during any sexual contact with females of childbearing potential even if they have undergone a successful vasectomy. • Avoid crowds; those with active infection. • Treatment may cause blood clots in the arms, legs, or lungs; report arm or leg pain/swelling, difficulty breathing, chest pain.

# lenvatinib

len-**va**-ti-nib
(Lenvima)
**Do not confuse lenvatinib with dasatinib, ibrutinib, imatinib.**

## ◆CLASSIFICATION

**PHARMACOTHERAPEUTIC:** Kinase inhibitor. **CLINICAL:** Antineoplastic.

## USES

Treatment of locally recurrent or metastatic, progressive, radioactive iodine–refractory differentiated thyroid cancer. Treatment of advanced renal cell carcinoma (RCC) after one course of another antineoplastic.

## PRECAUTIONS

**Contraindications:** Hypersensitivity to lenvatinib. **Cautions:** Electrolyte imbalance (hypokalemia, hypomagnesemia), hepatic/renal impairment. History of cardiac dysfunction (HF, pulmonary edema, right or left ventricular dysfunction), GI perforation/hemorrhage, hypertension, long-QT interval syndrome, medications that prolong QT interval, thromboembolic events (e.g., CVA, DVT), pituitary/thyroid disease.

## ACTION

Inhibits tyrosine kinase receptor activity of vascular endothelial growth factor (VEGF) receptors. Inhibits tumor angiogenesis, growth, progression. **Therapeutic Effect:** Inhibits tumor cell growth and metastasis.

## PHARMACOKINETICS

Readily absorbed. Metabolized in liver. Protein binding: 98%–99%. Peak plasma concentration: 1–4 hrs. Eliminated in feces (64%), urine (25%). Not removed by dialysis. **Half-life:** 28 hrs.

## ▧ LIFESPAN CONSIDERATIONS

**Pregnancy/Lactation:** Avoid pregnancy; may cause fetal harm. Female pts of reproductive potential must use effective contraception during treatment for at least 2 mos after discontinuation. Potentially distributed in breast milk. Must either discontinue drug or discontinue breastfeeding. Treatment may reduce fertility in both female and male pts. **Children:** Safety and efficacy not established. **Elderly:** No age-related precautions noted.

## INTERACTIONS

**DRUG: CYP3A4 inhibitors (e.g., ketoconazole, ritonavir)** may increase concentration/effect. **CYP3A4 inducers (e.g., carbamazepine, rifampin)** may decrease concentration/effect. **Amiodarone, ciprofloxacin, quinidine** may increase risk of QT interval prolongation. **Hormonal contraceptives** may increase risk of thromboembolic events. **HERBAL:** None significant. **FOOD:** None known. **LAB VALUES:** May increase serum alkaline phosphatase, ALT/AST, amylase, bilirubin, cholesterol, creatinine, lipase. May decrease serum albumin, glucose, magnesium; platelets. May increase or decrease serum calcium, potassium.

## AVAILABILITY (Rx)

**Capsules:** 4 mg, 10 mg.

## ADMINISTRATION/HANDLING

**PO**
• Give without regard to food. • Administer same time each day. • Do not cut, crush, divide, or open capsules.

## INDICATIONS/ROUTES/DOSAGE

### Thyroid Cancer

**PO: ADULTS, ELDERLY:** 24 mg once daily. Continue until disease progression or unacceptable toxicity.

### RCC

**PO: ADULTS, ELDERLY:** 18 mg once daily (in combination with everolimus).

### Dose Modification

Based on Common Terminology Criteria for Adverse Events (CTCAE).

| Adverse Reaction | Modification | Adjusted Dose |
|---|---|---|
| First occurrence | Interrupt until resolved to grade 0 or 1 or baseline | 20 mg once daily |
| Second occurrence | Interrupt until resolved to grade 0 or 1 or baseline | 14 mg once daily |
| Third occurrence | Interrupt until resolved to grade 0 or 1 or baseline | 10 mg once daily |

### Arterial Thrombotic Event

Discontinue treatment.

### Cardiac Dysfunction/Hemorrhagic Event

**PO: ADULTS, ELDERLY:** Interrupt treatment for grade 3 event until improved to grade 0 to 1 or baseline. Either resume at reduced dose or discontinue (depending on the severity and persistence). Discontinue for grade 4 event.

### GI Perforation/Fistula Formation

Discontinue treatment.

### Hypertension

**PO: ADULTS, ELDERLY:** Interrupt treatment for grade 3 hypertension that persists despite optimal antihypertensive therapy. Resume at reduced dose when hypertension is controlled at less than or equal to grade 2. Discontinue for life-threatening hypertension.

### Proteinuria

**PO: ADULTS, ELDERLY:** Interrupt treatment for greater than or equal to 2 g proteinuria/24 hrs. Resume at reduced dose when proteinuria less than 2 g/24 hrs. Discontinue if nephrotic syndrome occurs.

### QT Prolongation

**PO: ADULTS, ELDERLY:** Interrupt treatment for grade 3 or greater. Resume at reduced dose when QT prolongation resolved to grade 0 or 1 or baseline.

### Renal Failure/Impairment or Hepatotoxicity

**PO: ADULTS, ELDERLY:** Interrupt treatment for grade 3 or 4 renal failure/impairment or hepatotoxicity until resolved to grade 0 or 1 or baseline. Either resume at reduced dose or discontinue (depending on the severity and persistence). Discontinue if hepatic failure occurs.

### Reversible Posterior Leukoencephalopathy Syndrome (RPLS)

**PO: ADULTS, ELDERLY:** Interrupt treatment until fully resolved. Resume at reduced dose or discontinue (depending on the severity and persistence of neurologic symptoms).

### Other Adverse Reactions

**PO: ADULTS, ELDERLY:** Reduce dose according to dose modification table. Due to limited data, there are no recommendations on resuming treatment in pts with grade 4 adverse events that resolve.

### Dosage in Renal Impairment

**Mild to moderate impairment:** No dose adjustment. **Severe impairment:** 14 mg once daily.

### Dosage in Hepatic Impairment

**Mild to moderate impairment:** No dose adjustment. **Severe impairment:** 14 mg once daily.

---

## SIDE EFFECTS

**Frequent (73%–29%):** Hypertension, diarrhea, fatigue, asthenia, malaise, arthralgia, myalgia, decreased appetite, weight decreased, nausea, stomatitis, glossitis, mouth ulceration, mucosal inflammation, headache, vomiting, dysphonia, abdominal pain, constipation. **Occasional (25%–7%):** Oral pain, glossodynia, cough, peripheral edema, rash, dysgeusia, dry mouth, dizziness, dyspepsia, insomnia, alopecia, hypotension, dehydration, hyperkeratosis.

## ADVERSE EFFECTS/TOXIC REACTIONS

Serious adverse effects may include: arterial thromboembolic events (5% of pts); cardiac dysfunction (7% of pts); dental and oral infections including gingivitis, parotitis, pericoronitis, periodenitis, sialoadenitis, tooth abscess, tooth infection (10% of pts); GI perforation/fistula formation (2% of pts); hemorrhagic events (35% of pts); hepatotoxicity (4% of pts); hypertension (73% of pts); grade 3 or greater hypocalcemia (9% of pts); impairment of thyroid-stimulating hormone (57% of pts); palmar-plantar erythrodysesthesia (32% of pts); proteinuria (34% of pts); QT interval prolongation (9% of pts); renal failure (14% of pts); urinary tract infection (11% of pts). Reverse posterior leukoencephalopathy occurs rarely. The median onset of hypertension was 16 days. The most frequently reported hemorrhagic event was epistaxis. The primary risk factor for renal failure was dehydration and hypovolemia related to diarrhea and vomiting.

## NURSING CONSIDERATIONS

### BASELINE ASSESSMENT

Obtain baseline CBC, BMP, LFT; serum magnesium, phosphate, ionized calcium; urinalysis for proteinuria. Confirm negative pregnancy status before initiating treatment. Receive full medication history and screen for interactions. Question history of cardiac/pituitary/thyroid disease, CVA/DVT, hypertension, hepatic/renal impairment, long-QT interval syndrome. Assess oral cavity for lesions, poor dentation. Ensure B/P is controlled prior to initiation. Assess hydration status.

### INTERVENTION/EVALUATION

Monitor B/P after 1 wk, then every 2 wks for the first 2 mos, then at least monthly thereafter. Monitor LFT every 2 wks for the first 2 mos, then at least monthly thereafter. Monitor for proteinuria periodically. If urine dipstick proteinuria is greater than or equal to 2+, obtain a 24-hr urine protein test. Monitor blood calcium levels at least monthly and replace as needed depending on severity, presence of EKG changes, persistence of hypocalcemia. Monitor and correct other electrolyte abnormalities as needed. Initiate medical management for nausea, vomiting, diarrhea prior to any interruption or dose reduction. Reversible posterior leukoencephalopathy syndrome should be considered in pts with altered mental status, confusion, headache, seizures, visual disturbances. Immediately report abdominal pain, GI bleeding, hemoptysis (may indicate GI perforation/fistula formation). Obtain cardiac echocardiogram, EKG if cardiac decompensation is suspected.

### PATIENT/FAMILY TEACHING

• Blood levels will be monitored regularly. • Treatment may cause fetal harm. Female pts of childbearing potential should use effective contraception during treatment and up to 2 mos following discontinuation. Immediately report suspected pregnancy. • Therapy may reduce fertility in both female and male pts. • Report liver problems such as upper abdominal pain, bruising, dark or amber-colored urine, nausea, vomiting, or yellowing of the skin or eyes; heart problems such as chest tightness, dizziness, fainting, palpitations, shortness of breath; kidney problems such as dark-colored urine, decreased urine output, extremity swelling, flank pain; skin changes such as rash, skin bubbling, sloughing. • Neurologic changes including blurry vision, confusion, headache, one-sided weakness, seizures, trouble speaking may indicate high blood pressure crisis, stroke, or life-threatening brain swelling. • Report mouth ulceration, jaw pain. • Swallow capsules whole; do not chew, crush, cut, or open capsules. • Treatment may increase risk of GI bleeding, nosebleeds. • Drink plenty of fluids.

---

## letrozole     HIGH ALERT

let-roe-zole
(Apo-Letrozole ♣, Femara)
**Do not confuse Femara with Famvir, Femhrt, or Provera, or letrozole with anastrozole.**

### ◆CLASSIFICATION

**PHARMACOTHERAPEUTIC:** Aromatase inhibitor, hormone. **CLINICAL:** Antineoplastic.

### USES

First-line treatment of hormone receptor–positive or hormone receptor unknown locally advanced or metastatic breast cancer. Treatment of advanced breast cancer in postmenopausal women with disease progression following antiestrogen therapy. Postsurgical treatment for postmenopausal women with hormone receptor–positive early breast cancer. Extended treatment of early breast cancer after 5 yrs of tamoxifen. **OFF-LABEL:** Treatment of ovarian (epithelial), endometrial cancer.

### PRECAUTIONS

**Contraindications:** Hypersensitivity to letrozole, other aromatase inhibitors. Use in women who are or may become pregnant. **Cautions:** Hepatic impairment, hyperlipidemia.

### ACTION

Decreases circulating estrogen by inhibiting aromatase, an enzyme that catalyzes the final step in estrogen production. **Therapeutic Effect:** Inhibits growth of breast cancers stimulated by estrogens.

### PHARMACOKINETICS

Rapidly, completely absorbed. Metabolized in liver. Primarily eliminated in urine. Unknown if removed by hemodialysis. **Half-life:** Approximately 2 days.

### ⌛ LIFESPAN CONSIDERATIONS

**Pregnancy/Lactation:** Unknown if distributed in breast milk. May cause fetal harm. **Children:** Safety and efficacy not established. **Elderly:** No age-related precautions noted.

### INTERACTIONS

**DRUG: Tamoxifen** may reduce concentration. **HERBAL:** None significant. **FOOD:** None known. **LAB VALUES:** May increase serum calcium, cholesterol, GGT, ALT, AST, bilirubin.

### AVAILABILITY (Rx)

**Tablets:** 2.5 mg.

### ADMINISTRATION/HANDLING

**PO**
• Give without regard to food.

### INDICATIONS/ROUTES/DOSAGE

**Breast Cancer (Advanced)**
**PO: ADULTS, ELDERLY:** 2.5 mg/day. Continue until tumor progression is evident.

**Breast Cancer (Early–Adjuvant Treatment)**
**PO: ADULTS, ELDERLY: (Postmenopausal):** 2.5 mg/day for planned duration of 5 yrs. Discontinue at relapse.

**Breast Cancer (Early–Extended Adjuvant Treatment)**
**PO: ADULTS, ELDERLY: (Postmenopausal):** 2.5 mg/day for planned duration of 5 yrs (after 5 yrs of tamoxifen). Discontinue at relapse.

**L**

---

**Dosage in Renal Impairment**
No dose adjustment.

**Dosage in Severe Hepatic Impairment**
**PO: ADULTS, ELDERLY:** 2.5 mg every other day.

## SIDE EFFECTS

**Frequent (21%–9%):** Musculoskeletal pain (back, arm, leg), nausea, headache. **Occasional (8%–5%):** Constipation, arthralgia, fatigue, vomiting, hot flashes, diarrhea, abdominal pain, cough, rash, anorexia, hypertension, peripheral edema. **Rare (4%–1%):** Asthenia, drowsiness, dyspepsia, weight gain, pruritus.

## ADVERSE EFFECTS/ TOXIC REACTIONS

Pleural effusion, pulmonary embolism, bone fracture, thromboembolic disorder, MI occur rarely.

## NURSING CONSIDERATIONS

### BASELINE ASSESSMENT
Obtain baseline CBC, chemistries, renal function, LFT. Obtain pregnancy test prior to beginning therapy.

### INTERVENTION/EVALUATION
Monitor for, assist with ambulation if asthenia, dizziness occurs. Assess for headache. Offer antiemetic for nausea, vomiting. Monitor CBC, thyroid function, electrolytes, renal function, LFT. Monitor for evidence of musculoskeletal pain; offer analgesics for pain relief.

### PATIENT/FAMILY TEACHING
• Report if nausea, asthenia, hot flashes become unmanageable. • Discuss importance of negative pregnancy test prior to beginning therapy and nonhormonal methods of birth control. • Explain possible risk to fetus if pt is or becomes pregnant before or during therapy.

# leucovorin

loo-**koe**-vor-in
**Do not confuse leucovorin with Leukeran.**

## ◆CLASSIFICATION

**PHARMACOTHERAPEUTIC:** Folic acid antagonist. **CLINICAL:** Antidote.

## USES

Antidote for folic acid antagonists (methotrexate, trimethoprim, pyrimethoamine). Treatment of megaloblastic anemias when folate deficient. Palliative treatment of advanced colon cancer (with fluorouracil). IV rescue therapy after high-dose methotrexate for osteosarcoma or orally to diminish toxicity and impaired methotrexate elimination. **OFF-LABEL:** Adjunctive cofactor therapy in methanol toxicity. Prevents pyrimethamine hematologic toxicity in HIV-positive pts.

## PRECAUTIONS

**Contraindications:** Hypersensitivity to leucovorin. Pernicious anemia, other megaloblastic anemias secondary to vitamin $B_{12}$ deficiency. **Cautions:** Renal impairment.

## ACTION

Competes with methotrexate for same transport processes into cells (limits methotrexate action on normal cells). **Therapeutic Effect:** Reverses toxic effects of folic acid antagonists. Reverses folic acid deficiency.

## PHARMACOKINETICS

Readily absorbed from GI tract. Widely distributed. Metabolized in liver, intestinal mucosa. Primarily excreted in urine. **Half-life:** 15 min; metabolite, 30–35 min.

## ⧗ LIFESPAN CONSIDERATIONS

**Pregnancy/Lactation:** Unknown if drug crosses placenta or is distributed in breast milk. **Children:** May increase

---

risk of seizures by counteracting anticonvulsant effects of **barbiturates, hydantoins.** **Elderly:** Age-related renal impairment may require dosage adjustment when used for rescue from effects of high-dose methotrexate therapy.

## INTERACTIONS

**DRUG:** May decrease effects of **anticonvulsants (e.g., phenytoin).** May increase **5-fluorouracil** toxicity/effects when taken in combination. **HERBAL:** None significant. **FOOD:** None known. **LAB VALUES:** May decrease platelets, WBCs (when used in combination with 5-fluorouracil).

## AVAILABILITY (Rx)

**Injection, Powder for Reconstitution:** 50 mg, 100 mg, 200 mg, 350 mg, 500 mg. **Injection, Solution:** 10 mg/ml. **Tablets:** 5 mg, 10 mg, 15 mg, 25 mg.

## ADMINISTRATION/HANDLING

 **IV**

◀ALERT▶ Strict adherence to timing of 5-fluorouracil following leucovorin therapy must be maintained.

**Reconstitution** • Reconstitute each 50-mg vial with 5 ml Sterile Water for Injection or Bacteriostatic Water for Injection containing benzyl alcohol to provide concentration of 10 mg/ml. • Due to benzyl alcohol in 1-mg ampule and in Bacteriostatic Water for Injection, reconstitute doses greater than 10 mg/m² with Sterile Water for Injection. • Further dilute with 100–1,000 ml D₅W or 0.9% NaCl.

**Rate of Administration** • Do not exceed 160 mg/min if given by IV infusion (due to calcium content).

**Storage** • Store powdered vials for parenteral use at room temperature. • Refrigerate solution for injection vials. • Injection appears as clear, yellowish solution. • Use immediately if reconstituted with Sterile Water for Injection; stable for 7 days if reconstituted with Bacteriostatic Water for Injection. Diluted solutions stable for 24 hrs at room temperature or 4 days refrigerated.

**PO**
• Scored tablets may be crushed.

## 🔳 IV INCOMPATIBILITIES

Amphotericin B complex (Abelcet, AmBisome, Amphotec), droperidol (Inapsine), foscarnet (Foscavir).

## 🔳 IV COMPATIBILITIES

Cisplatin (Platinol AQ), cyclophosphamide (Cytoxan), doxorubicin (Adriamycin), etoposide (VePesid), filgrastim (Neupogen), 5-fluorouracil, gemcitabine (Gemzar), granisetron (Kytril), heparin, methotrexate, metoclopramide (Reglan), mitomycin (Mutamycin), piperacillin and tazobactam (Zosyn), vinblastine (Velban), vincristine (Oncovin).

## INDICATIONS/ROUTES/DOSAGE

**Rescue in High-Dose Methotrexate Therapy**
**PO, IV, IM: ADULTS, ELDERLY, CHILDREN:** 15 mg (approximately 10 mg/m²) started 24 hrs after starting methotrexate infusion; continue q6h for 10 doses, until methotrexate level is less than 0.05 micromole/L.

**Folic Acid Antagonist Overdose**
**PO: ADULTS, ELDERLY, CHILDREN:** 5–15 mg/day.

**Megaloblastic Anemia Secondary to Folate Deficiency**
**IM: ADULTS, ELDERLY, CHILDREN:** 1 mg or less per day.

**Colon Cancer**
◀ALERT▶ For rescue therapy in cancer chemotherapy, refer to specific protocols used for optimal dosage and sequence of leucovorin administration.
**IV: ADULTS, ELDERLY: (In Combination with 5-fluorouracil):** 200 mg/m² daily for 5 days. Repeat course at 4-wk intervals for 2 courses, then 4- to 5-wk intervals or

20 mg/m² daily for 5 days. Repeat course at 4-wk intervals for 2 courses, then 4- to 5-wk intervals.

**Dosage in Renal/Hepatic Impairment**
No dose adjustment.

## SIDE EFFECTS

**Frequent:** When combined with chemotherapeutic agents: diarrhea, stomatitis, nausea, vomiting, lethargy, malaise, fatigue, alopecia, anorexia. **Occasional:** Urticaria, dermatitis.

## ADVERSE EFFECTS/ TOXIC REACTIONS

Excessive dosage may negate chemotherapeutic effects of folic acid antagonists. Anaphylaxis occurs rarely. Diarrhea may cause rapid clinical deterioration.

## NURSING CONSIDERATIONS

### BASELINE ASSESSMENT
Obtain baseline CBC, LFT, renal function. Give as soon as possible, preferably within 1 hr, for treatment of accidental overdosage of folic acid antagonists.

### INTERVENTION/EVALUATION
Monitor for vomiting (may need to change from oral to parenteral therapy). Observe elderly, debilitated closely due to risk for severe toxicities. Assess CBC, BMP, LFT.

### PATIENT/FAMILY TEACHING
• Explain purpose of medication in treatment of cancer. • Report allergic reaction, vomiting.

---

## *leuprolide*    `HIGH ALERT`

**loo**-proe-lide
(Eligard, Lupron ✸, <u>Lupron Depot</u>, Lupron Depot-Ped)

### ◆CLASSIFICATION

**PHARMACOTHERAPEUTIC:** Gonadotropin-releasing hormone (GnRH) analogue. **CLINICAL:** Antineoplastic.

## USES

Palliative treatment of advanced prostate carcinoma. Management of endometriosis. Treatment of anemia caused by uterine leiomyomata (fibroids). Treatment of central precocious puberty. **OFF-LABEL:** Treatment of breast cancer, infertility.

## PRECAUTIONS

**Contraindications:** Hypersensitivity to leuprolide. Pregnancy, breastfeeding, undiagnosed vaginal bleeding. Eligard 7.5 mg is contraindicated in women, children; pts with hypersensitivity to GnRH, GnRH agonist analogues, or any of its components. 22.5 mg, 30 mg, 45 mg Lupron Depot contraindicated in women. **Cautions:** History of psychiatric illness, QTc prolongation or medications that prolong QTc interval, preexisting cardiac disease, chronic alcohol use, steroid therapy, seizures or medications that decrease seizures threshold.

## ACTION

Inhibits gonadotropin secretion; suppresses ovarian and testicular steroidgenesis due to decreased LH/FSH levels. Decreases testosterone and estrogen. **Therapeutic Effect:** Produces pharmacologic castration, decreases growth of abnormal prostate tissue in males; causes endometrial tissue to become inactive, atrophic in females; decreases rate of pubertal development in children with central precocious puberty.

## PHARMACOKINETICS

Rapidly, well absorbed after subcutaneous administration. Absorbed slowly after IM administration. Protein binding: 43%–49%. **Half-life:** 3–4 hrs.

## ⌛ LIFESPAN CONSIDERATIONS

**Pregnancy/Lactation:** **Depot:** Contraindicated in pregnancy. May cause spontaneous abortion. **Children:** Long-term safety not established. **Elderly:** No age-related precautions noted.

## INTERACTIONS

**DRUG:** None significant. **HERBAL:** None significant. **FOOD:** None known. **LAB VALUES:** May increase serum prostatic acid phosphatase (PAP). Initially increases, then decreases, serum testosterone. May increase serum ALT, AST, alkaline phosphatase, glucose, LDH, LDL, cholesterol, triglycerides. May decrease platelets, WBC.

## AVAILABILITY (Rx)

**Injection Depot Formulation: Eligard:** 7.5 mg, 22.5 mg, 30 mg, 45 mg. **Lupron Depot-Ped:** 7.5 mg, 11.25 mg (3-month), 11.25 (monthly), 15 mg, 30 mg. **Lupron Depot:** 3.75 mg, 11.25 mg, 22.5 mg, 30 mg, 45 mg. **Injection Solution (Lupron):** 5 mg/ml.

## ADMINISTRATION/HANDLING

◄ALERT► May be carcinogenic, mutagenic, teratogenic. Handle with extreme care during preparation/administration.

**IM**
**Lupron Depot** • Store at room temperature. • Protect from light, heat. • Do not freeze vials. • Reconstitute only with diluent provided. Follow manufacturer's instructions for mixing.
• Do not use needles less than 22 gauge; use syringes provided by the manufacturer (0.5-ml low-dose insulin syringes may be used as an alternative). • Administer immediately.
**Eligard** • Refrigerate. • Allow to warm to room temperature before reconstitution. • Follow manufacturer's instructions for mixing. • Following reconstitution, administer within 30 min.

**Subcutaneous**
**Lupron** • Refrigerate vials. • Injection appears clear, colorless. • Discard if discolored or precipitate forms. • Administer into deltoid muscle, anterior thigh, abdomen.

## INDICATIONS/ROUTES/DOSAGE

**Advanced Prostatic Carcinoma**
**IM** *(Lupron Depot):* **ADULTS, ELDERLY:** 7.5 mg q1mo, 22.5 mg q3mos, 30 mg q4mos, or 45 mg q6mos.
**SQ** *(Eligard):* **ADULTS, ELDERLY:** 7.5 mg every mo, 22.5 mg q3mos, 30 mg q4mos, or 45 mg q6mos.
**SQ** *(Lupron):* **ADULTS, ELDERLY:** 1 mg/day.

**Endometriosis**
**IM** *(Lupron Depot):* **ADULTS, ELDERLY:** 3.75 mg/mo for up to 6 mos or 11.25 mg q3mos for up to 2 doses.

**Uterine Leiomyomata**
**IM** *(with Iron [Lupron Depot]):* **ADULTS, ELDERLY:** 3.75 mg/mo for up to 3 mos or 11.25 mg as a single injection.

**Precocious Puberty**
**IM** *(Lupron Depot-Ped):* **CHILDREN GREATER THAN 37.5 KG:** 15 mg q mo. **GREATER THAN 25 KG TO 37.5 KG:** 11.25 mg q mo. **25 KG OR LESS:** 7.5 mg q mo. Titrate dose upward by 3.75 mg/mo if down regulation not achieved. **LUPRON DEPOT-PED (3 MOS):** 11.25 mg or 30 mg q12wks.
**SQ** *(Lupron):* **CHILDREN:** Initially, 50 mcg/kg/day. Titrate upward by 10 mcg/kg/day if down regulation is not achieved.

**Dosage in Renal/Hepatic Impairment**
No dose adjustment.

## SIDE EFFECTS

**Frequent:** Hot flashes (ranging from mild flushing to diaphoresis), migraines, hyperhidrosis. **Females:** Amenorrhea, spotting. **Occasional:** Arrhythmias, palpitations, blurred vision, dizziness, edema, headache, burning, pruritus, swelling at injection site, nausea, insomnia, weight gain. **Females:** Deepening voice, hirsutism, decreased libido, increased breast tenderness, vaginitis, altered mood. **Males:** Constipation, decreased testicle size, gynecomastia, impotence, decreased appetite, angina. **Rare: Males:** Thrombophlebitis.

**L**

## ADVERSE EFFECTS/ TOXIC REACTIONS

Occasionally, signs/symptoms of prostatic carcinoma worsen 1–2 wks after initial dosing (subsides during continued therapy). Increased bone pain and, less frequently, dysuria, hematuria, weakness, paresthesia of lower extremities may be noted. MI, pulmonary embolism occur rarely.

## NURSING CONSIDERATIONS

### BASELINE ASSESSMENT

Question for possibility of pregnancy before initiating therapy. Obtain serum testosterone, prostatic acid phosphates (PAP) periodically during therapy. Serum testosterone, PAP should increase during first wk of therapy. Serum testosterone then should decrease to baseline level or less within 2 wks, PAP within 4 wks.

### INTERVENTION/EVALUATION

Monitor for arrhythmias, palpitations. Assess for peripheral edema. Assess sleep pattern. Monitor for visual difficulties. Assist with ambulation if dizziness occurs. Offer antiemetics if nausea occurs.

### PATIENT/ FAMILY TEACHING

• Hot flashes tend to decrease during continued therapy. • Temporary exacerbation of signs/symptoms of disease may occur during first few wks of therapy. • Use contraceptive measures. • Report persistent, regular menstruation; pregnancy. • Avoid tasks that require alertness, motor skills until response to drug is established (potential for dizziness).

---

# levalbuterol

lee-val-**bue**-ter-ole
(Xopenex, Xopenex HFA)
**Do not confuse Xopenex with Xanax.**

## ◆CLASSIFICATION

**PHARMACOTHERAPEUTIC:** Sympathomimetic. **CLINICAL:** Bronchodilator.

## USES

Treatment, prevention of bronchospasm due to reversible obstructive airway disease (e.g., asthma, bronchitis, emphysema).

## PRECAUTIONS

**Contraindications:** History of hypersensitivity to albuterol or levalbuterol. **Cautions:** Cardiovascular disorders (cardiac arrhythmias, HF), seizures, hypertension, hyperthyroidism, diabetes mellitus, glaucoma, hypokalemia.

## ACTION

Stimulates beta$_2$-adrenergic receptors in lungs, resulting in relaxation of bronchial smooth muscle. **Therapeutic Effect:** Relieves bronchospasm, reduces airway resistance.

## PHARMACOKINETICS

| Route | Onset | Peak | Duration |
|---|---|---|---|
| Inhalation | 5–10 min | 1.5 hrs | 5–6 hrs |
| Nebulization | 10–17 min | 1.5 hrs | 5–8 hrs |

**Half-life:** 3.3–4 hrs.

## ⌛ LIFESPAN CONSIDERATIONS

**Pregnancy/Lactation:** Crosses placenta. Unknown if distributed in breast milk. **Pregnancy Category C. Children:** Safety and efficacy not established in those younger than 12 yrs. **Elderly:** Lower initial dosages recommended.

## INTERACTIONS

**DRUG: Beta blockers (e.g., carvedilol, metoprolol)** antagonize effects; may produce severe bronchospasm. May decrease **digoxin** concentration. **MAOIs (e.g., phenelzine, tranylcypromine), tricyclic antidepressants (e.g., amitriptyline, desipramine)** may potentiate cardiovascular effects. **Diuretics (e.g., furosemide, HCTZ)** may increase hypokalemia. **HERBAL:** None significant. **FOOD:** None known. **LAB VALUES:** May decrease serum potassium.

## AVAILABILITY (Rx)

**Inhalation Aerosol:** 45 mcg/activation. **Solution for Nebulization:** 0.31 in 3-ml vials, 0.63 mg in 3-ml vials, 1.25 mg in 3-ml vials, 1.25 mg in 0.5-ml vials.

## ADMINISTRATION/HANDLING

**Nebulization**

• No diluent necessary. • Protect from light, excessive heat. Store at room temperature. • Once foil is opened, use within 2 wks. • Use within 1 wk and protect from light after removal from pouch • Discard if solution is not colorless. • Do not mix with other medications. • Concentrated solution (1.25 mg in 0.5 ml) should be diluted with 2.5 ml 0.9% NaCl prior to use. • Give over 5–15 min.

**Inhalation**

• Shake well before inhalation. • Following first inhalation, wait 2 min before inhaling second dose (allows for deeper bronchial penetration). • Rinsing mouth with water immediately after inhalation prevents mouth/throat dryness.

## INDICATIONS/ROUTES/DOSAGE

**Treatment/Prevention of Bronchospasm**
**Nebulization: ADULTS, ELDERLY, CHILDREN 12 YRS AND OLDER:** Initially, 0.63 mg 3 times/day 6–8 hrs apart. May increase to 1.25 mg 3 times/day with dose monitoring. **CHILDREN 5–11 YRS:** Initially, 0.31 mg 3 times/day. **Maximum:** 0.63 mg 3 times/day. **CHILDREN 4 YRS OR YOUNGER:** 0.31–1.25 mg q4–6h as needed.
**Inhalation: ADULTS, ELDERLY, CHILDREN 4 YRS AND OLDER:** 1–2 inhalations q4–6h.

**Acute Asthma Exacerbation**
**Nebulization: ADULTS, ELDERLY, CHILDREN 12 YRS AND OLDER:** 1.25–2.5 mg q20min for 3 doses, then 1.25–5 mg q1–4h as needed. **CHILDREN YOUNGER THAN 12 YRS:** 0.075 mg/kg (minimum dose: 1.25 mg) q20min for 3 doses, then 0.075–0.15 mg/kg q1–4h as needed.
**Inhalation: ADULTS, ELDERLY, CHILDREN 12 YRS AND OLDER:** 4–8 puffs q20min for up to 4 hrs, then q1–4h. **CHILDREN**

**YOUNGER THAN 12 YRS:** 4–8 puffs q20min for 3 doses, then q1–4h.

**Dosage in Renal/Hepatic Impairment**
No dose adjustment.

## SIDE EFFECTS

**Occasional (11%–4%):** Nervousness, tremor, rhinitis, flu-like illness. **Rare (less than 3%):** Tachycardia, dizziness, anxiety, viral infection, dyspepsia, dry mouth, headache, chest pain.

## ADVERSE EFFECTS/ TOXIC REACTIONS

Excessive sympathomimetic stimulation may produce palpitations, premature heart contraction, tachycardia, chest pain, slight increase in B/P followed by substantial decrease, chills, diaphoresis, blanching of skin. Too-frequent or excessive use may decrease bronchodilating effectiveness, lead to severe, paradoxical bronchoconstriction.

## NURSING CONSIDERATIONS

### BASELINE ASSESSMENT

Offer emotional support (high incidence of anxiety due to difficulty in breathing, sympathomimetic response to drug). Assess lung sounds, pulse, B/P. Note color, amount of sputum.

### INTERVENTION/EVALUATION

Monitor rate, depth, rhythm, type of respiration; quality/rate of pulse, EKG, serum potassium, ABG determinations. Assess lung sounds for wheezing (bronchoconstriction), rales. Observe for paradoxical bronchospasm.

### PATIENT/ FAMILY TEACHING

• Increase fluid intake (decreases lung secretion viscosity). • Rinsing mouth with water immediately after inhalation may prevent mouth/throat dryness. • Avoid excessive use of caffeine derivatives (chocolate, coffee, tea, cola, cocoa). • Report if palpitations, tachycardia, chest pain, tremors, dizziness, headache occurs or shortness of breath is not relieved.

---

✦ Canadian trade name        Non-Crushable Drug        High Alert drug

# *levETIRAcetam

lee-ve-tye-ra-se-tam
(Apo-Levetiracetam ✚, Elepsia XR,
Keppra, Keppra XR, Spritam)
**Do not confuse Keppra with
Kaletra, Keflex, or Keppra XR,
or levetiracetam with levo-
floxacin.**

## ◆CLASSIFICATION

**PHARMACOTHERAPEUTIC:** Pyrro-
lidine derivative. **CLINICAL:** Anticonvulsant.

## USES

Adjunctive therapy in treatment of partial-onset, myoclonic, and/or primary
generalized tonic-clonic seizures.

## PRECAUTIONS

**Contraindications:** Hypersensitivity to
levetiracetam. **Cautions:** Renal impairment, pts with depression at high risk
for suicide.

## ACTION

Exact mechanism unknown. May inhibit
voltage-dependent calcium channels, facilitate GABA inhibitory transmission, reduce
potassium current, or bind to synaptic
proteins that modulate neurotransmitter
release. **Therapeutic Effect:** Prevents
seizure activity.

## PHARMACOKINETICS

Rapidly, completely absorbed following PO
administration. Protein binding: less than
10%. Metabolized primarily by enzymatic
hydrolysis. Primarily excreted in urine as
unchanged drug. **Half-life:** 6–8 hrs.

## ⌛ LIFESPAN CONSIDERATIONS

**Pregnancy/Lactation:** Distributed in
breast milk. Breastfeeding not recommended. **Children:** Safety and efficacy
not established in children 4 yrs or
younger. **Elderly:** Age-related renal impairment may require dosage adjustment.

## INTERACTIONS

**DRUG:** None significant. **HERBAL:** None significant. **FOOD:** None known. **LAB VALUES:**
May decrease Hgb, Hct, RBC, WBC counts.

## AVAILABILITY (Rx)

**Injection, Solution:** 100 mg/ml. **Oral
Solution:** 100 mg/ml. **Tablets:** 250 mg,
500 mg, 750 mg, 1,000 mg.

 **Tablets, Extended-Release:** 500 mg,
750 mg.

## ADMINISTRATION/HANDLING

### 🗄 IV

**Rate of Infusion** • Infuse over 15 min.
**Reconstitution** • Dilute with 100 ml
0.9% NaCl or D₅W.
**Storage** • Store at room temperature. • Stable for 24 hrs following
dilution.

## ▨ IV INCOMPATIBILITIES

Data not available.

## ▨ IV COMPATIBILITIES

Diazepam (Valium), lorazepam (Ativan),
valproate (Depacon).

### PO

• Give without regard to food. • Use
oral solution for pts weighing 20 kg or
less. • Use tablets or oral solution for
pts weighing more than 20 kg. • Oral
solution should be administered with a
calibrated measuring device. • Swallow
extended-release and immediate-release
tablets whole; do not break, crush, dissolve, or divide.

## INDICATIONS/ROUTES/DOSAGE

**Partial-Onset Seizures**
**IV/PO: ADULTS, ELDERLY, CHILDREN 17
YRS AND OLDER:** *(Immediate-Release):*
Initially, 500 mg q12h. May increase by
1,000 mg/day q2wks. **Maximum:** 3,000
mg/day in 2 divided doses. *Extended
Release:* 1,000 mg once daily. May increase in increments of 1,000 mg/day
q2wks. **Maximum:** 3,000 mg once daily.

---

**PO: CHILDREN 4–16 YRS:** 20 mg/kg/day in 2 divided doses. May increase q2wks by 10 mg/kg/dose. **Maximum:** 60 mg/kg/day in 2 divided doses. **CHILDREN 6 MOS TO YOUNGER THAN 4 YRS:** 20 mg/kg/day in 2 divided doses. May increase q2wks by 10 mg/kg/dose. **Maximum:** 50 mg/kg/day in 2 divided doses. **CHILDREN 1 MO TO YOUNGER THAN 6 MOS (ORAL SOLUTION):** 14 mg/kg/day in 2 divided doses. May increase q2wks by 7 mg/kg/dose. **Maximum:** 42 mg/kg/day in 2 divided doses.

**Myoclonic Seizures**
**PO/IV: ADULTS, ELDERLY, CHILDREN 12 YRS AND OLDER:** *(Immediate-Release):* Initially, 500 mg q12h. May increase by 1,000 mg/day q2wks. **Maximum:** 3,000 mg/day in 2 divided doses.

**Tonic-Clonic Seizures**
**PO: ADULTS, ELDERLY, CHILDREN 16 YRS AND OLDER:** *(Immediate-Release):* Initially, 500 mg twice daily. May increase by 1,000 mg/day q2wks up to recommended dose of 1,500 mg 2 times/day. **CHILDREN 6–15 YRS:** Initially, 10 mg/kg twice daily. May increase by 20 mg/kg/day q2wks up to recommended dose of 30 mg/kg 2 times/day.

**Dosage in Renal Impairment**
Dosage is modified based on creatinine clearance. **Note: CrCl less than 50 ml/min:** Not recommended with Elepsia XR.

| Creatinine Clearance | Dosage (Immediate-Release, IV) | Dosage (Extended-Release) |
|---|---|---|
| Greater than 80 ml/min: | 500–1,500 mg q12h | 1,000–3,000 mg q24h |
| 50–80 ml/min: | 500–1,000 mg q12h | 1,000–2,000 mg q24h |
| 30–49 ml/min: | 250–750 mg q12h | 500–1,500 mg q24h |
| Less than 30 ml/min: | 250–500 mg q12h | 500–1,000 mg q24h |

| Creatinine Clearance | Dosage (Immediate-Release, IV) | Dosage (Extended-Release) |
|---|---|---|
| End-stage renal disease using dialysis: | 500–1,000 mg q24h, after dialysis, a 250- to 500-mg supplemental dose is recommended | NA |
| CRRT | 250–750 mg q12h | |

**Dosage in Hepatic Impairment**
No dose adjustment.

## SIDE EFFECTS

**Frequent (15%–10%):** Drowsiness, asthenia, headache, infection. **Occasional (9%–3%):** Dizziness, pharyngitis, pain, depression, anxiety, vertigo, rhinitis, anorexia. **Rare (less than 3%):** Amnesia, emotional lability, cough, sinusitis, anorexia, diplopia.

## ADVERSE EFFECTS/ TOXIC REACTIONS

Acute psychosis, seizures have been reported. Sudden discontinuance increases risk of seizure activity. Serious dermatological reactions, including Steven-Johnson syndrome and toxic epidermal necrolysis, have been reported.

## NURSING CONSIDERATIONS

**BASELINE ASSESSMENT**
Review history of seizure disorder (intensity, frequency, duration, LOC). Initiate seizure precautions. Assess for hypersensitivity to levetiracetam. Obtain renal function test.

**INTERVENTION/EVALUATION**
Observe for recurrence of seizure activity. Assess for clinical improvement (decrease in intensity/frequency of seizures). Monitor renal function tests. Observe for suicidal ideation, depression, behavioral changes. Assist with ambulation if dizziness occurs.

L

## PATIENT/ FAMILY TEACHING

• Drowsiness usually diminishes with continued therapy. • Avoid tasks that require alertness, motor skills until response to drug is established. • Avoid alcohol. • Do not abruptly discontinue medication (may precipitate seizures). • Strict maintenance of drug therapy is essential for seizure control. • Report mood swings, hostile behavior, suicidal ideation, unusual changes in behavior.

---

## *levoFLOXacin   TOP 100

lee-voe-flox-a-sin
(Apo-Levofloxacin ✷, Levaquin, Quixin)

■ **BLACK BOX ALERT** ■ May increase risk of tendonitis, tendon rupture. (Risk increased with concurrent corticosteroids, organ transplant, pts older than 60 yrs.) May exacerbate myasthenia gravis.
**Do not confuse Levaquin with Levoxyl, Levsin/SL, or Lovenox, or levofloxacin with levetiracetam or levothyroxine.**

## ◆ CLASSIFICATION

**PHARMACOTHERAPEUTIC:** Fluoroquinolone. **CLINICAL:** Antibiotic.

## USES

Treatment of susceptible infections due to *S. pneumoniae, S. aureus, E. faecalis, H. influenzae, M. catarrhalis, Serratia marcescens, K. pneumoniae, E. coli, P. mirabilis, P. aeruginosa, C. pneumoniae, Legionella pneumophila, Mycoplasma pneumoniae,* including acute bacterial exacerbation of chronic bronchitis, acute bacterial sinusitis, community-acquired pneumonia, nosocomial pneumonia, complicated and uncomplicated UTI, acute pyelonephritis, complicated and uncomplicated mild to moderate skin/skin structure infections, prostatitis. Inhalation anthrax (post-exposure); plague. **Ophthalmic:** Treatment of superficial infections to conjunctiva (0.5%), cornea (1.5%). **OFF-LABEL:** Urethritis, traveler's diarrhea, diverticulitis, enterocolitis, Legionnaire's disease, peritonitis. Treatment of prosthetic joint infection.

## PRECAUTIONS

**Contraindications:** Hypersensitivity to levofloxacin, other fluoroquinolones. **Cautions:** Known or suspected CNS disorders, seizure disorder, renal impairment, bradycardia, rheumatoid arthritis, elderly, hypokalemia, hypomagnesemia, myasthenia gravis, severe cerebral arteriosclerosis, prolonged QT interval, medications that potentiate QT interval prolongation, diabetes.

## ACTION

Inhibits DNA enzyme gyrase in susceptible microorganisms, interfering with bacterial cell replication, repair. **Therapeutic Effect:** Bactericidal.

## PHARMACOKINETICS

Well absorbed after PO, IV administration. Protein binding: 50%. Widely distributed. Eliminated unchanged in urine. Partially removed by hemodialysis. **Half-life:** 6–8 hrs.

## ⧖ LIFESPAN CONSIDERATIONS

**Pregnancy/Lactation:** Distributed in breast milk. Avoid use in pregnancy. **Children:** Safety and efficacy not established in pts younger than 18 yrs. **Elderly:** Age-related renal impairment may require dosage adjustment.

## INTERACTIONS

**DRUG: Antacids, iron preparations, sucralfate, zinc** decrease absorption. **NSAIDs** may increase risk of CNS stimulation, seizures. **Medications that prolong QT interval (e.g., amiodarone, fluoxetine, haloperidol, sotalol, quinidine)** may increase risk of arrhythmias. May increase effects of **warfarin. HERBAL:** None significant. **FOOD:** None known. **LAB VALUES:** May alter serum glucose.

---

## AVAILABILITY (Rx)

**Infusion Premix:** 250 mg/50 ml, 500 mg/100 ml, 750 mg/150 ml. **Injection, Solution:** 25 mg/ml. **Ophthalmic Solution:** 0.5%. **Oral Solution:** 25 mg/ml. **Tablets:** 250 mg, 500 mg, 750 mg.

## ADMINISTRATION/HANDLING

 IV

**Reconstitution** • For infusion using single-dose vial, withdraw desired amount (10 ml for 250 mg, 20 ml for 500 mg). Dilute each 10 ml (250 mg) with minimum 40 ml 0.9% NaCl, D₅W, providing a concentration of 5 mg/ml.
**Rate of Administration** • Administer no less than 60 min for 250 mg or 500 mg; 90 min for 750 mg.
**Storage** • Available in single-dose 20-ml (500-mg) vials and premixed with D₅W, ready to infuse. • Diluted vials stable for 72 hrs at room temperature, 14 days if refrigerated.

### PO
• Do not administer antacids (aluminum, magnesium), sucralfate, iron or multivitamin preparations with zinc within 2 hrs of administration (significantly reduces absorption). • Give tablets without regard to food. • Give oral solution 1 hr before or 2 hrs after meals.

### Ophthalmic
• Place a gloved finger on lower eyelid and pull out until a pocket is formed between eye and lower lid. • Place prescribed number of drops into pocket. • Instruct pt to close eye gently (so medication will not be squeezed out of the sac) and to apply digital pressure to lacrimal sac for 1–2 min to minimize systemic absorption.

## ⊞ IV INCOMPATIBILITIES

Furosemide (Lasix), heparin, insulin, nitroglycerin, propofol (Diprivan).

## ⊞ IV COMPATIBILITIES

Dexmedetomidine (Precedex), dobutamine (Dobutrex), dopamine (Intropin), fentanyl (Sublimaze), lidocaine, lorazepam (Ativan), magnesium, morphine.

## INDICATIONS/ROUTES/DOSAGE

**Usual Dosage Range**
**PO, IV: ADULTS, ELDERLY:** 250–500 mg q24h; 750 mg q24h for severe or complicated infections.

**Bacterial Conjunctivitis**
**Ophthalmic: ADULTS, ELDERLY, CHILDREN 1 YR AND OLDER (QUIXIN) (0.5%):** 1–2 drops q2h for 2 days while awake (up to 8 times/day), then 1–2 drops q4h while awake up to 4 times/day.

**Dosage in Renal Impairment**
Normal renal function dosage of 250 mg/day:

| Creatinine Clearance | Dosage |
|---|---|
| 20–49 ml/min | No change |
| 10–19 ml/min | 250 mg initially, then 250 mg q48h |

Normal renal function dosage of 500 mg/day:

| Creatinine Clearance | Dosage |
|---|---|
| 50–80 ml/min | No change |
| 20–49 ml/min | 500 mg initially, then 250 mg q24h |
| 10–19 ml/min | 500 mg initially, then 250 mg q48h |

For pts undergoing dialysis, 500 mg initially, then 250 mg q48h.

Normal renal function dosage of 750 mg/day:

| Creatinine Clearance | Dosage |
|---|---|
| 50–80 ml/min | No change |
| 20–49 ml/min | Initially, 750 mg, then 750 mg q48h |
| 10–19 ml/min | Initially, 750 mg, then 500 mg q48h |

| Creatinine Clearance | Dosage |
|---|---|
| Dialysis | 500 mg q48h (administer after dialysis on dialysis days) |
| Continuous Renal Replacement Therapy | |
| CVVH | 500–750 mg once, then 250 mg q24h |
| CVVHD | 500–750 mg once, then 250–500 mg q24h |
| CVVHDT | 500–750 mg once, then 250–750 mg q24h |

**Dosage in Hepatic Impairment**
No dose adjustment.

## SIDE EFFECTS

**Occasional (3%–1%):** Diarrhea, nausea, abdominal pain, dizziness, drowsiness, headache. **Ophthalmic:** Local burning/discomfort, margin crusting, crystals/scales, foreign body sensation, ocular itching, altered taste. **Rare (less than 1%):** Flatulence; pain, inflammation, swelling in calves, hands, shoulder; chest pain, difficulty breathing, palpitations, edema, tendon pain. **Ophthalmic:** Corneal staining, keratitis, allergic reaction, eyelid swelling, tearing, reduced visual acuity.

## ADVERSE EFFECTS/ TOXIC REACTIONS

Antibiotic-associated colitis, other superinfections (abdominal cramps, severe watery diarrhea, fever) may occur. Superinfection (genital/anal pruritus, ulceration/changes in oral mucosa, moderate to severe diarrhea) may occur from altered bacterial balance in GI tract. Hypersensitivity reactions, including photosensitivity (rash, pruritus, blisters, edema, sensation of burning skin) have occurred in pts receiving fluoroquinolones.

## NURSING CONSIDERATIONS

### BASELINE ASSESSMENT

Question for hypersensitivity to levofloxacin, other fluoroquinolones. Question history as listed in Precautions. Receive full medication history and screen for interactions, esp. medications that prolong QT interval.

### INTERVENTION/EVALUATION

Monitor serum glucose, renal function, LFT. Monitor daily pattern of bowel activity, stool consistency. Report hypersensitivity reaction: skin rash, urticaria, pruritus, photosensitivity promptly. Be alert for superinfection: fever, vomiting, diarrhea, anal/genital pruritus, oral mucosal changes (ulceration, pain, erythema). Provide symptomatic relief for nausea. Evaluate food tolerance, altered taste.

### PATIENT/ FAMILY TEACHING

• Drink 6–8 glasses of fluid a day (prevents formation of urine crystals). • Avoid tasks that require alertness, motor skills until response to drug is established (may cause dizziness, drowsiness). • Report tendon pain/swelling, palpitations, chest pain, difficulty breathing, persistent diarrhea occurs. • Avoid exposure to direct sunlight. • Report use of warfarin.

# levothyroxine <sup>TOP 100</sup>

lee-voe-thy-**rox**-een
(Eltroxin ✶, Levoxyl, <u>Synthroid</u>, Tirosint, Unithroid)

■ **BLACK BOX ALERT** ■ Ineffective, potentially toxic for weight reduction. High doses increase risk of serious, life-threatening toxic effects, especially when used with some anorectic drugs.
**Do not confuse levothyroxine with levofloxacin or liothyronine, or Synthroid with Symmetrel.**

## FIXED-COMBINATION(S)

With liothyronine, $T_3$ **(Thyrolar).**

---

## ◆CLASSIFICATION

**PHARMACOTHERAPEUTIC:** Synthetic isomer of thyroxine. **CLINICAL:** Thyroid hormone ($T_4$).

## USES

**PO:** Treatment of hypothyroidism, pituitary thyroid-stimulating hormone (TSH) suppression. **IV:** Myxedema coma. **OFF-LABEL:** Management of hemodynamically unstable potential organ donors.

## PRECAUTIONS

**Contraindications:** Hypersensitivity to levothyroxine. Acute MI, untreated subclinical or overt thyrotoxicosis, uncorrected adrenal insufficiency. **Capsule:** Inability to swallow capsules. **Cautions:** Elderly, angina pectoris, hypertension, other cardiovascular disease, adrenal insufficiency, myxedema, diabetes mellitus and insipidus, swallowing disorders.

## ACTION

Converts to $T_3$, then binds to thyroid receptor proteins exerting metabolic effects through DNA and protein synthesis. **Therapeutic Effect:** Involved in normal metabolism, growth and development. Increases basal metabolic rate, enhances gluconeogenesis, stimulates protein synthesis.

## PHARMACOKINETICS

Variable, incomplete absorption from GI tract. Protein binding: greater than 99%. Widely distributed. Deiodinated in peripheral tissues, minimal metabolism in liver. Eliminated by biliary excretion. **Half-life:** 6–7 days.

## ⧖ LIFESPAN CONSIDERATIONS

**Pregnancy/Lactation:** Does not cross placenta. Minimal distribution in breast milk. **Children:** No age-related precautions noted. Caution in neonates in interpreting thyroid function tests. **Elderly:** May be more sensitive to thyroid effects; individualized dosage recommended.

## INTERACTIONS

**DRUG: Cholestyramine, colestipol, aluminum-** and **magnesium-containing antacids** may decrease absorption. **Estrogens** may cause decrease in serum-free thyroxine. May enhance effects of **oral anticoagulants (e.g, warfarin). Sympathomimetics (e.g., norepinephrine, phenylephrine)** may increase risk of coronary insufficiency, effects of levothyroxine. May decrease effects of **insulin, oral hypoglycemic agents. HERBAL:** None significant. **FOOD:** None known. **LAB VALUES:** None known.

## AVAILABILITY (Rx)

**Capsules (Tirosint):** 13 mcg, 25 mcg, 50 mcg, 75 mcg, 88 mcg, 100 mcg, 112 mcg, 125 mcg, 137 mcg, 150 mcg. **Injection, Powder for Reconstitution (Synthroid):** 100 mcg, 200 mcg, 500 mcg. **Tablets (Synthroid, Unithroid):** 25 mcg, 50 mcg, 75 mcg, 88 mcg, 100 mcg, 112 mcg, 125 mcg, 137 mcg, 150 mcg, 175 mcg, 200 mcg, 300 mcg.

## ADMINISTRATION/HANDLING

◀**ALERT▶** Do not interchange brands (known issues with bioequivalence between manufacturers).

 **IV**

**Reconstitution** • Reconstitute 200-mcg or 500-mcg vial with 5 ml 0.9% NaCl to provide concentration of 40 or 100 mcg/ml, respectively; shake until clear.
**Rate of Administration** • Use immediately; discard unused portions. • Give each 100 mcg or less over 1 min.
**Storage** • Store vials at room temperature.

**PO**
• Administer in the morning on an empty stomach, 30 min before food. • Administer before breakfast to prevent insomnia. • Tablets may be crushed. • Take 4 hrs apart from antacids, iron, calcium supplements.

L

---

## 🏶 IV INCOMPATIBILITIES

Do not use or mix with other IV solutions.

## INDICATIONS/ROUTES/DOSAGE

**Note:** IV dose is 50% of oral dose.

**Hypothyroidism**
**PO: ADULTS, CHILDREN IN WHOM GROWTH AND PUBERTY ARE COMPLETE, OLDER ADULTS RECENTLY TREATED FOR HYPOTHYROIDISM OR WHO HAVE BEEN HYPOTHYROID FOR ONLY A FEW MOS:** 1.7 mcg/kg/day as single daily dose. Usual maintenance: 100–125 mcg/day. **ADULTS YOUNGER THAN 50 YRS WITH CARDIAC DISEASE, OLDER THAN 50 YRS WITHOUT CARDIAC DISEASE:** Initially, 25–50 mcg/day. Adjust dose by 12.5–25 mcg at 6–8-wk intervals. **ADULTS (OLDER THAN 50 YRS WITH CARDIAC DISEASE):** Initially, 12.5–50 mcg/day. Adjust dose by 12.5–25 mcg/day at 4–8-wk intervals. **CHILDREN OLDER THAN 12 YRS, GROWTH AND PUBERTY INCOMPLETE:** 2–3 mcg/kg/day. **CHILDREN 6–12 YRS:** 4–5 mcg/kg/day. **CHILDREN 1–5 YRS:** 5–6 mcg/kg/day. **CHILDREN 6–12 MOS:** 6–8 mcg/kg/day. **CHILDREN 3–5 MOS:** 8–10 mcg/kg/day. **CHILDREN YOUNGER THAN 3 MOS:** 10–15 mcg/kg/day.

**Myxedema Coma**
**IV: ADULTS, ELDERLY:** Initially, 300–500 mcg, then 50–100 mcg once daily until able to tolerate PO administration.

**Pituitary Thyroid-Stimulating Hormone (TSH) Suppression**
**PO: ADULTS, ELDERLY:** Doses greater than 2 mcg/kg/day usually required to suppress TSH below 0.1 milliunits/L.

**Dosage in Renal/Hepatic Impairment**
No dose adjustment.

## SIDE EFFECTS

**Occasional:** Reversible hair loss at start of therapy in children. **Rare:** Dry skin, GI intolerance, rash, urticaria, pseudotumor cerebri, severe headache in children.

## ADVERSE EFFECTS/ TOXIC REACTIONS

Excessive dosage produces signs/symptoms of hyperthyroidism (weight loss, palpitations, increased appetite, tremors, anxiety, tachycardia, hypertension, headache, insomnia, menstrual irregularities). Cardiac arrhythmias occur rarely.

## NURSING CONSIDERATIONS

### BASELINE ASSESSMENT

Obtain baseline TSH, $T_3$, $T_4$, weight, vital signs. Signs/symptoms of diabetes mellitus, diabetes insipidus, adrenal insufficiency, hypopituitarism may become intensified. Treat with adrenocortical steroids before thyroid therapy in coexisting hypothyroidism and hypoadrenalism.

### INTERVENTION/EVALUATION

Monitor pulse for rate, rhythm (report pulse greater than 100 or marked increase). Observe for tremors, anxiety. Assess appetite, sleep pattern. **Children: (Undertreatment):** May decrease intellectual development, linear growth. **(Overtreatment):** Adversely affects brain maturation, accelerates bone age. Monitor thyroid function tests.

### PATIENT/ FAMILY TEACHING

• Do not discontinue drug therapy; replacement for hypothyroidism is lifelong. • Follow-up office visits, thyroid function tests are essential. • Take medication at the same time each day, preferably in the morning. • Monitor pulse for rate, rhythm; report irregular rhythm or pulse rate over 100 beats/min. • Promptly report chest pain, weight loss, anxiety, tremors, insomnia. • Children may have reversible hair loss, increased aggressiveness during first few mos of therapy. • Full therapeutic effect may take 1–3 wks.

# lidocaine

lye-doe-kane
(Lidoderm, Xylocaine)

## FIXED-COMBINATION(S)

**EMLA:** lidocaine/prilocaine (an anesthetic): 2.5%/2.5%. **Lidosite:** lidocaine/epinephrine (a sympathomimetic): 10%/0.1%. **Lidocaine with epinephrine:** lidocaine/epinephrine (a sympathomimetic): 2%/1:50,000, 1%/1:100,000, 1%/1:200,000, 0.5%/1:200,000. **Synéra:** lidocaine/tetracaine (an anesthetic): 70 mg/70 mg.

## ◆CLASSIFICATION

**PHARMACOTHERAPEUTIC:** Amide anesthetic. **CLINICAL:** Class 1B Antiarrhythmic, anesthetic.

## USES

**Antiarrhythmic:** Rapid control of acute ventricular arrhythmias following MI, cardiac catheterization, cardiac surgery. **Local Anesthetic:** Infiltration/nerve block for dental/surgical procedures, childbirth. **Topical Anesthetic:** Local skin disorders (minor burns, insect bites, prickly heat, skin manifestations of chickenpox, abrasions). Mucous membranes (local anesthesia of oral, nasal, laryngeal mucous membranes; local anesthesia of respiratory, urinary tracts; relief of discomfort of pruritus ani, hemorrhoids, pruritus vulvae). **Dermal patch:** Relief of chronic pain in postherpetic neuralgia, allodynia (painful hypersensitivity).

## PRECAUTIONS

**Contraindications:** Hypersensitivity to lidocaine. Adams-Stokes syndrome, hypersensitivity to amide-type local anesthetics, supraventricular arrhythmias, Wolff-Parkinson-White syndrome. Severe degree of SA, AV, or intraventricular heart block (except in pts with functioning pacemaker). **Cautions:** Hepatic disease, marked hypoxia, severe respiratory depression, hypovolemia, incomplete heart. History of malignant hyperthermia, shock, elderly, HF.

## ACTION

**Anesthetic:** Inhibits conduction of nerve impulses. **Therapeutic Effect:** Causes temporary loss of feeling/sensation. **Antiarrhythmic:** Suppresses automaticity of conduction tissue; increases electrical stimulation threshold of ventricle, His Purkinje system; and spontaneous depolarization of ventricle during diastole. **Therapeutic Effect:** Inhibits ventricular arrhythmias.

## PHARMACOKINETICS

| Route | Onset | Peak | Duration |
|---|---|---|---|
| IV | 30–90 sec | N/A | 10–20 min |
| Local anesthetic | 2.5 min | N/A | 30–60 min |

Completely absorbed after IM administration. Protein binding: 60%–80%. Widely distributed. Metabolized in liver. Primarily excreted in urine. Minimally removed by hemodialysis. **Half-life:** 1–2 hrs.

## ⌛ LIFESPAN CONSIDERATIONS

**Pregnancy/Lactation:** Crosses placenta. Distributed in breast milk. **Children:** No age-related precautions noted. **Elderly:** More sensitive to adverse effects. Dose, rate of infusion should be reduced. Age-related renal impairment may require dosage adjustment.

## INTERACTIONS

**DRUG: Class 1 antiarrhythmics** may increase cardiac effects. **HERBAL: St. John's wort** may decrease concentration. **FOOD:** None known. **LAB VALUES:** IM lidocaine may increase creatine kinase (CK) level. **Therapeutic serum level:** 1.5 to 6 mcg/ml; **toxic serum level:** greater than 6 mcg/ml.

## AVAILABILITY (Rx)

**Cream, Topical:** 4%. **Infusion Premix:** 0.4% (4 mg/ml in 250 ml, 500 ml); 0.8% (8 mg/ml in 250 ml, 500 ml). **Injection,**

**L**

Solution: 0.5% (5 mg/ml), 1% (10 mg/ml), 2% (20 mg/ml). Jelly, Topical: 2%. Solution, Topical: 4%. Solution, Viscous: 2%. Transdermal, Topical (Lidoderm): 5%.

## ADMINISTRATION/HANDLING

◄ALERT► Resuscitative equipment, drugs (including $O_2$) must always be readily available when administering lidocaine by any route.

### IV

◄ALERT► Use only lidocaine without preservative, clearly marked **for IV use**.
**Reconstitution** • For IV infusion, prepare solution by adding 2 g to 250–500 ml $D_5W$ or 0.9% NaCl to provide concentration of 8 mg/ml or 4 mg/ml, respectively. • Commercially available preparations of 0.4% and 0.8% may be used for IV infusion. **Maximum concentration:** 4 g/250 ml (16 mg/ml).
**Rate of Administration** • For IV push, use 1% (10 mg/ml) or 2% (20 mg/ml). • Administer IV push at rate of 25–50 mg/min. • Administer for IV infusion at rate of 1–4 mg/min (1–4 ml); use volume control IV set.
**Storage** • Store premix solutions at room temperature.

### Topical

• Not for ophthalmic use. • For skin disorders, apply directly to affected area or put on gauze or bandage, which is then applied to the skin. • For mucous membrane use, apply to desired area per manufacturer's insert. • Administer lowest dosage possible that still provides anesthesia.

### Dermal Patch

Patch may be cut to appropriate size.

### ▦ IV INCOMPATIBILITIES

Amphotericin B complex (Abelcet, AmBisome, Amphotec).

### ▦ IV COMPATIBILITIES

Amiodarone (Cordarone), calcium gluconate, dexmedetomidine (Precedex), digoxin (Lanoxin), diltiazem (Cardizem), dobutamine (Dobutrex), dopamine (Intropin), enalapril (Vasotec), furosemide (Lasix), heparin, insulin, nitroglycerin, potassium chloride.

## INDICATIONS/ROUTES/DOSAGE

### Ventricular Arrhythmias

**IV: ADULTS, ELDERLY:** Initially, 1–1.5 mg/kg. Refractory ventricular tachycardia, fibrillation: Repeat dose at 0.5–0.75 mg/kg q10–15min after initial dose for a maximum of 3 doses. Total dose not to exceed 3 mg/kg. Follow with continuous infusion (1–4 mg/min) after return of perfusion. Reappearance of arrhythmia during infusion: 0.5 mg/kg, reassess infusion. **CHILDREN, INFANTS:** Initially, 1 mg/kg (**maximum: 100 mg**). May repeat second dose of 0.5–1 mg/kg if start of infusion longer than 15 min. **Maintenance:** 20–50 mcg/kg/min as IV infusion.

### Local Anesthesia

**Infiltration, Nerve Block: ADULTS:** Local anesthetic dosage varies with procedure, degree of anesthesia, vascularity, duration. **Maximum dose:** 4.5 mg/kg. Do not repeat within 2 hrs.

### Topical Local Anesthesia

**Topical: ADULTS, ELDERLY:** Apply to affected areas as needed.

### Treatment of Localized Pain

◄ALERT► Transdermal patch may contain conducting metal (e.g., aluminum). Remove patch prior to MRI.
**Topical *(Dermal Patch):* ADULTS, ELDERLY:** Apply to intact skin over most painful area (up to 3 applications once for up to 12 hrs in a 24-hr period).

### Dosage in Renal Impairment

No dose adjustment.

### Dosage in Hepatic Impairment

Use with caution.

## SIDE EFFECTS

CNS effects generally dose-related and of short duration. **Occasional: IM:** Pain at injection site. **Topical:** Burning, stinging, tenderness at application site. **Rare:** Generally associated with high dose: Drowsiness, dizziness, disorientation, light-headedness, tremors, apprehension, euphoria, sensation of heat, cold, numbness; blurred or double vision, tinnitus, nausea.

## ADVERSE EFFECTS/ TOXIC REACTIONS

Serious adverse reactions to lidocaine are uncommon, but high dosage by any route may produce cardiovascular depression, bradycardia, hypotension, arrhythmias, heart block, cardiovascular collapse, cardiac arrest. Potential for malignant hyperthermia, CNS toxicity may occur, esp. with regional anesthesia use, progressing rapidly from mild side effects to tremors, drowsiness, seizures, vomiting, respiratory depression. Methemoglobinemia (evidenced by cyanosis) has occurred following topical application of lidocaine for teething discomfort and laryngeal anesthetic spray.

## NURSING CONSIDERATIONS

### BASELINE ASSESSMENT

Question for hypersensitivity to lidocaine, amide anesthetics. Obtain baseline B/P, pulse, respiratory rate, EKG, serum electrolytes.

### INTERVENTION/EVALUATION

Monitor EKG, vital signs closely during and following drug administration for cardiac performance. If EKG shows arrhythmias, prolongation of PR interval or QRS complex, inform physician immediately. Assess pulse for rhythm, rate, quality. Assess B/P for evidence of hypotension. Monitor for therapeutic serum level (1.5–6 mcg/ml). For lidocaine given by all routes, monitor vital signs, LOC. Drowsiness should be considered a warning sign of high serum levels of lidocaine. **Therapeutic serum level:** 1.5–6 mcg/ml; **toxic serum level:** greater than 6 mcg/ml.

### PATIENT/ FAMILY TEACHING

• **Local anesthesia:** Due to loss of feeling/sensation, protective measures may be needed until anesthetic wears off (no ambulation, including special positions for some regional anesthesia). • **Oral mucous membrane anesthesia:** Do not eat, drink, chew gum for 1 hr after application (swallowing reflex may be impaired, increasing risk of aspiration; numbness of tongue, buccal mucosa may lead to bite trauma). • **IV infusions:** Report dizziness, numbness, double vision, nausea, pain/burning, respiratory difficulty. • **Topical:** Report irritation, pain, numbness, swelling, blurred vision, tinnitus, respiratory difficulty.

# linaclotide

lin-a-**kloe**-tide
(Constella ✦, Linzess)

■ **BLACK BOX ALERT** ■ Contraindicated in pediatric pts 6 yrs of age and younger. Avoid use in pediatric patients 7 yrs through 17 yrs old.

## ◆CLASSIFICATION

**PHARMACOTHERAPEUTIC:** Guanylate cyclase-C (cGMP) agonist. **CLINICAL:** Anti-constipation agent.

## USES

Treatment of irritable bowel syndrome with constipation, chronic idiopathic constipation.

## PRECAUTIONS

**Contraindications:** Hypersensitivity to linaclotide. Pediatric patients 6 yrs and younger, known or suspected mechanical GI obstruction. **Cautions:** Diarrhea.

## ACTION

Binds on the luminal surface of GI epithelium. Increase cGMP which stimulates chloride and bicarbonate into intestinal lumen. **Therapeutic Effect:** Increase intestinal fluid, accelerates transit.

## PHARMACOKINETICS

Metabolized within GI tract. Minimal distribution beyond GI tissue. Minimal systemic absorption. **Half-life:** N/A.

## ⧗ LIFESPAN CONSIDERATIONS

**Pregnancy/Lactation:** Unknown if distributed in breast milk. **Children:** Avoid use in pediatric pts 7 yrs through 17 yrs. Contraindicated in pediatric pts 6 yrs and younger. **Elderly:** No age-related precautions noted.

## INTERACTIONS

**DRUG:** None significant. **HERBAL:** None significant. **FOOD:** None known. **LAB VALUES:** None significant.

## AVAILABILITY (Rx)

 **Capsules:** 145 mcg, 290 mcg.

## ADMINISTRATION/HANDLING

**PO**
• Give on empty stomach at least 30 min prior to first meal of day. • Do not break, crush, or open capsule.

## INDICATIONS/ROUTES/DOSAGE

**Irritable Bowel Syndrome With Constipation**
**PO: ADULTS 18 YRS AND OLDER, ELDERLY:** 290 mcg once daily.

**Chronic Idiopathic Constipation**
**PO: ADULTS 18 YRS AND OLDER, ELDERLY:** 145 mcg once daily.

**Dosage in Renal/Hepatic Impairment**
No dose adjustment.

## SIDE EFFECTS

**Frequent (16%):** Diarrhea (may begin within first 2 wks of initiation of treatment). **Occasional (7%–2%):** Abdominal pain, flatulence, headache, abdominal distention. **Rare (1% and Less):** Gastroesophageal reflux, vomiting.

## ADVERSE EFFECTS/ TOXIC REACTIONS

Severe diarrhea was reported in 2% of pts. Viral gastroenteritis was noted in 3% of pts. Fecal incontinence, dehydration was reported in 1%. Dose reduced or suspended secondary to diarrhea, other GI adverse reaction.

## NURSING CONSIDERATIONS

### BASELINE ASSESSMENT

Encourage adequate fluid intake. Assess bowel sounds for peristalsis. Assess for abdominal disturbances.

### INTERVENTION/EVALUATION

For pts with irritable bowel syndrome, assess for improvement in symptoms (relief from bloating, cramping, urgency, abdominal discomfort). Monitor daily bowel activity, stool consistency. Monitor serum electrolytes in pts with prolonged, frequent, or excessive use of medication.

### PATIENT/FAMILY TEACHING

• Institute measures to promote defecation: increase fluid intake, exercise, high-fiber diet. • Report new/worsening episodes of abdominal pain, severe diarrhea. • Do not break, crush, or open capsule. Take whole.

# linagliptin

lin-a-**glip**-tin
(Tradjenta)
**Do not confuse linagliptin with saxagliptin or sitagliptin.**

## FIXED-COMBINATION(S)

**Glyxambi:** linagliptin/empagliflozin (an antidiabetic): 5 mg/10 mg, 5 mg/25 mg. **Jentadueto:** linagliptin/ metformin (an antidiabetic): 2.5 mg/ 500 mg; 2.5 mg/850 mg; 2.5 mg/ 1,000 mg. **Jentadueto XR:** linagliptin/ metformin (extended-release): 2.5 mg/1,000 mg; 5 mg/1,000 mg.

## ♦CLASSIFICATION

**PHARMACOTHERAPEUTIC:** Dipeptidyl peptidase-4 (DDP-4) inhibitor (gliptan). **CLINICAL:** Antidiabetic agent.

## USES

Adjunctive treatment to diet and exercise to improve glycemic controls in pts with type 2 diabetes mellitus alone or in combination with other antidiabetic agents.

## PRECAUTIONS

**Contraindications:** Hypersensitivity to linagliptin, other DD4 inhibitors. **Cautions:** Concurrent use of other hypoglycemics. Not recommended for use in type 1 diabetes, diabetic ketoacidosis, history of pancreatitis, HF.

## ACTION

Slows inactivation of incretin hormones by inhibiting DDP-4 enzyme. **Therapeutic Effect:** Incretin hormones increase insulin synthesis/release from pancreas and decrease glucagon secretion. Lowers serum glucose levels.

## PHARMACOKINETICS

Rapidly absorbed following PO administration. Peak plasma concentration: 1.5 hrs. Extensive tissue distribution. Protein binding: 70%–99%. Minimal metabolism (90% excreted as unchanged metabolite). Excreted primarily in enterohepatic system (80%), urine (5%). **Half-life:** 12 hrs.

## ⌛ LIFESPAN CONSIDERATIONS

**Pregnancy/Lactation:** Unknown if distributed in breast milk. **Children:** Safety and efficacy not established. **Elderly:** No age-related precautions noted.

## INTERACTIONS

**DRUG: CYP3A4 inducers** (e.g., **rifampin**) may decrease concentration. **Insulin, metformin, saxagliptin, sitagliptin, sulfonylureas** may increase risk of hypoglycemia. **HERBAL: Ginseng, ginger, other herbs with hypoglycemic activity** may increase risk of hypoglycemia. **FOOD:** None known. **LAB VALUES:** Decreases serum glucose. May increase serum uric acid.

## AVAILABILITY (Rx)

**Tablets:** 5 mg.

## ADMINISTRATION/HANDLING

**PO**
• May give without regard to food.

## INDICATIONS/ROUTES/DOSAGE

**Note:** Dose reduction of insulin and/or insulin secretagogues may be needed.

**Type 2 Diabetes Mellitus**
**PO: ADULTS, ELDERLY:** 5 mg once daily.

**Dosage in Renal/Hepatic Impairment**
No dose adjustment.

## SIDE EFFECTS

**Occasional (5%):** Nasopharyngitis. **Rare (less than 2%):** Cough, headache.

## ADVERSE EFFECTS/ TOXIC REACTIONS

Hypoglycemia reported in 7% of pts. Concomitant use of hypoglycemic medication may increase hypoglycemic risk. Pancreatitis, hypersensitivity reactions (angioedema, rash, urticaria, pruritus, bronchospasm) occur rarely.

## NURSING CONSIDERATIONS

### BASELINE ASSESSMENT

Check blood glucose, hemoglobin A1c level. Assess pt's understanding of diabetes management, routine glucose monitoring. Receive full medication history including herbal products.

### INTERVENTION/EVALUATION

Monitor blood glucose, hemoglobin A1c level. Assess for hypoglycemia (diaphoresis, tremors, dizziness, anxiety, headache,

L

---

 ♦ Canadian trade name      Non-Crushable Drug     🔲HIGH ALERT High Alert drug tachycardia, perioral numbness, hunger, diplopia, difficulty concentrating), hyperglycemia (polyuria, polyphagia, polydipsia, nausea, vomiting, fatigue, Kussmaul breathing). Screen for glucose-altering conditions: fever, increased activity or stress, surgical procedures. Dietary consult for nutritional education.

### PATIENT/FAMILY TEACHING

• Diabetes mellitus requires lifelong control. • Diet and exercise is principal part of treatment; do not skip or delay meals. • Test blood glucose regularly. • When taking combination drug therapy or when glucose demands are altered (fever, infection, trauma, stress, heavy physical activity), have hypoglycemic treatment available (glucagon, oral dextrose). • Monitor daily calorie intake.

---

# linezolid

lin-**ez**-oh-lid
Apo-Linezolid ✦, (Zyvox, Zyvoxam ✦)
**Do not confuse Zyvox with Zosyn or Zovirax.**

### ◆CLASSIFICATION

**PHARMACOTHERAPEUTIC:** Oxazolidinone. **CLINICAL:** Antibiotic.

## USES

Treatment of susceptible infections due to aerobic and facultative, gram-positive microorganisms, including *E. faecium* (vancomycin-resistant strains only), *S. aureus* (including methicillin-resistant strains), *S. agalactiae, S. pneumoniae* (including multidrug-resistant strains), *S. pyogenes.* Treatment of pneumonia (community-acquired and hospital acquired), skin, soft tissue infections (including diabetic foot infections), bacteremia caused by susceptible vancomycin-resistant organisms. **OFF-LABEL:** Treatment of prosthetic joint infection. Septic arthritis.

## PRECAUTIONS

**Contraindications:** Hypersensitivity to linezolid. Concurrent use or within 2 wks of MAOIs. **Cautions:** History of seizures, preexisting myelosuppression, medications that may cause bone marrow depression, uncontrolled hypertension, pheochromocytoma, carcinoid syndrome, untreated hyperthyroidism, diabetes, chronic infection; concurrent use of SSRIs, SNRIs, tricyclic antidepressants, triptans, bupropion.

## ACTION

Binds to bacterial ribosomal RNA sites preventing formation of a complex essential for bacterial translation. **Therapeutic Effect:** Bacteriostatic against enterococci, staphylococci; bactericidal against streptococci.

## PHARMACOKINETICS

Rapidly, extensively absorbed after PO administration. Protein binding: 31%. Metabolized in liver by oxidation. Excreted in urine. **Half-life:** 4–5.4 hrs.

## ⧗ LIFESPAN CONSIDERATIONS

**Pregnancy/Lactation:** Unknown if distributed in breast milk. **Children:** Safety and efficacy not established. **Elderly:** No age-related precautions noted.

## INTERACTIONS

**DRUG: CYP3A4 inducers (e.g., carbamazepine, phenytoin)** may decrease concentration/effects. **Adrenergic medications (sympathomimetics)** may increase effects. **SSRIs** may increase risk of serotonin syndrome. **HERBAL:** Supplements containing **caffeine, tyrosine,** or **tryptophan** may precipitate hypertensive crisis. **FOOD:** Excessive amounts of **tyramine-containing foods, beverages** may cause significant hypertension. **LAB VALUES:** May decrease Hgb, neutrophils, platelets, WBC. May increase serum ALT, AST, alkaline phosphatase, amylase, bilirubin, BUN, creatinine, LDH, lipase.

---

## AVAILABILITY (Rx)

Injection Premix: 2 mg/ml in 100-ml, 300-ml bags. Powder for Oral Suspension: 100 mg/5 ml. Tablets: 600 mg.

## ADMINISTRATION/HANDLING

 IV

**Rate of Administration** • Infuse over 30–120 min. • Should be administered without further dilution.
**Storage** • Store at room temperature. • Protect from light. • Yellow color does not affect potency.

### PO

• Give without regard to meals. • Use suspension within 21 days after reconstitution. Gently invert 3–5 times before administration. • Do not shake.

## ▒ IV INCOMPATIBILITIES

Amphotericin B complex (Abelcet, AmBisome, Amphotec), co-trimoxazole (Bactrim), diazepam (Valium), erythromycin (Erythrocin), pentamidine (Pentam IV), phenytoin (Dilantin).

## ▒ IV COMPATIBILITIES

Calcium gluconate, dexmedetomidine (Precedex), heparin, magnesium, potassium chloride.

## INDICATIONS/ROUTES/DOSAGE

**Vancomycin-Resistant Infections (VRI)**
PO, IV: ADULTS, ELDERLY, CHILDREN OLDER THAN 11 YRS: 600 mg q12h for 14–28 days. CHILDREN 11 YRS AND YOUNGER: 10 mg/kg q8–12h for 14–28 days.

**Pneumonia, Complicated Skin/Skin Structure Infections**
PO, IV: ADULTS, ELDERLY, CHILDREN OLDER THAN 11 YRS: 600 mg q12h for 10–14 days. CHILDREN 11 YRS AND YOUNGER: 10 mg/kg q8h for 10–14 days.

**Uncomplicated Skin/Skin Structure Infections**
PO: ADULTS, ELDERLY: 400 mg q12h for 10–14 days. CHILDREN OLDER THAN 11 YRS: 600 mg q12h for 10–14 days. CHILDREN 5–11 YRS: 10 mg/kg/dose q12h for 10–14 days. CHILDREN YOUNGER THAN 5 YRS: 10 mg/kg q8h for 10–14 days.

**Usual Neonate Dosage**
PO, IV: NEONATES: 10 mg/kg/dose q8–12h.

**Dosage in Renal/Hepatic Impairment**
No dose adjustment. Administer after HD on dialysis days.

## SIDE EFFECTS

**Occasional (9%–2%):** Diarrhea, nausea, vomiting, insomnia, constipation, rash, dizziness, fever, headache. **Rare (less than 2%):** Altered taste, vaginal candidiasis, fungal infection, tongue discoloration.

## ADVERSE EFFECTS/ TOXIC REACTIONS

Thrombocytopenia, myelosuppression occur rarely. Antibiotic-associated colitis, other superinfections (abdominal cramps, severe watery diarrhea, fever) may result from altered bacterial balance in GI tract.

## NURSING CONSIDERATIONS

### BASELINE ASSESSMENT

Obtain appropriate culture specimens for sensitivity testing prior to therapy. Obtain baseline CBC, chemistries.

### INTERVENTION/EVALUATION

Monitor daily pattern of bowel activity, stool consistency. Mild GI effects may be tolerable, but increasing severity may indicate onset of antibiotic-associated colitis. Be alert for superinfection: fever, vomiting, diarrhea, anal/genital pruritus, oral mucosal changes (ulceration, pain, erythema). Monitor CBC, platelets, Hgb, chemistries.

### PATIENT/ FAMILY TEACHING

• Continue therapy for full length of treatment. • Doses should be evenly spaced. • May cause GI upset (may take with food, milk). • Excessive amounts of tyramine-containing foods (red wine, aged cheese) may cause severe reaction (severe headache, neck stiffness, diaphoresis, palpitations). • Avoid alcohol. • Report persistent diarrhea, nausea, vomiting.

# liraglutide

TOP 100

leer-a-gloo-tide
(Saxenda, Victoza)

■ BLACK BOX ALERT ■ Causes dose-dependent and treatment duration–dependent thyroid C-cell tumors, including medullary thyroid cancer.

## FIXED COMBINATION(S)

Xultophy: liraglutide 3.6 mg/ml and insulin degludec 100 units/ml.

## ◆CLASSIFICATION

PHARMACOTHERAPEUTIC: Antihyperglycemic (glucagon-like peptide-1 [GLP-1] receptor agonist). CLINICAL: Antidiabetic agent.

## USES

Saxenda: Adjunct to diet and increased physical activity for chronic weight management in adults with body mass index (BMI) of 30 kg/m$^2$ or greater, or 27 kg/m$^2$ or greater, with at least one co-morbid condition (e.g., hypertension, diabetes, dyslipidemia). Victoza: Adjunct to diet and exercise to improve glycemic control in adult pts with type 2 diabetes mellitus.

## PRECAUTIONS

Contraindications: Hypersensitivity to liraglutide. Personal or family history of medullary thyroid carcinoma (MTC), pts with multiple endocrine neoplasia syndrome type 2 (MEN2). (Saxenda): Pregnancy. Cautions: History of pancreatitis, cholelithiasis, alcohol abuse, renal/hepatic impairment. History of angioedema to other GLP-1 receptor agonists. Do not use in type 1 diabetes or diabetic ketoacidosis. Medications with narrow therapeutic index or requiring rapid GI absorption.

## ACTION

Stimulates release of insulin from pancreatic beta cells, mimics enhancement of glucose-dependent insulin secretion, suppresses elevated glucagon secretion, slows gastric emptying. Therapeutic Effect: Improves glycemic control by increasing postmeal insulin secretion, emptying, increasing satiety.

## PHARMACOKINETICS

Maximum concentration achieved in 8–12 hrs. Protein binding: 98%. Metabolized to large proteins without a specific organ as major route of elimination. Half-life: 13 hrs.

## ⏳ LIFESPAN CONSIDERATIONS

Pregnancy/Lactation: Unknown if distributed in breast milk. Children: Safety and efficacy not established. Elderly: No age-related precautions noted.

## INTERACTIONS

DRUG: Liraglutide has potential to alter absorption of concurrently administered oral medications. HERBAL: None significant. FOOD: None known. LAB VALUES: Decreases glucose serum levels (when used in combination with insulin secretagogues [e.g., sulfonylureas]).

## AVAILABILITY (Rx)

Subcutaneous, Solution (Prefilled Pen): (Victoza): 18 mg/3 ml. (Saxenda): (Prefilled Pen) 18 mg/3 ml. Delivers doses of 0.6 mg, 1.2 mg, 1.8 mg, 2.4 mg, or 3 mg.

## ADMINISTRATION/HANDLING

Subcutaneous
• May be given in thigh, abdomen, upper arm. • Rotation of injection sites is essential; maintain careful records. • Give at any time without regard to meals.
Storage • Refrigerate prefilled pens. • Discard if freezing occurs. • Discard pen 30 days after initial use.

## INDICATIONS/ROUTES/DOSAGE

Diabetes Mellitus (Victoza)
SQ: ADULTS, ELDERLY: Initial dose: 0.6 mg subcutaneously once per day for at

least 1 wk. (**Note:** This dose is intended to reduce GI symptoms during initial titration; it is not effective for glycemic control.) After 1 wk, increase dose to 1.2 mg. If 1.2-mg dose does not result in acceptable glycemic control, dose can be increased to 1.8 mg.

**Weight Management (Saxenda)**
**SQ: ADULTS, ELDERLY:** Initially, 0.6 mg daily for one week. Increase wkly by 0.6 mg/day to a target dose of 3 mg once daily. **Note:** Evaluate change in weight 16 wks after initiation. Discontinue if less than 4% of baseline weight not achieved.

**Dosage in Renal/Hepatic Impairment**
Use caution.

## SIDE EFFECTS

**Frequent (greater than 13%):** Headache, nausea, diarrhea, liraglutide antibody resistance. **Occasional (13%–6%):** Diarrhea, vomiting, dizziness, nervousness, dyspepsia. **Rare (less than 6%):** Weakness, decreased appetite.

## ADVERSE EFFECTS/ TOXIC REACTIONS

Serious hypoglycemia may occur when used concurrently with insulin analogue (e.g., sulfonylurea); consider lowering dose.

## NURSING CONSIDERATIONS

**BASELINE ASSESSMENT**
Check blood glucose concentration before administration. Discuss pt's lifestyle to determine extent of learning, emotional needs. Ensure follow-up instruction if pt/family does not thoroughly understand diabetes management or glucose testing technique. Dose is gradually increased to improve GI tolerance.

**INTERVENTION/EVALUATION**
Monitor blood glucose level, food intake. Assess for hypoglycemia (cool wet skin, tremors, dizziness, anxiety, headache, tachycardia, numbness in mouth, hunger, diplopia) or hyperglycemia (polyuria,

polyphagia, polydipsia, nausea, vomiting, dim vision, fatigue, deep rapid breathing). Be alert to conditions that alter glucose requirements (fever, increased activity/stress, surgical procedures). Consider lowering dose of insulin analogue to reduce risk of hypoglycemia.

**PATIENT/FAMILY TEACHING**
• Diabetes mellitus requires lifelong control. • Prescribed diet, exercise are principal parts of treatment; do not skip/delay meals. • Continue following dietary instructions, regular exercise program, regular testing of blood glucose level. • Serious hypoglycemia may occur when used concurrently with insulin analogue (e.g., sulfonylurea). • Have source of glucose available to treat symptoms of low blood sugar.

---

**TOP 100**

# lisdexamfetamine

lis-dex-am-**fet**-a-meen
(Vyvanse)

■ **BLACK BOX ALERT** ■ Potential for drug abuse dependency exists. **Do not confuse lisdexamfetamine with dextroamphetamine, or Vyvanse with Glucovance, Vivactil, or Vytorin.**

◆ **CLASSIFICATION**
**PHARMACOTHERAPEUTIC:** Amphetamine **(Schedule II). CLINICAL:** CNS stimulant.

## USES

Treatment of attention-deficit/hyperactivity disorder (ADHD), moderate to severe binge eating disorder (BED).

## PRECAUTIONS

**Contraindications:** Hypersensitivity to lisdexamfetamine, amphetamine products. Concurrent use or within 2 wks of use of MAOI. **Cautions:** Hyperthyroidism, glaucoma, agitated states, cardiovascular

---

conditions (hypertension, recent MI, ventricular arrhythmias), elderly, psychiatric/seizures, preexisting psychosis or bipolar disorder, Tourette syndrome. Avoid use in pts with serious structural cardiac abnormalities, cardiomyopathy, arrhythmias, CAD. History of alcohol or drug abuse.

## ACTION

Enhances action of dopamine, norepinephrine by blocking reuptake from synapses, increasing levels in extraneuronal space. **Therapeutic Effect:** Improves attention span in ADHD.

## PHARMACOKINETICS

Rapidly absorbed. Converted to dextroamphetamine. Excreted in urine. **Half-life:** Less than 1 hr.

## ⌛ LIFESPAN CONSIDERATIONS

**Pregnancy/Lactation:** Has potential for fetal harm. Unknown if distributed in breast milk. **Children:** Safety and efficacy not established in pts younger than 6 yrs. **Elderly:** No age-related precautions noted.

## INTERACTIONS

**DRUG: MAOIs** may prolong/intensify effects. May decrease sedative effect of **antihistamines (e.g., diphenhydramine).** May decrease hypotensive effects of **antihypertensives (e.g., amlodipine, lisinopril, valsartan).** Effects may be decreased by **chlorpromazine, haloperidol, lithium, urinary acidifying agents (ammonium chloride, sodium acid phosphate).** May increase absorption of **phenobarbital, phenytoin.** Tricyclic antidepressants **(e.g., amitriptyline, doxepin)** may increase cardiovascular effects. **HERBAL:** None significant. **FOOD:** None known. **LAB VALUES:** May increase plasma corticosteroid.

## AVAILABILITY (Rx)

**Capsules:** 10 mg, 20 mg, 30 mg, 40 mg, 50 mg, 60 mg, 70 mg.

## ADMINISTRATION/HANDLING

**PO**
• May be given in the morning without regard to food. • Administer capsule whole; pt must not chew. • Capsules may be opened and dissolved in water and taken immediately.

## INDICATIONS/ROUTES/DOSAGE

**ADHD**
**PO: ADULTS, CHILDREN 6 YRS AND OLDER:** Initially, 30 mg once daily in the morning. May increase dosage in increments of 10 or 20 mg/day at wkly intervals. **Maximum:** 70 mg/day.

**BED**
**PO: ADULTS, ELDERLY:** Initially, 30 mg once daily in morning. May increase by 20 mg/day at wkly intervals to a target dose of 50–70 mg once daily. **Maximum:** 70 mg/day.

**Dosage in Renal Impairment**
**CrCl 30 ml/min or greater: Maximum:** 70 mg/day. **CrCl 15–29 ml/min:** **Maximum:** 50 mg/day. **CrCl less than 15 ml/min or end-stage renal disease: Maximum:** 30 mg/day.

**Dosage in Hepatic Impairment**
No dose adjustment.

## SIDE EFFECTS

**Frequent (39%):** Decreased appetite. **Occasional (19%–9%):** Insomnia, upper abdominal pain, headache, irritability, vomiting, weight decrease. **Rare (6%–2%):** Nausea, dry mouth, dizziness, rash, affect change, fatigue, tic.

## ADVERSE EFFECTS/ TOXIC REACTIONS

Abrupt withdrawal following prolonged administration of high dosage may produce extreme fatigue (may last for wks). Prolonged administration to children with ADHD may produce a suppression of weight and/or height patterns. May produce cardiac irregularities, psychotic syndrome.

## NURSING CONSIDERATIONS

### BASELINE ASSESSMENT

Assess attention span, impulse control, interaction with others.

### INTERVENTION/EVALUATION

Monitor for CNS stimulation, increase in B/P, weight loss, pulse, sleep pattern, appetite. Observe for signs of hostility, aggression, depression.

### PATIENT/FAMILY TEACHING

• Take early in day. • May mask extreme fatigue. • Report pronounced dizziness, decreased appetite, dry mouth, weight loss, new or worsened psychiatric problems, palpitations, dyspnea.

---

# lisinopril    TOP 100

lye-**sin**-o-pril
(Apo-Lisinopril ♣, Prinivil, Qbrelis, Zestril)

■ **BLACK BOX ALERT** ■ May cause fetal injury, mortality. Discontinue as soon as possible once pregnancy is detected.
**Do not confuse lisinopril with fosinopril, or Prinivil with Plendil, Pravachol, Prevacid, Prilosec, Proventil, or Restoril, or Zestril with Desyrel, Restoril, Vistaril, Zetia, or Zostrix. Do not confuse lisinopril's combination form Zestoretic with Prilosec.**

## FIXED-COMBINATION(S)

**Prinzide/Zestoretic:** lisinopril/hydrochlorothiazide (a diuretic): 10 mg/12.5 mg, 20 mg/12.5 mg, 20 mg/25 mg.

## ◆CLASSIFICATION

**PHARMACOTHERAPEUTIC:** ACE inhibitor. **CLINICAL:** Antihypertensive.

## USES

Treatment of hypertension in adults and children 6 yrs and older. Used alone or in combination with other antihypertensives. Adjunctive therapy in management of heart failure. Treatment of acute MI within 24 hrs in hemodynamically stable pts to improve survival. Treatment of left ventricular dysfunction following MI.

## PRECAUTIONS

**Contraindications:** Hypersensitivity to lisinopril, other ACE inhibitors. History of angioedema from treatment with ACE inhibitors, idiopathic or hereditary angioedema. Concomitant use with aliskiren in pts with diabetes. **Cautions:** Renal impairment, unstented unilateral/bilateral renal artery stenosis, volume depletion, ischemic heart disease, cerebrovascular disease, severe aortic stenosis, hypertrophic cardiomyopathy, HF, systolic B/P less than 100, dialysis, hyponatremia; before, during, or immediately after major surgery. Concomitant use of potassium supplements.

## ACTION

Suppresses renin-angiotensin-aldosterone system (prevents conversion of angiotensin I to angiotensin II, a potent vasoconstrictor; may inhibit angiotensin II at local vascular, renal sites). Decreases plasma angiotensin II, increases plasma renin activity, decreases aldosterone secretion. **Therapeutic Effect:** Reduces blood pressure.

## PHARMACOKINETICS

| Route | Onset | Peak | Duration |
|-------|-------|------|----------|
| PO | 1 hr | 6 hrs | 24 hrs |

Incompletely absorbed from GI tract. Protein binding: 25%. Primarily excreted unchanged in urine. Removed by hemodialysis. **Half-life:** 12 hrs (increased in renal impairment).

##  LIFESPAN CONSIDERATIONS

**Pregnancy/Lactation:** Crosses placenta. Unknown if distributed in breast milk. **Children:** Safety and efficacy not established. **Elderly:** May be more sensitive to hypotensive effects.

---

**L**

## INTERACTIONS

**DRUG: Diuretics (e.g., furosemide, HCTZ)** may increase hypotensive effects. May increase concentration, risk of toxicity of **lithium. NSAIDs** may decrease effects. **Potassium-sparing diuretics (e.g., spironolactone, triamterene), potassium supplements** may cause hyperkalemia. May increase hypoglycemic effect of **oral hypoglycemic agents (e.g., glyburide, metformin).** **HERBAL: Ephedra, ginseng, licorice, yohimbe** may worsen hypertension. **Black cohosh, periwinkle** may increase antihypertensive effect. **FOOD:** None known. **LAB VALUES:** May increase serum BUN, alkaline phosphatase, bilirubin, creatinine, potassium, ALT, AST. May decrease serum sodium. May cause positive ANA titer.

## AVAILABILITY (Rx)

**Solution, Oral: (Qbrelis)** 1 mg/ml. **Tablets:** 2.5 mg, 5 mg, 10 mg, 20 mg, 30 mg, 40 mg.

## ADMINISTRATION/HANDLING

**PO**
• Give without regard to food. • Tablets may be crushed.

## INDICATIONS/ROUTES/DOSAGE

**Hypertension (Used Alone)**
**PO: ADULTS:** Initially, 10 mg/day. May increase by 5–10 mg/day at 1- to 2-wk intervals. Range: 10–40 mg/day. **ELDERLY:** Initially, 2.5–5 mg/day. May increase by 2.5–5 mg/day at 1- to 2-wk intervals. **Maximum:** 40 mg/day. **CHILDREN 6 YRS OR OLDER:** Initially, 0.07 mg/kg once daily (up to 5 mg). Titrate at 1- to 2-wk intervals. **Maximum:** 40 mg/day.

**Hypertension (in Combination with Other Antihypertensives)**
**◄ALERT►** If possible, discontinue diuretics 48–72 hrs prior to initiating lisinopril therapy.
**PO: ADULTS, ELDERLY:** Initially, 2.5–5 mg/day titrated to pt's needs. Range: 10–40 mg/day.

**HF**
**PO: ADULTS, ELDERLY:** Initially, 2.5–5 mg/day. May increase by no more than 10 mg/day at intervals of at least 2 wks to a target dose of 20–40 mg once daily.

**Improve Survival in Pts after MI**
**PO: ADULTS, ELDERLY:** Initially, 5 mg, then 5 mg after 24 hrs, 10 mg after 48 hrs, then 10 mg/day for 6 wks. For pts with low systolic B/P, give 2.5 mg/day for 3 days, then 2.5–5 mg/day. Discontinue if systolic B/P less than 90 mm Hg for more than 1 hr.

**Dosage in Renal Impairment**
**CrCl less than 30 ml/min:** Not recommended in children. Titrate to pt's needs after giving the following initial dose:

**Hypertension**

| Creatinine Clearance | Initial Dose |
|---|---|
| 10–30 ml/min | 5 mg |
| Less than 10 ml/min or Dialysis | 2.5 mg |

**HF**
**CrCl less than 30 ml/min or serum creatinine greater than 3 mg/dL:** Initial dose: 2.5 mg.

**Acute MI**
**Creatinine clearance 30 ml/min or less:** Initial dose: 2.5 mg.

**Dosage in Hepatic Impairment**
No dose adjustment.

## SIDE EFFECTS

**Frequent (12%–5%):** Headache, dizziness, postural hypotension. **Occasional (4%–2%):** Chest discomfort, fatigue, rash, abdominal pain, nausea, diarrhea, upper respiratory infection. **Rare (1% or less):** Palpitations, tachycardia, peripheral edema, insomnia, paresthesia, confusion, constipation, dry mouth, muscle cramps.

## ADVERSE EFFECTS/ TOXIC REACTIONS

Excessive hypotension ("first-dose syncope") may occur in pts with HF, severe salt/volume depletion. Angioedema (swelling of face and lips), hyperkalemia occur rarely. Agranulocytosis, neutropenia may be noted in pts with collagen vascular disease (scleroderma, systemic lupus erythematosus). Nephrotic syndrome may be noted in pts with history of renal disease.

## NURSING CONSIDERATIONS

### BASELINE ASSESSMENT

Obtain B/P, apical pulse immediately before each dose, in addition to regular monitoring (be alert to fluctuations). In pts with renal impairment, autoimmune disease, taking drugs that affect leukocytes or immune response, CBC and differential count should be performed before beginning therapy and q2wks for 3 mos, then periodically thereafter.

### INTERVENTION/EVALUATION

Assess for edema. Auscultate lungs for rales. Monitor I&O; weigh daily. Monitor daily pattern of bowel activity, stool consistency. Assist with ambulation if dizziness occurs. Monitor B/P, renal function tests, WBC, serum potassium. If excessive reduction in B/P occurs, place pt in supine position, feet slightly elevated.

### PATIENT/ FAMILY TEACHING

• To reduce hypotensive effect, go from lying to standing slowly. • Limit alcohol intake. • Report vomiting, diarrhea, diaphoresis, swelling of face/lips/tongue, difficulty in breathing, persistent cough. • Limit salt intake.

# lithium

**lith**-ee-um
(Apo-Lithium ✦, Lithobid)
■ **BLACK BOX ALERT** ■ Lithium toxicity is closely related to serum lithium levels and can occur at therapeutic doses. Routine determination of serum lithium levels is essential during therapy.
**Do not confuse Lithobid with Levbid or Lithostat.**

## ◆ CLASSIFICATION

**PHARMACOTHERAPEUTIC:** Psychotherapeutic. **CLINICAL:** Antimanic, antidepressant, vascular headache prophylactic.

## USES

Management of bipolar disorder. Treatment of mania in pts with bipolar disorder. **OFF-LABEL:** Augmenting agent for depression.

## PRECAUTIONS

**Contraindications:** Hypersensitivity to lithium. Severely debilitated pts, severe cardiovascular disease, severe dehydration, severe renal disease, severe sodium depletion or dehydration. **Cautions:** Mild to moderate cardiovascular disease, thyroid disease, elderly, mild to moderate renal impairment, medications altering sodium excretion, pregnancy, pts at risk for suicide, pts with significant fluid loss, pts receiving neuromuscular blocking agents.

## ACTION

Changes cation transport across cell membrane in nerve/muscle cells; influences reuptake of serotonin/norepinephrine. **Therapeutic Effect:** Produces antimanic, antidepressant effects.

## PHARMACOKINETICS

Rapidly, completely absorbed from GI tract. Protein binding: None. Primarily excreted unchanged in urine. Removed

L

---

by hemodialysis. **Half-life:** 18–24 hrs (increased in elderly).

## ⧖ LIFESPAN CONSIDERATIONS

**Pregnancy/Lactation:** Freely crosses placenta. Distributed in breast milk. **Children:** May increase bone formation or density (alter parathyroid hormone concentrations). **Elderly:** More susceptible to develop lithium-induced goiter or clinical hypothyroidism, CNS toxicity. Increased thirst, urination noted more frequently; lower dosage recommended.

## INTERACTIONS

**DRUG:** Diuretics (e.g., **furosemide**), **NSAIDs, metronidazole, ACE inhibitors** (e.g., **enalapril, lisinopril**), **angiotensin II antagonists, SSRIs, calcium channel blockers** (e.g., **losartan, valsartan**) may increase lithium concentration, risk of toxicity. **HERBAL:** None significant. **FOOD:** None known. **LAB VALUES:** May increase serum glucose, immunoreactive parathyroid hormone, calcium. **Therapeutic serum level:** 0.6–1.2 mEq/L; **toxic serum level:** greater than 1.5 mEq/L.

## AVAILABILITY (Rx)

**Capsules:** 150 mg, 300 mg, 600 mg. **Oral Solution:** 300 mg/5 ml. **Tablets:** 300 mg.

**Tablets (Extended-Release):** 300 mg, 450 mg.

## ADMINISTRATION/HANDLING

**PO**
• Administer with meals, milk to decrease GI upset. • Do not break, crush, dissolve, or divide extended-release tablets.

## INDICATIONS/ROUTES/DOSAGE

◄ALERT► During acute phase, a therapeutic serum lithium concentration of 0.6–1.2 mEq/L is required. For long-term control, desired level is 0.8–1 mEq/L. Monitor serum drug concentration, clinical response to determine proper dosage.

**Usual Dosage**
**PO: ADULTS, ELDERLY, CHILDREN OLDER THAN 12 YRS:** *(Immediate-Release):* 300 mg 3–4 times/day. *(Extended-Release):* 450 mg twice daily. Gradually increase based on response/tolerability. Usual dose: *(Immediate-Release):* 900–1,800 mg/day in 3–4 divided doses. *(Extended-Release):* 900–1,800 mg in 2 divided doses. **CHILDREN 6–12 YRS:** *(Immediate-Release):* 15–60 mg/kg/day in 3–4 divided doses not to exceed usual adult dose.

**Dosage in Renal Impairment**

| Creatinine Clearance | Dosage |
|---|---|
| 10–50 ml/min | 50%–75% normal dose |
| Less than 10 ml/min | 25%–50% normal dose |
| End-stage renal disease with HD | Dose after HD |

**Dosage in Hepatic Impairment**
No dose adjustment.

## SIDE EFFECTS

◄ALERT► Side effects are dose related and seldom occur at lithium serum levels less than 1.5 mEq/L. **Occasional:** Fine hand tremor, polydipsia, polyuria, mild nausea. **Rare:** Weight gain, bradycardia, tachycardia, acne, rash, muscle twitching, peripheral cyanosis, pseudotumor cerebri (eye pain, headache, tinnitus, vision disturbances).

## ADVERSE EFFECTS/ TOXIC REACTIONS

Lithium serum concentration of 1.5–2.0 mEq/L may produce vomiting, diarrhea, drowsiness, confusion, incoordination, coarse hand tremor, muscle twitching, T-wave depression on EKG. Lithium serum concentration of 2.0–2.5 mEq/L may result in ataxia, giddiness, tinnitus, blurred vision, clonic movements, severe hypotension. Acute toxicity may be characterized by seizures, oliguria, circulatory failure, coma, death.

## NURSING CONSIDERATIONS

### BASELINE ASSESSMENT

Assess mental status (e.g., mood, behavior). Serum lithium levels should be tested q3–4days during initial phase of therapy, q1–2mos thereafter, and wkly if there is no improvement of disorder or adverse effects occur.

### INTERVENTION/EVALUATION

Clinical assessment of therapeutic effect, tolerance to drug effect is necessary for correct dosing-level management. Assess behavior, appearance, emotional status, response to environment, speech pattern, thought content. Monitor serum lithium concentrations, CBC with differential, urinalysis, creatinine clearance. Monitor renal, hepatic, thyroid, cardiovascular function; serum electrolytes. Assess for increased urinary output, persistent thirst. Report polyuria, prolonged vomiting, diarrhea, fever to physician (may need to temporarily reduce or discontinue dosage). Monitor for signs of lithium toxicity. Assess for therapeutic response (interest in surroundings, improvement in self-care, increased ability to concentrate, relaxed facial expression). Monitor lithium levels q3–4days at initiation of therapy (then q1–2mos). Obtain lithium levels 8–12 hrs postdose. **Therapeutic serum level:** 0.6–1.2 mEq/L; **toxic serum level:** greater than 1.5 mEq/L.

### PATIENT/ FAMILY TEACHING

• Limit alcohol, caffeine intake. • Avoid tasks requiring coordination until CNS effects of drug are known. • May cause dry mouth. • Maintain steady salt, fluid intake (avoid dehydration). • Report vomiting, diarrhea, muscle weakness, tremors, drowsiness, ataxia. • Serum level monitoring is necessary to determine proper dose.

# lixisenatide

lix-i-sen-a-tide
(Adlyxin)
**Do not confuse lixisenatide with exenatide, liraglutide.**

### FIXED-COMBINATION(S)

**Soliqua:** lixisenatide 33 mcg/ml and insulin glargine 100 units/ml.

## ◆CLASSIFICATION

**PHARMACOTHERAPEUTIC:** Antihyperglycemic (glucagon-like peptide-1 [GLP-1]) receptor agonist. **CLINICAL:** Antidiabetic agent.

## USES

Adjunct to diet and exercise to improve glycemic controls in pts with type 2 diabetes mellitus.

## PRECAUTIONS

**Contraindications:** Hypersensitivity to lixisenatide. **Cautions:** Renal impairment, severe gastroparesis, history of pancreatitis. Not recommended in pts with diabetic ketoacidosis, type 1 diabetes mellitus. Not a substitute for insulin. Medications with narrow therapeutic index or requiring rapid GI absorption.

## ACTION

Increases glucose-dependent insulin secretion; decreases glucagon secretion. Slows gastric emptying. **Therapeutic Effect:** Improves glycemic control by lowering fasting glucose and postprandial blood glucose.

## PHARMACOKINETICS

Widely distributed. Protein binding: not specified. Peak plasma concentration: 1–3.5 hrs. Eliminated through glomerulus filtration and proteolytic degradation. **Half-life:** 3 hrs.

## ☒ LIFESPAN CONSIDERATIONS

**Pregnancy/Lactation:** Unknown if distributed in breast milk. **Children:** Safety and efficacy not established in pts younger than 18 yrs. **Elderly:** No age-related precautions noted.

## INTERACTIONS

**DRUG:** May increase hypoglycemic effect when added to **insulin or sulfonylureas.** May decrease the rate of absorption of **oral medications** due to delayed gastric emptying. **Oral contraceptive** should be taken 1 hr before or 11 hrs after lixisenatide. **HERBAL:** None significant. **FOOD:** None known. **LAB VALUES:** Expected to decreased serum glucose, Hgb A1c.

## AVAILABILITY (Rx)

**Prefilled Injector Pens:** 50 mcg/ml in 3 ml (for 14 preset doses of 10 mcg/dose), 100 mcg/ml in 3 ml (for 14 preset doses of 20 mcg/dose).

## ADMINISTRATION/HANDLING

**Subcutaneous**

**Preparation** • Follow instructions for preparation according to manufacturer guidelines. • Visually inspect for particulate matter or discoloration. Solution should appear clear and colorless. • Do not use if solution is cloudy or discolored or if visible particles are observed.

**Administration** • Administer within 1 hr before the first meal of the day, preferably the same time each day. If a dose is missed, administer within 1 hr prior to next meal. • Insert needle subcutaneously into upper arms, outer thigh, or abdomen and inject solution. • Do not inject into areas of active skin disease or injury such as sunburns, skin rashes, inflammation, skin infections, or active psoriasis. • Rotate injection sites.

**Storage** • Refrigerate unused injector pens. • Once injector pen is activated, store at room temperature for up to 14 days. • Do not freeze. • Protect from light.

## INDICATIONS/ROUTES/DOSAGE

**Type 2 Diabetes Mellitus**

**SQ: ADULTS, ELDERLY:** 10 mcg once daily for 14 days. **Maintenance:** Increase to 20 mcg once daily on day 15.

**Dosage in Renal Impairment**
Use caution.

**Dosage in Hepatic Impairment**
No dose adjustment.

## SIDE EFFECTS

**Frequent (25%–10%):** Nausea, vomiting. **Occasional (9%–1%):** Headache, diarrhea, dizziness, dyspepsia, constipation, abdominal distention, abdominal pain.

## ADVERSE EFFECTS/TOXIC REACTIONS

May increase risk of acute renal failure or worsening of chronic renal impairment (esp. in pts with vomiting, dehydration). May increase risk of hypoglycemia when used with other hypoglycemic agents or insulin. Anaphylaxis reported in less than 1% of pts. Other hypersensitivity reactions including angioedema, bronchospasm, laryngeal edema occur rarely. Acute pancreatitis, hemorrhagic or necrotizing pancreatitis were reported. Immunogenicity (auto-lixisenatide antibodies) occurred in 70% of pts.

## NURSING CONSIDERATIONS

### BASELINE ASSESSMENT

Obtain baseline fasting glucose level, Hgb A1c; BMP. Question history of renal impairment, gastroparesis, hypersensitivity reaction. Screen for use of other hypoglycemic agents or insulin. Assess pt's understanding of diabetes management, routine home glucose monitoring, medication self-administration. Assess hydration status. Obtain dietary consult for nutritional education.

### INTERVENTION/EVALUATION

Monitor capillary blood glucose levels, Hgb A1c; renal function test (esp. in pts with renal impairment who report diarrhea, gastroparesis, vomiting). Assess for hypoglycemia (anxiety, confusion, diaphoresis, diplopia, dizziness, headache, hunger, perioral numbness, tachycardia, tremors), hyperglycemia (confusion,

L

fatigue, Kussmaul breathing, nausea, polyuria, vomiting). Screen for glucose-altering conditions: fever, stress, surgical procedures, trauma. Monitor for hypersensitivity reactions; abdominal pain that radiates to the back. Encourage PO intake. Monitor I&Os.

**PATIENT/FAMILY TEACHING**

• Diabetes mellitus requires lifelong control. Diet and exercise is principal part of treatment; do not skip or delay meals. • Test blood sugar regularly. • Monitor daily calorie intake. • When taking additional medications to lower blood sugar or when glucose demands are altered (fever, infection, stress trauma), have low blood sugar treatment available (glucagon, oral dextrose). • Persistent, severe abdominal pain that radiates to the back (with or without vomiting) may indicate acute pancreatitis. • Report allergic reactions of any kind, esp. difficulty breathing, itching, rash, swelling of the face or throat. • Oral contraceptives should be taken at least 1 hr before or 11 hrs after dose. • Therapy may cause acute kidney injury or kidney failure; report decreased urine output, amber-colored urine, flank pain.

# lomitapide

lom-i-**ta**-pide
(Juxtapid)
**Do not confuse lomitapide with loperamide.**

■ **BLACK BOX ALERT** ■ May cause hepatotoxicity. May cause hepatic steatosis (increase in hepatic fat) regardless of serum ALT, AST elevation; may be risk factor for progressive hepatic disease, including steatohepatitis and cirrhosis.

## ◆CLASSIFICATION

**PHARMACOTHERAPEUTIC:** Microsomal triglyceride transfer protein inhibitor. **CLINICAL:** Antihyperlipidemic.

## USES

Treatment of homozygous familial hypercholesterolemia (HoFH) in combination with low-fat diet and other lipid-lowering therapies, including LDL-C apheresis, to reduce LDL, total cholesterol, apoprotein B, non–HDL-C.

## PRECAUTIONS

**Contraindications:** Hypersensitivity to lomitapide. Pregnancy, breastfeeding, moderate to severe hepatic impairment, active hepatic disease including unexplained persistent elevation of serum transaminases, concomitant use of strong CYP3A4 inhibitors (e.g., ketoconazole, protease inhibitors). **Cautions:** Mild to moderate renal impairment, end-stage renal disease, mild hepatic impairment, alcohol consumption. Avoid use in pts with history of glucose-galactose malabsorption, other agents having hepatotoxic potential (e.g., acetaminophen).

## ACTION

Inhibits microsomal triglyceride transfer protein in lumen of endoplasmic reticulum. Prevents assembly of apo-B-containing lipoproteins in enterocytes, hepatocytes; inhibits synthesis of chylomicrons, very low density lipoprotein (VLDL). **Therapeutic Effect:** Decreases plasma low-density lipoprotein cholesterol (LDL-C).

## PHARMACOKINETICS

Well absorbed in GI tract. Metabolized in liver. Protein binding: 99%. Peak plasma concentration: 6 hrs. Primarily excreted in feces. **Half-life:** 40 hrs.

## ⧖ LIFESPAN CONSIDERATIONS

**Pregnancy/Lactation:** Contraindicated in pregnancy. May cause fetal harm. Must use effective contraception in addition to barrier methods. Unknown if distributed in breast milk. Must either discontinue breastfeeding or discontinue therapy. **Children:** Safety and efficacy not established. **Elderly:** Increased risk for side effects, adverse reactions.

L

## INTERACTIONS

**DRUG:** **Acetaminophen, amiodarone, isotretinoin, methotrexate, tamoxifen, tetracycline** may increase risk for hepatotoxicity. **Strong CYP3A4 inhibitors (e.g., ketoconazole, protease inhibitors)** contraindicated due to increased risk for myopathy, rhabdomyolysis. Moderate **CYP3A4 inhibitors (e.g., atorvastatin, oral contraceptives)** may increase concentration. May increase concentration of **warfarin**. May increase effects of **P-glycoprotein substrates (e.g., digoxin, sitagliptin)**. **HERBAL:** None known. **FOOD: Grapefruit products** may increase absorption, toxicity. **LAB VALUES:** May increase serum alkaline phosphatase, bilirubin, ALT, AST.

## AVAILABILITY (Rx)

**Capsules:** 5 mg, 10 mg, 20 mg, 30 mg, 40 mg, 60 mg.

## ADMINISTRATION/HANDLING

**PO**
• Give with water only. • Administer without food (at least 2 hrs after evening meal). • Administer whole; do not break, crush, or open capsules.

## INDICATIONS/ROUTES/DOSAGE

◀ALERT▶ To reduce risk for fat-soluble nutrient deficiency, recommend supplemental coadministration: vitamin E 400 international units PO daily, linolenic acid 200 mg PO daily, alpha-linolenic acid (ALA) 210 mg PO daily, eicosapentaenoic acid (EPA) 110 mg PO daily, docosahexaenoic acid (DHA) 80 mg PO daily. Because of risk for myopathy, concurrent use of simvastatin should not exceed 20–40 mg/day.

**Homozygous Familial Hypercholesterolemia**
**PO: ADULTS, ELDERLY:** Initially, 5 mg once daily for minimum of 2 wks. Gradually increase dose at 4-wk (minimum) intervals to 10 mg once daily, then 20 mg once daily, then 40 mg once daily, then 60 mg once daily based on tolerability. **Maximum:** 60 mg/day.

**Dose Modification**
*Elevated Hepatic Enzymes*
If ALT, AST is between 3–5 times upper limit of normal (ULN), reduce dose until ALT, AST less than 3 times ULN. If ALT, AST is greater than 5 times ULN, withhold dose until less than 3 times ULN, then restart at reduced dose. If hepatotoxicity occurs or bilirubin level rises greater than 2 times ULN, discontinue treatment.
*End-Stage Renal Disease Receiving Dialysis, Mild Hepatic Impairment*
Do not exceed 40 mg/day.
*Concurrent Use of Weak CYP3A4 Inhibitors*
Do not exceed 30 mg/day.
*Concurrent Use of Oral Contraception*
Do not exceed 30 mg/day.

**Dosage in Renal Impairment**
No dose adjustment. **End-stage renal disease:** Maximum: 40 mg/day.

**Dosage in Hepatic Impairment**
**Mild impairment:** Maximum: 40 mg/day. **Moderate to severe impairment:** Contraindicated.

## SIDE EFFECTS

**Frequent (79%–65%):** Diarrhea, nausea. **Occasional (38%–10%):** Dyspepsia, vomiting, abdominal pain, weight loss, abdominal distention, constipation, flatulence, fatigue, back pain, gastric reflux, headache, dizziness.

## ADVERSE EFFECTS/ TOXIC REACTIONS

Progressive hepatic disease including steatohepatitis, cirrhosis has been reported in 6% of pts due to increased hepatic fat. May reduce absorption of fat-soluble nutrients; recommend daily supplemental replacement. Increased risk for myopathy including rhabdomyolysis (muscle pain/tenderness, weakness, dark or decreased urine output, elevated serum creatinine, CPK) when used with other antihyperlipidemics. May increase risk for supratherapeutic INR with warfarin. Infections including influenza, nasopharyngitis, gastroenteritis reported in 5% of pts. Palpitations, angina pectoris report in 3% of pts. Increased risk for dehydration/malabsorption with galactose intolerance hereditary disorder, pancreatic disease, diarrhea.

## NURSING CONSIDERATIONS

### BASELINE ASSESSMENT

Obtain detailed dietary history, esp. fat consumption. Confirm negative pregnancy test before initiating treatment. Obtain baseline laboratory studies: ALT, AST, alkaline phosphatase, bilirubin, serum cholesterol, triglycerides, PT/INR (if pt is on warfarin). Confirm positive history of homozygous familial hypercholesterolemia (HoFH). Receive full medication history including vitamins, minerals, herbal products. Screen for history of galactose intolerance, renal/hepatic impairment, angina.

### INTERVENTION/EVALUATION

Maintain hydration; offer fluids frequently. Monitor INR routinely (with anticoagulants). Monitor LFT with any dosage change, then every month for first year when maintenance goal reached, then every 3 mos. Obtain EKG for palpitations, shortness of breath, dizziness. Monitor for bruising, hematuria, jaundice, right upper abdominal pain, fever, lethargy, melena.

### PATIENT/FAMILY TEACHING

• Avoid pregnancy. • Use appropriate contraception measures, including barrier precautions. • If pregnancy occurs, inform physician immediately. • Diarrhea may decrease effectiveness of oral contraception. • Do not breastfeed. • Maintain low-fat diet. • Report yellowing of skin, bruising, black/tarry stool, right upper quadrant pain, fever, lethargy, chest pain, palpitations. • Avoid alcohol. • Avoid grapefruit products.

• Do not chew, crush, or open capsules. • Report any newly prescribed medications.

# loperamide

loe-**per**-a-myde
(Apo-Loperamide ✦, Diamode, Diarr-Eze ✦, Imodium A-D, Loperacap ✦, Novo-Loperamide ✦)
**Do not confuse Imodium with Indocin, or loperamide with furosemide.**

## FIXED-COMBINATION(S)

**Imodium Advanced:** loperamide/simethicone (an antiflatulent): 2 mg/125 mg.

## ◆CLASSIFICATION

**PHARMACOTHERAPEUTIC:** Antidiarrheal agent. **CLINICAL:** Antidiarrheal.

## USES

Controls, provides symptomatic relief of acute nonspecific diarrhea, chronic diarrhea associated with inflammatory bowel disease, reduce volume of ileostomy discharge. **OTC:** Control symptoms of diarrhea, including traveler's diarrhea. **OFF-LABEL:** Chemotherapy-induced diarrhea, irinotecan-induced delayed diarrhea.

## PRECAUTIONS

**Contraindications:** Hypersensitivity to loperamide. Abdominal pain without diarrhea, children younger than 2 yrs. **Cautions:** Hepatic impairment, use in young children. Avoid use when inhibition of peristalsis is undesirable (e.g., potential for ileus, megacolon).

## ACTION

Directly affects intestinal wall muscles through opioid receptor. **Therapeutic Effect:** Slows intestinal motility, prolongs transit time of intestinal contents by reducing fecal volume, diminishing loss

---

of fluid, electrolytes, increasing viscosity, bulk of stool. Increases tone of anal sphincter.

## PHARMACOKINETICS

Poorly absorbed from GI tract. Protein binding: 97%. Metabolized in liver. Excreted in feces (30%), urine (less than 2%). Not removed by hemodialysis. **Half-life:** 7–14 hrs.

## ⌛ LIFESPAN CONSIDERATIONS

**Pregnancy/Lactation:** Unknown if drug crosses placenta or is distributed in breast milk. **Children:** Not recommended for pts younger than 6 yrs (infants younger than 3 mos more susceptible to CNS effects). **Elderly:** May mask dehydration, electrolyte depletion.

## INTERACTIONS

**DRUG: Ritonavir** may increase concentration, side effects. May decrease concentration of **saquinavir. HERBAL:** None significant. **FOOD:** None known. **LAB VALUES:** None significant.

## AVAILABILITY (Rx)

**Capsules:** 2 mg. **Liquid:** 1 mg/5 ml, 1 mg/7.5 ml. **Suspension, Oral:** 1 mg/7.5 ml. **Tablet:** 2 mg. **Tablet, Chewable:** 2 mg.

## ADMINISTRATION/HANDLING

**Liquid**
• When administering to children, use accompanying plastic dropper to measure the liquid.

## INDICATIONS/ROUTES/DOSAGE

**Acute Diarrhea**
PO *(Capsules):* **ADULTS, ELDERLY:** Initially, 4 mg, then 2 mg after each unformed stool. **Maximum:** 16 mg/day. **CHILDREN 9–12 YRS, WEIGHING MORE THAN 30 KG:** Initially, 2 mg 3 times/day for 24 hrs. **CHILDREN 6–8 YRS, WEIGHING 20–30 KG:** Initially, 2 mg twice daily for 24 hrs. **CHILDREN 2–5 YRS, WEIGHING 13–20 KG:** Initially, 1 mg 3 times/day for 24 hrs.

**Maintenance:** 1 mg/10 kg only after loose stool but not exceeding initial dose.

**Chronic Diarrhea**
PO: **ADULTS, ELDERLY:** Initially, 4 mg, then 2 mg after each unformed stool until diarrhea is controlled. Average maintenance dose: 4–8 mg/day. **Maximum:** 16 mg/day. **CHILDREN:** 0.08–0.24 mg/kg/day in 2–3 divided doses. **Maximum:** 2 mg/dose.

**Traveler's Diarrhea**
PO: **ADULTS, ELDERLY:** Initially, 4 mg, then 2 mg after each loose bowel movement (LBM). **Maximum:** 8 mg/day for 2 days. **CHILDREN 9–11 YRS:** Initially, 2 mg, then 1 mg after each LBM. **Maximum:** 6 mg/day for 2 days. **CHILDREN 6–8 YRS:** Initially, 2 mg, then 1 mg after each LBM. **Maximum:** 4 mg/day for 2 days.

**Dosage in Renal/Hepatic Impairment**
No dose adjustment.

## SIDE EFFECTS

**Rare:** Dry mouth, drowsiness, abdominal discomfort, allergic reaction (rash, pruritus).

## ADVERSE EFFECTS/ TOXIC REACTIONS

Toxicity results in constipation, GI irritation (nausea, vomiting), CNS depression. Activated charcoal is used to treat loperamide toxicity.

## NURSING CONSIDERATIONS

### BASELINE ASSESSMENT
Do not administer in presence of bloody diarrhea, temperature greater than 101°F.

### INTERVENTION/EVALUATION
Encourage adequate fluid intake. Assess bowel sounds for peristalsis. Monitor daily pattern of bowel activity, stool consistency. Withhold drug, notify physician promptly in event of abdominal pain, distention, fever.

• Do not exceed prescribed dose. • May cause dry mouth. • Avoid alcohol. • Avoid tasks that require alertness, motor skills until response to drug is established. • Report diarrhea lasting more than 3 days, abdominal pain with distention, new-onset fever.

# lopinavir/ritonavir

loe-**pin**-a-veer/rit-**oh**-na-veer
(Kaletra)
**Do not confuse Kaletra with Keppra.**

## ◆CLASSIFICATION

**PHARMACOTHERAPEUTIC:** Protease inhibitor combination. **CLINICAL:** Antiretroviral.

## USES

In combination with other antiretroviral agents for treatment of HIV infection.

## PRECAUTIONS

**Contraindications:** Hypersensitivity to lopinavir, ritonavir. Concomitant use of potent CYP3A inducers: alfuzosin, ergot derivatives (causes vasospasm, peripheral ischemia of extremities), lovastatin, midazolam (oral), pimozide, rifampin, sildenafil (for treatment of pulmonary arterial hypertension), simvastatin, St. John's wort, triazolam (increased sedation, respiratory depression); co-administration of medications highly dependent on CYP3A for clearance and increased concentrations associated with serious adverse reactions. **Cautions:** Hepatic impairment, hepatitis B or C infection, cardiac disease with underlying conduction abnormalities or structural heart defects, ischemic heart disease, cardiomyopathies, congenital long QT syndrome or medications that prolong QT interval, hypokalemia, history of pancreatitis, diabetes.

## ACTION

Lopinavir inhibits activity of protease, an enzyme, late in HIV replication process; ritonavir increases plasma levels of lopinavir. **Therapeutic Effect:** Formation of immature, noninfectious viral particles.

## PHARMACOKINETICS

Readily absorbed after PO administration (absorption increased when taken with food). Protein binding: 98%–99%. Metabolized in liver. Eliminated primarily in feces. Not removed by hemodialysis. **Half-life:** 5–6 hrs.

## ⧗ LIFESPAN CONSIDERATIONS

**Pregnancy/Lactation:** Unknown if distributed in breast milk. Breastfeeding by HIV-infected mothers not recommended. **Children:** Safety and efficacy not established in pts younger than 6 mos. **Elderly:** Age-related renal/hepatic/cardiac impairment requires caution.

## INTERACTIONS

**DRUG:** May increase concentration/toxicity of **amiodarone, atorvastatin, bepridil, clarithromycin, cyclosporine, felodipine, fluticasone, ketoconazole, lidocaine, lovastatin, midazolam, nelfinavir, nicardipine, nifedipine, sildenafil, simvastatin, tacrolimus, trazodone, triazolam, warfarin.** May decrease concentration/effects of **oral contraceptives. CYP3A4 inducers** (e.g., **carbamazepine, phenytoin, rifampin**) may decrease concentration/effects. May cause disulfiram-like reaction with **metronidazole. HERBAL: St. John's wort** may decrease concentration/effects. **FOOD:** None known. **LAB VALUES:** May increase serum glucose, GGT, amylase, bilirubin, total cholesterol, triglycerides, uric acid, ALT, AST. May decrease platelets, serum sodium.

## AVAILABILITY (Rx)

**Oral Solution:** 80 mg/ml lopinavir/20 mg/ml ritonavir.

🔪 **Tablets:** 100 mg lopinavir/25 mg ritonavir, 200 mg lopinavir/50 mg ritonavir.

---

## ADMINISTRATION/HANDLING

### PO

• Give tablets whole; do not break, crush, dissolve, or divide. • Does not require refrigeration. • Give tablets without regard to food. • Solution should be given with food. • Administer solution using calibrated oral syringe.

## INDICATIONS/ROUTES/DOSAGE

### HIV Infection

Doses based on lopinavir component.
**PO: ADULTS:** 800 mg once daily or 400 mg twice daily. **Pregnant Women:** 400 mg twice daily. **CHILDREN 6 MOS–18 YRS, WEIGHING GREATER THAN 40 KG:** *(Oral Solution):* 400 mg twice daily. **WEIGHING 15–40 KG:** 10 mg/kg twice daily. **WEIGHING LESS THAN 15 KG:** 12 mg/kg twice daily. **CHILDREN 14 DAYS–6 MOS:** 16 mg/kg twice daily. *(Tablets):* **WEIGHING GREATER THAN 35 KG:** 400 mg twice daily. **WEIGHING 26–35 KG:** 300 mg twice daily. **WEIGHING 15–25 KG:** 200 mg twice daily. **WEIGHING LESS THAN 15 KG:** Not recommended.

### Dosage Adjustment for Combination Therapy

**Efavirenz, Fosamprenavir, Nelfinavir, Nevirapine: ADULTS, CHILDREN 6 MOS–18 YRS, WEIGHING GREATER THAN 45 KG:** 500 mg (533-mg solution) twice daily. *(Solution):* **15–45 KG:** 11 mg/kg twice daily. **LESS THAN 15 KG:** 13 mg/kg twice daily. *(Tablet):* **31–45 KG:** 400 mg twice daily. **21–30 KG:** 300 mg twice daily. **15–20 KG:** 200 mg twice daily. **LESS THAN 15 KG:** Not recommended.

### Dosage in Renal Impairment

No dose adjustment. Avoid once daily dosing in HD pts.

### Dosage in Hepatic Impairment

Use caution.

## SIDE EFFECTS

**Frequent (14%):** Mild to moderate diarrhea. **Occasional (6%–2%):** Nausea, asthenia. Abdominal pain, headache, vomiting. **Rare (less than 2%):** Insomnia, rash.

## ADVERSE EFFECTS/ TOXIC REACTIONS

Anemia, leukopenia, lymphadenopathy, deep vein thrombosis (DVT), Cushing's syndrome, pancreatitis, hemorrhagic colitis occur rarely.

## NURSING CONSIDERATIONS

### BASELINE ASSESSMENT

Obtain baseline CBC, renal function, LFT viral load, CD4 count, cell count. Obtain baseline weight.

### INTERVENTION/EVALUATION

Monitor daily pattern of bowel activity, stool consistency. Assess for opportunistic infections: onset of fever, oral mucosa changes, cough, other respiratory symptoms. Check weight at least 2 times/wk. Assess for nausea, vomiting. Observe for signs/symptoms of pancreatitis (nausea, vomiting, abdominal pain). Monitor electrolytes, serum glucose, cholesterol, LFT, CBC with differential, CD4 cell count, viral load.

### PATIENT/ FAMILY TEACHING

• Explain correct administration of medication. • Eat small, frequent meals to offset nausea, vomiting. • Lopinavir/ritonavir is not a cure for HIV infection, nor does it reduce risk of transmission to others. • Pt must continue practices to prevent HIV transmission. • Illnesses, including opportunistic infections, may still occur.

# loratadine

lor-**at**-a-deen
(Alavert, Apo-Loratadine ✿, Claritin, Claritin Reditabs, Loradamed)
**Do not confuse Claritin with clarithromycin.**

## FIXED-COMBINATION(S)

**Alavert Allergy and Sinus, Claritin-D:** loratadine/pseudoephedrine (a sympathomimetic): 5 mg/120 mg, 10 mg/240 mg.

## ◆CLASSIFICATION

**PHARMACOTHERAPEUTIC:** $H_1$ antagonist. **CLINICAL:** Antihistamine.

## USES

Relief of nasal, non-nasal symptoms of seasonal allergic rhinitis (hay fever). Treatment of itching due to hives (urticaria).

## PRECAUTIONS

**Contraindications:** Hypersensitivity to loratadine. **Cautions:** Renal/hepatic impairment.

## ACTION

Competes with histamine for $H_1$ receptor sites on effector cells. **Therapeutic Effect:** Prevents allergic responses mediated by histamine (e.g., rhinitis, urticaria, pruritus).

## PHARMACOKINETICS

| Route | Onset | Peak | Duration |
|---|---|---|---|
| PO | 1–3 hrs | 8–12 hrs | Longer than 24 hrs |

Rapidly, almost completely absorbed from GI tract. Protein binding: 97%; metabolite, 73%–77%. Distributed mainly to liver, lungs, GI tract, bile. Metabolized in liver. Eliminated in urine (40%) and feces (40%). Not removed by hemodialysis. **Half-life:** 8.4 hrs; metabolite, 28 hrs (increased in elderly, hepatic impairment).

## ⧖ LIFESPAN CONSIDERATIONS

**Pregnancy/Lactation:** Distributed in breast milk. **Children:** Safety and efficacy not established in pts younger than 2 yrs. **Elderly:** More sensitive to anticholinergic effects (e.g., dry mouth, nose, throat).

## INTERACTIONS

**DRUG: Clarithromycin, erythromycin, fluconazole, ketoconazole** may increase concentration. **HERBAL: St. John's wort** may decrease concentration/effects. **FOOD: All foods** delay absorption. **LAB VALUES:** May suppress wheal, flare reactions to antigen skin testing unless drug is discontinued 4 days before testing.

## AVAILABILITY (Rx)

**Capsule:** 5 mg. **Solution, Oral:** 5 mg/5 ml. **Syrup:** 5 mg/5 ml. **Tablets (Alavert, Claritin, Loradamed):** 10 mg. **Tablets, Chewable (Claritin):** 5 mg. **Tablets (Orally Disintegrating [Alavert]):** 5 mg, 10 mg.

## ADMINISTRATION/HANDLING

**PO**
• May take without regard for food.

**Orally Disintegrating Tablets**
• Place under tongue. • Disintegration occurs within seconds, after which tablet contents may be swallowed with or without water.

## INDICATIONS/ROUTES/DOSAGE

**Allergic Rhinitis, Urticaria**
**PO: ADULTS, ELDERLY, CHILDREN 6 YRS AND OLDER:** 10 mg once daily or 5 mg twice daily (Claritin Reditabs). **CHILDREN 2–5 YRS:** 5 mg once daily.

**Dosage in Renal Impairment (CrCl Less Than 30 ml/min)**
**PO: ADULTS, ELDERLY, CHILDREN 6 YRS AND OLDER:** 10 mg every other day. **CHILDREN 2–5 YRS:** No dose adjustment.

**Dosage in Hepatic Impairment**
No dose adjustment.

## SIDE EFFECTS

**Frequent (12%–8%):** Headache, fatigue, drowsiness. **Occasional (3%):** Dry mouth, nose, throat. **Rare:** Photosensitivity.

## ADVERSE EFFECTS/ TOXIC REACTIONS

None significant.

## NURSING CONSIDERATIONS

### BASELINE ASSESSMENT

Assess lung sounds for wheezing, skin for urticaria, other allergy symptoms.

### INTERVENTION/EVALUATION

For upper respiratory allergies, increase fluids to decrease viscosity of secretions,

 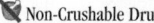

offset thirst, replenish loss of fluids from increased diaphoresis. Monitor symptoms for therapeutic response.

**PATIENT/FAMILY TEACHING**

• Drink plenty of water (may cause dry mouth). • Avoid alcohol. • Avoid tasks that require alertness, motor skills until response to drug is established (may cause drowsiness). • May cause photosensitivity reactions (avoid direct exposure to sunlight).

# *LORazepam

lor-**az**-e-pam
(Apo-Lorazepam ✦, <u>Ativan</u>, Lorazepam Intensol, Novo-Lorazem ✦)
**Do not confuse Ativan with Ambien or Atarax, or lorazepam with alprazolam, diazepam, Lovaza, temazepam, or Zolpidem.**

## ◆CLASSIFICATION

**PHARMACOTHERAPEUTIC:** Benzodiazepine **(Schedule IV). CLINICAL:** Antianxiety, sedative-hypnotic, antiemetic, skeletal muscle relaxant, amnesiac, anticonvulsant, antitremor.

## USES

**PO:** Management of anxiety disorders, short-term relief of symptoms of anxiety, anxiety associated with depressive symptoms. Insomnia due to anxiety or transient stress. **IV:** Status epilepticus, preanesthesia for amnesia, sedation. **OFF-LABEL:** Treatment of alcohol withdrawal, psychogenic catatonia, partial complex seizures, agitation (IV administration only), antiemetic for chemotherapy; rapid tranquilization of agitated pt, status epilepticus in children.

## PRECAUTIONS

**Contraindications:** Hypersensitivity to lorazepam, other benzodiazepines. Acute narrow-angle glaucoma, IV administration in pts with sleep apnea, severe respiratory depression (except during mechanical ventilation). **Cautions:** Neonates, renal/hepatic impairment, compromised pulmonary function, concomitant CNS depressant use, depression, history of drug dependence, alcohol abuse, or significant personality disorder, pts at risk for suicide.

## ACTION

Enhances action of inhibitory neurotransmitter gamma-aminobutyric acid (GABA) in CNS, affecting memory, motor, sensory, cognitive function. **Therapeutic Effect:** Produces anxiolytic, anticonvulsant, sedative, muscle relaxant, antiemetic effects.

## PHARMACOKINETICS

| Route | Onset | Peak | Duration |
|---|---|---|---|
| PO | 30–60 min | N/A | 6–8 hrs |
| IV | 5–20 min | N/A | 6–8 hrs |
| IM | 20–30 min | N/A | 6–8 hrs |

Well absorbed after PO, IM administration. Protein binding: 85%. Widely distributed. Metabolized in liver. Primarily excreted in urine. Not removed by hemodialysis. **Half-life:** 10–20 hrs.

## ⧗ LIFESPAN CONSIDERATIONS

**Pregnancy/Lactation:** May cross placenta. May be distributed in breast milk. May increase risk of fetal abnormalities if administered during first trimester of pregnancy. Chronic ingestion during pregnancy may produce fetal toxicity, withdrawal symptoms, CNS depression in neonates. **Children:** Safety and efficacy not established in pts younger than 12 yrs. **Elderly:** Use small initial doses with gradual increases to avoid ataxia, excessive sedation, or paradoxical CNS restlessness, excitement.

## INTERACTIONS

**DRUG: Valproic acid** may increase concentration/effects. **Alcohol, other CNS depressants (e.g., morphine, phenobarbital, zolpidem)** may increase CNS depression. **HERBAL: Gotu kola, kava kava, St. John's wort, valerian**

may increase CNS depression. **FOOD:** None known. **LAB VALUES:** None significant. **Therapeutic serum level:** 50–240 ng/ml; **toxic serum level:** unknown.

## AVAILABILITY (Rx)

**Injection Solution:** 2 mg/ml, 4 mg/ml. **Oral Solution (Lorazepam Intensol):** 2 mg/ml. **Tablets:** 0.5 mg, 1 mg, 2 mg.

## ADMINISTRATION/HANDLING

 **IV**

**Reconstitution** • Dilute with equal volume of Sterile Water for Injection, D₅W, or 0.9% NaCl.
**Rate of Administration** • Give by IV push into tubing of free-flowing IV infusion (0.9% NaCl, D₅W) at a rate not to exceed 2 mg/min.
**Storage** • Refrigerate parenteral form. • Do not use if discolored or precipitate forms. • Avoid freezing.

**IM**
• Give deep IM into large muscle mass.

**PO**
• Give with food. • Tablets may be crushed. • Dilute oral solution in water, juice, soda, or semisolid food.

## 🞥 IV INCOMPATIBILITIES

Aztreonam (Azactam), ondansetron (Zofran).

## 🞥 IV COMPATIBILITIES

Bumetanide (Bumex), cefepime (Maxipime), dexmedetomidine (Precedex), diltiazem (Cardizem), dobutamine (Dobutrex), dopamine (Intropin), heparin, labetalol (Normodyne, Trandate), milrinone (Primacor), norepinephrine (Levophed), piperacillin and tazobactam (Zosyn), potassium, propofol (Diprivan).

## INDICATIONS/ROUTES/DOSAGE

**Anxiety**
**PO: ADULTS:** Initially, 2–3 mg/day in 2–3 divided doses. Usual dose: 2–6 mg/day in divided doses. Range: 1–10 mg/day.

**ELDERLY:** Initially, 1–2 mg/day in divided doses. **Maximum:** 3 mg/day in divided doses.

**Insomnia Due to Anxiety**
**PO: ADULTS:** 2–4 mg at bedtime.

**Status Epilepticus**
**IV: ADULTS, ELDERLY, CHILDREN:** 0.1 mg/kg. **Maximum:** 4 mg over 2–5 min. May repeat in 5–10 min. **NEONATES:** 0.05 mg/kg over 2–5 min. May repeat in 10–15 min.

**Dosage in Renal/Hepatic Impairment**
**PO:** No dose adjustment. **IM/IV: Mild to moderate impairment:** Use caution. Not recommended in severe impairment.

## SIDE EFFECTS

**Frequent (16%–7%):** Drowsiness, dizziness. **Rare (less than 4%):** Weakness, ataxia, headache, hypotension, nausea, vomiting, confusion, injection site reaction.

## ADVERSE EFFECTS/ TOXIC REACTIONS

Abrupt or too-rapid withdrawal may result in pronounced restlessness, irritability, insomnia, hand tremor, abdominal cramping, muscle cramps, diaphoresis, vomiting, seizures. Overdose results in drowsiness, confusion, diminished reflexes, coma. **Antidote:** Flumazenil (see Appendix J for dosage).

## NURSING CONSIDERATIONS

### BASELINE ASSESSMENT

Offer emotional support to anxious pt. Pt must remain recumbent following parenteral administration to reduce hypotensive effect. Assess motor responses (agitation, trembling, tension), autonomic responses (cold or clammy hands, diaphoresis).

### INTERVENTION/EVALUATION

Monitor B/P, respiratory rate, heart rate. For those on long-term therapy, hepatic/renal function tests, CBC should be performed periodically. Assess for paradoxical reaction, particularly during

L

early therapy. Evaluate for therapeutic response: calm facial expression, decreased restlessness, insomnia, decrease in seizure-related symptoms. **Therapeutic serum level:** 50–240 ng/ml; **toxic serum level:** N/A.

### PATIENT/ FAMILY TEACHING

• Drowsiness usually subsides during continued therapy. • Avoid tasks that require alertness, motor skills until response to drug is established. • Smoking reduces drug effectiveness. • Do not abruptly discontinue medication after long-term therapy. • Do not use alcohol, CNS depressants. • Contraception recommended for long-term therapy. • Immediately report suspected pregnancy.

---

# lorcaserin

lor-**kas**-er-in
(Belviq, Belviq XR)

### ◆CLASSIFICATION

**PHARMACOTHERAPEUTIC:** Serotonin receptor agonist. **CLINICAL:** Weight loss agent.

## USES

Adjunct to reduced-calorie diet and increased physical activity for chronic weight management in adults with an initial body mass index (BMI) of 30 kg/m$^2$ or greater (obese), or 27 kg/m$^2$ or greater (overweight) with at least one weight-related comorbid condition (e.g., hypertension, dyslipidemia, type 2 diabetes).

## PRECAUTIONS

**Contraindications:** Hypersensitivity to lorcaserin, pregnancy. **Cautions:** Use in pts with severe renal impairment, end-stage renal disease is not recommended. Concurrent use with medications that affect serotonergic neurotransmitter system (particularly during initiation of therapy and dose increases). Moderate renal impairment, severe hepatic impairment, HF, pts predisposed to priapism

(e.g., leukemia). Pts at high risk for suicidal thoughts, behavior. Bradycardia, heart block, diabetes.

## ACTION

Activates 5HT$_{2O}$ receptors on anorexigenic neurons located in the hypothalamus. **Therapeutic Effect:** Decreases food consumption, promotes satiety.

## PHARMACOKINETICS

Rapidly absorbed from GI tract. Peak plasma concentration: 1.5–2h. Distributed in cerebrospinal fluid and CNS. Protein binding: 70%. Metabolized in liver. Primarily excreted in urine.

## ⧖ LIFESPAN CONSIDERATIONS

**Pregnancy/Lactation:** May cause fetal harm. Unknown if distributed in breast milk. **Children:** Not for use in this age group. **Elderly:** Age-related renal impairment may require dose adjustment.

## INTERACTIONS

**DRUG:** May increase concentration/effects of **CYP3D6** substrates (e.g., amitriptyline, metoprolol, venlafaxine). **Triptans, monoamine oxidase inhibitors (MAOIs, including linezolid), selective serotonin reuptake inhibitors (SSRIs), selective serotonin-norepinephrine reuptake inhibitors, dextromethorphan, tricyclic antidepressants, bupropion, lithium, tramadol, tryptophan** may increase risk for serotonin syndrome. **HERBAL: St. John's wort** increases potential for serotonin syndrome. **FOOD:** None known. **ALTERED LAB VALUES:** May lower Hgb, neutrophil count. May increase serum prolactin.

## AVAILABILITY (Rx)

▨ **Capsules, Extended-Release:** (Belviq XR) 20 mg. **Tablets, Film-Coated:** (Belviq) 10 mg.

## ADMINISTRATION/HANDLING

• Do not break, crush, dissolve, or divide film-coated tablet. May give without regard to food.

---

*"Tall Man" lettering    <u>underlined</u> – top prescribed drug

## INDICATIONS/ROUTES/DOSAGE

**Weight Management**
**PO: ADULTS, ELDERLY:** (Belviq) 10 mg twice daily. Do not exceed 10 mg twice daily. (Belviq XR) 20 mg once daily. Belviq should be discontinued if 5% weight loss is not achieved by week 12 of therapy.

**Dosage in Renal Impairment**
**Mild impairment:** No dose adjustment. **Moderate:** Use caution. **Severe impairment, end-stage renal disease:** Not recommended.

**Dosage in Hepatic Impairment**
**Mild to moderate impairment:** No dose adjustment. **Severe impairment:** Use caution.

## SIDE EFFECTS

**Note:** Side effects tend to be mild and transient in nature, gradually diminishing during treatment. **Frequent (16%–5%):** Headache, dizziness, fatigue, diarrhea, nausea, dry mouth, constipation. **Type 2 Diabetic Pts (29%–7%):** Hypoglycemia, headache, back pain, nasopharyngitis, nausea, cough, fatigue, dizziness. **Occasional (6%–2%):** Cough, oropharyngeal pain, sinus congestion, musculoskeletal pain, rash. **Rare (4%–2%): Type 2 Diabetic Pts:** Muscle spasm, peripheral edema, anxiety, insomnia, seasonal allergy, gastroenteritis, toothache, decreased appetite, depression.

## ADVERSE EFFECTS/ TOXIC REACTIONS

**Potential for Serotonin Syndrome** Serotonin syndrome symptoms including mental status changes (e.g., agitation, hallucinations, coma), autonomic instability (e.g., tachycardia, labile B/P, hyperthermia), neuromuscular changes (e.g., hyperreflexia, incoordination), and/or GI symptoms (e.g., nausea, vomiting, diarrhea) have been observed. Serotonin syndrome, in its most severe form, can resemble neuroleptic malignant syndrome, which includes hyperthermia, muscle rigidity, autonomic instability with possible rapid fluctuation of vital signs, and mental status changes. Urinary tract infection occurs in 9% of type 2 diabetic pts.

## NURSING CONSIDERATIONS

### BASELINE ASSESSMENT
Ensure negative pregnancy test prior to initiating treatment. Obtain baseline chemistries, particularly renal function, LFT. Obtain weight, BMI.

### INTERVENTION/EVALUATION
In trials, most patients lost at least 5% of their body weight over a year, and a further one third lost at least 10%. Pts who develop signs or symptoms of valvular cardiac disease, including dyspnea, dependent edema, HF, or a new cardiac murmur while on medication should be consistently monitored; discontinuation of treatment may be necessary.

### PATIENT/FAMILY TEACHING
• Discontinue therapy if 5% weight loss has not been achieved by 12 wks of treatment. • High-fiber, low-fat diet decreases fat evacuation. • Avoid tasks that require alertness, motor skills until response to drug is established. • Do not break, chew, dissolve, or divide tablets; swallow whole.

# losartan

loe-**sar**-tan
(Apo-Losartan ✦, Cozaar)
■ **BLACK BOX ALERT** ■ May cause fetal injury, mortality. Discontinue as soon as possible once pregnancy is detected.
**Do not confuse Cozaar with Colace, Coreg, Hyzaar, or Zocor, or losartan with lorcaserin, valsartan.**

## FIXED-COMBINATION(S)

**Hyzaar:** losartan/hydrochlorothiazide (a diuretic): 50 mg/12.5 mg, 100 mg/12.5 mg, 100 mg/25 mg.

## ✦CLASSIFICATION

**PHARMACOTHERAPEUTIC:** Angiotensin II receptor antagonist. **CLINICAL:** Antihypertensive.

## USES

Treatment of hypertension. Used alone or in combination with other antihypertensives. Treatment of diabetic nephropathy (in pts with type 2 diabetes and hypertension), prevention of stroke in pts with hypertension and left ventricular hypertrophy. **OFF-LABEL:** Slow rate of progression of aortic root dilation in children with Marfan's syndrome. HF in pts intolerant of ACE inhibitors.

## PRECAUTIONS

**Contraindications:** Hypersensitivity to losartan. Concomitant use of aliskiren in pts with diabetes. **Cautions:** Renal/hepatic impairment, unstented renal arterial stenosis, significant aortic/mitral stenosis. Concurrent use of potassium supplements. Pts with history of angioedema.

## ACTION

Blocks vasoconstrictor, aldosterone-secreting effects of angiotensin II, inhibiting binding of angiotensin II to $AT_1$ receptors. **Therapeutic Effect:** Causes vasodilation, decreases peripheral resistance, decreases B/P.

## PHARMACOKINETICS

| Route | Onset | Peak | Duration |
|-------|-------|------|----------|
| PO | N/A | 6 hrs | 24 hrs |

Well absorbed after PO administration. Protein binding: 98%. Metabolized in liver. Eliminated in urine (35%), feces (60%). Not removed by hemodialysis. **Half-life:** 2 hrs; metabolite, 6–9 hrs.

## ⧖ LIFESPAN CONSIDERATIONS

**Pregnancy/Lactation:** Has caused fetal/neonatal morbidity, mortality. Potential for adverse effects on breastfed infant. Breastfeeding not recommended. **Children:** Safety and efficacy not established. **Elderly:** No age-related precautions noted.

## INTERACTIONS

**DRUG: NSAIDs** may decrease effects. **Potassium-sparing diuretics (e.g., spironolactone, triamterene), potassium supplements** may increase serum potassium. **Diuretics (e.g., furosemide, HCTZ), antihypertensive medications (e.g., amlodipine, lisinopril, valsartan)** may produce additive hypotension. **HERBAL: Ephedra, ginseng, licorice, yohimbe** may worsen hypertension. **Black cohosh, periwinkle** may increase antihypertensive effect. **Garlic, ginger, ginseng** may increase hypoglycemic effect. **FOOD:** None known. **LAB VALUES:** May increase serum bilirubin, ALT, AST, Hgb, Hct. May decrease serum glucose.

## AVAILABILITY (Rx)

**Tablets:** 25 mg, 50 mg, 100 mg.

## ADMINISTRATION/HANDLING

**PO**
• May give without regard to food.

## INDICATIONS/ROUTES/DOSAGE

**Hypertension**
**PO: ADULTS, ELDERLY:** Initially, 50 mg once daily. **Maximum:** May be given once or twice daily, with total daily doses ranging from 25–100 mg. **CHILDREN 6–16 YRS:** 0.7 mg/kg once daily. **Maximum:** 50 mg/day.

**Diabetic Nephropathy**
**PO: ADULTS, ELDERLY:** Initially, 50 mg/day. May increase to 100 mg/day based on B/P response.

**Stroke Prevention (Hypertension with Left Ventricular Hypertrophy)**
**PO: ADULTS, ELDERLY:** 50 mg/day. **Maximum:** 100 mg/day.

**Renal Impairment**
Not recommended if glomerular filtration rate (GFR) less than 30 ml/min.

**Hepatic Impairment**
**PO: ADULTS, ELDERLY:** Initially, 25 mg/day. May increase up to 100 mg/day.

## SIDE EFFECTS

**Frequent (8%):** Upper respiratory tract infection. **Occasional (4%–2%):** Dizziness, diarrhea, cough. **Rare (1% or less):** Insomnia, dyspepsia, heartburn, back/leg pain, muscle cramps, myalgia, nasal congestion, sinusitis, depression.

## ADVERSE EFFECTS/ TOXIC REACTIONS

Overdosage may manifest as hypotension and tachycardia. Bradycardia occurs less often. Institute supportive measures.

## NURSING CONSIDERATIONS

### BASELINE ASSESSMENT

Obtain B/P, apical pulse immediately before each dose, in addition to regular monitoring (be alert to fluctuations). Question for possibility of pregnancy. Assess medication history (esp. diuretics).

### INTERVENTION/EVALUATION

Maintain hydration (offer fluids frequently). Assess for evidence of upper respiratory infection, cough. Monitor B/P, pulse. If excessive reduction in B/P occurs, place pt in supine position, feet slightly elevated. Assist with ambulation if dizziness occurs. Monitor daily pattern of bowel activity, stool consistency.

### PATIENT/FAMILY TEACHING

• Female pts of childbearing age should take measures to avoid pregnancy. • Report pregnancy as soon as possible. • Avoid tasks that require alertness, motor skills until response to drug is established (possible dizziness effect). • Report any sign of infection (sore throat, fever), chest pain. • Do not take OTC cold preparations, nasal decongestants. • Do not stop taking medication. • Limit salt intake.

# lovastatin

**loe**-va-stat-in
(Altoprev, Apo-Lovastatin ♣, Mevacor)
**Do not confuse lovastatin with atorvastatin, Leustatin, Lotensin, nystatin, pitavastatin, or pravastatin, or Mevacor with Benicar or Lipitor.**

## FIXED-COMBINATION(S)

**Advicor:** lovastatin/niacin: 20 mg/500 mg, 20 mg/750 mg, 20 mg/1,000 mg.

## ◆CLASSIFICATION

**PHARMACOTHERAPEUTIC:** HMG-CoA reductase inhibitor. **CLINICAL:** Antihyperlipidemic.

## USES

Decreases elevated serum total and LDL cholesterol in primary hypercholesterolemia; primary prevention of coronary artery disease. Slows progression of coronary atherosclerosis in pts with coronary heart disease. Adjunct to diet in adolescent pts (10–17 yrs) with heterozygous familial hypercholesterolemia.

## PRECAUTIONS

**Contraindications:** Hypersensitivity to lovastatin. Active hepatic disease, pregnancy, unexplained elevated LFT. Pregnancy, breastfeeding. Concomitant use of strong CYP3A4 inhibitors. **Cautions:** History of heavy/chronic alcohol use, renal impairment, hepatic disease; concomitant use of amiodarone, cyclosporine, fibrates, gemfibrozil, niacin, verapamil (increased risk of myopathy), elderly.

## ACTION

Inhibits HMG-CoA reductase, the enzyme that catalyzes the early step in cholesterol synthesis. **Therapeutic Effect:** Decreases LDL, VLDL, triglycerides; increases HDL.

L

## PHARMACOKINETICS

| Route | Onset | Peak | Duration |
|-------|-------|------|----------|
| PO (LDL, cholesterol reduction) | 3 days | N/A | N/A |

Incompletely absorbed from GI tract (increased on empty stomach). Protein binding: 95%. Hydrolyzed in liver. Primarily eliminated in feces. Not removed by hemodialysis. **Half-life:** 1.1–1.7 hrs.

## ⚕ LIFESPAN CONSIDERATIONS

**Pregnancy/Lactation:** Contraindicated in pregnancy (suppression of cholesterol biosynthesis may cause fetal toxicity) and lactation. Unknown if drug is distributed in breast milk. **Children:** Safety and efficacy not established. **Elderly:** No age-related precautions noted.

## INTERACTIONS

**DRUG: CYP3A4 inhibitors (e.g., ketoconazole, clarithromycin)** may increase concentration, risk of myopathy, rhabdomyolysis. **Cyclosporine, fibrates, gemfibrozil, niacin, amiodarone, verapamil** may increase risk of rhabdomyolysis, acute renal failure. **HERBAL: St. John's wort** may decrease concentration/effects. **FOOD:** Large quantities of **grapefruit juice** may increase risk of side effects (e.g., myalgia, weakness). **Red yeast rice** may increase concentration (2.4 mg lovastatin/600 mg rice). **LAB VALUES:** May increase serum creatine kinase (CK), transaminase.

## AVAILABILITY (Rx)

**Tablets (Mevacor):** 10 mg, 20 mg, 40 mg.

🔖 **Tablets (Extended-Release [Altoprev]):** 20 mg, 40 mg, 60 mg.

## ADMINISTRATION/HANDLING

**PO**
• Immediate-release tablet given with evening meal; extended-release at bedtime. • Avoid intake of large quantities of grapefruit juice (greater than 1 quart). • Do not break, crush, dissolve, or divide extended-release tablets.

## INDICATIONS/ROUTES/DOSAGE

**Hypercholesterolemia**
**PO (Immediate-Release): ADULTS, ELDERLY:** Initially, 20 mg/day. Adjust at 4-wk intervals. **Maintenance:** 10–80 mg once daily or in 2 divided doses. **Maximum:** 80 mg/day.
**PO (Extended-Release): ADULTS, ELDERLY:** Initially, 20–60 mg once daily at bedtime. Adjust at 4-wk intervals. **Maximum:** 60 mg once daily at bedtime.

**Heterozygous Familial Hypercholesterolemia**
**PO (Immediate-Release): CHILDREN 10–17 YRS:** Initially, 10–20 mg/day. Adjust at 4-wk intervals. **Range:** 10–40 mg daily.

**Dosage with Concurrent Medication**
**Amiodarone: Maximum:** 40 mg/day. **Diltiazem, Dronedarone, Verapamil: Maximum: (Immediate-Release):** 10 mg/day. **(Extended-Release):** 20 mg/day. **Lomitapide:** Consider reduction in dose.

**Dosage in Renal Impairment**
Use caution.

**Dosage in Hepatic Impairment**
No dose adjustment.

## SIDE EFFECTS

Generally well tolerated. Side effects usually mild and transient. **Frequent (9%–5%):** Headache, flatulence, diarrhea, abdominal pain, abdominal cramping, rash, pruritus. **Occasional (4%–3%):** Nausea, vomiting, constipation, dyspepsia. **Rare (2%–1%):** Dizziness, heartburn, myalgia, blurred vision, eye irritation.

## ADVERSE EFFECTS/ TOXIC REACTIONS

Potential for cataract development. Occasionally produces myopathy manifested as muscle pain, tenderness, weakness with elevated creatine kinase (CK). Severe myopathy may lead to rhabdomyolysis.

## NURSING CONSIDERATIONS

### BASELINE ASSESSMENT
Obtain dietary history. Question for possibility of pregnancy before initiating therapy. Assess baseline lab results: serum cholesterol, triglycerides, LFT.

### INTERVENTION/EVALUATION
Monitor daily pattern of bowel activity, stool consistency. Monitor for headache, dizziness, blurred vision. Assess for rash, pruritus. Monitor serum cholesterol, triglycerides for therapeutic response. Be alert for malaise, muscle cramping/weakness. Monitor LFT.

### PATIENT/FAMILY TEACHING
• Follow special diet (important part of treatment). • Periodic lab tests are essential part of therapy. • Maintain appropriate birth control measures. • Avoid grapefruit juice, alcohol. • Report severe gastric upset, vision changes, myalgia, weakness, changes in color of urine/stool, yellowing of eyes/skin, unusual bruising.

---

# lubiprostone

loo-bi-**pros**-tone
(Amitiza)

◆**CLASSIFICATION**
**PHARMACOTHERAPEUTIC:** Chloride channel activator. **CLINICAL:** Laxative.

## USES
Treatment of chronic idiopathic constipation in adults. Treatment of opioid-induced constipation. Treatment of irritable bowel syndrome (IBS) with constipation in women 18 yrs and older.

## PRECAUTIONS
**Contraindications:** Hypersensitivity to lubiprostone. History of mechanical GI obstruction. **Cautions:** Severe diarrhea.

## ACTION
Secretes fluid into abdominal lumen through activation of chloride channels in apical membranes of GI epithelium. **Therapeutic Effect:** Increases intestinal motility, thereby increasing passage of stool, alleviating symptoms associated with chronic idiopathic constipation.

## PHARMACOKINETICS
Rapidly, extensively metabolized within stomach and jejunum. Minimal distribution beyond GI tissue. Protein binding: 94%. Excreted in urine (60%), feces (30%). **Half-life:** 0.9–1.4 hrs.

## ⧗ LIFESPAN CONSIDERATIONS
May have potential for teratogenic effects. Unknown if distributed in breast milk. **Children:** Safety and efficacy not established. **Elderly:** No age-related precautions noted.

## INTERACTIONS
**DRUG:** None significant. **HERBAL:** None significant. **FOOD:** None known. **LAB VALUES:** None significant.

## AVAILABILITY (Rx)
**Capsules:** 8 mcg, 24 mcg.

## ADMINISTRATION/HANDLING
**PO**
• Give with food and water.

## INDICATIONS/ROUTES/DOSAGE
**Chronic Idiopathic Constipation, Opioid-Induced Constipation**
**PO: ADULTS, ELDERLY:** 24 mcg twice daily with food and water.

**IBS**
**PO: ADULTS, ELDERLY (FEMALES):** 8 mcg twice daily with food and water.

**Dosage in Renal Impairment**
No dose adjustment.

---

**Dosage in Hepatic Impairment**
**Mild impairment:** No dose adjustment.
**Moderate impairment: (IBS):** No dose adjustment. **(Constipation):** 16 mcg twice daily. May increase to 24 mcg twice daily.
**Severe impairment: (IBS):** 8 mcg once daily. May increase to 8 mcg twice daily. **(Constipation):** 8 mcg twice daily. May increase to 16–24 mcg twice daily.

## SIDE EFFECTS

**Frequent    (31%):** Nausea. **Occasional (13%–4%):** Headache, diarrhea, abdominal distention, abdominal pain, flatulence, vomiting, peripheral edema, dizziness. **Rare (3%–2%):** Dyspepsia, loose stools, fatigue, dry mouth, arthralgia, back pain, cough.

## ADVERSE EFFECTS/ TOXIC REACTIONS

UTI, upper respiratory tract infection occurs in 4% of pts.

## NURSING CONSIDERATIONS

### BASELINE ASSESSMENT

Confirm negative pregnancy test prior to beginning therapy and comply with effective contraceptive measures during therapy. Assess for diarrhea (avoid use in these pts). Question characteristics of bowel movements.

### INTERVENTION/EVALUATION

Assess for improvement in symptoms (relief from bloating, cramping, urgency, abdominal discomfort). Monitor daily pattern of bowel activity, stool consistency.

### PATIENT/FAMILY TEACHING

• Report new/worsening episodes of abdominal pain, severe diarrhea. • Avoid tasks that require alertness, motor skills until response to drug is established.

# lurasidone

loo-**ras**-i-done
(Latuda)

■ **BLACK BOX ALERT** ■ Elderly pts with dementia-related psychosis are at increased risk for mortality due to cardiovascular events, infectious diseases. Increased risk of suicidal thinking/behavior in children, adolescents, young adults.

## ◆CLASSIFICATION

**PHARMACOTHERAPEUTIC:** Dopamine, serotonin receptor antagonist. **CLINICAL:** Antipsychotic.

## USES

Treatment of schizophrenia. Depression associated with bipolar I disorder as monotherapy and as adjunctive therapy with lithium or valproate.

## PRECAUTIONS

**Contraindications:** Hypersensitivity to lurasidone. Concurrent use with strong CYP3A4 inhibitors (e.g., ketoconazole) and inducers (e.g., rifampin). **Cautions:** Cardiovascular disease (HF, history of MI, ischemia, conduction abnormalities), cerebrovascular disease (history of CVA in pts with dementia, seizure disorders), diabetes mellitus, Parkinson's disease, renal/hepatic impairment, pts at risk for aspiration pneumonia, pts at risk for suicide, disorders where CNS depression is a feature, pts at risk for hypotension, elderly, head trauma, alcoholism, medications that lower seizure threshold.

## ACTION

Antagonizes central dopamine type 2 and serotonin type 2 receptors. **Therapeutic Effect:** Diminishes symptoms of schizophrenia. Reduces incidence of extrapyramidal side effects.

## PHARMACOKINETICS

Absorbed in 1–3 hrs. Steady-state concentration occurs in 7 days. Well absorbed from GI tract (unaffected by food). Protein binding: 99%. Metabolized in liver. Excreted in feces (80%), urine (9%). Half-life: 18 hrs.

## ⌛ LIFESPAN CONSIDERATIONS

**Pregnancy/Lactation:** Unknown if distributed in breast milk. Breastfeeding not recommended. **Children:** Safety and efficacy not established. **Elderly:** More susceptible to postural hypotension. Increased risk of cerebrovascular events, mortality, including stroke, in elderly pts with psychosis.

## INTERACTIONS

**DRUG:** Alcohol, CNS depressants (e.g., lorazepam, morphine, zolpidem) may increase CNS depression. **Rifampin** decreases concentration/effects. **Diltiazem, ketoconazole, ritonavir** may increase concentration/effects. **HERBAL: Gotu kola, kava kava, St. John's wort, valerian** may increase CNS depression. **FOOD: Grapefruit products** may increase risk of torsades, orthostatic hypotension. **LAB VALUES:** May increase prolactin levels.

## AVAILABILITY (Rx)

**Tablets:** 20 mg, 40 mg, 80 mg, 120 mg.

## ADMINISTRATION/HANDLING

**PO**
• Give with food. • Tablets may be crushed.

## INDICATIONS/ROUTES/DOSAGE

**Schizophrenia**
**PO: ADULTS, ELDERLY:** 40 mg once daily with food. **Maximum:** 160 mg once daily with food.

**Depressive Episode Associated with Bipolar Disorder**
**PO: ADULTS, ELDERLY:** Initially, 20 mg once daily. **Maximum:** 120 mg/day. Titration not required.

**Concomitant Use of Moderate CYP3A4 Inhibitors**
**PO: ADULTS, ELDERLY:** Initially, 20 mg/day. **Maximum:** 80 mg/day.

**Moderate to Severe Renal Impairment**
**CrCl less than 50 ml/min:** Initially, 20 mg/day. **Maximum:** 80 mg/day.

**Hepatic Impairment**
**Mild impairment:** No dose adjustment. **Moderate impairment:** Initially, 20 mg/day. **Maximum:** 80 mg/day. **Severe impairment:** Initially, 20 mg/day. **Maximum:** 40 mg/day.

## SIDE EFFECTS

**Frequent (15%–7%):** Drowsiness, sedation, insomnia (paradoxical reaction). **Occasional (6%–3%):** Nausea, vomiting, dyspepsia, fatigue, back pain, akathisia, dizziness, agitation, anxiety. **Rare (2%–1%):** Restlessness, salivary hypersecretion, tongue spasm, torticollis, trismus.

## ADVERSE EFFECTS/ TOXIC REACTIONS

Extrapyramidal disorder (including cogwheel rigidity, drooling, bradykinesia, tardive dyskinesia, tremors) occurs in 5% of pts. Neuroleptic malignant syndrome (fever, muscle rigidity, irregular B/P or pulse, altered mental status, visual changes, dyspnea) occurs rarely.

## NURSING CONSIDERATIONS

### BASELINE ASSESSMENT

Assess behavior, appearance, emotional status, response to environment, speech pattern, thought content. Renal function, LFT should be obtained before therapy as dose adjustment is required when initiating therapy.

### INTERVENTION/EVALUATION

Supervise suicidal risk pt closely during early therapy (as depression lessens, energy level improves, increasing suicide potential). Monitor for potential neuroleptic malignant syndrome. Assess for therapeutic response (greater interest in surroundings, improved self-care, increased ability to concentrate, relaxed facial expression).

## PATIENT/FAMILY TEACHING

• Avoid tasks that may require alertness, motor skills until response to drug is established (may cause drowsiness, dizziness). • Avoid alcohol. • Report trembling in fingers, altered gait, unusual muscle/skeletal movements, palpitations, severe dizziness, fainting, visual changes, rash, difficulty breathing. • Report suicidal ideation, unusual changes in behavior.

# magnesium ⬛HIGH ALERT

mag-**nee**-zee-um

## magnesium chloride

(Mag-Delay, Slow-Mag)

## magnesium citrate

(Citroma, Citro-Mag ❧)

## magnesium hydroxide

(Milk of Magnesia)

## magnesium oxide

(Mag-Ox 400, Uro-Mag)

## magnesium sulfate

(Epsom salt, magnesium sulfate injection)
**Do not confuse magnesium sulfate with morphine sulfate.**

## FIXED-COMBINATION(S)

With aluminum and simethicone, an antiflatulent **(Mylanta).**

## ◆CLASSIFICATION

**CLINICAL:** Antacid, anticonvulsant, electrolyte, laxative.

## USES

**Magnesium chloride:** Dietary supplement. **Magnesium citrate:** Evacuation of bowel before surgical, diagnostic procedures. Relieves occasional constipation. **Magnesium hydroxide:** Short-term treatment of constipation, symptoms of hyperacidity, laxative. **Magnesium oxide:** Relief of acid indigestion and upset stomach, short-term relief of constipation. Dietary supplement. **Magnesium sulfate:** Treatment/prevention of hypomagnesemia; prevention and treatment of seizures in severe preeclampsia or eclampsia; pediatric acute nephritis, treatment of arrhythmias due to hypomagnesemia (ventricular fibrillation, ventricular tachycardia, or torsades de points). **OFF-LABEL: Magnesium sulfate:** Asthma exacerbation unresponsive to conventional treatment.

## PRECAUTIONS

**Contraindications: Antacid:** Appendicitis, symptoms of appendicitis, ileostomy, intestinal obstruction, severe renal impairment. **Laxative:** Appendicitis, HF, colostomy, hypersensitivity, ileostomy, intestinal obstruction, undiagnosed rectal bleeding. **Systemic:** Heart block, myocardial damage, IV use for preeclampsia/eclampsia during the 2 hrs prior to delivery. **Cautions:** Safety in children younger than 6 yrs not known. **Antacids:** Undiagnosed GI/rectal bleeding, ulcerative colitis, colostomy, diverticulitis, chronic diarrhea. **Laxative:** Diabetes mellitus, pts on low-salt diet (some products contain sugar, sodium). **Systemic:** Severe renal impairment. Myasthenia gravis or other neuromuscular diseases.

## ACTION

**Antacid:** Acts in stomach to neutralize gastric acid. **Therapeutic Effect:** Increases pH. **Laxative:** Osmotic effect primarily in small intestine, draws water into intestinal lumen. **Therapeutic Effect:** Promotes peristalsis, bowel evacuation. **Systemic (dietary supplement replacement):** Found primarily in intracellular fluids. **Therapeutic Effect:** Essential for enzyme activity, nerve conduction, muscle contraction. Maintains and restores magnesium levels. **Anticonvulsant:** Blocks neuromuscular transmission, amount of acetylcholine released at motor end plate. **Therapeutic Effect:** Produces seizure control.

M

## PHARMACOKINETICS

**Antacid, laxative:** Minimal absorption through intestine. Absorbed dose primarily excreted in urine. **Systemic:** Widely distributed. Primarily excreted in urine.

## ⧗ LIFESPAN CONSIDERATIONS

**Pregnancy/Lactation: Antacid:** Unknown if distributed in breast milk. **Parenteral:** Readily crosses placenta. Distributed in breast milk for 24 hrs after magnesium therapy is discontinued. Continuous IV infusion increases risk of magnesium toxicity in neonate. IV administration should not be used 2 hrs preceding delivery. **Children:** No age-related precautions noted. **Elderly:** Increased risk of developing magnesium deficiency (e.g., poor diet, decreased absorption, medications).

## INTERACTIONS

**DRUG:** May decrease absorption of **quinolones (e.g., ciprofloxacin, levofloxacin), tetracycline, bisphosphonates.** May increase effects of **antihypertensives (e.g., amlodipine, lisinopril). HERBAL:** None significant. **FOOD:** None known. **LAB VALUES: Antacid:** May increase gastrin production, pH. **Laxative:** May decrease serum potassium. **Systemic:** None significant.

## AVAILABILITY

MAGNESIUM CHLORIDE
**Tablets (Mag Delay, Slow-Mag):** 64 mg.
MAGNESIUM CITRATE
**Oral Solution (Citroma):** 290 mg/5 ml.
MAGNESIUM HYDROXIDE
**Oral Liquid (Milk of Magnesia):** 400 mg/ 5 ml, 1,200 mg/5 ml.
**Tablets (Chewable [Phillips Milk of Magnesia]):** 311 mg.
MAGNESIUM OXIDE
**Capsules (Uro-Mag):** 140 mg. **Tablets (Mag-Ox 400):** 400 mg.

MAGNESIUM SULFATE
**Infusion Solution:** 10 mg/ml, 20 mg/ml, 40 mg/ml, 80 mg/ml. **Injection Solution:** 125 mg/ml, 500 mg/ml.

## ADMINISTRATION/HANDLING

 **IV**

**Reconstitution** • Must dilute to maximum concentration of 20% for IV infusion. May give IV push, IV piggyback, or continuous infusion.
**Rate of Administration** • For IV push (diluted): Give no faster than 150 mg/min. For IV infusion, maximum rate of infusion is 2 g/hr.
**Storage** • Store at room temperature.

**IM**
• For adults, elderly, use 250 mg/ml (25%) or 500 mg/ml (50%) magnesium sulfate concentration. • For infants, children, do not exceed 200 mg/ml (20% diluted solution).

**PO (Antacid)**
• Shake suspension well before use.
• Chewable tablets should be chewed thoroughly before swallowing, followed by full glass of water.

**PO (Laxative)**
• Drink full glass of liquid (8 oz) with each dose (prevents dehydration).
• Flavor may be improved by following with fruit juice, citrus carbonated beverage. • Refrigerate citrate of magnesia (retains potency, palatability).

## ▨ IV INCOMPATIBILITIES

Amphotericin B complex (Abelcet, AmBisome, Amphotec), cefepime (Maxipime), lansoprazole (Prevacid), pantoprazole (Protonix).

## ▨ IV COMPATIBILITIES

Amikacin (Amikin), cefazolin (Ancef), ciprofloxacin (Cipro), dexmedetomidine (Precedex), dobutamine (Dobutrex), enalapril (Vasotec), gentamicin, heparin,

M

hydromorphone (Dilaudid), insulin, linezolid (Zyvox), metoclopramide (Reglan), milrinone (Primacor), morphine, piperacillin/tazobactam (Zosyn), potassium chloride, propofol (Diprivan), tobramycin (Nebcin), vancomycin (Vancocin).

## INDICATIONS/ROUTES/DOSAGE

**MAGNESIUM SULFATE**
**Hypomagnesemia**
**Mild Deficiency**
**IM: ADULTS, ELDERLY:** 1 g q6h for 4 doses.

**Severe Deficiency**
**IM: ADULTS, ELDERLY:** Up to 250 mg/kg over 4 hrs.
**IV: ADULTS, ELDERLY:** 1–2 g/hr for 3–6 hrs, then 0.5–1 g/hr as needed to correct deficiency. **CHILDREN:** 25–50 mg/kg/dose over 10–20 min. **Maximum single dose:** 2 g.

**Usual Dose for Neonates**
**IM/IV:** 25–50 mg/kg/dose q8–12h for 2–3 doses.

**Eclampsia/Preeclampsia**
**IV: ADULTS:** 4–5 g infusion, then 1–2 g/hr continuous infusion. **Maximum:** 40 g/24 hrs.

**MAGNESIUM CHLORIDE**
**Dietary Supplement**
**PO: ADULTS, ELDERLY:** 2 tablets once daily.

**MAGNESIUM CITRATE**
**Laxative**
**PO: ADULTS, ELDERLY, CHILDREN 12 YRS AND OLDER:** 195–300 ml once or in divided doses. **6–12 YRS:** 90–210 ml once or in divided doses. **2–5 YRS:** 60–90 ml once or in divided doses.

**MAGNESIUM HYDROXIDE**
**Antacid**
**PO: ADULTS, ELDERLY, CHILDREN 12 YRS AND OLDER:** *(400 mg/5 ml):* 5–15 ml as needed up to 4 times/day.

**Laxative**
**PO: ADULTS, ELDERLY, CHILDREN 12 YRS AND OLDER:** *(400 mg/5 ml):* 30–60 ml at HS or in divided doses. **CHILDREN 6–11 YRS:** 15–30 ml at HS. **CHILDREN 2–5 YRS:** 5–15 ml at HS.

**MAGNESIUM OXIDE**
**Antacid/Dietary Supplement**
**PO: ADULTS, ELDERLY:** 1–2 tablets daily.

**Dosage in Renal Impairment**
Use caution.

**Dosage in Hepatic Impairment**
No dose adjustment.

## SIDE EFFECTS

**Frequent: Antacid:** Chalky taste, diarrhea, laxative effect. **Occasional: Antacid:** Nausea, vomiting, stomach cramps. **Antacid, laxative:** Prolonged use or large doses in renal impairment may cause hypermagnesemia (dizziness, palpitations, altered mental status, fatigue, weakness). **Laxative:** Cramping, diarrhea, increased thirst, flatulence. **Systemic (dietary supplement, electrolyte replacement):** Reduced respiratory rate, decreased reflexes, flushing, hypotension, decreased heart rate.

## ADVERSE EFFECTS/ TOXIC REACTIONS

Magnesium as antacid, laxative has no known adverse reactions. Systemic use may produce prolonged PR interval, widening of QRS interval. Magnesium toxicity may cause loss of deep tendon reflexes, heart block, respiratory paralysis, cardiac arrest. **Antidote:** 10–20 ml 10% calcium gluconate (5–10 mEq of calcium).

## NURSING CONSIDERATIONS

**BASELINE ASSESSMENT**

Assess sensitivity to magnesium. **Antacid:** Assess GI pain (duration, location, quality, time of occurrence, relief with food, causative/exacerbative factors). **Laxative:** Assess for weight loss, nausea, vomiting, history of recent abdominal surgery. **Systemic:** Assess renal function, serum magnesium.

### INTERVENTION/EVALUATION

**Antacid:** Assess for relief of gastric distress. Monitor renal function (esp. if dosing is long term or frequent). **Laxative:** Monitor daily pattern of bowel activity, stool consistency. Maintain adequate fluid intake. **Systemic:** Monitor renal function, magnesium levels, EKG for cardiac function. Test patellar reflexes before giving repeated, rapid parenteral doses (used as indication of CNS depression; suppressed reflexes may be sign of impending respiratory arrest). Patellar reflex must be present, respiratory rate should be 16/min or over before each parenteral dose. Initiate seizure precautions.

### PATIENT/FAMILY TEACHING

• **Antacid:** Take at least 2 hrs apart from other medication. • Do not take longer than 2 wks unless directed by physician. • For peptic ulcer, take 1 and 3 hrs after meals and at bedtime for 4–6 wks. • Chew tablets thoroughly, followed by 8 oz of water; shake suspensions well. • Repeat dosing or large doses may have laxative effect. • **Laxative:** Drink full glass (8 oz) liquid to aid stool softening. • Use only for short term. Do not use if abdominal pain, nausea, vomiting is present. • **Systemic:** Report any signs of hypermagnesemia (dizziness, palpitations, altered mental status, fatigue, weakness).

---

# mannitol

man-it-ol
(Aridol, Osmitrol)
**Do not confuse Osmitrol with esmolol.**

■ **BLACK BOX ALERT** ■ May result in severe bronchospasm. Not recommended in pts with asthma.

### ◆CLASSIFICATION

**PHARMACOTHERAPEUTIC:** Polyol (sugar alcohol). **CLINICAL:** Osmotic diuretic.

## USES

Reduces increased ICP due to cerebral edema; IOP due to acute glaucoma. Promotes urinary excretion of toxic substances. **OFF-LABEL:** Improves renal transplant function. Severe, traumatic brain injury.

## PRECAUTIONS

**Contraindications:** Hypersensitivity to mannitol. Severe dehydration, active intracranial bleeding (except during craniotomy), severe pulmonary edema, congestion, severe renal disease (anuria), progressive HF. **Cautions:** Concurrent nephrotoxic agents, conditions increasing sensitivity to bronchoconstriction (e.g., recent abdominal, thoracic surgery), sepsis, preexisting renal disease, hypernatremia.

## ACTION

Elevates osmotic pressure of glomerular filtrate, inhibiting tubular reabsorption of water and electrolytes, resulting in increased urine output. Reduces intracranial pressure by decreasing blood viscosity, thereby increasing cerebral blood flow/oxygen transport. **Therapeutic Effect:** Produces diuresis; reduces intraocular pressure (IOP), intracranial pressure (ICP), cerebral edema.

## PHARMACOKINETICS

| Route | Onset | Peak | Duration |
|---|---|---|---|
| IV (diuresis) | 1–3 hrs | N/A | — |
| IV (reduced ICP) | 15–30 min | N/A | 1.5–6 hrs |

Remains in extracellular fluid. Primarily excreted unchanged in urine. Removed by hemodialysis. **Half-life:** 4.7 hrs.

## ⧖ LIFESPAN CONSIDERATIONS

**Pregnancy/Lactation:** Unknown if drug crosses placenta or is distributed in

---

breast milk. **Children:** Safety and efficacy not established in pts younger than 12 yrs. **Elderly:** Age-related renal impairment may require dosage adjustment.

## INTERACTIONS

**DRUG:** None significant. **HERBAL: Yohimbe** may decrease effects. **FOOD:** None known. **LAB VALUES:** May decrease serum phosphate, potassium, sodium.

## AVAILABILITY (Rx)

Injection Solution (Osmitrol): 20%, 25%.

## ADMINISTRATION/HANDLING

◀**ALERT**▶ Assess IV site for patency before each dose. Pain, thrombosis noted with extravasation. In-line filter (less than 5 microns) used for concentrations over 20%.

 **IV**

**Rate of Administration •** Administer test dose for pts with oliguria. • Give IV push over 3–5 min; over 30–60 min for cerebral edema, elevated ICP. Maximum concentration: 25%. • Do not add KCl or NaCl to mannitol 20% or greater. Do not add to whole blood for transfusion.
**Storage •** Store at room temperature. • If crystals are noted in solution, warm bottle in hot water, shake vigorously at intervals. Cool to body temperature before administration. Do not use if crystals remain after warming procedure.

## ▨ IV INCOMPATIBILITIES

Cefepime (Maxipime), filgrastim (Neupogen), imipenem-cilastatin (Primaxin).

## ▨ IV COMPATIBILITIES

Cisplatin (Platinol), furosemide (Lasix), linezolid (Zyvox), ondansetron (Zofran), propofol (Diprivan).

## INDICATIONS/ROUTES/DOSAGE

**Usual Dosage**
**Elevated Intracranial Pressure**
**IV: ADULTS, ELDERLY:** 0.25–1 g/kg/dose. May repeat q6–8h as needed. **CHILDREN:**

0.25–1 g/kg/dose; repeat to maintain serum osmolality <300–320 mOsm/kg.

**Dosage in Renal Impairment**
Contraindicated with severe impairment; caution with underlying renal disease.

**Dosage in Hepatic Impairment**
No dose adjustment.

## SIDE EFFECTS

**Frequent:** Dry mouth, thirst. **Occasional:** Blurred vision, increased urinary frequency/volume, headache, arm pain, backache, nausea, vomiting, urticaria, dizziness, hypotension, hypertension, tachycardia, fever, angina-like chest pain.

## ADVERSE EFFECTS/ TOXIC REACTIONS

Fluid, electrolyte imbalance may occur due to rapid administration of large doses or inadequate urine output resulting in overexpansion of extracellular fluid. Circulatory overload may produce pulmonary edema, HF. Excessive diuresis may produce hypokalemia, hyponatremia. Fluid loss in excess of electrolyte excretion may produce hypernatremia, hyperkalemia.

## NURSING CONSIDERATIONS

### BASELINE ASSESSMENT

Obtain baseline B/P, pulse. Assess skin turgor, mucous membranes, mental status, muscle strength. Obtain baseline weight, chemistry studies. Assess I&O.

### INTERVENTION/EVALUATION

Monitor urinary output to ascertain therapeutic response. Monitor serum electrolytes, serum osmolarity, ICP, renal function, LFT. Assess vital signs, skin turgor, mucous membranes. Weigh daily. Monitor for signs of hypernatremia. (confusion, drowsiness, thirst, dry mouth, cold/clammy skin); signs of hypokalemia (changes in muscle strength, tremors, muscle cramps, altered mental status, cardiac arrhythmias). Signs of hyperkalemia include colic, diarrhea, muscle

M

twitching followed by weakness, paralysis, arrhythmias.

**PATIENT/FAMILY TEACHING**

• Expect increased urinary frequency/volume. • May cause dry mouth.

# meclizine

**mek**-li-zeen
(Dramamine Less Drowsy)
**Do not confuse Antivert with Alavert or Axert.**

## ◆CLASSIFICATION

**PHARMACOTHERAPEUTIC:** Anticholinergic. **CLINICAL:** Antiemetic, antivertigo.

## USES

Prevention/treatment of vertigo due to motion sickness. Treatment of vertigo associated with diseases affecting vestibular system.

## PRECAUTIONS

**Contraindications:** Hypersensitivity to meclizine. **Cautions:** Narrow-angle glaucoma, asthma, CNS disorders where CNS depression is present; prostatic hyperplasia, pyloric/duodenal obstruction, bladder neck obstruction, elderly.

## ACTION

Reduces labyrinthine excitability, diminishes vestibular stimulation of labyrinth, blocks anticholinergic action of chemoreceptor trigger zone. **Therapeutic Effect:** Reduces nausea, vomiting, vertigo.

## PHARMACOKINETICS

| Route | Onset | Peak | Duration |
|-------|-------|------|----------|
| PO | 30–60 min | N/A | 8–24 hrs |

Well absorbed from GI tract. Widely distributed. Metabolized in liver. Primarily excreted in urine. **Half-life:** 6 hrs.

## ⌛ LIFESPAN CONSIDERATIONS

**Pregnancy/Lactation:** Unknown if drug crosses placenta or is distributed in breast milk (may produce irritability in nursing infants). **Children/Elderly:** May be more sensitive to anticholinergic effects (e.g., dry mouth).

## INTERACTIONS

**DRUG: Alcohol, CNS depressants (e.g., morphine, phenobarbital, zolpidem)** may increase CNS depressant effect. **HERBAL:** None significant. **FOOD:** None known. **LAB VALUES:** May produce false-negative results in antigen skin testing unless meclizine is discontinued 4 days before testing.

## AVAILABILITY (Rx)

**Tablets (Antivert):** 12.5 mg, 25 mg. **(Dramamine Less Drowsy):** 25 mg. **Tablets (Chewable):** 25 mg.

## ADMINISTRATION/HANDLING

**PO**

• Give without regard to meals. • Scored tablets may be crushed.

## INDICATIONS/ROUTES/DOSAGE

**Motion Sickness**

**PO: ADULTS, ELDERLY, CHILDREN 12 YRS AND OLDER:** 25–50 mg 1 hr before travel. May repeat q24h if needed.

**Vertigo**

**PO: ADULTS, ELDERLY, CHILDREN 12 YRS AND OLDER:** 25–100 mg/day in divided doses, as needed.

**Dosage in Renal/Hepatic Impairment**
No dose adjustment.

## SIDE EFFECTS

**Frequent:** Drowsiness. **Occasional:** Blurred vision, dry mouth, nose, throat.

## ADVERSE EFFECTS/TOXIC REACTIONS

Hypersensitivity reaction (eczema, pruritus, rash, cardiac disturbances, photosensitivity) may occur. Overdose may vary from CNS depression (sedation, apnea, cardiovascular collapse, death) to severe paradoxical reaction (hallucinations, tremor, seizures). Children may experience paradoxical reaction (restlessness, insomnia, euphoria, anxiety, tremors). Overdose in children may result in hallucinations, seizures, death.

## NURSING CONSIDERATIONS

### BASELINE ASSESSMENT
Assess degree of nausea/vomiting, degree of vertigo. Assess LOC.

### INTERVENTION/EVALUATION
Monitor B/P, esp. in elderly (increased risk of hypotension). Monitor children closely for paradoxical reaction. Monitor serum electrolytes in pts with severe vomiting. Assess skin turgor, mucous membranes to evaluate hydration status.

### PATIENT/FAMILY TEACHING
• Avoid tasks that require alertness, motor skills until response to drug is established. • Dry mouth, drowsiness, dizziness may be an expected response to drug. • Tolerance to sedative effect may occur. • Avoid alcohol. • Sugarless gum, sips of water may relieve dry mouth. • Coffee, tea may help reduce drowsiness.

# *medroxy-PROGESTERone

me-**drox**-ee-proe-**jes**-ter-one
(Apo-Medroxy ✦, Depo-Provera, Depo-SubQ Provera 104, Novo-Medrone ✦, Provera)

■ **BLACK BOX ALERT** ■ Prolonged use (over 2 yrs) of contraceptive injection form may result in loss of bone mineral density. Limit long-term use (more than 2 yrs). May increase risk of dementia in postmenopausal women. Increased risk of invasive breast cancer in postmenopausal women in combination with conjugated estrogens. **Do not confuse medroxyprogesterone with hydroxyprogesterone, methylprednisolone, or methyltestosterone, or Provera with Covera, Femara, Parlodel, or Premarin.**

## ◆ CLASSIFICATION

**PHARMACOTHERAPEUTIC:** Hormone. **CLINICAL:** Progestin, antineoplastic, contraceptive hormone.

## USES

**PO:** Reduction of endometrial hyperplasia in nonhysterectomized postmenopausal women (concurrently given with estrogen to women with intact uterus), treatment of secondary amenorrhea, abnormal uterine bleeding due to hormonal imbalance. **IM:** Adjunctive therapy, palliative treatment of inoperable, recurrent, metastatic endometrial carcinoma; prevention of pregnancy, endometriosis-associated pain. **OFF-LABEL:** Treatment of paraphilia/hypersexuality.

## PRECAUTIONS

**Contraindications:** Hypersensitivity to medroxyprogesterone. Carcinoma of breast, or other progesterone-dependent or estrogen-dependent neoplasm, history of or active thrombotic disorders (cerebral apoplexy, thrombophlebitis, thromboembolic disorders), known or suspected pregnancy, missed abortion, severe hepatic impairment, undiagnosed abnormal vaginal bleeding, cerebrovascular disease, use as pregnancy test. **Cautions:** Pts with conditions aggravated by fluid retention (asthma, seizures, migraine, cardiac/renal dysfunction), diabetes, history of mental depression, preexisting hypercholesterolemia, hypertriglyceridemia.

## ACTION

Inhibits secretion of pituitary gonadotropins. **Therapeutic Effect:** Prevents

M

follicular maturation, ovulation. Causes endometrial thinning.

## PHARMACOKINETICS

Well absorbed after PO administration. Slowly absorbed after IM administration. Protein binding: 90%. Metabolized in liver. Primarily excreted in urine. **Half-life: PO:** 12–17 hrs. **IM:** 40–50 days.

## ⧗ LIFESPAN CONSIDERATIONS

**Pregnancy/Lactation:** Avoid use during pregnancy, esp. first 4 mos (congenital heart, limb reduction defects may occur). Distributed in breast milk. **Children:** Safety and efficacy not established. **Elderly:** No age-related precautions noted.

## INTERACTIONS

**DRUG: CYP3A inducers (e.g., carbamazepine, phenytoin, rifampin)** may decrease effects. **HERBAL: St. John's wort** may decrease effect of progestin contraceptive. **FOOD:** None known. **LAB VALUES:** May alter serum thyroid, LFT, PT, HDL, total cholesterol, triglycerides; metapyrone test. May increase LDL.

## AVAILABILITY (Rx)

**Injection Suspension:** 104 mg/0.65 ml prefilled syringe (Depo-SubQ Provera 104), 150 mg/ml (Depo-Provera), 400 mg/ml (Depo-Provera). **Tablets (Provera):** 2.5 mg, 5 mg, 10 mg.

## ADMINISTRATION/HANDLING

**IM**
• Shake vial immediately before administering (ensures complete suspension).
• Administer deep IM into gluteal or deltoid muscle.

**SQ**
• Shake vigorously prior to administration. • Inject in upper thigh or abdomen (avoid bony areas and umbilicus). • Give over 5–7 sec; do not rub injection area.

**PO**
• Give with food.

## INDICATIONS/ROUTES/DOSAGE

**Endometrial Hyperplasia**
**PO: ADULTS:** 5–10 mg/day for 12–14 consecutive days each month starting on day 1 or 16 of cycle.

**Secondary Amenorrhea**
**PO: ADULTS:** 5–10 mg/day for 5–10 days, beginning at any time during menstrual cycle.

**Abnormal Uterine Bleeding**
**PO: ADULTS:** 5–10 mg/day for 5–10 days, beginning on calculated day 16 or day 21 of menstrual cycle.

**Endometrial Carcinoma**
**IM: ADULTS, ELDERLY:** Initially, 400–1,000 mg; repeat at 1-wk intervals. If improvement occurs and disease is stabilized, begin maintenance with as little as 400 mg/mo.

**Pregnancy Prevention**
**IM:** *(Depo-Provera):* **ADULTS:** 150 mg q3mos.
**SQ:** *(Depo-Subq Provera 104):* **ADULTS:** 104 mg q3mos (q12–14wks).

**Endometriosis-Associated Pain**
**SQ:** *(Depo-Subq Provera 104):* **ADULTS:** 104 mg q3mos (q12–14 wks) for up to 2 yrs.

**Dosage in Renal Impairment**
No dose adjustment.

**Dosage in Hepatic Impairment**
Contraindicated with severe impairment.

## SIDE EFFECTS

**Frequent:** Transient menstrual abnormalities (spotting, change in menstrual flow/cervical secretions, amenorrhea) at initiation of therapy. **Occasional:** Edema, weight change, breast tenderness, anxiety, insomnia, fatigue, dizziness. **Rare:** Alopecia, depression, dermatologic changes, headache, fever, nausea.

**M**

## ADVERSE EFFECTS/ TOXIC REACTIONS

Thrombophlebitis, pulmonary/cerebral embolism, retinal thrombosis occur rarely.

## NURSING CONSIDERATIONS

### BASELINE ASSESSMENT

Obtain usual menstrual history. Question for hypersensitivity to progestins, possibility of pregnancy before initiating therapy. Obtain baseline weight, serum glucose, B/P.

### INTERVENTION/EVALUATION

Check weight daily; report wkly gain of 5 lb or more. Assess B/P periodically. Assess skin for rash, urticaria. Report development of chest pain, sudden shortness of breath, sudden decrease in vision, migraine headache, pain (esp. with swelling, warmth, redness) in calves, numbness of arm/leg (thrombotic disorders) immediately.

### PATIENT/FAMILY TEACHING

• Report sudden loss of vision, severe headache, chest pain, coughing up of blood (hemoptysis), numbness in arm/leg, severe pain/swelling in calf, unusual heavy vaginal bleeding, severe abdominal pain/tenderness.
• Depo-Provera Contraceptive injection should be used as long-term birth control method (e.g., longer than 2 yrs) only if other birth control methods are inadequate.

---

## *megestrol*    HIGH ALERT

meh-**jes**-trol
(Megace, Megace ES, Megace OS ✤)
**Do not confuse megestrol with mesalamine.**

### ◆ CLASSIFICATION

**PHARMACOTHERAPEUTIC:** Synthetic hormone. **CLINICAL:** Antineoplastic, progestin.

## USES

Palliative treatment of advanced endometrial or breast carcinoma; treatment of anorexia, cachexia, unexplained significant weight loss in pts with AIDS.

## PRECAUTIONS

**Contraindications:** Hypersensitivity to megestrol. **Suspension:** Known or suspected pregnancy. **Cautions:** History of thrombophlebitis, elderly.

## ACTION

Antiestrogenic; interferes with normal estrogen cycle by decreasing release of luteinizing hormone (LH) from anterior pituitary gland by inhibiting pituitary function. May increase appetite by antagonizing metabolic effects of catabolic cytokines. **Therapeutic Effect:** Reduces tumor size. Increases appetite.

## PHARMACOKINETICS

Well absorbed from GI tract. Metabolized in liver. Excreted in urine. **Half-life:** 13–105 hrs (mean 34 hrs).

## ⧗ LIFESPAN CONSIDERATIONS

**Pregnancy/Lactation:** If possible, avoid use during pregnancy, esp. first 4 mos. Breastfeeding not recommended. **Children:** Safety and efficacy not established. **Elderly:** No age-related precautions noted.

## INTERACTIONS

**DRUG:** None significant. **HERBAL:** Avoid **black cohosh, dong quai** in estrogen-dependent tumors. Avoid **herbs with progestogenic properties (e.g., chasteberry);** may increase adverse effects. **FOOD:** None known. **LAB VALUES:** May alter serum thyroid, LFT, PT, HDL, total cholesterol, triglycerides. May increase LDL.

## AVAILABILITY (Rx)

**Oral Suspension:** 40 mg/ml (Megace), 625 mg/5 ml (Megace ES). **Tablets (Megace):** 20 mg, 40 mg.

## ADMINISTRATION/HANDLING

### PO

• Store tablets, oral suspension at room temperature. • Shake suspension well

**M**

---

before use. • Oral suspension compatible with water, orange juice, apple juice. • Administer without regard to food.

## INDICATIONS/ROUTES/DOSAGE

**Palliative Treatment of Advanced Breast Cancer**
**PO: ADULTS, ELDERLY:** 40 mg 4 times/day for at least 2 mos.

**Palliative Treatment of Advanced Endometrial Carcinoma**
**PO: ADULTS, ELDERLY:** 40–320 mg/day in divided doses for at least 2 mos.

**Anorexia, Cachexia, Weight Loss**
**PO:** *(Megace):* **ADULTS, ELDERLY:** (125 mg/ml suspension) 625 mg (5 ml) or (40 mg/ml suspension) 800 mg (20 ml)/day. **PO:** *(Megace ES):* **ADULTS, ELDERLY:** 625 mg/day.

**Dosage in Renal Impairment**
Use caution.

**Dosage in Hepatic Impairment**
No dose adjustment.

## SIDE EFFECTS

**Frequent:** Weight gain secondary to increased appetite. **Occasional:** Nausea, breakthrough menstrual bleeding, backache, headache, breast tenderness, carpal tunnel syndrome. **Rare:** Feeling of coldness.

## ADVERSE EFFECTS/ TOXIC REACTIONS

Thrombophlebitis, pulmonary embolism occur rarely.

## NURSING CONSIDERATIONS

### BASELINE ASSESSMENT

Question for possibility of pregnancy. Provide support to pt, family, recognizing this drug is palliative, not curative.

### INTERVENTION/EVALUATION

Monitor for tumor response. Monitor pt weight, caloric intake (appetite stimulant).

### PATIENT/FAMILY TEACHING

• Contraception is imperative. • Report lower leg (calf) pain, difficulty breathing, vaginal bleeding. • May cause headache, nausea, vomiting, breast tenderness, backache.

# meloxicam

mel-**ox**-i-kam
(Apo-Meloxicam ✹, Mobic, Vivolex)
■ **BLACK BOX ALERT** ■ Increased risk of serious cardiovascular thrombotic events, including myocardial infarction, CVA. Increased risk of severe GI reactions, including ulceration, bleeding, GI perforation.

## ◆CLASSIFICATION

**PHARMACOTHERAPEUTIC:** NSAID. **CLINICAL:** Anti-inflammatory, analgesic.

## USES

Relief of signs/symptoms of osteoarthritis, rheumatoid arthritis (RA). Treatment of juvenile idiopathic arthritis (JIA).

## PRECAUTIONS

**Contraindications:** Hypersensitivity to meloxicam. Pts with aspirin triad (asthma, rhinitis, aspirin intolerance). History of asthma, urticaria with NSAIDs, perioperative pain in setting of CABG surgery. **Cautions:** Renal/hepatic impairment, asthma, coagulation disorders, hypertension, history of GI disease (bleeding or ulcers), concurrent use of anticoagulants, fluid retention, HF, dehydration, smoking, alcohol use, elderly, debilitated.

## ACTION

Produces analgesic, antipyretic, anti-inflammatory effects by inhibiting prostaglandin synthesis. **Therapeutic Effect:** Reduces inflammatory response, intensity of pain.

## PHARMACOKINETICS

| Route | Onset | Peak | Duration |
|-------|-------|------|----------|
| PO (analgesic) | 30 min | 4–5 hrs | N/A |

Well absorbed after PO administration. Protein binding: 99%. Metabolized in liver. Eliminated equally in urine, feces. Not removed by hemodialysis. **Half-life:** 15–20 hrs.

## ⧖ LIFESPAN CONSIDERATIONS

**Pregnancy/Lactation:** Distributed in breast milk. **Children:** Safety and efficacy not established. **Elderly:** Age-related renal impairment may require dosage adjustment. More susceptible to GI toxicity; lower dosage recommended.

## INTERACTIONS

**DRUG:** May decrease antihypertensive effects of **ACE inhibitors (e.g., enalapril, lisinopril).** May increase risk of nephrotoxicity with **cyclosporine. Aspirin** may increase risk of epigastric distress (heartburn, indigestion). **Warfarin, aspirin** may increase risk of bleeding. May increase concentration, risk of toxicity of **lithium. HERBAL:** Cat's claw, **dong quai, evening primrose, feverfew, garlic, ginger, ginkgo, green tea, red clover, SAMe** may increase antiplatelet activity, risk of bleeding. **FOOD:** None known. **LAB VALUES:** May increase serum creatinine, ALT, AST.

## AVAILABILITY (Rx)

**Oral Suspension:** *(Mobic):* 7.5 mg/5 ml. **Tablets:** *(Mobic):* 7.5 mg, 15 mg. *(Vivolex):* 5 mg, 10 mg.

## ADMINISTRATION/HANDLING

**PO**
• Give with food or milk to minimize GI irritation. Shake oral suspension gently before administering.

## INDICATIONS/ROUTES/DOSAGE

**Osteoarthritis, Rheumatoid Arthritis (RA)**
**PO:** *(Mobic):* **ADULTS, ELDERLY:** Initially, 7.5 mg/day. **Maximum:** 15 mg/day (7.5 mg for pts on dialysis).

**Osteoarthritis**
**PO:** *(Vivolex):* **ADULTS, ELDERLY:** Initially, 5 mg once daily. May increase to 10 mg once daily.

**JIA**
**PO:** **CHILDREN, 2 YRS AND OLDER:** 0.125 mg/kg once daily. **Maximum:** 7.5 mg.

**Dosage in Renal Impairment**
Not recommended with severe impairment.

**Dosage in Hepatic Impairment**
No dose adjustment.

## SIDE EFFECTS

**Frequent (9%–7%):** Dyspepsia, headache, diarrhea, nausea. **Occasional (4%–3%):** Dizziness, insomnia, rash, pruritus, flatulence, constipation, vomiting. **Rare (less than 2%):** Drowsiness, urticaria, photosensitivity, tinnitus.

## ADVERSE EFFECTS/ TOXIC REACTIONS

In pts treated chronically, peptic ulcer, GI bleeding, gastritis, severe hepatic reaction (jaundice), nephrotoxicity (hematuria, dysuria, proteinuria), severe hypersensitivity reaction (bronchospasm, angioedema) occur rarely.

## NURSING CONSIDERATIONS

### BASELINE ASSESSMENT

Assess onset, type, location, duration of pain/inflammation. Inspect appearance of affected joints for immobility, deformities, skin condition. Question history of GI bleeding, gastric or duodenal ulcers, hepatic/renal impairment, asthma.

### INTERVENTION/EVALUATION

Monitor CBC, BMP, LFT. Assess skin for petechiae. Assess for therapeutic response: relief of pain, stiffness, swelling; increased joint mobility; reduced joint tenderness; improved grip strength. Monitor for abdominal pain, hematemesis.

### PATIENT/FAMILY TEACHING

• Take with food, milk to reduce GI upset. • Report tinnitus, persistent abdominal pain/cramping, severe nausea, vomiting, difficulty breathing, unusual bruising or bleeding, rash, peripheral edema, chest pain, palpitations.

---

## melphalan                    `HIGH ALERT`

mel-fa-lan
(Alkeran, Evomela)

■ **BLACK BOX ALERT** ■ Myelosuppression is common. Potentially mutagenic, leukemogenic. Hypersensitivity noted with IV administration. Must be administered by certified chemotherapy personnel.
**Do not confuse Alkeran with Leukeran or Myleran, or melphalan with Mephyton or Myleran.**

### ◆CLASSIFICATION

**PHARMACOTHERAPEUTIC:** Alkylating agent. **CLINICAL:** Antineoplastic.

### USES

Treatment of nonresectable epithelial ovarian carcinoma, multiple myeloma. **OFF-LABEL:** Hodgkin's lymphoma, malignant melanoma, neuroblastoma, induction regimen for bone marrow and stem cell transplantation, light chain amyloidosis, Ewing's sarcoma.

### PRECAUTIONS

**Contraindications:** Hypersensitivity to melphalan. Resistance to prior melphalan therapy. **Cautions:** Pre-existing bone marrow suppression, renal impairment, pregnancy, prior chemotherapy or irradiation.

### ACTION

Inhibits protein synthesis primarily by cross-linking strands of DNA, RNA. Cell cycle–phase nonspecific. **Therapeutic Effect:** Disrupts nucleic acid function, producing tumor cell death.

### PHARMACOKINETICS

Oral administration is highly variable. Incomplete intestinal absorption, variable first-pass metabolism, rapid hydrolysis may result. Protein binding: 60%–90%. Extensively metabolized in blood. Eliminated from plasma primarily by chemical hydrolysis. Partially excreted in feces; minimal elimination in urine. **Half-life: PO:** 1–1.25 hrs. **IV:** 1.5 hrs.

### 🖄 LIFESPAN CONSIDERATIONS

**Pregnancy/Lactation:** May cause fetal harm. Unknown if distributed in breast milk. **Children:** Safety and efficacy not established. **Elderly:** Age-related renal impairment may require dosage adjustment.

### INTERACTIONS

**DRUG: Bone marrow depressants** may increase myelosuppression. **Live virus vaccines** may potentiate virus replication, increase vaccine side effects, decrease pt's antibody response to vaccine. **HERBAL: Echinacea** may decrease effects. **FOOD:** None known. **LAB VALUES:** May increase serum uric acid.

### AVAILABILITY (Rx)

**Injection, Powder for Reconstitution:** 50 mg. **Tablets (Alkeran):** 2 mg.

### ADMINISTRATION/HANDLING
 IV

**Reconstitution** • Reconstitute 50-mg vial with diluent supplied by manufacturer to yield 5 mg/ml solution. • Further dilute with 0.9% NaCl to final concentration not exceeding 0.45 mg/ml.
**Rate of Administration** • Infuse over 15–30 min at rate not to exceed 10 mg/min (total infusion should be administered within 1 hr).
**Storage** • Store at room temperature; protect from light. • Once reconstituted, complete administration within 60 min.

---

## PO

• Store tablets in refrigerator; protect from light. • Give on empty stomach (1 hr before or 2 hrs after meals).

###  IV INCOMPATIBILITIES

Amphotericin B complex (Abelcet, AmBisome, Amphotec).

###  IV COMPATIBILITIES

Acyclovir, dexamethasone (Decadron), famotidine (Pepcid), furosemide (Lasix), lorazepam (Ativan), morphine.

### INDICATIONS/ROUTES/DOSAGE

**Note: WBC less than 3,000/mm³, platelets less than 100,000/mm³:** Withhold treatment until recovery.

**Ovarian Carcinoma**
**PO: ADULTS, ELDERLY:** 0.2 mg/kg/day for 5 successive days. Repeat at 4- to 5-wk intervals.

**Multiple Myeloma**
**PO: ADULTS:** Initially, 6 mg once daily for 2–3 wks, followed by up to 4 wks rest, then maintenance dose of 2 mg daily; or 0.15 mg/kg/day for 7 days with 2–6 wks rest, then maintenance dose of 0.05 mg/kg/day; or 0.25 mg/kg/day for 4 days, repeat at 4- to 6-wk intervals.
**IV: ADULTS:** 16 mg/m²/dose every 2 wks for 4 doses, then repeat monthly after hematologic recovery.

**Dosage in Renal Impairment**
**IV: BUN LEVEL GREATER THAN 30 MG/DL:** Decrease melphalan dosage by 50%.

**Dosage in Hepatic Impairment**
No dose adjustment.

### SIDE EFFECTS

**Frequent:** Nausea, vomiting (may be severe with large dose). **Occasional:** Diarrhea, stomatitis, rash, pruritus, alopecia.

### ADVERSE EFFECTS/ TOXIC REACTIONS

Myelosuppression manifested as hematologic toxicity (principally leukopenia, thrombocytopenia, and, to lesser extent, anemia, pancytopenia, agranulocytosis). Leukopenia may occur as early as 5 days after drug initiation. WBC, platelet counts return to normal during 5th wk after therapy, but leukopenia, thrombocytopenia may last more than 6 wks after discontinuing drug. Hyperuricemia noted by hematuria, crystalluria, flank pain.

### NURSING CONSIDERATIONS

#### BASELINE ASSESSMENT

Obtain CBC, then wkly thereafter. Dosage may be decreased or discontinued if WBC falls below 3,000/mm³ or platelet count falls below 100,000/mm³. Antiemetics may be effective in preventing/treating nausea, vomiting.

#### INTERVENTION/EVALUATION

Monitor CBC with differential, serum electrolytes. Monitor for stomatitis. Monitor for hematologic toxicity (fever, sore throat, signs of local infection, unusual bruising/bleeding from any site), symptoms of anemia (excessive fatigue, weakness), signs of hyperuricemia (hematuria, flank pain). Avoid IM injections, rectal temperatures, other traumas that may induce bleeding.

#### PATIENT/FAMILY TEACHING

• Increase fluid intake (may protect against hyperuricemia). • Maintain strict oral hygiene. • Hair loss is reversible, but new hair growth may have different color, texture. • Avoid crowds, those with infections. • Report fever, shortness of breath, cough, sore throat, bleeding, unusual bruising.

**M**

---

# memantine  <sup>TOP 100</sup>

me-**man**-teen
(Apo-Memantine ✦, Ebixa ✦, Namenda, Namenda XR)

---

**M**

## FIXED-COMBINATION(S)

Namzaric: memantine/donepazil (a cholinesterase inhibitor): 7 mg/10 mg; 14 mg/10 mg; 21 mg/ 10 mg; 28 mg/10 mg.

## ◆CLASSIFICATION

**PHARMACOTHERAPEUTIC:** Neurotransmitter inhibitor. **CLINICAL:** Anti-Alzheimer's agent.

## USES

Treatment of moderate to severe dementia of Alzheimer's type. **OFF-LABEL:** Treatment of mild to moderate vascular dementia.

## PRECAUTIONS

**Contraindications:** Hypersensitivity to memantine. **Cautions:** Moderate to severe renal impairment, severe hepatic impairment, cardiovascular disease, seizure disorder, GU conditions that raise urine pH level.

## ACTION

Decreases effects of glutamate, the principal excitatory neurotransmitter in the brain. Persistent CNS excitation by glutamate is thought to cause symptoms of Alzheimer's disease. **Therapeutic Effect:** May inhibit clinical deterioration in moderate to severe Alzheimer's disease.

## PHARMACOKINETICS

Rapidly, completely absorbed after PO administration. Protein binding: 45%. Undergoes little metabolism; most of dose is excreted unchanged in urine. **Half-life:** 60–80 hrs.

## ⧗ LIFESPAN CONSIDERATIONS

**Pregnancy/Lactation:** Unknown if drug crosses placenta or is distributed in breast milk. **Children:** Not prescribed for this pt population. **Elderly:** No age-related precautions noted, but use is not recommended in pts with severe renal impairment (CrCl less than 9 ml/min).

## INTERACTIONS

**DRUG: Urine alkalinizers (e.g., carbonic anhydrase inhibitors, sodium bicarbonate)** may decrease renal elimination. **HERBAL:** None significant. **FOOD:** None known. **LAB VALUES:** None significant.

## AVAILABILITY (Rx)

**Oral Solution:** 2 mg/ml. **Tablets:** 5 mg, 10 mg.

⧉ **Capsules (Extended-Release [Namenda XR]):** 7 mg, 14 mg, 21 mg, 28 mg.

## ADMINISTRATION/HANDLING

**PO**

• Give without regard to food. • Administer oral solution using syringe provided. Do not dilute or mix with other fluids. • Give extended-release capsules whole. Do not crush. May open capsule and sprinkle on applesauce; give immediately.

## INDICATIONS/ROUTES/DOSAGE

**Alzheimer's Disease**

**PO: ADULTS, ELDERLY (Immediate-Release):** Initially, 5 mg once daily. May increase dosage at intervals of at least 1 wk in 5-mg increments to 10 mg/day (5 mg twice daily), then 15 mg/day (5 mg and 10 mg as separate doses), and finally 20 mg/day (10 mg twice daily). Target dose: 20 mg/day. **(Extended-Release):** Initially, 7 mg once daily. May increase at intervals of at least 7 days in increments of 7 mg. **Maximum:** 28 mg once daily. Switching from immediate-release to extended-release: Begin the day following last dose of immediate release. 10 mg twice daily: 28 mg once daily. 5 mg twice daily: 14 mg once daily.

**Dosage in Renal Impairment**

| Creatinine Clearance | Dosage | |
|---|---|---|
| | Immediate-Release | Extended-Release |
| 30 ml/min or greater | No adjustments | No adjustments |
| 5–29 ml/min | 5 mg twice daily or 10 mg once daily | 14 mg once daily |

**Dosage in Hepatic Impairment**
**Mild to moderate impairment:** No dose adjustment. **Severe impairment:** Use caution.

## SIDE EFFECTS

**Occasional (7%–4%):** Dizziness, headache, confusion, constipation, hypertension, cough. **Rare (3%–2%):** Back pain, nausea, fatigue, anxiety, peripheral edema, arthralgia, insomnia.

## ADVERSE EFFECTS/ TOXIC REACTIONS

None known.

## NURSING CONSIDERATIONS

### BASELINE ASSESSMENT
Assess cognitive, behavioral, functional deficits of pt. Assess renal function.

### INTERVENTION/EVALUATION
Monitor cognitive, behavioral, functional status of pt. Monitor urine pH (alterations of urine pH toward the alkaline condition may lead to accumulation of the drug with possible increase in side effects). Monitor BUN, CrCl, serum creatinine lab values.

### PATIENT/FAMILY TEACHING
• Do not reduce or stop medication; do not increase dosage without physician direction. • Ensure adequate fluid intake. • If therapy is interrupted for several days, restart at lowest dose, titrate to current dose at minimum of 1-wk intervals. • Local chapter of Alzheimer's Disease Association can provide a guide to services.

---

## mepolizumab

me-poe-**liz**-ue-mab
(Nucala)
**Do not confuse mepolizumab with atezolizumab, certolizumab, eculizumab, omalizumab, pembrolizumab, or Nucala with Calan or Nucynta.**

## ◆CLASSIFICATION

**PHARMACOTHERAPEUTIC:** Interleukin-5 receptor antagonist. Monoclonal antibody. **CLINICAL:** Antiasthmatic.

## USES

Add-on maintenance treatment of pts with severe asthma and with an eosinophil phenotype.

## PRECAUTIONS

**Contraindications:** Hypersensitivity to mepolizumab. **Cautions:** History of herpes zoster infection, parasitic infection. Not indicated for treatment of other eosinophilic conditions; relief of acute bronchospasm, status asthmaticus, exercise-induced bronchospasm.

## ACTION

Inhibits signaling of interleukin-5 cytokine, reducing production and survival of eosinophils responsible for asthmatic inflammation and pathogenesis. **Therapeutic Effect:** Prevents inflammatory process; relieves signs/symptoms of asthma.

## PHARMACOKINETICS

Widely distributed. Degraded into small peptides and amino acids via proteolytic enzymes. Elimination not specified. **Half-life:** 16–22 days.

## LIFESPAN CONSIDERATIONS

**Pregnancy/Lactation:** Unknown if distributed in breast milk. However, human immunoglobulin G is present in breast milk and is known to cross placenta. **Children:** Safety and efficacy not established in pts younger than 12 yrs. **Elderly:** Safety and efficacy not established.

## INTERACTIONS

**DRUG:** None known. **HERBAL:** None significant. **FOOD:** None known. **LAB VALUES:** None known.

M

---

## AVAILABILITY (Rx)

**Injection Powder:** 100 mg.

## ADMINISTRATION/HANDLING

**Subcutaneous**

**Reconstitution** • Using a 2- or 3-ml syringe and 21G needle, reconstitute vial with 1.2 ml Sterile Water for Injection to a final concentration of 100 mg/ml. • Direct stream vertically onto center of the lyophilized cake. • Gently swirl in a circular motion for 10 secs at 15-sec intervals until fully dissolved (approx. 5 mins or more). • Do not shake (may cause foaming/precipitate formation). If mechanical reconstitution device is used, swirl at 450 rpm for up to 10 mins or at 1,000 rpm for up to 5 mins. • Visually inspect for particulate matter or discoloration. Solution should appear clear to opalescent, colorless to pale yellow or pale brown (essentially free of particles). Air bubbles are expected and allowed. • Do not use if solution is cloudy or discolored or if visible particles are observed.

**Administration** • Prior to administration, withdraw 1 ml of solution (100 mg) from vial. • Do not shake or agitate. • Using a polypropylene syringe fitted with a 21G–27G × 0.5 (13-mm) needle, subcutaneously insert needle into upper arms, outer thigh, or abdomen and inject solution. • Do not inject into areas of active skin disease or injury such as sunburns, skin rashes, inflammation, skin infections, or active psoriasis. • Rotate injection sites.

**Storage** • Store unused vials below 25°C (77°F). • Do not freeze. • Do not shake. • Protect from light. • May store reconstituted solution below 30°C (86°F) up to 8 hrs.

## INDICATIONS/ROUTES/DOSAGE

**Asthma (Severe)**

**SQ: ADULTS, ELDERLY, CHILDREN 12 YRS AND OLDER:** 100 mg once q4wks.

**Dosage in Renal/Hepatic Impairment**
No dose adjustment.

## SIDE EFFECTS

**Frequent (19%):** Headache. **Occasional (8%–3%):** Injection site reaction (pain, erythema, swelling, itching, burning sensation), back pain, fatigue, eczema, abdominal pain, pruritus, muscle spasms.

## ADVERSE EFFECTS/TOXIC REACTIONS

Hypersensitivity reactions including angioedema, bronchospasm, hypotension, urticaria, rash were reported. Hypersensitivity reactions typically occurred hrs to days after administration. Infections including herpes zoster, influenza, UTI may occur. Unknown if treatment will influence the immunological response to helminth (parasite) infection. Immunogenicity (auto-mepolizumab antibodies) reported in 6% of pts.

## NURSING CONSIDERATIONS

### BASELINE ASSESSMENT

Obtain apical pulse, oxygen saturation. Auscultate lung fields. Question history of herpes zoster infection, parasitic infection, hypersensitivity reaction. Pts with preexisting helminth (parasite) infection should be treated prior to initiation. Consider varicella vaccination before starting therapy. Inhaled or systemic corticosteroids should not be suddenly discontinued upon initiation. Corticosteroids that are not gradually reduced may cause withdrawal symptoms or unmask conditions that were originally suppressed with corticosteroid therapy.

### INTERVENTION/EVALUATION

Monitor rate, depth, rhythm of respirations. Assess lungs for wheezing, rales. Monitor oxygen saturation. Interrupt or discontinue treatment if hypersensitivity reaction, opportunistic infection (esp. parasite infection, herpes zoster infection); worsening of asthma-related symptoms (esp. in pts tapering off corticosteroids) occurs. Obtain pulmonary function test to assess disease improvement.

Monitor for increased use of rescue inhalers; may indicate deterioration of asthma.

### PATIENT/FAMILY TEACHING

• Not indicated for relief of acute asthmatic episodes. • Have a rescue inhaler readily available. • Increased use of rescue inhaler may indicate worsening of asthma. • Seek medical attention if asthma symptoms worsen or remain uncontrolled after starting treatment. • Immediately report allergic reactions such as difficulty breathing, itching, hives, rash, swelling of the face or tongue. • Report infections of any kind, esp. shingles (herpes zoster). • Do not stop corticosteroid therapy unless directed by prescriber.

# meropenem

mer-oh-**pen**-em
(Merrem)
**Do not confuse meropenem with doripenem, ertapenem, or imipenem.**

### ◆CLASSIFICATION

**PHARMACOTHERAPEUTIC:** Carbapenem. **CLINICAL:** Antibiotic.

## USES

Treatment of multidrug-resistant infections; meningitis in children 3 mos and older; intra-abdominal infections; complicated skin/skin structure infections caused by susceptible *S. aureus, S. pyogenes, S. agalactiae, S. pneumoniae, H. influenzae, N. meningitidis, M. catarrhalis, E. coli, Klebsiella, Enterobacter, Serratia, P. aeruginosa, B. fragilis.*
**OFF-LABEL:** Febrile neutropenia, liver abscess, otitis externa, prosthetic joint infection.

## PRECAUTIONS

**Contraindications:** Hypersensitivity to meropenem, other beta-lactams.

**Cautions:** Renal impairment, CNS disorders (particularly with history of seizures, concurrent use with valproic acid).

## ACTION

Binds to penicillin-binding proteins. Inhibits bacterial cell wall synthesis. **Therapeutic Effect:** Bactericidal.

## PHARMACOKINETICS

After IV administration, widely distributed into tissues and body fluids, including CSF. Protein binding: 2%. Primarily excreted unchanged in urine. Removed by hemodialysis. **Half-life:** 1 hr.

## ⧗ LIFESPAN CONSIDERATIONS

**Pregnancy/Lactation:** Unknown if distributed in breast milk. **Children:** Safety and efficacy not established in pts younger than 3 mos. **Elderly:** Age-related renal impairment may require dosage adjustment.

## INTERACTIONS

**DRUG:** May decrease effects of **valproic acid. HERBAL:** None significant. **FOOD:** None known. **LAB VALUES:** May increase serum BUN, alkaline phosphatase, LDH, ALT, AST, bilirubin. May decrease Hgb, Hct, WBC.

## AVAILABILITY (Rx)

**Injection, Powder for Reconstitution:** 500 mg, 1 g.

## ADMINISTRATION/HANDLING

 IV

**Reconstitution** • Reconstitute each 500 mg with 10 ml Sterile Water for Injection, 0.9% NaCl, or D₅W to provide concentration of 50 mg/ml. • Shake to dissolve until clear. • May further dilute with 0.9% NaCl or D₅W to a concentration of 1–20 mg/ml.
**Rate of Administration** • May give by IV push or IV intermittent infusion (piggyback). • If administering as IV

M

intermittent infusion (piggyback), give over 15–30 min (may also give over 3 hrs); if administered by IV push, give over 3–5 min (at a concentration not greater than 50 mg/ml).

**Storage** • Store vials at room temperature. • After reconstitution of vials with 0.9% NaCl, stable for 2 hrs at room temperature or 18 hrs if refrigerated (with D₅W, stable for 1 hr at room temperature, 8 hrs if refrigerated). IV infusion with 0.9% NaCl stable for 4 hrs at room temperature or 24 hrs if refrigerated (with D₅W, 1 hr at room temperature or 4 hrs if refrigerated).

## ▨ IV INCOMPATIBILITIES

Acyclovir (Zovirax), amphotericin B (Fungizone), diazepam (Valium), doxycycline (Vibramycin), metronidazole (Flagyl), ondansetron (Zofran).

## ▨ IV COMPATIBILITIES

Dexamethasone (Decadron), dobutamine (Dobutrex), dopamine (Intropin), furosemide (Lasix), heparin, magnesium, morphine.

## INDICATIONS/ROUTES/DOSAGE

**Usual Dosage**
IV: **ADULTS, ELDERLY:** 1.5–6 g/day in divided doses q8h. *(Extended-Infusion):* 0.5–2g over 3 hrs q8h. **CHILDREN, ADOLESCENTS WEIGHING MORE THAN 50 KG:** 1.5–6 g/day in divided doses q8h. **CHILDREN 3 MOS AND OLDER WEIGHING 50 KG OR LESS:** 30–120 mg/kg/day in divided doses q8h. **Maximum:** 6 g/day. **NEONATES:** 20 mg/kg/dose q8–12h.

**Meningitis**
IV: **ADULTS, ELDERLY, CHILDREN WEIGHING 50 KG OR MORE:** 2 g q8h. **CHILDREN 3 MOS AND OLDER WEIGHING LESS THAN 50 KG:** 40 mg/kg q8h. **Maximum:** 2 g/dose.

**Dosage in Renal Impairment**
Dosage and frequency are modified based on creatinine clearance.

| Creatinine Clearance | Dosage | Interval |
|---|---|---|
| 26–49 ml/min | Normal dose | q12h |
| 10–25 ml/min | 50% of normal dose | q12h |
| Less than 10 ml/min | 50% of normal dose | q24h |
| Hemodialysis: | 500 mg | q24h |
| Peritoneal dialysis: | Recommended dose (based on indication) | q24h |

**Continuous renal replacement therapy**

| | | |
|---|---|---|
| Continuous venovenous hemofiltration | 1 gram then 500 mg 1 gram | q8h OR q12h |
| Continuous venovenous hemodialysis/ continuous venovenous hemodiafiltration | 1 gram then 500 mg 1 gram | q6–8h OR q8–12h |

**Dosage in Hepatic Impairment**
No dose adjustment.

## SIDE EFFECTS

**Frequent (5%–3%):** Diarrhea, nausea, vomiting, headache, inflammation at injection site. **Occasional (2%):** Oral candidiasis, rash, pruritus. **Rare (less than 2%):** Constipation, glossitis.

## ADVERSE EFFECTS/ TOXIC REACTIONS

Antibiotic-associated colitis, other superinfections (abdominal cramps, severe watery diarrhea, fever) may result from altered bacterial balance in GI tract. Anaphylactic reactions have been reported. Seizures may occur in those with CNS disorders (e.g., brain lesions, history of seizures), bacterial meningitis, renal impairment.

## NURSING CONSIDERATIONS

### BASELINE ASSESSMENT

Question history of hypersensitivity, allergic reaction to penicillins, cephalosporins. Inquire about history of seizures.

### INTERVENTION/EVALUATION
Monitor daily pattern of bowel activity, stool consistency. Monitor for nausea, vomiting. Evaluate for inflammation at IV injection site. Assess skin for rash. Evaluate hydration status. Monitor I&O, renal function, LFT. Check mental status; be alert to tremors, possible seizures. Assess temperature, B/P twice daily, more often if necessary. Monitor serum electrolytes, esp. potassium.

### PATIENT/FAMILY TEACHING
• Report persistent diarrhea, abdominal cramps, fever.

# mesalamine

me-**sal**-a-meen
(Apriso, Asacol HD, Canasa, Delzicol, Lialda, Mesasal ✹, Pentasa, Rowasa, Salofalk ✹, sfRowasa)
**Do not confuse Asacol with Os-Cal, Lialda with Aldara, or mesalamine with megestrol, memantine, or methenamine.**

### ◆CLASSIFICATION
**PHARMACOTHERAPEUTIC:** Salicylic acid derivative. **CLINICAL:** Anti-inflammatory agent.

### USES
**PO:** Treatment, maintenance of remission of mild to moderate active ulcerative colitis. **Rectal:** Treatment of active mild to moderate distal ulcerative colitis, proctosigmoiditis or proctitis.

### PRECAUTIONS
**Contraindications:** Hypersensitivity to mesalamine, salicylates. **Cautions:** Sulfasalazine, active peptic ulcer, pyloric stenosis, pericarditis, myocarditis, renal/hepatic impairment, elderly.

### ACTION
Mechanism unknown. May modulate local mediators of inflammation, may inhibit tumor necrosis factor. **Therapeutic Effect:** Diminishes inflammation in colon.

### PHARMACOKINETICS
Poorly absorbed from colon. Moderately absorbed from GI tract. Metabolized in liver. Unabsorbed portion eliminated in feces; absorbed portion excreted in urine. Unknown if removed by hemodialysis. **Half-life:** 0.5–1.5 hrs; metabolite, 5–10 hrs.

### ⌛ LIFESPAN CONSIDERATIONS
**Pregnancy/Lactation:** Unknown if drug crosses placenta or is distributed in breast milk. **Children:** Safety and efficacy not established. **Elderly:** Age-related renal impairment may require dosage adjustment.

### INTERACTIONS
**DRUG:** None known. **HERBAL:** None significant. **FOOD:** None known. **LAB VALUES:** May increase serum alkaline phosphatase, ALT, AST, bilirubin.

### AVAILABILITY (Rx)
**Rectal Suspension (Rowasa, sfRowasa):** 4 g/60 ml. **Suppositories (Canasa):** 1 g.
🛡 **Capsules (Controlled-Release [Pentasa]):** 250 mg, 500 mg. **Capsules (Delayed-Release [Delzicol]):** 400 mg. 🛡 **Capsules (Extended-Release [Apriso]):** 375 mg. 🛡 **Tablets (Delayed-Release): (Asacol HD):** 800 mg. **(Lialda):** 1.2 g.

### ADMINISTRATION/HANDLING
◀**ALERT**▶ Store rectal suspension, suppository, oral forms at room temperature.

**PO**
• Have pt swallow whole; do not break outer coating of tablet. • Give without regard to food. **Apriso:** Do not administer with antacids. **Lialda:** Administer once daily with meal.

**Rectal**
• Shake bottle well. • Instruct pt to lie on left side with lower leg extended,

---

upper leg flexed forward. • Knee-chest position may also be used. • Insert applicator tip into rectum, pointing toward umbilicus. • Squeeze bottle steadily until contents are emptied. • Store suppositories at room temperature. Do not refrigerate.

## INDICATIONS/ROUTES/DOSAGE

**Treatment of Ulcerative Colitis**
**PO** *(Capsule [Pentasa]):* **ADULTS, ELDERLY:** 1 g 4 times daily. **CHILDREN:** 30–60 mg/kg/day divided q6–12h.
**PO** *(Capsule [Delzicol]):* **ADULTS, ELDERLY:** 800 mg 3 times daily. **CHILDREN 5 YRS AND OLDER, WEIGHING 54–90 KG:** 27–44 mg/kg/day in 2 divided doses. **Maximum:** 2,400 mg/day. **33–53 KG:** 37–61 mg/kg/day in 2 divided doses. **Maximum:** 2,000 mg/day. **17–32 KG:** 36–71 mg/kg/day in 2 divided doses. **Maximum:** 1,200 mg/day.
**PO** *(Tablet [Asacol HD]):* **ADULTS, ELDERLY:** 1.6 g 3 times daily. **CHILDREN:** 30–60 mg/kg/day divided q8–12h.
**PO** *(Tablet [Lialda]):* **ADULTS, ELDERLY:** 2.4–4.8 g once daily.

**Maintenance of Remission in Ulcerative Colitis**
**PO** *(Capsule [Pentasa]):* **ADULTS, ELDERLY:** 1 g 4 times daily.
**PO** *(Capsule [Delzicol]):* **ADULTS, ELDERLY:** 1.6 g/day in divided doses.
**PO** *(Capsule, Extended-Release [Apriso]):* **ADULTS, ELDERLY:** 1,500 mg once daily in the morning.
**PO** *(Tablet [Lialda]):* 2.4 g once daily with food.

**Distal Ulcerative Colitis, Proctosigmoiditis, Proctitis**
**Rectal** *(Retention Enema):* **ADULTS, ELDERLY:** 60 ml (4 g) at bedtime; retained overnight for approximately 8 hrs for 3–6 wks.
**Rectal** *(1 G Suppository):* **ADULTS, ELDERLY:** Once daily at bedtime. Continue therapy for 3–6 wks.
**◀ALERT▶** Suppository should be retained for 1–3 hrs for maximum benefit.

**Dosage of Renal/Hepatic Impairment**
Use caution.

## SIDE EFFECTS

Mesalamine is generally well tolerated, with only mild, transient effects. **Frequent (greater than 6%): PO:** Abdominal cramps/pain, diarrhea, dizziness, headache, nausea, vomiting, rhinitis, unusual fatigue. **Rectal:** Abdominal/stomach cramps, flatulence, headache, nausea. **Occasional (6%–2%): PO:** Hair loss, decreased appetite, back/joint pain, flatulence, acne. **Rectal:** Alopecia. **Rare (less than 2%): Rectal:** Anal irritation.

## ADVERSE EFFECTS/ TOXIC REACTIONS

Sulfite sensitivity may occur in susceptible pts, manifested as cramping, headache, diarrhea, fever, rash, urticaria, pruritus, wheezing. Discontinue drug immediately. Hepatitis, pancreatitis, pericarditis occur rarely with oral forms.

## NURSING CONSIDERATIONS

**BASELINE ASSESSMENT**
Obtain BUN, serum creatinine, LFT. Assess for abdominal pain, discomfort.

**INTERVENTION/EVALUATION**
Encourage adequate fluid intake. Assess bowel sounds for peristalsis. Monitor daily pattern of bowel activity, stool consistency; record time of evacuation. Assess for abdominal disturbances. Assess skin for rash, urticaria. Discontinue medication if rash, fever, cramping, diarrhea occurs.

**PATIENT/FAMILY TEACHING**
• Report rash, fever, abdominal pain, significant diarrhea. • Avoid tasks that require alertness, motor skills until response to drug is established. • May discolor urine yellow-brown. • Suppositories stain fabrics.

# mesna

**mess**-na
(Mesnex, Uromitexan ✦)

## ◆CLASSIFICATION

**PHARMACOTHERAPEUTIC:** Cytoprotective agent. **CLINICAL:** Antineoplastic adjunct, antidote.

## USES

Detoxifying agent used as protectant against hemorrhagic cystitis induced by ifosfamide. **OFF-LABEL:** Reduce incidence of cyclophosphamide-induced hemorrhagic cystitis with high-dose cyclophosphamide.

## PRECAUTIONS

**Contraindications:** Hypersensitivity to mesna. **Cautions:** Preexisting autoimmune disorders.

## ACTION

Binds with, detoxifies urotoxic metabolites of ifosfamide/cyclophosphamide. **Therapeutic Effect:** Inhibits ifosfamide/cyclophosphamide-induced hemorrhagic cystitis.

## PHARMACOKINETICS

Rapidly metabolized after IV administration to mesna disulfide, which is reduced to mesna in kidneys. Protein binding: 69%–75%. Excreted in urine. **Half-life:** 24 min; metabolite: 72 min.

## ⌛ LIFESPAN CONSIDERATIONS

**Pregnancy/Lactation:** Unknown if drug crosses placenta or is distributed in breast milk. **Children:** Safety and efficacy not established. **Elderly:** Information not available.

## INTERACTIONS

**DRUG:** None significant. **HERBAL:** None significant. **FOOD:** None known. **LAB VALUES:** May produce false-positive test result for urinary ketones.

## AVAILABILITY (Rx)

**Injection Solution:** 100 mg/ml. **Tablets:** 400 mg.

## ADMINISTRATION/HANDLING

 IV

**Reconstitution** • Dilute with $D_5W$ or 0.9% NaCl to concentration of 20 mg/ml. • May add to solutions containing ifosfamide or cyclophosphamide.
**Rate of Administration** • Administer by IV infusion over 15–30 min or by continuous infusion.
**Storage** • Store parenteral form at room temperature. • After dilution, in 0.9% NaCl or $D_5W$, stable for 48 hrs at room temperature (solutions of mesna and cyclophosphamide in $D_5W$ stable for 48 hrs if refrigerated or 6 hrs at room temperature). Discard unused medication.

**PO**
• Administer orally in either tablet formulation or parenteral solution. • Dilute mesna solution before PO administration to decrease sulfur odor. Can be diluted (1:1 to 1:10) in carbonated cola drinks, fruit juices, milk.

## ▦ IV INCOMPATIBILITIES

Amphotericin B complex (Abelcet, AmBisome, Amphotec), cisplatin (Platinol).

## ▦ IV COMPATIBILITIES

Allopurinol (Aloprim), docetaxel (Taxotere), doxorubicin (Adriamycin), etoposide (VePesid), gemcitabine (Gemzar), granisetron (Kytril), methotrexate, ondansetron (Zofran), paclitaxel (Taxol), vinorelbine (Navelbine).

## INDICATIONS/ROUTES/DOSAGE

**Prevention of Hemorrhagic Cystitis in Pts Receiving Ifosfamide**
**IV: ADULTS, ELDERLY:** 20% of ifosfamide dose at time of ifosfamide administration and 4 and 8 hrs after each dose of ifosfamide. **Total dose:** 60% of ifosfamide dosage. Range: 60%–160% of the daily ifosfamide dose.

M

**IV/PO:** 100% of ifosfamide dose, given as 20% at start time followed by 40% given orally 2 and 6 hrs after start of ifosfamide.

**Dosage in Renal/Hepatic Impairment**
No dose adjustment.

## SIDE EFFECTS

**Frequent (greater than 17%):** Altered taste, soft stools. **Large doses:** Diarrhea, myalgia, headache, fatigue, nausea, hypotension, allergic reaction.

## ADVERSE EFFECTS/ TOXIC REACTIONS

Hematuria occurs rarely.

## NURSING CONSIDERATIONS

### BASELINE ASSESSMENT
◄**ALERT**► Each dose must be administered with ifosfamide therapy.

### INTERVENTION/EVALUATION
Assess morning urine specimen for hematuria. If such occurs, dosage reduction or discontinuation may be necessary. Monitor daily pattern of bowel activity, stool consistency; record time of evacuation. Monitor B/P for hypotension.

### PATIENT/FAMILY TEACHING
• Report headache, myalgia, nausea.

---

**metFORMIN**    TOP 100   HIGH ALERT

met-**for**-min
(Apo-Metformin ❖, Fortamet, Glucophage, Glucophage XR, Glumetza, Glycon ❖, Riomet)

■ **BLACK BOX ALERT** ■ Lactic acidosis occurs very rarely, but mortality rate is 50%. Risk increases with degree of renal impairment, pt's age, those with diabetes, unstable or acute HF.

**Do not confuse Glucophage with Glucotrol, or metformin with metronidazole.**

## FIXED-COMBINATION(S)

**Actoplus Met:** metformin/pioglitazone (an antidiabetic): 500 mg/15 mg, 850 mg/15 mg. **Avandamet:** metformin/rosiglitazone (an antidiabetic): 500 mg/1 mg, 500 mg/2 mg, 500 mg/4 mg, 1,000 mg/2 mg, 1,000 mg/4 mg. **Glucovance:** metformin/glyburide (an antidiabetic): 250 mg/1.25 mg, 500 mg/2.5 mg, 500 mg/5 mg. **Invokamet:** metformin/canagliflozin (an antidiabetic): 500 mg/50 mg, 500 mg/150 mg, 1,000 mg/50 mg, 1,000 mg/150 mg. **Janumet, Janumet XR:** metformin/sitagliptin (an antidiabetic): 500 mg/50 mg, 1,000 mg/50 mg. **Jentadueto, Jentadueto XR:** metformin/linagliptin (an antidiabetic): 500 mg/2.5 mg; 1,000 mg/2.5 mg. 1,000 mg extended-release/2.5 mg; 1,000 mg extended-release/5 mg. **Kazano:** metformin/alogliptin (an antidiabetic): 500 mg/12.5 mg; 1,000 mg/12.5 mg. **Kombiglyze XR:** metformin/saxagliptin (an antidiabetic): 500 mg/5 mg, 1,000 mg/5 mg, 1,000 mg/2.5 mg. **Metaglip:** metformin/glipizide (an antidiabetic): 250 mg/2.5 mg, 500 mg/2.5 mg, 500 mg/5 mg. **PrandiMet:** metformin/repaglinide (an antidiabetic): 500 mg/1 mg, 500 mg/2 mg. **Synjardy:** metformin/empagliflozin (an antidiabetic): 500 mg/5 mg, 1,000 mg/5 mg, 500 mg/12.5 mg, 1,000 mg/12.5 mg.

## ◆CLASSIFICATION

**PHARMACOTHERAPEUTIC:** Biguanide; Antihyperglycemic. **CLINICAL:** Antidiabetic agent.

## USES

Management of type 2 diabetes mellitus as monotherapy or concomitantly with oral sulfonylurea or insulin. **OFF-LABEL:** Polycystic ovarian syndrome, gestational diabetes mellitus. Prevention of type 2 diabetes.

---

M

## PRECAUTIONS

◄ALERT► Lactic acidosis is a rare but potentially severe consequence of metformin therapy. Withhold in pts with conditions that may predispose to lactic acidosis (e.g., hypoxemia, dehydration, hypoperfusion, sepsis).
**Contraindications:** Hypersensitivity to metformin. Renal disease/dysfunction (serum creatinine 1.5 or greater in male pts or 1.4 or greater in female pts); abnormal CrCl from any cause including MI, acute HF, septicemia, or shock; acute or chronic metabolic acidosis, use within 48 hrs of IV contrast dye. **Cautions:** HF, hepatic impairment, excessive acute/chronic alcohol intake, elderly.

## ACTION

Decreases hepatic production of glucose. Decreases intestinal absorption of glucose, improves insulin sensitivity. **Therapeutic Effect:** Improves glycemic control, stabilizes/decreases body weight, improves lipid profile.

## PHARMACOKINETICS

Slowly, incompletely absorbed after PO administration. Food delays, decreases extent of absorption. Protein binding: Negligible. Primarily distributed to intestinal mucosa, salivary glands. Primarily excreted unchanged in urine. Removed by hemodialysis. **Half-life:** 9–17 hrs.

## LIFESPAN CONSIDERATIONS

**Pregnancy/Lactation:** Insulin is drug of choice during pregnancy. Distributed in breast milk in animals. **Children:** Safety and efficacy not established. **Elderly:** Age-related renal impairment or peripheral vascular disease may require dosage adjustment or discontinuation.

## INTERACTIONS

**DRUG: Furosemide** may increase concentration. **Cationic medications (e.g., digoxin, morphine, quinine, ranitidine, vancomycin)** may increase concentration/effects. **IV contrast dye** may increase risk of metformin-induced lactic acidosis, acute renal failure (discontinue metformin 24–48 hrs prior to and up to 72 hrs after contrast exposure). **HERBAL: Garlic** may cause hypoglycemia. **FOOD:** None known. **LAB VALUES:** May alter cholesterol, LDL, triglycerides, HDL.

## AVAILABILITY (Rx)

**Oral Solution (Riomet):** 100 mg/ml. **Tablets (Glucophage):** 500 mg, 850 mg, 1,000 mg.
**Tablets (Extended-Release):** 500 mg (Fortamet, Glucophage XR, Glumetza), 750 mg (Glucophage XR), 1,000 mg (Fortamet, Glumetza).

## ADMINISTRATION/HANDLING

**PO**
• Give extended-release tablets whole. Do not break, crush, dissolve, or divide extended-release tablets. • Give with meals (to decrease GI upset). Give Fortamet with glass of water.

## INDICATIONS/ROUTES/DOSAGE

◄ALERT► Allow 1–2 wks between dose titrations.
**Diabetes Mellitus**
**PO (Immediate-Release Tablets, Solution):** **ADULTS, ELDERLY:** Initially, 500 mg twice daily or 850 mg once daily. Titrate in increments of 500 mg wkly or 850 mg every other wk. **Maintenance:** 1,000–2,550 mg/day in 2–3 divided doses. **Maximum:** 2,550 mg/day. **CHILDREN 10–16 YRS:** Initially, 500 mg twice daily. **Maintenance:** Titrate in 500-mg increments wkly. **Maximum:** 2,000 mg/day.
**PO (Extended-Release Tablets [Glucophage XR]):** **ADULTS, ELDERLY:** Initially, 500 mg once daily. May increase by 500 mg at 1-wk intervals. **Maintenance:** 1,000–2,000 mg daily. **Maximum:** 2,000 mg/day.
**PO (Extended-Release Tablets [Glumetza]):** **ADULTS, ELDERLY:** Initially, 1,000 mg once daily. May increase by 500 mg at

M

1-wk intervals. **Maximum:** 2,000 mg/day. *[Fortamet]:* Initially, 500–1,000 mg once daily. May increase by 500 mg at 1-wk intervals. **Maximum:** 2,500 mg/day.

**Dosage in Renal Impairment**
Contraindicated in pts with serum creatinine greater than 1.5 mg/dL (males) or greater than 1.4 mg/dL (females). **Alternative Recommendation: CrCl 45–60 ml/min:** Continue use; monitor renal function q3–6 mos. **CrCl 30–44 ml/min:** Use caution. Consider dose reduction; monitor renal function q3mos. **CrCL less than 30 ml/min:** Discontinue use.

**Dosage in Hepatic Impairment**
Avoid use (risk factor for lactic acidosis).

## SIDE EFFECTS

**Occasional (greater than 3%):** GI disturbances (diarrhea, nausea, vomiting, abdominal bloating, flatulence, anorexia) that are transient and resolve spontaneously during therapy. **Rare (3%–1%):** Unpleasant/metallic taste that resolves spontaneously during therapy.

## ADVERSE EFFECTS/ TOXIC REACTIONS

Lactic acidosis occurs rarely (0.03 cases/1,000 pts) but is a serious and often fatal (50%) complication. Lactic acidosis is characterized by increase in blood lactate levels (greater than 5 mmol/L), decrease in blood pH, electrolyte disturbances. Symptoms include unexplained hyperventilation, myalgia, malaise, drowsiness. May advance to cardiovascular collapse (shock), acute HF, acute MI, prerenal azotemia.

## NURSING CONSIDERATIONS

**BASELINE ASSESSMENT**
Verify pt has not received IV contrast dye within last 48 hrs. Obtain CBC, renal function test, fasting serum glucose, Hgb A1c.

**INTERVENTION/EVALUATION**
Monitor fasting serum glucose, Hgb A1c, renal function, CBC. Monitor folic acid, renal function tests for evidence of early lactic acidosis. If pt is on concurrent oral sulfonylureas, assess for hypoglycemia (cool/wet skin, tremors, dizziness, anxiety, headache, tachycardia, numbness in mouth, hunger, diplopia). Be alert to conditions that alter glucose requirements: fever, increased activity, stress, surgical procedure.

**PATIENT/FAMILY TEACHING**
• Discontinue metformin, report immediately if evidence of lactic acidosis appears (unexplained hyperventilation, muscle aches, extreme fatigue, unusual drowsiness). • Prescribed diet is principal part of treatment; do not skip, delay meals. • Diabetes mellitus requires lifelong control. • Avoid alcohol. • Report persistent headache, nausea, vomiting, diarrhea or if skin rash, unusual bruising/bleeding, change in color of urine or stool occurs. • Do not take dose for at least 48 hrs after receiving IV contrast dye with radiologic testing.

# methadone

meth-a-done
(Dolophine, Metadol ✹, Methadone Disket, Methadone Intensol, Methadose)

■ **BLACK BOX ALERT** ■ May prolong QT interval. May cause respiratory depression. Monitor for signs of misuse, abuse, addiction. Prolonged maternal use may cause neonatal withdrawal syndrome.
**Do not confuse methadone with Mephyton, Metadate CD, Metadate ER, methylphenidate, or morphine.**

## ◆CLASSIFICATION

**PHARMACOTHERAPEUTIC:** Narcotic agonist **(Schedule II). CLINICAL:** Opioid analgesic.

## USES

Moderate to severe pain when a continuous around-the-clock analgesic is needed. Detoxification/maintenance treatment of opioid addiction in conjunction with social/medical services.

## PRECAUTIONS

**Contraindications:** Hypersensitivity to methadone. Severe respiratory depression, acute or severe asthma (in absence of resuscitative equipment or unmonitored setting), hypercarbia, known or suspected paralytic ileus, concurrent use of selegiline. **Caution:** Renal/hepatic impairment, elderly/debilitated, risk for QT prolongation, medications that prolong QT interval, conduction abnormalities, severe volume depletion, hypokalemia, hypomagnesemia, cardiovascular disease, depression, suicidal tendencies, history of drug abuse, respiratory disease, biliary tract dysfunction, acute pancreatitis, hypothyroidism, Addison's disease, head injury, increased intracranial pressure.

## ACTION

Binds with opioid receptors within CNS, causing inhibition of ascending pain pathways. **Therapeutic Effect:** Alters processes affecting analgesia, emotional response to pain; reduces withdrawal symptoms from other opioid drugs.

## PHARMACOKINETICS

| Route | Onset | Peak | Duration |
|---|---|---|---|
| PO | 0.5–1 hr | 1.5–2 hrs | 6–8 hrs |
| IM | 10–20 min | 1–2 hrs | 4–5 hrs |
| IV | N/A | 15–30 min | 3–4 hrs |

Well absorbed after IM injection. Protein binding: 85%–90%. Metabolized in liver. Primarily excreted in urine. Not removed by hemodialysis. **Half-life:** 7–59 hrs.

## ⏳ LIFESPAN CONSIDERATIONS

**Pregnancy/Lactation:** Crosses placenta. Distributed in breast milk. Respiratory depression may occur in neonate if mother received opiates during labor. Regular use of opiates during pregnancy may produce withdrawal symptoms in neonate (irritability, excessive crying, tremors, hyperactive reflexes, fever, vomiting, diarrhea, yawning, sneezing, seizures). **Children:** Paradoxical excitement may occur. Pts younger than 2 yrs more susceptible to respiratory depressant effects. **Elderly:** More susceptible to respiratory depressant effects. Age-related renal impairment may increase risk of urinary retention.

## INTERACTIONS

**DRUG: Alcohol, other CNS depressants (e.g., lorazepam, morphine, zolpidem)** may increase CNS effects, respiratory depression, hypotension. **CYP3A4 inducers (e.g., carbamazepine, phenobarbital)** may decrease concentration/effects. **CYP3A4 inhibitors (e.g., rifampin, clarithromycin)** may increase methadone level. **Amiodarone, erythromycin** may prolong QT interval. **MAOIs** may produce serotonin syndrome (reduce dose to ¼ of usual methadone dose). **HERBAL: Gotu kola, kava kava, St. John's wort, valerian** may increase CNS depression. **St. John's wort** may decrease concentration/effects. **FOOD: Grapefruit products** may alter concentration/effects. **LAB VALUES:** May increase serum amylase, lipase.

## AVAILABILITY (Rx)

**Injection Solution (Dolophine):** 10 mg/ml. **Oral Concentrate (Methadone Intensol, Methadose):** 10 mg/ml. **Oral Solution:** 5 mg/5 ml, 10 mg/5 ml. **Tablets (Dispersible [Methadose, Methadone Diskets]):** 40 mg. **Tablets (Dolophine):** 5 mg, 10 mg.

## ADMINISTRATION/HANDLING

**IM, SQ**

**◀ALERT▶** IM preferred over SQ route (SQ produces pain, local irritation, induration). • Do not use if solution appears cloudy or contains a precipitate.

---

• Administer slowly. • Those with circulatory impairment experience higher risk of overdosage due to delayed absorption of repeated administration.

**PO**
• Give without regard to meals. • Oral dose for detoxification and maintenance may be given in fruit juice or water. • Dispersible tablet should not be chewed or swallowed; add to liquid, allow to dissolve before swallowing.

## INDICATIONS/ROUTES/DOSAGE

**Analgesia**
**PO: ADULTS, ELDERLY:** Initially, 2.5 mg q8–12 hrs. May increase by 2.5 mg/dose or 5 mg/day q5–7 days. **CHILDREN:** 0.1–0.2 mg/kg/dose q4–8h for 2–3 doses then q6–12h as needed. **Maximum dose:** 10 mg.
**IV, IM, SQ: ADULTS, ELDERLY:** Initially, 2.5 mg q8–12h, then titrate slowly to desired effect. **CHILDREN:** 0.1 mg/kg q4–8h for 2–3 doses, then q4–12h. **Maximum:** 10 mg/dose.

**Dosage in Renal Impairment**
**CrCl less than 10 ml/min:** 50–75% normal dose. Avoid in severe hepatic disease.

**Dosage in Hepatic Impairment**
**Mild to moderate impairment:** No dose adjustment. **Severe Impairment:** Avoid use.

**Detoxification**
**PO: ADULTS, ELDERLY:** Initially, dose of 20–30 mg. An additional 5–10 mg may be provided if withdrawal symptoms have not been suppressed or if symptoms reappear after 2–4 hrs. Total daily dose not to exceed 40 mg. **Maintenance range:** Titrate to dose that prevents withdrawal symptoms for 24 hrs, prevents craving, reduces euphoria effect of self-administered opioids, while ensuring tolerance to sedative effects of methadone. Usual range: 80–120 mg/day. Withdrawal should be less than 10% of the maintenance dose

every 10–14 days. **Short-term:** Initially, titrate to 40 mg/day in 2 divided doses. Continue 40-mg dose for 2–3 days. After 2–3 days of stabilization at 40 mg, gradually decrease dose to level keeping withdrawal symptoms tolerable.

## SIDE EFFECTS
**Frequent:** Sedation, orthostatic hypotension, diaphoresis, facial flushing, constipation, dizziness, nausea, vomiting. **Occasional:** Confusion, urinary retention, palpitations, abdominal cramps, visual changes, dry mouth, headache, decreased appetite, anxiety, insomnia. **Rare:** Allergic reaction (rash, pruritus).

## ADVERSE EFFECTS/ TOXIC REACTIONS
Overdose results in respiratory depression, skeletal muscle flaccidity, cold/clammy skin, cyanosis, extreme drowsiness progressing to seizures, stupor, coma. Early sign of toxicity presents as increased sedation after being on a stable dose. Cardiac toxicity manifested as QT prolongation, torsades de pointes. Tolerance to analgesic effect, physical dependence may occur with repeated use. **Antidote:** Naloxone (see Appendix J for dosage).

## NURSING CONSIDERATIONS

### BASELINE ASSESSMENT
Assess type, location, intensity of pain. **Detoxification:** Assess pt for opioid withdrawal. Pt should be in recumbent position before drug administration by parenteral route. Obtain vital signs before giving medication. If respirations are 12/min or less (20/min or less in children), withhold medication, contact physician.

### INTERVENTION/EVALUATION
Monitor vital signs 15–30 min after SQ/IM dose, 5–10 min following IV dose. Oral medication is 50% as potent as parenteral. Assess for adequate voiding. Monitor daily pattern of bowel activity, stool consistency. Assess for clinical improvement, record onset of relief of pain.

Provide support to pt in detoxification program; monitor for withdrawal symptoms.

### PATIENT/FAMILY TEACHING

• Methadone may produce drug dependence, has potential for being abused. • Avoid alcohol. • Do not stop taking abruptly after prolonged use. • May cause dry mouth, drowsiness. • Avoid tasks that require alertness, motor skills until response to drug is established. • Report severe drowsiness, respiratory depression.

# methocarbamol

meth-oh-**kar**-ba-mal
(Robaxin, Robaxin-750)
**Do not confuse Robaxin with Skelaxin.**

## ◆CLASSIFICATION

**PHARMACOTHERAPEUTIC:** Autonomic agent, carbamate derivative of guaifenesin. **CLINICAL:** Skeletal muscle relaxant.

## USES

Adjunct to rest and physical therapy for relief of discomfort associated with acute, painful musculoskeletal conditions (e.g., tetanus).

## PRECAUTIONS

**Contraindications:** Hypersensitivity to methocarbamol. Renal impairment (injectable formulation). **Cautions:** Elderly, hepatic impairment, seizure disorders (injectable formulation).

## ACTION

Skeletal muscle relaxant action may be related to its CNS depressant effects. Does not directly relax skeletal muscle, motor end plate, or nerve fiber. **Therapeutic Effect:** Relieves musculoskeletal pain.

## PHARMACOKINETICS

Extensively distributed in tissues. Protein binding: 46%–50%. Converts to metabolites. Metabolized by dealkylation, hydroxylation; excreted in urine. **Half-life:** 1–2 hrs.

## ⧖ LIFESPAN CONSIDERATIONS

**Pregnancy/Lactation:** Unknown if distributed in breast milk. **Children:** Safety and efficacy not established in pts 16 yrs and younger. **Elderly:** May be more susceptible to CNS effects.

## INTERACTIONS

**DRUG: Alcohol, CNS depressants (e.g., lorazepam, morphine, zolpidem), tricyclic antidepressants (e.g., amitriptyline, doxepin)** may increase sedative effects. May inhibit effect of **pyridostigmine. HERBAL: St. John's wort, valerian, kava kava, gotu kola** may increase CNS depression. **FOOD: High-fat meals** may increase concentration. **LAB VALUES:** May decrease WBC count.

## AVAILABILITY (Rx)

**Injection, Solution:** 100 mg/ml.

🔖 **Tablets, Film-Coated:** 500 mg, 750 mg.

## ADMINISTRATION/HANDLING

**IM/IV**

**(IM)** • Maximum of 5 ml can be given into each gluteal region.
**(IV)** • May give undiluted at maximum rate of 3 ml/min. • May dilute with D₅W or 0.9% NaCl to concentration of 4 mg/ml. • Administer in recumbent position and remain in position for 10–15 min after IV administration.

**PO**

• Give without regard to food. • May crush or break tablets and mix with food or liquid.

## INDICATIONS/ROUTES/DOSAGE

**Muscle Spasm**
**PO: ADULTS, ELDERLY, CHILDREN 16 YRS AND OLDER:** 1.5 g 4 times/day for 2–3

M

---

 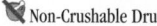

days, then 4–4.5 g/day in 3–6 divided doses.

**Usual Parenteral Dose (Muscle Spasms)**
**IM/IV: ADULTS, ELDERLY:** 1 g q8h for up to 3 days. **Maximum:** 3 g/day.

**Tetanus**
◀**ALERT**▶ Do not use for longer than 72 hrs.
**IV: ADULTS, ELDERLY:** Initially, 1–2 g by direct IV injection, then 1–2 g by IV infusion q6h until oral therapy possible. **Maximum:** 24 g/day. **CHILDREN:** 15 mg/kg/dose. May repeat q6h if needed. **Maximum:** 1.8 g/m²/day.

**Dosage in Renal/Hepatic Impairment**
No dose adjustment. Injection contraindicated in severe renal impairment; use caution in pts with cirrhosis.

## SIDE EFFECTS

**Occasional:** Dizziness, drowsiness, confusion, double vision, insomnia, headache, irritability, nausea, nervousness, dyspepsia, vomiting, metallic taste.

## ADVERSE EFFECTS/ TOXIC REACTIONS

Anaphylactic reaction (rash, pruritus, urticaria, angioneurotic edema, fever, bradycardia, hypotension, syncope) has occurred. Leukopenia, cholestatic jaundice, seizure occur rarely.

## NURSING CONSIDERATIONS

**BASELINE ASSESSMENT**
Record onset, type, location, duration of musculoskeletal pain, inflammation. Inspect appearance of affected joints for immobility, stiffness, swelling.

**INTERVENTION/EVALUATION**
Assist with ambulation at all times. Evaluate for therapeutic response: relief of pain, stiffness, swelling; improved mobility; reduced joint tenderness; improved grip strength.

**PATIENT/FAMILY TEACHING**
• Avoid tasks that require alertness, motor skills until response to drug is established. • Avoid alcohol. • May color urine brown, black, or green. • Medication intended for short-term use (3 wks). • Report severe sedation.

---

## *methotrexate*

meth-o-**trex**-ate
(Apo-Methotrexate ✤, Otrexup, Rasuvo, Rheumatrex, Trexall)
■ **BLACK BOX ALERT** ■ May cause fetal abnormalities, death. May produce potentially fatal chronic hepatotoxicity, dermatologic reactions, acute renal failure, pneumonitis, myelosuppression, malignant lymphoma, aplastic anemia, GI toxicity. Do not use for psoriasis or rheumatoid arthritis treatment in pregnant women.
**Do not confuse methotrexate with metolazone, methylprednisolone, or mitoxantrone. MTX is an error-prone abbreviation; do not use as an abbreviation.**

◆**CLASSIFICATION**

**PHARMACOTHERAPEUTIC:** Antimetabolite. **CLINICAL:** Antineoplastic, antiarthritic, antipsoriatic.

## USES

**Oncology-related:** Treatment of breast, head/neck, non–small-cell lung, small cell lung carcinomas; trophoblastic tumors, acute lymphocytic, meningeal leukemias; non-Hodgkin's lymphomas (lymphosarcoma, Burkitt's lymphoma), carcinoma of gastrointestinal tract, mycosis fungoides, osteosarcoma. **Non-oncology uses:** Psoriasis, rheumatoid arthritis (including juvenile idiopathic arthritis). **OFF-LABEL:** Treatment of acute myelocytic leukemia, bladder carcinoma, ectopic pregnancy, management of abortion, systemic lupus erythematosus, treatment of and maintenance of remission in Crohn's disease.

## PRECAUTIONS

**Contraindications:** Hypersensitivity to methotrexate. Breastfeeding. **Additional: For pts with psoriasis or rheumatoid arthritis:** Pregnancy, hepatic disease, alcoholism, immunodeficiency syndrome, preexisting blood dyscrasias. **Cautions:** Peptic ulcer, ulcerative colitis, preexisting myelosuppression, history of chronic hepatic disease, alcohol consumption, obesity, diabetes, hyperlipidemia, use with other hepatotoxic medications, concomitant use of proton pump inhibitors. Use of NSAIDs or aspirin with lower methotrexate doses for rheumatoid arthritis.

## ACTION

Competes with enzymes necessary to reduce folic acid to tetrahydrofolic acid, a component essential to DNA synthesis, repair, and cellular replication. **Therapeutic Effect:** Inhibits DNA, RNA, protein synthesis. Possesses anti-inflammatory and immune-modulating activity.

## PHARMACOKINETICS

Variably absorbed from GI tract. Completely absorbed after IM administration. Protein binding: 50%–60%. Widely distributed. Metabolized in liver. Primarily excreted in urine. Removed by hemodialysis but not by peritoneal dialysis. **Half-life:** 3–10 hrs (large doses, 8–15 hrs).

## ⏳ LIFESPAN CONSIDERATIONS

**Pregnancy/Lactation:** Avoid pregnancy during methotrexate therapy and minimum 3 mos after therapy in males or at least one ovulatory cycle after therapy in females. May cause fetal death, congenital anomalies. Distributed in breast milk. Breastfeeding not recommended. **Children/Elderly:** Renal/hepatic impairment may require dosage adjustment.

## INTERACTIONS

**DRUG: Alcohol, hepatotoxic medications** (e.g., acetaminophen, isoniazid, ketoconazole, simvastatin) may increase risk of hepatotoxicity. **Bone marrow depressants** may increase myelosuppression. **Live virus vaccines** may potentiate virus replication, increase vaccine side effects, decrease pt's antibody response to vaccine. **NSAIDs** may increase risk of toxicity. **Probenecid, salicylates (e.g., aspirin)** may increase concentration, risk of toxicity. **HERBAL: Cat's claw, echinacea** possess immunostimulant properties. **FOOD:** None known. **LAB VALUES:** May increase serum uric acid, AST.

## AVAILABILITY (Rx)

**Injection, Powder for Reconstitution:** 1 g. **Injection, Autoinjector (Rasuvo):** 7.5 mg, 10 mg, 12.5 mg, 15 mg, 17.5 mg, 20 mg, 22.5 mg, 25 mg, 27.5 mg, 30 mg. **Injection Solution:** 25 mg/ml. **Injection Syringe (Otrexup):** 7.5 mg/0.4 ml, 10 mg/0.4 ml, 15 mg/0.4 ml, 20 mg/0.4 ml, 25 mg/0.4 ml. **Tablets:** 2.5 mg (Rheumatrex), 5 mg (Trexall), 7.5 mg (Trexall), 10 mg (Trexall), 15 mg (Trexall).

## ADMINISTRATION/HANDLING

◀**ALERT**▶ May be carcinogenic, mutagenic, teratogenic. Handle with extreme care during preparation/administration. Wear gloves when preparing solution. If powder or solution comes in contact with skin, wash immediately, thoroughly with soap, water. May give IM, IV, intra-arterially, intrathecally.

 **IV**

**Reconstitution** • Reconstitute powder with $D_5W$ or 0.9% NaCl to provide concentration of 25 mg/ml or less. • For intrathecal use, dilute with preservative-free 0.9% NaCl to provide a concentration not greater than 2–4 mg/ml. **Rate of Administration** • Give IV push at rate of 10 mg/min. • Give IV

M

infusion at rate of 4–20 mg/hr (refer to specific protocol).

**Storage** • Store vials at room temperature. Diluted solutions stable for 24 hrs at room temperature.

## 🞑 IV INCOMPATIBILITIES

Droperidol (Inapsine), gemcitabine (Gemzar), idarubicin (Idamycin), midazolam (Versed), nalbuphine (Nubain).

## 🞑 IV COMPATIBILITIES

Cisplatin (Platinol AQ), cyclophosphamide (Cytoxan), daunorubicin (DaunoXome), doxorubicin (Adriamycin), etoposide (VePesid), 5-fluorouracil, granisetron (Kytril), leucovorin, mitomycin (Mutamycin), ondansetron (Zofran), paclitaxel (Taxol), vinblastine (Velban), vincristine (Oncovin), vinorelbine (Navelbine).

## INDICATIONS/ROUTES/DOSAGE

### Oncology Uses

◀ALERT▶ Refer to individual specific protocols for optimum dosage, sequence of administration.

### Head/Neck Cancer

**PO, IV, IM: ADULTS, ELDERLY:** 40 mg/m² once weekly.

### Breast Cancer

**IV: ADULTS, ELDERLY:** 40 mg/m² days 1 and 8 q3–4wks.

### Mycosis Fungoides

**IM, PO: ADULTS, ELDERLY:** 5–50 mg once weekly or 15–37.5 mg twice weekly.

### Rheumatoid Arthritis (RA)

**PO: ADULTS:** Initially, 7.5 mg once wkly or 2.5 mg q12h for 3 doses once wkly. Adjust dose gradually to optimal response. **SQ/IM:** Initially, 7.5 mg/wk. Adjust dose gradually to optimal response. **ELDERLY:** Initially, 5–7.5 mg/wk. **Maximum:** 20 mg/wk.

### Juvenile Rheumatoid Arthritis (JRA)

**PO, IM, SQ: CHILDREN:** Initially, 10 mg/m² once wkly, then 20–30 mg/m²/wk as a single dose.

### Psoriasis

**PO: ADULTS, ELDERLY:** Initially, 10–25 mg once wkly or 2.5–5 mg q12h for 3 doses once wkly. **IM/SQ:** 10–25 mg once wkly. Adjust dose gradually to optimal response. Titrate to lowest effective dose.

### Dosage in Renal Impairment

| Creatinine Clearance | Reduce Dose to |
|---|---|
| 61–80 ml/min | 75% of normal |
| 51–60 ml/min | 70% of normal |
| 10–50 ml/min | 30–50% of normal |
| Less than 10 ml/min | Avoid use |

### Dosage in Hepatic Impairment
Use caution.

## SIDE EFFECTS

**Frequent (10%–3%):** Nausea, vomiting, stomatitis, burning/erythema at psoriatic site (in pts with psoriasis). **Occasional (3%–1%):** Diarrhea, rash, dermatitis, pruritus, alopecia, dizziness, anorexia, malaise, headache, drowsiness, blurred vision.

## ADVERSE EFFECTS/ TOXIC REACTIONS

High potential for various, severe toxicities. GI toxicity may produce gingivitis, glossitis, pharyngitis, stomatitis, enteritis, hematemesis. Hepatotoxicity more likely to occur with frequent small doses than with large intermittent doses. Pulmonary toxicity characterized by interstitial pneumonitis. Hematologic toxicity, resulting from marked myelosuppression, may manifest as leukopenia, thrombocytopenia, anemia, hemorrhage. Dermatologic toxicity may produce rash, pruritus, urticaria, pigmentation, photosensitivity, petechiae, ecchymosis, pustules. Severe nephrotoxicity produces azotemia, hematuria, renal failure.

## NURSING CONSIDERATIONS

### BASELINE ASSESSMENT

**Rheumatoid arthritis:** Assess pain, range of motion. **Psoriasis:** Assess skin lesions. Question for possibility of pregnancy in pts with psoriasis, rheumatoid arthritis (RA). Obtain all functional tests before therapy, repeat throughout therapy. Antiemetics may prevent nausea, vomiting.

### INTERVENTION/EVALUATION

Monitor CBC, BMP, LFT, urinalysis, chest X-rays, serum uric acid. Monitor for hematologic toxicity (fever, sore throat, signs of local infection, unusual bruising/bleeding from any site), symptoms of anemia (excessive fatigue, weakness). Assess skin for evidence of dermatologic toxicity. Keep pt well hydrated, urine alkaline. Avoid rectal temperatures, traumas that induce bleeding. Apply 5 full min of pressure to IV sites.

### PATIENT/FAMILY TEACHING

• Maintain strict oral hygiene. • Do not have immunizations without physician's approval (drug lowers resistance). • Avoid crowds, those with infection. • Avoid alcohol, aspirin. • Avoid ultraviolet sunlight exposure. • Use contraceptive measures during therapy and for 3 mos (males) or 1 ovulatory cycle (females) after therapy. • Promptly report fever, sore throat, signs of local infection, unusual bruising/bleeding from any site, diarrhea. • Hair loss is reversible, but new hair growth may have different color, texture. • Report persistent nausea/vomiting.

# methylergonovine

meth-il-er-**goe**-noe-veen
(Methergine ♣)

## ◆CLASSIFICATION

**PHARMACOTHERAPEUTIC:** Ergot alkaloid. **CLINICAL:** Oxytocic agent, uterine stimulant.

## USES

Management of uterine atony, hemorrhage and subinvolution of uterus following delivery of placenta. Control uterine hemorrhage following delivery of anterior shoulder in second stage of labor.

## PRECAUTIONS

**Contraindications:** Hypersensitivity to methylergonovine. Hypertension, pregnancy, toxemia. **Cautions:** Renal/hepatic impairment, cardiovascular disease, concurrent use with CYP3A4 inhibitors (e.g., protease inhibitors), occlusive peripheral vascular disease, sepsis, second stage of labor.

## ACTION

Increases tone, rate, amplitude of contraction of uterine smooth muscle. **Therapeutic Effect:** Shortens third stage of labor, reduces blood loss.

## PHARMACOKINETICS

| Route | Onset | Peak | Duration |
|-------|-------|------|----------|
| PO | 5–10 min | N/A | 3 hrs |
| IV | Immediate | N/A | 45 min |
| IM | 2–5 min | N/A | 3 hrs |

Rapidly absorbed from GI tract after IM administration. Distributed rapidly to plasma, extracellular fluid, tissues. Metabolized in liver. Primarily excreted in urine. **Half-life:** 0.5–2 hrs.

## ⧗ LIFESPAN CONSIDERATIONS

**Pregnancy/Lactation:** Contraindicated during pregnancy. Small amounts distributed in breast milk. **Children/Elderly:** No information available.

## INTERACTIONS

**DRUG: Dopamine, norepinephrine, phenylephrine, vasopressin** may increase effects. **HERBAL:** None significant. **FOOD:** None known. **LAB VALUES:** May decrease serum prolactin.

M

## AVAILABILITY (Rx)

**Injection Solution:** 0.2 mg/ml. **Tablets:** 0.2 mg.

## ADMINISTRATION/HANDLING

**Reconstitution** • Dilute with 0.9% NaCl to volume of 5 ml.
**Rate of Administration** • Give over at least 1 min, carefully monitoring B/P.
**Storage** • Refrigerate ampules. • Initial dose may be given parenterally, followed by oral regimen. • IV use in life-threatening emergencies only.

## ▩ IV INCOMPATIBILITIES

None known.

## ▩ IV COMPATIBILITIES

Heparin, potassium.

## INDICATIONS/ROUTES/DOSAGE

**Prevention/Treatment of Postpartum, Postabortion Hemorrhage**
**PO: ADULTS:** 0.2 mg 3–4 times daily. Continue for up to 7 days.
**IV, IM: ADULTS:** Initially, 0.2 mg after delivery of anterior shoulder, after delivery of placenta, or during puerperium. May repeat q2–4h as needed.

**Dosage in Renal/Hepatic Impairment**
Use caution.

## SIDE EFFECTS

**Frequent:** Nausea, uterine cramping, vomiting. **Occasional:** Abdominal pain, diarrhea, dizziness, diaphoresis, tinnitus, bradycardia, chest pain. **Rare:** Allergic reaction (rash, pruritus), dyspnea, severe or sudden hypertension.

## ADVERSE EFFECTS/ TOXIC REACTIONS

Severe hypertensive episodes may result in CVA, serious arrhythmias, seizures. Hypertensive effects are more frequent with pt susceptibility, rapid IV administration, concurrent use of regional anesthesia, vasoconstrictors. Peripheral ischemia may lead to gangrene.

## NURSING CONSIDERATIONS

### BASELINE ASSESSMENT
Determine baseline serum calcium level, B/P, pulse. Assess for any evidence of bleeding before administration.

### INTERVENTION/EVALUATION
Monitor uterine tone, bleeding, B/P, pulse q15min until stable (about 1–2 hrs). Assess extremities for color, warmth, movement, pain. Report chest pain promptly. Provide support with ambulation if dizziness occurs.

### PATIENT/FAMILY TEACHING
• Avoid smoking: causes increased vasoconstriction. • Report increased cramping, bleeding, foul-smelling lochia. • Report pale, cold hands/feet (possibility of diminished circulation).

# methylnaltrexone

meth-il-nal-**trex**-own
(Relistor)
**Do not confuse methylnaltrexone with naltrexone.**

## ◆CLASSIFICATION

**PHARMACOTHERAPEUTIC:** Opioid receptor antagonist. **CLINICAL:** Laxative.

## USES

**Injection:** Treatment of opioid-induced constipation in pts with advanced illness who are receiving palliative care when response to laxative therapy is insufficient. **Injection/Tablets:** Treatment of opioid-induced constipation for chronic pain unrelated to cancer.

## PRECAUTIONS

**Contraindications:** Hypersensitivity to methylnaltrexone. Known or suspected GI obstruction. Pts at increased risk of recurrent obstruction due to potential of GI perforation. **Cautions:** Renal impairment, history of GI tract lesions (e.g., peptic ulcer disease, GI tract malignancies).

## ACTION

Blocks binding of opioids to peripheral opioid receptors within GI tract. **Therapeutic Effect:** Decreases constipating effect of opioids without reducing analgesic effect.

## PHARMACOKINETICS

Absorbed rapidly. Undergoes moderate tissue distribution. Protein binding: 11%–15%. Excreted in urine (50%), feces (35%) **Half-life:** 8 hrs.

## ⌛ LIFESPAN CONSIDERATIONS

**Pregnancy/Lactation:** Unknown if distributed in breast milk. **Children:** Safety and efficacy not established. **Elderly:** No age-related precautions noted.

## INTERACTIONS

**DRUG:** None significant. **HERBAL:** None significant. **FOOD:** None known. **LAB VALUES:** None significant.

## AVAILABILITY (Rx)

**Injection, Solution:** 8 mg/0.4 ml, 12 mg/0.6 ml. **Tablets:** 150 mg.

## ADMINISTRATION/HANDLING

**Subcutaneous**
• Inject into upper arm, abdomen, or thigh. Do not inject in tender, bruised, red, or hard areas.
**Storage** • Solution appears as clear and colorless to pale yellow. • If particulate matter is noted, discard. • Once solution is drawn into syringe, may be stored at room temperature. • Administer within 24 hrs.

## INDICATIONS/ROUTES/DOSAGE

◄ALERT► Usual schedule is once every other day, as needed, but no more frequently than once every 24 hrs.

**Constipation (Chronic Non-cancer Pain)**
**PO: ADULTS, ELDERLY:** 450 mg once daily in the morning. **SQ: ADULTS, ELDERLY:** 12 mg/day. **Note:** Discontinue all laxatives prior to use.

**Constipation (Advanced Illness)**
**SQ: ADULTS, ELDERLY WEIGHING 38 KG TO LESS THAN 62 KG:** 8 mg. **ADULTS, ELDERLY WEIGHING 62–114 KG:** 12 mg. **ADULTS, ELDERLY WHOSE WEIGHT FALLS OUTSIDE THESE RANGES:** Dose at 0.15 mg/kg (round dose up to nearest 0.1 ml of volume).

**Dosage in Severe Renal Impairment (CrCl Less Than 30 ml/min)**
**SQ: ADULTS, ELDERLY:** Administer 50% of recommended dose.

**Dosage in Hepatic Impairment**
No dose adjustment.

## SIDE EFFECTS

**Frequent (29%–12%):** Abdominal pain, flatulence, nausea. **Occasional (7%–5%):** Diarrhea, dizziness.

## ADVERSE EFFECTS/ TOXIC REACTIONS

None known.

M

### NURSING CONSIDERATIONS

**BASELINE ASSESSMENT**
30% of pts report defecation within 30 min after drug administration.

**INTERVENTION/EVALUATION**
Encourage fluid intake. Assess bowel sounds for peristalsis. Monitor daily pattern of bowel activity, stool consistency. If opioid medication is stopped, drug should be discontinued. Assess for abdominal disturbances.

**PATIENT/FAMILY TEACHING**
• Laxative effect usually occurs within 30 min but may take up to 24 hrs after medication administration. • Common side effects include transient abdominal pain, nausea, vomiting. • Report persistent or worsening symptoms, or if severe or persistent diarrhea occurs.

# methylphenidate

meth-il-**fen**-i-date
(Apo-Methylphenidate ✦, Aptensio XR, <u>Concerta</u>, Daytrana, Metadate CD, <u>Metadate ER</u>, Methylin, PMS-Methylphenidate ✦, Quillichew ER, Quillivant XR, Ritalin, Ritalin LA)

■ **BLACK BOX ALERT** ■ Chronic abuse can lead to marked tolerance, psychological dependence. Abrupt withdrawal from prolonged use may lead to severe depression, psychosis.

**Do not confuse Metadate ER with Metadate CD, Methylphenidate with methadone, or Ritalin with Rifadin.**

## ◆CLASSIFICATION

**PHARMACOTHERAPEUTIC:** CNS stimulant **(Schedule II). CLINICAL:** CNS stimulant.

## USES

Treatment of attention-deficit hyperactivity disorder (ADHD). Management of narcolepsy.     **OFF-LABEL:** Secondary mental depression (especially elderly, medically ill).

## PRECAUTIONS

**Contraindications:** Hypersensitivity to methylphenidate. Use of MAOIs within 14 days; marked anxiety, tension, agitation, motor tics; family history or diagnosis of Tourette's syndrome, glaucoma. **Metadate (additional):** Severe hypertension, heart failure, arrhythmia, hyperthyroidism, recent MI or angina. **Cautions:** Hypertension, seizures, acute stress reaction, emotional instability, history of drug dependence, HF, recent MI, hyperthyroidism, known structural cardiac abnormality, bipolar disorder, cardiomyopathy, arrhythmias, alcohol abuse.

## ACTION

Blocks reuptake of norepinephrine, dopamine into presynaptic neurons. **Therapeutic Effect:** Decreases motor restlessness, fatigue. Increases motor activity, attention span, mental alertness. Produces mild euphoria.

## PHARMACOKINETICS

| Onset | Peak | Duration |
|---|---|---|
| Immediate-release | 2 hrs | 3–6 hrs |
| Sustained-release | 4–7 hrs | 8 hrs |
| Extended-release | N/A | 12 hrs |
| Transdermal | 2 hrs | N/A |

Slowly, incompletely absorbed from GI tract. Protein binding: 15%. Metabolized in liver. Primarily excreted in urine. Unknown if removed by hemodialysis. **Half-life:** 2–4 hrs.

## ⏳ LIFESPAN CONSIDERATIONS

**Pregnancy/Lactation:** Unknown if drug crosses placenta or is distributed in breast milk. **Children:** May be more susceptible to developing anorexia, insomnia, stomach pain, decreased weight. Chronic use may inhibit growth. **Elderly:** No age-related precautions noted.

## INTERACTIONS

**DRUG:** **MAOIs** may increase effects. **Other CNS stimulants (e.g., caffeine, dextroamphetamine, phentermine)** may have additive effect. May inhibit metabolism of **warfarin, anticonvulsants (e.g., carbamazepine, phenytoin), antidepressants.** **HERBAL:** **Ephedra** may cause hypertension, arrhythmias. **Yohimbe** may increase CNS stimulation. **FOOD:** None known. **LAB VALUES:** None significant.

## AVAILABILITY (Rx)

**Oral Solution (Methylin):** 5 mg/5 ml, 10 mg/5 ml, 10 mg/1 ml. **Tablets (Chewable [Methylin]):** 2.5 mg, 5 mg, 10 mg. **Tablets (Methylin, Ritalin):** 5 mg, 10 mg, 20 mg. **Topical Patch (Daytrana):** 10 mg/9

M

hrs, 15 mg/9 hrs, 20 mg/9 hrs, 30 mg/9 hrs. **Powder for Suspension, Extended-Release (Quillivant XR):** 25 mg/5 ml.

💉 **Capsules (Extended-Release [Aptensio XR]):** 10 mg, 15 mg, 20 mg, 30 mg, 40 mg, 50 mg, 60 mg. **Capsules (Extended-Release [Metadate CD]):** 10 mg, 20 mg, 30 mg, 40 mg, 50 mg, 60 mg. 💉 **Capsules (Extended-Release [Ritalin LA]):** 10 mg, 20 mg, 30 mg, 40 mg. 💉 **Tablets (Extended-Release [Concerta]):** 18 mg, 27 mg, 36 mg, 54 mg, 72 mg. 💉 **Tablets (Extended-Release [Metadate ER, Methylin ER]):** 10 mg, 20 mg. **Tablets (Extended-Release [Quillichew ER]):** 20 mg, 30 mg, 40 mg. 💉 **Tablets (Sustained-Release [Ritalin SR]):** 20 mg.

## ADMINISTRATION/HANDLING

◀**ALERT**▶ Sustained-release, extended-release tablets may be given in place of regular tablets, once daily dose is titrated using regular tablets, and titrated dosage corresponds to sustained-release or extended-release tablet strength.

**PO**
• Do not give in afternoon or evening (may cause insomnia). • Do not crush, break extended-release capsules, extended- or sustained-release tablets. • Immediate-release tablets may be crushed. • Give dose 30–45 min before meals.
• **Concerta:** Administer once daily in morning. May take without regard to food but must be taken with water, milk, or juice.
• **Methylin Chewable:** Give with at least 8 oz of water or other fluid.
• **Metadate CD, Ritalin LA:** • May be opened, sprinkled on applesauce. • Instruct pt to swallow applesauce without chewing. Do not crush or chew capsule contents.
• **Quillivant XR:** Administer in morning with or without food. Shake bottle more than 10 sec prior to administration.

**Patch**
• To be worn daily for 9 hrs. • Replace daily in morning. • Apply to dry, clean area of hip. • Avoid applying to waistline (clothing may cause patch to rub off). • Alternate application site daily. • Press firmly in place for 30 sec to ensure patch is in good contact with skin. • Do not cut patch.

## INDICATIONS/ROUTES/DOSAGE
### ADHD
**PO: ADULTS:** *(Immediate-Release):* 5 mg twice daily, before breakfast and lunch. May increase by 5–10 mg/day at wkly intervals. **Maximum:** 60 mg/day in 2–3 divided doses. **CHILDREN 6 YRS AND OLDER:** Initially, 0.3 mg/kg/dose or 2.5–5 mg before breakfast and lunch. May increase by 5–10 mg/day at wkly intervals. **Usual dose:** 20–30 mg/day in 2–3 divided doses. **Maximum:** 60 mg/day if 50 kg or less; 100 mg if greater than 50 kg.
**PO** *(Concerta):* **CHILDREN 6 YRS AND OLDER, ADULTS UP TO 65 YRS OF AGE:** Initially, 18 mg once daily; may increase by 18 mg/day at wkly intervals. **Maximum:** 72 mg/day.
**PO** *(Metadate CD):* **CHILDREN 6 YRS AND OLDER:** Initially, 20 mg/day. May increase by 10–20 mg/day at wkly intervals. **Maximum:** 60 mg/day.
**PO:** *(Quillichew ER):* **CHILDREN 6 YRS AND OLDER:** Initially, 20 mg/day. May increase by 10 mg/15 mg or 20 mg/day at wkly intervals. **Maximum:** 60 mg/day.
**PO** *(Quillivant XR):* **CHILDREN 6 YRS AND OLDER:** Initially, 20 mg once daily in the morning. May increase in increments of 10–20 mg/day at wkly increments. **Maximum:** 60 mg/day.
**PO** *(Ritalin LA):* **CHILDREN 6 YRS AND OLDER:** Initially, 20 mg/day. May increase by 10 mg/day at wkly intervals. **Maximum:** 60 mg/day.
**PO** *(Metadate ER, Methylin ER):* **CHILDREN 6 YRS AND OLDER:** May replace regular tablets after daily dose is titrated and 8-hr dosage corresponds to sustained-release or extended-release tablet strength. **Maximum:** 60 mg/day.

**M**

**PATCH** *(Daytrana):* **CHILDREN 6–12 YRS, ADOLESCENTS:** Initially, 10 mg daily (applied and worn for 9 hrs). Dosage is titrated to desired effect. May increase dose no more frequently than every wk.

**Narcolepsy**
**PO: ADULTS, ELDERLY:** *(Immediate-Release):* Initially, 5 mg twice daily, before breakfast and lunch. May increase by 5–10 mg/day at wkly intervals. **Maximum:** 60 mg/day in 2–3 divided doses. *(Extended Release):* May give once immediate-release titrated. **Maximum:** 60 mg/day.

**Dosage in Renal/Hepatic Impairment**
No dose adjustment.

## SIDE EFFECTS

**Frequent:** Anxiety, insomnia, anorexia. **Occasional:** Dizziness, drowsiness, headache, nausea, abdominal pain, fever, rash, arthralgia, vomiting. **Rare:** Blurred vision, Tourette's syndrome (uncontrolled vocal outbursts, repetitive body movements, tics), palpitations, priapism.

## ADVERSE EFFECTS/ TOXIC REACTIONS

Prolonged administration to children with ADHD may delay normal weight gain pattern. Overdose may produce tachycardia, palpitations, arrhythmias, chest pain, psychotic episode, seizures, coma. Hypersensitivity reactions, blood dyscrasias occur rarely.

## NURSING CONSIDERATIONS

**BASELINE ASSESSMENT**

**ADHD:** Assess attention span, impulsivity, interaction with others, distractibility. **Narcolepsy:** Observe/assess frequency of episodes. Question history of seizures.

**INTERVENTION/EVALUATION**

Monitor B/P, pulse, changes in ADHD symptoms. CBC with differential should be performed routinely during therapy. If

paradoxical return of attention-deficit occurs, dosage should be reduced or discontinued. Monitor growth.

**PATIENT/FAMILY TEACHING**

• Avoid tasks that require alertness, motor skills until response to drug is established. • Sugarless gum, sips of water may relieve dry mouth. • Report any increase in seizures. • Take daily dose early in morning to avoid insomnia. • Report anxiety, palpitations, fever, vomiting, skin rash. • Report new or worsened symptoms (e.g., behavior, hostility, concentration ability). • Avoid caffeine. • Do not stop taking abruptly after prolonged use.

# *methylPREDNISolone

(Medrol)

# *methylPREDNISolone acetate

(DepoMedrol)

# *methylPREDNISolone sodium succinate

(Solu-Medrol)
meth-il-pred-**niss**-oh-lone
**Do not confuse DepoMedrol with Solu-Medrol, Medrol with Mebaral, or methylprednisolone with medroxyprogesterone or prednisolone.**

## ◆CLASSIFICATION

**PHARMACOTHERAPEUTIC:** Adrenal corticosteroid. **CLINICAL:** Anti-inflammatory.

## USES

Anti-inflammatory or immunosuppressant in treatment of hematologic, allergic, inflammatory, autoimmune, or neoplastic disorders. **OFF-LABEL:** Acute spinal cord injury.

## PRECAUTIONS

**Contraindications:** Hypersensitivity to methylprednisolone. Administration of live virus vaccines, systemic fungal infection. **IM (additional):** Idiopathic thrombocytopenia purpura. **Cautions:** Respiratory tuberculosis, untreated systemic infections, hypertension, HF, diabetes, GI disease (e.g., peptic ulcer), myasthenia gravis, renal/hepatic impairment, seizures, cataracts, glaucoma, following acute MI, thyroid disorder, thromboembolic tendencies, cardiovascular disease, elderly, psychiatric conditions, pts at risk for osteoporosis.

## ACTION

Suppresses migration of polymorphonuclear leukocytes, reverses increased capillary permeability. **Therapeutic Effect:** Decreases inflammation.

## PHARMACOKINETICS

| Route | Onset | Peak | Duration |
|-------|-------|------|----------|
| PO | Rapid | 1–2 hrs | 30–36 hrs |
| IM | Rapid | 4–8 days | 1–4 wks |
| IV | Rapid | N/A | N/A |

Well absorbed from GI tract after IM administration. Widely distributed. Metabolized in liver. Excreted in urine. Removed by hemodialysis. **Half-life:** 3.5 hrs.

## ⧗ LIFESPAN CONSIDERATIONS

**Pregnancy/Lactation:** Crosses placenta. Distributed in breast milk. May cause cleft palate (chronic use in first trimester). Breastfeeding not recommended. **Children:** Prolonged treatment or high dosages may decrease short-term growth rate, cortisol secretion. **Elderly:** No age-related precautions noted.

## INTERACTIONS

**DRUG:** May alter effects of **warfarin.** **Hepatic enzyme inducers (e.g.,**
**phenytoin, rifampin)** may decrease effects. **Live virus vaccines** may decrease pt's antibody response to vaccine, increase vaccine side effects, potentiate virus replication. **HERBAL: Cat's claw, echinacea** possess immunostimulant properties. **St. John's wort** may decrease concentration. **FOOD:** None known. **LAB VALUES:** May increase serum glucose, cholesterol, lipids, amylase, sodium. May decrease serum calcium, potassium, thyroxine, hypothalamic-pituitary-adrenal (HPA) axis.

## AVAILABILITY (Rx)

**Injection, Powder for Reconstitution (Solu-Medrol):** 40 mg, 125 mg, 500 mg, 1 g. **Injection Suspension (Depo-Medrol):** 40 mg/ml, 80 mg/ml. **Tablets (Medrol):** 2 mg, 4 mg, 8 mg, 16 mg, 32 mg. **(Medrol Dosepak):** 4 mg (21 tablets).

## ADMINISTRATION/HANDLING

◀**ALERT**▶ Do **not** give methylprednisolone acetate IV.

 **IV**

**Reconstitution** • For infusion, add to $D_5W$, 0.9% NaCl.
**Rate of Administration** • Give IV push over 3–15 min. • Give IV piggyback. Dose of 250 mg over 15–30 min; dose of 500–999 mg over at least 30 min; dose of 1g or greater over 1 hr.
**Storage** • Store vials at room temperature. Diluted solution is stable for 48 hrs at room temperature or refrigerated.

**IM**
• Methylprednisolone acetate should not be further diluted. • Methylprednisolone sodium succinate should be reconstituted with Bacteriostatic Water for Injection. • Give deep IM in gluteus maximus (avoid injection into deltoid muscle).

**PO**
• Give with food, milk.

**M**

## ▣ IV INCOMPATIBILITIES

Ciprofloxacin (Cipro), diltiazem (Cardizem), potassium chloride, propofol (Diprivan).

## ▣ IV COMPATIBILITIES

Dexmedetomidine (Precedex), dopamine (Intropin), heparin, midazolam (Versed), theophylline.

## INDICATIONS/ROUTES/DOSAGE

**Anti-Inflammatory, Immunosuppressive**
**IV: ADULTS, ELDERLY:** 10–40 mg. May repeat q4–6h as needed. **CHILDREN:** 0.5–1.7 mg/kg/day or 5–25 mg/m²/day in 2–4 divided doses.
**PO: ADULTS, ELDERLY:** 2–60 mg/day in 1–4 divided doses. **CHILDREN:** 0.5–1.7 mg/kg/day or 5–25 mg/m²/day in 2–4 divided doses.
**IM** *(Methylprednisolone Acetate):* **ADULTS, ELDERLY:** 10–80 mg q1–2wks.
**Intra-Articular, Intralesional: ADULTS, ELDERLY:** 20–60 mg q1–5wks.

**Dosage in Renal/Hepatic Impairment**
No dose adjustment.

## SIDE EFFECTS

**Frequent:** Insomnia, heartburn, anxiety, abdominal distention, diaphoresis, acne, mood swings, increased appetite, facial flushing, GI distress, delayed wound healing, increased susceptibility to infection, diarrhea, constipation. **Occasional:** Headache, edema, tachycardia, change in skin color, frequent urination, depression. **Rare:** Psychosis, increased blood coagulability, hallucinations.

## ADVERSE EFFECTS/ TOXIC REACTIONS

**Long-term therapy:** Hypocalcemia, hypokalemia, muscle wasting (esp. in arms, legs), osteoporosis, spontaneous fractures, amenorrhea, cataracts, glaucoma, peptic ulcer, HF. **Abrupt withdrawal after long-term therapy:** Anorexia, nausea, fever, headache, severe arthralgia, rebound inflammation, fatigue, weakness, lethargy, dizziness, orthostatic hypotension.

## NURSING CONSIDERATIONS

### BASELINE ASSESSMENT

Question for hypersensitivity to any of the corticosteroids, components. Obtain baselines for height, weight, B/P, serum glucose, electrolytes. Check results of initial tests (tuberculosis [TB] skin test, X-rays, EKG). Question history of diabetes.

### INTERVENTION/EVALUATION

Monitor I&O, daily weight; assess for edema. Monitor daily pattern of bowel activity, stool consistency. Check vital signs at least twice daily. Be alert for infection (sore throat, fever, vague symptoms). Monitor serum electrolytes, including B/P, glucose. Monitor for hypocalcemia (muscle twitching, cramps, positive Trousseau's or Chvostek's signs), hypokalemia (weakness, muscle cramps, numbness, tingling [esp. lower extremities], nausea/vomiting, irritability, EKG changes). Assess emotional status, ability to sleep. Check lab results for blood coagulability, clinical evidence of thromboembolism.

### PATIENT/FAMILY TEACHING

• Take oral dose with food, milk. • Do not change dose/schedule or stop taking drug; must taper off gradually under medical supervision. • Report fever, sore throat, muscle aches, sudden weight gain or loss, edema, loss of appetite, fatigue. • Maintain strict personal hygiene, avoid exposure to disease, trauma. • Severe stress (serious infection, surgery, trauma) may require increased dosage. • Follow-up visits, lab tests are necessary. • Children must be assessed for growth retardation. • Inform dentist, other physicians of methylprednisolone therapy now or within past 12 mos.

## metoclopramide

met-oh-**kloe**-pra-myde
(Apo-Metoclop ♣, Metozolv ODT, Reglan)

M

■ **BLACK BOX ALERT** ■ Prolonged use may cause tardive dyskinesia. **Do not confuse metoclopramide with metolazone or metoprolol, or Reglan with Renagel.**

♦ **CLASSIFICATION**

**PHARMACOTHERAPEUTIC:** Dopamine receptor antagonist. **CLINICAL:** GI emptying adjunct, peristaltic stimulant, antiemetic.

## USES

**ORAL:** Symptomatic treatment of diabetic gastroparesis, gastroesophageal reflux. **IV/IM:** Symptomatic treatment of diabetic gastroparesis, placement of enteral feeding tubes, prevent/treat nausea/vomiting with chemotherapy or after surgery.

## PRECAUTIONS

**Contraindications:** Hypersensitivity to metoclopramide. Concurrent use of medications likely to produce extrapyramidal reactions, GI hemorrhage, GI obstruction/perforation, history of seizure disorder, pheochromocytoma. **Cautions:** Renal impairment, HF, cirrhosis, hypertension, depression, Parkinson's disease, elderly.

## ACTION

Stimulates motility of upper GI tract. Blocks dopamine/serotonin receptors in chemoreceptor trigger zone. Enhances acetylcholine response in upper GI tract; increases lower esophageal sphincter tone. **Therapeutic Effect:** Accelerates intestinal transit, promotes gastric emptying. Relieves nausea, vomiting.

## PHARMACOKINETICS

| Route | Onset | Peak | Duration |
|---|---|---|---|
| PO | 30–60 min | N/A | 1–2 hrs |
| IV | 1–3 min | N/A | 1–2 hrs |
| IM | 10–15 min | N/A | 1–2 hrs |

Well absorbed from GI tract. Metabolized in liver. Protein binding: 30%. Primarily excreted in urine. Not removed by hemodialysis. **Half-life:** 4–6 hrs.

## ⧗ LIFESPAN CONSIDERATIONS

**Pregnancy/Lactation:** Crosses placenta. Distributed in breast milk. **Children:** More susceptible to having dystonic reactions. **Elderly:** More likely to have parkinsonian dyskinesias after long-term therapy.

## INTERACTIONS

**DRUG: Alcohol, other CNS depressants** may increase CNS depressant effect. **Anticholinergics (e.g., scopolamine), opioid analgesics (e.g., morphine, hydromorphone)** may decrease effects on GI motility. **HERBAL:** None significant. **FOOD:** None known. **LAB VALUES:** May increase serum aldosterone, prolactin.

## AVAILABILITY (Rx)

**Injection Solution:** 5 mg/ml. **Syrup:** 5 mg/5 ml. **Tablets:** 5 mg, 10 mg.

🔖 **Tablets, Orally Disintegrating:** 5 mg, 10 mg.

## ADMINISTRATION/HANDLING

 IV

**Reconstitution** • Dilute doses greater than 10 mg in 50 ml $D_5W$ or 0.9% NaCl. **Rate of Administration** • Infuse over 15–30 min. • May give undiluted slow IV push at rate of 10 mg over 1–2 min. • Too-rapid IV injection may produce intense feeling of anxiety, restlessness, followed by drowsiness.

**Storage** • Store vials at room temperature. • After dilution, IV infusion (piggyback) is stable for 24 hrs.

### PO

• Give 30 min before meals and at bedtime. • Tablets may be crushed. • Do not cut, divide, break orally disintegrating tablets. Place on tongue, swallow with saliva.

M

### ▨ IV INCOMPATIBILITIES

Allopurinol (Aloprim), cefepime (Maxipime), furosemide (Lasix), propofol (Diprivan).

### ▨ IV COMPATIBILITIES

Dexamethasone, dexmedetomidine (Precedex), diltiazem (Cardizem), diphenhydramine (Benadryl), fentanyl (Sublimaze), heparin, hydromorphone (Dilaudid), morphine, potassium chloride.

## INDICATIONS/ROUTES/DOSAGE

**Prevention of Chemotherapy-Induced Nausea/Vomiting**
**IV: ADULTS, ELDERLY, CHILDREN:** 1–2 mg/kg 30 min before chemotherapy; repeat q2h for 2 doses, then q3h as needed for total of 5 doses/day.

**Postop Nausea/Vomiting**
**IV: ADULTS, ELDERLY:** 10–20 mg near end of surgery.

**Gastroparesis**
**PO, IV: ADULTS:** 10 mg 30 min before meals and at bedtime for 2–8 wks.
**PO, IV: ELDERLY:** Initially, 5 mg 30 min before meals and at bedtime. May increase to 10 mg.
**IV: ADULTS:** 10 mg over 1–2 min.
**ELDERLY:** 5 mg over 1–2 min. May increase to 10 mg.

**Symptomatic Gastroesophageal Reflux Disease (GERD)**
**PO: ADULTS:** 10–15 mg up to 4 times/day, or single doses up to 20 mg as needed. **ELDERLY:** Initially, 5 mg 4 times/day. May increase to 10 mg. **CHILDREN:** 0.1–0.2 mg/kg/dose 4 times/day.

**Facilitate Small Bowel Intubation (Single Dose)**
**IV: ADULTS, ELDERLY:** 10 mg as a single dose. **CHILDREN 6–14 YRS:** 2.5–5 mg as a single dose. **CHILDREN YOUNGER THAN 6 YRS:** 0.1 mg/kg as a single dose.

**Dosage in Renal Impairment**
Dosage is modified based on creatinine clearance.

| Creatinine Clearance | Dosage |
|---|---|
| Less than 40 ml/min | 50% of normal dose |

**Dosage in Hepatic Impairment**
No dose adjustment.

## SIDE EFFECTS

◀**ALERT**▶ Doses of 2 mg/kg or greater, or increased length of therapy, may result in a greater incidence of side effects.
**Frequent (10%):** Drowsiness, restlessness, fatigue, lethargy. **Occasional (3%):** Dizziness, anxiety, headache, insomnia, breast tenderness, altered menstruation, constipation, rash, dry mouth, galactorrhea, gynecomastia. **Rare (less than 3%):** Hypotension, hypertension, tachycardia.

## ADVERSE EFFECTS/TOXIC REACTIONS

Extrapyramidal reactions occur most frequently in children, young adults (18–30 yrs) receiving large doses (2 mg/kg) during chemotherapy and usually are limited to akathisia (involuntary limb movement, facial grimacing, motor restlessness). Neuroleptic malignant syndrome (diaphoresis, fever, unstable B/P, muscular rigidity) has been reported.

### NURSING CONSIDERATIONS

**BASELINE ASSESSMENT**

**Antiemetic:** Assess for dehydration (poor skin turgor, dry mucous membranes, longitudinal furrows in tongue). Assess for nausea, vomiting, abdominal distention, bowel sounds.

**INTERVENTION/EVALUATION**

Monitor for anxiety, restlessness, extrapyramidal symptoms (EPS) during IV administration. Monitor daily pattern of bowel activity, stool consistency. Assess skin for rash. Evaluate for therapeutic response from gastroparesis (nausea, vomiting, bloating). Monitor renal function, B/P, heart rate.

**PATIENT/FAMILY TEACHING**

• Avoid tasks that require alertness, motor skills until response to drug is established. • Report involuntary eye, facial, limb movement (extrapyramidal reaction). • Avoid alcohol.

# *metOLazone

meh-**toe**-la-zone
(Zaroxolyn ✦)
**Do not confuse metolazone
with metaxalone, methotrexate,
metoclopramide, or metoprolol,
or Zaroxolyn with Zarontin.**

### ◆CLASSIFICATION

**PHARMACOTHERAPEUTIC:** Thiazide diuretic. **CLINICAL:** Diuretic, antihypertensive.

## USES

Treatment of mild to moderate hypertension, edema due to HF, nephrotic syndrome or impaired renal function.

## PRECAUTIONS

**Contraindications:** Hypersensitivity to metolazone. Anuria, hepatic coma/precoma. **Cautions:** History of hypersensitivity to sulfonamides, thiazide diuretics. Severe renal disease, severe hepatic impairment, gout, prediabetes or diabetes, elevated serum cholesterol, triglycerides.

## ACTION

Blocks reabsorption of sodium, potassium, chloride at distal convoluted tubule, increasing excretion of sodium, potassium, water. **Therapeutic Effect:** Reduces B/P, promotes diuresis.

## PHARMACOKINETICS

| Route | Onset | Peak | Duration |
|---|---|---|---|
| PO (diuretic) | 1 hr | — | 24 hrs |

Incompletely absorbed from GI tract. Protein binding: 95%. Primarily excreted unchanged in urine. Not removed by hemodialysis. **Half-life:** 20 hrs.

## ⌛ LIFESPAN CONSIDERATIONS

**Pregnancy/Lactation:** Crosses placenta. Small amount distributed in breast milk. Breastfeeding not recommended. **Children:** No age-related precautions noted. **Elderly:** May be more sensitive to hypotensive or electrolyte effects. Age-related renal impairment may require dosage adjustment.

## INTERACTIONS

**DRUG:** May increase risk of **digoxin** toxicity associated with metolazone-induced hypokalemia. May increase risk of **lithium** toxicity. **HERBAL:** **Ephedra, ginseng, licorice** may decrease effect. **Black cohosh, periwinkle** may enhance effect. **FOOD:** None known. **LAB VALUES:** May increase serum glucose, cholesterol, LDL, bilirubin, calcium, creatinine, uric acid, triglycerides. May decrease urinary calcium, serum magnesium, potassium, sodium.

## AVAILABILITY (Rx)

**Tablets:** 2.5 mg, 5 mg, 10 mg.

## ADMINISTRATION/HANDLING

**PO**
• May give with food, milk if GI upset occurs, preferably with breakfast (may prevent nocturia).

## INDICATIONS/ROUTES/DOSAGE

**Edema**
**PO: ADULTS:** 2.5–10 mg/day. May increase to 20 mg/day in edema associated with renal disease or heart failure.

**Hypertension**
**PO: ADULTS, ELDERLY:** Initially, 2.5–5 mg/day. Adjust dose to achieve maximum therapeutic effect.

**Usual Pediatric Dosage**
**PO:** 0.2–0.4 mg/kg/day in 1–2 divided doses.

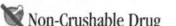

**Dosage in Renal Impairment**
**Mild to moderate impairment:** No dose adjustment. **Severe impairment:** Use caution.

**Dosage in Hepatic Impairment**
No dose adjustment. Contraindicated with hepatic coma or precoma.

## SIDE EFFECTS

**Expected:** Increased urinary frequency/volume. **Frequent (10%–9%):** Dizziness, light-headedness, headache. **Occasional (6%–4%):** Muscle cramps/spasm, drowsiness, fatigue, lethargy. **Rare (less than 2%):** Asthenia, palpitations, depression, nausea, vomiting, abdominal bloating, constipation, diarrhea, urticaria.

## ADVERSE EFFECTS/ TOXIC REACTIONS

Vigorous diuresis may lead to profound water loss and electrolyte depletion, resulting in hypokalemia, hyponatremia, dehydration. Acute hypotensive episodes may occur. Hyperglycemia may occur during prolonged therapy. Pancreatitis, paresthesia, blood dyscrasias, pulmonary edema, allergic pneumonitis, dermatologic reactions occur rarely. Overdose can lead to lethargy, coma without changes in electrolytes, hydration.

## NURSING CONSIDERATIONS

**BASELINE ASSESSMENT**

Check vital signs, esp. B/P for hypotension, before administration. Assess baseline serum electrolytes, particularly check for hypokalemia. Assess skin turgor, mucous membranes for hydration status. Assess for peripheral edema. Assess muscle strength, mental status. Note skin temperature, moisture. Obtain baseline weight. Monitor I&O.

**INTERVENTION/EVALUATION**

Continue to monitor B/P, vital signs, serum electrolytes, I&O, weight. Note extent of diuresis. Monitor for electrolyte disturbances (hypokalemia may result in weakness, tremors, muscle cramps, nausea, vomiting, altered mental status, tachycardia; hyponatremia may result in confusion, thirst, cold/clammy skin).

**PATIENT/FAMILY TEACHING**

• Expect increased urinary frequency/volume. • Slowly go from lying to standing to reduce hypotensive effect. • Avoid tasks requiring motor skills, mental alertness until response to drug is established. • Eat foods high in potassium, such as whole grains (cereals), legumes, meat, bananas, apricots, orange juice, potatoes (white, sweet), raisins.

---

## *metoprolol*

me-**toe**-pro-lol
(Apo-Metoprolol ✥, Lopressor, Toprol XL)
■ **BLACK BOX ALERT** ■ Abrupt withdrawal can produce acute tachycardia, hypertension, ischemia. Drug should be gradually tapered over 1–2 wks.
**Do not confuse metoprolol with atenolol, labetolol, nadolol, or stanozolol, or Toprol XL with Tegretol, Tegretol XR, or Topamax.**

## FIXED-COMBINATION(S)

**Dutoprol:** metoprolol/hydrochlorothiazide (a diuretic): 25 mg/12.5 mg, 50 mg/12.5 mg, 100 mg/12.5 mg. **Lopressor HCT:** metoprolol/hydro-chlorothiazide (a diuretic): 50 mg/25 mg, 100 mg/25 mg, 100 mg/50 mg.

## ◆CLASSIFICATION

**PHARMACOTHERAPEUTIC:** Beta$_1$-adrenergic blocker. **CLINICAL:** Antianginal, antihypertensive, MI adjunct.

## USES

**Lopressor:** Treatment of hemodynamically stable acute myocardial infarction

(AMI), angina pectoris, hypertension. **Toprol XL:** Treatment of angina pectoris, to reduce mortality or hospitalizations in pts with HF, already receiving ACE inhibitors, diuretics, and/or digoxin; hypertension. **OFF-LABEL:** Treatment of ventricular arrhythmias, migraine prophylaxis, essential tremor, aggressive behavior, prevent reinfarction post MI, prevent/treat atrial fibrillation/atrial flutter, hypertrophic cardiomyopathy, thyrotoxicosis.

## PRECAUTIONS

**Contraindications:** Hypersensitivity to metoprolol. *(Immediate-Release):* **MI:** Severe sinus bradycardia, MI with heart rate less than 45 beats/min or systolic B/P less than 100 mm Hg, moderate to severe HF, significant first-degree heart block, second- or third-degree heart block. *(Immediate-Release):* **HTN/Angina:** Sinus bradycardia, second- or third-degree heart block, cardiogenic shock, overt HF, sick sinus syndrome (except with pacemaker), severe peripheral arterial disease, pheochromocytoma. **Extended-Release:** Severe bradycardia, second- or third-degree heart block, cardiogenic shock, decompensated HF, sick sinus syndrome (except with functioning pacemaker). **Cautions:** Arterial obstruction, bronchospastic disease hepatic impairment, peripheral vascular disease, hyperthyroidism, diabetes mellitus, myasthenia gravis, psychiatric disease, history of severe anaphylaxis to allergens. **Extended-Release:** Compensated HF.

## ACTION

Selectively blocks beta$_1$-adrenergic receptors. **Therapeutic Effect:** Slows heart rate, decreases cardiac output, reduces B/P. Decreases myocardial ischemia severity.

## PHARMACOKINETICS

| Route | Onset | Peak | Duration |
|---|---|---|---|
| PO | 10–15 min | 1–2 hrs | N/A |
| PO (extended-release) | N/A | 6–12 hrs | N/A |
| IV | Immediate | 20 min | N/A |

Well absorbed from GI tract. Protein binding: 12%. Widely distributed. Metabolized in liver. Primarily excreted in urine. Removed by hemodialysis. **Half-life:** 3–7 hrs.

## ⧖ LIFESPAN CONSIDERATIONS

**Pregnancy/Lactation:** Crosses placenta; distributed in breast milk. Avoid use during first trimester. May produce bradycardia, apnea, hypoglycemia, hypothermia during delivery, low birth-weight infants. **Children:** Safety and efficacy not established. **Elderly:** Age-related peripheral vascular disease may increase susceptibility to decreased peripheral circulation.

## INTERACTIONS

**DRUG:** **Diuretics (e.g., furosemide, HCTZ), other antihypertensives (e.g., amlodipine, lisinopril, valsartan)** may increase hypotensive effect. May mask symptoms of hypoglycemia, prolong hypoglycemic effect of **insulin, oral hypoglycemics. NSAIDs** may decrease antihypertensive effect. **Sympathomimetics, xanthines** may mutually inhibit effects. Potent **CYP2D6 inhibitors (e.g., fluoxetine, cimetidine)** may increase concentration. **Digoxin, verapamil, diltiazem** may increase risk of bradycardia/heart block. **HERBAL:** **Ephedra, ginseng, yohimbe** may worsen hypertension. **Garlic** may increase antihypertensive effect. **FOOD:** None known. **LAB VALUES:** May increase serum antinuclear antibody titer (ANA), serum BUN, lipoprotein, LDH, alkaline phosphatase, bilirubin, creatinine, potassium, uric acid, ALT, AST, triglycerides.

**M**

---

✦ Canadian trade name    🌿 Non-Crushable Drug    ⬛ High Alert drug

## AVAILABILITY (Rx)

Injection Solution (Lopressor): 1 mg/ml.
Tablets (Lopressor): 25 mg, 50 mg,
100 mg.

 Tablets (Extended-Release [Toprol
XL]): 25 mg, 50 mg, 100 mg, 200 mg.

## ADMINISTRATION/HANDLING
### IV

**Rate of Administration** • May give
undiluted. • Administer IV injection
over 1 min. • May give by IV piggyback
(in 50 ml D$_5$W or 0.9% NaCl) over 30–
60 min. • Monitor EKG, B/P during
administration.
**Storage** • Store at room temperature.

### PO
• Tablets may be crushed; do not crush
extended-release tablets. • Extended-
release tablets may be divided in half.
• Give at same time each day. • May be
given with or immediately after meals
(enhances absorption).

### IV INCOMPATIBILITY

Amphotericin B complex (Abelcet, AmBisome, Amphotec), lidocaine, nitroglycerin.

### IV COMPATIBILITIES

Amiodarone, diltiazem, furosemide, heparin, morphine.

## INDICATIONS/ROUTES/DOSAGE

**Hypertension**
**PO** *(Immediate-Release):* **ADULTS,
ELDERLY:** Initially, 50 mg twice daily. Increase at wkly (or longer) intervals.
**Maintenance:** 100–450 mg/day in 2–3
divided doses. **CHILDREN:** Initially, 1–2
mg/kg/day in 2 divided doses. **Maximum:** 6 mg/kg/day in 2 divided doses
(200 mg).
**PO** *(Extended-Release):* **ADULTS, EL-
DERLY:** Initially, 25–100 mg/day as single
dose. May increase at least at wkly intervals until optimum B/P attained. **Maximum:** 400 mg/day. **CHILDREN 6 YRS OR
OLDER:** Initially, 1 mg/kg once daily.

**Maximum:** 50 mg. May increase to 2
mg/kg/day. **Maximum:** 200 mg/day.

**Angina Pectoris**
**PO** *(Immediate-Release):* **ADULTS:**
Initially, 50 mg twice daily. Increase at
wkly (or longer) intervals. Usual range:
50–200 mg twice daily. **Maximum:** 400
mg/day.
**PO** *(Extended-Release):* **ADULTS:** Initially, 100 mg/day as single dose. May
increase at least at wkly intervals until
optimum clinical response achieved.
**Maximum:** 400 mg/day.

**HF**
**PO** *(Extended-Release):* **ADULTS:** Initially, 25 mg/day. May double dose q2wks
up to target dose of 200 mg/day.

**Early Treatment of MI**
**IV:** **ADULTS:** 5 mg q5min for 3 doses,
followed by 25–50 mg orally q6–12h for
48–72 hrs. Transition over 2–3 days to
twice daily Lopressor or once daily Toprol XL. May increase up to a maximum of
200 mg/day.

**Dosage in Renal/Hepatic Impairment**
No dose adjustment.

## SIDE EFFECTS

Metoprolol is generally well tolerated,
with transient and mild side effects. **Frequent:** Diminished sexual function,
drowsiness, insomnia, unusual fatigue/
weakness. **Occasional:** Anxiety, diarrhea,
constipation, nausea, vomiting, nasal congestion, abdominal discomfort, dizziness,
difficulty breathing, cold hands/feet. **Rare:**
Altered taste, dry eyes, nightmares, paresthesia, allergic reaction (rash, pruritus).

## ADVERSE EFFECTS/
## TOXIC REACTIONS

Overdose may produce profound bradycardia, hypotension, bronchospasm.
Abrupt withdrawal may result in diaphoresis, palpitations, headache, tremulousness, exacerbation of angina, MI,

**M**

ventricular arrhythmias. May precipitate HF, MI in pts with heart disease, thyroid storm in those with thyrotoxicosis, peripheral ischemia in those with existing peripheral vascular disease. Hypoglycemia may occur in pts with previously controlled diabetes mellitus (may mask signs of hypoglycemia). **Antidote:** Glucagon (see Appendix J for dosage).

## NURSING CONSIDERATIONS

### BASELINE ASSESSMENT

Assess baseline renal function, LFT. Assess B/P, apical pulse immediately before drug administration (if pulse is 60/min or less or systolic B/P is less than 90 mm Hg, withhold medication, contact physician). **Antianginal:** Record onset, type (sharp, dull, squeezing), radiation, location, intensity, duration of anginal pain, precipitating factors (exertion, emotional stress).

### INTERVENTION/EVALUATION

Measure B/P near end of dosing interval (determines whether B/P is controlled throughout day). Monitor B/P for hypotension, respiration for shortness of breath. Assess pulse for quality, rate, rhythm. Assess for evidence of HF: dyspnea (esp. on exertion, lying down), night cough, peripheral edema, distended neck veins. Monitor I&O (increased weight, decreased urinary output may indicate HF). Therapeutic response to hypertension noted in 1–2 wks.

### PATIENT/FAMILY TEACHING

• Do not abruptly discontinue medication. • Compliance with therapy regimen is essential to control hypertension, arrhythmias. • If dose is missed, take next scheduled dose (do not double dose). • Go from lying to standing slowly. • Report excessive fatigue, dizziness. • Avoid tasks that require alertness, motor skills until response to drug is established. • Do not use nasal decongestants, OTC cold preparations (stimulants) without physician approval. • Monitor B/P, pulse before taking medication. • Restrict salt, alcohol intake.

## *metroNIDAZOLE

**me**-troe-**nye**-da-zole
(Flagyl, Flagyl ER, Metro, MetroCream, MetroGel, MetroGel-Vaginal, NidaGel ✦, Noritate, Vandazole)
**Do not confuse metronidazole with meropenum, metformin, methotrexate, or miconazole.**

### FIXED-COMBINATION(S)

**Helidac:** metronidazole/bismuth/tetracycline (an anti-infective): 250 mg/262 mg/500 mg. **Pylera:** metronidazole/bismuth/tetracycline (an anti-infective): 125 mg/140 mg/125 mg.

### ◆CLASSIFICATION

**PHARMACOTHERAPEUTIC:** Nitroimidazole derivative. **CLINICAL:** Antibacterial, antiprotozoal.

## USES

Treatment of anaerobic infections (skin/skin structure, CNS, lower respiratory tract, bone/joints, intra-abdominal, gynecologic, endocarditis, septicemia). Treatment of *H. pylori* (part of multidrug regimen); surgical prophylaxis (colorectal), trichomoniasis, amebiasis. Topical treatment of acne rosacea or inflammatory lesions. **Vaginal gel:** Treatment of bacterial vaginosis. **OFF-LABEL:** Crohn's disease, urethritis. Antibiotic-associated pseudomembranous colitis (AAPC) caused by *C. difficile*.

## PRECAUTIONS

**Contraindications:** Hypersensitivity to metronidazole. Pregnancy (first trimester with trichomoniasis), use of disulfiram

M

within 2 wks, use of alcohol during therapy or within 3 days of discontinuing metronidazole. **Cautions:** Blood dyscrasias, severe hepatic dysfunction, end-stage renal disease, history of seizures, HF, other sodium-retaining states, elderly.

## ACTION

Disrupts DNA, inhibiting nucleic acid synthesis. **Therapeutic Effect:** Produces bactericidal, antiprotozoal, amebicidal, trichomonacidal effects. Produces anti-inflammatory, immunosuppressive effects when applied topically.

## PHARMACOKINETICS

Well absorbed from GI tract; minimally absorbed after topical application. Protein binding: less than 20%. Widely distributed; crosses blood-brain barrier. Metabolized in liver. Excreted in urine (80%), feces (15%). Removed by hemodialysis. **Half-life:** 8 hrs (increased in cirrhosis, neonates). Active metabolite prolonged in renal failure.

## ⏳ LIFESPAN CONSIDERATIONS

**Pregnancy/Lactation:** Readily crosses placenta. Distributed in breast milk. Contraindicated during first trimester in those with trichomoniasis. Topical use during pregnancy, lactation discouraged. **Children:** Safety and efficacy of topical administration not established in pts younger than 21 yrs. **Elderly:** Age-related hepatic impairment may require dosage adjustment.

## INTERACTIONS

**DRUG: Alcohol** may cause disulfiram-type reaction (e.g., abdominal cramps, nausea, vomiting, headache, psychotic reactions). **Disulfiram** may increase risk of toxicity. May increase effects of **oral anticoagulants (e.g., warfarin).** **HERBAL:** None significant. **FOOD:** None known. **LAB VALUES:** May increase serum LDH, ALT, AST.

## AVAILABILITY (Rx)

**Capsules:** 375 mg. **Injection (Infusion):** 500 mg/100 ml. **Tablets (Flagyl):** 250

mg, 500 mg. **Topical Cream:** 0.75% (MetroCream), 1% (Noritate). **Topical Gel (MetroGel):** 0.75%, 1%. **Vaginal Gel (MetroGel-Vaginal, Vandazole):** 0.75%.

 Tablets (Extended-Release [Flagyl ER]): 750 mg.

## ADMINISTRATION/HANDLING

💧 IV

**Rate of Administration** • Infuse IV over 30–60 min. Do not give by IV bolus. **Storage** • Store at room temperature (ready-to-use infusion bags).

PO
• Give without regard to meals. Give with food to decrease GI irritation. • Extended-release tablet should be given on an empty stomach (1 hr before or 2 hrs after meals). • Do not crush extended-release tablets.

## ▒ IV INCOMPATIBILITIES

Amphotericin B complex (Abelcet, AmBisome, Amphotec).

## ▒ IV COMPATIBILITIES

Dexmedetomidine (Precedex), diltiazem (Cardizem), dopamine (Intropin), heparin, hydromorphone (Dilaudid), lorazepam (Ativan), magnesium sulfate, midazolam (Versed), morphine.

## INDICATIONS/ROUTES/DOSAGE

**Amebiasis**
**PO: ADULTS, ELDERLY:** 750 mg q8h for 5–10 days.

**Anaerobic Infections**
**PO, IV: ADULTS, ELDERLY:** 500 mg q6–8h. **Maximum:** 4 g/day.
**PO: CHILDREN, INFANTS:** 15–35 mg/kg/day in divided doses q8h. **Maximum:** 2,250 mg/day.
**IV: CHILDREN, INFANTS:** 30 mg/kg/day in 3 divided doses. **Maximum:** 1,500 mg/day.

**Intra-abdominal Infections**
**IV: ADULTS, ELDERLY:** 500 mg q8h. **Maximum:** 4 g/day.

### Pseudomembranous Colitis
**PO: ADULTS, ELDERLY:** 250–500 mg 3–4 times/day. **CHILDREN:** 30 mg/kg/day in divided doses q6h for 7–10 days. **Maximum:** 2 g/day.

### Bacterial Vaginosis
**Intravaginal: ADULTS:** 0.75% apply twice daily for 5 days. 1.3% apply once as a single dose.
◄**ALERT**► Centers for Disease Control and Prevention (CDC) does not recommend the use of topical agents during pregnancy.

### Rosacea
**Topical: ADULTS, ELDERLY: (1%):** Apply to affected area once daily. **(0.75%):** Apply to affected area twice daily.

### Dosage in Renal Impairment
No dose adjustment.

### Dosage in Hepatic Impairment
**Mild to moderate impairment:** Use caution. No dose adjustment. **Severe impairment:** Reduce dose by 50% for immediate-release; not recommended for extended-release.

## SIDE EFFECTS
**Frequent: Systemic:** Anorexia, nausea, dry mouth, metallic taste. **Vaginal:** Symptomatic cervicitis/vaginitis, abdominal cramps, uterine pain. **Occasional: Systemic:** Diarrhea, constipation, vomiting, dizziness, erythematous rash, urticaria, reddish-brown urine. **Topical:** Transient erythema, mild dryness, burning, irritation, stinging, tearing when applied too close to eyes. **Vaginal:** Vaginal, perineal, vulvar itching; vulvar swelling. **Rare:** Mild, transient leukopenia; thrombophlebitis with IV therapy.

## ADVERSE EFFECTS/ TOXIC REACTIONS
Oral therapy may result in furry tongue, glossitis, cystitis, dysuria, pancreatitis. Peripheral neuropathy (manifested as numbness, tingling of hands/feet) usually is reversible if treatment is stopped immediately upon appearance of neurologic symptoms. Seizures occur occasionally.

## NURSING CONSIDERATIONS

### BASELINE ASSESSMENT
Question for history of hypersensitivity to metronidazole, other nitroimidazole derivatives (and parabens with topical). Obtain specimens for diagnostic tests, cultures before giving first dose (therapy may begin before results are known).

### INTERVENTION/EVALUATION
Monitor daily pattern of bowel activity, stool consistency. Monitor I&O, assess for urinary problems. Be alert to neurologic symptoms (dizziness, paresthesia of extremities). Assess for rash, urticaria. Monitor for onset of superinfection (ulceration/change of oral mucosa, furry tongue, vaginal discharge, genital/anal pruritus).

### PATIENT/FAMILY TEACHING
• Urine may be red-brown or dark. • Avoid alcohol, alcohol-containing preparations (cough syrups, elixirs) for at least 48 hrs after last dose. • Avoid tasks that require alertness, motor skills until response to drug is established. • If taking metronidazole for trichomoniasis, refrain from sexual intercourse until full treatment is completed. • For amebiasis, frequent stool specimen checks will be necessary. • **Topical:** Avoid contact with eyes. • May apply cosmetics after application. • Metronidazole acts on erythema, papules, pustules but has no effect on rhinophyma (hypertrophy of nose), telangiectasia, ocular problems (conjunctivitis, keratitis, blepharitis). • Other recommendations for rosacea include avoidance of hot/spicy foods, alcohol, extremes of hot/cold temperatures, excessive sunlight.

M

# micafungin

mye-ka-**fun**-jin
(Mycamine)

## ◆CLASSIFICATION
**PHARMACOTHERAPEUTIC:** Echinocandin antifungal. **CLINICAL:** Antifungal.

---

## USES

Treatment of esophageal candidiasis, candidemia, candida peritonitis, abscesses, acute disseminated candidiasis, prophylaxis of *Candida* infection in pts undergoing hematopoietic stem cell transplant. **OFF-LABEL:** Treatment of infections due to *Aspergillus* spp.

## PRECAUTIONS

**Contraindications:** Hypersensitivity to micafungin. **Cautions:** Hepatic/renal impairment, concomitant hepatotoxic medications.

## ACTION

Inhibits synthesis of glucan (vital component of fungal cell formation), damaging fungal cell membrane. **Therapeutic Effect:** Decreased glucan content leads to cellular lysis.

## PHARMACOKINETICS

Slowly metabolized in liver. Protein binding: greater than 99%. Primarily excreted in feces. Not removed by hemodialysis. **Half-life:** 11–21 hrs.

## ⧗ LIFESPAN CONSIDERATIONS

**Pregnancy/Lactation:** May reduce sperm count. May be embryotoxic. Unknown if distributed in breast milk. **Children:** Safety and efficacy not established. **Elderly:** No age-related precautions noted.

## INTERACTIONS

**DRUG:** May increase concentration of **nifedipine, sirolimus, itraconazole.** **HERBAL:** None significant. **FOOD:** None known. **LAB VALUES:** May increase serum creatinine, alkaline phosphatase, LDH, ALT, AST.

## AVAILABILITY (Rx)

**Injection, Powder for Reconstitution:** 50 mg, 100 mg.

## ADMINISTRATION/HANDLING

 **IV**

**Reconstitution** • Add 5 ml 0.9% NaCl (without bacteriostatic agent) to each 50-mg vial (10 ml to 100-mg vial) to yield micafungin 10 mg/ml. • Gently swirl to dissolve; do not shake. • Further dilute in 0.9% NaCl or $D_5W$ to final concentration of 0.5–1.5 mg/ml. • Alternatively, $D_5W$ may be used for reconstitution and dilution. • Flush existing IV line with 0.9% NaCl or $D_5W$ before infusion.
**Rate of Administration** • Infuse over 60 min.
**Storage** • Reconstituted solution is stable for 24 hrs at room temperature. • Discard if precipitate is present.

## ▦ IV INCOMPATIBILITIES

Amiodarone, nicardipine.

## ▦ IV COMPATIBILITIES

Bumetanide (Bumex), calcium gluconate, heparin.

## INDICATIONS/ROUTES/DOSAGE

**Esophageal Candidiasis**
**IV: ADULTS, ELDERLY:** 150 mg/day for 10–30 days. **CHILDREN 4 MOS OR OLDER: (GREATER THAN 30 KG):** 2.5 mg/kg/day. (**Maximum:** 150 mg daily.) **(30 KG OR LESS):** 3 mg/kg/day.

**Candida Prophylaxis in Stem Cell Pts**
**IV: ADULTS, ELDERLY:** 50 mg/day. **CHILDREN 4 MOS OR OLDER:** 1 mg/kg/day. **Maximum:** 50 mg/day.

**Candidemia, Disseminated Candidiasis, Peritonitis, Abscesses**
**IV: ADULTS, ELDERLY:** 100 mg/day for 15 days. **CHILDREN 4 MOS OR OLDER:** 2 mg/kg/day. **Maximum:** 100 mg daily.

**Dosage in Renal/Hepatic Impairment**
No dose adjustment.

**M**

## SIDE EFFECTS

**Occasional (3%–2%):** Nausea, headache, diarrhea, vomiting, fever. **Rare (1%):** Dizziness, drowsiness, pruritus, abdominal pain, dyspepsia.

## ADVERSE EFFECTS/ TOXIC REACTIONS

Hypersensitivity reaction characterized by rash, pruritus, facial edema occurs rarely. Anaphylaxis, hemoglobinuria, hemolytic anemia have been reported.

## NURSING CONSIDERATIONS

### BASELINE ASSESSMENT

Determine baseline renal function, LFT and periodically thereafter.

### INTERVENTION/EVALUATION

Monitor serum chemistry results for evidence of hepatic/renal impairment.

---

## *midazolam* HIGH ALERT

mye-**da**-zoe-lam
(Apo-Midazolam , Versed)
■ **BLACK BOX ALERT** ■ May cause severe respiratory depression, respiratory arrest, apnea. Initial doses in elderly should be conservative. Do not administer by rapid IV injection in neonates (may cause severe hypotension/seizures).
**Do not confuse Versed with VePesid or Vistaril.**

## ◆CLASSIFICATION

**PHARMACOTHERAPEUTIC:** Benzodiazepine **(Schedule IV)**. **CLINICAL:** Sedative, anxiolytic.

## USES

Sedation, anxiolytic, amnesia before procedure or induction of anesthesia, conscious sedation before diagnostic/radiographic procedure, continuous IV sedation of intubated or mechanically ventilated pts. **OFF-LABEL:** Anxiety, status epilepticus, conscious sedation (intranasal route).

## PRECAUTIONS

**Contraindications:** Hypersensitivity to midazolam. Acute narrow-angle glaucoma, concurrent use of potent CYP3A4 inhibitors (e.g., atazanavir, ritonavir). **Cautions:** Renal/hepatic/pulmonary impairment, impaired gag reflex, HF, treated open-angle glaucoma, obese pts, concurrent CNS depressants, alcohol dependency, elderly, debilitated.

## ACTION

Enhances action of gamma-aminobutyric acid (GABA), one of the major inhibitory neurotransmitters in the brain. **Therapeutic Effect:** Produces anxiolytic, hypnotic, anticonvulsant, muscle relaxant, amnestic effects.

## PHARMACOKINETICS

| Route | Onset | Peak | Duration |
|-------|-------|------|----------|
| PO | 10–20 min | N/A | N/A |
| IV | 1–5 min | 5–7 min | 20–30 min |
| IM | 5–15 min | 30–60 min | 2–6 hrs |

Well absorbed after IM administration. Protein binding: 97%. Metabolized in liver. Primarily excreted in urine. Not removed by hemodialysis. **Half-life:** 1–5 hrs.

## ⧗ LIFESPAN CONSIDERATIONS

**Pregnancy/Lactation:** Crosses placenta. Unknown if drug is distributed in breast milk. **Children:** Neonates more likely to have respiratory depression. **Elderly:** Age-related renal impairment may require dosage adjustment.

## INTERACTIONS

**DRUG: Alcohol, other CNS depressants (e.g., lorazepam, morphine, zolpidem)** may increase CNS effects, respiratory depression, hypotensive effect. **CYP3A4 inhibitors (e.g., erythromycin)** may increase concentration/sedative effect. **HERBAL: Gotu kola, kava kava, St. John's wort, valerian** may increase CNS depression. **St. John's wort** may decrease concentration. **FOOD: Grapefruit products** increase oral absorption,

**M**

---

systemic availability. **LAB VALUES:** None significant.

## AVAILABILITY (Rx)

**Injection Solution:** 1 mg/ml, 5 mg/ml. **Syrup:** 2 mg/ml.

## ADMINISTRATION/HANDLING

 IV

**Rate of Administration** • May give undiluted or as infusion. • Resuscitative equipment, $O_2$ must be readily available before IV administration. • Administer by slow IV injection over at least 2–5 min at concentration of 1–5 mg/ml. • Reduce IV rate in those older than 60 yrs, debilitated pts with chronic disease states, pulmonary impairment. • Too-rapid IV rate, excessive doses, or single large dose increases risk of respiratory depression/arrest.
**Storage** • Store vials at room temperature.

**IM**
• Give deep IM into large muscle mass. **Maximum concentration:** 1 mg/ml.

**PO**
• Do not mix with grapefruit juice.

## ▓ IV INCOMPATIBILITIES

Albumin, amphotericin B complex (Abelcet, AmBisome, Amphotec), ampicillin (Polycillin), ampicillin and sulbactam (Unasyn), bumetanide (Bumex), co-trimoxazole (Bactrim), dexamethasone (Decadron), fosphenytoin (Cerebyx), furosemide (Lasix), hydrocortisone (Solu-Cortef), methotrexate, nafcillin (Nafcil), sodium bicarbonate.

## ▓ IV COMPATIBILITIES

Amiodarone (Cordarone), atropine, calcium gluconate, dexmedetomidine (Precedex), diltiazem (Cardizem), diphenhydramine (Benadryl), dobutamine (Dobutrex), dopamine (Intropin), etomidate (Amidate), fentanyl (Sublimaze), glycopyrrolate (Robinul), heparin, hydromorphone (Dilaudid), hydroxyzine (Vistaril), insulin, lorazepam (Ativan), milrinone (Primacor), morphine, nitroglycerin, norepinephrine (Levophed), potassium chloride, propofol (Diprivan).

## INDICATIONS/ROUTES/DOSAGE

**Preop Sedation**
**PO: CHILDREN:** 0.5–0.75 mg/kg. **Maximum:** 20 mg.
**IV: ADULTS, ELDERLY:** 0.02–0.04 mg/kg. Usual dose: 1–2.5 mg. **CHILDREN 6–12 YRS:** 0.025–0.05 mg/kg. **CHILDREN 6 MOS–5 YRS:** 0.05–0.1 mg/kg.
**IM: ADULTS, ELDERLY:** 0.07–0.08 mg/ kg 30–60 min before surgery. Usual dose: 5 mg. **CHILDREN:** 0.1–0.15 mg/kg 30–60 min before surgery. **Maximum:** 10 mg.

**Continuous Sedation During Mechanical Ventilation**
**IV: ADULTS, ELDERLY:** Initially, 0.01–0.05 mg/kg (1–5 mg in 70-kg adult). May repeat at 5- to 15-min intervals until adequate sedation achieved or continuous infusion rate of 0.02–0.1 mg/kg/hr and titrated to desired effect. **CHILDREN:** Initially, 0.05–0.2 mg/kg followed by continuous infusion of 0.06–0.12 mg/kg/hr (1–2 mcg/kg/min) titrated to desired effect. Usual range: 0.4–6 mcg/kg/min.

**Dosage in Renal Impairment**
No dose adjustment.

**Dosage in Hepatic Impairment**
Use caution.

## SIDE EFFECTS

**Frequent (10%–4%):** Decreased respiratory rate, tenderness at IM or IV injection site, pain during injection, oxygen desaturation, hiccups. **Occasional (3%–2%):** Hypotension, paradoxical CNS reaction. **Rare (less than 2%):** Nausea, vomiting, headache, coughing.

## ADVERSE EFFECTS/ TOXIC REACTIONS

Inadequate or excessive dosage, improper administration may result in cerebral hypoxia, agitation, involuntary movements, hyperactivity, combativeness. Too-rapid IV rate, excessive doses, or single large dose increases risk of respiratory depression/arrest. Respiratory depression/apnea may produce hypoxia, cardiac arrest.

## NURSING CONSIDERATIONS

### BASELINE ASSESSMENT

Resuscitative equipment, oxygen must be available. Obtain vital signs before administration.

### INTERVENTION/EVALUATION

Monitor respiratory rate, oxygen saturation continuously during parenteral administration for underventilation, apnea. Monitor vital signs, level of sedation q3–5min during recovery period.

---

# midodrine

mye-doe-dreen
(Amatine ✽, Apo-Midodrine ✽)
■ **BLACK BOX ALERT** ■ Can cause marked rise in supine blood pressure; use in pts for whom orthostatic hypotension significantly impairs daily life.
**Do not confuse Amatine with amantadine or protamine, or midodrine with Midrin.**

## ◆CLASSIFICATION

**PHARMACOTHERAPEUTIC:** Vasopressor. **CLINICAL:** Orthostatic hypotension adjunct.

## USES

Treatment of symptomatic orthostatic hypotension. **OFF-LABEL:** Vasovagal syncope, prevention of dialysis-induced hypotension.

## PRECAUTIONS

**Contraindications:** Hypersensitivity to midodrine. Acute renal failure, persistent supine hypertension, pheochromocytoma, severe cardiac disease, thyrotoxicosis, urinary retention. **Cautions:** Renal/hepatic impairment, history of visual problems, diabetes; concurrent administration with digoxin, beta blockers (e.g., metoprolol), vasoconstrictors (e.g., norepinephrine).

## ACTION

Forms active metabolite desglymidodrine, an alpha$_1$ agonist, increasing arteriolar and venous tone. **Therapeutic Effect:** Increases standing, sitting, and supine systolic B/P in pts with orthostatic hypotension.

## PHARMACOKINETICS

| Route | Onset | Peak | Duration |
|-------|-------|------|----------|
| PO | 1 hr | — | 2–3 hrs |

Rapid absorption from GI tract following PO administration. Protein binding: Low. Undergoes enzymatic hydrolysis (deglycination) in systemic circulation. Excreted in urine. **Half-life:** 0.5 hr.

## ⧗ LIFESPAN CONSIDERATIONS

**Pregnancy/Lactation:** Unknown if drug crosses placenta or is distributed in breast milk. **Children:** Safety and efficacy not established. **Elderly:** Age-related renal impairment may require dosage adjustment.

## INTERACTIONS

**DRUG: Digoxin** may have additive bradycardic effects. **Sodium-retaining steroids (e.g., fludrocortisone)** may increase sodium retention. **Vasoconstrictors (e.g., dopamine, norepinephrine)** may have additive effects. **HERBAL:** None significant. **FOOD:** None known. **LAB VALUES:** None significant.

## AVAILABILITY (Rx)

**Tablets:** 2.5 mg, 5 mg, 10 mg.

M

---

✽ Canadian trade name     🗽 Non-Crushable Drug     🔲 High Alert drug

## ADMINISTRATION/HANDLING

• Give without regard to food. • Last dose of day should be given 3–4 hrs before bedtime.

## INDICATIONS/ROUTES/DOSAGE

**Orthostatic Hypotension**
**PO: ADULTS, ELDERLY:** 10 mg 3 times/day (q3–4hrs). Give during the day when pt is upright, such as upon arising, midday, and late afternoon. Do not give later than 6 PM. **Maximum:** 30 mg/day.

**Dosage in Renal Impairment**
2.5 mg 3 times/day; increase gradually, as tolerated. **Hemodialysis:** Dose after HD unless used to prevent HD-induced hypotension.

**Dosage in Hepatic Impairment**
Use caution.

## SIDE EFFECTS

**Frequent (20%–7%):** Paresthesia, piloerection, pruritus, dysuria, supine hypertension. **Occasional (6%–1%):** Pain, rash, chills, headache, facial flushing, confusion, dry mouth, anxiety.

## ADVERSE EFFECTS/ TOXIC REACTIONS

Increased systolic arterial pressure has been noted.

## NURSING CONSIDERATIONS

### BASELINE ASSESSMENT

Assess sensitivity to midodrine, other medications (esp. digoxin, sodium-retaining vasoconstrictors). Assess medical history, esp. for renal impairment, severe hypertension, cardiac disease.

### INTERVENTION/EVALUATION

Monitor B/P, renal, hepatic, cardiac function.

### PATIENT/FAMILY TEACHING

• Do not take last dose of the day after evening meal or less than 4 hrs before bedtime. • Do not give if pt will be supine.

• Use caution with OTC medications that may affect B/P (e.g., cough and cold, diet medications).

# milnacipran

mil-**nay**-sip-ran
(Savella)

■ **BLACK BOX ALERT** ■ Increased risk of suicidal ideation and behavior in children, adolescents, and young adults 18–24 yrs with major depressive disorder, other psychiatric disorders.
**Do not confuse Savella with cevimeline or sevelamer.**

## ◆CLASSIFICATION

**PHARMACOTHERAPEUTIC:** Serotonin, norepinephrine reuptake inhibitor. **CLINICAL:** Fibromyalgia agent.

## USES

Management of fibromyalgia.

## PRECAUTIONS

**Contraindications:** Hypersensitivity to milnacipran. Concomitant use of MAOIs to treat psychiatric disorders (concurrently or within 5 days of discontinuing milnacipran or within 2 wks of discontinuing MAOI), uncontrolled narrow-angle glaucoma, initiation of milnacipran in pts receiving linezolid or IV methylene blue. **Cautions:** Pts with depression, pts at increased risk of suicide, other psychiatric disorders; elevated blood pressure or heart rate, history of seizures, pts with substantial alcohol use or chronic hepatic disease, pts with history of dysuria (e.g., prostatic hypertrophy, prostatitis), controlled narrow-angle glaucoma, renal impairment, cardiovascular disease, elderly.

## ACTION

Appears to inhibit serotonin and norepinephrine reuptake at CNS neuronal presynaptic membranes. **Therapeutic Effect:** Reduces chronic pain, fatigue, depression, sleep disorders associated with fibromyalgia syndrome; improves physical function.

## PHARMACOKINETICS

Well absorbed following PO administration. Protein binding: 13%. Eliminated unchanged in urine. Steady-state levels reached in 36–48 hrs. **Half-life:** 6–8 hrs.

## ⧖ LIFESPAN CONSIDERATIONS

**Pregnancy/Lactation:** Increased risk of fetal complications, including need for respiratory support, if given during third trimester. Unknown if distributed in breast milk. **Children:** Safety and efficacy not established in pts younger than 18 yrs. **Elderly:** Severe renal impairment requires dosage adjustment.

## INTERACTIONS

**DRUG:** **Lithium, MAOIs** may increase risk of serotonin syndrome. **Epinephrine, norepinephrine** may produce paroxysmal hypertension, arrhythmias. **Intravenous digoxin** may produce tachycardia, hypotension. May inhibit antihypertensive effect of **clonidine.** **HERBAL:** **Gotu kola, kava kava, St. John's wort, valerian** may increase CNS depression, increase risk of serotonin syndrome. **FOOD:** None known. **LAB VALUES:** May decrease serum sodium.

## AVAILABILITY (Rx)

 **Tablets, Film-Coated:** 12.5 mg, 25 mg, 50 mg, 100 mg.

## ADMINISTRATION/HANDLING

• Give without regard to food. • Do not break, crush, dissolve, or divide film-coated tablets.

## INDICATIONS/ROUTES/DOSAGE

**Fibromyalgia**
**PO: ADULTS, ELDERLY: Day 1:** 12.5 mg once. **Days 2–3:** 25 mg/day (12.5 mg twice daily). **Days 4–7:** 50 mg/day (25 mg twice daily). **After Day 7:** 100 mg/day (50 mg twice daily thereafter). Dose may be increased to 200 mg/day (100 mg twice daily).

**Dosage in Renal Impairment**
**Mild impairment:** No dose adjustment. **Moderate impairment:** Use caution. **Severe impairment:** Reduce maintenance dose by 50% to 50 mg/day (25 mg twice daily). Based on pt response, dose may be increased to 100 mg/day (50 mg twice daily). Not recommended in end-stage renal disease.

**Dosage in Hepatic Impairment**
**Mild to moderate impairment:** No dose adjustment. **Severe impairment:** Use caution.

## SIDE EFFECTS

**Frequent (37%–18%):** Nausea, headache. **Occasional (16%–5%):** Constipation, insomnia, hot flashes, dizziness, hyperhidrosis, palpitations, vomiting, URI. **Rare (Less Than 5%):** Dry mouth, increased B/P, anxiety, skin flushing, rash, blurred vision, abdominal pain, chest pain, chills, pruritus, paresthesia, tachycardia.

## ADVERSE EFFECTS/ TOXIC REACTIONS

Abrupt discontinuation may present withdrawal symptoms (dysphoria, irritability, agitation, dizziness, paresthesia, anxiety, confusion, headache, lethargy, emotional lability, tinnitus, seizures). Serotonin syndrome symptoms may include mental status changes (agitation, hallucinations), hyperreflexia, incoordination. May increase risk of bleeding events (e.g., ecchymoses, hematomas, epistaxis).

## NURSING CONSIDERATIONS

### BASELINE ASSESSMENT

Obtain baseline pain intensity scale, location(s) of pain, tenderness. Obtain

**M**

---

 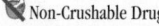

baseline B/P, heart rate. Question for history of changes in day-to-day pain intensity.

### INTERVENTION/EVALUATION

Control nausea with antiemetics. Treat complaint of headache, migraine with appropriate analgesics. Monitor for increase in B/P, pulse. Question for changes in visual acuity. Assess for clinical improvement and record onset of pain control, decreased fatigue, lessening of depressive symptoms, improvement in sleep pattern. Monitor for suicidal ideation.

### PATIENT/FAMILY TEACHING

• Avoid tasks that require alertness, motor skills until response to drug is established. • Do not abruptly discontinue medication. • Increase fluids, bulk to prevent constipation. • Report unusual changes in behavior, suicidal ideation; hot flushing that becomes intolerant, excessive sweating. • Caution about risk of bleeding associated with concomitant use of NSAIDs, aspirin.

---

## milrinone ~~HIGH ALERT~~

mil-ri-none
**Do not confuse Primacor with Primaxin.**

### ◆CLASSIFICATION

**PHARMACOTHERAPEUTIC:** Cardiac inotropic agent. **CLINICAL:** Vasodilator.

## USES

Short-term management of decompensated HF. **OFF-LABEL:** Inotropic therapy for pts unresponsive to other therapy, outpatient inotropic therapy for heart transplant candidates, palliation of symptoms in end-stage HF.

## PRECAUTIONS

**Contraindications:** Hypersensitivity to milrinone. **Cautions:** Severe obstructive aortic or pulmonic valvular disease, history of ventricular arrhythmias, atrial fibrillation/flutter, renal impairment. Not recommended in pts with acute MI.

## ACTION

Inhibits phosphodiesterase, which increases cyclic adenosine monophosphate (cAMP), potentiating delivery of calcium to myocardial contractile systems. **Therapeutic Effect:** Relaxes vascular muscle, causing vasodilation. Increases cardiac output, decreases pulmonary capillary wedge pressure, vascular resistance.

## PHARMACOKINETICS

| Route | Onset | Peak | Duration |
|-------|-------|------|----------|
| IV | 5–15 min | N/A | N/A |

Protein binding: 70%. Metabolized in liver. Primarily excreted in urine. **Half-life:** 1.7–2.7 hrs.

## ⧗ LIFESPAN CONSIDERATIONS

**Pregnancy/Lactation:** Unknown if drug crosses placenta or is distributed in breast milk. **Children:** Safety and efficacy not established. **Elderly:** Age-related renal impairment may require dosage adjustment.

## INTERACTIONS

**DRUG:** None significant. **HERBAL:** None significant. **FOOD:** None known. **LAB VALUES:** None significant.

## AVAILABILITY (Rx)

**Injection Solution (Primacor):** 1 mg/ml, 10-ml vial. **Injection Solution (Premix [Primacor]):** 200 mcg/ml (100 ml, 200 ml).

## ADMINISTRATION/HANDLING

 IV

**Reconstitution** • For IV infusion, dilute 20-mg (20-ml) vial with 80 ml 0.9% NaCl or D$_5$W to provide concentration of 0.2 mg/ml (200 mcg/ml).

**Rate of Administration** • For IV injection (loading dose), administer undiluted slowly over 10 min. • Monitor for arrhythmias, hypotension during IV therapy; reduce or temporarily discontinue infusion until condition stabilizes. IV infusion via infusion pump.

**Storage** • Diluted solutions stable for 72 hrs at room temperature.

### 🔲 IV INCOMPATIBILITIES

Furosemide (Lasix), imipenem-cilastatin (Primaxin), procainamide (Pronestyl).

### 🔲 IV COMPATIBILITIES

Calcium gluconate, dexamethasone (Decadron), dexmedetomidine (Precedex), digoxin (Lanoxin), diltiazem (Cardizem), dobutamine (Dobutrex), dopamine (Intropin), heparin, hydromorphone (Dilaudid), lidocaine, magnesium, midazolam (Versed), morphine, nitroglycerin, potassium, propofol (Diprivan).

### INDICATIONS/ROUTES/DOSAGE

**Management of HF**

**IV: ADULTS:** Initially, 50 mcg/kg over 10 min. Continue with maintenance infusion rate of 0.375–0.75 mcg/kg/min based on hemodynamic and clinical response.

**Dosage in Renal Impairment**

| Creatinine Clearance | Dosage |
| --- | --- |
| 50 ml/min | 0.43 mcg/kg/min |
| 40 ml/min | 0.38 mcg/kg/min |
| 30 ml/min | 0.33 mcg/kg/min |
| 20 ml/min | 0.28 mcg/kg/min |
| 10 ml/min | 0.23 mcg/kg/min |
| 5 ml/min | 0.2 mcg/kg/min |

**Dosage in Hepatic Impairment**
No dose adjustment.

### SIDE EFFECTS

**Occasional (3%–1%):** Headache, hypotension. **Rare (less than 1%):** Angina, chest pain.

### ADVERSE EFFECTS/ TOXIC REACTIONS

Supraventricular/ventricular arrhythmias (12%), nonsustained ventricular tachycardia (2%), sustained ventricular tachycardia (1%) may occur. Ventricular fibrillation (0.2%) has been documented.

### NURSING CONSIDERATIONS

#### BASELINE ASSESSMENT

Obtain baseline lab studies, esp. BN peptide. Offer emotional support (difficulty breathing may produce anxiety). Assess B/P, apical pulse rate before treatment begins and during IV therapy. Assess lung sounds; observe for edema.

#### INTERVENTION/EVALUATION

Monitor B/P, heart rate, cardiac output, EKG, serum potassium, renal function, signs/symptoms of HF.

## minocycline

mye-noe-**sye**-kleen
(Apo-Minocycline ✿, Minocin, Solodyn)
**Do not confuse Dynacin with Dyazide, DynaCirc, or Dynapen, or Minocin with Indocin, Mithracin, or niacin.**

### ◆ CLASSIFICATION

**PHARMACOTHERAPEUTIC:** Tetracycline. **CLINICAL:** Antibiotic.

### USES

Treatment of susceptible infections due to *Rickettsiae, M. pneumoniae, C. trachomatis, C. psittaci, H. ducreyi, Yersinia pestis, Francisella tularensis, Vibrio cholerae, Brucella* spp., gram-negative organisms, including prostate, urinary tract, CNS infections (not meningitis), uncomplicated gonorrhea, inflammatory acne, brucellosis, skin granulomas, cholera, trachoma, nocardiasis,

M

yaws, syphilis (when penicillins are contraindicated). **Solodyn:** Treatment of inflammatory lesions of moderate to severe non-nodular acne. **OFF-LABEL:** Treatment of nocardiosis, community-acquired MRSA infection, rheumatoid arthritis (RA), prosthetic joint infection.

## PRECAUTIONS

**Contraindications:** Hypersensitivity to minocycline, other tetracyclines. **Cautions:** Children younger than 8 yrs, renal impairment, hepatic impairment, sun/ultraviolet exposure (severe photosensitivity reaction). Avoid use in pregnancy.

## ACTION

Inhibits bacterial protein synthesis by binding to ribosomes. **Therapeutic Effect:** Bacteriostatic.

## PHARMACOKINETICS

Well absorbed from GI tract. Protein binding: 70%–75%. Partial elimination in feces; minimal excretion in urine. Not removed by hemodialysis. **Half-life:** 11–23 hrs.

## ⧖ LIFESPAN CONSIDERATIONS

**Pregnancy/Lactation:** Readily crosses placenta; distributed in breast milk. May inhibit fetal skeletal growth. **Children:** May cause permanent discoloration of teeth, enamel hypoplasia. Not recommended in pts younger than 8 yrs. **Elderly:** No age-related precautions noted.

## INTERACTIONS

**DRUG: Aluminum-, calcium-, magnesium-containing antacids** may decrease absorption, effect. **Ergot** may increase risk of ergotism. May decrease the effects of **estrogen-containing oral contraceptives. HERBAL: Dong quai, St. John's wort** may increase risk of photosensitivity. **FOOD:** None known. **LAB VALUES:** May increase serum alkaline phosphatase, amylase, bilirubin, ALT, AST, BUN.

## AVAILABILITY (Rx)

**Capsules:** 50 mg, 75 mg, 100 mg.
**Tablets:** 50 mg, 75 mg, 100 mg.

**Tablets (Extended-Release [Solodyn]):** 45 mg, 55 mg, 65 mg, 80 mg, 90 mg, 105 mg, 115 mg, 135 mg.

## ADMINISTRATION/HANDLING

### PO

• Take without regard to food. • Give with adequate fluid (reduces risk of esophageal irritation and ulceration). • Give pellet-filled capsules, extended-release tablets whole; do not cut, crush, dissolve, or divide.

## INDICATIONS/ROUTES/DOSAGE

**Usual Dosage**
**PO:** **ADULTS, ELDERLY:** Initially, 100–200 mg once, then 100 mg q12h or 50 mg 4 times/day. **CHILDREN OLDER THAN 8 YRS:** Initially, 4 mg/kg once, then 2 mg/kg q12h. **Maximum:** 100 mg/dose, 200 mg/day.

**Acne**
**PO** *(Solodyn):* **CHILDREN 12 YRS AND OLDER, WEIGHING 126–136 KG:** 135 mg once daily; **WEIGHING 111–125 KG:** 115 mg once daily; **WEIGHING 97–110 KG:** 105 mg once daily; **WEIGHING 85–96 KG:** 90 mg once daily; **WEIGHING 72–84 KG:** 80 mg once daily; **WEIGHING 60–71 KG:** 65 mg once daily; **WEIGHING 50–59 KG:** 55 mg once daily; **WEIGHING 45–49 KG:** 45 mg once daily. *(Capsule or Immediate-Release Tablet):* **ADULTS, ELDERLY:** 50–100 mg/twice daily.

**Dosage in Renal/Hepatic Impairment**
Use caution.

## SIDE EFFECTS

**Frequent:** Dizziness, light-headedness, diarrhea, nausea, vomiting, abdominal cramps, possibly severe photosensitivity, drowsiness, vertigo. **Occasional:** Altered pigmentation of skin, mucous membranes, rectal/genital pruritus, stomatitis.

---

## ADVERSE EFFECTS/ TOXIC REACTIONS

Superinfection (esp. fungal), anaphylaxis, increased ICP may occur. Bulging fontanelles occur rarely in infants.

## NURSING CONSIDERATIONS

### BASELINE ASSESSMENT

Question for history of allergies, esp. tetracyclines, sulfite.

### INTERVENTION/EVALUATION

Assess ability to ambulate (may cause vertigo, dizziness). Monitor daily pattern of bowel activity, stool consistency. Monitor renal function, LFT with long-term therapy. Assess skin for rash. Observe for signs of increased intracranial pressure (altered LOC, widened pulse pressure). Be alert for superinfection: fever, vomiting, diarrhea, anal/genital pruritus, oral mucosal changes (ulceration, pain, erythema).

### PATIENT/FAMILY TEACHING

• Continue antibiotic for full length of treatment. • Space doses evenly. • Drink full glass of water with capsules or tablets. • Avoid tasks that require alertness, motor skills until response to drug is established. • Report diarrhea, rash, other new symptoms. • Protect skin from sun exposure. • Advise female pts to use additional form of birth control (may decrease effectiveness of oral contraceptives).

## mipomersen

**mi**-poe-**mer**-sen
(Kynamro)
■ **BLACK BOX ALERT** ■ May cause hepatotoxicity. May cause hepatic steatosis (increase in hepatic fat) regardless of serum ALT, AST elevation; may be risk factor for progressive hepatic disease including steatohepatitis and cirrhosis. Monitor hepatic enzymes regularly. Treatment only available through restricted program under the Risk Evaluation and Mitigation Strategy (REMS) named KYNAMRO REMS PROGRAM.

## ◆CLASSIFICATION

**PHARMACOTHERAPEUTIC:** Oligonucleotide inhibitor. **CLINICAL:** Antihyperlipidemic.

## USES

Adjunct to lipid-lowering medications and diet to reduce low-density lipoprotein cholesterol (LDL-C), apolipoprotein B (apo-B), total cholesterol (TC), and non–high-density lipoprotein cholesterol (non-HDL-C) in pts with homozygous familial hypercholesterolemia (HoFH).

## PRECAUTIONS

**Contraindications:** Hypersensitivity to mipomersen. Moderate to severe hepatic impairment, active hepatic disease, hepatitis, unexplained persistent elevations of serum transaminases. **Cautions:** Alcohol dependency, other medications known to cause hepatotoxicity.

## ACTION

Prevents assembly of apo-B–containing lipoproteins by inhibiting translation of apo-B 100 human messenger ribonucleic acid (mRNA); the principle precursor of LDL. **Therapeutic Effect:** Decreases plasma low-density lipoprotein cholesterol (LDL-C) and total cholesterol.

## PHARMACOKINETICS

Readily absorbed following SQ administration. Metabolized in tissues by endonucleases. Protein binding: greater than 90%. Peak plasma concentration: 3–4 hrs. Steady state reached within 6 mos. Excreted primarily in urine. **Half-life:** 1–2 mos.

## ⏳ LIFESPAN CONSIDERATIONS

**Pregnancy/Lactation:** Unknown if distributed in breast milk. Must either

M

discontinue drug or discontinue breast-feeding. **Children:** Safety and efficacy not established. **Elderly:** May have increased risk of adverse reactions including hypertension, peripheral edema.

## INTERACTIONS

**DRUG: Hepatotoxic medications (e.g., acetaminophen, isoniazid, ketoconazole, simvastatin)** may increase risk of hepatotoxicity. **HERBAL: Black cohosh, kava kava** may increase risk of hepatotoxicity. **FOOD:** None known. **LAB VALUES:** May increase serum alkaline phosphatase, ALT, AST, bilirubin; urine protein.

## AVAILABILITY (Rx)

**Single-Use Prefilled Syringe:** 200 mg/ml (1 ml).

## ADMINISTRATION/HANDLING

**SQ**
• Allow syringe/vial to reach room temperature before administration. • Inspect for particulate matter. • Pinch approx. 1 inch of SQ tissue on abdomen, thigh, or upper arm between thumb and first finger. • Do not inject areas with sunburn, tattoos, psoriasis, or active inflammation. • Insert needle at proper angle and steadily inject. • Alternate injection sites.
**Storage** • Refrigerate until time of use. • Solution stored at room temperature expires after 14 days. • Solution should appear clear and colorless. • Protect from light.

## INDICATIONS/ROUTES/DOSAGE

**Homozygous Familial Hypercholesterolemia**
**SQ: ADULTS/ELDERLY:** 200 mg once wkly. (If dose is missed, the dose should be given at least 3 days from the next wkly dose.)

**Dose Modification**
If ALT, AST greater than 3 times upper limit of normal (ULN), withhold dose until resolution to below 3 times ULN and

investigate for other causes. If treatment resumed, monitor hepatic function test every 1–2 wks. Discontinue if symptomatic hepatotoxicity occurs or elevated ALT, AST does not resolve.

**Dosage in Renal/Hepatic Impairment**
No dose adjustment.

## SIDE EFFECTS

**Frequent (84%):** Injection site reactions (pain, swelling, erythema, pruritus, rash, induration, urticaria). **Occasional (14%–4%):** Fatigue, nausea, body aches, chills, headache, pyrexia, extremity pain, hypertension, chills, peripheral edema, vomiting, musculoskeletal pain. **Rare (3%):** Palpitations, abdominal pain, insomnia.

## ADVERSE EFFECTS/ TOXIC REACTIONS

Increased risk of progressive hepatic disease including steatohepatitis, cirrhosis due to increased hepatic fat. Elevated transaminases reported in 12% of pts. Alcohol may exacerbate hepatotoxicity. Increased risk of myopathy including rhabdomyolysis (muscle pain/tenderness, weakness, dark or decreased urine output, elevated serum creatinine or CPK level) when used with other antihyperlipidemics (statins). Angina pectoris reported in 4% of pts. Immunogenicity (autoantibodies) reported in 38% of pts. Neoplasms (benign and malignant) reported in 4% of pts.

## NURSING CONSIDERATIONS

### BASELINE ASSESSMENT

Obtain baseline lipid panel, LFT. Confirm positive history of HoFH. Receive full medication history including vitamins, minerals, herbal products. Screen for history of hepatic impairment, cardiovascular disease, alcohol dependency. Assess skin for appropriate injection sites.

### INTERVENTION/EVALUATION

Monitor lipid panel every 3 mos; hepatic function every mo for 12 mos, then every

3 mos. If serum ALT, AST elevations occur, obtain PT/INR and monitor for bruising, hematuria, jaundice, right upper abdominal pain, fever, lethargy, melena. Offer antiemetics for nausea/vomiting. Obtain EKG for chest pain, palpitations. Assess extremities for edema.

**PATIENT/FAMILY TEACHING**
• Diet and exercise are essential to treatment. • Blood levels will be routinely monitored. • Report signs of liver problems (yellowing of skin, bruising, black/tarry stool, right upper quadrant pain, fever, lethargy), chest pain, palpitations. • Avoid alcohol. • Most pts experience injection site reactions. • Flu-like symptoms (chills, fatigue, nausea, muscle pain) most likely occur within 2 days. • Inject medication into fatty tissue of upper arm, abdomen, thigh; do not inject into muscle.

---

# mirabegron

mir-a-**beg**-ron
(Myrbetriq)

◆**CLASSIFICATION**
**PHARMACOTHERAPEUTIC:** Beta$_3$-adrenergic agonist. **CLINICAL:** Smooth muscle relaxant.

## USES
Treatment of overactive bladder with symptoms of urinary incontinence, urgency, frequency.

## PRECAUTIONS
**Contraindications:** Hypersensitivity to mirabegron. **Cautions:** Bladder outlet obstruction, pts taking antimuscarinic medications (increases urinary retention), mild to moderate hepatic/renal impairment, history of QT-interval prolongation, medications known to prolong QT interval. Not recommended for use in pts with severe uncontrolled hypertension (SBP equal to or greater than 180 mm Hg and/or DBP equal to or greater than 110 mm Hg).

## ACTION
Relaxes detrusor smooth muscle of bladder through beta$_3$ stimulation during storage phase of urinary bladder fill–void cycle. **Therapeutic Effect:** Increases bladder capacity, reduces symptoms of urinary urgency, increased voiding frequency, urge incontinence, nocturia.

## PHARMACOKINETICS
Readily absorbed following PO administration; widely distributed. Protein binding: 71%. Renal elimination primarily through active tubular secretion along with glomerular filtration. Eliminated in urine (55%), feces (35%). **Half-life:** 50 hrs.

## ⧗ LIFESPAN CONSIDERATIONS
**Pregnancy/Lactation:** Unknown if distributed in breast milk. **Children:** Safety and efficacy not established. **Elderly:** No age-related precautions noted.

## INTERACTIONS
**DRUG:** May increase concentration of **desipramine, digoxin, metoprolol, thioridazine, flecainide, propafenone. HERBAL:** None significant. **FOOD:** None known. **LAB VALUES:** May increase GGT, LDH; temporarily increase ALT, AST.

## AVAILABILITY (RX)
⬚ **Tablets, Extended-Release:** 25 mg, 50 mg.

## ADMINISTRATION/HANDLING
**PO**
• Give without regard to meals. • Administer with water; instruct pt to swallow whole. • Do not break, crush, dissolve or divide film-coated tablets.

## INDICATIONS/ROUTES/DOSAGE
**Overactive Bladder**
**PO: ADULTS, ELDERLY:** Initially, 25 mg once daily. Efficacy seen within 8 wks for 25 mg dose. May increase to 50 mg once daily.

---

M

**Dosage in Renal Impairment**

**Mild to moderate impairment:** No dosage adjustment. **Severe impairment:** Do not exceed 25 mg once daily.

**Dosage in Hepatic Impairment**

**Mild impairment:** No dosage adjustment. **Moderate impairment:** Do not exceed 25 mg once daily. **Severe impairment:** Not recommended.

## SIDE EFFECTS

**Occasional (9%–4%):** Hypertension, headache, nasopharyngitis. **Rare (2%–1%):** Constipation, arthralgia, diarrhea, tachycardia, fatigue.

## ADVERSE EFFECTS/ TOXIC REACTIONS

Worsening of preexisting hypertension reported infrequently. Urinary tract infection occured in 6% of pts, influenza in 3%, and upper respiratory infection in 1.5%.

## NURSING CONSIDERATIONS

### BASELINE ASSESSMENT

Check B/P; assess for hypertension. Monitor EKG. Receive full medication history and screen for possible drug interactions. Monitor I&O (particularly in pts with history of urinary retention).

### INTERVENTION/EVALUATION

Monitor ALT, AST, LDH, GGT periodically. Palpate bladder for urinary retention. Measure B/P near end of dosing interval (determines whether B/P is controlled throughout day). Periodic B/P determinations are recommended, especially in hypertensive pts. For pts taking digoxin, monitor digoxin serum level for therapeutic effect (very narrow line between therapeutic and toxic level). Assess pulse for quality, irregular rate, bradycardia. Question for evidence of headache.

### PATIENT/FAMILY TEACHING

• Report urinary retention. • Do not use nasal decongestants, over-the-counter cold preparations without doctor approval.

Restrict salt, alcohol intake. • Take mirabegron with water; swallow tablet whole; do not chew, crush, dissolve, or divide tablet. • May take with or without food.

# mirtazapine

mir-**taz**-a-peen
(Apo-Mirtazapine ✱, Remeron, Remeron Soltab)
■ **BLACK BOX ALERT** ■ Increased risk of suicidal thinking and behavior in children, adolescents, young adults 18–24 yrs with major depressive disorder, other psychiatric disorders.
**Do not confuse Remeron with Premarin, Rozerem, or Zemuron.**

## ◆CLASSIFICATION

**PHARMACOTHERAPEUTIC:** Tetracyclic compound. **CLINICAL:** Antidepressant.

## USES

Treatment of depression.

## PRECAUTIONS

**Contraindications:** Hypersensitivity to mirtazapine. Use of MAOIs to treat psychiatric disorders (concurrently or within 14 days of discontinuing either MAOI or mirtazapine), initiation of mirtazapine in pts receiving linezolid or IV methylene blue. **Cautions:** Renal/hepatic impairment, elderly, high-risk pts for seizures, suicidal ideation or behavior, alcoholism, concurrent medications that lower seizure threshold, cardiovascular disease, pts at risk for QT prolongation, history of QT prolongation, medications known to prolong QT interval.

## ACTION

Acts as antagonist at presynaptic alpha$_2$-adrenergic receptors, increasing norepinephrine, serotonin neurotransmission. Has low anticholinergic activity. **Therapeutic Effect:** Relieves depression, produces sedative effects.

M

## PHARMACOKINETICS

Rapidly, completely absorbed after PO administration; absorption not affected by food. Protein binding: 85%. Metabolized in liver. Primarily excreted in urine. Unknown if removed by hemodialysis. **Half-life:** 20–40 hrs (longer in males [37 hrs] than females [26 hrs]).

## ☒ LIFESPAN CONSIDERATIONS

**Pregnancy/Lactation:** Unknown if distributed in breast milk. **Children:** Safety and efficacy not established. **Elderly:** Age-related renal impairment may require dosage adjustment.

## INTERACTIONS

**DRUG: Alcohol, CNS depressant medications (e.g., lorazepam, morphine, zolpidem)** may increase impairment of cognition, motor skills. **Serotonergic drugs (e.g., venlafaxine)** may increase risk of serotonin syndrome. **CYP3A4 inducers (e.g., phenytoin)** may decrease concentration/effects. **CYP3A4 inhibitors (e.g., ketoconazole)** may increase concentration/effects. **MAOIs** may increase risk of neuroleptic malignant syndrome, hypertensive crisis, severe seizures. **HERBAL: Gotu kola, kava kava, St. John's wort, valerian** may increase CNS depression. **St. John's wort** may decrease concentration/effects, may increase risk of serotonin syndrome. **FOOD:** None known. **LAB VALUES:** May increase serum cholesterol, triglycerides, ALT.

## AVAILABILITY (Rx)

**Tablets (Remeron):** 7.5 mg, 15 mg, 30 mg, 45 mg. **Tablets (Orally Disintegrating [Remeron Soltab]):** 15 mg, 30 mg, 45 mg.

## ADMINISTRATION/HANDLING

**PO**
• Give without regard to food. • May crush/break scored tablets.

**Orally Disintegrating Tablets**
• Give without regard to food. • Do not split tablet. • Place on tongue; dissolves without water.

## INDICATIONS/ROUTES/DOSAGE

**Depression**
**PO: ADULTS:** Initially, 15 mg at bedtime. May increase by 15 mg/day q1–2wks. **Maximum:** 45 mg/day. **ELDERLY:** Initially, 7.5 mg at bedtime. May increase by 7.5–15 mg/day q1–2wks. **Maximum:** 45 mg/day.

**Dosage in Renal/Hepatic Impairment**
Use caution.

## SIDE EFFECTS

**Frequent (54%–12%):** Drowsiness, dry mouth, increased appetite, constipation, weight gain. **Occasional (89%–4%):** Asthenia, dizziness, flu-like symptoms, abnormal dreams. **Rare:** Abdominal discomfort, vasodilation, paresthesia, acne, dry skin, thirst, arthralgia.

## ADVERSE EFFECTS/ TOXIC REACTIONS

Higher incidence of seizures than with tricyclic antidepressants (esp. in those with no history of seizures). Overdose may produce cardiovascular effects (severe orthostatic hypotension, dizziness, tachycardia, palpitations, arrhythmias). Abrupt discontinuation from prolonged therapy may produce headache, malaise, nausea, vomiting, vivid dreams. Agranulocytosis occurs rarely.

## NURSING CONSIDERATIONS

**BASELINE ASSESSMENT**
Assess mental status, appearance, behavior, speech pattern, level of interest, mood. Obtain baseline weight. For pts on long-term therapy, renal function, LFT, CBC should be performed periodically.

**INTERVENTION/EVALUATION**
Supervise suicidal-risk pt closely during early therapy (as depression lessens,

**M**

energy level improves, increasing suicide potential). Children, adolescents are at increased risk for suicidal thoughts/behavior and worsening of depression, esp. during first few mos of therapy. Assess appearance, behavior, speech pattern, level of interest, mood. Monitor for hypotension, arrhythmias.

**PATIENT/FAMILY TEACHING**

• Take as single bedtime dose. • Avoid alcohol, depressant/sedating medications. • Avoid tasks requiring alertness, motor skills until response to drug established. • Report worsening depression, suicidal ideation, unusual changes in behavior.

---

# *miSOPROStol

mis-oh-**pros**-tol
(Cytotec, Novo-Misoprostol ✸)

■ **BLACK BOX ALERT** ■ Pregnancy Category X. Use during pregnancy can cause abortion, premature birth, birth defects. Not recommended in women of childbearing potential unless pt is capable of complying with effective contraception.
**Do not confuse Cytotec with Cytoxan, or misoprostol with metoprolol or mifepristone.**

## FIXED-COMBINATION(S)

**Arthrotec:** misoprostol/diclofenac (an NSAID): 200 mcg/50 mg, 200 mcg/75 mg.

## ◆CLASSIFICATION

**PHARMACOTHERAPEUTIC:** Prostaglandin. **CLINICAL:** Antisecretory, gastric protectant.

## USES

Prevention of NSAID-induced gastric ulcers and in pts at high risk for developing gastric ulcer/gastric ulcer complications. Medical termination of pregnancy 49 days or less. (in conjunction with mifepristone). **OFF-LABEL:**

Cervical ripening, labor induction, treatment/prevention of postpartum hemorrhage, treatment of incomplete or missed abortion.

## PRECAUTIONS

**Contraindications:** Hypersensitivity to prostaglandins; pregnancy when used to reduce NSAID-induced ulcers (produces uterine contractions). **Cautions:** Renal impairment, cardiovascular disease, elderly.

## ACTION

Replaces protective prostaglandins consumed with prostaglandin-inhibiting therapies (e.g., NSAIDs). Induces uterine contractions. **Therapeutic Effect:** Reduces acid secretion from gastric parietal cells, stimulates bicarbonate production from gastric/duodenal mucosa.

## PHARMACOKINETICS

| Route | Onset | Peak | Duration |
|-------|-------|------|----------|
| PO | 30 min | 1–1.5 hrs | 3–6 hrs |

Rapidly absorbed from GI tract. Protein binding: 80%–90%. Rapidly converted to active metabolite. Primarily excreted in urine. Unknown if removed by hemodialysis. **Half-life:** 20–40 min.

## ⧗ LIFESPAN CONSIDERATIONS

**Pregnancy/Lactation:** Unknown if distributed in breast milk. Produces uterine contractions, uterine bleeding, expulsion of products of conception (abortifacient property). **Children:** Safety and efficacy not established. **Elderly:** No age-related precautions noted.

## INTERACTIONS

**DRUG: Antacids** may increase concentration. **HERBAL:** None significant. **FOOD:** None known. **LAB VALUES:** None significant.

## AVAILABILITY (Rx)

**Tablets:** 100 mcg, 200 mcg.

---

## ADMINISTRATION/HANDLING

### PO

- Give with or after meals (minimizes diarrhea).

## INDICATIONS/ROUTES/DOSAGE

**Prevention of NSAID-Induced Gastric Ulcer**

**PO: ADULTS:** 200 mcg 4 times/day with food (last dose at bedtime). Continue for duration of NSAID therapy. May reduce dosage to 100 mcg 4 times/day or 200 mcg 2 times/day with food. **ELDERLY:** 100–200 mcg 4 times/day with food.

**Chemical Termination of Pregnancy**
See manufacturer guidelines of mifepristone.

**Dosage in Renal/Hepatic Impairment**
No dose adjustment.

## SIDE EFFECTS

**Frequent (40%–20%):** Abdominal pain, diarrhea. **Occasional (3%–2%):** Nausea, flatulence, dyspepsia, headache. **Rare (1%):** Vomiting, constipation.

## ADVERSE EFFECTS/ TOXIC REACTIONS

Overdosage may produce sedation, tremor, seizures, dyspnea, palpitations, hypotension, bradycardia.

## NURSING CONSIDERATIONS

### BASELINE ASSESSMENT

Question for possibility of pregnancy before initiating therapy.

### PATIENT/FAMILY TEACHING

- Avoid magnesium-containing antacids (minimizes potential for diarrhea).
- Women of childbearing potential must not be pregnant before or during medication therapy (may result in hospitalization, surgery, infertility, fetal death).
- Incidence of diarrhea may be lessened by taking immediately following meals.

---

## *mitoMYcin    HIGH ALERT

mye-toe-**mye**-sin
(Mutamycin ✦)

■ **BLACK BOX ALERT** ■ Potent vesicant. Marked myelosuppression. Infiltration produces ulceration, necrosis, cellulitis, tissue sloughing. Hemolytic-uremic syndrome reported. Must be administered by certified chemotherapy personnel. **Do not confuse mitomycin with mithramycin or mitoxantrone.**

### ◆CLASSIFICATION

**PHARMACOTHERAPEUTIC:** Antibiotic. **CLINICAL:** Antineoplastic.

## USES

Treatment of disseminated adenocarcinoma of stomach, pancreas. **OFF-LABEL:** Treatment of bladder cancer, anal carcinoma; cervical, esophageal, gastric, non–small-cell lung cancer.

## PRECAUTIONS

**Contraindications:** Hypersensitivity to mitomycin. Coagulation disorders, other increased bleeding tendencies, thrombocytopenia. **Cautions:** Myelosuppression, renal (serum creatinine greater than 1.7 mg/dL)/hepatic impairment, pregnancy, prior radiation treatment.

## ACTION

Alkylating agent, cross-linking with strands of DNA. **Therapeutic Effect:** Inhibits DNA, RNA synthesis.

## PHARMACOKINETICS

Widely distributed. Does not cross blood-brain barrier. Primarily metabolized in liver. Excreted in urine. **Half-life:** 50 min.

## ⧖ LIFESPAN CONSIDERATIONS

**Pregnancy/Lactation:** If possible, avoid use during pregnancy, esp. first trimester. Breastfeeding not recommended. Safety in pregnancy not established. **Children:** No age-related precautions noted.

M

---

**Elderly:** Age-related renal impairment may require dosage adjustment.

## INTERACTIONS

**DRUG: Bone marrow depressants** may increase myelosuppression. **Live virus vaccines** may potentiate virus replication, increase vaccine side effects, decrease pt's antibody response to vaccine. **HERBAL:** Avoid **black cohosh, dong quai** in estrogen-dependent tumors. **FOOD:** None known. **LAB VALUES:** May increase serum BUN, creatinine.

## AVAILABILITY (Rx)

**Injection, Powder for Reconstitution:** 5 mg, 20 mg, 40 mg.

## ADMINISTRATION/HANDLING

◄ALERT► May be carcinogenic, mutagenic, teratogenic. Handle with extreme care during preparation/administration. Give via IV push, IV infusion. Extremely irritating to vein. Injection may produce pain with induration, thrombophlebitis, paresthesia.

 IV

**Reconstitution** • Reconstitute with Sterile Water for Injection to provide solution containing 0.5–1 mg/ml. • Do not shake vial to dissolve. • Allow vial to stand at room temperature until complete dissolution occurs. • For IV infusion, further dilute with 50–100 ml D₅W or 0.9% NaCl (concentration 20–40 mcg/ml).
**Rate of Administration** • Give slow IV push or by IV infusion over 15–30 min. • Extravasation may produce cellulitis, ulceration, tissue sloughing. Terminate administration immediately, inject ordered antidote. Apply ice intermittently for up to 72 hrs; keep area elevated.
**Storage** • Use only clear, blue-gray solutions. • Concentration of 0.5 mg/ml (reconstituted vial or syringe) is stable for 7 days at room temperature or 2 wks if refrigerated. Further diluted solution with D₅W is stable for 3 hrs, 12 hrs if diluted with 0.9% NaCl at room temperature.

## ⚙ IV INCOMPATIBILITIES

Aztreonam (Azactam), bleomycin (Blenoxane), cefepime (Maxipime), filgrastim (Neupogen), heparin, piperacillin/tazobactam (Zosyn), sargramostim (Leukine), vinorelbine (Navelbine).

## ⚙ IV COMPATIBILITIES

Cisplatin (Platinol AQ), cyclophosphamide (Cytoxan), doxorubicin (Adriamycin), 5-fluorouracil, granisetron (Kytril), leucovorin, methotrexate, ondansetron (Zofran), vinblastine (Velban), vincristine (Oncovin).

## INDICATIONS/ROUTES/DOSAGE

Refer to individual protocols.

**Stomach, Pancreatic Cancer**
**IV: ADULTS, ELDERLY, CHILDREN:** 20 mg/m² as single dose. Repeat q6–8wks.

**Bladder Cancer (non–muscle invasive)**
**Intravesicular Instillation: ADULTS, ELDERLY:** Low risk of recurrence: 40 mg as single dose postoperatively (retain in bladder for 1–2 hrs). High risk of recurrence: 20 mg/wk for 6 wks, then 20 mg qmo for 3 yrs (retain in bladder for 1–2 hrs).

**Dose Modification for Toxicity**

| | |
|---|---|
| Leukocytes 2,000 to less than 3,000/mm³ | Hold therapy until leukocytes 4,000 or more/mm³, reduce dose to 70% or more in subsequent cycles |
| Leukocyte less than 2,000/mm³ | Hold therapy until leukocytes 4,000 or more/mm³, reduce dose to 50% in subsequent cycles |
| Platelets 25,000 to less than 75,000/mm³ | Hold therapy until platelets 100,000 or more/mm³, reduce dose to 70% in subsequent cycles |
| Platelets less than 25,000/mm³ | Hold therapy until platelets 100,000 or more/mm³, reduce dose to 50% in subsequent cycles |

**Dosage in Renal Impairment**
**CrCl less than 10 ml/min:** Give 75% of normal dose.

**Dosage in Hepatic Impairment**
No dose adjustment.

## SIDE EFFECTS

**Frequent (Greater Than 10%):** Fever, anorexia, nausea, vomiting. **Occasional (10%–2%):** Stomatitis, paresthesia, purple colored bands on nails, rash, alopecia, unusual fatigue. **Rare (Less Than 1%):** Thrombophlebitis, cellulitis with extravasation.

## ADVERSE EFFECTS/ TOXIC REACTIONS

Marked myelosuppression results in hematologic toxicity manifested as leukopenia, thrombocytopenia, and, to a lesser extent, anemia (generally occurs within 2–4 wks after initial therapy). Renal toxicity may be evidenced by increased serum BUN, creatinine levels. Pulmonary toxicity manifested as dyspnea, cough, hemoptysis, pneumonia. Long-term therapy may produce hemolytic uremic syndrome, characterized by hemolytic anemia, thrombocytopenia, renal failure, hypertension.

## NURSING CONSIDERATIONS

**BASELINE ASSESSMENT**

Obtain CBC with differential, PT, bleeding time, before and periodically during therapy. Antiemetics before and during therapy may alleviate nausea/vomiting.

**INTERVENTION/EVALUATION**

Monitor hematologic status, renal function studies. Assess IV site for phlebitis, extravasation. Monitor for hematologic toxicity (fever, sore throat, signs of local infection, unusual bruising/bleeding from any site), symptoms of anemia (excessive fatigue, weakness). Assess for renal toxicity (foul odor from urine, elevated serum BUN, creatinine).

**PATIENT/FAMILY TEACHING**

• Maintain strict oral hygiene. • Immediately report stinging, burning, pain at injection site. • Do not have immunizations without physician's approval (drug lowers resistance to infection). • Avoid contact with those who have recently received live virus vaccine. • Hair loss is reversible, but new hair growth may have different color, texture. • Report nausea/vomiting, fever, sore throat, bruising, bleeding, shortness of breath, painful urination.

# modafinil

moe-**daf**-i-nil
(Alertec ♣, Apo-Modafinil ♣, Provigil)

## ◆CLASSIFICATION

**PHARMACOTHERAPEUTIC:** Alpha$_1$-agonist, CNS stimulant **(Schedule IV).**
**CLINICAL:** Wakefulness-promoting agent, antinarcoleptic.

## USES

Treatment of excessive daytime sleepiness associated with narcolepsy, shift work sleep disorder, adjunct therapy for obstructive sleep apnea/hypopnea syndrome. **OFF-LABEL:** Treatment of ADHD, multiple sclerosis–related fatigue.

## PRECAUTIONS

**Contraindications:** Hypersensitivity to modafinil, armodafinil. **Cautions:** History of clinically significant mitral valve prolapse, left ventricular hypertrophy, renal/hepatic impairment, angina, cardiac disease, myocardial ischemia, recent MI, preexisting psychosis or bipolar disorder, Tourette's syndrome.

## ACTION

Increases alpha activity, decreasing delta, theta, brain wave activity. **Therapeutic Effect:** Reduces number of sleep episodes, total daytime sleep.

## PHARMACOKINETICS

Well absorbed from GI tract. Protein binding: 60%. Widely distributed. Metabolized in liver. Excreted by kidneys. Unknown if removed by hemodialysis. **Half-life:** 15 hrs.

## ⧗ LIFESPAN CONSIDERATIONS

**Pregnancy/Lactation:** Unknown if drug is excreted in breast milk. Use caution if given to pregnant women. **Children:** Safety and efficacy not established in pts younger than 16 yrs. **Elderly:** Age-related renal/hepatic impairment may require decreased dosage.

## INTERACTIONS

**DRUG:** May decrease concentrations of **cyclosporine, oral contraceptives.** May increase concentrations of **tricyclic antidepressants (e.g., amitriptyline, doxepin), warfarin. Other CNS stimulants** may increase CNS stimulation. **HERBAL:** None significant. **FOOD:** None known. **LAB VALUES:** None significant.

## AVAILABILITY (Rx)

**Tablets (Provigil):** 100 mg, 200 mg.

## ADMINISTRATION/HANDLING

**PO**
• Give without regard to meals.

## INDICATIONS/ROUTES/DOSAGE

**Narcolepsy, Obstructive Sleep Apnea/ Hypopnea Syndrome**
**PO: ADULTS:** 200 mg/day in the morning. **ELDERLY:** 100 mg/day in the morning.

**Shift Work Sleep Disorder**
**PO: ADULTS:** 200 mg about 1 hr prior to start of work shift.

**Dosage in Renal Impairment**
No dose adjustment.

**Dosage in Hepatic impairment**
**Mild to moderate impairment:** No dose adjustment. Reduce dose 50% with severe impairment.

## SIDE EFFECTS

Generally well tolerated. **Occasional (5%):** Headache, nausea, dizziness, insomnia, palpitations, diarrhea.

## ADVERSE EFFECTS/ TOXIC REACTIONS

Agitation, excitation, increased B/P, insomnia may occur. Psychiatric disturbances (anxiety, hallucinations, suicidal ideation), serious allergic reactions (angioedema, Stevens-Johnson syndrome) have been noted.

## NURSING CONSIDERATIONS

### BASELINE ASSESSMENT

Obtain baseline evidence of narcolepsy or other sleep disorders, including pattern, environmental situations, length of sleep episodes. Question for sudden loss of muscle tone (cataplexy) precipitated by strong emotional responses before sleep episode. Assess frequency/severity of sleep episodes before drug therapy.

### INTERVENTION/EVALUATION

Monitor sleep pattern, evidence of restlessness during sleep, length of insomnia episodes at night. Assess for dizziness, anxiety; initiate fall precautions.

### PATIENT/FAMILY TEACHING

• Avoid alcohol. • Sugarless gum, sips of water may relieve dry mouth. • Do not increase dose without physician approval. • Use alternative contraceptives during therapy and 1 mo after discontinuing modafinil (reduces effectiveness of oral contraceptives).

---

# mometasone ᵀᴼᴾ¹⁰⁰

moe-**met**-a-sone
(Asmanex, Asmanex HFA, Elocon, Nasonex)

## FIXED-COMBINATION(S)

**Dulera:** mometasone/formoterol (beta-adrenergic agonist): 100 mcg/ 5 mcg, 200 mcg/5 mcg.

M

## ◆CLASSIFICATION

**PHARMACOTHERAPEUTIC:** Adreno-corticosteroid. **CLINICAL:** Anti-inflammatory.

## USES

**Nasal:** Treatment of nasal symptoms of seasonal/perennial allergic rhinitis in adults, children 2 yrs and older. Prophylaxis of nasal symptoms of seasonal allergic rhinitis in adults, adolescents 12 yrs and older. Treatment of nasal polyps in adults. **Inhalation:** Maintenance treatment of asthma as prophylactic therapy. **Topical:** Relief of inflammatory, pruritic manifestations of steroid-responsive dermatoses.

## PRECAUTIONS

**Contraindications:** Hypersensitivity to mometasone, milk proteins. Primary treatment of status asthmaticus or acute bronchospasm. **Cautions:** Thyroid/hepatic/renal impairment, elderly, diabetes, cardiovascular disease, glaucoma, cataracts, myasthenia gravis, pts at risk for osteoporosis, seizures, GI disease (e.g., ulcer, colitis); following MI. Untreated systemic fungal, viral, bacterial infections.

## ACTION

Inhibits release of mediators of inflammation. (e.g., histamine, kinins). **Therapeutic Effect:** Improves symptoms of asthma, rhinitis.

## PHARMACOKINETICS

Undetectable in plasma. Protein binding: 98%–99%. Swallowed portion undergoes extensive metabolism. Excreted through bile (74%), urine (8%). **Half-life:** 5 hrs.

## ⊠ LIFESPAN CONSIDERATIONS

**Pregnancy/Lactation:** Unknown if drug crosses placenta or is distributed in breast milk. **Children:** Prolonged treatment/high doses may decrease short-term growth rate, cortisol secretion. **Elderly:** No age-related precautions noted.

## INTERACTIONS

**DRUG: Ketoconazole** may increase concentration (inhalation). **HERBAL:** None significant. **FOOD:** None known. **LAB VALUES:** None significant.

## AVAILABILITY (Rx)

**Cream (Elocon):** 0.1%. **Lotion (Elocon):** 0.1%. **Nasal Spray (Nasonex):** 50 mcg/spray. **Ointment (Elocon):** 0.1%. **Powder for Oral Inhaler (Asmanex):** 110 mcg (delivers 100 mcg/actuation), 220 mcg (delivers 200 mcg/actuation). **(Asmanex HFA):** 100 mcg/actuation, 200 mcg/actuation.

## ADMINISTRATION/HANDLING

**Inhalation**
• Hold twisthaler straight up with pink portion (base) on bottom, remove cap. • Exhale fully. • Firmly close lips around mouthpiece and inhale a fast, deep breath. • Hold breath for 10 sec.

**Intranasal**
• Instruct pt to clear nasal passages as much as possible before use. • Tilt head slightly forward. • Insert spray tip into nostril, pointing toward nasal passages, away from nasal septum. • Spray into one nostril while pt holds other nostril closed, concurrently inspires through nose to permit medication as high into nasal passages as possible.

**Topical**
• Apply thin layer of cream, lotion, ointment to cover affected area. Rub in gently. • Do not cover area with occlusive dressing.

## INDICATIONS/ROUTES/DOSAGE

**Allergic Rhinitis**
**Nasal Spray: ADULTS, ELDERLY, CHILDREN 12 YRS AND OLDER:** 2 sprays in each nostril once daily. When used to prevent nasal rhinitis, begin 2–4 wks prior to

M

---

✦ Canadian trade name    ⬛ Non-Crushable Drug    ▣ High Alert drug start of pollen season. **CHILDREN 2–11 YRS:** 1 spray in each nostril once daily.

### Asthma

**Inhalation: ADULTS, ELDERLY, CHILDREN 12 YRS AND OLDER (Previous therapy with bronchodilators:** *(Asmanex):* Initially, inhale 220 mcg (1 puff) once daily. **Maximum:** 440 mcg/day as single or 2 divided doses. **(Previous therapy with inhaled corticosteroids):** *(Asmanex HFA):* Initially, 100–200 mcg twice daily. **Maximum:** 400 mcg twice daily. **(Previous therapy with oral corticosteroids):** *(Asmanex):* 440 mcg (2 puffs) twice daily. *(Asmanex HFA):* 400 mcg twice daily. Reduce prednisone no faster than 2.5 mg/day beginning after at least 1 wk of mometasone. **CHILDREN 4–11 YRS:** *(Asmanex):* 110 mcg once daily in evening.

### Skin Disease

**Topical: ADULTS, ELDERLY, CHILDREN 12 YRS AND OLDER:** Apply cream, lotion, or ointment sparingly to affected area once daily.

### Nasal Polyp

**Nasal Spray: ADULTS, ELDERLY:** 2 sprays (100 mcg) in each nostril twice daily. Total dose: 400 mcg.

### Dosage in Renal/Hepatic Impairment

No dose adjustment.

## SIDE EFFECTS

**Occasional: Inhalation:** Headache, allergic rhinitis, upper respiratory infection, muscle pain, fatigue. **Nasal:** Nasal irritation, stinging. **Topical:** Burning. **Rare: Inhalation:** Abdominal pain, dyspepsia, nausea. **Nasal:** Nasal/pharyngeal candidiasis. **Topical:** Pruritus.

## ADVERSE EFFECTS/ TOXIC REACTIONS

Acute hypersensitivity reaction (urticaria, angioedema, severe bronchospasm) occurs rarely. Transfer from systemic to local steroid therapy may unmask previously suppressed bronchial asthma condition.

## NURSING CONSIDERATIONS

### BASELINE ASSESSMENT

Question for hypersensitivity to any corticosteroids.

### INTERVENTION/EVALUATION

Teach proper use of nasal spray, oral inhaler. Instruct pt to clear nasal passages before use. Report if no improvement in symptoms, sneezing, nasal irritation occur. Assess lung sounds for wheezing, rales.

### PATIENT/FAMILY TEACHING

• Do not change dose schedule or stop taking drug; must taper off gradually under medical supervision. **Nasal:** Report if symptoms do not improve; sneezing, nasal irritation occur. • Clear nasal passages prior to use. **Inhalation:** Inhale rapidly, deeply; rinse mouth after inhalation. • Not indicated for acute asthma attacks. **Topical:** Do not cover affected area with bandage, dressing.

## montelukast

mon-**tee**-loo-kast
(Apo-Montelukast ✦, Singulair)
**Do not confuse Singulair with Sinequan.**

### ◆CLASSIFICATION

**PHARMACOTHERAPEUTIC:** Leukotriene receptor inhibitor. **CLINICAL:** Antiasthmatic.

## USES

Prophylaxis, chronic treatment of asthma. Prevention of exercise-induced bronchoconstriction. Treatment of seasonal allergic rhinitis (hay fever). Relief of perennial allergic rhinitis. **OFF-LABEL:** Urticaria.

## PRECAUTIONS

**Contraindications:** Hypersensitivity to montelukast. **Cautions:** Systemic corticosteroid treatment reduction during montelukast therapy. Concomitant use of CYP3A4 inducers. Not for use in acute asthma attacks.

## ACTION

Binds to cysteinyl leukotriene receptors, inhibiting effects of leukotrienes on bronchial smooth muscle. **Therapeutic Effect:** Decreases bronchoconstriction, vascular permeability, mucosal edema, mucus production.

## PHARMACOKINETICS

| Route | Onset | Peak | Duration |
|---|---|---|---|
| PO | N/A | N/A | 24 hrs |
| PO (chewable) | N/A | N/A | 24 hrs |

Rapidly absorbed from GI tract. Protein binding: 99%. Extensively metabolized in liver. Excreted almost exclusively in feces. **Half-life:** 2.7–5.5 hrs (slightly longer in elderly).

## ⏳ LIFESPAN CONSIDERATIONS

**Pregnancy/Lactation:** Unknown if distributed in breast milk. Use during pregnancy only if necessary. **Children/Elderly:** No age-related precautions noted in pts older than 6 yrs or the elderly.

## INTERACTIONS

**DRUG:** **CYP3A4 inducers (e.g., carbamazepine, phenobarbital, rifampin)** may decrease concentration/effects. **HERBAL:** **St. John's wort** may decrease concentration/effects. **FOOD:** None known. **LAB VALUES:** May increase serum ALT, AST, eosinophils.

## AVAILABILITY (Rx)

**Oral Granules:** 4 mg per packet. **Tablets:** 10 mg. **Tablets (Chewable):** 4 mg, 5 mg.

## ADMINISTRATION/HANDLING

**PO**
• May take without regard to food/meals. When treating asthma, administer in evening. • When treating allergic rhinitis, may individualize administration times. • Granules may be given directly in mouth or mixed with carrots, rice, applesauce, ice cream, baby formula, or breast milk (do not add to any other liquid or food). • Give within 15 min of opening packet.

## INDICATIONS/ROUTES/DOSAGE

**Bronchial Asthma**
**PO: ADULTS, ELDERLY, CHILDREN 15 YRS AND OLDER:** One 10-mg tablet daily, taken in the evening. **CHILDREN 6–14 YRS:** One 5-mg chewable tablet daily, taken in the evening. **CHILDREN 2–5 YRS:** One 4-mg chewable tablet daily, taken in the evening. **CHILDREN 6–23 MOS:** 4 mg (oral granules) once daily in the evening.

**Seasonal Allergic Rhinitis**
**PO: ADULTS, ELDERLY, CHILDREN 15 YRS AND OLDER:** One 10-mg tablet, taken in the evening. **CHILDREN 6–14 YRS:** One 5-mg chewable tablet, taken in the evening. **CHILDREN 2–5 YRS:** One 4-mg chewable tablet, taken in the evening.

**Perennial Allergic Rhinitis**
**PO: ADULTS, ELDERLY, CHILDREN 15 YRS AND OLDER:** One 10-mg tablet, taken in the evening. **CHILDREN 6–14 YRS:** One 5-mg chewable tablet, taken in the evening. **CHILDREN 2–5 YRS:** One 4-mg chewable tablet, taken in the evening. **CHILDREN 6–23 MOS:** 4 mg oral granules, taken in the evening.

**Exercise-Induced Bronchoconstriction Prevention**
**PO: ADULTS, ELDERLY, CHILDREN 15 YRS AND OLDER:** 10 mg 2 or more hrs before exercise. No additional doses within 24 hrs. **CHILDREN 6–14 YRS:** 5 mg (chew tab) 2 or more hrs prior to exercise. No additional doses within 24 hrs.

**Dosage in Renal/Hepatic Impairment**
No dose adjustment.

**M**

---

## SIDE EFFECTS

**ADULTS, CHILDREN 15 YRS AND OLDER:**
**Frequent (18%):** Headache. **Occasional (4%):** Influenza. **Rare (3%–2%):** Abdominal pain, cough, dyspepsia, dizziness, fatigue, dental pain. **CHILDREN 6–14 YRS: Rare (less than 2%):** Diarrhea, laryngitis, pharyngitis, nausea, otitis media, sinusitis, viral infection.

## ADVERSE EFFECTS/ TOXIC REACTIONS

Suicidal ideation and behavior, depression has been noted.

## NURSING CONSIDERATIONS

### BASELINE ASSESSMENT

Chewable tablet contains phenylalanine (component of aspartame); parents of phenylketonuric pts should be informed. Assess lung sounds for wheezing. Assess for allergy symptoms.

### INTERVENTION/EVALUATION

Monitor rate, depth, rhythm, type of respirations; quality/rate of pulse. Assess lung sounds for wheezing. Monitor for change in mood, behavior.

### PATIENT/FAMILY TEACHING

• Increase fluid intake (decreases lung secretion viscosity). • Take as prescribed, even during symptom-free periods as well as during exacerbations of asthma. • Do not alter/stop other asthma medications. • Drug is not for treatment of acute asthma attacks. • Report increased use or frequency of short-acting bronchodilators, changes in behavior, suicidal ideation.

---

## *morphine*    TOP 100    HIGH ALERT

mor-feen
(Astramorph PF, Duramorph, Infumorph, <u>Kadian</u>, M-Eslon , MS Contin, MSIR )

■ **BLACK BOX ALERT** ■ Be alert for signs of abuse, misuse, diversion.

---

*Epidural:* Monitor for delayed sedation. *Sustained-release:* Do not crush or chew. *MS Contin:* Use only in opioid-tolerant pts requiring over 400 mg/day. *Kadian:* Use only in opioid-tolerant pts. *Avinza:* Alcohol disrupts extended-release timing. *Duramorph:* Risk of severe and/or sustained cardiopulmonary depression.

**Do not confuse Avinza with Evista or Invanz, morphine with hydromorphone, morphine sulfate with magnesium sulfate, MS Contin with Oxycontin. MSO$_4$ and MS are error-prone abbreviations.**

## FIXED-COMBINATION(S)

**Embeda:** morphine/naloxone (an opioid antagonist): 20 mg/0.8 mg, 30 mg/1.2 mg, 50 mg/2 mg, 60 mg/2.4 mg, 80 mg/3.2 mg, 100 mg/4 mg.

## ◆CLASSIFICATION

**PHARMACOTHERAPEUTIC:** Narcotic agonist **(Schedule II). CLINICAL:** Opiate analgesic.

## USES

Relief of moderate to severe, acute, or chronic pain; analgesia during labor, pain due to MI, dyspnea from pulmonary edema not resulting from chemical respiratory irritant. **Infumorph:** Use in devices for managing intractable chronic pain. **Extended-release:** Use only when repeated doses for extended periods of time are required.

## PRECAUTIONS

**Contraindications: All Formulations:** Hypersensitivity to morphine. Acute or severe asthma, GI obstruction, known or suspected paralytic ileus, severe hepatic/renal impairment, severe respiratory depression. **Extended-Release:** GI obstruction, acute postoperative pain. **Injection:** HF due to lung disease; arrhythmias, head injury, seizures, acute alcoholism. Labor when premature birth expected. **Immediate-Release (Tablets, Oral Solution):** Hypercarbia. Extreme **Caution:** COPD, cor pulmonale, hypoxia, hypercapnia, preexisting respiratory depression, head injury, increased ICP, severe hypotension. **Cautions:** Biliary tract disease, pancreatitis, Addison's disease, cardiovascular disease, morbid obesity, adrenal insufficiency, elderly, hypothyroidism, urethral stricture, prostatic hyperplasia, debilitated pts, pts with CNS depression, toxic psychosis, seizure disorders, alcoholism.

## ACTION

Binds with opioid receptors within CNS, inhibiting ascending pain pathways. **Therapeutic Effect:** Alters pain perception, emotional response to pain.

## PHARMACOKINETICS

| Route | Onset | Peak | Duration |
|---|---|---|---|
| Oral solution | 30 min | 1 hr | 3–5 hrs |
| Tablets | 30 min | 1 hr | 3–5 hrs |
| Tablets (extended-release) | N/A | 3–4 hrs | 8–12 hrs |
| IV | Rapid | 0.3 hr | 3–5 hrs |
| IM | 5–30 min | 0.5–1 hr | 3–5 hrs |
| Epidural | 15–60 min | 1 hr | 12–20 hrs |
| SQ | 10–30 min | 1.1–5 hrs | 3–5 hrs |
| Rectal | 20–60 min | 0.5–1 hr | 3–7 hrs |

Variably absorbed from GI tract. Readily absorbed after IM, SQ administration. Protein binding: 20%–35%. Widely distributed. Metabolized in liver. Primarily excreted in urine. Removed by hemodialysis. **Half-life:** 2–4 hrs (increased in hepatic disease).

## ⚕ LIFESPAN CONSIDERATIONS

**Pregnancy/Lactation:** Crosses placenta. Distributed in breast milk. May prolong labor if administered in latent phase of first stage of labor or before cervical dilation of 4–5 cm has occurred. Respiratory depression may occur in neonate if mother received opiates during labor. Regular use of opiates during pregnancy may produce withdrawal symptoms in neonate (irritability, excessive crying, tremors, hyperactive reflexes, fever, vomiting, diarrhea, yawning, sneezing, seizures). **Children:** Paradoxical excitement may occur; those younger than 2 yrs are more susceptible to respiratory depressant effects. **Elderly:** Paradoxical excitement may occur. Age-related renal impairment may increase risk of urinary retention.

## INTERACTIONS

**DRUG: Alcohol, other CNS depressants** may increase CNS effects, respiratory depression, hypotension. **MAOIs** may produce serotonin syndrome. (Reduce dosage to ¼ of usual morphine dose). **HERBAL: Gotu kola, kava kava, St. John's wort, valerian** may increase CNS depression. **FOOD:** None known. **LAB VALUES:** May increase serum amylase, lipase.

## AVAILABILITY (Rx)

**Injection, Solution:** 2 mg/ml, 4 mg/ml, 5 mg/ml, 10 mg/ml, 15 mg/ml, 25 mg/ml, 50 mg/ml. **Injection, Solution (Epidural, Intrathecal, IV Infusion) (Astramorph PF, Duramorph):** 0.5 mg/ml, 1 mg/ml. **Injection, Solution (Epidural or Intrathecal) (Infumorph):** 10 mg/ml, 25 mg/ml. **Injection, Solution Patient-Controlled Analgesia (PCA) Pump:** 1 mg/ml, 5 mg/ml. **Solution Oral:** 20 mg/ml, 10 mg/5 ml, 20 mg/5 ml. **Suppository:** 5 mg, 10 mg, 20 mg, 30 mg. **Tablets:** 15 mg, 30 mg.

🗲 **Capsules, Extended-Release (Avinza):** 30 mg, 45 mg, 60 mg, 75 mg, 90 mg, 120 mg. 🗲 **Capsules, Sustained-Release (Kadian):** 10 mg, 20 mg, 30 mg, 50 mg, 60 mg, 80 mg, 100 mg, 200 mg. 🗲 **Tablets, Extended-Release (MS Contin):** 15 mg, 30 mg, 60 mg, 100 mg, 200 mg.

**M**

---

✦ Canadian trade name       🗲 Non-Crushable Drug       🄷🄸🄶🄷 High Alert drug

## ADMINISTRATION/HANDLING

 **IV**

**Reconstitution** • May give undiluted. • For IV injection, may dilute in Sterile Water for Injection or 0.9% NaCl to final concentration of 1–2 mg/ml. • For continuous IV infusion, dilute to concentration of 0.1–1 mg/ml in D₅W and give through controlled infusion device.

**Rate of Administration** • Always administer very slowly. Rapid IV increases risk of severe adverse reactions (apnea, chest wall rigidity, peripheral circulatory collapse, cardiac arrest, anaphylactoid effects).

**Storage** • Store at room temperature.

**IM, SQ**
• Administer slowly, rotating injection sites. • Pts with circulatory impairment experience higher risk of overdosage due to delayed absorption of repeated administration.

**PO**
• May give without regard to food. • Mix liquid form with fruit juice to improve taste. • Do not break, crush, dissolve, or divide extended-release capsule, tablets. • **Avinza, Kadian:** May mix with applesauce immediately prior to administration.

**Rectal**
• If suppository is too soft, chill for 30 min in refrigerator or run cold water over foil wrapper. • Moisten suppository with cold water before inserting well into rectum.

## ▨ IV INCOMPATIBILITIES

Amphotericin B complex (Abelcet, AmBisome, Amphotec), cefepime (Maxipime), doxorubicin (Doxil), phenytoin (Dilantin).

## ▨ IV COMPATIBILITIES

Amiodarone (Cordarone), atropine, bumetanide (Bumex), bupivacaine (Marcaine, Sensorcaine), dexmedetomidine (Precedex), diltiazem (Cardizem), diphenhydramine (Benadryl), dobutamine (Dobutrex), dopamine (Intropin), glycopyrrolate (Robinul), heparin, hydroxyzine (Vistaril), lidocaine, lorazepam (Ativan), magnesium, midazolam (Versed), milrinone (Primacor), nitroglycerin, potassium, propofol (Diprivan).

## INDICATIONS/ROUTES/DOSAGE

◄ALERT► Dosage should be titrated to desired effect.

**Analgesia**
**PO** *(Immediate-Release):* **ADULTS, ELDERLY:** 10–30 mg q4h as needed. *(Solution):* 10–20 mg q4h as needed. *(Tablet):* 15–30 mg q4h as needed. **CHILDREN:** 0.15–0.3 mg/kg q3–4h as needed.

◄ALERT► For the Avinza dosage below, be aware that this drug is to be administered once daily only.

◄ALERT► For the Kadian dosage information below, be aware that this drug is to be administered q12h or once daily.

◄ALERT► Be aware that pediatric dosages of extended-release preparations of Kadian and Avinza have not been established.

◄ALERT► For the MS Contin dosage information below, be aware that the daily dosage is divided and given q8h or q12h.

**PO** *(Extended-Release [Avinza]):* **ADULTS, ELDERLY:** Dosage requirement should be established using prompt-release formulations and is based on total daily dose. Avinza is given once daily only.

**PO** *(Extended-Release [Kadian]):* **ADULTS, ELDERLY:** Dosage requirement should be established using prompt-release formulations and is based on total daily dose. Dose is given once daily or divided and given q12h.

**PO** *(Extended-Release [MS Contin]):* **ADULTS, ELDERLY:** Dosage requirement should be established using prompt-release formulations and is based on total daily dose. Daily dose is divided and given q8h or q12h.

**IV: ADULTS, ELDERLY:** 2.5–5 mg q3–4h as needed. **Note:** Repeated doses (e.g., 1–2 mg) may be given more frequently (e.g., every hr) if needed. **CHILDREN:** 0.05–0.3 mg/kg q3–4h as needed. **NEONATES:** Initially, 0.05–0.1 mg/kg/dose q4–6h as needed.

**IV Continuous Infusion: ADULTS, ELDERLY:** 0.8–10 mg/hr. Range: Titrate up to 80 mg/hr. **CHILDREN:** Initially, 10–30 mcg/kg/hr. Titrate as needed to control pain. **NEONATES:** Initially, 0.01 mg/kg/hr (10 mcg/kg/hr). **Maximum:** 0.015–0.02 mg/kg/hr.

**Note:** IM injection not recommended **IM: ADULTS, ELDERLY:** 5–10 mg q3–4h as needed. **CHILDREN:** 0.1–0.2 mg/kg q3–4h as needed.

**Patient-Controlled Analgesia (PCA)**
**IV: ADULTS, ELDERLY: Usual concentration:** 1 mg/ml. **Demand dose:** 1 mg (range: 0.5–2.5 mg). **Lockout interval:** 5–10 min.

**Dosage in Renal Impairment**

| Creatinine Clearance | Dose |
|---|---|
| 10–50 ml/min, CRRT: | 75% of normal dose |
| less than 10 ml/min, HD, PD: | 50% of normal dose |

**Dosage in Hepatic Impairment**
No dose adjustment.

## SIDE EFFECTS

◄**ALERT**► Ambulatory pts, pts not in severe pain may experience nausea, vomiting more frequently than pts in supine position or who have severe pain. **Frequent:** Sedation, decreased B/P (including orthostatic hypotension), diaphoresis, facial flushing, constipation, dizziness, drowsiness, nausea, vomiting. **Occasional:** Allergic reaction (rash, pruritus), dyspnea, confusion, palpitations, tremors, urinary retention, abdominal cramps, vision changes, dry mouth, headache,

decreased appetite, pain/burning at injection site. **Rare:** Paralytic ileus.

## ADVERSE EFFECTS/ TOXIC REACTIONS

Overdose results in respiratory depression, skeletal muscle flaccidity, cold/clammy skin, cyanosis, extreme drowsiness progressing to seizures, stupor, coma. Tolerance to analgesic effect, physical dependence may occur with repeated use. Prolonged duration of action, cumulative effect may occur in those with hepatic/renal impairment. **Antidote:** Naloxone (see Appendix J for dosage).

## NURSING CONSIDERATIONS

### BASELINE ASSESSMENT

Pt should be in recumbent position before drug is given by parenteral route. Assess onset, type, location, duration of pain. Obtain vital signs before giving medication. If respirations are 12/min or less (20/min or less in children), withhold medication, contact physician. Effect of medication is reduced if full pain recurs before next dose.

### INTERVENTION/EVALUATION

Monitor vital signs 5–10 min after IV administration, 15–30 min after SQ, IM. Be alert for decreased respirations, B/P. Check for adequate voiding. Monitor daily pattern of bowel activity, stool consistency; avoid constipation. Initiate deep breathing, coughing exercises, particularly in those with pulmonary impairment. Assess for clinical improvement, record onset of pain relief. Consult physician if pain relief is not adequate.

### PATIENT/FAMILY TEACHING

• Discomfort may occur with injection. • Change positions slowly to avoid orthostatic hypotension. • Avoid tasks that require alertness, motor skills until response to drug is established.

- Avoid alcohol, CNS depressants.
- Tolerance, dependence may occur with prolonged use of high doses. • Report ineffective pain control, constipation, urinary retention.

# moxifloxacin

mox-i-**flox**-a-sin
(Avelox, Avelox IV, Moxeza, Vigamox)

■ **BLACK BOX ALERT** ■ May increase risk of tendonitis, tendon rupture (increased with concurrent corticosteroids, organ transplant recipients, those older than 60 yrs). May aggravate myasthenia gravis (avoid use).
**Do not confuse Avelox with Avonex.**

## ◆ CLASSIFICATION

**PHARMACOTHERAPEUTIC:** Fluoroquinolone. **CLINICAL:** Antibacterial, antibiotic.

## USES

Treatment of susceptible infections due to *S. pneumoniae, S. pyogenes, S. aureus, H. influenzae, M. catarrhalis, K. pneumoniae, M. pneumoniae, C. pneumoniae* including acute bacterial exacerbation of chronic bronchitis, acute bacterial sinusitis, intra-abdominal infection, community-acquired pneumonia, uncomplicated skin/skin structure infections. **Ophthalmic:** Topical treatment of bacterial conjunctivitis due to susceptible strains of bacteria. **OFF-LABEL:** Legionella, pneumonia, tuberculosis (second-line therapy).

## PRECAUTIONS

**Contraindications:** Hypersensitivity to moxifloxacin, other quinolones. **Cautions:** Renal/hepatic impairment, bradycardia, acute myocardial ischemia, myasthenia gravis, diabetes, rheumatoid arthritis, seizures, pts with prolonged QT interval, medications known to prolong QT interval, hypokalemia, hypomagnesemia,

elderly, pts with suspected CNS disorder, history of tendon disorders.

## ACTION

Inhibits two enzymes, topoisomerase II and IV, in susceptible microorganisms. **Therapeutic Effect:** Interferes with bacterial DNA replication. Prevents/delays emergence of resistant organisms. Bactericidal.

## PHARMACOKINETICS

Well absorbed from GI tract after PO administration. Protein binding: 50%. Widely distributed throughout body with tissue concentration often exceeding plasma concentration. Metabolized in liver. Excreted in urine (20%), feces (25%) unchanged. **Half-life: PO:** 12 hrs; **IV:** 15 hrs.

## ⏳ LIFESPAN CONSIDERATIONS

**Pregnancy/Lactation:** May be distributed in breast milk. May produce teratogenic effects. **Children:** Safety and efficacy not established. **Elderly:** No age-related precautions noted.

## INTERACTIONS

**DRUG: Antacids, iron preparations, sucralfate** may decrease absorption. **NSAIDs** may increase risks of CNS stimulation/seizures. **HERBAL:** None significant. **FOOD:** None known. **LAB VALUES:** None significant.

## AVAILABILITY (Rx)

**Injection Infusion (Avelox IV):** 400 mg (250 ml). **Ophthalmic Solution (Moxeza, Vigamox):** 0.5%. **Tablets (Avelox):** 400 mg.

## ADMINISTRATION/HANDLING

 IV

**Reconstitution** • Available in ready-to-use containers.
**Rate of Administration** • Give by IV infusion only. • Avoid rapid or bolus IV infusion. • Infuse over 60 min.

**Storage** • Store at room temperature. • Do not refrigerate.

**PO**

• Give without regard to meals. • Oral moxifloxacin should be administered 4 hrs before or 8 hrs after antacids, multivitamins, iron preparations, sucralfate, didanosine chewable/buffered tablets, pediatric powder for oral solution.

**Ophthalmic**

• Place gloved finger on lower eyelid and pull out until a pocket is formed between eye and lower lid. • Place prescribed number of drops into pocket. • Instruct pt to close eye gently (so medication will not be squeezed out of the sac) and to apply digital pressure to lacrimal sac at inner canthus for 1 min to minimize systemic absorption.

### ▓ IV INCOMPATIBILITIES

Do not add or infuse other drugs simultaneously through the same IV line. Flush line before and after use if same IV line is used with other medications.

### INDICATIONS/ROUTES/DOSAGE

**Usual Dose**
**PO, IV: ADULTS, ELDERLY:** 400 mg q24h. Duration dependent on severity of infection.

**Acute Bacterial Sinusitis**
**PO, IV: ADULTS, ELDERLY:** 400 mg q24h for 10 days.

**Acute Bacterial Exacerbation of Chronic Bronchitis**
**PO, IV: ADULTS, ELDERLY:** 400 mg q24h for 5 days.

**Community-Acquired Pneumonia**
**PO, IV: ADULTS, ELDERLY:** 400 mg q24h for 7–14 days.

**Intra-Abdominal Infection**
**PO, IV: ADULTS, ELDERLY:** 400 mg q24h for 5–14 days.

**Skin/Skin Structure Infection**
**PO, IV: ADULTS, ELDERLY:** 400 mg once daily for 7–21 days.

**Topical Treatment of Bacterial Conjunctivitis Due to Susceptible Strains of Bacteria**
**Ophthalmic: ADULTS, ELDERLY, CHILDREN 1 YR AND OLDER: (Vigamox):** 1 drop 3 times/day for 7 days. **(Moxeza):** 1 drop 2 times/day for 7 days.

**Dosage in Renal Impairment**
No dose adjustment.

**Dosage in Hepatic Impairment**
**Mild to moderate impairment:** No dose adjustment. **Severe impairment:** Use caution.

### SIDE EFFECTS

**Frequent (8%–6%):** Nausea, diarrhea. **Occasional: PO, IV (3%–2%):** Dizziness, headache, abdominal pain, vomiting. **Ophthalmic (6%–1%):** Conjunctival irritation, reduced visual acuity, dry eye, keratitis, eye pain, ocular itching, swelling of tissue around cornea, eye discharge, fever, cough, pharyngitis, rash, rhinitis. **Rare (1%):** Altered taste, dyspepsia, photosensitivity.

### ADVERSE EFFECTS/ TOXIC REACTIONS

Pseudomembranous colitis (severe abdominal cramps/pain, severe watery diarrhea, fever) may occur. Superinfection (anal/genital pruritus, moderate to severe diarrhea, stomatitis) may occur.

### NURSING CONSIDERATIONS

**BASELINE ASSESSMENT**

Question for history of hypersensitivity to moxifloxacin, quinolones.

**INTERVENTION/EVALUATION**

Monitor daily pattern of bowel activity, stool consistency. Assist with ambulation if dizziness occurs. Assess for headache, abdominal pain, vomiting, altered

**M**

 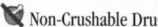

taste, dyspepsia. Monitor WBC, signs of infection.

**PATIENT/FAMILY TEACHING**
• May be taken without regard to food. • Drink plenty of fluids. • Avoid exposure to direct sunlight; may cause photosensitivity reaction. • Do not take antacids 4 hrs before or 8 hrs after dosing. • Take full course of therapy. • Report abdominal cramping/pain, persistent diarrhea.

# mupirocin

mue-peer-oh-sin
(Bactroban, Bactroban Nasal)
**Do not confuse Bactroban or Bactroban Nasal with bacitracin, baclofen, or Bactrim.**

## ◆CLASSIFICATION
**PHARMACOTHERAPEUTIC:** Antibacterial. **CLINICAL:** Topical antibiotic.

## USES
**Ointment:** Topical treatment of impetigo caused by *S. aureus, S. pyogenes.* **Cream:** Treatment of traumatic skin lesions due to *S. aureus, S. pyogenes.* **Intranasal ointment:** Eradication of *S. aureus* from nasal, perineal carriage sites. **OFF-LABEL:** Surgical prophylaxis to prevent wound infections (intranasal).

## PRECAUTIONS
**Contraindications:** Hypersensitivity to mupirocin. **Cautions:** Renal impairment, burn pts.

## ACTION
Inhibits bacterial protein, RNA synthesis. Less effective on DNA synthesis. **Nasal:** Eradicates nasal colonization of methicillin-resistant *Staphylococcus aureus* (MRSA). **Therapeutic Effect:** Prevents bacterial growth, replication. Bacteriostatic.

## PHARMACOKINETICS
Following topical administration, penetrates outer layer of skin (minimal through intact skin). Protein binding: 95%. Metabolized in liver. Excreted in urine. **Half-life:** 17–36 min.

## ⧗ LIFESPAN CONSIDERATIONS
**Pregnancy/Lactation:** Unknown if distributed in breast milk. Breastfeeding not recommended. **Children:** Safety and efficacy not established. **Elderly:** No age-related precautions noted.

## INTERACTIONS
**DRUG:** None significant. **HERBAL:** None significant. **FOOD:** None known. **LAB VALUES:** None significant.

## AVAILABILITY (Rx)
**Cream, Topical (Bactroban):** 2%. **Ointment, Intranasal (1-g single-use tube) (Bactroban Nasal):** 2%. **Ointment, Topical (Bactroban):** 2%.

## ADMINISTRATION/HANDLING
**Topical**
**Cream, Ointment** • For topical use only. • May cover with gauze dressing. • Avoid contact with eyes.

**Intranasal**
• Apply ½ of the ointment from single-use tube into each nostril. • Avoid contact with eyes.

## INDICATIONS/ROUTES/DOSAGE
**Usual Topical Dosage**
**Topical Cream: ADULTS, ELDERLY, CHILDREN 3 MOS AND OLDER:** Apply small amount 3 times/day for 10 days. **Topical Ointment: ADULTS, ELDERLY, CHILDREN 2 MOS AND OLDER:** Apply small amount 3 times/day for 5–14 days.

**Usual Nasal Dosage**
**Intranasal: ADULTS, ELDERLY, CHILDREN 12 YRS AND OLDER:** Apply small amount 2 times/day for 5–10 days.

M

## SIDE EFFECTS

**Frequent: Nasal (9%–3%):** Headache, rhinitis, upper respiratory congestion, pharyngitis, altered taste. **Occasional: Nasal (2%):** Burning, stinging, cough. **Topical (2%–1%):** Pain, burning, stinging, pruritus. **Rare: Nasal (less than 1%):** Pruritus, diarrhea, dry mouth, epistaxis, nausea, rash. **Topical (less than 1%):** Rash, nausea, dry skin, contact dermatitis.

## ADVERSE EFFECTS/ TOXIC REACTIONS

Superinfection may result in bacterial, fungal infections, esp. with prolonged, repeated therapy.

## NURSING CONSIDERATIONS

### BASELINE ASSESSMENT

Assess skin for type, extent of lesions.

### INTERVENTION/EVALUATION

Monitor healing of skin lesions. In event of skin reaction, stop applications, cleanse area gently, notify physician.

### PATIENT/FAMILY TEACHING

• For external use only. • Avoid contact with eyes. • Explain precautions to avoid spread of infection; teach how to apply medication. • Report skin reactions, irritation. • Report if no improvement is noted in 3–5 days.

# mycophenolate

mye-koe-**fen**-o-late
(Apo-Mycophenolate ✤, CellCept, Myfortic, Novo-Mycophenolate)

■ **BLACK BOX ALERT** ■ Increased risk of congenital malformation, spontaneous abortion. Increased risk for development of lymphoma, skin malignancy. Increased susceptibility to infections. Administer under supervision of physician experienced in immunosuppressive therapy.

## ◆ CLASSIFICATION

**PHARMACOTHERAPEUTIC:** Immunologic agent. **CLINICAL:** Immunosuppressant.

## USES

Should be used concurrently with cyclosporine and corticosteroids. **CellCept:** Prophylaxis of organ rejection in pts receiving allogeneic hepatic/renal/cardiac transplant. **Myfortic:** Renal transplants. **OFF-LABEL:** Treatment of hepatic transplant rejection in pts unable to tolerate tacrolimus or cyclosporine due to toxicity, mild heart transplant rejection, moderate to severe psoriasis, proliferative lupus nephritis, myasthenia gravis, graft-vs-host disease. Treatment of autoimmune hepatitis (refractory).

## PRECAUTIONS

**Contraindications:** Hypersensitivity to mycophenolic acid or polysorbate 80 (IV formulation). **Cautions:** Active severe GI disease, renal impairment, neutropenia, women of childbearing potential (use caution when handling).

## ACTION

Suppresses immunologically-mediated inflammatory response by inhibiting inosine monophosphate dehydrogenase, an enzyme that deprives lymphocytes of nucleotides necessary for DNA, RNA synthesis, thus inhibiting proliferation of T and B lymphocytes. **Therapeutic Effect:** Prevents transplant rejection.

## PHARMACOKINETICS

Rapidly, extensively absorbed after PO administration (food decreases drug plasma concentration but does not affect absorption). Protein binding: 97%. Completely hydrolyzed to active metabolite mycophenolic acid. Primarily excreted in urine. Not removed by hemodialysis. **Half-life:** 17.9 hrs.

M

---

## ⌛ LIFESPAN CONSIDERATIONS

**Pregnancy/Lactation:** Unknown if drug crosses placenta or is distributed in breast milk. Breastfeeding not recommended. Increased risk of miscarriage, birth defects. **Children:** Safety and efficacy not established. **Elderly:** Age-related renal impairment may require dosage adjustment.

## INTERACTIONS

**DRUG:** May increase concentrations of **acyclovir, ganciclovir** in pts with renal impairment. **Antacids (aluminum- and magnesium-containing), cholestyramine** may decrease absorption. **Live virus vaccines** may potentiate virus replication, increase vaccine side effects, decrease pt's antibody response to vaccine. **Other immunosuppressants (e.g., cyclophosphamide, cyclosporine, tacrolimus)** may increase risk of infection, lymphomas. **Probenecid** may increase concentration. **HERBAL: Cat's claw, echinacea** may decrease effects (have immunostimulant properties). **FOOD: All foods** may decrease concentration. **LAB VALUES:** May increase serum cholesterol, alkaline phosphatase, creatinine, ALT, AST. May alter serum glucose, lipids, calcium, potassium, phosphate, uric acid.

## AVAILABILITY (Rx)

**Capsules (CellCept):** 250 mg. **Injection, Powder for Reconstitution (CellCept):** 500 mg. **Oral Suspension (CellCept):** 200 mg/ml. **Tablets (CellCept):** 500 mg.

 **Tablets (Delayed-Release [Myfortic]):** 180 mg, 360 mg.

## ADMINISTRATION/HANDLING

### 📵 IV

**Reconstitution** • Reconstitute each 500-mg vial with 14 ml $D_5W$. Gently agitate. • For 1-g dose, further dilute with 140 ml $D_5W$; for 1.5-g dose further dilute with 210 ml $D_5W$, providing a concentration of 6 mg/ml.

**Rate of Administration** • Infuse over at least 2 hrs. • Begin infusion within 4 hrs of reconstitution.
**Storage** • Store at room temperature.

### PO

• Give on empty stomach (1 hr before or 2 hrs after food). • Do not break, crush, or open capsules or break, crush, dissolve, or divide delayed-release tablets. Avoid inhalation of powder in capsules, direct contact of powder on skin/mucous membranes. If contact occurs, wash thoroughly, with soap, water. Rinse eyes profusely with plain water. • May store reconstituted suspension in refrigerator or at room temperature. • Suspension is stable for 60 days after reconstitution. • Suspension can be administered orally or via an NG tube (minimum size 8 French).

## 🖥 IV INCOMPATIBILITIES

Mycophenolate is compatible only with $D_5W$. Do not infuse concurrently with other drugs or IV solutions.

## INDICATIONS/ROUTES/DOSAGE

**Prevention of Renal Transplant Rejection**
**PO, IV** *(Cellcept):* **ADULTS, ELDERLY:** 1 g twice daily. **PO: CHILDREN** *(Cellcept Suspension):* 600 mg/m²/dose twice daily. **Maximum:** 1 g twice daily.
**PO** *(Myfortic):* **ADULTS, ELDERLY:** 720 mg twice daily. **CHILDREN 5–16 YRS:** 400 mg/m² twice daily. **Maximum:** 720 mg twice daily.

**Prevention of Heart Transplant Rejection**
**PO, IV** *(Cellcept):* **ADULTS, ELDERLY:** 1.5 g twice daily.

**Prevention of Hepatic Transplant Rejection**
**PO** *(Cellcept):* **ADULTS, ELDERLY:** 1.5 g twice daily.
**IV** *(Cellcept):* **ADULTS, ELDERLY:** 1 g twice daily.

**Dosage in Renal/Hepatic Impairment**
No dose adjustment.

## SIDE EFFECTS

**Frequent (37%–20%):** UTI, hypertension, peripheral edema, diarrhea, constipation, fever, headache, nausea. **Occasional (18%–10%):** Dyspepsia, dyspnea, cough, hematuria, asthenia, vomiting, edema, tremors, abdominal, chest, back pain; oral candidiasis, acne. **Rare (9%–6%):** Insomnia, respiratory tract infection, rash, dizziness.

## ADVERSE EFFECTS/ TOXIC REACTIONS

Significant anemia, leukopenia, thrombocytopenia, neutropenia, leukocytosis may occur, particularly in those undergoing renal transplant rejection. Sepsis, infection occur occasionally. GI tract hemorrhage occurs rarely. There is an increased risk of developing neoplasms. Immunosuppression results in increased susceptibility to infection.

## NURSING CONSIDERATIONS

### BASELINE ASSESSMENT

Women of childbearing potential should have a negative serum or urine pregnancy test within 1 wk before initiation. Assess medical history, esp. renal function, existence of active digestive system disease, drug history, esp. other immunosuppressants.

### INTERVENTION/EVALUATION

CBC should be performed wkly during first mo of therapy, twice monthly during second and third mos of treatment, then monthly throughout the first yr. If rapid fall in WBC occurs, dosage should be reduced or discontinued. Assess particularly for delayed bone marrow suppression. Report any major change in assessment of pt.

### PATIENT/FAMILY TEACHING

• Effective contraception should be used before, during, and for 6 wks after discontinuing therapy, even if pt has a history of infertility, other than hysterectomy. • Two forms of contraception must be used concurrently unless abstinence is absolute. • Report unusual bleeding/bruising, sore throat, mouth sores, abdominal pain, fever. • Laboratory follow-up while taking medication is important part of therapy. • Malignancies may occur.

**M**

# nafcillin

naf-**sil**-in

## ◆CLASSIFICATION

**PHARMACOTHERAPEUTIC:** Penicillinase-resistant penicillin. **CLINICAL:** Antibiotic.

## USES

Treatment of respiratory tract, skin/skin structure infections, osteomyelitis, endocarditis, meningitis; perioperatively, esp. in cardiovascular, orthopedic procedures. Predominant treatment of infections caused by susceptible strains of staphylococci.

## PRECAUTIONS

**Contraindications:** Hypersensitivity to nafcillin, other penicillins. **Cautions:** History of allergies, particularly cephalosporins, severe renal/hepatic impairment, asthma, pts with HF.

## ACTION

Binds to bacterial membranes. **Therapeutic Effect:** Inhibits cell wall synthesis. Bactericidal.

## ⧖ LIFESPAN CONSIDERATIONS

**Pregnancy/Lactation:** Readily crosses placenta; appears in cord blood, amniotic fluid. Distributed in breast milk. May lead to rash, diarrhea, candidiasis in neonate, infant. **Children:** Immature renal function in neonate may delay renal excretion. **Elderly:** Age-related renal impairment may require dosage adjustment.

## INTERACTIONS

**DRUG:** High doses (2 g q4h) may decrease effects of **warfarin**. **HERBAL:** None significant. **FOOD:** None known. **LAB VALUES:** May cause false-positive Coombs' test.

## AVAILABILITY (Rx)

**Injection, Powder for Reconstitution:** 1 g, 2 g. **Infusion (Premix):** 1 g/50 ml, 2g/100 ml.

## ADMINISTRATION/HANDLING

◀**ALERT**▶ Space doses evenly around the clock.

 **IV**

**Reconstitution •** Reconstitute each vial with 10 ml Sterile Water for Injection or 0.9% NaCl. • For intermittent IV infusion (piggyback), further dilute with 50–100 ml 0.9% NaCl or D₅W.
**Rate of Administration •** Infuse over 30–60 min. • Because of potential for hypersensitivity/anaphylaxis, start initial dose at few drops per min, increase slowly to ordered rate; stay with pt first 10–15 min, then check q10min. • Limit IV therapy to less than 48 hrs, if possible. Stop infusion if pt complains of pain at IV site.
**Storage** *(IV infusion [piggyback])* • Diluted solution stable for 24 hrs at room temperature, 7 days if refrigerated. • Discard if precipitate forms.

**IM**
• Reconstitute each 500 mg with 1.7 ml Sterile Water for Injection or 0.9% NaCl to provide concentration of 250 mg/ml.
• Inject IM into large muscle mass.

## ▦ IV INCOMPATIBILITIES

Aztreonam (Azactam), diltiazem (Cardizem), droperidol (Inapsine), fentanyl, gentamicin, insulin, labetalol (Normodyne, Trandate), methylprednisolone (Solu-Medrol), midazolam (Versed), nalbuphine (Nubain), vancomycin (Vancocin), verapamil (Isoptin).

## ▦ IV COMPATIBILITIES

Acyclovir, famotidine (Pepcid), fluconazole (Diflucan), heparin, hydromorphone (Dilaudid), lidocaine, lipids, magnesium, morphine, potassium chloride, propofol (Diprivan).

## INDICATIONS/ROUTES/DOSAGE

**Usual Dosage**
**IV: ADULTS, ELDERLY:** 0.5–2 g q4–6h. **CHILDREN: Mild to Moderate Infections:** 100–150 mg/kg/day in divided

doses q6h. **Maximum:** 4 g/day. **Severe Infections:** 150–200 mg/kg/day in divided doses q4–6h. **Maximum:** 12 g/day. **NEONATES:** 25 mg/kg/dose in divided doses q6–12h.
**IM: ADULTS, ELDERLY:** 500 mg q4–6h.

**Dosage in Renal/Hepatic Impairment**
No dose adjustment.

### SIDE EFFECTS

**Frequent:** Mild hypersensitivity reaction (fever, rash, pruritus), GI effects (nausea, vomiting, diarrhea). **Occasional:** Hypokalemia with high IV dosages, phlebitis, thrombophlebitis (common in elderly). **Rare:** Extravasation with IV administration.

### ADVERSE EFFECTS/ TOXIC REACTIONS

Potentially fatal antibiotic-associated colitis, superinfections (abdominal cramps, severe watery diarrhea, fever) may result from altered bacterial balance in GI tract. Hematologic effects (esp. involving platelets, WBCs), severe hypersensitivity reactions, anaphylaxis occur rarely.

### NURSING CONSIDERATIONS

**BASELINE ASSESSMENT**
Question for history of allergies, esp. penicillins, cephalosporins.

**INTERVENTION/EVALUATION**
Hold medication, promptly report rash (possible hypersensitivity), diarrhea (fever, abdominal pain, mucus/blood in stool may indicate antibiotic-associated colitis). Evaluate IV site frequently for phlebitis (heat, pain, red streaking over vein), infiltration (potential extravasation). Monitor periodic CBC, urinalysis, BMP, LFT. Be alert for superinfection: fever, vomiting, diarrhea, anal/genital pruritus, oral mucosal changes (ulceration, pain, erythema).

**PATIENT/FAMILY TEACHING**
• Continue antibiotic for full length of treatment. • Doses should be evenly spaced. • Discomfort may occur with IM injection. • Report IV discomfort immediately. • Report diarrhea, rash, other new symptoms.

## nalbuphine    HIGH ALERT

**nal**-bue-feen
(Nubain ♣)

### ◆CLASSIFICATION

**PHARMACOTHERAPEUTIC:** Narcotic agonist, antagonist. **CLINICAL:** Opioid analgesic.

### USES

Relief of moderate to severe pain, preop analgesia, obstetric analgesia, adjunct to anesthesia. **OFF-LABEL:** Opioid-induced pruritus.

### PRECAUTIONS

**Contraindications:** Hypersensitivity to nalbuphine. **Cautions:** Hepatic/renal impairment, respiratory depression, recent MI, recent biliary tract impairment, pancreatitis, hypovolemia, head trauma, increased intracranial pressure (ICP), pregnancy, pts suspected of being opioid dependent, obesity, thyroid dysfunction, prostatic hyperplasia, urinary stricture, adrenal insufficiency, cardiovascular disease, elderly, debilitated.

### ACTION

Binds with opioid receptors within CNS, inhibiting ascending pain pathways. **Therapeutic Effect:** Alters pain perception, emotional response to pain.

### PHARMACOKINETICS

| Route | Onset | Peak | Duration |
|-------|-------|------|----------|
| IV | 2–3 min | 2–3 min | 3–4 hrs |
| IM | Less than 15 min | 30 min | 3–6 hrs |
| SQ | Less than 15 min | N/A | 3–6 hrs |

N

Well absorbed after IM, SQ administration. Metabolized in liver. Primarily eliminated in feces by biliary secretion. **Half-life:** 3.5–5 hrs.

## ⌛ LIFESPAN CONSIDERATIONS

**Pregnancy/Lactation:** Readily crosses placenta. Distributed in breast milk. Breastfeeding not recommended. May cause fetal, neonatal adverse effects during labor/delivery (e.g., fetal bradycardia). **Children:** Paradoxical excitement may occur. Pts younger than 2 yrs more susceptible to respiratory depression. **Elderly:** More susceptible to respiratory depression. Age-related renal impairment may increase risk of urinary retention.

## INTERACTIONS

**DRUG: Alcohol, other CNS depressants (e.g., lorazepam, morphine, zolpidem)** may increase CNS effects, respiratory depression, hypotension. **HERBAL: Gotu kola, kava kava, St. John's wort, valerian** may increase CNS depression. **FOOD:** None known. **LAB VALUES:** May increase serum amylase, lipase.

## AVAILABILITY (Rx)

**Injection Solution:** 10 mg/ml, 20 mg/ml.

## ADMINISTRATION/HANDLING

 IV

**Reconstitution** • May give undiluted. **Rate of Administration** • For IV push, administer each 10 mg over 3–5 min. **Storage** • Store parenteral form at room temperature.

**IM**
• Rotate IM injection sites.

## ▨ IV INCOMPATIBILITIES

Amphotericin B complex (Abelcet, AmBisome, Amphotec), cefepime (Maxipime), ketorolac (Toradol), nafcillin (Nafcil), piperacillin and tazobactam (Zosyn).

## ▨ IV COMPATIBILITIES

Dexmedetomidine (Precedex), diphenhydramine (Benadryl), droperidol (Inapsine), glycopyrrolate (Robinul), hydroxyzine (Vistaril), lidocaine, midazolam (Versed), prochlorperazine (Compazine), propofol (Diprivan).

## INDICATIONS/ROUTES/DOSAGE

**Analgesia**
**IV, IM, SQ: ADULTS, ELDERLY:** 10 mg q3–6h as needed. Do not exceed maximum single dose of 20 mg or daily dose of 160 mg. **CHILDREN 1 YR AND OLDER:** 0.1–0.2 mg/kg q3–4h as needed. **Maximum:** 20 mg/dose, 160 mg/day.

**Dosage in Renal/Hepatic Impairment**
Use caution.

## SIDE EFFECTS

**Frequent (36%):** Sedation. **Occasional (9%–3%):** Diaphoresis, cold/clammy skin, nausea, vomiting, dizziness, vertigo, dry mouth, headache. **Rare (less than 1%):** Restlessness, emotional lability, paresthesia, flushing, paradoxical reaction.

## ADVERSE EFFECTS/ TOXIC REACTIONS

Abrupt withdrawal after prolonged use may produce symptoms of narcotic withdrawal (abdominal cramping, rhinorrhea, lacrimation, anxiety, fever, piloerection [goose bumps]). Overdose results in severe respiratory depression, skeletal muscle flaccidity, cyanosis, extreme drowsiness progressing to seizures, stupor, coma. Tolerance to analgesic effect, physical dependence may occur with chronic use.

## NURSING CONSIDERATIONS

### BASELINE ASSESSMENT

Obtain vital signs before giving medication. If respirations are 12/min or less (20/min or less in children), withhold medication, contact physician. Assess

---

onset, type, location, duration of pain. Effect of medication is reduced if full pain recurs before next dose. Low abuse potential.

### INTERVENTION/EVALUATION

Monitor for change in respirations, B/P, rate/quality of pulse. Monitor daily pattern of bowel activity, stool consistency. Initiate deep breathing, coughing exercises, particularly in pts with pulmonary impairment. Assess for clinical improvement, record onset of relief of pain. Consult physician if pain relief is not adequate.

### PATIENT/FAMILY TEACHING

• Avoid alcohol. • Avoid tasks that require alertness, motor skills until response to drug is established. • May cause dry mouth. • May be habit forming.

# naloxone

nal-**ox**-own
(Evzio, Narcan, Narcan Nasal Spray)
**Do not confuse naloxone with Lanoxin or naltrexone.**

### FIXED-COMBINATION(S)

**Embeda:** naloxone/morphine (an opioid agonist): 0.8 mg/20 mg, 1.2 mg/30 mg, 2 mg/50 mg, 2.4 mg/60 mg, 3.2 mg/80 mg, 4 mg/100 mg. **Suboxone (sublingual film):** naloxone/buprenorphine (an analgesic): 0.5 mg/2 mg, 1 mg/4 mg, 2 mg/8 mg, 3 mg/12 mg. **Zubsolv:** naloxone/buprenorphine: 0.36 mg/1.4 mg, 1.4 mg/5.7 mg.

### ◆CLASSIFICATION

**PHARMACOTHERAPEUTIC:** Narcotic antagonist. **CLINICAL:** Antidote.

## USES

**Narcan:** Complete or partial reversal of opioid depression including respiratory depression. Diagnosis of suspected opioid tolerance or acute opioid overdose. **Evzio, Narcan Nasal Spray:** Emergency treatment of known or suspected opioid overdose. **OFF-LABEL:** Opioid-induced pruritus.

## PRECAUTIONS

**Contraindications:** Hypersensitivity to naloxone. **Cautions:** Cardiac/pulmonary disease. Medications with potential for adverse cardiovascular effects (e.g., hypotension, arrhythmias).

## ACTION

Displaces opioids at opioid-occupied receptor sites in CNS. **Therapeutic Effect:** Reverses opioid-induced sleep/sedation, increases respiratory rate, raises B/P to normal range.

## PHARMACOKINETICS

| Route | Onset | Peak | Duration |
|---|---|---|---|
| IV | 1–2 min | N/A | 20–60 min |
| IM | 2–5 min | N/A | 20–60 min |
| SQ | 2–5 min | N/A | 20–60 min |

Well absorbed after IM, SQ administration. Metabolized in liver. Primarily excreted in urine. **Half-life:** 60–100 min.

## ⧗ LIFESPAN CONSIDERATIONS

**Pregnancy/Lactation:** Unknown if drug crosses placenta or is distributed in breast milk. **Children/Elderly:** No age-related precautions noted.

## INTERACTIONS

**DRUG:** None significant. **HERBAL:** None significant. **FOOD:** None known. **LAB VALUES:** None significant.

## AVAILABILITY (Rx)

Injection, Autoinjector (Evzio): 0.4 mg/0.4 ml. Injection Solution: 0.4 mg/ml, 1 mg/ml. Narcan Nasal Spray: 4 mg/0.1 ml.

## ADMINISTRATION/HANDLING

 IV

**Reconstitution** • For IV push, may give undiluted (0.4 mg/ml or diluted with 9 ml 0.9% NaCl to concentration of 0.04 mg/ml). • For continuous IV infusion, dilute each 2 mg of naloxone with

500 ml of D$_5$W or 0.9% NaCl, producing solution containing 0.004 mg/ml (4 mcg/ml).
**Rate of Administration** • May give IV push over 30 sec.
**Storage** • Store parenteral form at room temperature. • Use mixture within 24 hrs; discard unused solution. • Protect from light. • Stable in D$_5$W or 0.9% NaCl at 4 mcg/ml for 24 hrs.

**IM**
• Give deep IM in large muscle mass.

## ▨ IV INCOMPATIBILITIES
Amphotericin B complex (Abelcet, AmBisome, Amphotec).

## ▨ IV COMPATIBILITIES
Heparin, ondansetron (Zofran), propofol (Diprivan).

## INDICATIONS/ROUTES/DOSAGE
**Opioid Overdose**
**IV, IM, SQ: ADULTS, ELDERLY:** 0.4–2 mg q2–3min as needed. May repeat doses q20–60min. **CHILDREN 5 YRS AND OLDER, WEIGHING 20 KG OR MORE:** 2 mg/dose; if no response, may repeat q2–3min. May need to repeat doses q20–60min. **CHILDREN YOUNGER THAN 5 YRS, WEIGHING LESS THAN 20 KG:** 0.1 mg/kg (**maximum:** 2 mg); if no response, repeat q2–3 min. May need to repeat doses q20–60 min. **NARCAN NASAL SPRAY: ADULTS, ELDERLY, CHILDREN:** Single spray into one nostril. May give q2–3min until emergency medical assistance arrives. *(Evzio):* **ADULTS, ELDERLY, CHILDREN:** 0.4 mg as a single dose; may repeat q2–3 min until emergency medical assistance becomes available.

**Reversal of Respiratory Depression with Therapeutic Opioid Dosing**
**IV, IM, SQ: ADULTS, ELDERLY:** Initially, 0.04–0.4 mg. May repeat until desired response achieved. **CHILDREN:** 0.001–0.015 mg/kg. Dose may be repeated as needed.

**Dosage in Renal/Hepatic Impairment**
No dose adjustment.

## SIDE EFFECTS
None known; little or no pharmacologic effect in absence of narcotics.

## ADVERSE EFFECTS/ TOXIC REACTIONS
Too-rapid reversal of narcotic-induced respiratory depression may result in agitation, nausea, vomiting, tremors, increased B/P, tachycardia. Excessive dosage in postop pts may produce significant reversal of analgesia, agitation, tremors. Hypotension or hypertension, ventricular tachycardia/fibrillation, pulmonary edema may occur in pts with cardiovascular disease.

## NURSING CONSIDERATIONS

### BASELINE ASSESSMENT
Maintain patent airway. Obtain weight of children to calculate drug dosage.

### INTERVENTION/EVALUATION
Monitor vital signs, esp. rate, depth, rhythm of respiration, during and frequently following administration. Carefully observe pt after satisfactory response (duration of opiate may exceed duration of naloxone, resulting in recurrence of respiratory depression). Assess for increased pain with reversal of opiate.

# naltrexone

nal-**trex**-own
(ReVia, Vivitrol)
**Do not confuse naltrexone with naloxone, or ReVia with Revatio or Revex.**

## FIXED COMBINATION(S)
**Troxyca ER:** naloxone/oxycodone (an opioid analgesic): 1.2 mg/10 mg, 2.4 mg/20 mg, 3.6 mg/30 mg, 4.8 mg/40 mg, 7.2 mg/60 mg, 9.6 ml/80 mg.

## ◆CLASSIFICATION
**PHARMACOTHERAPEUTIC:** Opioid receptor antagonist. **CLINICAL:** Narotic antagonist, alcohol antagonist antidote.

## USES

Treatment of alcohol dependence. Blocks effects of exogenously administered opioids.

## PRECAUTIONS

**Contraindications:** Hypersensitivity to naltrexone. Opioid dependence or current use of opioid analgesics, acute opioid withdrawal, failed naloxone challenge or positive urine screen for opioids. **Cautions:** Severe hepatic impairment, pts at high risk of suicide, thrombocytopenia, depression, history of bleeding disorders, concurrent anticoagulant therapy, moderate to severe renal impairment.

## ACTION

Blocks effects of endogenous opioid peptides by competitively binding at opioid receptors. **Therapeutic Effect: Alcohol deterrent:** Decreases craving, drinking days, relapse rate. **Antidote:** Blocks physical dependence of morphine, heroin, other opioids.

## PHARMACOKINETICS

| Route | Onset | Peak | Duration |
|-------|-------|------|----------|
| PO | N/A | N/A | 24–72 hrs |
| IM | N/A | 2 hrs | 2–4 wks |

Well absorbed following PO administration. Protein binding: 21%. Metabolized in liver. Reduction in first-pass hepatic metabolism when given by intramuscular route. Excreted primarily in urine. **Half-life: PO:** 4 hrs; **IM:** 5–10 days.

## ⧗ LIFESPAN CONSIDERATIONS

**Pregnancy/Lactation:** Unknown if drug crosses placenta or is distributed in breast milk. **Children:** Safety and efficacy not established in pts younger than 18 yrs. **Elderly:** No age-related precautions noted.

## INTERACTIONS

**DRUG:** May decrease effects of **opioid analgesics** (e.g., **morphine, hydrocodone, hydromorphone**). **HERBAL:** None significant. **FOOD:** None known. **LAB VALUES:** May increase serum transaminase, ALT, AST.

## AVAILABILITY (Rx)

**Injection Suspension, Extended-Release Kit (Vivitrol):** 380 mg/4 ml vial. **Tablets: (ReVia):** 50 mg.

## ADMINISTRATION/HANDLING

**◄ALERT►** In pts with narcotic dependence, do not attempt treatment until pt has remained opioid free for 7–10 days. Test urine for opioids for verification. Pt should not be experiencing withdrawal symptoms.

**IM**
• Give in deep muscle mass of gluteal region, alternating buttocks. • Vivitrol must be suspended only in diluent supplied in kit.
**Storage** • Store entire diluent supplied in the kit. • All components (microspheres, diluent, preparation needle, administration needle with safety device) are required for preparation administration. Spare administration needle is provided in case of clogging.

**PO**
• May take without regard to food. Administer with food or antacids or after meals to minimize adverse GI effects.

## INDICATIONS/ROUTES/DOSAGE

**Alcohol Dependence**
**PO: ADULTS, ELDERLY:** 50 mg once daily. Alternative maintenance regimens may be used (e.g., 50 mg/day Monday through Friday and 100 mg on Saturday, or 100 mg every other day, or 150 mg q3days.)
**IM: ADULTS, ELDERLY: (Vivitrol):** 380 mg once q4wks or once/mo.

**Opioid Dependence**
**PO: ADULTS, ELDERLY:** Initially, 25 mg. Observe for 1 hr. If no withdrawal signs appear, give 50 mg on day 2. Maintenance regimen is flexible, variable, and

**N**

individualized. May be given as 50 mg daily, 50 mg/day Monday through Friday and 100 mg on Saturday, 100 mg every other day, or 150 mg q3days for 12 wks. **IM: ADULTS, ELDERLY:** 380 mg q4wks.

**Dosage in Renal Impairment**
**Mild impairment:** No dose adjustment. **Moderate to severe impairment:** Use caution.

**Dosage in Hepatic Impairment**
No dose adjustment.

## SIDE EFFECTS

**Common: IM: (69%):** Injection site reaction (induration, tenderness, pain, nodules, swelling, pruritus, ecchymosis). **Frequent: Alcohol Deterrent: (33%–10%):** Nausea, headache, depression. **Narcotic Addiction (10%–5%):** Insomnia, anxiety, headache, low energy, abdominal cramps, nausea, vomiting, joint/muscle pain. **Occasional: Alcohol Deterrent (4%–2%):** Dizziness, anxiety, fatigue, insomnia, vomiting, suicidal ideation. **Narcotic Addiction (5% or less):** Irritability, increased energy, dizziness, anorexia, diarrhea, constipation, rash, chills, increased thirst.

## ADVERSE EFFECTS/ TOXIC REACTIONS

Signs/symptoms of opioid withdrawal include rhinorrhea, lacrimation, yawning, diaphoresis, tremor, vomiting, piloerection (goose bumps), feeling of temperature change, arthralgia, myalgia, abdominal cramps, formication (feeling of skin crawling). Accidental naltrexone overdosage produces withdrawal symptoms within 5 min of ingestion, lasts up to 48 hrs. Symptoms present as confusion, visual hallucinations, drowsiness, significant vomiting, diarrhea. Hepatotoxicity may occur with large doses.

## NURSING CONSIDERATIONS

### BASELINE ASSESSMENT

Treatment should not be instituted unless pt is opioid free for 7–10 days, alcohol free for 3–5 days before therapy begins. Obtain medication history (esp. opioids), other medical conditions (esp. hepatitis, other hepatic disease). If opioid dependence suspected, a naloxone challenge test should be performed (naloxone administered to verify opioid dependence and eligibility for admission to opioid treatment program).

### INTERVENTION/EVALUATION

Monitor for evidence of hepatotoxicity (abdominal pain that lasts longer than a few days, white bowel movements, dark urine, jaundice). Monitor serum ALT, AST, bilirubin.

### PATIENT/FAMILY TEACHING

• If heroin, other opiates are self-administered, there will be no effect. However, any attempt to overcome naltrexone's prolonged 24- to 72-hr blockade of opioid effect by taking large amounts of opioids is dangerous and may result in coma, serious injury, fatal overdose. • Naltrexone blocks effects of opioid-containing medicine (cough/cold preparations, antidiarrheal preparations, opioid analgesics). • Report abdominal pain lasting longer than 3 days, white bowel movement, dark-colored urine, yellowing of skin or eyes.

# naproxen

na-**prox**-en
(Aleve, Anaprox, Anaprox DS, Apo-Naproxen ✦, EC-Naprosyn, Naprelan, Naprosyn)

■ **BLACK BOX ALERT** ■ Increased risk of serious cardiovascular thrombotic events, including myocardial infarction, CVA. Increased risk of severe GI reactions, including ulceration, bleeding, perforation of stomach, intestines. **Do not confuse Aleve with Allese, or Anaprox with Anaspaz or Avapro.**

## ◆CLASSIFICATION

**PHARMACOTHERAPEUTIC:** NSAID. **CLINICAL:** Analgesic, anti-inflammatory.

## USES

Treatment of acute or long-term mild to moderate pain, primary dysmenorrhea, rheumatoid arthritis (RA), juvenile rheumatoid arthritis (JRA), osteoarthritis, ankylosing spondylitis, acute gouty arthritis, bursitis, tendonitis, fever. **OFF-LABEL:** Migraine prophylaxis.

## PRECAUTIONS

**Contraindications:** Hypersensitivity to aspirin, naproxen, other NSAIDs. Perioperative pain in setting of CABG surgery. **Cautions:** GI disease (bleeding, ulcers), fluid retention, renal/hepatic impairment, asthma, HF, concurrent use of anticoagulants, smoking, use of alcohol, elderly, debilitated.

## ACTION

Produces analgesic, anti-inflammatory effects by inhibiting prostaglandin synthesis. **Therapeutic Effect:** Reduces inflammatory response, intensity of pain.

## PHARMACOKINETICS

| Route | Onset | Peak | Duration |
|---|---|---|---|
| PO (analgesic) | 1 hr | 2–4 hrs | 7 hrs or less |
| PO (anti-inflammatory) | 2 wks | 2–4 wks | 12 hrs |

Completely absorbed from GI tract. Protein binding: 99%. Metabolized in liver. Primarily excreted in urine. Not removed by hemodialysis. **Half-life:** 13 hrs.

## ⌛ LIFESPAN CONSIDERATIONS

**Pregnancy/Lactation:** Crosses placenta. Distributed in breast milk. Avoid use during third trimester (may adversely affect fetal cardiovascular system: premature closing of ductus arteriosus). **Children:** Safety and efficacy not established in pts younger than 2 yrs. Children older than 2 yrs at increased risk for skin rash. **Elderly:** Age-related renal impairment may increase risk of hepatic/renal toxicity; reduced dosage recommended. More likely to have serious adverse effects with GI bleeding/ulceration.

## INTERACTIONS

**DRUG:** May decrease effects of **antihypertensives (e.g., amlodipine, lisinopril, valsartan), diuretics (e.g., furosemide, HCTZ). Aspirin, other salicylates** may increase risk of GI side effects, bleeding. **Bone marrow depressants** may increase risk of hematologic reactions. May increase risk of bleeding with **heparin, oral anticoagulants (e.g., warfarin), thrombolytics.** May increase concentration, risk of toxicity of **lithium.** May increase risk of **methotrexate** toxicity. **HERBAL:** Cat's claw, dong quai, evening primrose, feverfew, garlic, ginger, ginkgo, ginseng, horse chestnut, red clover possess antiplatelet activity, may increase risk of bleeding. **FOOD:** None known. **LAB VALUES:** May prolong bleeding time. May increase serum BUN, creatinine, ALT, AST, alkaline phosphatase. May decrease Hgb, Hct, leukocytes, platelets, uric acid.

## AVAILABILITY (Rx)

**Capsule (Aleve [OTC]):** 220 mg. **Oral Suspension (Naprosyn):** 125 mg/5 ml naproxen. **Tablets:** 220 mg, 250 mg, 275 mg, 375 mg, 500 mg, 550 mg.

 Tablets (Extended-Release): 375 mg, 500 mg, 750 mg.

N

## ADMINISTRATION/HANDLING

### PO

• Give controlled-release form whole. Do not break, crush, dissolve, or divide.
• Best taken with food or milk (decreases GI irritation). • Shake suspension well.

## INDICATIONS/ROUTES/DOSAGE

**Note:** Dosage expressed as naproxen base (200 mg naproxen base equivalent to 220 mg naproxen sodium).

### Rheumatoid Arthritis (RA), Osteoarthritis, Ankylosing Spondylitis

**PO: ADULTS, ELDERLY:** *(Immediate-Release):* 500–1,000 mg/day in 2 divided doses. May increase to 1,500 mg/day for limited time. *(Extended-Release):* Initially, 750–1,000 mg once daily. May increase temporarily to 1,500 mg once daily.

### Acute Gouty Arthritis

**PO: ADULTS, ELDERLY:** *(Immediate-Release):* Initially, 750 mg naproxen, then 250 mg naproxen q8h until attack subsides. **(Extended-Release):** Initially, 1,000–1,500 mg, then 1,000 mg once daily until attack subsides.

### Mild to Moderate Pain, Dysmenorrhea, Bursitis, Tendonitis

**PO: ADULTS, ELDERLY:** Initially, 500 mg, then 500 mg q12h or 250 mg q6–8h as needed. **Maximum:** 1,250 mg on day 1, then 1,000 mg once daily.

### Juvenile Idiopathic Arthritis (JIA)

**PO** *(Oral Suspension Recommended):* **CHILDREN OLDER THAN 2 YRS:** 10–15 mg/kg/day in 2 divided doses. **Maximum:** 1,000 mg/day.

### OTC Uses (Pain, Fever)

**PO: ADULTS 65 YRS AND YOUNGER, CHILDREN 12 YRS AND OLDER:** Initially, 400 mg once, then 200 mg q8–12h. **ADULTS OLDER THAN 65 YRS:** 200 mg q12h. **Maximum:** 400 mg in any 8–12-hr period or 600 mg/day.

### Dosage in Renal Impairment

Not recommended with CrCl less than 30 ml/min.

### Dosage in Hepatic Impairment

Use caution.

## SIDE EFFECTS

**Frequent (9%–4%):** Nausea, constipation, abdominal cramps/pain, heartburn, dizziness, headache, drowsiness. **Occasional (3%–1%):** Stomatitis, diarrhea, indigestion. **Rare (less than 1%):** Vomiting, confusion.

## ADVERSE EFFECTS/ TOXIC REACTIONS

Rare reactions with long-term use include peptic ulcer, GI bleeding, gastritis, severe hepatic reactions (cholestasis, jaundice), nephrotoxicity (dysuria, hematuria, proteinuria, nephrotic syndrome), and severe hypersensitivity reaction (fever, chills, bronchospasm).

## NURSING CONSIDERATIONS

### BASELINE ASSESSMENT

Assess onset, type, location, duration of pain/inflammation. Inspect appearance of affected joints for immobility, deformities, skin condition. Question history of GI bleeding, gastric or duodenal ulcers, hypertension.

### INTERVENTION/EVALUATION

Assist with ambulation if dizziness occurs. Monitor CBC, renal function, LFT, daily pattern of bowel activity, stool consistency. Evaluate for therapeutic response: relief of pain, stiffness, swelling; increased joint mobility, reduced joint tenderness, improved grip strength.

### PATIENT/FAMILY TEACHING

• Avoid tasks that require alertness, motor skills until response to drug is established.
• Take with food, milk. • Avoid aspirin, alcohol during therapy (increases risk of GI bleeding). • Report headache, rash, visual disturbances, weight gain, black or tarry stools, bleeding, persistent headache.

# naratriptan

nar-a-**trip**-tan
(Amerge)
**Do not confuse naratriptan with
eletriptan or almotriptan, or
Amerge with Altace or Amaryl.**

## ◆CLASSIFICATION

**PHARMACOTHERAPEUTIC:** Serotonin receptor agonist. **CLINICAL:** Antimigraine.

## USES

Treatment of acute migraine headache with or without aura in adults.

## PRECAUTIONS

**Contraindications:** Hypersensitivity to naratriptan. Basilar/hemiplegic migraine, cerebrovascular disease, peripheral vascular disease, coronary artery disease, ischemic heart disease (including angina pectoris, history of MI, silent ischemia, Prinzmetal's angina), severe hepatic impairment (Child-Pugh grade C), severe renal impairment (CrCl less than 15 ml/min), uncontrolled hypertension, use within 24 hrs of ergotamine-containing preparations or another serotonin receptor agonist, 5-HT agonist (e.g., sumatriptan), MAOI use within 14 days. **Cautions:** Mild to moderate renal/hepatic impairment, pt profile suggesting cardiovascular risks, elderly.

## ACTION

Binds selectively to serotonin receptors, producing vasoconstrictive effect on cranial blood vessels. **Therapeutic Effect:** Relieves migraine headache.

## PHARMACOKINETICS

Well absorbed after PO administration. Protein binding: 28%–31%. Metabolized in liver. Eliminated primarily in urine. **Half-life:** 6 hrs (increased in hepatic/renal impairment).

## ⧖ LIFESPAN CONSIDERATIONS

**Pregnancy/Lactation:** Unknown if drug is distributed in breast milk. **Children:** Safety and efficacy not established. **Elderly:** Not recommended in the elderly.

## INTERACTIONS

**DRUG: Ergotamine-containing medications** may produce vasospastic reaction. **SSRIs** and **SNRIs (e.g., fluoxetine, fluvoxamine, paroxetine, sertraline)** may produce serotonin syndrome. **HERBAL:** None significant. **FOOD:** None known. **LAB VALUES:** None significant.

## AVAILABILITY (Rx)

🔰 **Tablets:** 1 mg, 2.5 mg.

## ADMINISTRATION/HANDLING

**PO**

• Give without regard to food. • Do not break, crush, dissolve, or divide tablets. Swallow whole with water.

## INDICATIONS/ROUTES/DOSAGE

**Acute Migraine Attack**
**PO: ADULTS:** 1 or 2.5 mg. If headache improves but then returns, dose may be repeated after 4 hrs. **Maximum:** 5 mg/24 hrs.

**Dosage in Renal/Hepatic Impairment**

| Hepatic Failure | Creatinine Clearance | Dosage |
| --- | --- | --- |
| Mild to moderate | 15–39 ml/min | Initial, 1 mg Max: 2.5/24 hrs |
| Severe | Less than 15 ml/min | Contraindicated |

## SIDE EFFECTS

**Occasional (5%):** Nausea. **Rare (2%):** Paresthesia, dizziness, fatigue, drowsiness, feeling of pressure in throat, neck, jaw.

## ADVERSE EFFECTS/ TOXIC REACTIONS

Corneal opacities, other ocular defects may occur. Cardiac events (ischemia,

N

---

coronary artery vasospasm, MI), noncardiac vasospasm-related reactions (hemorrhage, cerebrovascular accident [CVA]) occur rarely, particularly in pts with hypertension, diabetes, strong family history of coronary artery disease, obese pts, smokers, males older than 40 yrs, postmenopausal women.

## NURSING CONSIDERATIONS

### BASELINE ASSESSMENT

Question for history of peripheral vascular disease, renal/hepatic impairment, possibility of pregnancy. Question pt regarding possible precipitating symptoms, onset, location, duration of migraine.

### INTERVENTION/EVALUATION

Assess for relief of migraine headache; potential for photophobia, phonophobia (sound sensitivity), nausea, vomiting.

### PATIENT/FAMILY TEACHING

- Do not chew, crush, dissolve, or divide tablet; swallow whole with water. • May repeat dose after 4 hrs (maximum of 5 mg/24 hrs). • May cause dizziness, fatigue, drowsiness. • Avoid tasks that require alertness, motor skills until response to drug is established. • Report any chest pain, palpitations, tightness in throat, rash, hallucinations, anxiety, panic.

# natalizumab

na-ta-**liz**-yoo-mab
(Tysabri)

■ **BLACK BOX ALERT** ■ Restricted distribution program (TOUCH), given only to program-qualified/enrolled pts. Increased risk of leukoencephalopathy (progressive, often fatal viral brain infection).

## ◆CLASSIFICATION

**PHARMACOTHERAPEUTIC:** Monoclonal antibody. **CLINICAL:** Multiple sclerosis agent, immunologic agent.

## USES

Treatment of relapsing forms of multiple sclerosis to reduce frequency of clinical exacerbations. Treatment of moderate to severe Crohn's disease in pts with inadequate response or unable to tolerate conventional Crohn's disease therapies.

## PRECAUTIONS

**Contraindications:** Hypersensitivity to natalizumab. Pts who have or have had progressive multifocal leukoencephalopathy (PML). **Cautions:** Chronic progressive multiple sclerosis, children younger than 18 yrs. Concomitant immunosuppressants (may increase risk of infection).

## ACTION

Binds to surface of leukocytes, inhibiting adhesion of leukocytes to vascular endothelial cells of GI tract, preventing migration of leukocytes across endothelium into inflamed parenchymal tissue. **Therapeutic Effect:** Inhibits inflammatory activity of activated immune cells, reduces clinical exacerbations of multiple sclerosis, Crohn's disease.

## PHARMACOKINETICS

Steady state reached in approximately 16–24 wks. **Half-life:** 11 days.

## ⧗ LIFESPAN CONSIDERATIONS

**Pregnancy/Lactation:** Unknown if drug crosses placenta or is distributed in breast milk. **Children:** Safety and efficacy not established in pts younger than 18 yrs. **Elderly:** No age-related precautions noted.

## INTERACTIONS

**DRUG: Antineoplastics, immunomodulating agents, immunosuppressants** may increase risk of PML. **HERBAL:** None significant. **FOOD:** None known. **LAB VALUES:** May increase basophils, lymphocytes, monocytes, eosinophils, red blood cells (usually reversible within 16 wks after last dose).

## AVAILABILITY (Rx)

**Injection Solution:** 300 mg/15 ml concentrate.

## ADMINISTRATION/HANDLING

 IV

**Reconstitution** • Withdraw 15 ml natalizumab from vial; inject concentrate into 100 ml 0.9% NaCl. • Invert solution to mix completely; do not shake. • Discard if solution is discolored or particulate forms.

**Rate of Administration** • Infuse over 1 hr. • Following completion of infusion, flush with 0.9% NaCl.

**Storage** • Refrigerate vials. • Do not shake, freeze. Protect from light. • After reconstitution, solution is stable for 8 hrs if refrigerated.

## ▓ IV INCOMPATIBILITIES

Do not mix with any other medications or diluent other than 0.9% NaCl.

## INDICATIONS/ROUTES/DOSAGE

**Relapsed Multiple Sclerosis, Crohn's Disease**
**IV Infusion: ADULTS 18 YRS AND OLDER, ELDERLY:** 300 mg q4wks.

**Dosage in Renal/Hepatic Impairment**
No dose adjustment. Discontinue with jaundice or signs/symptoms of hepatic injury.

## SIDE EFFECTS

**Frequent (35%–15%):** Headache, fatigue, depression, arthralgia. **Occasional (10%–5%):** Abdominal discomfort, rash, urinary urgency/frequency, irregular menstruation/dysmenorrhea, dermatitis. **Rare (4%–2%):** Pruritus, chest discomfort, local bleeding, rigors, tremor, syncope.

## ADVERSE EFFECTS/ TOXIC REACTIONS

UTI, lower respiratory tract infection, gastroenteritis, vaginitis, allergic reaction, tonsillitis, PMI.

## NURSING CONSIDERATIONS

### BASELINE ASSESSMENT
Obtain CBC, serum chemistries, LFT. Assess home situation for support of therapy.

### INTERVENTION/EVALUATION
Periodically monitor lab results. Assess for arthralgia, depression, urinary changes, menstrual irregularities. Assess skin for evidence of rash, pruritus, dermatitis. Monitor for signs/symptoms of UTI, respiratory infection.

---

# *nateglinide*

na-**te**-glye-nide
(Starlix)

## ◆CLASSIFICATION

**PHARMACOTHERAPEUTIC:** Antihyperglycemic. **CLINICAL:** Antidiabetic agent.

## USES
Treatment of type 2 diabetes mellitus as an adjunct to diet and exercise.

## PRECAUTIONS

**Contraindications:** Hypersensitivity to nateglinide. Diabetic ketoacidosis, type 1 diabetes mellitus. **Cautions:** Moderate to severe hepatic impairment, severe renal impairment, elderly, malnourished, adrenal/pituitary dysfunction.

## ACTION

Stimulates insulin release from beta cells of pancreas by depolarizing beta cells, leading to opening of calcium channels. Resulting calcium influx induces insulin secretion. **Therapeutic Effect:** Lowers serum glucose concentration.

## PHARMACOKINETICS

| Route | Onset | Peak | Duration |
|-------|-------|------|----------|
| PO | 20 min | 1 hr | 4 hrs |

Rapidly absorbed from GI tract. Protein binding: 98%. Extensive metabolism in

---

liver. Excreted in urine (83%), feces (10%). **Half-life:** 1.5 hrs.

## ⧖ LIFESPAN CONSIDERATIONS

**Pregnancy/Lactation:** Unknown if drug crosses placenta or is distributed in breast milk. **Children:** Safety and efficacy not established. **Elderly:** Increased susceptibility to hypoglycemia.

## INTERACTIONS

**DRUG:** Beta blockers (e.g., **carvedilol, metoprolol**) may mask symptoms of hypoglycemia. **Beta blockers (e.g., carvedilol, metoprolol), MAOIs, NSAIDs, salicylates** may increase hypoglycemic effect. **Corticosteroids (e.g., prednisone), sympathomimetics, thiazide diuretics (e.g., HCTZ), thyroid medications** may decrease hypoglycemic effect. **HERBAL:** Bilberry, garlic, ginger, ginseng may increase hypoglycemic effect. **St. John's wort** may decrease concentration/effects. **FOOD:** None known. **LAB VALUES:** Decrease in serum glucose expected.

## AVAILABILITY (Rx)

**Tablets:** 60 mg, 120 mg.

## ADMINISTRATION/HANDLING

**PO**
• Ideally, give within 15 min of a meal, but may be given immediately before a meal to as long as 30 min before a meal.

## INDICATIONS/ROUTES/DOSAGE

**Diabetes Mellitus**
**PO: ADULTS, ELDERLY: Initial/Maintenance:** 120 mg 3 times/day before meals. 60 mg 3 times/day may be given in pts close to HbA1C goal.

**Dosage in Renal Impairment**
**Mild to moderate impairment:** No dose adjustment. **Severe impairment:** Use caution.

**Dosage in Hepatic Impairment**
**Mild impairment:** No dose adjustment. **Moderate to severe impairment:** Use caution.

## SIDE EFFECTS

**Frequent (10%):** Upper respiratory tract infection. **Occasional (4%–3%):** Back pain, flu-like symptoms, dizziness, arthropathy, diarrhea. **Rare (2% or less):** Bronchitis, cough.

## ADVERSE EFFECTS/ TOXIC REACTIONS

Hypoglycemia occurs in less than 2% of pts.

## NURSING CONSIDERATIONS

### BASELINE ASSESSMENT

Check fasting serum glucose, Hgb (A1c) periodically to determine minimum effective dose. Discuss lifestyle to determine extent of learning, emotional needs. Ensure follow-up instruction if pt, family do not thoroughly understand diabetes management, glucose-testing technique. At least 1 wk should elapse to assess response to drug before new dose adjustment is made.

### INTERVENTION/EVALUATION

Monitor serum glucose, food intake. Assess for hypoglycemia (cool, wet skin, tremors, dizziness, anxiety, headache, tachycardia, numbness in mouth, hunger, diplopia), hyperglycemia (polyuria, polyphagia, polydipsia, nausea, vomiting, dim vision, fatigue, deep rapid breathing). Be alert to conditions that alter glucose requirements: fever, increased activity, stress, surgical procedures.

### PATIENT/FAMILY TEACHING

• Diabetes mellitus requires lifelong control. • Prescribed diet, exercise are principal parts of treatment; do not skip, delay meals. • Continue to adhere to dietary instructions, regular exercise program, regular testing of serum glucose.

# nebivolol

ne-**biv**-oh-lol
(Bystolic)
**Do not confuse nebivolol with nadolol or atenolol.**

## FIXED-COMBINATION(S)

**Byvalson:** nebivolol/valsartan (an ARB): 5 mg/80 mg.

## ◆CLASSIFICATION

**PHARMACOTHERAPEUTIC:** Beta-adrenergic blocker. **CLINICAL:** Antihypertensive.

## USES

Management of hypertension. Used alone or in combination with other antihypertensives. **OFF-LABEL:** HF.

## PRECAUTIONS

**Contraindications:** Hypersensitivity to nebivolol. Severe bradycardia, decompensated HF, cardiogenic shock, heart block greater than first degree, severe hepatic impairment, sick sinus rhythm (unless pt has pacemaker). **Cautions:** Diabetes mellitus, acute exacerbation of coronary artery disease, bronchospastic disease, peripheral vascular disease, Raynaud's syndrome, thyrotoxicosis, renal impairment; concomitant use of verapamil, digoxin.

## ACTION

Predominantly blocks beta$_1$-adrenergic receptors. Large doses block both beta$_1$ and beta$_2$ receptors. **Therapeutic Effect:** Lowers B/P.

## PHARMACOKINETICS

| | Onset | Peak | Duration |
|---|---|---|---|
| PO | 30 min | 1.5–4 hrs | 12 hrs |

Completely absorbed from GI tract. Protein binding: 98%. Metabolized in liver. Excreted in feces (44%), urine (38%). **Half-life:** 12 hrs (increased in severe renal impairment).

## ⊠ LIFESPAN CONSIDERATIONS

**Pregnancy/Lactation:** May cross placenta; appears to be distributed in breast milk. May produce low-birth-weight infants. **Children:** Safety and efficacy not established. **Elderly:** No age-related precautions noted.

## INTERACTIONS

**DRUG: Diuretics (e.g., furosemide, HCTZ), antihypertensives (e.g., amlodipine, lisinopril, valsartan)** may increase hypotensive effect. **CYP2D6 inhibitors (e.g., fluoxetine, paroxetine)** may increase concentration/effects. **HERBAL: Ephedra, ginseng, yohimbe, ginger, licorice** may worsen hypertension. **Black cohosh, periwinkle** may increase antihypertensive effect. **FOOD:** None known. **LAB VALUES:** May increase serum BUN, uric acid, ALT, AST, bilirubin, triglycerides. May decrease platelet count, serum HDL.

## AVAILABILITY (Rx)

**Tablets:** 2.5 mg, 5 mg, 10 mg, 20 mg.

## ADMINISTRATION/HANDLING

**PO**

• Give without regard to meals. • Do not break, crush, dissolve, or divide tablets.

## INDICATIONS/ROUTES/DOSAGE

**Hypertension**
**PO: ADULTS, ELDERLY:** Initially, 5 mg once daily. May increase at 2-wk intervals to maximum 40 mg once daily. Usual dose: 5–10 mg once daily.

**Dosage in Renal Impairment**
**Mild to moderate impairment:** No dose adjustment. **Severe impairment (CrCl less than 30 ml/min):** Initially, 2.5 mg once daily. Increase gradually.

**Dosage in Hepatic Impairment**
**Mild impairment:** No dose adjustment. **Moderate impairment:** Initially, 2.5 mg once daily. Increase cautiously. Contraindicated in severe impairment.

## SIDE EFFECTS

Generally well tolerated, with mild and transient side effects. **Occasional (9%):**

Headache. **Rare (2%–1%):** Fatigue, dizziness, diarrhea, nausea, insomnia, peripheral edema.

## ADVERSE EFFECTS/ TOXIC REACTIONS

Large doses may produce bradycardia, dyspnea, rash. Acute pulmonary edema, renal failure, AV block reported. **Antidote:** Glucagon (see Appendix J for dosage).

## NURSING CONSIDERATIONS

### BASELINE ASSESSMENT

Assess baseline renal function, LFT. Assess B/P, apical pulse immediately before drug administration (if pulse is 60/min or less, or systolic B/P is less than 90 mm Hg, withhold medication, contact physician).

### INTERVENTION/EVALUATION

Measure B/P near end of dosing interval (determines whether B/P is controlled throughout day). Monitor B/P for hypotension. Assess pulse for quality, regularity, bradycardia. Question for evidence of headache.

### PATIENT/FAMILY TEACHING

• Compliance with therapy regimen is essential to control hypertension. • Do not use nasal decongestants, OTC cold preparations (stimulants) without physician's approval. • Monitor B/P, pulse before taking medication. • Restrict salt, alcohol intake. • Do not chew, crush, dissolve, or divide tablets. Swallow whole.

# necitumumab

ne-si-**toom**-oo-mab
(Portrazza)

■ **BLACK BOX ALERT** ■ Cardiopulmonary arrest and/or sudden death reported in 3% of pts (when treated in combination with gemcitabine and cisplatin). Closely monitor serum electrolytes, esp. serum calcium, magnesium, potassium, and aggressively replace as appropriate.

Hypomagnesemia occurred in 83% of pts and was severe in 20%. Monitor pts for hypomagnesemia, hypocalcemia, hypokalemia prior to each dose, during treatment, and up to 8 wks after discontinuation. Withhold treatment for Grade 3 or 4 electrolyte abnormality.

**Do not confuse necitumumab with adalimumab, belimumab, daratumumab, ipilimumab, nivolumab, ofatumumab, or panitumumab.**

## ◆CLASSIFICATION

**PHARMACOTHERAPEUTIC:** Epidermal growth factor receptor (EGFR) inhibitor. Monoclonal antibody. **CLINICAL:** Antineoplastic.

## USES

First-line treatment of metastatic squamous non–small cell lung cancer (NSCLC) (in combination with gemcitabine and cisplatin).

## PRECAUTIONS

**Contraindications:** Severe hypersensitivity to necitumumab. **Cautions:** COPD, chronic arrhythmias, coronary artery disease, HF, recent MI (within 6 mos), pts at risk for electrolyte imbalance (e.g., adrenal insufficiency, alcoholism, renal failure, thyroid disorders, malnutrition, chronic diarrhea; concomitant use medication known to cause electrolyte abnormalities); history of venous or arterial thrombosis (e.g., CVA, DVT, MI, pulmonary embolism). Not indicated for treatment of non–squamous non–small cell lung cancer.

## ACTION

Binds to ligand-binding site of EGFR and prevents activation, expression, signaling of EGFR. **Therapeutic Effect:** Inhibits tumor cell growth and metastasis.

## PHARMACOKINETICS

Widely distributed. Metabolism not specified. Elimination not specified. **Half-life:** 14 days.

## LIFESPAN CONSIDERATIONS

**Pregnancy/Lactation:** Avoid pregnancy; may cause fetal harm. Female pts of reproductive potential should use effective contraception during treatment and for at least 3 mos after discontinuation. Unknown if distributed in breast milk. Breastfeeding not recommended during treatment and up to 3 mos after discontinuation. **Children:** Safety and efficacy not established. **Elderly:** May have increased risk of venous thromboembolism (including pulmonary embolism).

## INTERACTIONS

**DRUG:** None known. **HERBAL:** None known. **FOOD:** None known. **LAB VALUES:** May decrease serum calcium, magnesium, potassium.

## AVAILABILITY (Rx)

**Injection Solution:** 800 mg/50 ml (16 mg/ml).

## ADMINISTRATION/HANDLING

 **IV**

**Preparation** • Visually inspect for particulate matter or discoloration. • Solution should appear clear to slightly opalescent, colorless to slightly yellow in color. Discard if solution is cloudy or particulate matter is observed. • Dilute in 250 ml 0.9% NaCl bag. • Do not use solutions containing dextrose. • Gently invert to mix. Do not shake or agitate.

**Infusion Guidelines** • For pts with prior grade 1 or 2 infusion reaction, premedicate with diphenhydramine (or equivalent) before to each subsequent infusion. • For pts with recurrent grade 1 or 2 infusion reaction (despite administration of diphenhydramine), premedicate with dexamethasone (or equivalent), acetaminophen, diphenhydramine (or equivalent) before each subsequent infusion. • Once infusion complete, flush IV line with 0.9% NaCl only.

**Rate of Administration** • Infuse over 60 mins using infusion pump via dedicated line.

**Storage** • Refrigerate unused vials in original carton until time of use. • Protect from light. • May refrigerate diluted solution up to 24 hours or at room temperature up to 4 hrs.

## 🔳 IV INCOMPATABILITIES

Do not mix with dextrose-containing solutions. Do not infuse with other medications or electrolytes.

## INDICATIONS/ROUTES/DOSAGE

**Non–Small Cell Lung Cancer**
**IV: ADULTS, ELDERLY:** 800 mg on days 1 and 8 of each 3-wk cycle (in combination of gemcitabine and cisplatin). Continue until disease progression or unacceptable toxicity.

**Dose Modification**
Based on Common Terminology Criteria for Adverse Events (CTCAE).

**Infusion Reactions**
**Any grade 1 reaction:** Decrease rate by 50%. **Grade 2 reaction:** Interrupt infusion until resolved to Grade 1 or 0, then resume with rate reduced by 50% for all subsequent infusions. **Grade 3 reaction:** Permanently discontinue.

**Dermatological Toxicity**
**Grade 3 rash or acneiform rash:** Withhold treatment until resolved to grade 2 or better, then reduce dose to 400 mg for at least 1 treatment cycle. If tolerated, may increase dose to 600 mg and 800 mg for subsequent cycles. **Permanent Discontinuation:** Grade 3 rash or acneiform rash that does not resolve to Grade 2 or better within 6 wks; worsening of skin reaction or intolerance at 400 mg dose; Grade 3 skin induration or fibrosis; grade 4 dermatologic toxicity.

**Electrolyte Imbalance**
Withhold treatment for any Grade 3 or 4 electrolyte abnormalities. Resume once

**N**

abnormalities resolve to Grade 2 or better.

**Venous/Arterial Thrombosis**
**Any occurrence:** Permanently discontinue.

**Dosage in Renal Impairment**
No dose adjustment.

**Dosage in Hepatic Impairment**
**Mild to moderate impairment:** No dose adjustment. **Severe impairment:** Not specified; use caution.

## SIDE EFFECTS

**Frequent** **(44%–29%):** Rash, vomiting. **Occasional** **(16%–5%):** Diarrhea, dermatitis acneiform, decreased weight, stomatitis, headache, acne, pruritus, dry skin, paronychia, conjunctivitis, blurry vision, dry eye, reduced visual acuity, blepharitis, eye pain, increased lacrimation, ocular hyperemia, visual impairment, eye pruritus, skin fissures. **Rare** **(3%–1%):** Dysphagia, muscle spasm, oropharyngeal pain.

## ADVERSE EFFECTS/TOXIC REACTIONS

All cases were reported in combination with gemcitabine and cisplatin. Pts with severe hypomagnesemia, hypokalemia, hypocalcemia are at an increased risk for cardiac arrhythmias or sudden death. Cardiopulmonary arrest and/or sudden death occurred in 3% of pts. Most cases of cardiopulmonary arrest occurred with 30 days of the last dose and involved comorbidities including COPD, coronary artery disease, hypomagnesemia, hypertension. Hypomagnesemia reported in 83% of pts with median onset of approx. 6 wks. Severe hypomagnesemia (grade 3 or 4) reported in 20% of pts. Infusion reaction (any grade) reported in 1.5% of pts. Life-threatening venous and arterial thromboembolic events including pulmonary embolism (5% of pts), DVT (2% of pts), CVA (2% of pts), MI (1% of pts); thrombosis of mesenteric veins, pulmonary artery/vein, axillary vein, vena cava, subclavian vein; thrombophlebitis may occur. Hemoptysis reported in 10% of pts. Ocular toxicities including conjunctivitis, conjunctival hemorrhage, eye infections were reported. Severe skin toxicities occurred in 8% of pts. Immunogenicity (auto-necitumumab antibodies) occurred in 4% of pts.

## NURSING CONSIDERATIONS

### BASELINE ASSESSMENT
Obtain baseline BMP, serum magnesium, ionized calcium; vital signs prior to each dose. Obtain pregnancy test in female pts of reproductive potential. Receive full medication history and screen for drugs known to cause electrolyte imbalance. Assess nutritional status. Question history of CVA, DVT, pulmonary embolism, cardiac disease, recent MI; conditions known to cause electrolyte imbalance; prior hypersensitivity reaction to any drug in treatment regimen; prior infusion reaction. Offer emotional support. Conduct full dermatological exam.

### INTERVENTION/EVALUATION
Diligently monitor serum electrolytes, esp. serum magnesium, potassium, calcium, ionized calcium, during therapy and up to 8 wks after discontinuation. Monitor for symptoms of hypocalcemia, hypokalemia, hypomagnesemia. Obtain EKG, vital signs if arrhythmia, chest pain, palpitations, syncope occurs. Aggressively replete electrolytes as appropriate. Pts with sudden chest pain, dyspnea, hypoxia, tachycardia should be evaluated for pulmonary embolism. Monitor for symptoms of DVT (leg or arm pain/swelling), CVA (aphasia, altered LOC, hemiplegia, vision loss, headache, homonymous hemianopia [vision loss on the same side of both eyes]), MI (chest pain, dyspnea, syncope, diaphoresis, left arm pain, jaw pain). Monitor for hemoptysis. Assess skin for rash, hypersensitivity reaction; eyes for infection, subconjunctival hemorrhage.

• Blood levels will be routinely monitored. • Therapy may cause low levels of potassium, magnesium, calcium in the blood and may be life threatening. Replace electrolytes exactly as instructed. • Report symptoms of electrolyte imbalance such as fainting, fatigue, muscle cramps, palpations, paralysis, numbness or tingling, seizures, weakness. • Avoid pregnancy; treatment may cause birth defects. Female pts of child-bearing potential should use effective contraception during treatment and for at least 3 mos after last dose. Do not breastfeed during therapy and for at least 3 mos after last dose. • Treatment may cause blood clots in the arms, legs, lungs, brain, heart, or abdomen. Immediately report symptoms of stroke (difficulty speaking, confusion, paralysis, vision loss), heart attack (chest pain, shortness of breath, fainting, dizziness, profuse sweating, left arm or jaw pain), lung embolism (difficulty breathing, fast heart rate, chest pain), or blood clots in the arms or legs (pain/swelling). • Report skin rashes, allergic reactions, coughing up blood; eye problems such as infection, vision impairment, collection of blood in the whites of the eyes. • Avoid sunlight, tanning beds. Wear protect clothing, high SPF sunscreen, and lip balm when outdoors.

# niacin, nicotinic acid

TOP 100

nye-a-sin, nik-oh-**tin**-ik **as**-id
(Niacor, Niaspan, Slo-Niacin)
**Do not confuse niacin, Niacor, or Niaspan with minocin or Nitro-Bid.**

## FIXED-COMBINATION(S)

**Advicor:** niacin/lovastatin (HMG-CoA reductase inhibitor [statin]): 500 mg/20 mg, 750 mg/20 mg, 1,000 mg/20 mg. **Simcor:** niacin/simvastatin (HMG-CoA reductase inhibitor [statin]): 500 mg/20 mg, 500 mg/40 mg, 750 mg/20 mg, 1,000 mg/20 mg, 1,000 mg/40 mg.

## ◆CLASSIFICATION

**CLINICAL:** Antihyperlipidemic, water-soluble vitamin.

## USES

Treatment of dyslipidemias, lowers risk of recurrent MI (pts with history of MI/hyperlipidemia), slow progression of CAD, treatment of hypertriglyceridemia in pts at risk for pancreatitis, dietary supplement. **OFF-LABEL:** Treatment of pellagra.

## PRECAUTIONS

**Contraindications:** Hypersensitivity to niacin, nicotinic acid. Active peptic ulcer disease, arterial hemorrhage, significant or unexplained persistent elevations in hepatic transaminases, active hepatic disease. **Cautions:** Diabetes mellitus, gallbladder disease, unstable angina, MI, renal impairment, heavy alcohol use, concomitant use of anticoagulants, gout, history of jaundice/hepatic disease, inadequately treated hypothyroidism, elderly.

## ACTION

Component of two coenzymes needed for tissue respiration, lipid metabolism, glycogenolysis. May inhibit release of free fatty acids from adipose tissue; increase lipoprotein lipase activity. **Therapeutic Effect:** Reduces total, LDL, VLDL cholesterol levels and triglyceride levels; increases HDL cholesterol concentration.

## PHARMACOKINETICS

Readily absorbed from GI tract. Widely distributed. Protein binding: 20%. Metabolized in liver. Primarily excreted in urine. **Half-life:** 45 min.

N

## ⌛ LIFESPAN CONSIDERATIONS

**Pregnancy/Lactation:** Not recommended for use during pregnancy/lactation. Distributed in breast milk. **Children:** No age-related precautions noted. Not recommended in pts younger than 2 yrs. **Elderly:** No age-related precautions noted.

## INTERACTIONS

**DRUG: Alcohol** may increase risk of side effects. May increase effect of **antihypertensives. Lovastatin, pravastatin, simvastatin** may increase risk of acute renal failure, rhabdomyolysis. **Vasoactive drugs (e.g., calcium channel blockers, nitrates)** may increase hypotension. **HERBAL:** None significant. **FOOD:** None known. **LAB VALUES:** May increase serum uric acid, PT, amylase, bilirubin, fasting glucose, LDH, transaminase. May decrease platelets.

## AVAILABILITY (OTC)

**Tablets (Immediate-Release [Niacor]):** 50 mg, 100 mg, 250 mg, 500 mg.

🔖 **Capsules (Extended-Release):** 250 mg, 500 mg. 🔖 **Tablets (Extended-Release [Niaspan]):** 250 mg, 500 mg, 750 mg, 1,000 mg.

## ADMINISTRATION/HANDLING

**PO**

• For pts switching from immediate-release niacin to extended-release niacin, initiate extended-release form with low doses and titrate to therapeutic response. • Give with food. • Give aspirin 30 min before taking extended-release niacin to minimize flushing. • Do not break, crush, dissolve, or divide long-acting forms.

## INDICATIONS/ROUTES/DOSAGE

**Hyperlipidemia**

**PO** *(Immediate-Release):* **ADULTS, ELDERLY:** Initially, 250 mg once daily (with evening meal). May increase dose q4–7days up to 1.5–2 g/day in 2–3 divided doses. After 2 mos may increase at 2- to 4-wk intervals to 3 g/day in 3 divided

doses. **Maximum:** 6 g/day in 3 divided doses. Usual daily dose: 1.5–3 g/day.

**PO** *(Extended-Release):* **ADULTS, ELDERLY:** Initially, 500 mg/day at bedtime for 4 wks, then 1 g at bedtime for 4 wks. May increase by 500 mg q4wks up to maximum of 2 g/day. Usual daily dose: 1–2 g/day.

**Dosage for Hepatic Toxicity**

**Transaminases more than 3 times ULN:** Discontinue therapy.

**Dosage in Renal/Hepatic Impairment**

No dose adjustment.

## SIDE EFFECTS

**Frequent:** Flushing (esp. face, neck) occurring within 20 min of drug administration and lasting for 30–60 min, GI upset, pruritus. **Occasional:** Dizziness, hypotension, headache, blurred vision, burning/tingling of skin, flatulence, nausea, vomiting, diarrhea. **Rare:** Hyperglycemia, glycosuria, rash, hyperpigmentation, dry skin.

## ADVERSE EFFECTS/ TOXIC REACTIONS

Arrhythmias occur rarely.

## NURSING CONSIDERATIONS

### BASELINE ASSESSMENT

Obtain diet history, especially fat consumption. Question for history of hypersensitivity to niacin, tartrazine, aspirin. Obtain baseline serum cholesterol, triglyceride, glucose, LFT.

### INTERVENTION/EVALUATION

Evaluate flushing, degree of GI discomfort. Check for headache, dizziness, blurred vision. Monitor daily pattern of bowel activity, stool consistency. Monitor hepatic function, serum cholesterol, triglycerides. Check serum glucose carefully in pts on insulin, oral antihyperglycemics. Assess skin for rash, dryness. Monitor serum uric acid.

• Transient flushing of the skin, sensation of warmth, pruritus, tingling may occur. • Report dizziness (avoid sudden changes in posture). • Report nausea, vomiting, loss of appetite, yellowing of skin, dark urine, feeling of weakness. • If medically approved, take aspirin 30 min before taking extended-release niacin to minimize flushing. • Take at bedtime with low-fat snack. • Limit alcohol consumption.

# *niCARdipine

nye-**kar**-di-peen
(Cardene IV)
**Do not confuse Cardene SR with Cardizem SR or codeine, or nicardipine with nifedipine or nimodipine.**

## ◆CLASSIFICATION

**PHARMACOTHERAPEUTIC:** Calcium channel blocker. **CLINICAL:** Antianginal, antihypertensive.

## USES

**PO: Immediate-release:** Treatment of chronic stable (effort-associated) angina, hypertension. **Sustained-release:** Treatment of hypertension. **Parenteral:** Short-term treatment of hypertension when oral therapy not feasible or desirable. **OFF-LABEL:** Blood pressure control in acute ischemic stroke and intracranial hemorrhage.

## PRECAUTIONS

**Contraindications:** Hypersensitivity to nicardipine. Advanced aortic stenosis. **Cautions:** Cardiac/renal/hepatic dysfunction, HF, hypertrophic cardiomyopathy with outflow tract obstruction, aortic stenosis, coronary artery disease, portal hypertension.

## ACTION

Inhibits calcium ion movement across cell membranes, depressing contraction of cardiac, vascular smooth muscle. **Therapeutic Effect:** Increases heart rate, cardiac output, myocardial oxygen delivery. Decreases systemic vascular resistance, B/P.

## PHARMACOKINETICS

| Route | Onset | Peak | Duration |
|-------|-------|------|----------|
| PO | 0.5–2 hrs | — | 8 hrs |
| IV | 10 min | — | 8 hrs or less |

Rapidly, completely absorbed from GI tract. Protein binding: 95%. Metabolized in liver. Primarily excreted in urine. Not removed by hemodialysis. **Half-life:** 2–4 hrs.

## ⧗ LIFESPAN CONSIDERATIONS

**Pregnancy/Lactation:** Unknown if distributed in breast milk. **Children:** Safety and efficacy not established. **Elderly:** Age-related renal impairment may require dosage adjustment.

## INTERACTIONS

**DRUG:** May increase concentration of **cyclosporine. HERBAL:** Ephedra, ginger, ginseng, yohimbe may increase hypertension. **Licorice** may cause retention of sodium, water; may increase loss of potassium. **St. John's wort** may decrease levels. **FOOD: Grapefruit products** may alter absorption. **LAB VALUES:** None significant.

## AVAILABILITY (Rx)

**Capsules:** 20 mg, 30 mg. **Infusion, Ready to Use:** 20 mg/200 ml, 40 mg/200 ml. **Injection Solution (Cardene IV):** 2.5 mg/ml (10-ml vial).

 **Capsules (Sustained-Release [Cardene SR]):** 30 mg, 60 mg.

## ADMINISTRATION/HANDLING
🝪 IV

**Reconstitution** • Dilute 25-mg vial with 240 ml $D_5W$, 0.45% NaCl, or 0.9% NaCl to provide concentration of 0.1 mg/ml.
**Rate of Administration** • Give by slow IV infusion. • Change IV site q12h if administered peripherally.

N

**Storage** • Store at room temperature. • Diluted IV solution is stable for 24 hrs at room temperature.

**PO**
• Give without regard to food. • Do not break, crush, or open capsules. Give whole.

### 🔳 IV INCOMPATIBILITIES

Ampicillin (Principen), ampicillin/sulbactam (Unasyn), cefepime (Maxipime), ceftazidime (Fortaz), furosemide (Lasix), heparin, sodium bicarbonate.

### 🔳 IV COMPATIBILITIES

Diltiazem (Cardizem), dobutamine (Dobutrex), dopamine (Intropin), epinephrine, hydromorphone (Dilaudid), labetalol (Trandate), lorazepam (Ativan), midazolam (Versed), milrinone (Primacor), morphine, nitroglycerin, norepinephrine (Levophed), potassium chloride.

### INDICATIONS/ROUTES/DOSAGE

**Chronic Stable Angina**
**PO: ADULTS, ELDERLY:** Initially, 20 mg 3 times/day. Range: 20–40 mg 3 times/day (allow 3 days between dosage increases).

**Hypertension**
**PO: ADULTS, ELDERLY:** *(Immediate-Release):* Initially, 20 mg 3 times/day. Range: 20–40 mg 3 times/day (allow 3 days between dosage increases).
**PO** *(Extended-Release):* **ADULTS, ELDERLY:** Initially, 30 mg twice daily. Range: 30–60 mg twice daily.

**Acute Hypertension**
**IV: ADULTS, ELDERLY (GRADUAL B/P DECREASE):** Initially, 5 mg/hr. May increase by 2.5 mg/hr q5–15min. **Maximum:** 15 mg/hr. After B/P goal is achieved, decrease rate to 3 mg/hr.

**Dosage in Renal Impairment**
**ADULTS, ELDERLY: (PO):** Initially, give 20 mg q8h (30 mg twice daily [sustained-release capsules]), then titrate. **(IV):** No dose adjustment.

**Dosage in Hepatic Impairment**
**ADULTS, ELDERLY: (PO):** Initially, give 20 mg twice daily, then titrate. **(IV):** No dose adjustment.

### SIDE EFFECTS

**Frequent (10%–7%):** Headache, facial flushing, peripheral edema, light-headedness, dizziness. **Occasional (6%–3%):** Asthenia, palpitations, angina, tachycardia. **Rare (Less Than 2%):** Nausea, abdominal cramps, dyspepsia, dry mouth, rash.

### ADVERSE EFFECTS/ TOXIC REACTIONS

Overdose produces confusion, slurred speech, drowsiness, marked hypotension, bradycardia.

### NURSING CONSIDERATIONS

**BASELINE ASSESSMENT**
Concurrent therapy with sublingual nitroglycerin may be used for relief of anginal pain. Record onset, type (sharp, dull, squeezing), radiation, location, intensity, duration of anginal pain, precipitating factors (exertion, emotional stress).

**INTERVENTION/EVALUATION**
Monitor B/P during and following IV infusion. Assess for peripheral edema. Assess skin for facial flushing, dermatitis, rash. Question for asthenia, headache. Monitor LFT results. Assess EKG, pulse for tachycardia.

**PATIENT/FAMILY TEACHING**
• May take without regard to food. • Sustained-release capsule taken whole; do not break, chew, crush, or open. • Avoid alcohol, grapefruit products, limit caffeine. • Report if anginal pain not relieved or palpitations, shortness of breath, swelling, dizziness, constipation, nausea, hypotension occur. • Avoid tasks requiring motor skills, alertness until response to drug is established.

# nicotine

nik-o-teen
(Habitrol ✦, NicoDerm ✦, NicoDerm CQ, Nicorette, Nicorette Plus ✦, Nicotrol ✦, Nicotrol Inhaler, Nicotrol NS, Thrive)
**Do not confuse NicoDerm with Nitroderm.**

## ◆CLASSIFICATION

**PHARMACOTHERAPEUTIC:** Cholinergic-receptor agonist. **CLINICAL:** Smoking deterrent.

## USES

Treatment to aid smoking cessation for relief of nicotine withdrawal symptoms. **OFF-LABEL: Transdermal:** Management of ulcerative colitis.

## PRECAUTIONS

**Contraindications:** Hypersensitivity to nicotine. **Cautions:** Smoking post-MI period, severe or worsening angina, active temporomandibular joint disease (gum), pregnancy, hyperthyroidism, pheochromocytoma, insulin-dependent diabetes mellitus, severe renal impairment, eczematous dermatitis, oropharyngeal inflammation, esophagitis, peptic ulcer (delays healing in peptic ulcer disease), coronary artery disease, recent MI, serious cardiac arrhythmias, vasospastic disease, angina, hypertension, hepatic impairment, use of oral inhaler/nasal spray with bronchospastic disease.

## ACTION

Binds to acetylcholine receptors, producing both stimulating, depressant effects on peripheral, central nervous systems. **Therapeutic Effect:** Provides source of nicotine during nicotine withdrawal, reduces withdrawal symptoms.

## PHARMACOKINETICS

Absorbed slowly after transdermal administration. Protein binding: 5%. Metabolized in liver. Excreted primarily in urine. **Half-life:** 4 hrs.

## ⧖ LIFESPAN CONSIDERATIONS

**Pregnancy/Lactation:** Distributed in breast milk. Use of cigarettes, nicotine gum associated with decrease in fetal breathing movements. **Children:** Not recommended in this pt population. **Elderly:** Age-related decrease in cardiac function may require dosage adjustment.

## INTERACTIONS

**DRUG:** Smoking cessation, decreased dosage of nicotine may alter effects of **tricyclic antidepressants (e.g., amitriptyline, doxepin), theophylline. HERBAL:** None significant. **FOOD:** None known. **LAB VALUES:** None significant.

## AVAILABILITY (OTC)

**Chewing Gum (Nicorette, Thrive):** 2 mg, 4 mg. **Inhalation (Nicotrol Inhaler):** 10 mg cartridge. **Lozenges (Commit):** 2 mg, 4 mg. **Nasal Spray (Nicotrol NS):** 0.5 mg/spray. **Transdermal Patch (NicoDerm CQ):** 7 mg/24 hrs, 14 mg/24 hrs, 21 mg/24 hrs.

N

## ADMINISTRATION/HANDLING

### Gum

• Do not swallow. • Chew 1 piece when urge to smoke present. • Chew slowly and intermittently for 30 min. • Chew until distinctive nicotine taste (peppery) or slight tingling in mouth perceived, then stop; when tingling almost gone (about 1 min) repeat chewing procedure (this allows constant slow buccal absorption). • Too-rapid chewing may cause excessive release of nicotine, resulting in adverse effects similar to oversmoking (e.g., nausea, throat irritation).

### Inhaler

• Insert cartridge into mouthpiece. • Puff on nicotine cartridge mouthpiece for 20 min.

### Lozenge

• Do not chew or swallow. • Allow to dissolve slowly (20–30 min).

**Transdermal**
• Apply promptly upon removal from protective pouch (prevents evaporation, loss of nicotine). • Use only intact pouch. Do not cut patch. • Apply only once daily to hairless, clean, dry skin on upper body, outer arm. • Replace daily; rotate sites; do not use same site within 7 days; do not use same patch longer than 24 hrs. • Wash hands with water alone after applying patch (soap may increase nicotine absorption). • Discard used patch by folding patch in half (sticky side together), placing in pouch of new patch, and throwing away in such a way as to prevent child or pet accessibility. • Patch may contain conducting metal; remove prior to MRI.

## INDICATIONS/ROUTES/DOSAGE

**Smoking Cessation Aid to Relieve Nicotine Withdrawal Symptoms**
**PO:** *(Chewing Gum):* **ADULTS, ELDERLY:** 2 mg. Use 4 mg in pts who smoke first cigarette within 30 min of waking. Chew 1 piece of gum when urge to smoke, up to 24/day. Use following schedule: wks 1–6: q1–2h (at least 9 pieces/day); wks 7–9: q2–4h; wks 10–12: q4–8h.
**PO:** *(Lozenge):*
◄**ALERT**► For pts who smoke the first cigarette within 30 min of waking, administer the 4-mg lozenge; otherwise, administer the 2-mg lozenge.
**ADULTS, ELDERLY:** One 4-mg or 2-mg lozenge q1–2h for the first 6 wks (use at least 9 lozenges/day first 6 wks); 1 lozenge q2–4h for wks 7–9; and 1 lozenge q4–8h for wks 10–12. **Maximum:** 1 lozenge at a time, 5 lozenges/6 hrs, 20 lozenges/day.
**Transdermal:** ◄**ALERT**► Apply 1 new patch q24h. **ADULTS, ELDERLY WHO SMOKE 10 CIGARETTES OR MORE PER DAY:** Follow the guidelines below. **Step 1:** 21 mg/day for 6 wks. **Step 2:** 14 mg/day for 2 wks. **Step 3:** 7 mg/day for 2 wks. **ADULTS, ELDERLY WHO SMOKE LESS THAN 10 CIGARETTES PER DAY:** Follow the guidelines below. **Step 1:** 14 mg/day for 6 wks. **Step 2:** 7 mg/day for 2 wks.

**Nasal:** **ADULTS, ELDERLY:** Each dose (2 sprays, 1 spray in each nostril) = 1 mg nicotine. Initially, 1–2 doses/hr. **Maximum:** 5 doses/hr (10 sprays), 40 doses/day (80 sprays). For best results, take at least 8 doses/day (16 sprays).
**Inhaler** *(Nicotrol):* **ADULTS, ELDERLY:** Puff on nicotine cartridge mouthpiece for about 20 min as needed. **Maximum:** 16 cartridges/day.

**Dosage in Renal/Hepatic Impairment**
No dose adjustment.

## SIDE EFFECTS

**Frequent: All forms:** Hiccups, nausea. **Gum:** Mouth/throat soreness. **Transdermal:** Erythema, pruritus, burning at application site. **Occasional: All forms:** Eructation, GI upset, dry mouth, insomnia, diaphoresis, irritability. **Gum:** Hoarseness. **Inhaler:** Mouth/throat irritation, cough. **Rare: All forms:** Dizziness, myalgia, arthralgia.

## ADVERSE EFFECTS/ TOXIC REACTIONS

Overdose produces palpitations, tachyarrhythmias, seizures, depression, confusion, diaphoresis, hypotension, rapid/weak pulse, dyspnea. Lethal dose for adults is 40–60 mg. Death results from respiratory paralysis.

## NURSING CONSIDERATIONS

### BASELINE ASSESSMENT

Screen, evaluate those with coronary heart disease (history of MI, angina pectoris), serious cardiac arrhythmias, Buerger's disease, Prinzmetal's variant angina.

### INTERVENTION/EVALUATION

Monitor smoking habits, B/P, pulse, sleep pattern, skin for erythema, pruritus, burning at application site if transdermal system used.

### PATIENT/FAMILY TEACHING

• Follow guidelines for proper application of transdermal system. • Chew

**N**

gum slowly to avoid jaw ache, maximize benefit. • Report persistent rash, pruritus that occurs with patch. • Do not smoke while wearing patch.

# *NIFEdipine

nye-**fed**-i-peen
(Adalat CC, Adalat XL ✦,
Afeditab CR, Apo-Nifed ✦, Nifediac CC, Nifedical XL, Procardia, Procardia XL)
**Do not confuse nifedipine with nicardipine or nimodipine, or Procardia XL with Cartia XT.**

## ◆CLASSIFICATION

**PHARMACOTHERAPEUTIC:** Calcium channel blocker. **CLINICAL:** Antianginal, antihypertensive.

## USES

**Immediate-/extended-release:** Treatment of angina due to coronary artery spasm (Prinzmetal's variant angina), chronic stable angina (effort-associated angina). **Extended-release:** Treatment of hypertension. **OFF-LABEL:** Treatment of Raynaud's phenomenon, pulmonary hypertension, preterm labor, prevention/ treatment of high-altitude pulmonary edema.

## PRECAUTIONS

**Contraindications:** Hypersensitivity to nifedipine. Cardiogenic shock, concomitant administration with strong CYP3A4 inducers (e.g., rifampin), acute MI. **Cautions:** Renal/hepatic impairment, obstructive coronary disease, HF, severe aortic stenosis, edema, severe left ventricular dysfunction, hypertrophic cardiomyopathy, before major surgery, concurrent use with beta blockers or digoxin, CYP3A4 inhibitors/inducers.

## ACTION

Inhibits calcium ion movement across cell membranes, depressing contraction of cardiac, vascular smooth muscle. **Therapeutic Effect:** Increases heart rate, myocardial oxygen delivery, cardiac output. Decreases systemic vascular resistance, B/P.

## PHARMACOKINETICS

Rapidly, completely absorbed from GI tract. Protein binding: 92%–98%. Metabolized in liver. Primarily excreted in urine. Not removed by hemodialysis. **Half-life:** 2–5 hrs.

## ⧗ LIFESPAN CONSIDERATIONS

**Pregnancy/Lactation:** Insignificant amount distributed in breast milk. **Children:** Safety and efficacy not established. **Elderly:** Age-related renal impairment may require dosage adjustment.

## INTERACTIONS

**DRUG: Strong CYP3A4 inducers (e.g., rifampin, phenobarbital, phenytoin, carbamazepine)** may decrease concentration/effects. **CYP3A4 inhibitors (e.g., clarithromycin, ketoconazole)** may increase concentration. **Beta blockers (e.g., carvedilol, metoprolol)** may have additive effect. May increase **digoxin** concentration, risk of toxicity. **Hypokalemia-producing agents (e.g., furosemide, other diuretics)** may increase risk of arrhythmias. **HERBAL: Ephedra, garlic, ginseng, yohimbe** may increase hypertension. **Licorice** may cause retention of sodium, water; may increase loss of potassium. **St. John's wort** decreases concentration/effects. **FOOD: Grapefruit products** may increase risk for flushing, headache, tachycardia, hypotension. **LAB VALUES:** May cause positive ANA, direct Coombs' test.

## AVAILABILITY (Rx)

**Capsules:** 10 mg, 20 mg.

🔪 **Tablets, Extended-Release: (Adalat CC, Afeditab CR, Procardia XL):** 30 mg, 60 mg, 90 mg. **(Nifediac CC, Nifedical XL):** 30 mg, 60 mg.

N

## ADMINISTRATION/HANDLING

### PO
• Do not break, crush, dissolve, or divide extended-release tablets. • Give without regard to meals (Adalat CC, Nifediac CC should be taken on an empty stomach). • Grapefruit products may alter absorption; avoid use.

### Sublingual
• Capsules must be punctured, chewed, and/or squeezed to express liquid into mouth.

## INDICATIONS/ROUTES/DOSAGE

**Prinzmetal's Variant Angina, Chronic Stable (Effort-Associated) Angina**
**PO (Immediate-Release):** ADULTS, ELDERLY: Initially, 10 mg 3 times/day. Increase at 7- to 14-day intervals. **Maintenance:** 10 mg 3 times/day up to 30 mg 4 times/day. **Maximum:** 180 mg/day.
**PO (Extended-Release):** ADULTS, ELDERLY: Initially, 30–60 mg/day. May increase at 7- to 14-day intervals. **Maximum:** 120 mg/day.

**Hypertension**
**PO (Extended-Release):** ADULTS, ELDERLY: Initially, 30–60 mg/day. May increase at 7- to 14-day intervals. **Maximum:** 90–120 mg/day. **CHILDREN 1–17 YRS:** Initially, 0.2–0.5 mg/kg/day. **Maximum:** 3 mg/kg/day or 120 mg/day.

**Dosage in Renal/Hepatic Impairment**
No dose adjustment.

## SIDE EFFECTS

**Frequent (30%–11%):** Peripheral edema, headache, flushed skin, dizziness. **Occasional (12%–6%):** Nausea, shakiness, muscle cramps/pain, drowsiness, palpitations, nasal congestion, cough, dyspnea, wheezing. **Rare (5%–3%):** Hypotension, rash, pruritus, urticaria, constipation, abdominal discomfort, flatulence, sexual dysfunction.

## ADVERSE EFFECTS/ TOXIC REACTIONS

May precipitate HF, MI in pts with cardiac disease, peripheral ischemia. Overdose produces nausea, drowsiness, confusion, slurred speech. **Antidote:** Glucagon (see Appendix K for dosage).

## NURSING CONSIDERATIONS

### BASELINE ASSESSMENT
Concurrent therapy with sublingual nitroglycerin may be used for relief of anginal pain. Record onset, type (sharp, dull, squeezing), radiation, location, intensity, duration of anginal pain; precipitating factors (exertion, emotional stress). Check B/P for hypotension immediately before giving medication.

### INTERVENTION/EVALUATION
Assist with ambulation if light-headedness, dizziness occurs. Assess for peripheral edema. Assess skin for flushing. Monitor LFT. Observe for signs/symptoms of HF.

### PATIENT/FAMILY TEACHING
• Go from lying to standing slowly. • Report palpitations, shortness of breath, pronounced dizziness, nausea, exacerbations of angina. • Avoid alcohol; concomitant grapefruit product use.

## *nilotinib*

nye-**loe**-ti-nib
(Tasigna)
■ **BLACK BOX ALERT** ■ Prolongs QT interval; sudden deaths reported. Do not use in pts with hypokalemia, hypomagnesemia, prolonged QT syndrome.
**Do not confuse nilotinib with dasatinib, erlotinib, imatinib, nilutamide, sorafenib, sunitinib.**

## ◆CLASSIFICATION

**PHARMACOTHERAPEUTIC:** Protein-tyrosine kinase inhibitor. **CLINICAL:** Antineoplastic.

---

## SIDE EFFECTS

**Frequent (33%–21%):** Rash, nausea, headache, pruritus, fatigue, diarrhea, constipation, vomiting. **Occasional (18%–10%):** Arthralgia, cough, pharyngitis, asthenia, fever, myalgia, abdominal pain, peripheral edema, weight gain, bone pain, muscle spasm, back pain. **Rare (9%–1%):** Anorexia, insomnia, dizziness, paresthesia, vertigo, palpitations, flushing, hypertension, flatulence, alopecia, night sweats.

## ADVERSE EFFECTS/ TOXIC REACTIONS

Prolongation of QT interval producing ventricular tachycardia (torsades de pointes) may result in seizure, sudden death. Neutropenia, thrombocytopenia, anemia are expected response to drug. Respiratory toxicity manifested as dyspnea, pneumonia.

## NURSING CONSIDERATIONS

### BASELINE ASSESSMENT

Obtain CBC every 2 wks for the first 2 mos and then monthly thereafter. Hypokalemia or hypomagnesemia must be corrected prior to initiating therapy. Monitor LFT before treatment begins and monthly thereafter. Obtain baseline weight.

### INTERVENTION/EVALUATION

Monitor serum electrolytes periodically during therapy, particularly potassium, magnesium, sodium, lipase. Monitor for unexpected weight gain. Offer antiemetics to control nausea, vomiting. Monitor daily pattern of bowel frequency, stool consistency. Monitor CBC for evidence of neutropenia, thrombocytopenia; assess LFT for hepatotoxicity. Monitor closely for QT-interval prolongation.

### PATIENT/FAMILY TEACHING

• Avoid crowds, those with known infection. • Avoid contact with anyone who recently received live virus vaccine; do not receive vaccinations. • Do not ingest food less than 2 hours before and less than 1 hr after dose is taken. • Avoid grapefruit products.

# *niMODipine

nye-**mode**-i-peen
(Nimotop ✦, Nymalize)

■ **BLACK BOX ALERT** ■ Severe cardiovascular events, including fatalities, have resulted when capsule contents have been withdrawn by syringe and administered by IV injection rather than nasogastric tube.

**Do not confuse nimodipine with nicardipine or nifedipine.**

## ◆CLASSIFICATION

**PHARMACOTHERAPEUTIC:** Calcium channel blocker. **CLINICAL:** Cerebral vasospasm agent.

## USES

Improvement of neurologic deficits due to cerebral vasospasm following subarachnoid hemorrhage from ruptured intracranial aneurysms.

## PRECAUTIONS

**Contraindications:** Hypersensitivity to nimodipine. Concurrent use with strong CYP3A4 inhibitors. **Cautions:** Pts with cirrhosis, baseline hypotension.

## ⌛ LIFESPAN CONSIDERATIONS

**Pregnancy/Lactation:** Unknown if drug crosses placenta or is distributed in breast milk. **Children:** Safety and efficacy not established. **Elderly:** Age-related renal impairment may require dosage adjustment. May experience greater hypotensive response, constipation.

## ACTION

Inhibits movement of calcium ions across vascular smooth muscle cell membranes. Exerts greatest effect on cerebral arteries. **Therapeutic Effect:** Produces favorable effect on severity of neurologic deficits due to cerebral vasospasm. May prevent cerebral vasospasm.

## PHARMACOKINETICS

Rapidly absorbed from GI tract. Protein binding: 95%. Metabolized in liver. Excreted in bile (80%), urine (20%). Not removed by hemodialysis. **Half-life:** 1–2 hrs.

## INTERACTIONS

**DRUG: Beta blockers (e.g., metoprolol)** may have additive effect, increase depression of cardiac SA/AV conduction. May increase **digoxin** concentration. **Agents inducing hypokalemia (e.g., furosemide, HCTZ, high-dose or IV insulin)** may increase risk of arrhythmias. **CYP3A4 inhibitors (e.g., erythromycin, ketoconazole, protease inhibitors)** may inhibit metabolism. **CYP3A4 inducers (e.g., rifabutin, rifampin)** may increase metabolism. **HERBAL: Ephedra, garlic, ginseng, yohimbe** may increase hypertension. **Licorice** may cause retention of sodium, water; may increase loss of potassium. **St. John's wort** may decrease level/effects. **FOOD: Grapefruit products** may increase concentration, risk of toxicity. **LAB VALUES:** None significant.

## AVAILABILITY (Rx)

**Solution, Oral (Nymalize):** 60 mg/20 ml.

▼ **Capsules (Nimotop):** 30 mg.

## ADMINISTRATION/HANDLING

**PO**

• Administer 1 hr before or 2 hrs after meals. • If pt unable to swallow, place hole in both ends of capsule with 18-gauge needle to extract contents into syringe. Empty into NG tube; flush tube with 30 ml water.

## INDICATIONS/ROUTES/DOSAGE

**Subarachnoid Hemorrhage**
**PO: ADULTS, ELDERLY:** 60 mg q4h for 21 days. Begin within 96 hrs of subarachnoid hemorrhage.

**Dosage in Renal Impairment**
No dose adjustment.

**Dosage in Hepatic Impairment**
**PO: ADULTS, ELDERLY:** Reduce dose to 30 mg q4h in pts with cirrhosis.

## SIDE EFFECTS

**Occasional (6%–2%):** Hypotension, peripheral edema, diarrhea, headache. **Rare (Less Than 2%):** Allergic reaction (rash, urticaria), tachycardia, flushing of skin.

## ADVERSE EFFECTS/TOXIC REACTIONS

Overdose produces nausea, weakness, dizziness, drowsiness, confusion, slurred speech.

## NURSING CONSIDERATIONS

### BASELINE ASSESSMENT

Assess LOC, neurologic response, initially and throughout therapy. Monitor baseline LFT. Assess B/P, apical pulse immediately before drug administration (if pulse is 60/min or less or systolic B/P is less than 90 mm Hg, withhold medication, contact physician).

**N**

### INTERVENTION/EVALUATION

Monitor CNS response, heart rate, B/P for evidence of hypotension, signs/symptoms of HF. Monitor transcranial doppler results for evidence of vasospasm.

### PATIENT/FAMILY TEACHING

• Do not chew, crush, dissolve, or divide capsules. • Report palpitations, shortness of breath, swelling, constipation, nausea, dizziness. Immediately report headache, blurry vision, confusion (may indicate vasospasm).

## nitazoxanide

nye-ta-**zox**-a-nide
(Alinia)

◆**CLASSIFICATION**

**PHARMACOTHERAPEUTIC:** Antiparasitic. **CLINICAL:** Antiprotozoal agent.

## USES

Treatment of diarrhea caused by *Cryptosporidium parvum*, *Giardia lamblia* in children 12 mos and older, adults. **OFF-LABEL:** *C. difficile*-associated diarrhea.

## PRECAUTIONS

**Contraindications:** Hypersensitivity to nitazoxanide. **Cautions:** Caution with use of suspension in diabetic pts (due to sucrose content), hepatic/biliary disease, renal impairment.

## ACTION

Interferes with body's reaction to pyruvate ferredoxin oxidoreductase, an enzyme essential for anaerobic energy metabolism. **Therapeutic Effect:** Produces antiprotozoal activity, reducing/terminating diarrheal episodes.

## PHARMACOKINETICS

Rapidly hydrolyzed to active metabolite. Protein binding: 99%. Excreted in urine, bile, feces. **Half-life:** 2–4 hrs.

## ⌛ LIFESPAN CONSIDERATIONS

**Pregnancy/Lactation:** Unknown if distributed in breast milk. **Children:** Safety and efficacy not established in pts younger than 1 yr (suspension) and younger than 12 yrs (tablet). **Elderly:** Not for use in this age group.

## INTERACTIONS

**DRUG:** None significant. **HERBAL:** None significant. **FOOD:** None known. **LAB VALUES:** May increase serum creatinine, ALT.

## AVAILABILITY (Rx)

**Powder for Oral Suspension:** 100 mg/5 ml. **Tablets:** 500 mg.

## ADMINISTRATION/HANDLING

**PO (Oral Suspension)**
• Store unreconstituted powder at room temperature. • Reconstitute oral suspension with 48 ml water to provide concentration of 100 mg/5 ml. • Shake vigorously to suspend powder. • Reconstituted solution is stable for 7 days at room temperature. • Give with food.

**PO (Tablets)**
• Give with food.

## INDICATIONS/ROUTES/DOSAGE

**Diarrhea Caused by *C. Parvum*, *G. Lamblia***
**PO: ADULTS, ELDERLY, CHILDREN 12 YRS AND OLDER:** 500 mg q12h for 3 days. **CHILDREN 4–11 YRS:** 200 mg q12h for 3 days. **CHILDREN 1–3 YRS:** 100 mg q12h for 3 days.

**Dosage in Renal/Hepatic Impairment**
Use caution.

## SIDE EFFECTS

**Occasional (8%):** Abdominal pain. **Rare (2%–1%):** Diarrhea, vomiting, headache.

## ADVERSE EFFECTS/TOXIC REACTIONS

None known.

## NURSING CONSIDERATIONS

**BASELINE ASSESSMENT**
Establish baseline B/P, weight, serum glucose, electrolytes. Assess for dehydration.

**INTERVENTION/EVALUATION**
Evaluate serum glucose in diabetics, electrolytes (therapy generally reduces abnormalities). Weigh pt daily. Encourage adequate fluid intake. Assess bowel sounds for peristalsis. Monitor daily pattern of bowel activity, stool consistency.

**PATIENT/FAMILY TEACHING**
• Parents of children with diabetes should be aware that the oral suspension contains 1.48 g of sucrose per 5 ml. • Therapy should provide significant improvement of diarrhea.

## nitrofurantoin

**nye**-troe-fue-**ran**-toyn
(Apo-Nitrofurantoin ✦, Furadantin, Macrobid, Macrodantin, Novo-Furantoin ✦)

Do not confuse Macrobid with MicroK or Nitro-Bid, or nitrofurantoin with Neurontin or nitroglycerin.

## ◆ CLASSIFICATION

**PHARMACOTHERAPEUTIC:** Antibacterial. **CLINICAL:** Antibiotic, UTI prophylaxis.

## USES

Prevention/treatment of UTI caused by susceptible gram-negative, gram-positive organisms, including *E. coli, S. aureus, Enterococcus, Klebsiella, Enterobacter.*

## PRECAUTIONS

**Contraindications:** Hypersensitivity to nitrofurantoin. Anuria, oliguria, renal impairment (CrCl less than 60 ml/min), infants younger than 1 mo due to risk of hemolytic anemia. Pregnancy at term, during labor, or delivery, or when onset of labor is imminent. Pts with history of cholestatic jaundice or hepatic impairment with previous nitrofurantoin therapy **Cautions:** Renal impairment, diabetes mellitus, electrolyte imbalance, anemia, vitamin B deficiency, debilitated (greater risk of peripheral neuropathy), G6PD deficiency (greater risk of hemolytic anemia), elderly, prolonged therapy (may cause pulmonary toxicity).

## ACTION

Inhibits with bacterial enzyme systems, interfering with metabolism and cell wall synthesis. **Therapeutic Effect:** Bacteriostatic (bactericidal at high concentrations).

## PHARMACOKINETICS

Microcrystalline form rapidly, completely absorbed; macrocrystalline form more slowly absorbed. Food increases absorption. Protein binding: 60%. Primarily concentrated in urine, kidneys. Metabolized in most body tissues. Primarily excreted in urine. Removed by hemodialysis. **Half-life:** 20–60 min.

## ⧗ LIFESPAN CONSIDERATIONS

**Pregnancy/Lactation:** Readily crosses placenta. Distributed in breast milk. Contraindicated at term and during lactation when infant suspected of having G6PD deficiency. **Children:** No age-related precautions noted in pts older than 1 mo. **Elderly:** More likely to develop acute pneumonitis, peripheral neuropathy. Age-related renal impairment may require dosage adjustment.

## INTERACTIONS

**DRUG: Antacids containing magnesium trisilicate** may decrease absorption. **Probenecid** may increase concentration, risk of toxicity. **HERBAL:** None significant. **FOOD:** None known. **LAB VALUES:** May increase serum ALT, AST, phosphorus. May decrease Hgb.

## AVAILABILITY (Rx)

**Capsules (Macrocrystalline [Macrobid]):** 100 mg. **Capsules (Macrocrystalline [Macrodantin]):** 25 mg, 50 mg, 100 mg. **Oral Suspension (Microcrystalline [Furadantin]):** 25 mg/5 ml.

## ADMINISTRATION/HANDLING

**PO**
• Give with food, milk to enhance absorption, reduce GI upset. • May mix suspension with water, milk, fruit juice; shake well.

## INDICATIONS/ROUTES/DOSAGE

**UTI**
**PO:** *(Furadantin, Macrodantin):* **ADULTS, ELDERLY:** 50–100 mg q6h for 7 days or at least 3 days after obtaining sterile urine. **Maximum:** 400 mg/day. **CHILDREN, ADOLESCENTS:** 5–7 mg/kg/day in divided doses q6h for 7 days or at least 3 days after obtaining sterile urine. **Maximum:** 400 mg/day.
**PO:** *(Macrobid):* **ADULTS, ELDERLY, ADOLESCENTS:** 100 mg twice daily for 7 days.

**Long-Term Prevention of UTI**
**PO: ADULTS, ELDERLY:** 50–100 mg at bedtime. **CHILDREN OLDER THAN 1 MONTH:** 1–2 mg/kg/day in 2 divided doses. **Maximum:** 100 mg/day.

N

**Dosage in Renal Impairment**
Contraindicated in pts with CrCl less than 60 ml/min.

**Dosage in Hepatic Impairment**
No dose adjustment.

## SIDE EFFECTS

**Frequent:** Anorexia, nausea, vomiting, dark urine. **Occasional:** Abdominal pain, diarrhea, rash, pruritus, urticaria, hypertension, headache, dizziness, drowsiness. **Rare:** Photosensitivity, transient alopecia, asthmatic exacerbation in those with history of asthma.

## ADVERSE EFFECTS/ TOXIC REACTIONS

Superinfection, hepatotoxicity, peripheral neuropathy (may be irreversible), Stevens-Johnson syndrome, permanent pulmonary impairment, anaphylaxis occur rarely.

## NURSING CONSIDERATIONS

**BASELINE ASSESSMENT**
Question for history of asthma. Evaluate baseline renal function, LFT.

**INTERVENTION/EVALUATION**
Monitor CBC, BMP, LFT; I&O. Monitor daily pattern of bowel activity, stool consistency. Assess skin for rash, urticaria. Be alert for numbness/tingling, esp. of lower extremities (may signal onset of peripheral neuropathy). Observe for signs of hepatotoxicity (fever, rash, arthralgia, hepatomegaly). Monitor respiratory status, esp. in pts with asthma.

**PATIENT/ FAMILY TEACHING**
• Urine may become dark yellow/ brown. • Take with food, milk for best results, reduce GI upset. • Complete full course of therapy. • Avoid sun, ultraviolet light; use sunscreen, wear protective clothing. • Report cough, fever, chest pain, difficulty breathing, numbness/tingling of fingers, toes. • Rare occurrence of alopecia is transient.

# nitroglycerin

nye-troe-**glis**-er-in
(Minitran, Nitro-Bid, Nitro-Dur, Nitrolingual, NitroMist, Nitrostat, Nitro-Time, Rectiv, Trinipatch ❖)
**Do not confuse Nitro-Bid with Macrobid or Nicobid, Nitro-Dur with Nicoderm, nitroglycerin with nitrofurantoin or nitroprusside, or Nitrostat with Nilstat or Nystatin.**

## ◆CLASSIFICATION

**PHARMACOTHERAPEUTIC:** Nitrate.
**CLINICAL:** Antianginal, antihypertensive, coronary vasodilator.

## USES

Treatment/prevention of angina pectoris. Extended-release, topical forms used for prophylaxis, long-term angina management. IV form used in treatment of HF, acute MI, perioperative hypertension, induction of intraoperative hypotension. **OFF-LABEL:** Short-term management of pulmonary hypertension, esophageal spastic disorders, uterine relaxation, treatment of sympathomimetic vasopressor extravasation.

## PRECAUTIONS

**Contraindications:** Hypersensitivity to nitroglycerin. Allergy to adhesives (transdermal); increased ICP; severe anemia; concurrent use of sildenafil, tadalafil, vardenafil (PDE5 inhibitors). **(Additional) IV:** Restrictive cardiomyopathy, pericardial tamponade, constrictive pericarditis. **Sublingual, Rectal:** Increased intracranial pressure, severe anemia. **Cautions:** Blood volume depletion, severe hypotension (systolic B/P less than 90 mm Hg), bradycardia (less than 50 beats/min), inferior wall MI and suspected right ventricular involvement.

## ACTION

Dilates coronary arteries, improves collateral blood flow to ischemic areas within myocardium. IV form produces peripheral vasodilation. **Therapeutic Effect:** Decreases myocardial oxygen demand. Reduces left ventricular preload, afterload.

## PHARMACOKINETICS

| Route | Onset | Peak | Duration |
|---|---|---|---|
| Sublingual | 1–3 min | 4–8 min | 30–60 min |
| Translingual spray | 2 min | 4–10 min | 30–60 min |
| Buccal tablet | 2–5 min | 4–10 min | 2 hrs |
| PO (extended-release) | 20–45 min | 45–120 min | 4–8 hrs |
| Topical | 15–60 min | 30–120 min | 2–12 hrs |
| Transdermal patch | 40–60 min | 60–180 min | 18–24 hrs |
| IV | 1–2 min | Immediate | 3–5 min |

Well absorbed after PO, sublingual, topical administration. Metabolized in liver, by enzymes in bloodstream. Protein binding: 60%. Excreted in urine. Not removed by hemodialysis. **Half-life:** 1–4 min.

## ⧖ LIFESPAN CONSIDERATIONS

**Pregnancy/Lactation:** Unknown if drug crosses placenta or is distributed in breast milk. **Children:** Safety and efficacy not established. **Elderly:** More susceptible to hypotensive effects. Age-related renal impairment may require dosage adjustment.

## INTERACTIONS

**DRUG:** **Alcohol, other antihypertensives (e.g., amlodipine, lisinopril, valsartan), vasodilators** may increase risk of orthostatic hypotension. Concurrent use of **sildenafil, tadalafil, vardenafil** (PDE5 inhibitors) produces significant hypotension. **HERBAL:** **Ephedra, ginger, ginseng, licorice** may increase hypertension. **Black cohosh, goldenseal, hawthorne** may cause hypotension. **FOOD:** None known. **LAB VALUES:** May increase serum methemoglobin, urine catecholamine concentrations.

## AVAILABILITY (Rx)

**Infusion, Pre-Mix:** 25 mg/250 ml, 50 mg/500 ml, 50 mg/250 ml, 100 mg/250 ml. **Injection, Solution:** 5 mg/ml. **Ointment (Nitro-Bid):** 2%. **Translingual Spray (Nitrolingual):** 0.4 mg/spray. **Transdermal Patch (Minitran, Nitro-Dur):** 0.1 mg/hr, 0.2 mg/hr, 0.4 mg/hr, 0.6 mg/hr.

🍃 **Capsules, Extended-Release (Nitro-Time):** 2.5 mg, 6.5 mg, 9 mg. 🍃 **Tablets, Sublingual (Nitrostat):** 0.4 mg.

## ADMINISTRATION/HANDLING

◀ALERT▶ Cardioverter/defibrillator must not be discharged through paddle electrode overlying nitroglycerin (transdermal, ointment) system (may cause burns to pt or damage to paddle via arcing).

 **IV**

**Reconstitution** • Available in ready-to-use injectable containers. • Dilute vials in $D_5W$ or 0.9% NaCl. Maximum concentration: 400 mcg/ml. • Use glass bottles.

**Rate of Administration** • Use microdrop or infusion pump.

**Storage** • Store at room temperature. • Reconstituted solutions stable for 48 hrs at room temperature or 7 days if refrigerated.

**PO**

• Do not break, crush, or open extended-release capsules. • Do not shake oral aerosol canister before lingual spraying.

**Sublingual**

• Instruct pt to not swallow. • Dissolve under tongue. • Administer while seated. • Slight burning sensation under tongue may be lessened by placing tablet in buccal pouch. • Keep sublingual tablets in original container.

**Topical**
• Spread thin layer on clean, dry, hairless skin of upper arm or body (not below knee or elbow), using applicator or dose-measuring papers. Do not use fingers; do not rub/massage into skin.

**Transdermal**
• Apply patch on clean, dry, hairless skin of upper arm or body (not below knee or elbow). • May keep patch on when bathing/showering. • Do not cut/trim to adjust dose.

## ▨ IV INCOMPATIBILITIES

Alteplase (Activase), phenytoin (Dilantin).

## ▨ IV COMPATIBILITIES

Amiodarone (Cordarone), dexmedetomidine (Precedex), diltiazem (Cardizem), dobutamine (Dobutrex), dopamine (Intropin), epinephrine, famotidine (Pepcid), fentanyl (Sublimaze), furosemide (Lasix), heparin, hydromorphone (Dilaudid), insulin, labetalol (Trandate), lidocaine, lipids, lorazepam (Ativan), midazolam (Versed), milrinone (Primacor), morphine, nicardipine (Cardene), nitroprusside (Nipride), norepinephrine (Levophed), propofol (Diprivan).

## INDICATIONS/ROUTES/DOSAGE

**Angina, CAD**
**Translingual Spray:** ADULTS, ELDERLY: 1–2 sprays onto or under tongue q3–5min until relief is noted (no more than 3 sprays in 15-min period).
**Sublingual:** ADULTS, ELDERLY: One tablet under tongue. If chest pain has not improved in 5 min, call 911. After the call, may take additional tablet. A third tablet may be taken 5 min after second dose (maximum of 3 tablets).
**PO *(Extended-Release):* ADULTS, ELDERLY:** 2.5–6.5 mg 3–4 times/day. **Maximum:** 26 mg 4 times/day.
**Topical:** ADULTS, ELDERLY: Initially, ½ inch upon waking and ½ inch 6 hr later. May double dose to 1 inch and double again to 2 inches. **Maximum:** 2 doses/day including nitrate-free interval of 10–12 hrs.

**Transdermal Patch:** ADULTS, ELDERLY: Initially, 0.2–0.4 mg/hr. **Maintenance:** 0.4–0.8 mg/hr. Consider patch on for 12–14 hrs, patch off for 10–12 hrs (prevents tolerance).

**HF, Acute MI**
**IV:** ADULTS, ELDERLY: Initially, 5 mcg/min via infusion pump. Increase in 5-mcg/min increments at 3- to 5-min intervals until B/P response is noted or until dosage reaches 20 mcg/min, then increase by 10–20 mcg/min q3–5min. Dosage may be further titrated according to clinical, therapeutic response up to 400 mcg/min.

**Dosage in Renal/Hepatic Impairment**
No dose adjustment.

## SIDE EFFECTS

**Frequent:** Headache (possibly severe; occurs mostly in early therapy, diminishes rapidly in intensity, usually disappears during continued treatment), transient flushing of face/neck, dizziness (esp. if pt is standing immobile or is in a warm environment), weakness, orthostatic hypotension. **Sublingual:** Burning, tingling sensation at oral point of dissolution. **Ointment:** Erythema, pruritus. **Occasional:** GI upset. **Transdermal:** Contact dermatitis.

## ADVERSE EFFECTS/TOXIC REACTIONS

Discontinue drug if blurred vision, dry mouth occurs. Severe orthostatic hypotension may occur, manifested by syncope, pulselessness, cold/clammy skin, diaphoresis. Tolerance may occur with repeated, prolonged therapy; minor tolerance may occur with intermittent use of sublingual tablets. High doses tend to produce severe headache.

## NURSING CONSIDERATIONS

### BASELINE ASSESSMENT

Record onset, type (sharp, dull, squeezing), radiation, location, intensity, duration of anginal pain; precipitating factors (exertion, emotional stress). Assess B/P, apical pulse before administration and periodically following dose. Pt must have continuous EKG monitoring for IV administration. Rule out right-sided MI, if applicable (may precipitate life-threatening hypotension).

### INTERVENTION/EVALUATION

Monitor B/P, heart rate. Assess for facial, neck flushing. Cardioverter/defibrillator must not be discharged through paddle electrode overlying nitroglycerin (transdermal, ointment) system (may cause burns to pt or damage to paddle via electrical arcing). Consider NS boluses for hypotension.

### PATIENT/FAMILY TEACHING

• Go from lying to standing slowly. • Take oral form on empty stomach (however, if headache occurs during therapy, take medication with meals). • Use spray only when lying down. • Dissolve sublingual tablet under tongue; do not swallow. • Take at first sign of angina. • May take additional dose q5min if needed up to a total of 3 doses. • If not relieved within 5 min, contact physician or immediately go to emergency room. • Do not change brands. • Keep container away from heat, moisture. • Do not inhale lingual aerosol but spray onto or under tongue (avoid swallowing after spray is administered). • Expel from mouth any remaining lingual, sublingual, intrabuccal tablet after pain is completely relieved. • Place transmucosal tablets under upper lip or buccal pouch (between cheek and gum); do not chew/swallow tablet. • Avoid alcohol (intensifies hypotensive effect). If alcohol is ingested soon after taking nitroglycerin, possible acute hypotensive episode (marked drop in B/P, vertigo, diaphoresis, pallor) may occur. • Do not use within 48 hrs of sildenafil, tadalafil, vardenafil (PDE$_5$ inhibitors); may cause acute hypotensive episode.

# nitroprusside

nye-troe-**prus**-ide
(Nipride ✦, Nitropress)

■ **BLACK BOX ALERT** ■ Must dilute with D$_5$W. Can cause sharp decrease in B/P; may lead to irreversible ischemia, death. Unless used briefly or at low infusion rate (less than 2 mcg/kg/min), potentially lethal levels of cyanide may result. Do not use maximum dose for longer than 10 min.
**Do not confuse nitroprusside with nitroglycerin or Nitrostat.**

## ◆CLASSIFICATION

**PHARMACOTHERAPEUTIC:** Vasodilator. **CLINICAL:** Antihypertensive, vasodilator, antidote.

## USES

Immediate reduction of B/P in hypertensive crisis. Produces controlled hypotension in surgical procedures to reduce bleeding. Treatment of acute HF. **OFF LABEL:** Management of hypertension during acute ischemic stroke.

## PRECAUTIONS

**Contraindications:** Hypersensitivity to nitroprusside. Treatment of compensatory hypertension (AV shunt, coarctation of aorta), congenital (Leber's) optic atrophy, to produce controlled hypotension during surgery in pts with inadequate cerebral circulation, moribund pts requiring emergency surgery, tobacco amblyopia (dim vision). High-output HF associated with reduced systemic vascular resistance. **Cautions:** Severe hepatic/renal impairment, hypothyroidism, hyponatremia, elderly, increased intracranial pressure.

## ACTION

Direct vasodilating action on arterial, venous smooth muscle. Decreases peripheral vascular resistance, preload, afterload; improves cardiac output. **Therapeutic Effect:** Dilates coronary

N

arteries, decreases oxygen consumption, relieves persistent chest pain.

## PHARMACOKINETICS

| Route | Onset | Peak | Duration |
|-------|-------|------|----------|
| IV | Less than 2 min | Dependent on infusion rate | 1–10 min |

Reacts with Hgb in erythrocytes, producing cyanmethemoglobin, cyanide ions. Primarily excreted in urine. **Half-life:** Less than 10 min.

## ⧗ LIFESPAN CONSIDERATIONS

**Pregnancy/Lactation:** Unknown if drug crosses placenta or is distributed in breast milk. **Children:** Safety and efficacy not established. **Elderly:** More sensitive to hypotensive effect. Age-related renal impairment may require dosage adjustment.

## INTERACTIONS

**DRUG: Antihypertensives (e.g., amlodipine, lisinopril, valsartan)** may increase hypotensive effect. **HERBAL: Yohimbe** may decrease effects. **FOOD:** None known. **LAB VALUES:** None significant.

## AVAILABILITY (Rx)

**Injection Solution:** 25 mg/ml (2-ml vial).

## ADMINISTRATION/HANDLING

 IV

**Reconstitution** • Dilute with 250–1,000 ml D₅W to provide concentration of 200 mcg, 50 mcg/ml, respectively. **Maximum concentration:** 200 mg/250 ml. • Wrap infusion bottle in aluminum foil immediately after mixing.
**Rate of Administration** • Give by IV infusion only, using infusion rate chart provided by manufacturer or protocol. • Administer using IV infusion pump. • Be alert for extravasation (produces severe pain, sloughing).
**Storage** • Protect from light. • Solution should appear very faint brown. • Use

only freshly prepared solution. Once prepared, do not keep or use longer than 24 hrs. • Deterioration evidenced by color change from brown to blue, green, dark red. • Discard unused portion.

## ▨ IV INCOMPATIBILITY

Insulin (regular).

## ▨ IV COMPATIBILITIES

Cisatracurium (Nimbex), dexmedetomidine (Precedex), diltiazem (Cardizem), dobutamine (Dobutrex), dopamine (Intropin), enalapril (Vasotec), heparin, labetalol (Normodyne, Trandate), lidocaine, midazolam (Versed), milrinone (Primacor), nitroglycerin, propofol (Diprivan).

## INDICATIONS/ROUTES/DOSAGE

**Acute Hypertension**
**IV Infusion: ADULTS, ELDERLY, CHILDREN:** Initially, 0.3–0.5 mcg/kg/min. May increase by 0.5 mcg/kg/min to desired hemodynamic effect or appearance of headache, nausea. Usual dose: 3 mcg/kg/min. Doses greater than 4 mcg/kg/min rarely needed. **Maximum:** 10 mcg/kg/min.

**Acute HF**
**IV Infusion: ADULTS, ELDERLY:** Initially, 5–10 mcg/min. Titrate rapidly to achieve desired hemodynamic effect. Range: 5–300 mcg/min.

**Dosage in Renal/Hepatic Impairment**
No dose adjustment. Limit use. Use caution.

## SIDE EFFECTS

**Occasional:** Flushing of skin, pruritus, pain/redness at injection site.

## ADVERSE EFFECTS/ TOXIC REACTIONS

Too-rapid IV infusion rate reduces B/P too quickly. Nausea, vomiting, diaphoresis, apprehension, headache, restlessness, muscle twitching, dizziness, palpitations, retrosternal pain, abdominal pain may occur. Symptoms disappear rapidly if rate of administration is slowed or temporarily discontinued. Overdose produces metabolic acidosis, tolerance to therapeutic effect.

## NURSING CONSIDERATIONS

### BASELINE ASSESSMENT

Check with physician for desired B/P parameters (B/P is normally maintained approximately 30%–40% below pretreatment levels). Medication should be discontinued if therapeutic response is not achieved within 10 min after IV infusion at 10 mcg/kg/min.

### INTERVENTION/EVALUATION

Monitor EKG, B/P continuously. Monitor blood acid-base balance, electrolytes, laboratory results, I&O. Assess for metabolic acidosis (weakness, disorientation, headache, nausea, hyperventilation, vomiting). Assess for therapeutic response to medication. Monitor B/P for potential rebound hypertension after infusion is discontinued.

---

# nivolumab

nye-**vol**-ue-mab
(Opdivo)
**Do not confuse nivolumab with denosumab, adalimumab, or palivizumab.**

## ◆CLASSIFICATION

**PHARMACOTHERAPEUTIC:** Monoclonal antibody. **CLINICAL:** Antineoplastic.

## USES

Treatment of unresectable or metastatic melanoma as a single agent in pts with disease progression following ipilimumab and, if BRAF V600 mutation positive, a BRAF inhibitor; or in combination with ipilimumab in pts with BRAF V600 wild-type melanoma. Treatment of metastatic non–small cell lung cancer with progression on or after platinum-based chemotherapy. Treatment of advanced renal cell cancer in pts receiving prior antiangiogenic therapy. Classical Hodgkin lymphoma (cHL) that relapsed or progressed following autologous hematopoietic stem cell transplant (HSCT) and post-brentuximab. Recurrent or metastatic squamous cell carcinoma of the head and neck.

## PRECAUTIONS

**Contraindications:** Hypersensitivity to nivolumab. **Cautions:** Thyroid/pituitary disease, hepatic/renal impairment, interstitial lung disease, electrolyte imbalance.

## ACTION

Binds PD-1 ligands to PD-1 receptor found on T cells, blocking its interaction with the ligands (PD-L1 and PD-L2). Releases PD-1 pathway–mediated inhibition of immune response (including antitumor immune response). **Therapeutic Effect:** Inhibits T-cell proliferation and cytokine production. Inhibits tumor cell growth and metastasis.

## PHARMACOKINETICS

Information on metabolism and elimination is not available. Steady-state concentration: 12 wks. **Half-life:** 26.7 days.

## ⏳ LIFESPAN CONSIDERATIONS

**Pregnancy/Lactation:** Avoid pregnancy; may cause fetal harm. Unknown if distributed in breast milk. Must either discontinue drug or discontinue breast-feeding. Females of reproductive potential should use effective contraception during treatment and up to 5 mos after discontinuation. **Children:** Safety and efficacy not established. **Elderly:** May have increased risk of endocrine/hepatic/pulmonary/optic/renal injury due to age-related diseases.

## INTERACTIONS

**DRUG:** None known. **HERBAL:** None significant. **FOOD:** None known. **LAB VALUES: Single Therapy:** May increase serum alkaline phosphatase, ALT, AST, potassium. May decrease serum sodium. **Combo Therapy:** May increase serum alkaline phosphatase, ALT, AST, amylase, creatinine, lipase. May decrease RBC, Hct, Hgb, lymphocytes, neutrophils, platelets; serum calcium, sodium, magnesium. May increase or decrease serum calcium, potassium.

## AVAILABILITY (Rx)

**Injection Solution:** 40 mg/4 ml, 100 mg/10 ml single-use vial.

## ADMINISTRATION/HANDLING

 IV

**Preparation** • Visually inspect solution for particulate matter or discoloration. Solution should appear opalescent, colorless to pale yellow. Discard if solution is cloudy or contains particulate matter other than a few translucent to white, proteinaceous particles. • Do not shake vial. • Withdraw required dose volume and dilute in 0.9% NaCl or 5% Dextrose injection. Final concentration will equal 1–10 mg/ml based on volume of diluent. • Mix by gentle inversion. • Do not shake. • Discard partial used or empty vials.
**Rate of Administration** • Infuse over 60 min using sterile, nonpyrogenic, low-protein-binding, 0.2- to 1.2-micron in-line filter. • Flush IV line upon completion.
**Storage** • Refrigerate diluted solution up to 24 hrs or store at room temperature for no more than 4 hrs (includes time of preparation and infusion). • Do not freeze.

## ▓ IV INCOMPATABILITIES

Do not infuse with other medications.

## INDICATIONS/ROUTES/DOSAGE

**Melanoma**
**IV ADULTS, ELDERLY:** *(Single Agent):* 240 mg every 2 wks until disease progression or unacceptable toxicity. *(In combination with ipilimumab):* 1 mg/kg, followed by ipilimumab on the same day, every 3 wks

for 4 doses. Subsequent single-agent therapy dose is 240 mg every 2 wks until disease progression or unacceptable toxicity.

**Metastatic Non–Small Cell Lung Cancer**
**IV: ADULTS, ELDERLY:** 240 mg q2wks until disease progression or unacceptable toxicity.

**Renal Cell Carcinoma**
**IV: ADULTS, ELDERLY:** 240 mg q2wks until disease progression or unacceptable toxicity.

**cHL**
**IV: ADULTS, ELDERLY:** 3 mg/kg q2wks until disease progression or unacceptable toxicity.

**Head and Neck Carcinoma**
**IV: ADULTS, ELDERLY:** 3 mg/kg q2wks.

**Dose Modification**
Based on Common Terminology Criteria for Adverse Events (CTCAE).
*Withhold Treatment for Any of the Following Adverse Events:*
Grade 2 or 3 diarrhea or colitis; single-agent therapy–associated colitis; grade 2 pneumonitis; serum AST or ALT greater than 3–5 times upper limit of normal (ULN) or serum bilirubin 1.5–3 times ULN; grade 2 or 3 hypophysitis; grade 2 adrenal insufficiency; serum creatinine greater than 1.5–6 times ULN; grade 3 rash; first occurrence of any other grade 3 adverse reaction. When nivolumab is administered in combination with ipilimumab and nivolumab is withheld, then ipilimumab should also be withheld.
*Restarting Therapy:*
Resume when adverse reactions return to grade 0 or 1.
*Permanently Discontinue for Any of the Following Adverse Events:*
Combo-agent therapy (ipilimumab)–associated colitis; grade 3 or 4 pneumonitis; serum AST or ALT greater than 5 times ULN or serum bilirubin 3 times ULN; pts with liver metastasis who begin treatment with baseline grade 2 serum ALT or AST

N

elevation who experience serum ALT or AST elevation greater than or equal to 50% from baseline that persists for at least 1 wk; grade 4 hypophysitis; grade 3 or 4 adrenal insufficiency; serum creatinine greater than 6 times ULN; grade 4 rash; recurrence of any other grade 3 adverse reaction; any life-threatening or grade 4 adverse reaction; requirement for prednisone 10 mg/day or greater (or equivalent) for more than 12 wks; persistent grade 2 or 3 adverse reaction lasting longer than 12 wks.

**Dosage in Renal Impairment**
No dose adjustment.

**Dosage in Hepatic Impairment**
**Mild to moderate impairment:** No dose adjustment. **Severe impairment:** Not specified; use caution.

## SIDE EFFECTS

**Note:** Percentage of side effects may vary depending on the use of single or combination therapy. **Frequent (50%–24%):** Fatigue, dyspnea, musculoskeletal pain, decreased appetite, cough, nausea, headache, constipation. **Occasional (19%–10%):** Vomiting, asthenia, diarrhea, edema, pyrexia, cough, dehydration, rash, abdominal pain, chest pain, arthralgia, decreased weight, blurred vision, pruritus, peripheral edema, generalized pain.

## ADVERSE EFFECTS/TOXIC REACTIONS

Anemia, lymphopenia, neutropenia, thrombocytopenia is an expected response to therapy. May cause severe immune-mediated events including interstitial lung disease or pneumonitis (3%–10% of pts), colitis (21%–57% of pts), hepatitis (15%–28% of pts), hypophysitis (13% of pts), renal failure or nephritis (1%–2% of pts), hyperthyroidism (1% of pts), hypothyroidism (3%–19% of pts), rash (up to 37% of pts). Other adverse events including autoimmune nephropathy, demyelination, diabetic ketoacidosis, duodenitis, erythema multiforme, exfoliative dermatitis, facial and abducens nerve paresis, gastritis, iridocyclitis, motor dysfunction, pancreatitis, psoriasis, sarcoidosis, uveitis, vasculitis, ventricular arrhythmia, vitiligo reported in less than 2% of pts. Severe infusion-related reactions reported in less than 1% of pts. Occurrence of events are dependent on use of single or combination therapy. Upper respiratory tract infections including nasopharyngitis, pharyngitis, rhinitis reported in 11% of pts. Immunogenicity (auto-nivolumab antibodies) occurred in 8.5% of pts.

## NURSING CONSIDERATIONS

### BASELINE ASSESSMENT
Obtain baseline CBC, BMP, ionized calcium, LFT, TSH; vital signs; urine pregnancy. Record weight in kg. Screen for history of arrhythmias, pituitary/pulmonary/thyroid disease, autoimmune disorders, diabetes mellitus, hepatic/renal impairment; allergy to prednisone. Along with routine assessment, conduct full dermatologic exam, ophthalmologic exam/visual acuity. Receive full medication history and screen for interactions.

### INTERVENTION/EVALUATION
Monitor CBC, LFT, serum electrolytes; thyroid panel if applicable. Diligently monitor for immune-mediated adverse events as listed in Adverse Effects/Toxic Reactions. Notify physician if any CTCAE toxicities occur (see Appendix M) and initiate proper treatment. Obtain chest X-ray if interstitial lung disease, pneumonitis suspected. Screen for tumor lysis syndrome in pts with high tumor burden. Monitor I&Os, daily weight. If prednisone therapy is initiated for immune-mediated events, monitor capillary blood glucose and screen for corticosteroid side effects.

### PATIENT/FAMILY TEACHING
• Blood levels will be routinely monitored. • Avoid pregnancy; treatment may cause birth defects or miscarriage. Do not breastfeed. Females of childbearing

potential should use effective contraception during treatment and for at least 5 mos after discontinuation • Serious adverse reactions may affect lungs, GI tract, kidneys, or hormonal glands; anti-inflammatory medication may need to be started. • Immediately contact physician if serious or life-threatening inflammatory reactions occur in the following body systems: colon (severe abdominal pain or diarrhea); kidney (decreased or dark-colored urine, flank pain); lung (chest pain, cough, shortness of breath); liver (bruising easily, dark-colored urine, clay-colored/tarry stools, yellowing of skin or eyes); pituitary (persistent or unusual headache, dizziness, extreme weakness, fainting, vision changes); thyroid (trouble sleeping, high blood pressure, fast heart rate [overactive thyroid]), (fatigue, goiter, weight gain [underactive thyroid]).

# nizatidine

nye-**za**-ti-deen
(Apo-Nizatidine ✿, Axid, Axid AR
Novo-Nizatidine ✿)
**Do not confuse Axid with
Ansaid.**

## ◆CLASSIFICATION

**PHARMACOTHERAPEUTIC:** $H_2$ receptor antagonist. **CLINICAL:** Antiulcer, gastric acid secretion inhibitor.

## USES

Short-term treatment of active duodenal ulcer, active benign gastric ulcer. Prevention of duodenal ulcer recurrence. Treatment of gastroesophageal reflux disease (GERD), including erosive esophagitis. **OFF-LABEL:** Part of multidrug therapy for *H. pylori* eradication used to reduce risk of duodenal ulcer recurrence.

## PRECAUTIONS

**Contraindications:** Hypersensitivity to nizatidine, other $H_2$ antagonists. **Cautions:** Renal impairment.

## ACTION

Inhibits histamine action at histamine-2 ($H_2$) receptors of gastric parietal cells. **Therapeutic Effect:** Inhibits basal/nocturnal gastric acid secretion.

## PHARMACOKINETICS

Rapidly, well absorbed from GI tract. Protein binding: 35%. Metabolized in liver. Primarily excreted in urine. Not removed by hemodialysis. **Half-life:** 1–2 hrs (increased in renal impairment).

## ⌛ LIFESPAN CONSIDERATIONS

**Pregnancy/Lactation:** Unknown if drug crosses placenta or is distributed in breast milk. **Children:** Safety and efficacy not established in pts younger than 12 yrs. **Elderly:** No age-related precautions noted.

## INTERACTIONS

**DRUG:** None significant. **HERBAL:** None significant. **FOOD:** None known. **LAB VALUES:** Interferes with skin tests using allergen extracts. May increase serum alkaline phosphatase, ALT, AST.

## AVAILABILITY (Rx)

**Capsules (Axid):** 150 mg, 300 mg. **Oral Solution (Axid):** 15 mg/ml. **Tablet (Axid AR):** 75 mg.

## ADMINISTRATION/HANDLING

**PO**
• Give without regard to meals. Best given after meals or at bedtime. • Do not administer within 1 hr of magnesium- or aluminum-containing antacids (decreases absorption). • May give immediately before eating for heartburn prevention.

## INDICATIONS/ROUTES/DOSAGE

**Active Duodenal Ulcer**
**PO: ADULTS, ELDERLY:** 300 mg at bedtime or 150 mg twice daily.

**Prevention of Duodenal Ulcer Recurrence**
**PO: ADULTS, ELDERLY:** 150 mg at bedtime.

**Gastroesophageal Reflux Disease (GERD)**
**PO: ADULTS, ELDERLY:** 150 mg twice daily.

**Active Benign Gastric Ulcer**
**PO: ADULTS, ELDERLY:** 150 mg twice daily or 300 mg at bedtime.

**Dosage in Renal Impairment**
Dosage adjustment is based on creatinine clearance.

| Creatinine Clearance | Active Ulcer | Maintenance Therapy |
|---|---|---|
| 20–50 ml/min | 150 mg at bedtime | 150 mg every other day |
| Less than 20 ml/min | 150 mg every other day | 150 mg q3days |

**Dosage in Hepatic Impairment**
No dose adjustment.

## SIDE EFFECTS

**Occasional (2%):** Drowsiness, fatigue.
**Rare (1%):** Hyperhidrosis, rash.

## ADVERSE EFFECTS/ TOXIC REACTIONS

Asymptomatic ventricular tachycardia, hyperuricemia not associated with gout, nephrolithiasis occur rarely.

### NURSING CONSIDERATIONS

**INTERVENTION/EVALUATION**

Assess for abdominal pain, GI bleeding (overt blood in emesis/stool, tarry stools). Monitor LFT (hepatocellular injury).

**PATIENT/FAMILY TEACHING**

• Avoid tasks that require alertness, motor skills until response to drug is established. • Avoid alcohol, aspirin, smoking, excessive amounts of caffeine. • Report symptoms of heartburn, acid indigestion, sour stomach persisting after 2 wks of continuous use of nizatidine.

# norepinephrine

**nor**-ep-i-**nef**-rin
(Levophed)

■ **BLACK BOX ALERT** ■ Extravasation may produce severe tissue necrosis, sloughing. Using fine hypodermic needle, liberally infiltrate area with 10–15 ml saline solution containing 5–10 mg phentolamine.
**Do not confuse Levophed with Levaquin or levofloxacin, or norepinephrine with epinephrine.**

## ◆CLASSIFICATION

**PHARMACOTHERAPEUTIC:** Sympathomimetic. **CLINICAL:** Vasopressor.

## USES

Severe hypotension, treatment of shock persisting after fluid volume replacement.

## PRECAUTIONS

**Contraindications:** Hypersensitivity to norepinephrine. Hypotension related to hypovolemia (except in emergency to maintain coronary/cerebral perfusion until volume replaced), mesenteric/peripheral vascular thrombosis (unless it is lifesaving procedure). **Cautions:** Concurrent use of MAOIs.

## ACTION

Stimulates beta$_1$-adrenergic receptors, alpha-adrenergic receptors, increasing contractility, heart rate and producing vasoconstriction. **Therapeutic Effect:** Increases systemic B/P, coronary blood flow.

## PHARMACOKINETICS

| Route | Onset | Peak | Duration |
|---|---|---|---|
| IV | Rapid | 1–2 min | N/A |

Localized in sympathetic tissue. Metabolized in liver. Primarily excreted in urine.

## ⌛ LIFESPAN CONSIDERATIONS

**Pregnancy/Lactation:** Readily crosses placenta. May produce fetal anoxia

N

due to uterine contraction, constriction of uterine blood vessels. **Children/ Elderly:** No age-related precautions noted.

## INTERACTIONS

**DRUG: MAOIs, antidepressants (tricyclic)** may prolong hypertension. **HERBAL:** None significant. **FOOD:** None known. **LAB VALUES:** None significant.

## AVAILABILITY (Rx)

Injection Solution: 1 mg/ml.

## ADMINISTRATION/HANDLING

 IV

**Reconstitution** • Add 4 ml (4 mg) to 250 ml D₅W (16 mcg/ml). **Maximum concentration:** 32 ml (32 mg) to 250 ml (128 mcg/ml).

**Rate of Administration** • Closely monitor IV infusion flow rate (use infusion pump). • Monitor B/P q2min during IV infusion until desired therapeutic response is achieved, then q5min during remaining IV infusion. • Never leave pt unattended. • Maintain B/P at 90–100 mm Hg in previously normotensive pts, and 30–40 mm Hg below preexisting B/P in previously hypertensive pts. • Reduce IV infusion gradually. Avoid abrupt withdrawal. • If using peripherally inserted catheter, it is imperative to check the IV site frequently for free flow and infused vein for blanching, hardness to vein, coldness, pallor to extremity. • If extravasation occurs, area should be infiltrated with 10–15 ml sterile saline containing 5–10 mg phentolamine (does not alter pressor effects of norepinephrine).

**Storage** • Do not use if solution is brown or contains precipitate. • Store at room temperature. Diluted solution stable for 24 hrs at room temperature.

## IV INCOMPATIBILITIES

Pantoprazole (Protonix), regular insulin.

## IV COMPATIBILITIES

Amiodarone (Cordarone), calcium gluconate, dexmedetomidine (Precedex), diltiazem (Cardizem), dobutamine (Dobutrex), dopamine (Intropin), epinephrine, esmolol (Brevibloc), fentanyl (Sublimaze), furosemide (Lasix), haloperidol (Haldol), heparin, hydromorphone (Dilaudid), labetalol (Trandate), lipids, lorazepam (Ativan), magnesium, midazolam (Versed), milrinone (Primacor), morphine, nicardipine (Cardene), nitroglycerin, potassium chloride, propofol (Diprivan).

## INDICATIONS/ROUTES/DOSAGE

◀ALERT▶ If possible, blood, fluid volume depletion should be corrected before drug is administered.

**Acute Hypotension Unresponsive to Fluid Volume Replacement**

**IV INFUSION: ADULTS, ELDERLY:** Initially, administer at 8–12 mcg/min. Adjust rate of flow to desired response. Average maintenance range: 2–4 mcg/min (varies greatly based on clinical situation). **CHILDREN:** Initially, 0.05–0.1 mcg/kg/min; titrate to desired effect. **Maximum:** 2 mcg/kg/min.

**Dosage in Renal/Hepatic Impairment**
No dose adjustment.

## SIDE EFFECTS

Norepinephrine produces less pronounced, less frequent side effects than epinephrine. **Occasional (5%–3%):** Anxiety, bradycardia, palpitations. **Rare (2%–1%):** Nausea, anginal pain, shortness of breath, fever.

## ADVERSE EFFECTS/ TOXIC REACTIONS

Extravasation may produce tissue necrosis, sloughing. Overdose manifested as severe hypertension with violent headache (may be first clinical sign of overdose), arrhythmias, photophobia, retrosternal or pharyngeal pain, pallor, diaphoresis, vomiting. Prolonged therapy may result in plasma volume depletion. Hypotension may recur if plasma volume is not maintained.

## NURSING CONSIDERATIONS

### BASELINE ASSESSMENT

Assess EKG, B/P continuously (be alert to precipitous B/P drop). Never leave pt alone during IV infusion. Be alert to pt complaint of headache.

### INTERVENTION/EVALUATION

Monitor IV flow rate diligently. Assess for extravasation characterized by blanching of skin over vein, coolness (results from local vasoconstriction); color, temperature of IV site extremity (pallor, cyanosis, mottling). Assess nailbed capillary refill. Monitor I&O; measure output hourly, report urine output less than 30 ml/hr. Once B/P parameter has been reached, IV infusion should not be restarted unless systolic B/P falls below 90 mm Hg.

# nortriptyline

nor-**trip**-ti-leen
(Apo-Nortriptyline ✦, Aventyl ✦, Norventyl ✦, Pamelor)

■ **BLACK BOX ALERT** ■ Increased risk of suicidal thinking and behavior in children, adolescents, young adults 18–24 yrs with major depressive disorder, other psychiatric disorders.
**Do not confuse Aventyl with Bentyl, or nortriptyline with amitriptyline, desipramine, or Norpramin.**

## ◆CLASSIFICATION

**PHARMACOTHERAPEUTIC:** Tricyclic compound. **CLINICAL:** Antidepressant.

## USES

Treatment of symptoms of depression. **OFF-LABEL:** Adjunctive therapy for smoking cessation, myofascial pain, postherpetic pain, orofacial pain, chronic pain, irritable bowel syndrome.

## PRECAUTIONS

**Contraindications:** Hypersensitivity to nortriptyline. Acute recovery period after MI, MAOI use within 14 days, initiation of nortriptyline in pt receiving linezolid or methylene blue. **Cautions:** Prostatic hyperplasia, history of urinary retention/obstruction, narrow-angle glaucoma, diabetes mellitus, history of seizures, hyperthyroidism, cardiac/hepatic/renal disease, psychosis, increased intraocular pressure, pts at high risk for suicide, elderly.

## ACTION

Blocks reuptake of neurotransmitters (norepinephrine, serotonin) at neuronal presynaptic membranes, increasing their availability at postsynaptic receptor sites. **Therapeutic Effect:** Relieves depression, anxiety disorders, nocturnal enuresis.

## INTERACTIONS

**DRUG: Alcohol, other CNS depressants** may increase CNS effects, respiratory depression, hypotensive effects. **Cimetidine** may increase concentration, risk of toxicity. **MAOIs** may increase risk of neuroleptic malignant syndrome, seizures, hyperpyrexia, hypertensive crisis. **HERBAL: Gotu kola, kava kava, St. John's wort, valerian** may increase CNS depression and risk of serotonin syndrome. **FOOD: Grape juice, carbonated beverages** may decrease effectiveness. **Grapefruit products** may increase risk of side effects. **LAB VALUES:** May alter serum glucose, EKG readings. **Therapeutic peak serum level:** 6–10 mcg/ml; **therapeutic trough serum level:** 0.5–2 mcg/ml. **Toxic peak serum level:** greater than 12 mcg/ml; **toxic trough serum level:** greater than 2 mcg/ml.

N

## AVAILABILITY (Rx)

Capsules (Pamelor): 10 mg, 25 mg, 50 mg, 75 mg. **Oral Solution:** 10 mg/5 ml.

## ADMINISTRATION/HANDLING

◄**ALERT►** At least 14 days must elapse between use of MAOIs and nortriptyline.

**PO**
• Give with food, milk if GI distress occurs. • Dilute oral solution in water, milk, or fruit juice. Give immediately. (Do not mix with grape juice/carbonated beverages.)

## INDICATIONS/ROUTES/DOSAGE

**Depression**
**PO: ADULTS:** Initially, 25 mg 3–4 times/ day up to 150 mg/day. Adjust dose based on response and tolerability. **ELDERLY:** Initially, 30–50 mg at bedtime. May increase by 25 mg every 3–7 days. **Maximum:** 150 mg/day.

**Enuresis**
**PO: CHILDREN OLDER THAN 11 YRS:** 25–35 mg/day. **8–11 YRS:** 10–20 mg/day. **6–7 YRS:** 10 mg/day.

**Dosage in Renal Impairment**
No dose adjustment.

**Dosage in Hepatic Impairment**
Use caution.

## SIDE EFFECTS

**Frequent:** Drowsiness, fatigue, dry mouth, blurred vision, constipation, delayed micturition, orthostatic hypotension, diaphoresis, impaired concentration, increased appetite, urinary retention. **Occasional:** GI disturbances (nausea, GI distress, metallic taste), photosensitivity. **Rare:** Paradoxical reactions (agitation, restlessness, nightmares, insomnia), extrapyramidal symptoms (particularly fine hand tremor).

## ADVERSE EFFECTS/ TOXIC REACTIONS

High dosage may produce cardiovascular effects (severe orthostatic hypotension, dizziness, tachycardia, palpitations, arrhythmias), altered temperature regulation (hyperpyrexia, hypothermia). Abrupt discontinuation from prolonged therapy may produce headache, malaise, nausea, vomiting, vivid dreams.

## NURSING CONSIDERATIONS

### BASELINE ASSESSMENT
Assess for suicidal ideation/tendencies, behavior, thought content, appearance. Obtain baseline glucose, cholesterol levels. For pts on long-term therapy, hepatic/renal function tests, blood counts should be performed periodically.

### INTERVENTION/EVALUATION
Supervise suicidal-risk pt closely during early therapy (as depression lessens, energy level improves, increasing suicide potential). Assess appearance, behavior, speech pattern, level of interest, mood. Monitor daily pattern of bowel activity, stool consistency. Avoid constipation with increased fluids, bulky foods. Monitor B/P, pulse for hypotension, arrhythmias, weight. Assess for urinary retention. Therapeutic peak serum level: 6–10 mcg/ml; trough serum level: 0.5–2 mcg/ ml. Toxic peak serum level: greater than 12 mcg/ml; toxic trough: greater than 2 mcg/ml.

### PATIENT/FAMILY TEACHING
• Slowly go from lying to standing to avoid hypotensive effect; tolerance to postural hypotension, sedative, anticholinergic effects usually develops during early therapy. • Avoid alcohol. • Avoid tasks that require alertness, motor skills until response to drug is established. • Therapeutic effect may be noted in 2 wks or longer. • Photosensitivity to sun may occur; use sunscreen, protective

clothing. • Dry mouth may be relieved by sugarless gum, sips of water. • Report visual disturbances, worsening depression, suicidal ideation, unusual changes in behavior (esp. at initiation of therapy or with changes in dosage). • Do not abruptly discontinue medication.

# nystatin

nye-**stat**-in
(Candistatin ✦, Nystop, Pedi-Dri)
**Do not confuse nystatin with atorvastatin, fluvastatin, lovastatin, Nitrostat, pitavastatin, pravastatin, rosuvastatin, or simvastatin.**

## FIXED-COMBINATION(S)

**Mycolog, Myco-Triacet:** nystatin/triamcinolone (a steroid): 100,000 units/0.1%.

## ◆CLASSIFICATION

**PHARMACOTHERAPEUTIC:** Polyene antifungal antibiotic. **CLINICAL:** Antifungal.

## USES

Treatment of cutaneous, intestinal, oral cavity, infections caused by *Candida* spp.

## PRECAUTIONS

**Contraindications:** Hypersensitivity to nystatin. **Cautions:** None known.

## ACTION

Binds to sterols in cell membrane, increasing fungal cell membrane permeability, permitting loss of potassium, other cellular components. **Therapeutic Effect:** Fungistatic.

## PHARMACOKINETICS

**PO:** Poorly absorbed from GI tract. Eliminated unchanged in feces. **Topical:** Not absorbed systemically from intact skin.

## ⧖ LIFESPAN CONSIDERATIONS

**Pregnancy/Lactation:** Unknown if distributed in breast milk. Vaginal applicators may be contraindicated, requiring manual insertion of tablets during pregnancy. **Children:** No age-related precautions noted for suspension, topical use. Lozenges not recommended in pts younger than 5 yrs. **Elderly:** No age-related precautions noted.

## INTERACTIONS

**DRUG:** None significant. **HERBAL:** None significant. **FOOD:** None known. **LAB VALUES:** None significant.

## AVAILABILITY (Rx)

**Cream:** 100,000 units/g. **Ointment:** 100,000 units/g. **Oral Suspension:** 100,000 units/ml. **Tablets:** 500,000 units. **Topical Powder (Nystop, Pedi-Dri):** 100,000 units/g.

## ADMINISTRATION/HANDLING

**PO**
• Shake suspension well before administration. • Place and hold suspension in mouth or swish throughout mouth as long as possible before swallowing. • For neonates and infants, paint into recesses of the mouth.

## INDICATIONS/ROUTES/DOSAGE

**Intestinal Infection**
**PO: ADULTS, ELDERLY:** 500,000–1,000,000 units q8h.

**Oral Candidiasis**
**PO: ADULTS, ELDERLY, CHILDREN:** 400,000–600,000 units 4 times/day. **INFANTS:** 200,000 units 4 times/day. **PREMATURE INFANTS:** 100,000 units 4 times/day.

**Cutaneous Candidal Infections**
**Topical: ADULTS, ELDERLY, CHILDREN:** Apply 2–3 times/day.

**Dosage in Renal/Hepatic Impairment**
No dose adjustment.

N

✦ Canadian trade name      🗡 Non-Crushable Drug      🔲 High Alert drug

## SIDE EFFECTS

**Occasional: PO:** None known. **Topical:** Skin irritation. **Vaginal:** Vaginal irritation.

## ADVERSE EFFECTS/ TOXIC REACTIONS

High dosages of oral form may produce nausea, vomiting, diarrhea, GI distress.

## NURSING CONSIDERATIONS

### BASELINE ASSESSMENT

Confirm cultures, histologic tests were obtained for accurate diagnosis. Inspect oral mucous membranes.

### INTERVENTION/EVALUATION

Assess for increased skin irritation with topical, increased vaginal discharge with vaginal application.

### PATIENT/FAMILY TEACHING

• Do not miss doses; complete full length of treatment (continue vaginal use during menses). • Report nausea, vomiting, diarrhea, stomach pain. • **Vaginal:** Insert high in vagina. • Check with physician regarding douching, sexual intercourse. • **Topical:** Rub well into affected areas. • Avoid contact with eyes. • Use cream (sparingly) or powder on erythematous areas. • Keep areas clean, dry; wear light clothing for ventilation. • Separate personal items in contact with affected areas.

N

# obinutuzumab

oh-bi-nue-**tooz**-ue-mab
(Gazyva)

■ **BLACK BOX ALERT** ■ Hepatitis B virus reactivation, resulting in hepatic failure, fulminant hepatitis, and death have occurred. Screen all pt for hepatitis B infection before initiating treatment. Progressive multifocal leukoencephalopathy (PML) including fatal PML reported.

◆**CLASSIFICATION**

**PHARMACOTHERAPEUTIC:** Monoclonal antibody. **CLINICAL:** Antineoplastic.

## USES

Treatment of previously untreated chronic lymphocytic leukemia (CLL), in combination with chlorambucil. Treatment of follicular lymphoma (in combination with bendamustine) in pts who relapsed after, or are refractory to, a rituximab-containing regimen.

## PRECAUTIONS

**Contraindications:** Hypersensitivity to obinutuzumab. **Cautions:** Pts showing evidence of prior HBV infection, preexisting cardiac/pulmonary impairment; hematologic abnormalities (e.g., leukopenia, thrombocytopenia); electrolyte imbalance; avoid with active infection.

## ACTION

Targets CD20 antigen expressed on surface of B lymphocytes. Mediates B-cell lysis, cellular cytotoxicity, and antibody-dependant cellular phagocytosis (macrophage ingestion). **Therapeutic Effect:** Inhibits tumor cell growth and proliferation in chronic lymphocytic leukemia.

## PHARMACOKINETICS

Metabolism and elimination not specified. **Half-life:** 28 days.

## ⌛ LIFESPAN CONSIDERATIONS

**Pregnancy/Lactation:** Unknown if distributed in breast milk. Must either discontinue drug or discontinue breastfeeding. **Children:** Safety and efficacy not established. **Elderly:** May have increased risk of adverse reactions.

## INTERACTIONS

**DRUG: ACE inhibitors (e.g., enalapril), angiotensin receptor blockers (e.g., losartan), beta blockers (e.g., metoprolol)** may increase risk of hypotension. **HERBAL:** None significant. **FOOD:** None known. **LAB VALUES:** May increase serum alkaline phosphatase, ALT, AST, bilirubin, creatinine, uric acid. May decrease albumin, Hgb, Hct, lymphocytes, neutrophils, platelets, serum potassium, sodium.

## AVAILABILITY (Rx)

**Solution, Injection:** 1,000 mg/40 ml (25 mg/ml) single-use vial.

## ADMINISTRATION/HANDLING

◀**ALERT**▶ Administer via dedicated line. Do not administer IV push or bolus. Withhold hypertensive medications at least 12 hrs before and 1 hr after administration. Do not mix with dextrose-containing fluids.

 **IV**

**Reconstitution** • Visually inspect for particulate matter or discoloration. • For 100-mg dose: withdraw 40 ml solution from vial and dilute only 4 ml (100 mg) in 100 ml 0.9% NaCl for immediate administration. Dilute remaining 36 ml (900 mg) into 250 ml 0.9% NaCl at same time and refrigerate for up to 24 hrs for cycle 1: day 2. For remaining infusions (Day 8 and 15 of cycle 1), and day 1 of cycles 2–6, dilute 40 ml (1,000 mg) solution in 250 ml NaCl infusion bag. • Gently mix by inversion. • Do not shake.
**Rate of Administration** • **Day 1 of Cycle 1 (100 mg):** Infuse over 4 hrs (25 mg/hr). • Do not increase infusion

**O**

---

rate. • **Day 2 of Cycle 1 (900 mg):** Infuse at 50 mg/hr. • May increase by 50 mg/hr every 30 min to maximum rate of 400 mg/hr. • **Day 8 and Day 15 of Cycle 1, and Day 1 of Cycles 2–6 (1,000 mg):** Start at 100 mg/hr. May increase by 100 mg/hr every 30 min to maximum rate of 400 mg/hr. • Increase rate based on tolerability.

**Storage** • Solution should appear clear, colorless to slightly brown. • May refrigerate diluted solution up to 24 hrs.

## INDICATIONS/ROUTES/DOSAGE

### Chronic Lymphocytic Leukemia (CLL)

◀ALERT▶ Premedicate with glucocorticoid, acetaminophen, and antihistamine to decrease severity of infusion reaction. Consider premedication with antihyperuricemics (allopurinol) 12–24 hrs for pts with high tumor burden or high circulating absolute lymphocyte count greater than $25 \times 10^9$/L. Recommend antimicrobial prophylaxis throughout treatment for pts with neutropenia.
**IV: ADULTS/ELDERLY:** Six treatment cycles of 28 day cycle. **Day 1 of Cycle 1:** 100 mg. **Day 2 of Cycle 1:** 900 mg. **Day 8 and Day 15 of Cycle 1 and Day 1 of Cycles 2–6:** 1,000 mg. Discontinue treatment if any severe to life-threatening infusion reactions occur.

### Follicular Lymphoma

**IV: ADULTS, ELDERLY: Six treatment cycles of 28 days (in combination with bendamustine). Cycle 1:** 1,000 mg on days 1, 8, 15. **Cycles 2–6:** 1,000 mg on day 1. If achieves stable disease, complete or partial response, continue obinutuzumab (as monotherapy) 1,000 mg q2mos for 2 yrs.

### Dosage in Renal/Hepatic Impairment

No dose adjustment.

## SIDE EFFECTS

**Frequent (69%):** Infusion reactions (pruritis, flushing, urticaria). **Occasional (10%):** Pyrexia, cough.

## ADVERSE EFFECTS/ TOXIC REACTIONS

Thrombocytopenia, neutropenia, leukopenia, lymphopenia (47%–80% of pts) is an expected response to therapy, but more severe reactions including bone marrow failure, febrile neutropenia, opportunistic infection may result in life-threatening events. Hepatitis B virus reactivation may occur. Infusion reactions including hypotension, tachycardia, dyspnea, bronchospasm, wheezing, laryngeal edema, nausea, vomiting, flushing, pyrexia may occur during infusion. Tumor lysis syndrome may present as acute renal failure, hypocalcemia, hyperuricemia, hyperphosphatemia within 12–24 hrs of infusion. Immunogenicity (autoantibodies) occurred in 13% of pts. Progressive multifocal leukoencephalopathy (PML) occurred rarely and may include weakness, paralysis, vision loss, aphasia, cognition impairment.

## NURSING CONSIDERATIONS

### BASELINE ASSESSMENT

Obtain baseline CBC, BMP, ionized calcium, phosphate, uric acid; vital signs. Screen for history of anemia, asthma, arrhythmias, COPD, diabetes mellitus, GI bleeding, hypertension, hepatitis B infection, hepatic/renal impairment, peripheral edema. Receive full medication history esp. hypertension, anticoagulant medications. Perform baseline visual acuity.

### INTERVENTION/EVALUATION

Monitor CBC, serum electrolytes, LFT, vital signs. Monitor all pts for cardiovascular alterations, respiratory distress. If respiratory reactions occur, consider administration of oxygen, epinephrine, albuterol treatments. Locate rapid-sequence intubation kit if respiratory compromise occurs. Monitor strict I&O, hydration status. If PML suspected, consult neurologist for proper management. Obtain EKG for palpitations, severe hypokalemia, hyponatremia.

• Blood levels will be routinely monitored. • Avoid pregnancy. • Report any yellowing of skin or eyes, abdominal pain, bruising, black/tarry stools, amber or bloody urine. • Fever, cough, burning with urination, body aches, chills may indicate acute infection. • Avoid use of live virus vaccines. • Avoid alcohol. • Immediately report difficult breathing, severe coughing, chest tightness, wheezing. • Paralysis, vision changes, impaired speech, altered mental status may indicate life-threatening neurologic event.

# octreotide

ock-**tree**-oh-tide
(Sandostatin, Sandostatin LAR Depot)
**Do not confuse Sandostatin with Sandimmune, Sandostatin LAR, sargramostim, or simvastatin.**

## ◆CLASSIFICATION

**PHARMACOTHERAPEUTIC:** Somatostatin analogue. **CLINICAL:** Secretory inhibitory, growth hormone suppressant; antidiarrheal.

## USES

Controls diarrhea and flushing in pts with metastatic carcinoid tumors, treatment of watery diarrhea associated with vasoactive intestinal peptic-secreting tumors (VIPomas), acromegaly. **OFF-LABEL:** Control of bleeding esophageal varices, treatment of AIDS-associated secretory diarrhea, diarrhea, diarrhea associated with graft-vs-host disease chemotherapy-induced diarrhea, insulinomas, small-bowel fistulas, Zollinger-Ellison syndrome, Cushing's syndrome, hypothalamic obesity, malignant bowel obstruction, postgastrectomy dumping syndrome, islet cell tumors, sulfonylurea-induced hypoglycemia.

## PRECAUTIONS

**Contraindications:** Hypersensitivity to octreotide. **Cautions:** Diabetic pts with gastroparesis, renal failure, hepatic impairment, HF, concomitant medications altering heart rate or rhythm. Concurrent use of medications that prolong QT interval, elderly.

## ACTION

Suppresses secretion of serotonin, gastrin, VIP, insulin, glucagon, secretin, pancreatic polypeptide. **Therapeutic Effect:** Prolongs intestinal transit time.

## PHARMACOKINETICS

| Route | Onset | Peak | Duration |
|-------|-------|------|----------|
| SQ | N/A | N/A | Up to 12 hrs |

Rapidly, completely absorbed from injection site. Protein binding: 65%. Metabolized in liver. Excreted in urine. Removed by hemodialysis. **Half-life:** 1.7–1.9 hrs.

## ⌛ LIFESPAN CONSIDERATIONS

**Pregnancy/Lactation:** Unknown if distributed in breast milk. **Children:** Safety and efficacy not established. **Elderly:** No age-related precautions noted.

## INTERACTIONS

**DRUG:** May decrease effectiveness of **cyclosporine. Glucagon, growth hormone, insulin, oral antidiabetics (e.g., glipizide, metformin)** may alter glucose concentrations. **HERBAL:** Avoid herbs that have hypoglycemic activity **(e.g., garlic, ginger, ginseng).** **FOOD:** None known. **LAB VALUES:** May decrease serum thyroxine ($T_4$). May increase serum alkaline phosphatase, ALT, AST, GGT.

## AVAILABILITY (Rx)

**Injection Solution (Sandostatin):** 50 mcg/ml, 100 mcg/ml, 200 mcg/ml, 500 mcg/ml, 1,000 mcg/ml. **Injection Suspension (Sandostatin LAR):** 10-mg, 20-mg, 30-mg vials.

## ADMINISTRATION/HANDLING

**◄ALERT►** Sandostatin may be given IV, IM, SQ. Sandostatin LAR Depot may be given only IM. Refrigerate.

### IM

• Give immediately after mixing. • Administer deep IM in large muscle mass at 4-wk intervals. • Avoid deltoid injections.

### SQ

• Do not use if discolored or particulates form. • Avoid multiple injections at same site within short periods.

 **IV**

• Dilute in 50–100 ml 0.9% NaCl or D₅W and infuse over 15–30 min. In emergency, may give IV push over 3 min. Following dilution, stable for 96 hrs at room temperature when diluted with 0.9% NaCl (24 hrs with D₅W). Infuse over 15–30 min.

## INDICATIONS/ROUTES/DOSAGE

**Carcinoid Tumor**
**IV, SQ** *(Sandostatin):* **ADULTS, ELDERLY:** Initial 2 wks, 100–600 mcg/day in 2–4 divided doses. Range: 50–750 mcg.
**IM** *(Sandostatin Lar):* **ADULTS, ELDERLY:** Must be stabilized on SQ octreotide for at least 2 wks. 20 mg q4wks for 2 mos, then modify based on response.

**Vasoactive Intestinal Peptic-Secreting Tumor (VIPoma)**
**IV, SQ** *(Sandostatin):* **ADULTS, ELDERLY:** Initial 2 wks, 200–300 mcg/day in 2–4 divided doses. Range: 150–750 mcg.
**IM** *(Sandostatin Lar):* **ADULTS, ELDERLY:** Must be stabilized on SQ octreotide for at least 2 wks; 20 mg q4wks for 2 mos, then modify based on response.

**Esophageal Varices**
**IV** *(Sandostatin):* **ADULTS, ELDERLY:** Bolus of 25–100 mcg followed by IV infusion of 25–50 mcg/hr for 2–5 days.

**Acromegaly**
**IV, SQ** *(Sandostatin):* **ADULTS, ELDERLY:** Initially, 50 mcg 3 times/day. Increase as needed. Range: 300–1,500 mcg/day. Usual effective dose: 100–200 mcg 3 times/day.
**IM** *(Sandostatin Lar):* **ADULTS, ELDERLY:** Must be stabilized on SQ octreotide for at least 2 wks. 20 mg q4wks for 3 mos, then modify based on response. **Maximum:** 40 mg q4wks.

**Dosage in Renal/Hepatic Impairment**
No dose adjustment.

## SIDE EFFECTS

**Frequent (10%–6%; 58%–30% in Acromegaly Pts):** Diarrhea, nausea, abdominal discomfort, headache, injection site pain. **Occasional (5%–1%):** Vomiting, flatulence, constipation, alopecia, facial flushing, pruritus, dizziness, fatigue, arrhythmias, ecchymosis, blurred vision. **Rare (Less Than 1%):** Depression, diminished libido, vertigo, palpitations, dyspnea.

## ADVERSE EFFECTS/ TOXIC REACTIONS

Increased risk of cholelithiasis. Prolonged high-dose therapy may produce hypothyroidism. GI bleeding, hepatitis, seizures occur rarely.

## NURSING CONSIDERATIONS

### BASELINE ASSESSMENT

Establish baseline B/P, weight, thyroid function, serum glucose, electrolytes.

### INTERVENTION/EVALUATION

Monitor serum glucose, electrolytes, thyroid function. In acromegaly, monitor growth hormone levels. Weigh every 2–3 days, report over 5-lb gain per wk. Monitor B/P, pulse, respirations periodically during treatment. Be alert for decreased urinary output, peripheral edema. Monitor daily pattern of bowel activity, stool consistency.

• Therapy should provide significant improvement of severe, watery diarrhea.

# ofatumumab

oh-fa-**tue**-mue-mab
(Arzerra)

■ **BLACK BOX ALERT** ■ Hepatitis B virus (HBV) reactivation may occur, resulting in hepatitis, hepatic failure, death. Progressive multifocal leukoencephalopathy (PML), resulting in death may occur.
**Do not confuse ofatumumab with omalizumab.**

## ◆CLASSIFICATION

**PHARMACOTHERAPEUTIC:** Monoclonal antibody. **CLINICAL:** Antineoplastic.

## USES

Treatment of chronic lymphocytic leukemia (CLL) in pts previously untreated, relapsed, or require extended therapy. Treatment of CLL refractory to fludarabine and alemtuzumb.

## PRECAUTIONS

**Contraindications:** Hypersensitivity to ofatumumab. **Cautions:** Carriers of hepatitis B virus.

## ACTION

Binds to CD20 molecule, the antigen on surface of B-cell lymphocytes; inhibits early-stage B-lymphocyte activation. **Therapeutic Effect:** Controls tumor growth, triggers cell death.

## PHARMACOKINETICS

Eliminated through both a target-independent route and a B-cell–mediated route. Due to depletion of B cells, clearance is decreased substantially after subsequent infusions compared to first infusion. **Half-life:** 12–16 days.

## ⧗ LIFESPAN CONSIDERATIONS

**Pregnancy/Lactation:** Unknown if distributed in breast milk. **Children:**
Safety and efficacy not established. **Elderly:** No age-related precautions noted.

## INTERACTIONS

**DRUG: Bone marrow depressants** may increase myelosuppression. **Live virus vaccines** may potentiate virus replication, increase vaccine side effects, decrease pt's antibody response to vaccine. **HERBAL: Echinacea** may decrease concentration/effects. **FOOD:** None known. **LAB VALUES:** May decrease WBC, platelets.

## AVAILABILITY (Rx)

**Solution for Injection:** 100 mg/5 ml single-use vial.

## ADMINSTRATION/HANDLING

 IV

◄**ALERT**► Do not give by IV push or bolus. Use in-line filter supplied with product.
**Reconstitution • 300-mg dose:** Withdraw and discard 15 ml from 1,000 ml 0.9% NaCl. • Withdraw 5 ml from each of 3 vials and add to bag. • Gently invert. • **2,000-mg dose:** Withdraw and discard 100 ml from 1,000 ml 0.9% NaCl. • Withdraw 5 ml from each of 2 vials and add to bag. • Gently invert.
**Rate of Administration • Dose 1:** Initiate infusion at rate of 3.6 mg/hr (12 ml/hr). • **Dose 2:** Initiate infusion at rate of 24 mg/hr (12 ml/hr). • **Dose 3–12:** Initiate infusion at rate of 50 mg/hr (25 ml/hr). • If no infusion toxicity, rate of infusion may be increased every 30 min, using following table:

| Interval After Start of Infusion (min) | Dose 1 (ml/hr) | Dose 2 (ml/hr) | Doses 3–12 (ml/hr) |
|---|---|---|---|
| 0–30 | 12 | 12 | 25 |
| 31–60 | 25 | 25 | 50 |
| 61–90 | 50 | 50 | 100 |
| 91–120 | 100 | 100 | 200 |
| Over 120 | 200 | 200 | 400 |

**Storage** • Refrigerate vials. • After dilution, solution should be used within first 12 hrs; discard preparation after 24 hrs. • Discard if discoloration is present, but solution may contain visible, translucent-to-white particulates (will be removed by in-line filter).

## ▨ IV COMPATIBILITIES

Prepare all doses with 0.9% NaCl. Do not mix with dextrose solutions or any other medications.

## INDICATIONS/ROUTES/DOSAGE

◄ALERT► Premedicate 30 min to 2 hrs before each infusion with acetaminophen, an antihistamine, and a corticosteroid as prophylaxis for infusion reaction. Flush IV line with 0.9% NaCl before and after each dose. Interrupt infusion if infusion reaction of any severity occurs (do not resume for grade 4 reaction).

**Chronic Lymphocytic Leukemia (Untreated)**
**IV Infusion: ADULTS, ELDERLY:** Cycle 1: 300 mg, then 1,000 mg on day 8. Subsequent cycles: 1,000 mg on day 1 q28days. Continue for at least 3 cycles or a maximum of 12 cycles (in combination with chlorambucil).

**Chronic Lymphocytic Leukemia (Refractory)**
**IV Infusion: ADULTS, ELDERLY:** Recommended dosage is 12 doses given on the following schedule: 300 mg initial dose (dose 1), followed 1 wk later by 2,000 mg wkly for 7 doses (doses 2–8), followed 4 wks later by 2,000 mg every 4 wks for 4 doses (doses 9–12).

**Chronic Lymphocytic Leukemia (Relapsed)**
**IV Infusion: ADULTS, ELDERLY:** 300 mg once on day 1, then 1,000 mg on day 8, then 1,000 mg on day 1 of subsequent 28-day cycles for a maximum of 6 cycles.

**Extended Treatment of CLL**
**IV Infusion: ADULTS, ELDERLY:** 300 mg once on day 1, then 1,000 mg on day 8, then 1,000 mg 7 wks later and q8wks thereafter up to a maximum of 2 yrs.

**Dosage in Renal/Hepatic Impairment**
No dose adjustment.

## SIDE EFFECTS

**Frequent (20%–14%):** Fever, cough, diarrhea, fatigue, rash. **Occasional (13%–5%):** Nausea, bronchitis, peripheral edema, nasopharyngitis, urticaria, insomnia, headache, sinusitis, muscle spasm, hypertension.

## ADVERSE EFFECTS/ TOXIC REACTIONS

Most common serious adverse reactions were bacterial, viral, fungal infections (including pneumonia and sepsis), septic shock, neutropenia, thrombocytopenia. Infusion reactions occur more frequently with first 2 infusions. Severe infusion reactions manifested as angioedema, bronchospasm, dyspnea, fever, chills, back pain, hypotension. Progressive multifocal leukoencephalopathy may occur. Small bowel obstruction has been noted.

## NURSING CONSIDERATIONS

### BASELINE ASSESSMENT
Screen pts at high risk of hepatitis B virus. Assess baseline CBC prior to therapy.

### INTERVENTION/EVALUATION
Monitor CBC for evidence of myelosuppression during therapy, and increase frequency of monitoring in pts who develop grade 3 or 4 cytopenia. Monitor for blood dyscrasias (fever, sore throat, signs of local infection, unusual bruising/bleeding from any site), symptoms of anemia (excessive fatigue, weakness). Closely monitor for infusion reactions.

### PATIENT/FAMILY TEACHING
• Do not have immunizations without physician's approval (lowers body's resistance). • Avoid contact with those who have recently received live virus vaccine. • Avoid crowds, those with infection. • Promptly report fever, sore throat, signs of infection. • Report symptoms of infusion reactions (e.g., fever, chills, breathing problems, rash); bleeding, bruising, petechiae, worsening weakness or fatigue; new neurologic

symptoms (e.g., confusion, loss of balance, vision problems); symptoms of hepatitis (e.g., fatigue, yellow discoloration of skin/eyes); worsening abdominal pain, nausea.

# *OLANZapine

oh-**lan**-za-peen
(Apo-Olanzapine ✦, Zyprexa, Zyprexa Relprevv, Zyprexa Zydis)

■ **BLACK BOX ALERT** ■ Elderly pts with dementia-related psychosis are at increased risk for mortality due to cerebrovascular events. Sedation (including coma), delirium reported following use of Zyprexa Relprevv. **Do not confuse olanzapine with olsalazine or quetiapine, or Zyprexa with Celexa or Zyrtec.**

## FIXED-COMBINATION(S)

**Symbyax:** olanzapine/fluoxetine (an antidepressant): 6 mg/25 mg, 6 mg/50 mg, 12 mg/25 mg, 12 mg/50 mg.

## ◆CLASSIFICATION

**PHARMACOTHERAPEUTIC:** Dibenzazepine derivative. **CLINICAL:** Antipsychotic.

## USES

**PO:** Management of manifestations of schizophrenia. Treatment of acute mania associated with bipolar disorder as monotherapy or in combination with lithium or valproate). In combination with fluoxetine: treatment of depressive episodes associated with bipolar I disorder and treatment of treatment-resistant bipolar depression. **IM: Zyprexa Intramuscular:** Controls agitation in schizophrenia and bipolar mania. **Relprevv:** Long-acting antipsychotic for IM injection for treatment of schizophrenia. **OFF-LABEL:** Prevention of chemotherapy-induced nausea/vomiting. Acute treatment of delirium. Treatment of anorexia nervosa, Tourette syndrome, tic disorder.

## PRECAUTIONS

**Contraindications:** Hypersensitivity to olanzapine. **Cautions:** Disorders where CNS depression is prominent; cardiac disease, hemodynamic instability, prior MI, ischemic heart disease; hyperlipidemia, pts at risk for aspiration pneumonia, decreased GI motility, urinary retention, BPH, narrow-angle glaucoma, diabetes, elderly, pts at risk for suicide, Parkinson's disease, severe renal/hepatic impairment, predisposition to seizures.

## ACTION

Antagonizes alpha₁-adrenergic, dopamine, histamine, muscarinic, serotonin receptors. Produces anticholinergic, histaminic, CNS depressant effects. **Therapeutic Effect:** Diminishes psychotic symptoms.

## PHARMACOKINETICS

Well absorbed after PO administration. Rapid absorption following IM administration. Protein binding: 93%. Widely distributed. Excreted in urine (57%), feces (30%). Not removed by dialysis. **Half-life:** 21–54 hrs.

## ⧗ LIFESPAN CONSIDERATIONS

**Pregnancy/Lactation:** Unknown if drug crosses placenta or is distributed in breast milk. **Children:** Safety and efficacy not established. **Elderly:** No age-related precautions noted.

## INTERACTIONS

**DRUG: Alcohol, CNS depressants (e.g., lorazepam, morphine, zolpidem)** may increase CNS depressant effects. **Anticholinergics** may increase anticholinergic effects. **Hepatotoxic medications (e.g., acetaminophen, simvastatin)** may increase risk of hepatotoxicity. **HERBAL: Dong quai, St. John's wort** may increase photosensitization. **Gotu kola, kava kava, St. John's wort, valerian** may increase CNS depression. **FOOD:** None known. **LAB VALUES:** May increase serum GGT, cholesterol, prolactin, ALT, AST.

 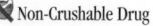

O

## AVAILABILITY (Rx)

Injection, Powder for Reconstitution (Zyprexa): 10 mg. Suspension for IM Injection (Relprevv): 210 mg, 300 mg, 405 mg. Tablets (Zyprexa): 2.5 mg, 5 mg, 7.5 mg, 10 mg, 15 mg, 20 mg. Tablets (Orally Disintegrating [Zyprexa Zydis]): 5 mg, 10 mg, 15 mg, 20 mg.

## ADMINISTRATION/HANDLING

### PO
• Give without regard to meals.

### Orally Disintegrating
• Remove by peeling back foil (do not push through foil). • Place in mouth immediately. • Tablet dissolves rapidly with saliva and may be swallowed with or without liquid.

### IM (Zyprexa Intramuscular)
• Reconstitute 10-mg vial with 2.1 ml Sterile Water for Injection to provide concentration of 5 mg/ml. • Use within 1 hr following reconstitution. • Discard unused portion.

### IM (Relprevv)
• Dilute to final concentration of 150 mg/ml. • Shake vigorously to mix. • Store at room temperature for up to 24 hrs.

## INDICATIONS/ROUTES/DOSAGE

### Schizophrenia
**PO: ADULTS, ELDERLY:** Initially, 5–10 mg once daily. May increase to 10 mg/day within 5–7 days. If further adjustments are indicated, may increase by 5 mg/day at 7-day intervals. **Maintenance:** 10–20 mg/day. **Maximum:** 20 mg/day. **CHILDREN:** Initially, 2.5–5 mg/day. Titrate in 2.5- or 5-mg increments at wkly intervals. Target dose: 10 mg/day. **Maximum:** 20 mg/day. IM *(Long-Acting [Relprevv]):* **ADULTS, ESTABLISHED ON 10 MG/DAY ORALLY:** 210 mg q2wks for 4 doses or 405 mg q4wks for 2 doses. **Maintenance:** 150 mg q2wks or 300 mg q4wks. **ESTABLISHED ON 15 MG/DAY ORALLY:** 300 mg q2wks for 4 doses. **Maintenance:** 210 mg q2wks

or 405 mg q4wks. **ESTABLISHED ON 20 MG/DAY ORALLY:** 300 mg q2wks.

### Depression Associated with Bipolar Disorder (with fluoxetine)
**PO: ADULTS, ELDERLY:** Initially, 5 mg in evening. Range: 5–12.5 mg/day. **CHILDREN 10–17 yrs:** Initially, 2.5 mg once daily. Adjust dose as tolerated.

### Treatment-Resistant Depression (with fluoxetine)
**PO: ADULTS, ELDERLY:** Initially, 5 mg in evening. Range: 5–20 mg/day.

### Bipolar Mania
**PO: ADULTS, ELDERLY:** (Monotherapy) Initially, 10–15 mg/day. May increase by 5 mg/day at intervals of at least 24 hrs. Range: 5–20 mg/day. **Maximum:** 20 mg/day. *(In Combination with Lithium or Valproate):* Initially, 10 mg/day. Range: 5–20 mg/day. **CHILDREN 13 YRS OF AGE AND OLDER:** Initially, 2.5–5 mg/day. Adjust dose by 2-5-5 mg daily to target dose of 10 mg/day. Range: 2.5–20 mg/day.

### Dosage for Elderly, Debilitated Pts, Pts Predisposed to Hypotensive Reactions
Initial dosage: 5 mg/day.

### Control of Agitation
**IM: ADULTS, ELDERLY:** *(Short-Acting):* Initially, 5–10 mg. 2 hrs after first dose, additional dose may be considered. 4 hrs after, second dose should be allowed to evaluate response. **Maximum:** 30 mg/day.

### Dosage in Renal/Hepatic Impairment
No dose adjustment.

## SIDE EFFECTS

**Frequent (26%–10%):** Drowsiness, agitation, insomnia, headache, nervousness, hostility, dizziness, rhinitis. **Occasional (9%–5%):** Anxiety, constipation, nonaggressive atypical behavior, dry mouth, weight gain, orthostatic hypotension, fever, arthralgia, restlessness, cough, pharyngitis, visual changes (dim vision). **Rare:** Tachycardia; back, chest, abdominal, or extremity pain; tremor.

## ADVERSE EFFECTS/ TOXIC REACTIONS

Rare reactions include seizures, neuroleptic malignant syndrome, a potentially fatal syndrome characterized by hyperpyrexia, muscle rigidity, irregular pulse or B/P, tachycardia, diaphoresis, cardiac arrhythmias. Extrapyramidal symptoms (EPS), dysphagia may occur. Overdose (300 mg) produces drowsiness, slurred speech.

## NURSING CONSIDERATIONS

### BASELINE ASSESSMENT

Obtain baseline LFT, serum glucose, weight, lipid profile before initiating treatment. Assess behavior, appearance, emotional status, response to environment, speech pattern, thought content.

### INTERVENTION/EVALUATION

Monitor B/P, serum glucose, lipids, LFT. Assess for tremors, changes in gait, abnormal muscular movements, behavior. Supervise suicidal-risk pt closely during early therapy (as depression lessens, energy level improves, increasing suicide potential). Assess for therapeutic response (interest in surroundings, improvement in self-care, increased ability to concentrate, relaxed facial expression). Assist with ambulation if dizziness occurs. Assess sleep pattern. Notify physician if extrapyramidal symptoms (EPS) occur.

### PATIENT/FAMILY TEACHING

• Avoid dehydration, particularly during exercise, exposure to extreme heat, concurrent use of medication causing dry mouth, other drying effects. • Sugarless gum, sips of water may relieve dry mouth. • Report suspected pregnancy. • Take medication as prescribed; do not stop taking or increase dosage. • Slowly go from lying to standing. • Avoid alcohol. • Avoid tasks that require alertness, motor skills until response to drug is established. • Monitor diet, exercise program to prevent weight gain.

# olaparib

oh-**lap**-a-rib
(Lynparza)

## ◆CLASSIFICATION

**PHARMACOTHERAPEUTIC:** Polymerase inhibitor. **CLINICAL:** Antineoplastic.

## USES

Treatment of deleterious or suspected deleterious germline BRCA-mutated advanced ovarian cancer in pts who have been treated with three or more prior lines of chemotherapy.

## PRECAUTIONS

**Contraindications:** Hypersensitivity to olaparib. **Cautions:** Baseline anemia, neutropenia, lymphopenia, thrombocytopenia. History of pulmonary disease. Avoid concomitant use of strong or moderate CYP3A inhibitors, strong or moderate CYP3A inducers.

## ACTION

Inhibits poly (ADP-ribose) polymerase enzymes, involved in normal cellular hemostasis (e.g., DNA transcription, cell cycle regulation, and DNA repair). Disrupts cellular homeostasis, resulting in cell death. **Therapeutic Effect:** Inhibits tumor cell growth and metastasis.

## PHARMACOKINETICS

Rapidly absorbed. Metabolized in liver. Protein binding: 82%. Peak plasma concentration: 1–3 hrs. Steady-state concentration: 3–4 days. Eliminated in urine (44%), feces (42%). **Half-life:** 11.9 hrs.

## ⧖ LIFESPAN CONSIDERATIONS

**Pregnancy/Lactation:** Avoid pregnancy; may cause fetal harm. Females of reproductive potential should use effective contraception during treatment and up to 1 mo after discontinuation. Unknown if distributed in breast milk. Must either

0

discontinue drug or discontinue breast-feeding. **Children:** Safety and efficacy not established. **Elderly:** No age-related precautions noted.

## INTERACTIONS

**DRUG:** **Strong CYP3A inhibitors (e.g., clarithromycin, ketoconazole, ritonavir), moderate CYP3A inhibitors (e.g., atazanavir, ciprofloxacin)** may increase concentration/effect. **Strong CYP3A inducers (e.g., carbamazepine), moderate CYP3A inducers (e.g., nafcillin)** may decrease concentration/effect. **HERBAL: St. John's wort** may decrease concentration/effect. **FOOD: Grapefruit products, Seville oranges** may increase concentration/effect. **High-fat food** may delay absorption. **LAB VALUES:** May increase mean corpuscular volume, serum creatinine. May decrease Hct, Hgb, lymphocytes, neutrophils, RBC.

## AVAILABILITY (Rx)

**Capsules:** 50 mg.

## ADMINISTRATION/HANDLING

**PO**
• Give without regard to meals. • Administer capsules whole; do not break, cut, crush, or open.

## INDICATIONS/ ROUTES/DOSAGE

**Ovarian Cancer**
**PO: ADULTS, ELDERLY:** 400 mg twice daily. Continue until disease progression or unacceptable toxicity.

**Dose Modification**
*Dose Reduction for Adverse Reactions*
**PO: ADULTS, ELDERLY:** Interrupt treatment until resolved. Then, decrease to 200 mg twice daily. If further dose reduction is indicated, decrease to 100 mg twice daily.
*Concomitant Use of Strong CYP3A Inhibitors*
**PO: ADULTS, ELDERLY:** 150 mg twice daily.

*Concomitant Use of Moderate CYP3A Inhibitors*
**PO: ADULTS, ELDERLY:** 200 mg twice daily.

**Dosage in Renal Impairment**
**Mild impairment:** No dose adjustment. **Moderate to severe impairment:** Not specified; use caution.

**Dosage in Hepatic Impairment**
Not specified; use caution.

## SIDE EFFECTS

**Frequent (66%–21%):** Fatigue, asthenia, nausea, vomiting, abdominal pain, diarrhea, dyspepsia, decreased appetite, headache, back pain, rash, myalgia, arthralgia, musculoskeletal pain, dysgeusia, cough.

## ADVERSE EFFECTS/TOXIC REACTIONS

Myelodysplastic syndrome/acute myeloid leukemia reported in 2% of pts. Pneumonitis, including fatal cases, occurred in less than 1% of pts. Respiratory tract infections including nasopharyngitis, pharyngitis, upper respiratory tract infection occurred in 43% of pts.

## NURSING CONSIDERATIONS

### BASELINE ASSESSMENT

Obtain baseline CBC. Do not initiate therapy until pts have recovered from hematologic toxicities caused by previous chemotherapy. Question history of pulmonary disease. Receive full medication history and screen for interactions.

### INTERVENTION/EVALUATION

Monitor CBC monthly. For prolonged hematologic toxicities, interrupt treatment and monitor CBC wkly until recovery. If hematologic levels have not recovered to Common Terminology Criteria for Adverse Events (CTCAE) grade 1 or 0 after 4 wks of treatment interruption, consider hematology consultation for further investigations such as bone marrow analysis and blood sample for cytogenetics.

Monitor for myelodysplastic syndrome/acute myeloid leukemia, pneumonitis.

### PATIENT/FAMILY TEACHING

• Report bleeding or bruising easily, bloody urine or stool, frequent infections, fatigue, shortness of breath, weakness, weight loss; may indicate acute bone marrow suppression or acute leukemia. • Report new or worsening respiratory symptoms such as cough, difficulty breathing, fever, wheezing; may indicate severe lung inflammation. • Do not ingest grapefruit product, Seville oranges. • Do not take herbal products. • Avoid pregnancy; treatment may cause birth defects or miscarriage. Do not breastfeed. Females of childbearing potential should use effective contraception during treatment and for at least 1 mos after stopping therapy.

---

# olmesartan

ol-me-**sar**-tan
(Benicar, Olmetec ✦)
■ **BLACK BOX ALERT** ■ May cause fetal injury, mortality. Discontinue as soon as possible once pregnancy is detected.
**Do not confuse Benicar with Mevacor.**

### FIXED-COMBINATION(S)

**Azor:** olmesartan/amlodipine (calcium channel blocker): 20 mg/5 mg, 40 mg/5 mg, 20 mg/10 mg, 40 mg/10 mg. **Benicar HCT:** olmesartan/hydrochlorothiazide (a diuretic): 20 mg/12.5 mg, 40 mg/12.5 mg, 40 mg/25 mg. **Tribenzor:** olmesartan/hydrochlorothiazide/amlodipine: 20 mg/12.5 mg/5 mg, 40 mg/12.5 mg/5 mg, 40 mg/25 mg/5 mg, 40 mg/12.5 mg/10 mg, 40 mg/25 mg/10 mg.

### ◆CLASSIFICATION

**PHARMACOTHERAPEUTIC:** Angiotensin II receptor antagonist. **CLINICAL:** Antihypertensive.

## USES

Treatment of hypertension alone or in combination with other antihypertensives.

## PRECAUTIONS

**Contraindications:** Hypersensitivity to olmesartan. Concomitant use with aliskiren in pts with diabetes. **Cautions:** Renal impairment, unstented unilateral or bilateral renal arterial stenosis, significant aortic/mitral stenosis. Concurrent potassium supplements; pts who are volume depleted.

## ACTION

Blocks vasoconstrictor, aldosterone-secreting effects of angiotensin II by inhibiting binding of angiotensin II to $AT_1$ receptors in vascular smooth muscle. **Therapeutic Effect:** Causes vasodilation, decreases peripheral resistance, decreases B/P.

## PHARMACOKINETICS

Moderately absorbed after PO administration. Hydrolyzed in GI tract to olmesartan. Protein binding: 99%. Eliminated in urine (35%–50%), remainder in feces. Not removed by hemodialysis. **Half-life:** 13 hrs.

## 🔲 LIFESPAN CONSIDERATIONS

**Pregnancy/Lactation:** Unknown if distributed in breast milk. **Children:** Safety and efficacy not established. **Elderly:** No age-related precautions noted.

## INTERACTIONS

**DRUG: NSAIDs** may decrease antihypertensive effect. **HERBAL: Ephedra, ginseng, yohimbe** may worsen hypertension. **Garlic** may increase antihypertensive effect. **FOOD:** None known. **LAB VALUES:** May slightly decrease Hgb, Hct. May increase serum BUN, creatinine, bilirubin, hepatic enzymes.

## AVAILABILITY (Rx)

**Tablets:** 5 mg, 20 mg, 40 mg.

---

## ADMINISTRATION/HANDLING

### PO
• Give without regard to meals.

## INDICATIONS/ROUTES/DOSAGE

**Hypertension**
**PO: ADULTS, ELDERLY:** Initially, 20 mg/day. May increase to 40 mg/day after 2 wks. Lower initial dose may be necessary in pts receiving volume-depleting medications (e.g., diuretics). **CHILDREN 6–16 YRS, WEIGHING 20 TO LESS THAN 35 KG:** Initially, 10 mg once daily. Range: 10–20 mg once daily. **WEIGHING 35 KG OR GREATER:** Initially, 20 mg once daily. Range: 20–40 mg once daily. Use with caution.

## SIDE EFFECTS

**Occasional (3%):** Dizziness. **Rare (less than 2%):** Headache, diarrhea, upper respiratory tract infection.

**Dosage in Renal/Hepatic Impairment**
Use caution.

## ADVERSE EFFECTS/ TOXIC REACTIONS

Overdosage may manifest as hypotension, tachycardia. Bradycardia occurs less often. Rare cases of rhabdomyolysis have been reported.

## NURSING CONSIDERATIONS

### BASELINE ASSESSMENT
Obtain B/P, apical pulse immediately before each dose in addition to regular monitoring (be alert to fluctuations). If excessive reduction in B/P occurs, place pt in supine position, feet slightly elevated. Question for possibility of pregnancy. Assess medication history (esp. diuretics).

### INTERVENTION/EVALUATION
Maintain hydration. Assess for evidence of upper respiratory infection. Assist with ambulation if dizziness occurs. Monitor serum potassium level. Assess B/P for hypertension, hypotension.

### PATIENT/FAMILY TEACHING
• Maintain adequate hydration. • Avoid pregnancy. • Avoid tasks that require alertness, motor skills until response to drug is established (possible dizziness effect). • Report any signs of infection (sore throat, fever). • Therapy requires lifelong control, diet, exercise.

# olodaterol

oh-loe-**da**-ter-ol
(Striverdi Respimat)
■ **BLACK BOX ALERT** ■ Long-acting beta$_2$-adrenergic agonists (LABA) increase risk of asthma-related deaths. Not indicated for treatment of asthma.
**Do not confuse olodaterol with albuterol, indacaterol, formoterol, salmeterol.**

## FIXED-COMBINATION(S)

**Stiolto Respimat:** olodaterol/ tiotropium (bronchodilator): 2.5 mcg/2.5 mcg.

## ◆CLASSIFICATION

**PHARMACOTHERAPEUTIC:** Sympathomimetic (beta$_2$-adrenergic agonist). **CLINICAL:** Bronchodilator.

## USES

Long-term, once daily, maintenance bronchodilator treatment of airflow obstruction in pts with chronic obstructive pulmonary disease (COPD), including chronic bronchitis and emphysema. Not indicated in asthma, acute deterioration of COPD.

## PRECAUTIONS

**Contraindications:** Hypersensitivity to olodaterol. Asthma without use of long-term asthma control medication, history of hypersensitivity to sympathomimetics. **Cautions:** Diabetes mellitus, ketoacidosis, cardiovascular disorders (e.g., coronary insufficiency, arrhythmias, hypertension, hypertrophic obstructive cardiomyopathy), seizure disorder, hyperthyroidism; history of severe bronchospasm, long QT syndrome, electrolyte imbalance.

## ACTION

Stimulates beta$_2$-adrenergic receptors in lungs, resulting in relaxation of bronchial smooth muscle. **Therapeutic Effect:** Relieves bronchospasm, reduces airway resistance, improves bronchodilation.

## PHARMACOKINETICS

Rapidly absorbed following inhalation. Extensively distributed in tissue. Metabolized in liver. Protein binding: 60%. Peak plasma concentration: 10–20 min. Eliminated in urine. **Half-life:** 45 hrs.

## ☒ LIFESPAN CONSIDERATIONS

**Pregnancy/Lactation:** Excretion into breast milk is probable. Breastfeeding not recommended. May interfere with uterine contractility. **Children:** Safety and efficacy not established. **Elderly:** No age-related precaution noted.

## INTERACTIONS

**DRUG:** **Beta blockers (e.g., metoprolol)** may decrease therapeutic effect, cause bronchospasms. **Beta$_2$-adrenergic agonists (e.g., salmeterol)** may potentiate sympathomimetic effects. **Xanthine derivatives (e.g., theophylline), steroids (e.g., methylprednisolone), non–potassium-sparing diuretics (e.g., furosemide)** may increase risk of hypokalemia. **Drugs that prolong QT interval, MAOIs,** and **tricyclic antidepressants (e.g., amitriptyline, doxepin)** may potentiate cardiovascular effects. **HERBAL: Caffeine, green tea, guarana** may increase sympathomimetic effects. **FOOD:** None known. **LAB VALUES:** May increase serum glucose. May decrease serum potassium.

## AVAILABILITY (Rx)

**Inhalation Spray (2.5 mcg/actuation):** 28 metered actuations/cartridge with inhaler, 60 metered actuations/cartridge with inhaler.

## ADMINISTRATION/HANDLING

### Inhalation

**Preparation** • With yellow cap closed, press safety catch while pulling off clear base. • Do not touch piercing element at bottom of base. • Write discard date on inhaler label (3 mos from cartridge insertion). • Push narrow end of cartridge into inhaler (base of cartridge will not be flush with inhaler). • May push cartridge on firm surface to ensure fit (1/8th of cartridge will remain visible). • Do not remove cartridge once inserted. • Put clear base back into place (do not remove again until cartridge empty and replaced).

**Priming For First Time Use** • Hold inhaler upright, with yellow cap closed, to avoid accidental release of dose. • Turn clear base in direction of black arrows on label until it clicks (half a turn). • Flip yellow cap open. • Point inhaler toward ground (away from face) and press dose release button. • Repeat all priming steps until spray is visible. • Once spray is visible, repeat all priming steps again 3 more times to ensure inhaler is ready for use. (The repeat of priming steps for first time use will not affect number of doses prescribed.)

**Daily Dosing** • Hold inhaler upright, with yellow cap closed, to avoid accidental release of dose. • Turn clear base in direction of black arrows on label until it clicks (half a turn). • Flip yellow cap open and close lips around mouthpiece. • While taking slow, deep breath through mouth, press release button and continue slow inhalation for as long as possible. • Hold breath for at least 10 sec and exhale. • Close yellow cap. • Dose indicator on left of inhaler will enter red area of scale when 7 days (30-dose product) or 3 days (14-dose product) remains.

**Repriming Guidelines:** • Do not reprime if inhaler is used daily. • If inhaler is not used for more than 3 days, spray 1 puff toward ground for preparation. • If more than 21 days has passed, repeat all first-time priming steps until spray is visible. • Then repeat all priming steps 3 more times to prepare inhaler for use.

## INDICATIONS/ROUTES/DOSAGE

### COPD

**Inhalation: ADULTS, ELDERLY:** Two inhalations (2.5 mcg per/inhalation for total of 5 mcg) once daily, at same time each day. **Maximum:** 5 mcg within 24-hr period.

**Dosage in Renal Impairment**
No dose adjustment.

**Dosage in Hepatic Impairment**
**Mild to moderate impairment:** No dose adjustment. **Severe impairment:** Use caution.

## SIDE EFFECTS

**Occasional (11%–4%):** Nasopharyngitis, upper respiratory tract infection, bronchitis, cough, back pain. **Rare (3%–2%):** Dizziness, insomnia, dry mouth, arthalgia, urinary retention.

## ADVERSE REACTIONS/TOXIC EFFECTS

Life-threatening asthma-related events, bronchospasm, or worsening of COPD-related symptoms have been reported. Serious cardiovascular events including arrhythmias, angina pectoris, cardiac arrest, hypertension, tachycardia; flattening of T wave, prolongation of QTc interval, ST segment depression have occurred. All beta-adrenergic agonists carry risk of hyperglycemia or significant hypokalemia. Pts with severe COPD or hypokalemia have additional increased risk of adverse effects related to hypoxia and concomitant medications.

## NURSING CONSIDERATIONS

### BASELINE ASSESSMENT

Obtain ABG, capillary glucose, $O_2$ saturation, serum potassium level, vital signs; EKG, pulmonary function test if applicable. Assess respiratory rate, depth, rhythm. Assess lung sounds for wheezing, rales. Receive full medication history and screen for drug interactions. Question history of asthma, cardiovascular disease, diabetes mellitus, long QT syndrome, seizure disorder. Teach proper inhaler priming and administration techniques.

### INTERVENTION/EVALUATION

Routinely monitor capillary glucose, $O_2$ saturation, serum potassium level, vital signs. Auscultate lung sounds. Obtain EKG for palpitation, tachycardia; symptomatic hypokalemia. Recommend discontinuation of short-acting beta$_2$-agonists (use only for symptomatic relief of acute respiratory symptoms). Monitor for hypoglycemia.

### PATIENT/FAMILY TEACHING

• Refill prescription when dose indicator on left of inhaler reaches red area of scale. • Follow manufacturer guidelines for proper use of inhaler. • Drink plenty of fluids (decreases lung secretion viscosity). • Rinse mouth with water after inhalation to decrease mouth/throat irritation. • Avoid excessive use of caffeine derivatives (chocolate, coffee, tea, cola). • Report fever, productive cough, body aches, difficulty breathing; may indicate lung infection or worsening of COPD.

# olsalazine

ole-**sal**-a-zeen
(Dipentum)
**Do not confuse Dipentum with Dilantin, or olsalazine with olanzapine.**

## ◆CLASSIFICATION

**PHARMACOTHERAPEUTIC:** Salicylic acid derivative. **CLINICAL:** Anti-inflammatory.

## USES

Maintenance of remission of ulcerative colitis in pts intolerant of sulfasalazine medication.

## PRECAUTIONS

**Contraindications:** Hypersensitivity to olsalazine. History of hypersensitivity to salicylates. **Cautions:** Renal/hepatic impairment, elderly, severe allergies, asthma.

## ACTION

Converted to mesalamine in colon by bacterial action. Blocks local chemical mediators of inflammatory response. **Therapeutic Effect:** Reduces colonic inflammation.

## PHARMACOKINETICS

Small amount absorbed. Protein binding: 99%. Metabolized by bacteria in colon. Minimal elimination in urine, feces. **Half-life:** 0.9 hr.

## ⏳ LIFESPAN CONSIDERATIONS

**Pregnancy/Lactation:** Crosses placenta; distributed in breast milk. **Children:** Safety and efficacy not established. **Elderly:** Age-related renal impairment may require dosage adjustment.

## INTERACTIONS

**DRUG:** May increase risk of bleeding with **warfarin, heparin.** May increase risk of myelosuppression with **mercaptopurine, thioguanine. HERBAL:** None significant. **FOOD:** None known. **LAB VALUES:** May increase serum ALT, AST.

## AVAILABILITY (Rx)

**Capsules:** 250 mg.

## ADMINISTRATION/HANDLING

**PO**
• Give with food.

## INDICATIONS/ ROUTES/DOSAGE

**Maintenance of Controlled Ulcerative Colitis**
**PO: ADULTS, ELDERLY:** 1 g/day in 2 divided doses, preferably q12h.

**Dosage in Renal/Hepatic Impairment**
No dose adjustment.

## SIDE EFFECTS

**Frequent (10%–5%):** Headache, diarrhea, abdominal pain/cramps, nausea. **Occasional (4%–2%):** Depression, fatigue, dyspepsia, upper respiratory tract infection, decreased appetite, rash, pruritus, arthralgia. **Rare (1%):** Dizziness, vomiting, stomatitis.

## ADVERSE EFFECTS/ TOXIC REACTIONS

Sulfite sensitivity may occur in susceptible pts (manifested as cramping, headache, diarrhea, fever, rash, urticaria, pruritus, wheezing). Discontinue drug immediately. Excessive diarrhea associated with extreme fatigue is rarely noted.

## NURSING CONSIDERATIONS

### INTERVENTION/EVALUATION

Encourage adequate fluid intake. Assess bowel sounds for peristalsis. Monitor daily pattern of bowel activity, stool consistency. Assess for abdominal disturbances. Assess skin for rash, urticaria. Medication should be discontinued if rash, fever, cramping, diarrhea occur.

### PATIENT/FAMILY TEACHING

• Report if diarrhea, cramping continues or worsens or if rash, fever, pruritus occur.

# omacetaxine

oh-ma-se-**tax**-een
(Synribo)

## ◆CLASSIFICATION

**PHARMACOTHERAPEUTIC:** Protein synthesis inhibitor. **CLINICAL:** Antineoplastic.

## USES

Treatment of adult pts with chronic or accelerated phase chronic myeloid leukemia (CML) with resistance and/or intolerance to two or more tyrosine kinase inhibitors.

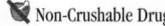

## PRECAUTIONS

**Contraindications:** Hypersensitivity to omacetaxine. **Cautions:** Glucose intolerance, poorly controlled diabetes, elderly, recent GI bleeding. Avoid all use of anticoagulants, aspirin, NSAIDs; all pts with baseline platelets less than 50,000/mm$^3$.

## ACTION

Inhibits protein synthesis of Bcr-Abl tyrosine kinase, a translocation-created enzyme, created by the Philadelphia chromosome abnormality noted in chronic myeloid leukemia (CML). **Therapeutic Effect:** Inhibits tumor proliferation and growth during accelerated and chronic stages of CML.

## PHARMACOKINETICS

Rapidly absorbed following SQ administration. Maximum concentration: 30 min. Protein binding: Less than 50%. Hydrolyzed via plasma esterases. **Half-life:** 6 hrs.

## ⧖ LIFESPAN CONSIDERATIONS

**Pregnancy/Lactation:** May cause fetal harm. Not recommended in nursing mothers. Unknown if distributed in breast milk. **Children:** Safety and efficacy not established. **Elderly:** Increased risk for toxicity (e.g., hematologic).

## INTERACTIONS

**DRUG:** NSAIDs, anticoagulants **(e.g., heparin, warfarin), antiplatelets (e.g., clopidogrel),** may increase risk for bleeding. **HERBAL:** None significant. **FOOD:** None known. **LAB VALUES:** May decrease platelets, Hgb, Hct, leukocytes, lymphocytes. May increase serum ALT.

## AVAILABILITY (Rx)

**Injection, Powder for Reconstitution:** 3.5-mg vial.

## ADMINISTRATION/HANDLING

**◀ALERT▶** Must be administered by health care workers trained in proper chemotherapy handling and disposal procedures.

**SQ**
**Reconstitution** • Reconstitute with 1 ml 0.9% NaCl. • Gently swirl until powder is completely dissolved. • Inspect vial for particular matter or discoloration. • Reconstituted vial will provide a concentration of 3.5 mg/ml. • Avoid contact with skin.
**Storage** • Solution should appear clear. • May store solution at room temperature for up to 12 hrs or may refrigerate up to 24 hrs. • Discard unused solution.

## INDICATIONS/ROUTES/DOSAGE

**Chronic or Accelerated Myeloid Leukemia**
**SQ: ADULTS, ELDERLY: Induction dose:** 1.25 mg/m$^2$ twice daily for 14 consecutive days every 28 days, over 28-day cycle. Continue induction dose until hematologic response achieved. **Maintenance dose:** 1.25 mg/m$^2$ twice daily for 7 consecutive days every 28 days of a 28-day cycle. Continue until no longer achieving clinical treatment benefit.

**Dosage Modification**
**Hematologic Toxicity:** If neutrophils less than 500/mm$^3$ or platelet less than 50,000/mm$^3$, interrupt therapy. Restart when neutrophil count greater than or equal to 1000/mm$^3$ or platelet count greater than or equal to 50,000/mm$^3$ and reduce number of dosing days by 2. **Nonhematologic Toxicity:** Interrupt therapy until toxicity/adverse effects resolved. Continue indefinitely until pt no longer benefits from therapy.

**Dosage in Renal/Hepatic Impairment**
No dose adjustment.

## SIDE EFFECTS

**Chronic Phase**
**Frequent (45%–25%):** Diarrhea, nausea, fatigue, pyrexia, asthenia. **Occasional (20%–11%):** Headache, arthralgia, cough, epistaxis, alopecia, constipation, abdominal pain, peripheral edema, vomiting, back pain, insomnia, rash.

O

---

**Accelerated Phase**
**Occasional (19%–7%):** Diarrhea, nausea, fatigue, pyrexia, asthenia, vomiting, cough, abdominal pain, chills, anorexia, headache. **Rare (7% or Less):** Dyspnea, epistaxis.

## ADVERSE EFFECTS/ TOXIC REACTIONS

Thrombocytopenia, neutropenia, leukopenia, lymphopenia, or myelosuppression is an expected response to therapy, but more severe reactions including bone marrow failure, febrile neutropenia may result in life-threatening events. Pts with neutropenia are at increased risk for infection. Thrombocytopenia may increase risk for intracranial hemorrhage, GI bleeding. Hyperglycemic events including hyperglycemic hyperosmolar nonketotic syndrome (HHNK) may occur. Pts with uncontrolled diabetes are at increased risk for hyperglycemic emergency.

## NURSING CONSIDERATIONS

### BASELINE ASSESSMENT

Obtain baseline serum chemistries, CBC, PT/INR if on anticoagulants. Question for possibility of pregnancy, current breast-feeding status. Obtain negative urine pregnancy before initiating treatment. Obtain full medication history including vitamins, supplements, herbal products, anticoagulants. Question for history of diabetes mellitus, GI bleeding.

### INTERVENTION/EVALUATION

Monitor CBC wkly, then every 2 wks during maintenance phase. Obtain frequent blood glucose levels, especially in diabetic pts. Do not initiate therapy until negative urine pregnancy confirmed. Monitor LFT if hepatic impairment suspected. If drug exposure occurs, immediately wash affected area with soap and water. Consider isolation protocol if pt develops neutropenia.

### PATIENT/FAMILY TEACHING

• Serum lab studies will be routinely monitored. • Report if pregnant or planning to become pregnant. • Use barrier methods during sexual activity. • Strictly avoid pregnancy. • May cause male infertility. • Immediately report yellowing of skin or eyes, abdominal pain, bruising, black/tarry stools, dark urine, dehydration, GI bleeding, nausea, vomiting, rash. • Report fever, cough, night sweats, flu-like symptoms, skin changes. • Shortness of breath, pale skin, weakness may indicate bleeding or severe myelosuppression. • Avoid tasks that require alertness, motor skills until response to drug is established.

# omalizumab

oh-ma-**liz**-ue-mab
(Xolair)

■ **BLACK BOX ALERT** ■ Anaphylaxis (severe bronchospasm, hypotension, angioedema, syncope, urticaria) has occurred after first dose, and in some cases, after 1 yr of regular treatment.
**Do not confuse omalizumab with ofatumumab.**

## ◆CLASSIFICATION

**PHARMACOTHERAPEUTIC:** Monoclonal antibody. **CLINICAL:** Antiasthmatic.

## USES

Treatment of moderate to severe persistent asthma in pts reactive to perennial allergens and inadequately controlled asthma symptoms with inhaled corticosteroids. Chronic idiopathic urticaria in adults and children 12 yrs and older.

## PRECAUTIONS

**Contraindications:** Hypersensitivity to omalizumab. Acute bronchospasm, status asthmaticus. **Cautions:** Pts at risk for parasitic infections.

## ACTION

Selectively binds to human immunoglobulin E (IgE). Inhibits binding of IgE on surface of mast cells, basophiles. **Therapeutic Effect:** Prevents/reduces number of asthmatic attacks.

## PHARMACOKINETICS

Absorbed slowly after SQ administration, with peak concentration in 7–8 days. Excreted primarily via hepatic degradation. **Half-life:** 26 days.

## ⧗ LIFESPAN CONSIDERATIONS

**Pregnancy/Lactation:** Because IgE is present in breast milk, omalizumab is expected to be present in breast milk. Use only if clearly needed. **Children:** Safety and efficacy not established in pts younger than 12 yrs. **Elderly:** No age-related precautions noted.

## INTERACTIONS

**DRUG:** None significant. **HERBAL:** Echinacea may decrease effects. **FOOD:** None known. **LAB VALUES:** May increase serum IgE levels.

## AVAILABILITY (Rx)

**Injection, Powder for Reconstitution:** 150 mg/1.2 ml after reconstitution.

## ADMINISTRATION/HANDLING

**SQ**
**Reconstitution** • Use only Sterile Water for Injection to prepare for SQ administration. • Medication takes 15–20 min to dissolve. • Draw 1.4 ml Sterile Water for Injection into 3-ml syringe with 1-inch, 18-gauge needle; inject contents into powdered vial. • Swirl vial for approximately 1 min (do not shake) and again swirl vial for 5–10 sec every 5 min until no gel-like particles appear in the solution. • Do not use if contents do not dissolve completely within 40 min.

• Invert vial for 15 sec (allows solution to drain toward the stopper). • Using new 3-ml syringe with 1-inch 18-gauge needle, obtain required 1.2-ml dose, replace 18-gauge needle with 25-gauge needle for SQ administration.
**Rate of Administration** • SQ administration may take 5–10 sec to administer due to its viscosity.
**Storage** • Use only clear or slightly opalescent solution; solution is slightly viscous. • Refrigerate. • Reconstituted solution is stable for 8 hrs if refrigerated or within 4 hrs of reconstitution when stored at room temperature.

## INDICATIONS/ ROUTES/DOSAGE

◄**ALERT**► Dosage and frequency of administration is based upon total IgE levels and body weight (see table). IgE levels should be measured prior to initiating treatment and not during treatment. Pts should be observed a minimum of 2 hrs following each omalizumab treatment.

**Asthma**
**SQ: ADULTS, ELDERLY, CHILDREN 6 YRS AND OLDER:** 75–375 mg every 2 or 4 wks; dose and dosing frequency are individualized based on body weight and pretreatment IgE level (as shown below). (Consult specific product labeling.)

**Chronic Idiopathic Urticaria**
**SQ: ADULTS, CHILDREN 12 YRS AND OLDER:** 150 mg or 300 mg q4wks. Dosing not dependent on IgE level or body weight.

**Dosage in Renal/Hepatic Impairment**
No dose adjustment.

**4-Wk Dosing Table**

| Pretreatment Serum IgE Levels (units/ml) | Weight 30–60 kg | Weight 61–70 kg | Weight 71–90 kg | Weight 91–150 kg |
|---|---|---|---|---|
| 30–100 | 150 mg | 150 mg | 150 mg | 300 mg |
| 101–200 | 300 mg | 300 mg | 300 mg | See next table |
| 201–300 | 300 mg | See next table | See next table | See next table |

**2-Wk Dosing Table**

| Pretreatment Serum IgE Levels (units/ml) | Weight 30–60 kg | Weight 61–70 kg | Weight 71–90 kg | Weight 91–150 kg |
|---|---|---|---|---|
| 101–200 | See preceding table | See preceding table | See preceding table | 225 mg |
| 201–300 | See preceding table | 225 mg | 225 mg | 300 mg |
| 301–400 | 225 mg | 225 mg | 300 mg | Do not dose |
| 401–500 | 300 mg | 300 mg | 375 mg | Do not dose |
| 501–600 | 300 mg | 375 mg | Do not dose | Do not dose |
| 601–700 | 375 mg | Do not dose | Do not dose | Do not dose |

## SIDE EFFECTS

**Frequent (45%–11%):** Injection site ecchymosis, redness, warmth, stinging, urticaria, viral infection, sinusitis, headache, pharyngitis. **Occasional (8%–3%):** Arthralgia, leg pain, fatigue, dizziness. **Rare (2%):** Arm pain, earache, dermatitis, pruritus.

## ADVERSE EFFECTS/ TOXIC REACTIONS

Anaphylaxis, occurring within 2 hrs of first dose or subsequent doses, occurs in 0.1% of pts. Malignant neoplasms occur in 0.5% of pts.

## NURSING CONSIDERATIONS

### BASELINE ASSESSMENT

Obtain baseline serum total IgE level before initiation of treatment (dosage is based on pretreatment levels). Drug is not for treatment of acute exacerbations of asthma, acute bronchospasm, status asthmaticus.

### INTERVENTION/EVALUATION

Monitor rate, depth, rhythm, type of respirations, quality/rate of pulse. Assess lung sounds for rhonchi, wheezing, rales. Observe lips, fingernails for cyanosis.

### PATIENT/FAMILY TEACHING

• Increase fluid intake (decreases viscosity of pulmonary secretions). • Do not alter/stop other asthma medications. • Report allergic reactions (e.g., breathing difficulty, swelling of throat/tongue).

# ombitasvir, paritaprevir, ritonavir

om-**bit**-as-vir/**par**-i-ta-pre-vir/rit-**oh**-na-vir
(Technivie)
**Do not confuse ombitasvir with daclatasvir, or paritaprevir with boceprevir or simeprevir, or ritonavir with Retrovir, lopinavir, darunavir, or saquinavir.**

## ◆CLASSIFICATION

**PHARMACOTHERAPEUTIC:** NS5A inhibitor, protease inhibitor, CYP3A inhibitor. **CLINICAL:** Antiviral.

## USES

Treatment of genotype 4 chronic hepatitis C virus (HCV) infection without cirrhosis, in combination with ribavirin.

## PRECAUTIONS

**Contraindications:** Hypersensitivity to any component. Severe hepatic impairment; decompensated hepatic cirrhosis; contraindication or known hypersensitivity to ribavirin; concomitant use of strong or moderate CYP3A inducers; drugs highly dependent on CYP3A for clearance and for which elevated plasma concentrations are associated with serious and/or life-threatening events. Concurrent use of alfuzosin, carbamazepine, efavirenz, ergotamine, dihydroergotamine, ethinyl estradiol–containing drugs including combined oral contraceptives, lovastatin, midazolam (oral), phenytoin, phenobarbital, pimozide, rifampin, sildenafil (when used to treat pulmonary arterial hypertension), simvastatin, St. John's wort, triazolam. **Cautions:** History of anemia, hepatitis B virus infection, HIV infection. Not recommended in pts with moderate hepatic impairment.

## ACTION

Ombitasvir inhibits HCV NS5A needed for viral RNA replication and virion assembly. Paritaprevir inhibits HCV protease needed for cleavage of HCV-encoded polyproteins and viral replication. Ritonavir inhibits CYP3A clearance; increases plasma concentrations of paritaprevir. **Therapeutic Effect:** Inhibits viral replication of hepatitis C virus.

## PHARMACOKINETICS

Readily absorbed. Paritaprevir and ritonavir metabolized in liver. Ombitasvir metabolized by amide hydrolysis. Protein binding: ombitasvir: greater than 99%, paritaprevir: 97%–99%, ritonavir: 99%. Peak plasma concentration: 4–5 hrs. Steady-state concentration: 12 days. Elimination: ombitasvir: feces (92%), urine (2%); paritaprevir: feces (88%), urine (9%); ritonavir: feces (86%), urine (11%). **Half-life:** ombitasvir: 21–25 hrs; paritaprevir: 5.5 hrs; ritonavir: 4 hrs.

## ⌛ LIFESPAN CONSIDERATIONS

**Pregnancy/Lactation:** Avoid pregnancy; may cause fetal harm. When administered with ribavirin, therapy is contraindicated in pregnant women and in men whose female partners are pregnant. Unknown if distributed in breastmilk. Concomitant use of ethinyl estradiol–containing drugs are contraindicated. Alternative contraception methods including progestin-only drugs, barrier methods, abstinence are recommended. **Children:** Safety and efficacy not established in

pts younger than 18 yrs. **Elderly:** No age-related precautions noted.

## INTERACTIONS

**DRUG:** May increase concentration/effects of **antiarrhythmics** (e.g., **amiodarone, quinidine**), **antifungals** (e.g., **itraconazole**), **calcium channel blockers** (e.g., **amlodipine, nifedipine**), **corticosteroids** (e.g., **fluticasone**), **immunosuppressants** (e.g., **cyclosporine**), **digoxin, HIV-antiretrovirals** (e.g., **paritaprevir, rilpivirine**), **phosphodiesterase-5 inhibitors** (e.g., **sildenafil**), **sedative/hypnotics** (e.g., **midazolam, triazolam**), **statins** (e.g., **atorvastatin, simvastatin**), **sirolimus, tacrolimus. Anticonvulsants** (e.g., **carbamazepine, phenytoin**), **dexamethasone, efavirenz, omeprazole, rifampin** may decrease concentration/effect. **HERBAL: St. John's wort, garlic** may decrease concentration/effect. **Kava kava** may increase risk of hepatotoxicity. **Red yeast** may increase risk of myopathy, rhabdomyolysis. **FOOD: Grapefruit products, Seville oranges** may increase concentration/effect. **LAB VALUES:** May increase serum alkaline phosphatase, ALT, INR. May decrease Hct, Hgb.

## AVAILABILITY (Rx)

**Fixed-Dose Combination Tablets:** ombitasvir 12.5 mg/paritaprevir 75 mg/ritonavir 50 mg.

## ADMINISTRATION/HANDLING

**PO**
• Give with food.

## INDICATIONS/ROUTES/DOSAGE

**Hepatitis C Virus Infection (Genotype 4)**
**PO: ADULTS, ELDERLY:** 2 tablets once daily, in combination with ribavirin for 12 wks. Therapy without ribavirin may be considered if unable to tolerate ribavirin. **Recommended dose of ribavirin based on weight in kg:** Less than 75 kg: 1,000 mg/day in 2 divided doses. 75 kg or greater: 1,200 mg/day in 2 divided doses. For ribavirin dose modifications, refer to prescribing information.

**Dosage in Hepatic Impairment**
**Mild impairment:** No dose adjustment.
**Moderate to severe impairment:** Contraindicated. Avoid use in cirrhosis.

**Dosage in Renal Impairment**
No dose adjustment.

## SIDE EFFECTS

**Frequent (29%):** Asthenia. **Occasional (15%–7%):** Fatigue, nausea, insomnia, pruritus, rash, erythema, eczema, allergic dermatitis, photosensitivity reaction, urticaria, skin exfoliation, skin ulcer.

## ADVERSE EFFECTS/TOXIC REACTIONS

Serum ALT greater than 5 times upper limit of normal (ULN) reported in 1% of pts (usually occurred during the first 4 wks of treatment). Elevations of serum ALT were significantly higher in female pts using ethinyl estradiol–containing drugs such as contraceptive patches, combined oral contraceptives, vaginal rings. May increase risk of drug resistance in HCV/HIV-1 co-infected pts using HIV-1 protease inhibitors. Hypersensitivity reactions including angioedema may occur.

## NURSING CONSIDERATIONS

### BASELINE ASSESSMENT

Obtain baseline CBC, LFT, HCV-RNA level, urine pregnancy. Confirm HCV genotype. Receive full medication history and screen for contraindications/interactions. Ethinyl estradiol–containing contraceptive drugs should be discontinued prior to initiation. Question history of hepatic impairment, HIV. To reduce risk of HIV-1 protease inhibitor drug resistance, consider suppressive antiretroviral drug therapy upon initiation.

### INTERVENTION/EVALUATION

Monitor LFT periodically during the first 4 wks of treatment, then as clinically indicated thereafter. Discontinue treatment for serum ALT persistently greater than

10 times ULN; serum ALT elevation associated with increase in serum alkaline phosphatase, bilirubin, INR; hepatic injury. Periodically monitor CBC for anemia, HCV-RNA level for treatment effectiveness. Reinforce birth control compliance. Monitor for abdominal pain, bruising, jaundice, nausea, vomiting; may indicate hepatic injury. Ethinyl estradiol–containing contraceptives may be restarted approx. 2 wks after discontinuation.

### PATIENT/FAMILY TEACHING

• Treatment must be used in combination with ribavirin. • Take with meals. • Inform pt of contraindications/adverse effects of therapy. • Do not take newly prescribed medication unless approved by doctor who originally started treatment. Do not take herbal products. • Pregnancy should be avoided when combination regimen is given with ribavirin. Females pts of childbearing potential must use reliable forms of birth control such as progestin-containing contraception, barrier methods, abstinence. Immediately report suspected pregnancy. Do not breastfeed. • Report abdominal pain, bruising easily, dark-colored urine, fatigue, yellowing of the skin or eyes. • Avoid alcohol. • Report skin changes such as rash, peeling, ulcers; allergic reactions such as difficulty breathing, itching, hives, tongue swelling.

O

# ombitasvir, paritaprevir, ritonavir, dasabuvir

om-**bit**-as-vir/**par**-i-**ta**-pre-vir/
rit-**oh**-na-vir/da-**sa**-bue-vir
(Viekira Pak, Viekira XR)
**Do not confuse ombitasvir with daclatasvir, or paritaprevir with boceprevir or simeprevir, or ritonavir with Retrovir, lopinavir, darunavir, or saquinavir, or dasabuvir with sofosbuvir.**

---

## ◆CLASSIFICATION

**PHARMACOTHERAPEUTIC:** NS5A inhibitor, protease inhibitor, CYP3A inhibitor, non-nucleoside inhibitor. **CLINICAL:** Antiviral.

## USES

Treatment of genotype 1 chronic hepatitis C virus (HCV) infection including those with compensated hepatic cirrhosis, with or without ribavirin.

## PRECAUTIONS

**Contraindications:** Hypersensitivity to any component. Severe hepatic impairment; decompensated hepatic cirrhosis; contraindication or known hypersensitivity to ribavirin; concomitant use of strong CYP3A inducers, strong CYP2C8 inducers or strong CYP2C8 inhibitors; drugs highly dependent on CYP3A for clearance and for which elevated plasma concentrations are associated with serious and/or life-threatening events. Concurrent use of alfuzosin, carbamazepine, colchicine, efavirenz, ergotamine, dihydroergotamine, ethinyl estradiol–containing drugs including combined oral contraceptives, gemfibrozil, lovastatin, midazolam (oral), phenytoin, phenobarbital, pimozide, rifampin, sildenafil (when used for pulmonary arterial hypertension), simvastatin, St. John's wort, triazolam. **Cautions:** History of anemia, hepatitis B virus infection, HIV infection. Not recommended in pts with moderate hepatic impairment.

## ACTION

Ombitasvir inhibits HCV NS5A needed for essential RNA replication and virion assembly. Paritaprevir inhibits HCV protease needed for cleavage of HCV-encoded polyproteins and viral replication. Ritonavir inhibits CYP3A clearance; increases plasma concentrations of paritaprevir. Dasabuvir inhibits HCV RNA-dependent RNA polymerase needed for replication of viral genome. **Therapeutic Effect:** Inhibits viral replication of hepatitis C virus.

## PHARMACOKINETICS

Readily absorbed. Paritaprevir, ritonavir, dasabuvir metabolized in liver. Ombitasvir metabolized by amide hydrolysis. Protein binding: ombitasvir: greater than 99%, paritaprevir: 97%–99%, ritonavir: 99%, dasabuvir: 99% Peak plasma concentration: 4–5 hrs. Steady state concentration: 12 days. Elimination: ombitasvir: feces (92%), urine (2%); paritaprevir: feces (88%), urine (9%); ritonavir: feces (86%), urine (11%); dasabuvir: feces (94%), urine (2%). **Half-life:** ombitasvir: 21–25 hrs; paritaprevir: 5.5 hrs; ritonavir: 4 hrs; dasabuvir: 5.5–6 hrs.

## ⧗ LIFESPAN CONSIDERATIONS

**Pregnancy/Lactation:** Avoid pregnancy; may cause fetal harm. When administered with ribavirin, therapy is contraindicated in pregnant women and in men whose female partners are pregnant. Unknown if distributed in breastmilk. Concomitant use of ethinyl estradiol-containing drugs are contraindicated. Alternative contraception methods including progestin-only drugs, barrier methods, abstinence are recommended. **Children:** Safety and efficacy not established in pts younger than 18 yrs. **Elderly:** No age-related precautions noted.

## INTERACTIONS

**DRUG:** May increase concentration/effects of **antiarrhythmics** (e.g., amiodarone), **antifungals** (e.g., itraconazole), **calcium channel blockers** (e.g., amlodipine, nifedipine), **corticosteroids** (e.g., fluticasone), **immunosuppressants** (e.g., cyclosporine), **digoxin**, **HIV antiretrovirals** (e.g., paritaprevir, rilpivirine), **phosphodiesterase-5 inhibitors** (e.g., sildenafil), **sedative/hypnotics** (e.g., temazepam), **statins** (e.g., atorvastatin, simvastatin), **sirolimus, tacrolimus.** Anticonvulsants (e.g., **carbamazepine, phenytoin**), **dexamethasone, efavirenz, omeprazole, rifampin** may decrease concentration/effect. **HERBAL:** **St. John's wort** may decrease concentration/effect. **Kava kava** may increase risk of hepatotoxicity. **Red yeast** may increase risk of myopathy, rhabdomyolysis. **Meals** increase absorption. **FOOD: Grapefruit products, Seville oranges** may increase concentration/effect. **LAB VALUES:** May increase serum alkaline phosphatase, ALT, INR. May decrease Hct, Hgb.

## AVAILABILITY (Rx)

**Fixed-Dose Combination Tablets (co-packaged with dasabuvir tablets): (Viekira Pak):** ombitasvir 12.5 mg/paritaprevir 75 mg/ritonavir 50 mg; dasabuvir 250 mg. **(Viekira XR):** ombitasvir 8.33 mg/ paritaprevir 50 mg, ritonavir 33.3 mg, dasabuvir 200 mg.

## ADMINISTRATION/HANDLING

### PO
• Give with food. Do not cut, crush, break, or divide XR tablets.

## INDICATIONS/ROUTES/DOSAGE

**Hepatitis C Virus Infection**
**PO: ADULTS, ELDERLY: (Viekira Pak):** 2 tablets of ombitasvir, paritaprevir, ritonavir once daily, plus 1 tablet of dasabuvir twice daily with or without ribavirin. **(Viekira XR):** 3 tablets once daily.

**Treatment Regimen and Duration**
**Genotype 1a, without cirrhosis:** Fixed combination regimen with ribavirin for 12 wks. **Genotype 1a, with cirrhosis:** Fixed combination regimen with ribavirin for 24 wks. Consider duration of 12 wks in pts with prior treatment history. **Genotype 1b, without cirrhosis:** Fixed combination regimen for 12 wks. **Genotype 1b, with cirrhosis:** Fixed combination regimen (with ribivarin) for 12 wks. **Recommended dose of ribavirin based on weight in kg: LESS THAN 75 KG:** 1,000 mg/day in 2 divided doses. **75 KG OR GREATER:** 1,200 mg/day in 2 divided doses. For ribavirin dose modifications, refer to prescribing information.

**Dose Modification**
*Liver Transplant Recipients*
**PO: ADULTS, ELDERLY:** 2 tablets of ombitasvir, paritaprevir, ritonavir once daily, plus 1 tablet of dasabuvir twice daily with ribavirin for 24 wks, irrespective of HCV genotype 1 subtype in pts with normal hepatic function and mild fibrosis.
*HCV/HIV-1 Co-infection*
Follow dose recommendations as listed in Treatment Regimen and Duration. Consider suppressive antiretroviral drug therapy during treatment.

**Dosage in Renal Impairment**
No dose adjustment.

**Dosage in Hepatic Impairment**
**Mild impairment:** No dose adjustment. **Moderate impairment:** Treatment not recommended. **Severe impairment:** Treatment contraindicated.

## SIDE EFFECTS

**Frequent (34%–22%):** Fatigue, nausea. **Occasional (18%–14%):** Pruritus, rash, erythema, eczema, allergic dermatitis, skin exfoliation, urticaria, photosensitivity reaction, skin ulcer, insomnia, asthenia.

## ADVERSE EFFECTS/TOXIC REACTIONS

Serum ALT greater than 5 times upper limit of normal (ULN) reported in 1% of pts (usually occurred during the first 4 wks of treatment). Elevations of serum ALT were significantly higher in female pts using ethinyl estradiol–containing drugs such as contraceptive patches, combined oral contraceptives, vaginal rings. May increase risk of drug resistance in HCV/ HIV-1 co-infected pts using HIV-1 protease inhibitors. Hypersensitivity reaction including angioedema may occur.

## NURSING CONSIDERATIONS

### BASELINE ASSESSMENT
Obtain baseline CBC, LFT, HCV-RNA level, urine pregnancy. Confirm HCV genotype. Receive full medication history and screen for contraindications/interactions. Ethinyl estradiol–containing contraceptive drugs should be discontinued prior to initiation. Question history of hepatic impairment, HIV.

**O**

To reduce risk of HIV-1 protease inhibitor drug resistance, consider suppressive antiretroviral drug therapy upon initiation.

**INTERVENTION/EVALUATION**

Monitor LFT periodically during the first 4 wks of treatment, then as clinically indicated thereafter. Discontinue treatment for serum ALT persistently greater than 10 times ULN; serum ALT elevation associated with increase in serum alkaline phosphatase, bilirubin, or INR; hepatic injury. Periodically monitor CBC for anemia, HCV-RNA level for treatment effectiveness. Reinforce birth control compliance. Monitor for abdominal pain, bruising, jaundice, nausea, vomiting; may indicate hepatic injury. Ethinyl estradiol–containing contraceptives may be restarted approx. 2 wks after discontinuation.

**PATIENT/FAMILY TEACHING**

• Treatment must be used in combination with ribavirin. • Take with meals. • Inform pt of contraindications/adverse effects of therapy. • Do not take newly prescribed medication unless approved by doctor who originally started treatment. Do not take herbal products. • Pregnancy should be avoided when combination regimen is given with ribavirin. Female pts of childbearing potential must use reliable forms of birth control such as progestin-containing contraception, barrier methods, abstinence. Immediately report suspected pregnancy. Do not breastfeed. • Report abdominal pain, bruising easily, dark-colored urine, fatigue, yellowing of the skin or eyes. • Avoid alcohol. • Report skin changes such as rash, peeling, ulcers; allergic reactions such as difficulty breathing, itching, hives, tongue swelling.

---

# omega-3 acid-ethyl esters

oh-**may**-ga 3 **as**-id **eth**-il **es**-ters
(Lovaza, Epanova, Omtryg, Vascepa)
**Do not confuse Lovaza with lorazepam.**

◆**CLASSIFICATION**

**PHARMACOTHERAPEUTIC:** Omega-3 fatty acid. **CLINICAL:** Antihypertriglyceride agent.

## USES

Adjunct to diet to reduce very high (500 mg/dL or higher) serum triglyceride levels in adult pts. Dietary supplement for pts with early risk of CAD. **OFF-LABEL:** Treatment of IgA nephropathy.

## PRECAUTIONS

**Contraindications:** Hypersensitivity to omega-3 fatty acids. **Cautions:** Known sensitivity, allergy to fish.

## ACTION

Inhibits esterification of fatty acids, prevents hepatic enzymes from catalyzing final step of triglyceride synthesis. **Therapeutic Effect:** Reduces serum triglyceride levels.

## PHARMACOKINETICS

Well absorbed following PO administration. Incorporated into phospholipids. **Half-life:** N/A.

## ⧗ LIFESPAN CONSIDERATIONS

**Pregnancy/Lactation:** Unknown if distributed in breast milk. **Children:** Safety and efficacy not established in pts younger than 18 yrs. **Elderly:** No age-related precautions noted.

## INTERACTIONS

**DRUG:** May increase bleeding time with **anticoagulants (e.g., heparin, warfarin). HERBAL:** None significant. **FOOD:** None known. **LAB VALUES:** May increase serum ALT, LDL.

## AVAILABILITY (Rx)

**Capsules:** 200 mg, 300 mg, 500 mg, 600 mg, 1000 mg, 1,200 mg.

## ADMINISTRATION/HANDLING

**PO**

• Give without regard to meals.

## INDICATIONS/ROUTES/DOSAGE

◄**ALERT►** Before initiating therapy, pt should be on standard cholesterol-lowering diet for minimum of 3–6 mos. Continue diet throughout therapy.

**Usual Dosage**
**PO: ADULTS, ELDERLY:** 4 g/day, given as a single dose (4 capsules), or 2 capsules twice daily.

**Dosage in Renal/Hepatic Impairment**
No dose adjustment.

## SIDE EFFECTS

**Occasional (5%–3%):** Eructation, altered taste, dyspepsia. **Rare (2%–1%):** Rash, back pain.

## ADVERSE EFFECTS/ TOXIC REACTIONS

None known.

### NURSING CONSIDERATIONS

**BASELINE ASSESSMENT**
Assess baseline serum triglyceride level, LFT. Obtain diet history, esp. fat consumption.

**INTERVENTION/EVALUATION**
Monitor serum triglyceride levels for therapeutic response. Monitor serum ALT, LDL periodically during therapy. Discontinue therapy if no response after 2 mos of treatment.

**PATIENT/FAMILY TEACHING**
• Continue to adhere to lipid-lowering diet (important part of treatment). • Periodic lab tests are essential part of therapy to determine drug effectiveness.

---

# omeprazole

oh-**mep**-ra-zole
(Apo-Omeprazole ✖, Losec ✖, Prilosec, Prilosec OTC)
**Do not confuse omeprazole with aripiprazole, pantoprazole or esomeprazole, or Prilosec**

with Plendil, Prevacid, Prinivil, or Prozac.

## FIXED-COMBINATION(S)

**Yosprala:** omeprazole/aspirin (a platelet aggregation inhibitor): 40 mg/81 mg, 40 mg/325 mg. **Zegerid:** omeprazole/sodium bicarbonate (an antacid): 20 mg/1,100 mg, 40 mg/ 1,100 mg. **Zegerid Powder:** 20 mg/ 1,680 mg, 40 mg/1,680 mg.

## ◆CLASSIFICATION

**PHARMACOTHERAPEUTIC:** Benz-imidazole. **CLINICAL:** Proton pump inhibitor.

## USES

Short-term treatment (4–8 wks) of erosive esophagitis (diagnosed by endoscopy), symptomatic gastroesophageal reflux disease (GERD) poorly responsive to other treatment. *H. pylori*–associated duodenal ulcer (with amoxicillin and clarithromycin). Long-term treatment of pathologic hypersecretory conditions, treatment of active duodenal ulcer or active benign gastric ulcer. Maintenance healing of erosive esophagitis. **OTC, short-term:** Treatment of frequent, uncomplicated heartburn occurring 2 or more days/wk. **OFF-LABEL:** Prevention/treatment of NSAID-induced ulcers, stress ulcer prophylaxis in critically ill pts.

## PRECAUTIONS

**Contraindications:** Hypersensitivity to omeprazole, other proton pump inhibitors. **Cautions:** May increase risk of fractures, gastrointestinal infections. Hepatic impairment, pts of Asian descent.

## ACTION

Inhibits hydrogen-potassium adenosine triphosphatase ($H^+/K^+$ ATP pump), an enzyme on the surface of gastric parietal cells. **Therapeutic Effect:** Increases gastric pH, reduces gastric acid production.

O

---

✖ Canadian trade name          🗡 Non-Crushable Drug          🔲 High Alert drug

## PHARMACOKINETICS

| Route | Onset | Peak | Duration |
|-------|-------|------|----------|
| PO | 1 hr | 2 hrs | 72 hrs |

Rapidly absorbed from GI tract. Protein binding: 95%. Primarily distributed into gastric parietal cells. Metabolized in liver. Primarily excreted in urine. Unknown if removed by hemodialysis. **Half-life:** 0.5–1 hr (increased in hepatic impairment).

## ⧗ LIFESPAN CONSIDERATIONS

**Pregnancy/Lactation:** Unknown if drug crosses placenta or is distributed in breast milk. **Children:** Safety and efficacy not established. **Elderly:** No age-related precautions noted.

## INTERACTIONS

**DRUG:** May decrease concentration/ effects of **atazanavir, clopidogrel.** May increase concentration/effects of **diazepam, oral anticoagulants (e.g., warfarin), phenytoin.** **HERBAL:** **St. John's wort** may decrease concentration/ effects. **FOOD:** None known. **LAB VALUES:** May increase serum alkaline phosphatase, ALT, AST.

## AVAILABILITY (Rx)

**Granules for Oral Suspension:** 2.5 mg/ packet, 10 mg/packet. **Powder for Oral Suspension:** 2 mg/ml.

🖊 **Capsules (Delayed-Release [Prilosec]):** 10 mg, 20 mg, 40 mg. 🖊 **Tablets (Delayed-Release [Prilosec OTC]):** 20 mg.

## ADMINISTRATION/HANDLING

**PO**
• Give before meals (breakfast preferred). • Give whole. Do not break, crush, dissolve, or divide delayed-release forms. • May open capsule, mix with applesauce and give immediately.

**PO (Suspension)**
• Following reconstitution, allow to thicken (2–3 min). • Administer within 30 min.

## INDICATIONS/ROUTES/DOSAGE

**Active Duodenal Ulcer**
**PO: ADULTS, ELDERLY:** 20 mg/day for 4–8 wks.

**Symptomatic GERD**
**PO: ADULTS, ELDERLY, CHILDREN WEIGHING 20 KG OR MORE:** 20 mg/day for up to 4 wks. **10–19 KG:** 10 mg/day. **5–9 KG:** 5 mg/day.

**Erosive Esophagitis**
**PO: ADULTS, ELDERLY:** 20 mg/day for 4–8 wks. **Maintenance:** 20 mg/day for up to 12 mos (including treatment period).

**Pathologic Hypersecretory Conditions**
**Note:** Doses more than 80 mg in divided doses. **PO: ADULTS, ELDERLY:** Initially, 60 mg/day up to 120 mg 3 times/day.

**H. Pylori Duodenal Ulcer**
**PO: ADULTS, ELDERLY:** 40 mg once daily (with clarithromycin) for 14 days or 20 mg twice daily (with amoxicillin and clarithromycin) for 10 days. Presence of ulcer at initiation may need 20 mg/day (monotherapy) for 14–18 days following combination therapy.

**Gastric Ulcer**
**PO: ADULTS, ELDERLY:** 40 mg/day for 4–8 wks.

**OTC Use (Frequent Heartburn)**
**PO: ADULTS, ELDERLY:** 20 mg/day for 14 days. May repeat after 4 mos if needed.

**Dosage in Renal/Hepatic Impairment**
No dose adjustment.

## SIDE EFFECTS

**Frequent (7%):** Headache. **Occasional (3%–2%):** Diarrhea, abdominal pain, nausea. **Rare (2%):** Dizziness, asthenia (loss of strength, energy), vomiting, constipation, upper respiratory tract infection, back pain, rash, cough.

## ADVERSE EFFECTS/ TOXIC REACTIONS

Pancreatitis, hepatotoxicity, interstitial nephritis occur rarely.

---

underlined – top prescribed drug

## NURSING CONSIDERATIONS

### INTERVENTION/EVALUATION
Evaluate for therapeutic response (relief of GI symptoms). Question if GI discomfort, nausea, diarrhea occurs.

### PATIENT/FAMILY TEACHING
• Report headache, onset of black, tarry stools, diarrhea, abdominal pain. • Avoid alcohol. • Swallow capsules whole; do not chew, crush, dissolve, or divide. • Take before eating.

---

# ondansetron

on-**dan**-se-tron
(Apo-Ondansetron ❦, Zofran, Zofran ODT, Zuplenz)
**Do not confuse ondansetron with dolasetron, granisetron, or palonosetron, or Zofran with Zantac or Zosyn.**

## ◆CLASSIFICATION

**PHARMACOTHERAPEUTIC:** Selective serotonin and 5-HT₃ receptor antagonist. **CLINICAL:** Antinausea, antiemetic.

## USES
Prevention/treatment of nausea/vomiting due to cancer chemotherapy (including high-dose cisplatin). Prevention and treatment of postop nausea, vomiting. Prevention of radiation-induced nausea, vomiting. **OFF-LABEL:** Breakthrough treatment of nausea and vomiting associated with chemotherapy, hyperemesis gravidarum.

## PRECAUTIONS
**Contraindications:** Hypersensitivity to ondansetron, other $HT_3$ antagonists. Use of apomorphine. **Cautions:** Mild to moderate hepatic impairment, pts at risk for QT prolongation or ventricular arrhythmia (congenital long QT prolongation, medications prolonging QT interval, hypokalemia, hypomagnesemia).

## ACTION
Blocks serotonin, both peripherally on vagal nerve terminals and centrally in chemoreceptor trigger zone. **Therapeutic Effect:** Prevents nausea/vomiting.

## PHARMACOKINETICS
Readily absorbed from GI tract. Protein binding: 70%–76%. Metabolized in liver. Primarily excreted in urine. Unknown if removed by hemodialysis. **Half-life:** 3–6 hrs (increased in hepatic impairment).

## ⧗ LIFESPAN CONSIDERATIONS
**Pregnancy/Lactation:** Unknown if drug crosses placenta or is distributed in breast milk. **Children:** Safety and efficacy not established. **Elderly:** No age-related precautions noted.

## INTERACTIONS
**DRUG: Apomorphine** may cause profound hypotension, altered LOC. **HERBAL: St. John's wort** may decrease concentration. **FOOD:** None known. **LAB VALUES:** May transiently increase serum bilirubin, ALT, AST.

## AVAILABILITY (Rx)
**Injection Solution (Zofran):** 2 mg/ml. **Oral Soluble Film (Zuplenz):** 4 mg, 8 mg. **Oral Solution (Zofran):** 4 mg/5 ml. **Tablets (Zofran):** 4 mg, 8 mg, 24 mg. **Tablets (Orally Disintegrating [Zofran ODT]):** 4 mg, 8 mg.

## ADMINISTRATION/HANDLING
 IV

**Reconstitution** • May give undiluted. • For IV infusion, dilute with 50 ml D₅W or 0.9% NaCl before administration. **Rate of Administration** • Give IV push over 2–5 min. • Give IV infusion over 15–30 min. **Storage** • Store at room temperature. • Stable for 48 hrs at room temperature following dilution.

---

❦ Canadian trade name        Non-Crushable Drug        High Alert drug

**IM**
• Inject undiluted into large muscle mass.

**PO**
• Give without regard to food.

**Orally Disintegrating Tablets**
• Do not remove from blister until needed. • Peel backing off; do not push through. • Place tablet on tongue; allow to dissolve. • Swallow with saliva.

**Oral Soluble Film**
• Keep film in pouch until ready to use. • Remove film strip from pouch and place on top of tongue, allow to dissolve. • Swallow after film dissolves. Do not chew or swallow film whole. • If using more than one, each should be allowed to dissolve before administering the next one.

### ▨ IV INCOMPATIBILITIES

Acyclovir (Zovirax), allopurinol (Aloprim), amphotericin B (Fungizone), amphotericin B complex (Abelcet, AmBisome, Amphotec), ampicillin (Polycillin), ampicillin and sulbactam (Unasyn), cefepime (Maxipime), 5-fluorouracil, lorazepam (Ativan), meropenem (Merrem IV), methylprednisolone (Solu-Medrol).

### ▨ IV COMPATIBILITIES

Carboplatin (Paraplatin), cisplatin (Platinol), cyclophosphamide (Cytoxan), cytarabine (Cytosar), dacarbazine (DTIC-Dome), daunorubicin (Cerubidine), dexmedetomidine (Precedex), dexamethasone (Decadron), diphenhydramine (Benadryl), docetaxel (Taxotere), dopamine (Intropin), etoposide (VePesid), gemcitabine (Gemzar), heparin, hydromorphone (Dilaudid), ifosfamide (Ifex), magnesium, mannitol, mesna (Mesnex), methotrexate, metoclopramide (Reglan), mitomycin (Mutamycin), mitoxantrone (Novantrone), morphine, paclitaxel (Taxol), potassium chloride, teniposide (Vumon), topotecan (Hycamtin), vinblastine (Velban), vincristine (Oncovin), vinorelbine (Navelbine).

### INDICATIONS/ROUTES/DOSAGE

**Chemotherapy-Induced Nausea/Vomiting**
**IV: ADULTS, ELDERLY, CHILDREN 6 MOS AND OLDER:** 0.15 mg/kg (**maximum:** 16 mg/dose) 3 times/day beginning 30 min before chemotherapy, followed by subsequent doses 4 and 8 hrs after the first dose.
**PO: ADULTS, ELDERLY, CHILDREN 12 YRS AND OLDER:** (highly emetogenic) 24 mg 30 min before start of chemotherapy, (moderately emetogenic) 8 mg repeat dose 8 hrs after initial dose, then q12h beginning 30 min before chemotherapy and continuing for 1–2 days after completion of chemotherapy. **CHILDREN 4–11 YRS:** 4 mg 30 min before chemotherapy, repeat 4 and 8 hrs after initial dose then q8h for 1–2 days after chemotherapy completed.

**Prevention of Postop Nausea/Vomiting**
**IV, IM: ADULTS, ELDERLY, CHILDREN OLDER THAN 12 YRS:** 4 mg as a single dose. **CHILDREN 1 MO–12 YRS, WEIGHING MORE THAN 40 KG:** 4 mg as a single dose. **CHILDREN 1 MO–12 YRS, WEIGHING 40 KG OR LESS:** 0.1 mg/kg as a single dose.
**PO: ADULTS, ELDERLY:** 16 mg 1 hr before induction of anesthesia.

**Prevention of Radiation-Induced Nausea/Vomiting**
**PO: ADULTS, ELDERLY:** (total body irradiation) 8 mg 1–2 hrs daily before each fraction of radiotherapy, (single high-dose radiotherapy to abdomen) 8 mg 1–2 hrs before irradiation, then 8 mg q8h after first dose for 1–2 days after completion of radiotherapy (daily fractionated radiotherapy to abdomen) 8 mg 1–2 hrs before irradiation, then 8 mg 8 hrs after first dose for each day of radiotherapy. **Zuplenz:** 8 mg q8h.

**Dosage in Renal Impairment**
No dose adjustment.

**Dosage in Hepatic Impairment**
**Mild to moderate impairment:** No dose adjustment. **Severe impairment: Maximum daily dose:** 8 mg.

## SIDE EFFECTS

**Frequent (13%–5%):** Anxiety, dizziness, drowsiness, headache, fatigue, constipation, diarrhea, hypoxia, urinary retention. **Occasional (4%–2%):** Abdominal pain, xerostomia, fever, feeling of cold, redness/pain at injection site, paresthesia, asthenia (loss of strength, energy). **Rare (1%):** Hypersensitivity reaction (rash, pruritus), blurred vision.

## ADVERSE EFFECTS/ TOXIC REACTIONS

Hypertension, acute renal failure, GI bleeding, respiratory depression, coma, extrapyramidal effects occur rarely.

## NURSING CONSIDERATIONS

### BASELINE ASSESSMENT

Assess degree of nausea, vomiting. Assess for dehydration if excessive vomiting occurs (poor skin turgor, dry mucous membranes, longitudinal furrows in tongue). Provide emotional support.

### INTERVENTION/EVALUATION

Monitor EKG in pts with electrolyte abnormalities (e.g., hypokalemia, hypomagnesemia), HF, bradyarrhythmias, concurrent use of other medications that may cause QT prolongation, pts receiving high doses or frequent doses. Provide supportive measures. Assess mental status. Assess bowel sounds for peristalsis. Monitor daily pattern of bowel activity, stool consistency. Record time of evacuation.

### PATIENT/FAMILY TEACHING

• Relief from nausea/vomiting generally occurs shortly after drug administration. • Avoid alcohol, barbiturates. • Report persistent vomiting. • Avoid tasks that require alertness, motor skills until response to drug is established (may cause drowsiness, dizziness).

# oritavancin

or-**it**-a-van-sin
(Orbactiv)
**Do not confuse oritavancin with dalbavancin or telavancin.**

## ◆ CLASSIFICATION

**PHARMACOTHERAPEUTIC:** Lipoglycopeptide (antibacterial). **CLINICAL:** Antibiotic (bactericidal).

## USES

Treatment of adult pts with acute bacterial skin and skin structure infections (ABSSSI) caused by susceptible strains of gram-positive microorganisms including *Staphylococcus aureus* (including methicillin-susceptible and methicillin-resistant strains), *Streptococcus agalactiae*, *Streptococcus anginosus* group (including *S. anginosus*, *S. intermedius*, *S. constellatus*), *Streptococcus dysgalactiae*, *Streptococcus pyogenes*, and *Enterococcus faecalis* (vancomycin-susceptible strains only).

## PRECAUTIONS

**Contraindications:** Hypersensitivity to oritavancin. Concomitant use of IV unfractionated heparin sodium within 48 hrs of oritavancin dose. **Cautions:** Severe hepatic impairment, history of hypersensitivity reaction to glycopeptides (e.g., vancomycin), recent *Clostridium difficile* infection or antibiotic-associated colitis.

## ACTION

Inhibits cell wall synthesis by binding to bacterial cell membrane, disrupting membrane integrity. **Therapeutic Effect:** Bactericidal.

## PHARMACOKINETICS

Widely distributed. Not metabolized. Protein binding: 85%. Eliminated unchanged in feces, urine. Not removed by hemodialysis. **Half-life:** 10.2 days.

O

---

## ⧗ LIFESPAN CONSIDERATIONS

**Pregnancy/Lactation:** Unknown if distributed in breast milk. **Children:** Safety and efficacy not established in pts younger than 18 yrs. **Elderly:** No age-related precautions noted.

## INTERACTIONS

**DRUG:** Use of **heparin** within 48 hrs of dose contraindicated. May increase risk of bleeding with **warfarin. Concomitant use of other antibiotics** may increase risk of antibiotic-associated colitis. **HERBAL:** None significant. **FOOD:** None known. **LAB VALUES:** May prolong aPTT, PT/INR. May increase ALT, AST, bilirubin, uric acid. May decrease glucose.

## AVAILABILITY (Rx)

**Sterile Powder for Injection:** 400 mg/vial.

## ADMINISTRATION/HANDLING

 IV

◀**ALERT**▶ No preservatives or bacteriostatic agent is present in product. Aseptic technique must be used when preparing solution. Must be reconstituted with Sterile Water for Injection and subsequently diluted with 5% Dextrose in Water only.
**Reconstitution** • Obtain three 400-mg vials to equal required 1,200-mg dose. • Add 40 ml of Sterile Water for Injection to each vial for final concentration of 10 mg/ml per vial. • To avoid foaming, gently swirl until contents completely dissolved. • Visually inspect each vial for particulate matter or discoloration.
**Dilution** • Using D₅W, withdraw 120 ml from 1,000-ml bag and discard. • Withdraw 40 ml from each vial and mix into D₅W to provide a final concentration of 1.2 mg/ml.
**Rate of Administration** • Administer over 3 hrs.
**Storage** • Reconstituted solution should appear clear, colorless to pale yellow. • Infuse diluted solution within 6 hrs when stored at room temperature or 12 hrs when refrigerated. • Combined storage time and 3 hr infusion time should not exceed 6 hrs if at room temperature or 12 hrs if refrigerated.

## ▨ IV INCOMPATIBILITIES

Dilute using 5% Dextrose in Water only. Dilution with normal saline may cause precipitate formation. Infuse via dedicated line only. Do not piggyback through maintenance IV line.

## INDICATIONS/ROUTES/DOSAGE

**Acute Bacterial Skin and Skin Structure Infection**
**IV: ADULTS, ELDERLY:** 1,200 mg as single dose.

**Dosage in Renal/Hepatic Impairment**
**Mild to moderate impairment:** No dose adjustment. **Severe impairment:** Use caution.

## SIDE EFFECTS

**Occasional (10%–5%):** Nausea, headache, vomiting. **Rare (4%–3%):** Diarrhea, dizziness, tachycardia.

## ADVERSE EFFECTS/TOXIC REACTIONS

Serious hypersensitivity reactions including anaphylaxis, angioedema, bronchospasm, severe skin reactions, wheezing have been reported with glycopeptide antibacterial agents. *C. difficile*–associated diarrhea with severity ranging from mild diarrhea to fatal colitis has occurred. Treatment in the absence of proven or strongly suspected bacterial infection may increase risk of drug-resistant bacteria. Infusion site reactions phlebitis, irritation, abscess, rash, pruritus have occurred. Increased incidence of osteomyelitis has been reported.

## NURSING CONSIDERATIONS

### BASELINE ASSESSMENT

Obtain baseline CBC (WBC), BMP, LFT, wound culture and sensitivity, vital signs. Question history of recent *C. difficile* infection, hepatic/renal impairment, hypersensitivity reaction. Assess skin wound characteristics, hydration status. Question pt's usual stool characteristics (color, frequency, consistency).

### INTERVENTION/EVALUATION

Assess skin infection/wound for improvement. Monitor daily pattern of bowel activity, stool consistency; increasing severity may indicate antibiotic-associated colitis. If frequent diarrhea occurs, obtain *C. difficile* toxin screen and initiate isolation precautions until result confirmed. Encourage PO intake. Monitor I&O. If osteomyelitis suspected, other antimicrobial agents may be required. Screen for hypersensitivity reaction.

### PATIENT/FAMILY TEACHING

• Treatment will consist of a single infusion only. • Report episodes of diarrhea, esp. following weeks after treatment completion. Frequent diarrhea, fever, abdominal pain, blood-streaked stool may indicate *C. difficile* infection, which may be contagious to others. • Report abdominal pain, black/tarry stools, bruising, yellowing of skin or eyes; dark urine, decreased urine output; or allergic reactions including difficulty breathing, itching, hives, tongue swelling, wheezing • Do not breastfeed. • Drink plenty of fluids. • Report symptoms of bone pain; may indicate bone infection.

# orlistat

or-lye-stat
(Alli, Xenical)
**Do not confuse Xenical with Xeloda.**

### ◆CLASSIFICATION

**PHARMACOTHERAPEUTIC:** Gastric/pancreatic lipase inhibitor. **CLINICAL:** Obesity management agent.

## USES

Management of obesity, including weight loss/maintenance, when used in conjunction with reduced-calorie diet. Reduces risk of weight regain after previous weight loss. Indicated for pts with initial BMI of 30 kg/m$^2$ or greater or 27 kg/m$^2$ or greater with other risk factors (e.g., diabetes, dyslipidemia, hypertension).

## PRECAUTIONS

**Contraindications:** Hypersensitivity to orlistat. Cholestasis, chronic malabsorption syndrome, pregnancy. **Cautions:** History of hyperoxaluria or calcium oxalate nephrolithiasis.

## ACTION

Inhibits absorption of dietary fats by inhibiting gastric and pancreatic lipases. **Therapeutic Effect:** Resulting caloric deficit may have positive effects on weight control.

## PHARMACOKINETICS

Minimal absorption after administration. Protein binding: 99%. Metabolized within GI wall. Primarily eliminated in feces. Unknown if removed by hemodialysis. **Half-life:** 1–2 hrs.

## ⧗ LIFESPAN CONSIDERATIONS

**Pregnancy/Lactation:** Unknown if distributed in breast milk. Not recommended during pregnancy. Breastfeeding not recommended. **Children:** Safety and efficacy not established. **Elderly:** No age-related precautions noted.

## INTERACTIONS

**DRUG:** May decrease concentration/effects of **cyclosporine, levothyroxine.** May reduce absorption of **vitamin E.** May alter effect of **warfarin** by altering vitamin K level. **HERBAL:** None significant. **FOOD:** None known. **LAB VALUES:** May decrease serum glucose, cholesterol, LDL.

## AVAILABILITY (Rx)

**Capsules (Alli):** 60 mg. **(Xenical):** 120 mg.

O

---

## ADMINISTRATION/HANDLING

**PO**

• Multivitamin supplements containing fat-soluble vitamins should be taken once daily at least 2 hrs before or after taking orlistat. • Distribute daily fat intake over 3 main meals (GI effects may increase when taken with any 1 meal very high in fat). Administer during or up to 1 hr after each meal containing fat.

## INDICATIONS/ROUTES/DOSAGE

**Weight Reduction**
**PO: ADULTS, ELDERLY, CHILDREN 12–16 YRS:**
*(Xenical):* 120 mg 3 times/day. *(Alli):* 60 mg 3 times/day with each main meal containing fat (do not take if meal is occasionally missed or contains no fat).

**Dosage with Other Medication**
*(Cyclosporine):* Give 3 hrs after orlistat. *(Levothyroxine):* Give at least 4 hrs apart. Monitor thyroid function.

**Dosage in Renal/Hepatic Impairment**
No dose adjustment.

## SIDE EFFECTS

**Frequent (30%–20%):** Headache, abdominal discomfort, flatulence, fecal urgency, fatty/oily stool. **Occasional (14%–5%):** Back pain, menstrual irregularity, nausea, fatigue, diarrhea, dizziness. **Rare (Less Than 4%):** Anxiety, rash, myalgia, dry skin, vomiting.

## ADVERSE EFFECTS/ TOXIC REACTIONS

Hypersensitivity reaction occurs rarely.

### NURSING CONSIDERATIONS

**BASELINE ASSESSMENT**
Obtain baseline laboratory tests. Obtain pt weight.

**INTERVENTION/EVALUATION**
Monitor serum cholesterol, LDL, glucose, changes in coagulation parameters. Monitor weight wkly.

**PATIENT/FAMILY TEACHING**
• Maintain nutritionally balanced, reduced-calorie diet. • Daily intake of fat, carbohydrates, protein to be distributed over 3 main meals.

# oseltamivir

TOP 100

oh-sel-**tam**-i-veer
(Tamiflu)
**Do not confuse Tamiflu with Thera-flu.**

## ◆CLASSIFICATION

**PHARMACOTHERAPEUTIC:** Neuraminidase inhibitor. **CLINICAL:** Antiviral.

## USES

Symptomatic treatment of uncomplicated acute illness caused by influenza A or B virus in adults and children 2 wks of age and older who are symptomatic no longer than 2 days. Prevention of influenza in adults, children 3 mos and older.

## PRECAUTIONS

**Contraindications:** Hypersensitivity to oseltamivir. **Cautions:** Renal impairment.

## ACTION

Selective inhibitor of influenza virus neuraminidase, an enzyme essential for viral replication. Acts against influenza A and B viruses. **Therapeutic Effect:** Suppresses spread of infection within respiratory system, reduces duration of clinical symptoms.

## PHARMACOKINETICS

Readily absorbed after PO administration. Protein binding: 3%. Metabolized in liver. Primarily excreted in urine. **Half-life:** 6–10 hrs.

## ⧗ LIFESPAN CONSIDERATIONS

**Pregnancy/Lactation:** Unknown if distributed in breast milk. **Children:** Safety and efficacy not established in pts younger than 1 yr. **Elderly:** No age-related precautions noted.

## INTERACTIONS

**DRUG: Live attenuated influenza virus vaccine intranasal** may interfere with effect. **HERBAL:** None significant. **FOOD:** None known. **LAB VALUES:** None significant.

## AVAILABILITY (Rx)

**Capsules:** 30 mg, 45 mg, 75 mg. **Powder for Oral Suspension:** 6 mg/ml.

## ADMINISTRATION/HANDLING

**PO**

• Give without regard to food. • May open capsules and mix with sweetened liquid. • Oral suspension stable for 10 days following reconstitution.

## INDICATIONS/ROUTES/DOSAGE

**Treatment of Influenza**

**Note:** Hospitalized pts may require longer treatment course. Initiate within 48 hrs of onset of symptoms. Consider duration longer than 5 days in pts with severe or complicated influenza.

**PO: ADULTS, ELDERLY, CHILDREN 13 YRS AND OLDER:** 75 mg twice daily for 5 days. **CHILDREN 1–12 YRS, WEIGHING MORE THAN 40 KG:** 75 mg twice daily for 5 days. **CHILDREN WEIGHING 24–40 KG:** 60 mg twice daily for 5 days. **CHILDREN WEIGHING 16–23 KG:** 45 mg twice daily for 5 days. **CHILDREN WEIGHING 15 KG OR LESS:** 30 mg twice daily for 5 days. **CHILDREN 2 WKS TO YOUNGER THAN 1 YR:** 3 mg/kg twice daily for 5 days.

**Prevention of Influenza**

**Note:** Initiate within 48 hrs of contact with an infected individual. **PO: ADULTS, ELDERLY, CHILDREN 13 YRS AND OLDER:** 75 mg once daily. **CHILDREN 1–12 YRS, WEIGHING MORE THAN 40 KG:** 75 mg once daily. **WEIGHING 24–40 KG:** 60 mg once daily. **WEIGHING 15–23 KG:** 45 mg once daily. **WEIGHING LESS THAN 15 KG:** 30 mg once daily. **9–11 mos:** 3.5 mg/kg/dose. **3–8 mos:** 3 mg/kg/dose.

**Dosage in Renal Impairment**

**CrCl 31–60 ml/min:** Treatment: 30 mg twice daily. Prevention: 30 mg once daily. **CrCl 11–30 ml/min:** Treatment: 30 mg once daily. Prevention: 30 mg every other day. **End-stage renal disease:** Not recommended.

**Dosage in Hepatic Impairment**

No dose adjustment.

## SIDE EFFECTS

**Frequent (10%–7%):** Nausea, vomiting, diarrhea. **Rare (2%–1%):** Abdominal pain, bronchitis, dizziness, headache, cough, insomnia, fatigue, vertigo.

## ADVERSE EFFECTS/ TOXIC REACTIONS

Colitis, pneumonia, tympanic membrane disorder, fever occur rarely.

## NURSING CONSIDERATIONS

### BASELINE ASSESSMENT

Obtain baseline laboratory tests as indicated. Confirm presence of influenza A or B virus.

### INTERVENTION/EVALUATION

Monitor serum glucose, renal function in pts with influenza symptoms, diabetes.

### PATIENT/FAMILY TEACHING

• Begin as soon as possible from first appearance of flu symptoms (recommended within 2 days from symptom onset). • Avoid contact with those who are at high risk for influenza. • Not a substitute for flu shot.

# osimertinib

**oh**-sim-**er**-ti-nib
(Tasgrisso)
**Do not confuse osimertinib with afatinib, dasatinib, erlotinib, ibrutinib, imatinib, olaparib, or ospemifene, or Tasgrisso with Targretin or Tasigna.**

## ◆CLASSIFICATION

**PHARMACOTHERAPEUTIC:** Tyrosine kinase inhibitor (TKI). **CLINICAL:** Antineoplastic.

## USES

Treatment of pts with metastatic epidermal growth factor receptor (EGFR) T790M mutation-positive non–small-cell lung cancer (NSCLC), as detected by FDA-approved test, who have progressed on or after EGFR TKI therapy.

## PRECAUTIONS

**Contraindications:** Hypersensitivity to osimertinib. **Cautions:** Baseline anemia, lymphopenia, neutropenia, thrombocytopenia; COPD, heart disease (bradycardia, cardiomyopathy, heart block, HF, recent MI), pts at risk for QTc interval prolongation or ventricular arrhythmia (congenital long QT syndrome, history for QT prolongation, medications that prolong QT interval, hypokalemia, hypomagnesemia); history of CVA, pulmonary embolism. Concomitant use of CYP3A inducers.

## ACTION

Exhibits antitumor activity by irreversibly binding to mutant forms of EGFR. **Therapeutic Effect:** Inhibits tumor cell growth and metastasis.

## PHARMACOKINETICS

Widely distributed. Metabolized in liver. Protein binding: Likely high. Peak plasma concentration: 3–24 hrs (median: 6 hrs). Steady state reached in 15 days. Eliminated in feces (68%), urine (14%). **Half-life:** 48 hrs.

## ⌛ LIFESPAN CONSIDERATIONS

**Pregnancy/Lactation:** Avoid pregnancy; may cause fetal harm. Female pts of reproductive potential should use effective contraception during treatment and for at least 6 wks after discontinuation. Male pts with female partners of reproductive potential must use effective barrier methods during treatment and at least 4 mos after discontinuation. Unknown if distributed in breast milk. Breastfeeding not recommended during treatment and up to 2 wks after discontinuation. May impair fertility in both females and males. **Children:** Safety and efficacy not established. **Elderly:** May have increased risk of grade 3 or 4 adverse events. May require more frequent dose modifications.

## INTERACTIONS

**DRUG: QTc interval-prolonging medications (e.g., amiodarone, fluoxetine, haloperidol, sotalol)** may increase risk of QTc prolongation. **Strong CYP3A inducers (e.g., carbamazepine, phenytoin, rifampin)** may decrease concentration/effect. **Strong CYP3A inhibitors (e.g., clarithromycin, ketoconazole, ritonavir)** may increase concentration/risk of adverse effects. **Osimertinib** may alter concentration of medications that are sensitive substrates of CYP3A, breast cancer resistance protein (BCRP), or CYP1A2 (e.g., carbamazepine, cyclosporine, phenytoin). **HERBAL: St. John's wort** may decrease concentration/effect. **FOOD:** None known. **LAB VALUES:** May decrease serum sodium, magnesium; Hgb, Hct, lymphocytes, neutrophils, platelets, RBCs. May decrease diagnostic effect of *Coccidioides immitis* skin test.

## AVAILABILITY (Rx)

**Tablets:** 40 mg, 80 mg.

## ADMINISTRATION/HANDLING

**PO**

• Tablets are hazardous; use cytotoxic precautions during handling and disposal. Recommend single gloving when handling intact tablets; double gloving, protective gown when handling liquid preparations. • Do not divide, crush, cut, or ultrasonicate tablets. • Give without regard to food. • If a dose is missed, skip missed dose and administer the next dose on schedule. • **Pts with dysphagia:** Disperse tablet in 60 ml of water (noncarbonated) only. • Stir until dissipated into small pieces (does not completely dissolve). • Deliver orally or via gastric tube. • Rinse container with 120–240 ml of water and administer any remaining drug residue. After oral administration of residue, instruct pt to thoroughly rinse mouth with water and swallow.

## INDICATIONS/ROUTES/DOSAGE

### Non–Small-Cell Lung Cancer

**PO: ADULTS, ELDERLY:** 80 mg once daily. Continue until disease progression or unacceptable toxicity.

### Dose Modification

Based on Common Terminology Criteria for Adverse Events (CTCAE).

### Cardiac Toxicity

**QTc interval greater than 500 msec on at least two separate ECGs:** Withhold treatment until QTc interval is less than 481 msec or recovers to baseline. Once resolved, resume at 40 mg once daily.

**QTc interval prolongation with symptoms of life-threatening arrhythmia:** Permanently discontinue.

**Asymptomatic, absolute decrease in left ventricular ejection fraction (LVEF) of 10% from baseline and below 50%:** Withhold treatment for up to 4 wks. Resume treatment if improved to baseline. If not improved to baseline, permanently discontinue.

### Pulmonary Toxicity

**Interstitial lung disease/pneumonitis:** Permanently discontinue.

### Other Toxicities

**Any grade 3 or higher reaction:** Withhold treatment for up to 3 wks. Resume treatment at 80 mg once daily or 40 mg once daily if improved to grade 2 or lower within 3 wks. If not improved within 3 wks, permanently discontinue.

**Concomitant use of strong CYP3A4 inducers:** Start dose at 160 mg once daily. May decrease dose to 80 mg once daily if strong CYP3A4 inducer has been discontinued for at least 3 wks.

### Dosage in Renal/Hepatic Impairment

**Mild to moderate impairment:** No dose adjustment. **Severe impairment:** Not specified; use caution.

## SIDE EFFECTS

**Frequent (42%–17%):** Diarrhea, rash (generalized, erythematous, macular, maculopapular, papular, pustular), erythema, folliculitis, acne, dermatitis, acneiform dermatitis, dry skin, eczema, skin fissures, xerosis, nail disorders (inflammation, tenderness, discoloration, dystrophy, infection, ridging, onychoclasis, onycholysis, onychomadesis, paronychia), dry eye, blurry vision, keratitis, cataract, eye irritation, blepharitis, eye pain, increased lacrimation, vitreous floaters, nausea. **Occasional (16%–10%):** Decreased appetite, constipation, pruritus, cough, fatigue, back pain, stomatitis, headache.

## ADVERSE EFFECTS/TOXIC REACTIONS

Anemia, leukopenia, neutropenia, thrombocytopenia are expected responses to therapy. Interstitial lung disease/pneumonitis reported in 3% of pts. May cause QTc interval prolongation (up to 3% of pts); cardiac toxicities including cardiomyopathy (1% of pts), decreased LVEF (2% of pts); other adverse effects including CVA, intracranial hemorrhage; pneumonia (4% of pts); venous thromboembolism including pulmonary embolism, jugular venous thrombosis, DVT (7% of pts).

## NURSING CONSIDERATIONS

### BASELINE ASSESSMENT

Obtain CBC, BMP, serum magnesium; vital signs; EKG. Confirm presence of T790M mutation in tumor specimen prior to initiation. Obtain pregnancy test in female pts of reproductive potential.

Receive full medication history and screen for interactions. Question history of CVA, DVT, pulmonary embolism, pulmonary disease, cardiac disease. Obtain baseline echocardiogram to assess LVEF. Obtain visual acuity. Screen for active infection. Offer emotional support.

### INTERVENTION/EVALUATION

Monitor CBC for cytopenias; BMP, serum magnesium for electrolyte abnormalities.

Pts with cough, dyspnea, fever, worsening of respiratory status should be investigated for interstitial lung disease/pneumonitis. Pts with sudden chest pain, dyspnea, hypoxia, tachycardia should be evaluated for pulmonary embolism. Monitor for symptoms of DVT (leg or arm pain/swelling); CVA, intracranial hemorrhage (aphasia, altered LOC, facial droop, headache, hemiplegia, homonymous hemianopsia [vision loss on the same side of both eyes], seizures). Assess LVEF by echocardiogram q3mos during therapy, or more frequently in pts suspected of HF, congestive HF. Assess for eye pain, visual changes. Monitor for skin rash/toxicities, hypersensitivity reaction. Diligently monitor for infection. Monitor daily stool pattern, consistency.

### PATIENT/FAMILY TEACHING

• Blood levels, echocardiograms will be routinely monitored. • Treatment may cause life-threatening adverse effects. Report symptoms of abnormal heart beats (dizziness, fainting, lightheadedness, palpitations), heart failure (shortness of breath, fast or slow heart rate, exercise intolerance, swelling of the ankles or legs), severe lung inflammation (difficulty breathing, cough with fever, lung pain). • Avoid pregnancy; treatment may cause birth defects. Female pts of childbearing potential should use effective contraception during treatment and for at least 6 wks after last dose. Male pts with female partners of childbearing potential should use condoms, abstinence during treatment and for at least 4 mos after last dose. Do not breastfeed during therapy and for at least 2 wks after last dose. • Treatment may cause blood clots in the arms, legs, lungs, or brain. Immediately report symptoms of stroke (difficulty speaking, confusion, paralysis, vision loss), lung embolism (difficulty breathing, fast heart rate, chest pain), blood clots in the arms or legs (pain/swelling). • Do not take any newly prescribed medications unless approved by doctor who originally started treatment. • Avoid crowds, people with active infection. • Do not take herbal supplements.

## oxaliplatin          HIGH ALERT

ox-**al**-i-**pla**-tin
(Eloxatin)

■ **BLACK BOX ALERT** ■ Anaphylactic-like reaction may occur within minutes of administration; may be controlled with epinephrine, corticosteroids, antihistamines.

**Do not confuse oxaliplatin with Aloxi, carboplatin, or cisplatin.**

### ◆CLASSIFICATION

**PHARMACOTHERAPEUTIC:** Platinum-containing complex. **CLINICAL:** Antineoplastic.

### USES

Treatment of stage III colon cancer after complete resection of primary tumor; treatment of advanced colon cancer. **OFF-LABEL:** Treatment of ovarian cancer, pancreatic cancer, hepatobiliary cancer, testicular cancer, esophageal cancer, gastric cancer, non-Hodgkin's lymphoma, chronic lymphocytic leukemia.

### PRECAUTIONS

**Contraindications:** History of allergy to oxaliplatin, other platinum compounds. **Cautions:** Previous therapy with other antineoplastic agents; radiation, renal impairment, pregnancy, immunosuppression, presence or history of peripheral neuropathy, elderly.

## ACTION

Inhibits DNA replication by cross-linking with DNA strands. Cell cycle–phase non-specific. **Therapeutic Effect:** Prevents cell division.

## PHARMACOKINETICS

Rapidly distributed. Protein binding: 90%. Undergoes rapid, extensive nonenzymatic biotransformation. Excreted in urine. **Half-life:** 391 hrs.

## ⧖ LIFESPAN CONSIDERATIONS

**Pregnancy/Lactation:** If possible, avoid use during pregnancy, esp. first trimester. May cause fetal harm. Breast-feeding not recommended. **Children:** Safety and efficacy not established. **Elderly:** Increased incidence of diarrhea, dehydration, hypokalemia, fatigue.

## INTERACTIONS

**DRUG: Bone marrow depressants** may increase myelosuppression, GI effects. **Live virus vaccines** may potentiate virus replication, increase vaccine side effects, decrease pt's antibody response to vaccine. **Nephrotic medications** may increase concentration. **HERBAL: Echinacea** may decrease effects. **FOOD:** None known. **LAB VALUES:** May increase serum creatinine, bilirubin, ALT, AST.

## AVAILABILITY (Rx)

Injection, Solution: 5 mg/ml (20-ml, 40-ml vials).

## ADMINISTRATION/HANDLING

◀ALERT▶ Wear protective gloves during handling of oxaliplatin. If solution comes in contact with skin, wash skin immediately with soap, water. Do not use aluminum needles or administration sets that may come in contact with drug; may cause degradation of platinum compounds.

◀ALERT▶ Pt should avoid ice, drinking cold beverages, touching cold objects during infusion and for 5 days thereafter (can exacerbate acute neuropathy).

 **IV**

**Reconstitution** • Dilute with 250–500 ml $D_5W$ (never dilute with sodium chloride solution or other chloride-containing solutions) to final concentration of 0.2–0.6 mg/ml.
**Rate of Administration** • Infuse over 2–6 hrs.
**Storage** • Do not freeze. • Protect from light. • Store vials at room temperature. • After dilution, solution is stable for 6 hrs at room temperature, 24 hrs if refrigerated.

## ▦ IV INCOMPATIBILITIES

Do not infuse oxaliplatin with alkaline medications.

## ▦ IV COMPATIBILITIES

Dexamethasone, diphenhydramine (Benadryl), granisetron (Kytril), ondansetron (Zofran), palonosetron (Aloxi).

## INDICATIONS/ROUTES/DOSAGE

Refer to individual protocols.
◀ALERT▶ Pretreat pt with antiemetics. Repeat courses should not be given more frequently than every 2 wks.

**Advanced Colorectal Cancer**
IV: **ADULTS:** 85 mg/m² q2wks until disease progression or unacceptable toxicity (in combination with fluorouracil/leucovorin).

**Stage III Colon Cancer**
IV: **ADULTS:** 85 mg/m² q2wks for total of 6 months (in combination with fluorouracil/leucovorin).

**Dosage in Renal Impairment**
**CrCl less than 30 ml/min:** Reduce dose to 65 mg/m².

**Dosage in Hepatic Impairment**
No dose adjustment.

## SIDE EFFECTS

**Frequent (76%–20%):** Peripheral/sensory neuropathy (usually occurs in hands,

**O**

feet, perioral area, throat but may present as: jaw spasm, abnormal tongue sensation, eye pain, chest pressure, difficulty walking, swallowing, writing), nausea, fatigue, diarrhea, vomiting, constipation, abdominal pain, fever, anorexia. **Occasional (14%–10%):** Stomatitis, earache, insomnia, cough, difficulty breathing, backache, edema. **Rare (7%–3%):** Dyspepsia, dizziness, rhinitis, flushing, alopecia.

## ADVERSE EFFECTS/ TOXIC REACTIONS

Peripheral/sensory neuropathy can occur without any prior event by drinking or holding a glass of cold liquid during IV infusion. Pulmonary fibrosis (characterized as nonproductive cough, dyspnea, crackles, radiologic pulmonary infiltrates) may warrant drug discontinuation. Hypersensitivity reaction (rash, urticaria, pruritus) occurs rarely.

## NURSING CONSIDERATIONS

### BASELINE ASSESSMENT

Obtain baseline renal function, WBC, platelet count.

### INTERVENTION/EVALUATION

Monitor for decrease in WBC, platelets (myelosuppression is minimal). Monitor daily pattern of bowel activity, stool consistency. Monitor for diarrhea, GI bleeding (bright red, black tarry stool), signs of neuropathy. Pt should avoid ice or drinking, holding glass of cold liquid during IV infusion and for 5 days following completion of infusion; may precipitate/exacerbate neurotoxicity (occurs within hrs or 1–2 days of dosing, lasts up to 14 days). Maintain strict I&O. Assess oral mucosa for stomatitis.

### PATIENT/FAMILY TEACHING

• Promptly report fever, sore throat, signs of local infection, unusual bruising/bleeding from any site, persistent diarrhea, difficulty breathing. • Do not have immunizations without physician's approval (drug lowers resistance). • Avoid contact with those who have recently taken oral polio vaccine. • Avoid cold drinks, ice, cold objects (may produce neuropathy).

# *OXcarbazepine

ox-kar-**baz**-e-peen
(Oxtellar XR, Trileptal)
**Do not confuse oxcarbazepine with carbamazepine, or Trileptal with TriLipix.**

## ◆CLASSIFICATION

**PHARMACOTHERAPEUTIC:** Carboxamide derivative, anticonvulsant. **CLINICAL:** Anticonvulsant.

## USES

**Trileptal:** Monotherapy, adjunctive therapy in treatment of partial seizures in adults. Monotherapy in children 4 yrs and older, adjunctive therapy in children 2 yrs and older. **Oxtellar XR:** Adjunctive therapy in treatment of partial seizures in children 6–17 yrs. **OFF-LABEL:** Treatment of neuropathic pain, bipolar disorder.

## PRECAUTIONS

**Contraindications:** Hypersensitivity to oxcarbazepine. **Cautions:** Renal impairment, sensitivity to carbamazepine, pts at increased risk for suicide.

## ACTION

Blocks sodium channels, stabilizing hyperexcited neural membranes, inhibiting repetitive neuronal firing, diminishing synaptic impulses. **Therapeutic Effect:** Prevents seizures.

## PHARMACOKINETICS

Completely absorbed from GI tract. Metabolized in liver. Protein binding: 40%. Primarily excreted in urine. **Half-life:** 2 hrs; metabolite, 6–10 hrs.

## ⧖ LIFESPAN CONSIDERATIONS

**Pregnancy/Lactation:** Crosses placenta. Distributed in breast milk. **Children:** No age-related precautions in those older than 4 yrs. **Elderly:** Age-related renal impairment may require dosage adjustment.

## INTERACTIONS

**DRUG: Alcohol, CNS depressants (e.g., lorazepam, morphine, zolpidem)** may have additive sedative effect. May decrease effectiveness of **felodipine, oral contraceptives, verapamil.** May increase concentration, risk of toxicity of **phenobarbital, phenytoin. HERBAL: Gotu kola, kava kava, St. John's wort, valerian** may increase CNS depression. **Evening primrose** may decrease seizure threshold. **St. John's wort** may decrease concentration. **FOOD:** None known. **LAB VALUES:** May increase serum alkaline phosphatase, ALT, AST. May decrease serum sodium.

## AVAILABILITY (Rx)

**Oral Suspension (Trileptal):** 300 mg/5 ml. **Tablets (Trileptal):** 150 mg, 300 mg, 600 mg.

 **Tablets, Extended-Release (Oxtellar XR):** 150 mg, 300 mg, 600 mg.

## ADMINISTRATION/HANDLING

### PO
• Give without regard to food. Do not break, crush, dissolve, or divide extended-release tablets. Swallow whole.

## INDICATIONS/ROUTES/DOSAGE

**Adjunctive Treatment of Seizures**
**PO: ADULTS, ELDERLY:** *(Immediate-Release):* Initially, 600 mg/day in 2 divided doses. May increase by up to 600 mg/day at wkly intervals. **Maximum:** 2,400 mg/day. **Usual maintenance dose:** 600 mg twice daily. **CHILDREN 4–16 YRS:** Initially, 8–10 mg/kg in 2 divided doses. **Maximum:** 600 mg/day. Increase dose slowly over 2 wks. **Maintenance (based on weight): CHILDREN WEIGHING MORE THAN 39 KG:** 1,800 mg/day in 2 divided doses; **CHILDREN WEIGHING 29.1–39 KG:** 1,200 mg/day in 2 divided doses; **CHILDREN WEIGHING 20–29 KG:** 900 mg/day

in 2 divided doses. **CHILDREN 2–3 YRS:** Initially, 8–10 mg/kg/day in 2 divided doses. **Maximum:** 600 mg/day in 2 divided doses. Increase dose slowly over 2 wks up to a **maximum** of 60 mg/kg/day in 2 divided doses. *(Extended-Release):* **ADULTS:** Initially, 600 mg once daily. May increase by 600 mg/day at wkly intervals. Range: 1,200–2,400 mg/day. **ELDERLY:** Initially, 300–450 mg/day. May increase by 300–450 mg/day at wkly intervals to desired clinical response. Range: Up to 2,400 mg/day.

**Conversion to Monotherapy**
**PO: ADULTS, ELDERLY:** *(Immediate-Release):* 600 mg/day in 2 divided doses (while decreasing concomitant anticonvulsant over 3–6 wks). May increase by 600 mg/day at wkly intervals up to 2,400 mg/day. **CHILDREN 4–16 YRS:** Initially, 8–10 mg/kg/day in 2 divided doses with simultaneous initial reduction of dose of concomitant antiepileptic over 3–6 wks. May increase by maximum of 10 mg/kg/day at wkly intervals (see below for recommended daily dose by weight).

**Initiation of Monotherapy**
**PO: ADULTS, ELDERLY:** *(Immediate-Release):* 600 mg/day in 2 divided doses. May increase by 300 mg/day every 3 days up to 1,200 mg/day. **CHILDREN 4–16 YRS:** Initially, 8–10 mg/kg/day in 2 divided doses. Increase at 3-day intervals by 5 mg/kg/day to achieve maintenance dose by weight as follows:

| Weight | Dosage |
|---|---|
| 70+ kg | 1,500–2,100 mg/day |
| 60–69 kg | 1,200–2,100 mg/day |
| 50–59 kg | 1,200–1,800 mg/day |
| 41–49 kg | 1,200–1,500 mg/day |
| 35–40 kg | 900–1,500 mg/day |
| 25–34 kg | 900–1,200 mg/day |
| 20–24 kg | 600–900 mg/day |

**Dosage in Renal Impairment**
**Mild to moderate impairment:** No dose adjustment. **CrCl less than 30 ml/min:** Give 50% of normal starting dose, then titrate slowly to desired dose.

**O**

**Dosage in Hepatic Impairment**
**Mild to moderate impairment:** No dose adjustment. **Severe impairment:** Use caution with immediate-release, not recommended with extended-release.

## SIDE EFFECTS

**Frequent (22%–13%):** Dizziness, nausea, headache. **Occasional (7%–5%):** Vomiting, diarrhea, ataxia muscular incoordination, nervousness, dyspepsia, constipation. **Rare (4%):** Tremor, rash, back pain, epistaxis, sinusitis, diplopia.

## ADVERSE EFFECTS/ TOXIC REACTIONS

Clinically significant hyponatremia may occur, manifested as leg cramping, hypotension, cold/clammy skin, increased pulse rate, headache, nausea, vomiting, diarrhea. Suicidal ideation occurs rarely.

## NURSING CONSIDERATIONS

### BASELINE ASSESSMENT

Review history of seizure disorder (type, onset, intensity, frequency, duration, LOC), drug history (esp. other anticonvulsants). Provide safety precautions; quiet, dark environment.

### INTERVENTION/EVALUATION

Assist with ambulation if dizziness, ataxia occur. Assess for visual abnormalities, headache. Monitor serum sodium. Assess for signs of hyponatremia (nausea, malaise, headache, lethargy, confusion). Assess for clinical improvement (decrease in intensity, frequency of seizures). Monitor for worsening depression, suicidal ideation.

### PATIENT/FAMILY TEACHING

• Do not abruptly stop taking medication (may increase seizure activity). • Report rash, nausea, headache, dizziness occurs. • May need periodic blood tests. • Avoid tasks that require alertness, motor skills until response to drug is established. • Avoid alcohol. • May decrease effectiveness of oral contraceptives.

# oxybutynin

ox-i-**bue**-ti-nin
(Apo-Oxybutynin ✦, Ditropan XL, Gelnique, Oxytrol for Women)
**Do not confuse Ditropan with Detrol, diazepam, or Diprivan, or oxybutynin with OxyContin.**

## ◆CLASSIFICATION

**PHARMACOTHERAPEUTIC:** Anticholinergic. **CLINICAL:** Antispasmodic.

## USES

**Immediate-Release:** Relief of symptoms (urgency, incontinence, frequency, nocturia, urge incontinence) associated with uninhibited neurogenic bladder, reflex neurogenic bladder. **Extended-Release (additional):** Treatment of symptoms associated with detrusor overactivity due to neurologic disorder (e.g., spina bifida).

## PRECAUTIONS

**Contraindications:** Hypersensitivity to oxybutynin. Pts with or at risk for uncontrolled narrow-angle glaucoma, urinary retention, gastric retention, or conditions with severely decreased GI motility. **Cautions:** Renal/hepatic impairment, pts with bladder outflow obstruction, treated narrow-angle glaucoma, hyperthyroidism, coronary artery disease, HF, hypertension, arrhythmias, prostatic hyperplasia, myasthenia gravis, reduced GI motility, GI obstructive disorder, gastroesophageal reflux.

## ACTION

Direct antispasmodic effect on smooth muscle; inhibits action of acetylcholine on smooth muscle. **Therapeutic Effect:** Increases bladder capacity, delays desire to void. Decreases urgency and frequency.

## PHARMACOKINETICS

| Route | Onset | Peak | Duration |
|-------|-------|------|----------|
| PO | 0.5–1 hr | 3–6 hrs | 6–10 hrs |

---

Rapidly, well absorbed from GI tract. Metabolized in liver. Primarily excreted in urine. Unknown if removed by hemodialysis. **Half-life:** 1–2.3 hrs; metabolite, 7–8 hrs.

## ⧗ LIFESPAN CONSIDERATIONS

**Pregnancy/Lactation:** Unknown if drug crosses placenta or is distributed in breast milk. **Children:** No age-related precautions noted in those older than 5 yrs. **Elderly:** May be more sensitive to anticholinergic effects (e.g., dry mouth, urinary retention).

## INTERACTIONS

**DRUG: Medications with anticholinergic action (e.g., antihistamines)** may increase anticholinergic effects. **Clarithromycin, erythromycin, itraconazole, ketoconazole** may alter pharmacokinetic parameters. **HERBAL:** None significant. **FOOD:** None known. **LAB VALUES:** None significant.

## AVAILABILITY (Rx)

**Syrup:** 5 mg/5 ml. **Tablets:** 5 mg. **Topical Gel (Gelnique):** 100 mg/unit dose sachet. **(3% Gel):** 30 mg/ml. **Transdermal (Oxytrol for Women):** 3.9 mg.

---

🔰 **Tablets (Extended-Release [Ditropan XL]):** 5 mg, 10 mg, 15 mg.

## ADMINISTRATION/HANDLING

### PO

• Give without regard to meals. • Extended-release tablet must be swallowed whole; do not break, crush, dissolve, or divide.

### Transdermal

• Apply patch to dry, intact skin on abdomen, hip, buttock. • Use new application site for each new patch; avoid reapplication to same site within 7 days.

### Topical Gel

• *(Gelnique):* Apply contents of 1 sachet once daily to dry, intact skin on abdomen, upper arms/shoulders, or thighs. • Do not bathe/shower until 1 hr after gel is applied. • *(3% Gel):* Apply 3 ml to thigh, upper arm, or shoulder.

## INDICATIONS/ROUTES/DOSAGE

### Neurogenic Bladder

**PO** *(Immediate-Release):* **ADULTS:** 5 mg 2–3 times/day. May increase 5 mg 4 times/day. **ELDERLY:** 2.5–5 mg 2–3 times/day. **CHILDREN OLDER THAN 5 YRS:** 5 mg twice daily. May increase 5 mg 3 times/day. **CHILDREN 1–5 YRS:** 0.2 mg/kg/dose 2–4 times/day.

**PO** *(Extended-Release):* **ADULTS, ELDERLY:** 5–10 mg/day. May increase 30 mg/day. **CHILDREN 6 YRS AND OLDER:** Initially, 5–10 mg once daily. May increase in 5–10 mg increments. **Maximum:** 20 mg/day.

**Transdermal: ADULTS:** 3.9 mg applied twice wkly. Apply every 3–4 days.

**Topical Gel: ADULTS, ELDERLY:** 100 mg once daily.

**Gel 3%:** Apply 3 ml (84 mg) once daily.

### Dosage in Renal/Hepatic Impairment

No dose adjustment.

## SIDE EFFECTS

**Frequent:** Constipation, dry mouth, drowsiness, decreased perspiration. **Occasional:** Decreased lacrimation/salivation, impotence, urinary hesitancy/retention, suppressed lactation, blurred vision, mydriasis, nausea/vomiting, insomnia.

## ADVERSE EFFECTS/ TOXIC REACTIONS

Overdose produces CNS excitation (nervousness, restlessness, hallucinations, irritability), hypotension/hypertension, confusion, tachycardia, facial flushing, respiratory depression.

## NURSING CONSIDERATIONS

### BASELINE ASSESSMENT

Assess degree of dysuria, urgency, frequency, incontinence.

### INTERVENTION/EVALUATION

Monitor for symptomatic relief. Monitor I&O; palpate bladder for urine retention. Monitor daily pattern of bowel activity, stool consistency.

## PATIENT/FAMILY TEACHING

• Avoid alcohol. • May cause dry mouth (sugarless candy/gum may reduce effect). • Avoid tasks that require alertness, motor skills until response to drug is established (may cause drowsiness). • Avoid strenuous activity in warm environment.

---

# *oxyCODONE    TOP 100    HIGH ALERT

ox-ee-**koe**-done
(Oxaydo, <u>OxyContin</u>, OxyIR , Roxicodone, Supeudol , Xtampza)

■ **BLACK BOX ALERT** ■ **OxyContin (controlled-release):** Not intended as an "as needed" analgesic or for immediate postop pain control. Extended-release should not be crushed, broken, or chewed (otherwise leads to rapid release and absorption of potentially fatal dose). Be alert to signs of abuse, misuse, and diversion. May cause potentially life-threatening respiratory depression. Prolonged use during pregnancy can cause neonatal withdrawal syndrome. Use of CYP3A4 inhibitors may increase effects/cause fatal respiratory depression. **Do not confuse oxycodone with hydrocodone, oxybutynin, or oxymorphone, OxyContin with MS Contin or oxybutynin, or Roxicodone with Roxanol.**

## FIXED-COMBINATION(S)

**Combunox:** oxycodone/ibuprofen (an NSAID): 5 mg/400 mg. **Endocet:** oxycodone/acetaminophen (a non-narcotic analgesic): 5 mg/325 mg, 7.5 mg/325 mg, 7.5 mg/500 mg, 10 mg/325 mg, 10 mg/650 mg. **Magnacet:** oxycodone/acetaminophen (a non-narcotic analgesic): 2.5 mg/400 mg, 7.5 mg/400 mg, 10 mg/400 mg. **Percocet:** oxycodone/acetaminophen: 2.5 mg/325 mg, 5 mg/325 mg, 5 mg/500 mg, 7.5 mg/325 mg, 7.5 mg/500 mg, 10 mg/325 mg, 10 mg/650 mg. **Percocet, Roxicet, Tylox:** oxycodone/acetaminophen (a non-narcotic analgesic): 5 mg/500 mg. **Percodan:** oxycodone/aspirin (a non-narcotic analgesic): 2.25 mg/325 mg, 4.5 mg/325 mg. **Targiniq ER:** oxycodone/naloxone (opioid antagonist): 10 mg/5 mg; 20 mg/10 mg; 40 mg/20 mg. **Troxyca ER:** oxycodone/naltrexone (an opioid antagonist): 10 mg/1.2 mg, 20 mg/2.4 mg, 30 mg/3.6 mg, 40 mg/4.8 mg, 60 mg/7.2 mg, 9.6 mg/80 mg. **Xartemis XR:** oxycodone/acetaminophen (non-narcotic analgesic): 7.5 mg/325 mg.

## ◆CLASSIFICATION

**PHARMACOTHERAPEUTIC:** Opioid analgesic **(Schedule II). CLINICAL:** Narcotic analgesic.

## USES

Relief of moderate to severe pain (usually in combination with nonopioid analgesics). **Extended-Release:** Around-the-clock management of moderate to severe pain when continuous analgesic is needed.

## PRECAUTIONS

**Contraindications:** Hypersensitivity to oxycodone. Acute or severe bronchial asthma, hypercarbia, paralytic ileus, GI obstruction, significant respiratory depression. **Extreme Caution:** CNS depression, anoxia, hypercapnia, respiratory depression, seizures, acute alcoholism, shock, untreated myxedema, respiratory dysfunction. **Cautions:** Elevated ICP, hepatic/renal impairment, coma, debilitated pts, head injury, biliary tract disease, toxic psychosis, acute abdominal conditions, hypothyroidism, prostatic hypertrophy, Addison's disease, urethral stricture, COPD, history of substance abuse, elderly.

## ACTION

Binds with opioid receptors within CNS, causing inhibition of ascending pain pathway. **Therapeutic Effect:** Alters perception of and emotional response to pain.

---

## PHARMACOKINETICS

| Route | Onset | Peak | Duration |
|-------|-------|------|----------|
| PO (immediate-release) | 10–15 min | 0.5–1 hr | 3–6 hrs |
| PO (controlled-release) | 10–15 min | 0.5–1 hr | Up to 12 hrs |

Moderately absorbed from GI tract. Protein binding: 38%–45%. Widely distributed. Metabolized in liver. Excreted in urine. Unknown if removed by hemodialysis. **Half-life:** 2–3 hrs (5 hrs controlled-release).

## ⧖ LIFESPAN CONSIDERATIONS

**Pregnancy/Lactation:** Readily crosses placenta. Distributed in breast milk. Respiratory depression may occur in neonate if mother received opiates during labor. Regular use of opiates during pregnancy may produce withdrawal symptoms in neonate (irritability, excessive crying, tremors, hyperactive reflexes, fever, vomiting, diarrhea, yawning, sneezing, seizures). **Children:** Paradoxical excitement may occur. Pts younger than 2 yrs are more susceptible to respiratory depressant effects. **Elderly:** Age-related renal impairment may increase risk of urinary retention. May be more susceptible to respiratory depressant effects.

## INTERACTIONS

**DRUG:** **Alcohol, other CNS depressants** may increase CNS effects, respiratory depression, hypotension. **CYP3A4 inhibitors (clarithromycin, ketoconazole)** may increase concentration, toxicity. **CYP3A4 inducers (carbamazepine, rifampin)** may decrease concentration/effects. **MAOIs** may produce serotonin syndrome, a severe, sometimes fatal reaction (administer ¼ of usual oxycodone dose). **HERBAL: Gotu kola, kava kava, St. John's wort, valerian** may increase CNS depression. **FOOD: Grapefruit products** may increase potential for respiratory depression.

**LAB VALUES:** May increase serum amylase, lipase.

## AVAILABILITY (Rx)

◄ALERT► New formulation of controlled-release intended to prevent medication from being cut, broken, chewed, crushed, or dissolved to reduce risk of overdose due to tampering, snorting, or injection. **Capsules:** 5 mg. **Oral Concentrate:** 20 mg/ml. **Oral Solution:** 5 mg/5 ml. **Tablets:** 5 mg, 10 mg, 15 mg, 20 mg, 30 mg. **Tablets, Abuse Deterrent (Oxaydo):** 5 mg, 7.5 mg.

⧖ **Capsules (Extended-Release [Xtampza]):** 9 mg, 13.5 mg, 18 mg, 27 mg, 36 mg. **Tablets (Controlled-Release [Oxycontin]):** 10 mg, 15 mg, 20 mg, 30 mg, 40 mg, 60 mg, 80 mg.

## ADMINISTRATION/HANDLING

### PO

• Give without regard to meals. • **Controlled-release:** Swallow whole; do not break, crush, dissolve, or divide.

## INDICATIONS/ROUTES/DOSAGE

**Note:** All doses should be titrated to desired effect.

### Analgesia

**PO (Immediate-Release): ADULTS, ELDERLY:** Initially, 5–15 mg q4–6h as needed. Range: 5–20 mg/dose. **CHILDREN, 6–18 YRS:** 0.1–0.2 mg/kg/dose q4–6h as needed.

### Opioid Naive

**PO (Controlled-Release): ADULTS, ELDERLY:** Initially, 10 mg q12h.
◄ALERT► To convert from other opioids or nonopioid analgesics to oxycodone controlled-release, refer to OxyContin package insert. Dosages are reduced in pts with severe hepatic disease.

### Dosage in Renal/Hepatic Impairment

Use caution. Titrate carefully.

---

## SIDE EFFECTS

◀ALERT▶ Effects are dependent on dosage amount. Ambulatory pts, pts not in severe pain may experience dizziness, nausea, vomiting, hypotension more frequently than those in supine position or having severe pain. **Frequent:** Drowsiness, dizziness, hypotension (including orthostatic hypotension), anorexia. **Occasional:** Confusion, diaphoresis, facial flushing, urinary retention, constipation, dry mouth, nausea, vomiting, headache. **Rare:** Allergic reaction, depression, paradoxical CNS hyperactivity, nervousness in children, paradoxical excitement, restlessness in elderly, debilitated pts.

## ADVERSE EFFECTS/ TOXIC REACTIONS

Overdose results in respiratory depression, skeletal muscle flaccidity, cold/ clammy skin, cyanosis, extreme drowsiness progressing to seizures, stupor, coma. Hepatotoxicity may occur with overdose of acetaminophen component of fixed-combination product. Tolerance to analgesic effect, physical dependence may occur with repeated use. **Antidote:** Naloxone (see Appendix J for dosage).

## NURSING CONSIDERATIONS

### BASELINE ASSESSMENT

Assess onset, type, location, duration of pain. Effect of medication is reduced if full pain recurs before next dose. Obtain vital signs before giving medication. If respirations are 12/min or less (20/min or less in children), withhold medication, contact physician.

### INTERVENTION/EVALUATION

Palpate bladder for urinary retention. Monitor daily pattern of bowel activity, stool consistency. Initiate deep breathing, coughing exercises, esp. in pts with pulmonary impairment. Monitor pain relief, respiratory rate, mental status, B/P, LOC.

### PATIENT/FAMILY TEACHING

• May cause dry mouth, drowsiness.
• Avoid tasks that require alertness, motor skills until response to drug is established. • Avoid alcohol. • May be habit forming. • Do not chew, crush, dissolve, or divide controlled-release tablets. • Report severe constipation, absence of pain relief.

## *oxyMORphone     HIGH ALERT

ox-ee-**mor**-fone
(Opana, Opana ER)

■ **BLACK BOX ALERT** ■ Has abuse liability. Concern about increased risk of abuse, misuse, or diversion. Prolonged use during pregnancy can cause neonatal withdrawal syndrome.
**Do not confuse oxymorphone with oxycodone.**

## ◆CLASSIFICATION

**PHARMACOTHERAPEUTIC:** Opioid agonist **(Schedule II). CLINICAL:** Narcotic analgesic, antianxiety, preop anesthetic.

## USES

**Injection:** Relief of moderate to severe acute pain. **PO (Immediate-release):** Relief of moderate to severe acute pain. **(Extended-release):** Relief of moderate to severe pain in pts requiring continuous treatment for extended period of time.

## PRECAUTIONS

**Contraindications:** Hypersensitivity to oxymorphone, morphine, acute severe bronchial asthma, severe respiratory depression, paralytic ileus, moderate to severe hepatic function impairment, hypercarbia. **Extreme Cautions:** Anoxia, hypercapnia, seizures, acute alcoholism, shock, untreated myxedema. **Cautions:** Hypothyroidism, prostatic hypertrophy, Addison's disease, urethral stricture, prostatic hyperplasia, toxic psychosis, renal impairment, COPD, biliary tract disease, acute pancreatitis, head injury, increased ICP, morbid obesity, mild hepatic dysfunction, history of substance abuse.

## ACTION

Binds to opiate receptor sites within CNS, causing inhibition of ascending pain pathways. **Therapeutic Effect:** Reduces intensity of pain stimuli, alters pain perception, emotional response to pain.

## PHARMACOKINETICS

| Route | Onset | Peak | Duration |
|-------|-------|------|----------|
| Parenteral | 5–10 min | N/A | 3–6 hrs |

Well absorbed. Protein binding: 10%. Widely distributed. Metabolized in liver. Excreted in urine. **Half-life:** 7–9 hrs; **extended-release:** 9–11 hrs.

## LIFESPAN CONSIDERATIONS

**Pregnancy/Lactation:** Unknown if distributed in breast milk. May prolong labor if administered in latent phase of first stage of labor or before cervical dilation of 4–5 cm has occurred. Respiratory depression may occur in neonate if mother received opiates during labor. Regular use of opiates during pregnancy may produce withdrawal symptoms in the neonate (irritability, excessive crying, tremors, hyperactive reflexes, fever, vomiting, diarrhea, yawning, sneezing, seizures). **Children:** Safety and efficacy not established in those younger than 18 yrs. **Elderly:** May be more susceptible to respiratory depression, may cause paradoxical excitement. Age-related hepatic impairment, debilitation may require dosage adjustment.

## INTERACTIONS

**DRUG: Alcohol, other CNS depressants** may increase CNS effects, respiratory depression, hypotension. **Anticholinergics** may increase risk of urinary retention, severe constipation (may lead to paralytic ileus). **Propofol** increases risk of bradycardia. Decreased effect when given concurrently with **phenothiazines. HERBAL: Gotu kola, kava,** kava, **St. John's wort, valerian** may produce CNS depressant effects. **FOOD:** None known. **LAB VALUES:** May increase serum amylase, lipase.

## AVAILABILITY (Rx)

**Injection:** 1 mg/ml. **Tablets:** 5 mg, 10 mg.

 **Tablets (Extended-Release):** 5 mg, 7.5 mg, 10 mg, 15 mg, 20 mg, 30 mg, 40 mg.

## ADMINISTRATION/HANDLING

**IV**

**Rate of Administration** • Administer IV push very slowly. • Rapid IV increases risk of severe adverse reactions (chest wall rigidity, apnea, peripheral circulatory collapse, anaphylactoid effects, cardiac arrest).

**IM/SQ**

• Inject deep IM, preferably in upper, outer quadrant of buttock. • Use short 30-gauge needle for SQ injection. • Administer slowly, rotating injection sites. • Pts with circulatory impairment experience higher risk of overdosage due to delayed absorption of repeated administration.

**Storage** • Store parenteral form at room temperature. Refrigerate suppository form. • Discard parenteral form if discolored or particulate forms.

**PO**

• Give 1 hr before or 2 hrs after meals. • Do not break, crush, dissolve, or divide extended-release tablet.

## IV COMPATIBILITIES

Glycopyrrolate, hydroxyzine, ranitidine.

## INDICATIONS/ROUTES/DOSAGE

**Analgesia**

**IV: ADULTS 18 YRS AND OLDER, ELDERLY:** Initially, 0.5 mg. Dose may be cautiously increased until satisfactory response is achieved.

◄**ALERT►** IM preferred over SQ route (SQ rate of absorption is less reliable).

 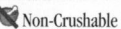

**IM/SQ: ADULTS 18 YRS AND OLDER, ELDERLY:** Initially, 1–1.5 mg every 4–6 hrs as needed.
**PO: ADULTS, ELDERLY: (IMMEDIATE-RELEASE):** 5–10 mg q4–6h. **(EXTENDED-RELEASE):** Initially, 5 mg q12h. May increase by 5–10 mg q12h at intervals of every 3–7 days.

**Dosage in Renal Impairment**
Reduce initial dose with CrCl less than 50 ml/min.

**Dosage in Hepatic impairment**
Reduce initial dose with mild impairment (contraindicated in moderate to severe impairment).

## SIDE EFFECTS

**Note:** Effects are dependent on dosage amount, route of administration. Ambulatory pts, pts not in severe pain may experience dizziness, nausea, vomiting, hypotension more frequently than those in supine position or having severe pain. **Frequent (10% or higher):** Drowsiness, hypotension, dizziness, nausea, vomiting, constipation, weakness. **Occasional (9%–2%):** Nervousness, headache, restlessness, malaise, confusion, anorexia, abdominal cramps, dry mouth, decreased urinary output, ureteral spasm, pain at injection site. **Rare (1% or less):** Depression, paradoxical CNS stimulation, hallucinations, rash, urticaria.

## ADVERSE EFFECTS/ TOXIC REACTIONS

Overdose results in respiratory depression, skeletal muscle flaccidity, cold/clammy skin, cyanosis, extreme drowsiness progressing to convulsions, stupor, coma. Tolerance to analgesic effect, physical dependence may occur with repeated use. Prolonged duration of action, cumulative effect may occur in those with hepatic/renal impairment.

## NURSING CONSIDERATIONS

### BASELINE ASSESSMENT

Assess onset, type, location, duration of pain. Obtain vital signs before giving medication. If respirations are 12/min or lower, withhold medication, contact physician. Effect of medication is reduced if full pain recurs before next dose.

### INTERVENTION/EVALUATION

Monitor vital signs 5–10 min after IV administration, 15–30 min after SQ, IM. Be alert for decreased respirations, B/P. To prevent pain cycles, instruct pt to request pain medication as soon as discomfort begins. Assess for clinical improvement, record onset of pain relief. Consult physician if pain relief is not adequate.

### PATIENT/FAMILY TEACHING

• Discomfort may occur with injection. • Slowly go from lying to standing to avoid postural hypotension. • Avoid tasks that require alertness, motor skills until response to drug is established. • Avoid alcohol. • Tolerance/dependence may occur with prolonged use of high doses.

---

## oxytocin    HIGH ALERT

ox-ee-**toe**-sin
(Pitocin)

■ **BLACK BOX ALERT** ■ Not to be given for elective labor induction, but when medically indicated.
**Do not confuse Pitocin with Pitressin.**

### ◆CLASSIFICATION

**PHARMACOTHERAPEUTIC:** Uterine smooth muscle stimulant. **CLINICAL:** Oxytocic agent.

## USES

**Antepartum:** Induction of labor in pts with medical indication (e.g., at or near term), stimulate reinforcement of labor, adjunct in managing incomplete or inevitable abortion. **Postpartum:** Produce uterine contractions during third stage of labor and control postpartum bleeding/hemorrhage.

## PRECAUTIONS

**Contraindications:** Hypersensitivity to oxytocin. Adequate uterine activity that fails to progress, cephalopelvic disproportion, fetal distress without imminent delivery, grand multiparity, hyperactive or hypertonic uterus, obstetric emergencies that favor surgical intervention, prematurity, unengaged fetal head, unfavorable fetal position/presentation, when vaginal delivery is contraindicated (e.g., active genital herpes infection, invasive cervical cancer, placenta previa, cord presentation). **Cautions:** Induction of labor should be for medical, not elective, reasons. Generally not recommended in: fetal distress, hydramnios, partial placental previa, predisposition to uterine rupture.

## ACTION

Activates receptors that trigger increase in intracellular calcium levels in uterine myofibrils; increases prostaglandin production. **Therapeutic Effect:** Stimulates uterine contractions.

## PHARMACOKINETICS

| Route | Onset | Peak | Duration |
|-------|-------|------|----------|
| IV | Immediate | N/A | 1 hr |
| IM | 3–5 min | N/A | 2–3 hrs |

Rapidly absorbed through nasal mucous membranes. Protein binding: 30%. Distributed in extracellular fluid. Metabolized in liver, kidney. Primarily excreted in urine. **Half-life:** 1–6 min.

## ⧗ LIFESPAN CONSIDERATIONS

**Pregnancy/Lactation:** Used as indicated, not expected to present risk of fetal abnormalities. Small amounts in breast milk. Breastfeeding not recommended. **Children/Elderly:** Not used in these pt populations.

## INTERACTIONS

**DRUG: Caudal block anesthetics, vasopressors** may increase pressor effects. **Other oxytocics** may cause cervical lacerations, uterine hypertonus, uterine rupture. **HERBAL:** None significant. **FOOD:** None known. **LAB VALUES:** None significant.

## AVAILABILITY (Rx)

**Injection (Pitocin):** 10 units/ml. **Injection, Solution:** 30 units/500 ml.

## ADMINISTRATION/HANDLING

 IV

**Reconstitution** • Dilute 10–40 units (1–4 ml) in 1,000 ml of 0.9% NaCl, lactated Ringer's, or D₅W to provide concentration of 10–40 milliunits/ml solution. **Rate of Administration** • Give by IV infusion (use infusion device to carefully control rate of flow as ordered by physician). **Storage** • Store at room temperature.

## ▧ IV INCOMPATIBILITIES

No known incompatibilities via Y-site administration.

## ▧ IV COMPATIBILITIES

Heparin, insulin (regular), multivitamins, potassium chloride, zidovudine.

## INDICATIONS/ROUTES/DOSAGE

**Induction or Stimulation of Labor**
**IV: ADULTS:** 0.5–1 milliunit/min. May gradually increase in increments of 1–2 milliunits/min. Rates of 9–10 milliunits/min are rarely required.

**Abortion**
**IV: ADULTS: (Midterm elective abortion):** 10–20 milliunits/min. **Maximum:** 30 units/12-hr dose. **(Incomplete, inevitable abortion):** 10 units or IV infusion after suction or a sharp curettage.

**Control of Postpartum Bleeding**
**IV Infusion: ADULTS:** 10–40 units in 1,000 ml IV fluid at rate sufficient to

sustain uterine contractions and control uterine atony.

**IM: ADULTS:** 10 units (total dose) after delivery.

**Dosage in Renal/Hepatic Impairment**
No dose adjustment.

## SIDE EFFECTS

**Occasional:** Tachycardia, premature ventricular contractions, hypotension, nausea, vomiting. **Rare: Nasal:** Lacrimation/tearing, nasal irritation, rhinorrhea, unexpected uterine bleeding/contractions.

## ADVERSE EFFECTS/ TOXIC REACTIONS

Hypertonicity may occur with tearing of uterus, increased bleeding, abruptio placentae (i.e., placental abruption), cervical/vaginal lacerations. **Fetal:** Bradycardia, CNS/brain damage, trauma due to rapid propulsion, low Apgar score at 5 min, retinal hemorrhage occur rarely. Prolonged IV infusion of oxytocin with excessive fluid volume has caused severe water intoxication with seizures, coma, death.

## NURSING CONSIDERATIONS

### BASELINE ASSESSMENT

Assess baselines for vital signs, B/P, fetal heart rate. Determine frequency, duration, strength of contractions.

### INTERVENTION/EVALUATION

Monitor B/P, pulse, respirations, fetal heart rate, intrauterine pressure, contractions (duration, strength, frequency) q15min. Notify physician of contractions that last longer than 1 min, occur more frequently than every 2 min, or stop. Maintain careful I&O; be alert to potential water intoxication. Check for blood loss.

### PATIENT/FAMILY TEACHING

• Keep pt, family informed of labor progress.

O

# *PAClitaxel

HIGH ALERT

pak-li-**tax**-el
(Abraxane, Apo-Paclitaxel ✦)

■ **BLACK BOX ALERT** ■ Myelosuppression is major dose-limiting toxicity. Must be administered by certified chemotherapy personnel. Severe hypersensitivity reactions reported. **Do not confuse paclitaxel with docetaxel, paroxetine, or Paxil.**

## ◆ CLASSIFICATION

**PHARMACOTHERAPEUTIC:** Taxoid, antimitotic agent. **CLINICAL:** Antineoplastic.

## USES

Treatment of breast cancer, ovarian cancer, AIDS-related Kaposi's sarcoma, non-small-cell lung cancer (NSCLC). **Abraxane:** Treatment of breast cancer after failure of combination chemotherapy or relapse within 6 mos of adjuvant chemotherapy. First-line treatment of metastatic adenocarcinoma of pancreas. Treatment of locally advanced or metastatic NSCLC. **OFF-LABEL:** Bladder, cervical, small-cell lung, head and neck cancers. Treatment of adenocarcinoma. **Abraxane:** Recurrent/persistent ovarian, fallopian tube, primary peritoneal cancers.

## PRECAUTIONS

**Contraindications:** Hypersensitivity to paclitaxel. Hypersensitivity to drugs developed with Cremophor EL (polyoxyethylated castor oil). Treatment of solid tumors with baseline neutrophil count less than 1,500/mm³; treatment of Kaposi sarcoma with baseline neutrophil count less than 1,000/mm³. **Cautions:** Hepatic impairment, severe neutropenia, peripheral neuropathy.

## ACTION

Increases action of tubulin dimers; stabilizes existing microtubules; inhibits their disassembly; interferes with late $G_2$ mitotic phase. **Therapeutic Effect:** Inhibits cellular mitosis, replication.

## PHARMACOKINETICS

Does not readily cross blood-brain barrier. Protein binding: 89%–98%. Metabolized in liver. Eliminated bile/feces (71%), urine (14%). Not removed by hemodialysis. **Half-life:** 3-hr infusion: 13.1–20.2 hrs; 24-hr infusion: 15.7–52.7 hrs.

## ⧗ LIFESPAN CONSIDERATIONS

**Pregnancy/Lactation:** May cause fetal harm. Unknown if distributed in breast milk. Avoid use in pregnancy. **Children:** Safety and efficacy not established. **Elderly:** No age-related precautions noted.

## INTERACTIONS

**DRUG: CYP3A4, CYP2C8 inhibitors (e.g., ritonavir, clarithromycin, ketoconazole)** may increase concentration/effects. **CYP3A4, CYP2C8 inducers (e.g., rifampin, carbamazepine)** may decrease effects. **Bone marrow depressants** may increase myelosuppression. **Live virus vaccines** may potentiate virus replication, increase vaccine side effects, decrease pt's antibody response to vaccine. **HERBAL:** Avoid **black cohosh, dong quai** in estrogen-dependent tumors. **Gotu kola, kava kava, St. John's wort, valerian** may increase CNS depression. **St. John's wort** may decrease concentration. **FOOD:** None known. **LAB VALUES:** May elevate serum alkaline phosphatase, bilirubin, ALT, AST, triglycerides.

## AVAILABILITY (Rx)

**Injection, Powder for Reconstitution (Abraxane):** 100-mg vial. **Injection Solution:** 6 mg/ml (5-ml, 16.7-ml, 25-ml, 50-ml vials).

## ADMINISTRATION/HANDLING

 IV

◄**ALERT**► Wear gloves during handling; if contact with skin occurs, wash hands thoroughly with soap, water. If contact with mucous membranes occurs, flush with water.

---

P

**Paclitaxel**

**Reconstitution** • Dilute with 250–1,000 ml 0.9% NaCl, D₅W to final concentration of 0.3–1.2 mg/ml.

**Rate of Administration** • Administer at rate per protocol (range: 1–96 hrs) through in-line filter not greater than 0.22 microns. • Monitor vital signs during infusion, esp. during first hour. • Discontinue administration if severe hypersensitivity reaction occurs.

**Storage** • Store unopened vials at room temperature. • Reconstituted solution is stable at room temperature for 72 hrs. • Store diluted solutions in bottles or plastic bags. Administer through polyethylene-lined administration sets (avoid plasticized PVC equipment or devices).

**Abraxane (Paclitaxel—Protein Bound)**

**Reconstitution** • Reconstitute each vial with 20 ml 0.9% NaCl to provide concentration of 5 mg/ml. • Slowly inject onto inside wall of vial; gently swirl over 2 min to avoid foaming. • Inject appropriate amount into empty PVC-type bag.

**Rate of Administration** • Infuse over 30 min. Do not use in-line filter.

**Storage** • Store unopened vials at room temperature • Once reconstituted, use immediately but may refrigerate for up to 8 hrs.

### 🔲 IV INCOMPATIBILITIES

◀ALERT▶ **IV compatibility:** Data for Abraxane not known; avoid mixing with other medication. Amphotericin B complex (Abelcet, AmBisome, Amphotec), doxorubicin liposomal (Doxil), hydroxyzine (Vistaril), methylprednisolone (Solu-Medrol), mitoxantrone (Novantrone).

### 🔲 IV COMPATIBILITIES

Carboplatin (Paraplatin), cisplatin (Platinol AQ), cyclophosphamide (Cytoxan), cytarabine (Cytosar), dacarbazine (DTIC-Dome), dexamethasone (Decadron), diphenhydramine (Benadryl), doxorubicin (Adriamycin), etoposide (VePesid), gemcitabine (Gemzar), granisetron (Kytril), hydromorphone (Dilaudid), lipids, magnesium sulfate, mannitol, methotrexate, morphine, ondansetron (Zofran), potassium chloride, vinblastine (Velban), vincristine (Oncovin).

## INDICATIONS/ROUTES/DOSAGE

**Note:** Premedication with dexamethasone, diphenhydramine, and cimetidine, famotidine, or ranitidine recommended. Refer to individual protocols.

**Paclitaxel**
**Ovarian Cancer**
**IV: ADULTS, ELDERLY: (Previously Treated):** 135–175 mg/m²/dose over 3 hrs q3wks. **(Previously Untreated):** 175 mg/m² over 3 hrs q3wks (in combination with cisplatin) or 135 mg/m² over 24 hrs q3wks (in combination with cisplatin).

**Breast Cancer (Adjuvant)**
**IV: ADULTS, ELDERLY:** 175 mg/m² over 3 hrs for 4 cycles (give sequentially following anthracycline-containing regimen).

**Breast Cancer (Metastatic/Relapsed)**
**IV: ADULTS, ELDERLY:** 175 mg/m² over 3 hrs q3wks.

**Non–Small-Cell Lung Cancer**
**IV: ADULTS, ELDERLY:** 135 mg/m² over 24 hrs (in combination with cisplatin).

**Kaposi's Sarcoma (AIDS Related)**
**IV: ADULTS, ELDERLY:** 135 mg/m²/dose over 3 hrs q3wks or 100 mg/m²/dose over 3 hrs q2wks.

**Dosage in Renal Impairment**
No dose adjustment.

**Dosage in Hepatic Impairment**

| Transaminase Level | Bilirubin | Dose |
|---|---|---|
| **24-HR INFUSION** | | |
| Less than 2 times ULN | 1.5 mg/dL or less | 135 mg/m² |
| 2 to less than 10 times ULN | 1.5 mg/dL or less | 100 mg/m² |

**P**

| Transaminase Level | Bilirubin | Dose |
|---|---|---|
| Less than 10 times ULN | 1.6–7.5 mg/dL or less | 50 mg/m² |
| **3-HR INFUSION** | | |
| Less than 10 times ULN | 1.25 mg/dL or less | 175 mg/m² |
| Less than 10 times ULN | 1.26–2 times ULN | 135 mg/m² |
| Less than 10 times ULN | 2.01–5 times ULN | 90 mg/m² |
| 10 times ULN or greater | Greater than 5 times ULN | Avoid use |

ULN: upper limit of normal

**Dosage Modification**
Courses of paclitaxel should be withheld until neutrophil count is 1,500 cells/mm³ or more and platelet count is 100,000 cells/mm³ or more.

**Abraxane**
**Breast Cancer (Metastatic)**
**IV Infusion: ADULTS, ELDERLY:** 260 mg/m² q3wks. For pts who experience severe neutropenia (neutrophils less than 500 cells/mm³ for a wk or longer) or severe sensory neuropathy, reduce dosage to 220 mg/m² for subsequent courses. For recurrence of severe neutropenia or severe sensory neuropathy, reduce dosage to 180 mg/m² q3wks for subsequent courses. For grade 3 sensory neuropathy, hold until resolution to grade 1 or 2, followed by reduced dose for subsequent courses. Dosage of Abraxane for bilirubin greater than 1.5 mg/dL is not known.

**NSCLC (Locally Advanced or Metastatic)**
**IV: ADULTS, ELDERLY:** 100 mg/m² on days 1, 8, 15 of each 21-day cycle (in combination with carboplatin).

**Adenocarcinoma of Pancreas (Metastatic) (in combination with gemcitabine)**
**IV: ADULTS, ELDERLY:** 125 mg/m² on days 1, 8, 15 of each 28-day cycle. (Administer gemcitabine immediately after Abraxane.)

**Dosage in Renal Impairment**
No dose adjustment.

**Dosage in Hepatic Impairment**

| | Mild Impairment (AST Less Than 10 Times Upper Limit of Normal [ULN], Bilirubin 1.25 Times ULN or Less) | Moderate Impairment (AST Less Than 10 Times ULN, Bilirubin 1.26–2 Times ULN) | Severe Impairment | |
|---|---|---|---|---|
| | | | (AST Less Than 10 Times ULN, Bilirubin 2.01–5 Times ULN) | (AST More Than 10 Times ULN or Bilirubin > 5 Times ULN) |
| Breast cancer | No adjustment | Reduce dose to 200 mg/m² | Reduce dose to 130 mg/m² (may increase to 200 mg/m² in subsequent cycles) | Not recommended |
| NSCLC | No adjustment | Reduce dose to 75 mg/m² | Reduce dose to 50 mg/m² (may increase to 75 mg/m² in subsequent cycles) | Not recommended |
| Pancreatic | No adjustment | Not recommended | Not recommended | Not recommended |

P

## SIDE EFFECTS

**Expected (90%–70%):** Diarrhea, alopecia, nausea, vomiting. **Frequent (48%–46%):** Myalgia, arthralgia, peripheral neuropathy. **Occasional (20%–13%):** Mucositis, hypotension during infusion, pain/redness at injection site. **Rare (3%):** Bradycardia.

## ADVERSE EFFECTS/ TOXIC REACTIONS

Neutropenic nadir occurs at median of 11 days. Anemia, leukopenia occur commonly; thrombocytopenia occurs occasionally. Severe hypersensitivity reaction (dyspnea, severe hypotension, angioedema, generalized urticaria) occurs rarely.

## NURSING CONSIDERATIONS

### BASELINE ASSESSMENT

Offer emotional support. Use strict asepsis, protect pt from infection. Check blood counts, particularly neutrophil, platelet count, before each course of therapy or as clinically indicated.

### INTERVENTION/EVALUATION

Monitor CBC, LFT, vital signs. Monitor for hematologic toxicity (fever, sore throat, signs of local infections, unusual bleeding/bruising), symptoms of anemia (excessive fatigue, weakness). Assess response to medication. Monitor daily pattern of bowel activity, stool consistency; report diarrhea. Avoid IM injections, rectal temperatures, other traumas that may induce bleeding. Hold pressure to injection sites for full 5 min.

### PATIENT/FAMILY TEACHING

• Hair loss is reversible, but new hair may have different color, texture. • Do not have immunizations without physician's approval (drug lowers resistance). • Avoid crowds, persons with known infections. • Report signs of infection at once (fever, flu-like symptoms). • Report persistent nausea/vomiting. • Be alert for signs of peripheral neuropathy. • Avoid pregnancy. • Avoid tasks that may require alertness, motor skills until response to drug is established.

# palbociclib

**pal**-boe-**sye**-klib
(Ibrance)

## ◆CLASSIFICATION

**PHARMACOTHERAPEUTIC:** Kinase inhibitor. **CLINICAL:** Antineoplastic.

## USES

Used in combination with letrozole for treatment of postmenopausal women with estrogen receptor–positive, human epidermal growth factor receptor 2 (*HER2*)–negative advanced breast cancer as initial endocrine-based therapy for metastatic disease or in combination with fulvestrant in women with disease progression following endocrine therapy.

## PRECAUTIONS

**Contraindications:** Hypersensitivity to palbociclib. **Cautions:** Baseline anemia, lymphopenia, neutropenia, thrombocytopenia. History of pulmonary embolism. Avoid concomitant use of strong or moderate CYP3A inhibitors, strong or moderate CYP3A inducers.

## ACTION

Inhibits proliferation of tumor cells that overexpress *HER2* by blocking cellular progression from G1 into S phase of cell cycle. Promotes cellular death (apoptosis). **Therapeutic Effect:** Inhibits tumor cell growth and metastasis.

## PHARMACOKINETICS

Readily absorbed. Widely distributed. Metabolized in liver. Protein binding: 85%. Peak plasma concentration: 6–12 hrs. Steady state reached in 8 days. Eliminated in feces (74%), urine (18%). **Half-life:** 29 hrs.

## ⧗ LIFESPAN CONSIDERATIONS

**Pregnancy/Lactation:** Treatment is indicated for postmenopausal women. However, treatment may cause fetal

P

harm when administered during pregnancy. Females of reproductive potential should use effective contraception during treatment and up to 2 wks after discontinuation. Unknown if distributed in breast milk. Must either discontinue drug or discontinue breastfeeding. **Children:** Safety and efficacy not established. Not indicated in this population. **Elderly:** No age-related precautions noted.

## INTERACTIONS

**DRUG:** Strong CYP3A inhibitors (e.g., clarithromycin, ketoconazole, ritonavir), moderate CYP3A inhibitors (e.g., atazanavir, ciprofloxacin) may increase concentration/effect; avoid use. Strong CYP3A inducers (e.g., carbamazepine, rifampicin), moderate CYP3A inducers (e.g., nafcillin) may decrease concentration/effect; avoid use. May increase concentration/effects of **medications with a narrow therapeutic index (e.g., cyclosporine, ergotamine, tacrolimus). HERBAL:** St. John's wort may decrease concentration/effect. **FOOD:** Grapefruit products may increase concentration/effect. **LAB VALUES:** May decrease Hgb, lymphocytes, neutrophils, platelets, WBC.

## AVAILABILITY (Rx)

**Capsules:** 75 mg, 100 mg, 125 mg.

## ADMINISTRATION/HANDLING

**PO**
• Give with food. • Administer whole; do not break, crush, cut, or open capsule. • If vomiting occurs after dosing, do not readminister dose; give next at next scheduled time.

## INDICATIONS/ROUTES/DOSAGE

**Breast Cancer**
**PO: ADULTS, ELDERLY:** 125 mg once daily for 21 days, followed by a 7-day rest period to complete a 28-day cycle. Use in combination with letrozole 2.5 mg once

daily throughout 28-day cycle or with fulvestrant 500 mg on days 1, 15, 29 and once monthly thereafter.

**Dose Reduction for Adverse Events**

| Dose Level | Dose |
|---|---|
| Recommended starting dose | 125 mg/day |
| First dose reduction | 100 mg/day |
| Second dose reduction | 75 mg/day |
| Unable to tolerate 75 mg/day | Permanently discontinue |

**Dose Modification**
Based on Common Terminology Criteria for Adverse Events (CTCAE).

**Hematologic Toxicities**
**Grade 1 or 2:** No dose adjustment. **Grade 3 (except lymphopenia unless associated with clinical events (e.g., opportunistic infection):** No dose adjustment. Withhold treatment until recovery to less than grade 2. **Grade 3, ANC 500–1000/mm³** plus fever that is greater than or equal to 38.5°C and/or active infection: Interrupt treatment (and initiation of the next cycle) until recovery to grade 2 or less. Resume at reduced dose upon starting.

**Nonhematologic Toxicities**
**Grade 1 or 2:** No dose adjustment. **Grade 3 or greater (if persistent despite optimal medical management):** Interrupt treatment until resolved to grade 1 or less; grade 2 or less if the event is not considered a serious medical risk. Resume at reduced dose upon starting.

**Concomitant Use of Strong CYP3A Inhibitors**
**PO: ADULTS, ELDERLY:** 75 mg once daily if unable to use alternative drug with minimal CYP3A inhibition. If CYP3A inhibitor is discontinued, increase palbociclib dose (after 3–5 half-lives of CYP3A inhibitor have elapsed) to the dose used prior to initiating strong CYP3A inhibitor.

P

Dosage in Renal Impairment
**Mild to moderate impairment:** No dose adjustment. **Severe impairment:** Not studied; use caution.

Dosage in Hepatic Impairment
**Mild impairment:** No dose adjustment. **Moderate to severe impairment:** Not studied; use caution.

## SIDE EFFECTS

**Frequent (41%–21%):** Fatigue, nausea, alopecia, diarrhea. **Occasional (16%–13%):** Decreased appetite, vomiting, asthenia.

## ADVERSE EFFECTS/TOXIC REACTIONS

Anemia, leukopenia, neutropenia, thrombocytopenia is an expected response to therapy. CTCAE grade 3 neutropenia reported in 57% of pts. The median onset of neutropenia was 15 days. Pulmonary embolism (5% of pts); upper respiratory tract infections including influenza, laryngitis, nasopharyngitis, pharyngitis, rhinitis, sinusitis (31% of pts); peripheral neuropathy (31% of pts); cheilitis, glossitis, glossodynia, mouth ulceration, stomatitis (25% of pts); epistaxis (11% of pts) were reported.

## NURSING CONSIDERATIONS

### BASELINE ASSESSMENT

Monitor baseline ANC, CBC. Confirm estrogen receptor–positive, *HER2*-negative status. Verify pregnancy status before start of each cycle. Screen for history of pulmonary embolism. Receive full medication history and screen for interactions. Assess hydration status. Screen for active infection.

### INTERVENTION/EVALUATION

Monitor ANC, CBC at start of each cycle and on day 14 on the first two cycles. If any grade 3 or 4 hematologic toxicity occurs, repeat CBC 7 days after interruption of therapy and at start of next cycle. If neutropenia occurs specifically, recommend treatment interruption, dose reduction, or delay in starting treatment for next cycle. Monitor for neurotoxicity (peripheral neuropathy), epistaxis. If chest pain, dyspnea, tachycardia occurs, provide supplemental $O_2$ and obtain radiologic testing to rule out pulmonary embolism.

### PATIENT/FAMILY TEACHING

• Blood levels will monitored regularly. • Treatment may cause fetal harm. Women of childbearing potential should use effective contraception during treatment and up to 2 wks following discontinuation. Immediately report suspected pregnancy. Do not breastfeed. • Immediately report chest pain, difficult breathing, fast heart rate, rapid breathing; may indicate life-threatening blood clot in the lungs. • Report symptoms of bone marrow suppression or infection such as bruising easily, chills, cough, dizziness, fainting, fever, shortness of breath, weakness. • Swallow capsules whole; do not chew, crush, cut, or open capsules. • Take each dose with food. • Treatment may increase risk of infection, nosebleeds. • Drink plenty of fluids. • Do not ingest grapefruit products or herbal supplements. • Avoid crowds; those with active infection.

# paliperidone     <sub>TOP 100</sub>

pal-ee-**per**-i-done
(Invega, Invega Sustenna, Invega Trinza)

■ **BLACK BOX ALERT** ■ Elderly pts with dementia-related psychosis are at increased risk for mortality due to cerebrovascular events.

## ◆CLASSIFICATION

**PHARMACOTHERAPEUTIC:** Benzisoxazole derivative. **CLINICAL:** Antipsychotic.

## USES

**Oral:** Treatment of schizophrenia. Acute treatment of schizoaffective disorder as monotherapy or as adjunct to mood stabilizers and/or antidepressants. **Injection:** Acute and maintenance treatment of schizophrenia. **OFF-LABEL:** Treatment of irritability associated with autistic disorder.

## PRECAUTIONS

**Contraindications:** Sensitivity to paliperidone, risperidone. **Cautions:** History of cardiac arrhythmias, mild renal impairment (not recommended in moderate to severe impairment), diabetes mellitus, HF, active seizures or predisposition to seizures, history of seizures, cardiovascular disease, congenital long QT syndrome, concomitant use with other medications that prolong QT interval (e.g., amiodarone, quinidine), pts at risk for aspiration pneumonia. May increase risk of stroke in pts with dementia-related psychosis. CNS depression, medications for hypertension, hypovolemia or dehydration, high risk for suicide. Pts with breast cancer, other prolactin-dependent tumors, children, adolescents.

## ACTION

Exact mechanism of action is unknown, but may antagonize dopamine and serotonin receptors. **Therapeutic Effect:** Suppresses behavioral response in psychosis.

## PHARMACOKINETICS

Absorbed from GI tract. Metabolized in liver. Primarily excreted in urine. **Half-life:** 23 hrs.

## ⧗ LIFESPAN CONSIDERATIONS

**Pregnancy/Lactation:** Unknown if drug crosses placenta or is distributed in breast milk. **Children:** Safety and efficacy not established. **Elderly:** Potential for orthostatic hypotension. Age-related renal impairment may require dosage adjustment.

## INTERACTIONS

**DRUG:** May decrease effects of **dopamine agonists, levodopa.** Alcohol, **CNS depressants (e.g., lorazepam, morphine, zolpidem)** may increase CNS depression. **HERBAL:** None significant.

**FOOD:** None known. **LAB VALUES:** May increase serum creatine phosphatase, uric acid, triglycerides, ALT, AST, prolactin. May decrease serum potassium, sodium, protein, glucose.

## AVAILABILITY (Rx)

**Injection Suspension (Invega Sustenna):** 39 mg/0.25 ml, 78 mg/0.5 ml, 117 mg/0.75 ml, 156 mg/ml, 234 mg/1.5 ml. **(Invega Trinza):** 273 mg, 410 mg, 546 mg, 819 mg.

🐾 **Tablets, Extended-Release:** 1.5 mg, 3 mg, 6 mg, 9 mg.

## ADMINISTRATION/HANDLING

**PO**
• May give without regard to food.
• Do not break, crush, dissolve, or divide extended-release tablets.

**IM**
• Administer 2 initial injections in deltoid muscle (helps attain therapeutic concentration rapidly). • Maintenance doses may be given in gluteal or deltoid muscle.

## INDICATIONS/ROUTES/DOSAGE

**Treatment of Schizophrenia**
**PO: ADULTS, ELDERLY:** Initially, 6 mg once daily in the morning. May increase dose in increments of 3 mg/day at intervals of more than 5 days. Range: 3–12 mg/day. **ADOLESCENTS (51 KG OR GREATER):** Initially, 3 mg once daily. Range: 3–12 mg/day. **(50 KG OR LESS):** Initially, 3 mg once daily. Range: 3–6 mg/day.
**IM:** *(Invega Sustenna):* **ADULTS, ELDERLY:** Initially, 234 mg on day 1 followed by 156 mg 1 wk later (second dose may be given 4 days before or after the wkly time point). **Maintenance:** Following the 1-wk initiation regimen, begin 117 mg monthly. Range: 39–234 mg. Monthly maintenance dose may be given 7 days before or after the monthly time point. *(Invega Trinza):* 273 mg to 819 mg q3mos (based on last dose of Invega Sustenna). Three-month IM used only after monthly IM dose established for at least 4 mos. The last 2 mos of monthly IM

should be the same dosage strength before starting 3-mo injections.

**Schizoaffective Disorder**
**PO: ADULTS, ELDERLY:** 6 mg once daily in the morning. May increase in increments of 3 mg/day at intervals of more than 4 days. Range: 3–12 mg/day. **IM: ADULTS, ELDERLY:** Initially, 234 mg, then 156 mg 1 wk later. **Maintenance range:** 78–234 mg monthly. May be given 7 days before or after the monthly time point.

**Dosage in Renal Impairment**

| Creatinine Clearance | Oral Dosage | IM Dosage |
|---|---|---|
| 50–80 ml/min | 6 mg/day maximum | 156 mg on day 1, then 117 mg 1 wk later Maintenance: 78 mg once monthly |
| 10–49 ml/min | 3 mg/day maximum | Not recommended |

**Dosage in Hepatic Impairment**
No dose adjustment.

## SIDE EFFECTS

**Occasional (14%–4%):** Tachycardia, headache, drowsiness, akathisia, anxiety, dizziness, dyspepsia, nausea.

## ADVERSE EFFECTS/ TOXIC REACTIONS

Neuroleptic malignant syndrome (NMS), hyperpyrexia, muscle rigidity, change in mental status, unstable pulse or B/P, tachycardia, diaphoresis, cardiac arrhythmias, rhabdomyolysis, acute renal failure, tardive dyskinesia (protrusion of tongue, puffing of cheeks, chewing/ puckering of mouth) may occur rarely. May prolong QT interval.

## NURSING CONSIDERATIONS

### BASELINE ASSESSMENT

Obtain baseline renal function tests. Assess behavior, appearance, emotional status, response to environment, speech pattern, thought content. Screen for comorbidities as listed in Precautions.

### INTERVENTION/EVALUATION

Monitor B/P, heart rate, weight, renal function tests, EKG. Monitor for fine tongue movement (may be first sign of tardive dyskinesia). Supervise suicidal-risk pt closely during early therapy (as depression lessons, energy level improves, increasing suicide potential). Assess for therapeutic response (greater interest in surroundings, improved self-care, increased ability to concentrate, relaxed facial expression). Monitor for potential neuroleptic malignant syndrome (fever, muscle rigidity, unstable B/P or pulse, altered mental status).

### PATIENT/FAMILY TEACHING

• Avoid tasks that may require alertness, motor skills until response to drug is established. • Use caution when changing position from lying or sitting to standing. • Report trembling in fingers, altered gait, unusual muscle/skeletal movements, palpitations, severe dizziness, fainting, swelling/pain in breasts, visual changes, rash, difficulty in breathing.

# palonosetron

pal-oh-**noe**-se-tron
(Aloxi)
**Do not confuse Aloxi with Eloxatin or oxaliplatin, or palonosetron with dolasetron, granisetron, or ondansetron.**

## FIXED-COMBINATION(S)

**Akynzeo:** palonosetron/netupitant (a substance P/neurokinin receptor antagonist): 0.5 mg/300 mg.

## ◆CLASSIFICATION

**PHARMACOTHERAPEUTIC:** 5-HT$_3$ receptor antagonist. **CLINICAL:** Antiemetic.

## USES

Prevention of acute and delayed nausea/vomiting associated with initial/repeated courses of moderately or highly emetogenic chemotherapy. Prevention of postop nausea/vomiting for up to 24 hrs following surgery.

## PRECAUTIONS

**Contraindications:** Hypersensitivity to palonosetron. **Cautions:** History of cardiovascular disease; congenital long QT syndrome, risk factors for QT prolongation (hypokalemia, hypomagnesemia), medications that prolong QT interval or reduce potassium/magnesium levels, pts at risk for ventricular arrhythmias.

## ACTION

Acts centrally in chemoreceptor trigger zone, peripherally at vagal nerve terminals. **Therapeutic Effect:** Prevents nausea/vomiting associated with chemotherapy.

## PHARMACOKINETICS

Protein binding: 52%. Metabolized in liver. Eliminated in urine. **Half-life:** 40 hrs.

## ⧗ LIFESPAN CONSIDERATIONS

**Pregnancy/Lactation:** Unknown if distributed in breast milk. **Children:** Safety and efficacy not established. **Elderly:** No age-related precautions noted.

## INTERACTIONS

**DRUG:** Fentanyl, lithium, MAOIs, SNRIs (e.g., duloxetine, venlafaxine), SSRIs (e.g., citalopram, fluoxetine, sertraline), tricyclic antidepressants (e.g., amitriptyline, doxepin) may increase risk of serotonin syndrome. **HERBAL:** None significant. **FOOD:** None known. **LAB VALUES:** May transiently increase serum bilirubin, ALT, AST.

## AVAILABILITY (Rx)

**Injection Solution:** 0.25 mg/5 ml.

## ADMINISTRATION/HANDLING

 **IV**

**Reconstitution •** Give undiluted as IV push.
**Rate of Administration •** Give IV push over 30 sec. Children: Infuse over 15 min. • Flush infusion line with 0.9% NaCl before and following administration.
**Storage •** Store at room temperature. Solution should appear colorless, clear. Discard if cloudy precipitate forms.

## ▦ IV COMPATIBILITIES

Famotidine (Pepcid), lorazepam (Ativan), midazolam (Versed), potassium chloride.

## INDICATIONS/ROUTES/DOSAGE

**Chemotherapy-Induced Nausea/Vomiting**
IV: **ADULTS, ELDERLY:** 0.25 mg as single dose 30 min before starting chemotherapy. **CHILDREN 1 MO TO YOUNGER THAN 17 YRS:** 20 mcg/kg as single dose 30 min before starting chemotherapy. **Maximum:** 1.5 mg.

**Postop Nausea/Vomiting**
IV: **ADULTS, ELDERLY:** 0.075 mg over 10 sec immediately before induction of anesthesia.

**Dosage in Renal/Hepatic Impairment**
No dose adjustment.

## SIDE EFFECTS

**Occasional (9%–5%):** Headache, constipation. **Rare (Less Than 1%):** Diarrhea, dizziness, fatigue, abdominal pain, insomnia.

## ADVERSE EFFECTS/TOXIC REACTIONS

Overdose may produce combination of CNS stimulation, depressant effects. May prolong QT interval. 5-HT$_3$ receptor antagonists are known to potentiate serotonin syndrome, esp. in pts taking serotonergic medications.

**P**

---

## NURSING CONSIDERATIONS

### BASELINE ASSESSMENT

Obtain BMP, serum magnesium in pts at risk for hypokalemia, hypomagnesemia. Assess for signs of dehydration due to excessive vomiting (poor skin turgor, dry mucous membranes). Question history of cardiac disease, long QT syndrome, cardiac arrhythmias. Screen for concomitant home medications that prolong QT interval, increase risk of serotonin syndrome. Provide emotional support.

### INTERVENTION/EVALUATION

Obtain BMP, serum magnesium; EKG in pts suspected of arrhythmia, QT interval prolongation. Assess for symptoms of serotonin syndrome (e.g., altered mental status, tachycardia, labile B/P, diaphoresis, hyperthermia, tremor, hyperreflexia, diarrhea, seizures). Monitor for hypersensitivity reaction. Monitor pt for signs of dehydration. Provide supportive measures. Assess mental status. Monitor daily pattern of bowel activity, stool consistency.

### PATIENT/FAMILY TEACHING

• Relief from nausea/vomiting generally occurs shortly after drug administration. • Avoid alcohol, barbiturates. • Report persistent vomiting. • Report palpitations, lightheadedness, fainting; allergic reactions of any kind.

---

# pamidronate

pam-id-**roe**-nate
(Aredia♣)
**Do not confuse Aredia with Adriamycin, or pamidronate with alendronate, ibandronate, or risedronate.**

### ◆CLASSIFICATION

**PHARMACOTHERAPEUTIC:** Bisphosphonate. **CLINICAL:** Hypocalcemic.

## USES

Treatment of moderate to severe hypercalcemia associated with malignancy (with/without bone metastases). Treatment of moderate to severe Paget's disease, osteolytic bone lesions of multiple myeloma or metastatic breast cancer. **OFF-LABEL:** Inhibits bone resorption in osteogenesis imperfecta, treatment of bone metastases of thyroid cancer, prevention of bone loss associated with androgen deprivation treatment in prostate cancer.

## PRECAUTIONS

**Contraindications:** Hypersensitivity to pamidronate, other bisphosphonates (e.g., etidronate, tiludronate, risedronate, alendronate). **Cautions:** Renal impairment, concurrent use with other nephrotoxic medications, history of thyroid surgery. Preexisting anemia, leukopenia, thrombocytopenia.

## ACTION

Inhibits bone resorption, decreases mineralization by disrupting activity of osteoclasts. **Therapeutic Effect:** Lowers serum calcium concentration.

## PHARMACOKINETICS

| Route | Onset | Peak | Duration |
|-------|-------|------|----------|
| IV | 24–48 hrs | 3–7 days | N/A |

After IV administration, rapidly absorbed by bone. Slowly excreted unchanged in urine. Unknown if removed by hemodialysis. **Half-life:** 21–35 hrs.

## ⌛ LIFESPAN CONSIDERATIONS

**Pregnancy/Lactation:** No adequate, well-controlled studies in pregnant women; unknown if fetal harm can occur. Unknown if distributed in breast milk. **Children:** Safety and efficacy not established. **Elderly:** May become overhydrated. Careful monitoring of fluid and electrolytes indicated; recommend dilution in smaller volume.

## INTERACTIONS

**DRUG:** **Nephrotoxic medications (e.g., acyclovir, amphotericin B, diclofenac, gentamicin, IV contrast dye, NSAIDs, vancomycin)** may increase potential for nephrotoxicity. **HERBAL:** None significant. **FOOD:** None known. **LAB VALUES:** None significant.

## AVAILABILITY (Rx)

**Injection, Powder for Reconstitution:** 30 mg, 90 mg. **Injection Solution:** 3 mg/ml, 6 mg/ml, 9 mg/ml.

## ADMINISTRATION/HANDLING

 IV

**Reconstitution** • Reconstitute each vial with 10 ml Sterile Water for Injection to provide concentration of 3 mg/ml or 9 mg/ml. • Allow drug to dissolve before withdrawing. • Further dilute with 250–1,000 ml sterile 0.45% or 0.9% NaCl or D$_5$W (1,000 ml for hypercalcemia of malignancy, 500 ml for Paget's disease, multiple myeloma, 250 ml for breast cancer). **Rate of Administration** • Adequate hydration is essential in conjunction with pamidronate therapy (avoid overhydration in pts with potential for HF). • Administer as IV infusion over 2–24 hrs for treatment of hypercalcemia; over 2 hrs for breast cancer; over 4 hrs for Paget's disease or multiple myeloma. **Storage** • Store parenteral form at room temperature. • Reconstituted vial is stable for 24 hrs if refrigerated; IV solution is stable for 24 hrs after dilution.

## ▨ IV INCOMPATIBILITIES

Calcium-containing IV fluids.

## INDICATIONS/ROUTES/DOSAGE

**Hypercalcemia**
**IV Infusion:** ADULTS, ELDERLY: **Moderate hypercalcemia (corrected serum calcium level 12–13.5 mg/dL):** 60–90 mg as a single dose over 2–24 hrs. **Severe hypercalcemia (corrected serum calcium level greater than 13.5 mg/dL):** 90 mg as a single dose over 2–24 hrs.

**Paget's Disease**
**IV Infusion:** ADULTS, ELDERLY: 30 mg/day over 4 hrs for 3 consecutive days.

**Osteolytic Bone Lesion (Multiple Myeloma)**
**IV Infusion:** ADULTS, ELDERLY: 90 mg over 4 hrs once monthly.

**Osteolytic Bone Lesion (Breast Cancer)**
**IV Infusion:** ADULTS, ELDERLY: 90 mg over 2 hrs q3–4wks.

**Dosage in Renal Impairment**
Not recommended.

**Dosage in Hepatic Impairment**
No dose adjustment.

## SIDE EFFECTS

**Frequent (27%–18%):** Temperature elevation (at least 1°C) 24–48 hrs after administration; erythema, swelling, induration, pain at catheter site in pts receiving 90 mg; anorexia, nausea, fatigue. **Occasional (10%–1%):** Constipation, rhinitis.

## ADVERSE EFFECTS/ TOXIC REACTIONS

Hypophosphatemia, hypokalemia, hypomagnesemia, hypocalcemia occur more frequently with higher dosages. Anemia, hypertension, tachycardia, atrial fibrillation, drowsiness occur more frequently with 90-mg doses. GI hemorrhage occurs rarely.

## NURSING CONSIDERATIONS

### BASELINE ASSESSMENT

Obtain CBC, serum calcium, ionized calcium, magnesium, phosphate; renal function test level prior to therapy. Determine hydration status.

### INTERVENTION/EVALUATION

Monitor serum calcium, ionized calcium, potassium, magnesium, creatinine, CBC.

P

Provide adequate hydration; assess overhydration. Monitor I&O carefully; assess lungs for rales, dependent body parts for edema. Monitor B/P, temperature, pulse. Assess catheter site for redness, swelling, pain. Monitor food intake, daily pattern of bowel activity, stool consistency. Be alert for potential GI hemorrhage with 90-mg dosage.

**PATIENT/FAMILY TEACHING**

• Report symptoms of low blood calcium levels, including confusion, muscle twitching/ cramps, numbness, seizures, tingling. • Immediately report GI bleeding.

# pancrelipase

pan-kree-**lye**-pace
(Creon, Pancreaze, Zenpep, Pertyze, Ultresa, Viokace)

## ◆CLASSIFICATION

**PHARMACOTHERAPEUTIC:** Digestive enzyme. **CLINICAL:** Pancreatic enzyme replenisher.

## USES

**Creon, Pancreaze, Pertyze, Ultresa Zenpep:** Treatment of exocrine pancreatic insufficiency (EPI) due to cystic fibrosis or other conditions. **Creon:** Chronic pancreatitis, pancreatectomy. **Viokace: (with a proton pump inhibitor):** Chronic pancreatitis, pancreatectomy.

## PRECAUTIONS

**Contraindications:** Hypersensitivity to pancrelipase. **Cautions:** Gout, hyperuricemia, renal impairment, hypersensitivity to pork proteins.

## ACTION

Replaces endogenous pancreatic enzymes. **Therapeutic Effect:** Assists in digestion of protein, starch, fats.

## INTERACTIONS

**DRUG:** May decrease absorption of **iron supplements. HERBAL:** None significant.

**FOOD:** None known. **LAB VALUES:** May increase serum uric acid.

## AVAILABILITY (Rx)

**Capsules,    Delayed-Release: (Creon):** 3,000 units lipase; 9,500 units protease; 15,000 units amylase. 6,000 units lipase; 19,000 units protease; 30,000 units amylase. 12,000 units lipase; 38,000 units protease; 60,000 units amylase. 24,000 units lipase; 76,000 units protease; 120,000 units amylase. **(Pancreaze):** 4,200 units lipase; 10,000 units protease; 17,500 units amylase; 10,500 units lipase; 25,000 units protease; 43,750 units amylase; 16,800 units lipase; 40,000 units protease; 70,000 units amylase; 21,000 units lipase; 37,000 units protease; 61,000 units amylase. **(Zenpep):** 3,000 units lipase; 10,000 units protease; 16,000 units amylase; 5,000 units lipase; 17,000 units protease; 27,000 units amylase. 10,000 units lipase; 34,000 units protease; 55,000 units amylase. 15,000 units lipase; 51,000 units protease; 82,000 units amylase. 20,000 units lipase; 68,000 units protease; 109,000 units amylase. 25,000 units lipase; 85,000 units protease; 136,000 units amylase. **Pertyze:** 8,000 units lipase; 28,750 units protease; 30,250 units amylase. 16,000 units lipase; 57,500 units protease; 60,500 units amylase. **Ultresa:** 13,800 units lipase; 27,600 units protease; 27,600 units amylase. 20,700 units lipase; 41,400 units protease; 41,400 units amylase. 23,000 units lipase; 46,000 units protease; 46,000 units amylase. ◆ **Tablets, Viokace:** 10,440 units lipase; 39,150 units protease; 39,150 units amylase. 20,880 units lipase; 78,300 units protease; 78,300 units amylase.

## ADMINISTRATION/HANDLING

### PO

• Give capsules whole with generous amount of liquid. • If pt unable to swallow intact capsule, contents may be given without crushing/chewing, followed by fluid. Contents may be sprinkled on soft acidic food such as applesauce.

- Swallow immediately after mixing. Give tablets whole, do not break, crush, dissolve, or divide. • **Viokace:** must be given with a proton pump inhibitor.

## INDICATIONS/ROUTES/DOSAGE

◀**ALERT**▶ Dosage expressed as lipase units/kg. Individualize dose based on clinical symptoms, degree of steatorrhea, fat content in diet.

**Pancreatic Insufficiency (Due to Conditions Such as Cystic Fibrosis)**
**PO: ADULTS, ELDERLY, CHILDREN 4 YRS AND OLDER:** Initially, 500 units/kg lipase/kg/meal up to 2,500 units lipase/kg/meal (or less than or equal to 10,000 lipase units/kg/day) or less than 4,000 lipase units/g of fat ingested/day. **CHILDREN OLDER THAN 12 MOS AND YOUNGER THAN 4 YRS:** Initially, 1,000 units lipase/kg/meal up to 2,500 units lipase/kg/meal (or less than or equal to 10,000 lipase units/kg/day) or less than 4,000 lipase units/g of fat ingested/day. **INFANTS UP TO 12 MOS:** 2,000–4,000 units lipase per 120 ml of formula or per breastfeeding. Do not mix Creon or Zenpep capsule contents directly into formula or breast milk prior to administration.

**Pancreatic Insufficiency (Due to Chronic Pancreatitis or Pancreatectomy)**
**PO: ADULTS, ELDERLY: (Cream):** 72,000 units/meal, while consuming 100 g or more of fat daily. **(Viokace):** 500 units/kg/meal. Range: 500–2,500 units/kg/meal.

**Dosage in Renal/Hepatic Impairment**
No dose adjustment.

## SIDE EFFECTS

**Rare:** Allergic reaction, mouth irritation, shortness of breath, wheezing.

## ADVERSE EFFECTS/ TOXIC REACTIONS

Excessive dosage may produce nausea, cramping, diarrhea. Hyperuricosuria, hyperuricemia reported with extremely high dosages.

## NURSING CONSIDERATIONS

### INTERVENTION/EVALUATION
Question for therapeutic relief from GI symptoms. Do not change brands without consulting physician.

### PATIENT/FAMILY TEACHING
- Do not chew capsules. • Instruct pts with trouble swallowing to open capsules, spread contents over applesauce, mashed fruit, rice cereal or follow with glass of water or juice to ensure swallowing. • Do not break, crush, dissolve, or divide tablets. Swallow whole.

---

# panitumumab

pan-i-**toom**-ue-mab
(Vectibix)
■ **BLACK BOX ALERT** ■ 90% of pts experience dermatologic toxicities (dermatitis acneiform, pruritus, erythema, rash, skin exfoliation, skin fissures, abscess). Severe infusion reactions (anaphylaxis, bronchospasm, fever, chills, hypotension), fatal reactions have occured.

## ◆CLASSIFICATION
**PHARMACOTHERAPEUTIC:** Monoclonal antibody. **CLINICAL:** Antineoplastic.

## USES
Treatment of wild-type KRAS metastatic colorectal cancer either as first-line therapy in combination with FOLFOX or as monotherapy following disease progression after prior treatment with fluoropyrimidine-, oxaliplatin-, or irinotecan-based regimens.

## PRECAUTIONS
**Contraindications:** Hypersensitivity to panitumumab. **Cautions:** Interstitial pneumonitis, pulmonary fibrosis, pulmonary infiltrates, renal impairment, baseline electrolyte imbalance. Not indicated in pts with *RAS*-mutant metastatic colorectal cancer or for whom *RAS* mutation status is unknown.

P

## ACTION

Binds specifically to epidermal growth factor receptor (EGFR) and competitively inhibits binding of epidermal growth factor. **Therapeutic Effect:** Prevents cell growth, proliferation, transformation, survival.

## PHARMACOKINETICS

Clearance varies by body weight, gender, tumor burden. **Half-life:** 3–10 days.

## ⧖ LIFESPAN CONSIDERATIONS

**Pregnancy/Lactation:** Teratogenic. Potential for fertility impairment. May decrease fetal body weight; increase risk of skeletal fetal abnormalities. Breast-feeding not recommended. **Children:** Safety and efficacy not established. **Elderly:** No age-related precautions noted.

## INTERACTIONS

**DRUG:** None significant. **HERBAL:** None significant. **FOOD:** None known. **LAB VALUES:** May decrease serum magnesium, calcium.

## AVAILABILITY (Rx)

**Injection Solution:** 20 mg/ml vial (5-ml, 20-ml vials).

## ADMINISTRATION/HANDLING

### 🖫 IV

◀**ALERT**▶ Do not give by IV push or bolus. Use low protein-binding 0.2- or 0.22-micron in-line filter. Flush IV line before and after chemotherapy administration with 0.9% NaCl.
**Reconstitution** • Dilute in 100–150 ml 0.9% NaCl to provide concentration of 10 mg/ml or less. • Do not shake solution. Invert gently to mix. • Discard any unused portion.
**Rate of Administration** • Give as IV infusion over 60 min. • Infuse doses greater than 1,000 mg over 90 min.
**Storage** • Refrigerate vials. • After dilution, solution may be stored for up to 6 hrs at room temperature, up to 24 hrs if refrigerated. • Discard if discolored but solution may contain visible, translucent-to-white particulates (will be removed by in-line filter).

## 🖩 IV INCOMPATIBILITIES

Do not mix with dextrose solutions or any other medications.

## INDICATIONS/ROUTES/DOSAGE

◀**ALERT**▶ Stop infusion immediately in pts experiencing severe infusion reactions.

**Metastatic Colorectal Cancer**
**IV Infusion: ADULTS, ELDERLY:** 6 mg/kg given over 60 min once every 14 days. Doses greater than 1,000 mg should be infused over 90 min.

**Dose Modification**
**Infusion Reactions**
**Mild to moderate reactions:** Reduce infusion rate by 50% for remainder of infusion. **Severe reactions:** Discontinue infusion. Depending on severity, consider permanent discontinuation.

**Skin Toxicity**
For all grade 3 skin toxicities, withhold treatment for 1–2 doses until improved to better than grade 3. Then, reduce dose as follows: **First occurrence of grade 3:** Resume at same dose. **Second occurrence of grade 3:** Reduce dose to 80% of initial dose. **Third occurrence of grade 3:** Reduce dose to 60% of initial dose. **Fourth occurrence of grade 3:** Permanently discontinue.

**Dosage in Renal/Hepatic Impairment**
No dose adjustment.

## SIDE EFFECTS

**Common (65%–57%):** Erythema, acneiform dermatitis, pruritus. **Frequent (26%–20%):** Fatigue, abdominal pain, skin exfoliation, paronychia (soft tissue infection around nailbed), nausea, rash, diarrhea, constipation, skin fissures. **Occasional (19%–10%):** Vomiting, acne, cough, peripheral edema, dry skin. **Rare**

(7%–2%): Stomatitis, mucosal inflammation, eyelash growth, conjunctivitis, increased lacrimation.

## ADVERSE EFFECTS/ TOXIC REACTIONS

Pulmonary fibrosis, severe dermatologic toxicity (complicated by infectious sequelae) occur rarely. Severe infusion reactions manifested as bronchospasm, fever, chills, hypotension occur rarely. Hypomagnesemia occurs in 39% of pts. Life-threatening and/or fatal bullous fasciitis, abscess, sepsis were reported. Severe dehydration and diarrhea may increase risk of acute renal failure. Exposure to sunlight may exacerbate skin toxicities. May cause ocular toxicities including keratitis, ulcerative keratitis, corneal ulceration.

## NURSING CONSIDERATIONS

### BASELINE ASSESSMENT

Assess baseline serum magnesium, calcium prior to therapy, periodically during therapy, and for 8 wks after completion of therapy. Assess *KRAS* mutational status in colorectal tumors and confirm the absence of a *RAS* mutation.

### INTERVENTION/EVALUATION

Assess for skin, ocular, mucosal, pulmonary toxicity, report effects. Median time to development of skin/ocular toxicity is 14–15 days; resolution after last dosing is 84 days. Monitor serum electrolytes for hypomagnesemia, hypocalcemia. Offer antiemetic if nausea/vomiting occurs. Monitor daily pattern of bowel activity, stool consistency.

### PATIENT/FAMILY TEACHING

• Do not have immunizations without physician's approval (drug lowers resistance). • Avoid contact with those who have recently received a live virus vaccine. • Avoid crowds, those with infection. • There is a potential risk for development of fetal abnormalities if pregnancy occurs; take measures to prevent pregnancy. • Report skin reactions including rash, sloughing, blisters, erosions. • Report difficulty breathing, fever with cough, lung pain; may indicate life-threatening lung inflammation. • Limit sun, UV exposure. Wear protective sunscreen, hats, and clothing while outdoors.

# panobinostat

**pan**-oh-**bin**-oh-stat
(Farydak)

■ **BLACK BOX ALERT** ■ Severe cases of diarrhea reported in 25% of pts. If diarrhea occurs, interrupt treatment, initiate antidiarrheal therapy, and then reduce or discontinue treatment. Severe and/or fatal cases of cardiac arrhythmias, cardiac ischemic events, EKG changes may occur. Electrolyte abnormalities may increase risk of arrhythmias. Obtain EKG, serum electrolytes at baseline and monitor during treatment.
**Do not confuse panobinostat with febuxostat or pentostatin.**

## ◆CLASSIFICATION

**PHARMACOTHERAPEUTIC:** Histone deacetylase inhibitor. **CLINICAL:** Antineoplastic.

P

## USES

Used in combination with bortezomib and dexamethasone, for treatment of pts with multiple myeloma who have received at least 2 prior regimens, including bortezomib and an immunomodulatory agent.

## PRECAUTIONS

**Contraindications:** Hypersensitivity to panobinostat. **Cautions:** Congenital long QT syndrome, concurrent medications that prolong QT interval, electrolyte abnormalities (hypokalemia, hypomagnesemia), renal impairment. Not recommended in pts with recent MI or unstable angina, severe hepatic impairment. Concurrent use of strong CYP3A inhibitors and/or CYP3A inducers, CYP2D6 substrates not recommended. Preexisting myelosuppression. Avoid use in pts with active infection.

## ACTION

Inhibits enzymatic activity of histone deacetylase. Increases acetylation of histone proteins, resulting in cell cycle arrest and/or cellular death (apoptosis). **Therapeutic Effect:** Inhibits tumor growth and metastasis. Promotes tumor cell death.

## PHARMACOKINETICS

Widely distributed. Extensively metabolized. Protein binding: 90%. Peak plasma concentration: 2 hrs. Eliminated in feces (44%–77%), urine (29–51%). **Half-life:** 37 hrs.

## ⌛ LIFESPAN CONSIDERATIONS

**Pregnancy/Lactation:** Avoid pregnancy; may cause fetal harm/malformations. Females of reproductive potential should use effective contraception during treatment and up to 1 mo after discontinuation. Unknown if distributed in breast milk. Must either discontinue drug or discontinue breastfeeding. **Males:** Males should use condoms during sexual activity during treatment and up to 3 mos after discontinuation. **Children:** Safety and efficacy not established. **Elderly:** May have increased risk of adverse effects (e.g., cardiac/GI/hematologic toxicities).

## INTERACTIONS

**DRUG:** Strong CYP3A inhibitors (e.g., **clarithromycin, ketoconazole, ritonavir**) may increase concentration/effect. **Strong CYP3A inducers** (e.g., **carbamazepine, rifampicin**) may decrease concentration/effect. May increase concentration/effects of **CYP2D6 substrates** (e.g., **metoprolol, venlafaxine**). Concurrent medications prolonging QT interval (e.g., **amiodarone, clarithromycin**) not recommended. **HERBAL: St. John's wort** may decrease concentration/effect. **FOOD: High-fat meals** may delay absorption.

**Grapefruit products** may increase concentration/effect. **LAB VALUES:** May decrease Hct, Hgb, leukocytes, lymphocytes, neutrophils, platelets; serum albumin, calcium, potassium, sodium. May increase serum bilirubin, creatinine, magnesium. May increase or decrease phosphate.

## AVAILABILITY (Rx)

**Capsules:** 10 mg, 15 mg, 20 mg.

## ADMINISTRATION/HANDLING

**PO**
• May give without regard to food; avoid grapefruit products (dexamethasone should be given with food to decrease GI upset). • Administer capsule whole; do not break, cut, crush, or open. • If vomiting occurs after dosing, do not readminister dose; give dose at next scheduled time.

## INDICATIONS/ROUTES/DOSAGE

**Multiple Myeloma**
**PO: ADULTS, ELDERLY:** 20 mg once every other day for 3 doses/wk during wk 1 and 2 of each 21-day cycle for up to 8 cycles, in combination with bortezomib and dexamethasone. Consider continuing treatment for additional 8 cycles based on tolerability. **Total duration:** Up to 16 cycles (48 wks). **Recommended dose of bortezomib:** 1.3 mg/m² as injection/day per dosing schedule. **Recommended dose of dexamethasone:** 20 mg orally/day on a full stomach per dosing schedule.

**Dosing Schedule for Cycles 1–8 of 21-Day Cycle**
**Week 1:** Panbinostat: days 1, 3, 5. Bortezomib: days 1, 4. Dexamethasone: days 1, 2, 4, 5.
**Week 2:** Panbinostat: days 8, 10, 12. Bortezomib: days 8, 11. Dexamethasone: days 8, 9, 11, 12.
**Week 3:** Rest period (all 3 drugs).

**Dosing Schedule for Cycles 9–16 of 21-Day Cycle**
**Week 1:** Panbinostat: days 1, 3, 5. Bortezomib: day 1 only. Dexamethasone: days 1, 2.

**Week 2:** Panbinostat: days 8, 10, 12. Bortezomib: day 8 only. Dexamethasone: days 8, 9.

**Week 3:** Rest period (all 3 drugs).

### Dose Reduction for Adverse Events

If reduction required, reduce panobinostat in increments of 5 mg. If the reduced dose is less than 10 mg 3 times/wk, discontinue treatment. Keep same schedule (21-day cycle) when dose reduced.

### Dose Modification for Clinical Toxicities

Based on Common Terminology Criteria for Adverse Events (CTCAE).

### Thrombocytopenia

**Grade 3:** No dose adjustment. **Bortezomib:** No dose adjustment. **Grade 3 with bleeding/grade 4:** Interrupt treatment until platelet count 50,000/mm$^3$ or greater, then resume at reduced dose. **Bortezomib:** Interrupt bortezomib until platelet count 75,000/mm$^3$ or greater. If only 1 dose was held prior to resolution of platelet count, resume bortezomib at same dose. If more than 2 doses were held consecutively, resume bortezomib at reduced dose.

### Neutropenia

**Grade 3:** No dose adjustment. **Bortezomib:** No dose adjustment. **Two or more occurrences of grade 3:** Interrupt treatment until ANC 1,000/mm$^3$ or greater, then resume at same dose. **Bortezomib:** No dose adjustment. **Grade 3 with febrile neutropenia/grade 4:** Interrupt treatment until febrile neutropenia resolves and ANC is 1,000/mm$^3$ or greater, then resume at reduced dose. **Bortezomib:** Interrupt bortezomib until febrile neutropenia resolves and ANC is 1,000/mm$^3$ or greater. If only 1 dose was held prior resolution of platelet count, resume bortezomib at same dose. If more than 2 doses were held consecutively, resume bortezomib at reduced dose.

### Anemia

**Grade 3:** Interrupt panobinostat until Hgb greater than or equal to 10 g/dL, then resume at reduced dose. **Bortezomib:** Not specified.

### Diarrhea

**Grade 2:** Interrupt treatment until resolved, then resume at same dose. **Bortezomib:** Consider interruption of bortezomib until resolved, then resume at same dose. **Grade 3 or hospitalization/administration of IV fluids:** Interrupt until resolved, then resume at reduced dose. **Bortezomib:** Interrupt until resolved, then resume bortezomib at reduced dose. **Grade 4:** Permanently discontinue panobinostat and bortezomib.

### Nausea/Vomiting

**Grade 3 or 4:** Interrupt until resolved, then resume at reduced dose. **Bortezomib:** Not specified.

### Other Toxicities (Other CTCAE Grades)

**Any grade 2 recurrence, any other grade 3 or 4:** Interrupt until resolved to grade 1 or 0, then resume at reduced dose. **Bortezomib:** Not specified. **Any other grade 3 or 4 recurrence:** Consider further dose reduction once resolved to grade 1 or 0.

### Concomitant Use of Strong CYP3A Inhibitors

**PO: ADULTS, ELDERLY:** 10 mg per dosing schedule.

### Dosage in Renal Impairment

No dose adjustment.

### Dosage in Hepatic Impairment

**PO: ADULTS, ELDERLY: Mild impairment:** 15 mg per dosing schedule. **Moderate impairment:** 10 mg per dosing schedule. **Severe impairment:** Treatment not recommended.

## SIDE EFFECTS

**Frequent (60%-2%):** Fatigue, asthenia, lethargy, diarrhea, nausea, peripheral edema, decreased appetite, vomiting, pyrexia. **Occasional (12%):** Decreased weight.

## ADVERSE EFFECTS/TOXIC REACTIONS

Anemia, leukopenia, neutropenia, thrombocytopenia is an expected response to therapy. Diarrhea occurred in 68% of pts. Severe cases of diarrhea occurred in 25% of pts. Cardiac toxicities such of cardiac ischemic events, ST-segment depression, T-wave abnormalities were reported. Cardiac arrhythmias including atrial fibrillation, atrial flutter, bradycardia, SVT, atrial/ventricular/sinus tachycardia occurred in 12% of pts. Severe thrombocytopenia may increase risk of fatal hemorrhage. Infectious processes such as bacterial infections, invasive fungal infections, pneumonia, sepsis, viral infections were reported. Severe and/or fatal infections occurred in 31% of pts.

## NURSING CONSIDERATIONS

### BASELINE ASSESSMENT

Obtain CBC, BMP, LFT; serum magnesium, phosphate; EKG, vital signs. Correct electrolyte imbalances prior to each cycle. Verify platelet count is at least 100,000/mm³, ANC is 1,500/mm³, QTc interval is less than 450 msec on EKG prior to each cycle. Verify pregnancy status. Assess hydration status; usual stool characteristics. Question history if acute MI, unstable angina, arrhythmia. Screen for active infection.

### INTERVENTION/EVALUATION

Monitor CBC, BMP; serum magnesium, phosphate wkly; LFT as indicated; vital signs. Monitor EKG periodically. If QTc interval increases to greater than 480 msec on EKG, interrupt treatment and correct any electrolyte abnormalities. If QT prolongation does not resolve, permanently discontinue treatment. Initiate medical management for nausea, vomiting, diarrhea prior to any interruption or dose reduction. Consider blood transfusion in pts with severe anemia, thrombocytopenia. Diligently monitor daily pattern bowel activity, stool consistency. Start antidiarrheal therapy at first sign of loose stool/diarrhea. Obtain 2D cardiac echocardiogram, EKG if cardiac decompensation is suspected. Monitor for infection.

### PATIENT/FAMILY TEACHING

• Blood levels will be monitored regularly. • Treatment may cause fetal harm. Women of childbearing potential should use effective contraception during treatment and up to 1 mo following discontinuation. Immediately report suspected pregnancy. Do not breastfeed. • Therapy may reduce fertility in both female and male pts. • Male pts must use condoms during sexual activity. • Report liver problems such as upper abdominal pain, bruising, dark or amber-colored urine, nausea, vomiting, or yellowing of the skin or eyes; heart problems such as chest tightness, dizziness, fainting, palpitations, shortness of breath; kidney problems such as dark-colored urine, decreased urine output, extremity swelling, flank pain; skin changes such as rash, redness. • Report mouth ulceration, jaw pain. • Swallow capsules whole; do not chew, crush, cut, or open capsules. • Treatment may increase risk of bleeding, nosebleeds. • Drink plenty of fluids. • Report the first signs of abdominal cramping, loose stool, diarrhea.

---

# pantoprazole TOP 100

pan-**toe**-pra-zole
(Apo-Pantoprazole , <u>Protonix</u>)
**Do not confuse pantoprazole with aripiprazole.**

## ◆CLASSIFICATION

**PHARMACOTHERAPEUTIC:** Benzimidazole. **CLINICAL:** Proton pump inhibitor.

---

## USES

**PO:** Treatment, maintenance of healing of erosive esophagitis associated with gastroesophageal reflux disease (GERD). Reduction of relapse rate of heartburn symptoms in GERD. Treatment of hypersecretory conditions including Zollinger-Ellison syndrome. **IV:** Short-term treatment of erosive esophagitis associated with GERD, treatment of hypersecretory conditions. **OFF-LABEL:** Peptic ulcer disease, active ulcer bleeding (injection), adjunct in treatment of *H. pylori*, stress ulcer prophylaxis in critically ill pts.

## PRECAUTIONS

**Contraindications:** Hypersensitivity to pantoprazole, other proton pump inhibitors (e.g., omeprazole). **Cautions:** May increase risk of fractures, GI infections.

## ACTION

Irreversibly binds to, inhibits hydrogen-potassium adenosine triphosphate, an enzyme on surface of gastric parietal cells. Inhibits hydrogen ion transport into gastric lumen. **Therapeutic Effect:** Increases gastric pH, reduces gastric acid production.

## PHARMACOKINETICS

| Route | Onset | Peak | Duration |
|-------|-------|------|----------|
| PO | N/A | N/A | 24 hrs |

Well absorbed from GI tract. Protein binding: 98% (primarily albumin). Primarily distributed into gastric parietal cells. Metabolized in liver. Primarily excreted in urine. Not removed by hemodialysis. **Half-life:** 1 hr.

## LIFESPAN CONSIDERATIONS

**Pregnancy/Lactation:** Unknown if drug crosses placenta or is distributed in breast milk. **Children:** Safety and efficacy not established. **Elderly:** No age-related precautions noted.

## INTERACTIONS

**DRUG:** May increase effects of **warfarin.** May decrease effects of **atazanavir,** **captopril, clopidogrel, dasatinib, nelfinavir. HERBAL: Ginger, goldenseal** may decrease effect. **FOOD:** None known. **LAB VALUES:** May increase serum creatinine, cholesterol, uric acid, glucose, lipoprotein, ALT.

## AVAILABILITY (Rx)

**Granules for Suspension:** 40 mg/packet. **Injection, Powder for Reconstitution (Protonix):** 40 mg.

 **Tablets (Delayed-Release [Protonix]):** 20 mg, 40 mg.

## ADMINISTRATION/HANDLING

### IV

**Reconstitution** • Mix 40-mg vial with 10 ml 0.9% NaCl injection. • May be further diluted with 100 ml D₅W, 0.9% NaCl.

**Rate of Administration** • Infuse 10 ml solution over at least 2 min. • Infuse 100 ml solution over at least 15 min. • Flush IV line after administration.

**Storage** • Store undiluted vials at room temperature. • Once diluted with 10 ml 0.9% NaCl, stable for 96 hrs at room temperature; when further diluted with 100 ml, stable for 96 hrs at room temperature.

### PO

• May be given without regard to food. Best given before breakfast. • Do not break, crush, dissolve, or divide tablets; give whole. • Administer oral suspension only in apple juice or applesauce. Best taken 30 min before a meal.

## IV COMPATIBILITIES

Dopamine, epinephrine, furosemide (Lasix), insulin (regular), potassium chloride, vasopressin.

## IV INCOMPATIBILITY

Dobutamine.

## INDICATIONS/ROUTES/DOSAGE

**Erosive Esophagitis**
**PO: ADULTS, ELDERLY:** 40 mg/day for up to 8 wks. If not healed after 8 wks, may

**P**

continue an additional 8 wks. **CHILDREN 5 YRS AND OLDER: (WEIGHING 40 KG OR MORE):** 40 mg/day for up to 8 wks. **(15–39 KG):** 20 mg/day for up to 8 wks.
**IV: ADULTS, ELDERLY:** 40 mg/day for 7–10 days.

**Maintenance of Healing of Erosive Esophagitis**
**PO: ADULTS, ELDERLY:** 40 mg once daily.

**Hypersecretory Conditions**
**PO: ADULTS, ELDERLY:** Initially, 40 mg twice daily. May increase to 240 mg/day.
**IV: ADULTS, ELDERLY:** 80 mg twice daily. May increase to 80 mg q8h.

**Prevention of Re-bleeding in Peptic Ulcer Bleed (Unlabeled)**
**IV: ADULTS, ELDERLY:** 80 mg followed by 8 mg/hr infusion for 72 hrs or 80 mg then 40 mg q12h for 72 hrs.

**Dosage in Renal/Hepatic Impairment**
No dose adjustment.

## SIDE EFFECTS

**Rare (less than 2%):** Diarrhea, headache, dizziness, pruritus, rash.

## ADVERSE EFFECTS/ TOXIC REACTIONS

Hyperglycemia occurs rarely. May increase risk of *C.difficile*–associated diarrhea.

## NURSING CONSIDERATIONS

### BASELINE ASSESSMENT

Question history of GI disease, ulcers, GERD.

### INTERVENTION/EVALUATION

Evaluate for therapeutic response (relief of GI symptoms). Question if GI discomfort, nausea occur. Monitor for abdominal pain, diarrhea (with or without fever).

### PATIENT/FAMILY TEACHING

• Report abdominal pain; diarrhea (with or without fever) that does not resolve; may indicate colon infection.

• Avoid alcohol. • Swallow tablets whole; do not chew, crush, dissolve, or divide. • Best if given before breakfast. May give without regard to food.

## *PARoxetine

par-**ox**-e-teen
(Apo-Paroxetine ✦, Brisdelle, Novo-Paroxetine ✦, Paxil, Paxil CR, Pexeva)
■ **BLACK BOX ALERT** ■ Increased risk of suicidal thinking and behavior in children, adolescents, young adults 18–24 yrs with major depressive disorder, other psychiatric disorders.
**Do not confuse paroxetine with piroxicam, fluoxetine or pyridoxine, or Paxil with Doxil, Plavix, Prozac, or Taxol.**

## ◆CLASSIFICATION

**PHARMACOTHERAPEUTIC:** Serotonin uptake inhibitor. **CLINICAL:** Antidepressant, antiobsessive-compulsive, antianxiety.

## USES

Treatment of major depressive disorder (MDD). Treatment of panic disorder, obsessive-compulsive disorder (OCD). Treatment of social anxiety disorder (SAD), generalized anxiety disorder (GAD), premenstrual dysphoric disorder (PMDD), post-traumatic stress disorder (PTSD). **(Brisdelle):** Treatment of moderate to severe vasomotor symptoms associated with menopause. **OFF-LABEL:** Social anxiety disorder in children, self-injurious behavior, treatment of depression and OCD in children.

## PRECAUTIONS

**Contraindications:** Hypersensitivity to paroxetine. Use of MAOIs with or within 14 days, initiation in pts treated with linezolid or methylene blue; concomitant use with thioridazine, pimozide. **(Brisdelle):** Pregnancy. **Cautions:** History of seizures, renal/hepatic impairment, pts with suicidal tendencies, elderly, narrow-angle glaucoma; avoid use in first trimester of pregnancy, alcohol use.

## ACTION

Selectively blocks uptake of neurotransmitter serotonin at CNS neuronal presynaptic membranes, increasing its availability at postsynaptic receptor sites. **Therapeutic Effect:** Relieves depression, reduces obsessive-compulsive behavior, decreases anxiety.

## PHARMACOKINETICS

Well absorbed from GI tract. Protein binding: 95%. Widely distributed. Metabolized in liver. Excreted in urine. Not removed by hemodialysis. **Half-life:** 24 hrs.

## ⧗ LIFESPAN CONSIDERATIONS

**Pregnancy/Lactation:** May impair reproductive function. Not distributed in breast milk. May increase risk of congenital malformations. **Children:** Safety and efficacy not established. **Elderly:** Age-related renal impairment may require dosage adjustment.

## INTERACTIONS

**DRUG:** May increase concentration, risk of toxicity of **tricyclic antidepressants (e.g., amitriptyline, doxepin).** Triptans, lithium, tramadol may increase risk of serotonin syndrome. **Aspirin, NSAIDs, warfarin** may increase risk of bleeding. **MAOIs** may cause confusion, agitation, severe seizures; increase risk of serotonin syndrome, hypertensive crises. **Thioridazine** may prolong QT interval. **HERBAL: Kava kava, St. John's wort, valerian** may increase CNS depression, risk of serotonin syndrome. **FOOD:** None known. **LAB VALUES:** May decrease Hgb, Hct, WBC count.

## AVAILABILITY (Rx)

**Capsules (Brisdelle):** 7.5 mg. **Oral Suspension (Paxil):** 10 mg/5 ml. **Tablets (Paxil, Pexeva):** 10 mg, 20 mg, 30 mg, 40 mg.

⧉ **Tablets (Controlled-Release [Paxil CR]):** 12.5 mg, 25 mg, 37.5 mg.

## ADMINISTRATION/HANDLING

### PO
• May give without regard to food.
• Give with food, milk if GI distress occurs. • Scored tablet may be crushed.
• Do not crush, break, dissolve, or divide controlled-release tablets.

## INDICATIONS/ROUTES/DOSAGE

### Depression
**PO:** *(Immediate-Release):* **ADULTS:** Initially, 20 mg/day. May increase by 10 mg/day at intervals of more than 1 wk. **Maximum:** 50 mg/day.
**PO:** *(Controlled-Release):* **ADULTS:** Initially, 25 mg/day. May increase by 12.5 mg/day at intervals of more than 1 wk. **Maximum:** 62.5 mg/day.

### Generalized Anxiety Disorder (GAD)
**PO: ADULTS:** Initially, 20 mg/day. May increase by 10 mg/day at intervals of more than 1 wk. Range: 20–50 mg/day.

### Obsessive-Compulsive Disorder (OCD)
**PO: ADULTS:** Initially, 20 mg/day. May increase by 10 mg/day at intervals of more than 1 wk. Range: 20–60 mg/day. Recommended dose: 40 mg/day.

### Panic Disorder
**PO: ADULTS:** Initially, 10–20 mg/day. May increase by 10 mg/day at intervals of more than 1 wk. Range: 10–60 mg/day.
**PO** *(Controlled-Release):* **ADULTS, ELDERLY:** Initially, 12.5 mg once daily. May increase by 12.5 mg/day at wkly intervals. **Maximum:** 75 mg/day.

### Social Anxiety Disorder (SAD)
**PO: ADULTS:** Initially 20 mg/day. Range: 20–60 mg/day.
**PO** *(Controlled-Release):* **ADULTS, ELDERLY:** Initially, 12.5 mg once daily. May increase by 12.5 mg/day at wkly intervals. **Maximum:** 37.5 mg/day.

### Post-Traumatic Stress Disorder (PTSD)
**PO: ADULTS:** Initially, 20 mg/day. May increase by 10 mg/day at intervals of more than 1 wk. Range: 20–50 mg/day.

**P**

**Premenstrual Dysphoric Disorder (PMDD)**
**PO:** *(Controlled-Release):* **ADULTS:** Initially, 12.5 mg/day. May increase by 12.5 mg at wkly intervals. **Maximum:** 25 mg/day.

**Vasomotor Symptoms**
**PO: ADULTS:** *(Brisdelle):* 7.5 mg once daily at bedtime.

**Usual Elderly Dosage**
**PO:** Initially, 10 mg/day. May increase by 10 mg/day at intervals of more than 1 wk. **Maximum:** 40 mg/day.
**PO** *(Controlled-Release):* Initially, 12.5 mg/day. May increase by 12.5 mg/day at intervals of more than 1 wk. **Maximum:** 50 mg/day.

**Dosage Renal/Hepatic Impairment**
CrCl less than 30 ml/min, severe hepatic impairment. **Immediate-Release:** Initially, 10 mg/day. May increase by 10 mg/dose at wkly intervals. **Maximum:** 40 mg/day. **Extended-Release:** Initially, 12.5 mg/day. May increase by 12.5/day at wkly intervals. **Maximum:** 50 mg/day. **Brisdelle:** No dosage adjustment.

## SIDE EFFECTS

**Frequent (26%–8%):** Nausea, drowsiness, headache, dry mouth, asthenia, constipation, dizziness, insomnia, diarrhea, diaphoresis, tremor. **Occasional (6%–3%):** Decreased appetite, respiratory disturbance (e.g., increased cough), anxiety, flatulence, paresthesia, yawning, decreased libido, sexual dysfunction, abdominal discomfort. **Rare:** Palpitations, vomiting, blurred vision, altered taste, confusion.

## ADVERSE EFFECTS/ TOXIC REACTIONS

Hyponatremia, seizures have been reported. Serotonin syndrome (agitation, confusion, diaphoresis, hallucinations, hyperreflexia) occurs rarely.

## NURSING CONSIDERATIONS

### BASELINE ASSESSMENT
Assess appearance, behavior, speech pattern, level of interest, mood.

### INTERVENTION/EVALUATION
For pts on long-term therapy, CBC, LFT, renal function test should be performed periodically. Assess mental status for depression, suicidal ideation (esp. at beginning of therapy or change in dosage), anxiety, social functioning, panic attacks. Assess appearance, behavior, speech pattern, level of interest, mood.

### PATIENT/FAMILY TEACHING
• May cause dry mouth. • Avoid alcohol, St. John's wort. • Therapeutic effect may be noted within 1–4 wks. • Do not abruptly discontinue medication. • Avoid tasks that require alertness, motor skills until response to drug is established. • May impair reproductive function. • Inform physician of intention for pregnancy or if pregnancy occurs. • Report worsening depression, suicidal ideation, unusual changes in behavior.

# patiromer

pa-**tir**-oh-mer
(Veltassa)

■ **BLACK BOX ALERT** ■ May reduce absorption and effectiveness of some oral medications (due to binding effect). Administer other oral medications at least 6 hrs before or 6 hrs after dose. If adequate drug separation is not possible, choose whether to give patiromer or other oral medications.

**Do not confuse patiromer with glatiramer, Levemir, or Veltassa with Pentasa, Valturna, or Voltaren.**

## ◆CLASSIFICATION

**PHARMACOTHERAPEUTIC:** Cation exchange polymer. **CLINICAL:** Antihyperkalemic, potassium binder.

## USES

Treatment of hyperkalemia.

## PRECAUTIONS

**Contraindications:** Hypersensitivity to patiromer. **Cautions:** Baseline hypomagnesemia, conditions predisposing to hypomagnesemia (alcohol abuse, chronic diarrhea, hypercalcemia, hyperaldosteronism, malnutrition). Avoid use in pts with acute bowel obstruction, bowel impaction; postoperative GI motility disorders, severe constipation. Not indicated for emergent or life-threatening hyperkalemia due to delayed onset of action.

## ACTION

Increases fecal excretion of potassium by binding to free potassium in GI tract. **Therapeutic Effect:** Decreases serum potassium levels.

## PHARMACOKINETICS

Not absorbed systemically. Onset: 7 hrs. Eliminated in feces. **Half-life:** Not specified.

## ⧗ LIFESPAN CONSIDERATIONS

**Pregnancy/Lactation:** Not absorbed systemically. Not expected to result in exposure during pregnancy or breastfeeding. **Children:** Safety and efficacy not established. **Elderly:** May have higher incidence of GI side effects.

## INTERACTIONS

**DRUG:** Decreases effectiveness of **other oral medications. HERBAL:** None significant. **FOOD:** None known. **LAB VALUES:** Expected to decrease serum potassium. May decrease serum magnesium.

## AVAILABILITY (Rx)

**Packets, Oral:** 8.4 g, 16.8 g, 25.2 g.

## ADMINISTRATION/HANDLING

### PO

**Preparation** • Measure ⅓ cup (~80 ml) of water and pour half into empty container. • Add packet contents and stir. • Add remaining water to mixture and stir. • Powder will not dissolve (mixture will look cloudy). • Additional water may be added for desired consistency. **Administration** • Give with food. • Do not administer in dry powder form. • Do not heat (e.g., microwave) or add heated liquids or foods. • If powder remains in container after initial administration, add more water, stir, and give immediately (repeat until full dose is ingested). • Give oral medications at least 6 hrs before or 6 hrs after dose.

## INDICATIONS/ROUTES/DOSAGE

**Hyperkalemia**
**PO: ADULTS, ELDERLY:** 8.4 g once daily. Adjust dose in increments of 8.4 g at 1-wk intervals (or longer) based on desired target range of serum potassium level. **Maximum:** 25.2 g/day.

**Dosage in Renal Impairment**
No dose adjustment.

**Dosage in Hepatic Impairment**
Use caution (not studied).

## SIDE EFFECTS

**Occasional (7%–4%):** Constipation, diarrhea. **Rare (2%):** Nausea, flatulence.

## ADVERSE EFFECTS/TOXIC REACTIONS

Hypomagnesemia, hypokalemia reported in 5% of pts. Hypomagnesemia, hypokalemia may result in cardiac arrhythmias. Hypersensitivity reaction, including lip edema, occurs rarely.

## NURSING CONSIDERATIONS

### BASELINE ASSESSMENT

Obtain serum potassium, magnesium; EKG. Obtain full medication history and decide whether to give patiromer or other oral medications. Question history of GI motility disorders, chronic constipation, bowel obstruction. Therapy does not rapidly correct severe hyperkalemia. If medical emergency occurs, consider other measures to treat severe hyperkalemia

**P**

(IV calcium, IV sodium bicarbonate, IV glucose, IV insulin; nebulized albuterol treatment; dialysis).

### INTERVENTION/EVALUATION

Monitor serum potassium, magnesium; EKG. Monitor for symptoms of hypokalemia including confusion, delayed thought process, fatigue, irritability, weakness; EKG changes (prolonged QT interval; widening, flattening, or inversion of T wave; biphasic T wave, prominent U wave). Monitor for symptoms of hypomagnesemia including coma, numbness, nystagmus, seizures, tremors, weakness; EKG changes (prolonged PR interval, widened QRS complex, prolonged QT interval, depressed T wave, premature ventricular contractions, torsades de pointes). If hypomagnesemia occurs, consider magnesium supplementation. Monitor daily pattern of bowel activity, stool consistency. Monitor I&Os.

### PATIENT/FAMILY TEACHING

• Patiromer binds to some oral medications and can reduce their effectiveness. Oral medications must be taken at least 6 hrs before or at least 6 hrs after dose. • Take with food. • Do not heat in microwave or add heated liquids or foods. • Report symptoms of low potassium such as confusion, fatigue, muscle cramps/twitching, palpitations, weakness; or symptoms of low magnesium such as coma, fatigue, muscle twitching, palpitations, seizures, tremors, weakness. • Therapy relies on fecal excretion; report severe constipation or severe diarrhea. • Drink plenty of fluids.

---

# *PAZOPanib

paz-**oh**-pa-nib
(Votrient)
■ **BLACK BOX ALERT** ■ Severe, fatal hepatotoxicity has been observed.

## ◆CLASSIFICATION

**PHARMACOTHERAPEUTIC:** Tyrosine kinase inhibitor. **CLINICAL:** Antineoplastic.

## USES

Treatment of advanced renal cell carcinoma (RCC), advanced soft-tissue sarcoma (STS) (in pts previously treated with chemotherapy). **OFF-LABEL:** Advanced thyroid cancer.

## PRECAUTIONS

**Contraindications:** Hypersensitivity to pazopanib. **Cautions:** Avoid use of strong CYP3A4 inhibitors (e.g., clarithromycin, ketoconazole) or CYP3A inducers (carbamazepine, rifampin), and grapefruit products. Cautious use in pts with increased risk or history of arterial thrombotic events (e.g., angina, MI, ischemic stroke), QT prolongation, hypokalemia, hypomagnesemia, hypertension, severe hepatic impairment, history of hemoptysis, cerebral hemorrhage or significant GI hemorrhage. Concomitant use of medications that may prolong QT interval not recommended.

## ACTION

Inhibits cell surface vascular endothelial growth factor receptors. **Therapeutic Effect:** Inhibits angiogenesis, blocks tumor growth.

## PHARMACOKINETICS

Peak concentration occurs 2–4 hrs following oral administration. Metabolized in liver. Protein binding: greater than 99%. Eliminated in feces (60%), urine (23%). **Half-life:** 31 hrs.

## ⧖ LIFESPAN CONSIDERATIONS

**Pregnancy/Lactation:** May cause fetal harm. Unknown if distributed in breast milk. **Children:** Safety and efficacy not established in pts younger than 18 yrs. **Elderly:** No age-related precautions noted.

## INTERACTIONS

**DRUG:** Famotidine, proton pump inhibitors (e.g., omeprazole, pantoprazole) may decrease effect. **QT interval-prolonging medications** (e.g., amiodarone, citalopram, dasatinib, haloperidol, **levofloxacin, ondanse-tron**) may prolong QT interval. **CYP3A4 inhibitors** (e.g., **clarithromycin, keto-conazole, ritonavir**) may increase concentration. **CYP3A4 inducers** (e.g., **car-bamazepine, phenytoin, rifampin**) may decrease concentration. **Simvastatin** may increase serum ALT. **Medications that increase gastric pH** may decrease concentration/effect. **HERBAL:** St. John's **wort** decreases concentration. **FOOD:** Food may increase concentration. **Grapefruit products** may increase concentration, po-tential for torsades de pointes, myelotoxicity. **LAB VALUES:** May decrease serum phos-phorus, sodium, magnesium, glucose, WBC count. May increase serum ALT, AST.

## AVAILABILITY (Rx)

✎ Tablets: 200 mg.

## ADMINISTRATION/HANDLING

**PO**
• Give at least 1 hr before or 2 hrs after ingestion of food. • Give tablets whole; do not break, crush, dissolve, or divide.

## INDICATIONS/ROUTES/DOSAGE

**Renal Cell Carcinoma, Soft-Tissue Sarcoma**
**PO: ADULTS, ELDERLY:** 800 mg once daily. Initial dose of 400 mg/day with concomi-tant strong CYP3A4 inhibitors.

**Dose Adjustment for Toxicity**
Prior to   dose reduction, temporarily discontinue therapy if 24-hr urine pro-tein 3 g or more or for other toxicities. Initial dose reduction: Renal cell carci-noma: 400 mg/day. Soft tissue sarcoma: 600 mg/day. Further dose adjustment: 200 mg/day.

**Dosage in Renal Impairment**
No dose adjustment.

**Dosage in Hepatic Impairment**
**Mild impairment:** No dose adjustment. **Moderate impairment:** Reduce dose to 200 mg/day. **Severe impairment:** Not recommended.

## SIDE EFFECTS

**Frequent (52%–19%):** Diarrhea, hyperten-sion, hair color changes, nausea, fatigue, anorexia, vomiting. **Occasional (14%–10%):** Asthenia, abdominal pain, headache. **Rare (Less Than 10%):** Alopecia, chest pain, al-tered taste, dyspepsia, proteinuria, rash, decreased weight.

## ADVERSE EFFECTS/ TOXIC REACTIONS

Hepatotoxicity, manifested as increase in serum bilirubin, ALT, AST, has been ob-served and may be fatal. Hemorrhagic events (hematuria, epistaxis, hemoptysis, GI bleeding or perforation, intracranial hemorrhage) have been noted and may be fatal. Hypertension (B/P greater than 150/100 mmHg) is common (47%), usually occurring early in the first 18 wks of treatment. Hypothyroidism has been reported occasionally. Arterial throm-botic events (MI, CVA), QT prolongation, torsades de pointes have been seen rarely.

## NURSING CONSIDERATIONS

### BASELINE ASSESSMENT
Obtain baseline EKG, CBC, serum chem-istries, LFT. Assess medical history, esp. hepatic impairment. Question history of hepatic impairment, arterial or venous thromboembolism, GI bleeding. Receive full medication history and screen for interactions.

### INTERVENTION/EVALUATION
Monitor B/P, LFT periodically for eleva-tions. Monitor CBC, serum chemistries for changes from baseline. Observe for hepa-totoxicity (jaundice, dark-colored urine, unusual fatigue, right upper quadrant abdominal pain). Observe EKG for QT-interval prolongation. Monitor for evidence of bleeding, hemorrhage. Monitor daily pattern of bowel activity, stool consistency.

### PATIENT/FAMILY TEACHING
• Avoid crowds, those with known infec-tion. • Avoid contact with anyone who

**P**

---

recently received live virus vaccine; do not receive vaccinations. • Swallow tablets whole; do not chew, crush, dissolve, or divide. • No food should be taken at least 1 hr before and 2 hrs after dose is taken. • Avoid grapefruit products. • Report diarrhea, abdominal pain, yellowing of skin or sclera, discolored urine, fatigue. • Report bleeding of any kind; esp. bloody stools, nosebleeds, coughing up blood. • Treatment may increase risk of heart attack, stroke, blood clots, or heart arrhythmias.

# pegaspargase

peg-ah-**spar**-jase
(Oncaspar)
**Do not confuse pegaspargase with asparaginase.**

## ◆ CLASSIFICATION

**PHARMACOTHERAPEUTIC:** Enzyme, immunomodulator. **CLINICAL:** Antineoplastic.

## USES

Treatment of acute lymphoblastic leukemia (ALL).

## PRECAUTIONS

**Contraindications:** Hypersensitivity reaction to pegaspargase, history of hemorrhage, pancreatitis, or thrombosis with L-asparaginase therapy. **Cautions:** Pts with diabetes mellitus, underlying coagulopathy, hepatic impairment, concurrent hepatotoxic medications, previous hematologic complications with asparaginase. Concomitant use of aspirin, NSAIDs, anticoagulation therapy.

## ACTION

Inhibits protein synthesis by deaminating asparagine in plasma and extracellular fluid. **Therapeutic Effect:** Deprives tumor cells of amino acids necessary for protein synthesis, thereby inhibiting tumor cell growth.

## PHARMACOKINETICS

Slowly absorbed following IM administration. Primarily excreted in urine elimination. **Half-life:** 6 days.

## 🕱 LIFESPAN CONSIDERATIONS

**Pregnancy/Lactation:** Unknown if distributed in breast milk. Must either discontinue drug or discontinue breastfeeding. **Children:** Safety and efficacy not established. **Elderly:** No age-related precautions noted.

## INTERACTIONS

**DRUG:** **Anticoagulants** (e.g., heparin, warfarin), **antiplatelets** (e.g., clopidogrel), **NSAIDs** may increase risk of coagulopathy, bleeding. **HERBAL:** **Echinacea** may decrease concentration/effects. **FOOD:** None known. **LAB VALUES:** May increase serum ALT, AST, bilirubin, glucose.

## AVAILABILITY (Rx)

**Injection Solution:** 3,750 international units/5 ml (750 international unit/ml).

## ADMINISTRATION/HANDLING

**Note:** Refrigerate unused vial.

**IM**
• Visually inspect for particulate matter. • Do not inject volume greater than 2 ml for single injection site. • Use multiple sites if injecting more than 2 ml of volume.

 **IV**

**Reconstitution** • Withdraw appropriate volume and dilute in 100 ml bag of NaCl or D₅W. • Gently mix bag by inversion. • Do not shake or agitate.
**Rate of Administration** • Infuse over 1–2 hrs.
**Storage** • Solution should appear clear, colorless. • May refrigerate diluted solution up to 48 hrs. • Protect infusion bag from direct sunlight.

## ⚙ IV INCOMPATIBILITIES

Do not mix with other intravenous medications.

## INDICATIONS/ROUTES/DOSAGE

**Acute Lymphoblastic Leukemia (ALL)**
**IM/IV: ADULTS/ELDERLY/CHILDREN:** 2,500 international units/m² every 14 days (of 28-day cycle) (in combination with other chemotherapeutic agents).

**Dosage in Renal/Hepatic Impairment**
No dose adjustment.

## SIDE EFFECTS

**Occasional:** Nausea, headache.

## ADVERSE EFFECTS/ TOXIC REACTIONS

Hypersensitivity reactions including anaphylactic reaction may include angioedema, dyspnea, flushing, hypotension, laryngeal edema, urticaria, wheezing. Central nervous system thrombosis including acute CVA occurred in 3% of pts. Pancreatitis may result in septic shock, acute respiratory distress syndrome (ARDS), hypotension, or death. Coagulopathy may increase risk of fatal bleeding. Immunogenicity (autoantibody formation) reported in 2%–10% of pts.

## NURSING CONSIDERATIONS

### BASELINE ASSESSMENT

Obtain baseline serum chemistries, PT/INR, capillary blood glucose. Question history of hepatic impairment, pancreatitis, prior hypersensitivity, DVT, MI, CVA. Receive full medication history.

### INTERVENTION/EVALUATION

Monitor serum LFT, capillary blood glucose, PT/INR regularly. Monitor pt for hypersensitivity reaction for at least 1 hr after administration. If anaphylactic reaction occurs, consider treatment with antihistamine, intravenous steroids, racemic epinephrine; locate rapid sequence intubation kit. If pancreatitis suspected (abdominal pain, Grey Turner's sign, intractable vomiting), contact physician to obtain serum chemistries, amylase and lipase levels, possible radiologic testing. Immediately report dyspnea, chest pain, hypoxia, unilateral peripheral edema/pain (may indicate thromboembolic event).

### PATIENT/FAMILY TEACHING

• Treatment may induce allergic reaction (difficulty breathing, itching, wheezing, rash, dizziness). • Increased urination, thirst, confusion, dehydration, fruity breath may indicate elevated blood sugar levels. • Immediately report flank bruising, vomiting, abdominal pain (may indicate pancreatitis). • Report difficulty breathing, chest pain, extremity pain swelling. • Report abdominal pain, yellowing of skin or eyes, dark-amber urine, clay-colored stools, fatigue, loss of appetite; may indicate liver problems.

# pegfilgrastim  TOP 100

peg-fil-**gras**-tim
(Neulasta, Neulasta Onpro)
**Do not confuse Neulasta with Lunesta, Neumega, or Neupogen.**

## ◆CLASSIFICATION

**PHARMACOTHERAPEUTIC:** Colony-stimulating factor. **CLINICAL:** Hematopoietic, antineutropenic.

## USES

Decreases incidence of infection manifested by febrile neutropenia in cancer pts receiving myelosuppressive chemotherapy associated with febrile neutropenia. To increase survival in pts acutely exposed to myelosuppressive doses of radiation.

## PRECAUTIONS

**Contraindications:** Hypersensitivity to pegfilgrastim, filgrastim. **Cautions:** Any malignancy with myeloid characteristics, sickle cell disease. The 6-mg fixed dose not to be used in infants, children, or adolescents weighing less than 45 kg. Do not administer within 14 days before and 24 hrs after cytotoxic chemotherapy.

## ACTION

Regulates production of neutrophils within bone marrow. A glycoprotein, primarily affects neutrophil progenitor proliferation, differentiation, selected end-cell functional activation. **Therapeutic Effect:** Increases phagocytic ability, antibody-dependent destruction; decreases incidence of infection.

## PHARMACOKINETICS

Readily absorbed after SQ administration. **Half-life:** 15–80 hrs.

## ⌛ LIFESPAN CONSIDERATIONS

**Pregnancy/Lactation:** Unknown if drug crosses placenta or is distributed in breast milk. **Children:** Safety and efficacy not established in children younger than 12 yrs. **Elderly:** No age-related precautions noted.

## INTERACTIONS

**DRUG:** None significant. **HERBAL:** None significant. **FOOD:** None known. **LAB VALUES:** May increase serum LDH, alkaline phosphatase, uric acid.

## AVAILABILITY (Rx)

**Injection Solution:** 6 mg/0.6 ml syringe.

## ADMINISTRATION/HANDLING

**SQ**

**Storage** • Store in refrigerator. Warm to room temperature prior to administering injection. Discard if left at room temperature for more than 48 hrs. • Protect from light. • Avoid freezing; but if accidentally frozen, may allow to thaw in refrigerator before administration. Discard if freezing takes place a second time. • Discard if discolored or precipitate forms.

## INDICATIONS/ROUTES/DOSAGE

**Neutropenia (Chemotherapy-Induced)**
**SQ: ADULTS, ELDERLY, CHILDREN 12–17 YRS, WEIGHING MORE THAN 45 KG:** Give as single 6-mg injection once per chemotherapy cycle beginning 24–72 hrs after completion of chemotherapy.

**◀ALERT▶** Do not administer between 14 days before and 24 hrs after cytotoxic chemotherapy. Do not use in infants, children, adolescents weighing less than 45 kg.

**Radiation Injury Syndrome**
**SQ: ADULTS, ELDERLY, CHILDREN WEIGHING 45 KG OR MORE:** 6 mg once wkly for 2 doses. **31–44 KG:** 4 mg once wkly for 2 doses. **21–30 KG:** 2.5 mg once wkly for 2 doses. **10–20 KG:** 1.5 mg once wkly for 2 doses. **LESS THAN 10 KG:** 0.1 mg/kg once wkly for 2 doses.

**Dosage in Renal/Hepatic Impairment**
No dose adjustment.

## SIDE EFFECTS

**Frequent (72%–15%):** Bone pain, nausea, fatigue, alopecia, diarrhea, vomiting, constipation, anorexia, abdominal pain, arthralgia, generalized weakness, peripheral edema, dizziness, stomatitis, mucositis, neutropenic fever.

## ADVERSE EFFECTS/ TOXIC REACTIONS

Allergic reactions (anaphylaxis, rash, urticaria) occur rarely. Cytopenia resulting from antibody response to growth factors occurs rarely. Splenomegaly occurs rarely. Severe sickle cell crisis reported in pts with sickle cell disease. Glomerulonephritis, capillary leak syndrome, tumor growth stimulatory effect on malignant cells, acute respiratory distress syndrome may occur.

## NURSING CONSIDERATIONS

### BASELINE ASSESSMENT

CBC should be obtained before initiating therapy and routinely thereafter. Question history of sickle cell disease, glomerulo-nephritis, splenic disease, hypersensitivity reaction to acrylic adhesive (injector uses acrylic adhesive).

### INTERVENTION/EVALUATION

Monitor for allergic reactions. Assess for peripheral edema. Assess mucous membranes for evidence of stomatitis, mucositis. Assess muscle strength. Monitor daily pattern of bowel activity, stool consistency. Adult respiratory distress syndrome (ARDS) may occur in septic pts.

### PATIENT/FAMILY TEACHING

• Inform pt of possible side effects, signs/symptoms of allergic reaction. • Counsel pt on importance of compliance with pegfilgrastim treatment, including regular monitoring of blood counts. • Report unusual fever or chills, severe bone pain, chest pain or palpitations.

# peginterferon alfa-2a

peg-in-ter-**feer**-on
(Pegasys)

■ **BLACK BOX ALERT** ■ Can cause or aggravate fatal or life-threatening autoimmune disorders, neuropsychiatric disorders (depression, suicidal ideation/behaviors), and infectious disorders. Combination with ribavirin can cause fetal mortality, birth defects, hemolytic anemia. May be carcinogenic. Avoid pregnancy in female pts and female partners of male pts.

**Do not confuse peginterferon alfa-2a with interferon alfa-2b, interferon alfa-n3, or peginterferon alfa-2b.**

### ◆CLASSIFICATION

**PHARMACOTHERAPEUTIC:** Immunomodulator. **CLINICAL:** Immunologic agent.

## USES

Treatment of chronic hepatitis C virus (HCV) infection alone or in combination with ribavirin (unless contraindicated or significant intolerance to ribavirin) in pts 5 yrs or older who have compensated hepatic disease. Treatment of adults coinfected with HCV and clinically stable HIV disease. Treatment of chronic hepatitis B virus infection with compensated hepatic disease and evidence of viral replication and hepatic inflammation.

## PRECAUTIONS

**Contraindications:** Hypersensitivity to peginterferon alfa-2a. Autoimmune hepatitis, decompensated hepatic disease with cirrhosis, or pts with chronic HCV and co-infected with HIV; infants, neonates. **Extreme Caution:** History of neuropsychiatric disorders, depression. **Cautions:** Renal impairment (CrCl less than 30 ml/min), elderly, pulmonary disorders, compromised CNS function, cardiac diseases, autoimmune disorders, endocrine abnormalities (e.g., diabetes, thyroid disorders), colitis, ophthalmologic disorders, myelosuppression.

## ACTION

Binds to specific membrane receptors on virus-infected cell surface, inhibiting viral replication. Suppresses cell proliferation, producing reversible decreases in leukocyte, platelet counts. **Therapeutic Effect:** Inhibits viral hepatitis.

## PHARMACOKINETICS

Readily absorbed after SQ administration. Excreted by kidneys. **Half-life:** 50–140 hrs.

## ⌛ LIFESPAN CONSIDERATIONS

**Pregnancy/Lactation:** May have abortifacient potential. Unknown if distributed in breast milk. **Children:** Safety and efficacy not established in pts younger than 18 yrs. **Elderly:** CNS, cardiac, systemic effects may be more severe in the elderly, particularly in those with renal impairment.

P

---

## INTERACTIONS

**DRUG: Didanosine** may cause hepatic failure, peripheral neuropathy, pancreatitis, lactic acidosis. May increase concentration, risk of toxicity of **methadone, theophylline.** Concurrent use of **ribavirin** may increase risk of hemolytic anemia. **HERBAL:** None significant. **FOOD:** None known. **LAB VALUES:** May increase serum ALT. May decrease absolute neutrophil count, platelet.

## AVAILABILITY (Rx)

**Injection, Prefilled Syringe:** 135 mcg/0.5 ml, 180 mcg/0.5 ml. **Injection Solution:** 180 mcg/ml.

## ADMINISTRATION/HANDLING

**SQ**
• Refrigerate. • Vials are for single use only; discard unused portion. • Give subcutaneously in abdomen, thigh.

## INDICATIONS/ROUTES/DOSAGE

**NOTE:** Duration of therapy based on genotype.
**Hepatitis C**
**SQ: ADULTS 18 YRS AND OLDER, ELDERLY:** 180 mcg injected in abdomen or thigh once wkly as monotherapy or in combination with ribavirin. **CHILDREN 5 YRS AND OLDER:** 180 mcg/m² × body surface area once wkly. **Maximum:** 180 mcg (with ribavirin).

**Chronic Hepatitis B**
**SQ: ADULTS, ELDERLY:** 180 mcg once wkly for 48 wks.

**Dosage in Renal Impairment**
For pts who require hemodialysis or CrCl less than 30 ml/min, dosage is 135 mg injected in abdomen or thigh once wkly.

**Dosage in Hepatic Impairment**
For pts with progressive ALT elevation above baseline values, dosage is 135 mcg injected in abdomen or thigh once wkly.

## SIDE EFFECTS

**Frequent (54%):** Headache. **Occasional (23%–13%):** Alopecia, nausea, insomnia, anorexia, dizziness, diarrhea, abdominal pain, flu-like symptoms, psychiatric reactions (depression, irritability, anxiety), injection site reaction. **Rare (8%–5%):** Impaired concentration, diaphoresis, dry mouth, nausea, vomiting.

## ADVERSE EFFECTS/TOXIC REACTIONS

Serious, acute hypersensitivity reactions (urticaria, angioedema, bronchoconstriction, anaphylaxis), pancreatitis, colitis, endocrine disorders (diabetes mellitus, hyperthyroidism, hypothyroidism), ophthalmologic disorders, pulmonary abnormalities occur rarely.

## NURSING CONSIDERATIONS

### BASELINE ASSESSMENT
CBC, urinalysis, renal function, LFT, EKG should be performed before initial therapy and routinely thereafter. Pts with diabetes, hypertension should have ophthalmologic exam before treatment begins.

### INTERVENTION/EVALUATION
Monitor for evidence of depression. Offer emotional support. Monitor for abdominal pain, melena as evidence of colitis. Assess for pulmonary impairment. Monitor chest X-ray for pulmonary infiltrates. Encourage ample fluid intake, particularly during early therapy. Assess serum hepatitis C virus RNA levels after 24 wks of treatment.

### PATIENT/FAMILY TEACHING
• Clinical response occurs in 1–3 mos. • Flu-like symptoms tend to diminish with continued therapy. • Immediately report symptoms of depression, suicidal ideation. • Avoid tasks requiring alertness, motor skills until response to drug is established. • Avoid alcohol.

# peginterferon alfa-2b

peg-in-ter-**feer**-on
(PEG-Intron, PEG-Intron RediPen, Sylatron)

■ **BLACK BOX ALERT** ■ Can cause or aggravate fatal or life-threatening autoimmune disorder, neuropsychiatric disorder (depression, suicidal ideation/behaviors), and infectious disorders. Combination with ribavirin can cause fetal mortality, birth defects, hemolytic anemia. May be carcinogenic. Avoid pregnancy in female pts and female partners of male pts.

**Do not confuse peginterferon alfa-2b with interferon alfa-2b, interferon alfa-n3, or peginterferon alfa-2a.**

## ◆CLASSIFICATION

**PHARMACOTHERAPEUTIC:** Immunomodulator. **CLINICAL:** Immunologic agent.

## USES

**PEG-Intron:** As monotherapy or in combination with ribavirin for treatment of chronic hepatitis C virus infection in pts not previously treated with interferon alfa who have compensated hepatic disease and are older than 18 yrs. **Sylatron:** Treatment of melanoma or gross nodal involvement within 84 days of definitive surgical resection including complete lymphadenectomy.

## PRECAUTIONS

**Contraindications:** Hypersensitivity to peginterferon alfa-2b. Autoimmune hepatitis, decompensated hepatic disease with cirrhosis. Hypersensitivity to interferon alfa-2b, other alfa interferons. **Cautions:** Renal impairment (CrCl less than 50 ml/min), elderly, pulmonary disorders, history of psychiatric disorders, compromised CNS function, cardiac diseases, autoimmune disorders, endocrine disorders (diabetes, hyperthyroidism,

hypothyroidism), ophthalmologic disorders, myelosuppression.

## ACTION

Inhibits viral replication in virus-infected cells, suppresses cell proliferation, increases phagocytic action of macrophages, augments specific cytotoxicity of lymphocytes for target cells. **Therapeutic Effect:** Inhibits viral hepatitis.

## PHARMACOKINETICS

Bioavailability is increased after multiple wkly doses. Excreted in urine. **Half-life:** 22–60 hrs.

## ⌛ LIFESPAN CONSIDERATIONS

**Pregnancy/Lactation:** May have abortifacient potential. Unknown if distributed in breast milk. **Children:** Safety and efficacy not established in pts younger than 18 yrs. **Elderly:** CNS, cardiac, systemic effects may be more severe in the elderly, particularly in those with renal impairment.

## INTERACTIONS

**DRUG:** None significant. **HERBAL:** None significant. **FOOD:** None known. **LAB VALUES:** May increase serum ALT. May decrease neutrophil, platelet counts.

## AVAILABILITY (Rx)

**Prefilled Syringe (RediPen):** 50 mcg, 80 mcg, 120 mcg, 150 mcg. **Sylatron:** 200 mcg, 400 mcg, 600 mcg.

## ADMINISTRATION/HANDLING

### SQ

**Reconstitution** • To reconstitute, add 0.7 ml Sterile Water for Injection (supplied) to vial. • Gently swirl. Use immediately. Reconstituted solution may be refrigerated for up to 24 hrs before use. • Prefilled Syringe (RediPen): Hold cartridge upright, press two halves together until "click" is heard. • Gently invert to mix.
**Storage** • Store at room temperature. • Refrigerate RediPen. Once reconstituted, both products stable for 24 hrs if refrigerated.

## INDICATIONS/ROUTES/DOSAGE

**Melanoma**
SQ: **ADULTS, ELDERLY:** (Sylatron): 6 mcg/kg/wk for 8 doses, then 3 mcg/kg/wk for up to 5 yrs.

**Chronic Hepatitis C, Monotherapy**
SQ: **ADULTS 18 YRS AND OLDER, ELDERLY:** (PEG-Intron): Initially, 1 mcg/kg/wk. Administer appropriate dosage (see chart below) once wkly for 1 yr on same day each wk.

| Weight (kg) | mcg* |
|---|---|
| 45 or less | 40 |
| 46–56 | 50 |
| 57–72 | 64 |
| 73–88 | 80 |
| 89–106 | 96 |
| 107–136 | 120 |
| 137–160 | 150 |

*Of peginterferon alfa-2b to administer.

**Chronic Hepatitis C with Ribavirin**
SQ: **COMBINATION THERAPY WITH RIBAVIRIN: ADULTS, ELDERLY:** Initially, 1.5 mcg/kg/wk. **CHILDREN 3 YRS AND OLDER:** 60 mcg/m² once wkly.

| Weight | Dosage |
|---|---|
| Less than 40 kg | 50 mcg |
| 40–50 kg | 64 mcg |
| 51–60 kg | 80 mcg |
| 61–75 kg | 96 mcg |
| 76–85 kg | 120 mcg |
| 86–105 kg | 150 mcg |
| Greater than 105 kg | 1.5 mcg/kg/wk |

◄ALERT► Do not use in pts with CrCl less than 50 ml/min. Dosage adjustments needed for hematologic toxicity (Hgb, WBCs, neutrophils, platelets) and depression.

**Dosage in Renal Impairment**
Monotherapy:

| Creatinine Clearance | Dose |
|---|---|
| 30–50 ml/min | Reduce dose by 25% |
| 10–29 ml/min | Reduce dose by 50% |

**Combination: ADULTS: CrCl less than 50 ml/min:** Not recommended. **CHILDREN: Serum creatinine more than 2 mg/dL:** Discontinue.

**Dosage in Hepatic Impairment**
Use is contraindicated.

## SIDE EFFECTS

**Frequent (50%–47%):** Flu-like symptoms; inflammation, bruising, pruritus, irritation at injection site. **Occasional (29%–18%):** Psychiatric reactions (depression, anxiety, emotional lability, irritability), insomnia, alopecia, diarrhea. **Rare:** Rash, diaphoresis, dry skin, dizziness, flushing, vomiting, dyspepsia.

## ADVERSE EFFECTS/ TOXIC REACTIONS

Serious, acute hypersensitivity reactions (urticaria, angioedema, bronchoconstriction, anaphylaxis), pulmonary disorders, endocrine disorders (diabetes mellitus, hypothyroidism, hyperthyroidism) pancreatitis occur rarely. Ulcerative colitis may occur within 12 wks of starting treatment.

## NURSING CONSIDERATIONS

### BASELINE ASSESSMENT

CBC, urinalysis, renal function, LFT, EKG should be performed before initial therapy and routinely thereafter. Pts with diabetes, hypertension should have ophthalmologic exam before treatment begins.

### INTERVENTION/EVALUATION

Monitor for abdominal pain, bloody diarrhea as evidence of colitis. Assess for pulmonary impairment. Monitor chest X-ray for pulmonary infiltrates. Encourage adequate fluid intake, particularly during early therapy. Assess serum hepatitis C virus RNA levels after 24 wks of treatment. Monitor for depression, suicidal ideation.

### PATIENT/FAMILY TEACHING

• Maintain adequate hydration. • Avoid alcohol. • May experience flu-like syndrome (nausea, body aches, headache). • Report persistent abdominal pain, bloody diarrhea, fever, signs of depression, suicidal ideation, or infection, unusual bruising/bleeding.

# peginterferon beta-1a

peg-in-ter-**feer**-on
(Plegridy)
**Do not confuse peginterferon beta with peginterferon alfa or interferon beta.**

## ◆CLASSIFICATION

**PHARMACOTHERAPEUTIC:** Biologic response modifier. **CLINICAL:** Multiple sclerosis agent.

## USES

Treatment of relapsing forms of multiple sclerosis.

## PRECAUTIONS

**Contraindications:** History of hypersensitivity reaction to natural or recombinant interferon beta or peginterferon. **Cautions:** Pts with severe psychiatric disorders, history of depression, high risk for suicide. Pts with active/history of hepatic disease, alcohol consumption, or increased ALT at baseline; bone marrow suppression; preexisting cardiac disease (e.g., angina, arrhythmias, HF); seizure disorder.

## ACTION

Exact mechanism of action unknown. May alter expression/response to surface antigens and enhance immune cell activity. **Therapeutic Effect:** Decreases progression of multiple sclerosis.

## PHARMACOKINETICS

Peak plasma concentration: 24–36 hrs. Not extensively metabolized in liver. Eliminated primarily in urine. **Half-life:** 78 hrs.

## ⧖ LIFESPAN CONSIDERATIONS

**Pregnancy/Lactation:** Unknown if distributed in breast milk. **Children:** Safety and efficacy not established. **Elderly:** No age-related precautions noted.

## INTERACTIONS

**DRUG:** None known. **HERBAL:** None significant. **FOOD:** None known. **LAB VALUES:** May increase serum ALT, AST, GGT. May decrease neutrophils, platelets, WBC.

## AVAILABILITY (Rx)

**Prefilled Injector Pens, Prefilled Syringes:** 63 mcg/0.5 ml, 95 mcg/0.5 ml, 125 mcg/0.5 ml.

## ADMINISTRATION/HANDLING

**SQ**
**Premedication** • Prophylactic and concurrent use of analgesics and/or antipyretics may prevent or lessen flu-like symptoms.
**Administration** • If refrigerated, allow pen/syringe to warm to room temperature for 30 min before using. • Administer any time of day, without regard to meals, at same time each administration day. • Subcutaneously insert needle into abdomen, thigh, or back of upper arm. • Do not inject where skin is bruised, infected, reddened, or scarred. • Do not reuse pens/syringes. • Rotate injection sites.
**Storage** • Refrigerate in original carton. • Do not freeze. • May store at room temperature for up to 30 days (if cooling unavailable). • If carton returned to refrigerator, total combined time out of refrigeration may not exceed 30 days. • Protect from light.

## INDICATIONS/ROUTES/DOSAGE

**Note:** Analgesics and/or antipyretics may decrease flu-like symptoms on treatment days.

**Multiple Sclerosis**
**SQ: ADULTS, ELDERLY: Treatment initiation: Dose 1:** 63 mcg on day 1. **Dose 2:** 94 mcg on day 15 (14 days later).

P

**Dose 3:** 125 mcg on day 29. **Maintenance:** 125 mcg every 14 days thereafter.

**Dosage in Renal/Hepatic Impairment**
No dose adjustment.

## SIDE EFFECTS

**Frequent (47%–44%):** Flu-like symptoms, pyrexia, headache. **Occasional (19%–4%):** Myalgia, chills, asthenia, arthralgia, nausea, vomiting, hyperthermia, pruritus. **Injection Site Reactions: Frequent (62%):** Erythema. **Occasional (15%–2%):** Pain, pruritus, edema, warmth, hematoma, rash.

## ADVERSE EFFECTS/ TOXIC REACTIONS

Hepatic injury including autoimmune hepatitis, hepatitis, hepatic failure, or elevation of LFT greater than 5 times upper limit of normal (ULN) occurred in 2% of pts. Depression and/or suicidal ideation reported in 8% of pts. Serious hypersensitivity reactions including anaphylaxis, angioedema, urticaria have been reported. Cardiomyopathy, HF occurred in 7% of pts. Treatment may decrease blood counts across all cell lines; may cause anemia, lymphopenia, neutropenia, pancytopenia, thrombocytopenia. Approximately 7% of pts developed neutralizing antibodies to peginterferon. Injection site reactions occurred in 66% of pts and may rarely include necrosis of injection site. Seizures occurred in less than 1% of pts.

## NURSING CONSIDERATIONS

### BASELINE ASSESSMENT

Obtain CBC, LFT, urine or serum pregnancy test. Assess pt's understanding of proper self-injection techniques. Question history of depression or suicidal ideation, heart disease, hematologic abnormalities, hypersensitivity reactions, renal impairment. Question plans for breastfeeding.

### INTERVENTION/EVALUATION

Monitor CBC for hematologic abnormalities. Be alert for worsening depression, suicidal ideation. If pt develops loss of treatment effectiveness, consider testing for anti-peginterferon antibodies. Check injection site after 2 hrs for redness, swelling, or tenderness. Due to increased drug exposure, monitor pts with renal impairment for adverse reactions.

### PATIENT/FAMILY TEACHING

• Report changes in mood or behavior, thoughts of suicide, self-destructive behavior. • A health care provider will show you how to properly inject your medication. You must demonstrate correct injection technique before using at home. • Inject under skin (subcutaneously); do not inject into muscle or vein. • Rotate injection sites. • Injection site reactions such as itching, swelling, redness are common. • Report generalized rash, itching, hives; may indicate allergic reaction. • Discard used needles using regulated sharps container. • Treatment may cause worsening of autoimmune or liver disease. • Report any upper abdominal pain, body aches, bruising, dark-colored urine, fever, yellowing of skin or eyes. • Protect drug from light. • Do not freeze medication. • Do not breastfeed.

# pegloticase

peg-**loe**-ti-kase
(Krystexxa)

■ **BLACK BOX ALERT** ■ Severe infusion reactions, anaphylaxis (bronchospasm, stridor, urticaria, hypotension, dyspnea, flushing, circumoral swelling) have occurred, especially within 2 hrs of first infusion. Premedicate pt with corticosteroids, antihistamines. Should be administered in health care setting by health care providers prepared to manage infusion reactions.

**Do not confuse pegloticase with Activase, cholinesterase, or pegaspargase.**

## ◆ CLASSIFICATION

**PHARMACOTHERAPEUTIC:** Uric acid enzyme. **CLINICAL:** Antigout agent.

## USES

Treatment of chronic gout in adult pts refractory to conventional therapy. Not recommended for treatment of asymptomatic hyperuricemia.

## PRECAUTIONS

**Contraindications:** Hypersensitivity to pegloticase. Glucose-6-phosphate dehydrogenase (G6PD) deficiency due to hemodialysis, methemoglobinemia. **Cautions:** History of HF, elderly, debilitated.

## ACTION

Decreases uric acid production by catalyzing oxidation of uric acid to allantoin, lowering serum uric acid. **Therapeutic Effect:** Lowers serum uric acid concentration.

## PHARMACOKINETICS

Catalyzes oxidation of uric acid to allantoin, an inert and water-soluble purine metabolite. Readily eliminated, primarily by renal excretion. **Half-life:** 14.5 days.

## ⧗ LIFESPAN CONSIDERATIONS

**Pregnancy/Lactation:** Unknown if drug crosses placenta or is distributed in breast milk. **Children:** Safety and efficacy not established in pts younger than 18 yrs. **Elderly:** No age-related precautions noted.

## INTERACTIONS

**DRUG:** None significant. **HERBAL:** None significant. **FOOD:** None known. **LAB VALUES:** Decreases serum uric acid (expected).

## AVAILABILITY (Rx)

**Injection Solution:** 2-ml (8 mg/ml) single-use vials.

## ADMINISTRATION/HANDLING

 IV

**Reconstitution** • Withdraw 1 ml from single-use vial and inject into 250 ml 0.9% NaCl or 0.45% NaCl. • Invert infusion bag a number of times to ensure thorough mixing; do not shake.
**Rate of Administration** • Infuse slowly over no less than 120 min.
**Storage** • Store in refrigerator. • Solution should appear clear; discard if particulate is present. • Allow diluted solution to reach room temperature prior to infusion. • Following dilution, solution remains stable for 4 hrs if refrigerated or at room temperature.

## INDICATIONS/ROUTES/DOSAGE

◀**ALERT**▶ Give by IV infusion; do not give as IV push or IV bolus. Pt to be pretreated with corticosteroids, antihistamines to reduce risk of infusion reaction, anaphylaxis.

**Gout**
**Note:** Discontinue oral agents prior to initiating pegloticase and do not initiate during course of therapy.
**IV Infusion: ADULTS, ELDERLY:** 8 mg every 2 wks.

**Dosage in Renal/Hepatic Impairment**
No dose adjustment.

## SIDE EFFECTS

**Occasional (12%–9%):** Nausea, ecchymosis at IV site, nasopharyngitis. **Rare (6%–5%):** Constipation, vomiting.

## ADVERSE EFFECTS/ TOXIC REACTIONS

Exacerbation of HF has been noted. Infusion-related reaction (urticaria, dyspnea, chest discomfort, chest pain, erythema, pruritus) occurs in 26% of pts; anaphylaxis occurs in 7% of pts. Increase in gout flares is frequently noted upon initiation of antihyperuricemic therapy due to changing serum uric acid levels.

## NURSING CONSIDERATIONS

### BASELINE ASSESSMENT

If gout flare occurs during treatment, prophylaxis with an NSAID or colchicine is recommended. Pts at higher risk for

G6PD deficiency (e.g., pts of African or Mediterranean ancestry) should be screened for G6PD deficiency before starting therapy. Obtain serum uric acid levels prior to each infusion. If levels reach greater than 6 mg/dL, particularly when 2 consecutive levels greater than 6 mg/dL are observed, treatment should be discontinued.

### INTERVENTION/EVALUATION

Monitor closely for infusion reaction during therapy and for 2 hrs post treatment. If infusion reaction occurs during administration, infusion may be slowed, or stopped and restarted at slower rate. If severe infusion reaction occurs, discontinue infusion and institute treatment as needed. Assess for therapeutic response (reduced joint tenderness, swelling, redness, limitation of motion).

### PATIENT/FAMILY TEACHING

• Educate pts on the most common signs and symptoms of infusion reaction (rash, redness of skin, difficulty breathing, flushing, chest discomfort, chest pain). • Advise pts to seek medical care immediately if they experience any symptoms of allergic reaction during or at any time after infusion.

# pembrolizumab

**pem**-broe-**liz**-ue-mab
(Keytruda)
**Do not confuse pembrolizumab with palivizumab.**

### ◆CLASSIFICATION

**PHARMACOTHERAPEUTIC:** Monoclonal antibody. **CLINICAL:** Antineoplastic.

## USES

Treatment of unresectable or metastatic melanoma. Treatment of metastatic head and neck squamous cell carcinoma (HNSCC) with disease progression on or after platinum-containing chemotherapy.

Treatment of metastatic non–small-cell lung (NSCL) cancer in pts with PD-L1–expressing tumors with disease progression on or after platinum-containing chemotherapy.

## PRECAUTIONS

**Contraindications:** Hypersensitivity to pembrolizumab. **Cautions:** Thyroid disease, hepatic/renal impairment, interstitial lung disease, electrolyte imbalance, hypertriglyceridemia.

## ACTION

Binds PD-1 ligands to PD-1 receptor found on T cells, blocking its interaction with the ligands (PD-L1 and PD-L2). Releases PD-1 pathway–mediated inhibition of immune response (including antitumor immune response). **Therapeutic Effect:** Inhibits T-cell proliferation and cytokine production.

## PHARMACOKINETICS

Information on metabolism and elimination not available. Steady-state concentration: 18 wks. **Half-life:** 26 days.

## ⌛ LIFESPAN CONSIDERATIONS

**Pregnancy/Lactation:** Avoid pregnancy; may cause fetal harm. Unknown if distributed in breast milk. Must either discontinue drug or discontinue breastfeeding. Recommended effective contraception during treatment and up to 4 mos after discontinuation. **Children:** Safety and efficacy not established. **Elderly:** No age-related precautions noted.

## INTERACTIONS

**DRUG:** None known. **HERBAL:** None significant. **FOOD:** None known. **LAB VALUES:** May increase serum AST, glucose, triglycerides. May decrease albumin, serum calcium, sodium.

## AVAILABILITY (Rx)

**Injection, Lyophilized Powder for Reconstitution:** 50 mg/vial. **Injection solution:** 100 mg/4 ml.

## ADMINISTRATION/HANDLING

**IV**

◀**ALERT**▶ Use 0.2–0.5 micron in-line filter.

**Reconstitution** • Verify weight in kg. • Inject 2.3 ml of Sterile Water for Injection against glass wall of vial. Do not inject directly onto lyophilized powder. • Gently swirl contents until completely dissolved; do not shake. • Allow vial to stand for up to 5 min for bubbles to clear. • Visually inspect for particulate matter. • Do not use if extraneous particulate matter other than translucent to white protein-like particles observed. • Final concentration of reconstituted vial equals 25 mg/ml. • Withdraw required dose and mix into 0.9% NaCl infusion bag (diluent volume depends on dose required) • Final concentration of diluent bag should equal 1–10 mg/ml. • Allow refrigerated solution to warm to room temperature before infusing.

**Rate of Administration** • Infuse via dedicated line over 30 min using a 0.2–0.5 micron filter.

**Storage** • Reconstituted solution should appear clear to slightly opalescent, colorless to slightly yellow. Refrigerate reconstituted or diluted solution up to 24 hrs, or at room temperature up to 4 hrs. Store time should not exceed total combined time of reconstitution, dilution, storage, and infusion.

## INDICATIONS/ROUTES/DOSAGE

**Metastatic or Unresectable Melanoma**
**IV: ADULTS, ELDERLY:** 2 mg/kg every 21 days until disease progression or unacceptable toxicity.

**NSCL, HNSCC**
**IV: ADULTS, ELDERLY:** 200 mg q3wks.

**Dose Modification**
Based on Common Terminology Criteria for Adverse Events (CTCAE).
**Withhold Treatment for Any of the Following Adverse Events:** ALT or AST greater than 3–5 times upper limit of normal (ULN) or bilirubin 1.5–3 times ULN, grade 2 or 3 colitis, grade 3 hyperthyroidism, grade 2 nephritis, grade 2 pneumonitis, symptomatic hypophysitis; any grade 3 treatment-related adverse reaction. **Permanently Discontinue for Any of the Following Adverse Events:** ALT or AST greater than 5 times ULN or bilirubin 3 times ULN (or pts with liver metastasis who begin treatment with grade 2 ALT, AST, if ALT or AST increases greater than or equal to 50% from baseline and lasts for at least 1 wk), grade 3 or 4 infusion-related reaction, grade 3 or 4 nephritis, grade 3 or 4 pneumonitis; inability to reduce corticosteroid dose to 10 mg/day or less (or prednisone equivalent) after last dose; persistent grade 2 or 3 adverse reaction that does not recover to grade 0–1 within 12 wks after last dose; any severe or grade 3 treatment-related adverse reaction that reoccurs.

**Dosage in Renal Impairment**
No dose adjustment.

**Dosage in Hepatic Impairment**
**Mild impairment:** No dose adjustment. **Moderate to severe impairment:** Not studied, use caution.

## SIDE EFFECTS

**Frequent (47–20%):** Fatigue, nausea, cough, pruritus, rash, decreased appetite, constipation, diarrhea, arthralgia. **Occasional (18%–11%):** Dyspnea, extremity pain, peripheral edema, vomiting, headache, chills, insomnia, myalgia, abdominal pain, back pain, pyrexia, vitiligo, dizziness, upper respiratory tract infection.

## ADVERSE REACTIONS/ TOXIC EFFECTS

May cause severe immune-mediated events such as pneumonitis (2.9% of pts), colitis (1% of pts), hepatitis (0.5% of pts), hypophysitis (0.5% of pts), renal failure or nephritis (0.7% of pts), hyperthyroidism (1.2% of pts), hypothyroidism (8.3% of pts). Other reported events include adrenal insufficiency, arthritis, cellulitis, exfoliative dermatitis, hemolytic anemia, myositis, myasthenic syndrome,

**P**

pancreatitis, partial seizures, pneumonia, optic neuritis, rhabdomyolysis, sepsis. Immunogenicity (anti-pembrolizumab antibody formation) may occur.

## NURSING CONSIDERATIONS

### BASELINE ASSESSMENT

Obtain baseline CBC, BMP, ionized calcium, LFT, TSH, free T4, vital signs, urine pregnancy. Obtain weight in kg. Screen for history of adrenal/pituitary/pulmonary/thyroid disease, autoimmune disorders, hepatic/renal impairment, allergy to prednisone. Question possibility of pregnancy, plans for breastfeeding. Along with routine assessment, conduct full dermatologic exam, visual acuity.

### INTERVENTION/EVALUATION

Monitor CBC, LFT, serum electrolytes; thyroid panel if applicable. Monitor for immune-mediated adverse events. Notify physician if any CTCAE toxicities occur (see Appendix M) and initiate proper treatment. Obtain chest X-ray if pneumonitis suspected. Screen for tumor lysis syndrome in pts with high tumor burden. Offer antiemetics if nausea vomiting occurs. Monitor I&Os, daily weight. If prednisone therapy initiated, monitor capillary blood glucose and screen for corticosteroid side effects.

### PATIENT/FAMILY TEACHING

• Blood levels will be routinely monitored. • Avoid pregnancy; treatment may cause birth defects or miscarriage. Do not breastfeed. • Serious adverse reactions may affect lungs, GI tract, kidneys, or hormonal glands and prednisone therapy may need to be started. • Immediately contact physician if serious or life-threatening inflammatory reactions occur in following body systems: lung (chest pain, cough, shortness of breath); colon (severe abdominal pain or diarrhea); liver (bruising, clay-colored/tarry stools, yellowing of skin or eyes); pituitary (persistent or unusual headache, dizziness, extreme weakness, fainting, vision changes); kidney (decreased or dark-colored urine, flank pain), thyroid (insomnia, hypertension, tachycardia [overactive thyroid]), (fatigue, goiter, weight gain [underactive thyroid]).

---

## *PEMEtrexed TOP 100 HIGH ALERT

pem-e-**trex**-ed
(Alimta)
**Do not confuse pemetrexed with methotrexate or pralatrexate.**

### ◆ CLASSIFICATION

**PHARMACOTHERAPEUTIC:** Antimetabolite. **CLINICAL:** Antineoplastic.

## USES

Treatment of unresectable malignant pleural mesothelioma in combination with cisplatin. Initial treatment of locally advanced or metastatic non–squamous non–small-cell lung cancer (NSCLC) in combination with cisplatin. Single-agent maintenance treatment of NSCLC in pts whose disease has not progressed following 4 cycles of platinum-based first-line chemotherapy. **OFF-LABEL:** Treatment of bladder, cervical, ovarian, thymic malignancies; malignant pleural mesothelioma.

## PRECAUTIONS

**Contraindications:** Severe hypersensitivity to pemetrexed. **Cautions:** Hepatic/renal impairment, concurrent use of nephrotoxic medications, preexisting myelosuppresion. Not indicated for squamous cell NSCLC.

## ACTION

Disrupts folate-dependent enzymes essential for cell replication. **Therapeutic Effect:** Inhibits growth of mesothelioma cell lines.

## PHARMACOKINETICS

Protein binding: 81%. Not metabolized. Excreted in urine. **Half-life:** 3.5 hrs.

---

## LIFESPAN CONSIDERATIONS

**Pregnancy/Lactation:** Unknown if drug crosses placenta or is distributed in breast milk. Breastfeeding not recommended. May cause fetal harm. Not recommended during pregnancy. **Children:** Safety and efficacy not established in pts younger than 18 yrs. **Elderly:** Higher incidence of fatigue, leukopenia, neutropenia, thrombocytopenia in pts 65 yrs and older.

## INTERACTIONS

**DRUG: NSAIDs** may increase concentration/effects. **Bone marrow depressants** may increase risk of myelosuppression. **Live virus vaccines** may potentiate virus replication, increase vaccine side effects, decrease pt's antibody response to vaccine. **HERBAL: Echinacea** may decrease effects. **FOOD:** None known. **LAB VALUES:** May increase serum ALT, AST, creatinine.

## AVAILABILITY (Rx)

**Injection, Powder for Reconstitution:** 100 mg; 500 mg.

## ADMINISTRATION/HANDLING

 **IV Infusion**

**Reconstitution** • Dilute 500-mg vial with 20 ml (4.2 ml to 100-mg vial) 0.9% NaCl to provide concentration of 25 mg/ml. • Gently swirl each vial until powder is completely dissolved. • Solution appears clear and ranges in color from colorless to yellow or green-yellow. • Further dilute reconstituted solution with 100 ml 0.9% NaCl.
**Rate of Administration** • Infuse over 10 min.
**Storage** • Store at room temperature. • Diluted solution is stable for up to 24 hrs at room temperature or if refrigerated.

##  IV INCOMPATIBILITIES

Use only 0.9% NaCl to reconstitute; flush line prior to and following infusion.

Do not add any other medications to IV line.

## INDICATIONS/ROUTES/DOSAGE

Refer to individual protocols.
◄**ALERT**► Pretreatment with dexamethasone (or equivalent) will reduce risk, severity of cutaneous reaction; treatment with folic acid and vitamin $B_{12}$ beginning 1 wk before treatment and continuing for 21 days after last pemetrexed dose will reduce risk of side effects. Do not begin new treatment cycles unless ANC 1,500/$mm^3$ or greater, platelets 100,000/$mm^3$ or greater, and CrCl 45 ml/min or greater.

**Malignant Pleural Mesothelioma**
**IV: ADULTS, ELDERLY:** 500 mg/$m^2$ on day 1 of each 21-day cycle in combination with cisplatin.

**Non–Squamous Non–Small-Cell Lung Cancer (NSCLC)**
**IV: ADULTS, ELDERLY:** Initial treatment 500 mg/$m^2$ on day 1 of each 21-day cycle (in combination with cisplatin). **Maintenance or second-line treatment:** 500 mg/$m^2$ on day 1 of each 21-day cycle (as single agent).

**Dose Modification for Toxicity**
*Hematologic Toxicity*
**Nadir ANC less than 500/$mm^3$ and platelets 50,000/$mm^3$ or more:** Reduce dose to 75% of previous dose. **Nadir platelets less than 50,000/$mm^3$ without bleeding:** Reduce dose to 75% of previous dose. **Nadir platelets less than 50,000/$mm^3$ with bleeding:** Reduce dose to 50% of previous dose. **Nonhematologic toxicity grade 3 or greater (excluding neurotoxicity):** Reduce dose to 75% of previous dose (excluding mucositis). **Grade 3 or 4 mucositis:** Reduce dose to 50% of previous dose.

**Dosage in Renal Impairment**
Not recommended with CrCl less than 45 ml/min.

**P**

**Dosage in Hepatic Impairment**
**Grade 3 (5.1–20 times upper level normal) or grade 4 (greater than 20 times upper level normal):** 75% of previous dose.

## SIDE EFFECTS

**Frequent (12%–10%):** Fatigue, nausea, vomiting, rash, desquamation. **Occasional (8%–4%):** Stomatitis, pharyngitis, diarrhea, anorexia, hypertension, chest pain. **Rare (Less Than 3%):** Constipation, depression, dysphagia.

## ADVERSE EFFECTS/ TOXIC REACTIONS

Myelosuppression, characterized as grade 1–4 neutropenia, thrombocytopenia, anemia was reported.

## NURSING CONSIDERATIONS

### BASELINE ASSESSMENT

Question for possibility of pregnancy before initiating therapy. Obtain CBC, serum chemistry tests before therapy and at regular intervals throughout therapy.

### INTERVENTION/EVALUATION

Monitor Hgb, Hct, WBC, platelet count, renal/hepatic function. Monitor for hematologic toxicity (fever, sore throat, signs of local infection, unusual bruising/bleeding from any site), symptoms of anemia (excessive fatigue, weakness). Assess skin for evidence of dermatologic toxicity. Keep pt well hydrated, urine alkaline. Monitor WBC count for nadir, recovery.

### PATIENT/FAMILY TEACHING

• Maintain strict oral hygiene. • Do not have immunizations without physician's approval (drug lowers resistance). • Avoid crowds, those with infection. • Use contraceptive measures during therapy. • Promptly report fever, sore throat, signs of local infection, unusual bruising/bleeding from any site. • Do not breastfeed.

# penicillin G potassium

pen-i-**sil**-in G po-**tas**-ee-um
(Crystapen ✦, Pfizerpen)
**Do not confuse penicillin with penicillamine.**

## ◆CLASSIFICATION

**PHARMACOTHERAPEUTIC:** Penicillin.
**CLINICAL:** Antibiotic.

## USES

Treatment of susceptible infections including sepsis, meningitis, endocarditis, pneumonia. Active against gram-positive organisms (except *S. aureus*), some gram-negative organisms (e.g., *N. gonorrhoeae*), and some anaerobes and spirochetes.

## PRECAUTIONS

**Contraindications:** Hypersensitivity to any penicillin. **Cautions:** Renal/hepatic impairment, seizure disorder, hypersensitivity to cephalosporins, pts with asthma.

## ACTION

Inhibits bacterial cell wall synthesis by binding to one or more of the penicillin-binding proteins of bacteria. **Therapeutic Effect:** Bactericidal.

## PHARMACOKINETICS

Protein binding: 60%. Widely distributed (poor CNS penetration). Metabolized in liver. Primarily excreted in urine. **Half-life:** 0.5–1 hr (increased in renal impairment).

## ⏳ LIFESPAN CONSIDERATIONS

**Pregnancy/Lactation:** Readily crosses placenta; distributed in breast milk. **Children:** May delay renal excretion in neonates, young infants. **Elderly:** Age-related renal impairment may require dosage adjustment.

## INTERACTIONS

**DRUG: Probenecid** increases concentration. **HERBAL:** None significant. **FOOD:**

**Food, milk** decrease absorption. **LAB VALUES:** May cause positive Coombs' test. May increase serum ALT, AST, alkaline phosphatase, LDH. May decrease WBC count.

## AVAILABILITY (Rx)

**Injection, Powder for Reconstitution:** 5 million units.

## ADMINISTRATION/HANDLING

 IV

**Reconstitution** • After reconstitution, further dilute with 50–100 ml $D_5W$ or 0.9% NaCl for final concentration of 100,000–500,000 units/ml (50,000 units/ml for infants, neonates).
**Rate of Administration** • Infuse over 15–30 min.
**Storage** • Reconstituted solution is stable for 7 days if refrigerated.

### ▦ IV INCOMPATIBILITIES

Dopamine (Intropin), sodium bicarbonate.

### ▦ IV COMPATIBILITIES

Amiodarone (Cordarone), calcium gluconate, diltiazem (Cardizem), heparin, magnesium sulfate, potassium chloride.

## INDICATIONS/ROUTES/DOSAGE

**Usual Dosage**
**IV, IM: ADULTS, ELDERLY:** 6–24 million units/day in divided doses q4–6h. **CHILDREN:** 100,000–400,000 units/kg/day in divided doses q4–6h. **Maximum:** 24 million units/day. **NEONATES:** 25,000–50,000 units/kg/dose q8–12h.

**Dosage in Renal Impairment**
Dosage interval is modified based on creatinine clearance.

| Creatinine Clearance | Dosage |
|---|---|
| Greater than 50 ml/min | No dose adjustment |
| 10–50 ml/min | 75% normal dose |
| Less than 10 ml/min | 20%–50% normal dose |
| Hemodialysis: | 50%–100% normal dose q8–12h |

| Creatinine Clearance | Dosage |
|---|---|
| Continuous renal replacement therapy | |
| Continuous venovenous hemofiltration: | Loading dose 4 million units, then 2 million units q4–6h |
| Continuous venovenous hemodialysis: | Loading dose 4 million units, then 2–3 million units q4–6h |
| Continuous venovenous hemodiafiltration: | Loading dose 4 million units, then 2–4 million units q4–6h |

**Dosage in Hepatic Impairment**
No dose adjustment.

## SIDE EFFECTS

**Occasional:** Lethargy, fever, dizziness, rash, electrolyte imbalance, diarrhea, thrombophlebitis. **Rare:** Seizures, interstitial nephritis.

## ADVERSE EFFECTS/ TOXIC REACTIONS

Hypersensitivity reactions ranging from rash, fever, chills to anaphylaxis occur occasionally.

### NURSING CONSIDERATIONS

#### BASELINE ASSESSMENT
Question for history of allergies, particularly penicillins, cephalosporins.

#### INTERVENTION/EVALUATION
Promptly report rash (hypersensitivity), diarrhea (with fever, abdominal pain, mucus, or blood in stool, may indicate antibiotic-associated colitis). Monitor I&O, urinalysis electrolytes, renal function tests for nephrotoxicity.

# penicillin V potassium

pen-i-**sil**-in V po-**tas**-ee-um
(Apo-Pen-VK ✦, Novo-Pen-VK ✦, NuPen VK ✦)

P

## ◆CLASSIFICATION

**PHARMACOTHERAPEUTIC:** Penicillin. **CLINICAL:** Antibiotic.

## USES

Treatment of infections of respiratory tract, skin/skin structure, otitis media, necrotizing ulcerative gingivitis; prophylaxis for rheumatic fever, dental procedures. **OFF-LABEL:** Prosthetic joint infection.

## PRECAUTIONS

**Contraindications:** Hypersensitivity to any penicillin. **Cautions:** Severe renal impairment, history of allergies (particularly cephalosporins), history of seizures, asthma.

## ACTION

Inhibits cell wall synthesis by binding to bacterial cell membranes. **Therapeutic Effect:** Bactericidal.

## PHARMACOKINETICS

Moderately absorbed from GI tract. Protein binding: 80%. Widely distributed. Metabolized in liver. Primarily excreted in urine. Half-life: 1 hr (increased in renal impairment).

## ⧗ LIFESPAN CONSIDERATIONS

**Pregnancy/Lactation:** Readily crosses placenta; appears in cord blood, amniotic fluid. Distributed in breast milk in low concentrations. May lead to allergic sensitization, diarrhea, candidiasis, skin rash in infant. **Children:** Use caution in neonates and young infants (may delay renal elimination). **Elderly:** Age-related renal impairment may require dosage adjustment.

## INTERACTIONS

**DRUG: ACE inhibitors (e.g., enalapril, lisinopril), potassium-sparing diuretics (e.g., spironolactone), potassium supplements** may increase risk of hyperkalemia. May increase **methotrexate** concentration, toxicity. **Probenecid** may increase concentration, risk of toxicity. **HERBAL:** None significant. **FOOD:** None known. **LAB VALUES:** May cause positive Coombs' test. May increase serum ALT, AST, alkaline phosphatase, LDH. May decrease WBC count.

## AVAILABILITY (Rx)

**Powder for Oral Solution:** 125 mg/5 ml, 250 mg/5 ml. **Tablets:** 250 mg, 500 mg.

## ADMINISTRATION/HANDLING

**PO**
- Give on empty stomach 1 hr before or 2 hrs after meals (increases absorption).
- After reconstitution, oral solution is stable for 14 days if refrigerated. • Space doses evenly around the clock.

## INDICATIONS/ROUTES/DOSAGE

**Usual Dosage**
**PO: ADULTS, ELDERLY, CHILDREN 12 YRS AND OLDER:** 125–500 mg q6–8h. **CHILDREN YOUNGER THAN 12 YRS:** 25–75 mg/kg/day in divided doses q6–8h. **Maximum:** 3 g/day.

**Dosage in Renal/Hepatic Impairment**
No dose adjustment.

## SIDE EFFECTS

**Frequent:** Mild hypersensitivity reaction (chills, fever, rash), nausea, vomiting, diarrhea. **Rare:** Bleeding, allergic reaction.

## ADVERSE EFFECTS/ TOXIC REACTIONS

Severe hypersensitivity reactions, including anaphylaxis, may occur. Nephrotoxicity, antibiotic-associated colitis, other superinfections (abdominal cramps, severe watery diarrhea, fever) may result from high dosages, prolonged therapy.

## NURSING CONSIDERATIONS

### BASELINE ASSESSMENT

Question for history of allergies, particularly penicillins, cephalosporins.

P

## INTERVENTION/EVALUATION

Hold medication, promptly report rash (hypersensitivity), diarrhea (with fever, abdominal pain, mucus or blood in stool may indicate antibiotic-associated colitis). Be alert for superinfection: fever, vomiting, diarrhea, anal/genital pruritus, oral mucosal change (ulceration, pain, erythema). Review Hgb levels; check for bleeding (overt/occult bleeding, ecchymosis, swelling of tissue). Monitor I&O, urinalysis, renal function tests for nephrotoxicity.

## PATIENT/FAMILY TEACHING

• Continue antibiotic for full length of treatment. • Space doses evenly. • Report immediately if rash, diarrhea, bleeding, bruising, other new symptoms occur.

# pentamidine

pen-**tam**-i-deen
(NebuPent, Pentam)

## ◆CLASSIFICATION

**PHARMACOTHERAPEUTIC:** Anti-infective. **CLINICAL:** Antiprotozoal, antifungal agent.

## USES

**IM/IV:** Treatment of pneumonia caused by *Pneumocystis jiroveci* (PCP). **Inhalation:** Prevention of PCP in high-risk HIV-infected pts either with history of PCP or with a CD4+ count 200/mm³ or less. **OFF-LABEL:** Treatment of African trypanosomiasis, cutaneous/visceral leishmaniasis. Prevention of PCP in non–HIV-infected pts.

## PRECAUTIONS

**Contraindications:** Hypersensitivity to pentamidine. **Cautions:** Diabetes mellitus, hepatic impairment, hypertension/hypotension, anemia, thrombocytopenia, preexisting cardiac disease, hypocalcemia, prolonged QT interval, congenital long QT syndrome, medications that prolong QT interval, ventricular tachycardia, severe renal impairment, concurrent use of other nephrotoxic drugs, history of seizures or pancreatic disease, or elevated amylase/lipase levels, hematologic disorders. Pts with Stevens-Johnson syndrome.

## ACTION

Interferes with nuclear metabolism, incorporation of nucleotides, inhibiting DNA, RNA, phospholipid, protein synthesis. **Therapeutic Effect:** Produces antibacterial, antiprotozoal effects.

## PHARMACOKINETICS

Well absorbed after IM administration; minimally absorbed after inhalation. Widely distributed. Primarily excreted in urine. Minimally removed by hemodialysis. **Half-life:** 6.4–9.4 hrs (increased in renal impairment).

## ⧗ LIFESPAN CONSIDERATIONS

**Pregnancy/Lactation:** Unknown if drug crosses placenta or is distributed in breast milk. **Children:** No age-related precautions noted. **Elderly:** No age-related information available.

## INTERACTIONS

**DRUG: Nephrotoxic medications** may increase risk of nephrotoxicity. **HERBAL:** None significant. **FOOD:** None known. **LAB VALUES:** May increase serum alkaline phosphatase, bilirubin, BUN, creatinine, ALT, AST. May decrease serum calcium, magnesium. May alter serum glucose.

## AVAILABILITY (Rx)

**Injection, Powder for Reconstitution (Pentam):** 300 mg. **Powder for Nebulization (NebuPent):** 300 mg.

## ADMINISTRATION/HANDLING

◀**ALERT**▶ Pt must be in supine position during IM, IV administration, with frequent B/P checks until stable (potential for life-threatening hypotensive reaction). Have resuscitative equipment immediately available.

**P**

---

**IV**

**Reconstitution** • For intermittent IV infusion (piggyback), reconstitute each vial with 3–5 ml D₅W or Sterile Water for Injection. • Withdraw desired dose; further dilute with 50–250 ml D₅W to concentration not to exceed 6 mg/ml.
**Rate of Administration** • Infuse over 60–120 min. • Do not give by IV injection or rapid IV infusion (increases potential for severe hypotension).
**Storage** • Store vials at room temperature. • After reconstitution, IV solution is stable for 48 hrs at room temperature (24 hrs if reconstituted with D₅W). • Discard unused portion.

**IM**
• Reconstitute 300-mg vial with 3 ml Sterile Water for Injection to provide concentration of 100 mg/ml. • Administer deep IM.

**Aerosol (Nebulizer)**
• Aerosol stable for 48 hrs at room temperature. • Reconstitute 300-mg vial with 6 ml Sterile Water for Injection. Avoid NaCl (may cause precipitate). • Do not mix with other medication in nebulizer reservoir.

### ▦ IV INCOMPATIBILITIES

Cefazolin (Ancef), cefotaxime (Claforan), ceftazidime (Fortaz), ceftriaxone (Rocephin), fluconazole (Diflucan), foscarnet (Foscavir), interleukin (Proleukin).

### ▦ IV COMPATIBILITIES

Diltiazem (Cardizem), total parenteral nutrition (TPN), zidovudine (Retrovir).

### INDICATIONS/ROUTES/DOSAGE

**Treatment of *Pneumocystis Jiroveci* Pneumonia (PCP)**
**IV, IM:** **ADULTS, ELDERLY, CHILDREN OLDER THAN 4 MOS:** 4 mg/kg/day once daily for 14–21 days.

**Prevention of PCP**
**Inhalation:** **ADULTS, ELDERLY, CHILDREN 5 YRS AND OLDER:** 300 mg once q4wks.

**Dosage in Rena/Hepatic Impairment**
Use caution.

### SIDE EFFECTS

**Frequent: Injection (Greater Than 10%):** Abscess, pain at injection site. **Inhalation (Greater Than 5%):** Fatigue, metallic taste, shortness of breath, decreased appetite, dizziness, rash, cough, nausea, vomiting, chills. **Occasional: Injection (10%–1%):** Nausea, decreased appetite, hypotension, fever, rash, altered taste, confusion. **Inhalation (5%–1%):** Diarrhea, headache, anemia, muscle pain. **Rare: Injection (less than 1%):** Neuralgia, thrombocytopenia, phlebitis, dizziness.

### ADVERSE EFFECTS/ TOXIC REACTIONS

Life-threatening/fatal hypotension, arrhythmias, hypoglycemia, leukopenia, nephrotoxicity, renal failure, anaphylactic shock, Stevens-Johnson syndrome, toxic epidural necrolysis occur rarely. Hyperglycemia, insulin-dependent diabetes mellitus (often permanent) may occur even mos after therapy has stopped.

### NURSING CONSIDERATIONS

**BASELINE ASSESSMENT**
Avoid concurrent use of nephrotoxic drugs. Establish baseline for B/P, serum glucose. Obtain specimens for diagnostic tests before giving first dose. Screen for concomitant medications that increase risk of QT interval prolongation or nephrotoxicity.

**INTERVENTION/EVALUATION**
Monitor B/P during administration until stable for both IM and IV administration (pt should remain supine). Check serum glucose levels; observe for clinical signs of hypoglycemia (diaphoresis, anxiety, tremor, tachycardia, palpitations, dizziness, headache, numbness of lips, double vision, incoordination), hyperglycemia (polyuria, polyphagia, polydipsia, malaise, visual changes, abdominal pain, headache, nausea/vomiting). Evaluate IM

sites for pain, redness, induration; IV sites for phlebitis (heat, pain, red streaking over vein). Monitor renal, hepatic, hematology test results. Assess skin for rash. Evaluate equilibrium during ambulation. Be alert for respiratory difficulty when administering by inhalation route.

## PATIENT/FAMILY TEACHING

• Remain flat in bed during administration of medication; get up slowly with assistance only when B/P stable. • Immediately report profuse sweating, shakiness, dizziness, palpitations. • Drowsiness, increased urination, thirst, anorexia may develop in mos following therapy. • Maintain adequate fluid intake. • Report fever, cough, shortness of breath. • Avoid alcohol.

---

# perampanel

per-**am**-pa-nel
(Fycompa)

■ **BLACK BOX ALERT** ■ Risk for serious neuropsychiatric events, including irritability, aggression, anger, anxiety, paranoia, euphoric mood, agitation, mental status changes. Some of these events reported as serious and life-threatening. Violent thoughts or threatening behavior were also observed. Immediately report any changes in mood or behavior that are not typical for the patient are observed. Health care professionals should closely monitor patients during titration period when higher doses are used.

## ◆CLASSIFICATION

**PHARMACOTHERAPEUTIC:** Noncompetitive AMPA glutamate receptive antagonist. **CLINICAL:** Anticonvulsant.

## USES

Adjunctive therapy for the treatment of partial-onset seizures with or without secondary generalized seizures. Adjunctive therapy for the treatment of primary generalized tonic-clonic seizures.

## PRECAUTIONS

**Contraindications:** Hypersensitivity to perampanel. **Cautions:** Elderly (increased falls, dizziness, gait disturbances), severe renal/hepatic impairment, dialysis, concurrent use of CNS depressants, pts at risk for suicidal behavior.

## ACTION

Noncompetitive antagonist of AMPA glutamate receptors, a primary excitatory neurotransmitter on postsynaptic neurons. **Therapeutic Effect:** Reduces neuronal over excitation.

## PHARMACOKINETICS

Rapidly, completely absorbed. Peak concentration: 0.5–2.5 hrs. Protein binding: 95%–96%. Steady-state reached in 2–3 wks. Metabolized via oxidation/glucuronidation. Excreted in feces (48%), urine (22%). **Half-life:** 105 hrs.

## ⧖ LIFESPAN CONSIDERATIONS

**Pregnancy/Lactation:** Unknown if distributed in breast milk. Use caution when breastfeeding. **Children:** Safety and efficacy not established in pts less than 12 yrs. **Elderly:** Owing to greater likelihood for adverse reactions in the elderly, dosing titration should proceed very slowly.

P

## INTERACTIONS

**DRUG: CYP450 inducers (e.g., carbamazepine, oxcarbazepine, phenytoin)** may decrease concentration/effects. May decrease effectiveness of **hormonal contraceptives containing levonorgestrel. Alcohol, other CNS depressants (e.g., lorazepam, morphine, zolpidem)** may increase CNS depression. **HERBAL: St. John's wort, kava kava, valerian** may increase CNS depression. **Evening primrose** may decrease seizure threshold. **FOOD:** None known. **LAB VALUES:** None significant.

---

## AVAILABILITY (Rx)

Suspension, Oral: 0.5 mg/ml. Tablets, Film-Coated: 2 mg, 4 mg, 6 mg, 8 mg, 10 mg, 12 mg.

## ADMINISTRATION/HANDLING

**PO**
• Give at bedtime. • Give tablet whole; do not break, crush, dissolve, or divide tablet. • Measure oral suspension using provided adapter and dosing syringe.

## INDICATIONS/ROUTES/DOSAGE

◄ **ALERT** ► Initial starting dose should be increased when enzyme-inducing anticonvulsants are given concurrently. Individual dosing based on clinical response, tolerability. Do not use in severe hepatic/renal impairment, pts on hemodialysis.

**Partial-Onset Seizures, Generalized Tonic-Clonic Seizures in Absence of an Enzyme-Inducing Anticonvulsant**
**PO: ADULTS, ELDERLY, CHILDREN 12 YRS AND OLDER:** Initially, 2 mg once daily at bedtime. May titrate in 2-mg increments at wkly intervals (in elderly, no more frequently than every 2 wks). **Recommended maintenance dose:** (Partial Seizures): 8–12 mg/day at bedtime. (Tonic-Clonic Seizures): 8 mg/day at bedtime.

**Partial-Onset Seizures, Generalized Tonic-Clonic Seizures (Concurrently Taking an Enzyme-Inducing Anticonvulsant)**
**PO: ADULTS, ELDERLY, CHILDREN 12 YRS AND OLDER:** Initially, 4 mg once daily at bedtime. May titrate in 2-mg increments at wkly intervals (in elderly, no more frequently than every 2 wks). **Recommended maintenance dose:** 8–12 mg/day at bedtime.

**Dosage in Renal Impairment**
**CrCl less than 30 ml/min:** Not recommended.

**Dosage in Hepatic Impairment**
**PO: ADULTS, ELDERLY, CHILDREN 12 YRS AND OLDER:** 2 mg once daily with wkly increase of 2 mg daily every 2 wks until target dose is achieved. **Mild impairment: Maximum:** 6 mg. **Moderate impairment: Maximum:** 4 mg. **Severe impairment:** Not recommended.

## SIDE EFFECTS

**Frequent (32%–11%):** Dizziness, sleepiness, headache. **Occasional (8%–3%):** Fatigue, irritability, nausea, balance disorder, weight gain, gait disturbance, vertigo, blurred vision, vomiting, arthralgia, anxiety. **Rare (2%–1%):** Constipation, back pain, extremity pain, asthenia, oropharyngeal pain, aggression.

## ADVERSE EFFECTS/ TOXIC REACTIONS

Irritability, aggression, anger, anxiety, affect lability, agitation occurred rarely (2% of pts). Increased risk for seizures when anticonvulsants are withdrawn abruptly.

## NURSING CONSIDERATIONS

### BASELINE ASSESSMENT

Review history of seizure disorder (intensity, frequency, duration, LOC). Initiate seizure precautions. Obtain medication history (esp. use of other anticonvulsant therapy; dosage based on concurrent seizure medication). Observe clinically. Assist with ambulation until response to drug is established (32% of pts experience dizziness).

### INTERVENTION/EVALUATION

Assess mental status, cognitive abilities, behavioral changes. Monitor for clinical response, tolerability to medication, dosing level during treatment and for at least 1 mo after last therapy dose. Report persistent, severe, or worsening psychiatric symptoms or behaviors. Assess for clinical improvement (decrease in intensity, frequency of seizures).

### PATIENT/FAMILY TEACHING

• Avoid alcohol (greater risk for adverse effects). • The combination of alcohol and perampanel may significantly worsen

---

mood, increase anger. • Counsel pts, families, and caregivers of need to monitor for emergence of anger, aggression, hostility, unusual changes in mental status. • Avoid tasks that require alertness, motor skills until response to drug is established (greater risk for dizziness, sleepiness).

# pertuzumab

per-**tue**-zue-mab
(Perjeta)

■ **BLACK BOX ALERT** ■ Can result in embryo-fetal death, birth defects. Pts must be made aware of danger to fetus, need for effective contraception. May result in cardiac failure. Assess left ventricular ejection fraction.

## ◆CLASSIFICATION

**PHARMACOTHERAPEUTIC:** *HER2* receptor antagonist. **CLINICAL:** Antineoplastic.

## USES

Treatment of *HER2*-positive metastatic breast cancer who have not received prior anti-*HER2* therapy or chemotherapy for metastatic disease in combination with trastuzumab and docetaxel. Neoadjuvant treatment of pts with *HER2*-positive, locally advanced inflammatory, or early-stage breast cancer in combination with trastuzumab and docetaxel.

## PRECAUTIONS

**Contraindications:** Hypersensitivity to pertuzumab. **Cautions:** Conditions that may impair left ventricular function (e.g., uncontrolled hypertension, recent MI, severe cardiac arrhythmia), history of infusion-related reaction. Prior anthracycline therapy or irradiation.

## ACTION

Targets human epidermal growth factor 2 (*HER2*), blocking ligand-initiated intercellular signaling, which can result in cell growth arrest and cell death. **Therapeutic Effect:** Inhibits proliferation of tumor cells.

## PHARMACOKINETICS

Peak plasma concentration reached after first maintenance dose. **Half-life:** 18 days.

## ⧗ LIFESPAN CONSIDERATIONS

**Pregnancy/Lactation:** May cause embryo-fetal harm. Must use effective contraception in addition to barrier methods. Unknown if distributed in breast milk. **Children:** Safety and efficacy not established. **Elderly:** No age-related precautions noted.

## INTERACTIONS

**DRUG:** None significant. **HERBAL:** None significant. **FOOD:** None known. **LAB VALUES:** None significant.

## AVAILABILITY (Rx)

**Injection Solution:** 420 mg/14 ml (30 mg/ml) vial.

## ADMINISTRATION/HANDLING
 IV

**Reconstitution** • Withdraw ordered volume of solution from vial. • Dilute into 250 ml 0.9% NaCl only (do not use D₅W). • Gently invert solution (do not shake).
**Rate of Administration** • Initial dose to be infused over 60 min. • Subsequent doses may be infused over 30–60 min.
**Storage** • Refrigerate vials. Store vials in outside cartons (protects from light). • Once diluted, use immediately or refrigerate for up to 24 hrs. • Do not use if solution appears cloudy or contains particulate.

## ▦ IV INCOMPATIBILITIES

Do not mix with any other medications.

## INDICATIONS/ROUTES/DOSAGE

◀**ALERT**▶ Give as an IV infusion only. Do not give by IV push or bolus. If diluted solution is not used immediately, may refrigerate for up to 24 hrs.

---

 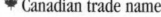

**Breast Carcinoma**
**IV  Infusion: ADULTS/ELDERLY:** Initially, 840 mg given over 60 min, followed every 3 wks thereafter by 420 mg given as a 30–60 min infusion for 3–6 cycles in combination with trastuzumab and docetaxel. Continue until disease progression or unacceptable toxicity.

**Breast Cancer (Neoadjuvant)**
**IV Infusion: ADULTS, ELDERLY:** 840 mg once followed by 420 mg q3wks for 3–6 cycles. May be administered as: 4 preoperative cycles of pertuzumab, trastuzumab, docetaxel, then 3 postoperative cycles of 5-fluorouracil, epirubicin, and cyclophosphamide (FEC) **or** 3 preoperative cycles of FEC alone, then 3 preoperative cycles of pertuzumab, trastuzumab, docetaxel **or** 6 cycles of pertuzumab, trastuzumab, docetaxel, and carboplatin. **Note:** Continue trastuzumab postoperatively to complete 1 yr of treatment.

**Dosage in Renal/Hepatic Impairment**
No dose adjustment.

## SIDE EFFECTS

**Frequent (67%–21%):** Diarrhea, alopecia, nausea, fatigue, rash, peripheral neuropathy, anorexia, asthenia, mucosal inflammation, vomiting, peripheral edema, myalgia, nail disorder, headache. **Occasional (19%–12%):** Stomatitis, pyrexia, dysgeusia, arthralgia, constipation, increased lacrimation, pruritus, insomnia, dizziness. **Rare (10%–7%):** Nasopharyngitis, dry skin, paronychia.

## ADVERSE EFFECTS/ TOXIC REACTIONS

Neutropenia occurs in 53% of pts, anemia occurs in 23% of pts, and leukopenia occurs in 18% of pts. Upper respiratory tract infection occurs in 17% of pts. Dyspnea, febrile neutropenia occurs in 14% of pts. Pleural effusion occurs in 5% of pts, left ventricular dysfunction occurs in 4% of pts.

## NURSING CONSIDERATIONS

**BASELINE ASSESSMENT**
Negative pregnancy test must be confirmed before initiating treatment. Obtain *HER2* testing by an FDA-approved laboratory. Assess daily serum blood chemistries, CBC.

**INTERVENTION/EVALUATION**
Monitor daily ANC. Monitor left ventricular ejection fraction (LVEF) and withhold dosing if ordered. Assess skin, IV site for infusion-associated reactions, hypersensitivity reactions, anaphylaxis. If a significant infusion-associated reaction occurs, slow or interrupt infusion and administer appropriate medical treatment. If a reaction is noted, the most common is pyrexia. Chills, fatigue, headache, asthenia, or vomiting usually occurs during the infusion or on the same day as the infusion. Observe pt closely for 60 min after the first infusion and for 30 min after subsequent infusions. Offer antiemetics if nausea occurs.

**PATIENT/FAMILY TEACHING**
• Avoid pregnancy. • Use effective contraceptive measures, including condoms during treatment and for 6 mos after treatment in women of childbearing potential. • If pregnancy occurs, inform physician immediately. • Do not breastfeed. • Alopecia is reversible, but new hair growth may have different color, texture.

# phenazopyridine

fen-**ay**-zoe-**pir**-i-deen
(Azo-Gesic, Pyridium)
**Do not confuse phenazopyridine with pyridoxine, or Pyridium with Dyrenium or Perdiem.**

## ◆CLASSIFICATION

**PHARMACOTHERAPEUTIC:** Interstitial cystitis agent. **CLINICAL:** Urinary tract analgesic.

## USES

Symptomatic relief of pain, burning, urgency, frequency resulting from lower urinary tract mucosa irritation (may be caused by infection, trauma, surgery).

## PRECAUTIONS

**Contraindications:** Hypersensitivity to phenazopyridine. Renal impairment (CrCl less than 50 ml/min). **Cautions:** Renal impairment (CrCl 50–80 ml/min).

## ACTION

Exerts topical analgesic effect on urinary tract mucosa. **Therapeutic Effect:** Relieves urinary pain, burning, urgency, frequency.

## PHARMACOKINETICS

Well absorbed from GI tract. Partially metabolized in liver. Primarily excreted in urine. **Half-life:** Unknown.

## ⌛ LIFESPAN CONSIDERATIONS

**Pregnancy/Lactation:** Unknown if drug crosses placenta or is distributed in breast milk. **Children:** No age-related precautions noted in pts older than 6 yrs. **Elderly:** Age-related renal impairment may increase toxicity.

## INTERACTIONS

**DRUG:** None significant. **HERBAL:** None significant. **FOOD:** None known. **LAB VALUES:** May interfere with urinalysis tests based on color reactions (e.g., urinary glucose, ketones, protein, 17-ketosteroids).

## AVAILABILITY (Rx)

**Tablets:** (Azo-Gesic, Azo-Standard, Uristat): 95 mg. **(Pyridium):** 100 mg, 200 mg.

## ADMINISTRATION/HANDLING

**PO**
• Give with meals.

## INDICATIONS/ROUTES/DOSAGE

**Urinary Analgesic**
**PO: ADULTS, ELDERLY, CHILDREN 12 YRS AND OLDER:** *(Rx):* 200 mg 3 times/day

for 2 days. *(OTC):* 190 mg 3 times/day for 2 days.

**Dosage in Renal Impairment**
Use contraindicated in pts with CrCl less than 50 ml/min.

**Dosage in Hepatic Impairment**
No dose adjustment.

## SIDE EFFECTS

**Occasional:** Headache, GI disturbance, rash, pruritus.

## ADVERSE EFFECTS/TOXIC REACTIONS

Overdose in pts with renal impairment, severe hypersensitivity may lead to hemolytic anemia, nephrotoxicity, hepatotoxicity. Methemoglobinemia generally occurs as result of massive, acute overdose.

## NURSING CONSIDERATIONS

### BASELINE ASSESSMENT

Assess pt for dysuria, urinary urgency or frequency.

### INTERVENTION/EVALUATION

Monitor for therapeutic response: relief of dysuria (pain, burning), urgency, frequency of urination.

### PATIENT/FAMILY TEACHING

• Reddish orange discoloration of urine should be expected. • May stain fabric. • Take with meals (reduces possibility of GI upset).

## *PHENobarbital

**fee**-noe-**bar**-bi-tal
**Do not confuse phenobarbital with Phenergan or phenytoin.**

### FIXED-COMBINATION(S)

**Donnatal:** phenobarbital/atropine (an anticholinergic)/hyoscyamine (an anticholinergic)/scopolamine (an anticholinergic): 16.2 mg/0.0194 mg/0.1037 mg/0.0065 mg.

## ◆ CLASSIFICATION

**PHARMACOTHERAPEUTIC:** Barbiturate **(Schedule IV). CLINICAL:** Anticonvulsant, hypnotic.

## USES

Management of generalized tonic-clonic (grand mal) seizures, partial seizures, control of acute seizure episodes (status epilepticus. **OFF-LABEL:** Treatment of alcohol withdrawal, sedative/hypnotic withdrawal.

## PRECAUTIONS

**Contraindications:** Hypersensitivity to phenobarbital, other barbiturates, porphyria, dyspnea or airway obstruction, use in nephritic pts, severe hepatic impairment. Pts with history of sedative/hypnotic addiction. **Cautions:** Renal/hepatic impairment, acute/chronic pain, depression, suicidal tendencies, history of drug abuse, elderly, debilitated, children, hemodynamically unstable pts, hypoadrenalism, respiratory disease.

## ACTION

Depresses sensory cortex, decreases motor activity, alters cerebellar function. **Therapeutic Effect:** Induces drowsiness, sedation, anticonvulsant activity.

## PHARMACOKINETICS

| Route | Onset | Peak | Duration |
|-------|-------|------|----------|
| PO | 20–60 min | N/A | 6–10 hrs |
| IV | 5 min | 30 min | 4–10 hrs |

Well absorbed after PO, parenteral administration. Protein binding: 20%–45%. Rapidly and widely distributed. Metabolized in liver. Primarily excreted in urine. Removed by hemodialysis. **Half-life:** 53–140 hrs.

## ⧗ LIFESPAN CONSIDERATIONS

**Pregnancy/Lactation:** Readily crosses placenta. Distributed in breast milk. Produces respiratory depression in neonates during labor. May cause postpartum hemorrhage, hemorrhagic disease in newborn. Withdrawal symptoms may appear in neonates born to women receiving barbiturates during last trimester of pregnancy. Lowers serum bilirubin in neonates. **Children:** May cause paradoxical excitement. **Elderly:** May exhibit excitement, confusion, mental depression.

## INTERACTIONS

**DRUG: Alcohol, other CNS depressants (e.g., lorazepam, morphine)** may increase effects. May decrease effects of **warfarin, oral contraceptives. Valproic acid** may increase concentration, risk of toxicity. **HERBAL: Evening primrose** may decrease seizure threshold. **Gotu kola, kava kava, St. John's wort, valerian** may increase CNS depression. **FOOD:** None known. **LAB VALUES:** May decrease serum bilirubin. **Therapeutic serum level:** 10–40 mcg/ml; **toxic serum level:** greater than 40 mcg/ml.

## AVAILABILITY (Rx)

**Elixir:** 20 mg/5 ml. **Oral Solution:** 20 mg/5 ml. **Injection, Solution:** 65 mg/ml, 130 mg/ml. **Tablets:** 15 mg, 30 mg, 60 mg, 100 mg.

## ADMINISTRATION/HANDLING

 **IV**

**Reconstitution** • May give undiluted or may dilute with NaCl.
**Rate of Administration** • Adequately hydrate pt before and immediately after drug therapy (decreases risk of adverse renal effects). • Do not inject IV faster than 30 mg/min for children and 60 mg/min for adults. Too-rapid IV may produce severe hypotension, marked respiratory depression. • Inadvertent intra-arterial injection may result in arterial spasm with severe pain, tissue necrosis. Extravasation in SQ tissue may produce redness, tenderness, tissue necrosis.
**Storage** • Store vials at room temperature.

**IM**

• Do not inject more than 5 ml in any one IM injection site (produces tissue irritation). • Inject deep IM into large muscle mass.

P

### PO

• Give without regard to meals. • Tablets may be crushed. • Elixir may be mixed with water, milk, fruit juice.

### ▦ IV INCOMPATIBILITIES

Amphotericin B complex (Abelcet, AmBisome, Amphotec).

### ▦ IV COMPATIBILITIES

Calcium gluconate, enalapril (Vasotec), fosphenytoin (Cerebyx), propofol (Diprivan).

### INDICATIONS/ROUTES/DOSAGE

**Status Epilepticus**
**IV: ADULTS, ELDERLY, CHILDREN:** 20 mg/kg. May repeat once in 10 min with a dose of 5–10 mg/kg.

**Seizure Control (Maintenance)**
**PO, IV: ADULTS, ELDERLY, CHILDREN OLDER THAN 12 YRS:** 1–3 mg/kg/day or 50–100 mg 2–3 times daily. **CHILDREN 5–12 YRS:** 4–6 mg/kg/day. **CHILDREN 1–5 YRS:** 6–8 mg/kg/day. **CHILDREN YOUNGER THAN 1 YR:** 5–8 mg/kg/day in 1–2 divided doses. **NEONATES:** 3–4 mg/kg/day given once daily.

**Dosage in Renal/Hepatic Impairment**
No dose adjustment.

### SIDE EFFECTS

**Occasional (3%–1%):** Drowsiness. **Rare (less than 1%):** Confusion, paradoxical CNS reactions (hyperactivity, anxiety in children; excitement, restlessness in elderly, generally noted during first 2 wks of therapy, particularly in presence of uncontrolled pain).

### ADVERSE EFFECTS/TOXIC REACTIONS

Abrupt withdrawal after prolonged therapy may produce increased dreaming, nightmares, insomnia, tremor, diaphoresis, vomiting, hallucinations, delirium, seizures, status epilepticus. Skin eruptions appear as hypersensitivity reaction. Blood dyscrasias, hepatic disease, hypocalcemia occur rarely. Overdose produces cold/clammy skin, hypothermia, severe CNS depression, cyanosis, tachycardia, Cheyne-Stokes respirations. Toxicity may result in severe renal impairment.

## NURSING CONSIDERATIONS

### BASELINE ASSESSMENT

Assess B/P, pulse, respirations immediately before administration. **Hypnotic:** Raise bed rails, provide environment conducive to sleep (back rub, quiet environment, low lighting). **Seizures:** Review history of seizure disorder (length, presence of auras, LOC). Observe for recurrence of seizure activity. Initiate seizure precautions.

### INTERVENTION/EVALUATION

Monitor CNS status, seizure activity, hepatic/renal function, respiratory rate, heart rate, B/P. Monitor for therapeutic serum level. **Therapeutic serum level:** 10–40 mcg/ml; **toxic serum level:** greater than 40 mcg/ml.

### PATIENT/FAMILY TEACHING

• Avoid alcohol, limit caffeine. • May be habit forming. • Do not discontinue abruptly. • May cause dizziness/drowsiness; avoid tasks that require alertness, motor skills until response to drug is established.

## *phenylephrine* ▪HIGH ALERT

fen-il-**ef**-rin
(AK-Dilate, Mydfrin, Neo-Synephrine, Sudafed PE)

■ **BLACK BOX ALERT** ■ Intravenous use should be administered by adequately trained individuals familiar with its use.
**Do not confuse Mydfrin with Midrin, or Sudafed PE with Sudafed.**

### ◆CLASSIFICATION

**PHARMACOTHERAPEUTIC:** Sympathomimetic, alpha-receptor stimulant. **CLINICAL:** Nasal decongestant, mydriatic, vasopressor.

## USES

**Nasal decongestant:** Topical application to nasal mucosa reduces nasal secretion, promoting drainage of sinus secretions. **Ophthalmic:** Topical application to conjunctiva relieves congestion, itching, minor irritation; whitens sclera of eye. **Parenteral:** Vascular failure in shock, supraventricular tachycardia, hypotension.

## PRECAUTIONS

**Contraindications:** Hypersensitivity to phenylephrine. **Injection:** Severe hypertension, ventricular tachycardia. **Oral:** Use within 14 days of MAOI therapy. **Cautions: Injection:** Elderly, hyperthyroidism, bradycardia, partial heart block, cardiac disease, HF, cardiogenic shock, hypertension. **Oral:** Asthma, bowel obstruction, cardiac disease, ischemic heart disease, hypertension, increased intraocular pressure, elderly, prostatic hyperplasia.

## ACTION

Acts on alpha-adrenergic receptors of vascular smooth muscle. Causes vasoconstriction of arterioles of nasal mucosa/conjunctiva; produces systemic arterial vasoconstriction. **Therapeutic Effect:** Decreases mucosal blood flow, relieves congestion. Increases B/P. Reduces heart rate due to decrease in cardiac output.

## PHARMACOKINETICS

| Route | Onset | Peak | Duration |
|---|---|---|---|
| IV | Immediate | N/A | 15–20 min |
| IM | 10–15 min | N/A | 0.5–2 hrs |
| SQ | 10–15 min | N/A | 1 hr |

Minimal absorption after intranasal, ophthalmic administration. Metabolized in liver, GI tract. Primarily excreted in urine. **Half-life:** 2.5 hrs.

## ⧗ LIFESPAN CONSIDERATIONS

**Pregnancy/Lactation:** Crosses placenta. Distributed in breast milk. **Children:** May exhibit increased absorption, toxicity with nasal preparation. No age-related precautions noted with systemic use.

**Elderly:** More likely to experience adverse effects.

## INTERACTIONS

**DRUG: MAOIs (e.g., phenelzine, selegiline)** may increase vasopressor effects. **Tricyclic antidepressants (e.g., amitriptyline, doxepin)** may increase cardiovascular effects. **HERBAL: Ephedra, yohimbe** may increase CNS stimulation. **FOOD:** None known. **LAB VALUES:** None significant.

## AVAILABILITY (OTC)

**Injection, Solution:** 10 mg/ml. **Solution, Nasal Drops (Neo-Synephrine):** 0.125%, 0.25%. **Solution, Nasal Spray (Neo-Synephrine):** 0.25%, 0.5%. **Solution, Oral:** 2.5 mg/5 ml. **Tablets (Sudafed PE):** 10 mg.

## ADMINISTRATION/HANDLING

 **IV**

**Reconstitution** • For IV push, dilute 1 ml of 10 mg/ml solution with 9 ml Sterile Water for Injection to provide concentration of 1 mg/ml. • For IV infusion, dilute 10–100 mg with 500 ml 0.9% NaCl or D₅W.
**Rate of Administration** • For IV push, give over 20–30 sec. • For IV infusion, titrate dose to maintain systolic B/P greater than 90 mm Hg.
**Storage** • Store vials at room temperature.

**Nasal**
• Instruct pt to blow nose prior to administering medication. • With head tilted back, apply drops in 1 nostril. Wait 5 min before applying drops in other nostril. • Sprays should be administered into each nostril with head erect. • Pt should sniff briskly while squeezing container, then wait 3–5 min before blowing nose gently. • Rinse tip of spray bottle.

## ▦ IV INCOMPATIBILITY

Furosemide (Lasix).

### ✜ IV COMPATIBILITIES

Amiodarone (Cordarone), dexmedetomidine (Precedex), dobutamine (Dobutrex), lidocaine, potassium chloride, propofol (Diprivan), vasopressin.

### INDICATIONS/ROUTES/DOSAGE

**Nasal Decongestant**

**◀ALERT▶** Do not use for more than 3 days.

**Intranasal: ADULTS, ELDERLY, CHILDREN 12 YRS AND OLDER:** 1–2 drops or 1–2 sprays of 0.25%–0.5% solution into each nostril q4h as needed. **CHILDREN 6–11 YRS:** 1–2 drops or 1–2 sprays of 0.25% solution into each nostril q4h as needed. **CHILDREN 2–5 YRS:** 1 drop of 0.125% solution (dilute 0.5% solution with 0.9% NaCl to achieve 0.125%) in each nostril. Repeat q2–4h as needed.

**PO: ADULTS, ELDERLY, CHILDREN 13 YRS AND OLDER:** 10 mg q4h as needed for up to 7 days. **CHILDREN 6–11 YRS:** 5 mg q4h as needed for up to 7 days. **CHILDREN 4–5 YRS:** 2.5 mg q4h as needed for up to 7 days.

**Hypotension, Shock**

**IV Bolus: ADULTS, ELDERLY:** 100–500 mcg (0.1–0.5 mg)/dose q10–15min as needed. **CHILDREN:** 5–20 mcg/kg/dose q10–15min as needed.

**IV Infusion: ADULTS, ELDERLY:** 100–180 mcg/min or 0.5 mcg/kg/min. Titrate to desired response. **CHILDREN:** 0.1–0.5 mcg/kg/min. Titrate to desired effect.

### SIDE EFFECTS

**Frequent: Nasal:** Rebound nasal congestion due to overuse, esp. when used longer than 3 days. **Occasional:** Mild CNS stimulation (restlessness, nervousness, tremors, headache, insomnia, particularly in those hypersensitive to sympathomimetics, such as elderly pts). **Nasal:** Stinging, burning, drying of nasal mucosa. **Ophthalmic:** Transient burning/stinging, brow ache, blurred vision.

### ADVERSE EFFECTS/TOXIC REACTIONS

Large doses may produce tachycardia, palpitations (particularly in pts with cardiac disease), dizziness, nausea, vomiting. Overdose in pts older than 60 yrs may result in hallucinations, CNS depression, seizures. Prolonged nasal use may produce chronic swelling of nasal mucosa, rhinitis. If phenylephrine 10% ophthalmic is instilled into denuded/damaged corneal epithelium, corneal clouding may result.

### NURSING CONSIDERATIONS

**BASELINE ASSESSMENT**

Obtain baseline symptomology, vital signs. Question history of hypertension, cardiac disease, asthma, recent use of MAOI therapy.

**INTERVENTION/EVALUATION**

Monitor B/P, heart rate. For severe hypotension or shock states, monitor central venous pressure.

**PATIENT/FAMILY TEACHING**

• Discontinue drug if adverse reactions occur. • Do not use for nasal decongestion for longer than 3 days (rebound congestion). • Discontinue drug if insomnia, dizziness, weakness, tremor, palpitations occur. • **Nasal:** Stinging/burning of nasal mucosa may occur. • **Ophthalmic:** Blurring of vision with eye instillation generally subsides with continued therapy. • Discontinue medication if redness/swelling of eyelids, itching occurs.

## phenytoin

fen-i-toyn
(Dilantin, Novo-Phenytoin ✜, Phenytek)

■ **BLACK BOX ALERT** ■ Do not exceed IV rate of 50 mg/min in adults and 1–3 mg/kg/min in pediatric pts. **Do not confuse Dilantin with Dilaudid or diltiazem, or phenytoin with phenelzine or fosphenytoin.**

P

### ◆CLASSIFICATION

**PHARMACOTHERAPEUTIC:** Hydantoin. **CLINICAL:** Anticonvulsant, antiarrhythmic.

## USES

Management of generalized tonic-clonic seizures (grand mal), complex partial seizures, status epilepticus. Prevention of seizures following head trauma/neurosurgery. **OFF-LABEL:** Prevention of early posttraumatic seizures following traumatic brain injury.

## PRECAUTIONS

**Contraindications:** Hypersensitivity to phenytoin, other hydantoins. Concurrent use of delavirdine, IV (additional), second- and third-degree AV block, sinoatrial block, sinus bradycardia, Adams-Stokes syndrome. **Cautions:** Porphyria, renal/hepatic impairment, those at increased risk of suicidal behavior/thoughts, elderly/debilitated pts, low serum albumin, cardiac disease, hypothyroidism, pts of Asian descent.

## ACTION

**Anticonvulsant:** Stabilizes neuronal membranes in motor cortex. Decreases influx of sodium during generation of nerve impulses. **Therapeutic Effect:** Decreases seizure activity.

## PHARMACOKINETICS

Slowly, variably absorbed after PO administration. Protein binding: 90%–95%. Widely distributed. Metabolized in liver. Primarily excreted in urine. Not removed by hemodialysis. **Half-life:** 7–42 hrs.

## ⧖ LIFESPAN CONSIDERATIONS

**Pregnancy/Lactation:** Crosses placenta; distributed in small amount in breast milk. Fetal hydantoin syndrome (craniofacial abnormalities, nail/digital hypoplasia, prenatal growth deficiency) has been reported. Increased frequency of seizures in pregnant women due to altered absorption of metabolism of phenytoin.

May increase risk of hemorrhage in neonate, maternal bleeding during delivery. **Children:** More susceptible to gingival hyperplasia, coarsening of facial hair; excess body hair. **Elderly:** No age-related precautions noted but lower dosages recommended.

## INTERACTIONS

**DRUG: Alcohol, other CNS depressants (e.g., lorazepam, morphine, zolpidem)** may increase CNS depression. **Amiodarone, cimetidine, disulfiram, fluoxetine, isoniazid, sulfonamides** may increase concentration/ effects, risk of toxicity. **Calcium-containing antacids** may decrease absorption. May decrease effects of **glucocorticoids (e.g., dexamethasone, prednisone), anticoagulants (e.g., heparin, warfarin), oral contraceptives. Lidocaine, propranolol** may increase cardiac depressant effects. **Valproic acid** may decrease metabolism, increase concentration. May increase metabolism, decrease effects of **xanthines. HERBAL: Evening primrose** may decrease seizure threshold. **Gotu kola, kava kava, St. John's wort, valerian** may increase CNS depression. **FOOD:** None known. **LAB VALUES:** May increase serum glucose, GGT, alkaline phosphatase. **Therapeutic serum level:** 10–20 mcg/ml; **toxic serum level:** greater than 20 mcg/ml.

## AVAILABILITY (Rx)

**Capsules, Extended-Release:** 30 mg, 100 mg, 200 mg, 300 mg. **Injection, Solution:** 50 mg/ml. **Suspension, Oral:** 125 mg/5 ml. **Tablets, Chewable:** 50 mg.

## ADMINISTRATION/HANDLING

 **IV**

◄**ALERT►** Give by IV push or IV piggyback. IV push very painful (chemical irritation of vein due to alkalinity of solution). To minimize effect, flush vein with sterile saline solution through same IV needle and catheter after each IV push.

**Reconstitution** • May give undiluted or may dilute with 0.9% NaCl to a concentration of 5 mg/ml or more.

**Rate of Administration** • Administer 50 mg over 1 min in adults, 20 mg/min in elderly, pts with preexisting cardiovascular conditions. In neonates, administer at rate not exceeding 1–3 mg/kg/min. • Severe hypotension, cardiovascular collapse occur if rate of IV injection exceeds 50 mg/min for adults. • IV toxicity characterized by CNS depression, cardiovascular collapse.

**Storage** • Precipitate may form if parenteral form is refrigerated (will dissolve at room temperature). • Slight yellow discoloration of parenteral form does not affect potency, but do not use if solution is cloudy or precipitate forms. Discard if not used within 4 hrs of preparation.

**PO**

• Give with food if GI distress occurs.
• Tablets may be chewed. • Shake oral suspension well before using. • Separate administration of phenytoin with antacids or tube feeding by 2 hrs.

## ▦ IV INCOMPATIBILITIES

Diltiazem (Cardizem), dobutamine (Dobutrex), enalapril (Vasotec), heparin, hydromorphone (Dilaudid), insulin, lidocaine, morphine, nitroglycerin, norepinephrine (Levophed), potassium chloride, propofol (Diprivan).

## INDICATIONS/ROUTES/ DOSAGE

**Status Epilepticus**

**IV: ADULTS, ELDERLY, ADOLESCENTS:** Loading dose: 20 mg/kg at maximum rate of 50 mg/min. May repeat in 10 min with dose of 5–10 mg/kg. **INFANTS, CHILDREN:** Loading dose: 20 mg/kg at maximum rate of 1 mg/kg/min. May give additional dose of 5–10 mg/kg after loading dose.

**Seizure Control**

**PO: ADULTS, ELDERLY:** Initially, 100 mg 3 times/day. Adjust dose at 7–10-day intervals. Maintenance: 300–400 mg/day.

May increase up to 600 mg/day. **CHILDREN:** Initially, 5 mg/kg/day in 2–3 divided doses. Adjust dose at 7–10-day intervals. **Maintenance:** 4–8 mg/kg/day. **Maximum:** 300 mg/day.

**Dosage in Renal/Hepatic Impairment**
No dose adjustment.

## SIDE EFFECTS

**Frequent:** Drowsiness, lethargy, confusion, slurred speech, irritability, gingival hyperplasia, hypersensitivity reaction (fever, rash, lymphadenopathy), constipation, dizziness, nausea. **Occasional:** Headache, hirsutism, coarsening of facial features, insomnia, muscle twitching.

## ADVERSE EFFECTS/ TOXIC REACTIONS

Abrupt withdrawal may precipitate status epilepticus. Blood dyscrasias, lymphadenopathy, osteomalacia (due to interference of vitamin D metabolism) may occur. Toxic phenytoin blood concentration (25 mcg/ml or more) may produce ataxia, nystagmus, diplopia. As level increases, extreme lethargy to comatose state occurs.

## NURSING CONSIDERATIONS

**BASELINE ASSESSMENT**

**Anticonvulsant:** Review history of seizure disorder (intensity, frequency, duration, LOC). Initiate seizure precautions. LFT, CBC should be performed before beginning therapy and periodically during therapy. Repeat CBC 2 wks following initiation of therapy and 2 wks following administration of maintenance dose.

**INTERVENTION/EVALUATION**

Observe frequently for recurrence of seizure activity. Assess for clinical improvement (decrease in intensity/frequency of seizures). Monitor for signs/symptoms of depression, suicidal tendencies, unusual behavior. Monitor CBC with differential, renal function, LFT, B/P (with IV use). Assist with ambulation if drowsiness, lethargy occurs. Monitor for therapeutic

**P**

serum level (10–20 mcg/ml). **Therapeutic serum level:** 10–20 mcg/ml; **toxic serum level:** greater than 20 mcg/ml. **Free unbound levels: Therapeutic:** 1–2 mcg/ml; **toxic:** more than 2 mcg/ml.

**PATIENT/FAMILY TEACHING**

• Pain may occur with IV injection. • To prevent gingival hyperplasia (bleeding, tenderness, swelling of gums), maintain good oral hygiene, gum massage, regular dental visits. • Serum levels should be performed every mo for 1 yr after maintenance dose is established and q3mos thereafter. • Report sore throat, fever, glandular swelling, skin reaction (hematologic toxicity). • Drowsiness usually diminishes with continued therapy. • Avoid tasks that require alertness, motor skills until response to drug is established. • Do not abruptly withdraw medication after long-term use (may precipitate seizures). • Strict maintenance of drug therapy is essential for seizure control, arrhythmias. • Avoid alcohol. • Report any unusual changes in behavior.

# phosphates potassium sodium

fos-fates

## ◆CLASSIFICATION

**PHARMACOTHERAPEUTIC:** Electrolyte supplement. **CLINICAL:** Mineral.

## USES

Prevention and treatment of hypophosphatemia.

## PRECAUTIONS

**Contraindications:** Hyperkalemia, hypernatremia, hyperphosphatemia, hypocalcemia. **Cautions:** Renal impairment, concomitant use of potassium-sparing drugs, acid-base alteration, digitalized pts, cardiac disease, metabolic alkalosis.

## ACTION

Active in bone deposition, calcium metabolism, utilization of B complex vitamins. Acts as buffers in maintaining acid-base balance. Exerts osmotic effect in small intestine. **Therapeutic Effect:** Corrects hypophosphatemia, acidifies urine, prevents calcium deposits in urinary tract, promotes peristalsis in GI tract.

## PHARMACOKINETICS

Poorly absorbed after PO administration. PO form excreted in feces; IV form excreted in urine.

## ⧗ LIFESPAN CONSIDERATIONS

**Pregnancy/Lactation:** Use caution in pregnant women with other medical conditions (e.g., preeclampsia). **Children:** Increased risk of dehydration in pts younger than 12 yrs. **Elderly:** No age-related precautions noted.

## INTERACTIONS

**DRUG: ACE inhibitors (e.g., enalapril, lisinopril), NSAIDs, potassium-containing medications, potassium-sparing diuretics (e.g., spironolactone, triamterene), salt substitutes containing potassium phosphate** may increase serum potassium. **Antacids** may decrease absorption. **Calcium-containing medications** may increase risk of calcium deposition in soft tissues, decrease phosphate absorption. **HERBAL:** None significant. **FOOD:** None known. **LAB VALUES:** None significant.

## AVAILABILITY (Rx)

**Injection Solution (Potassium Phosphate):** 3 mmol phosphate and 4.4 mEq potassium per ml. **Injection Solution (Sodium Phosphate):** 3 mmol phosphate and 4 mEq sodium per ml.

## ADMINISTRATION/HANDLING

 IV

**Reconstitution** • Must be diluted. Soluble in all commonly used IV solutions.

**Rate of Administration** • Infuse over minimum of 4 hrs (usually over 6 hrs). Maximum rate: 0.06 mmol/kg/hr.
**Storage** • Store at room temperature.

## 🕮 IV INCOMPATIBILITY

Amiodarone, dobutamine (Dobutrex), pantoprazole (Protonix).

## 🕮 IV COMPATIBILITIES

Diltiazem (Cardizem), enalapril (Vasotec), famotidine (Pepcid), metoclopramide (Reglan), nicardipine (Cardene).

## INDICATIONS/ROUTES/ DOSAGE

### Hypophosphatemia

**Potassium/Sodium Phosphate:** (Phosphate level 2.3–3 mg/dL): 0.16–0.32 mmol/kg over 4–6 hr. (Phosphate level 1.6–22 mg/dL): 0.32–0.64 mmol/kg over 4–6 hr. (Phosphate level <1.5 mg/dL): 0.64–1 mmol/kg over 8–12 hr.

## SIDE EFFECTS

**Frequent:** Mild laxative effect (in first few days of therapy). **Occasional:** Diarrhea, nausea, abdominal pain, vomiting. **Rare:** Headache, dizziness, confusion, heaviness of lower extremities, fatigue, muscle cramps, paresthesia, peripheral edema, arrhythmias, weight gain, thirst.

## ADVERSE EFFECTS/ TOXIC REACTIONS

Hyperphosphatemia may produce extraskeletal calcification.

## NURSING CONSIDERATIONS

### INTERVENTION/EVALUATION

Routinely monitor serum calcium, phosphorus, potassium, sodium, ALT, AST, alkaline phosphatase, bilirubin.

### PATIENT/FAMILY TEACHING

• Report diarrhea, nausea, vomiting.

# pimavanserin

pim-a-**van**-ser-in
(Nuplazid)

■ **BLACK BOX ALERT** ■ Increased risk of mortality in elderly pts with dementia-related psychosis. Not approved for dementia-related psychosis unrelated to the hallucinations and delusions associated with Parkinson's disease psychosis.
**Do not confuse pimavanserin with eplivanserin, flibanserin, or pravastatin, or Nuplazid with Neulasta or Neupogen.**

## ◆ CLASSIFICATION

**PHARMACOTHERAPEUTIC:** Second-generation (atypical) antipsychotic. **CLINICAL:** Antipsychotic.

## USES

Treatment of hallucinations and delusions associated with Parkinson's disease psychosis.

## PRECAUTIONS

**Contraindications:** Hypersensitivity to pimavanserin. **Cautions:** Concomitant use of strong CYP3A4 inhibitors, strong CYP3A4 inducers. History of orthostatic hypotension, hepatic impairment. Avoid use in pts with history of cardiac arrhythmias, symptomatic bradycardia; conditions predisposing to sudden cardiac failure, torsades de pointes (congenital long QT syndrome, medications known to prolong QT interval, HF; hypokalemia, hypomagnesemia). Not approved for dementia-related psychosis unrelated to the hallucinations and delusions associated with Parkinson's disease psychosis.

## ACTION

Exact mechanism unknown. Displays agonist and antagonist activity with high affinity for 5-HT$_{2A}$ receptors and low affinity to 5-HT$_{2C}$ receptors. **Therapeutic Effect:** Produces tranquilizing effect. Reduces symptoms of psychosis.

P

## PHARMACOKINETICS

Widely distributed. Metabolized in liver. Protein binding: 95%. Peak plasma concentration: 6 hrs (range: 4–24 hrs). Eliminated in feces (less than 2%), urine (less than 1%). **Half-life:** 57 hrs.

## ⚖ LIFESPAN CONSIDERATIONS

**Pregnancy/Lactation:** Unknown if distributed in breast milk. **Children:** Safety and efficacy not established. **Elderly:** No age-related precautions noted.

## INTERACTIONS

**DRUG:** QT interval–prolonging medications (e.g., **amiodarone, fluoxetine, haloperidol, moxifloxacin, sotalol**) may increase risk of QT interval prolongation. **Strong CYP3A inducers** (e.g., **carbamazepine, phenobarbital, rifampin**) may decrease concentration/effect. **Strong CYP3A inhibitors** (e.g., **clarithromycin, ketoconazole, ritonavir**) may increase concentration/effects. **HERBAL: St. John's wort** may decrease concentration/effect. **FOOD:** None known. **LAB VALUES:** None known.

## AVAILABILITY (Rx)

**Tablets:** 17 mg.

## ADMINISTRATION/HANDLING

**PO**
• Give without regard to food.

## INDICATIONS/ROUTES/DOSAGE

**Parkinson's Disease Psychosis**
**PO: ADULTS, ELDERLY:** 34 mg (two 17-mg tablets) once daily.

**Dose Modification**
**Concomitant use of strong CYP3A4 inhibitors:** 17 mg once daily.
**Concomitant use of strong CYP3A4 inducers:** 34 mg once daily (dosage increase may be necessary due to reduced effectiveness).

**Dosage in Renal Impairment**
**Mild to moderate impairment:** No dose adjustment. **Severe impairment:** Not recommended.

**Dosage in Hepatic Impairment**
Not recommended.

## SIDE EFFECTS

**Occasional (7%–4%):** Peripheral edema, confusion, hallucinations (auditory, tactile, somatic, visual), constipation. **Rare (2%):** Gait disturbance.

## ADVERSE EFFECTS/TOXIC REACTIONS

May increase risk of death in pts with dementia-related psychosis. Drug-related deaths were reported in 5% of pts and were mainly cardiovascular (e.g., sudden death, cardiac failure) or infectious (e.g., pneumonia) in nature. May prolong QT interval. May increase risk cardiac arrhythmias.

## NURSING CONSIDERATIONS

### BASELINE ASSESSMENT

Obtain vital signs. Assess behavior, appearance, emotional status, response to environment, speech pattern, thought content. Therapy is intended only for Parkinson's disease psychosis. Screen pts for dementia-related psychosis. Receive full medication history and screen for interactions. Question history of cardiac arrhythmias, symptomatic bradycardia, HF, QT interval prolongation, heart block.

### INTERVENTION/EVALUATION

Monitor pulse rate; EKG. Obtain orthostatic vital signs. Assess for therapeutic response (interest in surroundings, improvement in self-care, increased ability to concentrate, relaxed facial expressions). Monitor for chest pain, sudden dizziness, syncopy. Monitor EKG for cardiac arrhythmias, QT interval prolongation, torsades de pointes. Obtain serum potassium, magnesium in pts with EKG abnormalities and replace electrolytes as appropriate. Monitor for reduced effectiveness in pts taking concomitant CYP3A4 inducers.

### PATIENT/FAMILY TEACHING

• Do not abruptly withdraw from long-term therapy. • Drowsiness may subside after continued therapy. • Avoid tasks that require alertness, motor skills until response to drug established. • Go slowly from lying to standing. • Avoid alcohol. • Use caution when taking other drugs that depress the central nervous system. • Do not take newly prescribed medications unless approved by prescriber that originally started therapy. • Do not take herbal products. • Therapy may cause life-threatening cardiac arrhythmias. Seek immediate medical attention if chest pain, dizziness, fainting, palpitations, or feelings of impending doom occur. • Report continued hallucinations or delirium.

---

## *pioglitazone* HIGH ALERT

pye-oh-**glit**-a-zone
(Actos, Apo-Pioglitazone ✦)

■ **BLACK BOX ALERT** ■ May cause or exacerbate HF.
**Do not confuse Actos with Actidose or Actonel.**

### FIXED-COMBINATION(S)

**Actoplus Met:** pioglitazone/metformin (an antidiabetic): 15 mg/500 mg, 15 mg/850 mg. **Duetact:** pioglitazone/glimepiride (an antidiabetic): 30 mg/2 mg, 30 mg/4 mg. **Oseni:** pioglitazone/alogliptin (an antidiabetic): 15 mg/25 mg, 30 mg/25 mg, 45 mg/25 mg, 15 mg/12.5 mg, 30 mg/12.5 mg, 45 mg/12.5 mg.

### ◆CLASSIFICATION

**PHARMACOTHERAPEUTIC:** Thiazolidinedione antihyperglycemic. **CLINICAL:** Antidiabetic agent.

## USES

Adjunct to diet and exercise to lower serum glucose in those with type 2 non–insulin-dependent diabetes mellitus (NIDDM). Used as monotherapy or combination therapy.

## PRECAUTIONS

**Contraindications:** Hypersensitivity to pioglitazone. NYHA class III/IV HF (at initiation of therapy). **Cautions:** Hepatic impairment, anemia, pts with edema; avoid in pts with bladder cancer. For premenopausal, anovulatory women may result in ovulation resumption, increased risk of pregnancy. NYHA class I/II HF.

## ACTION

Improves target-cell response to insulin without increasing pancreatic insulin secretion. Action dependent on presence of insulin. **Therapeutic Effect:** Lowers serum glucose concentration.

## PHARMACOKINETICS

Rapidly absorbed. Protein binding: 99%. Metabolized in liver. Excreted in urine. Unknown if removed by hemodialysis. **Half-life:** 16–24 hrs.

## ⧗ LIFESPAN CONSIDERATIONS

**Pregnancy/Lactation:** Unknown if drug crosses placenta or is distributed in breast milk. Not recommended in pregnant or breastfeeding women. **Children:** Safety and efficacy not established. **Elderly:** No age-related precautions noted.

## INTERACTIONS

**DRUG:** CYP2C8 inhibitors (e.g., **gemfibrozil**) may increase concentration/effects. **CYP2C8 inducers** (e.g., **rifampin**) may decrease concentration. **HERBAL:** Garlic, ginger, ginseng may cause hypoglycemia. **FOOD:** None known. **LAB VALUES:** May increase serum creatine kinase (CK). May decrease Hgb (by 2%–4%). May increase serum alkaline phosphatase, bilirubin, ALT. Less than 1% of pts experience ALT values 3 times the normal level.

**P**

## AVAILABILITY (Rx)

**Tablets:** 15 mg, 30 mg, 45 mg.

## ADMINISTRATION/HANDLING

**PO**
• Give without regard to meals.

## INDICATIONS/ROUTES/DOSAGE

**Diabetes Mellitus**
**PO: ADULTS, ELDERLY:** 15–30 mg once daily.
**Maximum:** 45 mg once daily.

**Dosage Adjustment in HF**
**Note:** Not recommended in pts with symptomatic HF.
**PO: ADULTS, ELDERLY:** 15 mg once daily.

**Dosage in Renal/Hepatic Impairment**
No dose adjustment. **Note:** Hepatic injury has been associated with use. Use caution.

## SIDE EFFECTS

**Frequent (13%–9%):** Headache, upper respiratory tract infection. **Occasional (6%–5%):** Sinusitis, myalgia, pharyngitis, aggravated diabetes mellitus, edema.

## ADVERSE EFFECTS/
## TOXIC REACTIONS

Hepatotoxicity occurs rarely. May cause/worsen macular edema. Increased risk of HF. May increase risk of fractures. Pts with ischemic heart disease are at high risk of MI.

## NURSING CONSIDERATIONS

### BASELINE ASSESSMENT

Obtain baseline chemistries, esp. LFT, before initiating therapy and periodically thereafter.

### INTERVENTION/EVALUATION

Monitor serum glucose, Hgb A1c, LFT. Assess for hypoglycemia (cool/wet skin, tremors, dizziness, anxiety, headache, tachycardia, numbness in mouth, hunger, diplopia), hyperglycemia (polyuria, polyphagia, polydipsia, nausea, vomiting, dim vision, fatigue, deep rapid breathing).

Be alert to conditions that alter serum glucose requirements: fever, increased activity, trauma, stress, surgical procedures. Monitor for signs/symptoms of HF.

### PATIENT/FAMILY TEACHING

• Be alert for signs/symptoms of hypoglycemia and take measures to manage it. • Avoid alcohol. • Report chest pain, palpitations, abdominal pain, fever, rash, hypoglycemic reactions, yellowing of skin/eyes, dark urine, light stool, nausea, vomiting. • Report any change in vision. • Report rapid weight gain, edema, difficulty breathing. • Ensure follow-up instruction if pt, family do not thoroughly understand diabetes management, glucose-testing technique.

# piperacillin sodium/tazobactam sodium

pye-per-a-**sil**-in/tay-zoe-**bak**-tam
(Tazocin ✦, Zosyn)
**Do not confuse Zosyn with Zofran or Zyvox.**

## ◆CLASSIFICATION

**PHARMACOTHERAPEUTIC:** Penicillin.
**CLINICAL:** Antibiotic.

## USES

Treatment of moderate to severe bacterial infections, including community-acquired/nosocomial pneumonia, intraabdominal, pelvic, skin, and skin structure infections. Tazobactam expands piperacillin activity to include beta-lactamase-producing strains of *S. aureus, H. influenzae, Bacteroides*. **OFF-LABEL:** Surgical prophylaxis, complicated intra-abdominal infections.

## PRECAUTIONS

**Contraindications:** Hypersensitivity to piperacillin/tazobactam, any penicillin. **Cautions:** History of allergies (esp.

cephalosporins, other drugs), renal impairment, preexisting seizure disorder.

## ACTION

**Piperacillin:** Inhibits cell wall synthesis by binding to bacterial cell membranes. **Therapeutic Effect:** Bactericidal. **Tazobactam:** Inactivates bacterial beta-lactamase. **Therapeutic Effect:** Protects piperacillin from enzymatic degradation, extends its spectrum of activity, prevents bacterial overgrowth.

## PHARMACOKINETICS

Protein binding: 16%–30%. Widely distributed. Primarily excreted unchanged in urine. Removed by hemodialysis. **Half-life:** 0.7–1.2 hrs (increased in hepatic cirrhosis, renal impairment).

## ⧗ LIFESPAN CONSIDERATIONS

**Pregnancy/Lactation:** Readily crosses placenta; appears in cord blood, amniotic fluid. Distributed in breast milk in low concentrations. May lead to allergic sensitization, diarrhea, candidiasis, skin rash in infant. **Children:** Dosage not established for pts younger than 12 yrs. **Elderly:** Age-related renal impairment may require dosage adjustment.

## INTERACTIONS

**DRUG:** Concurrent use of **aminoglycosides (e.g., gentamicin, tobramycin)** may cause mutual inactivation (must give at least 1 hr apart). May increase concentration, toxicity of **methotrexate. Probenecid** may increase concentration, risk of toxicity. High-dose piperacillin may increase risk of bleeding with **heparin, NSAIDs, platelet inhibitors (e.g., aspirin, clopidogrel), thrombolytic agents (e.g., alteplase), warfarin. HERBAL:** None significant. **FOOD:** None known. **LAB VALUES:** May increase serum sodium, alkaline phosphatase, bilirubin, LDH, ALT, AST, BUN, creatinine, PT, PTT. May decrease serum potassium. May cause positive Coombs' test.

## AVAILABILITY (Rx)

◀**ALERT**▶ Piperacillin/tazobactam is a combination product in an 8:1 ratio of piperacillin to tazobactam. **Injection Powder:** 2.25 g, 3.375 g, 4.5 g. **Premix Ready to Use:** 2.25 g (50 ml), 3.375 g (50 ml), 4.5 g (100 ml).

## ADMINISTRATION/HANDLING

 **IV**

**Reconstitution** • Reconstitute each 1 g with 5 ml D5W or 0.9% NaCl. Shake vigorously to dissolve. • Further dilute with at least 50 ml D5W or 0.9% NaCl. **Rate of Administration** • Infuse over 30 min. Expanded infusion over 3–4 hrs. **Storage** • Reconstituted vial is stable for 24 hrs at room temperature or 48 hrs if refrigerated. • After further dilution, stable for 24 hrs at room temperature or 7 days if refrigerated.

## ▨ IV INCOMPATIBILITIES

Amphotericin B (Fungizone), amphotericin B complex (Abelcet, AmBisome, Amphotec), famotidine (Pepcid), haloperidol (Haldol), hydroxyzine (Vistaril), vancomycin (Vancocin).

## ▨ IV COMPATIBILITIES

Bumetanide (Bumex), calcium gluconate, dexmedetomidine (Precedex), diphenhydramine (Benadryl), dopamine (Intropin), enalapril (Vasotec), furosemide (Lasix), granisetron (Kytril), heparin, hydrocortisone (Solu-Cortef), hydromorphone (Dilaudid), lorazepam (Ativan), magnesium sulfate, methylprednisolone (Solu-Medrol), metoclopramide (Reglan), morphine, ondansetron (Zofran), potassium chloride.

## INDICATIONS/ROUTES/DOSAGE

**Note:** Extended Infusion: ADULTS, ELDERLY: 3.375–4.5 g over 4 hrs q8h.

**Usual Dosage**
**IV: ADULTS, ELDERLY, CHILDREN 12 YRS AND OLDER WEIGHING MORE THAN 40 KG:** 4.5 g

**P**

q6–8h or 3.375 g q6h. **Maximum:** 18 g daily. **CHILDREN 9 MOS AND OLDER AND 40 KG OR LESS:** 100 mg piperacillin component/kg/dose q8h. **Maximum:** 16 g/day. **CHILDREN 2–8 MOS:** 80 mg piperacillin component/kg/dose q8h. **NEONATES:** 75–100 mg piperacillin component/kg/dose q6–12h.

| Creatinine Clearance | Dosage |
|---|---|
| 20–40 ml/min | 2.25 g q6h (3.375 g q6h for nosocomial pneumonia) |
| Less than 20 ml/min | 2.25 g q8h (2.25 g q6h for nosocomial pneumonia) |
| | Extended Infusion 3.375 g q12h |

**Dosage for Hemodialysis**
**IV: ADULTS, ELDERLY:** 2.25 g q8–12h with additional dose of 0.75 g after each dialysis session.

**Dosage for CRRT**

| CVVH | 2.25–3.375 g q6–8h |
|---|---|
| CVVHD | 2.25–3.375 g q6h |
| CVVHDF | 3.375 g q6h |

**Dosage in Renal Impairment**
Dosage and frequency are modified based on creatinine clearance.

**Dosage in Hepatic Impairment**
No dose adjustment.

## SIDE EFFECTS

**Frequent:** Diarrhea, headache, constipation, nausea, insomnia, rash. **Occasional:** Vomiting, dyspepsia, pruritus, fever, agitation, candidiasis, dizziness, abdominal pain, edema, anxiety, dyspnea, rhinitis.

## ADVERSE EFFECTS/ TOXIC REACTIONS

Antibiotic-associated colitis, other super-infections (abdominal cramps, severe watery diarrhea, fever) may result from altered bacterial balance in GI tract. Overdose, more often with renal impairment, may produce seizures, neurologic reactions. Severe hypersensitivity reactions, including anaphylaxis, occur rarely.

## NURSING CONSIDERATIONS

### BASELINE ASSESSMENT
Question for history of allergies, esp. to penicillins, cephalosporins.

### INTERVENTION/EVALUATION
Monitor daily pattern of bowel activity, stool consistency; mild GI effects may be tolerable, but increasing severity may indicate onset of antibiotic-associated colitis. Be alert for superinfection: fever, vomiting, diarrhea, anal/genital pruritus, oral mucosal changes (ulceration, pain, erythema). Monitor I&O, urinalysis. Monitor serum electrolytes, esp. potassium, renal function tests.

# piroxicam

peer-**ox**-i-kam
(Apo-Piroxicam ✤, Feldene)
■ **BLACK BOX ALERT** ■ May increase risk of serious, potentially fatal cardiovascular thrombotic events, MI, stroke. Increased risk of serious GI events (bleeding, ulceration, perforation).
**Do not confuse Feldene with fluoxetine, or piroxicam with paroxetine.**

## ◆CLASSIFICATION
**PHARMACOTHERAPEUTIC:** NSAID. **CLINICAL:** Anti-inflammatory, analgesic.

## USES

Management of acute or chronic rheumatoid arthritis (RA), osteoarthritis. **OFF-LABEL:** Treatment of juvenile idiopathic arthritis.

## PRECAUTIONS

**Contraindications:** Hypersensitivity to piroxicam. Perioperative pain in setting of CABG surgery, history of hypersensitivity to aspirin/NSAIDs, active GI bleeding. Pts with aspirin triad (asthma, rhinitis, and aspirin intolerance). **Cautions:** Advanced renal disease, hepatic impairment, asthma, coagulation disorders, concomitant use of anticoagulants, poor CYP2C9 metabolizers. History of GI bleeding or ulcers, alcohol abuse. Avoid use in late pregnancy.

## ACTION

Produces analgesic, anti-inflammatory effects by inhibiting prostaglandin synthesis. **Therapeutic Effect:** Reduces inflammatory response, intensity of pain.

## PHARMACOKINETICS

| Route | Onset | Peak | Duration |
|-------|-------|------|----------|
| PO | 1 hr | 3–5 hrs | — |

Well absorbed following PO administration. Protein binding: 99%. Metabolized in liver. Primarily excreted in urine; small amount eliminated in feces. **Half-life:** 50 hrs.

## ⧗ LIFESPAN CONSIDERATIONS

**Pregnancy/Lactation:** Crosses placenta; distributed in breast milk. Avoid use during third trimester (may adversely affect fetal cardiovascular system: premature closing of ductus arteriosus). **Children:** Safety and efficacy not established. **Elderly:** Age-related renal impairment may increase risk of hepatotoxicity, renal toxicity; reduced dosage recommended. More likely to have serious adverse effects with GI bleeding/ulceration.

## INTERACTIONS

**DRUG:** May decrease effects of **antihypertensives (e.g., amlodipine, lisinopril, valsartan), diuretics (e.g., furosemide, HCTZ). Aspirin, other salicylates** may increase risk of GI side effects, bleeding. May increase effects of **heparin, oral anticoagulants (e.g., rivaroxaban, warfarin), thrombolytics (e.g., alteplase).** May increase concentration, risk of toxicity of **lithium, methotrexate. HERBAL:** **Cat's claw, dong quai, evening primrose, feverfew, garlic, ginger, ginkgo, ginseng, horse chestnut, red clover** possess antiplatelet activity, may increase risk of bleeding. **St. John's wort** may increase risk of phototoxicity. **FOOD:** None known. **LAB VALUES:** May increase serum BUN, creatinine, LDH, alkaline phosphatase, ALT, AST. May decrease serum uric acid, Hgb, Hct, platelets, leukocytes.

## AVAILABILITY (Rx)

🗳 **Capsules:** 10 mg, 20 mg.

## ADMINISTRATION/HANDLING

**PO**

• Do not break, crush, or open capsules. • May give with food, milk, antacids if GI distress occurs.

## INDICATIONS/ROUTES/DOSAGE

**Rheumatoid Arthritis (RA), Osteoarthritis**
**PO: ADULTS, ELDERLY:** Initially, 10–20 mg/day as a single dose or in divided doses. **Maximum:** 20 mg/day. **CHILDREN: (Juvenile Idiopathic Arthritis)** 0.2–0.4 mg/kg/day. **Maximum:** 15 mg/day.

**Dosage in Renal Impairment**
**Mild to moderate impairment:** No dose adjustment. **Severe impairment:** Not recommended.

**Dosage in Hepatic Impairment**
No dose adjustment.

## SIDE EFFECTS

**Frequent (9%–4%):** Dyspepsia, nausea, dizziness. **Occasional (3%–1%):** Diarrhea, constipation, abdominal cramps/pain, flatulence, stomatitis. **Rare (less than 1%):** Hypertension, urticaria, dysuria, ecchymosis, blurred vision, insomnia, phototoxicity.

P

## ADVERSE EFFECTS/ TOXIC REACTIONS

Peptic ulcer, GI bleeding, gastritis, severe hepatic reaction (cholestasis, jaundice) occur rarely. Nephrotoxicity (dysuria, hematuria, proteinuria, nephrotic syndrome), hematologic toxicity (anemia, leukopenia, eosinophilia, thrombocytopenia), severe hypersensitivity reaction (fever, chills, bronchospasm) occur rarely with long-term treatment.

## NURSING CONSIDERATIONS

### BASELINE ASSESSMENT

Assess onset, type, location, duration of pain/inflammation. Inspect appearance of affected joints for immobility, deformities, skin condition.

### INTERVENTION/EVALUATION

Monitor daily pattern of bowel activity, stool consistency. Monitor for evidence of nausea, GI distress. Assess for therapeutic response: relief of pain, stiffness, swelling; increased joint mobility; reduced joint tenderness; improved grip strength. Monitor CBC, renal/hepatic function tests.

### PATIENT/FAMILY TEACHING

• Avoid aspirin, alcohol during therapy (increases risk of GI bleeding). • If GI upset occurs, take with food, milk, antacids. • Avoid tasks that require alertness until response to drug is established.

## pitavastatin

pit-**av**-a-**stat**-in
(Livalo)
**Do not confuse pitavastatin with atorvastatin, lovastatin, pravastatin, or simvastatin.**

### ◆CLASSIFICATION

**PHARMACOTHERAPEUTIC:** HMG-CoA reductase inhibitor. **CLINICAL:** Antihyperlipidemic.

## USES

Reduces elevated total cholesterol, low-density lipoproteins (LDLs), apolipoprotein B, triglycerides; increases low high-density lipoproteins (HDLs) in primary hyperlipidemia and mixed dyslipidemia. **OFF-LABEL:** Primary and secondary prevention of atherosclerotic cardiovascular disease.

## PRECAUTIONS

**Contraindications:** Hypersensitivity to pitavastatin. Active hepatic disease, persistent or unexplained elevations of LFT; concurrent cyclosporine use, pregnancy, breastfeeding. **Cautions:** History of hepatic disease, substantial alcohol consumption, moderate renal impairment. Withholding/ discontinuing pitavastatin may be necessary when pt at risk for renal failure. Pts at risk for myopathy: elderly, renal impairment, inadequately treated hypothyroidism.

## ACTION

Interferes with cholesterol biosynthesis by inhibiting conversion of HMG-CoA reductase to a precursor to cholesterol. **Therapeutic Effect:** Lowers total cholesterol, LDL cholesterol, apolipoprotein B (Apo B), plasma triglycerides; increases HDL cholesterol.

## PHARMACOKINETICS

Poorly absorbed from GI tract. Protein binding: greater than 99%. Metabolized in liver. Primarily excreted in feces. **Half-life:** 12 hrs.

## ⧖ LIFESPAN CONSIDERATIONS

**Pregnancy/Lactation:** Contraindicated in pregnancy (suppression of cholesterol biosynthesis may cause fetal toxicity) and lactation. Unknown if drug is distributed in breast milk (risk of serious adverse reactions in nursing infants). **Children:** Safety and efficacy not established in pts younger than 18 yrs. **Elderly:** No age-related precautions noted.

## INTERACTIONS:

**DRUG:** Increased risk of rhabdomyolysis, acute renal failure with **gemfibrozil, niacin, other fibrates. Cyclosporine, erythromycin, rifampin** may increase serum pitavastatin levels. **HERBAL:** None significant. **FOOD:** None known. **LAB VALUES:** May increase serum creatine kinase (CPK), ALT, AST concentrations.

## AVAILABILITY (Rx)

**Tablets:** 1 mg, 2 mg, 4 mg.

## ADMINISTRATION/HANDLING

### PO

• Give without regard to meals or time of day.

## INDICATIONS/ROUTES/ DOSAGE

◀ALERT▶ Before initiating therapy, pt should be on standard cholesterol-lowering diet for minimum of 3–6 mos. Continue diet throughout pitavastatin therapy.

**Usual Dosage**
**PO: ADULTS:** Initially, 2 mg/day. **Maximum:** 4 mg/day. Range: 1–4 mg/day. **Maximum dosage with erythromycin:** 1 mg/day; **with rifampin:** 2 mg/day.

**Dosage in Renal Impairment**
**CrCl 30–59, 15–60 ml/min not receiving hemodialysis, or end-stage renal disease in pts on hemodialysis:** Initially, 1 mg/day. **Maximum:** 2 mg/day.

**Dosage in Hepatic Impairment**
See contraindications.

## SIDE EFFECTS

Generally well tolerated. Side effects usually mild and transient. **Rare (Less Than 4%):** Myalgia, constipation/diarrhea, back/extremity pain, arthralgia, headache, nasopharyngitis.

## ADVERSE EFFECTS/ TOXIC REACTIONS

Hypersensitivity (rash, pruritus, urticaria) occurs rarely.

## NURSING CONSIDERATIONS

### BASELINE ASSESSMENT

Obtain LFT, serum cholesterol, triglycerides. Question for possibility of pregnancy before initiating therapy.

### INTERVENTION/EVALUATION

Monitor cholesterol and triglyceride levels; LFT. Monitor daily pattern of bowel activity, stool consistency. Check for myalgia, arthralgia, headache. Assess for rash, pruritus. Be alert for malaise, muscle cramping/weakness.

### PATIENT/FAMILY TEACHING

• Follow special diet (important part of treatment). • Periodic lab tests are essential part of therapy. • Report promptly any muscle pain/weakness. • Use non-hormonal contraception.

# plerixafor

pler-**ix**-a-for
(Mozobil)

### ◆CLASSIFICATION

**PHARMACOTHERAPEUTIC:** Chemokine receptor inhibitor. **CLINICAL:** Hematopoietic stem cell mobilizer.

## USES

Indicated in combination with granulocyte colony-stimulating factor (G-CSF) to mobilize stem cells to peripheral blood for collection and transplantation in pts with non-Hodgkin's lymphoma and multiple myeloma.

## PRECAUTIONS

**Contraindications:** Hypersensitivity to plerixafor. **Cautions:** Avoid use in leukemic pts, in pts with neutrophil count greater than 50,000/mm$^3$, those with moderate to severe renal impairment.

## ACTION

Immobilizes hematopoietic stem cells in bone marrow. Once in the marrow,

P

acts to help anchor these cells to marrow matrix through induction of adhesion molecules. **Therapeutic Effect:** Results in leukocytosis, elevation in circulating hematopoietic progenitor cells in peripheral blood system.

## PHARMACOKINETICS

Readily absorbed after SQ administration. Generally confines to extravascular fluid space. Protein binding: 58%. Peak plasma concentration: 30–60 min. Eliminated in urine. Clearance reduced with renal impairment. **Half-life:** 3–5 hrs.

## ⌛ LIFESPAN CONSIDERATIONS

**Pregnancy/Lactation:** Potential for teratogenic effects. May cause fetal harm. **Children:** Safety and efficacy not established. **Elderly:** Age-related renal impairment may require dosage adjustment.

## INTERACTIONS

**DRUG:** None significant. **HERBAL:** None significant. **FOOD:** None known. **LAB VALUES:** May increase WBC count. May decrease platelet count.

## AVAILABILITY (Rx)

**Injection Solution:** 24 mg/1.2 ml vial.

## ADMINISTRATION/ HANDLING

### SQ

• Aspirate syringe before injection (avoid intra-arterial administration). **Storage** • Store at room temperature. • Discard if particulate matter is present or if solution is discolored. • Use single-dose vial; discard unused drug.

## INDICATIONS/ROUTES/ DOSAGE

◀ALERT▶ Begin therapy after pt has received daily morning doses of G-CSF, 10 mcg/kg once daily for 4 days prior to the first evening dose of plerixafor and approximately 11 hrs prior to the

initiation of apheresis for up to 4 consecutive days.

**Daily Dosage**
**SQ: ADULTS, ELDERLY (WEIGHING MORE THAN 83 KG):** 0.24 mg/kg once daily (about 11 hrs prior to apheresis) for up to 4 consecutive days. **Maximum:** 40 mg/day. **(83 KG or LESS):** 20 mg fixed dose or 0.24 mg/kg once daily for up to 4 consecutive days.

**Dosage in Moderate to Severe Renal Impairment (CrCl Equal to or Less Than 50 ml/min):**
**SQ: ADULTS, ELDERLY (WEIGHING MORE THAN 83 KG):** Decrease dose to 0.16 mg/kg, not to exceed 27 mg/day. **(83 KG OR LESS):** 13 mg fixed dose or 0.16 mg/kg once daily.

**Dosage in Hepatic Impairment**
No dose adjustment.

## SIDE EFFECTS

**Frequent (37%–22%):** Diarrhea, nausea, injection site irritation, fatigue, headache. **Occasional (13%–7%):** Arthralgia, dizziness, vomiting, insomnia, flatulence.

## ADVERSE EFFECTS/ TOXIC REACTIONS

Thrombocytopenia may occur. Dyspnea, hypoxia, vasovagal reaction, periorbital edema, urticaria have been noted; may resolve spontaneously, generally responds to antihistamines, corticosteroids.

## NURSING CONSIDERATIONS

### BASELINE ASSESSMENT

Obtain CBC, renal function test in pts with renal impairment.

### INTERVENTION/EVALUATION

Monitor WBC, platelet count. Assess for potential systemic reaction (periorbital edema, dyspnea, urticaria), orthostatic hypotension during or shortly after injection. Advise female pt with reproductive potential to use effective contraceptive method.

**PATIENT/FAMILY TEACHING**
• Manage gastrointestinal disorders; report severe diarrhea, nausea, vomiting.
• Report upper quadrant pain or scapular/shoulder pain.

# polyethylene glycol

# polyethylene glycol-electrolyte solution (PEG-ES) (CoLyte, GoLYTELY)

pol-ee-**eth**-il-een-**glye**-kol
(CoLyTELY, GoLYTELY, Klean-Prep ♣, MiraLax, NuLytely, Peglyte ♣, TriLyte)
**Do not confuse MiraLax with Mirapex.**

## ◆CLASSIFICATION

**PHARMACOTHERAPEUTIC:** Osmotic/laxative. **CLINICAL:** Bowel evacuant.

## USES

**Polyethylene glycol-electrolyte solution:** Bowel cleansing before GI examination, colon surgery. **Polyethylene glycol:** Treatment of occasional constipation.

## PRECAUTIONS

**Contraindications:** Hypersensitivity to polyethylene glycol. Bowel perforation, gastric retention, GI obstruction, megacolon, toxic colitis, toxic ileus. **Cautions: (Propylene glycol):** Renal impairment. **(Propylene glycol–electrolyte solution):** Ulcerative colitis, medications altering electrolytes, hyponatremia, cardiac arrhythmias, impaired gag reflex, history of seizures, elderly.

## ACTION

Osmotic effect. **Therapeutic Effect:** Induces diarrhea, cleanses bowel without depleting electrolytes.

## PHARMACOKINETICS

| Route | Onset | Peak | Duration |
|---|---|---|---|
| PO (bowel cleansing) | 1–2 hrs | N/A | N/A |
| PO (constipation) | 2–4 days | N/A | N/A |

## ⌛ LIFESPAN CONSIDERATIONS

**Pregnancy/Lactation:** Unknown if drug crosses placenta or is distributed in breast milk. **Children/Elderly:** No age-related precautions noted.

## INTERACTIONS

**DRUG:** May decrease absorption of **oral medications** if given within 1 hr (may be flushed from GI tract). **HERBAL:** None significant. **FOOD:** None known. **LAB VALUES:** None significant.

## AVAILABILITY (Rx)

**Powder for Oral Solution: Propylene glycol (MiraLax):** 17 g/dose. **Propylene glycol–electrolyte solution (CoLyte, GoLYTELY):** See individual product for specific ingredients.

## ADMINISTRATION/HANDLING

**PO**
*Polyethylene Glycol-Electrolyte Solution*
• Refrigerate reconstituted solutions; use within 48 hrs. • May use tap water to prepare solution. Shake vigorously for several min to ensure complete dissolution of powder. • Fasting should occur for more than 3 hrs prior to ingestion of solution (always avoid solid food less than 2 hrs prior to administration). • Only clear liquids permitted after administration. • May give via NG tube. • Rapid drinking preferred. Chilled solution is more palatable.

---

**P**

*Polyethylene Glycol*
• Add to 4- to 8-oz beverage.

## INDICATIONS/ROUTES/DOSAGE

**Bowel Evacuant**
**PO: ADULTS, ELDERLY:** Before GI examination: 240 ml (8 oz) q10min until 4 L consumed or rectal effluent clear. NG tube: 20–30 ml/min until 4 L given. **CHILDREN 6 MOS AND OLDER:** 25 ml/kg/hr until rectal effluent clear. **Maximum:** 4 L.

**Constipation**
**PO** *(Miralax):* **ADULTS:** 17 g or 1 heaping tbsp/day. **CHILDREN 6 MOS AND OLDER:** 0.5–1.5 g/kg/day. **Maximum:** 17 g/day.

**Dosage in Renal/Hepatic Impairment**
No dose adjustment.

## SIDE EFFECTS

**Frequent (50%):** Some degree of abdominal fullness, nausea, bloating. **Occasional (10%–1%):** Abdominal cramping, vomiting, anal irritation. **Rare (less than 1%):** Urticaria, rhinorrhea, dermatitis.

## ADVERSE EFFECTS/ TOXIC REACTIONS

None known.

## NURSING CONSIDERATIONS

**BASELINE ASSESSMENT**
Do not give oral medication within 1 hr of start of therapy (may not adequately be absorbed before GI cleansing).

**INTERVENTION/EVALUATION**
Assess bowel sounds for peristalsis. Monitor daily pattern of bowel activity, stool consistency. Assess for abdominal disturbances. Monitor serum electrolytes.

**PATIENT/FAMILY TEACHING**
• May take 2–4 days to produce a bowel movement. • Report unusual cramps, bloating, diarrhea.

# pomalidomide

poe-ma-**lid**-oh-mide
(Pomalyst)

■ **BLACK BOX ALERT** ■ May cause life-threatening birth defects. Pregnancy contraindicated. Exclude pregnancy before initiating treatment. Females of reproductive potential must use two reliable forms of contraception or continuously abstain during treatment and for 4 wks after treatment. Deep vein thrombosis and pulmonary embolism may occur. Consider venous thromboembolism (VTE) prophylaxis during treatment.

## ◆CLASSIFICATION

**PHARMACOTHERAPEUTIC:** Thalidomide analogue. **CLINICAL:** Antineoplastic.

## USES

Treatment of multiple myeloma in pts who have received at least two prior therapies including lenalidomide and bortezomib and have demonstrated disease progression on or within 60 days of completion of the last therapy.

## PRECAUTIONS

◄**ALERT**► Do not donate blood products.
**Contraindications:** Hypersensitivity to pomalidomide. **Cautions:** Anemia, HF, hepatic/renal impairment, smoking, breastfeeding, or prior history of CVA, MI, DVT, PE.

## ACTION

Inhibits tumor cell proliferation and induces apoptosis (cell death) of hematopoietic cells. Enhances T-cell– and natural killer (NK) cell–mediated immunity. Inhibits proinflammatory cytokines. **Therapeutic Effect:** Inhibits tumor cell growth and metastasis. Promotes tumor cell death.

## PHARMACOKINETICS

Readily absorbed following PO administration. Metabolized in liver. Protein binding: 12%–44%. Peak plasma concentration: 2–3 hrs. Eliminated in urine (73%), feces (15%). **Half-life:** 8–10 hrs.

## ⌛ LIFESPAN CONSIDERATIONS

**Pregnancy/Lactation:** Pregnancy/breastfeeding contraindicated. May cause fetal harm. Unknown if distributed in breast milk. Do not breastfeed. Must verify negative pregnancy status before initiation. Must use two reliable forms of birth control (intrauterine device [IUD], tubal ligation) plus barrier methods. Avoid pregnancy for at least 4 wks after discontinuation. **Males:** Must use condoms during treatment and up to 1 mo after treatment, despite prior history of vasectomy. Do not donate sperm. **Children:** Safety and efficacy not established. **Elderly:** May have increased risk of serious adverse effects, renal failure, electrolyte imbalance.

## INTERACTIONS

**DRUG:** CYP3A4, P-glycoprotein inhibitors (e.g., **erythromycin, ketoconazole**) may increase concentration/effects. CYP3A4, P-glycoprotein inducers (e.g., **carbamazepine, rifampin**) may decrease concentration/effects. **HERBAL:** None significant. **FOOD:** All foods may reduce absorption/concentration. **LAB VALUES:** May decrease Hgb, Hct, neutrophils, platelets, leukocytes, lymphocytes, serum calcium, potassium, sodium. May increase serum calcium, creatinine, glucose.

## AVAILABILITY (Rx)

🐾 **Capsules:** 1 mg, 2 mg, 3 mg, 4 mg.

## ADMINISTRATION/HANDLING

**PO**

- Do not break, crush, or open capsule.
- Give on empty stomach; must administer at least 2 hrs before or 2 hrs after meal.

## INDICATIONS/ROUTES/DOSAGE

**Note:** Absolute neutrophil count (ANC) should be 500 cells/mm³ or greater and platelets 50,000 cells/mm³ or greater prior to starting new cycles of therapy.

### Multiple Myeloma

**PO: ADULTS/ELDERLY:** 4 mg once daily on days 1–21 of 28-day cycle (in combination with dexamethasone).

### Dose Modification
#### Neutropenia

**ANC less than 500/mm³ or febrile neutropenia:** Interrupt treatment until ANC is greater than 500/mm³, then reduce dose to 3 mg once daily. **Any subsequent drop of ANC less than 500/mm³ after prior reduction:** Interrupt treatment until ANC is greater than 500/mm³, then reduce dose at 1 mg less than previous dose. Discontinue if 1-mg dose is intolerable.

#### Thrombocytopenia

**Platelet count less than 25,000/mm³:** Interrupt treatment until platelet count greater than 50,000/mm³, then reduce dose to 3 mg once daily. **Any subsequent platelet drop to less than 25,000/mm³:** Interrupt treatment until platelet count greater than 50,000-mm³, then reduce dose at 1 mg less than previous dose. Discontinue if 1-mg dose is intolerable.

### Dosage in Renal Impairment

Avoid use in pts with serum creatinine more than 3 mg/dL or CrCl less than 45 ml/min.

### Dosage in Hepatic Impairment

Avoid use with bilirubin more than 2 mg/dL and ALT, AST more than 3 times upper limit of normal (ULN).

## SIDE EFFECTS

**Frequent (55%–22%):** Fatigue, constipation, nausea, diarrhea, dyspnea, back pain, peripheral edema, musculoskeletal chest pain, anorexia, rash. **Occasional (20%–7%):** Dizziness, pyrexia, muscle spasms, arthralgia, pruritus, vomiting,

P

cough, weight loss, headache, bone pain, muscular weakness, anxiety, musculoskeletal pain, peripheral neuropathy, chills, dry skin, tremor, insomnia. **Rare (6%–1%):** Hyperhidrosis, extremity pain, back pain, night sweats, constipation.

## ADVERSE EFFECTS/ TOXIC REACTIONS

Neutropenia, leukopenia, thrombocytopenia is an expected outcome of therapy; may increase risk of infection such as pneumonia, upper respiratory tract infection, UTI. Neurologic events such as acute confusion, dizziness reported. Peripheral neuropathy occurred in 18% of pts. Venous thromboembolism including DVT, PE occurred in 3% of pts. Epistaxis occurred in 15% of pts. Increased risk of secondary malignancies reported. Acute renal failure reported in 16% of pts. Additional adverse events may include interstitial lung disease (ILD), neutropenic sepsis, *Pneumocystis jiroveci* pneumonia, respiratory syncytial virus infection, urinary retention, vertigo.

## NURSING CONSIDERATIONS

### BASELINE ASSESSMENT

Obtain vital signs, CBC with differential, serum chemistries, esp. magnesium, phosphate, ionized calcium, PT/INR, urinalysis. Confirm negative pregnancy status 10–14 days before and 24 hrs before starting treatment. Receive full medication history. Obtain baseline neurologic exam. Question history of diabetes mellitus, electrolyte imbalance, hepatic/renal impairment, pulmonary disease, thromboembolism, smoking.

### INTERVENTION/EVALUATION

Monitor CBC, serum chemistries, PT/INR. Offer antiemetics for nausea, vomiting. Monitor pregnancy status every mo during treatment and for at least 4 mos after discontinuation. Obtain EKG for palpitation, chest pain, hypokalemia, hyperkalemia, hypocalcemia, bradycardia, ventricular arrhythmias. Immediately report dyspnea, chest pain, hypoxia, unilateral peripheral edema/pain (may indicate thromboembolic event). Consider sequential compression device (SCD) for immobilized pts. Perform routine neurologic assessments to screen for confusion, delirium. Monitor urine output, frequency.

### PATIENT/FAMILY TEACHING

• Blood levels will be routinely monitored. • May cause birth defects or miscarriage. Do not breastfeed. Consult with gynecologist for appropriate birth control methods. Female pts must use contraception during treatment and for at least 1 mo after treatment. Immediately report suspected pregnancy. Male pts must use condoms with spermicide during sexual activity, despite history of vasectomy. • Do not donate blood. • Swallow capsules whole; do not break, crush, or open. • Go from lying to standing slowly (prevents postural hypotension, dizziness). Avoid tasks that require alertness, motor skills until response to drug is established. • Do not smoke. • Do not eat 2 hrs before or 2 hrs after dose. • Avoid alcohol. • Report difficulty breathing, chest pain, extremity pain or swelling, dizziness, confusion.

# posaconazole

poe-sa-**kon**-a-zole
(Noxafil, Posanol ✦)
**Do not confuse Noxafil with minoxidil.**

## ◆CLASSIFICATION

**PHARMACOTHERAPEUTIC:** Azole derivative. **CLINICAL:** Antifungal.

## USES

Prophylaxis of invasive *Aspergillus* and *Candida* infections in pts 13 yrs and older who are at high risk for developing these infections due to severely immunocompromised conditions. Treatment of oropharyngeal candidiasis. **OFF-LABEL:** Salvage therapy of refractory invasive fungal infections, mucomycosis, pulmonary infections.

## PRECAUTIONS

**Contraindications:** Hypersensitivity to posaconazole, other azole antifungals. Co-administration with pimozide, quinidine (may cause QT prolongation, torsades de pointes), HMG-CoA reductase inhibitors metabolized by CYP3A4 (e.g., atorvastatin, simvastatin), sirolimus, ergot alkaloids. **Cautions:** Renal/hepatic impairment, hypokalemia, hypomagnesemia, pts at increased risk of arrhythmias. Concomitant administration of medications that prolong QT interval, pts with long QT syndrome.

## ACTION

Inhibits synthesis of ergosterol, a vital component of fungal cell wall formation. **Therapeutic Effect:** Damages fungal cell wall membrane, altering its function.

## PHARMACOKINETICS

Moderately absorbed following PO administration. Absorption increased if drug is taken with food. Widely distributed. Protein binding: 98%. Not significantly metabolized. Primarily excreted in feces. **Half-life:** 20–66 hrs.

## ⧖ LIFESPAN CONSIDERATIONS

**Pregnancy/Lactation:** May cause fetal harm. Breastfeeding not recommended. **Children:** Safety and efficacy not established in pts younger than 13 yrs. **Elderly:** No age-related precautions noted.

## INTERACTIONS

**DRUG:** May increase concentrations of **atorvastatin, cyclosporine, ergot alkaloids, felodipine, midazolam, phenytoin, pimozide, quinidine, rifabutin, simvastatin, sirolimus, tacrolimus, vinblastine, vincristine. Cimetidine, phenytoin** may decrease concentration. **HERBAL:** None significant. **FOOD:** Concentration higher when given with **food or nutritional supplements. Grapefruit products** may decrease concentration/effects. **LAB VALUES:** May decrease WBC, RBC, Hgb, Hct, platelets, serum calcium, potassium, magnesium. May increase serum glucose, bilirubin, ALT, AST, alkaline phosphatase.

## AVAILABILITY (Rx)

**Injection Solution:** 300 mg/16.7 ml (18 mg/ml). **Oral Suspension:** 40 mg/ml. ⧯ **Tablets (Delayed-Release):** 100 mg.

## ADMINISTRATION/HANDLING

**IV**

**Reconstitution •** Transfer 300 mg (16.7 ml) posaconazole into 150 ml D₅W or 0.9% NaCl bag.
**Rate of Administration •** Infuse over 90 min via central venous line.
**Storage •** Refrigerate vials. Once diluted, use immediately. May refrigerate solution up to 24 hrs if not used immediately.

**PO**

• Administer with or within 20 min of full meal, liquid nutritional supplement, or acidic carbonated beverage (e.g., ginger ale) (enhances absorption).
• Store oral suspension at room temperature. • Shake suspension well before use. **Tablets •** Swallow whole; do not crush, cut, dissolve, or divide. Administer with food.

## INDICATIONS/ROUTES/DOSAGE

**Prophylaxis of Invasive *Aspergillus* and *Candida***
**PO: ADULTS, ELDERLY, CHILDREN 13 YRS AND OLDER:** *(Oral Suspension):* 200 mg (5 ml) 3 times/day, given with full meal or liquid nutritional supplement. *(Delayed-Release):* 300 mg twice daily on first day, then 300 mg once daily **IV:** 300 mg twice daily on first day, then 300 mg once daily thereafter.

**Oropharyngeal Candidiasis**
**PO: ADULTS, ELDERLY, CHILDREN 13 YRS AND OLDER:** 100 mg twice daily for 1 day, then 100 mg once daily for 13 days.

**Refractory Oropharyngeal Candidiasis**
**PO: ADULTS, ELDERLY:** 400 mg twice daily for 3 days, then 400 mg once daily for up to

P

28 days. **HIV-Infected Pts:** 400 mg twice daily on day 1, then 400 mg once daily for 7–14 days (28 days in azole refractory pts).

**Dosage in Renal Impairment**
**PO:** No dose adjustment. **IV:** Avoid use in pts with CrCl less than 50 ml/min.

**Dosage in Hepatic Impairment**
No dose adjustment.

## SIDE EFFECTS

**Common (42%–24%):** Diarrhea, nausea, vomiting, headache, abdominal pain, cough. **Frequent (20%–15%):** Constipation, rigors, rash, hypertension, fatigue, insomnia, mucositis, musculoskeletal pain, edema of lower extremities, herpes simplex, anorexia. **Occasional (14%–8%):** Hypotension, epistaxis, tachycardia, pharyngitis, dizziness, pruritus, arthralgia, dyspepsia, back pain, generalized edema, weakness.

## ADVERSE EFFECTS/ TOXIC REACTIONS

Bacteremia occurs in 18% of pts; upper respiratory tract infection occurs in 7%. Allergic/hypersensitivity reactions, QT prolongation, hemolytic uremic syndrome, thrombotic thrombocytopenic purpura, pulmonary embolus have been reported.

## NURSING CONSIDERATIONS

### BASELINE ASSESSMENT

Obtain BMP, LFT. Receive full medication history and screen for interactions (esp. drugs known to prolong QT interval).

### INTERVENTION/EVALUATION

Monitor LFT periodically. Monitor daily pattern of bowel activity, stool consistency. Obtain order for antiemetic if excessive vomiting occurs. Monitor B/P for hypertension, hypotension. Assess for lower extremity edema.

### PATIENT/FAMILY TEACHING

• Take each dose with full meal or liquid nutritional supplement. • Report severe diarrhea, vomiting, chest pain, yellowing of skin/eyes. • Maintain strict oral hygiene.

## potassium acetate
**HIGH ALERT**

## potassium bicarbonate/citrate

(Effer-K, <u>Klor-Con EF</u>)

## potassium chloride

(Apo-K ✤, Kaon-Cl, Klor-Con, <u>Klor-Con M10</u>, <u>Klor-Con M20</u>, Micro-K)
poe-**tass**-ee-um
**Do not confuse Micro-K with Macrobid or Micronase.**

## ◆CLASSIFICATION

**PHARMACOTHERAPEUTIC:** Electrolyte. **CLINICAL:** Potassium replenisher.

## USES

**Potassium acetate, potassium bicarbonate/citrate:** Treatment, prevention of hypokalemia when necessary to avoid chloride or acid/base imbalance (requires bicarbonate). **Potassium chloride:** Treatment, prevention of hypokalemia.

## PRECAUTIONS

**Contraindications:** Severe renal impairment, hyperkalemia. Solid oral dosage form in pts where there is structural, pathologic cause for delay in passage through GI tract. **Cautions:** Cardiac disease, acid-base disorders, potassium-altering disorders, digitalized pts, concomitant therapy that increases serum potassium (e.g., ACE inhibitors), renal impairment. Do not administer IV undiluted.

## ACTION

Necessary for multiple cellular metabolic processes. Primary action is intracellular. **Therapeutic Effect:** Required for nerve impulse conduction, contraction of cardiac, skeletal, smooth muscle; maintains normal renal function, acid-base balance.

## PHARMACOKINETICS

Well absorbed from GI tract. Enters cells by active transport from extracellular fluid. Primarily excreted in urine.

## ⏳ LIFESPAN CONSIDERATIONS

**Pregnancy/Lactation:** Unknown if drug crosses placenta or is distributed in breast milk. **Children:** No age-related precautions noted. **Elderly:** May be at increased risk for hyperkalemia. Age-related ability to excrete potassium is reduced.

## INTERACTIONS

**DRUG: ACE inhibitors (e.g., enalapril, lisinopril), potassium-containing medications, potassium-sparing diuretics (e.g., spironolactone, triamterene), salt substitutes** may increase serum potassium concentration. **HERBAL:** None significant. **FOOD:** None known. **LAB VALUES:** None known.

## AVAILABILITY (Rx)

POTASSIUM ACETATE
**Injection, Solution:** 2 mEq/ml.
POTASSIUM BICARBONATE AND POTASSIUM CITRATE
**Tablets for Solution: (Effer-K):** 10 mEq, 20 mEq, 25 mEq. **(Klor-Con EF):** 25 mEq.
POTASSIUM CHLORIDE
**Injection, Solution:** 2 mEq/ml. **Oral Solution:** 20 mEq/15 ml, 40 mEq/15 ml. **Powder for Oral Solution:** 20 mEq/packet, 25 mEq/packet.

🗸 **Capsules, Extended-Release (Micro-K):** 8 mEq, 10 mEq. 🗸 **Tablets, Extended-Release:** 8 mEq, 10 mEq, 15 mEq, 20 mEq.

## ADMINISTRATION/HANDLING

### 💉 IV

**Reconstitution** • For IV infusion only, must dilute before administration, mix well, infuse slowly. • Avoid adding potassium to hanging IV.

**Rate of Administration** • Routinely, give at concentration of no more than 40 mEq/L, no faster than 10 mEq/hr for peripheral infusion, 40 mEq/hr for central infusion. • Check IV site closely during infusion for evidence of phlebitis (heat, pain, red streaking of skin over vein, hardness to vein), extravasation (swelling, pain, cool skin, little/no blood return).

**Storage** • Store at room temperature. Use admixtures within 24 hrs.

### PO

• Take with or after meals, with full glass of water (decreases GI upset). • Liquids, powder, effervescent tablets: Mix, dissolve with juice, water before administering. • Do not break, crush, dissolve, or divide tablets; give whole.

## 🔲 IV INCOMPATIBILITIES

Amphotericin B complex (Abelcet, AmBisome, Amphotec), phenytoin (Dilantin).

## 🔲 IV COMPATIBILITIES

Amiodarone (Cordarone), atropine, aztreonam (Azactam), calcium gluconate, cefepime (Maxipime), ciprofloxacin (Cipro), clindamycin (Cleocin), dexamethasone (Decadron), dexmedetomidine (Precedex), digoxin (Lanoxin), diltiazem (Cardizem), diphenhydramine (Benadryl), dobutamine (Dobutrex), dopamine (Intropin), enalapril (Vasotec), famotidine (Pepcid), fluconazole (Diflucan), furosemide (Lasix), granisetron (Kytril), heparin, hydrocortisone (Solu-Cortef), insulin, lidocaine, lorazepam (Ativan), magnesium sulfate, methylprednisolone (Solu-Medrol), metoclopramide (Reglan), midazolam (Versed), milrinone (Primacor), morphine, norepinephrine (Levophed), ondansetron (Zofran), oxytocin (Pitocin), piperacillin and tazobactam (Zosyn), procainamide (Pronestyl), propofol (Diprivan), propranolol (Inderal).

## INDICATIONS/ROUTES/DOSAGE

**Treatment of Hypokalemia**
**PO: ADULTS, ELDERLY:** 40–100 mEq/day in divided doses (generally limit amount

per dose to 20–25 mEq to avoid GI discomfort); further doses based on laboratory values. **CHILDREN:** Initially, 1–2 mEq/kg; further doses based on laboratory values.

**IV: ADULTS, ELDERLY:** 5–10 mEq/hr. **Maximum:** 200 mEq/day. **CHILDREN:** 0.5–1 mEq/kg per dose. **Maximum dose:** 40 mEq per dose to infuse at 0.3–0.5 mEq/kg/hr.

**Dosage in Renal/Hepatic Impairment**
No dose adjustment. Use caution with potassium acetate (may increase serum aluminum and/or potassium).

## SIDE EFFECTS

**Occasional:** Nausea, vomiting, diarrhea, flatulence, abdominal discomfort with distention, phlebitis with IV administration (particularly when potassium concentration of greater than 40 mEq/L is infused). **Rare:** Rash.

## ADVERSE EFFECTS/ TOXIC REACTIONS

Hyperkalemia (more common in elderly, pts with renal impairment) manifested as paresthesia, feeling of heaviness in lower extremities, cold skin, grayish pallor, hypotension, confusion, irritability, flaccid paralysis, cardiac arrhythmias.

## NURSING CONSIDERATIONS

### BASELINE ASSESSMENT

Assess for hypokalemia (weakness, fatigue, polyuria, polydipsia). PO should be given with food or after meals with full glass of water, fruit juice (minimizes GI irritation).

### INTERVENTION/EVALUATION

Monitor serum potassium (particularly in renal impairment). If GI disturbance is noted, dilute preparation further or give with meals. Be alert to decreased urinary output (may be indication of renal insufficiency). Monitor daily pattern of bowel activity, stool consistency. Assess I&O

diligently during diuresis, IV site for extravasation, phlebitis. Be alert to evidence of hyperkalemia (skin pallor/coldness, complaints of paresthesia, feeling of heaviness of lower extremities).

### PATIENT/FAMILY TEACHING

• Foods rich in potassium include beef, veal, ham, chicken, turkey, fish, milk, bananas, dates, prunes, raisins, avocados, watermelon, cantaloupe, apricots, molasses, beans, yams, broccoli, Brussels sprouts, lentils, potatoes, spinach. • Report paresthesia, feeling of heaviness of lower extremities, tarry or bloody stools, weakness, unusual fatigue.

# *PRALAtrexate

pral-a-**trex**-ate
(Folotyn)
**Do not confuse Folotyn with Focalin, or pralatrexate with methotrexate or pemetrexed.**

## ◆CLASSIFICATION

**PHARMACOTHERAPEUTIC:** Antimetabolite. **CLINICAL:** Antineoplastic.

## USES

Treatment of relapsed or refractory peripheral T-cell lymphoma (PTCL). **OFF-LABEL:** Treatment of relapsed/refractory cutaneous T-cell lymphoma.

## PRECAUTIONS

**Contraindications:** Hypersensitivity to pralatrexate. **Cautions:** Moderate to severe renal impairment, hepatic impairment. Avoid use in end-stage renal disease.

## ACTION

Folate analogue metabolic inhibitor that competes with enzymes necessary for tumor cell reproduction. Inhibits DNA, RNA, protein synthesis. **Therapeutic Effect:** Inhibits tumor growth.

## PHARMACOKINETICS

Protein binding: 67%. Partially excreted in urine. **Half-life:** 12–18 hrs.

## ⧗ LIFESPAN CONSIDERATIONS

**Pregnancy/Lactation:** May cause fetal harm. Unknown if drug is distributed in breast milk. **Children:** Safety and efficacy not established. **Elderly:** No age-related precautions noted.

## INTERACTIONS

**DRUG: NSAIDs, probenecid, trimethoprim/sulfamethoxazole** may delay clearance, increase concentration. **HERBAL:** Echinacea may decrease concentration/effects. **FOOD:** None known. **LAB VALUES:** May decrease RBC, WBC, Hgb, Hct, platelet count, serum potassium. May increase serum ALT, AST.

## AVAILABILITY (Rx)

**Injection Solution:** 20 mg/ml.

## ADMINISTRATION/HANDLING

◀**ALERT▶** May be carcinogenic, mutagenic, teratogenic. Handle with extreme care during preparation/administration. Wear gloves when preparing solution. If powder or solution comes in contact with skin, wash immediately, thoroughly with soap, water.

◀**ALERT▶** Pt should begin taking oral folic acid (1 mg) daily starting 10 days prior to first IV pralatrexate dose and continue for 30 days after last dose. Pt should also receive vitamin $B_{12}$ (1 mg) IM injection no more than 10 wks prior to first IV pralatrexate dose and every 8–10 wks thereafter.

 **IV**

**Reconstitution** • Withdraw calculated dose into syringe for immediate use. • Intended for single use only. • Do not dilute.
**Rate of Administration** • Administer as IV push over 3–5 min into IV infusion of 0.9% NaCl.

**Storage** • Refrigerate vials until use, protect from light. Stable at room temperature for 72 hrs. • Discard vial if solution is discolored (solution should appear clear to yellow) or particulate matter is present.

## ▦ IV INCOMPATIBILITIES

Do not mix with any other medication.

## INDICATIONS/ROUTES/DOSAGE

◀**ALERT▶** Prior to any dose, mucositis should be no higher than grade 1, platelets 100,000/mm$^3$ or greater for first dose and 50,000/mm$^3$ or greater for subsequent doses, and absolute neutrophil count (ANC) 1,000/mm$^3$ or greater.

**Refractory/Relapsed Peripheral T-Cell Lymphoma**
**IV: ADULTS, ELDERLY:** 30 mg/m$^2$ administered once wkly for 6 wks in 7-wk cycles. Dose may be decreased to 20 mg/m$^2$ to manage adverse reactions. Continue until disease progression or unacceptable toxicity.

**Dosage in Renal Impairment**
Monitor for toxicities. Avoid use in end-stage renal disease.

**Dosage in Hepatic Impairment**
**Grade 3:** Withhold dose; decrease to 20 mg/m$^3$ when grade 2 or less.
**Grade 4:** Discontinue.

## SIDE EFFECTS

**Common (70%–36%):** Mucositis, nausea, fatigue. **Frequent (34%–10%):** Constipation/diarrhea, pyrexia, edema, cough, epistaxis, vomiting, dyspnea, anorexia, rash, throat/abdominal/back pain, night sweats, asthenia, tachycardia, upper respiratory infection.

## ADVERSE EFFECTS/TOXIC REACTIONS

Hematologic toxicity, resulting from blood dyscrasias, may manifest as thrombocytopenia (41% of pts), anemia (34%

---

of pts), neutropenia (24% of pts), leuko-penia (11% of pts). High potential for development of mucositis (70% of pts). Mucositis is less severe when folic acid, vitamin $B_{12}$ therapy is ongoing. Sepsis, pyrexia, febrile neutropenia, dehydration have occurred. Overdosage requires general supportive care. Prompt administration of leucovorin should be considered in case of overdose, based on mechanism of action of pralatrexate.

## NURSING CONSIDERATIONS

### BASELINE ASSESSMENT

Evaluate baseline CBC with differential, renal function, LFT, serum potassium level. Question for possibility of pregnancy before initiating therapy. Assess baseline vital signs, temperature. Antiemetics before and during therapy may alleviate nausea/vomiting. Initiate folic acid, vitamin $B_{12}$ administration prior to and throughout therapy.

### INTERVENTION/EVALUATION

Prior to any dose: mucositis should be grade 1 or less. Platelet count 100,000/$mm^3$ or greater for first dose (50,000/$mm^3$ or greater for all subsequent doses). Absolute neutrophil count (ANC) 1,000/$mm^3$ or greater. Assess for signs of mucositis (oropharyngeal ulcers, oral/throat pain, local infection). Monitor for signs of hematologic toxicity, sepsis (fever, signs of local infection, altered CBC results). Monitor hepatic/renal function. Monitor for hypokalemia (muscle cramps, weakness, EKG changes).

### PATIENT/FAMILY TEACHING

• Explain importance of folic acid, vitamin $B_{12}$ therapy to reduce adverse effects. • Maintain strict oral hygiene. • Do not have immunizations without physician's approval (drug lowers body's resistance). • Avoid crowds, those with infection. • Promptly report fever, sore throat, signs of local infection, unusual bruising/bleeding from any site. • Use nonhormonal contraception. • Report persistent nausea/vomiting.

# pramipexole

pram-i-**pex**-ole
(Apo-Pramipexole ✦, Mirapex, Mirapex ER)
**Do not confuse Mirapex with Mifeprex or MiraLax.**

## ◆CLASSIFICATION

**PHARMACOTHERAPEUTIC:** Dopamine receptor agonist. **CLINICAL:** Antiparkinson agent.

## USES

**Mirapex:** Treatment of signs/symptoms of idiopathic Parkinson's disease, restless legs syndrome. **Mirapex ER:** Treatment of Parkinson's disease. **OFF-LABEL: (Immediate-Release):** Depression (due to bipolar disorder), fibromyalgia.

## PRECAUTIONS

**Contraindications:** Hypersensitivity to pramipexole. **Cautions:** History of orthostatic hypotension, pts at risk for hypotension, syncope, hallucinations, renal impairment (extended release not recommended with CrCl less than 30 ml/min), concomitant use of CNS depressants, preexisting dyskinesia, elderly.

## ACTION

Stimulates dopamine receptors in striatum and substantia nigra. **Therapeutic Effect:** Relieves signs/symptoms of Parkinson's disease.

## PHARMACOKINETICS

Rapidly, extensively absorbed after PO administration. Protein binding: 15%. Widely distributed. Steady-state concentrations achieved within 2 days. Primarily eliminated in urine. Not removed by hemodialysis. **Half-life:** 8 hrs (12 hrs in pts older than 65 yrs).

## ⌛ LIFESPAN CONSIDERATIONS

**Pregnancy/Lactation:** Unknown if drug is distributed in breast milk.

**Children:** Safety and efficacy not established. **Elderly:** Increased risk of hallucinations.

## INTERACTIONS

**DRUG:** May increase plasma concentrations of **carbidopa, levodopa. HERBAL: Gotu kola, kava kava, St. John's wort, SAMe, valerian** may increase CNS depression, risk of serotonin syndrome. **FOOD: All foods** delay peak drug plasma levels by 1 hr (extent of absorption not affected). **LAB VALUES:** None significant.

## AVAILABILITY (Rx)

**Tablets:** 0.125 mg, 0.25 mg, 0.5 mg, 0.75 mg, 1 mg, 1.5 mg.

 Tablets (Extended-Release [Mirapex ER]): 0.375 mg, 0.75 mg, 1.5 mg, 2.25 mg, 3 mg, 3.75 mg, 4.5 mg.

## ADMINISTRATION/HANDLING

**PO (Mirapex)**
• Give without regard to food.

**PO (Mirapex ER)**
• Give once daily, without regard to food.
• Give whole; do not break, crush, dissolve, or divide tablets.

## INDICATIONS/ROUTES/DOSAGE

**Parkinson's Disease (Mirapex)**
**PO:** *(Immediate-Release):* **ADULTS, ELDERLY:** Initially, 0.125 mg 3 times/day. Increase no more frequently than every 5–7 days. **Maintenance:** 0.5–1.5 mg 3 times/day.

*(Extended-Release):* Initially, 0.375 mg once daily. May increase to 0.75 mg, then by 0.75-mg increments no more frequently than 5–7 days. **Maximum:** 4.5 mg once daily. **Note:** May switch overnight from immediate-release to extended-release at same daily dose.

**Restless Legs Syndrome**
**PO: ADULTS, ELDERLY:** *(Immediate-Release):* Initially, 0.125 mg once daily 2–3 hrs before bedtime. May increase to 0.25 mg after 4–7 days, then to 0.5 mg after 4–7 days (interval is 14 days in pts

with renal impairment). **Maximum:** 0.5 mg/day.

**Dosage in Renal Impairment**
Dosage and frequency are modified based on creatinine clearance.

**(Parkinson's Disease)**
*Immediate-Release*

| Creatinine Clearance | Dosage | |
|---|---|---|
| | Initial | Maximum |
| 30–50 ml/min | 0.125 mg twice daily | 0.75 mg 3 times/day |
| 15–29 ml/min | 0.125 mg once daily | 1.5 mg once daily |

*Extended-Release*
**CrCl 30–50 ml/min:** Initially, 0.375 mg every other day. May increase by 0.375 mg/day in 7 days or longer. **Maximum:** 2.25 mg once daily. **CrCl less than 30 ml/min:** Not recommended.

**Restless Legs Syndrome**
No dose adjustment.

**Dosage in Hepatic Impairment**
No dose adjustment.

## SIDE EFFECTS

**Frequent: Early Parkinson's disease (28%–10%):** Nausea, asthenia, dizziness, drowsiness, insomnia, constipation. **Advanced Parkinson's disease (53%–17%):** Orthostatic hypotension, extrapyramidal reactions, insomnia, dizziness, hallucinations. **Occasional: Early Parkinson's disease (5%–2%):** Edema, malaise, confusion, amnesia, akathisia, anorexia, dysphagia, peripheral edema, vision changes, impotence. **Advanced Parkinson's disease (10%–7%):** Asthenia, drowsiness, confusion, constipation, abnormal gait, dry mouth. **Rare: Advanced Parkinson's disease (6%–2%):** General edema, malaise, angina, amnesia, tremor, urinary frequency/incontinence, dyspnea, rhinitis, vision changes. **Restless legs syndrome: Frequent (16%):** Headache, nausea. **Occasional (13%–9%):** Insomnia,

P

fatigue. **Rare (6%–3%):** Drowsiness, constipation, diarrhea, dry mouth.

## ADVERSE EFFECTS/ TOXIC REACTIONS

Vascular disease, atrial fibrillation, arrhythmias, pulmonary embolism, impulsive/compulsive behavior (pathological gambling, hypersexuality, binge eating) have been reported.

## NURSING CONSIDERATIONS

### BASELINE ASSESSMENT

**Parkinson's disease:** Assess for tremor, muscle weakness and rigidity, ataxia. **Restless legs syndrome:** Assess frequency of symptoms, sleep pattern.

### INTERVENTION/EVALUATION

Assess for clinical improvement. Assist with ambulation if dizziness occurs. Assess for constipation; encourage fiber, fluids, exercise.

### PATIENT/FAMILY TEACHING

• Inform pt that hallucinations may occur, esp. in the elderly. • Go from lying to standing slowly. • Avoid tasks that require alertness, motor skills until response to drug is established. • If nausea occurs, take medication with food. • Avoid abrupt withdrawal. • Avoid alcohol. • Report new or increased impulsive/compulsive behaviors (e.g., gambling, sexual urges, compulsive eating or buying).

## *pramlintide*    HIGH ALERT

**pram**-lin-tide
(SymlinPen 60, SymlinPen 120)

■ **BLACK BOX ALERT** ■ Increased risk of severe hypoglycemia; usually occurs within 3 hrs of injection. Coadministration with insulin may increase incidence.

### ◆CLASSIFICATION

**PHARMACOTHERAPEUTIC:** Antihyperglycemic. **CLINICAL:** Antidiabetic agent.

## USES

Adjunctive treatment in pts with type 1 or type 2 diabetes who use mealtime insulin therapy and who have failed to achieve desired glucose control despite optimal insulin therapy.

## PRECAUTIONS

**Contraindications:** Hypersensitivity to pramlintide. Diagnosed gastroparesis, hypoglycemia unawareness. **Cautions:** Coadministration with insulin may induce severe hypoglycemia (usually within 3 hrs following administration); concurrent use of other glucose-lowering agents may increase risk of hypoglycemia. History of nausea, visual or dexterity impairment, poor compliance with insulin monitoring or current insulin therapy, pts with hemoglobin $A_{1c}$ greater than 9%, pts with conditions or taking concurrent medications likely to impair gastric motility (e.g., anticholinergics), pts requiring medication to stimulate gastric emptying.

## ACTION

Cosecreted with insulin by pancreatic beta cells, reduces postprandial glucose increases by slowing gastric emptying time, reducing postprandial glucagon secretion, reducing caloric intake through centrally mediated appetite suppression. **Therapeutic Effect:** Improves glycemic control by reducing postprandial glucose concentrations in pts with type 1, type 2 diabetes mellitus.

## PHARMACOKINETICS

|    | Onset | Peak | Duration |
|----|-------|------|----------|
| SQ | NA | 20 min | 3 hrs |

Metabolized primarily by kidneys. Protein binding: 60%. Excreted in urine. **Half-life:** 48 min.

## ⧗ LIFESPAN CONSIDERATIONS

**Pregnancy/Lactation:** Unknown if distributed in breast milk. **Children:** Safety and efficacy not established. **Elderly:** No age-related precautions noted.

## INTERACTIONS

**DRUG: Anticholinergics (e.g., dicyclomine, glycopyrrolate, scopolamine)** may cause additive impairment of gastric motility. **HERBAL: Garlic** may increase hypoglycemia. **FOOD: Ethanol** may increase risk of hypoglycemia. **LAB VALUES:** None significant.

## AVAILABILITY (Rx)

**Injection, Solution (SymlinPen 120):** Delivers fixed doses of 120 mcg. **(Symlin-Pen 60):** Delivers fixed doses of 60 mcg.

## ADMINISTRATION/HANDLING

**SQ**

• Administer immediately before each major meal (350 or more kcal or containing 30 g or more carbohydrate). • Give in abdomen or thigh; do not give in arm (variable absorption). • Injection site should be distinct from insulin injection site. • Rotation of injection sites is essential. • Use U-100 insulin syringe for accuracy. • Always give pramlintide and insulin as separate injections.

**Storage** • Store unopened vials in refrigerator. • Discard if freezing occurs. • Vials that have been opened (punctured) may be stored in refrigerator or kept at room temperature for up to 30 days.

## INDICATIONS/ROUTES/ DOSAGE

**◀ALERT▶** Initially, current insulin dosage in all pts with type 1, type 2 diabetes mellitus should be reduced by 50%. This includes preprandial, rapid-acting, short-acting, fixed-mixed insulins.

**Type 1 Diabetes Mellitus**
**SQ: ADULTS, ELDERLY:** Initially, 15 mcg immediately before each major meal. Titrate in 15-mcg increments every 3 days (if no significant nausea occurs) to target dose of 30–60 mcg.

**Type 2 Diabetes Mellitus**
**SQ: ADULTS, ELDERLY:** Initially, 60 mcg immediately before each major meal. After 3–7 days, increase to 120 mcg if no significant nausea occurs (if nausea occurs at 120 mcg dose, reduce to 60 mcg).

**Dosage in Renal/Hepatic Impairment**
No dose adjustment.

## SIDE EFFECTS

**TYPE 1 DIABETES MELLITUS**
**Frequent (48%):** Nausea. **Occasional (17%–11%):** Anorexia, vomiting. **Rare (7%–5%):** Fatigue, arthralgia, allergic reaction, dizziness.
**TYPE 2 DIABETES MELLITUS**
**Frequent (28%):** Nausea. **Occasional (13%–8%):** Headache, anorexia, vomiting, abdominal pain. **Rare (7%–5%):** Fatigue, dizziness, cough, pharyngitis.

## ADVERSE EFFECTS/ TOXIC REACTIONS

Overdose produces severe nausea, vomiting, diarrhea, vasodilation, dizziness. No hypoglycemia was reported. Increased risk of severe hypoglycemia when given concurrently with nontitrated insulin.

## NURSING CONSIDERATIONS

### BASELINE ASSESSMENT

Check serum glucose concentration before administration, both before and after meals and at bedtime. Discuss lifestyle to determine extent of learning, emotional needs. Ensure follow-up instruction if pt, family does not thoroughly understand diabetes management, glucose testing technique.

### INTERVENTION/EVALUATION

Risk for hypoglycemia occurs within first 3 hrs following drug administration if given concurrently with insulin. Assess for hypoglycemia (diaphoresis, tremors, dizziness, anxiety, headache, tachycardia, numbness in mouth, hunger, diplopia, difficulty concentrating). Be alert to conditions that alter glucose requirements (fever, increased activity, stress, surgical procedures).

**P**

 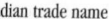

## PATIENT/FAMILY TEACHING

• Diabetes mellitus requires lifelong control. • Prescribed diet, exercise are principal parts of treatment; do not skip/delay meals. • Continue to adhere to dietary instructions, regular exercise program, regular testing of serum glucose. • When taking combination drug therapy, have source of glucose available to treat symptoms of low blood sugar.

---

# prasugrel

pra-soo-grel
(Effient)

■ **BLACK BOX ALERT** ■ Serious, sometimes fatal, hemorrhage may occur.
**Do not confuse Effient with Effexor, or prasugrel with praziquantel.**

## ◆CLASSIFICATION

**PHARMACOTHERAPEUTIC:** Thienopyridine derivative inhibitor. **CLINICAL:** Antiplatelet agent.

## USES

Reduction of thrombotic cardiovascular events (MI, CVA, stent thrombosis) in pts with acute coronary syndrome (unstable angina, non–ST-segment elevation MI, ST-segment MI) who are to be managed with percutaneous coronary intervention (PCI). **OFF-LABEL:** Initial treatment of unstable angina, STEMI in pts undergoing PCI with allergy or major GI intolerance to aspirin.

## PRECAUTIONS

**Contraindications:** Hypersensitivity to prasugrel. Active bleeding, prior transient ischemic attack (TIA), CVA. **Cautions:** Pts who undergo coronary artery bypass graft (CABG) after receiving prasugrel, pts at risk for bleeding (age 75 yrs or older, body weight less than 60 kg, recent trauma/surgery, recent GI bleeding or active peptic ulcer disease, severe hepatic impairment).

## ACTION

Inhibits binding of the enzyme adenosine phosphate (ADP) to its platelet receptor and subsequent ADP-mediated activation of a glycoprotein complex. **Therapeutic Effect:** Inhibits platelet aggregation.

## PHARMACOKINETICS

Rapidly absorbed, with peak concentration occurring 30 min following administration. Metabolized in liver. Protein binding: 98%. Eliminated in urine (68%), feces (27%). **Half-life:** 7 hrs.

## ☒ LIFESPAN CONSIDERATIONS

**Pregnancy/Lactation:** Unknown if drug crosses placenta or is distributed in breast milk. **Children:** Safety and efficacy not established. **Elderly:** May have increased risk for intracranial hemorrhage; caution advised in pts 75 yrs and older.

## INTERACTIONS

**DRUG:** Aspirin, NSAIDs, warfarin may increase risk of bleeding. **HERBAL:** Cat's claw, dong quai, evening primrose, feverfew, garlic, ginger, ginseng, green tea, horse chestnut, red clover may have additive platelet effects. **Ginkgo biloba** may increase risk of bleeding. **FOOD:** None known. **LAB VALUES:** May decrease Hgb, Hct, WBC, platelet count. May increase bleeding time, serum cholesterol, ALT, AST.

## AVAILABILITY (Rx)

🏷 **Tablets:** 5 mg, 10 mg.

## ADMINISTRATION/HANDLING

**PO**
• Give without regard to food. • Do not crush tablet.

## INDICATIONS/ROUTES/DOSAGE

**Acute Coronary Syndrome**
◀**ALERT**▶ Consider 5 mg once daily for pts weighing less than 60 kg. Not recommened in pts 75 yrs and older.
**PO: ADULTS, ELDERLY:** Initially, 60-mg loading dose, then 10 mg once daily (in combination with aspirin) for at least 12 mos.

**Dosage in Renal/Hepatic Impairment**
No dose adjustment.

## SIDE EFFECTS

**Occasional (8%–4%):** Hypertension, minor bleeding, headache, back pain, dyspnea, nausea, dizziness. **Rare (Less Than 4%):** Cough, hypotension, fatigue, noncardiac chest pain, bradycardia, rash, pyrexia, peripheral edema, extremity pain, diarrhea.

## ADVERSE EFFECTS/ TOXIC REACTIONS

Major bleeding (intracranial hemorrhage, epistaxis, GI bleeding, hemoptysis, SQ hematoma, postprocedural hemorrhage, retroperitoneal hemorrhage, retinal hemorrhage) has been reported. Severe thrombocytopenia, anemia, abnormal hepatic function, anaphylactic reaction, angioedema, atrial fibrillation occur rarely. Overdosage may require platelet transfusion to restore clotting ability.

## NURSING CONSIDERATIONS

### BASELINE ASSESSMENT

Obtain baseline vital signs, CBC, EKG, LFT. Question history of intracranial hemorrhage, GI bleeding, ulcers, recent surgery or trauma.

### INTERVENTION/EVALUATION

Monitor vital signs for changes in B/P, pulse. Assess for signs of unusual bleeding or hemorrhage, pain. Monitor platelet count, LFT, EKG for changes from baseline.

### PATIENT/FAMILY TEACHING

• It may take longer to stop minor bleeding during drug therapy. Report unusual bleeding/bruising, blood noted in stool or urine, chest/back pain, extremity pain, symptoms of stroke. • Monitor for dyspnea. • Report fever, weakness, extreme skin paleness, purple skin patches, yellowing of skin or eyes, changes in mental status. • Do not discontinue drug therapy without physician approval. • Inform physicians, dentists before undergoing any invasive procedure or surgery.

# pravastatin

**pra**-va-sta-tin
(Apo-Pravastatin ♣, Pravachol)
**Do not confuse pravastatin with atorvastatin, lovastatin, nystatin, pitavastatin, or simvastatin, or Pravachol with Prevacid, Prinivil, or propranolol.**

## FIXED-COMBINATION(S)

**Pravigard:** pravastatin/aspirin (anticoagulant): 20 mg/81 mg, 40 mg/81 mg, 80 mg/81 mg, 20 mg/325 mg, 40 mg/325 mg, 80 mg/325 mg.

## ◆CLASSIFICATION

**PHARMACOTHERAPEUTIC:** Hydroxymethylglutaryl CoA (HMG-CoA) reductase inhibitor. **CLINICAL:** Antihyperlipidemic.

## USES

Treatment of primary hyperlipidemias and mixed dyslipidemias to reduce total cholesterol, LDL cholesterol, apolipoprotein B, triglycerides; increase HDL cholesterol. Reduces risk of MI, revascularization, and mortality in hypercholesterolemia without clinically evident CHD. Reduces mortality risk in pts with CHD. Reduces elevated triglycerides in hypertriglyceridemia. Treatment of heterozygous familial hypercholesterolemia in pediatric pts 8–18 yrs.

## PRECAUTIONS

**Contraindications:** Hypersensitivity to pravastatin. Active hepatic disease or unexplained, persistent elevations of hepatic function test results. Pregnancy, breastfeeding. **Cautions:** History of hepatic disease, substantial alcohol consumption. Withholding/discontinuing pravastatin may be necessary when pt is at risk for renal failure secondary to rhabdomyolysis, elderly.

## ACTION

Interferes with cholesterol biosynthesis by preventing conversion of HMG-CoA reductase to mevalonate, a precursor to cholesterol. **Therapeutic Effect:** Lowers LDL, VLDL cholesterol, plasma triglycerides; increases HDL.

## PHARMACOKINETICS

Rapidly absorbed from GI tract. Protein binding: 50%. Metabolized in liver. Primarily excreted in feces via biliary system. Not removed by hemodialysis. **Half-life:** 2–3 hrs. (Half-life including all metabolites: 77 hrs.)

## ⧖ LIFESPAN CONSIDERATIONS

**Pregnancy/Lactation:** Contraindicated in pregnancy (suppression of cholesterol biosynthesis may cause fetal toxicity) and lactation. Unknown if drug is distributed in breast milk, but there is risk of serious adverse reactions in breastfeeding infants. **Children:** Safety and efficacy not established. **Elderly:** No age-related precautions noted.

## INTERACTIONS

**DRUG: Cyclosporine, clarithromycin, colchicine, erythromycin, gemfibrozil, immunosuppressants, niacin** increase risk of myopathy, rhabdomyolysis. **HERBAL: St. John's wort** may decrease concentration. **FOOD: Red yeast rice** contains 2.4 mg **lovastatin** per 600 mg rice. **LAB VALUES:** May increase serum creatine kinase (CK), transaminase.

## AVAILABILITY (Rx)

**Tablets:** 10 mg, 20 mg, 40 mg, 80 mg.

## ADMINISTRATION/HANDLING

**PO**
• Give without regard to meals.

## INDICATIONS/ROUTES/DOSAGE

◀**ALERT**▶ Prior to initiating therapy, pt should be on standard cholesterol-lowering diet for 3–6 mos. Low-cholesterol diet should be continued throughout pravastatin therapy.

**Hyperlipidemia, Prevention of Coronary/Cardiovascular Events**
**PO: ADULTS, ELDERLY:** Initially, 40 mg/day. Titrate to desired response. Range: 10–80 mg/day.

**Heterozygous Familial Hypercholesterolemia**
**PO: CHILDREN 14–18 YRS:** 40 mg/day. **CHILDREN 8–13 YRS:** 20 mg/day.

**Dosage with Clarithromycin**
**Maximum:** 40 mg/day.

**Dosage with Cyclosporine**
**ADULTS, ELDERLY:** Initially, 10 mg/day. **Maximum:** 20 mg/day.

**Dosage in Renal Impairment**
For adults, give 10 mg/day initially. Titrate to desired response.

**Dosage in Hepatic Impairment**
See contraindications.

## SIDE EFFECTS

Pravastatin is generally well tolerated. Side effects are usually mild and transient. **Occasional (7%–4%):** Nausea, vomiting, diarrhea, constipation, abdominal pain, headache, rhinitis, rash, pruritus. **Rare (3%–2%):** Heartburn, myalgia, dizziness, cough, fatigue, flu-like symptoms, depression, photosensitivity.

## ADVERSE EFFECTS/TOXIC REACTIONS

Potential for malignancy, cataracts. Hypersensitivity, myopathy occur rarely. Rhabdomyolysis has been reported.

## NURSING CONSIDERATIONS

### BASELINE ASSESSMENT

Obtain dietary history, esp. fat consumption. Question for possibility of pregnancy before initiating therapy. Assess baseline serum lab results (cholesterol, triglycerides, LFT).

### INTERVENTION/EVALUATION

Monitor serum cholesterol, triglyceride lab results for therapeutic response. Monitor LFT, CPK. Monitor daily pattern of bowel activity, stool consistency. Assess for headache, dizziness (provide assistance as needed). Assess for rash, pruritus. Be alert for malaise, muscle cramping/weakness; if accompanied by fever, may require discontinuation of medication.

### PATIENT/FAMILY TEACHING

• Follow special diet (important part of treatment). • Periodic lab tests are essential part of therapy. • Report promptly any muscle pain/weakness, esp. if accompanied by fever, malaise. • Avoid tasks that require alertness, motor skills until response to drug is established (potential for dizziness). • Use nonhormonal contraception. • Avoid direct exposure to sunlight.

## *prednisoLONE

pred-**niss**-oh-lone
(Millipred, Novo-Prednisolone ✦, Omnipred, Orapred ODT, Pediapred, Pred Forte, Pred Mild, Prelone, Veripred)
**Do not confuse Pediapred with Pediazole, prednisolone with prednisone or primidone, or Prelone with Prozac.**

### FIXED-COMBINATION(S)

**Blephamide:** prednisolone/sulfacetamide (an anti-infective): 0.2%/10%. **Vasocidin:** prednisolone/sulfacetamide: 0.25%/10%.

## ◆CLASSIFICATION

**PHARMACOTHERAPEUTIC:** Adrenal corticosteroid. **CLINICAL:** Glucocorticoid.

## USES

**Systemic:** Endocrine, rheumatic, hematologic disorders; collagen, respiratory, neoplastic, GI diseases; allergic states; acute or chronic solid organ rejection. **Ophthalmic:** Treatment of conjunctivitis, corneal injury (from chemical/thermal burns, foreign body).

## PRECAUTIONS

**Contraindications:** Hypersensitivity to prednisolone. Acute superficial herpes simplex keratitis, systemic fungal infections, varicella, live or attenuated virus vaccines. **Cautions:** Hyperthyroidism, cirrhosis, ocular herpes simplex, respiratory tuberculosis, untreated systemic infections, renal/hepatic impairment, diabetes, cataracts, glaucoma, history of seizure disorder, peptic ulcer disease, osteoporosis, myasthenia gravis, hypertension, HF, ulcerative colitis, thromboembolic disorders, elderly.

## ACTION

Inhibits accumulation of inflammatory cells at inflammation sites, phagocytosis, lysosomal enzyme release/synthesis, release of mediators of inflammation. **Therapeutic Effect:** Prevents/suppresses cell-mediated immune reactions. Decreases/prevents tissue response to inflammatory process.

## PHARMACOKINETICS

Protein binding: 65%–91%. Metabolized in liver. Excreted in urine. **Half-life:** 3.6 hrs.

## ⧖ LIFESPAN CONSIDERATIONS

**Pregnancy/Lactation:** Crosses placenta. Distributed in breast milk. Fetal cleft palate often occurs with chronic, first-trimester use. Breastfeeding not recommended. **Children:** Prolonged treatment or high dosages may decrease short-term growth rate, cortisol secretion. **Elderly:** May be more susceptible to developing hypertension or osteoporosis.

## INTERACTIONS

**DRUG:** Hepatic enzyme inducers (e.g., **phenobarbital, phenytoin, rifampin**) may decrease effects. **Live virus vaccines** increase vaccine side effects, potentiate virus replication, decrease pt's antibody response to vaccine. May increase effect of **warfarin**. **HERBAL:** St. John's wort may decrease concentration. Cat's claw, echinacea have immunostimulant properties. Echinacea may decrease level/effects. **FOOD:** None known. **LAB VALUES:** May increase serum glucose, lipids, sodium, uric acid. May decrease serum calcium, WBC, hypothalamic pituitary adrenal (HPA) axis function, potassium.

## AVAILABILITY (Rx)

**Solution, Ophthalmic:** 1%. **Solution, Oral:** 15 mg/5 ml. **(Pediapred):** 5 mg/5 ml. **(Millipred):** 10 mg/5 ml. **(Veripred):** 20 mg/5 ml. **Suspension, Ophthalmic (Pred Forte):** 1%; **(Pred Mild):** 0.12%. **Syrup (Prelone):** 15 mg/5 ml. **Tablets:** 5 mg.

 **Tablets, Orally Disintegrating:** 10 mg, 15 mg, 30 mg.

## ADMINISTRATION/HANDLING

**PO**
• Give with food or fluids to decrease GI side effects.

**Orally Disintegrating Tablets**
• Do not break, crush, or divide tablets. • Remove from blister just prior to giving, place on tongue. • Pt may swallow whole or allow to dissolve in mouth with/without water.

**Ophthalmic**
• For ophthalmic solution, shake well before using. • Instill drops into conjunctival sac, as prescribed. • Avoid touching applicator tip to conjunctiva to avoid contamination.

## INDICATIONS/ROUTES/DOSAGE

**Usual Dosage**
**PO: ADULTS, ELDERLY:** 5–60 mg/day in divided doses. **CHILDREN:** 0.1–2 mg/kg/day in 1–4 divided doses.

**Treatment of Conjunctivitis, Corneal Injury**
**Ophthalmic: ADULTS, ELDERLY, CHILDREN:** 1–2 drops every hr during day and q2h during night. After response, decrease dosage to 1 drop q4h, then 1 drop 3–4 times/day.

**Dosage in Renal/Hepatic Impairment**
No dose adjustment.

## SIDE EFFECTS

**Frequent:** Insomnia, heartburn, nervousness, abdominal distention, diaphoresis, acne, mood swings, increased appetite, facial flushing, delayed wound healing, increased susceptibility to infection, diarrhea, constipation. **Occasional:** Headache, edema, change in skin color, frequent urination. **Rare:** Tachycardia, allergic reaction (rash, urticaria), psychological changes, hallucinations, depression. **Ophthalmic:** Stinging/burning, posterior subcapsular cataracts.

## ADVERSE EFFECTS/ TOXIC REACTIONS

**Long-term therapy:** Hypocalcemia, hypokalemia, muscle wasting (esp. arms, legs) osteoporosis, spontaneous fractures, amenorrhea, cataracts, glaucoma, peptic ulcer, HF. **Abrupt withdrawal following long-term therapy:** Anorexia, nausea, fever, headache, severe/sudden joint pain, rebound inflammation, fatigue, weakness, lethargy, dizziness, orthostatic hypotension. Sudden discontinuance may be fatal.

## NURSING CONSIDERATIONS

### BASELINE ASSESSMENT

Question medical history as listed in Precautions. Obtain baselines for height, weight, B/P, serum glucose, electrolytes. Check results of initial tests (tuberculosis [TB] skin test, X-rays, EKG).

### INTERVENTION/EVALUATION

Monitor B/P, weight, serum electrolytes, glucose, results of bone mineral density test, height, weight in children. Be alert to infection (sore throat, fever, vague symptoms); assess oral cavity daily for signs of candida infection.

### PATIENT/FAMILY TEACHING

• Report fever, sore throat, muscle aches, sudden weight gain, swelling, loss of appetite, fatigue. • Avoid alcohol, limit caffeine. • Maintain fastidious oral hygiene. • Do not abruptly discontinue without physician's approval. • Avoid exposure to chickenpox, measles.

---

## *predniSONE

pred-ni-sone
(Apo-Prednisone ✦, Prednisone Intensol, Rayos, Winpred ✦)
**Do not confuse prednisone with methylprednisolone, prazosin, prednisolone, Prilosec, primidone, or promethazine.**

### ◆CLASSIFICATION

**PHARMACOTHERAPEUTIC:** Adrenal corticosteroid. **CLINICAL:** Glucocorticoid.

## USES

**Substitution therapy in deficiency states:** Acute or chronic adrenal insufficiency, congenital adrenal hyperplasia, adrenal insufficiency secondary to pituitary insufficiency. **Nonendocrine disorders:** Arthritis, rheumatic carditis; allergic, collagen, intestinal tract, multiple sclerosis exacerbations; liver, ocular, renal, skin diseases; bronchial asthma, cerebral edema, malignancies. **OFF-LABEL:** Prevention of postherpetic neuralgia, relief of acute pain in pts with herpes zoster, autoimmune hepatitis.

## PRECAUTIONS

**Contraindications:** Hypersensitivity to prednisone. Acute superficial herpes simplex keratitis, systemic fungal infections, varicella, administration of live or attenuated virus vaccines. **Cautions:** Hyperthyroidism, cirrhosis, ocular herpes simplex, respiratory tuberculosis, untreated systemic infections, renal/hepatic impairment; following acute MI, diabetes, cataracts, glaucoma, seizures, peptic ulcer disease, osteoporosis, myasthenia gravis, hypertension, HF, ulcerative colitis, thromboembolic disorders, elderly.

## ACTION

Inhibits accumulation of inflammatory cells at inflammation sites, phagocytosis, lysosomal enzyme release/synthesis, release of mediators of inflammation. **Therapeutic Effect:** Prevents/suppresses cell-mediated immune reactions. Decreases/prevents tissue response to inflammatory process.

## PHARMACOKINETICS

Well absorbed from GI tract. Protein binding: 70%–90%. Widely distributed. Metabolized in liver, converted to prednisolone. Primarily excreted in urine. Not removed by hemodialysis. **Half-life:** 2.5–3.5 hrs.

## ⌛ LIFESPAN CONSIDERATIONS

**Pregnancy/Lactation:** Crosses placenta. Distributed in breast milk. Fetal cleft palate often occurs with chronic, first trimester use. Breastfeeding not recommended. **Children:** Prolonged treatment or high dosages may decrease short-term growth rate, cortisol secretion. **Elderly:** May be more susceptible to developing hypertension or osteoporosis.

## INTERACTIONS

**DRUG: Hepatic enzyme inducers (e.g., phenobarbital, phenytoin, rifampin)** may decrease effects. **Live virus vaccines** may increase vaccine side effects, potentiate virus replication, decrease pt's antibody response to vaccine. May increase effect of **warfarin. HERBAL: St. John's wort** may

---

P

decrease concentration. **Cat's claw, echinacea** have immunostimulant properties. **FOOD:** None known. **LAB VALUES:** May increase serum glucose, lipids, sodium, uric acid. May decrease serum calcium, potassium, WBC, hypothalamic pituitary adrenal (HPA) axis function.

## AVAILABILITY (Rx)

**Solution, Oral:** 1 mg/ml. **Solution, Oral Concentrate (Prednisone Intensol):** 5 mg/ml. **Tablets:** 1 mg, 2.5 mg, 5 mg, 10 mg, 20 mg, 50 mg.

🌿 **Tablet: (Delayed-Release [Rayos]):** 1 mg, 2 mg, 5 mg.

## ADMINISTRATION/HANDLING

**PO**
• Give with food or fluids to decrease GI side effects. • Give single doses before 9 AM, multiple doses at evenly spaced intervals. • Give delayed-release tablet whole; do not break, crush, dissolve, or divide.

## INDICATIONS/ROUTES/DOSAGE

**Note:** Dose dependent upon condition treated, pt response rather than by rigid adherence to age, weight, or body surface area.

**Usual Dosage**
**PO: ADULTS, ELDERLY:** 5–60 mg/day in divided doses. **CHILDREN:** 0.05–2 mg/kg/day in 1–4 divided doses.

**Dosage in Renal/Hepatic Impairment**
No dose adjustment.

## SIDE EFFECTS

**Frequent:** Insomnia, heartburn, nervousness, abdominal distention, diaphoresis, acne, mood swings, increased appetite, facial flushing, delayed wound healing, increased susceptibility to infection, diarrhea, constipation. **Occasional:** Headache, edema, change in skin color, frequent urination. **Rare:** Tachycardia, allergic reaction (rash, urticaria), psychological changes, hallucinations, depression.

## ADVERSE EFFECTS/TOXIC REACTIONS

**Long-term therapy:** Muscle wasting (esp. in arms, legs), osteoporosis, spontaneous fractures, amenorrhea, cataracts, glaucoma, peptic ulcer, HF. **Abrupt withdrawal following long-term therapy:** Anorexia, nausea, fever, headache, rebound inflammation, fatigue, weakness, lethargy, dizziness, orthostatic hypotension. Sudden discontinuance may be fatal.

## NURSING CONSIDERATIONS

### BASELINE ASSESSMENT

Question medical history as listed in Precautions. Obtain baselines for height, weight, B/P, serum glucose, electrolytes. Check results of initial tests (tuberculosis [TB] skin test, X-rays, EKG).

### INTERVENTION/EVALUATION

Monitor B/P, serum electrolytes, glucose, results of bone mineral density test, height, weight in children. Be alert to infection (sore throat, fever, vague symptoms); assess oral cavity daily for signs of candida infection.

### PATIENT/FAMILY TEACHING

• Report fever, sore throat, muscle aches, sudden weight gain, swelling, loss of appetite, or fatigue. • Avoid alcohol, minimize use of caffeine. • Maintain fastidious oral hygiene. • Do not abruptly discontinue without physician's approval. • Avoid exposure to chickenpox, measles.

# pregabalin `TOP 100`

pre-**gab**-a-lin
(Apo-Pregabalin ✦, Lyrica)

## ◆CLASSIFICATION

**CLINICAL:** Anticonvulsant, antineuralgic, analgesic **(Schedule V).**

## USES

Adjunctive therapy in treatment of partial-onset seizures. Management of neuropathic pain associated with diabetic peripheral neuropathy or spinal cord injury. Management of postherpetic neuralgia. Management of fibromyalgia.

## PRECAUTIONS

**Contraindications:** Hypersensitivity to pregabalin. **Cautions:** HF, renal impairment, cardiovascular disease, diabetes, history of angioedema, pts at risk for suicide. Concurrent use of thiazolidine antidiabetics (e.g., Actos).

## ACTION

Binds to calcium channel sites in CNS tissue, inhibiting excitatory neurotransmitter release. Exerts antinociceptive, anticonvulsant activity. **Therapeutic Effect:** Decreases symptoms of painful peripheral neuropathy; decreases frequency of partial seizures.

## PHARMACOKINETICS

Well absorbed following PO administration. Eliminated in urine unchanged. **Half-life:** 6 hrs.

## ⌛ LIFESPAN CONSIDERATIONS

**Pregnancy/Lactation:** Increased risk of fetal skeletal abnormalities. Unknown if distributed in breast milk. **Children:** Safety and efficacy not established. **Elderly:** Age-related renal impairment may require dosage adjustment.

## INTERACTIONS

**DRUG:** Alcohol, barbiturates, narcotic analgesics, other sedative agents may increase sedative effect. **HERBAL:** Gotu kola, kava kava, St. John's wort, valerian may increase CNS depression. **FOOD:** None known. **LAB VALUES:** May increase CPK. May cause mild PR interval prolongation. May decrease platelet count.

## AVAILABILITY (Rx)

**Solution, Oral:** 20 mg/ml.

🥄 **Capsules (Lyrica):** 25 mg, 50 mg, 75 mg, 100 mg, 150 mg, 200 mg, 225 mg, 300 mg.

## ADMINISTRATION/HANDLING

• Give without regard to food. • Do not break, crush, or open capsule.

## INDICATIONS/ROUTES/DOSAGE

**Partial-Onset Seizures**
**PO: ADULTS, ELDERLY:** Initially, 75 mg twice daily or 50 mg 3 times/day. May increase dose based on tolerability/effect. **Maximum:** 600 mg/day.

**Neuropathic Pain (Diabetes-Associated)**
**PO: ADULTS, ELDERLY:** Initially, 50 mg 3 times/day. **Maximum:** 300 mg/day in 3 divided doses.

**Postherpetic Neuralgia, Neuropathic Pain Associated with Spinal Cord Injury**
**PO: ADULTS, ELDERLY:** Initially, 75 mg twice daily or 50 mg 3 times/day. May increase to 300 mg/day within 1 wk. May further increase to 600 mg/day after 2–4 wks. **Maximum:** 600 mg/day.

**Fibromyalgia**
**PO: ADULTS, ELDERLY:** Initially, 75 mg twice daily. May increase to 150 mg twice daily within 1 wk. **Maximum:** 225 mg twice daily.

**Dosage in Renal Impairment**

| Creatinine Clearance | Daily Dosage |
| --- | --- |
| 30–60 ml/min | 75–300 mg in 2–3 divided doses |
| 15–29 ml/min | 25–150 mg in 1 or 2 doses |
| Less than 15 ml/min | 25–75 mg once daily |

**Dosage for Hemodialysis**
◀ **ALERT** ▶ Take supplemental dose immediately following dialysis.

| Daily Dosage | Supplemental Dosage |
| --- | --- |
| 25 mg | Single dose of 25 mg or 50 mg |
| 25–50 mg | Single dose of 50 mg or 75 mg |
| 75 mg | Single dose of 100 mg or 150 mg |

**Dosage in Hepatic Impairment**
No dose adjustment.

P

## SIDE EFFECTS

**Frequent (32%–12%):** Dizziness, drowsiness, ataxia, peripheral edema. **Occasional (12%–5%):** Weight gain, blurred vision, diplopia, difficulty with concentration, attention, cognition; tremor, dry mouth, headache, constipation, asthenia. **Rare (4%–2%):** Abnormal gait, confusion, incoordination, twitching, flatulence, vomiting, edema, myopathy.

## ADVERSE EFFECTS/ TOXIC REACTIONS

Abrupt withdrawal increases risk of seizure frequency in pts with seizure disorders; withdraw gradually over a minimum of 1 wk.

## NURSING CONSIDERATIONS

### BASELINE ASSESSMENT

**Seizure:** Review history of seizure disorder (type, onset, intensity, frequency, duration, LOC). **Pain:** Assess onset, type, location, and duration of pain.

### INTERVENTION/EVALUATION

Provide safety measures as needed. Assess for seizure activity. Assess for clinical improvement; record onset of relief of pain. Assess for evidence of peripheral edema behind medial malleolus (usually first area of edema). Question for changes in visual acuity.

### PATIENT/FAMILY TEACHING

• Do not abruptly stop taking drug; seizure frequency may be increased. • Avoid tasks that require alertness, motor skills until response to drug is established. • Avoid alcohol. • Carry identification card, bracelet to note seizure disorder, anticonvulsant therapy.

# primidone

**prim**-i-done
(Apo-Primidone ❖, Mysoline)
**Do not confuse primidone with prednisone or pyridoxine.**

## ◆CLASSIFICATION

**PHARMACOTHERAPEUTIC:** Barbiturate. **CLINICAL:** Anticonvulsant.

## USES

Management of partial seizures, generalized tonic-clonic (grand mal) seizures, focal seizures. **OFF-LABEL:** Treatment of essential tremor (familial tremor).

## PRECAUTIONS

**Contraindications:** Hypersensitivity to primidone, phenobarbital; porphyria. **Cautions:** Renal/hepatic impairment, pulmonary insufficiency, elderly, debilitated, children, hypoadrenalism, pts at risk for suicidal thoughts/behavior, depression, history of drug abuse.

## ACTION

Decreases neuron excitability. **Therapeutic Effect:** Reduces seizure activity.

## PHARMACOKINETICS

Rapidly, usually completely absorbed following PO administration. Protein binding: 99%. Metabolized in liver to phenobarbital. Minimal excretion in urine. **Half-life:** 3–6 hrs. (Phenobarbital: 2–5 days.)

## ⏳ LIFESPAN CONSIDERATIONS

**Pregnancy/Lactation:** Crosses placenta; distributed in breast milk. **Children, Elderly:** May produce paradoxical excitement, restlessness.

## INTERACTIONS

**DRUG: Alcohol, other CNS depressants (e.g., lorazepam, morphine, zolpidem)** may increase effects. **Valproic acid** increases concentration, risk of toxicity. **HERBAL: Evening primrose** may decrease seizure threshold. **Gotu kola, kava kava, St. John's wort, valerian** may increase CNS depression. **FOOD:** None known. **LAB VALUES:** May decrease serum bilirubin. **Therapeutic serum level:** 4–12 mcg/ml; **toxic serum level:** greater than 12 mcg/ml.

## AVAILABILITY (Rx)

**Tablets:** 50 mg, 250 mg.

## ADMINISTRATION/HANDLING

**PO**
• Give with food to minimize GI effects.

## INDICATIONS/ROUTES/DOSAGE

**Seizure Control**

**PO: ADULTS, ELDERLY, CHILDREN 8 YRS AND OLDER:** Initially, 100–125 mg/day at bedtime for days 1–3. **Days 4–6:** 100–125 mg twice daily. **Days 7–9:** 100–125 mg 3 times/day. **Usual dose:** 750–1,500 mg/day. **Maximum:** 2 g/day. **CHILDREN YOUNGER THAN 8 YRS:** Initially, 50 mg/day at bedtime for days 1–3. **Days 4–6:** 50 mg twice daily. **Days 7–9:** 100 mg twice daily. **Usual dose:** 10–25 mg/kg/day (375–750 mg) in 3–4 divided doses. **NEONATES:** 12–20 mg/kg/day in divided doses 2–4 times/day.

**Dosage in Renal Impairment**

| Creatine Clearance | Interval |
|---|---|
| 50 ml/min or greater | q12h |
| 10–49 ml/min | q12–24h |
| Less than 10 ml/min | q24h |
| Hemodialysis (HD) | Administer dose post-HD |

**Dosage in Hepatic Impairment**
No dose adjustment.

## SIDE EFFECTS

**Frequent:** Ataxia, dizziness. **Occasional:** Anorexia, drowsiness, altered mental status, nausea, vomiting, paradoxical excitement. **Rare:** Rash.

## ADVERSE EFFECTS/ TOXIC REACTIONS

Abrupt withdrawal after prolonged therapy may produce effects ranging from markedly increased dreaming, nightmares, insomnia, tremor, diaphoresis, vomiting to hallucinations, delirium, seizures, status epilepticus. Skin eruptions may appear as hypersensitivity reaction. Blood dyscrasias, hepatic disease, hypocalcemia occur rarely. Overdose produces cold/clammy skin, hypothermia, severe CNS depression, followed by high fever, coma.

## NURSING CONSIDERATIONS

### BASELINE ASSESSMENT

Review history of seizure disorder (intensity, frequency, duration, LOC). Observe frequently for recurrence of seizure activity. Initiate seizure precautions.

### INTERVENTION/EVALUATION

Monitor for changes in behavior, depression, suicidal ideation. Monitor CBC, neurologic status (frequency, duration, severity of seizures). Monitor for **therapeutic serum level:** 4–12 mcg/ml; **toxic serum level:** more than 12 mcg/ml.

### PATIENT/FAMILY TEACHING

• Do not abruptly discontinue medication after long-term use (may precipitate seizures). • Strict maintenance of drug therapy is essential for seizure control. • Avoid tasks that require alertness, motor skills until response to drug is established; drowsiness usually disappears during continued therapy. • Slowly go from lying to standing. • Avoid alcohol. • Report depression, thoughts of suicide, unusual changes in behavior.

# prochlorperazine

proe-klor-**per**-a-zeen
(Apo-Prochlorperazine ♣, Compazine, Compro)

■ **BLACK BOX ALERT** ■ Increased risk for death in elderly with dementia-related psychosis.
**Do not confuse prochlorperazine with chlorpromazine.**

## ◆CLASSIFICATION

**PHARMACOTHERAPEUTIC:** Phenothiazine. **CLINICAL:** Antiemetic, antipsychotic.

P

## USES

Management of nausea/vomiting. Treatment of acute or chronic psychosis, nonpsychotic anxiety. **OFF-LABEL:** Behavior syndromes in dementia, psychosis/agitation related to Alzheimer's dementia.

## PRECAUTIONS

**Contraindications:** Hypersensitivity to prochlorperazine. Severe CNS depression, coma, children younger than 2 yrs or less than 9 kg. Postoperative nausea/vomiting following pediatric surgery. **Cautions:** History of seizures, Parkinson's disease, elderly, pts at risk for pneumonia, severe renal/hepatic impairment, decreased GI motility, urinary retention, visual problems, narrow angle glaucoma, paralytic ileus, myasthenia gravis, cerebrovascular/cardiovascular disease.

## ACTION

Acts centrally to inhibit/block dopamine receptors in brain. **Therapeutic Effect:** Relieves nausea/vomiting.

## PHARMACOKINETICS

| Route | Onset* | Peak | Duration |
|-------|--------|------|----------|
| PO | 30–40 min | N/A | 3–4 hrs |
| IM | 10–20 min | N/A | 4–6 hrs |
| Rectal | 60 min | N/A | 12 hrs |

*As an antiemetic.

Variably absorbed after PO administration. Widely distributed. Metabolized in liver, GI mucosa. Primarily excreted in urine. Unknown if removed by hemodialysis. **Half-life:** PO: 3–5 hrs, IV: 7 hrs.

## ⌛ LIFESPAN CONSIDERATIONS

**Pregnancy/Lactation:** Crosses placenta. Distributed in breast milk. **Children:** Safety and efficacy not established in pts weighing less than 9 kg or younger than 2 yrs. **Elderly:** More susceptible to orthostatic hypotension, anticholinergic effects (e.g., dry mouth), sedation, extrapyramidal symptoms (EPS); lower dosage recommended.

## INTERACTIONS

**DRUG:** **Alcohol, other CNS depressants** (e.g,. **lorazepam, morphine, zolpidem**) may increase CNS, respiratory depression, hypotensive effects. **Extrapyramidal symptom (EPS)– producing medications** (e.g., **haloperidol metoclopramide, SSRIs**) may increase EPS. **Lithium** may decrease absorption, produce adverse neurologic effects. **MAOIs, tricyclic antidepressants** (e.g., **amitriptyline, doxepin**) may increase anticholinergic, sedative effects. **HERBAL:** **Dong quai, St. John's wort** may increase photosensitization. **Gotu kola, kava kava, St. John's wort, valerian** may increase CNS depression. **FOOD:** None known. **LAB VALUES:** None significant.

## AVAILABILITY (Rx)

**Injection Solution:** 5 mg/ml. **Suppositories (Compro):** 25 mg. **Tablets:** 5 mg, 10 mg.

## ADMINISTRATION/HANDLING

 **IV**

**Rate of Administration** • May give by IV push slowly. Maximum rate: 5 mg/min. **Storage** • Store at room temperature. • Protect from light. • Clear or slightly yellow solutions may be used.

**IM**
• Inject deep IM into outer quadrant of buttocks.

**PO**
• Should be administered with food or water.

**Rectal**
• Moisten suppository with cold water before inserting well into rectum.

## ▦ IV INCOMPATIBILITIES

Furosemide (Lasix), hydrocortisone, hydromorphone (Dilaudid), midazolam (Versed).

## ✦ IV COMPATIBILITIES

Calcium gluconate, dexmedetomidine (Precedex), diphenhydramine (Benadryl), fentanyl, heparin, metoclopramide (Reglan), morphine, potassium chloride, promethazine (Phenergan), propofol (Diprivan).

## INDICATIONS/ROUTES/DOSAGE

### Nausea/Vomiting

**PO: ADULTS, ELDERLY:** 5–10 mg 3–4 times/day. **CHILDREN: GREATER THAN 39 KG:** 5–10 mg q6–8h. **Maximum:** 40 mg/day. **18 KG TO 39 KG:** 2.5 mg q8h or 5 mg q12h. **Maximum:** 15 mg/day. **13 KG TO 18 KG:** 2.5 mg q8–12h. **Maximum:** 10 mg/day. **9–13 KG:** 2.5 mg q12–24h. **Maximum:** 7.5 mg/day.

**IV: ADULTS, ELDERLY:** 2.5–10 mg. May repeat q3–4h. **Maximum:** 10 mg/dose or 40 mg/day.

**IM: ADULTS, ELDERLY:** 5–10 mg q3–4h. **CHILDREN:** 0.1–0.15 mg/kg/dose q8–12h. **Maximum:** 40 mg/day.

**Rectal: ADULTS, ELDERLY:** 25 mg twice daily.

### Psychosis

**PO: ADULTS, ELDERLY:** 5–10 mg 3–4 times/day. **Maximum:** 150 mg/day. **CHILDREN 2–12 YRS:** 2.5 mg 2–3 times/day. **Maximum daily dose:** 25 mg for children 6–12 yrs; 20 mg for children 2–5 yrs.

**IM: ADULTS, ELDERLY:** 10–20 mg q4h. **CHILDREN:** 0.13 mg/kg/dose.

### Dosage in Renal/Hepatic Impairment

No dose adjustment.

## SIDE EFFECTS

**Frequent:** Drowsiness, hypotension, dizziness, fainting (commonly occurring after first dose, occasionally after subsequent doses, rarely with oral form). **Occasional:** Dry mouth, blurred vision, lethargy, constipation, diarrhea, myalgia, nasal congestion, peripheral edema, urinary retention.

## ADVERSE EFFECTS/TOXIC REACTIONS

Extrapyramidal symptoms (EPS) appear dose related and are divided into three categories: akathisia (e.g., inability to sit still, tapping of feet), parkinsonian symptoms (mask-like face, tremors, shuffling gait, hypersalivation), acute dystonias (torticollis [neck muscle spasm], opisthotonos [rigidity of back muscles], oculogyric crisis [rolling back of eyes]). Dystonic reaction may produce diaphoresis, pallor. Tardive dyskinesia (tongue protrusion, puffing of cheeks, puckering of mouth) occurs rarely and may be irreversible. Abrupt withdrawal after long-term therapy may precipitate nausea, vomiting, gastritis, dizziness, tremors. Blood dyscrasias, particularly agranulocytosis, mild leukopenia, may occur. May lower seizure threshold.

## NURSING CONSIDERATIONS

### BASELINE ASSESSMENT

Avoid skin contact with solution (contact dermatitis). **Antiemetic:** Assess for dehydration (poor skin turgor, dry mucous membranes, longitudinal furrows in tongue). **Antipsychotic:** Assess behavior, appearance, emotional status, response to environment, speech pattern, thought content.

### INTERVENTION/EVALUATION

Monitor B/P for hypotension. Assess for EPS. Monitor WBC, differential count for blood dyscrasias. Monitor for fine tongue movement (may be early sign of tardive dyskinesia). Supervise suicidal-risk pt closely during early therapy (as depression lessens, energy level improves, increasing suicide potential). Assess for therapeutic response (interest in surroundings, improvement in self-care, increased ability to concentrate, relaxed facial expression or relief of nausea, vomiting).

### PATIENT/FAMILY TEACHING

• Limit caffeine. • Avoid alcohol. • Avoid tasks requiring alertness, motor skills until response to drug is established (may cause drowsiness, impairment).

P

---

✦ Canadian trade name     🔰 Non-Crushable Drug     🔲 High Alert drug

# progesterone

pro-**jes**-te-rone
(Crinone, Endometrin Vaginal
Insert, Prochieve, Prometrium)

■ **BLACK BOX ALERT** ■ Not indicated to prevent coronary heart disease. Risk of dementia may be increased in postmenopausal women.

◆**CLASSIFICATION**

**PHARMACOTHERAPEUTIC:** Progestin.
**CLINICAL:** Hormone.

## USES

**PO:** Prevent endometrial hyperplasia in nonhysterectomized, postmenopausal women receiving conjugated estrogens, secondary amenorrhea. **IM:** Amenorrhea, abnormal uterine bleeding due to hormonal imbalance. **Vaginal gel:** Treatment of infertility, secondary amenorrhea. **Vaginal insert:** Treatment of infertility. **OFF-LABEL:** Reduce risk of recurrent preterm birth.

## PRECAUTIONS

**Contraindications:** Hypersensitivity to progesterone. History of or suspected carcinoma of breast, active breast cancer; thromboembolic disorders, thrombophlebitis, missed abortion or ectopic pregnancy, severe hepatic dysfunction, undiagnosed abnormal vaginal bleeding, use as a pregnancy test. **Cautions:** Diabetes, conditions aggravated by fluid retention (e.g., asthma, epilepsy, migraine, cardiac/renal dysfunction), history of mental depression.

## ACTION

Promotes mammary gland development, relaxes uterine smooth muscle, induces secretory changes in the endometrium, blocks follicular maturation and ovulation, maintains pregnancy. **Therapeutic Effect:** Decreases abnormal uterine bleeding; transforms endometrium from proliferative to secretory in estrogen-primed endometrium.

## PHARMACOKINETICS

Protein binding: 96%–99%. Metabolized in liver. Excreted in bile, urine. **Half-life (vaginal gel):** 5–20 min.

## ⧖ LIFESPAN CONSIDERATIONS

**Pregnancy/Lactation:** Distributed in breast milk. Avoid use during pregnancy. None established for vaginal gel, vaginal insert, or injection. **Children:** Safety and efficacy not established. **Elderly:** No age-related precautions noted.

## INTERACTIONS

**DRUG: CYP3A4 inducers (e.g., carbamazepine, phenobarbital, phenytoin, rifampin)** may decrease effects. **HERBAL: St. John's wort** may decrease effect. **FOOD:** None known. **LAB VALUES:** May alter HDL, cholesterol, triglycerides, LDL. May increase hepatic function values.

## AVAILABILITY (Rx)

**Capsules (Prometrium):** 100 mg, 200 mg. **Injection Oil:** 50 mg/ml. **Vaginal Gel (Crinone, Prochieve):** 4% (45 mg/dose), 8% (90 mg/dose). **Vaginal Insert (Endometrin Vaginal Insert):** 100 mg. **Vaginal suppository:** 25 mg, 50 mg, 100 mg, 200 mg, 400 mg.

## ADMINISTRATION/HANDLING

**IM**
• Store at room temperature. • Administer only deep IM in large muscle mass.

**PO**
• If given in morning, administer 2 hrs after breakfast with full glass of water.

**Vaginal Gel**
• Remove applicator from sealed wrapper. Do not remove twist-off tab at this time. • Hold applicator by thick end. Shake down several times (like a thermometer) to ensure contents are at thin end. • Hold applicator by flat section of thick end and twist off tab at other end. Do not squeeze thick end while twisting tab (could force some gel to be released before insertion).

• Insert applicator into vagina either in sitting position or lying on back with knees bent. • Insert thin end well into vagina. • Squeeze thick end of applicator to deposit gel. • Remove applicator, discard.

## INDICATIONS/ROUTES/DOSAGE

**Amenorrhea**
PO: **ADULTS:** 400 mg daily in evening for 10 days.
IM: **ADULTS:** 5–10 mg for 6–8 days. Withdrawal bleeding expected in 48–72 hrs if ovarian activity produced proliferative endometrium.
**Vaginal: ADULTS:** Apply 45 mg (4% gel) every other day for 6 or fewer doses. If response inadequate, may increase to 8% gel at same schedule.

**Abnormal Uterine Bleeding**
IM: **ADULTS:** 5–10 mg/day for 6 days. When estrogen given concomitantly, begin progesterone after 2 wks of estrogen therapy; discontinue when menstruation begins.

**Prevention of Endometrial Hyperplasia**
PO: **ADULTS:** 200 mg in evening for 12 days per 28-day cycle, in combination with daily conjugated estrogen.

**Infertility**
**Vaginal Gel: ADULTS:** 90 mg (8% gel) once daily (twice daily in women with partial or complete ovarian failure). If pregnancy occurs, may continue up to 10–12 wks. **Vaginal Insert:** 100 mg 2–3 times/day starting at oocyte retrieval and continuing for up to 10 wks.

**Dosage in Renal Impairment**
No dose adjustment.

**Dosage in Hepatic Impairment**
Contraindicated.

## SIDE EFFECTS

**Frequent:** Breakthrough bleeding/spotting at beginning of therapy, amenorrhea, change in menstrual flow, breast tenderness. **Gel:** Drowsiness. **Occasional:** Edema, weight gain/loss, rash, pruritus, photosensitivity, skin pigmentation. **Rare:** Pain/swelling at injection site, acne, depression, alopecia, hirsutism.

## ADVERSE EFFECTS/TOXIC REACTIONS

Thrombophlebitis, cerebrovascular disorders, retinal thrombosis, pulmonary embolism occur rarely.

## NURSING CONSIDERATIONS

### BASELINE ASSESSMENT
Question for possibility of pregnancy, hypersensitivity to progestins before initiating therapy. Obtain baseline weight, serum glucose level, B/P.

### INTERVENTION/EVALUATION
Check weight daily; report wkly gain over 5 lbs. Assess skin for rash, urticaria. Immediately report development of chest pain, sudden shortness of breath, sudden decrease in vision, migraine headache, pain (esp. with swelling, warmth, redness) in calves, numbness of arm/leg (thrombotic disorders). Check B/P periodically. Note progesterone therapy on pathology specimens.

### PATIENT/FAMILY TEACHING
• Use sunscreen, protective clothing to protect from sunlight, ultraviolet light until tolerance determined. • Report abnormal vaginal bleeding, other related symptoms. • Stop taking medication, contact physician at once if pregnancy suspected. • If using vaginal gel, avoid tasks that require alertness, motor skills until response to drug is established.

## promethazine

proe-**meth**-a-zeen
(Phenadoz, Phenergan, Promethegan)

■ **BLACK BOX ALERT** ■ Fatalities due to respiratory depression reported in children 2 yrs and younger.

Severe tissue injury, including gangrene, may occur with intravenous injection (preferred route is deep intramuscular). Be alert for signs and symptoms of tissue injury including burning or pain at injection site, phlebitis, swelling, blistering. Risk reduced by diluting promethazine with 10–20 ml 0.9% NaCl or diluting in a minibag (piggyback); administer slowly over 10–15 min; use large veins or central venous site (no hand or wrist veins).

**Do not confuse Phenergan with phenelzine, or promethazine with chlorpromazine or prednisone.**

### FIXED-COMBINATION(S)

**Phenergan with codeine:** promethazine/codeine (a cough suppressant): 6.25 mg/10 mg/5 ml. **Phenergan VC:** promethazine/phenylephrine (a vasoconstrictor): 6.25 mg/5 mg/5 ml. **Phenergan VC with codeine:** promethazine/phenylephrine/codeine: 6.25 mg/5 mg/10 mg/5 ml.

### ◆CLASSIFICATION

**PHARMACOTHERAPEUTIC:** Phenothiazine. **CLINICAL:** Antihistamine, antiemetic, sedative-hypnotic.

### USES

Treatment of allergic conditions, motion sickness, nausea, vomiting. May be used as mild sedative. Adjunct to postoperative analgesia. **OFF-LABEL:** Nausea/vomiting related to pregnancy.

### PRECAUTIONS

**Contraindications:** Hypersensitivity to promethazine, other phenothiazines. Children 2 yrs and younger (may cause fatal respiratory depression), severe CNS depression, coma, treatment of lower respiratory tract symptoms including asthma. **Cautions:** Cardiovascular/hepatic or respiratory impairment, narrow-angle glaucoma, prostatic hypertrophy, GI/GU obstruction, urinary retention, visual problems, decreased GI motility, myasthenia gravis,

Parkinson's disease, elderly, bone marrow depression, asthma, peptic ulcer, history of seizures, sleep apnea, pts suspected of Reye's syndrome.

### ACTION

Block postsynaptic dopaminergic receptors; competes with histamine for histamine receptors; possesses muscarinic blocking effect. **Therapeutic Effect:** Prevents allergic responses mediated by histamine (urticaria, pruritus). Prevents, relieves nausea/vomiting. Produces mild sedative effect.

### PHARMACOKINETICS

| Route | Onset | Peak | Duration |
|-------|-------|------|----------|
| PO | 20 min | N/A | 2–8 hrs |
| IV | 3–5 min | N/A | 2–8 hrs |
| IM | 20 min | N/A | 2–8 hrs |
| Rectal | 20 min | N/A | 2–8 hrs |

Well absorbed from GI tract after IM administration. Protein binding: 83%. Widely distributed. Metabolized in liver. Primarily excreted in urine. Not removed by hemodialysis. **Half-life:** 9–16 hrs.

### ⧗ LIFESPAN CONSIDERATIONS

**Pregnancy/Lactation:** Readily crosses placenta. Unknown if drug is distributed in breast milk. May inhibit platelet aggregation in neonates if taken within 2 wks of birth. May produce jaundice, extrapyramidal symptoms (EPS) in neonates if taken during pregnancy. **Children:** May experience increased excitement. Not recommended for pts younger than 2 yrs. **Elderly:** More sensitive to dizziness, sedation, confusion, hypotension, hyperexcitability, anticholinergic effects (e.g., dry mouth).

### INTERACTIONS

**DRUG: Alcohol, CNS depressants** (e.g., **lorazepam, morphine, zolpidem**) may increase CNS depressant effects. **Anticholinergics** (e.g., **dicyclomine, glycopyrrolate, scopolamine**) may increase anticholinergic effects. **MAOIs** (e.g., **phenelzine, selegiline**)

P

may prolong, intensify anticholinergic, CNS depressant effects. **HERBAL: Gotu kola, kava kava, St. John's wort, valerian** may increase CNS depression. **FOOD:** None known. **LAB VALUES:** May suppress wheal/flare reactions to antigen skin testing unless discontinued 4 days before testing.

## AVAILABILITY (Rx)

**Injection Solution:** 25 mg/ml, 50 mg/ml. **Solution, Oral:** 6.25 mg/5 ml. **Suppositories:** 12.5 mg, 25 mg, 50 mg. **Syrup:** 6.25 mg/5 ml. **Tablets:** 12.5 mg, 25 mg, 50 mg.

## ADMINISTRATION/HANDLING

◄**ALERT**► IM is preferred route; avoid IV if possible. Significant tissue necrosis may occur if given subcutaneously. Inadvertent intra-arterial injection may produce significant arteriospasm, resulting in severe circulation impairment.

 **IV**

**Reconstitution** • Dilute with 10–20 ml 0.9% NaCl or prepare minibag.
**Rate of Administration** • Administer slowly over 10–15 min. • Use large vein or central venous site (no hand or wrist veins). • Too-rapid rate of infusion may result in transient fall in B/P, producing orthostatic hypotension, reflex tachycardia, serious tissue injury.
**Storage** • Store at room temperature.

**IM**
• Inject deep IM.

**PO**
• Give with food or fluids to reduce GI distress. • Scored tablets may be crushed.

**Rectal**
• Refrigerate suppository. • Moisten suppository with cold water before inserting well into rectum.

## ▦ IV INCOMPATIBILITIES

Allopurinol (Aloprim), amphotericin B complex (Abelcet, AmBisome, Amphotec), heparin, ketorolac (Toradol), nalbuphine (Nubain), piperacillin and tazobactam (Zosyn).

## ▦ IV COMPATIBILITIES

Dexmedetomidine (Precedex), diphenhydramine (Benadryl), hydromorphone (Dilaudid), midazolam (Versed), morphine.

## INDICATIONS/ROUTES/DOSAGE

◄**ALERT**► Contraindicated in children 2 yrs and younger.

**Allergic Symptoms**
**PO: ADULTS, ELDERLY:** 6.25–12.5 mg 3 times/day plus 25 mg at bedtime. **CHILDREN:** 0.1 mg/kg/dose (**Maximum:** 12.5 mg) 4 times/day plus 0.5 mg/kg/dose (**Maximum:** 25 mg) at bedtime.
**IV, IM: ADULTS, ELDERLY:** 25 mg. May repeat in 2 hrs.

**Motion Sickness**
**PO: ADULTS, ELDERLY:** 25 mg 30–60 min before departure; may repeat in 8–12 hrs, then every morning on rising and before evening meal. **CHILDREN:** 0.5 mg/kg 30–60 min before departure; may repeat in 8–12 hrs, then every morning on rising and before evening meal. **Maximum:** 25 mg twice daily.

**Prevention of Nausea/Vomiting**
**PO, IV, IM, Rectal: ADULTS, ELDERLY:** 12.5–25 mg q4–6h as needed. **CHILDREN:** 0.25–1 mg/kg q4–6h as needed. **Maximum:** 25 mg/dose.

**Sedative**
**PO, IV, IM, Rectal: ADULTS, ELDERLY:** 12.5–50 mg/dose. **CHILDREN:** 12.5–25 mg/dose.

**Dosage in Renal Impairment**
No dose adjustment.

**Dosage in Hepatic Impairment**
Use caution.

**P**

## SIDE EFFECTS

**Frequent:** Drowsiness, dry mouth, nose, throat; urinary retention, thickening of bronchial secretions. **Occasional:** Epigastric distress, flushing, visual disturbances, hearing disturbances, wheezing, paresthesia, diaphoresis, chills, disorientation, hypotension, confusion, syncope in elderly. **Rare:** Dizziness, urticaria, photosensitivity, nightmares.

## ADVERSE EFFECTS/ TOXIC REACTIONS

Paradoxical reaction (particularly in children) manifested as excitation, anxiety, tremor, hyperactive reflexes, seizures. Long-term therapy may produce extrapyramidal symptoms (EPS) noted as dystonia (abnormal movements), pronounced motor restlessness (most frequently in children), parkinsonism (esp. noted in elderly). Blood dyscrasias, particularly agranulocytosis, occur rarely.

## NURSING CONSIDERATIONS

### BASELINE ASSESSMENT

Assess allergy symptoms. Assess B/P, pulse for bradycardia, tachycardia if pt is given parenteral form. If used as antiemetic, assess for dehydration (poor skin turgor, dry mucous membranes, longitudinal furrows in tongue). Assess LOC.

### INTERVENTION/EVALUATION

Monitor serum electrolytes in pts with severe vomiting. Assist with ambulation if drowsiness, dizziness occurs. Monitor for relief of nausea, vomiting, allergic symptoms.

### PATIENT/FAMILY TEACHING

• Drowsiness, dry mouth may be expected response to drug. • Avoid tasks that require alertness, motor skills until response to drug is established. • Sugarless gum, sips of water may relieve dry mouth. • Coffee, tea may help reduce drowsiness. • Report visual disturbances, involuntary movements, restlessness. • Avoid alcohol, other CNS depressants. • Avoid prolonged exposure to sunlight.

# propafenone

proe-**paf**-e-nown
(Apo-Propafenone ✦, Rythmol, Rythmol SR)

■ **BLACK BOX ALERT** ■ Mortality or nonfatal cardiac arrest rate (7.7%) in asymptomatic non–life-threatening ventricular arrhythmia pts with recent MI (more than 6 days but less than 2 years prior) reported.

## ◆CLASSIFICATION

**PHARMACOTHERAPEUTIC:** Class 1c antiarrhythmic. **CLINICAL:** Antiarrhythmic.

## USES

Treatment of life-threatening ventricular arrhythmias (e.g., sustained ventricular tachycardias). Treatment of paroxysmal atrial fibrillation/flutter (PAF) or paroxysmal supraventricular tachycardia (PSVT) in pts with disabling symptoms and without structural heart disease. **Rythmol SR:** Prolong the time to recurrence of atrial fibrillation/flutter or paroxysmal supraventricular tachycardia in pts with disabling symptoms without structural heart disease. **OFF-LABEL:** Treatment following cardioversion of recent-onset atrial fibrillation; supraventricular tachycardia in pts with Wolff-Parkinson-White syndrome.

## PRECAUTIONS

**Contraindications:** Hypersensitivity to propafenone. Bradycardia, bronchospastic disorders, cardiogenic shock, electrolyte imbalance, sinoatrial, AV, intraventricular impulse generation or conduction disorders (e.g., sick sinus syndrome, AV block) without pacemaker, uncontrolled HF, hypotension. **Cautions:** Renal/hepatic impairment, myasthenia gravis, concurrent use of other medications that prolong QT interval, hypokalemia, hypomagnesemia.

## ACTION

Decreases fast sodium current in Purkinje/myocardial cells. Decreases excitability, automaticity; prolongs conduction velocity, refractory period. **Therapeutic Effect:** Suppresses arrhythmias.

## PHARMACOKINETICS

Nearly completely absorbed following PO administration. Protein binding: 85%–97%. Metabolized in liver. Primarily excreted in feces. **Half-life:** 2–10 hrs.

## ⧗ LIFESPAN CONSIDERATIONS

**Pregnancy/Lactation:** Unknown if drug crosses placenta or is distributed in breast milk. **Children:** Safety and efficacy not established. **Elderly:** No age-related precautions noted.

## INTERACTIONS

**DRUG: Amiodarone** may affect cardiac conduction, repolarization. May increase **digoxin** concentration. May increase effects of **warfarin. CYP3A4 inhibitors (e.g., ketoconazole, erythromycin)** may increase concentration/toxicity. **HERBAL: St. John's wort** may decrease concentration/effect. **Ephedra** may worsen arrhythmias. **FOOD: Grapefruit products** may increase concentration. **LAB VALUES:** May cause EKG changes (e.g., QRS widening, PR interval prolongation), positive ANA titer.

## AVAILABILITY (Rx)

Tablets (Rythmol): 150 mg, 225 mg, 300 mg.

🦫 Capsules (Extended-Release [Rythmol SR]): 225 mg, 325 mg, 425 mg.

## ADMINISTRATION/HANDLING

**PO**
• May take without regard to meals.
• Give whole; do not break, crush, divide, or open capsules.

## INDICATIONS/ROUTES/DOSAGE

**Ventricular Arrhythmias, PAT, PSVT**
**PO** *(Immediate-Release):* **ADULTS, ELDERLY:** Initially, 150 mg q8h. May increase at 3- to 4-day intervals to 225 mg q8h, then to 300 mg q8h. **Maximum:** 900 mg/day.

**Atrial Fibrillation (Prevention of Recurrence)**
**PO** *(Immediate-Release):* **ADULTS, ELDERLY:** Initially, 150 mg q8h. May increase at 3- to 4-day intervals to 225 mg q8h, then to 300 mg q8h. **Maximum:** 900 mg/day. *(Extended-Release):* **ADULTS, ELDERLY:** Initially, 225 mg q12h. May increase at 5-day intervals to 325 mg q12h. **Maximum:** 425 mg q12h.

**Dosage in Renal Impairment**
No dose adjustment.

**Dosage in Hepatic Impairment**
Use caution.

## SIDE EFFECTS

**Frequent (13%–7%):** Dizziness, nausea, vomiting, altered taste, constipation. **Occasional (6%–3%):** Headache, dyspnea, blurred vision, dyspepsia. **Rare (Less Than 2%):** Rash, weakness, dry mouth, diarrhea, edema, hot flashes.

## ADVERSE EFFECTS/ TOXIC REACTIONS

May produce, worsen arrhythmias. Overdose may produce hypotension, drowsiness, bradycardia, atrioventricular conduction disturbances.

## NURSING CONSIDERATIONS

### BASELINE ASSESSMENT

Correct electrolyte imbalance before administering medication. Obtain baseline EKG. Screen for cardiac contraindications.

### INTERVENTION/EVALUATION

Assess pulse for quality, rhythm, rate. Monitor EKG for cardiac performance or changes, particularly widening of QRS, prolongation of PR interval. Question for visual disturbances, headache, GI upset. Monitor fluid, serum electrolyte levels. Monitor daily pattern of bowel activity, stool consistency. Assess for dizziness, unsteadiness. Monitor LFT. Monitor for therapeutic serum level (0.06–1 mcg/ml).

P

## PATIENT/FAMILY TEACHING

• Compliance with therapy regimen is essential to control arrhythmias. • Altered taste sensation may occur. • Report headache, blurred vision. • Avoid tasks that require alertness, motor skills until response to drug is established. • Report chest pain, difficulty breathing, palpitations.

---

# propofol

**HIGH ALERT**

proe-poe-fol
(Diprivan, Fresenius Propoven)
**Do not confuse Diprivan with Diflucan or Ditropan, or propofol with fospropofol.**

## ◆CLASSIFICATION

**PHARMACOTHERAPEUTIC:** Rapid-acting general anesthetic. **CLINICAL:** Sedative-hypnotic.

## USES

Induction/maintenance of anesthesia. Continuous sedation in intubated and respiratory controlled adult pts in ICU. **OFF-LABEL:** Postop antiemetic, refractory status epilepticus.

## PRECAUTIONS

**Contraindications:** Hypersensitivity to propofol, eggs, egg products, soybean or soy products. **Cautions:** Hemodynamically unstable pts, hypovolemia, severe cardiac/respiratory disease, elevated ICP, impaired cerebral circulation, preexisting pancreatitis, hyperlipidemia, history of epilepsy, seizure disorder, elderly, debilitated, pts allergic to peanuts.

## ACTION

Cause CNS depression through agonist action of GABA receptors. **Therapeutic Effect:** Produces hypnosis rapidly.

## PHARMACOKINETICS

| Route | Onset | Peak | Duration |
|-------|-------|------|----------|
| IV | 40 sec | N/A | 3–10 min |

Rapidly, extensively distributed. Protein binding: 97%–99%. Metabolized in liver. Primarily excreted in urine. Unknown if removed by hemodialysis. Rapid awakening can occur 10–15 min after discontinuation. **Half-life:** 3–12 hrs.

## ▧ LIFESPAN CONSIDERATIONS

**Pregnancy/Lactation:** Unknown if drug crosses placenta. Distributed in breast milk. Not recommended for obstetrics, breastfeeding mothers. **Pregnancy Category B. Children:** Safety and efficacy not established. FDA approved for use in those 2 mos and older. **Elderly:** No age-related precautions noted; lower dosages recommended.

## INTERACTIONS

**DRUG: Alcohol, CNS depressants (e.g., lorazepam, morphine, zolpidem)** may increase CNS, respiratory depression, hypotensive effects. **Antihypertensive medications (e.g. amlodipine, lisinopril, valsartan)** may increase hypotensive effects. **HERBAL:** None significant. **FOOD:** None known. **LAB VALUES:** May increase serum triglycerides.

## AVAILABILITY (Rx)

**Injection Emulsion:** 10 mg/ml.

## ADMINISTRATION/HANDLING

▧ **IV**

◀**ALERT**▶ Do not give through same IV line with blood or plasma.
**Reconstitution** • May give undiluted, or dilute only with D₅W. • Do not dilute to concentration less than 2 mg/ml (4 ml D₅W to 1 ml propofol yields 2 mg/ml).
**Rate of Administration** • Too-rapid IV administration may produce marked severe hypotension, respiratory depression, irregular muscular movements. • Observe for signs of extravasation (pain, discolored skin patches, white or blue color to peripheral IV site area, delayed onset of drug action).

---

**Storage** • Store at room temperature. • Discard unused portions. • Do not use if emulsion separates. • Shake well before using.

## 🔲 IV INCOMPATIBILITIES

Amikacin (Amikin), amphotericin B complex (Abelcet, AmBisome, Amphotec), bretylium (Bretylol), calcium chloride, ciprofloxacin (Cipro), diazepam (Valium), digoxin (Lanoxin), doxorubicin (Adriamycin), gentamicin (Garamycin), methylprednisolone (Solu-Medrol), minocycline (Minocin), phenytoin (Dilantin), tobramycin (Nebcin), verapamil (Isoptin).

## 🔲 IV COMPATIBILITIES

Acyclovir (Zovirax), bumetanide (Bumex), calcium gluconate, ceftazidime (Fortaz), dexmedetomidine (Precedex), dobutamine (Dobutrex), dopamine (Intropin), enalapril (Vasotec), fentanyl, heparin, insulin, labetalol (Normodyne, Trandate), lidocaine, lorazepam (Ativan), magnesium, milrinone (Primacor), nitroglycerin, norepinephrine (Levophed), potassium chloride, vancomycin (Vancocin).

## INDICATIONS/ROUTES/ DOSAGE

### Anesthesia

**IV: ADULTS, ELDERLY:** Induction, 2–2.5 mg/kg (approximately 40 mg q10sec until onset of anesthesia). **Maintenance:** Initially, 100–200 mcg/kg/min or 6–12 mg/kg/hr for 10–15 min. Usual maintenance infusion: 50–100 mcg/kg/min or 3–6 mg/kg/hr. **CHILDREN 3–16 YRS:** Induction, 2.5–3.5 mg/kg over 20–30 sec, then infusion of 125–300 mcg/kg/min or 7.5–18 mg/kg/hr.

### Sedation in ICU

**IV: ADULTS, ELDERLY:** Initially, 5 mcg/kg/min (0.3 mg/kg/hr) for 5 min, then titrate to 5–80 mcg/kg/min (0.3–4.8 mg/kg/hr) in 5–10 mcg/kg/min (0.3–0.6 mg/kg/hr) increments allowing minimum of 5 min between dose adjustments. **Usual maintenance:** 5–50 mcg/kg/min (0.3–3 mg/kg/hr).

**Dosage in Renal/Hepatic Impairment**
No dose adjustment.

## SIDE EFFECTS

**Frequent:** Involuntary muscle movements, apnea (common during induction; often lasts longer than 60 sec), hypotension, nausea, vomiting, IV site burning/stinging. **Occasional:** Twitching, thrashing, headache, dizziness, bradycardia, hypertension, fever, abdominal cramps, paresthesia, coldness, cough, hiccups, facial flushing, green-tinted urine. **Rare:** Rash, dry mouth, agitation, confusion, myalgia, thrombophlebitis.

**Dosage in Renal/Hepatic Impairment**
No dose adjustment.

## ADVERSE EFFECTS/ TOXIC REACTIONS

Continuous infusion or repeated intermittent infusions of propofol may result in extreme drowsiness, respiratory depression, circulatory depression, delirium. Too-rapid IV administration may produce severe hypotension, respiratory depression, involuntary muscle movements. Pt may experience acute allergic reaction, characterized by abdominal pain, anxiety, restlessness, dyspnea, erythema, hypotension, pruritus, rhinitis, urticaria.

## NURSING CONSIDERATIONS

### BASELINE ASSESSMENT

Resuscitative equipment, suction, $O_2$ must be available. Obtain vital signs before administration.

### INTERVENTION/EVALUATION

Observe pt for signs of wakefulness, agitation. Monitor respiratory rate, B/P, heart rate, $O_2$ saturation, ABGs, depth of sedation, serum lipid, triglycerides (if used longer than 24 hrs). May change urine color to green.

P

## propranolol

proe-**pran**-oh-lol
(Apo-Propranolol ✿, Hemangeol,
<u>Inderal LA</u>, Inderal XL,
<u>InnoPran XL</u>, Novo-Pranol ✿)

■ **BLACK BOX ALERT** ■ Severe angina exacerbation, MI, ventricular arrhythmias may occur in angina pts after abrupt discontinuation; must taper gradually over 1–2 wks. **Do not confuse Inderal LA with Adderall, Imdur, Isordil, or Toradol, or propranolol with Pravachol.**

### FIXED-COMBINATION(S)

**Inderide:** propranolol/hydrochlorothiazide (a diuretic): 40 mg/25 mg, 80 mg/25 mg. **Inderide LA:** propranolol/hydrochlorothiazide (a diuretic): 80 mg/50 mg, 120 mg/50 mg, 160 mg/50 mg.

### ◆CLASSIFICATION

**PHARMACOTHERAPEUTIC:** Beta-adrenergic blocker. **CLINICAL:** Antihypertensive, antianginal, antiarrhythmic, antimigraine.

### USES

Treatment of angina pectoris, supraventricular arrhythmias, essential tremors, hypertension, ventricular tachycardia, obstructive hypertrophic cardiomyopathy, treatment of proliferating infantile hemangioma requiring systemic therapy, migraine headache, pheochromocytoma, prevention of MI. **Hemangeol:** Treatment of proliferating infantile hemangioma needing systemic therapy. **OFF-LABEL:** Treatment adjunct for anxiety, tremor due to Parkinson's disease, alcohol withdrawal, aggressive behavior, schizophrenia, antipsychotic-induced akathisia, variceal hemorrhage, acute panic.

### PRECAUTIONS

**Contraindications:** Hypersensitivity to propranolol. Bronchial asthma, severe sinus bradycardia, cardiogenic shock, COPD, sick sinus syndrome, heart block other than first-degree (unless pt has functional pacemaker), uncompensated HF. **Hemangeol (Additional):** Premature infants with corrected age younger than 5 wks, infants weighing less than 2 kg; asthma, history of bronchospasm, bradycardia (less than 80 beats/min), greater than first-degree heart block, decompensated HF; B/P less than 50/30 mmHg, pheochromocytoma. **Cautions:** Diabetes, renal/hepatic impairment, Raynaud's disease, hyperthyroidism, myasthenia gravis, psychiatric disease, bronchospastic disease, elderly, history of severe anaphylaxis to allergens.

### ACTION

Blocks beta₁-, beta₂-adrenergic receptors. **Therapeutic Effect:** Slows heart rate; decreases B/P, myocardial contractility, myocardial oxygen demand.

### PHARMACOKINETICS

| Route | Onset | Peak | Duration |
|-------|-------|------|----------|
| PO | 1–2 hrs | N/A | 6 hrs |

Well absorbed from GI tract. Protein binding: 93%. Widely distributed. Metabolized in liver. Primarily excreted in urine. Not removed by hemodialysis. **Half-life:** 4–6 hrs.

### 🅧 LIFESPAN CONSIDERATIONS

**Pregnancy/Lactation:** Crosses placenta. Distributed in breast milk. Avoid use during first trimester. May produce low birth-weight infants, bradycardia, apnea, hypoglycemia, hypothermia during delivery. **Children:** No age-related precautions noted. **Elderly:** Age-related peripheral vascular disease may increase susceptibility to decreased peripheral circulation.

### INTERACTIONS

**DRUG:** Diuretics (e.g., furosemide, HCTZ), other antihypertensives (e.g., amlodipine, lisinopril, valsartan) may increase hypotensive effect. May mask symptoms of hypoglycemia, prolong hypoglycemic effect of **insulin, oral hypoglycemics (e.g., glipizide, metformin). Digoxin** may increase risk for bradycardia. **NSAIDs** may decrease antihypertensive effect. **HERBAL: Ephedra, ginger, licorice, ginseng, yohimbe** may worsen hypertension. **Licorice** may increase water retention. **Garlic, periwinkle** have antihypertensive effects. **FOOD:** None known. **LAB VALUES:** May increase serum antinuclear antibody (ANA) titer, serum BUN, LDH, lipoprotein, alkaline phosphatase, potassium, uric acid, ALT, AST, triglycerides.

## AVAILABILITY (Rx)

Injection Solution: 1 mg/ml. Oral Solution: 20 mg/5 ml, 40 mg/5 ml. Oral Solution (Hemangeol): 4.28 mg/ml. Tablets: 10 mg, 20 mg, 40 mg, 60 mg, 80 mg.

 Capsules (Extended-Release [Inno-Pran XL]): 80 mg, 120 mg.  Capsules (Sustained-Release [Inderal LA]): 60 mg, 80 mg, 120 mg, 160 mg.

## ADMINISTRATION/HANDLING

### 🔲 IV

**Reconstitution** • Give undiluted for IV push. • For IV infusion, may dilute each 1 mg in 10 ml $D_5W$.
**Rate of Administration** • Do not exceed 1 mg/min injection rate. • For IV infusion, give over 30 min.
**Storage** • Store at room temperature. • Once diluted, stable for 24 hrs at room temperature.

### PO

• May crush scored tablets. • Do not break, crush, or open extended- or sustained-release capsules. • Give immediate-release tablets on empty stomach. • Give extended-release, sustained-release without regard to food.

### ▦ IV INCOMPATIBILITIES

Amphotericin B complex (Abelcet, AmBisome, Amphotec).

### ▦ IV COMPATIBILITIES

Alteplase (Activase), heparin, milrinone (Primacor), potassium chloride, propofol (Diprivan).

## INDICATIONS/ROUTES/ DOSAGE

**Hypertension**
**PO: ADULTS, ELDERLY:** *(Immediate Release):* Initially, 40 mg twice daily. May increase dose q3–7days. Usual dose: 120–240 mg/day in 2–3 divided doses. **Maximum:** 640 mg/day. **CHILDREN:** Initially, 1–2 mg/kg/day in 2–3 divided doses. May increase at 3- to 5-day intervals. Usual dose: 4 mg/kg/day. **Maximum:** 4 mg/kg/day.
**PO ADULTS, ELDERLY:** *(Sustained-Release): (Inderal LA):* Initially, 80 mg once daily. **Maintenance:** 120–160 mg/day.
*(Extended-Release):* Initially, 80 mg at bedtime. May increase at 2- to 3-wk intervals. **Maximum:** 120 mg.

**Angina**
**PO: ADULTS, ELDERLY:** *(Immediate Release):* 80–320 mg/day in 2–4 divided doses.
**PO** *(Extended-Release):* Initially, 80 mg/day. **Maximum:** 320 mg/day.

**Arrhythmia**
**IV: ADULTS, ELDERLY:** 1–3 mg. Repeat q2–5min up to total of 5 mg. **CHILDREN:** 0.01–0.1 mg/kg. **Maximum:** Infants, 1 mg; children, 3 mg.
**PO: ADULTS, ELDERLY:** *(Immediate Release):* 10–30 mg q6–8h or 10–40 mg 3–4 times/day. **CHILDREN:** Initially, 0.5–1 mg/kg/day in divided doses q6–8h. May increase q3days. Usual dosage: 2–6 mg/kg/day. **Maximum:** 16 mg/kg/day or 60 mg/day.

**Obstructive Hypertrophic Cardiomyopathy**
**PO: ADULTS, ELDERLY:** *(Immediate Release):* 20–40 mg 3–4 times/day or 80–160 mg once daily as extended-release capsule.

**P**

**Adjunct to Alpha-Blocking Agents to Treat Pheochromocytoma**
PO: **ADULTS, ELDERLY:** 30–60 mg/day in divided doses.

**Migraine Headache**
PO: **ADULTS, ELDERLY:** *(Immediate Release):* Initially, 80 mg/day in 3–4 divided doses or 80 mg once daily as extended-release capsule. May increase by 20–40 mg/dose q3–4wks up to 160–240 mg/day in divided doses. **CHILDREN WEIGHING 35 KG OR LESS:** 10–20 mg 3 times/day. **CHILDREN WEIGHING OVER 35 KG:** 20–40 mg 3 times/day.
**Extended-Release** *(Inderal LA):* **ADULTS, ELDERLY:** Initially, 80 mg daily. Effective range: 160–240 mg/day.

**Reduction of Cardiovascular Mortality, Reinfarction in Pts with Previous MI**
PO: **ADULTS, ELDERLY:** *(Immediate Release):* Initially, 40 mg 3 times/day. Range: 180–240 mg/day in 3–4 divided doses.

**Essential Tremor**
PO: **ADULTS, ELDERLY:** Initially, 40 mg twice daily increased up to 120–320 mg/day in 3 divided doses.

**Infantile Hemangioma**
**Note:** Separate doses by at least 9 hrs during or after feeding.
PO: **INFANTS 5 WKS TO 5 MOS:** Initially, 0.15 ml/kg (0.6 mg/kg) twice daily. After 1 wk, increase to 0.3 ml/kg (1.1 mg/kg) twice daily. After 2 wks, increase to maintenance dose of 0.4 ml/kg (1.7 mg/kg) twice daily.

**Dosage in Renal/Hepatic Impairment**
Use caution.

## SIDE EFFECTS

**Frequent:** Diminished sexual function, drowsiness, difficulty sleeping, unusual fatigue/weakness. **Occasional:** Bradycardia, depression, sensation of coldness in extremities, diarrhea, constipation, anxiety, nasal congestion, nausea, vomiting. **Rare:** Altered taste, dry eyes, pruritus, paresthesia.

## ADVERSE EFFECTS/TOXIC REACTIONS

Overdose may produce profound bradycardia, hypotension. Abrupt withdrawal may result in diaphoresis, palpitations, headache, tremulousness. May precipitate HF, MI in pts with cardiac disease, thyroid storm in pts with thyrotoxicosis, peripheral ischemia in pts with existing peripheral vascular disease. Hypoglycemia may occur in pts with previously controlled diabetes. **Antidote:** Glucagon (see Appendix K for dosage).

## NURSING CONSIDERATIONS

### BASELINE ASSESSMENT

Assess baseline renal function, LFT. Assess B/P, apical pulse immediately before administering drug (if pulse is 60/min or less or systolic B/P is less than 90 mm Hg, withhold medication, contact physician). **Angina:** Record onset, quality, radiation, location, intensity, duration of anginal pain, precipitating factors (exertion, emotional stress).

### INTERVENTION/EVALUATION

Assess pulse for quality, regularity, bradycardia. Monitor EKG for cardiac arrhythmias. Assess fingers for color, numbness (Raynaud's). Assess for evidence of HF (dyspnea [particularly on exertion or lying down], night cough, peripheral edema, distended neck veins). Monitor I&O (increase in weight, decrease in urinary output may indicate HF). Assess for rash, fatigue, behavioral changes. Therapeutic response time ranges from a few days to several wks. Measure B/P near end of dosing interval (determines if B/P is controlled throughout day).

### PATIENT/FAMILY TEACHING

• Do not abruptly discontinue medication. • Compliance with therapy

---

regimen is essential to control hypertension, arrhythmia, anginal pain. • To avoid hypotensive effect, slowly go from lying to standing. • Avoid tasks that require alertness, motor skills until response to drug is established. • Report excessively slow pulse rate (less than 50 beats/min), peripheral numbness, dizziness. • Do not use nasal decongestants, OTC cold preparations (stimulants) without physician approval. • Restrict salt, alcohol intake.

# propylthiouracil

proe-pil-thye-oh-ure-a-sil
(Propyl-Thyracil ✦)

■ **BLACK BOX ALERT** ■ May cause severe hepatic injury, acute hepatic failure, death.

**Do not confuse propylthiouracil with purinethol.**

## ◆CLASSIFICATION

**PHARMACOTHERAPEUTIC:** Thiourea derivative. **CLINICAL:** Antithyroid agent.

## USES

Palliative treatment of hyperthyroidism; adjunct to ameliorate hyperthyroidism in preparation for surgical treatment, radioactive iodine therapy. **OFF-LABEL:** Management of thyrotoxic crises, Graves' disease, thyroid storm.

## PRECAUTIONS

**Contraindications:** Hypersensitivity to propylthiouracil. **Cautions:** In combination with other agranulocytosis-inducing drugs.

## ACTION

Blocks oxidation of iodine in thyroid gland, blocks synthesis of thyroxine, triiodothyronine. **Therapeutic Effect:** Inhibits synthesis of thyroid hormone.

## PHARMACOKINETICS

Readily absorbed from GI tract. Protein binding: 80%. Metabolized in liver.

Excreted in urine. **Half-life:** 1.5–5 hrs.

## INTERACTIONS

**DRUG:** May increase concentration of **digoxin** (as pt becomes euthyroid). May increase effect of **oral anticoagulants** (e.g., **apixaban, warfarin**). **HERBAL:** None significant. **FOOD:** None known. **LAB VALUES:** May increase LDH, serum alkaline phosphatase, bilirubin, ALT, AST, prothrombin time.

## AVAILABILITY (Rx)

**Tablets:** 50 mg.

## ADMINISTRATION/HANDLING

**PO**
• Give with food.

## INDICATIONS/ROUTES/DOSAGE

**Hyperthyroidism**
**PO: ADULTS, ELDERLY:** Initially, 300–400 mg/day (**ELDERLY:** 150–300 mg/day) in divided doses q8h. **Maintenance:** 100–150 mg/day in divided doses q8–12h.

**Dosage in Renal/Hepatic Impairment**
No dose adjustment.

## SIDE EFFECTS

**Frequent:** Urticaria, rash, pruritus, nausea, skin pigmentation, hair loss, headache, paresthesia. **Occasional:** Drowsiness, lymphadenopathy, vertigo. **Rare:** Drug fever, lupus-like syndrome.

## ADVERSE EFFECTS/ TOXIC REACTIONS

Agranulocytosis (may occur as long as 4 mos after therapy), pancytopenia, fatal hepatitis have occurred.

## NURSING CONSIDERATIONS

### BASELINE ASSESSMENT
Obtain baseline weight, pulse.

### INTERVENTION/EVALUATION
Monitor pulse, weight daily. Check for skin eruptions, pruritus, swollen lymph glands.

P

Be alert for signs, symptoms of hepatic injury, hepatitis (nausea, vomiting, drowsiness, jaundice). Monitor hematology results for bone marrow suppression; observe for signs of infection, bleeding.

### PATIENT/FAMILY TEACHING

• Space doses evenly around the clock. • Take resting pulse daily. • Report pulse rate less than 60 beats/min. • Seafood, iodine products may be restricted. • Report fever, sore throat, yellowing of skin/eyes, unusual bleeding/bruising immediately. • Report sudden or continuous weight gain, cold intolerance, depression.

---

# pseudoephedrine

soo-doe-e-**fed**-rin
(Balminil Decongestant ✤, Nexafed, PMS-Pseudoephedrine ✤, Robidrine ✤, Sudafed, Sudafed 12 Hour, Sudafed 24 Hour, Sudafed Children's)

### FIXED-COMBINATION(S)

**Advil Cold, Motrin Cold:** pseudoephedrine/ibuprofen (an NSAID): 30 mg/200 mg, 15 mg/100 mg per 5 ml. **Allegra-D:** pseudoephedrine/fexofenadine (an antihistamine): 120 mg/60 mg. **Allegra-D 24 Hour:** pseudoephedrine/fexofenadine: 240 mg/180 mg. **Claritin-D:** pseudoephedrine/loratadine (an antihistamine): 120 mg/5 mg, 240 mg/10 mg. **Clarinex-D 24-Hour:** pseudoephedrine/desloratadine (an antihistamine): 240 mg/5 mg. **Clarinex-D 12-Hour:** pseudoephedrine/desloratadine: 120 mg/2.5 mg. **Rezira:** pseudoephedrine/hydrocodone (an opioid analgesic): 60 mg/5 mg per 5 ml. **Zyrtec-D:** pseudoephedrine/cetirizine (an antihistamine): 120 mg/5 mg.

### ◆CLASSIFICATION

**PHARMACOTHERAPEUTIC:** Sympathomimetic. **CLINICAL:** Nasal decongestant.

## USES

Temporary relief of nasal congestion due to common cold, upper respiratory allergies, sinusitis. Enhances nasal, sinus drainage.

## PRECAUTIONS

**Contraindications:** Hypersensitivity to pseudoephedrine. Use of MAOIs within 14 days. Severe hypertension, coronary artery disease. **Cautions:** Elderly, hyperthyroidism, diabetes, ischemic heart disease, prostatic hypertrophy, mild to moderate hypertension, arrhythmias, renal impairment, seizure disorder, increased intraocular pressure.

## ACTION

Directly stimulates alpha-adrenergic, beta-adrenergic receptors. **Therapeutic Effect:** Produces vasoconstriction; causes bronchial relaxation, increased heart rate/contractility.

## PHARMACOKINETICS

| Route | Onset | Peak | Duration |
|---|---|---|---|
| PO (tablets, syrup) | 15–30 min | 30–60 min | 4–6 hrs |
| PO (extended-release) | N/A | N/A | 8–12 hrs |

Well absorbed from GI tract. Partially metabolized in liver. Primarily excreted in urine. Not removed by hemodialysis. **Half-life:** 9–16 hrs.

## ⧗ LIFESPAN CONSIDERATIONS

**Pregnancy/Lactation:** Crosses placenta. Distributed in breast milk. **Children:** Safety and efficacy not established in pts younger than 2 yrs. **Elderly:** Age-related prostatic hypertrophy may require dosage adjustment.

## INTERACTIONS

**DRUG:** May decrease effects of **antihypertensives** (e.g., amlodipine, lisinopril, valsartan), **beta blockers** (e.g., carvedilol, metoprolol), **diuretics** (e.g., furosemide, HCTZ). **HERBAL: Ephedra, yohimbe** may cause hypertension.

FOOD: None known. **LAB VALUES:** None significant.

## AVAILABILITY (OTC)

**Liquid:** 15 mg/5 ml, 30 mg/5 ml. **Syrup:** 30 mg/5 ml. **Tablets:** 30 mg.

🔋 **Tablets, Extended-Release:** (12 Hour): 120 mg. 🔋 **Tablets, Extended-Release:** (24 Hour): 240 mg.

◀**ALERT**▶ Pseudoephedrine is key ingredient in synthesizing methamphetamine. Many pharmacies have moved pseudoephedrine behind the counter due to concerns about its purchase and theft for purposes of methamphetamine manufacture.

## ADMINISTRATION/HANDLING

**PO**
• Administer with water or milk to decrease GI upset. • Do not break, crush, dissolve, or divide extended-release forms; give whole.

## INDICATIONS/ROUTES/ DOSAGE

**Decongestant**
**PO: ADULTS, ELDERLY, CHILDREN 12 YRS AND OLDER:** 30–60 mg q4–6h. **Maximum:** 240 mg/day. **CHILDREN 6–11 YRS:** 30 mg q4–6h. **Maximum:** 120 mg/day. **CHILDREN 4–5 YRS:** 15 mg q4–6h. **Maximum:** 60 mg/day.

**PO** *(Extended-Release):* **ADULTS, CHILDREN 12 YRS AND OLDER:** 120 mg q12h or 240 mg once daily.

**Dosage in Renal/Hepatic Impairment**
No dose adjustment.

## SIDE EFFECTS

**Occasional (10%–5%):** Nervousness, restlessness, insomnia, tremor, headache. **Rare (4%–1%):** Diaphoresis, weakness.

## ADVERSE EFFECTS/ TOXIC REACTIONS

Large doses may produce tachycardia, palpitations (particularly in pts with cardiac disease), light-headedness, nausea, vomiting. Overdose in those older than 60 yrs may result in hallucinations, CNS depression, seizures.

## NURSING CONSIDERATIONS

### PATIENT/FAMILY TEACHING

• Discontinue drug if adverse reactions occur. • Report insomnia, dizziness, tremors, tachycardia, palpitations.

# psyllium

sil-ee-yum
(Konsyl, Metamucil, Multihealth Fiber)
**Do not confuse Fiberall with Feverall.**

## ◆CLASSIFICATION

**PHARMACOTHERAPEUTIC:** Bulk-forming agent. **CLINICAL:** Laxative.

## USES

Treatment of occasional constipation. Dietary fiber supplement. Reduce risk of CHD.

## PRECAUTIONS

**Contraindications:** Hypersensitivity to psyllium, difficulty swallowing. **Cautions:** Esophageal strictures, ulcers, stenosis, intestinal adhesions, difficulty swallowing, management of irritable bowel syndrome (IBS), elderly. Pts with or prone to fecal impaction or GI obstruction. Avoid use in pts with nausea, vomiting, or abdominal pain.

## ACTION

Dissolves and swells in water providing increased bulk, moisture content in stool. **Therapeutic Effect:** Promotes peristalsis, bowel motility.

## PHARMACOKINETICS

| Route | Onset | Peak | Duration |
|-------|-------|------|----------|
| PO | 12–24 hrs | 2–3 days | N/A |

Acts in small, large intestines.

P

## ⌛ LIFESPAN CONSIDERATIONS

**Pregnancy/Lactation:** Safe for use in pregnancy. **Children:** Safety and efficacy not established in pts younger than 6 yrs. **Elderly:** No age-related precautions noted.

## INTERACTIONS

**DRUG:** None significant. **HERBAL:** None significant. **FOOD:** None known. **LAB VALUES:** May increase serum glucose. May decrease serum potassium.

## AVAILABILITY (OTC)

**Capsules:** 500 mg. **Powder:** 300 g, 450 g bulk powder.

## ADMINISTRATION/HANDLING

### PO

• Administer at least 2 hrs before or after other medication. • All doses should be followed with 8 oz liquid. • Drink 6–8 glasses of water/day (aids stool softening). • Do not swallow in dry form; mix with at least 1 full glass (8 oz) of liquid.

## INDICATIONS/ROUTES/DOSAGE

**Constipation**
Refer to specific dosing guidelines on product labeling.
**PO: ADULTS, ELDERLY:** (2.5–30 g/day in divided doses) 2–5 capsules/dose up to 3 times/day. 1 rounded tsp or 1 tbsp of powder up to 3 times/day. **CHILDREN 6–11 YRS:** (1.25–15 g/day in divided doses). Approximately ½ adult dose up to 3 times/day.

**Reduce Risk of CHD**
**PO: ADULTS, ELDERLY:** 7 g or more daily.

## SIDE EFFECTS

**Rare:** Some degree of abdominal discomfort, nausea, mild abdominal cramps, griping, faintness.

## ADVERSE EFFECTS/ TOXIC REACTIONS

Esophageal/bowel obstruction may occur if administered with insufficient liquid (less than 250 ml).

## NURSING CONSIDERATIONS

### INTERVENTION/EVALUATION

Encourage adequate fluid intake. Assess bowel sounds for peristalsis. Monitor daily pattern of bowel activity, stool consistency. Monitor serum electrolytes in pts exposed to prolonged, frequent, excessive use of medication.

### PATIENT/FAMILY TEACHING

• Take each dose with full glass (250 ml) of water. • Inadequate fluid intake may cause GI obstruction. • Institute measures to promote defecation (increase fluid intake, exercise, high-fiber diet).

# pyrazinamide

peer-a-**zin**-a-mide
(Tebrazid ✦)

## FIXED-COMBINATION(S)

**Rifater:** pyrazinamide/isoniazid/ rifampin (an antitubercular): 300 mg/50 mg/120 mg.

## ◆CLASSIFICATION

**PHARMACOTHERAPEUTIC:** Synthetic pyrazine analogue. **CLINICAL:** Antitubercular.

## USES

Treatment of clinical tuberculosis in conjunction with other antitubercular agents.

## PRECAUTIONS

**Contraindications:** Hypersensitivity to pyrazinamide. Acute gout, severe hepatic dysfunction. **Cautions:** Diabetes mellitus, porphyria, renal impairment, history of gout, history of alcoholism, concurrent medication associated with hepatotoxicity.

## ACTION

Exact mechanism unknown. May disrupt mycobacterium tuberculosis membrane transport. **Therapeutic Effect:** Bacteriostatic or bactericidal, depending on drug concentration at infection site, susceptibility of infecting bacteria.

## PHARMACOKINETICS

Well absorbed from GI tract. Protein binding: 5%–10%. Widely distributed. Metabolized in liver. Excreted in urine. **Half-life:** 9–10 hrs.

## ⏳ LIFESPAN CONSIDERATIONS

**Pregnancy/Lactation:** Unknown if drug crosses placenta or is distributed in breast milk. **Children:** Safety and efficacy not established. **Elderly:** No age-related precautions noted.

## INTERACTIONS

**DRUG:** None significant. **HERBAL:** None significant. **FOOD:** None known. **LAB VALUES:** May increase serum ALT, AST, uric acid.

## AVAILABILITY (Rx)

**Tablets:** 500 mg.

## INDICATIONS/ROUTES/DOSAGE

**Tuberculosis (in Combination With Other Antituberculars)**
**PO: ADULTS:** Based on lean body weight. **40–55 KG:** 1,000 mg daily; **56–75 KG:** 1,500 mg daily; **76–90 KG:** 2,000 mg (**maximum dose** regardless of weight). **CHILDREN:** 15–30 mg/kg/day in 1 or 2 doses. **Maximum:** 2 g/day.

**Dosage in Renal/Hepatic Impairment**
**CrCl less than 30 ml/min or receiving HD:** 25–35 mg/kg/dose 3 times/wk (give after dialysis). Contraindicated in severe hepatic impairment.

## SIDE EFFECTS

**Frequent:** Arthralgia, myalgia (usually mild, self-limited). **Rare:** Hypersensitivity reaction (rash, pruritus, urticaria), photosensitivity, gouty arthritis.

## ADVERSE EFFECTS/ TOXIC REACTIONS

Hepatotoxicity, gouty arthritis, thrombocytopenia, anemia occur rarely.

## NURSING CONSIDERATIONS

### BASELINE ASSESSMENT

Question for hypersensitivity to pyrazinamide, isoniazid, ethionamide, niacin. Ensure collection of specimens for culture, sensitivity. Obtain CBC, LFT, serum uric acid levels.

### INTERVENTION/EVALUATION

Monitor LFT results; be alert for hepatic reactions: jaundice, malaise, fever, abdominal (RUQ) tenderness, anorexia, nausea, vomiting (stop drug, notify physician promptly). Check serum uric acid levels; assess for hot, painful, swollen joints, esp. big toe, ankle, knee (gout). Evaluate serum blood glucose levels, diabetic status carefully (pyrazinamide makes management difficult). Assess for rash, skin eruptions. Monitor CBC for thrombocytopenia, anemia.

### PATIENT/FAMILY TEACHING

• Do not skip doses; complete full length of therapy (may be mos or yrs). • Office visits, lab tests are essential part of treatment. • Take with food to reduce GI upset. • Avoid excessive exposure to sun, ultraviolet light until photosensitivity is determined. • Report any new symptom, immediately for jaundice (yellowing sclera of eyes/skin); unusual fatigue; fever; loss of appetite; hot, painful, swollen joints.

# pyridostigmine

peer-id-oh-**stig**-meen
(Mestinon, Mestinon SR ✦, Regonol)
**Do not confuse pyridostigmine with physostigmine, or Regonol with Reglan or Renagel.**

## ◆CLASSIFICATION

**PHARMACOTHERAPEUTIC:** Anticholinesterase. **CLINICAL:** Cholinergic muscle stimulant.

## USES

Improvement of muscle strength in control of myasthenia gravis, reversal of effects of nondepolarizing neuromuscular blocking agents after surgery.

## PRECAUTIONS

**Contraindications:** Hypersensitivity to pyridostigmine. Mechanical GI/urinary tract obstruction. **Cautions:** Bronchial asthma, bradycardia, seizure disorder, hyperthyroidism, cardiac arrhythmias, peptic ulcer, renal impairment.

## ACTION

Prevents destruction of acetylcholine by inhibiting the enzyme acetylcholinesterase, enhancing impulse transmission across myoneural junction. **Therapeutic Effect:** Produces miosis; increases intestinal, skeletal muscle tone; stimulates salivary, sweat gland secretions.

## PHARMACOKINETICS

Poorly absorbed from GI tract. Metabolized in liver. Excreted primarily unchanged in urine. **Half-life:** 1–2 hrs.

## LIFESPAN CONSIDERATIONS

**Pregnancy/Lactation:** Unknown if drug crosses placenta or is distributed in breast milk. **Children:** Safety and efficacy not established. **Elderly:** No age-related precautions noted.

## INTERACTIONS

**DRUG:** Antagonizes effects of **neuromuscular blockers (e.g., succinylcholine, vecuronium). Anticholinergics (e.g., dicyclomine, glycopyrrolate, scopolamine)** prevent, reverse effects. **Cholinesterase inhibitors (e.g., donepezil, tacrine)** may increase risk of toxicity. **HERBAL:** None significant. **FOOD:** None known. **LAB VALUES:** None significant.

## AVAILABILITY (Rx)

**Injection Solution (Regonol):** 5 mg/ml. **Syrup (Mestinon):** 60 mg/5 ml. **Tablets (Mestinon):** 60 mg.

 **Tablets (Extended-Release [Mestinon Timespan]):** 180 mg.

## ADMINISTRATION/HANDLING

### IV, IM

• Give large parenteral doses concurrently with 0.6–1.2 mg atropine sulfate IV to minimize side effects.

### PO

• Give with food, milk. • Tablets may be crushed. Do not chew, crush extended-release tablets (may be broken). • Give larger dose at times of increased fatigue (e.g., for those with difficulty in chewing, 30–45 min before meals).

### IV INCOMPATIBILITIES

Do not mix with any other medications.

## INDICATIONS/ROUTES/DOSAGE

**Note:** Highly individualized dosing ranges.

**Myasthenia Gravis**
**PO: ADULTS, ELDERLY:** *(Immediate-Release):* Initially, 60 mg 3 times/day. Dosage increased at 48-hr intervals. **Maintenance:** 60 mg–1.5 g/day divided into 5–6 doses/day. (Usual dose: 600 mg/day.) **CHILDREN:** Initially, 1 mg/kg/dose q4–6h. **Maximum:** 7 mg/kg/24 hr divided into 5–6 doses. Usual dose: 600 mg/day.
**PO** *(Extended-Release):* **ADULTS, ELDERLY:** 180–540 mg 1–2 times/day with at least a 6-hr interval between doses.
**IV, IM: ADULTS, ELDERLY:** 2 mg or 1/30th of oral dose q2–3h. **CHILDREN:** 0.05–0.15 mg/kg/dose. **Maximum single dose:** 10 mg.

**Dosage in Renal/Hepatic Impairment**
No dose adjustment.

## SIDE EFFECTS

**Frequent:** Miosis, increased GI/skeletal muscle tone, bradycardia, constriction of bronchi/ureters, diaphoresis, increased salivation. **Occasional:** Headache, rash, temporary decrease in diastolic B/P with mild reflex tachycardia, short periods of atrial fibrillation (in hyperthyroid pts), marked drop in B/P (in hypertensive pts).

## ADVERSE EFFECTS/ TOXIC REACTIONS

Overdose may produce cholinergic crisis, manifested as increasingly severe descending muscle weakness (appears first in muscles involving chewing, swallowing, followed by muscle weakness of shoulder girdle, upper extremities), respiratory muscle paralysis, followed by pelvis girdle/leg muscle paralysis. Requires withdrawal of all cholinergic drugs and immediate use of 1–4 mg atropine sulfate IV for adults, 0.01 mg/kg for infants and children younger than 12 yrs.

## NURSING CONSIDERATIONS

### BASELINE ASSESSMENT

Larger doses should be given at time of greatest fatigue. Assess muscle strength before testing for diagnosis of myasthenia gravis and following drug administration. Avoid large doses in pts with megacolon, reduced GI motility.

### INTERVENTION/EVALUATION

Have facial tissues readily available at pt's bedside. Monitor respirations closely during myasthenia gravis testing or if dosage is increased. Assess diligently for cholinergic reaction, bradycardia in myasthenic pt in crisis. Coordinate dosage time with periods of fatigue and increased/decreased muscle strength. Monitor for therapeutic response to medication (increased muscle strength, decreased fatigue, improved chewing/swallowing functions).

### PATIENT/FAMILY TEACHING

• Report nausea, vomiting, diarrhea, diaphoresis, profuse salivary secretions, palpitations, muscle weakness, severe abdominal pain, difficulty breathing.

# pyridoxine (vitamin B$_6$)

peer-i-**dox**-een
(Pyri-500)
**Do not confuse pyridoxine with paroxetine, pralidoxime, or Pyridium.**

## ◆CLASSIFICATION

**PHARMACOTHERAPEUTIC:** Coenzyme. **CLINICAL:** Vitamin (B$_6$).

## USES

Prevention/treatment of vitamin B$_6$ deficiency. **OFF-LABEL:** Pyridoxine-dependent seizures in infants, drug-induced neuritis (e.g., associated with isoniazid). Treatment of peripheral neuropathy associated with isoniazid; nausea and vomiting of pregnancy.

## PRECAUTIONS

**Contraindications:** Hypersensitivity to pyridoxine. **Cautions:** Impaired renal function, neonates.

## ACTION

Coenzyme for various metabolic functions, including metabolism of proteins, carbohydrates, fats. Aids in breakdown of glycogen and in synthesis of gamma-aminobutyric acid (GABA) in CNS. **Therapeutic Effect:** Prevents pyridoxine deficiency. Increases excretion of certain drugs (e.g., isoniazid) that are pyridoxine antagonists.

## PHARMACOKINETICS

Readily absorbed, primarily in jejunum. Stored in liver, muscle, brain. Metabolized in liver. Primarily excreted in urine. Removed by hemodialysis. **Half-life:** 15–20 days.

## ⧗ LIFESPAN CONSIDERATIONS

**Pregnancy/Lactation:** Crosses placenta. Distributed in breast milk. High dosages in utero may produce seizures

P

in neonates. **Children/Elderly:** No age-related precautions noted.

## INTERACTIONS

**DRUG:** Decreases effects of **levodopa. HERBAL:** None significant. **FOOD:** None known. **LAB VALUES:** None significant.

## AVAILABILITY (OTC)

**Capsules:** 250 mg. **Injection Solution:** 100 mg/ml. **Tablets:** 25 mg, 50 mg, 100 mg, 250 mg, 500 mg. **Tablet, Extended-Release:** 200 mg.

## ADMINISTRATION/HANDLING

◄ALERT► Give PO unless nausea, vomiting, malabsorption occurs. Avoid IV use in cardiac pts.

 **IV**

• Give undiluted or may be added to IV solutions and given as infusion.

**PO**

• Give without regard to food.

## ✳ IV INCOMPATIBILITIES

Do not mix with any other medications.

## INDICATIONS/ROUTES/DOSAGE

**Pyridoxine Deficiency**
**PO/IM/IV: ADULTS, ELDERLY:** 10–20 mg/day for 3 wks, followed by oral therapy up to 600 mg/day.

## SIDE EFFECTS

**Occasional:** Stinging at IM injection site. **Rare:** Headache, nausea, drowsiness, sensory neuropathy (paresthesia, unstable gait, clumsiness of hands) with high doses.

## ADVERSE EFFECTS/ TOXIC REACTIONS

Long-term megadoses (2–6 g for longer than 2 mos) may produce sensory neuropathy (reduced deep tendon reflexes, profound impairment of sense of position in distal limbs, gradual sensory ataxia). Toxic symptoms subside when drug is discontinued. Seizures have occurred after IV megadoses.

## NURSING CONSIDERATIONS

### INTERVENTION/EVALUATION

Observe for improvement of deficiency symptoms, glossitis. Evaluate for nutritional adequacy.

### PATIENT/FAMILY TEACHING

• Discomfort may occur with IM injection. • Consume foods rich in pyridoxine (legumes, soybeans, eggs, sunflower seeds, hazelnuts, organ meats, tuna, shrimp, carrots, avocados, bananas, wheat germ, bran).

# *QUEtiapine

kwet-**eye**-a-peen
(Apo-Quetiapine ✦, Seroquel,
Seroquel XR)

■ **BLACK BOX ALERT** ■ Increased risk of suicidal ideation and behavior in children, adolescents, young adults 18–24 yrs with major depressive disorder, other psychiatric disorders. Elderly with dementia-related psychosis are at increased risk for death.
**Do not confuse quetiapine with olanzapine, or Seroquel with Sinequan.**

## ◆CLASSIFICATION

**PHARMACOTHERAPEUTIC:** Dibenzapine derivative. **CLINICAL:** Antipsychotic.

## USES

Treatment of schizophrenia. Treatment of acute manic episodes associated with bipolar disorder (alone or in combination with lithium or valproate). Maintenance treatment of bipolar disorder as an adjunct to lithium or valproic acid. Treatment of acute depressive episodes associated with bipolar disorder. Adjunctive treatment to antidepressants in major depressive disorder (MDD). **OFF-LABEL:** Delirium in critically ill pts, psychosis/agitation related to Alzheimer's dementia. Treatment of autism, treatment-resistant obsessive compulsive disorder.

## PRECAUTIONS

**Contraindications:** Hypersensitivity to quetiapine. **Cautions:** Renal/hepatic impairment, preexisting abnormal lipid profile, pts at risk for aspiration pneumonia, cardiovascular disease (e.g., HF, history of MI), cerebrovascular disease, dehydration, hypovolemia, history of drug abuse/dependence, seizures, hypothyroidism, pts at risk for suicide, Parkinson's disease, decreased GI motility, urinary retention, narrow-angle glaucoma, diabetes,

visual problems, elderly, pts at risk for orthostatic hypotension. Avoid use in pts at risk for torsades de pointes (hypokalemia, hypomagnesemia, history of cardiac arrhythmias, congenital prolongation QT interval, concurrent medications that prolong QT interval).

## ACTION

Antagonizes dopamine, serotonin, histamine, alpha$_1$-adrenergic receptors. **Therapeutic Effect:** Diminishes symptoms associated with schizophrenia/bipolar disorders.

## PHARMACOKINETICS

Rapidly absorbed. Protein binding: 83%. Widely distributed in tissues; CNS concentration exceeds plasma concentration. Metabolized in liver. Primarily excreted in urine. **Half-life:** 6 hrs.

## ⧗ LIFESPAN CONSIDERATIONS

**Pregnancy/Lactation:** Unknown if drug is distributed in breast milk. Not recommended for breastfeeding mothers. **Children:** Safety and efficacy not established. **Elderly:** No age-related precautions noted, but lower initial and target dosages may be necessary.

## INTERACTIONS

**DRUG: Medications prolonging QT interval (e.g., amiodarone, citalopram, dasatinib, haloperidol, levofloxacin, ondansetron)** may increase risk of QT prolongation. **Alcohol, other CNS depressants (e.g., lorazepam, morphine, zolpidem)** may increase CNS depression. May increase hypotensive effects of **antihypertensives. CYP3A4 inducers (e.g., phenytoin)** may increase clearance. **CYP3A4 inhibitors (e.g., clarithromycin, erythromycin, fluconazole, itraconazole)** may increase effects. **HERBAL: St. John's wort** may decrease concentration. **Gotu kola, kava kava, St. John's wort, valerian** may increase CNS depression. **FOOD:** None known. **LAB VALUES:** May decrease total free thyroxine (T$_4$) serum levels. May

Q

increase serum cholesterol, triglycerides, ALT, AST, WBC, GGT. May produce false-positive pregnancy test result.

## AVAILABILITY (Rx)

**Tablets:** 25 mg, 50 mg, 100 mg, 200 mg, 300 mg, 400 mg.

 **Tablets, Extended-Release:** 50 mg, 150 mg, 200 mg, 300 mg, 400 mg.

## ADMINISTRATION/HANDLING

**PO**
• Give immediate-release tablets without regard to food. • Do not break, crush, dissolve, or divide extended-release tablets. • Extended-release tablets should be given without regard to food or with a light meal in evening.

## INDICATIONS/ROUTES/DOSAGE

**Note:** When restarting pts who have been off quetiapine for less than 1 wk, titration is not required and maintenance dose can be reinstituted. • When restarting pts who have been off quetiapine for longer than 1 wk, follow initial titration schedule.

### Schizophrenia

**PO:** *(Immediate-Release):* **ADULTS, ELDERLY:** Initially, 25 mg twice daily, then increase in 25–50-mg increments divided 2–3 times/day on the second and third days, up to 300–400 mg/day in 2–3 divided doses by the fourth day. Further adjustments of 25–50 mg twice daily may be made at intervals of 2 days or longer. **Maintenance:** 150–750 mg/day (adults); 50–200 mg/day (elderly). *(Extended-Release):* Initially, 300 mg/day. May increase at intervals as short as 1 day up to 300 mg/day. Range: 400–800 mg/day. *(Immediate-Release):* **CHILDREN 13 YRS AND OLDER:** Initially, 25 mg twice daily on day 1, 50 mg twice daily on day 2, then increase by 100 mg/day to target dose of 400 mg twice daily on day 5. May further increase to 800 mg/day in increments of 100 mg or less daily. Range: 400–800 mg/day. **Maximum:** 800 mg. Total dose in 3 divided doses. *(Extended-Release):* Initially, 50 mg once daily on day 1, 100 mg on day 2, until 400 mg once daily is reached on day 5. Range: 400–800 mg/day. **Maximum:** 800 mg/day.

### Mania in Bipolar Disorder

**PO:** *(Immediate-Release):* **ADULTS, ELDERLY:** Initially, 50 mg twice daily for 1 day. May increase in increments of 100 mg/day to 200 mg twice daily on day 4. May further increase in increments of 200 mg/day to 800 mg/day on day 6. Range: 400–800 mg/day. *(Extended-Release):* Initially, 300 mg on day 1 in the evening; 600 mg on day 2 and adjust between 400–800 mg/day thereafter. *(Immediate-Release):* **CHILDREN 10 YRS AND OLDER:** 25 mg twice daily on day 1, 50 mg twice daily on day 2, then increase by 100 mg/day until target dose of 400 mg/day reached on day 5. May increase up to 600 mg/day. Range: 400–600 mg/day. *(Extended-Release):* 50 mg on day 1; 100 mg on day 2; further increases of 100 mg/day until 400 mg once daily is reached on day 4; Usual range: 400–600 mg once daily.

### Depression in Bipolar Disorder

**PO:** *(Immediate-Release):* **ADULTS, ELDERLY:** Initially, 50 mg/day on day 1, increase to 100 mg/day on day 2, then increase by 100 mg/day up to target dose of 300 mg/day. *(Extended-Release):* Initially, 50 mg on day 1 in the evening, 100 mg on day 2, 200 mg on day 3, 300 mg on day 4 and thereafter.

### Adjunctive Therapy in MDD

**PO:** **ADULTS, ELDERLY:** *(Extended-Release):* Initially, 50 mg on days 1 and 2; then 150 mg on days 3 and 4; then 150–300 mg/day thereafter.

### Dosage in Hepatic Impairment

*(Immediate-Release):* Initially, 25 mg/day. Increase by 25–50 mg/day to effective dose.

Q

*(Extended-Release):* Initially, 50 mg/day, increase by 50 mg/day until effective dose.

**Dosage in Renal Impairment**
No dose adjustment.

## SIDE EFFECTS

**Frequent (19%–10%):** Headache, drowsiness, dizziness. **Occasional (9%–3%):** Constipation, orthostatic hypotension, tachycardia, dry mouth, dyspepsia, rash, asthenia, abdominal pain, rhinitis. **Rare (2%):** Back pain, fever, weight gain.

## ADVERSE EFFECTS/ TOXIC REACTIONS

Overdose may produce heart block, hypotension, hypokalemia, tachycardia.

## NURSING CONSIDERATIONS

### BASELINE ASSESSMENT

Assess behavior, appearance, emotional status, response to environment, speech pattern, thought content. Obtain baseline CBC, hepatic enzyme levels before initiating treatment and periodically thereafter. Question medical history as listed in Precautions.

### INTERVENTION/EVALUATION

Monitor mental status, onset of extrapyramidal symptoms. Assist with ambulation if dizziness occurs. Supervise suicidal-risk pt closely during early therapy (as psychosis, depression lessens, energy level improves, increasing suicide potential). Monitor B/P for hypotension, lipid profile, blood glucose, CBC, or worsening depression, unusual behavior. Assess pulse for tachycardia (esp. with rapid increase in dosage). Monitor daily pattern of bowel activity, stool consistency. Assess for therapeutic response (improved thought content, increased ability to concentrate, improvement in self-care). Eye exam to detect cataract formation should be obtained q6mos during treatment.

### PATIENT/ FAMILY TEACHING

• Avoid exposure to extreme heat. • Drink fluids often, esp. during physical activity. • Take medication as ordered; do not stop taking or increase dosage. • Drowsiness generally subsides during continued therapy. • Avoid tasks that require alertness, motor skills until response to drug is established. • Avoid alcohol. • Slowly go from lying to standing. • Report suicidal ideation, unusual changes in behavior.

# quinapril

kwin-a-pril
(Accupril, Apo-Quinapril ✦)
■ **BLACK BOX ALERT** ■ May cause fetal injury, mortality. Discontinue as soon as possible once pregnancy detected.
**Do not confuse Accupril with Accolate, Accutane, Aciphex, or Monopril.**

## FIXED-COMBINATION(S)

**Accuretic:** quinapril/hydrochlorothiazide (a diuretic): 10 mg/12.5 mg, 20 mg/12.5 mg, 20 mg/25 mg.

## ◆CLASSIFICATION

**PHARMACOTHERAPEUTIC:** Angiotensin-converting enzyme (ACE) inhibitor. **CLINICAL:** Antihypertensive.

## USES

Treatment of hypertension. Used alone or in combination with other antihypertensives. Adjunctive therapy in management of HF. **OFF-LABEL:** Treatment of pediatric hypertension.

## PRECAUTIONS

**Contraindications:** Hypersensitivity to quinapril. History of angioedema from previous treatment with ACE inhibitors, concomitant use with aliskiren in pts with diabetes. **Cautions:** Renal impairment, hypertrophic cardiomyopathy with outflow tract obstruction, major surgery, HF, hypovolemia, unstented bilateral renal artery stenosis, hyperkalemia, concurrent potassium supplements, severe aortic stenosis, ischemic heart disease, cerebrovascular disease.

## ACTION

Suppresses renin-angiotensin-aldosterone system, preventing conversion of angiotensin I to angiotensin II, a potent vasoconstrictor; may inhibit angiotensin II at local vascular renal sites. **Therapeutic Effect:** Reduces peripheral arterial resistance, B/P, pulmonary capillary wedge pressure; improves cardiac output.

## PHARMACOKINETICS

| Route | Onset | Peak | Duration |
|-------|-------|------|----------|
| PO | 1 hr | N/A | 24 hrs |

Readily absorbed from GI tract. Protein binding: 97%. Rapidly hydrolyzed to active metabolite. Primarily excreted in urine. Minimal removal by hemodialysis. **Half-life:** 1–2 hrs; metabolite, 3 hrs (increased in renal impairment).

## ⌛ LIFESPAN CONSIDERATIONS

**Pregnancy/Lactation:** Crosses placenta. Unknown if distributed in breast milk. May cause fetal, neonatal mortality or morbidity. **Children:** Safety and efficacy not established. **Elderly:** May be more sensitive to hypotensive effects.

## INTERACTIONS

**DRUG: Alcohol, antihypertensives** (e.g., **amlodipine, lisinopril, valsartan**), **diuretics** (e.g., **furosemide, HCTZ**) may increase effects. May increase concentration, risk of toxicity of **lithium. NSAIDs** may decrease effects. **Potassium-sparing diuretics** (e.g., **spironolactone, triamterene**), **potassium supplements** may cause hyperkalemia. **HERBAL: Black cohosh, periwinkle** may increase antihypertensive effect. **Ginseng, yohimbe, licorice** may worsen hypertension. **FOOD:** None known. **LAB VALUES:** May increase serum BUN, alkaline phosphatase, bilirubin, creatinine, potassium, ALT, AST. May decrease serum sodium. May cause positive antinuclear antibody (ANA) titer.

## AVAILABILITY (Rx)

**Tablets:** 5 mg, 10 mg, 20 mg, 40 mg.

## ADMINISTRATION/HANDLING

**PO**
• Give without regard to food. • Tablets may be crushed.

## INDICATIONS/ROUTES/DOSAGE

**Hypertension (Monotherapy)**
**PO: ADULTS:** Initially, 10–20 mg/day. May adjust dosage at intervals of at least 2 wks or longer. **Maintenance:** 10–40 once daily. **ELDERLY:** Initially, 10 mg once daily. Titrate to optimal response.

**Hypertension (Combination Diuretic Therapy)**
**PO: ADULTS, ELDERLY:** Initially, 5 mg/day titrated to pt's needs.

**Adjunct to Manage HF**
**PO: ADULTS, ELDERLY:** Initially, 5 mg twice daily. Titrate at wkly intervals to 20–40 mg/day in 2 divided doses.

**Dosage in Renal Impairment**
*Hypertension*

| Creatinine Clearance | Initial Dose |
|----------------------|--------------|
| More than 60 ml/min | 10 mg |
| 30–60 ml/min | 5 mg |
| 10–29 ml/min | 2.5 mg |

*HF*

| Creatinine Clearance | Initial Dose |
|----------------------|--------------|
| Greater than 30 ml/min | 5 mg |
| 10–30 ml/min | 2.5 mg |

**Dosage in Hepatic Impairment**
No dose adjustment.

## SIDE EFFECTS

**Frequent (7%–5%):** Headache, dizziness. **Occasional (4%–2%):** Fatigue, vomiting, nausea, hypotension, chest pain, cough, syncope. **Rare (less than 2%):** Diarrhea, cough, dyspnea, rash, palpitations, impotence, insomnia, drowsiness, malaise.

## ADVERSE EFFECTS/ TOXIC REACTIONS

Excessive hypotension ("first-dose syncope") may occur in pts with HF, those who are severely salt/volume depleted. Angioedema, hyperkalemia occur rarely. Agranulocytosis, neutropenia may be noted in those with collagen vascular disease (scleroderma, systemic lupus erythematosus), renal impairment. Nephrotic syndrome may be noted in those with history of renal disease.

## NURSING CONSIDERATIONS

### BASELINE ASSESSMENT

Obtain B/P immediately before each dose in addition to regular monitoring (be alert to fluctuations). If excessive reduction in B/P occurs, place pt in supine position with legs slightly elevated. Renal function tests should be performed before beginning therapy. In pts with prior renal disease, urine test for protein by dipstick method should be made with first urine of day before beginning therapy and periodically thereafter. In pts with renal impairment, autoimmune disease, or taking drugs that affect leukocytes or immune response, CBC, differential count should be performed before beginning therapy and q2wks for 3 mos, then periodically thereafter.

### INTERVENTION/EVALUATION

Monitor B/P, renal function, serum potassium, WBC. Assist with ambulation if dizziness occurs. Question for evidence of headache. Noncola carbonated beverage, unsalted crackers, dry toast may relieve nausea.

### PATIENT/ FAMILY TEACHING

• Go from lying to standing slowly. • Full therapeutic effect may take 1–2 wks. • Report any sign of infection (sore throat, fever). • Skipping doses or voluntarily discontinuing drug may produce severe rebound hypertension. • Avoid tasks that require alertness, motor skills until response to drug is established. • Avoid alcohol.

## *RABEprazole  `TOP 100`

ra-**bep**-ra-zole
(Aciphex, Aciphex Sprinkle,
Apo-Rabeprazole)
**Do not confuse Aciphex
with Accupril or Aricept, or
rabeprazole with aripiprazole,
lansoprazole, omeprazole, or
raloxifene.**

### ◆CLASSIFICATION

**PHARMACOTHERAPEUTIC:** Proton
pump inhibitor. **CLINICAL:** Gastric acid
inhibitor.

## USES

Short-term treatment (4–8 wks), maintenance of erosive or ulcerative gastroesophageal reflux disease (GERD). Treatment of daytime/nighttime heartburn,
other symptoms of GERD. Short-term
treatment (4 wks or less) in healing,
symptomatic relief of duodenal ulcers.
Long-term treatment of pathologic hypersecretory conditions, including Zollinger-
Ellison syndrome. Treatment of *H. pylori*
(in combination with other medication).
Sprinkle dose form approved for treatment
of GERD in children 1–11 yrs. **OFF-LABEL:**
Maintenance of healing and prevention of
relapse of duodenal ulcers. Treatment of
NSAID-induced ulcers.

## PRECAUTIONS

**Contraindications:** Hypersensitivity to rabeprazole, other proton pump inhibitors
(e.g., omeprazole). **Cautions:** Severe hepatic impairment. May increase risk of
bone fractures, GI infections.

## ACTION

Suppresses gastric acid secretion by
inhibiting $H^+/K^+$–ATP pump. **Therapeutic Effect:** Increases gastric pH, reducing gastric acid production.

## PHARMACOKINETICS

Rapidly absorbed from GI tract after
passing through stomach relatively intact
as delayed-release tablet. Protein binding: 96%. Metabolized in liver. Primarily
excreted in urine. **Half-life:** 1–2 hrs
(increased with hepatic impairment).

## ⧗ LIFESPAN CONSIDERATIONS

**Pregnancy/Lactation:** Unknown if drug
crosses placenta or is distributed in breast
milk. **Children:** Safety and efficacy not
established. **Elderly:** No age-related precautions noted.

## INTERACTIONS

**DRUG:** May increase concentration/effects
of **cyclosporine, warfarin.** May decrease concentration of **ketoconazole,
clopidogrel, atazanavir. HERBAL: St.
John's wort** may decrease concentration/
effects. **FOOD:** None known. **LAB VAL-
UES:** May increase serum ALT, AST, thyroid stimulating hormone (TSH).

## AVAILABILITY (Rx)

 **Tablets (Delayed-Release):** 20 mg.
**Capsule, Sprinkle:** 5 mg, 10 mg.

## ADMINISTRATION/HANDLING

**PO**
• May give without regard to meals; best
taken after breakfast. • Do not break,
crush, dissolve, or divide tablet; give
whole.

**Sprinkle**
• May give with antacid. • Administer
30 min before a meal. • Open capsule,
sprinkle on soft food. Take within 15 min
of preparation. • Do not chew, crush.

## INDICATIONS/ROUTES/DOSAGE

**Gastroesophageal Reflux Disease (GERD)**
**PO: ADULTS, ELDERLY: (Erosive or ul-
cerative):** 20 mg/day for 4–8 wks.
**Maintenance:** 20 mg/day. **(Symptomatic):** 20 mg/day for 4 wks.

**Short-Term Treatment of GERD**
**PO: CHILDREN 12 YRS AND OLDER:** 20 mg/
day for 4 wks. If inadequate response,
may repeat additional 4 wks. **CHILDREN,
1–11 YRS (15 KG OR GREATER):** 10 mg once

R

daily for up to 12 wks. **(LESS THAN 15 KG):** 5 mg once daily for up to 12 wks; may increase to 10 mg once daily.

**Duodenal Ulcer**
**PO: ADULTS, ELDERLY:** 20 mg/day after morning meal for 4 wks.

**Pathologic Hypersecretory Conditions**
**PO: ADULTS, ELDERLY:** Initially, 60 mg once daily. May increase to 60 mg twice daily.

**H. Pylori Infection**
**PO: ADULTS, ELDERLY:** 20 mg twice daily for 10–14 days (given with amoxicillin 1,000 mg and clarithromycin 500 mg).

**Dosage in Renal Impairment**
No dose adjustment.

**Dosage in Hepatic Impairment**
**Mild to moderate impairment:** No dose adjustment. **Severe impairment:** Use caution.

## SIDE EFFECTS

**Rare (less than 2%):** Headache, nausea, dizziness, rash, diarrhea, malaise.

## ADVERSE EFFECTS/ TOXIC REACTIONS

Hyperglycemia, hypokalemia, hyponatremia, hyperlipemia occur rarely.

## NURSING CONSIDERATIONS

### BASELINE ASSESSMENT

Obtain baseline lab values, esp. serum chemistries.

### INTERVENTION/EVALUATION

Monitor ongoing laboratory results. Evaluate for therapeutic response (relief of GI symptoms). Question if GI discomfort, nausea, diarrhea, headache occurs. Assess skin for evidence of rash. Observe for evidence of dizziness; utilize appropriate safety precautions.

### PATIENT/FAMILY TEACHING
• Swallow tablets whole; do not break, chew, dissolve, or divide tablets. • Report headache.

# raloxifene

ra-**lox**-i-feen
(Evista, Apo-Raloxifene ✦)

■ **BLACK BOX ALERT** ■ Increases risk of deep vein thrombosis, pulmonary embolism. Women with coronary heart disease or pts at risk for coronary events are at increased risk for death due to stroke.
**Do not confuse Evista with Avinza.**

## ◆CLASSIFICATION

**PHARMACOTHERAPEUTIC:** Selective estrogen receptor modulator. **CLINICAL:** Osteoporosis preventive.

## USES

Prevention/treatment of osteoporosis in postmenopausal women. Reduces risk of invasive breast cancer in postmenopausal women with osteoporosis and postmenopausal women at high risk for invasive breast cancer.

## PRECAUTIONS

**Contraindications:** Hypersensitivity to raloxifene. Active or history of venous thromboembolic events, such as deep vein thrombosis (DVT), pulmonary embolism, retinal vein thrombosis; women who are or may become pregnant, breastfeeding. **Cautions:** Cardiovascular disease, renal/hepatic impairment, risk for venous thromboembolism, unexplained uterine bleeding, elevated triglycerides in response to oral estrogen therapy.

## ACTION

Selective estrogen receptor modulator (SERM) that binds to estrogen receptors, increasing bone mineral density. Blocks

R

estrogen effects in breast/uterus. **Therapeutic Effect:** Reduces bone resorption, increases bone mineral density, reduces incidence of fractures.

## PHARMACOKINETICS

Rapidly absorbed after PO administration. Protein binding: 95%. Metabolized in liver. Excreted primarily in feces. Unknown if removed by hemodialysis. **Half-life:** 27.7–32.5 hrs.

## ⏳ LIFESPAN CONSIDERATIONS

**Pregnancy/Lactation:** Unknown if distributed in breast milk. Not recommended for breastfeeding mothers. **Children:** Not used in this population. **Elderly:** No age-related precautions noted.

## INTERACTIONS

**DRUG: Cholestyramine** reduces peak levels, extent of absorption. Do not use concurrently with **hormone replacement therapy, systemic estrogen.** May decrease effect of **warfarin** (decreases INR). **HERBAL:** None significant. **FOOD:** None known. **LAB VALUES:** May lower serum total cholesterol, LDL. May decrease platelet count, serum inorganic phosphate, albumin, calcium, protein.

## AVAILABILITY (Rx)

**Tablets:** 60 mg.

## ADMINISTRATION/HANDLING

**PO**
• Give without regard to meals.

## INDICATIONS/ROUTES/DOSAGE

**Note:** Discontinue at least 72 hrs prior to and during prolonged immobilization (may increase risk for DVT/PE).

**Prophylaxis/Treatment of Osteoporosis, Breast Cancer Risk Reduction**
**PO: ADULTS, ELDERLY:** 60 mg/day.

**Dosage in Renal/Hepatic Impairment**
No dose adjustment.

## SIDE EFFECTS

**Frequent (25%–10%):** Hot flashes, flu-like symptoms, arthralgia, sinusitis. **Occasional (9%–5%):** Weight gain, nausea, myalgia, pharyngitis, cough, dyspepsia, leg cramps, rash, depression. **Rare (4%–3%):** Vaginitis, UTI, peripheral edema, flatulence, vomiting, fever, migraine, diaphoresis.

## ADVERSE EFFECTS/ TOXIC REACTIONS

Pneumonia, gastroenteritis, chest pain, vaginal bleeding, breast pain occur rarely.

## NURSING CONSIDERATIONS

### BASELINE ASSESSMENT

Question for possibility of pregnancy. Drug should be discontinued 72 hrs before and during prolonged immobilization (postop recovery, prolonged bed rest). Therapy may be resumed only after pt is fully ambulatory. Determine serum total, LDL cholesterol before therapy and routinely thereafter.

### INTERVENTION/EVALUATION

Monitor serum total cholesterol, total calcium, inorganic phosphate, total protein, albumin, bone mineral density, platelet count.

### PATIENT/FAMILY TEACHING

• Avoid prolonged restriction of movement during travel (increased risk of venous thromboembolic events). • Take supplemental calcium, vitamin D if daily dietary intake is inadequate. • Engage in regular weight-bearing exercise. • Modify, discontinue habits of cigarette smoking, alcohol consumption.

## raltegravir

ral-**teg**-ra-veer
(Isentress)

## ◆CLASSIFICATION

**PHARMACOTHERAPEUTIC:** Integrase inhibitor. **CLINICAL:** Antiviral.

## USES

Treatment of HIV-1 infection in adults and children 4 wks and older and weighing at least 3 kg. Used in combination with at least two other antiretroviral agents. **OFF-LABEL:** Postexposure prophylaxis for occupational exposure to HIV.

## PRECAUTIONS

**Contraindications:** Hypersensitivity to raltegravir. **Cautions:** Elderly, pts at risk for creatine kinase (CK) elevations and/or skeletal muscle abnormalities.

## ACTION

Inhibits activity of HIV-1 integrase, an enzyme that incorporates viral DNA into host cell. **Therapeutic Effect:** Prevents integration and replication of viral HIV-1.

## PHARMACOKINETICS

Variably absorbed following PO administration. Protein binding: 83%. Metabolized in liver. Eliminated in feces (51%), urine (32%). **Half-life:** 9 hrs.

## ⧗ LIFESPAN CONSIDERATIONS

**Pregnancy/Lactation:** May cross placenta. Breastfeeding not recommended. **Children:** Safety and efficacy not established in pts younger than 16 yrs. **Elderly:** Age-related hepatic, renal, cardiac impairment requires strict monitoring.

## INTERACTIONS

**DRUG: Proton pump inhibitors (e.g., omeprazole, pantoprazole)** may increase concentration. **HERBAL: St. John's wort** may decrease concentration/effects. **FOOD:** None known. **LAB VALUES:** May increase serum glucose, bilirubin, aminotransferase, alkaline phosphatase, amylase, lipase, creatine kinase. May decrease lymphocytes, neutrophil count (ANC), Hgb, platelets.

## AVAILABILITY (Rx)

**Packet, Oral:** 100 mg. **Tablets, Chewable:** 25 mg, 100 mg.

🔪 **Tablets, Film-Coated:** 400 mg.

## ADMINISTRATION/HANDLING

**PO**
• Give without regard to food. • Do not break, crush, dissolve, or divide film-coated tablets. • Chewable tablets may be chewed or taken whole. • **Oral Packet:** Mix with 5 ml water. Once mixed, measure dose with oral syringe. Give within 30 min of mixing.

## INDICATIONS/ROUTES/DOSAGE

**HIV Infection**
**PO: ADULTS, ELDERLY, CHILDREN 12 YRS AND OLDER:** 400 mg twice daily. Dosage increased to 800 mg twice daily when given with rifampin. **CHILDREN 2–11 YRS (CHEWABLE TABLETS): 40 KG OR GREATER:** 300 mg twice daily. **28–39 KG:** 200 mg twice daily. **20–27 KG:** 150 mg twice daily. **(ORAL PACKET): 14–19 KG:** 100 mg twice daily. **11–13 KG:** 80 mg twice daily. **8–10 KG:** 60 mg twice daily. **6–7 KG:** 40 mg twice daily. **4–5 KG:** 30 mg twice daily. **3–4 KG:** 20 mg twice daily.

**Dosage in Renal/Hepatic Impairment**
No dose adjustment.

## SIDE EFFECTS

**Frequent (17%–10%):** Diarrhea, nausea, headache. **Occasional (5%):** Fever. **Rare (2%–1%):** Vomiting, abdominal pain, fatigue, dizziness.

## ADVERSE EFFECTS/ TOXIC REACTIONS

Hypersensitivity reactions, anemia, neutropenia, MI, gastritis, hepatitis, herpes simplex, toxic nephropathy, renal failure, chronic renal failure, renal tubular necrosis occur rarely.

## NURSING CONSIDERATIONS

### BASELINE ASSESSMENT

Obtain baseline CBC, BMP, LFT, CD4 count, viral load beginning therapy and at periodic intervals during therapy. Offer emotional support. Obtain medication history.

**R**

### INTERVENTION/EVALUATION

Closely monitor for evidence of GI discomfort. Monitor daily pattern of bowel activity, stool consistency. Monitor serum chemistry tests for marked laboratory abnormalities. Assess for opportunistic infections: onset of fever, cough, other respiratory symptoms.

### PATIENT/FAMILY TEACHING

• Report fever, abdominal pain, yellowing of skin/eyes, dark urine. • Avoid tasks that require alertness, motor skills until response to drug is established. • Raltegravir is not a cure for HIV infection, nor does it reduce risk of transmission to others. • Pt may continue to experience illnesses, including opportunistic infections.

---

# ramelteon

ra-**mel**-tee-on
(Rozerem)
**Do not confuse ramelteon with Remeron, or Rozerem with Razadyne or Remeron.**

### ◆CLASSIFICATION

**PHARMACOTHERAPEUTIC:** Melatonin receptor agonist. **CLINICAL:** Hypnotic.

## USES

Treatment of insomnia in pts who experience difficulty with sleep onset.

## PRECAUTIONS

**Contraindications:** Hypersensitivity to ramelteon. Concurrent fluvoxamine therapy, history of angioedema with previous ramelteon therapy. **Cautions:** Depression, other psychiatric conditions, alcohol consumption, other CNS depressants, moderate hepatic impairment, severe sleep apnea, COPD; concomitant strong CYP1A2 inhibitors (e.g., fluvoxamine).

## ACTION

Selectively targets melatonin receptors thought to be involved in maintenance of circadian rhythm underlying normal sleep-wake cycle. **Therapeutic Effect:** Prevents insomnia characterized by difficulty with sleep onset.

## PHARMACOKINETICS

Rapidly absorbed following PO administration. Protein binding: 82%. Substantial tissue distribution. Metabolized in liver. Excreted in urine (84%), feces (4%). **Half-life:** 2–5 hrs.

## ⧗ LIFESPAN CONSIDERATIONS

**Pregnancy/Lactation:** Unknown if distributed in breast milk. Breastfeeding not recommended. **Children:** Safety and efficacy not established. **Elderly:** Age-related hepatic impairment may require dosage adjustment.

## INTERACTIONS

**DRUG:** Concurrent use with **alcohol** may produce additive effect. **Fluconazole, ketoconazole** may increase serum concentration/effects. **Donepezil, doxepin, fluvoxamine** may cause marked increase in serum level, toxicity. **Rifampin** may decrease serum level, effects. **HERBAL:** Gotu kola, kava kava, St. John's wort, valerian may increase CNS depression. **FOOD:** Onset of action may be reduced if taken with or immediately after a **high-fat meal. LAB VALUES:** May decrease serum cortisol.

## AVAILABILITY (Rx)

Tablets, Film-Coated: 8 mg (Rozerem).

## ADMINISTRATION/HANDLING

**PO**
• Administer within 30 min before bedtime. • Do not give with, or immediately following, a high-fat meal. • Do not break, crush, dissolve, or divide tablet.

## INDICATIONS/ROUTES/DOSAGE

**Insomnia**
**PO: ADULTS, ELDERLY:** 8 mg 30 min before bedtime.

**Dosage in Renal Impairment**
No dose adjustment.

**Dosage in Hepatic Impairment**
**Mild to moderate impairment:** No dose adjustment. **Severe impairment:** Not recommended.

## SIDE EFFECTS

**Frequent (7%–5%):** Headache, dizziness, drowsiness (expected effect). **Occasional (4%–3%):** Fatigue, nausea, exacerbated insomnia. **Rare (2%):** Diarrhea, myalgia, depression, altered taste, arthralgia.

## ADVERSE EFFECTS/ TOXIC REACTIONS

May affect reproductive hormones in adults (decreased testosterone levels, increased prolactin levels), resulting in unexplained amenorrhea, galactorrhea, decreased libido, impaired fertility.

## NURSING CONSIDERATIONS

### BASELINE ASSESSMENT

Assess B/P, pulse, respirations. Raise bed rails, provide call light. Provide environment conducive to sleep (quiet environment, low/no lighting, TV off).

### INTERVENTION/EVALUATION

Assess sleep pattern of pt. Evaluate for therapeutic response: rapid induction of sleep onset, decrease in number of nocturnal awakenings.

### PATIENT/FAMILY TEACHING

• Take within 30 min before going to bed; confine activities to those necessary to prepare for bed. • Avoid tasks that require alertness, motor skills until response to drug is established. • Avoid alcohol. • Do not take medication with or immediately after a high-fat meal.

# ramipril

**ram-i-pril**
(Altace, Apo-Ramipril ✦)
■ **BLACK BOX ALERT** ■ May cause fetal injury, mortality. Discontinue as soon as possible once pregnancy is detected.
**Do not confuse Altace with alteplase, Amaryl, or Artane, or ramipril with enalapril or Monopril.**

## ◆ CLASSIFICATION

**PHARMACOTHERAPEUTIC:** Renin-angiotensin system antagonist. **CLINICAL:** Antihypertensive.

## USES

Treatment of hypertension. Used alone or in combination with other antihypertensives. Treatment of HF following MI. Reduce risk of heart attack, stroke in pts at increased risk of developing major cardiovascular events. **OFF-LABEL:** HF. Delay progression of nephropathy, reduce risks of cardiovascular events in hypertensive pts with type 1 or type 2 diabetes.

## PRECAUTIONS

**Contraindications:** Hypersensitivity to ramipril, other ACE inhibitors. History of ACE-inhibitor induced angioedema, concomitant use with aliskiren in pts with diabetes. **Cautions:** Renal impairment, elderly, collagen vascular disease, hyperkalemia, hypertrophic cardiomyopathy with outflow tract obstruction; unstented unilateral, bilateral renal artery stenosis; severe aortic stenosis; before, during, or immediately after major surgery, concomitant potassium supplements.

## ACTION

Suppresses renin-angiotensin-aldosterone system. Decreases plasma angiotensin II, increases plasma renin activity, decreases aldosterone secretion. **Therapeutic Effect:** Reduces peripheral arterial resistance, decreasing B/P.

R

## PHARMACOKINETICS

| Route | Onset | Peak | Duration |
|-------|-------|------|----------|
| PO | 1–2 hrs | 3–6 hrs | 24 hrs |

Well absorbed from GI tract. Protein binding: 73%. Metabolized in liver. Primarily excreted in urine. Not removed by hemodialysis. **Half-life:** 5.1 hrs.

## ⧗ LIFESPAN CONSIDERATIONS

**Pregnancy/Lactation:** Crosses placenta. Distributed in breast milk. May cause fetal or neonatal mortality or morbidity. **Children:** Safety and efficacy not established. **Elderly:** May be more sensitive to hypotensive effects.

## INTERACTIONS

**DRUG:** Alcohol, **antihypertensives** (e.g., **amlodipine, lisinopril, valsartan**), **diuretics** (e.g., **furosemide, HCTZ**) may increase effects. May increase **lithium** concentration, risk of toxicity. **NSAIDs** may decrease effects. **Potassium-sparing diuretics** (e.g., **spironolactone, triamterene**), **potassium supplements** may cause hyperkalemia. **HERBAL:** Black cohosh, periwinkle may increase antihypertensive effect. **Ginseng, ginger, licorice, yohimbe** may worsen hypertension. **FOOD:** None known. **LAB VALUES:** May increase serum BUN, alkaline phosphatase, bilirubin, creatinine, potassium, ALT, AST. May decrease serum sodium. May cause positive antinuclear antibody (ANA) titer.

## AVAILABILITY (Rx)

**Capsules:** 1.25 mg, 2.5 mg, 5 mg, 10 mg.

## ADMINISTRATION/HANDLING

**PO**
• Give without regard to food. • May mix with water, apple juice/sauce.

## INDICATIONS/ROUTES/DOSAGE

**Hypertension (Monotherapy)**
**PO: ADULTS, ELDERLY:** Initially, 2.5 mg/day. Usual dose: 5–10 mg/day.

**Hypertension (in Combination with Other Antihypertensives)**
**PO: ADULTS, ELDERLY:** Initially, 1.25 mg/day titrated to pt's needs.

**HF Following MI**
**PO: ADULTS, ELDERLY:** Initially, 1.25–2.5 mg twice daily. Continue for 1 wk, then titrate upward q3wks to target dose of 5 mg twice daily.

**Risk Reduction for MI/Stroke**
**PO: ADULTS, ELDERLY:** Initially, 2.5 mg/day for 7 days, then 5 mg/day for 21 days, then 10 mg/day as a single dose or in divided doses.

**Dosage in Renal Impairment**
**CrCl equal to or less than 40 ml/min:** 25% of normal dose.

**Renal Failure and Hypertension**
Initially, 1.25 mg/day titrated upward. **Maximum:** 5 mg/day.
**Renal Failure and HF:** Initially, 1.25 mg/day, titrated up to 2.5 mg twice daily.

**Dosage in Hepatic Impairment**
No dose adjustment. Discontinue for jaundice or marked elevation of hepatic enzymes.

## SIDE EFFECTS

**Frequent (12%–5%):** Cough, headache. **Occasional (4%–2%):** Dizziness, fatigue, nausea, asthenia. **Rare (less than 2%):** Palpitations, insomnia, nervousness, malaise, abdominal pain, myalgia.

## ADVERSE EFFECTS/ TOXIC REACTIONS

Excessive hypotension ("first-dose syncope") may occur in pts with HF, severely salt or volume depleted. Angioedema, hyperkalemia occur rarely. Agranulocytosis, neutropenia may be noted in pts with collagen vascular disease (scleroderma, systemic lupus erythematosus), renal impairment. Nephrotic syndrome may be noted in those with history of renal disease.

# NURSING CONSIDERATIONS

## BASELINE ASSESSMENT

Obtain B/P immediately before each dose, in addition to regular monitoring (be alert to fluctuations). If excessive reduction in B/P occurs, place pt in supine position with legs elevated. Renal function tests should be performed before beginning therapy. In pts with prior renal disease, urine test for protein (by dipstick method) should be made with first urine of day before beginning therapy and periodically thereafter. In pts with renal impairment, autoimmune disease, or taking drugs that affect leukocytes or immune response, CBC, differential count should be performed before beginning therapy and q2wks for 3 mos periodically thereafter. Question history of hypersensitivity reaction, angioedema.

## INTERVENTION/EVALUATION

Monitor B/P, renal function, serum potassium, WBC. Assess for cough (frequent effect). Assist with ambulation if dizziness occurs. Assess lung sounds for rales, wheezing in pts with HF. Monitor urinalysis for proteinuria. Monitor serum potassium in pts on concurrent diuretic therapy.

## PATIENT/FAMILY TEACHING

• Do not discontinue medication without physician's approval. • Slowly go from lying to standing to minimize hypotensive effect. • Report palpitations, cough, chest pain. • Dizziness may occur in first few days. • Avoid tasks that require alertness, motor skills until response to drug is established. • Avoid alcohol. • Report swelling of the face, lips, or tongue.

# ramucirumab

ra-mue-**sir**-ue-mab
(Cyramza)

■ **BLACK BOX ALERT** ■ May increase risk of severe, and sometimes fatal, hemorrhagic events. Permanently discontinue if severe bleeding occurs.

**Do not confuse ramucirumab with ranibizumab.**

## ◆CLASSIFICATION

**PHARMACOTHERAPEUTIC:** Vascular endothelial growth factor 2 antagonist. **CLINICAL:** Antineoplastic.

## USES

As a single agent or in combination with paclitaxel, for treatment of advanced or metastatic gastric or gastroesophageal junction adenocarcinoma with disease progression on or after prior fluoropyrimidine- or platinum-containing chemotherapy. In combination with docetaxel, for treatment of metastatic non small cell lung cancer (NSCLC) with disease progression on or after platinum based chemotherapy. In combination with FOLFIRI, for treatment of metastatic colorectal cancer with disease progression on or after therapy with bevacizumab, oxaliplatin, and a fluoropyrimidine.

## PRECAUTIONS

**Contraindications:** Hypersensitivity to ramucirumab. **Cautions:** History of arterial/venous thromboembolism (e.g., MI, cardiac arrest, CVA, cerebral ischemia) hepatic cirrhosis, electrolyte imbalance, hypertension, GI bleeding/perforation, chronic/unhealed wounds; baseline neutropenia, thrombocytopenia.

## ACTION

Binds vascular endothelial growth factor (VEGF) receptor 2 and blocks binding of VEGF ligands, VEGF-A, VEGF-C, and VEGF-D. **Therapeutic Effect:** Inhibits/reduces tumor vascularity and growth.

## PHARMACOKINETICS

Metabolism not specified. Elimination not specified.

## ⧖ LIFESPAN CONSIDERATIONS

**Pregnancy/Lactation:** May cause fetal harm. Contraception recommended during treatment and up to 3 mos after

R

discontinuation. Must either discontinue drug or discontinue breastfeeding. Unknown if distributed in breast milk. **Children:** Safety and efficacy not established. **Elderly:** No age-related precautions noted.

## INTERACTIONS

**DRUG:** None known (no studies conducted). **HERBAL:** None significant. **FOOD:** None known. **LAB VALUES:** May increase urine protein. May decrease neutrophils, serum sodium.

## AVAILABILITY (Rx)

**Injection Solution:** 100 mg/10 ml, 500 mg/50 ml.

## ADMINISTRATION/HANDLING

 IV

• Do not administer IV push or bolus. • Recommend premedication with IV histamine $H_1$ antagonist (e.g., diphenhydramine) prior to each infusion. Pts with prior grade 1 or grade 2 infusion reaction should be also premedicated with dexamethasone (or equivalent) and acetaminophen prior to each infusion. • Thoroughly flush IV with 0.9% NaCl upon infusion completion.

**Reconstitution** • Calculate dose, required solution volume, and number of vials needed using weight in kg • Vials contain either 100 mg/10 ml or 500 ml/50 ml at concentration of 10 mg/ml. • Visually inspect for particulate matter. Discard if particulate matter or discoloration observed. • Using 250 ml 0.9% NaCl bag, withdraw and discard a volume equal to the total calculated volume of solution. • Slowly add required dose to diluent bag for final volume of 250 ml. Gently invert bag to mix; do not shake.

**Rate of Administration** • Infuse over 60 min using 0.22-micron in-line filter via dedicated line.

**Storage** • Refrigerate vials in original carton until time of use. • Do not freeze. • Diluted solution may be refrigerated up to 24 hrs or stored at room temperature for up to 4 hrs. • Protect from light.

## ⬛ IV INCOMPATABILITIES

Do not dilute in dextrose-containing fluids or infuse concomitantly with other electrolytes or medications.

## INDICATIONS/ROUTES/DOSAGE

**Gastric or Gastroesophageal Junction Cancer**
**IV: ADULTS, ELDERLY:** 8 mg/kg every 14 days, either as a single agent or in combination with paclitaxel. Continue until disease progression or unacceptable toxicity.

**NSCLC**
**IV: ADULTS, ELDERLY:** 10 mg/kg on day 1 of a 21-day cycle in combination with docetaxel. Continue until disease progression or unacceptable toxicity.

**Colorectal Cancer**
**IV: ADULTS, ELDERLY:** 8 mg/kg q2wks, in combination with FOLFIRI (irinotecan, leucovorin, 5-fluorouracil). Continue until disease progression or unacceptable toxicity.

**Dose Modification**
Based on Common Terminology Criteria for Adverse Events (CTCAE).
**Infusion-related reaction:** Reduce infusion rate by 50% for grade 1 or grade 2 reaction. Permanently discontinue for grade 3 or grade 4 reaction.
**Severe hypertension:** Interrupt treatment until controlled with medical management. Permanently discontinue for severe hypertension that is not controlled with antihypertensive therapy.
**Proteinuria:** Interrupt treatment for urine protein level greater than or equal to 2 g/24 hrs. Restart treatment at reduced dose of 6 mg/kg every 14 days once urine protein level returns to less than 2 g/24 hrs. If level greater than or equal 2 g/24 hrs reoccurs, interrupt treatment and reduce dose to 5 mg/kg every 14 days once level returns to less than

R

2 mg/24 hrs. Permanently discontinue for urine protein level greater than 3 g/24 hrs or in the setting of nephrotic syndrome.

**Wound healing complications:** Interrupt treatment prior to scheduled surgery until wound is fully healed.

**Arterial thromboembolic events, GI perforation, or grade 3 or grade 4 bleeding:** Permanently discontinue.

**Dosage in Renal Impairment**
No dose adjustment.

**Dosage in Hepatic Impairment**
**Mild to moderate impairment:** No dose adjustment. **Severe impairment:** Use caution.

## SIDE EFFECTS

**Occasional (16%–9%):** Hypertension, diarrhea, headache.
**Ramucirumab plus Paclitaxel: Frequent (57%–20%):** Fatigue, diarrhea, peripheral edema, hypertension, stomatitis.

## ADVERSE EFFECTS/ TOXIC REACTIONS

Severe, and sometimes fatal, hemorrhagic events including GI bleeding occurred in 3.4% of pts receiving single agent and in 4.3% of pts receiving combo therapy. GI perforations occurred in 0.7% of pts receiving single agent and in 1.2% of pts receiving combo therapy. Thromboembolic events including arterial thromboembolism, CVA, MI reported in 1.7% of pts. Severe hypertension occurred in 8% of pts receiving single agent and in 15% of pts receiving combo therapy despite medical management. Severe infusion-related reactions such as back pain/spasms, bronchospasm, chest pain, chills, dyspnea, flushing, hypotension, hypoxia, paresthesia, rigors/tremors, supraventricular tachycardia, wheezing occurred in 16% of pts. May cause ineffective wound healing or wound dehiscence requiring medical intervention. Reversible posterior leukoencephalopathy syndrome (RPLS) reported in less than 1% of pts. Proteinuria may indicate nephrotic syndrome. Clinical deterioration of hepatic cirrhosis, manifested by new-onset or worsening encephalopathy, ascites, or hepatorenal syndrome, was reported in pts receiving single agent. Other adverse reactions include epistaxis, intestinal obstruction neutropenia, severe rash, thrombocytopenia. Immunogenicity (anti-ramucirumab antibodies) occurred in 6% of pts.

## NURSING CONSIDERATIONS

### BASELINE ASSESSMENT

Obtain CBC, BMP, urinalysis, urine protein, vital signs. Assess skin for open wounds. Question possibility of pregnancy, current breastfeeding status. Receive full medication history including vitamins, herbal products. Question history of CVA, hepatic impairment/cirrhosis hypertension, MI, prior hypersensitivity reaction.

### INTERVENTION/EVALUATION

Monitor CBC, electrolytes, urinalysis, urine protein. Routinely assess vital signs and report hypertension. Persistent diastolic hypertension may indicate hypertensive emergency. Obtain EKG for arrhythmia, chest pain palpitation. Consider RPLS in pts with altered mental status, confusion, headache, seizure, visual disturbances. Encourage PO intake. Screen for GI bleeding, GI perforation. Notify physician if any CTCAE toxicities occur (see Appendix M). Monitor for hypersensitivity reaction. Once infusion completed, IV access must be flushed with NS.

### PATIENT/FAMILY TEACHING

• Blood levels will be routinely monitored. • Treatment may cause severe allergic reaction or infusion-related reaction. • Avoid pregnancy; treatment may cause birth defects or miscarriage. Do not breastfeed. Contraception should be taken during treatment and up to 3 mos after discontinuation. • Neurologic changes, including altered mental status, headache, seizures, trouble speaking, may indicate high blood pressure crisis or

R

life-threatening brain swelling. • Immediately report abdominal pain, GI bleeding, vomiting blood; may indicate gastrointestinal tear. • Therapy may cause severe blood-clotting events such as heart attack or stroke.

# *raNITIdine

ra-**nit**-i-deen
(Apo-Ranitidine ❦, Deprizine FusePaq, Zantac, Zantac-75, Zantac-150 Maximum Strength)
**Do not confuse ranitidine with amantadine or rimantadine, or Zantac with Xanax, Ziac, Zofran, or Zyrtec.**

## ◆CLASSIFICATION

**PHARMACOTHERAPEUTIC:** Histamine $H_2$ receptor antagonist. **CLINICAL:** Antiulcer.

## USES

Short-term treatment of active duodenal ulcer. Prevention of duodenal ulcer recurrence. Treatment of active benign gastric ulcer, pathologic GI hypersecretory conditions, acute gastroesophageal reflux disease (GERD), including erosive esophagitis. Maintenance of healed erosive esophagitis. **OTC:** Relieve heartburn, acid indigestion, sour stomach. **OFF-LABEL:** Treatment of upper GI bleeding. Prevention of stress-induced ulcers in ICU. Anaphylaxis (adjunct therapy). Premedication to prevent taxane hypersensitivity.

## PRECAUTIONS

**Contraindications:** Hypersensitivity to ranitidine. **Cautions:** Renal/hepatic impairment, elderly, history of acute porphyria.

## ACTION

Inhibits histamine action at histamine 2 receptors of gastric parietal cells.

**Therapeutic Effect:** Inhibits gastric acid secretion. Reduces gastric volume, hydrogen ion concentration of gastric juice.

## PHARMACOKINETICS

Rapidly absorbed from GI tract. Protein binding: 15%. Widely distributed. Metabolized in liver. Primarily excreted in urine. Not removed by hemodialysis. **Half-life: PO:** 2.5 hrs; **IV:** 2–2.5 hrs (increased with renal impairment).

## ⌛ LIFESPAN CONSIDERATIONS

**Pregnancy/Lactation:** Unknown if drug crosses placenta or is distributed in breast milk. **Children:** No age-related precautions noted. **Elderly:** Confusion more likely with hepatic/renal impairment.

## INTERACTIONS

**DRUG: Magnesium or aluminum antacids** may decrease absorption. May decrease absorption of **atazanavir, itraconazole, ketoconazole. HERBAL:** None significant. **FOOD:** None known. **LAB VALUES:** Interferes with skin tests using allergen extracts. May increase serum ALT, AST, GGT, creatinine.

## AVAILABILITY (Rx)

**Capsules:** 150 mg, 300 mg. **Injection Solution:** 25 mg/ml. **Syrup:** 15 mg/ml. **Suspension (Deprizine FusePaq):** 22.4 mg/ml. **Tablets:** 75 mg, 150 mg, 300 mg.

## ADMINISTRATION/HANDLING

 IV

**Reconstitution** • For IV push, dilute each 50 mg with 20 ml 0.9% NaCl, $D_5W$. • For intermittent IV infusion (piggyback), dilute each 50 mg with 0.9% NaCl, $D_5W$ to a maximum concentration of 0.5 mg/ml. • For IV infusion, dilute with 0.9% NaCl, $D_5W$ to a maximum concentration of 2.5 mg/ml.
**Rate of Administration** • Administer IV push over minimum of 5 min (prevents arrhythmias, hypotension). • Infuse IV piggyback over 15–20 min. • Infuse IV infusion over 24 hrs.

R

**Storage** • IV solutions appear clear, colorless to yellow (slight darkening does not affect potency). • IV infusion (piggyback) is stable for 48 hrs at room temperature (discard if discolored or precipitate forms).

### IM

• May be given undiluted. • Give deep IM into large muscle mass.

### PO

• Give without regard to meals (best given with meals or at bedtime). • Do not administer within 1 hr of magnesium- or aluminum-containing antacids (decreases absorption).

### 🅥 IV INCOMPATIBILITIES

Amphotericin B complex (Abelcet, AmBisome, Amphotec).

### 🅥 IV COMPATIBILITIES

Dexmedetomidine (Precedex), diltiazem (Cardizem), dobutamine (Dobutrex), dopamine (Intropin), heparin, hydromorphone (Dilaudid), insulin, lidocaine, lorazepam (Ativan), morphine, norepinephrine (Levophed), potassium chloride, propofol (Diprivan).

## INDICATIONS/ROUTES/DOSAGE

**Duodenal Ulcer**
**PO: ADULTS, ELDERLY: Treatment:** 150 mg twice daily or 300 mg once daily. **Maintenance:** 150 mg once daily at bedtime. **CHILDREN 1 MO TO 16 YRS: Treatment:** 4–8 mg/kg/day in 2 divided doses. **Maximum:** 300 mg. **Maintenance:** 2–4 mg/kg/day once daily. **Maximum:** 150 mg/day.

**Gastric Ulcer (Benign)**
**PO: ADULTS, ELDERLY: Treatment:** 150 mg 2 times/day. **Maintenance:** 150 mg once daily at bedtime. **CHILDREN 1 MO–16 YRS: Treatment:** 4–8 mg/kg/day in 2 divided doses. **Maximum:** 300 mg/day. **Maintenance:** 2–4 mg/kg/day once daily. **Maximum (healing):** 150 mg/day.

**Hypersecretory Conditions**
**PO: ADULTS, ELDERLY:** 150 mg twice daily up to 6 g/day. **IV Infusion:** Initially, 1 mg/kg/hr. May increase by 0.5 mg/kg/hr up to 2.5 mg/kg/hr.

**GERD**
**PO: ADULTS, ELDERLY:** 150 mg twice daily. **CHILDREN 1 MO TO 16 YRS:** 5–10 mg/kg/day in 2 divided doses. **Maximum:** 300 mg/day.

**Erosive Esophagitis**
**PO: ADULTS, ELDERLY: Treatment:** 150 mg 4 times/day. **Maintenance:** 150 mg twice daily. **CHILDREN 1 MO TO 16 YRS: Treatment:** 5–10 mg/kg/day in 2 divided doses. **Maximum:** 600 mg/day.

**Prevention of Heartburn**
**PO: ADULTS, ELDERLY, CHILDREN 12 YRS AND OLDER:** 75–150 mg 30–60 min before eating or drinking beverages that cause heartburn. **Maximum:** 2 doses/day. Do not use more than 14 days.

**Usual Parenteral Dosage**
**IV: ADULTS, ELDERLY:** 50 mg q6–8h. **CHILDREN:** 2–4 mg/kg/day in divided doses q6–8h. **Maximum:** 200 mg/day. **IV Infusion:** 6.25 mg/hr.

**Usual Neonatal Dosage**
**PO: NEONATES:** 2 mg/kg/day in divided doses q8–12h.
**IV: NEONATES:** Initially, 1.5 mg/kg/dose, then 1.5–2 mg/kg/day in divided doses q8h. **IV Infusion: NEONATES:** Loading dose: 1.5 mg/kg, then 1–2 mg/kg/day (0.04–0.08 mg/kg/hr).

**Dosage in Renal Impairment**
**CrCl less than 50 ml/min:** Give 150 mg PO q24h or 50 mg IV q18–24h.

**Dosage in Hepatic Impairment**
No dose adjustment.

## SIDE EFFECTS

**Occasional (2%):** Diarrhea. **Rare (1%):** Constipation, headache (may be severe).

R

## ADVERSE EFFECTS/ TOXIC REACTIONS

Reversible hepatitis, blood dyscrasias occur rarely.

## NURSING CONSIDERATIONS

### BASELINE ASSESSMENT

Obtain history of epigastric/abdominal pain. Obtain baseline renal function in pts with renal impairment.

### INTERVENTION/EVALUATION

Assess mental status in elderly. Question present abdominal pain, GI distress.

### PATIENT/FAMILY TEACHING

• Smoking decreases effectiveness of medication. • Do not take medicine within 1 hr of magnesium- or aluminum-containing antacids. • Transient burning/ pruritus may occur with IV administration. • Report headache. • Avoid alcohol, aspirin.

---

# ranolazine

ra-**noe**-la-zeen
(Ranexa)
**Do not confuse Ranexa with Celexa.**

## ◆CLASSIFICATION

**PHARMACOTHERAPEUTIC:** Sodium current inhibitor. **CLINICAL:** Antianginal, anti-ischemic.

## USES

Treatment of chronic angina.

## PRECAUTIONS

**Contraindications:** Hypersensitivity to ranolazine. Hepatic cirrhosis, concurrent use of strong CYP3A inhibitors (e.g., rifampin, carbamazepine) or CYP3A inducers (e.g., ketoconazole, itraconazole, fluconazole, clarithromycin, erythromycin). **Cautions:** Renal/hepatic impairment. Preexisting QT prolongation, concurrent use with medications known to prolong QT interval, pts 75 yrs of age or older, hypokalemia, hypomagnesemia.

## ACTION

Inhibits inward current of sodium channel during cardiac repolarization, thereby reducing calcium influx. Decreased influx of calcium reduces ventricular tension, myocardial oxygen demand. Does not reduce heart rate, B/P. **Therapeutic Effect:** Exerts antianginal, anti-ischemic effects on cardiac tissue.

## PHARMACOKINETICS

Absorption highly variable. Peak plasma concentration: 2–5 hrs. Rapidly, extensively metabolized in intestine, liver. Protein binding: 62%. Eliminated in urine (75%), feces (25%). **Half-life:** 7 hrs.

## ⧗ LIFESPAN CONSIDERATIONS

**Pregnancy/Lactation:** Unknown if drug crosses placenta or is distributed in breast milk. **Children:** Safety and efficacy not established. **Elderly:** No age-related precautions noted.

## INTERACTIONS

**DRUG:** See contraindications. **Diltiazem, verapamil** may increase serum concentration. May increase concentration of **cyclosporine, digoxin, simvastatin, sirolimus, tacrolimus.** Antiarrhythmic agents, **dofetilide, quinidine, sotalol, thioridazine, ziprasidone** may increase risk of QT prolongation. **HERBAL: St. John's wort** may decrease concentration/ effects. **FOOD: Grapefruit products** may increase plasma concentration, risk of QT prolongation. **LAB VALUES:** May slightly elevate serum BUN, creatinine.

## AVAILABILITY (Rx)

🐚 Tablets (Extended-Release): 500 mg, 1,000 mg.

## ADMINISTRATION/HANDLING

### PO

• May give without regard to food.
• Do not break, crush, dissolve, or divide extended-release tablets.

---

*"Tall Man" lettering                    underlined – top prescribed drug

## INDICATIONS/ROUTES/DOSAGE

### Chronic Angina

**PO: ADULTS, ELDERLY:** Initially, 500 mg twice daily. May increase to 1,000 mg twice daily, based on clinical response. Dose should not exceed 500 mg twice daily when used concurrently with moderate CYP3A inhibitors (e.g., diltiazem, verapamil).

### Dosage in Renal/Hepatic Impairment

No dose adjustment (discontinue if acute renal failure develops). Contraindicated in pts with cirrhosis.

## SIDE EFFECTS

**Occasional (6%–4%):** Dizziness, headache, constipation, nausea. **Rare (2%–1%):** Peripheral edema, abdominal pain, dry mouth, vomiting, tinnitus, vertigo, palpitations.

## ADVERSE EFFECTS/TOXIC REACTIONS

Overdose manifested as confusion, diplopia, dizziness, paresthesia, syncope.

## NURSING CONSIDERATIONS

### BASELINE ASSESSMENT

Receive full medication history and screen for contraindications. Question history of hepatic impairment, long QT syndrome. Record onset, type (sharp, dull, squeezing), radiation, location, intensity, duration of anginal pain, precipitating factors (exertion, emotional stress). Obtain baseline EKG.

### INTERVENTION/EVALUATION

Assist with ambulation if dizziness occurs. Give with food if nausea occurs. Assess for relief of anginal pain. Monitor EKG, pulse for irregularities.

### PATIENT/FAMILY TEACHING

• Avoid grapefruit products. • Do not chew, crush, dissolve, or divide extended-release tablets. • Avoid tasks requiring alertness, motor skills until response to drug is established.

# rasagiline

ra-**sa**-ji-leen
(Azilect)
**Do not confuse Azilect with Aricept.**

## ◆CLASSIFICATION

**PHARMACOTHERAPEUTIC:** MAOI.
**CLINICAL:** Antiparkinson agent.

## USES

Treatment of signs/symptoms of Parkinson's disease as initial monotherapy or as adjunct therapy with or without levodopa.

## PRECAUTIONS

**Contraindications:** Hypersensitivity to rasagiline. Concurrent use with methadone, tramadol, dextromethorphan, St. John's wort, cyclobenzaprine, meperidine, MAOIs within 14 days of rasagiline. **Cautions:** Hepatic impairment (avoid use in moderate to severe impairment); cardiovascular, cerebrovascular disease, pts with hypotension. Avoid foods high in tyramine. Do not use within 5 wks of stopping fluoxetine; do not start tricyclic, SSRI, or SNRI within 2 wks of stopping rasagiline. History of major psychotic disorder.

## ACTION

Inhibits monoamine oxidase type B, an enzyme that plays a major role in catabolism of dopamine. Inhibition of dopamine depletion reduces symptomatic motor deficits of Parkinson's disease. **Therapeutic Effect:** Reduces symptoms of Parkinson's disease, appears to delay disease progression.

## PHARMACOKINETICS

Rapidly absorbed following PO administration. Protein binding: 88%–94%. Metabolized in liver. Eliminated in urine (62%), feces (7%). **Half-life:** 1.3–3 hrs.

R

## ⌛ LIFESPAN CONSIDERATIONS

**Pregnancy/Lactation:** Unknown if distributed in breast milk. **Children:** Safety and efficacy not established. **Elderly:** No age-related precautions noted.

## INTERACTIONS

**DRUG: Amphetamines, other MAOIs (e.g., phenelzine, tranylcypromine), sympathomimetics (e.g., dopamine, phenylephrine, pseudoephedrine)** may cause hypertensive crisis. **Anorexiants (e.g., dexfenfluramine, fenfluramine, sibutramine), CNS stimulants (e.g., methylphenidate), cyclobenzaprine, dextromethorphan, meperidine, methadone, mirtazapine, serotonin or norepinephrine reuptake inhibitors (e.g., citalopram, sertraline, venlafaxine), sibutramine, tramadol, trazodone, tricyclic antidepressants (e.g., amitriptyline, doxepin), venlafaxine** may cause serotonin syndrome. May increase risk of **atomoxetine, bupropion** toxicity. **Ciprofloxacin, entacapone, tolcapone** may increase concentration (reduced dosage recommended). **Levodopa** may cause hypertensive/hypotensive reaction. **HERBAL: Kava kava, SAMe, St. John's wort, valerian** may increase risk of serotonin syndrome, excessive sedation. **FOOD: Caffeine, foods/beverages containing tyramine** may result in hypertensive reaction, hypertensive crisis. **LAB VALUES:** May increase serum alkaline phosphatase, bilirubin, ALT, AST. May cause leukopenia.

## AVAILABILITY (Rx)

**Tablets:** 0.5 mg, 1 mg.

## ADMINISTRATION/HANDLING

**PO**
• Give without regard to food. • Avoid food, beverages containing tyramine (e.g., cheese, sour cream, yogurt, pickled herring, liver, figs, raisins, bananas, avocados, soy sauce, broad beans, yeast extracts, meat tenderizers, red wine, beer), excessive amounts of caffeine (e.g., coffee, tea).

## INDICATIONS/ROUTES/DOSAGE

◀**ALERT▶** When used in combination with levodopa, dosage reduction of levodopa should be considered.

**Parkinson's Disease**
**PO: ADULTS, ELDERLY, MONOTHERAPY:** 1 mg once daily.
**PO: ADULTS, ELDERLY, ADJUNCTIVE THERAPY WITH LEVODOPA:** Initially, 0.5 mg once daily. If therapeutic response is not achieved, dose may be increased to 1 mg once daily. **ADJUNCTIVE THERAPY WITHOUT LEVODOPA:** 1 mg once daily.

**Dosage in Hepatic Impairment**
**Mild impairment, concurrent use of ciprofloxacin, other CYP1A2 inhibitors:** 0.5 mg once daily. **Moderate to severe impairment:** Not recommended.

**Dosage in Renal Impairment**
No dose adjustment.

## SIDE EFFECTS

**Frequent (14%–12%):** Headache, nausea. **Occasional (9%–5%):** Orthostatic hypotension, weight loss, dyspepsia, dry mouth, arthralgia, depression, hallucinations, constipation. **Rare (4%–2%):** Fever, vertigo, ecchymosis, rhinitis, neck pain, arthritis, paresthesia.

## ADVERSE EFFECTS/ TOXIC REACTIONS

Increase in dyskinesia (impaired voluntary movement), dystonia (impaired muscular tone) occur in 18% of pts, angina occurs in 9%. Gastroenteritis, conjunctivitis occur rarely (3% of pts).

## NURSING CONSIDERATIONS

**BASELINE ASSESSMENT**
Obtain baseline LFT, blood pressure. Receive full medication history and screen for interactions. Question history of severe hepatic impairment, cardiovascular disease.

R

## INTERVENTION/EVALUATION

Give with food if nausea occurs. Monitor B/P. Instruct pt to slowly go from lying to standing to prevent orthostatic hypotension. Assess for clinical reversal of symptoms (improvement of tremor of head/hands at rest, mask-like facial expression, shuffling gait, muscular rigidity). If hallucinations or dyskinesia occur, symptoms may be eliminated if levodopa dosage is reduced. Hallucinations generally are accompanied by confusion and, to a lesser extent, insomnia.

## PATIENT/FAMILY TEACHING

• Orthostatic hypotension may occur more frequently during initial therapy. • Avoid tasks that require alertness, motor skills until response to drug is established. • Hallucinations may occur (more so in the elderly with Parkinson's disease), typically within first 2 wks of therapy. • Avoid foods that contain tyramine (cheese, sour cream, beer, wine, pickled herring, liver, figs, raisins, bananas, avocados, soy sauce, yeast extracts, yogurt, papaya, broad beans, meat tenderizers), excessive amounts of caffeine (coffee, tea, chocolate), OTC preparations for hay fever, colds, weight reduction (may produce significant rise in B/P). • Do not take any newly prescribed medications unless approved by prescriber who originally started therapy.

# rasburicase

ras-**bure**-i-kase
(Elitek, Fasturtec ✦)

■ **BLACK BOX ALERT** ■ Severe hypersensitivity reactions including anaphylaxis reported. May cause severe hemolysis in pts with glucose-6-phosphate dehydrogenase (G6PD) deficiency. Screen pts at high risk for G6PD (African or Mediterranean descent) prior to therapy. Methemoglobinemia has been reported. Blood samples left at room temperature may interfere

with uric acid measurements. Must collect blood samples in prechilled tubes containing heparin and immediately immerse in ice water bath. Assay plasma samples within 4 hrs of collection. Elitek enzymatically degrades uric acid in blood samples left at room temperature.

## ◆CLASSIFICATION

**PHARMACOTHERAPEUTIC:** Urate-oxidase inhibitor. **CLINICAL:** Antihyperuricemic.

## USES

Initial management of uric acid levels in pts with leukemia, lymphoma, and solid tumor malignancies who are receiving chemotherapy expected to result in tumor lysis and subsequent elevation of plasma uric acid.

## PRECAUTIONS

**Contraindications:** History of anaphylaxis or severe hypersensitivity to rasburicase. Prior drug reaction including hypersensitivity reactions, hemolysis, methemoglobinemia; G6PD deficiency. **Cautions:** Pts at high risk for G6PD deficiency (e.g., African, Mediterranean, or Southeast Asian descent).

## ACTION

Catalyzes enzymatic oxidation of poorly soluble uric acid into soluble, inactive metabolites by converting uric acid into allantoin. Does not inhibit formation of uric acid. **Therapeutic Effect:** Decreases uric acid levels.

## PHARMACOKINETICS

**Half-life:** 16–23 hrs.

## ⌛ LIFESPAN CONSIDERATIONS

**Pregnancy/Lactation:** Unknown if distributed in breast milk. Unknown if crosses placenta. May cause fetal harm. **Children/Elderly:** No age-related precautions noted.

R

---

✦ Canadian trade name          🔪 Non-Crushable Drug          ᴴᴵᴳᴴ High Alert drug

## INTERACTIONS

**DRUG:** None significant. **HERBAL:** None significant. **FOOD:** None known. **LAB VALUES:** May increase serum bilirubin, ALT. May decrease serum phosphate.

## AVAILABILITY (Rx)

**Injection, Powder for Reconstitution:** 1.5 mg/vial, 7.5 mg/vial.

## ADMINISTRATION/HANDLING

 IV

**Reconstitution** • Must use diluent provided in carton. • Reconstitute 1.5-mg vial with 1 ml of diluent or 7.5-mg vial with 5 ml of diluent to provide concentration of 1.5 mg/ml. • Gently swirl to mix. Do not shake. • Inspect for particulate matter or discoloration. • Inject calculated dose into appropriate volume of 0.9% NaCl to achieve a final volume of 50 ml.
**Rate of Administration** • Infuse over 30 min. • Do not use filter during reconstitution or infusion.
**Storage** • Refrigerate solution until time of use. • Discard after 24 hrs following reconstitution.

## IV INCOMPATIBILITIES

Do not mix with other IV medications.

## INDICATIONS/ROUTES/DOSAGE

**Management of Hyperuricemia**
**IV: ADULTS, ELDERLY, CHILDREN:** 0.2 mg/kg once daily up to 5 days.

**Dosage in Renal/Hepatic Impairment**
No dose adjustment.

## SIDE EFFECTS

**Frequent (50%–46%):** Vomiting, fever. **Occasional (27%–13%):** Nausea, headache, abdominal pain, constipation, diarrhea, mucositis, rash.

## ADVERSE EFFECTS/ TOXIC REACTIONS

Hypersensitivity reactions occurred in 4.3% of pts including injection irritation, peripheral edema, urticaria, pruritus. Anaphylaxis, hemolysis, methemoglobinemia occurred in less than 1%. Pulmonary hemorrhage, respiratory failure, supraventricular arrhythmias, ischemic coronary artery disorders, sepsis, abdominal, gastrointestinal infections occurred in greater than 2% of pts. Clinical tumor lysis syndrome (TLS), manifested by hyperuricemia, hyperkalemia, hyperphosphatemia, seizure, increased serum creatinine, renal failure reported in 3% of pts. Anti-rasburicase antibodies reported.

## NURSING CONSIDERATIONS

### BASELINE ASSESSMENT

Obtain CBC, BMP, LFT, serum phosphate, uric acid level; urine pregnancy if applicable. Question for history of prior hypersensitivity reactions. Assess G6PD deficiency risk in potential candidates.

### INTERVENTION/EVALUATION

Offer antiemetics to control nausea, vomiting. Monitor CBC, BMP, LFT, serum phosphate. If hypersensitivity reaction occurs, stop infusion and immediately notify physician. Screen for clinical tumor lysis syndrome, hemolysis, methemoglobinemia. Follow strict procedure when collecting uric acid levels. Obtain EKG for chest pain/tightness, hyperkalemia, dyspnea. Assess skin for rash.

### PATIENT/FAMILY TEACHING

• Report any allergic reaction, bronchospasm, chest pain or tightness, cough, difficulty breathing, dizziness, fainting, rash or itching.

## regorafenib

re-goe-**raf**-e-nib
(Stivarga)

■ **BLACK BOX ALERT** ■ Severe, sometimes fatal, hepatotoxicity reported. Monitor hepatic function prior to and during treatment. Interrupt, reduce, or discontinue therapy if hepatotoxicity or hepatocellular necrosis occurs.

## ◆CLASSIFICATION

**PHARMACOTHERAPEUTIC:** Multikinase inhibitor. **CLINICAL:** Antineoplastic.

## USES

Treatment of metastatic colorectal cancer in pts who have been previously treated with fluoropyrimidine/oxaliplatin/irinotecan-based chemotherapy, anti-VEGF or anti-EGFR therapy. Locally advanced, unresectable or metastatic GI stromal tumor previously treated with imatinib and sunitinib.

## PRECAUTIONS

**Contraindications:** Hypersensitivity to regorafenib. **Cautions:** Mild to moderate hepatic impairment (not recommended with severe hepatic impairment), hypertension (not recommended with severe or uncontrolled hypertension), recent surgical/dental procedures, chronic open wounds/ulcers, hemoptysis, concomitant warfarin therapy, cardiovascular disease, recent MI.

## ACTION

Inhibits tyrosine kinase activity involved with tumor angiogenesis, oncogenesis, and maintenance of tumor microenvironment. **Therapeutic Effect:** Inhibits colorectal tumor cell growth and metastasis.

## PHARMACOKINETICS

Readily absorbed following PO administration. Metabolized in liver. Protein binding: 99.5%. Peak plasma concentration: 4 hrs. Excreted in feces (71%), urine (19%). Half-life: 28 hrs (Range: 14–58 hrs).

## ⊠ LIFESPAN CONSIDERATIONS

**Pregnancy/Lactation:** May cause fetal harm. Not recommended in nursing mothers. Unknown if distributed in breast milk. Contraception recommended during treatment and up to 2 mos after discontinuation of therapy. **Children:** Safety and efficacy not established in pts younger than 18 yrs. **Elderly:** No age-related precautions noted.

## INTERACTIONS

**DRUG:** Strong **CYP3A4 inducers (e.g., carbamazepine, phenytoin)** may decrease concentration/effects. Strong **CYP3A4 inhibitors (e.g., clarithromycin, ketoconazole)** may increase concentration/effects. **HERBAL:** St. John's wort may decrease concentration/effects. **FOOD:** **Grapefruit products** may increase concentration/effects. **High-fat meal** may increase absorption/concentration. **LAB VALUES:** May decrease lymphocytes, neutrophils, platelets, serum calcium, phosphorus, potassium, sodium. May increase serum bilirubin, ALT, AST, lipase, amylase, INR, urine protein.

## AVAILABILITY (Rx)

⬗ **Tablets:** 40 mg.

## ADMINISTRATION/HANDLING

**PO**
• Take at same time each day with low-fat (less than 30%) breakfast. • Give whole; do not break, crush, dissolve, or divide tablet.

## INDICATIONS/ROUTES/DOSAGE

**Metastatic Colorectal Cancer, GI Stromal Tumor**
**PO: ADULTS/ELDERLY:** 160 mg once daily for first 21 days, of each 28-day cycle. Continue until disease progression or unacceptable toxicity.

**Dosage Modification**
*Symptomatic Hypertension, Toxic Skin Reactions, Severe Side Effects (Grades 3–4)*
**PO: ADULTS/ELDERLY:** Reduce dose to 120 mg once daily. If recovery does not occur within 7 days (despite dose reduction), interrupt treatment for minimum of 7 days and reassess. If recovery does not occur after interruption, reduce dose to 80 mg once daily. Discontinue for intolerance of 80-mg dose, serum ALT or AST greater than 20 times upper limit of normal (ULN), serum ALT/AST greater than 3 times

**R**

ULN and bilirubin greater than 2 times ULN or recurrent serum ALT/AST greater than 5 times ULN despite dose of 120 mg. Recovery failure of grade 3 or 4 side effects, toxic skin reaction.

**Dosage in Renal Impairment**
No dose adjustment.

**Dosage in Hepatic Impairment**
**Mild to moderate impairment:** No dose adjustment. **Severe impairment:** Not recommended.

## SIDE EFFECTS

**Frequent (64%–26%):** Asthenia/fatigue, anorexia, diarrhea, mucositis, weight loss, hypertension, dysphonia, generalized pain, fever, rash. **Occasional (10%–5%):** Headache, alopecia, dysgeusia, musculoskeletal stiffness, dry mouth. **Rare (2% or Less):** Tremor, gastric reflux.

## ADVERSE EFFECTS/ TOXIC REACTIONS

May cause GI perforation, GI fistula formation. Hemorrhaging of respiratory, GI, genitourinary tracts reported in 21% of pts. Hypertension (30% of pts) may lead to hypertensive crisis. May cause ineffective wound healing or wound dehiscence requiring medical intervention. Palmar-plantar erythrodysesthesia syndrome (PPES), a chemotherapy-induced skin condition that presents with redness, swelling, numbness, skin sloughing of hands, feet (45% of pts). Reversible posterior leukoencephalopathy syndrome (RPLS) reported in less than 1% of pts. May induce cardiac ischemia and/or MI. Severe, sometimes fatal, hepatotoxicity including hepatocellular necrosis reported in less than 1%. Various, unspecified infections reported in 31% of pts (most likely due to neutropenia).

## NURSING CONSIDERATIONS

### BASELINE ASSESSMENT

Obtain baseline vital signs, CBC with differential, serum magnesium, phosphate, ionized calcium, urinalysis, urine pregnancy, urine protein, LFT, amylase, lipase, PT/INR. Assess recent surgical/dental procedures. Question possibility of pregnancy, current breastfeeding status. Obtain full medication history including vitamins, herbal products. Question for history of hypertension, hepatic impairment, cardiovascular disease. Assess skin for open/unhealed wounds.

### INTERVENTION/EVALUATION

Monitor CBC, electrolytes, urinalysis. Monitor LFT q2wks for 2 mos, then monthly; or every wk if elevated. Persistent diastolic hypertension may indicate hypertensive emergency. Obtain EKG for palpitation, chest pain, hypokalemia, hyperkalemia, hypocalcemia, bradycardia, ventricular arrhythmias. Reverse Posterior Leukoencephalopathy Syndrome (RPLS) should be considered in pts with seizure, headache, visual disturbances, altered mental status, malignant hypertension. Assess hydration status. Encourage PO intake. Immediately report any hemorrhaging, bloody stools, hematuria, abdominal pain, hemoptysis (may indicate GI perforation/fistula formation).

### PATIENT/FAMILY TEACHING

• Blood levels will be routinely monitored. • Avoid pregnancy. Contraception should be practiced during treatment and up to 2 mos after last dose. • Report any yellowing of skin or eyes, abdominal pain, bruising, black/tarry stools, dark urine, decreased urine output, skin changes. • Report neurologic changes including confusion, seizures, vision loss, high blood pressure crisis (may indicate RPLS). • Do no take herbal products. • Notify physician before any planned surgical/dental procedures. • Do not ingest grapefruit products. • Take with low-fat food only. • Drink liquids often if diarrhea occurs (may lead to dehydration). • Immediately report bleeding of any kind. • Swallow tablet whole; do not chew, crush, dissolve, or divide.

# *repaglinide* HIGH ALERT

re-**pag**-li-nide
(Apo-Repaglinide ✦, GlucoNorm ✦, Prandin)
**Do not confuse Prandin with Avandia.**

## FIXED-COMBINATION(S)

**Prandimet:** repaglinide/metformin (an antidiabetic): 1 mg/500 mg, 2 mg/500 mg.

## ◆CLASSIFICATION

**PHARMACOTHERAPEUTIC:** Antihyperglycemic. **CLINICAL:** Antidiabetic agent.

## USES

Adjunct to diet and exercise to lower serum glucose in pts with type 2 diabetes mellitus. Used as monotherapy or in combination with metformin, pioglitazone, rosiglitazone.

## PRECAUTIONS

**Contraindications:** Hypersensitivity to repaglinide. Diabetic ketoacidosis, type 1 diabetes mellitus, concurrent gemfibrozil therapy. **Cautions:** Hepatic/renal impairment, elderly, malnourished, adrenal/pituitary dysfunction.

## ACTION

Stimulates release of insulin from beta cells of pancreas by depolarizing beta cells, leading to opening of calcium channels. Resulting calcium influx induces insulin secretion. **Therapeutic Effect:** Lowers serum glucose concentration.

## PHARMACOKINETICS

Rapidly, completely absorbed from GI tract. Protein binding: 98%. Metabolized in liver. Excreted in feces (90%), urine (8%). Unknown if removed by hemodialysis. **Half-life:** 1 hr.

## ⏳ LIFESPAN CONSIDERATIONS

**Pregnancy/Lactation:** Unknown if drug is distributed in breast milk. **Children:** Safety and efficacy not established. **Elderly:** No age-related precautions noted, but hypoglycemia may be more difficult to recognize.

## INTERACTIONS

**DRUG: CYP3A4 inhibitors (e.g., ketoconazole, erythromycin), CYP2C8 inhibitors (e.g., gemfibrozil)** may increase concentration/toxicity. **CYP3A4 inducers (e.g., carbamazepine, rifampin)** may decrease effects. **Beta blockers (e.g., carvedilol, metoprolol), NSAIDs** may increase hypoglycemic effect. **HERBAL: St. John's wort** may decrease concentration. **Garlic, ginger, ginseng** may cause hypoglycemia. **FOOD: Food** decreases concentration. **LAB VALUES:** Serum alkaline phosphatase, ALT, AST may be elevated.

## AVAILABILITY (Rx)

**Tablets:** 0.5 mg, 1 mg, 2 mg.

## ADMINISTRATION/HANDLING

### PO

• Ideally, give within 15 min of a meal but may be given immediately before a meal to as long as 30 min before a meal.

## INDICATIONS/ROUTES/DOSAGE

**Diabetes Mellitus**
**PO: ADULTS, ELDERLY: (Pts not previously treated or whose Hgb A1c is less than 8%):** 0.5 mg before each meal. **(Pts previously treated whose Hgb A1c is greater than 8%):** 1–2 mg before each meal. May adjust dose by at least 1-wk intervals. **Range:** 0.5–4 mg 2–4 times/day. **Maximum:** 16 mg/day.

**Dosage in Renal Impairment**
**CrCl 20–40 ml/min:** Initially, 0.5 mg with meals, titrate carefully.

**Dosage in Hepatic Impairment**
Use caution.

R

---

✦ Canadian trade name    🅝 Non-Crushable Drug    **HIGH ALERT** High Alert drug

## SIDE EFFECTS

**Frequent (10%–6%):** Upper respiratory tract infection, headache, rhinitis, bronchitis, back pain. **Occasional (5%–3%):** Diarrhea, dyspepsia, sinusitis, nausea, arthralgia, UTI. **Rare (2%):** Constipation, vomiting, paresthesia, allergy.

## ADVERSE EFFECTS/ TOXIC REACTIONS

Hypoglycemia occurs in 16% of pts. Chest pain occurs rarely.

## NURSING CONSIDERATIONS

### BASELINE ASSESSMENT

Check fasting serum glucose, glycosylated Hgb A1c levels periodically to determine minimum effective dose.

### INTERVENTION/EVALUATION

Monitor fasting serum glucose, glycosylated Hgb A1c levels, food intake. Assess for hypoglycemia (cool/wet skin, tremors, dizziness, anxiety, headache, tachycardia, numbness in mouth, hunger, diplopia), hyperglycemia (polyuria, polyphagia, polydipsia, nausea, vomiting, dim vision, fatigue, deep or rapid breathing). Be alert to conditions that alter glucose requirements (fever, increased activity/stress, surgical procedures). Ensure follow-up instruction if pt, family do not thoroughly understand diabetes management, glucose-testing technique. At least 1 wk should elapse to assess response to drug before new dosage adjustment is made.

### PATIENT/FAMILY TEACHING

• Diabetes mellitus requires lifelong control. • Prescribed diet, exercise is principal part of treatment; do not skip, delay meals. • Continue to adhere to dietary instructions, regular exercise program, regular testing of urine or serum glucose. • When taking combination drug therapy with a sulfonylurea or insulin, have source of glucose available to treat symptoms of low blood sugar.

# reslizumab

res-li-zoo-mab
(Cinqair)

■ **BLACK BOX ALERT** ■ Life-threatening anaphylaxis was reported in less than 1% of pts and occurred as early as second dose. Pts should be monitored for an appropriate time period by health care professionals who are trained and readily prepared to manage anaphylactic reactions. Immediately discontinue in pts experiencing anaphylaxis.

**Do not confuse reslizumab with certolizumab, daclizumab, eculizumab, efalizumab, mepolizumab, natalizumab, omalizumab, pembrolizumab, tocilizumab, or vedolizumab, or Cinqair with Cinryze, Cinolar, Cinobac, Sinemet, Singulair, or Sinequan.**

## ◆CLASSIFICATION

**PHARMACOTHERAPEUTIC:** Interleukin-5 receptor antagonist. Monoclonal antibody. **CLINICAL:** Antiasthmatic.

## USES

Add-on maintenance treatment of pts with severe asthma, aged 18 yrs and older, and with an eosinophil phenotype.

## PRECAUTIONS

**Contraindications:** Hypersensitivity to reslizumab. **Cautions:** History of helminth (parasite) infection; long-term use of corticosteroids. Not indicated for treatment of other eosinophilic conditions; relief of acute bronchospasm, status asthmaticus, exercise-induced bronchospasm. History of anaphylaxis.

## ACTION

Exact mechanism unknown. Inhibits signaling of interleukin-5 cytokine, reducing production and survival of eosinophils responsible for asthmatic inflammation

R

and pathogenesis. **Therapeutic Effect:** Prevents inflammatory process; relieves signs/symptoms of asthma.

## PHARMACOKINETICS

Widely distributed. Degraded into small peptides and amino acids via proteolytic enzymes. Peak plasma concentration: reached by end of infusion. Elimination not specified. **Half-life:** 24 days.

## ⧖ LIFESPAN CONSIDERATIONS

**Pregnancy/Lactation:** Unknown if distributed in breast milk. However, human immunoglobulin G is present in breast milk and is known to cross placenta. **Children:** Safety and efficacy not established in pts younger than 18 yrs. **Elderly:** No age-related precautions noted.

## INTERACTIONS

**DRUG:** None known. **HERBAL:** None significant. **FOOD:** None known. **LAB VALUES:** May increase creatine phosphokinase (CPK).

## AVAILABILITY (Rx)

**Injection Solution:** 100 mg/10 ml (10 mg/ml).

## ADMINISTRATION/HANDLING

 IV

**Preparation** • Allow vial to warm to room temperature. • Visually inspect for particulate matter or discoloration. Solution should appear clear to slightly opalescent, colorless to pale yellow. • Proteinaceous particles may be present. • Air bubbles are expected and allowed. • Do not use if solution is cloudy or discolored or if foreign particles are observed. • Do not shake. • Withdraw proper dose volume from vial and dilute in 50 ml 0.9% NaCl bag. • Gently invert to mix. Do not shake (may cause foaming/precipitate formation). • Infuse via dedicated line. • After infusion is complete, flush IV line with 0.9% NaCl.
**Rate of Administration** • Infuse over 20–50 mins (depending on total volume of infusion) using an in-line, low-protein-binding filter (pore size: 0.2 micron).

**Storage** • Refrigerate unused vials. • Do not freeze. • Diluted solution may be refrigerated or stored at room temperature for up to 16 hrs. • If refrigerated, allow diluted solution to warm to room temperature before use. • Protect from light.

## IV INCOMPATIBILITIES

Do not mix or infuse with other medications.

## INDICATIONS/ROUTES/DOSAGE

**Asthma (Severe)**
**IV:** **ADULTS, ELDERLY:** 3 mg/kg once q4wks.

**Dosage in Renal/Hepatic Impairment**
Not specified; use caution.

## SIDE EFFECTS

**Rare (3%–1%):** Oropharyngeal pain, myalgia.

## ADVERSE EFFECTS/TOXIC REACTIONS

Life-threatening anaphylaxis reported in less than 1% of pts. Hypersensitivity reactions including bronchospasm, dyspnea, hypoxia, rash, urticaria, vomiting usually occurred during infusion or within 20 mins after completion. Less than 1% of pts reported at least one malignant neoplasm within 6 mos of initiation. Unknown if treatment will influence the immunologic response to helminth (parasite) infection. Immunogenicity (auto-mepolizumab antibodies) reported in 5% of pts.

## NURSING CONSIDERATIONS

### BASELINE ASSESSMENT

Obtain serum CPK. Verify presence of eosinophil phenotype. Question history of hypersensitivity reaction of any kind. Therapy should be administered in a health care setting by medical professionals who are trained and prepared to readily manage anaphylaxis. Have anaphylactic medications (e.g., antihistamine, bronchodilator, corticosteroid, epinephrine, H$_2$

R

receptor antagonist), intubation kit, supplemental oxygen readily available before initiation. Inhaled or systemic corticosteroids should not be suddenly discontinued upon initiation. Corticosteroids that are not gradually reduced may cause withdrawal symptoms or unmask conditions that were originally suppressed with corticosteroid therapy. Pts with preexisting helminth infection should be treated prior to initiation.

### INTERVENTION/EVALUATION

Obtain serum CPK in pts complaining of myalgia. Diligently observe for hypersensitivity/anaphylactic reaction during infusion and directly after completion. If anaphylaxis occurs, discontinue infusion and provide immediate resuscitation support. Early detection is vital. Assess rate, depth, rhythm of respirations, oxygen saturation for therapeutic effectiveness. Assess lungs for wheezing, rales. Obtain pulmonary function test to assess disease improvement. Interrupt or discontinue therapy if helminth infection occurs; if worsening of asthma-related symptoms occurs (esp. in pts tapering off corticosteroids). Monitor for increased use of rescue inhalers; may indicate deterioration of asthma. Monitor for primary malignancies.

### PATIENT/FAMILY TEACHING

• Treatment may cause life-threatening anaphylaxis. Immediately report allergic reactions such as difficulty breathing, hives, itching, low blood pressure, rash, swelling of the face or tongue, sudden coughing, vomiting, wheezing during infusion or immediately after infusion. • Therapy not indicated for relief of acute asthma or bronchospasm. • Have a rescue inhaler readily available. • Increased use of rescue inhalers may indicate worsening of asthma. • Seek medical attention if asthma symptoms worsen or remain uncontrolled. • Do not stop corticosteroid therapy unless directed by prescriber. • Treatment may increase risk of new cancers or alter the body's immune response to parasite infections.

# ribavirin

rye-ba-**vye**-rin
(Copegus, Rebetol, Ribasphere, Virazole)

■ **BLACK BOX ALERT** ■ Significant teratogenic/embryocidal effects. Hemolytic anemia is significant toxicity, usually occurring within 1–2 wks. May worsen cardiac disease and lead to fatal or nonfatal MI. Inhalation may interfere with safe and effective assisted ventilation. Monotherapy not effective for chronic hepatitis C virus infection.
**Do not confuse ribavirin with riboflavin, rifampin, or Robaxin.**

## FIXED-COMBINATION(S)

With interferon alfa 2b (**Rebetron**). Individually packaged.

## ◆CLASSIFICATION

**PHARMACOTHERAPEUTIC:** Synthetic nucleoside. **CLINICAL:** Antiviral.

## USES

**Inhalation:** Treatment of respiratory syncytial virus (RSV) infections (esp. in pts with underlying compromising conditions such as chronic lung disorders, congenital heart disease, recent transplant recipients). **Capsule/tablet/oral solution:** Treatment of chronic hepatitis C virus infection in pts with compensated hepatic disease in combination with other medications.

## PRECAUTIONS

**Contraindications:** Hypersensitivity to ribavirin. **(Additional) Inhalation:** Women who are pregnant or may become pregnant. **Oral formulations:** Hemoglobinopathies (e.g., sickle cell anemia), men whose female partner is pregnant, women of childbearing age who are pregnant or may become pregnant. Concomitant use of didanosine. **Ribasphere, Rebetol only:** CrCl less than 50 ml/min. **Cautions: Inhalation:** Pts requiring assisted ventilation, COPD, asthma. **PO:** Cardiac or pulmonary disease, elderly, history of psychiatric disorders, renal impairment, pts with sarcoidosis, pts with baseline risk of severe anemia.

## ACTION

Inhibits replication of viral RNA, DNA, influenza virus RNA polymerase activity, interferes with expression of messenger RNA. **Therapeutic Effect:** Inhibits viral protein synthesis.

## PHARMACOKINETICS

Readily absorbed. Peak concentrations: (Inhalation): At end of inhalation period. (Capsules): 3 hrs. (Tablet): 2 hrs. Protein binding: None. Metabolized in liver and intracellularly. Primarily excreted in urine. **Half-life:** (Inhalation): 6.5–11 hrs. (Capsule): 298 hr at steady state. (Tablet): 120–170 hrs.

## ⧗ LIFESPAN CONSIDERATIONS

**Pregnancy/Lactation:** Contraindicated in pregnancy. Unknown if excreted in breast milk. **Children/Elderly:** No age-related precautions noted.

## INTERACTIONS

**DRUG: Didanosine** may increase risk of pancreatitis, peripheral neuropathy. May decrease effects of **didanosine. Nucleoside analogues** (e.g., adefovir, didanosine, lamivudine, stavudine, zalcitabine, zidovudine) may increase risk of lactic acidosis. **HERBAL:** None significant. **FOOD:** None known. **LAB VALUES:** None significant.

## AVAILABILITY (Rx)

**Capsules** (Rebetol, Ribasphere): 200 mg. **Powder for Solution, Nebulization** (Virazole): 6 g. **Solution, Oral** (Rebetol): 40 mg/ml. **Tablet** (Copegus): 200 mg. (Ribasphere): 200 mg, 400 mg, 600 mg.

## ADMINISTRATION/HANDLING

**PO**
• Capsules may be taken without regard to food. • Do not break, crush, or open capsules. • Use oral solution in children 5 yrs or younger, those 47 kg or less, or those unable to swallow. • Give capsules with food when combined with peginterferon alfa-2b. • Tablets should be given with food.

**Inhalation**
◀**ALERT**▶ May be given via nasal or oral inhalation.
• Solution appears clear, colorless; is stable for 24 hrs at room temperature. • Discard solution for nebulization after 24 hrs. • Discard if discolored or cloudy. • Add 50–100 ml Sterile Water for Injection or Inhalation to 6-g vial. • Transfer to a flask, serving as reservoir for aerosol generator. • Further dilute to final volume of 300 ml, giving solution concentration of 20 mg/ml. • Use only aerosol generator available from manufacturer of drug. • Do not give concomitantly with other drug solutions for nebulization. • Discard reservoir solution when fluid levels are low and at least q24h. • Only experienced personnel should administer drug.

## INDICATIONS/ROUTES/DOSAGE

**Chronic Hepatitis C Virus Infection**
*Rebetol, Ribasphere (Oral Capsule or Solution) (In Combination with Peginterferon alfa-2b)*
**PO: ADULTS, ELDERLY: (More than 105 kg):** 1,400 mg daily (600 mg in morning, 800 mg in evening); **(85–105 kg):** 1,200 mg daily (600 mg in morning and evening); **(66–80 kg):** 1,000 mg daily (400 mg in morning, 600 mg in evening); **(less than 66 kg):** 800 mg daily (400 mg in morning and evening). **CHILDREN 3 YRS OR OLDER: (More than 73 kg):** 1,200 mg daily (600 mg in morning and evening); **(60–73 kg):** 1,000 mg daily (400 mg in morning, 600 mg in evening); **(47–59 kg):** 800 mg daily (400 mg in morning and evening); **(less than 47 kg):** 15 mg/kg/day in 2 divided doses as oral solution.

*Rebetol, Ribasphere (Oral Capsule/
Solution) (In Combination with Interferon
alfa-2b)*
PO: ADULTS, ELDERLY: **(More than 75kg):**
1,200 mg daily (600 mg in morning and
evening); **(75 kg or less):** 1,000 mg daily
(400 mg in morning, 600 mg in evening).
*Copegus, Ribasphere (Oral Tablet) (In
Combination with Peginterferon alfa-2b)*
PO: ADULTS, ELDERLY: **Genotype 1, 4
(more than 75kg):** 1,200 mg daily (600
mg in morning and evening); **(75 kg or
less):** 1,000 mg daily (400 mg in morning, 600 mg in evening). Duration: 48 wks.
**Genotype 2, 3:** 800 mg daily (400 mg in
morning and evening). Duration: 24 wks.
CHILDREN 5 YRS AND OLDER: **(75 kg or
greater):** 1,200 mg daily (600 mg in
morning and evening); **(60–74 kg):**
1000 mg daily (400 mg in morning, 600
mg in evening; **(47–59 kg):** 800 mg daily
(400 mg in morning and evening); **(34–
46 kg):** 600 mg daily (200 mg in morning, 400 mg in evening; **(23–33 kg):** 400
mg daily (200 mg in morning and evening). Duration: 24 wks for genotypes 2, 3;
48 wks for genotypes 1, 4.

**Dosage in Renal Impairment**
*Rebetol Capsules/Oral Solution;
Ribasphere Capsules*
ADULTS: **CrCl less than 50 ml/min:**
Contraindicated. CHILDREN: **Serum cre-
atinine more than 2 mg/dL:** Discon-
tinue treatment.
*Ribasphere Tablets*
ADULTS: **CrCl less than 50 ml/min:**
Not recommended.
*Copegus Tablets*
**CrCl 30–50 ml/min:** Alternate 200 mg
and 400 mg every other day. **CrCl less
than 30 ml/min, end-stage renal
disease:** 200 mg once daily.

**Dosage in Hepatic Impairment**
Contraindicated.

**Severe Lower Respiratory Tract Infection
Caused by Respiratory Syncytial Virus (RSV)**
Inhalation: CHILDREN, INFANTS: Use with
Viratek small-particle aerosol generator at
concentration of 20 mg/ml (6 g reconstituted with 300 ml Sterile Water for Injection) over 12–18 hrs/day for 3–7 days.

## SIDE EFFECTS

**Frequent (greater than 10%):** Hemolytic
anemia, dizziness, headache, fatigue, fever, insomnia, irritability, depression,
emotional lability, impaired concentration, alopecia, rash, pruritus, nausea,
anorexia, dyspepsia, vomiting, decreased
hemoglobin, hemolysis, arthralgia, musculoskeletal pain, dyspnea, sinusitis, flu-
like symptoms. **Occasional (10%–1%):**
Nervousness, altered taste, weakness.

## ADVERSE EFFECTS/
TOXIC REACTIONS

Cardiac arrest, apnea, ventilator dependence, bacterial pneumonia, pneumonia,
pneumothorax occur rarely. If treatment
exceeds 7 days, anemia may occur.

## NURSING CONSIDERATIONS

### BASELINE ASSESSMENT

Obtain sputum specimens before giving
first dose or at least during first 24 hrs
of therapy. Assess respiratory status for
baseline. **PO:** Obtain CBC with differential, pretreatment and monthly pregnancy
test for women of childbearing age.

### INTERVENTION/EVALUATION

Monitor Hgb, Hct, platelets, LFT, I&O,
fluid balance carefully. Check hematology reports for anemia due to reticulocy-
tosis when therapy exceeds 7 days. For
ventilator-assisted pts, watch for "rain-
out" in tubing and empty frequently; be
alert to impaired ventilation/gas exchange due to drug precipitate. Assess
skin for rash. Monitor B/P, respirations;
assess lung sounds.

### PATIENT/FAMILY TEACHING

• Report immediately any difficulty
breathing, itching/swelling/redness of
eyes, severe abdominal pain, bloody diarrhea, unusual bleeding/bruising. • Female pts should take measures to avoid

R

pregnancy. • Male pts must use condoms during sexual activity.

# rifabutin

rif-a-**bue**-tin
(Mycobutin)
**Do not confuse rifabutin with rifampin.**

## ◆CLASSIFICATION

**PHARMACOTHERAPEUTIC:** Antitubercular, antibiotic. **CLINICAL:** Antibacterial, antibiotic (antimycobacterial).

## USES

Prevention of disseminated *Mycobacterium avium* complex (MAC) disease in those with advanced HIV infection. **OFF-LABEL:** Part of multidrug regimen for treatment of MAC. Alternative to rifampin as prophylaxis for latent tuberculosis infection, part of multidrug regimen for treatment of active tuberculosis infection.

## PRECAUTIONS

**Contraindications:** Hypersensitivity to rifabutin, other rifamycins (e.g., rifampin). **Cautions:** Severe renal impairment. Avoid use in renal/hepatic impairment for prophylaxis in pts with active TB.

## ACTION

Inhibits DNA-dependent RNA polymerase. **Therapeutic Effect:** Prevents MAC disease.

## PHARMACOKINETICS

Readily absorbed from GI tract. Protein binding: 85%. Widely distributed. Crosses blood-brain barrier. Extensive intracellular tissue uptake. Metabolized in liver. Excreted in urine (53%), feces (30%). Unknown if removed by hemodialysis. **Half-life:** 16–69 hrs.

## ⧖ LIFESPAN CONSIDERATIONS

**Pregnancy/Lactation:** Unknown if drug crosses placenta or is distributed in breast milk. **Children/Elderly:** No age-related precautions noted.

## INTERACTIONS

**DRUG:** May decrease effectiveness of **oral contraceptives, clarithromycin, itraconazole.** May decrease concentration/effects of **non-nucleoside reverse transcriptase inhibitors (e.g., delavirdine, efavirenz, nevirapine), protease inhibitors (e.g., amprenavir, indinavir, ritonavir, saquinavir).** **HERBAL:** None significant. **FOOD:** **High-fat meals** may delay absorption. **LAB VALUES:** May increase serum alkaline phosphatase, ALT, AST.

## AVAILABILITY (Rx)

**Capsules:** 150 mg.

## ADMINISTRATION/HANDLING

**PO**
• May take with meals to reduce nausea/vomiting.

## INDICATIONS/ROUTES/DOSAGE

**Prevention of MAC (Advanced HIV Infection)**
**PO: ADULTS, ELDERLY:** 300 mg once daily or 150 mg twice daily to reduce gastrointestinal upset. **CHILDREN, INFANTS:** 5 mg/kg once daily. **Maximum:** 300 mg once daily.

**Dosage in Renal Impairment**
If CrCl is less than 30 ml/min, reduce dosage by 50%.

**Dosage in Hepatic Impairment**
No dose adjustment.

## SIDE EFFECTS

**Frequent (30%):** Red-orange or red-brown discoloration of urine, feces, saliva, skin, sputum, sweat, tears. **Occasional (11%–3%):** Rash, nausea, abdominal pain, diarrhea, dyspepsia, belching, headache, altered taste, uveitis, corneal deposits. **Rare (Less Than 2%):** Anorexia, flatulence, fever, myalgia, vomiting, insomnia.

R

## ADVERSE EFFECTS/ TOXIC REACTIONS

Hepatitis, anemia, thrombocytopenia, neutropenia occur rarely.

## NURSING CONSIDERATIONS

### BASELINE ASSESSMENT

Obtain chest X-ray; sputum, blood cultures. Biopsy of suspicious node(s) must be done to rule out active tuberculosis. Obtain baseline CBC, serum hepatic function tests.

### INTERVENTION/EVALUATION

Monitor serum LFT, platelet count, Hgb, Hct. Avoid IM injections, rectal temperatures, other trauma that may induce bleeding. Check temperature; notify physician of flu-like syndrome, rash, GI intolerance.

### PATIENT/FAMILY TEACHING

• Urine, feces, saliva, sputum, perspiration, tears, skin may be discolored brown-orange. • Soft contact lenses may be permanently discolored. • Rifabutin may decrease efficacy of oral contraceptives; nonhormonal methods should be considered. • Avoid crowds, those with infection. • Report flu-like symptoms, nausea, vomiting, dark urine, unusual bruising/bleeding from any site, any visual disturbances.

R

## *rifAMPin

rif-**am**-pin
(Rifadin, Rofact ✦)
**Do not confuse Rifadin with Rifater or Ritalin, or rifampin with ribavirin, rifabutin, Rifamate, rifapentine, rifaximin, or Ritalin.**

## FIXED-COMBINATION(S)

**Rifamate:** rifampin/isoniazid (an antitubercular): 300 mg/150 mg. **Rifater:** rifampin/isoniazid/pyrazinamide (an antitubercular): 120 mg/50 mg/300 mg.

## ◆CLASSIFICATION

**PHARMACOTHERAPEUTIC:** Antitubercular, antibiotic. **CLINICAL:** Antibiotic, antitubercular, anti-infective.

## USES

In combination with other antitubercular agents for initial treatment, re-treatment of active tuberculosis. Eliminates meningococci from nasopharynx of asymptomatic carriers. **OFF-LABEL:** Prophylaxis of *H. influenzae* type b infection, *Legionella* pneumonia, serious infections caused by *Staphylococcus* spp. (in combination with other agents). Treatment of prosthetic joint infection.

## PRECAUTIONS

**Contraindications:** Concomitant therapy with amprenavir, atazanavir, darunavir, saquinavir, ritonavir, tipranavir; hypersensitivity to rifampin, other rifamycins. **Cautions:** Hepatic impairment, active or treated alcoholism, porphyria. Concurrent medications associated with hepatotoxicity.

## ACTION

Interferes with bacterial RNA synthesis by binding to DNA-dependent RNA polymerase, preventing attachment to DNA, thereby blocking RNA transcription. **Therapeutic Effect:** Bactericidal in susceptible microorganisms.

## PHARMACOKINETICS

Well absorbed from GI tract (food delays absorption). Protein binding: 80%. Widely distributed. Metabolized in liver. Primarily eliminated by biliary system. Not removed by hemodialysis. **Half-life:** 3–5 hrs (increased in hepatic impairment).

## ⧗ LIFESPAN CONSIDERATIONS

**Pregnancy/Lactation:** Crosses placenta. Distributed in breast milk. **Children/ Elderly:** No age-related precautions noted.

## INTERACTIONS

**DRUG:** Alcohol, hepatotoxic medications (e.g., **acetaminophen, isoniazid, methotrexate, ketoconazole**), **ritonavir, saquinavir** may increase risk of hepatotoxicity. May decrease effects of **digoxin, disopyramide, fluconazole, methadone, mexiletine, oral anticoagulants** (e.g., **apixaban, warfarin**), **oral antidiabetics** (e.g., **glipizide, metformin**), **oral contraceptives, tacrolimus, tricyclic antidepressants, phenytoin, quinidine, tocainide, verapamil.** **HERBAL:** St. John's wort may decrease concentration. **FOOD:** Food decreases extent of absorption. **LAB VALUES:** May increase serum alkaline phosphatase, bilirubin, uric acid, ALT, AST.

## AVAILABILITY (Rx)

**Capsules (Rifadin):** 150 mg, 300 mg. **Injection, Powder for Reconstitution:** 600 mg.

## ADMINISTRATION/HANDLING

 IV

**Reconstitution •** Reconstitute 600-mg vial with 10 ml Sterile Water for Injection to provide concentration of 60 mg/ml. • Withdraw desired dose and further dilute with 0.9% NaCl or $D_5W$ to concentration not to exceed 6 mg/ml. **Rate of Administration •** For IV infusion only. Avoid IM, SQ administration. • Avoid extravasation (local irritation, inflammation). • Infuse over 30 min to 3 hrs. **Storage •** Reconstituted vial is stable for 24 hrs. • Once reconstituted vial is further diluted, it is stable for 4 hrs in $D_5W$ or 24 hrs in 0.9% NaCl.

**PO**
• Preferably give 1 hr before or 2 hrs following meals with 8 oz of water (may give with food to decrease GI upset; will delay absorption). • For pts unable to swallow capsules, contents may be mixed with applesauce, jelly. • Administer at least 1 hr before antacids, esp. those containing aluminum.

## ▦ IV INCOMPATIBILITY

Diltiazem (Cardizem).

## ▦ IV COMPATIBILITY

$D_5W$ if infused within 4 hrs (risk of precipitation beyond this time period).

## INDICATIONS/ROUTES/DOSAGE

**Tuberculosis**
**Note:** A four-drug regimen is preferred for initial, empiric treatment.
**PO, IV: ADULTS, ELDERLY:** 10 mg/kg/day. **Maximum:** 600 mg/day. **CHILDREN:** 10–20 mg/kg/day usually as a single dose. **Maximum:** 600 mg/day.

**Dosage in Renal/Hepatic Impairment**
No dose adjustment.

## SIDE EFFECTS

**Frequent:** Red-orange or red-brown discoloration of urine, feces, saliva, skin, sputum, sweat, tears. **Occasional (5%–3%):** Hypersensitivity reaction (flushing, pruritus, rash). **Rare (2%–1%):** Diarrhea, dyspepsia, nausea, oral candida (sore mouth, tongue).

## ADVERSE EFFECTS/ TOXIC REACTIONS

Hepatotoxicity (risk is increased when rifampin is taken with isoniazid), hepatitis, blood dyscrasias, Stevens-Johnson syndrome, antibiotic-associated colitis occur rarely.

R

## NURSING CONSIDERATIONS

### BASELINE ASSESSMENT

Obtain CBC, renal function test, LFT. Screen for concomitant medications known to cause hepatotoxicity. Question for hypersensitivity to rifampin, rifamycins. Ensure collection of diagnostic specimens.

### INTERVENTION/EVALUATION

Assess IV site at least hourly during infusion; restart at another site at the first sign of irritation or inflammation. Monitor

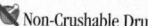

LFT, assess for hepatitis: jaundice, anorexia, nausea, vomiting, fatigue, weakness (hold rifampin, inform physician at once). Report hypersensitivity reactions promptly: any type of skin eruption, pruritus, flu-like syndrome with high dosage. Monitor daily pattern of bowel activity, stool consistency (potential for antibiotic-associated colitis). Monitor CBC results for blood dyscrasias, be alert for infection (fever, sore throat), unusual bruising/bleeding, unusual fatigue/weakness.

**PATIENT/FAMILY TEACHING**

• Preferably take on empty stomach with 8 oz of water 1 hr before or 2 hrs after meal (with food if GI upset). • Avoid alcohol. • Do not take any other medications without consulting physician, including antacids; must take rifampin at least 1 hr before antacid. • Urine, feces, sputum, sweat, tears may become red-orange; soft contact lenses may be permanently stained. • Report any new symptom immediately such as yellow eyes/skin, fatigue, weakness, nausea/vomiting, sore throat, fever, flu, unusual bruising/bleeding. • If taking oral contraceptives, check with physician (reliability may be affected).

---

## *rifAXIMin

rif-**ax**-i-min
(Xifaxan)
**Do not confuse rifaximin with rifampin.**

### ◆ CLASSIFICATION

**PHARMACOTHERAPEUTIC:** Anti-infective. **CLINICAL:** Site-specific antibiotic.

## USES

Treatment of traveler's diarrhea caused by noninvasive strains of *E. coli*. Reduction of risk for recurrence of overt hepatic encephalopathy. Treatment of irritable bowel syndrome with diarrhea (IBS-D) in adults. **OFF-LABEL:** Treatment of hepatic encephalopathy. Treatment of *C. difficile*–associated diarrhea.

## PRECAUTIONS

**Contraindications:** Hypersensitivity to rifaximin, other rifamycin antibiotics. **Cautions:** Severe hepatic impairment.

## ACTION

Inhibits bacterial RNA synthesis by binding to a subunit of bacterial DNA-dependent RNA polymerase. **Therapeutic Effect:** Bactericidal.

## PHARMACOKINETICS

Less than 0.4% absorbed after PO administration. Primarily eliminated in feces. **Half-life:** 5.85 hrs.

## ⌛ LIFESPAN CONSIDERATIONS

**Pregnancy/Lactation:** Unknown if drug is distributed in breast milk. **Children:** Safety and efficacy not established in pts younger than 12 yrs. **Elderly:** No age-related precautions noted.

## INTERACTIONS

**DRUG:** None significant. **HERBAL:** None significant. **FOOD:** None known. **LAB VALUES:** None significant.

## AVAILABILITY (Rx)

🔖 **Tablets:** 200 mg, 550 mg.

## ADMINISTRATION/HANDLING

**PO**
• Give without regard to food. • Do not break, crush, dissolve, or divide film-coated tablets.

## INDICATIONS/ROUTES/DOSAGE

**Traveler's Diarrhea**
**PO: ADULTS, ELDERLY, CHILDREN 12 YRS AND OLDER:** 200 mg 3 times/day for 3 days.

**Hepatic Encephalopathy**
**PO: ADULTS, ELDERLY:** 550 mg 2 times/day.

---

### IBS-D

**PO: ADULTS, ELDERLY:** 550 mg 3 times/day for 14 days. May repeat up to 2 times if symptoms recur.

**Dosage in Renal/Hepatic Impairment**
No dose adjustment.

### SIDE EFFECTS

**Occasional (11%–5%):** Flatulence, headache, abdominal discomfort, rectal tenesmus, defecation urgency, nausea. **Rare (4%–2%):** Constipation, fever, vomiting.

### ADVERSE EFFECTS/ TOXIC REACTIONS

Hypersensitivity reaction, superinfection occur rarely.

### NURSING CONSIDERATIONS

#### BASELINE ASSESSMENT

Check baseline hydration status: skin turgor, mucous membranes for dryness, urinary status. Assess stool frequency, consistency.

#### INTERVENTION/EVALUATION

Encourage adequate fluid intake. Assess bowel sounds for peristalsis. Monitor daily pattern of bowel activity, stool consistency. Assess for GI disturbances, blood in stool.

#### PATIENT/FAMILY TEACHING

• Report if diarrhea worsens or if blood occurs in stool, fever develops within 48 hrs.

## rilpivirine

**ril**-pi-**vir**-een
(Edurant)
**Do not confuse rilpivirine with delavirdine, etravirine, or nevirapine.**

### FIXED-COMBINATION(S)

**Complera:** rilpivirine/emtricitabine (an antiretroviral)/tenofovir (TDF) (an antiretroviral): 25 mg/200 mg/300 mg. **Odefsey:** rilpivirine/emtricitabine/tenofovir (TAF): 25 mg/200 mg/25 mg.

### ◆CLASSIFICATION

**PHARMACOTHERAPEUTIC:** Non-nucleoside reverse transcriptase inhibitor. **CLINICAL:** Antiretroviral.

### USES

Used in combination with at least two other antiretroviral agents for treatment of HIV-1 infection in treatment-naive pts with HIV-1 RNA 100,000 copies/ml or less.

### PRECAUTIONS

**Contraindications:** Hypersensitivity to rilpivirine. Concurrent use of carbamazepine, dexamethasone (greater than 1 dose), oxcarbazepine, phenobarbital, phenytoin, proton pump inhibitors (see drug classification), rifabutin, rifampin, rifapentine, St. John's wort. **Cautions:** Severe depressive disorders, medications that increase risk of prolongation of QT interval (torsades de pointes), hypokalemia, hypomagnesemia, pts with significant transaminase elevations, hepatitis B or C virus infection. Not for treatment-experienced pts.

### ACTION

Inhibits HIV-1 replication by binding to HIV-1 reverse transcriptase. **Therapeutic Effect:** Interferes with HIV replication, slowing progression of HIV infection.

### PHARMACOKINETICS

Readily absorbed after PO administration. Peak concentration: 4–5 hrs. Protein binding: 99.7%. Metabolized in liver. Excreted primarily in feces. **Half-life:** 50 hrs.

### ⌛ LIFESPAN CONSIDERATIONS

**Pregnancy/Lactation:** Unknown if distributed in breast milk. HIV-infected mothers should not breastfeed infants due to risk of postnatal HIV transmission.

**R**

**Children:** Safety and efficacy not established. **Elderly:** Caution due to higher risk of impaired renal/hepatic function.

## INTERACTIONS

**DRUG:** **CYP3A4 inducers (e.g., carbamazepine, phenobarbital, phenytoin, proton pump inhibitors, rifabutin, rifampin)** may significantly decrease effectiveness. **Antacids, H₂-receptor antagonists (e.g., cimetidine, famotidine)** may decrease plasma concentration. **CYP3A4 inhibitors (e.g., clarithromycin, ketoconazole, verapamil)** may increase plasma concentration. **HERBAL: St. John's wort** may decrease concentration/effects. **FOOD: Grapefruit products** may increase potential for torsades de pointes. **LAB VALUES:** May increase serum creatinine, ALT, AST, bilirubin, cholesterol, triglycerides.

## AVAILABILITY (Rx)

**Tablets:** 25 mg.

## ADMINISTRATION/HANDLING

**PO**
• Give with a meal. Administer antacids 2 hrs before or 4 hrs after rilpivirine; H₂-receptor antagonist 12 hrs before or 4 hrs after rilpivirine.

## INDICATIONS/ROUTES/DOSAGE

**HIV Infection (in Combination with Other Antiretrovirals)**
**PO: ADULTS, ELDERLY, CHILDREN 12 YRS AND OLDER:** 25 mg once daily with a meal. With rifabutin: increase to 50 mg once daily.

**Dosage in Renal/Hepatic Impairment**
No dose adjustment. Use caution with severe renal impairment.

## SIDE EFFECTS

**Occasional (3%):** Headache, insomnia, rash. **Rare (1%):** Nausea, vomiting, abdominal pain, fatigue, dizziness, abnormal dreams.

## ADVERSE EFFECTS/ TOXIC REACTIONS

Psychiatric disorders including depression, dysphoria, altered mood, suicidal ideation reported in 3% of pts. May prolong QT interval. May develop redistribution/accumulation of body fat (lipodystrophy) or immune reconstitution syndrome.

## NURSING CONSIDERATIONS

### BASELINE ASSESSMENT
Obtain CBC, BMP, LFT, lipid panel, CD4 count, viral load. Receive full medication history including herbal products. Question for history of prolonged QT interval, torsades de pointes, psychiatric disorder.

### INTERVENTION/EVALUATION
Closely monitor for evidence of rash. Monitor CBC, renal function, LFT.

### PATIENT/FAMILY TEACHING
• Offer emotional support. • Take with food (optimizes absorption). • Report any signs of depression, thoughts of suicide, decreased urine output, abdominal pain, yellowing of skin, darkened urine, clay-colored stools, chest tightness, difficulty breathing, palpitations. • Report any newly prescribed medications. • Rilpivirine does not cure HIV infection nor reduce risk of transmission to others. • Continue to practice safe sex with barrier methods or practice abstinence.

## risedronate

ris-**ed**-roe-nate
(<u>Actonel</u>, Atelvia, Apo-Risedronate ✱)
**Do not confuse Actonel with Actos, or risedronate with alendronate.**

### FIXED-COMBINATION(S)
**Actonel with Calcium:** risedronate/calcium: 35 mg/6 × 500 mg.

## ◆CLASSIFICATION

**PHARMACOTHERAPEUTIC:** Bisphosphonate. **CLINICAL:** Calcium regulator.

## USES

**Actonel:** Treatment of Paget's disease of bone. Treatment/prevention of osteoporosis in postmenopausal women, glucocorticoid-induced osteoporosis. Treatment of osteoporosis in men. **Atelvia:** Treatment of osteoporosis in postmenopausal women.

## PRECAUTIONS

**Contraindications:** Hypersensitivity to risedronate, other bisphosphonates (e.g., alendronate); inability to stand or sit upright for at least 30 min; abnormalities of esophagus that delay esophageal emptying. **Cautions:** GI diseases (duodenitis, dysphagia, esophagitis, gastritis, ulcers [drug may exacerbate these conditions]), severe renal impairment (CrCl less than 30 ml/min), hypocalcemia.

## ACTION

Inhibits bone resorption by action on osteoclasts or osteoclast precursors. **Therapeutic Effect:** Decreases bone resorption (indirectly increases bone mineral density). **Paget's Disease:** Inhibition of bone resorption causes a decrease (but more normal architecture) in bone formation.

## PHARMACOKINETICS

Rapidly absorbed. Bioavailability decreased when administered with food. Protein binding: 24%. Not metabolized. Excreted unchanged in urine, feces. Not removed by hemodialysis. **Half-life:** 1.5 hrs (initial); 480 hrs (terminal).

## ⊠ LIFESPAN CONSIDERATIONS

**Pregnancy/Lactation:** Unknown if distributed in breast milk. **Children:** Not indicated for use in this pt population. **Elderly:** No age-related precautions noted.

## INTERACTIONS

**DRUG: Antacids containing aluminum, calcium, magnesium; vitamin D** may decrease absorption (avoid administration within 30 min of **risedronate**). **HERBAL:** None significant. **FOOD:** None known. **LAB VALUES:** None significant.

## AVAILABILITY (Rx)

 Tablets (Actonel): 5 mg, 30 mg, 35 mg, 150 mg. **Tablets, Delayed-Release (Atelvia):** 35 mg.

## ADMINISTRATION/HANDLING

### PO

**Actonel:** • Administer 30–60 min before any food, drink, other oral medications to avoid interference with absorption. • Give on empty stomach with full glass of plain water (not mineral water). • Pt must avoid lying down for at least 30 min after swallowing tablet (assists with delivery to stomach, reduces risk of esophageal irritation). • Give whole; do not break, crush, dissolve, or divide tablet.

**Atelvia:** • Take in morning immediately following breakfast with at least 4 oz water. • Remain upright for 30 min after taking dose.

## INDICATIONS/ROUTES/DOSAGE

**Paget's Disease**

**PO:** *(Actonel):* **ADULTS, ELDERLY:** 30 mg/day for 2 mos. Retreatment may occur after 2-mo post-treatment observation period.

**Prophylaxis, Treatment of Postmenopausal Osteoporosis**

**PO:** *(Actonel):* **ADULTS, ELDERLY:** 5 mg/day or 35 mg once wkly or 150 mg once monthly.

**Treatment of Postmenopausal Osteoporosis**

**PO:** *(Atelvia):* **ADULTS, ELDERLY:** 35 mg once wkly.

**Treatment of Male Osteoporosis**

**PO:** *(Actonel):* **ADULTS, ELDERLY:** 35 mg once wkly.

**R**

---

**Glucocorticoid-Induced Osteoporosis**
**PO:** *(Actonel):* **ADULTS, ELDERLY:** 5 mg/
day.

**Dosage in Renal Impairment**
Not recommended with CrCl less than
30 ml/min.

**Dosage in Hepatic Impairment**
No dose adjustment.

## SIDE EFFECTS

**Frequent (30%):** Arthralgia. **Occasional
(12%–8%):** Rash, diarrhea, constipation,
nausea, abdominal pain, dyspepsia, flu-
like symptoms, peripheral edema. **Rare
(5%–3%):** Bone pain, sinusitis, asthenia,
dry eye, tinnitus.

## ADVERSE EFFECTS/
## TOXIC REACTIONS

Overdose produces hypocalcemia, hypophosphatemia, significant GI disturbances,
osteonecrosis of jaw.

## NURSING CONSIDERATIONS

### BASELINE ASSESSMENT

Assess symptoms of Paget's disease
(bone pain, bone deformities). Hypocalcemia, vitamin D deficiency must be
corrected before therapy begins. Obtain
baseline laboratory studies, esp. serum
electrolytes, renal function. Verify pt is
able to stand or sit upright for at least 30
min.

### INTERVENTION/EVALUATION

Check serum electrolytes (esp. calcium,
ionized calcium, phosphorus, alkaline
phosphatase levels). Monitor I&O, BUN,
creatinine in pts with renal impairment.

### PATIENT/FAMILY TEACHING

• Expected benefits occur only when
medication is taken with full glass (6–8
oz) of plain water, first thing in the morning and at least 30 min before first food,
beverage, medication of the day. Any other
beverage (mineral water, orange juice,
coffee) significantly reduces absorption of

medication. • Do not lie down for at least
30 min after taking medication (potentiates
delivery to stomach, reduces risk of esophageal irritation). • Report swallowing difficulties, pain when swallowing, chest pain,
new/worsening heartburn. • Consider
weight-bearing exercises, modify behavioral
factors (cigarette smoking, alcohol consumption). • Report jaw pain, incapacitat-
ing bone, joint, or muscle pain.

## *risperiDONE

ris-**per**-i-done
(Apo-Risperidone ✦, Risperdal,
Risperdal Consta, Risperdal M-Tabs,
Risperidone M-Tab)
■ **BLACK BOX ALERT** ■ Increased
risk of mortality in elderly pts with
dementia-related psychosis, mainly
due to pneumonia, HF.
**Do not confuse Risperdal with
Restoril, or risperidone with
ropinirole.**

## ◆CLASSIFICATION

**PHARMACOTHERAPEUTIC:**
Benzisoxazole derivative. **CLINICAL:**
Antipsychotic.

## USES

**(Oral):** Treatment of schizophrenia, irri-
tability/aggression associated with autistic
disease in children. Treatment of acute
mania associated with bipolar disorder
(monotherapy in children and adults; in
combination with lithium or valproate in
adults). **(IM):** Management of schizophrenia, maintenance treatment of bipolar
1 disorder (monotherapy or in combination with lithium or valproate in adults).
**OFF-LABEL:** Tourette's syndrome. Post-
traumatic stress syndrome. Major depressive disorder.

## PRECAUTIONS

**Contraindications:** Hypersensitivity to
risperidone. **Cautions:** Renal/hepatic
impairment, seizure disorders, cardiac

disease, recent MI, breast cancer or other prolactin-dependent tumors, suicidal pts, pts at risk for aspiration pneumonia. Parkinson's disease, pts at risk for orthostatic hypotension, elderly, diabetes, decreased GI motility, urinary retention, BPH, xerostomia, visual problems, pts exposed to temperature extremes, preexisting myelosuppression, narrow-angle glaucoma; pts with high risk of suicide.

## ACTION

May antagonize dopamine, serotonin receptors in both CNS and periphery. **Therapeutic Effect:** Suppresses psychotic behavior.

## PHARMACOKINETICS

Well absorbed from GI tract; unaffected by food. Protein binding: 90%. Metabolized in liver. Primarily excreted in urine. **Half-life:** 3–20 hrs; metabolite, 21–30 hrs (increased in elderly). **Injection:** 3–6 days.

## ⌛ LIFESPAN CONSIDERATIONS

**Pregnancy/Lactation:** Unknown if drug crosses placenta or is distributed in breast milk. Breastfeeding not recommended. **Children:** Safety and efficacy not established. **Elderly:** More susceptible to postural hypotension. Age-related renal/hepatic impairment may require dosage adjustment.

## INTERACTIONS

**DRUG: Alcohol, other CNS depressants** (e.g., **lorazepam, morphine, zolpidem**) may increase CNS depression. **Carbamazepine** may decrease concentration. May decrease effects of **dopamine agonists, levodopa. Paroxetine, fluoxetine** may increase concentration, risk of extrapyramidal symptoms (EPS). **Antihypertensives** (e.g., **amlodipine, lisinopril, valsartan**), **beta blockers** (e.g., **carvedilol, metoprolol**), **calcium channel blockers** (e.g., **diltiazem, verapamil**) **diuretics** (e.g., **furosemide, HCTZ**); **doxepin, pramipexole, prazosin, sildenafil. Antihypertensives,**

**hypotension-producing medications** may increase hypotensive effect. **HERBAL: Gotu kola, kava kava, St. John's wort, valerian** may increase CNS depression. **FOOD:** None known. **LAB VALUES:** May increase serum prolactin. May cause EKG changes.

## AVAILABILITY (Rx)

**Injection, Powder for Reconstitution (Risperdal Consta):** 12.5 mg, 25 mg, 37.5 mg, 50 mg. **Oral Solution (Risperdal):** 1 mg/ml. **Tablets (Risperdal):** 0.25 mg, 0.5 mg, 1 mg, 2 mg, 3 mg, 4 mg.

🖋 **Tablets (Orally Disintegrating [Risperdal M-Tabs, Risperidone M-Tab]):** 0.25 mg, 0.5 mg, 1 mg, 2 mg, 3 mg, 4 mg.

## ADMINISTRATION/HANDLING

◄**ALERT►** Do not administer via IV route.

### IM

**Reconstitution** • Use only diluent and needle supplied in dose pack. • Prepare suspension according to manufacturer's directions. • May be given up to 6 hrs after reconstitution, but immediate administration is recommended. • If 2 min pass between reconstitution and injection, shake upright vial vigorously back and forth to resuspend solution.
**Rate of Administration** • Inject IM into upper outer quadrant of gluteus maximus or into deltoid muscle in upper arm.
**Storage** • Store at room temperature.

### PO

• Give without regard to food. • May mix oral solution with water, coffee, orange juice, low-fat milk. Do not mix with cola, tea.

### Orally Disintegrating Tablet

• Remove from blister pack immediately before administration. • Using gloves, place immediately on tongue. • Tablet dissolves in seconds. • Pt may swallow with or without liquid. • Do not split or chew.

---

## INDICATIONS/ROUTES/DOSAGE

### Schizophrenia

**PO: ADULTS:** Initially, 1 mg twice daily. May increase gradually (1–2 mg/day at intervals of at least 24 hrs) to target dose of 6 mg/day. Range: 4–8 mg/day. **Maintenance:** Target dose of 4 mg once daily (range: 2–8 mg/day). **ELDERLY:** Initially, 0.5 mg twice daily. May increase slowly at increments of no more than 0.5 mg twice daily. Range: 2–6 mg/day. **CHILDREN 13–17 YRS:** Initially, 0.5 mg/day (as single daily dose). May increase by 0.5–1 mg/day at intervals of greater than 24 hrs to recommended dose of 3 mg/day.

**IM: ADULTS, ELDERLY:** Initially, 12.5–25 mg q2wks. **Maximum:** 50 mg q2wks. Dosage adjustments should not be made more frequently than every 4 wks.

### Bipolar Mania

**PO: ADULTS, ELDERLY:** Initially, 2–3 mg as a single daily dose. May increase by 1 mg/day at 24-hr intervals. Range: 1–6 mg/day.

**PO: CHILDREN 10–17 YRS:** Initially, 0.5 mg/day. May increase by 0.5 mg/day at intervals of greater than 24 hrs to recommended dose of 2.5 mg/day. **IM: ADULTS, ELDERLY:** 25 mg q2wks. **Maximum:** 50 mg q2wks. Dosage adjustments should not be made more frequently than every 4 wks.

### Autism

**CHILDREN 5 YRS AND OLDER WEIGHING MORE THAN 19 KG:** Initially, 0.5 mg/day. May increase to 1 mg after 4 days. May further increase dose by 0.5 mg/day in greater than 2-wk intervals. Range: 0.5–3 mg/day. **CHILDREN 5 YRS AND OLDER WEIGHING 15–19 KG:** Initially, 0.25 mg/day. May increase to 0.5 mg/day after 4 days. May further increase dose by 0.25 mg/day in greater than 2-wk intervals. Range: 0.5–3 mg/day.

### Dosage in Renal/Hepatic Impairment

**Mild to moderate impairment:** No dose adjustment. **Severe impairment:** Initial dosage for adults, elderly pts is 0.25–0.5 mg twice daily. Dosage is titrated slowly to desired effect.

## SIDE EFFECTS

**Frequent (26%–13%):** Agitation, anxiety, insomnia, headache, constipation. **Occasional (10%–4%):** Dyspepsia, rhinitis, drowsiness, dizziness, nausea, vomiting, rash, abdominal pain, dry skin, tachycardia. **Rare (3%–2%):** Visual disturbances, fever, back pain, pharyngitis, cough, arthralgia, angina, aggressive behavior, orthostatic hypotension, breast swelling.

## ADVERSE EFFECTS/ TOXIC REACTIONS

Rare reactions include tardive dyskinesia (characterized by tongue protrusion, puffing of the cheeks, chewing or puckering of mouth), neuroleptic malignant syndrome (marked by hyperpyrexia, muscle rigidity, altered mental status, irregular pulse or B/P, tachycardia, diaphoresis, cardiac arrhythmias, rhabdomyolysis, acute renal failure). Hyperglycemia, in some cases, life-threatening events such as ketoacidosis, hyperosmolar coma, death, has been reported.

## NURSING CONSIDERATIONS

### BASELINE ASSESSMENT

Renal function test, LFT should be performed before therapy begins. Assess behavior, appearance, emotional status, response to environment, speech pattern, thought content, baseline weight. Obtain fasting serum glucose.

### INTERVENTION/EVALUATION

Monitor B/P, heart rate, weight, LFT, EKG. Monitor for fine tongue movement (may be first sign of tardive dyskinesia, which may be irreversible). Monitor for suicidal ideation. Assess for therapeutic response (greater interest in surroundings, improved self-care, increased ability to concentrate, relaxed facial expression). Monitor for potential neuroleptic malignant syndrome: fever, muscle rigidity, irregular B/P or pulse, altered mental status. Monitor fasting serum glucose periodically during therapy.

### PATIENT/FAMILY TEACHING

• Avoid tasks that may require alertness, motor skills until response to drug is established (may cause dizziness/drowsiness). • Avoid alcohol. • Go from lying to standing slowly. • Report trembling in fingers, altered gait, unusual muscular/skeletal movements, palpitations, severe dizziness/fainting, swelling/pain in breasts, visual changes, rash, difficulty breathing.

---

# ritonavir

rit-**oh**-na-veer
(Norvir)

■ **BLACK BOX ALERT** ■ Concurrent use with other medications (nonsedating antihistamines, sedative hypnotics, antiarrhythmics, ergot alkaloids) may result in potentially serious, life-threatening events.
**Do not confuse Norvir with Norvasc, or ritonavir with Retrovir.**

## ◆CLASSIFICATION

**PHARMACOTHERAPEUTIC:** Protease inhibitor. **CLINICAL:** Antiviral.

## USES

Treatment of HIV infection in combination with other antiretroviral agents. May be used as "booster" for other protease inhibitors.

## PRECAUTIONS

**Contraindications:** Hypersensitivity to ritonavir. Due to potential serious and/or life-threatening drug interactions (e.g., arrhythmias, hematologic abnormalities, seizures), the following medications should not be given concomitantly with ritonavir: alfuzosin, amiodarone, dihydroergotamine, ergotamine, ergonovine, flecainide, lovastatin, methylergonovine, midazolam (oral), pimozide, propafenone, quinidine, sildenafil (when used for pulmonary arterial hypertension), simvastatin, St. John's wort, triazolam, voriconazole (when ritonavir dose 800 mg or greater/day). **Cautions:** Hepatic impairment, cardiomyopathy, ischemic heart disease, preexisting cardiac conduction abnormalities, structural heart disease, pts with increased triglycerides, hemophilia A and B, diabetes, hepatitis B or C virus infection, medications that prolong PR interval, diabetes.

## ACTION

Inhibits HIV-1 and HIV-2 proteases, rendering these enzymes incapable of processing polypeptide precursors leading to production of noninfectious, immature HIV particles. **Therapeutic Effect:** Slows HIV replication, reducing progression of HIV infection.

## PHARMACOKINETICS

Well absorbed (absorption increased with food). Protein binding: 98%–99%. Metabolized in liver. Primarily eliminated in feces. Unknown if removed by hemodialysis. **Half-life:** 2.7–5 hrs.

## ⌛ LIFESPAN CONSIDERATIONS

**Pregnancy/Lactation:** Breastfeeding not recommended (possibility of HIV transmission). **Pregnancy Category B. Children:** No age-related precautions noted in those older than 2 yrs. **Elderly:** None known.

## INTERACTIONS

**DRUG:** See contraindications. May increase concentration of **clarithromycin, fluticasone, ketoconazole, protease inhibitors, sildenafil, statins.** May decrease concentration/effects of **methadone, phenytoin, warfarin. Rifampin** may decrease concentration/effects. **HERBAL:** St. John's wort may decrease concentration/effects. **FOOD:** None known. **LAB VALUES:** May increase serum creatine kinase (CK), GGT, triglycerides, uric acid, ALT, AST, glucose. May decrease Hgb, Hct, WBC, neutrophils.

---

## AVAILABILITY (Rx)

**Capsules:** 100 mg. **Oral Solution:** 80 mg/ml.

**Tablets:** 100 mg.

## ADMINISTRATION/HANDLING

### PO

• Store capsules in refrigerator. Store tablets, oral solution at room temperature. • Protect from light. • Give without regard to meals (preferably give with food). • Give tablets whole; do not break, crush, dissolve, or divide. • May improve taste of oral solution by mixing with chocolate milk, Ensure, Advera, Boost within 1 hr of dosing.

## INDICATIONS/ROUTES/DOSAGE

**Note:** Not recommended as primary protease inhibitor in any regimen.

**Treatment of HIV Infection**
**PO: ADULTS, CHILDREN 12 YRS AND OLDER:** 600 mg twice daily. If nausea occurs at this dosage, give 300 mg twice daily for 1 day, then increase by 100 mg twice daily every 2–3 days to recommended dose of 600 mg twice daily. **CHILDREN 1 MO–11 YRS:** Initially, 250 mg/m²/dose twice daily. Increase by 50 mg/m²/dose q2–3days up to 350–400 mg/m²/dose. **Maximum:** 600 mg/dose twice daily.

**Booster Therapy**
**PO: ADULTS, ELDERLY:** 100–400 mg/day (usually as 100–200 mg 1–2 times/day.)

**Dosage in Renal Impairment**
No dose adjustment.

**Dosage in Hepatic Impairment**
**Mild to moderate impairment:** No dose adjustment. **Severe impairment:** Not recommended.

## SIDE EFFECTS

**Frequent:** GI disturbances (abdominal pain, anorexia, diarrhea, nausea, vomiting), circumoral and peripheral paresthesia, altered taste, headache, dizziness, fatigue, asthenia. **Occasional:** Allergic reaction, flu-like symptoms, hypotension. **Rare:** Diabetes mellitus, hyperglycemia.

## ADVERSE EFFECTS/ TOXIC REACTIONS

Hepatitis, pancreatitis occur rarely.

## NURSING CONSIDERATIONS

### BASELINE ASSESSMENT

Pts beginning combination therapy with ritonavir and nucleosides may promote GI tolerance by beginning ritonavir alone, then subsequently adding nucleosides before completing 2 wks of ritonavir monotherapy. Obtain baseline laboratory testing, esp. LFT, triglycerides before beginning ritonavir therapy and at periodic intervals during therapy. Offer emotional support. Obtain full medication history and screen for contraindications/interactions.

### INTERVENTION/EVALUATION

Closely monitor for evidence of GI disturbances, neurologic abnormalities (particularly paresthesia). Monitor LFT, serum glucose, CD4 cell count, plasma levels of HIV RNA.

### PATIENT/FAMILY TEACHING

• Continue therapy for full length of treatment. • Doses should be evenly spaced. • Ritonavir is not a cure for HIV infection, nor does it reduce risk of transmission to others. • Pts may continue to acquire illnesses associated with advanced HIV infection. • If possible, take ritonavir with food. • Taste of solution may be improved when mixed with chocolate milk, Ensure, Advera, Boost. • Report increased thirst, frequent urination, nausea, vomiting, abdominal pain.

**R**

# *riTUXimab

ri-**tux**-i-mab
(Rituxan)

■ **BLACK BOX ALERT** ■ Profound, occasionally fatal infusion-related reactions reported during first 30–120 min of first infusion. Tumor lysis syndrome leading to acute renal failure may occur 12–24 hrs following first dose. Severe, sometimes fatal, mucocutaneous reactions resulting in multifocal leukoencephalopathy (PML) and death reported.
**Do not confuse Rituxan with Remicade, or rituximab with bevacizumab or infliximab, brentuximab, ruxolitinib.**

## ◆CLASSIFICATION

**PHARMACOTHERAPEUTIC:** Monoclonal antibody. **CLINICAL:** Antineoplastic.

## USES

Treatment of CD20-positive non-Hodgkin's lymphomas (NHL): Relapsed or refractory, low-grade, or follicular B-cell NHL; follicular B-cell NHL (previously untreated); nonprogressive, low-grade B-cell NHL; diffuse large B-cell NHL, previously untreated. Treatment of CD20-positive chronic lymphocytic leukemia (CLL). Treatment of moderate to severe active rheumatoid arthritis (RA) in combination with methotrexate. Treatment of granulomatosis with polyangitis (GPA). Treatment of microscopic polyangitis (MPA). **OFF-LABEL:** Treatment of autoimmune hemolytic anemia, chronic immune thrombocytopenic purpura (ITP), systemic autoimmune disease (other than rheumatoid arthritis), Burkitt's lymphoma, CNS lymphoma, Hodgkin's lymphoma.

## PRECAUTIONS

**Contraindications:** Hypersensitivity to rituximab, murine proteins. **Cautions:** Pts at risk for tumor lysis syndrome. Cardiac disease, elderly, pulmonary disease, renal impairment, severe active infection; history of hepatitis B virus infection.

## ACTION

Binds to CD20, the antigen found on surface of B lymphocytes, B-cell non-Hodgkin's lymphoma (NHL). Activates B-cell cytotoxicity. **Therapeutic Effect:** Produces cytotoxicity, reduces tumor size. Signs/symptoms of rheumatoid arthritis are reduced; structural damage delayed.

## PHARMACOKINETICS

Rapidly depletes B cells. **Half-life:** 59.8 hrs after first infusion, 174 hrs after fourth infusion.

## ⌛ LIFESPAN CONSIDERATIONS

**Pregnancy/Lactation:** Has potential to cause fetal B-cell depletion. Unknown if distributed in breast milk. Female pts of reproductive potential should use effective contraception during treatment and up to 12 mos after discontinuation. **Children:** Safety and efficacy not established. **Elderly:** No age-related precautions noted.

## INTERACTIONS

**DRUG:** None significant. **HERBAL:** **Echinacea** may decrease therapeutic effect. **Garlic, ginger, ginseng** may increase hypoglycemic effect. **FOOD:** None known. **LAB VALUES:** May increase creatinine, LDH. May decrease Hgb, Hct, neutrophils, platelets, B-cell counts, immunoglobulin concentrations.

## AVAILABILITY (Rx)

**Injection Solution:** 10 mg/ml (10 ml, 50 ml).

## ADMINISTRATION/HANDLING

⊞ IV

◀**ALERT**▶ Do not give by IV push or bolus.

**Reconstitution •** Dilute with 0.9% NaCl or D₅W to provide final concentration of 1–4 mg/ml into infusion bag.

---

**Rate of Administration** • Initially infuse at rate of 50 mg/hr. If no hypersensitivity or infusion-related reaction, may increase infusion rate in 50 mg/hr increments q30min to maximum 400 mg/hr. • Subsequent infusion can be given at 100 mg/hr and increased by 100 mg/hr increments q30min to maximum 400 mg/hr.

**Storage** • Refrigerate vials. • Diluted solution is stable for 24 hrs if refrigerated or at room temperature.

## ❀ IV INCOMPATIBILITIES

Do not mix with any other medications.

## INDICATIONS/ROUTES/DOSAGE

**Note:** Refer to specific protocols.

**NHL (Relapsed/Refractory, Low-Grade or Follicular CD20-Positive B-cell)**
**IV: ADULTS:** 375 mg/m$^2$ wkly for 4 or 8 doses.

**NHL (Diffuse Large B-cell)**
**IV: ADULTS:** 375 mg/m$^2$ on day 1 of each cycle up to 8 doses.

**NHL (Follicular, CD20-Positive, B-cell, Previously Untreated)**
**IV: ADULTS:** 375 mg/m$^2$ on day 1 of each cycle up to 8 doses. **Maintenance (single agent):** 375 mg/m$^2$ q8 wks for 12 doses.

**NHL (Nonprogressive, CD20-Positive, B-cell Following 6–8 Cycles of Cyclophosphamide, Vincristine, and Prednisolone [CVP Therapy])**
**IV: ADULTS:** 375 mg/m$^2$ once wkly for 4 doses q6 mos. **Maximum:** 16 doses.

**NHL (Combination with Ibritumomab)**
**IV: ADULTS:** 250 mg/m$^2$ day 1; repeat in 7–9 days with ibritumomab.

**Rheumatoid Arthritis**
**IV: ADULTS:** 1,000 mg every 2 wks times 2 doses in combination with methotrexate. May repeat course q24 wks (if needed, no sooner than 16 wks).

**CLL**
**IV: ADULTS:** 375 mg/m$^2$ in first cycle (on day prior to fludarabine/cyclophosphamide) and 500 mg/m$^2$ on day 1 in cycles 2–6, administered every 28 days.

**GPA, MPA**
**IV: ADULTS:** 375 mg/m$^2$ once wkly for 4 wks (in combination with methylprednisolone IV for 1–3 days, then daily prednisone).

**Dosage in Renal/Hepatic Impairment**
No dose adjustment.

## SIDE EFFECTS

**Frequent (49%–10%):** Fever, chills, nausea, asthenia, headache, angioedema, hypotension, rash/pruritus. **Occasional (less than 10%):** Myalgia, dizziness, weakness, abdominal pain, throat irritation, vomiting, neutropenia, rhinitis, bronchospasm, urticaria.

## ADVERSE EFFECTS/ TOXIC REACTIONS

Hypersensitivity reaction produces hypotension, bronchospasm, angioedema. Arrhythmias may occur, particularly in pts with history of preexisting cardiac conditions.

## NURSING CONSIDERATIONS

### BASELINE ASSESSMENT

Pretreatment with acetaminophen and diphenhydramine before each infusion may prevent infusion-related effects. CBC should be obtained at regular intervals during therapy.

### INTERVENTION/EVALUATION

Monitor CBC, renal function, LFT. Diligently monitor for tumor lysis syndrome in pts with high tumor burden. Monitor for an infusion-related symptoms complex consisting mainly of fever, chills, rigors that generally occurs within 30 min–2 hrs of beginning first infusion. Slowing infusion resolves symptoms.

**R**

• Report fever, sore throat, abdominal pain, yellowing of eyes/skin, unusual bruising/bleeding.

# rivaroxaban

TOP
100

rye-va-**rox**-a-ban
(Xarelto)

■ **BLACK BOX ALERT** ■ Epidural/spinal hematomas may occur in pts receiving neuraxial anesthesia or spinal puncture, resulting in long-term or permanent paralysis. Factors increasing risk of epidural/spinal hematoma include indwelling epidural catheters, concomitant drugs such as NSAIDs, platelet inhibitors, other anticoagulants; history of traumatic or repeated spinal or epidural punctures, history of spinal deformity or spinal surgery. Monitor for signs and symptoms of neurologic impairment. Consider benefits and risks before neuraxial intervention in anticoagulated pts or planned thromboprophylaxis. Increased risk of stroke may occur in pts with atrial fibrillation when discontinuing for reasons other than bleeding.
**Do not confuse rivaroxaban with argatroban.**

◆**CLASSIFICATION**

**PHARMACOTHERAPEUTIC:** Factor Xa inhibitor. **CLINICAL:** Anticoagulant.

## USES

Prophylaxis of deep vein thrombosis (DVT) in pts undergoing knee or hip replacement surgery. Prevents stroke/systemic embolism in pts with nonvalvular atrial fibrillation. Treatment of DVT/PE. Reduces risk of recurrent DVT/PE following 6 mos of treatment.

## PRECAUTIONS

**Contraindications:** Hypersensitivity to rivaroxaban. Active major bleeding. **Cautions:** Renal/hepatic impairment, pts at increased risk of bleeding (e.g., thrombocytopenia, stroke, severe uncontrolled hypertension), elderly; avoid use with heparin, low molecular weight heparin (LMWH), aspirin, warfarin, NSAIDs.

## ACTION

Selectively blocks active site of factor Xa, a key factor in the intrinsic and extrinsic pathway of blood coagulation cascade. Inhibits platelet activation and fibrin clot formation. **Therapeutic Effect:** Inhibits blood coagulation.

## PHARMACOKINETICS

Rapidly absorbed after PO administration. Peak plasma concentration: 2–4 hrs. Absorption dependent on site of drug release within GI tract. Avoid administration into small intestine due to reduced absorption. Protein binding: 92%–95%. Metabolized in liver. Excreted in urine (66%), feces (28%). **Half-life:** 5–9 hrs, 11–13 hrs (elderly).

## ⧖ LIFESPAN CONSIDERATIONS

**Pregnancy/Lactation:** Unknown if excreted in breast milk. **Children:** Safety and efficacy not established. **Elderly:** May be at increased risk for bleeding due to age-related renal impairment.

## INTERACTIONS

**DRUG: CYP3A4 inhibitors (e.g., ketoconazole, clarithromycin, ritonavir)** may increase concentration, risk of bleeding. **Anticoagulants (e.g., heparin, warfarin), antiplatelets (e.g., aspirin, clopidogrel), NSAIDs** may increase bleeding risk. **HERBAL: St. John's wort** may decrease effect. **FOOD: Grapefruit products** may increase risk of bleeding. **LAB VALUES:** May decrease platelets. May increase serum ALT, AST, bilirubin.

## AVAILABILITY (Rx)

**Tablets:** 10 mg, 15 mg, 20 mg.

R

## ADMINISTRATION/HANDLING

### PO

• **DVT prophylaxis (knee, hip):** Give without regard to meals. • **Nonvalvular atrial fibrillation:** Give with evening meal. • **Treatment DVT/PE:** Give with food. • **Risk reduction DVT/PE:** Give with food.

## INDICATIONS/ROUTES/DOSAGE

### DVT Prophylaxis, Knee Replacement

**PO: ADULTS:** 10 mg daily for minimum 10–14 days up to 35 days. Initiate at least 6–10 hrs after surgery once hemostasis established. **CrCl less than 30 ml/min:** Avoid use.

### DVT Prophylaxis, Hip Replacement

**PO: ADULTS:** 10 mg daily for 10–14 days (minimum) up to 35 days. Initiate at least 6–10 hrs after surgery once hemostasis established. **CrCl less than 30 ml/min:** Avoid use.

### Nonvalvular Atrial Fibrillation

**PO: ADULTS: CrCl greater than 50 ml/min:** 20 mg daily. **CrCl 15–50 ml/min:** 15 mg daily. **CrCl less than 15 ml/min:** Avoid use.

### Treatment of DVT/PE

**PO: ADULTS, ELDERLY:** 15 mg twice daily for 3 wks, then 20 mg once daily.

### Reduce Risk of DVT/PE (After 6 mos Treatment)

**PO: ADULTS, ELDERLY:** 20 mg once daily up to 6–12 mos.

### Dosage in Renal Impairment

**CrCl less than 30 ml/min:** Avoid use in DVT/PE; postoperative thromboprophylaxis. *Nonvalvular atrial fibrillation:* **CrCl 15–50 ml/min:** 15 mg once daily with evening meal. **CrCl less than 15 ml/min:** Avoid use.

### Dosage in Hepatic Impairment

**Mild impairment:** No dose adjustment. **Moderate to severe impairment:** Avoid use.

## SIDE EFFECTS

**Rare (3%–1%):** Wound secretion/oozing, extremity pain, muscle spasm, syncope, pruritus.

## ADVERSE EFFECTS/TOXIC REACTIONS

Increased risk of bleeding/hemorrhagic events including retroperitoneal hemorrhage, cerebral hemorrhage, subdural hematoma, epidural/spinal hematoma (esp. with epidural catheters, spinal trauma). Serious reactions including jaundice, cholestasis, cytolytic hepatitis, Stevens-Johnson syndrome, hypersensitivity reaction, anaphylaxis reported.

## NURSING CONSIDERATIONS

### BASELINE ASSESSMENT

Obtain CBC, serum chemistries, PT/INR, vital signs, urine pregnancy if applicable. Obtain EKG for pts with a history of atrial fibrillation. Question for history of bleeding disorders, recent surgery, spinal punctures, intracranial hemorrhage, bleeding ulcers, open wounds, anemia, renal/hepatic impairment. Receive full medication history including herbal products.

### INTERVENTION/EVALUATION

Monitor CBC, serum chemistries, renal function, occult urine/stool. Be alert for complaints of abdominal/back pain, headache, confusion, weakness, vision change (may indicate hemorrhage). Question for increased menstrual bleeding/discharge. Assess peripheral pulses; skin for ecchymosis, petechiae. Check for excessive bleeding from minor cuts, scratches. Assess urine output for hematuria. Immediately report suspected pregnancy.

### PATIENT/FAMILY TEACHING

• Do not take/discontinue any medication except on advice of physician. • Avoid alcohol, aspirin, NSAIDs. • Consult physician before surgery, dental work. • Use electric razor, soft toothbrush to prevent

R

bleeding. • Report any unusual bleeding/ bruising, spinal/epidural hematomas (e.g., tingling, numbness, muscular weakness). • Report if pregnant or planning to become pregnant. • Avoid grapefruit products.

# rivastigmine

riv-a-**stig**-meen
(Apo-Rivastigmine ✦, Exelon, Novo-Rivastigmine ✦)

### ◆CLASSIFICATION

**PHARMACOTHERAPEUTIC:** Cholinesterase inhibitor. **CLINICAL:** Anti-Alzheimer's dementia agent.

## USES

Treatment of mild to severe dementia of Alzheimer's or mild to moderate dementia of Parkinson's disease. **OFF-LABEL:** Lewy body dementia.

## PRECAUTIONS

**Contraindications:** Hypersensitivity to rivastigmine, other carbamate derivatives (e.g., neostigmine), history of application site reactions with rivastigmine. **Cautions:** Peptic ulcer disease, concurrent use of NSAIDs, sick sinus syndrome, bradycardia or supraventricular conduction defects, urinary obstruction, seizure disorders, asthma, COPD, pts with body weight less than 50 kg.

## ACTION

Increases acetylcholine in CNS by inhibiting hydrolysis by cholinesterase. **Therapeutic Effect:** Slows progression of symptoms of Alzheimer's disease, dementia of Parkinson's disease.

## PHARMACOKINETICS

Rapidly, completely absorbed. Protein binding: 40%. Widely distributed throughout body. Rapidly, extensively metabolized. Primarily excreted in urine. **Half-life:** 1.5 hrs.

## ⌛ LIFESPAN CONSIDERATIONS

**Pregnancy/Lactation:** Unknown if distributed in breast milk. **Children:** Not indicated for use in this pt population. **Elderly:** No age-related precautions noted.

## INTERACTIONS

**DRUG:** May interfere with **anticholinergics (e.g., dicyclomine, glycopyrrolate, scopolamine)** effects. May have additive effect with **bethanechol.** NSAIDs may increase GI effects, irritation. **HERBAL:** Ginkgo biloba may increase cholinergic effects. **FOOD:** None known. **LAB VALUES:** None significant.

## AVAILABILITY (Rx)

**Transdermal Patch:** 4.6 mg/24 hrs, 9.5 mg/24 hrs, 13.3 mg/24 hrs.

🏷 **Capsules:** 1.5 mg, 3 mg, 4.5 mg, 6 mg.

## ADMINISTRATION/HANDLING

### PO

• Give morning and evening doses with food. • Give capsule whole.

### Transdermal Patch

• May apply the day following the last oral dose. • Apply to upper or lower back, upper arm, or chest. • Avoid reapplication to same spot of skin for 14 days. • Do not apply to red, irritated, or broken skin. • Avoid eye contact. • After removal, fold patch to press adhesive together and discard.

## INDICATIONS/ROUTES/DOSAGE

### Alzheimer's Dementia (Mild to Moderate)

**PO: ADULTS, ELDERLY:** Initially, 1.5 mg twice daily. May increase at intervals of at least 2 wks to 3 mg twice daily, then 4.5 mg twice daily, and finally 6 mg twice daily. **Maximum:** 6 mg twice daily. **Transdermal:** Initially, 4.6 mg/24 hrs. May increase at intervals of at least 4 wks to 9.5 mg/24 hrs and then to 13.3 mg/24 hrs.

**R**

---

**Alzheimer's Dementia (Severe)**
**Transdermal: ADULTS, ELDERLY:** Initially, 4.6 mg/24 hrs. May increase at intervals of at least 4 wks to 9.5 mg/24 hrs and then to 13.3 mg/24 hrs.

**Parkinson's Dementia**
**PO: ADULTS, ELDERLY:** Initially, 1.5 mg twice daily. May increase at intervals of at least 4 wks to 3 mg twice daily, then 4.5 mg twice daily, and finally 6 mg twice daily. **Maximum:** 6 mg twice daily.
**Transdermal Dosage: Note:** Initially, 4.6 mg/24 hrs. May increase after 4 wks to 9.5 mg/24 hrs and then to 13.3 mg/24 hrs.

**Dosage in Renal Impairment**
No dose adjustment.

**Dosage in Hepatic Impairment**
**Oral:** No dose adjustment. **Transdermal:** Maximum dose: 4.6 mg/24 hrs.

## SIDE EFFECTS

**Frequent (47%–17%):** Nausea, vomiting, dizziness, diarrhea, headache, anorexia. **Occasional (13%–6%):** Abdominal pain, insomnia, dyspepsia (heartburn, indigestion, epigastric pain), confusion, UTI, depression. **Rare (5%–3%):** Anxiety, drowsiness, constipation, malaise, hallucinations, tremor, flatulence, rhinitis, hypertension, flu-like symptoms, weight loss, syncope.

## ADVERSE EFFECTS/ TOXIC REACTIONS

Overdose can produce cholinergic crisis, characterized by severe nausea/vomiting, increased salivation, diaphoresis, bradycardia, hypotension, respiratory depression, seizures.

## NURSING CONSIDERATIONS

### BASELINE ASSESSMENT

Obtain baseline vital signs. Assess history for peptic ulcer, urinary obstruction, asthma, COPD, cardiac disease. Assess cognitive, behavioral, functional deficits.

### INTERVENTION/EVALUATION

Monitor for cholinergic reaction: GI discomfort/cramping, feeling of facial warmth, excessive salivation, diaphoresis, lacrimation, pallor, urinary urgency, dizziness. Monitor for nausea, diarrhea, headache, insomnia.

### PATIENT/ FAMILY TEACHING

• Take with meals (at breakfast, dinner). • Swallow capsule whole. Do not break, chew, or divide capsules. • Report nausea, vomiting, diarrhea, diaphoresis, increased salivary secretions, severe abdominal pain, dizziness.

# rizatriptan

**rye**-za-trip-tan
(Apo-Rizatriptan ✦, Maxalt, Maxalt-MLT, Maxalt RPD ✦)

## ◆CLASSIFICATION

**PHARMACOTHERAPEUTIC:** Serotonin receptor agonist. **CLINICAL:** Antimigraine.

## USES

Treatment of acute migraine headache with or without aura.

## PRECAUTIONS

**Contraindications:** Hypersensitivity to rizatriptan. Basilar or hemiplegic migraine, history of stroke or transient ischemic attack; severe cardiovascular disease, coronary artery vasospasm, peripheral vascular disease, ischemic bowel disease, uncontrolled hypertension, use within 24 hrs of ergotamine-containing preparations or another serotonin receptor agonist, MAOI use within 14 days. **Cautions:** Mild to moderate renal/hepatic impairment, dialysis pts, elderly, pt profile suggesting cardiovascular risks (e.g., hypertension, diabetes, hypercholesterolemia).

## ACTION

Binds selectively to serotonin receptors in cranial arteries producing vasoconstriction. **Therapeutic Effect:** Relieves migraine headache.

## PHARMACOKINETICS

Well absorbed after PO administration. Protein binding: 14%. Crosses blood-brain barrier. Metabolized by liver. Eliminated primarily in urine (82%), feces (12%). **Half-life:** 2–3 hrs.

## ⌛ LIFESPAN CONSIDERATIONS

**Pregnancy/Lactation:** Unknown if drug is distributed in breast milk. **Children:** Safety and efficacy not established. **Elderly:** No age-related precautions noted.

## INTERACTIONS

**DRUG: Ergotamine-containing medications** may produce vasospastic reaction. **Fluoxetine, fluvoxamine, paroxetine, sertraline** may produce hyperreflexia, incoordination, weakness. **MAOIs, propranolol** may dramatically increase concentration (avoid concurrent use). **HERBAL:** None significant. **FOOD: All foods** delay peak drug concentration by 1 hr. **LAB VALUES:** None significant.

## AVAILABILITY (Rx)

**Tablets (Maxalt):** 5 mg, 10 mg. **Tablets (Orally Disintegrating [Maxalt-MLT]):** 5 mg, 10 mg.

## ADMINISTRATION/HANDLING

### PO

• Orally disintegrating tablet is packaged in individual aluminum pouch. • Open packet with dry hands. • Place tablet onto tongue, allow to dissolve, swallow with saliva. Administration with water is not necessary.

## INDICATIONS/ROUTES/DOSAGE

**Acute Migraine Headache**
**PO: ADULTS OLDER THAN 18 YRS, ELDERLY:** 5–10 mg. If significant improvement is not attained, dose may be repeated after 2 hrs. **Maximum:** 30 mg/24 hrs.

(Use 5 mg/dose in pts taking propranolol with maximum of 15 mg/24 hrs.) **CHILDREN 6–17 YRS: 40 KG OR GREATER:** 10 mg as single dose. (Maximum 5 mg as single dose with propranolol.) **LESS THAN 40 KG:** 5 mg as a single dose. (Not recommended if taking propranolol.)

**Dosage in Renal/Hepatic Imapirment**
No dose adjustment.

## SIDE EFFECTS

**Frequent (9%–7%):** Dizziness, drowsiness, paresthesia, fatigue. **Occasional (6%–3%):** Nausea, chest pressure, dry mouth. **Rare (2%):** Headache; neck, throat, jaw pressure; photosensitivity.

## ADVERSE EFFECTS/ TOXIC REACTIONS

Cardiac reactions (ischemia, coronary artery vasospasm, MI), noncardiac vasospasm-related reactions (hemorrhage, CVA) occur rarely, particularly in pts with hypertension, diabetes, strong family history of coronary artery disease, obesity, smokers, males older than 40 yrs, postmenopausal women.

## NURSING CONSIDERATIONS

### BASELINE ASSESSMENT

Question for history of peripheral vascular disease, renal/hepatic impairment. Question pt regarding onset, location, duration of migraine, possible precipitating symptoms.

### INTERVENTION/EVALUATION

Monitor for evidence of dizziness. Assess for photophobia, phonophobia (sound sensitivity, nausea, vomiting), relief of migraine headache.

### PATIENT/FAMILY TEACHING

• Take single dose as soon as symptoms of an actual migraine headache appear. • Medication is intended to relieve migraine, not to prevent or reduce number of attacks. • Avoid tasks that require alertness, motor skills until response to

R

drug is established. • Report immediately if palpitations, pain/tightness in chest/throat, pain/weakness of extremities occurs. • Do not remove orally disintegrating tablet from blister pack until just before dosing. • Use protective measures against exposure to UV light, sunlight (sunscreen, protective clothing).

# roflumilast

roe-**floo**-mi-last
(Daliresp, Daxas ✦)

## ◆CLASSIFICATION

**PHARMACOTHERAPEUTIC:** Phosphodiesterase 4 (PDE4) inhibitor. **CLINICAL:** Anti-COPD agent.

## USES

Adjunct to bronchodilator therapy for maintenance treatment of severe COPD-associated with chronic bronchitis and history of exacerbations.

## PRECAUTIONS

**Contraindications:** Hypersensitivity to roflumilast. Moderate to severe hepatic impairment. Not indicated as bronchodilator or relief of acute bronchospasm. **Cautions:** Mild hepatic impairment, history of depression, suicidal ideation.

## ACTION

Selectively inhibits PDE4, causing an accumulation of cyclic AMP within inflammatory/structural cells necessary in pathogenesis of COPD. Produces anti-inflammatory effects. **Therapeutic Effect:** Reduces risk of exacerbation of COPD/chronic bronchitis.

## PHARMACOKINETICS

Readily absorbed after PO administration. Maximum plasma concentration: 0.5–2 hrs. Protein binding: 99%. Metabolized in liver. Primarily excreted in urine (70%). **Half-life:** 17 hrs.

## ⧗ LIFESPAN CONSIDERATIONS

**Pregnancy/Lactation:** Unknown if distributed in breast milk. Not recommended for nursing mothers. **Children:** Safety and efficacy not established. **Elderly:** No age-related precautions noted.

## INTERACTIONS

**DRUG: CYP3A4 inducers (e.g., carbamazepine, phenytoin, rifampin)** may decrease efficacy. **CYP3A4 inhibitors (e.g., erythromycin, ketoconazole)** may increase concentration. **HERBAL:** None significant. **FOOD:** None known. **LAB VALUES:** None significant.

## AVAILABILITY (Rx)

**Tablets:** 500 mcg.

## ADMINISTRATION/HANDLING

**PO**
• Give without regard to food.

## INDICATIONS/ROUTES/DOSAGE

**Adjunct in Severe COPD**
**PO: ADULTS, ELDERLY:** 500 mcg once daily.

**Dosage in Renal Impairment**
No dose adjustment.

**Dosage in Hepatic Impairment**
**Mild impairment:** No dose adjustment. **Moderate to severe impairment:** Contraindicated.

## SIDE EFFECTS

**Occasional (10%–4%):** Diarrhea, nausea, headache. **Rare (3%–2%):** Back pain, flu-like symptoms, insomnia, dizziness, decreased appetite, vomiting, abdominal pain, rhinitis, muscle spasm, tremor, dyspepsia.

## ADVERSE EFFECTS/ TOXIC REACTIONS

Psychiatric events including worsening depression, suicidal ideation, anxiety reported in less than 2%. Moderate to severe weight loss may result in discontinuation.

R

## NURSING CONSIDERATIONS

### BASELINE ASSESSMENT

Assess vital signs, O₂ saturation, lungs sounds, body weight. Question for history of depression, anxiety, suicidal ideation, dehydration, COPD, hepatic impairment. Assess plans of breastfeeding. Obtain full medication history.

### INTERVENTION/EVALUATION

Monitor vital signs, O₂ saturation, mental status, body weight. Assess for dehydration if diarrhea occurs (skin turgor, mucous membranes, decreased urine output, dizziness, dry mouth).

### PATIENT/FAMILY TEACHING

• Report changes in mood or behavior, thoughts of suicide, insomnia, anxiety. • Report any weight loss. • Increase fluid intake if dehydration suspected. • Worsening cough, fever, difficulty breathing may indicate exacerbation/infection. • Immediately report if pregnancy is suspected.

---

# rolapitant

roe-**la**-pi-tant
(Varubi)
**Do not confuse rolapitant with aprepitant, fosaprepitant.**

### ◆CLASSIFICATION

**PHARMACOTHERAPEUTIC:** Substance P/neurokinin (P/NK) receptor antagonist. **CLINICAL:** Antinausea, antiemetic.

## USES

Prevention of delayed nausea and vomiting associated with initial and repeat courses of emetogenic cancer chemotherapy, including, but not limited to, highly emetogenic chemotherapy, in combination with other antiemetic agents.

## PRECAUTIONS

**Contraindications:** Hypersensitivity to rolapitant. Concomitant use of thioridazine.

**Cautions:** Mild to moderate hepatic impairment, pts at risk for QT interval prolongation or ventricular arrhythmia (congenital long QT syndrome, medications that prolong QT interval, hypokalemia, hypomagnesemia). Not recommended in severe hepatic impairment.

## ACTION

Antagonizes human substance P/NK 1 receptors. **Therapeutic Effect:** Decreases nausea and vomiting associated with chemotherapy.

## PHARMACOKINETICS

Readily absorbed. Widely distributed. Metabolized in liver. Protein binding: greater than 99%. Peak plasma concentration: 4 hrs. Eliminated in urine (14%), feces (73%). **Half-life:** 158 hrs.

## ⧖ LIFESPAN CONSIDERATIONS

**Pregnancy/Lactation:** Unknown if distributed in breast milk. **Children:** Safety and efficacy not established. **Elderly:** No age-related precautions noted.

## INTERACTIONS

**DRUG: Thioridazine** may increase risk of torsades de pointes, QT internal prolongation (contraindicated). **Strong CYP3A inducers (e.g., rifampin)** may decrease concentration/effect. May increase concentration/effect of **BCRP substrates (e.g., methotrexate, rosuvastatin), CYP2D6 substrates (e.g., pimozide), P-gp substrates (e.g., digoxin).** **HERBAL: St. John's wort** may decrease concentration/effect. **FOOD:** None significant. **LAB VALUES:** May decrease Hct, Hgb, neutrophils, RBC.

## AVAILABILITY (Rx)

**Tablets:** 90 mg.

## ADMINISTRATION/HANDLING

### PO

• Administer approx. 1–2 hrs prior to chemotherapy. • Give without regard to meals. Administer prior to initiation of each chemotherapy cycle at no less than 2-wk intervals.

---

◆ Canadian trade name　　　　🔪 Non-Crushable Drug　　　　🈴 High Alert drug

R

## INDICATIONS/ROUTES/DOSAGE

**Chemotherapy-Associated Nausea/ Vomiting**
**PO: ADULTS, ELDERLY:** 180 mg once on day 1. Do not give at less than 2-wk intervals.

**Dosage in Renal Impairment**
**Mild to moderate impairment:** No dose adjustment. **Severe impairment:** Not specified; use caution.

**Dosage in Hepatic Impairment**
**Mild to moderate impairment:** No dose adjustment. **Severe impairment:** Treatment not recommended.

## SIDE EFFECTS

**Occasional (9%–6%):** Decreased appetite, hiccups, dizziness. **Rare (4%–3%):** Abdominal pain.

## ADVERSE EFFECTS/TOXIC REACTIONS

Torsades de pointes, QT prolongation reported in pts taking thioridazine concomitantly; avoid use. Baseline electrolyte imbalance may increase risk of arrhythmias.

### NURSING CONSIDERATIONS

**BASELINE ASSESSMENT**

Obtain CBC, BMP, serum magnesium. Question history of arrhythmias, hepatic impairment, congenital long QT syndrome. Receive mediation history and screen for interactions. Assess hydration status. Obtain EKG in pts taking concomitant drugs that prolong QT interval.

**INTERVENTION/EVALUATION**

Periodically monitor CBC, BMP. Monitor hydration, nutritional status, I&O. Correct electrolyte imbalances prior to each dose. If CYP2D6 substrate medications cannot be withheld, diligently monitor for QT interval prolongation, ventricular arrhythmias. Assist with ambulation if dizziness occurs. Assess for anemia-related symptoms.

• Therapy may alter effectiveness of other drugs. Do not take any newly prescribed medications unless approved by doctor who originally started treatment. • Report symptoms of arrhythmias such as chest pain, dizziness, fainting, fatigue, palpitations, shortness of breath. • Do not take herbal products or ingest grapefruit products. • Report persistent nausea, vomiting despite treatment.

## *romiDEPsin

roe-mi-**dep**-sin
(Istodax)
**Do not confuse romidepsin with romiplostim.**

### ◆CLASSIFICATION

**PHARMACOTHERAPEUTIC:** Histone deacetylase inhibitor. **CLINICAL:** Antineoplastic.

## USES

Treatment of refractory cutaneous T-cell lymphoma (CTCL) or refractory peripheral T-cell lymphoma (PTCL).

## PRECAUTIONS

**Contraindications:** Hypersensitivity to romidepsin. **Cautions:** Moderate or severe hepatic impairment, end-stage renal impairment, preexisting cardiac disease, pts with QT interval prolongation, concomitant administration of medications prolonging QT interval, hypokalemia, hypomagnesemia. Avoid concomitant strong CYP3A4 inhibitors/inducers; caution with moderate CYP3A4 inhibitors or P-glycoprotein inhibitors.

## ACTION

Inhibits histone deacetylase resulting in acetyl group accumulation, which alters chromatin structure, terminating cell growth. **Therapeutic Effect:** Induces cell cycle arrest, cell death.

---

## PHARMACOKINETICS

Extensively metabolized. Protein binding: 92%–94%. **Half-life:** 3 hrs.

## ⏳ LIFESPAN CONSIDERATIONS

**Pregnancy/Lactation:** May cause fetal harm. Unknown if distributed in breast milk. **Children:** Safety and efficacy not established. **Elderly:** No age-related precautions noted.

## INTERACTIONS

**DRUG: Coumarin-derivative anticoagulants** prolong PT, INR. **Strong CYP3A4 inhibitors (e.g., clarithromycin, itraconazole, ritonavir)** may increase concentration. Potent **CYP3A4 inducers (e.g., carbamazepine, phenobarbital, rifabutin, rifampin)** may decrease concentration. **HERBAL: St. John's wort** may increase metabolism and decrease concentration. **FOOD: Grapefruit products** may increase concentration/effects. **LAB VALUES:** May decrease Hgb, Hct, WBC count, platelets, serum magnesium, calcium, potassium, sodium, albumin, phosphates. May increase serum glucose, ALT, AST, uric acid. May alter serum magnesium.

## AVAILABILITY (Rx)

**Injection, Powder for Reconstitution, 2-Vial Kit:** 10 mg.

## ADMINISTRATION/HANDLING

**Reconstitution** • Reconstitute powder with 2 ml of supplied diluent (80% propylene glycol, 20% dehydrated alcohol). • Swirl contents gently to dissolve powder. • Reconstituted solution provides 5 mg/ml. Further dilute in 500 ml 0.9% NaCl.
**Rate of Administration** • Infuse over 4 hrs.
**Storage** • Reconstituted solution is stable for at least 24 hrs at room temperature. • Solution appears clear, colorless. Discard if precipitate is present or solution is discolored.

## INDICATIONS/ROUTES/DOSAGE

**CTCL, PTCL**
**IV: ADULTS, ELDERLY:** 14 mg/m² administered over 4 hrs on days 1, 8, and 15 of a 28-day cycle. Repeat cycles every 28 days if pt continues to benefit from and tolerates therapy.

**Dose Modification for Toxicity**
*Hematologic Toxicity*
**Grade 3 or 4 neutropenia or thrombocytopenia:** Delay treatment until ANC 1,500/mm³ or more and/or platelets 75,000/mm³ less or more (or baseline); restart at 14 mg/m².
**Grade 4 neutropenia or thrombocytopenia requiring platelet transfusion:** Delay treatment until Grade 1 or better (or baseline); permanently reduce dose to 10 mg/m².
*Nonhematolic Toxicity (Excluding Alopecia)*
**Grade 2 or 3:** Delay treatment until toxicity returns to grade 1 or better (or baseline); may restart at 14 mg/m².
**Grade 4, recurrent grade 3:** Delay treatment until toxicity returns to grade 1 or better (or baseline); permanently reduce dose to 10 mg/m².
**Recurrent grade 3 or 4 toxicity (with dose reduction):** Permanently discontinue.

**Dosage in Renal Impairment**
No dose adjustment. Use caution in end-stage-renal disease.

**Dosage in Hepatic Impairment**
**Mild impairment:** No dose adjustment. **Moderate to severe impairment:** Use caution.

## SIDE EFFECTS

**Frequent (57%–23%):** Nausea, fatigue, vomiting, anorexia. **Occasional (20%–7%):** Diarrhea, fever, distorted sense of taste, constipation, hypotension, pruritus. **Rare (4%–2%):** Dermatitis, T-wave and ST-wave changes on EKG.

R

---

## ADVERSE EFFECTS/ TOXIC REACTIONS

Infection is very common (47% of pts), including sepsis, arrhythmias, acute respiratory distress syndrome, acute renal failure. Anemia occurs in 19% of pts, thrombocytopenia in 17% of pts, neutropenia in 11% of pts.

## NURSING CONSIDERATIONS

### BASELINE ASSESSMENT

Provide emotional support. Baseline CBC, BMP, LFT, PT/INR, serum magnesium, ionized calcium; capillary blood glucose; EKG should be obtained prior to therapy at baseline and routinely thereafter. Inform women of childbearing potential of risk to fetus if pregnancy occurs.

### INTERVENTION/EVALUATION

Calculate daily absolute neutrophil count (ANC). Closely monitor hematologic, chemistry parameters, EKG. Diligently monitor for fever and obtain blood cultures times 2 if occurs. Provide antiemetics to control nausea/vomiting.

### PATIENT/FAMILY TEACHING

• Diarrhea may cause dehydration, electrolyte depletion. • Do not have immunizations without physician's approval (lowers body's resistance). • Avoid contact with those who recently received live virus vaccine. • Avoid crowds, those with infection. • May reduce effectiveness of estrogen-containing contraceptives. • Report excessive nausea or vomiting, palpitations, chest pain, shortness of breath. Seek immediate medical attention if unusual bleeding occurs.

## *romiPLOStim

roe-mye-**ploe**-stim
(Nplate)
**Do not confuse romiplostim with romidepsin.**

## ◆CLASSIFICATION

**PHARMACOTHERAPEUTIC:** Recombinant fusion protein, thrombopoietin receptor agonist. **CLINICAL:** Hematologic agent.

## USES

Treatment of thrombocytopenia in pts with chronic immune (idiopathic) thrombocytopenic purpura (ITP) who have had an insufficient response to corticosteroids, immunoglobulins, or splenectomy.

## PRECAUTIONS

**Contraindications:** Hypersensitivity to romiplostim. **Cautions:** Myelodysplastic syndrome, hematologic malignancy, hepatic impairment, history of cerebrovascular disease, concurrent anticoagulants or antiplatelet medication.

## ACTION

Binds and activates thrombopoietin (TPO) receptors on hematopoietic cells. **Therapeutic Effect:** Increases platelet production.

## PHARMACOKINETICS

Concentration is dependent on dose and baseline platelet count. Peak concentration occurs in 7–50 hrs (median, 14 hrs). **Half-life:** 1–34 days (median, 3.5 days).

## ⏳ LIFESPAN CONSIDERATIONS

**Pregnancy/Lactation:** Studies suggest drug crosses placenta, is distributed in breast milk. **Children:** Safety and efficacy not established in pts younger than 18 yrs. **Elderly:** Age-related renal, hepatic, cardiac abnormalities may require dosage adjustment.

## INTERACTIONS

**DRUG: Anticoagulants (e.g., apixaban, heparin, warfarin), antiplatelets (e.g., aspirin, clopidogrel)** may increase risk of bleeding. **HERBAL:** None significant. **FOOD:** None known. **LAB VALUES:** Increases platelet count.

## AVAILABILITY (Rx)

**Injection, Powder for Reconstitution:** 250-mcg, 500-mcg single-use vial.

## ADMINISTRATION/HANDLING

**◄ALERT►** Use syringe with 0.01-ml graduations for reconstitution.

### SQ

**Reconstitution** • Reconstitute 0.72 ml Sterile Water for Injection to 250-mcg single-use vial for final concentration of 500 mcg/ml. • Reconstitute 1.2 ml Sterile Water for Injection to 500-mcg single-use vial for final concentration of 500 mcg/ml. • Gently swirl and invert vial to reconstitute; do not shake. • Dissolution takes less than 2 min. • Inject at abdomen, thigh, upper arm. • Do not inject at sites that are bruised, red, tender, or indurated. **Storage** • Refrigerate unreconstituted vial. • Reconstituted solution can be kept at room temperature or refrigerated for up to 24 hrs. • Protect reconstituted solution from light. • Do not use if discolored or particulate is present. • Discard unused portion.

## INDICATIONS/ROUTES/DOSAGE

**Thrombocytopenia**
**SQ: ADULTS, ELDERLY:** Initially, 1 mcg/kg once wkly based on actual body weight. Adjust wkly doses by increments of 1 mcg/kg to achieve platelet count 50,000/mm³ or greater and reduce risk of bleeding. **Maximum:** 10 mcg/kg wkly.

**Dosage Adjustments**

| Platelet Count | Dose |
|---|---|
| Less than 50,000/mm³ | Increase by 1 mcg/kg |
| Greater than 200,000/mm³ for 2 consecutive wks | Reduce by 1 mcg/kg |
| Greater than 400,000/mm³ | Hold dose |

**Dosage in Renal/Hepatic Impairment**
No dose adjustment.

## SIDE EFFECTS

**Frequent (35%–26%):** Headache, arthralgia. **Occasional (17%–6%):** Dizziness, insomnia, myalgia, extremity pain, abdominal pain, shoulder pain, paresthesia, dyspepsia.

## ADVERSE EFFECTS/ TOXIC REACTIONS

Reticulin fiber deposits within the bone marrow, progressing to bone marrow fibrosis may occur. Worsening thrombocytopenia may be noted. Discontinuation of therapy may result in thrombocytopenia of greater severity than baseline, increasing risk of bleeding. Thromboembolic effects may occur. Increases risk of hematologic malignancies.

## NURSING CONSIDERATIONS

### BASELINE ASSESSMENT

Establish baseline CBC with differential prior to initiation, wkly during therapy and for 2 wks following discontinuation. Assess extent of RBC, WBC abnormalities.

### INTERVENTION/EVALUATION

Monitor CBC with differential wkly during dose adjustment phase and then monthly following establishment of a stable dose.

### PATIENT/FAMILY TEACHING

• Report if bruising, bleeding occur. • Essential to receive drug therapy at scheduled times or risk of bleeding may occur.

## *rOPINIRole

roe-**pin**-i-role
(Requip, Requip XL)
**Do not confuse ropinirole with Risperdal or risperidone.**

### ◆CLASSIFICATION

**PHARMACOTHERAPEUTIC:** Dopamine agonist. **CLINICAL:** Antiparkinson agent.

## USES

Treatment of signs/symptoms of idiopathic Parkinson's disease. **Immediate-release**

R

---

only: Treatment of moderate to severe primary restless legs syndrome (RLS).

## PRECAUTIONS

**Contraindications:** Hypersensitivity to ropinirole. **Cautions:** History of orthostatic hypotension, cardiovascular or cerebrovascular disease, syncope, hallucinations (esp. in elderly), concurrent use of CNS depressants, preexisting dyskinesia, hepatic or severe renal dysfunction (endstage renal disease [ESRD]), major psychotic disorder, elderly.

## ACTION

Stimulates postsynaptic dopamine receptors in caudate putamen in the brain. **Therapeutic Effect:** Relieves signs/symptoms of Parkinson's disease.

## PHARMACOKINETICS

Rapidly absorbed after PO administration. Protein binding: 40%. Widely distributed. Extensively metabolized. Steady-state concentrations achieved within 2 days. Eliminated in urine. Unknown if removed by hemodialysis. **Half-life:** 6 hrs.

## ⌛ LIFESPAN CONSIDERATIONS

**Pregnancy/Lactation:** Distributed in breast milk. Drug activity possible in breastfeeding infant. **Children:** Safety and efficacy not established. **Elderly:** No age-related precautions noted, but hallucinations may occur more frequently.

## INTERACTIONS

**DRUG: Ciprofloxacin** may increase concentration. **Alcohol, CNS depressants (e.g., lorazepam, morphine, zolpidem)** may increase CNS depressant effects. **HERBAL: Gotu kola, kava kava, St. John's wort, valerian** may increase CNS depression. **FOOD: All foods** delay peak plasma levels by 1 hr but do not affect drug absorption. **LAB VALUES:** May increase serum alkaline phosphatase.

## AVAILABILITY (Rx)

**Tablets:** 0.25 mg, 0.5 mg, 1 mg, 2 mg, 3 mg, 4 mg, 5 mg.

**Tablets, Extended-Release:** 2 mg, 4 mg, 6 mg, 8 mg, 12 mg.

## ADMINISTRATION/HANDLING

### PO
• May give without regard to meals.
• Do not break, crush, dissolve, or divide extended-release tablets.

## INDICATIONS/ROUTES/DOSAGE

**Parkinson's Disease**
**PO (Immediate-Release): ADULTS, ELDERLY:** Initially, 0.25 mg 3 times/day based on individual pt response. Dosage should be titrated with wkly increments as noted:
**Week 1:** 0.25 mg 3 times/day; total daily dose: 0.75 mg.
**Week 2:** 0.5 mg 3 times/day; total daily dose: 1.5 mg.
**Week 3:** 0.75 mg 3 times/day; total daily dose: 2.25 mg.
**Week 4:** 1 mg 3 times/day; total daily dose: 3 mg.
After week 4, may increase dose by 1.5 mg/day on wkly basis up to dose of 9 mg/day. May then further increase by 3 mg/day on wkly basis up to total dose of 24 mg/day (ESRD: 18 mg).
**(Extended-Release):** Initially, 2 mg once daily for 1–2 wks. May increase by 2 mg/day at 1 wk or longer interval. **Maximum:** 24 mg/day. ESRD: 18 mg.

**Discontinuation Taper**
Gradually taper over 7 days as follows: Decrease frequency from 3 times/day to twice daily for 4 days, then decrease from twice daily to once daily for remaining 3 days.

**Restless Legs Syndrome**
**PO (Immediate-Release): ADULTS, ELDERLY:** 0.25 mg for days 1 and 2. May increase to 0.5 mg for days 3–7 and after 7 days to 1 mg daily. May further titrate upward in 0.5-mg increments q7days until reaching daily dose of 3 mg during week 6. Daily dose may be increased to maximum of 4 mg beginning week 7. Give all doses 1–3 hrs before bedtime. ESRD: 3 mg maximum.

R

**Dosage in Renal/Hepatic Impairment**
No dose adjustment. Use caution with severe renal impairment. Titrate cautiously in pts with hepatic impairment.

## SIDE EFFECTS

**Frequent (60%–40%):** Nausea, dizziness, extreme drowsiness. **Occasional (12%–5%):** Syncope, vomiting, fatigue, viral infection, dyspepsia, diaphoresis, asthenia (loss of strength, energy), orthostatic hypotension, abdominal discomfort, pharyngitis, abnormal vision, dry mouth, hypertension, hallucinations, confusion. **Rare (Less Than 4%):** Anorexia, peripheral edema, memory loss, rhinitis, sinusitis, palpitations, impotence.

## ADVERSE EFFECTS/ TOXIC REACTIONS

Dyskinesia, impulsive/compulsive behavior (pathologic gambling, hypersexuality, binge eating) occur rarely.

## NURSING CONSIDERATIONS

### BASELINE ASSESSMENT
**Parkinson's disease:** Assess signs/ symptoms (e.g., tremor, gait). **Restless legs syndrome:** Assess frequency of symptoms, sleep pattern.

### INTERVENTION/EVALUATION
Assess for clinical improvement, clinical reversal of symptoms (improvement of tremors of head/hands at rest, mask-like facial expression, shuffling gait, muscular rigidity). Assist with ambulation if dizziness occurs. Monitor B/P, daytime alertness.

### PATIENT/FAMILY TEACHING
• Drowsiness, dizziness may be an initial response to drug. • Postural hypotension may occur more frequently during initial therapy. Slowly go from lying to standing. • Avoid tasks that require alertness, motor skills until response to drug is established. • If nausea occurs, take medication with food. • Hallucinations may occur, more so in the elderly than in younger pts with Parkinson's disease.

• Report occurrence of falling asleep during activities of daily living, new or worsening symptoms, changes in B/P, fainting, unusual urges. • Avoid alcohol.

---

# *rosiglitazone* **HIGH ALERT**

roe-zi-**glit**-a-zone
(Avandia)
■ **BLACK BOX ALERT** ■ May cause or exacerbate heart failure.
**Do not confuse Avandia with Avalide or Avinza, or Avandaryl with Benadryl.**

## FIXED-COMBINATION(S)

**Avandamet:** rosiglitazone/metformin: 1 mg/500 mg, 2 mg/500 mg, 4 mg/500 mg, 2 mg/1 g, 4 mg/1 g. **Avandaryl:** rosiglitazone/glimepiride (an antidiabetic): 4 mg/1 mg, 4 mg/2 mg, 4 mg/4 mg.

## ◆CLASSIFICATION

**PHARMACOTHERAPEUTIC:** Thiazolidinedione. **CLINICAL:** Antidiabetic agent.

## USES

Adjunct to diet/exercise to lower serum glucose in pts with type 2 non–insulin-dependent diabetes mellitus (NIDDM). Used as monotherapy or in combination with metformin, sulfonylurea to improve glycemic control.

## PRECAUTIONS

**Contraindications:** Hypersensitivity to rosiglitazone. NYHA class III or IV HF. **Cautions:** Hepatic impairment, pre-existing macular edema or diabetic retinopathy, pts at risk for cardiovascular events, edema, anemia, premenopausal or anovulatory women.

## ACTION

Improves target-cell response to insulin without increasing pancreatic insulin secretion. Decreases hepatic glucose output, increases insulin-dependent glucose utilization in skeletal muscle. **Therapeutic Effect:** Lowers serum glucose.

## PHARMACOKINETICS

Rapidly absorbed. Protein binding: 99%. Metabolized in liver. Excreted in urine (64%), feces (23%). Not removed by hemodialysis. **Half-life:** 3–4 hrs.

## ⧗ LIFESPAN CONSIDERATIONS

**Pregnancy/Lactation:** Unknown if drug crosses placenta or is distributed in breast milk. Not recommended in pregnant or breastfeeding women. **Children:** Safety and efficacy not established. **Elderly:** No age-related precautions noted.

## INTERACTIONS

**DRUG: Rifampin** may decrease concentration/effects. **Gemfibrozil** may increase concentration, toxicity. **HERBAL: Garlic, ginger, ginseng** may cause hypoglycemia. **FOOD:** None known. **LAB VALUES:** May increase serum ALT, AST, cholesterol, HDL, LDL. May decrease Hgb, Hct.

## AVAILABILITY (Rx)

**Tablets:** 2 mg, 4 mg, 8 mg.

## ADMINISTRATION/HANDLING

**PO**
• Give without regard to meals.

## INDICATIONS/ROUTES/DOSAGE

**Note:** Do not initiate with active hepatic disease or ALT greater than 2.5 times upper limit of normal (ULN).

**Diabetes Mellitus**
**PO: ADULTS, ELDERLY:** Initially, 4 mg as single daily dose or in divided doses twice daily. May increase to 8 mg/day after 12 wks of therapy if fasting glucose level is not adequately controlled.

**Dosage in Renal/Hepatic Impairment**
No dose adjustment. Do not initiate with active hepatic disease or elevated transaminases at baseline.

## SIDE EFFECTS

**Frequent (9%):** Upper respiratory tract infection. **Occasional (4%–2%):** Headache, edema, back pain, fatigue, sinusitis, diarrhea.

## ADVERSE EFFECTS/ TOXIC REACTIONS

Hepatotoxicity occurs rarely. Increased risk of HF. May cause or worsen macular edema. May increase risk of fractures. Pts with ischemic heart disease are at high risk of MI.

## NURSING CONSIDERATIONS

### BASELINE ASSESSMENT

Obtain LFT before initiation of therapy and periodically thereafter. Ensure follow-up instruction if pt, family do not thoroughly understand diabetes management, glucose-testing technique.

### INTERVENTION/EVALUATION

Monitor Hgb, serum glucose, LFT. Assess for hypoglycemia (cool/wet skin, tremors, dizziness, anxiety, headache, tachycardia, numbness in mouth, hunger, diplopia), hyperglycemia (polyuria, polyphagia, polydipsia, nausea, vomiting, dim vision, fatigue, deep/rapid breathing). Be alert to conditions that alter glucose requirements (fever, increased activity/stress, trauma, surgical procedures).

### PATIENT/ FAMILY TEACHING

• Diabetes mellitus requires lifelong control. • Prescribed diet, exercise are principal parts of treatment; do not skip/ delay meals. • Wear medical alert identification. • Continue to adhere to dietary instructions, regular exercise program, regular testing of urine or blood glucose. • When taking combination drug therapy with a sulfonylurea or insulin, have source of glucose available to treat symptoms of low blood sugar. • Report rapid increase in weight, edema, shortness of breath, chest pain, abdominal pain, yellowing of skin/eyes.

# rosuvastatin

roe-**soo**-va-**sta**-tin
(Apo-Rosuvastatin ✦, Crestor)
**Do not confuse rosuvastatin with atorvastatin, lovastatin, nystatin, pitavastatin, or simvastatin.**

## ◆CLASSIFICATION

**PHARMACOTHERAPEUTIC:** HMG-CoA reductase inhibitor. **CLINICAL:** Antihyperlipidemic.

## USES

Adjunct to diet therapy in pts with primary hyperlipidemia and mixed dyslipidemia; to decrease elevated total, LDL cholesterol, serum triglyceride levels; increases HDL. Adjunct to diet to slow progression of atherosclerosis in pts with elevated cholesterol. Treatment of primary dysbetalipoproteinemia, homozygous familial hypercholesterolemia (FH). Treatment of pts ages 10–17 yrs with heterozygous familial hypercholesterolemia (HeFH) to reduce elevated total cholesterol, LDL cholesterol, and apolipoprotein B. Primary prevention of cardiovascular disease (risk reduction of MI, stroke, arterial revascularization) without clinically evident CAD, but with multiple risk factors.

## PRECAUTIONS

**Contraindications:** Hypersensitivity to rosuvastatin. Active hepatic disease, breastfeeding, pregnancy, unexplained, persistent elevations of hepatic enzymes. **Cautions:** Anticoagulant therapy, hepatic impairment, substantial alcohol consumption, elective major surgery, renal impairment, acute renal failure, uncontrolled hypothyroidism, elderly.

## ACTION

Interferes with cholesterol biosynthesis by inhibiting conversion of the enzyme HMG-CoA to mevalonate, a precursor to cholesterol. **Therapeutic Effect:** Decreases LDL, VLDL, plasma triglyceride levels; increases HDL concentration.

## PHARMACOKINETICS

Protein binding: 88%. Minimal hepatic metabolism. Primarily eliminated in feces. **Half-life:** 19 hrs (increased in severe renal dysfunction).

## ⌛ LIFESPAN CONSIDERATIONS

**Pregnancy/Lactation:** Contraindicated in pregnancy (suppression of cholesterol biosynthesis may cause fetal toxicity), lactation. Risk of serious adverse reactions in breastfeeding infants. **Children:** Safety and efficacy not established. **Elderly:** No age-related precautions noted.

## INTERACTIONS

**DRUG: Aluminum- and magnesium-containing antacids** may decrease concentration/effects. Increased risk of myopathy with **cyclosporine, fibrate, gemfibrozil, niacin.** May increase concentrations of **estradiol, ethinyl, norgestrel.** Enhances anticoagulant effect of **warfarin. HERBAL:** None significant. **FOOD: Red yeast rice** contains 2.4 mg **lovastatin** per 600 mg rice. **LAB VALUES:** May increase serum alkaline phosphatase, bilirubin, creatinine phosphokinase, glucose, transaminases. May produce hematuria, proteinuria.

## AVAILABILITY (Rx)

**Tablets:** 5 mg, 10 mg, 20 mg, 40 mg.

## ADMINISTRATION/HANDLING

**PO**
• Give without regard to meals. May give at any time of day.

## INDICATIONS/ROUTES/DOSAGE

**Hyperlipidemia, Dyslipidemia, Atherosclerosis, Dysbetalipoproteinemia, Primary Prevention of Cardiovascular Disease**
**PO: ADULTS, ELDERLY:** Usual starting dosage is 10 mg/day, with adjustments based on lipid levels; monitor q2–4wks

R

until desired level is achieved. Lower starting dose of 5 mg is recommended in pts of Asian ancestry. **Maximum:** 40 mg/day. Range: 5–40 mg/day.

### FH
PO: **ADULTS, ELDERLY:** Initially, 20 mg/day. **Maximum:** 40 mg/day.

### HeFH
PO: **CHILDREN 10–17 YRS:** Initially, 20 mg once daily. Range: 5–20 mg once daily. **8–9 YRS:** 5–10 mg once daily.

### Concurrent Cyclosporine Use
PO: **ADULTS, ELDERLY:** 5 mg/day maximum.

### Concurrent Gemfibrozil, Atazanavir/Ritonavir, or Lopinavir/Ritonavir Therapy
PO: **ADULTS, ELDERLY:** Initially, 5 mg/day. 10 mg/day maximum.

### Dosage in Renal Impairment (CrCl Less Than 30 ml/min)
PO: **ADULTS, ELDERLY:** 5 mg/day; do not exceed 10 mg/day.

### Dosage in Hepatic Impairment
Contraindicated in active in liver disease.

## SIDE EFFECTS

Generally well tolerated. Side effects are usually mild, transient. **Occasional (9%–3%):** Pharyngitis, headache, diarrhea, dyspepsia, nausea, depression. **Rare (less than 3%):** Myalgia, asthenia, back pain.

## ADVERSE EFFECTS/ TOXIC REACTIONS

Potential for ocular lens opacities. Hypersensitivity reaction, hepatitis, rhabdomyolysis occur rarely.

## NURSING CONSIDERATIONS

### BASELINE ASSESSMENT
Obtain dietary history, esp. fat consumption. Question for possibility of pregnancy before initiating therapy. Assess baseline lab results: serum cholesterol, triglycerides, LFT.

### INTERVENTION/EVALUATION
Monitor serum cholesterol, triglycerides for therapeutic response. Lipid levels should be monitored within 2–4 wks of initiation of therapy or change in dosage. Monitor LFT at 12 wks following initiation of therapy, at any elevation of dose, and periodically (e.g., semiannually) thereafter. Monitor CPK if myopathy is suspected. Monitor daily pattern of bowel activity, stool consistency. Assess for headache, sore throat. Be alert for myalgia, weakness.

### PATIENT/FAMILY TEACHING
• Use appropriate contraceptive measures. • Periodic lab tests are essential part of therapy. • Maintain appropriate diet (important part of treatment). • Report unexplained muscle pain, tenderness, weakness, esp. if associated with fever, malaise.

# rufinamide

rue-**fin**-a-myde
(Banzel)

◆**CLASSIFICATION**
**PHARMACOTHERAPEUTIC:** Triazole derivative. **CLINICAL:** Anticonvulsant.

## USES

Adjunctive therapy in treatment of seizures associated with Lennox-Gastaut syndrome in adults and children 1 yr and older.

## PRECAUTIONS

**Contraindications:** Hypersensitivity to rufinamide. Familial short QT syndrome. **Cautions:** Other drugs that shorten QT interval, clinical depression, pts at high risk for suicide, mild to moderate hepatic impairment (not recommended in pts with severe hepatic impairment), concurrent use with hormonal contraceptives.

## ACTION

Modulates activity of sodium channels. Prolongs inactive state of the sodium channel in cortical neurons, limits sustained repetitive firing of sodium-dependent action potential, inhibiting excitatory neurotransmitter release. **Therapeutic Effect:** Exerts anticonvulsant activity.

## PHARMACOKINETICS

Well absorbed following PO administration. Protein binding: 34%. Extensively metabolized. Eliminated primarily in urine. **Half-life:** 6–10 hrs.

## ⧖ LIFESPAN CONSIDERATIONS

**Pregnancy/Lactation:** May produce fetal skeletal abnormalities. May be distributed in breast milk. **Children:** Safety and efficacy not established in pts younger than 4 yrs. **Elderly:** Age-related renal, hepatic, or cardiac impairment may require initiation of therapy at low end of dosing range.

## INTERACTIONS

**DRUG:** May increase concentration of phenobarbital, phenytoin. May decrease concentration of carbamazepine, lamotrigine. **Valproate** may increase concentration. May decrease effects of estradiol, norethindrone. **Alcohol, CNS depressants (e.g., lorazepam, morphine, zolpidem)** may increase CNS depressant effect. **HERBAL: Evening primrose** may decrease seizure threshold. **FOOD:** None known. **LAB VALUES:** May decrease WBC count.

## AVAILABILITY (Rx)

**Oral Suspension:** 40 mg/ml. **Tablets, Film-Coated:** 200 mg, 400 mg.

## ADMINISTRATION/HANDLING

**PO**
• Give with food. • Film-coated tablets may be cut or crushed for dosing flexibility. • Shake oral suspension well before each dose; use bottle adapter and dosing syringes provided.

## INDICATIONS/ROUTES/DOSAGE

**Lennox-Gastaut Seizures**
**PO:** **ADULTS, ELDERLY:** Initially, 400–800 mg/day, given in 2 equally divided doses. Dose should be increased by 400–800 mg/day every 2 days. **Maximum:** 3,200 mg/day, administered in 2 equally divided doses. **CHILDREN 1 YR AND OLDER:** Treatment should be initiated at a daily dose of 10 mg/kg/day, given in 2 equally divided doses. Increase by 10-mg/kg increments every other day to a target dose of 45 mg/kg/day or 3,200 mg/day, whichever is less, administered in 2 equally divided doses.

**Dosage in Renal Impairment**
No dose adjustment.

**Dosage in Hepatic Impairment**
**Mild to moderate impairment:** Use caution. **Severe impairment:** Not recommended.

## SIDE EFFECTS

**CHILDREN: Frequent (27%–11%):** Headache, dizziness, fatigue, nausea, drowsiness, diplopia. **Occasional (6%–4%):** Tremor, nystagmus, blurred vision, vomiting. **Rare (3%):** Ataxia, upper abdominal pain, anxiety, constipation, dyspepsia, back pain, gait disturbance, vertigo.

**ADULTS: Frequent (17%–7%):** Lethargy, vomiting, headache, fatigue, dizziness, nausea. **Occasional (5%–4%):** Influenza, nasopharyngitis, anorexia, rash, ataxia, diplopia. **Rare (3%):** Bronchitis, sinusitis, psychomotor hyperactivity, upper abdominal pain, aggression, ear infection, inattention, pruritus.

## ADVERSE EFFECTS/ TOXIC REACTIONS

Suicidal ideation or behavior occur rarely, noted as early as 1 wk after initiation of therapy and persisting for at least 24 wks. Shortening of the QT interval (up to 20 msec), hypersensitivity reaction (rash, fever, urticaria) have been noted. Abrupt withdrawal may precipitate seizure, status epilepticus.

R

## NURSING CONSIDERATIONS

### BASELINE ASSESSMENT

Review history of seizure disorder (intensity, frequency, duration, level of consciousness). Initiate seizure precautions.

### INTERVENTION/EVALUATION

Provide safety measures as needed. Observe frequently for recurrence of seizure activity. Assess for clinical improvement (decrease in intensity, frequency of seizures). Assist with ambulation if drowsiness, lethargy occur. Question for evidence of headache.

### PATIENT/FAMILY TEACHING

• Do not abruptly withdraw medication (may precipitate seizures). • Avoid tasks that require alertness, motor skills until response to drug is established. • Strict maintenance of drug therapy is essential for seizure control. • Avoid alcohol. • Female pts of childbearing age should be informed that concurrent use of rufinamide with hormonal contraceptives may render contraceptive less effective; non-hormonal forms of contraception are recommended. • Be alert for any unusual changes in mood/behavior (may increase risk of suicidal ideation/behavior).

# ruxolitinib

rux-oh-li-ti-nib
(Jakafi)

### ◆CLASSIFICATION

**PHARMACOTHERAPEUTIC:** Kinase inhibitor. **CLINICAL:** Antineoplastic.

## USES

Treatment of intermediate or high-risk myelofibrosis, including primary myelofibrosis, post–polycythemia vera myelofibrosis, post–essential thrombocythemia myelofibrosis. Treatment of polycythemia vera.

## PRECAUTIONS

**Contraindications:** Hypersensitivity to ruxolitinib. **Cautions:** Pts at risk for developing bacterial, fungal, or viral infections, renal/hepatic impairment, concomitant use of strong CYP3A4 inhibitors, history of bradycardia, conduction disturbances, ischemic heart disease, HF.

## ACTION

Inhibits Janus-associated kinases (JAKs) JAK1 and JAK2, which mediate the signaling of cytokines and growth factor important for hematopoiesis and immune function. **Therapeutic Effect:** Reduces symptoms of myelofibrosis, including enlarged spleen.

## PHARMACOKINETICS

Rapidly absorbed after PO administration. Widely distributed. Protein binding: 97%. Metabolized in liver. Excreted in urine (74%), feces (22%). **Half-life:** 3–5 hrs.

## ⧗ LIFESPAN CONSIDERATIONS

**Pregnancy/Lactation:** Unknown if distributed in breast milk. Not recommended in nursing mothers. Must either discontinue drug or discontinue breastfeeding. **Children:** Safety and efficacy not established. **Elderly:** No age-related precautions noted.

## INTERACTIONS

**DRUG: Strong CYP3A4 inhibitors (e.g., clarithromycin, cyclosporine, HIV protease inhibitors, ketoconazole)** may increase concentration/effects. **HERBAL:** None known. **FOOD: Grapefruit products** may increase concentration. **LAB VALUES:** May decrease platelets, RBC, Hgb, Hct, WBC. May increase serum bilirubin, ALT, AST, cholesterol.

## AVAILABILITY (Rx)

**Tablets:** 5 mg, 10 mg, 15 mg, 20 mg, 25 mg.

## ADMINISTRATION/HANDLING

### PO

• Give without regard to food.

## FEEDING TUBE

• Suspend tablet in 40 ml water and stir for 10 min. • May administer suspension within 6 hrs after tablet has dispersed. • Flush with 75 ml water after administration.

## INDICATIONS/ROUTES/DOSAGE

### Myelofibrosis
**PO: ADULTS:** 20 mg twice daily if platelets greater than 200,000/mm$^3$, or 15 mg twice daily if platelets 100,000–200,000/mm$^3$, or 5 mg twice daily if platelets 50,000 to less than 100,000/mm$^3$. Dose reduction based on platelet response. **Maximum:** 25 mg twice daily.

### Polycythemia Vera
**PO: ADULTS, ELDERLY:** Initially, 10 mg bid. Doses titrated based on safety/efficacy.

### Dosage in Renal/Hepatic Impairment
Initial dose 5 mg bid.

### Dosage in Renal Impairment

| CrCl | Platelets | |
|---|---|---|
| CrCl 15–59 ml/min | Platelets 100,000–150,000/mm$^3$ | 10 mg twice daily |
| CrCl 15–59 ml/min | Platelets less than 100,000/mm$^3$ | Avoid use |
| End-stage renal disease (ESRD) on dialysis | Platelets 100,000–200,000/mm$^3$ | 15 mg after dialysis on days of dialysis |
| ESRD on dialysis | Platelets greater than 200,000/mm$^3$ | 20 mg after dialysis on days of dialysis |
| ESRD not requiring dialysis | | Avoid use |

### Dosage in Hepatic Impairment

| Hepatic impairment | Platelets 100,000–150,000/mm$^3$ | 10 mg twice daily |
|---|---|---|
| Hepatic impairment | Platelets less than 100,000/mm$^3$ | Avoid use |

## SIDE EFFECTS

**Frequent (23%–14%):** Bruising, dizziness, vertigo, labyrinthitis, headache. **Occasional (9%–7%):** Weight gain, flatulence.

## ADVERSE EFFECTS/ TOXIC REACTIONS

May cause severe thrombocytopenia (70%), anemia (96%), neutropenia (18%), which may improve with reduced dose or temporarily withholding regimen. Anemic pts may require blood transfusions. Increased risk of developing opportunistic bacterial, mycobacterial, fungal, viral infections including herpes zoster, urinary tract infection, urosepsis, renal infection, pyuria. Increased risk of bleeding disorders including ecchymosis, hematoma, injection site hematoma, periorbital hematoma, petechiae, purpura.

## NURSING CONSIDERATIONS

### BASELINE ASSESSMENT

Obtain CBC, serum chemistries, renal function, LFT, urinalysis, cholesterol level. Assess recent vaccinations status. Receive full medication history including herbal products. Question for possibility of pregnancy, renal/hepatic impairment, HIV.

### INTERVENTION/EVALUATION

Monitor CBC (every 2–4 wks until doses stabilized), serum chemistries, renal function, LFT, cholesterol. Obtain urinalysis with reflex culture for suspected UTI. Routinely assess vital signs, I&O, breath sounds, gait. Monitor temperature; be alert for fever, infectious process. Avoid IM injections, rectal temperatures, other traumas that induce bleeding. Assess skin for petechiae, hematoma, purpura.

### PATIENT/FAMILY TEACHING

• Report any new bruising/bleeding, bloody stools or urine, fever, chills, rash, painful urination, suspected infection, fatigue, shortness of breath. • Do not breastfeed. • Avoid grapefruit products. • Open skin lesions, blisters may signal herpes infection. • Blood work will be routinely monitored; if on dialysis, take only following dialysis.

R

◆ Canadian trade name    ⚑ Non-Crushable Drug    [HIGH ALERT] High Alert drug

# sacubitril-valsartan

sak-**ue**-bi-tril
(Entresto)

■ **BLACK BOX ALERT** ■ May cause fetal harm, mortality. Discontinue as soon as pregnancy detected.

## ◆CLASSIFICATION

**PHARMACOTHERAPEUTIC:** Combination of sacubitril, a neprilysin inhibitor and valsartan, an angiotensin II receptor blocker. **CLINICAL:** Reduces risk of complications in HF.

## USES

To reduce the risk of cardiovascular death and hospitalization in pts with chronic HF (NYHA class II-IV) and reduced ejection fraction.

## PRECAUTIONS

**Contraindications:** Hypersensitivity to sacubitril or valsartan; history of angioedema related to angiotensin-converting enzyme (ACE) inhibitor or angiotensin receptor blockers (ARB); concomitant use or within 36 hrs of ACE inhibitors; concomitant use of aliskiren in pts with diabetes. **Cautions:** Baseline anemia, dehydration, hypovolemia, sodium depletion; concomitant use of potassium-sparing diuretics or potassium supplements; hepatic/renal impairment, unstented bilateral/unilateral renal artery stenosis, significant aortic/mitral stenosis. Pts with orthostatic hypotension.

## ACTION

Sacubitril inhibits neprilysin, increasing peptide levels that are degraded by neprilysin (e.g., natriuretic peptides). Valsartan directly antagonizes angiotensin II receptors; blocks vasoconstrictor, aldosterone secreting effects of angiotensin II, inhibiting binding of angiotensin II to AT$_1$ receptors. **Therapeutic Effect:** Decreases risk of mortality in pts with chronic HF; produces vasodilation; decreases peripheral resistance; decreases B/P.

## PHARMACOKINETICS

Widely distributed. Sacubitril is converted by esterases; not significantly metabolized after conversion. Valsartan is minimally metabolized in liver. Protein binding (both): 94%–97%. Peak plasma concentration: sacubitril: 30 min, valsartan: 1.5 hrs. Steady-state concentration: 3 days. Elimination: sacubitril: urine (52%–68%), feces (37%–48%); valsartan: feces (86%), urine (13%). **Half-life:** sacubitril: 1.4 hrs; valsartan: 9.9 hrs.

## ⌛ LIFESPAN CONSIDERATIONS

**Pregnancy/Lactation:** Avoid pregnancy; may cause fetal harm/mortality. Unknown if distributed in breast milk. Must either discontinue drug or discontinue breastfeeding. **Children:** Safety and efficacy not established. **Elderly:** No age-related precautions noted.

## INTERACTIONS

**DRUG: ACE inhibitors (e.g., enalapril, ramipril)** may increase risk of angioedema (contraindicated). **Potassium-sparing diuretics (e.g., spironolactone)** may increase risk of hyperkalemia. **NSAIDs (e.g., ibuprofen, naproxen)** may worsen renal function. May increase concentration/effect of **lithium. HERBAL: Ginger, ginseng, licorice** may worsen hypertension. **FOOD:** None known. **LAB VALUES:** May increase serum BUN, creatinine, potassium. May decrease Hct, Hgb.

## AVAILABILITY (Rx)

**Fixed-dose Combination Tablets:** sacubitril/valsartan: 24 mg/26 mg, 49 mg/51 mg, 97 mg/103 mg.

## ADMINISTRATION/HANDLING

**PO**
- Give without regard to food.

S

## INDICATIONS/ROUTES/DOSAGE

### HF

**NOTE:** Allow a 36-hr washout period when switching from or to an ACE inhibitor. After initial dose, may double dose as tolerated q2–4wks to target dose of 97 mg/105 mg.
**PO: ADULTS, ELDERLY:** (Previously taking high dose of ACE Inhibitor or ARB): Initially, 49 mg/51 mg twice daily. (Previously taking low dose of ACE inhibitor or ARB): 24 mg/26 mg twice daily. (Not currently taking an ACE inhibitor or ARB): 24 mg/26 mg twice daily.

### Dosage in Renal Impairment

**PO: ADULTS, ELDERLY: Mild to moderate impairment:** No dose adjustment. **Severe impairment:** Initially, 24 mg/26 mg twice daily. **Maintenance:** May double each dose every 2–4 wks up to 97 mg/103 mg twice daily based on tolerability.

### Dosage in Hepatic Impairment

**PO: ADULTS, ELDERLY: Mild impairment:** No dose adjustment. **Moderate impairment:** Initially, 24 mg/26 mg twice daily. **Maintenance:** May double each dose every 2–4 wks up to 97 mg/103 mg twice daily based on tolerability. **Severe impairment:** Treatment not recommended.

## SIDE EFFECTS

**Occasional (9%):** Cough, dizziness.

## ADVERSE EFFECTS/TOXIC REACTIONS

Angioedema (less than 1% of pts), hypotension (18% of pts), orthostatic hypotension (2% of pts), impaired/decrease renal function due to inhibition of renin-angiotensin-aldosterone system (5% of pts), elevation of serum creatinine greater than 50% from baseline (1.4% of pts), renal impairment including oliguria, azotemia, acute renal failure (5% of pts), hyperkalemia (12% of pts), serum potassium elevation greater than 5.5 mEq/L (4% of pts) have occurred.

## NURSING CONSIDERATIONS

### BASELINE ASSESSMENT

Obtain baseline BMP; CBC in pts with baseline anemia. Obtain B/P, HP immediately before each dose, in addition to regular monitoring (be alert for fluctuations). Assess hydration status. Correct hydration/sodium depletion prior to initiation. Receive medication history and screen for interactions, esp. concomitant use of aliskiren, ACE inhibitors, ARBs, potassium-sparing diuretics, potassium supplements. Verify negative pregnancy status. Question history of hepatic/renal impairment, renal artery stenosis; angioedema, hypersensitivity reaction.

### INTERVENTION/EVALUATION

Monitor BMP esp. serum BUN, creatinine, potassium. Monitor for hyperkalemia, hypotension. If hypotension occurs, place pt in supine position, feet slightly elevated; consider interrupting treatment or altering dose of diuretic, antihypertensive drugs and screen for dehydration/serum sodium depletion. If pt positive for dehydration, be cautious with PO/IV administration. Overhydration may exacerbate HF. Assist with ambulation if dizziness occurs. Monitor for hypersensitivity reaction including angioedema. If angioedema occurs, interrupt treatment and institute therapy to protect airway patency.

### PATIENT/FAMILY TEACHING

• Go slowly from lying to standing. • Be cautious of fluid intake. Overhydration may lead to worsening of HF, while underhydration may lead to low blood pressure. • Report urine changes such as darkened urine, decreased output. • Immediately report allergic reactions such as difficulty breathing, itching, rash, tongue swelling; symptoms of high potassium levels such as extreme fatigue, muscle weakness, palpitations; suspected pregnancy. • Do not breastfeed. • Diuretics (water pills) may increase risk of low pressure or low potassium levels.

S

# salmeterol

sal-**met**-er-all
(Serevent Diskhaler Disk ❦,
Serevent Diskus)

■ **BLACK BOX ALERT** ■ Long-acting beta₂-adrenergic agonists may increase risk of asthma-related deaths and asthma-related hospitalizations in pediatric and adolescents. Use only as adjuvant therapy. **Do not confuse salmeterol with Solu-Medrol, or Serevent with Atrovent, Combivent, Serentil, or Sinemet.**

## FIXED-COMBINATION(S)

**Advair Diskus:** salmeterol/fluticasone (a corticosteroid): 50 mcg/100 mcg, 50 mcg/250 mcg, 50 mcg/500 mcg. **Advair HFA:** salmeterol/fluticasone (a corticosteroid): 21 mcg/45 mcg, 21 mcg/115 mcg, 21 mcg/230 mcg.

## ◆CLASSIFICATION

**PHARMACOTHERAPEUTIC:** Sympathomimetic (adrenergic agonist). **CLINICAL:** Bronchodilator.

## USES

Prevention of exercise-induced bronchospasm, bronchospasm; maintenance treatment of asthma and prevention of bronchospasm in pts with reversible obstructive airway disease including those with symptoms of nocturnal asthma. Long-term maintenance treatment of bronchospasm associated with COPD.

## PRECAUTIONS

**Contraindications:** Hypersensitivity to salmeterol. Status asthmaticus, acute episodes of asthma or COPD. Use as monotherapy in treatment of asthma without concomitant long-term asthma control medication (e.g., inhaled corticosteroids). **Cautions:** Not for acute symptoms; may cause paradoxical bronchospasm, severe asthma. Cardiovascular disorders (coronary insufficiency, arrhythmias, hypertension), seizure disorders, diabetes, hyperthyroidism, hepatic impairment, hypokalemia.

## ACTION

Stimulates beta₂-adrenergic receptors in lungs, resulting in relaxation of bronchial smooth muscle. **Therapeutic Effect:** Relieves bronchospasm, reducing airway resistance.

## PHARMACOKINETICS

| Route | Onset | Peak | Duration |
|---|---|---|---|
| Inhalation (asthma) | 30–45 min | 2–4 hrs | 12 hrs |
| Inhalation (COPD) | 2 hrs | 3.25–4.75 hrs | 12 hrs |

Low systemic absorption; acts primarily in lungs. Protein binding: 95%. Metabolized in liver. Eliminated in urine (25%), feces (60%). **Half-life:** 5.5 hrs.

## ⧖ LIFESPAN CONSIDERATIONS

**Pregnancy/Lactation:** Unknown if distributed in breast milk. **Children:** No age-related precautions in pts older than 4 yrs. **Elderly:** Lower dosages may be needed (may be more susceptible to tachycardia, tremors).

## INTERACTIONS

**DRUG:** Beta blockers (e.g., **carvedilol, metoprolol**) may reduce effect; may produce bronchospasm. **CYP3A4 inhibitors** (e.g., **ketoconazole, protease inhibitors**) may increase concentration, risk of QT prolongation. **MAOIs** (e.g., **phenelzine, selegiline**), tricyclic antidepressants (e.g., **amitriptyline, doxepin**) may increase concentration/effects (wait 14 days after stopping MAOIs, tricyclic antidepressants before starting salmeterol). **HERBAL:** None significant. **FOOD:** None known. **LAB VALUES:** May decrease serum potassium. May increase serum glucose.

## AVAILABILITY (Rx)

**Powder for Oral Inhalation:** 50 mcg/inhalation.

## ADMINISTRATION/HANDLING

**Inhalation**

• Shake container well, instruct pt to exhale completely through mouth; place mouthpiece between lips, holding inhaler upright. • Inhale deeply through mouth while fully depressing top of canister. Pt should hold breath as long as possible before exhaling slowly. • Allow at least 2 min before second dose (allows for deeper bronchial penetration). • Rinse mouth with water immediately after inhalation (prevents mouth/throat dryness).

## INDICATIONS/ROUTES/DOSAGE

**Maintenance and Prevention Therapy for Asthma**

**Inhalation:** *(Diskus):* **ADULTS, ELDERLY, CHILDREN 4 YRS AND OLDER:** 1 inhalation (50 mcg) q12h (used in combination with inhaled corticosteroids not as monotherapy).

**Prevention of Exercise-Induced Bronchospasm**

**Inhalation:** *(Diskus):* **ADULTS, ELDERLY, CHILDREN 4 YRS AND OLDER:** 1 inhalation at least 30 min before exercise. Additional doses should not be given for 12 hrs. Do not administer if already giving salmeterol twice daily.

**Maintenance Therapy for COPD**

**Inhalation:** *(Diskus):* **ADULTS, ELDERLY:** 1 inhalation (50 mcg) q12h.

**Dosage in Renal/Hepatic Impairment**

No dose adjustment.

## SIDE EFFECTS

**Frequent (28%):** Headache. **Occasional (7%–3%):** Cough, tremor, dizziness, vertigo, throat dryness/irritation, pharyngitis. **Rare (less than 3%):** Palpitations, tachycardia, nausea, heartburn, GI distress, diarrhea.

## ADVERSE EFFECTS/ TOXIC REACTIONS

May prolong QT interval (can precipitate ventricular arrhythmias). Hypokalemia, hyperglycemia may occur.

## NURSING CONSIDERATIONS

### BASELINE ASSESSMENT

Question history of cardiac disease, hepatic impairment, seizure disorder. Screen for concomitant medications known to prolong QT interval. Assess lung sounds; vital signs.

### INTERVENTION/EVALUATION

Monitor rate, depth, rhythm, type of respiration; quality/rate of pulse, B/P. Assess lungs for wheezing, rales, rhonchi. Periodically evaluate serum potassium levels.

### PATIENT/FAMILY TEACHING

• Not for relief of acute episodes. • Keep canister at room temperature (cold decreases effects). • Do not stop medication or exceed recommended dosage. • Report chest pain, dizziness. • Wait at least 1 full min before second inhalation. • Administer dose 30–60 min before exercise when used to prevent exercise-induced bronchospasm. • Avoid excessive use of caffeine derivatives (coffee, tea, colas, chocolate).

# sargramostim

sar-**gra**-moe-stim
(Leukine)
**Do not confuse Leukine with leucovoran or Leukerin.**

## ◆CLASSIFICATION

**PHARMACOTHERAPEUTIC:** Colony-stimulating factor. **CLINICAL:** Hematopoietic, antineutropenic agent.

## USES

**Acute Myelogenous Leukemia (AML: following induction chemotherapy):** Shortens time to neutrophil recovery;

reduces incidence of severe infections. **Bone Marrow Transplant (allogenic or autologous):** For graft failure, engraftment delay. **Myeloid reconstitution** following allogenic or autologous bone marrow transplant. **Peripheral stem cell transplant (allogenic or autogolous):** Mobilizes hematopoietic progenitor cells. **OFF-LABEL:** Primary prophylaxis of neutropenia; treatment of radiation-induced myelosuppression.

## PRECAUTIONS

**Contraindications:** Hypersensitivity to sargramostim. Concurrent (24 hrs preceding or following) myelosuppressive chemotherapy or radiation, pts with excessive leukemic myeloid blasts in bone marrow or peripheral blood (greater than 10%), known hypersensitivity to yeast-derived products. **Cautions:** Preexisting HF, fluid retention, cardiovascular disease, pulmonary disease (hypoxia, pulmonary infiltrates), renal/hepatic impairment.

## ACTION

Stimulates proliferation/differentiation and functional activity of eosinophils, monocytes, neutrophils, and macrophages. **Therapeutic Effect:** Assists bone marrow in making new WBCs, increases their chemotactic, antifungal, antiparasitic activity. Increases cytoneoplastic cells, activates neutrophils to inhibit tumor cell growth.

## PHARMACOKINETICS

| Route | Onset | Peak | Duration |
|---|---|---|---|
| IV (increase WBCs) | 7–14 days | N/A | 1 wk |

Detected in serum within 5 min after SQ administration. **Peak serum levels:** 1–3 hrs. **Half-life: IV:** 1 hr; **SQ:** 3 hrs.

## ⏳ LIFESPAN CONSIDERATIONS

**Pregnancy/Lactation:** Unknown if drug crosses placenta or is distributed in breast milk. **Children:** Safety and efficacy not established. **Elderly:** No age-related precautions noted.

## INTERACTIONS

**DRUG:** None significant. **HERBAL:** None significant. **FOOD:** None known. **LAB VALUES:** May increase serum ALT, AST, bilirubin, creatinine. May decrease serum albumin.

## AVAILABILITY (Rx)

**Injection, Powder for Reconstitution:** 250 mcg.

## ADMINISTRATION/HANDLING

 IV

**Reconstitution •** To 250-mcg vial, add 1 ml Sterile Water for Injection (preservative free) or Bactiostatic Water for Injection. Direct diluent to side of vial, gently swirl contents to avoid foaming; do not shake or vigorously agitate. • After reconstitution, further dilute in 25–50 ml 0.9% NaCl to a concentration of 10 mcg/ml or greater. If final concentration less than 10 mcg/ml, add 1 mg albumin/ml 0.9% NaCl to provide a final albumin concentration of 0.1% (e.g., 1 ml 5% albumin per 50 ml 0.9% NaCl).

**◀ALERT▶** Albumin is added before addition of sargramostim (prevents drug adsorption to components of drug delivery system).

**Rate of Administration •** Give each single dose over 30 min, 2 hr, 6 hr, or continuous infusion.

**Storage •** Refrigerate powder, reconstituted solution, diluted solution for injection. • Do not shake. • Reconstituted solutions are clear, colorless. • Use within 6 hrs; discard unused portions. • Use 1 dose per vial; do not reenter vial.

## 🔲 IV INCOMPATIBILITIES

Amphotericin B complex (Abelcet, AmBisome, Amphotec), ondansetron (Zofran).

## 🔲 IV COMPATIBILITIES

Dexamethasone (Decadron), diphenhydramine (Benadryl), famotidine (Pepcid), granisetron (Kytril), heparin, metoclopramide (Reglan), promethazine (Phenergan).

## INDICATIONS/ROUTES/DOSAGE

**Neutrophil Recovery Following Chemotherapy in AML**
IV Infusion: ADULTS, ELDERLY: 250 mcg/m²/day (as 4-hr infusion) starting approximately 4 days following completion of induction chemotherapy. Continue until ANC is greater than 1,500 cells/mm³ for 3 consecutive days to a maximum of 42 days.

**Myeloid Recovery Following Bone Marrow Transplant (BMT)**
IV Infusion: ADULTS, ELDERLY: Usual parenteral dosage: 250 mcg/m²/day (as 2-hr infusion). Begin 2–4 hrs after autologous bone marrow infusion and not less than 24 hrs after last dose of chemotherapy or last radiation treatment. Continue until ANC greater than 1,500 cells/mm³ for 3 consecutive days. Discontinue if blast cells appear or underlying disease progresses.

**Bone Marrow Transplant Failure, Engraftment Delay**
IV Infusion: ADULTS, ELDERLY: 250 mcg/m²/day for 14 days. Infuse over 2 hrs. May repeat after 7 days off therapy if engraftment has not occurred. A third course with 500 mcg/m²/day for 14 days may be tried if engraftment still has not occurred.

**Stem Cell Transplant, Mobilization**
IV, SQ: ADULTS: 250 mcg/m²/day IV (as 24-hr infusion) or SQ once daily. Continue same dose throughout peripheral blood progenitor cell collection. If WBC greater than 50,000/mm³, reduce dose by 50%.

**Stem Cell Transplant, Post-transplant**
IV, SQ: ADULTS, ELDERLY: 250 mcg/m²/day IV (as 24-hr infusion) or SQ once daily beginning immediately following infusion of progenitor cells. Continue until ANC greater than 1,500/mm³ for 3 consecutive days.

**Dosage in Renal/Hepatic Impairment**
No dose adjustment.

## SIDE EFFECTS

**Frequent:** GI disturbances (nausea, diarrhea, vomiting, stomatitis, anorexia, abdominal pain), arthralgia or myalgia, headache, malaise, rash, pruritus. **Occasional:** Peripheral edema, weight gain, dyspnea, asthenia, fever, leukocytosis, capillary leak syndrome (fluid retention, irritation at local injection site, peripheral edema). **Rare:** Tachycardia, arrhythmias, thrombophlebitis.

## ADVERSE EFFECTS/ TOXIC REACTIONS

Pleural/pericardial effusion occurs rarely after infusion.

## NURSING CONSIDERATIONS

### BASELINE ASSESSMENT
Obtain CBC, BMP, LFT; vital signs. Question history of cardiac/pulmonary disease, renal/hepatic impairment.

### INTERVENTION/EVALUATION
Monitor CBC with differential, serum renal/hepatic function, pulmonary function, vital signs, weight. Monitor for supraventricular arrhythmias during administration (particularly in pts with history of cardiac arrhythmias). Assess closely for dyspnea during and immediately following infusion (particularly in pts with history of lung disease). If dyspnea occurs during infusion, cut infusion rate by half. If dyspnea continues, stop infusion immediately. If neutrophil count exceeds 20,000 cells/mm³ or platelet count exceeds 500,000/mm³, stop infusion or reduce dose by half, based on clinical condition of pt. Blood counts return to normal or baseline 3–7 days after discontinuation of therapy.

### PATIENT/FAMILY TEACHING
• Report difficulty breathing, esp. during or immediately after infusion. • May increase risk of cardiac arrhythmias;

**S**

---

report dizziness, fainting, palpitations.
• Treatment may cause edema; fluid collection in the lungs or around the heart.

# *sAXagliptin

sax-a-**glip**-tin
(Onglyza)
**Do not confuse saxagliptin with sitagliptin or sumatriptan.**

### FIXED-COMBINATION(S)

**Kombiglyze XR:** saxagliptin/metformin (an antidiabetic): 2.5 mg/1,000 mg, 5 mg/500 mg, 5 mg/1,000 mg.

### ◆CLASSIFICATION

**PHARMACOTHERAPEUTIC:** DDP-4 inhibitor (gliptins). **CLINICAL:** Antidiabetic agent.

## USES

Adjunctive treatment to diet and exercise to improve glycemic control in pts with type 2 diabetes mellitus as monotherapy or in combination with other antidiabetic agents.

## PRECAUTIONS

**Contraindications:** Hypersensitivity to saxagliptin. **Cautions:** Concurrent use of other glucose-lowering agents may increase risk of hypoglycemia, moderate to severe renal impairment, end-stage renal disease requiring hemodialysis, concurrent use of strong CYP3A4 inhibitors (e.g., clarithromycin).

## ACTION

Slows the inactivation of incretin hormones by inhibiting DDP-4 enzyme. Incretin hormones increase insulin synthesis/release from pancreas and decrease glucagon secretion. **Therapeutic Effect:** Regulates glucose homeostasis.

## PHARMACOKINETICS

| Route | Onset | Peak | Duration |
|-------|-------|------|----------|
| Oral  | —     | —    | 24 hrs   |

Rapidly absorbed following PO administration. Extensively metabolized. Eliminated by both renal and hepatic pathways. **Half-life:** 2.5 hrs; metabolite, 3.1 hrs.

## 🕱 LIFESPAN CONSIDERATIONS

**Pregnancy/Lactation:** Unknown if distributed in breast milk. **Children:** Safety and efficacy not established. **Elderly:** Age-related renal impairment may require dosage adjustment.

## INTERACTIONS

**DRUG:** CYP3A4 inhibitors (e.g., clarithromycin, ketoconazole) may increase concentration. **CYP3A4 inducers (e.g., rifampin)** may decrease concentration. **HERBAL: Herbal supplements** that have hypoglycemic effects increase risk of hypoglycemia. **FOOD: Grapefruit products** may increase concentration. **LAB VALUES:** May slightly decrease WBCs, lymphocytes. May increase serum creatinine.

## AVAILABILITY (Rx)

🖋 Tablets, Film-Coated: 2.5 mg, 5 mg.

## ADMINISTRATION/HANDLING

**PO**
• May give without regard to food.
• Do not break, crush, dissolve, or divide film-coated tablets.

## INDICATIONS/ROUTES/DOSAGE

**Type 2 Diabetes Mellitus**
**PO: ADULTS OVER 18 YRS, ELDERLY:** 2.5 or 5 mg once daily. **Concurrent Strong CYP3A4 Inhibitors (e.g., ketoconazole):** 2.5 mg once daily. **Hemodialysis:** Give dose after dialysis.

**Dosage in Renal Impairment**
**Mild impairment:** No dose adjustment. **Moderate to severe impairment: CrCl**

**less than 50 ml/min:** 2.5 mg once daily.

**Dosage in Hepatic Impairment**
No dose adjustment.

### SIDE EFFECTS

**Occasional (7%):** Headache. **Rare (3%–1%):** Peripheral edema, sinusitis, abdominal pain, gastroenteritis, vomiting, rash.

### ADVERSE EFFECTS/ TOXIC REACTIONS

Lymphopenia, rash occur rarely. Upper respiratory tract infection, urinary tract infection occur in approximately 7% of pts.

## NURSING CONSIDERATIONS

### BASELINE ASSESSMENT

Check serum blood glucose before administration. Discuss lifestyle to determine extent of learning, emotional needs. Ensure follow-up instruction if pt or family does not thoroughly understand diabetes management or glucose-testing technique.

### INTERVENTION/EVALUATION

Assess for hypoglycemia (diaphoresis, tremors, dizziness, anxiety, headache, tachycardia, perioral numbness, hunger, diplopia, difficulty concentrating), hyperglycemia (polyuria, polyphagia, polydipsia, nausea, vomiting, dim vision, fatigue, deep, rapid breathing). Be alert to conditions that alter glucose requirements (fever, increased activity or stress, surgical procedures).

### PATIENT/FAMILY TEACHING

• Diabetes mellitus requires lifelong control. Prescribed diet and exercise are principal parts of treatment; do not skip or delay meals. • Continue to adhere to dietary instructions, regular exercise program, regular testing of blood glucose. • When taking combination drug therapy or when glucose demands are altered (fever, infection, trauma, stress, heavy physical activity), have a source of glucose available to treat symptoms of hypoglycemia.

# scopolamine

skoe-**pol**-a-meen
(Trans-Derm Scop, Transderm-V ♣)

### FIXED-COMBINATION(S)

**Donnatal:** scopolamine/atropine (anticholinergic)/hyoscyamine (anticholinergic)/phenobarbital (sedative): 0.0065 mg/0.0194 mg/0.1037 mg/16.2 mg.

### ◆CLASSIFICATION

**PHARMACOTHERAPEUTIC:** Anticholinergic. **CLINICAL:** Antinausea, antiemetic.

### USES

Prevention of motion sickness, postop nausea/vomiting. **OFF-LABEL:** Breakthrough treatment of nausea/vomiting associated with chemotherapy.

### PRECAUTIONS

**Contraindications:** Hypersensitivity to scopolamine. Narrow-angle glaucoma. **Cautions:** Hepatic/renal impairment, cardiac disease (hypertension, HF), seizures, psychoses, coronary artery disease, prostatic hyperplasia, urinary retention, reflux esophagitis, ulcerative colitis, hyperthyroidism, GI obstruction, hiatal hernia, elderly.

### ACTION

Competitively inhibits action of acetylcholine at muscarinic receptors. Reduces excitability of labyrinthine receptors, depressing conduction in vestibular cerebellar pathway. **Therapeutic Effect:** Prevents motion-induced nausea/vomiting.

### ⧖ LIFESPAN CONSIDERATIONS

**Pregnancy/Lactation:** Crosses placenta; unknown if distributed in breast milk. **Children:** May be more susceptible to adverse effects. **Elderly:** Dizziness, hallucinations, confusion may require dosage adjustment.

S

## INTERACTIONS

**DRUG: Anticholinergics** (e.g., dicyclomine, glycopyrrolate), **antihistamines** (e.g., diphenhydramine), **tricyclic antidepressants** (e.g., amitriptyline, doxepin) may increase anticholinergic effects. **CNS depressants** (e.g., lorazepam, morphine, zolpidem) may increase CNS depression. **HERBAL:** None significant. **FOOD: Grapefruit products** may increase concentration/effects. **LAB VALUES:** May interfere with gastric secretion test.

## AVAILABILITY (Rx)

**Transdermal System (Trans-Derm Scop):** 1.5 mg.

## ADMINISTRATION/HANDLING

**Transdermal**
• Apply patch to hairless area behind one ear. • If dislodged or on for more than 72 hrs, replace with fresh patch.

## INDICATIONS/ROUTES/DOSAGE

**Prevention of Motion Sickness**
**Transdermal: ADULTS:** One system at least 4 hrs prior to exposure (best if 12 hrs before) and q72h as needed.

**Postop Nausea/Vomiting**
**Transdermal: ADULTS, ELDERLY:** 1 system no sooner than 1 hr before surgery and removed 24 hrs after surgery.

**Dosage in Renal/Hepatic Impairment**
No dose adjustment.

## SIDE EFFECTS

**Frequent (Greater Than 15%):** Dry mouth, drowsiness, blurred vision. **Rare (5%–1%):** Dizziness, restlessness, hallucinations, confusion, difficulty urinating, rash.

## ADVERSE EFFECTS/ TOXIC REACTIONS

None known.

## NURSING CONSIDERATIONS

### BASELINE ASSESSMENT

Assess for use of other CNS depressants, drugs with anticholinergic action, history of narrow-angle glaucoma.

### INTERVENTION/EVALUATION

Monitor for dehydration. Observe for improvement of symptoms.

### PATIENT/FAMILY TEACHING

• Avoid tasks requiring alertness, motor skills until response to drug is established (may cause drowsiness, disorientation, confusion). • Use only 1 patch at a time; do not cut. • Wash hands after administration.

# secukinumab

**sek**-ue-**kin**-ue-mab
(Cosentyx, Cosentyx Sensor Pen)
**Do not confuse secukinumab with canakinumab, ranibizumab, trastuzumab, ustekinumab**

## ◆CLASSIFICATION

**PHARMACOTHERAPEUTIC:** Human interleukin-17A antagonist. **CLINICAL:** Antipsoriasis agent.

## USES

Treatment of moderate to severe plaque psoriasis in adult pts who are candidates for systemic therapy or phototherapy, active psoriatic arthritis (PsA), active ankylosing spondylitis (AS).

## PRECAUTIONS

**Contraindications:** Hypersensitivity to secukinumab. **Cautions:** Elderly, active Crohn's disease, HIV infection, concomitant immunosuppressants, conditions predisposing to infections (e.g., diabetes), hypersensitivity to latex (injector pen/prefilled syringe), preexisting or recent-onset CNS demyelinating disorders (e.g., multiple sclerosis, polyneuropathy), pts with chronic or recurrent infection or who have been exposed to tuberculosis, hematologic cytopenias. Concomitant use of live vaccine not recommended.

## ACTION

Binds to and inhibits interaction of interleukin-17A receptor, a cytokine that is involved in inflammatory and immune response. May reduce epidermal neutrophils in psoriatic plaques. **Therapeutic Effect:** Alters biologic immune response; reduces inflammation.

## PHARMACOKINETICS

Widely distributed. Degraded into small peptides and amino acids via catabolic pathway. Peak plasma concentration: 6 days. Steady state reached in 24 wks. Elimination not defined. **Half-life:** 22–31 days.

## ⧖ LIFESPAN CONSIDERATIONS

**Pregnancy/Lactation:** Unknown if distributed in breast milk. **Children:** Safety and efficacy not established. **Elderly:** No age-related precautions noted.

## INTERACTIONS

**DRUG:** May decrease efficacy/immune response of **live vaccines. HERBAL:** None significant. **FOOD:** None known. **LAB VALUES:** May significant.

## AVAILABILITY (Rx)

**Injector Pen:** 150 mg/ml solution. **Prefilled Syringe:** 150 mg/ml solution. **Injection, Lyophilized Powder:** 150-mg vials.

## ADMINISTRATION/HANDLING

### SQ

**Injector Pen/Prefilled Syringe** • Follow instructions for reconstitution and preparation according to manufacturer guidelines.
**Reconstitution (Vial)** • Inject 1 ml Sterile Water for Injection into each vial. • Gently roll vial to mix (approx. 1 min). Do not shake or agitate. • Allow vial to stand for 10 min at room temperature to allow dissolution. Foaming may occur. • Repeat

gentle rolling of vial to further mix (approx. 1 min). Do not shake or agitate. • Allow vial to stand undisturbed at room temperature for additional 5 min. • Visually inspect for particulate matter or discoloration. Solution should appear slight opalescent, colorless to slightly yellow in color. Do not use is particulates or discoloration is observed. • Final concentration will equal 150 mg/ml.
**Administration** • Insert needle subcutaneously into upper arms, outer thigh, or abdomen and inject solution. • Do not inject into areas of active skin disease or injury such as sunburns, skin rashes, inflammation, skin infections, or active psoriasis. • Rotate injection sites.
**Storage** • Refrigerate until time of use. • Allow injector pen/prefilled syringe/vial to warm to room temperature before use (15–30 min). Do not freeze.

## INDICATIONS/ROUTES/DOSAGE

**Plaque Psoriasis**
**SQ: ADULTS, ELDERLY:** 300 mg every wk for 5 wks, then 300 mg q4wks. Each 300 mg dose is given as 2 separate injections of 150 mg each.

**PsA, AS**
**Note:** With coexistent plaque psoriasis, use dose for plaque psoriasis.
**SQ: ADULTS, ELDERLY:** Initially, 150 mg at wks 0, 1, 2, 3, and 4, then q4wks or 150 mg q4wks. For PsA, may consider dose of 300 mg.

**Dosage in Renal/Hepatic Impairment**
Not studied; use caution.

## SIDE EFFECTS:

**Rare (4%–1%):** Diarrhea, urticaria, rhinorrhea.

## ADVERSE EFFECTS/TOXIC REACTIONS

May increase risk of infection including tuberculosis. Infection processes including nasopharyngitis (11% of pts), upper respiratory tract infection (2.5% of pts), mucocutaneous infection with candida

S

(1.2% of pts), rhinitis, pharyngitis, oral herpes (1% of pts) have occurred. May cause exacerbation of Crohn's disease. Hypersensitivity reactions including anaphylaxis were reported. Immunogenicity (auto-secukinumab antibodies) occurred in less than 1% of pts.

## NURSING CONSIDERATIONS

### BASELINE ASSESSMENT

Obtain baseline vital signs. Pts should be evaluated for active tuberculosis and tested for latent infection prior to initiating treatment and periodically during therapy. Induration of 5 mm or greater with tuberculin skin testing should be considered a positive test result when assessing if treatment for latent tuberculosis is necessary. Antifungal therapy should be considered for those who reside or travel to regions where mycoses are endemic. Do not initiate therapy during active infection. Question history of active Crohn's disease, hepatitis B or C virus infection, HIV infection, demyelinating disorders, cardiovascular disease; concomitant use of immunosuppressive agents.

### INTERVENTION/EVALUATION

Monitor for symptoms of tuberculosis, including those who tested negative for latent tuberculosis infection prior to initiating therapy. Interrupt or discontinue treatment if serious infection, opportunistic infection, or sepsis occurs and appropriate antimicrobial therapy. Monitor skin for disease improvement. Monitor for hypersensitivity reaction.

### PATIENT/FAMILY TEACHING

• Treatment may lower your immune system response and reduce your ability to fight infection. • Report symptoms of infection such as body aches, chills, cough, fatigue, fever. • Do not receive live vaccines. • Expect frequent tuberculosis screening. • Report travel plans to possible endemic areas. • Avoid

those with active infection. • Injector pen/prefilled syringe should not be used by pts with latex allergy. • Immediately report itching, hive, rash, swelling of the face or tongue; may indicate allergic reaction. • Treatment may cause worsening of Crohn's disease.

# selegiline

se-le-ji-leen
(Apo-Selegiline ✳, Eldepryl, Emsam, Zelapar)
■ **BLACK BOX ALERT** ■ Transdermal: Increased risk of suicidal thinking and behavior in children, adolescents, young adults 18–24 yrs with major depressive disorder, other psychiatric disorders. **Do not confuse Eldepryl with Elavil or enalapril, selegiline with Salagen, sertraline, or Stelazine, or Zelapar with Zaleplon, Zemplar, or Zyprexa.**

## ◆CLASSIFICATION

**PHARMACOTHERAPEUTIC:** MAOI. **CLINICAL:** Antiparkinson agent.

## USES

**Oral:** Adjunct to levodopa/carbidopa in treatment of Parkinson's disease. **Transdermal:** Treatment of major depressive disorder (MDD). **OFF-LABEL:** Treatment of ADHD, early Parkinson's disease.

## PRECAUTIONS

**Contraindications:** Hypersensitivity to selegiline. Concurrent use of meperidine. **Orally disintegrating tablet (additional):** Concurrent use of dextromethorphan, methadone, tramadol, oral selegiline, other MAOIs. **Transdermal (additional):** Pheochromocytoma; concurrent use of bupropion, selective serotonin reuptake inhibitors (e.g., fluoxetine), dual serotonin/norepinephrine reuptake inhibitors (e.g., duloxetine), tricyclic antidepressants, buspirone, tramadol, methadone, dextromethorphan, St. John's wort, mirtazapine, cyclobenzaprine, oral selegiline, other MAOIs, carbamazepine, oxcarbazepine. Elective surgery requiring general anesthesia, local anesthesia containing sympathomimetics; foods high in tyramine content. **Cautions:** Renal/hepatic impairment, depression, elderly, major psychiatric disorder; pts at high risk of suicide; pts at high risk of hypotension (cerebrovascular disease, cardiovascular disease, hypovolemia).

## ACTION

Irreversibly inhibits activity of monoamine oxidase type B (enzyme that breaks down dopamine), thereby increasing dopaminergic action. **Therapeutic Effect:** Relieves signs/symptoms of Parkinson's disease (tremor, akinesia, posture/equilibrium disorders, rigidity).

## PHARMACOKINETICS

| Route | Onset | Peak | Duration |
|-------|-------|------|----------|
| PO | 1 hr | — | 24–72 hrs |

Rapidly absorbed from GI tract. Crosses blood-brain barrier. Protein binding: 90%. Metabolized in liver. Primarily excreted in urine. **Half-life: PO:** 10 hrs. **Transdermal:** 18–25 hrs.

## ⌛ LIFESPAN CONSIDERATIONS

**Pregnancy/Lactation:** Unknown if drug crosses placenta or is distributed in breast milk. **Children:** Safety and efficacy not established. **Elderly:** No age-related precautions noted.

## INTERACTIONS

**DRUG: Fluoxetine, fluvoxamine, paroxetine, sertraline, venlafaxine** may cause mania, serotonin syndrome (altered mental status, restlessness, diaphoresis, diarrhea, fever). **Meperidine** may cause serotonin syndrome reaction (e.g., excitation, diaphoresis, rigidity, hypertension/hypotension, coma, death). **Tricyclic antidepressants (e.g., amitriptyline, doxepin)** may cause

diaphoresis, hypertension, syncope, altered mental status, hyperpyrexia, seizures, tremors (wait 14 days between stopping selegiline and starting tricyclic antidepressants). **HERBAL: Kava kava, SAMe, St. John's wort, valerian** may increase risk of serotonin syndrome, excessive sedation. **FOOD: Tyramine-rich foods** may produce hypertensive reactions. **LAB VALUES:** None significant.

## AVAILABILITY (Rx)

**Capsules (Eldepryl):** 5 mg. **Tablets:** 5 mg. **Tablets (Orally Disintegrating [Zelapar]):** 1.25 mg. **Transdermal (Emsam):** 6 mg/24 hrs, 9 mg/24 hrs, 12 mg/24 hrs.

## ADMINISTRATION/HANDLING

**PO**
• Give without regard to meals. • Avoid tyramine-containing foods, large quantities of caffeine-containing beverages.

**PO (Orally Disintegrating Tablets)**
• Give in morning before breakfast and without liquid. • Peel off backing with dry hands (do not push tablets through foil). • Immediately place on top of tongue, allow to disintegrate. • Avoid food, liquids for 5 min before and after taking selegiline.

**Transdermal**
• Apply to dry, intact skin on upper torso or thigh, outer surface of upper arm. • Avoid exposure to external heat source.

## INDICATIONS/ROUTES/DOSAGE

**Adjunctive Treatment of Parkinson's Disease**
**PO: ADULTS:** *(Eldepryl):* 10 mg/day in divided doses, such as 5 mg at breakfast and lunch, given concomitantly with each dose of carbidopa and levodopa. **ELDERLY:** Initially, 5 mg in the morning. May increase up to 10 mg/day. **ADULTS, ELDERLY:** *(Zelapar):* Initially, 1.25 mg daily for at least 6 wks. May increase to maximum of 2.5 mg/day.

S

**Major Depressive Disorder**
**Transdermal: ADULTS:** Initially, 6 mg/24 hrs. May increase in 3 mg/24 hrs increments at minimum of 2 wks. **Maximum:** 12 mg/24 hrs. **ELDERLY:** 6 mg/24 hrs.

**Dosage in Renal/Hepatic Impairment**
**Orally disintegrating tablet:** Not recommended in severe impairment.
**Oral:** Use caution.
**Transdermal:** No dose adjustment.

## SIDE EFFECTS

**Frequent (10%–4%):** Nausea, dizziness, light-headedness, syncope, abdominal discomfort. **Occasional (3%–2%):** Confusion, hallucinations, dry mouth, vivid dreams, dyskinesia. **Rare (1%):** Headache, myalgia, anxiety, diarrhea, insomnia.

## ADVERSE EFFECTS/ TOXIC REACTIONS

Symptoms of overdose may vary from CNS depression (sedation, apnea, cardiovascular collapse, death) to severe paradoxical reactions (hallucinations, tremor, seizures). Impaired motor coordination, (loss of balance, blepharospasm, facial grimaces, feeling of heaviness in lower extremities), depression, nightmares, delusions, overstimulation, sleep disturbance, anger, hallucinations, confusion may occur.

## NURSING CONSIDERATIONS

### BASELINE ASSESSMENT

Obtain accurate medication history, diet history. Assess current state of mental health.

### INTERVENTION/EVALUATION

Be alert to neurologic effects (headache, lethargy, mental confusion, agitation). Monitor for evidence of dyskinesia (difficulty with movement). Assess for clinical reversal of symptoms (improvement of tremors of head/hands at rest, mask-like facial expression, shuffling gait, muscular rigidity). Monitor for unusual behavior, worsening depression, suicidal ideation, especially at initiation of therapy or with changes in dosage.

### PATIENT/FAMILY TEACHING

• Tolerance to dizziness, light-headedness develops during therapy. • To reduce hypotensive effect, slowly go from lying to standing. • Avoid tasks that require alertness, motor skills until response to drug is established. • Dry mouth, drowsiness, dizziness may be an expected response to drug. • Avoid alcohol during therapy. • Coffee, tea may help reduce drowsiness. • Report worsening depression, unusual behavior, thoughts of suicide. • Avoid tyramine-rich foods.

# sertraline

ser-tra-leen
(Apo-Sertraline ✦, PMS-Sertraline ✦, Zoloft)

■ **BLACK BOX ALERT** ■ Increased risk of suicidal ideation and behavior in children, adolescents, young adults 18–24 yrs with major depressive disorder, other psychiatric disorders.

**Do not confuse sertraline with selegiline, Serentil, or Serevent, or Zoloft with Zocor.**

## ◆CLASSIFICATION

**PHARMACOTHERAPEUTIC:** Serotonin reuptake inhibitor. **CLINICAL:** Antidepressant, anxiolytic, obsessive-compulsive disorder adjunct.

## USES

Treatment of major depressive disorders, panic disorder, obsessive-compulsive disorder (OCD), post-traumatic stress disorder (PTSD), premenstrual dysphoric disorder (PMDD), social anxiety disorder. **OFF-LABEL:** Eating disorders, bulimia nervosa, generalized anxiety disorder (GAD).

## PRECAUTIONS

**Contraindications:** Hypersensitivity to sertraline. MAOI use within 14 days (concurrently or within 14 days of stopping an MAOI or sertraline). Concurrent use of oral concentrate with disulfiram. Concurrent use with pimozide; initiation in pts treated with linezolid or methylene blue. **Cautions:** Seizure disorders, hepatic impairment, pts at risk for uric acid nephropathy, elderly, pts in third trimester of pregnancy, pts at high risk for suicide, family history of bipolar disorder or mania, pts with risk factors for QT prolongation (e.g., hypokalemia, hypomagnesemia), alcoholism. Pts in whom weight loss is undesirable.

## ACTION

Blocks reuptake of the neurotransmitter serotonin at CNS neuronal presynaptic membranes, increasing availability at postsynaptic receptor sites. **Therapeutic Effect:** Relieves depression, reduces obsessive-compulsive behavior, decreases anxiety.

## PHARMACOKINETICS

Incompletely, slowly absorbed from GI tract; food increases absorption. Protein binding: 98%. Widely distributed. Metabolized in liver. Excreted in urine (45%), feces (45%). Not removed by hemodialysis. **Half-life:** 26 hrs.

## ☒ LIFESPAN CONSIDERATIONS

**Pregnancy/Lactation:** Unknown if drug crosses placenta or is distributed in breast milk. **Children:** Children and adolescents are at increased risk for suicidal ideation and behavior or worsening of depression, esp. during the first few mos of therapy. **Elderly:** No age-related precautions noted, but lower initial dosages recommended.

## INTERACTIONS

**DRUG:** May increase risk of bleeding with **aspirin, NSAIDs, warfarin.** May increase concentration, risk of toxicity of **highly protein-bound medications (e.g., digoxin, warfarin). MAOIs (e.g., phenelzine, selegiline)** may

cause neuroleptic malignant syndrome, serotonin syndrome. Concomitant use of other **serotonergic drugs** may cause serotonin syndrome. May increase concentration, toxicity of **tricyclic antidepressants (e.g., amitriptyline, doxepin). HERBAL: Gotu kola, kava kava, St. John's wort, valerian** may increase CNS depression. **St. John's wort** may increase risk of serotonin syndrome. **FOOD:** None known. **LAB VALUES:** May increase total serum cholesterol, triglycerides, ALT, AST. May decrease serum uric acid.

## AVAILABILITY (Rx)

**Oral Concentrate:** 20 mg/ml. **Tablets:** 25 mg, 50 mg, 100 mg.

## ADMINISTRATION/HANDLING

**PO**

• Give with food, milk if GI distress occurs. • Oral concentrate must be diluted before administration. Mix with 4 oz water, ginger ale, lemon/lime soda, or orange juice *only*. Give immediately after mixing.

## INDICATIONS/ROUTES/DOSAGE

**Depression**
**PO: ADULTS:** Initially, 50 mg/day. May increase by 50 mg/day at 7-day intervals up to 200 mg/day. **ELDERLY:** Initially, 25 mg/day. May increase by 25–50 mg/day at 7-day intervals up to 200 mg/day.

**Obsessive-Compulsive Disorder (OCD)**
**PO: ADULTS, CHILDREN 13–17 YRS:** Initially, 50 mg/day with morning or evening meal. May increase by 50 mg/day at 7-day intervals up to 200 mg/day. **ELDERLY, CHILDREN 6–12 YRS:** Initially, 25 mg/day. May increase by 25–50 mg/day at 7-day intervals. **Maximum:** 200 mg/day.

**Panic Disorder, Post-Traumatic Stress Disorder (PTSD), Social Anxiety Disorder (SAD)**
**PO: ADULTS, ELDERLY:** Initially, 25 mg/day. May increase by 50 mg/day at 7-day

**S**

intervals. Range: 50–200 mg/day. **Maximum:** 200 mg/day.

**Premenstrual Dysphoric Disorder (PMDD)**
**PO: ADULTS:** Initially, 50 mg/day either daily throughout menstrual cycle or limited to luteal phase of menstrual cycle. May increase up to 150 mg/day per menstrual cycle in 50-mg increments when dosing throughout menstrual cycle or 100 mg/day when dosing during luteal phase only.

**Dosage in Renal Impairment**
No dose adjustment.

**Dosage in Hepatic Impairment**
Use caution.

## SIDE EFFECTS

**Frequent (26%–12%):** Headache, nausea, diarrhea, insomnia, drowsiness, dizziness, fatigue, rash, dry mouth. **Occasional (6%–4%):** Anxiety, nervousness, agitation, tremor, dyspepsia, diaphoresis, vomiting, constipation, sexual dysfunction, visual disturbances, altered taste. **Rare (less than 3%):** Flatulence, urinary frequency, paresthesia, hot flashes, chills.

## ADVERSE EFFECTS/ TOXIC REACTIONS

Serotonin syndrome (seizures, arrhythmias, high fever), neuroleptic malignant syndrome (muscle rigidity, cognitive changes), suicidal ideation have occurred.

## NURSING CONSIDERATIONS

### BASELINE ASSESSMENT

Assess appearance, behavior, speech patterns, level of interest, mood. For pts on long-term therapy, CBC, renal function, LFT should be performed periodically.

### INTERVENTION/EVALUATION

Assess mental status for depression, suicidal ideation (esp. at beginning of therapy or change in dosage), anxiety, social function, panic attack. Monitor daily pattern of bowel activity, stool consistency. Assist with ambulation if dizziness occurs.

### PATIENT/FAMILY TEACHING

• Dry mouth may be relieved by sugarless gum, sips of water. • Report headache, fatigue, tremor, sexual dysfunction. • Avoid tasks that require alertness, motor skills until response to drug is established (may cause dizziness, drowsiness). • Take with food if nausea occurs. • Inform physician if pregnancy occurs. • Avoid alcohol. • Do not take OTC medications without consulting physician. • Report worsening of depression, suicidal ideation.

---

# sevelamer

se-**vel**-a-mer
(<u>Renagel</u>, <u>Renvela</u>)
**Do not confuse Renagel with Reglan, Regonol, or Renvela, or sevelamer with Savella.**

## ◆CLASSIFICATION

**PHARMACOTHERAPEUTIC:** Polymeric phosphate binder. **CLINICAL:** Electrolyte modifier, antihyperphosphatemia agent.

## USES

Reduction of serum phosphorus in pts with chronic renal disease on hemodialysis.

## PRECAUTIONS

**Contraindications:** Hypersensitivity to sevelamer. Bowel obstruction. **Cautions:** Dysphagia, severe GI tract motility disorders, major GI tract surgery.

## ACTION

Binds with dietary phosphorus in GI tract, allowing phosphorus to be eliminated through normal digestive process, decreasing serum phosphorus level. **Therapeutic Effect:** Decreases incidence of hypercalcemic episodes in pts receiving calcium acetate treatment.

## PHARMACOKINETICS

Not absorbed systemically. Unknown if removed by hemodialysis.

## ⧗ LIFESPAN CONSIDERATIONS

**Pregnancy/Lactation:** Not distributed in breast milk. **Children:** Safety and efficacy not established. **Elderly:** No age-related precautions noted.

## INTERACTIONS

**DRUG:** May decrease concentration/effect of **fluoroquinolones (e.g., levofloxacin)**. **HERBAL:** None significant. **FOOD:** None known. **LAB VALUES:** Expected to decrease serum phosphate.

## AVAILABILITY (Rx)

**Powder for Oral Suspension (Renvela):** 0.8 g/pack, 2.4 g/pack.

🥄 **Tablets (Renagel):** 400 mg, 800 mg. **(Renvela):** 800 mg.

## ADMINISTRATION/HANDLING

### PO

• Give with meals. • Space other medication by at least 1 hr before or 3 hrs after sevelamer. • Give tablets whole; do not break, crush, dissolve, or divide. • **Oral Suspension:** Mix 0.8 g with 30 ml water (2.4 g with 60 ml water). Stir vigorously to suspend (does not dissolve) just prior to drinking.

## INDICATIONS/ROUTES/DOSAGE

### Hyperphosphatemia

**PO: ADULTS, ELDERLY:** 800–1,600 mg with each meal, depending on severity of hyperphosphatemia (5.5–7.4 mg/dL: 800 mg 3 times/day; 7.5–8.9 mg/dL: 1,200–1,600 mg 3 times/day; 9 mg/dL or greater: 1,600 mg 3 times/day). **Maintenance:** Based on serum phosphorus concentrations. Goal range: 3.5–5.5 mg/dL.

| Serum Phosphorus Concentration | Dosage |
|---|---|
| Greater than 5.5 mg/dL | Increase by 400–800 mg per meal at 2-wk intervals |
| 3.5–5.5 mg/dL | Maintain current dosage |
| Less than 3.5 mg/dL | Decrease by 400–800 mg per meal |

**Dosage in Renal/Hepatic Impairment**
No dose adjustment.

## SIDE EFFECTS

**Frequent (20%–11%):** Infection, pain, hypotension, diarrhea, dyspepsia, nausea, vomiting. **Occasional (10%–1%):** Headache, constipation, hypertension, increased cough.

## ADVERSE EFFECTS/ TOXIC REACTIONS

Thrombosis occurs rarely.

## NURSING CONSIDERATIONS

### BASELINE ASSESSMENT

Obtain baseline chemistries, esp serum calcium, phosphate; assess for bowel obstruction.

### INTERVENTION/EVALUATION

Monitor serum phosphorus, bicarbonate, chloride, calcium.

### PATIENT/FAMILY TEACHING

• Take with meals, swallow tablets whole; do not chew, crush, dissolve, or divide tablets. • Report persistent headache, nausea, vomiting, diarrhea, hypotension.

# simeprevir

sim-**e**-pre-veer
**(Galexos ✦, Olysio)**
**Do not confuse simeprevir with sofosbuvir.**

**S**

---

✦ Canadian trade name          🥄 Non-Crushable Drug          [HIGH ALERT] High Alert drug

## ◆CLASSIFICATION

**PHARMACOTHERAPEUTIC:** Protease inhibitor. **CLINICAL:** Antiviral.

## USES

Treatment of chronic hepatitis C virus infection, in combination with sofosbuvir, for genotype 1 without cirrhosis or with compensated cirrhosis; or, in combination with peginterferon alfa and ribavirin, for genotypes 1 and 4 without cirrhosis or with compensated cirrhosis.

## PRECAUTIONS

**Contraindications:** Hypersensitivity to simeprevir. Pregnancy, male partners of pregnant women, breastfeeding, any contraindications to other antihepacivirals used in combination for treatment of chronic hepatitis C. **Cautions:** Pts of East Asian ancestry, sulfa allergy, or history of HIV, sun exposure, severe hepatic impairment. Do not use as monotherapy. Combination with ribavirin is contraindicated with pregnancy. Avoid use in combination with peginterferon and ribavirin with decompensated cirrhosis.

## ACTION

Inhibits hepatitis C virus (HCV) protease needed for cleavage of HCV-encoded polyproteins by binding to active serine protease sites. **Therapeutic Effect:** Inhibits viral replication of hepatitis C virus.

## PHARMACOKINETICS

Well absorbed after PO administration. Metabolized in liver. Protein binding: 99.9%. Peak plasma concentration: 4–6 hrs. Excreted primarily in feces via biliary route (91%). **Half-life:** 10–13 hrs.

## ⧗ LIFESPAN CONSIDERATIONS

**Pregnancy/Lactation:** Strictly avoid pregnancy. May cause birth defects or fetal demise. Women of child-bearing age must use two different forms of reliable of birth control during treatment and for at least 6 mos after discontinuation. Do not initiate therapy until negative pregnancy test confirmed.

Unknown if distributed in breast milk. Breastfeeding contraindicated. **Children:** Safety and efficacy not established. **Elderly:** No age-related precautions noted. **Race:** Pts of East Asian ancestry may have increased risk of adverse reactions due to increased drug exposure/sensitivity.

## INTERACTIONS

**DRUG:** May increase concentration/effects of **antiarrhythmics** (e.g., amiodarone, quinidine), **calcium channel blockers** (e.g., felodipine, nifedipine), **cyclosporine, digoxin, sedative/hypnotics** (e.g., midazolam, triazolam), **statins** (e.g., atorvastatin, simvastatin), **sildenafil, vardenafil.** May decrease concentration/effects of **sirolimus, tacrolimus. CYP3A4 inducers** (e.g., carbamazepine, rifampin) may decrease concentration/effects. **CYP3A4 inhibitors** (e.g., itraconazole, fluconazole, clarithromycin, ritonavir) may increase concentration/effects. **HERBAL: St. John's wort** may decrease concentration/effects. **Milk thistle (silybum marianum)** may increase concentration/effects. **FOOD:** None known. **LAB VALUES:** May increase serum alkaline phosphatase, bilirubin.

## AVAILABILITY (Rx)

🖢 **Capsules:** 150 mg.

## ADMINISTRATION/HANDLING

**PO**

• Administer with food. • Administer capsule whole; do not break, crush, or open.

## INDICATIONS/ROUTES/DOSAGE

◄**ALERT**► Must use in combination with other antihepacivirals. Not recommended as monotherapy. Dose reduction of simeprevir not recommended.

**Chronic Hepatitis C Infection (with Peginterferon Alfa and Ribavirin)**
**PO: ADULTS/ELDERLY:** 150 mg daily with food for 12 wks (with peginterferon alfa and ribavirin).

*Treatment Naïve, Prior Relapsers (Including Cirrhosis):* Extend peginterferon alfa and ribavirin therapy for additional 12 wks after completing 12-wk triple therapy (24 wks total).

*Prior Nonresponders (Including Cirrhosis):* Extend peginterferon alfa and ribavirin therapy for additional 36 wks after completing 12-wk triple therapy (48 wks total).

**Chronic Hepatitis C Infection (with Sofosbuvir)**

PO: ADULTS, ELDERLY: **(Treatment naive or treatment experienced without cirrhosis):** 150 mg daily with food for 12 wks. **(Treatment naive or treatment experienced with cirrhosis):** 150 mg daily with food for 24 wks.

**Treatment Futility**

If HCV RNA viral load greater than or equal to 25 IU/ml at wk 4, discontinue simeprevir, peginterferon alfa, and ribavirin. If HCV RNA viral load greater than or equal to 25 IU/ml at wk 12 or 24, discontinue peginterferon alfa and ribavirin (simeprevir already completed at wk 12). Discontinue therapy if serious adverse effects occur.

**Dosage in Renal Impairment**

No dose adjustment.

**Dosage in Hepatic Impairment**

Not recommended in moderate to severe impairment.

## SIDE EFFECTS

**Frequent (28%–22%):** Rash, pruritus, nausea. **Occasional (16%–12%):** Myalgia, dyspnea.

## ADVERSE EFFECTS/ TOXIC REACTIONS

Increased risk of thromboembolic events associated with peginterferon alfa. Dermatologic events/photosensitivity including generalized rash, erythema, eczema, maculopapular rash, dermatitis, skin exfoliation, rash erythematosus, urticaria, allergic dermatitis, cutaneous vasculitis, skin eruption, photodermatosis, sunburn reported. Mild to moderate dyspnea reported in 12% of pts. Pts of East Asian ancestry may have increased risk of photosensitivity.

## NURSING CONSIDERATIONS

### BASELINE ASSESSMENT

Obtain baseline vital signs, CBC, HCV-RNA level, complete metabolic panel, liver function test. Confirm hepatitis C genotype. Receive full history of home medications including herbal products. Screen for contraindications to peginterferon alfa and ribavirin. Confirm negative pregnancy test before initiating treatment. Question history of anemia, HIV, hepatitis B, liver transplantation, pulmonary disease, renal impairment. Conduct dermatologic exam, noting baseline skin characteristics, moles, lesions.

### INTERVENTION/EVALUATION

Assess vital signs routinely. Monitor CBC, HCV-RNA levels, electrolytes accordingly. Obtain urine pregnancy every mo and for 6 mos after discontinuation in female pts of childbearing age. Reinforce birth control compliance. Monitor for intrauterine device failures if applicable. Monitor international normalized ratio (INR) level if on warfarin. Monitor for bruising, dyspnea, hematuria, DVT, pulmonary embolism. Encourage nutritional intake and assess for anorexia, weight loss.

### PATIENT/FAMILY TEACHING

• Treatment must be used in combination with peginterferon, ribavirin. Inform pts of side effects/contraindications of triple-medication regimen. Periodic lab tests are an essential part of therapy.
• Report any newly prescribed medications. • Do not take herbal products.
• Women of childbearing age must use two different forms of reliable birth control during treatment and for at least 6 mos after treatment. Do not breastfeed.

S

---

Notify physician if female partner becomes pregnant. • Report difficulty breathing, weakness, dizziness, weight loss. • Avoid alcohol. • Take with meals. Do not use tanning beds. Limit sun exposure; use protective UV measures. Immediately report any changes to skin including rash, skin peeling, ulcers, or new moles/lesions.

# simvastatin
**TOP 100**

**sim**-va-sta-tin
(Apo-Simvastatin ✱, <u>Zocor</u>)
**Do not confuse simvastatin with atorvastatin, lovastatin, nystatin, pitavastatin, or pravastatin, or Zocor with Cozaar, Lipitor, Zoloft, or Zyrtec.**

## FIXED-COMBINATION(S)

**Juvisync:** simvastatin/sitagliptin (an antidiabetic agent): 10 mg/100 mg, 20 mg/100 mg, 40 mg/100 mg. **Simcor:** simvastatin/niacin (an antilipemic agent): 20 mg/500 mg, 40 mg/500 mg, 20 mg/750 mg, 20 mg/1,000 mg, 40 mg/1,000 mg. **Vytorin:** simvastatin/ezetimibe (a cholesterol absorption inhibitor): 10 mg/10 mg, 20 mg/10 mg, 40 mg/10 mg, 80 mg/10 mg.

## ◆CLASSIFICATION

**PHARMACOTHERAPEUTIC:** Hydroxymethylglutaryl-CoA (HMG-CoA) reductase inhibitor. **CLINICAL:** Antihyperlipidemic.

## USES

Secondary prevention of cardiovascular events in pts with hypercholesterolemia and coronary heart disease (CHD) or at high risk for CHD. Treatment of hyperlipidemias to reduce elevations in total serum cholesterol, LDL-C, apolipoprotein B, triglycerides, VLDL-C and increase HDL-C. Treatment of homozygous familial hypercholesterolemia. Treatment of heterozygous familial hypercholesterolemia in adolescents (10–17 yrs, females more than 1 yr postmenarche).

## PRECAUTIONS

**Contraindications:** Hypersensitivity to simvastatin. Active hepatic disease or unexplained, persistent elevations of hepatic function test results, pregnancy, breastfeeding, concurrent use of strong CYP3A4 inhibitors (e.g., clarithromycin cyclosporine, gemfibrozil). **Cautions:** History of hepatic disease, diabetes, severe renal impairment, substantial alcohol consumption. Withholding or discontinuing simvastatin may be necessary when pt is at risk for renal failure secondary to rhabdomyolysis. Concomitant use of other medications associated with myopathy.

## ACTION

Interferes with cholesterol biosynthesis by inhibiting conversion of the enzyme HMG-CoA to mevalonate. **Therapeutic Effect:** Decreases LDL, cholesterol, VLDL, triglyceride levels; increase in HDL concentration.

## PHARMACOKINETICS

Well absorbed from GI tract. Protein binding: 95%. Metabolized in liver. Excreted in feces (60%), urine (13%). Unknown if removed by hemodialysis.

| Route | Onset | Peak | Duration |
|---|---|---|---|
| PO (to reduce cholesterol) | 3 days | 14 days | N/A |

## ⧗ LIFESPAN CONSIDERATIONS

**Pregnancy/Lactation:** Contraindicated in pregnancy (suppression of cholesterol biosynthesis may cause fetal toxicity), lactation. Risk of serious adverse reactions in breastfeeding infants. **Children:** Safety and efficacy not established in children less than 10 yrs of age or in premenarcheal girls. **Elderly:** No age-related precautions noted.

S

## INTERACTIONS

**DRUG:** Cyclosporine, CYP3A4 inhibitors (e.g., ketoconazole, erythromycin), amiodarone, calcium channel blockers (e.g., diltiazem, verapamil), colchicine, fibrates, gemfibrozil, niacin, ranolazine may increase risk of acute renal failure, rhabdomyolysis. **HERBAL:** St. John's wort may decrease concentration. **FOOD:** Grapefruit products may increase concentration, toxicity. **Red yeast rice** contains 2.4 mg lovastatin per 600 mg rice. **LAB VALUES:** May increase serum creatine kinase (CK), transaminase.

## AVAILABILITY (Rx)

**Tablets:** 5 mg, 10 mg, 20 mg, 40 mg, 80 mg.

## ADMINISTRATION/HANDLING

**PO**

• Give without regard to meals. • Administer in evening for maximum efficacy.

## INDICATIONS/ROUTES/DOSAGE

**Note:** Limit 80 mg dose to pts taking simvastatin longer than 12 months without evidence of myopathy.

**Prevention of Cardiovascular Events**
**PO: ADULTS, ELDERLY:** 20–40 mg once daily. Range: 5–40 mg/day.

**Hyerlipidemias**
**PO: ADULTS, ELDERLY:** Initially, 10–20 mg once daily. (Pts with CHD or CHD risk equivalents): Initially, 40 mg/day. Range: 5–40 mg/day.

**Homozygous Familial Hypercholesterolemia**
**PO: ADULTS, ELDERLY:** 40 mg once daily in evening.

**Heterozygous Familial Hypercholesterolemia**
**PO: CHILDREN 10–17 YRS:** 10 mg once daily in evening. Range: 10–40 mg/day.

**Dosing Adjustment with Medications**
**Cyclosporine, gemfibrozil:** Do not exceed 10 mg/day. **Amiodarone, amlodipine, ranolazine:** Do not exceed 20 mg/day. **Diltiazem, verapamil:** Do not exceed 10 mg/day.

**Dosage In Renal Impairment**
**CrCl less than 30 ml/min:** Initially, 5 mg/day.

**Dosage in Hepatic Impairment**
Contraindicated with active hepatic disease.

## SIDE EFFECTS

Generally well tolerated. Side effects are usually mild and transient. **Occasional (3%–2%):** Headache, abdominal pain/cramps, constipation, upper respiratory tract infection. **Rare (less than 2%):** Diarrhea, flatulence, asthenia, nausea/vomiting, depression.

## ADVERSE EFFECTS/ TOXIC REACTIONS

Potential for ocular lens opacities. Hypersensitivity reaction, hepatitis occur rarely. Myopathy (muscle pain, tenderness, weakness with elevated serum creatine kinase [CK], sometimes taking the form of rhabdomyolysis) has occurred.

## NURSING CONSIDERATIONS

### BASELINE ASSESSMENT

Obtain dietary history, esp. fat consumption. Question for possibility of pregnancy before initiating therapy. Question for history of hypersensitivity to simvastatin. Assess baseline lab results: serum cholesterol, triglycerides, LFT.

### INTERVENTION/EVALUATION

Monitor serum cholesterol, triglyceride lab results for therapeutic response. Monitor LFT. Monitor daily pattern of bowel activity, stool consistency. Assess for headache, myopathy.

### PATIENT/FAMILY TEACHING

• Use appropriate contraceptive measures. • Periodic lab tests are essential part of therapy. • Maintain appropriate diet. Avoid grapefruit products. • Report unexplained muscle pain, tenderness, weakness.

S

# sirolimus

sir-**oh**-li-mus
(Rapamune)

■ **BLACK BOX ALERT** ■ Increased susceptibility to infection and potential for development of lymphoma. Not recommended for liver or lung transplant pts. Use only by physicians experienced in immunosuppressive therapy and management of transplant pts.

**Do not confuse Rapamune with Rapaflo, or sirolimus with everolimus, pimecrolimus, tacrolimus, or temsirolimus.**

◆**CLASSIFICATION**

**PHARMACOTHERAPEUTIC:** Immunosuppressant. **CLINICAL:** Immunosuppressant.

## USES

Prophylaxis of organ rejection in pts receiving renal transplant. Treatment of lymphangioleiomyomatosis. **OFF-LABEL:** Prophylaxis of organ rejection in heart transplant recipients. Prevention of acute graft-vs-host disease in allogenic stem cell transplantation. Treatment of refractory acute or chronic graft-vs-host disease. Rescue agent for acute and chronic organ rejection.

## PRECAUTIONS

**Contraindications:** Hypersensitivity to sirolimus. **Cautions:** Cardiovascular disease (HF, hypertension); pulmonary disease, hepatic impairment, renal impairment, hyperlipidemia, perioperative period due to increased chance of surgical complications from impaired wound and tissue healing. Concurrent use with medications that may alter renal function.

## ACTION

Inhibits T-lymphocyte activation and proliferation in response to antigenic and cytokine stimulation, and inhibits antibody production. **Therapeutic Effect:** Inhibits acute rejection of allografts and prolongs graft survival.

## PHARMACOKINETICS

Rapidly absorbed from GI tract. Protein binding: 92%. Extensively metabolized in liver. Primarily eliminated in feces (91%). **Half-life:** 57–63 hrs.

## ⧗ LIFESPAN CONSIDERATIONS

**Pregnancy/Lactation:** Unknown if drug crosses placenta or is distributed in breast milk. **Children:** Safety and efficacy not established in pts younger than 13 yrs. **Elderly:** No age-related precautions noted.

## INTERACTIONS

**DRUG:** **CYP3A4 inducers** (e.g., **carbamazepine, rifabutin, rifampin**) may decrease concentration/effects. **CYP3A4 inhibitors** (e.g., **clarithromycin, erythromycin, itraconazole, verapamil**) may increase concentration, toxicity. May increase concentration/effects of **cyclosporine. HERBAL:** **St. John's wort** may decrease concentration. **Cat's claw, echinacea** possess immunostimulant properties. **Garlic, ginger, ginseng** may increase hypoglycemia. **FOOD:** **Grapefruit products** may increase risk of myelotoxicity, nephrotoxicity. **LAB VALUES:** May increase serum ALT, AST, alkaline phosphatase, LDH, BUN, creatine phosphate, cholesterol, triglycerides, creatinine. May alter WBC, serum glucose, calcium. May decrease Hgb, Hct.

## AVAILABILITY (Rx)

**Oral Solution:** 1 mg/ml.

🖉 **Tablets:** 0.5 mg, 1 mg, 2 mg.

## ADMINISTRATION/HANDLING

• Doses should be taken 4 hrs after cyclosporine. • Take consistently with or without food. • Do not break, crush, dissolve, or divide tablets. • Mix oral solution with only water or orange juice, stir vigorously, drink immediately.

## INDICATIONS/ROUTES/DOSAGE

◀ ALERT ▶ Tablets and oral solution are not bioequivalent.

**Prevention of Organ Transplant Rejection (Low to Moderate Risk)**
PO: **ADULTS, CHILDREN 13 YRS AND OLDER WEIGHING MORE THAN 40 KG:** Loading dose: 6 mg on day 1. **Maintenance:** 2 mg/day. **ADULTS, CHILDREN 13 YRS AND OLDER WEIGHING LESS THAN 40 KG:** Loading dose: 3 mg/m² on day 1. **Maintenance:** 1 mg/m²/day.

**Prevention of Organ Transplant Rejection (High Risk)**
PO: **ADULTS:** Loading dose: Up to 15 mg on day 1. **Maintenance:** 5 mg/day. Obtain trough between 5–7 days. Continue therapy for 1 yr following transplantation. Further adjustments based on clinical status.

**Lymphangioleiomyomatosis**
PO: **ADULTS, ELDERLY:** Initially, 2 mg/day with dosage adjustment to maintain concentration between 5–15 ng/ml.

**Dosage in Renal Impairment**
No dose adjustment.

**Dosage in Hepatic Impairment**
Loading dose: No change. **Maintenance dose: Mild to moderate impairment:** Reduce dose by 33%. **Severe impairment:** Reduce dose by 50%.

## SIDE EFFECTS

**Occasional:** Hypercholesterolemia, hyperlipidemia, hypertension, rash. **High doses (5 mg/day):** Anemia, arthralgia, diarrhea, hypokalemia, thrombocytopenia. **Rare:** Peripheral edema.

## ADVERSE EFFECTS/ TOXIC REACTIONS

Hepatotoxicity occurs rarely. Skin carcinoma (including basal cell, squamous cell, melanoma) has been observed.

## NURSING CONSIDERATIONS

### BASELINE ASSESSMENT

Obtain LFT. Assess for pregnancy, lactation. Question for medication usage (esp. cyclosporine, diltiazem, ketoconazole, rifampin). Determine if pt has chickenpox, herpes zoster, malignancy, infection.

### INTERVENTION/EVALUATION

Monitor serum renal function, LFT periodically. Monitor serum cholesterol, triglycerides, platelets; Hgb.

### PATIENT/FAMILY TEACHING

• Avoid those with colds, other infections. • Avoid grapefruit products. • Avoid exposure to sunlight, artificial light sources. • Strict monitoring is essential in identifying, preventing symptoms of organ rejection. • Do not chew, crush, dissolve, or divide tablets.

---

## *SITagliptin

sit-a-**glip**-tin
(Januvia)
**Do not confuse Januvia with Enjuvia, Jantoven, or Janumet, or sitagliptin with saxagliptin or sumatriptan.**

### FIXED-COMBINATION(S)

**Janumet, Janumet XR:** sitagliptin/metformin (an antidiabetic): 50 mg/500 mg, 50 mg/1,000 mg. **Juvisync:** sitagliptin/simvastatin (an antilipidemic agent): 100 mg/10 mg, 100 mg/20 mg, 100 mg/40 mg.

### ◆ CLASSIFICATION

**PHARMACOTHERAPEUTIC:** DPP-4 inhibitors (gliptins). **CLINICAL:** Antidiabetic agent.

### USES

Adjunctive treatment to diet, exercise to improve glycemic control in pts with type 2

S

---

diabetes mellitus as monotherapy or in combination with other antidiabetic agents.

## PRECAUTIONS

**Contraindications:** Hypersensitivity to sitagliptin. **Cautions:** Type I diabetes, diabetic ketoacidosis, renal impairment, end-stage renal disease, history of pancreatitis, angioedema with other DPP-4 inhibitors. Concurrent use of other glucose-lowering agents may increase risk of hypoglycemia.

## ACTION

Inhibits DPP-4 enzyme, causing prolonged active incretin levels. Incretin regulates glucose homeostasis. **Therapeutic Effect:** Increases synthesis and release of insulin from pancreatic cells; lowers glucagon secretion from pancreas, decreases hepatic glucose production.

## PHARMACOKINETICS

| Route | Onset | Peak | Duration |
|-------|-------|------|----------|
| PO | N/A | 1–4 hrs | 24 hrs |

Rapidly absorbed. Protein binding: 38%. Eliminated in urine (87%), feces (13%). **Half-life:** 12 hrs.

## ⏳ LIFESPAN CONSIDERATIONS

**Pregnancy/Lactation:** Unknown if distributed in breast milk. **Children:** Safety and efficacy not established. **Elderly:** No age-related precautions noted.

## INTERACTIONS

**DRUG:** None known. **HERBAL:** None significant. **FOOD:** None known. **LAB VALUES:** May slightly increase WBCs, particularly neutrophil count. May increase serum creatinine.

## AVAILABILITY (Rx)

🏷 **Tablets (Film-Coated):** 25 mg, 50 mg, 100 mg.

## ADMINISTRATION/HANDLING

**PO**
• May give without regard to food.
• Do not break, crush, dissolve, or divide film-coated tablets.

## INDICATIONS/ROUTES/DOSAGE

**Type 2 Diabetes**
**PO: ADULTS OVER 18 YRS, ELDERLY:** 100 mg once daily.

**Dosage in Renal Impairment**
**Moderate impairment: CrCl equal to or greater than 30 ml/min to less than 50 ml/min:** 50 mg once daily. **Severe impairment: CrCl less than 30 ml/min: Dialysis:** 25 mg once daily.

**Dosage in Hepatic Impairment**
No dose adjustment.

## SIDE EFFECTS

**Occasional (5% and greater):** Headache, nasopharyngitis. **Rare (3%–1%):** Diarrhea, abdominal pain, nausea.

## ADVERSE EFFECTS/ TOXIC REACTIONS

Hypersensitivity reactions including angioedema, Stevens-Johnson syndrome reported. Acute pancreatitis occurs rarely.

## NURSING CONSIDERATIONS

### BASELINE ASSESSMENT

Check serum glucose concentration before administration. Assess renal function. Discuss lifestyle to determine extent of learning, emotional needs. Ensure follow-up instruction if pt, family do not thoroughly understand diabetes management, glucose-testing technique.

### INTERVENTION/EVALUATION

Monitor serum glucose, Hgb A1c, BUN, creatinine. Assess for hypoglycemia (diaphoresis, tremor, dizziness, anxiety, headache, tachycardia, perioral numbness, hunger, diplopia, difficulty concentrating),

**S**

hyperglycemia (polyuria, polyphagia, polydipsia, nausea, vomiting, dim vision, fatigue, deep, rapid breathing). Be alert to conditions that alter glucose requirements (fever, increased activity, stress, trauma, surgical procedures).

### PATIENT/FAMILY TEACHING

• Diabetes mellitus requires lifelong control. • Prescribed diet, exercise are principal part of treatment; do not skip, delay meals. • Continue to adhere to dietary instructions, regular exercise program, regular testing of serum glucose. • When taking combination drug therapy or when glucose demands are altered (fever, infection, trauma, stress, heavy physical activity), have source of glucose available to treat symptoms of hypoglycemia. • Report nausea, vomiting, anorexia, severe abdominal pain, pancreatitis.

---

# sodium bicarbonate

**soe**-dee-um bye-**kar**-boe-nate

## ◆CLASSIFICATION

**PHARMACOTHERAPEUTIC:** Alkalinizing agent. **CLINICAL:** Antacid electrolyte, urinary/systemic alkalinizer.

## USES

Management of metabolic acidosis, gastric hyperacidity. Alkalinization agent for urine; hyperkalemia treatment; management of overdose of tricyclic antidepressants and aspirin. **OFF-LABEL:** Prevention of contrast-induced nephropathy.

## PRECAUTIONS

**Contraindications:** Hypersensitivity to sodium bicarbonate. Hypernatremia, alkalosis, unknown abdominal pain, hypocalcemia, severe pulmonary edema. **Cautions:** HF, edematous states, renal insufficiency, cirrhosis.

## ACTION

Dissociates to provide bicarbonate ion. **Therapeutic Effect:** Neutralizes hydrogen ion concentration, raises blood, urinary pH.

## PHARMACOKINETICS

| Route | Onset | Peak | Duration |
|-------|-------|------|----------|
| PO | 15 min | N/A | 1–3 hrs |
| IV | Immediate | N/A | 8–10 min |

Well absorbed following PO administration, sodium bicarbonate dissociates to sodium and bicarbonate ions. With increased hydrogen ion concentrations, bicarbonate ions combine with hydrogen ions to form carbonic acid, which then dissociates to $CO_2$, which is excreted by the lungs. Plasma concentration regulated by kidney (ability to form, excrete bicarbonate).

## ⧖ LIFESPAN CONSIDERATIONS

**Pregnancy/Lactation:** May produce hypernatremia, increase tendon reflexes in neonate or fetus whose mother is administered chronically high doses. May be distributed in breast milk. **Children:** No age-related precautions noted. Do not use as antacid in pts younger than 6 yrs. **Elderly:** Age-related renal impairment may require dosage adjustment.

## INTERACTIONS

**DRUG:** May increase concentration, toxicity of **quinidine, quinine.** May decrease effects of **lithium. HERBAL:** None significant. **FOOD: Milk, other dairy products** may result in milk-alkali syndrome. **LAB VALUES:** May increase serum, urinary pH.

## AVAILABILITY

**Injection Solution (Rx):** 0.5 mEq/ml (4.2%), 1 mEq/ml (8.4%). **Tablets (OTC):** 325 mg, 650 mg.

## ADMINISTRATION/HANDLING

 **IV**

◀**ALERT**▶ For direct IV administration in neonates or infants, use 0.5 mEq/ml concentration.

**Reconstitution** • May give undiluted.
**Rate of Administration** • For IV push, give up to 1 mEq/kg over 1–3 min for cardiac arrest. • For IV infusion, do not exceed rate of infusion of 1 mEq/kg/hr. • For children younger than 2 yrs, premature infants, neonates, administer by slow infusion, up to 10 mEq/min.
**Storage** • Store at room temperature.

**PO**
• Give 1–3 hrs after meals.

### 🔲 IV INCOMPATIBILITIES

Amiodarone (Cordarone), ascorbic acid, calcium chloride, diltiazem (Cardizem), dobutamine (Dobutrex), dopamine (Intropin), hydromorphone (Dilaudid), magnesium sulfate, midazolam (Versed), norepinephrine (Levophed), ondansetron (Zofran).

### 🔲 IV COMPATIBILITIES

Dexmedetomidine (Precedex), furosemide (Lasix), heparin, insulin, lidocaine, mannitol, milrinone (Primacor), morphine, phenylephrine (Neo-Synephrine), potassium chloride, propofol (Diprivan), vancomycin (Vancocin).

### INDICATIONS/ROUTES/DOSAGE

◀ALERT▶ May give by IV push, IV infusion, or orally. Dose individualized based on severity of acidosis, laboratory values, pt age, weight, clinical conditions. Do not fully correct bicarbonate deficit during the first 24 hrs (may cause metabolic alkalosis).

**Cardiac Arrest**
◀ALERT▶ Routine use not recommended.
**IV: ADULTS, ELDERLY:** Initially, 1 mEq/kg. May repeat with 0.5 mEq/kg in 10 min one time during continued cardiopulmonary arrest. Use in postresuscitation phase is based on arterial blood pH, partial pressure of carbon dioxide in arterial blood ($PaCO_2$), base deficit calculation. **CHILDREN, INFANTS:** Initially, 0.5–1 mEq/kg. Repeat in 10 min one time, or as indicated by pt's acid-base status.

**Metabolic Acidosis (Mild to Moderate)**
**IV: ADULTS, ELDERLY, CHILDREN:** 2–5 mEq/kg over 4–8 hrs. May repeat based on acid-base status.

**Prevention of Contrast-Induced Nephropathy**
**IV Infusion: ADULTS, ELDERLY:** 154 mEq/L sodium bicarbonate in $D_5W$ solution: 3 ml/kg/hr 1 hr immediately before contrast injection, then 1 ml/kg/hr during contrast exposure and for 6 hrs after procedure.

**Metabolic Acidosis (Associated with Chronic Renal Failure)**
**PO: ADULTS, ELDERLY:** Initially, 20–36 mEq/day in divided doses. Titrate to bicarbonate level of 18–20 mEq/L. **CHILDREN:** 1–3 mEq/kg/day.

**Renal Tubular Acidosis (Distal)**
**PO: ADULTS, ELDERLY:** 0.5–2 mEq/kg/day in 4–6 divided doses. **CHILDREN:** 2–3 mEq/kg/day in divided doses.

**Renal Tubular Acidosis (Proximal)**
**PO: ADULTS, ELDERLY, CHILDREN:** 5–10 mEq/kg/day in divided doses. Maintenance dose to maintain serum bicarbonate in normal range.

**Urine Alkalinization**
**PO: ADULTS, ELDERLY:** Initially, 4 g, then 1–2 g q4h. **Maximum:** 16 g/day (8g/day in adults older than 60 yrs). **CHILDREN:** 1–10 mEq/kg/day in divided doses q4–6h.

**Antacid**
**PO: ADULTS, ELDERLY:** 300 mg–2 g 1–4 times/day.

**Hyperkalemia**
**IV: ADULTS, ELDERLY:** 50 mEq over 5 min.

### SIDE EFFECTS

**Frequent:** Abdominal distention, flatulence, belching.

---

S

## ADVERSE EFFECTS/ TOXIC REACTIONS

Excessive, chronic use may produce metabolic alkalosis (irritability, twitching, paresthesia, cyanosis, slow or shallow respirations, headache, thirst, nausea). Fluid overload results in headache, weakness, blurred vision, behavioral changes, incoordination, muscle twitching, elevated B/P, bradycardia, tachypnea, wheezing, coughing, distended neck veins. Extravasation may occur at the IV site, resulting in tissue necrosis, ulceration.

## NURSING CONSIDERATIONS

### BASELINE ASSESSMENT

Assess for signs and symptoms of acidosis, alkalosis. Do not give PO medication within 1 hr of antacids.

### INTERVENTION/EVALUATION

Monitor serum, urinary pH, $CO_2$ level, serum electrolytes, plasma bicarbonate levels. Watch for signs of metabolic alkalosis, fluid overload. Assess for clinical improvement of metabolic acidosis (relief from hyperventilation, weakness, disorientation). Monitor daily pattern of bowel activity, stool consistency. Monitor serum phosphate, calcium, uric acid levels. Assess for relief of gastric distress.

## *sodium chloride*

so-dee-um **klor**-ide
(Muro 128, Nasal Moist, Ocean, SalineX)

### ◆CLASSIFICATION

**PHARMACOTHERAPEUTIC:** Salt. **CLINICAL:** Electrolyte, isotonic volume expander, ophthalmic adjunct, bronchodilator.

## USES

**Parenteral:** Source of hydration; prevention/treatment of sodium, chloride deficiencies (hypertonic for severe deficiencies). Prevention of muscle cramps, heat prostration occurring with excessive perspiration. **Nasal:** Restores moisture, relieves dry, inflamed nasal membranes. **Ophthalmic:** Therapy in reduction of corneal edema, diagnostic aid in ophthalmoscopic exam.

## PRECAUTIONS

**Contraindications:** Hypersensitivity to sodium chloride. Fluid retention, hypernatremia, hypertonic uterus. **Cautions:** HF, renal impairment, cirrhosis, hypertension, edema. Do not use sodium chloride preserved with benzyl alcohol in neonates.

## ACTION

Sodium is a major cation of extracellular fluid. **Therapeutic Effect:** Controls water distribution, fluid and electrolyte balance, osmotic pressure of body fluids; maintains acid-base balance.

## PHARMACOKINETICS

Well absorbed from GI tract. Widely distributed. Primarily excreted in urine and, to a lesser degree, in sweat, tears, saliva.

## ⏳ LIFESPAN CONSIDERATIONS

**Children/Elderly:** No age-related precautions noted.

## INTERACTIONS

**DRUG:** May decrease effect of **lithium. HERBAL:** None significant. **FOOD:** None known. **LAB VALUES:** None significant.

## AVAILABILITY

Injection (Concentrate) **(Rx):** 23.4% (4 mEq/ml). **Injection Solution (Rx):** 0.45%, 0.9%, 3%. **Irrigation (Rx):** 0.45%, 0.9%. **Nasal Gel (Nasal Moist) (OTC):** 0.65%. **Nasal Solution (OTC):** 0.4% (SalineX), 0.65% (Nasal Moist, Ocean). **Ophthalmic Ointment (OTC [Muro 128]):** 5%. **Ophthalmic Solution (OTC [Muro 128]):** 2%, 5%.

🔖 Tablets **(OTC):** 1 g.

---

## ADMINISTRATION/HANDLING

### ⬚ IV

• Hypertonic solutions (3% or 5%) are administered via large vein; avoid infiltration; do not exceed 100 ml/hr. • Vials containing 2.5–4 mEq/ml (concentrated NaCl) must be diluted with $D_5W$ or $D_{10}W$ before administration.

### PO

• Do not crush/break enteric-coated or extended-release tablets. • Administer with full glass of water.

### Nasal

• Instruct pt to begin inhaling slowly just before releasing medication into nose. • Instruct pt to inhale slowly, then release air gently through mouth. • Continue technique for 20–30 sec.

### Ophthalmic

• Place gloved finger on lower eyelid and pull out until pocket is formed between eye and lower lid. • Place prescribed number of drops (or ¼–½ inch of ointment) into pocket. • Instruct pt to close eye gently for 1–2 min so that medication will not be squeezed out of sac. • When lower lid is released, have pt keep eye open without blinking for at least 30 sec for solution; for ointment have pt close eye, roll eyeball around to distribute medication. • When using drops, apply gentle finger pressure to lacrimal sac at inner canthus for 1 min to minimize systemic absorption.

## INDICATIONS/ROUTES/DOSAGE

◄ALERT► Dosage based on age, weight, clinical condition; fluid, electrolyte, acid-base balance status.

### Usual Parenteral Dosage

**IV: ADULTS, ELDERLY, CHILDREN:** Determined by laboratory determinations (mEq). Dosage varies widely based on clinical conditions.

### Usual Oral Dosage

**PO: ADULTS, ELDERLY:** 1–2 g 3 times/day.

### Usual Nasal Dosage

**Intranasal: ADULTS, ELDERLY, CHILDREN:** 2–3 sprays as needed.

### Usual Ophthalmic Dosage

**Ophthalmic Solution: ADULTS, ELDERLY:** Apply 1–2 drops q3–4h.
**Ophthalmic Ointment: ADULTS, ELDERLY:** Apply once daily or as directed.

## SIDE EFFECTS

**Frequent:** Facial flushing. **Occasional:** Fever; irritation, phlebitis, extravasation at injection site. **Ophthalmic:** Temporary burning, irritation.

## ADVERSE EFFECTS/ TOXIC REACTIONS

Too-rapid administration may produce peripheral edema, HF, pulmonary edema. Excessive dosage may produce hypokalemia, hypervolemia, hypernatremia.

## NURSING CONSIDERATIONS

### BASELINE ASSESSMENT

Obtain baseline serum electrolyte studies. Assess fluid balance (I&O, daily weight, lung sounds, edema).

### INTERVENTION/EVALUATION

Monitor fluid balance (I&O, daily weight, lung sounds, edema), IV site for extravasation. Monitor serum electrolytes, acid-base balance, B/P. Hypernatremia associated with edema, weight gain, elevated B/P; hyponatremia associated with muscle cramps, nausea, vomiting, dry mucous membranes.

### PATIENT/FAMILY TEACHING

• Temporary burning, irritation may occur upon instillation of eye medication. • Discontinue eye medication and report severe pain, headache, rapid change in vision (peripheral, direct), sudden appearance of floating spots, acute redness of eyes, pain on exposure to light, double vision occurs.

# sodium polystyrene sulfonate

so-dee-um pol-ee-**stye**-reen
(Kayexalate, Kionex, PMS-Sodium
Polystyrene Sulfonate ✤, SPS)
**Do not confuse Kayexalate with
Kaopectate.**

## ◆CLASSIFICATION

**PHARMACOTHERAPEUTIC:** Cation
exchange resin. **CLINICAL:** Antihyperkalemic.

## USES

Treatment of hyperkalemia.

## PRECAUTIONS

**Contraindications:** Hypersensitivity to sodium polystyrene sulfonate. Hypokalemia,
neonates with reduced GI motility, intestinal
obstruction/perforation. **Cautions:** Severe
HF, hypertension, edema. Use in premature
or low-birth-weight infants, use in children
when administering rectally. Avoid use in
pts at risk for constipation/impaction.

## ACTION

Releases sodium ions in exchange primarily for potassium ions. **Therapeutic Effect:** Moves potassium from blood into
intestine to be expelled from the body.

## PHARMACOKINETICS

Onset: 2–24 hrs. Eliminated only in feces.

## ⌛ LIFESPAN CONSIDERATIONS

**Pregnancy/Lactation:** Unknown if
drug crosses placenta or is distributed in
breast milk. **Children:** No age-related precautions noted. **Elderly:** Increased risk for
fecal impaction.

## INTERACTIONS

**DRUG:** Cation-donating antacids,
laxatives (e.g., magnesium hydroxide) may decrease effect; may cause
systemic alkalosis in pts with renal impairment. **HERBAL:** None significant.

**FOOD:** None known. **LAB VALUES:** May
decrease serum calcium, magnesium,
potassium. May increase serum sodium.

## AVAILABILITY (Rx)

**Powder for Suspension (Kayexalate, Ki-
onex):** 15 g/4 level tsp (480 g). **Suspension (SPS):** 15 g/60 ml.

## ADMINISTRATION/HANDLING

**PO**
• Shake suspension well prior to administration. • Do not mix with orange
juice. • Chilling suspension will increase palatability.

**Rectal**
• After initial cleansing enema, insert
large rubber tube into rectum well into
sigmoid colon, tape in place. • Introduce suspension (with 100 ml sorbitol)
via gravity. • Flush with 50–100 ml
fluid and clamp. • Pt must retain for
several hrs if possible. • Irrigate colon
with non–sodium-containing solution to
remove resin.

## INDICATIONS/ROUTES/DOSAGE

**Hyperkalemia**
**PO: ADULTS, ELDERLY:** 60 ml (15 g) 1–4
times/day. **CHILDREN:** 1 g/kg/dose q6h.
**Rectal: ADULTS, ELDERLY:** 30–50 g as
needed q6h. **CHILDREN:** 1 g/kg/dose q2–6h.

**Dosage in Renal/Hepatic Impairment**
No dose adjustment.

## SIDE EFFECTS

**Frequent: High dosage:** Anorexia, nausea, vomiting, constipation. **High dosage
in elderly:** Fecal impaction (severe
stomach pain with nausea/vomiting).
**Occasional:** Diarrhea, sodium retention
(decreased urination, peripheral edema,
increased weight).

## ADVERSE EFFECTS/
TOXIC REACTIONS

Potassium deficiency may occur. Early
signs of hypokalemia include confusion,
delayed thought processes, extreme

**S**

weakness, irritability, EKG changes (often associated with prolonged QT interval; widening, flattening, or inversion of T wave; prominent U waves). Hypocalcemia, manifested by abdominal/muscle cramps, occurs occasionally. Arrhythmias, severe muscle weakness may be noted.

## NURSING CONSIDERATIONS

### BASELINE ASSESSMENT

Does not rapidly correct severe hyperkalemia (may take hrs to days). Consider other measures in medical emergency (IV calcium, IV sodium bicarbonate/glucose/insulin, dialysis).

### INTERVENTION/EVALUATION

Monitor serum potassium levels frequently. Assess pt's clinical condition, EKG (valuable in determining when treatment should be discontinued). Also monitor serum magnesium, calcium levels. Monitor daily pattern of bowel activity, stool consistency (fecal impaction may occur in pts on high dosages, particularly in elderly).

## sofosbuvir

soe-**fos**-bue-veer
(Sovaldi)
**Do not confuse sofosbuvir with fosamprenavir or simeprevir.**

### FIXED-COMBINATION(S)

**Harvoni:** Sofosbuvir/ledipasvir (a hepatitis C virus NS5A inhibitor): 400 mg/90 mg.

### ◆CLASSIFICATION

**PHARMACOTHERAPEUTIC:** Nucleotide polymerase inhibitor. **CLINICAL:** Antiviral.

## USES

Treatment of chronic hepatitis C virus (HCV) infection, in combination with peginterferon alfa and/or ribavirin or simeprevir. Indicated for HCV genotype 1,

2, 3, or 4 infection, including pts with hepatocellular carcinoma that meet Milan criteria (awaiting liver transplantation), and pts with HCV/HIV-1 co-infection.

## PRECAUTIONS

**Contraindications:** Hypersensitivity to sofosbuvir. All contraindications to peginterferon alfa or ribavirin including pregnancy, male partners of pregnant women. **Cautions:** Concurrent use of potent P-glycoprotein inducers (e.g., rifampin, St. John's wort) may decrease concentration/effects. Do not use as monotherapy.

## ACTION

Inhibits viral replication of viral-infected cells. Suppresses cell proliferation by interrupting polymerase activity, resulting in chain termination. **Therapeutic Effect:** Inhibits viral replication of hepatitis C virus.

## PHARMACOKINETICS

Well absorbed after PO administration. Metabolized in liver. Protein binding: 61%–65%. Peak plasma concentration: 2–4 hrs. Excreted in urine (80%), feces (14%), expired air (2.5%). Approximately 18% of dose removed by dialysis. **Half-life:** 27 hrs.

## ⌛ LIFESPAN CONSIDERATIONS

**Pregnancy/Lactation:** Strictly avoid pregnancy. May cause birth defects or fetal demise. Women of childbearing age must use two different forms of reliable birth control during treatment and for at least 6 mos after discontinuation. Do not initiate therapy until negative pregnancy test confirmed. Unknown if distributed in breast milk. Breastfeeding contraindicated. **Children:** Safety and efficacy not established in pts younger than 18 yrs. **Elderly:** No age-related precautions noted.

## INTERACTIONS

**DRUG: P-glycoprotein inducers (e.g., rifampin)** may decrease concentration/effects. **HERBAL:** St. John's wort may decrease concentration/effects. **FOOD:** None

S

known. **LAB VALUES:** May decrease Hgb, Hct, platelets, neutrophils, leukocytes. May increase serum ALT, AST, bilirubin, creatine kinase, lipase.

## AVAILABILITY (Rx)

Tablets (Film-Coated): 400 mg.

## ADMINISTRATION/HANDLING

**PO**
• Give without regard to meals.

## INDICATIONS/ROUTES/DOSAGE

◀**ALERT**▶ Must use in combination with peginterferon alfa and/or ribavirin or simeprevir. Not recommended as monotherapy. Dose reduction of sofosbuvir not recommended.

### Chronic Hepatitis C Infection

**PO: ADULTS/ELDERLY: (Genotype 1): (with simeprevir)** 400 mg daily with food for 12 wks (without cirrhosis), for 24 wks (with cirrhosis). **(Genotype 1 or 4):** 400 mg daily with food for 12 wks (with peginterferon alfa and ribavirin). If pt ineligible to receive peginterferon alfa, may consider extending ribavirin regimen to 24 wks. If serious adverse reactions occur, consider dose reduction of peginterferon alfa and/or ribavirin. **(Genotype 2):** 400 mg daily with food for 12 wks (with ribavirin only). If serious adverse reactions occur, consider dose reduction of ribavirin. **(Genotype 3):** 400 mg daily with food for 24 wks (with ribavirin only). If serious adverse reaction occurs, consider dose reduction of ribavirin.

### Ribavirin Dose Modification for Adverse Effects

**History of Noncardiac Disease:** Reduce ribavirin dose to 600 mg/day if Hgb less than 10 g/dL. Discontinue ribavirin if Hgb less than 8.5 g/dL. **History of Stable Cardiac Disease:** Reduce ribavirin dose to 600 mg/day if Hgb decreases greater than or equal to 2 g/dL during any 4-wk treatment period. Discontinue ribavirin if Hgb less than 12 g/dL despite 4 wks at reduced dose.

### Chronic Hepatitis C with Hepatocellular Carcinoma (Awaiting Liver Transplantation)

**PO: ADULTS/ELDERLY:** 400 mg daily with food for 48 wks (with peginterferon alfa and ribavirin) or until liver transplantation occurs.

### Dosage in Renal/Hepatic Impairment
No dose adjustment.

## SIDE EFFECTS

**(With ribavirin): Frequent (38%–22%):** Fatigue, headache, nausea. **Occasional (15%–6%):** Insomnia, pruritus, irritability, diarrhea, rash, asthenia, anorexia, myalgia. **Rare (4%–2%):** Pyrexia, body aches, chills. **(With peginterferon alfa and ribavirin): Frequent (55%–29%):** Fatigue, headache, nausea, insomnia, pruritus. **Occasional (18%–14%):** Rash, anorexia, chills, body aches, diarrhea, myalgia, irritability, pyrexia. **Rare (3%):** Asthenia.

## ADVERSE EFFECTS/ TOXIC REACTIONS

Increased risk of thromboembolic events associated with peginterferon alfa. Anemia may cause discontinuation of therapy. Severe depression, suicidal ideation occurs rarely.

## NURSING CONSIDERATIONS

### BASELINE ASSESSMENT

Obtain baseline vital signs, CBC, serum CPK, complete metabolic panel, LFT, lipase level. Confirm hepatitis C virus genotype. Receive full history of home medications including herbal products. Screen for contraindications to peginterferon alfa/ribavirin. Confirm negative pregnancy test before initiating treatment for female pts of childbearing potential. Question history of anemia, pancytopenia, dialysis, hepatitis B infection, HIV infection, liver transplantation, renal impairment, pancreatitis.

### INTERVENTION/EVALUATION

Assess vital signs, O₂ saturation routinely. Monitor CBC routinely or with any dosage

S

change. Obtain monthly pregnancy tests; monitor for intrauterine device failures if applicable. Reinforce birth control compliance. Assess for anemia-related dizziness, exertional dyspnea, fatigue, weakness, syncope. Report decreases in Hgb, Hct, platelets, neutrophils. Monitor for acute infection (fever, diaphoresis, lethargy, oral mucosal changes, productive cough), bloody stools, bruising, DVT, hematuria, pulmonary embolism. Encourage nutritional intake; assess for anorexia, weight loss. Observe for signs of dyspnea or depression, suicidal ideation.

### PATIENT/FAMILY TEACHING

• Periodic lab testing is an essential part of therapy. • Treatment must be used in combination with peginterferon, ribavirin. Inform pt of side effects/contraindications of multi-medication regimen. • Report any newly prescribed medications. • Do not take herbal products. • Women of childbearing age must use two different forms of reliable birth control during treatment and for at least 6 mos after treatment. Do not breastfeed. Notify physician if female partner becomes pregnant. • May alter taste of food or decrease appetite. • Report bloody stool/urine, increased bruising, difficulty breathing, weakness, dizziness, palpitations, weight loss. • Avoid alcohol. • Report signs of depression or suicidal ideation.

# sofosbuvir/ velpatasvir

soe-**fos**-bue-vir/vel-**pat**-as-vir
(Epclusa)
**Do not confuse sofosbuvir with boceprevir, dasabuvir, fosamprenavir, or simeprevir, or velpatasvir with daclatasvir, grazoprevir, or paritaprevir.**

## ◆ CLASSIFICATION

**PHARMACOTHERAPEUTIC:** Nucleotide analog NS5B polymerase inhibitor, NS5A inhibitor. **CLINICAL:** Antiviral.

## USES

Treatment of chronic hepatitis C virus (HCV) genotype 1, 2, 3, 4, 5, or 6 infection in adults pts without cirrhosis, or with compensated cirrhosis, or in combination with ribavirin in pts with decompensated cirrhosis.

## PRECAUTIONS

**Contraindications:** Hypersensitivity to sofosbuvir, velpatasvir. Contraindication or hypersensitivity to ribavirin. **Cautions:** Anemia (when used with ribavirin), renal impairment, end-stage renal disease requiring hemodialysis, hepatic disease unrelated to HCV infection, HIV infection. Concomitant use of amiodarone (with or without beta blockers) in pts with underlying cardiac disease. Concomitant use of P-glycoprotein inducers, moderate CYP2B6 inducers, strong CYP2C8 inducers, moderate or strong CYP3A4 inducers not recommended.

## ACTION

Inhibits viral replication of viral-infected cells. Suppresses cell proliferation by interrupting RNA polymerase activity, resulting in chain termination. **Therapeutic Effect:** Inhibits viral replication of hepatitis C virus.

## PHARMACOKINETICS

Rapidly absorbed following oral administration. Widely distributed. Metabolized in liver. Protein binding: sofosbuvir: 61%–68%; velpatasvir: greater than 99.5%. Peak plasma concentration: sofosbuvir: 0.5–1 hr; velpatasvir: 3 hrs. Elimination: sofosbuvir: urine (80%), feces (14%); velpatasvir: urine (94%), feces (0.4%). **Half-life:** sofosbuvir: 0.5 hr; velpatasvir: 15 hrs.

## ⌛ LIFESPAN CONSIDERATIONS

**Pregnancy/Lactation:** When used with ribavirin, therapy is contraindicated in pregnant women and in men whose female partners are pregnant. Female and male pts of reproductive potential must use effective contraception for at least 6 mos following discontinuation (if therapy includes ribavirin). Unknown if distributed in breast milk. **Children:** Safety and efficacy not established. **Elderly:** No age-related precautions noted.

## INTERACTIONS

**DRUG: Moderate or potent inducers of CYP2B6, CYP2C8, CYP3A4, P-glycoprotein (e.g., carbamazepine, phenytoin, oxcarbazepine, rifampicin)** may decrease concentration/effect of sofosbuvir/velpatasvir. **Amiodarone (with or without beta blockers [e.g., carvedilol, metoprolol])** may significantly increase risk of symptomatic bradycardia. **HERBAL: St. John's wort** may decrease concentration/effect of sofosbuvir/velpatasvir. **FOOD:** None known. **LAB VALUES:** May increase **serum bilirubin (indirect), creatine phosphokinase (CPK), lipase.**

## AVAILABILITY (Rx)

**Tablets (Fixed-Dose):** sofosbuvir 400 mg/velpatasvir 100 mg.

## ADMINISTRATION/HANDLING

**PO**
• Give without regard to food.

## INDICATIONS/ROUTES/DOSAGE

**Hepatitis C Virus Infection**
**PO: ADULTS, ELDERLY:** 1 tablet (sofosbuvir/velpatasvir) once daily.

**Treatment Regimen and Duration**
**Pts without cirrhosis or pts with compensated cirrhosis (Child-Pugh A):** 1 tablet once daily for 12 wks.
**Pts with decompensated cirrhosis (Child-Pugh B or C):** 1 tablet once daily with ribavirin for 12 wks.

**Dosage in Renal Impairment**
**Mild to moderate impairment (CrCl greater than or equal to 30 ml/min):** No dose adjustment. **Severe impairment (CrCl less than 30 ml/min, end-stage renal disease):** Not specified; use caution.

**Dosage in Hepatic Impairment**
**Mild to severe impairment:** No dose adjustment.

## SIDE EFFECTS

**Frequent (22%–15%):** Headache, fatigue. **Occasional (9%–5%):** Nausea, asthenia, insomnia, irritability. **Rare (2%):** Rash.

## ADVERSE EFFECTS/TOXIC REACTIONS

Symptomatic bradycardia requiring pacemaker intervention was reported in pts taking amiodarone and sofosbuvir, in combination with daclatasvir or simeprevir. Cardiac arrest was reported in a pt taking amiodarone, in combination with sofosbuvir and ledipasvir. Bradycardia usually occurred within hrs to days, but may occur up 2 wks after initiation (when used with amiodarone). Pts with underlying cardiac disease or advanced hepatic disease or taking concomitant beta blockers are at an increased risk for bradycardia when used concomitantly with amiodarone. Depression reported in 1% of pts.

## NURSING CONSIDERATIONS

### BASELINE ASSESSMENT

Obtain CBC (when used with ribavirin), renal function test, LFT, HCV-RNA level; serum lipase, CPK; pregnancy test in female pts of reproductive potential. Confirm hepatitis C virus genotype. Question history renal impairment, hepatic disease unrelated to HCV infection; HIV infection or use of antiretroviral therapy. Receive full medication history and screen for interactions (esp. concomitant use of amiodarone).

### INTERVENTION/EVALUATION

Monitor serum lipase, CPK. Periodically monitor HCV-RNA level for treatment effectiveness. If unable to discontinue amiodarone, recommend in-patient cardiac monitoring for at least 48 hrs, followed by outpatient or self-monitoring of HR for at least 2 wks after initiation.

S

Cardiac monitoring is also recommended in pts who discontinue amiodarone just prior to initiation. Reinforce birth control compliance and obtain monthly pregnancy tests in female pts of reproductive potential taking concomitant ribavirin. Encourage nutritional intake.

**PATIENT/FAMILY TEACHING**

• Pts who take amiodarone during therapy may require inpatient and outpatient cardiac monitoring (and in some cases, pacemaker implantation) due to an increased risk of slow heart beats or cardiac arrest. If amiodarone cannot be interrupted or discontinued, immediately report symptoms of slow heartbeat such as chest pain, confusion, dizziness, fainting, lightheadedness, memory problems, palpitations, weakness. • Treatment may be used in combination with ribavirin. Inform pt of contraindications/adverse effects of ribavirin therapy. If therapy includes ribavirin, female pts of reproductive potential should avoid pregnancy during treatment and up to 6 mos after last dose. • Immediately report suspected pregnancy. • Do not breastfeed. • Do not take newly prescribed medications unless approved by prescriber who originally started treatment. • Do not take herbal products. • Avoid alcohol. • Maintain proper nutritional intake.

---

# solifenacin

**sol**-i-**fen**-a-sin
(VESIcare)

## ◆CLASSIFICATION

**PHARMACOTHERAPEUTIC:** Anticholinergic agent, muscarinic receptor antagonist. **CLINICAL:** Urinary antispasmodic.

## USES

Treatment of overactive bladder with symptoms of urinary incontinence, urgency, frequency.

## PRECAUTIONS

**Contraindications:** Hypersensitivity to solifenacin. GI obstruction, uncontrolled narrow-angle glaucoma, urinary retention. **Cautions:** Bladder outflow obstruction, GI obstructive disorders, decreased GI motility, controlled narrow-angle glaucoma, renal/hepatic impairment, congenital or acquired QT prolongation, concurrent medications that prolong QT interval, hypokalemia, hypomagnesemia, hot weather and/or exercise.

## ACTION

Inhibits muscarinic receptors. **Therapeutic Effect:** Decreases urinary bladder contractions, increases residual urine volume, decreases detrusor muscle pressure.

## PHARMACOKINETICS

Well absorbed. Protein binding: 98%. Metabolized in liver. Excreted in urine (69%), feces (23%). **Half-life:** 40–68 hrs.

## ⧗ LIFESPAN CONSIDERATIONS

**Pregnancy/Lactation:** Unknown if drug crosses placenta or is distributed is breast milk. **Children:** Safety and efficacy not established. **Elderly:** No age-related precautions noted.

## INTERACTIONS

**DRUG: CYP3A4 inhibitors (e.g., ketoconazole, erythromycin, azole antifungals, clarithromycin)** may increase concentration/effects. **HERBAL: St. John's wort** may decrease concentration/effects. **FOOD: Grapefruit products** may increase effects. **LAB VALUES:** None known.

## AVAILABILITY (Rx)

**Tablets:** 5 mg, 10 mg.

## ADMINISTRATION/HANDLING

**PO**

• Give without regard to food. Swallow tablets whole, with liquids.

---

## INDICATIONS/ROUTES/DOSAGE

**Overactive Bladder**
**PO: ADULTS, ELDERLY:** 5 mg/day; if tolerated, may increase to 10 mg/day.

**Dosage with CYP3A4 Inhibitors**
**Maximum:** 5 mg/day.

**Dosage in Renal/Hepatic Impairment**
**Severe renal impairment: (CrCl less than 30 ml/min) or moderate hepatic impairment:** Maximum dosage is 5 mg/day. Not recommended in severe hepatic impairment.

## SIDE EFFECTS

**Frequent (28%–13%):** Dry mouth, constipation. **Occasional (5%–3%):** Blurred vision, UTI, dyspepsia, nausea. **Rare (2%–1%):** Dizziness, dry eyes, fatigue, depression, edema, hypertension, epigastric pain, vomiting, urinary retention.

## ADVERSE EFFECTS/ TOXIC REACTIONS

Angioneurotic edema, GI obstruction occur rarely. Overdose can result in severe anticholinergic effects.

## NURSING CONSIDERATIONS

### BASELINE ASSESSMENT

Assess symptoms of overactive bladder before beginning the drug. Question history of narrow-angle glaucoma, urinary retention, GI obstruction. Screen for concomitant medications known to prolong QT interval.

### INTERVENTION/EVALUATION

Monitor I&O, anticholinergic effects, creatinine clearance. Assess for decrease in symptoms.

### PATIENT/FAMILY TEACHING

• Avoid tasks requiring alertness, motor skills until response to drug is established. • Anticholinergic side effects include constipation, urinary retention, blurred vision, heat prostration in hot environment. • Use caution during exercise, exposure to heat.

# somatropin

soe-ma-**troe**-pin
(Genotropin, Genotropin Miniquick, Humatrope, Norditropin, Nutropin, Nutropin AQ, Omnitrope, Saizen, Serostim, Zomacton, Zorbtive)
**Do not confuse somatropin with sumatriptan.**

## ◆CLASSIFICATION

**PHARMACOTHERAPEUTIC:** Polypeptide hormone. **CLINICAL:** Growth hormone.

## USES

**Adults:** Growth deficiency due to pituitary disease, hypothalamic disease, surgery, radiation, or trauma; AIDS-related wasting or cachexia. **Zorbtive:** Short bowel syndrome. **Children:** Long-term treatment of growth failure due to lack of or inadequate endogenous growth hormone secretion; chronic renal insufficiency; short stature associated with Turner's syndrome, Noonan's syndrome, or homeobox gene deficiency; idiopathic short stature. **OFF-LABEL:** Treatment of pediatric HIV pts with wasting/cachexia; HIV adipose redistribution syndrome.

## PRECAUTIONS

**Contraindications:** Hypersensitivity to growth hormone. Pts with Prader-Willi syndrome with growth hormone deficiency who are severely obese or have severe respiratory impairment, Prader-Willi syndrome without growth hormone deficiency, children with closed epiphyses, acute critical illness due to complications after open heart or abdominal surgery, multiple accidental trauma, acute respiratory failure, active neoplasia, diabetic retinopathy. Active malignancy, progression of active growing intracranial lesion or tumor. **Cautions:** Diabetes mellitus, elderly.

**S**

## ACTION

Stimulates cartilaginous growth areas of long bones; increases number, size of skeletal muscle cells; influences size of organs; increases RBC mass by stimulating erythropoietin. Influences metabolism of carbohydrates (decreases insulin sensitivity), fats (mobilizes fatty acids), minerals (retains phosphorus, sodium, potassium by promotion of cell growth), proteins (increases protein synthesis). **Therapeutic Effect:** Stimulates growth.

## PHARMACOKINETICS

Well absorbed after SQ, IM administration. Localized primarily in kidneys, liver. **Half-life: IV:** 20–30 min; **SQ, IM:** 3–5 hrs.

## ⌛ LIFESPAN CONSIDERATIONS

**Pregnancy/Lactation:** Unknown if drug is distributed in breast milk. **Children/Elderly:** No age-related precautions noted.

## INTERACTIONS

**DRUG: Corticosteroids (e.g., hydrocortisone, prednisone)** may inhibit growth response. **Oral estrogens** may decrease response to somatropin. **HERBAL:** None significant. **FOOD:** None known. **LAB VALUES:** May increase serum alkaline phosphatase, inorganic phosphorus, parathyroid hormone. May decrease glucose tolerance. May slightly decrease thyroid function.

## AVAILABILITY (Rx)

Injection, Powder for Reconstitution (**Genotropin**): 5 mg, 12 mg. (**Genotropin Miniquick**): 0.2 mg, 0.4 mg, 0.6 mg, 0.8 mg, 1 mg, 1.2 mg, 1.4 mg, 1.6 mg, 1.8 mg, 2 mg. (**Humatrope**): 6 mg, 12 mg, 24 mg. (**Nutropin**): 5 mg, 10 mg. (**Omnitrope**): 5.8 mg. (**Saizen**): 5 mg, 8.8 mg. (**Serostim**): 4 mg, 5 mg, 6 mg. (**Zomacton**): 5 mg, 10 mg. (**Zorbitive**): 8.8 mg. Injection Solution: (**Norditropin**): 5 mg/1.5 ml, 10 mg/1.5 ml, 15 mg/1.5 ml. (**Nutropin AQ**): 5 mg/ml. (**Omnitrope**): 5 mg/1.5 ml,

10 mg/1.5 ml. (**Norditropin FlexPro Pen**): 5 mg/1.5 ml, 10 mg/1.5 ml, 30 mg/3 ml.

## ADMINISTRATION/HANDLING

◄**ALERT**► **Neonate:** Benzyl alcohol as a preservative has been associated with fatal toxicity (gasping syndrome) in premature infants. Reconstitute with Sterile Water for Injection only. Use only 1 dose per vial. Discard unused portion.

**Reconstitution**
**Genotropin, Genotropin Miniquick:** Reconstitute with diluent provided.
**Humatrope:** Reconstitute with 1.5–5 ml diluent provided, swirl gently, do not shake.
**Humatrope Cartridge:** Dilute with solution provided with cartridge only.
**Nutropin:** Reconstitute each 5 mg with 1.5–5 ml diluent, swirl gently, do not shake.
**Omnitrope:** Reconstitute with diluents provided, swirl gently, do not shake.
**Saigen:** 5 mg: Reconstitute with 1–3 ml diluent provided, swirl gently, do not shake. 8.8 mg: Reconstitute with 2–3 ml diluent provided, swirl gently, do not shake.
**Serostim:** Reconstitute with Sterile Water for Injection.
**Zorbitive:** Reconstitute with 1–2 ml Bacteriostatic Water for Injection.

**Storage**
**Long-term storage:** Refrigerate all products except Zorbitive. Once reconstituted, Humatrope, Nutropin, Saigen, Zorbitive stable for 14 days, Genotropin for 21 days, Humatrope Cartridge for 28 days. **Genotropin Miniquick:** Refrigerate, use within 24 hrs.

## INDICATIONS/ROUTES/DOSAGE

**Growth Hormone Deficiency**
**SQ:**     *(Genotropin,     Omnitrope):* **ADULTS:** 0.04 mg/kg wkly divided into 6–7 equal doses/wk. May increase at 4- to 8-wk intervals to maximum of 0.08 mg/kg/wk. **CHILDREN:** 0.16–0.24 mg/kg wkly divided into daily doses.
**SQ:** *(Humatrope):* **ADULTS:** 0.006 mg/kg once daily. May increase to maximum

---

of 0.0125 mg/kg/day. **CHILDREN:** 0.18–0.3 mg/kg wkly divided into alternate-day doses or 6 doses/wk.

**SQ:** *(Norditropin):* **ADULTS:** 0.004 mg/kg/day. May increase after 6 wks up to 0.016 mg/kg/day. **CHILDREN:** 0.024–0.036 mg/kg/dose 6–7 times/wk.

**SQ:** *(Nutropin):* **ADULTS:** 0.006 mg/kg once daily. May increase to maximum of 0.025 mg/kg/day (younger than 35 yrs) or 0.0125/kg/day (35 yrs and older). **CHILDREN:** 0.3–0.7 mg/kg wkly divided into daily doses.

**SQ:** *(Nutropin AQ):* **ADULTS:** 0.006 mg/kg once daily. May increase to maximum of 0.0125 mg/kg/day.

**SQ:** *(Saizen):* **ADULTS:** 0.005 mg/kg/day. May increase up to 0.01 mg/kg/day after 4 wks. **CHILDREN:** 0.06 mg/kg 3 times/wk.

**Chronic Renal Insufficiency**
**SQ:** *(Nutropin, Nutropin AQ):* **CHILDREN:** 0.35 mg/kg wkly divided into daily doses.

**Turner's Syndrome**
**SQ:** *(Humatrope, Nutropin, Nutropin AQ):* **CHILDREN:** 0.375 mg/kg wkly divided into equal doses 3–7 times/wk. *(Genotropin, Omnitrope):* 0.33 mg/kg wkly divided into 6–7 doses. *(Norditropin):* Up to 0.067 mg/kg/day.

**AIDS-Related Wasting**
**SQ:** *(Serostim):* **ADULTS WEIGHING MORE THAN 55 KG:** 6 mg once daily at bedtime. **ADULTS WEIGHING 45–55 KG:** 5 mg once daily at bedtime. **ADULTS WEIGHING 35–44 KG:** 4 mg once daily at bedtime. **ADULTS WEIGHING LESS THAN 35 KG:** 0.1 mg/kg once daily at bedtime.

**Short Bowel Syndrome**
**SQ:** *(Zorbitive):* **ADULTS:** 0.1 mg/kg/day. **Maximum:** 8 mg/day.

**Dosage in Renal/Hepatic Impairment**
No dose adjustment.

## SIDE EFFECTS

**Frequent:** Otitis media, other ear disorders (with Turner's syndrome). **Occasional:** Carpal tunnel syndrome, gynecomastia, myalgia, peripheral edema, fatigue, asthenia. **Rare:** Rash, pruritus, visual changes, headache, nausea, vomiting, injection site pain/swelling, abdominal pain, hip/knee pain.

## ADVERSE EFFECTS/ TOXIC REACTIONS

Pancreatitis occurs rarely.

## NURSING CONSIDERATIONS

### BASELINE ASSESSMENT
Obtain baseline lab chemistries, thyroid function, serum glucose level. Obtain full medical history (drug has multiple contraindications).

### INTERVENTION/EVALUATION
Monitor bone growth, growth rate in relation to pt's age. Monitor serum calcium, glucose, phosphorus levels; renal, parathyroid, thyroid function. Observe for decreased muscle wasting in AIDS pts.

### PATIENT/FAMILY TEACHING
• Follow correct procedure to reconstitute drug for administration, safe handling/disposal of needles. • Regular follow-up with physician is important part of therapy. • Report development of severe headache, visual changes, pain in hip/knee, limping.

**S**

# sonidegib

**soe**-ni-**deg**-ib
(Odomzo)

■ **BLACK BOX ALERT** ■ May cause embryo-fetal death/severe malformations when given during pregnancy. Verify pregnancy status before initiation. Female patients of reproductive potential must use effective contraception during treatment and for at least 20 mos after discontinuation. Due to the potential risk of exposure through semen, male patients must use condoms during sexual activity (even after a vasectomy) during treatment and for at least 8 mos after discontinuation. **Do not confuse sonidegib with vismodegib.**

## ◆CLASSIFICATION

**PHARMACOTHERAPEUTIC:** Hedgehog pathway inhibitor. **CLINICAL:** Antineoplastic.

## USES

Treatment of adult pts with locally advanced basal cell carcinoma that has recurred following surgery or radiation therapy, or those who are not candidates for surgery or radiation.

## PRECAUTIONS

**Contraindications:** Hypersensitivity to sonidegib. **Cautions:** Renal/hepatic impairment. Avoid concomitant use of strong or moderate CYP3A inhibitors, strong or moderate CYP3A inducers.

## ACTION

Inhibits cell migration, proliferation, survival of tumor cells. Binds to and inhibits Smoothened, a transmembrane protein involved in Hedgehog signal transduction. **Therapeutic Effect:** Inhibits tumor cell growth and metastasis of basal cell carcinoma.

## PHARMACOKINETICS

Poorly absorbed after PO administration (less than 10%). Metabolized in liver. Protein binding: greater than 97%. Peak plasma concentration: 2–4 hrs. Steady state reached in 4 mos. Eliminated in feces (70%), urine (30%). **Half-life:** 28 days.

## ⌛ LIFESPAN CONSIDERATIONS

**Pregnancy/Lactation:** May cause fetal death/malformations. Unknown if distributed in breast milk. Must either discontinue drug or discontinue breastfeeding. Female patients of reproductive potential must use effective contraception during treatment and up to 20 mos after discontinuation. May compromise female fertility. **Males:** Male patients must use condoms during sexual activity (after a vasectomy) during treatment and up to 8 mos after discontinuation. **Children:** Safety and efficacy not established. **Elderly:** May have increased risk of severe musculoskeletal adverse events (e.g., muscle spasms, myopathy).

## INTERACTIONS

**DRUG: Strong CYP3A inhibitors (e.g., clarithromycin, ketoconazole), moderate CYP3A inhibitors (e.g., atazanavir, fluconazole)** may increase concentration/effect. **Strong CYP3A inducers (e.g., carbamazepine, phenytoin, rifampin)** may decrease concentration/effect. **Statins (e.g., simvastatin)** may increase risk of rhabdomyolysis. **HERBAL: St. John's wort** may decrease concentration/effect. **FOOD: High-fat meals** may increase absorption/concentration. **LAB VALUES:** May increase serum ALT/AST, amylase, creatinine, CK, glucose, lipase. May decreased Hct, Hgb, lymphocytes.

## AVAILABILITY (Rx)

**Capsules:** 200 mg.

## ADMINISTRATION/HANDLING

**PO**
• Give on an empty stomach at least 1 hr before or 2 hrs after a meal.

## INDICATIONS/ROUTES/DOSAGE

**Basal Cell Carcinoma**
**PO: ADULTS, ELDERLY:** 200 mg once daily. Continue until disease progression or unacceptable toxicity.

**Dose Modification**
Interrupt therapy for severe or intolerable musculoskeletal adverse reactions; first occurrence of serum CK level 2.5–10 times upper limit of normal (ULN); recurrent serum CK level 2.5–5 times ULN. Once resolved, resume at 200 mg once daily.

### Discontinuation

Permanently discontinue treatment for serum CK level greater than 2.5 times ULN with worsening renal function; serum CK level greater than 10 times ULN; recurrent serum CK level greater than 5 times ULN; recurrent severe or intolerable musculoskeletal adverse reactions.

### Renal Impairment

No dose adjustment.

### Hepatic Impairment

**Mild impairment:** No dose adjustment. **Moderate to severe impairment:** Not studied; use caution.

## SIDE EFFECTS

**Frequent (54%–23%):** Muscle spasm, alopecia, dysgeusia, fatigue, nausea, diarrhea, musculoskeletal pain, decreased appetite. **Occasional (19%–10%):** Myalgia, abdominal pain, headache, generalized pain, vomiting, pruritus.

## ADVERSE EFFECTS/TOXIC REACTIONS

Musculoskeletal events occurred in 68% of pts. Common Terminology Criteria for Adverse Events (CTCAE) grade 3 or 4 musculoskeletal events (9% of pts) may require administration of muscle relaxants, analgesics/narcotics, magnesium supplementation, IV hydration. Serum CK level elevations usually occur before musculoskeletal pain or spasms. Increased serum CK levels reported in 61% of pts. The median onset of serum CK elevation was approx. 12 wks. May increase risk of rhabdomyolysis. Amenorrhea lasting longer than 18 mos has occurred.

## NURSING CONSIDERATIONS

### BASELINE ASSESSMENT

Obtain baseline capillary blood glucose, CBC, LFT, serum CK level, renal function test. Verify negative pregnancy status before initiation. Question current breastfeeding status. Receive medication history and screen for interactions. Assess hydration status.

### INTERVENTION/EVALUATION

Monitor renal function, serum CK levels periodically and with any musculoskeletal adverse events. If musculoskeletal adverse reactions occur with serum CK levels greater than 2.5 times ULN, obtain serum CK level at least wkly until resolution. Offer antiemetics for nausea/vomiting. Monitor urine color, output. Serum CK level elevation or worsening of renal function may indicate rhabdomyolysis. Monitor pregnancy status during therapy.

### PATIENT/FAMILY TEACHING

• Treatment may cause severe muscle damage, which may cause kidney damage. • Report dark-colored urine or decreased urine output despite hydration. • Immediately report musculoskeletal symptoms such as muscle pain/spasms/tenderness/weakness. • Do not donate blood or blood products during treatment and up to 20 mos after discontinuation. • Males must use condoms during sexual activity during treatment and up to 8 mos following discontinuation. • Treatment may cause birth defects or miscarriage. • Immediately report suspected pregnancy. • Hair loss is an expected side effect. • Swallow capsules whole; do not chew, crush, cut or open. • Take on empty stomach at least 1 hr before or 2 hrs after a meal.

# *SORAfenib

S

soe-**raf**-e-nib
(Nexavar)
**Do not confuse Nexavar with Nexium, or sorafenib with imatinib or sunitinib.**

## ◆CLASSIFICATION

**PHARMACOTHERAPEUTIC:** Multikinase inhibitor. **CLINICAL:** Antineoplastic.

## USES

Treatment of advanced renal cell carcinoma, unresectable hepatocellular carcinoma, locally recurrent or metastatic progressive differentiated thyroid carcinoma refractory to radioactive iodine treatment. **OFF-LABEL:** Recurrent or metastatic angiosarcoma, resistant gastrointestinal stromal tumor.

## PRECAUTIONS

**Contraindications:** Hypersensitivity to sorafenib. Use in combination with carboplatin and paclitaxel in pts with squamous cell lung cancer. **Cautions:** Underlying or poorly controlled hypertension, pts with congenital long QT syndrome, medications that prolong QT interval, electrolyte imbalance (hypokalemia, hypomagnesemia), unstable coronary artery disease, recent MI, HF, concurrent use with strong CYP3A4 inducers.

## ACTION

Decreases tumor cell proliferation by interacting with multiple intracellular, cell surface kinases. **Therapeutic Effect:** Inhibits tumor growth.

## PHARMACOKINETICS

Metabolized in liver. Protein binding: 99.5%. Eliminated mainly in feces, with lesser amount excreted in urine. **Half-life:** 25–48 hrs.

## ☒ LIFESPAN CONSIDERATIONS

**Pregnancy/Lactation:** May cause fetal harm. Adequate contraception should be used during therapy and for at least 2 wks after therapy completion. Unknown if distributed in breast milk. Breastfeeding not recommended. **Children:** Safety and efficacy not established. **Elderly:** No age-related precautions noted.

## INTERACTIONS

**DRUG: Strong CYP3A4 inducers (e.g., carbamazepine, phenobarbital, rifampin)** may decrease concentration. **HERBAL: St. John's wort** may decrease concentration. **FOOD: High-fat meals** decrease effectiveness. **LAB**

**VALUES:** May increase serum lipase, amylase, bilirubin, alkaline phosphatase, transaminases. May decrease serum phosphorus, lymphocytes, WBCs, Hgb, Hct.

## AVAILABILITY (Rx)

🗌 **Tablets:** 200 mg (Nexavar).

## ADMINISTRATION/HANDLING

**PO**
- Give 1 hr before or 2 hrs after eating (high-fat meal reduces effectiveness).
- Swallow tablet whole; do not break, crush, dissolve, or divide tablet.

## INDICATIONS/ROUTES/DOSAGE

**Renal Cell Carcinoma, Hepatocellular Carcinoma, Thyroid Carcinoma**
**PO: ADULTS, ELDERLY:** 400 mg (2 tablets) twice daily without food. Continue until disease progression or unacceptable toxicity.

**Dosage in Renal Impairment**

| Creatinine Clearance | Dosage |
| --- | --- |
| 40–59 ml/min | 400 mg twice daily |
| 20–39 ml/min | 200 mg twice daily |
| Hemodialysis | 200 mg once daily |

**Dosage in Hepatic Impairment**
**Bilirubin greater than 1 to 1.5 times upper limit of normal (ULN) and/or AST greater than ULN:** 400 mg twice daily. **Bilirubin greater than 1.5 to 3 times ULN and any AST:** 200 mg twice daily. **Albumin less than 2.5 g/dL (any bilirubin/AST):** 200 mg once daily.

## SIDE EFFECTS

**Frequent (43%–16%):** Diarrhea, rash, fatigue, exfoliative dermatitis, alopecia, nausea, pruritus, hypertension, anorexia, vomiting. **Occasional (15%–10%):** Constipation, minor bleeding, dyspnea, sensory neuropathy, cough, abdominal pain, dry skin, weight loss, joint pain, headache. **Rare (9%–1%):** Acne, flushing, stomatitis, mucositis, dyspepsia, arthralgia, myalgia, hoarseness.

## ADVERSE EFFECTS/ TOXIC REACTIONS

Anemia, neutropenia, thrombocytopenia, leukopenia occur in less than 10% of pts. Pancreatitis, gastritis, erectile dysfunction occur occasionally. Hemorrhage, cardiac ischemia/infarction, hypertensive crisis occur rarely.

## NURSING CONSIDERATIONS

### BASELINE ASSESSMENT

Monitor B/P wkly during first 6 wks of therapy and routinely thereafter. CBC, serum chemistries including electrolytes, renal function, LFT, chest X-ray should be performed before therapy begins and routinely thereafter.

### INTERVENTION/EVALUATION

Determine serum amylase, lipase, phosphorus concentrations frequently during therapy. Monitor CBC for evidence of myelosuppression. Monitor for blood dyscrasias (fever, sore throat, signs of local infection, unusual bruising/bleeding from any site), symptoms of anemia (excessive fatigue, weakness). Monitor for signs of neuropathy (gait disturbances, fine motor control difficulties, numbness).

### PATIENT/FAMILY TEACHING

• Report any episode of chest pain. • Do not have immunizations without physician's approval (drug lowers resistance). Avoid contact with those who have recently taken live virus vaccine. • Promptly report fever, sore throat, signs of local infection, unusual bruising/bleeding from any site. • Swallow whole; do not chew, crush, dissolve, or divide tablet. • Avoid administration after high-fat meals.

## sotalol  HIGH ALERT

soe-ta-lol
(Apo-Sotalol ✦, Betapace, Betapace AF, Novo-Sotalol ✦, Sorine, Sotylize)

■ BLACK BOX ALERT ■ Initiation, titration to occur in a hospital setting with continuous EKG to monitor potential onset of life-threatening arrhythmias. Betapace should not be substituted for Betapace AF.
**Do not confuse Betapace with Betapace AF, or sotalol with Stadol or Sudafed.**

### ◆ CLASSIFICATION

**PHARMACOTHERAPEUTIC:** Beta-adrenergic blocking agent. **CLINICAL:** Antiarrhythmic.

### USES

**Betapace, Sorine, Sotylize:** Treatment of documented, life-threatening ventricular arrhythmias. **Betapace AF:** Maintain normal sinus rhythm in pts with symptomatic atrial fibrillation/flutter. **OFF-LABEL:** Fetal tachycardia, treatment of atrial fibrillation with hypertrophic cardiomyopathy.

### PRECAUTIONS

**Contraindications:** Hypersensitivity to sotalol. Cardiogenic shock, congenital or acquired long QT syndrome, second- or third-degree heart block (unless functioning pacemaker is present), sinus bradycardia, uncontrolled HF, bronchial asthma. **Betapace AF, Sotylize:** (additional): Baseline QT interval greater than 450 msec, bronchospastic conditions, CrCl less than 40 ml/min, serum potassium less than 4 mEq/L, sick sinus syndrome. **Cautions:** Pts with history of ventricular tachycardia, ventricular fibrillation, cardiomegaly, compensated HF, diabetes mellitus, QT interval prolongation, concurrent medications that prolong QT interval, hypokalemia, hypomagnesemia, renal impairment, within first 2 wks post MI, peripheral vascular disease, Raynaud's syndrome, myasthenia gravis, psychiatric disease, bronchospastic disease. Concurrent use of digoxin, verapamil, diltiazem, history of severe anaphylaxis to allergens.

S

## ACTION

Prolongs cardiac action potential, effective refractory period, QT interval. Decreases heart rate, AV node conduction; increases AV node refractoriness. **Therapeutic Effect:** Produces antiarrhythmic activity.

## PHARMACOKINETICS

| Route | Onset | Peak | Duration |
|-------|-------|------|----------|
| PO | 1–2 hrs | 2.5–4 hrs | 8–16 hrs |

Well absorbed from GI tract. Protein binding: None. Widely distributed. Primarily excreted unchanged in urine. Removed by hemodialysis. **Half-life:** 12 hrs (increased in elderly, renal impairment).

## LIFESPAN CONSIDERATIONS

**Pregnancy/Lactation:** Crosses placenta. Distributed in breast milk. **Children:** Safety and efficacy not established. **Elderly:** Age-related peripheral vascular disease may increase susceptibility to decreased peripheral circulation. Age-related renal impairment may require dosage adjustment.

## INTERACTIONS

**DRUG: Calcium channel blockers (e.g., diltiazem, verapamil)** may increase effect on AV conduction, B/P. May mask symptoms of hypoglycemia, prolong hypoglycemic effects of **insulin, oral hypoglycemics (e.g., glipizide, metformin).** **QT prolonging medications (e.g., amiodarone, ciprofloxacin, haloperidol, ketoconazole, ondansetron)** may increase risk of prolonged QT interval. **HERBAL: Ephedra** may worsen arrhythmias. **FOOD:** None known. **LAB VALUES:** May increase serum BUN, glucose, alkaline phosphatase, LDH, lipoprotein, ALT, AST, triglycerides, potassium, uric acid.

## AVAILABILITY (Rx)

**Solution, Intravenous:** 150 mg/10 ml. **Solution, Oral (Sotylize):** 5 mg/ml. **Tablets:** 80 mg (Betapace, Betapace AF, Sorine), 120 mg (Betapace, Betapace AF, Sorine), 160 mg (Betapace, Betapace AF, Sorine), 240 mg (Sorine).

## ADMINISTRATION/HANDLING

**PO**
• Give without regard to food. • Give at same time each day.

## INDICATIONS/ROUTES/DOSAGE

**Ventricular Arrhythmias**
**PO *(Betapace, Sorine, Sotylize):*** **ADULTS, ELDERLY:** Initially, 80 mg twice daily. May increase in 80-mg increments at 3-day intervals. Range: 160–320 mg/day in 2–3 divided doses. **Maximum:** 640 mg/day in life-threatening refractive arrhythmias.
**IV:** Initially, 75 mg infused over 5 hrs twice daily. Range: 75–150 mg twice daily. Maximum: 300 mg twice daily.

**Atrial Fibrillation, Atrial Flutter**
**PO *(Betapace AF, Sotylize):*** **ADULTS, ELDERLY:** Initially, 80 mg twice daily. May increase to 120–160 mg twice daily.
**IV:** Initially, 75 mg infused over 5 hrs twice daily. Usual dose: 112.5 mg twice daily. Maximum: 150 mg twice daily.

**Usual Dosage for Children**
**PO:** Initially, 90 mg/m$^2$/day in 3 divided doses. May incrementally increase up to a maximum of 180 mg/m$^2$/day.

**Dosage in Renal Impairment**
Dosage interval is modified based on creatinine clearance.

### BETAPACE, SORINE

| Creatinine Clearance | Dosage |
|----------------------|--------|
| 31–60 ml/min | 24 hrs |
| 10–30 ml/min | 36–48 hrs |
| Less than 10 ml/min | Individualized |

### BETAPACE AF

| Creatinine Clearance | Dosage |
|----------------------|--------|
| Greater than 60 ml/min | 12 hrs |
| 40–60 ml/min | 24 hrs |
| Less than 40 ml/min | Contraindicated |

**Dosage in Hepatic Impairment**
No dose adjustment.

## SIDE EFFECTS

**Frequent:** Diminished sexual function, drowsiness, insomnia, asthenia. **Occasional:** Depression, cold hands/feet, diarrhea, constipation, anxiety, nasal congestion, nausea, vomiting. **Rare:** Altered taste, dry eyes, pruritus, paresthesia of fingers, toes, scalp.

## ADVERSE EFFECTS/ TOXIC REACTIONS

Bradycardia, HF, hypotension, bronchospasm, hypoglycemia, prolonged QT interval, torsades de pointes, ventricular tachycardia, premature ventricular complexes may occur.

## NURSING CONSIDERATIONS

### BASELINE ASSESSMENT

Pt must be on continuous cardiac monitoring upon initiation of therapy. Do not administer without consulting physician if pulse is 60 beats/min or less. Assess creatinine clearance before dosing.

### INTERVENTION/EVALUATION

Diligently monitor for arrhythmias. Assess B/P for hypotension, pulse for bradycardia. Assess for HF: dyspnea, peripheral edema, jugular vein distention, increased weight, rales in lungs, decreased urinary output.

### PATIENT/FAMILY TEACHING

• Do not discontinue, change dose without physician approval. • Avoid tasks requiring alertness, motor skills until response to drug is established (may cause drowsiness). • Periodic lab tests, EKGs are essential part of therapy. • Report rapid heartbeat, chest pain, swelling of ankles/legs, difficulty breathing.

# spironolactone

spir-**on**-oh-**lak**-tone
(Aldactone)
■ **BLACK BOX ALERT** ■ Has been shown to produce tumors in chronic toxicity studies.

**Do not confuse Aldactone with Aldactazide.**

### FIXED-COMBINATION(S)

**Aldactazide:** spironolactone/hydrochlorothiazide (a thiazide diuretic): 25 mg/25 mg, 50 mg/50 mg.

## ◆CLASSIFICATION

**PHARMACOTHERAPEUTIC:** Aldosterone antagonist. **CLINICAL:** Potassium-sparing diuretic, antihypertensive, antihypokalemic.

## USES

Management of edema associated with excessive aldosterone excretion or with HF; hypertension; hypokalemia, nephrotic syndrome, severe HF; primary hyperaldosteronism. **OFF-LABEL:** Treatment of edema, hypertension in children, female acne, female hirsutism. Ascites, due to cirrhosis.

## PRECAUTIONS

**Contraindications:** Hypersensitivity to spironolactone. Acute renal insufficiency, significant impairment of renal excretory function, anuria, hyperkalemia, Addison's disease, concomitant use with eplerenone. **Cautions:** Dehydration, hyponatremia, concurrent use of supplemental potassium, elderly, mild renal impairment, declining renal function, ACE inhibitors or angiotensin receptor blockers.

## ACTION

Interferes with sodium reabsorption by competitively inhibiting action of aldosterone in distal tubule, promoting sodium and water excretion, increasing potassium retention. **Therapeutic Effect:** Produces diuresis, lowers B/P.

## PHARMACOKINETICS

Well absorbed from GI tract (absorption increased with food). Protein binding: 91%–98%. Metabolized in liver to active metabolite. Primarily excreted in urine. Unknown if removed by hemodialysis. **Half-life:** 78–84 min.

S

## ⌛ LIFESPAN CONSIDERATIONS

**Pregnancy/Lactation:** Active metabolite excreted in breast milk. Breastfeeding not recommended. **Children:** No age-related precautions noted. **Elderly:** May be more susceptible to developing hyperkalemia. Age-related renal impairment may require dosage adjustment.

## INTERACTIONS

**DRUG: ACE inhibitors (e.g., captopril, lisinopril), angiotensin receptor blockers (e.g., valsartan), potassium-containing medications, potassium supplements** may increase risk of hyperkalemia. May increase half-life of **digoxin. NSAIDs** may decrease antihypertensive effect. **HERBAL:** Avoid **natural licorice** (possesses mineralocorticoid activity). **FOOD: Food** increases absorption. **LAB VALUES:** May increase urinary calcium excretion, serum BUN, glucose, creatinine, magnesium, potassium, uric acid. May decrease serum sodium.

## AVAILABILITY (Rx)

**Tablets:** 25 mg, 50 mg, 100 mg.

## ADMINISTRATION/HANDLING

**PO**
• Take with food to reduce GI irritation and increase absorption.

## INDICATIONS/ROUTES/ DOSAGE

**Edema**
PO: **ADULTS, ELDERLY:** 25–200 mg/day as single dose or in 2 divided doses. **CHILDREN:** 1–3.3 mg/kg/day in divided doses q6–12h. **Maximum:** 100 mg. **NEONATES:** 1–3 mg/kg/day in divided doses q12–24h.

**Hypertension**
PO: **ADULTS, ELDERLY:** 25–50 mg/day in 1–2 doses/day. **CHILDREN:** 1–3.3 mg/kg/day in divided doses q6–12h. **Maximum:** 100 mg.

**Hypokalemia**
PO: **ADULTS, ELDERLY:** 25–100 mg/day as single dose or in 2 divided doses.

**Primary Aldosteronism**
PO: **ADULTS, ELDERLY:** 400 mg/day for 4 days up to 3–4 wks, then maintenance dose of 100–400 mg/day as single dose or in 2 divided doses. **CHILDREN:** 100–400 mg/m$^2$/day as single dose or in 2 divided doses.

**HF**
PO: **ADULTS, ELDERLY:** 12.5–25 mg/day adjusted based on pt response, evidence of hyperkalemia. **Maximum:** 50 mg.

**Dosage in Renal Impairment**
**CrCl 50 ml/min or greater:** Initially, 12.5–25 mg once daily. **Maintenance:** 25 mg once or twice daily. **CrCl 30–49 ml/min:** Initially, 12.5 mg once daily or every other day. **Maintenance:** 12.5–25 mg once daily. **CrCl less than 30 ml/min:** Not recommended.

**Dosage in Hepatic Impairment**
No dose adjustment.

## SIDE EFFECTS

**Frequent:** Hyperkalemia (in pts with renal insufficiency, those taking potassium supplements), dehydration, hyponatremia, lethargy. **Occasional:** Nausea, vomiting, anorexia, abdominal cramps, diarrhea, headache, ataxia, drowsiness, confusion, fever. **Male:** Gynecomastia, impotence, decreased libido. **Female:** Menstrual irregularities (amenorrhea, postmenopausal bleeding), breast tenderness. **Rare:** Rash, urticaria, hirsutism.

## ADVERSE EFFECTS/ TOXIC REACTIONS

Severe hyperkalemia may produce arrhythmias, bradycardia, EKG changes (tented T waves, widening QRS complex, ST segment depression). May proceed to cardiac standstill, ventricular fibrillation. Cirrhosis pts at risk for hepatic decompensation if dehydration, hyponatremia occurs. Pts with primary aldosteronism may experience rapid weight loss, severe fatigue during high-dose therapy.

## NURSING CONSIDERATIONS

### BASELINE ASSESSMENT

Weigh pt; initiate strict I&O. Evaluate hydration status by assessing mucous membranes, skin turgor. Obtain baseline serum electrolytes, renal/hepatic function, urinalysis. Assess for edema; note location, extent. Check baseline vital signs, note pulse rate/regularity.

### INTERVENTION/EVALUATION

Monitor serum electrolyte values, esp. for increased potassium, BUN, creatinine. Monitor B/P. Monitor for hyponatremia: mental confusion, thirst, cold/clammy skin, drowsiness, dry mouth. Monitor for hyperkalemia: colic, diarrhea, muscle twitching followed by weakness/paralysis, arrhythmias. Obtain daily weight. Note changes in edema, skin turgor.

### PATIENT/FAMILY TEACHING

• Expect increase in volume, frequency of urination. • Therapeutic effect takes several days to begin and can last for several days when drug is discontinued. This may not apply if pt is on a potassium-losing drug concomitantly (diet, use of supplements should be established by physician). • Report irregular or slow pulse, symptoms of electrolyte imbalance (see previous Intervention/Evaluation). • Avoid foods high in potassium, such as whole grains (cereals), legumes, meat, bananas, apricots, orange juice, potatoes (white, sweet), raisins. • Avoid alcohol. • Avoid tasks that require alertness, motor skills until response to drug is established (may cause drowsiness).

## sucralfate

soo-**kral**-fate
(Apo-Sucralfate ✱, Carafate, Novo-Sucralate ✱)

**Do not confuse Carafate with Cafergot, or sucralfate with salsalate.**

### ◆ CLASSIFICATION

**PHARMACOTHERAPEUTIC:** Gastrointestinal agent. **CLINICAL:** Antiulcer.

### USES

Short-term treatment (up to 8 wks) of duodenal ulcer. Maintenance therapy of duodenal ulcer after healing of acute ulcers.

### PRECAUTIONS

**Contraindications:** Hypersensitivity to sucralfate. **Cautions:** Renal failure (due to accumulation of aluminum).

### ACTION

Forms ulcer-adherent complex with proteinaceous exudate (e.g., albumin) at ulcer site. Forms viscous, adhesive barrier on surface of intact mucosa of stomach, duodenum. **Therapeutic Effect:** Protects damaged mucosa from further destruction by absorbing gastric acid, pepsin, bile salts.

### PHARMACOKINETICS

Minimally absorbed from GI tract. Eliminated in feces, with small amount excreted in urine. Not removed by hemodialysis.

### ⧗ LIFESPAN CONSIDERATIONS

**Pregnancy/Lactation:** Unknown if drug crosses placenta or is distributed in breast milk. **Children:** Safety and efficacy not established. **Elderly:** No age-related precautions noted.

### INTERACTIONS

**DRUG:** May decrease absorption of **digoxin, ketoconazole, levothyroxine, phenytoin, quinidine, quinolones (e.g., ciprofloxacin), ranitidine, tetracycline, theophylline.** **HERBAL:** None significant. **FOOD:** None known. **LAB VALUES:** None known.

S

## AVAILABILITY (Rx)

**Oral Suspension:** 1 g/10 ml. **Tablets:** 1 g.

## ADMINISTRATION/HANDLING

### PO

• Administer 1 hr before meals and at bedtime. • Tablets may be crushed and dissolved in water. • Avoid antacids for 30 min before or after giving sucralfate. • Shake suspension well before using.

## INDICATIONS/ROUTES/DOSAGE

**Active Duodenal Ulcers**
**PO: ADULTS, ELDERLY:** 1 g 4 times/day (before meals and at bedtime) for up to 8 wks.

**Maintenance Therapy of Duodenal Ulcers**
**PO: ADULTS, ELDERLY:** 1 g twice daily.

**Dosage in Renal/Hepatic Impairment**
No dose adjustment. Use caution in chronic renal failure.

## SIDE EFFECTS

**Frequent (2%):** Constipation. **Occasional (less than 2%):** Dry mouth, backache, diarrhea, dizziness, drowsiness, nausea, indigestion, rash, urticaria, pruritus, abdominal discomfort.

## ADVERSE EFFECTS/ TOXIC REACTIONS

Bezoars (compacted, undigestible material that does not pass into intestine) have been reported.

## NURSING CONSIDERATIONS

### INTERVENTION/EVALUATION

Monitor daily pattern of bowel activity, stool consistency.

### PATIENT/FAMILY TEACHING

• Take medication on an empty stomach. • Antacids may be given as an adjunct but should not be taken for 30 min before or after sucralfate (formation of sucralfate gel is activated by stomach acid). • Dry mouth may be relieved by sour hard candy, sips of tepid water.

# sulfamethoxazole-trimethoprim

**sul**-fa-meth-**ox**-a-zole-trye-**meth**-oh-prim
(Apo-Sulfatrim ✦, Bactrim, Bactrim DS, Sulfatrim)
**Do not confuse Bactrim with bacitracin or Bactroban.**

## FIXED-COMBINATION(S)

**Bactrim, Septra:** sulfa-methoxa-zole/trimethoprim: 5:1 ratio remains constant in all dosage forms (e.g., 400 mg/80 mg).

## ◆CLASSIFICATION

**PHARMACOTHERAPEUTIC:** Sulfonamide/folate antagonist. **CLINICAL:** Antibiotic.

## USES

Treatment of susceptible infections due to *S. pneumoniae, H. influenzae, E. coli, Klebsiella* spp., *Enterobacter* spp., *M. morganii, P. mirabilis, P. vulgaris, S. flexneri, Pneumocystis jiroveci* including acute or complicated and recurrent or chronic UTI, *Pneumocystis jiroveci* pneumonia (PCP), shigellosis, enteritis, otitis media, chronic bronchitis, traveler's diarrhea. Prophylaxis of PCP. **OFF-LABEL:** Chronic prostatitis, prophylaxis for UTI, MRSA infections, prosthetic joint infection.

## PRECAUTIONS

**Contraindications:** Hypersensitivity to any sulfa medication, trimethoprim. History of drug-induced immune thrombocytopenia with sulfonamides or trimethoprim, infants younger than 2 mos, megaloblastic anemia due to folate deficiency, severe hepatic/renal impairment. **Cautions:** Pts with G6PD deficiency, impaired renal/hepatic function, porphyria, pts with allergies or asthma, elderly, alcoholism, thyroid dysfunction, concurrent anticonvulsant therapy.

S

## ACTION

Blocks bacterial folic acid synthesis and growth. **Therapeutic Effect:** Bactericidal in susceptible microorganisms.

## PHARMACOKINETICS

Rapidly, well absorbed from GI tract. Protein binding: 45%–60%. Widely distributed. Metabolized in liver. Excreted in urine. Minimally removed by hemodialysis. **Half-life:** sulfamethoxazole, 6–12 hrs; trimethoprim, 6–17 hrs (increased in renal impairment).

## ⧗ LIFESPAN CONSIDERATIONS

**Pregnancy/Lactation:** Contraindicated during pregnancy at term and during lactation. Readily crosses placenta. Distributed in breast milk. May produce kernicterus in newborn. **Children:** Contraindicated in pts younger than 2 mos; may increase risk of kernicterus in newborn. **Elderly:** Increased risk for severe skin reaction, myelosuppression, decreased platelet count.

## INTERACTIONS

**DRUG:** May increase/prolong effects, increase adverse effects of **phenytoin, digoxin, oral hypoglycemics (e.g., glipizide, metformin), warfarin.** May increase effects of **methotrexate. HERBAL:** Dong quai, St. John's wort may increase photosensitization reaction. **FOOD:** None known. **LAB VALUES:** May increase serum BUN, creatinine, ALT, AST, bilirubin.

## AVAILABILITY (Rx)

◀**ALERT**▶ All dosage forms have same 5:1 ratio of sulfamethoxazole (SMZ) to trimethoprim (TMP). **Injection Solution:** SMZ 80 mg and TMP 16 mg per ml. **Oral Suspension:** SMZ 200 mg and TMP 40 mg per 5 ml. **Tablets (Bactrim):** SMZ 400 mg and TMP 80 mg. **Tablets (Double Strength [Bactrim DS, Septra DS]):** SMZ 800 mg and TMP 160 mg.

## ADMINISTRATION/HANDLING

 **IV**

**Reconstitution** • For IV infusion (piggyback), dilute each 5 ml with 75–125 ml $D_5W$. • Do not mix with other drugs or solutions.
**Rate of Administration** • Infuse over 60–90 min. Must avoid bolus or rapid infusion. • Do not give IM. • Ensure adequate hydration.
**Storage** • IV infusion (piggyback) stable for 2 hrs (5 ml/75 ml $D_5W$), 4 hrs (5 ml/100 ml $D_5W$), 6 hrs (5 ml/125 ml $D_5W$). • Discard if cloudy or precipitate forms.

**PO**
• Store tablets, suspension at room temperature. • Administer without regard to meals. • Give with at least 8 oz water.

## ▦ IV INCOMPATIBILITIES

Fluconazole (Diflucan), foscarnet (Foscavir), midazolam (Versed), vinorelbine (Navelbine).

## ▦ IV COMPATIBILITIES

Dexmedetomidine (Precedex), diltiazem (Cardizem), heparin, hydromorphone (Dilaudid), lorazepam (Ativan), magnesium sulfate, morphine, nicardipine (Cardene).

## INDICATIONS/ROUTES/DOSAGE

**Usual Adult/Elderly Dosage Range**
**PO:** 1–2 double-strength tablets q12–24h. **IV:** 8–20 mg/kg/day as trimethoprim in divided doses q6–12h.

**Usual Dosage Range, Children Older Than 2 Mos Mild to Moderate Infection**
**PO: CHILDREN:** 8 mg/kg/day as trimethoprim in divided doses q12h.

**Severe Infections**
**PO: CHILDREN:** 15–20 mg/kg/day as trimethoprim in divided doses q6h.
**IV: CHILDREN:** 8–12 mg/kg/day as trimethoprim in divided doses q6–12h.

**S**

### Dosage in Renal Impairment

| Creatinine Clearance | Dosage |
| --- | --- |
| 15–30 ml/min | 50% of usual dosage |
| Less than 15 ml/min | Not recommended |
| HD | 2.5–10 mg/kg trimethoprim q24h (or 5–20 mg/kg 3 times/wk) (give after HD) |
| CRRT | 2.5–7.5 mg/kg trimethoprim q12h |

### Dosage in Hepatic Impairment
No dose adjustment.

## SIDE EFFECTS

**Frequent:** Anorexia, nausea, vomiting, rash (generally 7–14 days after therapy begins), urticaria. **Occasional:** Diarrhea, abdominal pain, pain/irritation at IV infusion site. **Rare:** Headache, vertigo, insomnia, seizures, hallucinations, depression.

## ADVERSE EFFECTS/ TOXIC REACTIONS

Rash, fever, sore throat, pallor, purpura, cough, shortness of breath may be early signs of serious adverse effects. Fatalities are rare but have occurred in sulfonamide therapy following Stevens-Johnson syndrome, toxic epidermal necrolysis, fulminant hepatic necrosis, agranulocytosis, aplastic anemia, other blood dyscrasias. Myelosuppression, decreased platelet count, severe dermatologic reactions may occur, esp. in the elderly.

## NURSING CONSIDERATIONS

### BASELINE ASSESSMENT

Obtain history for hypersensitivity to trimethoprim or any sulfonamide, sulfite sensitivity, bronchial asthma. Determine serum renal, hepatic, hematologic baselines.

### INTERVENTION/EVALUATION

Monitor daily pattern of bowel activity, stool consistency. Assess skin for rash, pallor, purpura. Check IV site, flow rate. Monitor renal, hepatic, hematology function. Assess I&O. Check for CNS symptoms (headache, vertigo, insomnia, hallucinations). Monitor vital signs at least twice daily. Monitor for cough, shortness of breath. Assess for overt bleeding, ecchymosis, edema.

### PATIENT/FAMILY TEACHING

• Continue medication for full length of therapy. • Space doses evenly around the clock. • Take oral doses with 8 oz water and drink several extra glasses of water daily. • Report immediately any new symptoms, esp. rash, other skin changes, bleeding/bruising, fever, sore throat, diarrhea. • Avoid prolonged exposure to UV, direct sunlight.

## *sulfaSALAzine

**sul**-fa-**sal**-a-zeen
(Apo-Sulfasalazine ✣, Azulfidine, Azulfidine EN-tabs, Salazopyrin ✣, Salazopyrin EN-Tabs ✣)
**Do not confuse Azulfidine with Augmentin or azathioprine, or sulfasalazine with sulfadiazine or sulfisoxazole.**

## ◆CLASSIFICATION

**PHARMACOTHERAPEUTIC:** Sulfonamide. **CLINICAL:** Anti-inflammatory.

## USES

Treatment of mild to moderate ulcerative colitis, adjunctive therapy in severe ulcerative colitis, rheumatoid arthritis (RA), juvenile rheumatoid arthritis. **OFF-LABEL:** Treatment of ankylosing spondylitis, Crohn's disease, psoriasis, psoriatic arthritis.

## PRECAUTIONS

**Contraindications:** Hypersensitivity to sulfasalazine, sulfa, salicylates; porphyria; GI or GU obstruction. **Cautions:** Severe allergies, bronchial asthma, impaired hepatic/renal function, G6PD deficiency, blood dyscrasias, history of recurring or chronic infections.

## ACTION

Modulates local mediators of inflammatory response. **Therapeutic Effect:** Decreases inflammatory response, interferes with GI secretion. Effect appears topical rather than systemic.

## PHARMACOKINETICS

Poorly absorbed from GI tract. Cleaved, absorbed in colon by intestinal bacteria, forming sulfapyridine and mesalamine (5-ASA). Widely distributed. Metabolized via colonic intestinal flora. Primarily excreted in urine. **Half-life:** 5.7–10 hrs.

## ⌛ LIFESPAN CONSIDERATIONS

**Pregnancy/Lactation:** May produce infertility, oligospermia in men while taking medication. Readily crosses placenta; if given near term, may produce jaundice, hemolytic anemia, kernicterus in newborn. Distributed in breast milk. Pt should not breastfeed premature infant or those with hyperbilirubinemia or G6PD deficiency. **Children:** No age-related precautions noted in pts older than 2 yrs. **Elderly:** No age-related precautions noted.

## INTERACTIONS

**DRUG: Hepatotoxic medications** (e.g., acetaminophen, isoniazid, ketoconazole, simvastatin, SSRIs) may increase risk of hepatotoxicity. **HERBAL: Dong quai, St. John's wort** may increase photosensitization. **FOOD:** None known. **LAB VALUES:** None significant.

## AVAILABILITY (Rx)

Tablets (Azulfidine): 500 mg.

🔪 Tablets (Delayed-Release [Azulfidine EN-tabs]): 500 mg.

## ADMINISTRATION/HANDLING

**PO**

• Space doses evenly (intervals not to exceed 8 hrs). • Administer after meals or with food. • Swallow enteric-coated tablets whole; do not break, crush, dissolve, or divide. • Give with 8 oz of water; encourage several glasses of water between meals.

## INDICATIONS/ROUTES/DOSAGE

**Ulcerative Colitis**
**PO: ADULTS, ELDERLY:** Initially, 1 g 3–4 times/day in divided doses q4–6h. **Maximum:** 6 g/day. **Maintenance:** 2 g/day in divided doses at intervals less than or equal to q8h. **CHILDREN 6 YRS AND OLDER:** Initially, 40–60 mg/kg/day in 4–6 divided doses. **Maximum** (initial dose): 4 g/day. **Maintenance:** 30 mg/kg/day in 4 divided doses at intervals less than or equal to q8h. **Maximum (maintenance dose):** 2 g/day.

**Rheumatoid Arthritis (RA)**
**PO:** *(Delayed-Release Tablets):* **ADULTS, ELDERLY:** Initially, 0.5–1 g/day for 1 wk. Increase by 0.5 g/wk, up to 2 g/day in 2 divided doses. **Maximum:** 3 g/day (if response to 2 g/day is inadequate after 12 wks of treatment).

**Juvenile Rheumatoid Arthritis (JRA)**
**PO:** *(Delayed-Release Tablets):* **CHILDREN:** Initially, 10 mg/kg/day. May increase by 10 mg/kg/day at wkly intervals. **Range:** 30–50 mg/kg/day. **Maximum:** 2 g/day.

**Dosage in Renal/Hepatic Impairment**
Use caution.

## SIDE EFFECTS

**Frequent (33%):** Anorexia, nausea, vomiting, headache, oligospermia (generally reversed by withdrawal of drug). **Occasional (3%):** Hypersensitivity reaction (rash, urticaria, pruritus, fever, anemia). **Rare (Less Than 1%):** Tinnitus, hypoglycemia, diuresis, photosensitivity.

## ADVERSE EFFECTS/ TOXIC REACTIONS

Anaphylaxis, Stevens-Johnson syndrome, hematologic toxicity (leukopenia,

**S**

agranulocytosis), hepatotoxicity, nephrotoxicity occur rarely.

## NURSING CONSIDERATIONS

### BASELINE ASSESSMENT
Question for hypersensitivity to medications. Check initial urinalysis, CBC, serum renal function, LFT.

### INTERVENTION/EVALUATION
Monitor I&O, urinalysis, renal function tests; ensure adequate hydration (minimum output 1,500 ml/24 hrs) to prevent nephrotoxicity. Assess skin for rash (discontinue drug, notify physician at first sign). Monitor daily pattern of bowel activity, stool consistency. (Dosage increase may be needed if diarrhea continues, recurs.) Monitor CBC closely; assess for and report immediately any hematologic effects (bleeding, ecchymoses, fever, pharyngitis, pallor, weakness, purpura). Monitor LFT; observe for jaundice.

### PATIENT/FAMILY TEACHING
• May cause orange-yellow discoloration of urine, skin. • Space doses evenly around the clock. • Take after or with food with 8 oz of water; drink several glasses of water between meals. • Swallow enteric-coated tablets whole; do not chew, crush, dissolve, or divide tablets. • Continue for full length of treatment; may be necessary to take drug even after symptoms relieved. • Routinely monitor blood levels. • Inform dentist, surgeon of sulfasalazine therapy. • Avoid exposure to sun, ultraviolet light until photosensitivity determined (may last for mos after last dose).

## *SUMAtriptan

soo-ma-**trip**-tan
(Alsuma, Apo-Sumatriptan ✦,
<u>Imitrex</u>, Onzetra, Sumavel DosePro,
<u>Zecuity</u>, Zembrace SymTouch)

**Do not confuse sumatriptan with saxagliptin, sitagliptin, somatropin, or zolmitriptan.**

### FIXED-COMBINATION(S)
**Treximet:** sumatriptan/naproxen (an NSAID): 85 mg/500 mg, 10 mg/60 mg.

### ◆CLASSIFICATION
**PHARMACOTHERAPEUTIC:** Serotonin 5-HT$_1$ receptor agonist. **CLINICAL:** Antimigraine.

## USES
**PO, SQ, Intranasal, Transdermal:** Acute treatment of migraine headache with or without aura. **SQ:** Treatment of cluster headaches.

## PRECAUTIONS
**Contraindications:** Hypersensitivity to sumatriptan. Management of hemiplegic or basilar migraine, peripheral vascular disease, CVA, ischemic heart disease (including angina pectoris, history of MI, silent ischemia, Prinzmetal's angina), severe hepatic impairment, transient ischemic attack, uncontrolled hypertension, MAOI use within 14 days, use within 24 hrs of ergotamine preparations or another 5-HT$_1$ agonist. **Cautions:** Mild to moderate hepatic impairment, history of seizure disorder, controlled hypertension, elderly.

## ACTION
Binds selectively to serotonin receptors in cranial arteries, producing vasoconstrictive effect on cranial blood vessels. **Therapeutic Effect:** Relieves migraine headache.

## PHARMACOKINETICS

| Route | Onset | Peak | Duration |
|-------|-------|------|----------|
| Nasal | 15 min | N/A | 24–48 hrs |
| PO | 30 min | 2 hrs | 24–48 hrs |
| SQ | 10 min | 1 hr | 24–48 hrs |

S

Rapidly absorbed after SQ administration. Absorption after PO administration is incomplete; significant amounts undergo hepatic metabolism, resulting in low bioavailability (about 14%). Protein binding: 10%–21%. Widely distributed. Undergoes first-pass metabolism in liver. Excreted in urine. **Half-life:** 2 hrs.

## ⌛ LIFESPAN CONSIDERATIONS

**Pregnancy/Lactation:** Unknown if distributed in breast milk. **Children:** Safety and efficacy not established. **Elderly:** No age-related precautions noted.

## INTERACTIONS

**DRUG: Ergotamine-containing medications** may produce vasospastic reaction. **MAOIs** may increase concentration, half-life. **SSRIs** and **SNRI antidepressants** may increase risk of serotonin syndrome. **HERBAL:** None significant. **FOOD:** None known. **LAB VALUES:** None significant.

## AVAILABILITY (Rx)

**Injection, Prefilled Autoinjector (Alsuma):** 6 mg/0.5 ml. **(Zembrace SymTouch):** 3-mg prefilled syringe. **Injection Solution (Imitrex):** 4 mg/0.5 ml, 6 mg/0.5 ml. **(Sumavel DosePro):** 4 mg/0.5 ml, 6 mg/0.5 ml. **Nasal Powder (Onzetra, Xsail): Capsules:** 11 mg (to be used with Xsail breath powdered nasal device). **Nasal Spray (Imitrex Nasal):** 5 mg/actuation, 20 mg/actuation. **Tablets (Imitrex):** 25 mg, 50 mg, 100 mg. **Transdermal (Zecuity):** Delivers 6.5 mg over 4 hrs.

## ADMINISTRATION/HANDLING

### SQ

• Follow manufacturer's instructions for autoinjection device use. • Administer needleless (Sumavel DosePro) only to abdomen or thigh.

### PO

• Swallow tablets whole. Do not break, crush, dissolve, or divide. • Take with full glass of water.

### Nasal

• Unit contains only one spray—do not test before use. • Instruct pt to gently blow nose to clear nasal passages. • With head upright, close one nostril with index finger, breathe out gently through mouth. • Have pt insert nozzle into open nostril about ½ inch, close mouth and, while taking a breath through nose, release spray dosage by firmly pressing plunger. • Instruct pt to remove nozzle from nose and gently breathe in through nose and out through mouth for 10–20 sec; do not breathe in deeply.

### Transdermal

• Apply to dry, intact, nonirritated skin on upper arm or thigh. • After applying, push activate button (red LED); light will turn off when dosing complete and patch can be removed. • Do not swim, bathe, or shower while wearing patch.

## INDICATIONS/ROUTES/DOSAGE

**Acute Migraine Headache**

**PO: ADULTS, ELDERLY:** 25–100 mg. Dose may be repeated after at least 2 hrs. **Maximum:** 100 mg/single dose; 200 mg/24 hrs.

**SQ: ADULTS, ELDERLY:** Up to 6 mg. **Maximum:** Up to two 6-mg injections/24 hrs (separated by at least 1 hr). **(Zembrace SymTouch):** 3-mg single dose. **Maximum:** 12 mg/24 hrs. Separate dose by at least 1 hr.

**Intranasal: ADULTS, ELDERLY: (Spray):** 5–20 mg; may repeat in 2 hrs. **Maximum:** 40 mg/24 hrs. **(Nasal Powder):** 11 mg in each nostril. **Maximum:** 44 mg/24 hrs separated by at least 2 hrs.

**Transdermal: ADULTS, ELDERLY:** 6.5 mg (over 4 hrs). May repeat no sooner than 2 hrs after activation of first patch. **Maximum:** 2 patches in any 24-hr period.

**Dosage in Renal Impairment**
No dose adjustment.

S

**Dosage in Hepatic Impairment**
**Mild to moderate impairment: Maximum PO dose:** 50 mg. **Severe impairment:** Contraindicated.

## SIDE EFFECTS

**Frequent: PO (10%–5%):** Tingling, nasal discomfort. **SQ (greater than 10%):** Injection site reactions, tingling, warm/hot sensation, dizziness, vertigo. **Nasal (greater than 10%):** Altered taste, nausea, vomiting. **Occasional: PO (5%–1%):** Flushing, asthenia, visual disturbances. **SQ (10%–2%):** Burning sensation, numbness, chest discomfort, drowsiness, asthenia. **Nasal (5%–1%):** Nasopharyngeal discomfort, dizziness. **Rare: PO (less than 1%):** Agitation, eye irritation, dysuria. **SQ (less than 2%):** Anxiety, fatigue, diaphoresis, muscle cramps, myalgia. **Nasal (less than 1%):** Burning sensation.

## ADVERSE EFFECTS/ TOXIC REACTIONS

Excessive dosage may produce tremors, redness of extremities, reduced respirations, cyanosis, seizures, paralysis. Serious arrhythmias occur rarely, esp. in pts with hypertension, obesity, smokers, diabetes, strong family history of coronary artery disease. Serotonin syndrome may occur (agitation, confusion, hallucinations, hyper-reflexia, myoclonus, shivering, tachycardia).

## NURSING CONSIDERATIONS

### BASELINE ASSESSMENT

Receive full medical history, medication history and screen for contraindications. Obtain pregnancy test in female pts of reproductive potential. Question regarding onset, location, duration of migraine, possible precipitating symptoms.

### INTERVENTION/EVALUATION

Evaluate for relief of migraine headache and resulting photophobia, phonophobia (sound sensitivity), nausea, vomiting.

### PATIENT/FAMILY TEACHING

• Follow proper technique for loading of autoinjector, injection technique, discarding of syringe. • Do not use more than 2 injections during any 24-hr period and allow at least 1 hr between injections. • Report immediately if wheezing, palpitations, skin rash, facial swelling, pain/tightness in chest/throat occur.

---

## *SUNitinib    `HIGH ALERT`

soo-**nit**-in-ib
(Sutent)

■ **BLACK BOX ALERT** ■ Hepatotoxicity may be severe and/or result in fatal liver failure.
**Do not confuse sunitinib with imatinib or sorafenib.**

## ◆CLASSIFICATION

**PHARMACOTHERAPEUTIC:** Tyrosine kinase inhibitor, vascular endothelial growth factor. **CLINICAL:** Antineoplastic.

## USES

Treatment of GI stromal tumor after disease progression while on or demonstrating intolerance to imatinib. Treatment of advanced renal cell carcinoma. Treatment of pancreatic neuroendocrine tumor (PNET). **OFF-LABEL:** Non-GI stromal tumor, soft tissue sarcomas, advanced thyroid cancer.

## PRECAUTIONS

**Contraindications:** Hypersensitivity to sunitinib. **Cautions:** Cardiac dysfunction, bradycardia, electrolyte imbalance, bleeding tendencies, hypertension, history of prolonged QT interval, medications that prolong QT interval, hypokalemia, hypomagnesemia, concurrent use of strong CYP3A4 inducers or inhibitors, HF, renal/hepatic impairment.

## ACTION

Inhibitory action against multiple kinases, growth factor receptors, stem cell

---

S

factor receptors, colony-stimulating factor receptors, glial cell-line neurotrophic factor receptors. **Therapeutic Effect:** Prevents tumor cell growth, produces tumor regression, inhibits metastasis.

## PHARMACOKINETICS

Metabolized in liver. Protein binding: 95%. Excreted in feces (61%), urine (16%). **Half-life:** 40–60 hrs.

## ⌛ LIFESPAN CONSIDERATIONS

**Pregnancy/Lactation:** Has potential for embryotoxic, teratogenic effects. Breastfeeding not recommended. **Children:** Safety and efficacy not established. **Elderly:** No age-related precautions noted.

## INTERACTIONS

**DRUG: Strong CYP3A4 inhibitors (e.g., clarithromycin, itraconazole, ketoconazole, voriconazole)** may increase concentration, toxicity. **Strong CYP3A4 inducers (e.g., carbamazepine, phenobarbital, phenytoin, rifampin)** may decrease concentration/effects. **HERBAL: St. John's wort** may decrease concentration. **FOOD: Grapefruit products** may increase concentration, potential for torsades de pointes, myelotoxicity. **LAB VALUES:** May increase serum alkaline phosphatase, bilirubin, amylase, lipase, creatinine, ALT, AST. May alter serum potassium, sodium, uric acid. May produce thrombocytopenia, neutropenia. May decrease serum phosphate, thyroid function levels.

## AVAILABILITY (Rx)

**Capsules:** 12.5 mg, 25 mg, 50 mg.

## ADMINISTRATION/HANDLING

**PO**
• Give without regard to food. Avoid grapefruit products.

## INDICATIONS/ROUTES/DOSAGE

**GI Stromal Tumor, Renal Cell Carcinoma**
**PO: ADULTS, ELDERLY:** 50 mg once daily for 4 wks, followed by 2 wks off of 6-wk cycle.

**Pancreatic Neuroendocrine Tumor**
**PO: ADULTS, ELDERLY:** 37.5 mg once daily continuously without a scheduled off-treatment period.

**Dose Modification**
**PO: ADULTS, ELDERLY:** Dosage increase or reduction in 12.5-mg increments is recommended based on safety and tolerability.

**Dosage in Renal Impairment**
No initial dose adjustment; subsequent adjustment may be needed.

**Dosage in Hepatic Impairment**
No dose adjustment initially; grade 3 or 4 hepatotoxicity during treatment: withhold/discontinue if hepatotoxicity does not resolve.

## SIDE EFFECTS

**Stromal tumor: Common (42%–30%):** Fatigue, diarrhea, anorexia, abdominal pain, nausea, hyperpigmentation. **Frequent (29%–18%):** Mucositis/stomatitis, vomiting, asthenia, altered taste, constipation, fever. **Occasional (15%–8%):** Hypertension, rash, myalgia, headache, arthralgia, back pain, dyspnea, cough. **Renal carcinoma: Common (74%–43%):** Fatigue, diarrhea, nausea, mucositis/stomatitis, dyspepsia, altered taste. **Frequent (38%–20%):** Rash, vomiting, constipation, hyperpigmentation, anorexia, arthralgia, dyspnea, hypertension, headache, abdominal pain. **Occasional (18%–11%):** Limb pain, peripheral/periorbital edema, dry skin, hair color change, myalgia, cough, back pain, dizziness, fever, tongue pain, flatulence, alopecia, dehydration.

S

## ADVERSE EFFECTS/ TOXIC REACTIONS

Palmar-plantar erythrodysesthesia syndrome (PPES) occurs occasionally (14%), manifested as blistering/rash/ peeling of skin on palms of hands, soles of feet. Bleeding, decrease in left ventricular ejection fraction, deep vein thrombosis (DVT), pancreatitis, neutropenia, seizures occur rarely.

## NURSING CONSIDERATIONS

### BASELINE ASSESSMENT

Question possibility of pregnancy. Obtain baseline CBC, BMP, LFT before beginning therapy and prior to each treatment. Obtain baseline EKG, thyroid function tests.

### INTERVENTION/EVALUATION

Assess eye area, lower extremities for early evidence of fluid retention. Offer antiemetics to control nausea, vomiting. Monitor daily pattern of bowel activity, stool consistency. Monitor CBC for evidence of neutropenia, thrombocytopenia; assess LFT for hepatotoxicity. Monitor for PPES.

### PATIENT/FAMILY TEACHING

• Avoid crowds, those with known infection. • Avoid contact with anyone who recently received live virus vaccine. • Do not have immunizations without physician's approval (drug lowers resistance). • Avoid pregnancy; use effective contraceptive measures. • Promptly report fever, unusual bruising/bleeding from any site.

## suvorexant

**soo**-voe-**rex**-ant
(Belsomra)

### ◆CLASSIFICATION

**PHARMACOTHERAPEUTIC:** Orexin receptor antagonist. **CLINICAL:** Sedative-hypnotic.

## USES

Treatment of insomnia, characterized by difficulties with sleep onset and/or sleep maintenance.

## PRECAUTIONS

**Contraindications:** Hypersensitivity to suvorexant. History of narcolepsy. **Cautions:** History of COPD, depression, debilitation, drug dependency, obstructive sleep apnea, respiratory disease, pts at high risk of suicide; concomitant use of CNS depressants, strong CYP3A4 inhibitors/inducers. Concomitant use of other insomnia medications not recommended.

## ACTION

Suppresses wake drive of the orexin neuropeptide signaling system, the central promoter of wakefulness. Blocks binding of orexin neuropeptides orexin A and orexin B to receptors of OX1R and OX2R. **Therapeutic Effect:** Induces sleep with fewer nighttime awakenings; improves sleep pattern.

## PHARMACOKINETICS

Rapidly absorbed. Metabolized in liver. Protein binding: greater than 99%. Peak plasma concentration: 2 hrs. Eliminated in feces (66%), urine (23%). **Half-life:** 12 hrs.

## ⌛ LIFESPAN CONSIDERATIONS

**Pregnancy/Lactation:** Unknown if distributed in breast milk. **Children:** Safety and efficacy not established. **Elderly:** No age-related precautions noted.

## INTERACTIONS

**DRUG:** Alcohol, **CNS depressants (e.g., lorazepam, morphine, zolpidem)** may increase CNS depression. **Moderate CYP3A4 inhibitors (e.g., ciprofloxacin, diltiazem), strong CYP3A4 inhibitors (e.g., ketoconazole, clarithromycin)** may increase concentration/effect, CNS depression.

S

CYP3A4 inducers (e.g., rifampin, phenytoin) may decrease concentration/effect. May increase concentration/effect of digoxin. HERBAL: Gotu kola, kava kava, valerian may increase CNS depression. St. John's wort may decrease concentration/effect. FOOD: Meals may decrease absorption/effect. Grapefruit products may increase concentration/effect. LAB VALUES: May increase serum cholesterol.

## AVAILABILITY (Rx)

Tablets: 5 mg, 10 mg, 15 mg, 20 mg.

## ADMINISTRATION/HANDLING

### PO

• Administer no more than once per night, within 30 min of bedtime. • Do not administer unless 7 hrs or greater is dedicated for sleep. • For faster sleep onset, do not give with or immediately after meal.

## INDICATIONS/ROUTES/DOSAGE

### Insomnia

PO: ADULTS, ELDERLY: 10 mg once at bedtime. May increase to 20 mg at bedtime.

### Dose Modification

Concomitant use with other CNS depressants, moderate CYP3A4 inhibitors: Decrease starting dose to 5 mg once at bedtime. May increase to 10 mg once at bedtime. Concomitant use of strong CYP3A4 inhibitors: Not recommended. Daytime somnolence: Decrease dose or discontinue if daytime somnolence.

### Dosage in Renal Impairment

No dose adjustment.

### Dosage in Hepatic Impairment

Mild to moderate impairment: No dose adjustment. Severe impairment: Not recommended.

## SIDE EFFECTS

Occasional (7%): Headache, somnolence. Rare (3%–2%): Dizziness, diarrhea, dry mouth, upper respiratory tract infection, abnormal dreams, cough.

## ADVERSE EFFECTS/ TOXIC REACTIONS

Obese pts and female pts may have increased exposure-related effects compared to nonobese pts and male pts, respectively. May impair daytime wakefulness even when taken as prescribed. Impairment can occur in the absence of symptoms and may not be reliably detected by ordinary clinical exam. CNS depression may persist for up to several days. May increase risk of falling asleep while driving. Abnormal thinking and behavioral changes such as amnesia, anxiety, lowered sexual inhibition, hallucinations, "sleep driving," preparing and eating meals, making phone calls have been reported. May increase risk of suicidal ideation, worsening of depression. Sleep paralysis (inability to move or speak for up to several min during sleep-wake transitions, and hypnagogic/hypnopompic hallucinations including vivid and disturbing perceptions) may occur.

## NURSING CONSIDERATIONS

### BASELINE ASSESSMENT

Assess sleep pattern, ability to fall asleep. Provide environment conductive to restful sleep. Initiate fall precautions. Raise bed rails, provide call light. Receive full medication history including herbal products and screen medication interactions. Question history of co-morbidities esp. mental health disorders, substance abuse.

### INTERVENTION/EVALUATION

Monitor sleep pattern. Evaluate for therapeutic response: decrease in number of nocturnal awakenings, increase

S

in length of sleep. Diligently monitor for daytime somnolence and CNS depressant effects regardless of compliance. Worsening of insomnia, emergence of new cognitive or behavioral abnormalities, or treatment failure after 7–10 days may indicate underlying psychiatric disorder.

### PATIENT/FAMILY TEACHING

• Report nighttime episodes of sleep-driving, preparing food, making phone calls, or having sex while not fully awake. • Do not abruptly discontinue medication after long-term use. • Avoid tasks that require alertness, motor skills until drug response established. • Treatment may cause next-day impairment, drowsiness, or falling asleep while driving despite taking medication as prescribed (esp. pts taking higher doses). • Do not ingest alcohol or grapefruit products. • Do not take drug unless a full night can be dedicated to sleep. • Immediately report worsening of depression or thoughts of suicide.

# tacrolimus

ta-**kroe**-li-mus
(Advagraf ✦, Astagraf XL, Envarsus XR, <u>Prograf</u>, Protopic)

■ **BLACK BOX ALERT** ■ Increased susceptibility to infection and potential for development of lymphoma. Extended-release associated with increased mortality in female liver transplant recipients. Topical form associated with rare cases of malignancy. Topical form should be used only for short-term and intermittent treatment. Use in children less than 2 yrs of age not recommended. Use only 0.03% ointment for children 2–15 yrs of age. Administer under supervision of physician experienced in immunosuppressive therapy.

**Do not confuse Protopic with Protonix, or tacrolimus with everolimus, pimcrolimus, sirolimus, or temsirolimus.**

## ◆CLASSIFICATION

**PHARMACOTHERAPEUTIC:** Immunologic agent. **CLINICAL:** Immunosuppressant.

## USES

**PO/injection:** Prevention of organ rejection in pts receiving allogeneic liver, kidney, heart transplant. Should be used concurrently with adrenal corticosteroids. In heart and kidney transplants pts, should be used in conjunction with azathioprine or mycophenolate. **Topical:** Moderate to severe atopic dermatitis in immunocompetent pts. **OFF-LABEL:** Prevention of organ rejection in lung, small bowel recipients; prevention and treatment of graft-vs-host disease in allogeneic hematopoietic stem cell transplantation.

## PRECAUTIONS

**Contraindications:** Hypersensitivity to tacrolimus. **Cautions:** Hypersensitivity to HCO-60 polyoxyl 60 hydrogenated castor oil (used in solution for injection).

Renal/hepatic impairment, concurrent use with other nephrotoxic drugs (e.g., cyclosporine). Concurrent use of strong CYP3A4 inhibitors or inducers. Avoid use of potassium-sparing diuretics. Pts at risk for pure red cell aplasia (e.g., concurrent use of mycophenolate); pts at risk for QT prolongation, hypokalemia, hypomagnesemia. **Topical:** Exposure to sunlight.

## ACTION

Inhibits T-lymphocyte activation by binding to intracellular proteins, forming a complex, inhibiting phosphatase activity. **Therapeutic Effect:** Suppresses immunologically mediated inflammatory response; prevents organ transplant rejection.

## PHARMACOKINETICS

Variably absorbed after PO administration (food reduces absorption). Protein binding: 99%. Metabolized in liver. Primarily eliminated in feces. Not removed by hemodialysis. **Half-life:** 21–61 hrs.

## ⧗ LIFESPAN CONSIDERATIONS

**Pregnancy/Lactation:** Crosses placenta. Hyperkalemia, renal dysfunction noted in neonates. Distributed in breast milk. Breastfeeding not recommended. **Children:** May require higher dosages (decreased bioavailability, increased clearance). May make post-transplant lymphoproliferative disorder more common, esp. in pts younger than 3 yrs. **Elderly:** Age-related renal impairment may require dosage adjustment.

## INTERACTIONS

**DRUG: Aluminium-containing antacids** may increase concentration. **Strong CYP3A4 inhibitors (e.g., erythromycin, ketoconazole), protease inhibitors, calcium channel blockers (e.g., diltiazem)** may increase concentration/effects. **Strong CYP3A4 inducers (e.g., rifampin)** may decrease concentration/effects. May increase concentration of **cyclosporine. HERBAL: Echinacea,**

T

---

**St. John's wort** may decrease concentration/effects. **FOOD: Food** decreases rate/extent of absorption. **Grapefruit products** may increase concentration, toxicity (potential for nephrotoxicity). **LAB VALUES:** May increase serum glucose, BUN, creatinine, potassium, triglycerides, cholesterol, bilirubin, amylase, ALT, AST. May decrease serum magnesium, Hgb, Hct, platelets. May alter leukocytes.

## AVAILABILITY (Rx)

**Capsules (Prograf):** 0.5 mg, 1 mg, 5 mg. **Injection Solution (Prograf):** 5 mg/ml. **Ointment (Protopic):** 0.03%, 0.1%.

**Capsule, Extended-Release (Astagraf XL):** 0.5 mg, 1 mg, 5 mg. **Tablet, Extended-Release (Envarsus XR):** 0.75 mg, 1 mg, 4 mg.

## ADMINISTRATION/HANDLING

 IV

**Reconstitution** • Dilute with appropriate amount (250–1,000 ml, depending on desired dose) 0.9% NaCl or $D_5W$ to provide concentration between 0.004 and 0.02 mg/ml.
**Rate of Administration** • Give as continuous IV infusion. • Continuously monitor pt for anaphylaxis for at least 30 min after start of infusion. • Stop infusion immediately at first sign of hypersensitivity reaction.
**Storage** • Store diluted infusion solution in glass or polyethylene containers and discard after 24 hrs. • Do not store in PVC container (decreased stability, potential for extraction).

### PO

• Avoid grapefruit products. • **Immediate-Release:** Administer without regard to food. Be consistent with timing of administration.
• **Extended-Release.** Administer at least 1 hr before or 2 hrs after a meal. Do not crush, cut, dissolve, or divide; swallow whole.

### Topical

• For external use only. • Do not cover with occlusive dressing. • Rub gently, completely onto clean, dry skin.

## 🚫 IV INCOMPATIBILITY

Acyclovir.

## 🔷 IV COMPATIBILITIES

Calcium gluconate, dexamethasone (Decadron), diphenhydramine (Benadryl), dobutamine (Dobutrex), dopamine (Intropin), furosemide (Lasix), heparin, hydromorphone (Dilaudid), insulin, leucovorin, lorazepam (Ativan), morphine, nitroglycerin, potassium chloride.

## INDICATIONS/ROUTES/DOSAGE

**Note:** Give initial postoperative dose no sooner than 6 hrs after liver and heart transplants and within 24 hrs of kidney transplant.

**Prevention of Liver Transplant Rejection**
**PO: ADULTS, ELDERLY:** *(Immediate-Release):* 0.1–0.15 mg/kg/day in 2 divided doses 12 hrs apart. Titrate to target trough concentration. **CHILDREN:** 0.15–0.2 mg/kg/day in 2 divided doses 12 hrs apart. Titrate to target trough concentration.
**IV: ADULTS, ELDERLY, CHILDREN:** 0.03–0.05 mg/kg/day as continuous infusion.

**Prevention of Kidney Transplant Rejection**
**PO: ADULTS, ELDERLY:** *(Immediate-Release):* 0.2 mg/kg/day (in combination with azathioprine) in 2 divided doses 12 hrs apart or 0.1 mg/kg/day (in combination with mycophenolate). Titrate to target trough concentration. *(Extended-Release): (With Basiliximab Induction):* (Prior to or within 48 hrs of transplant completion): 0.15 mg/kg once daily (in combination with corticosteroids and mycophenolate). Titrate to target trough concentration. *(Without Basiliximab Induction):* Preoperative dose: 0.1 mg/kg (administer within 12 hrs prior to reperfusion).

T

Postoperative dosing: 0.2 mg/kg once daily (in combination with corticosteroids and mycophenolate). Give at least 4 hrs after preoperative dose and within 12 hrs of reperfusion. Titrate to target trough concentration.
**IV: ADULTS, ELDERLY:** 0.03–0.05 mg/kg/day as continuous infusion.

**Prevention of Heart Transplant Rejection**
**Note:** Recommend in combination with azathioprine or mycophenolate.
**PO: ADULTS, ELDERLY:** Initially, 0.075 mg/kg/day in 2 divided doses 12 hrs apart. Titrate to target trough concentration.
**IV: ADULTS, ELDERLY:** 0.01 mg/kg/day as continuous infusion.

**Atopic Dermatitis**
**Topical: ADULTS, ELDERLY, CHILDREN 15 YRS AND OLDER:** Apply 0.03% or 0.1% ointment to affected area twice daily. **CHILDREN 2–15 YRS:** Use 0.03% ointment. Continue treatment for 1 wk after symptoms have resolved. If no improvement within 6 wks, re-examine to confirm diagnosis.

## SIDE EFFECTS

**Frequent (greater than 30%):** Headache, tremor, insomnia, paresthesia, diarrhea, nausea, constipation, vomiting, abdominal pain, hypertension. **Occasional (29%–10%):** Rash, pruritus, anorexia, asthenia, peripheral edema, photosensitivity.

## ADVERSE EFFECTS/ TOXIC REACTIONS

Nephrotoxicity (characterized by increased serum creatinine, decreased urinary output), neurotoxicity (tremor, headache, altered mental status), pleural effusion occur commonly. Thrombocytopenia, leukocytosis, anemia, atelectasis, sepsis, infection occur occasionally.

## NURSING CONSIDERATIONS

### BASELINE ASSESSMENT

Assess medical history, esp. renal function; medication history, use of other immunosuppressants. Have aqueous solution of epinephrine 1:1,000, $O_2$ available at bedside before beginning IV infusion. Assess pt continuously for first 30 min following start of infusion and at frequent intervals thereafter.

### INTERVENTION/EVALUATION

Closely monitor pts with renal impairment. Monitor lab values, esp. serum creatinine, potassium levels, CBC with differential, LFT. Monitor I&O closely. CBC should be performed wkly during first mo of therapy, twice monthly during second and third mos of treatment, then monthly throughout the first yr. Report any major change in pt assessment.

### PATIENT/FAMILY TEACHING

• Avoid crowds, those with infection. • Report decreased urination, chest pain, headache, dizziness, respiratory infection, rash, unusual bleeding/bruising. • Avoid exposure to sun, artificial light (may cause photosensitivity reaction). • Do not take within 2 hrs of taking antacids. Do not take with grapefruit products.

## *tamoxifen* 🔲 HIGH ALERT

ta-**mox**-fen
(Apo-Tamox ✦, Nolvadex-D ✦, Soltamox)

■ **BLACK BOX ALERT** ■ Serious, possibly life-threatening stroke, pulmonary emboli, uterine malignancy (endometrial adenocarcinoma, uterine sarcoma) have occurred.
**Do not confuse tamoxifen with pentoxifylline, tamsulosin, or temazepam.**

### ◆ CLASSIFICATION

**PHARMACOTHERAPEUTIC:** Nonsteroidal antiestrogen. **CLINICAL:** Antineoplastic.

## USES

Adjunct treatment in advanced breast cancer after primary treatment with

**T**

surgery and radiation, reduce risk of breast cancer in women at high risk, reduce risk of invasive breast cancer in women with ductal carcinoma *in situ* (DCIS), metastatic breast cancer in women and men. **OFF-LABEL:** Ovarian cancer (advanced and/or recurrent), treatment of endometrial cancer; risk reduction in women with Paget's disease of the breast.

## PRECAUTIONS

**Contraindications:** Hypersensitivity to tamoxifen. Concomitant warfarin therapy when used in treatment of breast cancer in high-risk women, history of deep vein thrombosis (DVT) or pulmonary embolism (in high-risk women for breast cancer and in women with DCIS). **Cautions:** Thrombocytopenia, pregnancy, history of thromboembolic events, hyperlipidemia, concomitant strong CYP2D6 inhibitors and/or moderate CYP2D6 inhibitors.

## ACTION

Competes with estradiol for estrogen-receptor binding sites in breast, uterus, vaginal cells. **Therapeutic Effect:** Inhibits DNA synthesis, estrogen response.

## PHARMACOKINETICS

Well absorbed from GI tract. Metabolized in liver. Primarily eliminated in feces. **Half-life:** 7 days.

## ⌛ LIFESPAN CONSIDERATIONS

**Pregnancy/Lactation:** If possible, avoid use during pregnancy, esp. first trimester. May cause fetal harm. Unknown if distributed in breast milk. Breastfeeding not recommended. **Children:** Safe and effective in girls 2–10 yrs with McCune Albright syndrome, precocious puberty. **Elderly:** No age-related precautions noted.

## INTERACTIONS

**DRUG:** May increase effects of **warfarin.** May decrease effects of **anastrozole.** **Cytotoxic agents** may increase risk of thromboembolic events. **Moderate/strong CYP2D6 inhibitors (e.g., fluoxetine, sertraline)** may decrease efficacy and increase risk of breast cancer. **HERBAL:** Avoid **black cohosh, dong quai** in estrogen-dependent tumors. **St. John's wort** may decrease concentration/effects. **FOOD:** None known. **LAB VALUES:** May increase serum cholesterol, calcium, triglycerides, AST, ALT.

## AVAILABILITY (Rx)

**Solution, Oral (Soltamox):** 10 mg/5 ml.
**Tablets:** 10 mg, 20 mg.

## ADMINISTRATION/HANDLING

**PO**
• Give without regard to food. • Use supplied dosing cup for oral solution.

## INDICATIONS/ROUTES/DOSAGE

**Metastatic Breast Cancer**
**(Males and Females)**
**PO: ADULTS, ELDERLY:** 20–40 mg/day. Give doses greater than 20 mg/day in 2 divided doses.

**Breast Cancer Treatment**
**PO: ADJUVANT THERAPY (FEMALES), PRE-MENOPAUSAL WOMEN:** 20 mg once daily for 5 yrs.
**POSTMENOPAUSAL WOMEN:** Duration of 2–3 yrs, followed by an aromatase inhibitor to complete 5 yrs.

**Ductal Carcinoma *in Situ* (DCIS)**
**PO: ADULTS, ELDERLY:** 20 mg once daily for 5 yrs.

**Breast Cancer Risk Reduction**
**PO: ADULTS, ELDERLY:** 20 mg once daily for 5 yrs.

**Dosage in Renal/Hepatic Impairment**
No dose adjustment.

## SIDE EFFECTS

**Frequent: Women (greater than 10%):** Hot flashes, nausea, vomiting. **Occasional: Women (9%–1%):** Changes in menstruation, genital itching, vaginal discharge, endometrial hyperplasia, polyps. **Men:** Impotence, decreased libido. **Men and women:** Headache, nausea, vomiting, rash, bone pain, confusion, weakness, drowsiness.

## ADVERSE EFFECTS/ TOXIC REACTIONS

Retinopathy, corneal opacity, decreased visual acuity noted in pts receiving extremely high dosages (240–320 mg/day) for longer than 17 mos.

## NURSING CONSIDERATIONS

### BASELINE ASSESSMENT

Obtain estrogen receptor assay prior to therapy. Obtain baseline breast and gynecologic exams, mammogram results. CBC, serum calcium levels should be checked before and periodically during therapy.

### INTERVENTION/EVALUATION

Be alert to increased bone pain; ensure adequate pain relief. Monitor I&O, weight. Observe for edema, esp. of dependent areas, signs and symptoms of DVT. Assess for hypercalcemia (increased urinary volume, excessive thirst, nausea, vomiting, constipation, hypotonicity of muscles, deep bone/flank pain, renal stones).

### PATIENT/FAMILY TEACHING

• Report vaginal bleeding/discharge/ itching, leg cramps, weight gain, shortness of breath, weakness. • May initially experience increase in bone, tumor pain (appears to indicate good tumor response). • Report persistent nausea, vomiting. • Nonhormonal contraceptives are recommended during treatment.

# tamsulosin

tam-**soo**-loe-sin
(<u>Flomax</u>, Apo-Tamsulosin ✽)
**Do not confuse Flomax with Flonase, Flovent, Foltx, Fosamax, or Volmax, or tamsulosin with tamoxifen or terazosin.**

## FIXED-COMBINATION(S)

**Jalyn:** tamsulosin/dutasteride (an androgen hormone inhibitor): 0.4 mg/0.5 mg.

## ◆CLASSIFICATION

**PHARMACOTHERAPEUTIC:** Alpha$_1$-adrenergic blocker. **CLINICAL:** Benign prostatic hyperplasia agent.

## USES

Treatment of symptoms of benign prostatic hyperplasia (BPH), alone or in combination with dutasteride (Avodart). **OFF-LABEL:** Treatment of bladder outlet obstruction or dysfunction. Facilitate expulsion of ureteral stones (distal).

## PRECAUTIONS

**Contraindications:** Hypersensitivity to tamsulosin. **Cautions:** Concurrent use of phosphodiesterase (PDE5) inhibitors (e.g., sildenafil, tadalafil, vardenafil), pts with orthostatic hypotension.

## ACTION

Antagonist of alpha receptors in prostate. **Therapeutic Effect:** Relaxes smooth muscle, in bladder neck and prostate, improves urinary flow, symptoms of prostatic hyperplasia.

## PHARMACOKINETICS

Well absorbed, widely distributed. Protein binding: 94%–99%. Metabolized in liver. Primarily excreted in urine. Unknown if removed by hemodialysis. **Half-life:** 9–13 hrs.

## ⏳ LIFESPAN CONSIDERATIONS

**Pregnancy/Lactation:** Not indicated for use in women. **Children:** Not indicated in this pt population. **Elderly:** No age-related precautions noted.

## INTERACTIONS

**DRUG:** Other alpha-adrenergic blocking agents (e.g., doxazosin, prazosin, terazosin) may increase alpha-blockade effects. **Sildenafil, tadalafil,**

T

✽ Canadian trade name     🛇 Non-Crushable Drug     🄷🄸 High Alert drug vardenafil may cause symptomatic hypotension. **CYP3A4 inhibitors (e.g., ketoconazole)** may increase concentration. **HERBAL:** Avoid **saw palmetto** (limited experience with this combination). **Black cohosh, periwinkle** may increase hypotensive effect. **St. John's wort** may decrease concentration/effects. **FOOD: Grapefruit products** may increase potential for orthostatic hypotension. **LAB VALUES:** None known.

## AVAILABILITY (Rx)

**Capsules:** 0.4 mg.

## ADMINISTRATION/HANDLING

**PO**
• Give at same time each day, 30 min after the same meal. • Do not break, crush, or open capsule.

## INDICATIONS/ROUTES/DOSAGE

**Benign Prostatic Hyperplasia (BPH)**
**PO: ADULTS:** 0.4 mg once daily, approximately 30 min after same meal each day. May increase dosage to 0.8 mg if inadequate response in 2–4 wks.

**Dosage in Renal/Hepatic Impairment**
No dose adjustment.

## SIDE EFFECTS

**Frequent (9%–7%):** Dizziness, drowsiness. **Occasional (5%–3%):** Headache, anxiety, insomnia, orthostatic hypotension. **Rare (less than 2%):** Nasal congestion, pharyngitis, rhinitis, nausea, vertigo, impotence.

## ADVERSE EFFECTS/ TOXIC REACTIONS

First-dose syncope (hypotension with sudden loss of consciousness) may occur within 30–90 min after initial dose. May be preceded by tachycardia (pulse rate of 120–160 beats/min).

## NURSING CONSIDERATIONS

### BASELINE ASSESSMENT

Assess history of prostatic hyperplasia (difficulty initiating urine stream, dribbling, sense of urgency, leaking). Question for sensitivity to tamsulosin, or use of other alpha-adrenergic blocking agents. Obtain vital signs.

### INTERVENTION/EVALUATION

Assist with ambulation if dizziness occurs. Monitor renal function, I&O, weight changes, peripheral edema, B/P. Monitor for first-dose syncope.

### PATIENT/FAMILY TEACHING

• Take at same time each day, 30 min after the same meal. • Go from lying to standing slowly. • Avoid tasks that require alertness, motor skills until response to drug is established. • Do not break, crush, open capsule.

# tapentadol

ta-**pen**-ta-dol
(Nucynta, Nucynta ER, Nucynta IR ✦)
**Do not confuse tapentadol with tramadol.**

## ◆CLASSIFICATION

**PHARMACOTHERAPEUTIC:** Centrally acting synthetic analgesic. **CLINICAL:** Analgesic.

## USES

**Nucynta:** Relief of moderate to severe acute pain in adults 18 yrs and older. **Nucynta ER:** Management of moderate to severe chronic or neuropathic pain associated with diabetic peripheral neuropathy when around-the-clock analgesic needed for extended period.

## PRECAUTIONS

**Contraindications:** Hypersensitivity to tapentadol. Severe respiratory depression, acute or severe bronchial asthma, hypercapnia in uncontrolled settings, known or suspected paralytic ileus, concurrent use or ingestion within 14 days of MAOI use. **Cautions:** Respiratory disease or respiratory compromise (e.g., hypoxia, hypercapnia, or decreased respiratory reserve), asthma, COPD, severe obesity, sleep apnea syndrome, CNS depression, pts with head injury, intracranial lesions, pancreatic or biliary disease, renal or hepatic impairment, history of seizures, conditions that increase risk of seizures, pts at risk for hypotension, adrenal insufficiency, concurrent use with serotonergic agents, elderly, debilitated or cachetic pts.

## ACTION

Binds to mu-opioid receptors in the central nervous system, causing inhibition of ascending pain pathways; increases norepinephrine by inhibiting its reabsorption into nerve cells. **Therapeutic Effect:** Produces analgesia.

## PHARMACOKINETICS

Metabolized in liver. Primarily excreted in the urine. Widely distributed. Protein binding: 20%. **Half-life:** 4 hrs.

## ⧗ LIFESPAN CONSIDERATIONS

**Pregnancy/Lactation:** Unknown if drug crosses placenta or is distributed in breast milk. **Children:** Not recommended for use in this pt population. **Elderly:** Age-related renal impairment may increase risk of side effects.

## INTERACTIONS

**DRUG:** Alcohol, **CNS depressants** (e.g., lorazepam, morphine, zolpidem) may increase CNS depression, respiratory depression. **MAOIs, SSRIs** (e.g., fluoxetine), tricyclic antidepressants (e.g., amitriptyline), triptans (e.g., sumatriptan) may increase risk of serotonin syndrome. **HERBAL:** Kava kava, St. John's wort, valerian may increase CNS depression. **St. John's wort** may increase risk for serotonin

syndrome. **FOOD:** None known. **LAB VALUES:** None significant.

## AVAILABILITY (Rx)

**Tablets:** 50 mg, 75 mg, 100 mg.

🍋 **Tablets, Extended-Release:** 50 mg, 100 mg, 150 mg, 200 mg, 250 mg.

## ADMINISTRATION/HANDLING

**PO**
• Give without regard to food. • Tablets may be crushed. • Give extended-release tablets whole; do not break, crush, dissolve, or divide.

## INDICATIONS/ROUTES/DOSAGE

**Note:** Not recommended in severe renal or hepatic impairment.

**Pain Control**
**PO: ADULTS, ELDERLY: Nucynta:** 50–100 mg q4–6h as needed. **Maximum:** 600 mg/day (700 mg on day 1). **Nucynta ER:** Initially, 50 mg twice daily (12 hrs apart). May increase by 50 mg twice daily q3days to effective dose. Range: 100–250 mg twice daily. **Maximum:** 500 mg/day.

**Conversion To Extended-Release**
**Oral Opioids:** Discontinue all other opioids when extended-release tapentadol is initiated. Begin with a dose that is 50% of estimated tapentadol needed with immediate-release rescue medications as a supplement.
**Immediate-Release tapentadol:** Use same total daily dose but divide into 2 equal doses given twice daily. Maximum dose: 500 mg daily.

**Dosage in Renal Impairment**
**CrCl 30 ml/min or greater:** No adjustment. **CrCl less than 30 ml/min:** Not recommended.

**Dosage in Hepatic Impairment**
**Immediate-release:** Moderate impairment: 50 mg q8h. **Maximum:** 3 doses/24 hrs. **Extended-release:** Initially, 50 mg/day. **Maximum:** 100 mg/day.

T

## SIDE EFFECTS

**Frequent (greater than 10%):** Nausea, dizziness, vomiting, sleepiness, headache.

## ADVERSE EFFECTS/ TOXIC REACTIONS

Respiratory depression, serotonin syndrome have been reported.

## NURSING CONSIDERATIONS

### BASELINE ASSESSMENT

Assess onset, type, location, and duration of pain. Obtain vital signs before giving medication. If respirations are 12/min or lower, withhold medication, contact physician. Question history of hepatic impairment.

### INTERVENTION/EVALUATION

Be alert for decreased respirations or B/P. Initiate deep breathing and coughing exercises, particularly in pts with impaired pulmonary function. Assess for clinical improvement and record onset of pain relief.

### PATIENT/FAMILY TEACHING

• Avoid tasks that require alertness, motor skills until response to drug is established. • Avoid alcohol, CNS depressants. • Report nausea, vomiting, shortness of breath, difficulty breathing.

# tedizolid

**ted**-eye-**zoe**-lid
(Sivextro)
**Do not confuse tedizolid with linezolid.**

## ◆CLASSIFICATION

**PHARMACOTHERAPEUTIC:** Oxazolidinone-class antibacterial. **CLINICAL:** Antibiotic.

## USES

Treatment of adult pts with acute bacterial skin and skin structure infections (ABSSSI) caused by susceptible strains of gram-positive microorganisms including *Staphylococcus aureus* (including methicillin-susceptible and methicillin-resistant strains), *Streptococcus agalactiae, Streptococcus anginosus* group (including *S. anginosus, S. intermedius, S. constellatus), Streptococcus pyogenes*, and *Enterococcus faecalis*.

## PRECAUTIONS

**Contraindications:** Hypersensitivity to tedizolid. **Cautions:** History of *Clostridium difficile* infection or antibiotic-associated colitis, myelosuppression, neutropenia, peripheral/optic neuropathy.

## ACTION

Inhibits cellular protein synthesis by binding to 50S subunit of bacterial ribosome. **Therapeutic Effect:** Antibiotic.

## PHARMACOKINETICS

Readily absorbed following PO administration. Protein binding: 70%–90%. Peak plasma concentration: PO: 3 hrs; IV: end of infusion. Eliminated in feces (82%), urine (18%). Minimally removed by hemodialysis. **Half-life:** 12 hrs.

## ⌛ LIFESPAN CONSIDERATIONS

**Pregnancy/Lactation:** Unknown if distributed in breast milk. **Children:** Safety and efficacy not established in pts less than 18 yrs. **Elderly:** No age-related precautions noted.

## INTERACTIONS

**DRUG:** None significant. **HERBAL:** None significant. **FOOD:** None known. **LAB VALUES:** May decrease Hgb, platelets, neutrophils. May increase serum ALT, AST.

## AVAILABILITY (Rx)

**Lyophilized Powder for Injection:** 200 mg/vial. **Tablets:** 200 mg.

## ADMINISTRATION/HANDLING
💧 IV

• Vials contain no preservatives or bacteriostatic agents. • Must reconstitute with Sterile Water for Injection and subsequently dilute with 0.9% NaCl only. • Do not inject as IV push or bolus.

**Reconstitution** • Reconstitute vial with 4 ml of Sterile Water for Injection. • To avoid foaming, alternate between gentle swirling and inversion until powder completely dissolved. If foaming occurs, let vial stand until foam dispersed. • Visually inspect for particulate matter or discoloration. Do not use if particulate matter observed. • Withdraw 4 ml of solution with vial in upright position; do not invert vial during draw-up. • Further dilute in 250 ml 0.9% NaCl. • Gently invert bag to mix; do not shake.

**Rate of Administration** • Infuse over 1 hr via dedicated line.

**Storage** • Reconstituted solution should appear clear, colorless to yellow. • Administer within 24 hrs of reconstitution. • May refrigerate or store solution at room temperature up to 24 hrs.

**PO**
• Give without regard to meal.

### ▨ IV INCOMPATIBILITIES

Any solutions containing divalent cations (e.g., $Ca^{2+}$, $Mg^{2+}$), lactated Ringer's injection. Do not infuse with other medications.

### INDICATIONS/ROUTES/DOSAGE

**Acute Bacterial Skin and Skin Structure Infection**
**PO/IV: ADULTS, ELDERLY:** 200 mg once daily for 6 days.

**Dosage in Renal/Hepatic Impairment**
No dose adjustment.

### SIDE EFFECTS

**Occasional (8%–3%):** Nausea, headache, diarrhea, vomiting. **Rare (2%):** Dizziness, dermatitis, insomnia.

### ADVERSE EFFECTS/ TOXIC REACTIONS

Safety and efficacy in pts with neutropenia not established. Antibacterial activity may be reduced in the absence of granulocytes. *C. difficile*–associated diarrhea with severity ranging from mild diarrhea to fatal colitis has been reported for up to 2 mos following administration. Treatment in the absence of proven or strongly suspected bacterial infection may increase risk of drug-resistant bacteria. Infusion/hypersensitivity reactions (pruritus, urticaria, flushing, hypertension palpitation, tachycardia), optic disorders (asthenopia, blurry vision, neuropathy, visual impairment, vitreous floaters), neurologic disorders (hypoesthesia, paresthesia, peripheral neuropathy, cranial nerve VII paralysis), infections (oral candidiasis, vulvovaginal mycotic infection) occur rarely.

### NURSING CONSIDERATIONS

#### BASELINE ASSESSMENT

Obtain baseline CBC (note WBC, bands), wound culture/sensitivity, vital signs. Question history of recent *C. difficile* infection, hypersensitivity reaction. Assess skin wound characteristics; hydration status. Question pt's usual stool characteristics (color, frequency, consistency).

#### INTERVENTION/EVALUATION

Monitor skin infection/wound for improvement. Monitor daily pattern of bowel activity, stool consistency; increasing severity may indicate antibiotic-associated colitis. If frequent diarrhea occurs, obtain *C. difficile* toxin screen and initiate isolation precautions until result confirmed. Encourage PO intake. Monitor I&O. Monitor for infusion-related/hypersensitivity reaction.

#### PATIENT/FAMILY TEACHING

• It is essential to complete drug therapy despite symptom improvement. Early discontinuation may result in antibacterial resistance or an increased risk of recurrent infection. • Report episodes of diarrhea, esp. following wks after treatment completion. Frequent abdominal pain, blood-streaked stool, diarrhea, fever, may indicate *C. difficile* infection, which may be contagious. • Drink plenty of fluids.

T

# teduglutide

te-due-**gloo**-tide
(Gattex)
**Do not confuse teduglutide with liraglutide or albiglutide, or Gattex with Gas-X.**

## ◆CLASSIFICATION

**PHARMACOTHERAPEUTIC:** Human glucagon-like peptide-II. **CLINICAL:** Short bowel syndrome (short gut syndrome, short gut) agent.

## USES

Treatment of adults with short bowel syndrome (SBS) who are dependent on parenteral support.

## PRECAUTIONS

**Contraindications:** Hypersensitivity to teduglutide. **Cautions:** Cardiovascular disease, HF, pts at increased risk for malignancy, biliary tract (gallbladder, pancreatic) disease, hypervolemia, stenosis, renal impairment.

## ACTION

Analogue of naturally occurring peptide secreted by L cells of distal intestine, known to increase intestinal, portal blood flow, and inhibit gastric secretion. **Therapeutic Effect:** Improves intestinal absorption.

## PHARMACOKINETICS

Degrades into small peptides, amino acids via catabolic pathway. Primarily excreted in urine. Bioavailability: 86–89% following SQ injection. Peak plasma concentration: 3–5 hrs. **Half-life:** 1.3–2 hrs.

## ⧗ LIFESPAN CONSIDERATIONS

**Pregnancy/Lactation:** Unknown if distributed in breast milk. **Children:** Safety and efficacy not established. **Elderly:** No age-related precautions noted.

## INTERACTIONS

**DRUG:** May increase absorption of any **concomitant oral medication. HERBAL:** None significant. **FOOD:** None known. **LAB VALUES:** None significant.

## AVAILABILITY (Rx)

**Injection, Powder for Reconstitution:** 5 mg (delivers maximum of 0.38 ml containing 3.8 mg teduglutide).

## ADMINISTRATION/HANDLING

**SQ**

**Reconstitution** • If diluent syringe (contains 0.5 ml Sterile Water for Injection) has a white snap-off cap, snap or twist off white cap. • If diluent syringe has a gray screw top, unscrew top counter clockwise. • Push prefilled syringe into vial containing teduglutide. • After all diluent has gone into vial, remove syringe, needle and discard. • Allow vial to sit for 30 sec. • Gently roll vial for 15 sec (do not shake) and let stand for 2 min. • Withdraw prescribed dose, discard remaining fluid. • Use within 3 hrs following reconstitution. • Use abdomen, thighs, upper arms for injection. • Avoid injection sites where skin is tender, bruised, red, or hard.

**Storage** • Store kit in refrigerator. • Reconstituted solution should appear as a clear, colorless to light straw-colored liquid. • Discard if particulate is present. • Drug should be completely dissolved before solution is withdrawn from vial.

## INDICATIONS/ROUTES/DOSAGE

**Short Bowel Syndrome**
**SQ: ADULTS/ELDERLY:** 0.05 mg/kg/day.

**Dosage in Moderate to Severe Renal Impairment**
**SQ: ADULTS/ELDERLY: CrCl less than 50 ml/min:** 50% dose reduction.

**Dosage in Hepatic Impairment**
No dose adjustment.

## SIDE EFFECTS

**Frequent (30%–22%):** Abdominal pain, nausea, injection site reactions. **Occasional (18%–14%):** Headache, abdominal distention, vomiting. **Rare (9%):** Flatulence, hypersensitivity, appetite disorders, sleep disturbances.

## ADVERSE EFFECTS/ TOXIC REACTIONS

Upper respiratory tract infection occurs in 12% of pts. Fluid overload (hypervolemia) has been noted in 7% of pts. Potential for hypovolemia is increased in pts with cardiovascular disease, HF. Therapy increases risk for acceleration for neoplastic growth. Cholecystitis, cholangitis, cholelithiasis, pancreatitis has been reported.

## NURSING CONSIDERATIONS

### BASELINE ASSESSMENT

Obtain baseline serum chemistries, LFT, lipase, amylase. Colonoscopy (or alternate imaging) with removal of polyps should be completed within 5 mos prior to initiating treatment.

### INTERVENTION/EVALUATION

Follow-up colonoscopy (or alternate imaging) is recommended at the end of 1 year. If no polyp is found, subsequent colonoscopies should be done no less frequently than every 5 years. If a polyp is found, adherence to current polyp follow-up guidelines is recommended. Discovery of intestinal obstruction, intestinal malignancy necessitates discontinuation of treatment. Subsequent laboratory assessments, LFT is recommended every 6 mos. If clinically meaningful elevation is seen, further diagnostic workup is recommended as clinically indicated.

### PATIENT/FAMILY TEACHING

• Teach proper use and administration of medication. • Be aware of need for any new supplies. • Instruct pt in preparation of medication and observe correct administration technique. • Report yellowing of skin or eyes, dark urine, changes in stool color or consistency, severe abdominal pain, nausea, vomiting, sudden weight gain, swelling, or difficulty breathing.

# telavancin

tel-a-**van**-sin
(Vibativ)

■ **BLACK BOX ALERT** ■ Pts with preexisting renal impairment (CrCl less than 50 mL/min) who are treated for hospital-acquired pneumonia may have increased mortality risk when compared to vancomycin. May cause new or worsening renal impairment. May cause fetal harm (low birth weight, limb malformations). Women of childbearing potential should have pregnancy test before treatment; avoid use during pregnancy unless benefit to pt outweighs fetal risk.
**Do not confuse telavancin with dalbavancin or oritavancin; or Vibativ with Vibra-Tabs or vigabatrin.**

## ◆CLASSIFICATION

**PHARMACOTHERAPEUTIC:** Lipoglycopeptide antibacterial. **CLINICAL:** Antibiotic.

## USES

Treatment of complicated skin, soft tissue infections (cSSSI) caused by gram-positive microorganisms, including methicillin-susceptible or methicillin-resistant *S. aureus*, vancomycin-susceptible *Enterococcus*. Treatment of hospital-acquired and ventilator-associated bacterial pneumonia (HABP/VABP) caused by susceptible isolates of *S. aureus*.

## PRECAUTIONS

**Contraindications:** Prior hypersensitivity reactions to telavancin. Concomitant use of IV unfractionated heparin. **Cautions:** Renal impairment, concurrent therapy with other nephrotoxic medications (e.g.,

**T**

NSAIDs, ACE inhibitors, aminoglycosides). Avoid use in pts with history of congenital QT syndrome, known prolongation of QT interval, uncompensated HF, severe left ventricular hypertrophy, or receiving treatment with other drugs known to prolong QT interval, hypokalemia, hypomagnesemia, known vancomycin hypersensitivity.

## ACTION

Inhibits bacterial cell wall synthesis by blocking polymerization and cross-linking of peptidoglycan. Disrupts membrane potential and changes cell wall permeability. **Therapeutic Effect:** Bactericidal. Antibiotic.

## PHARMACOKINETICS

Not metabolized in liver; pathway unspecified. Protein binding: 90%. Primarily excreted unchanged in urine. Not removed by hemodialysis. **Half-life:** 8–9 hrs.

## ⌛ LIFESPAN CONSIDERATIONS

**Pregnancy/Lactation:** May cause fetal harm at regular dosage. Unknown if distributed in breast milk. **Children:** Safety and efficacy not established. **Elderly:** Age-related renal impairment may increase risk of nephrotoxicity; dosage adjustment recommended.

## INTERACTIONS

**DRUG:** Telavancin may increase levels/effects of **dronedarone, nilotinib, pimozide, quinine, tetrabenazine, thioridazine, ziprasidone. Cipro-floxacin** may increase concentration/effects. **HERBAL:** None significant. **FOOD:** None known. **LAB VALUES:** May alter serum potassium. May increase serum bilirubin, ALT, AST, BUN, creatinine; PT, aPTT, INR. May decrease Hgb, Hct, WBC count.

## AVAILABILITY (Rx)

**Injection, Powder for Reconstitution:** 250 mg, 750 mg.

## ADMINISTRATION/HANDLING

**IV**

◀ **ALERT** ▶ Give by intermittent IV infusion (piggyback). Do not give by IV push (may result in hypotension).
**Reconstitution** • Reconstitute with 45 ml Sterile Water for Injection, D$_5$W, or 0.9% NaCl to provide concentration of 15 mg/ml (total volume approximately 50 ml). • Prior to administration, further dilute with D$_5$W or 0.9% NaCl to final concentration of 0.6–8 mg/ml. • Do not shake.
**Rate of Administration** • Infuse over at least 60 min. Flush line with D$_5$W or 0.9% NaCl before and after administration.
**Storage** • Discard if particulate is present. • Following reconstitution, drug is stable for 4 hrs at room temperature or 72 hrs if refrigerated in vial or infusion bag.

## ▦ IV INCOMPATIBILITIES

Amphotericin, colistimethate, levofloxacin (Levaquin), micafungin (Mycomine).

## ▦ IV COMPATIBILITIES

Azithromycin, caspofungin, cefepime, ceftazidime, ceftriaxone, ciprofloxacin, doripenem, doxycycline, gentamicin, ertapenem, fluconazole, meropenem, tobramycin, pantoprazole, piperacillin-tazobactam, tigecycline.

## INDICATIONS/ROUTES/DOSAGE

**Usual Parenteral Dosage**
**IV Infusion: ADULTS, ELDERLY:** 10 mg/kg once every 24 hrs for 7–14 days (cSSSI); 14–21 days (HABP/VABP). Duration based on severity, infection site, and clinical progress of pt.

**Dosage in Renal Impairment**

| Creatinine Clearance | Dosage |
|---|---|
| 50 ml/min or greater | 10 mg/kg every 24 hrs |
| 30–49 ml/min | 7.5 mg/kg every 24 hrs |
| 10–29 ml/min | 10 mg/kg every 48 hrs |
| Less than 10 ml/min | No dose adjustment (not studied) |

T

**Dosage in Hepatic Impairment**

No dose adjustment (unless concomitant renal impairment).

## SIDE EFFECTS

**Frequent (33%–27%):** Altered taste, nausea. **Occasional (14%–6%):** Vomiting, foamy urine, diarrhea, dizziness, pruritus. **Rare (4%–2%):** Rigors, rash, infusion site pain, anorexia, infusion site erythema.

## ADVERSE EFFECTS/ TOXIC REACTIONS

Nephrotoxicity (acute kidney injury, acute tubular necrosis, renal failure), diarrhea due to *C. difficile* may occur. "Red-man syndrome" (characterized by erythema on face, neck, upper torso), tachycardia, hypotension, myalgia, angioedema may occur from too-rapid rate of infusion.

## NURSING CONSIDERATIONS

### BASELINE ASSESSMENT

Obtain pregnancy test prior to treatment. Obtain baseline serum BUN, creatinine, creatinine clearance prior to initiating therapy, every 48–72 hrs, and after treatment is completed. Obtain culture and sensitivity tests before giving first dose (therapy may begin before results are known).

### INTERVENTION/EVALUATION

Monitor renal function tests, I&O. Assess skin for rash. Avoid rapid infusion ("red-man syndrome"). Monitor daily pattern of bowel activity, stool consistency. Obtain *C. Difficile* PCR test if diarrhea occurs.

### PATIENT/FAMILY TEACHING

• Use effective contraception during treatment. • Report rash, signs/symptoms of nephrotoxicity, diarrhea. • Blood levels will be monitored routinely.

# telmisartan

tel-mi-**sar**-tan
(Micardis)

■ **BLACK BOX ALERT** ■ May cause fetal injury, mortality. Discontinue as soon as possible once pregnancy is detected.

## FIXED-COMBINATION(S)

**Micardis HCT:** telmisartan/ hydrochlorothiazide (a diuretic): 40 mg/12.5 mg, 80 mg/12.5 mg. **Twynsta:** telmisartan/amlodipine (a calcium channel blocker): 40 mg/5 mg, 40 mg/10 mg, 80 mg/5 mg, 80 mg/10 mg.

## ◆CLASSIFICATION

**PHARMACOTHERAPEUTIC:** Angiotensin II receptor antagonist. **CLINICAL:** Antihypertensive.

## USES

Treatment of hypertension alone or in combination with other antihypertensives. Reduces cardiovascular risk in pts 55 yrs of age and older unable to take ACE inhibitors and at high risk of major cardiovascular event (e.g., MI, stroke).

## PRECAUTIONS

**Contraindications:** Hypersensitivity to telmisartan. Concurrent use with aliskiren in pts with diabetes. **Cautions:** Hypovolemia, hepatic/renal impairment, renal artery stenosis (unilateral, bilateral), biliary obstructive disease, significant aortic/mitral stenosis. Concurrent use with ramipril not recommended. Avoid potassium supplements.

## ACTION

Blocks vasoconstrictor and aldosterone-secreting effects of angiotensin II, inhibiting binding of angiotensin II to $AT_1$ receptors. **Therapeutic Effect:** Causes vasodilation, decreases peripheral resistance, decreases B/P.

T

## PHARMACOKINETICS

| Route | Onset | Peak | Duration |
|---|---|---|---|
| PO (reduce B/P) | 1–2 hrs | — | 24 hrs |

Rapidly, completely absorbed. Protein binding: greater than 99%. Metabolized in liver. Excreted in feces. Unknown if removed by hemodialysis. **Half-life:** 24 hrs.

## ⌛ LIFESPAN CONSIDERATIONS

**Pregnancy/Lactation:** May cause fetal harm. Unknown if drug is distributed in breast milk. **Children:** Safety and efficacy not established. **Elderly:** No age-related precautions noted.

## INTERACTIONS

**DRUG: NSAIDs** may decrease antihypertensive effect. May increase **digoxin** concentration, risk of toxicity. **HERBAL: Ephedra, ginger, licorice, ginseng, yohimbe** may worsen hypertension. **Black cohosh, periwinkle** may increase antihypertensive effect. **FOOD:** None known. **LAB VALUES:** May increase serum BUN, creatinine, uric acid, cholesterol. May decrease Hgb, Hct.

## AVAILABILITY (Rx)

**Tablets:** 20 mg, 40 mg, 80 mg.

## ADMINISTRATION/HANDLING

**PO**
• Give without regard to meals.

## INDICATIONS/ROUTES/DOSAGE

**Hypertension**
**PO: ADULTS, ELDERLY:** Initially, 40 mg once daily. Usual range: 40–80 mg/day.

**Cardiovascular Risk Reduction**
**PO: ADULTS, ELDERLY:** 80 mg once daily.

**Dosage in Renal Impairment**
No dose adjustment.

**Dosage in Hepatic Impairment**
Use with caution.

## SIDE EFFECTS

**Occasional (7%–3%):** Upper respiratory tract infection, sinusitis, back/leg pain, diarrhea. **Rare (1%):** Dizziness, headache, fatigue, nausea, heartburn, myalgia, cough, peripheral edema.

## ADVERSE EFFECTS/ TOXIC REACTIONS

Overdosage may manifest as hypotension, tachycardia; bradycardia occurs less often.

## NURSING CONSIDERATIONS

### BASELINE ASSESSMENT

Obtain B/P, apical pulse immediately before each dose, in addition to regular monitoring (be alert to fluctuations). If excessive reduction in B/P occurs, place pt in supine position, feet slightly elevated. Assess medication history (esp. diuretics). Question for history of hepatic/renal impairment, renal artery stenosis. Obtain serum BUN, creatinine, Hgb, Hct, vital signs (particularly B/P, pulse rate).

### INTERVENTION/EVALUATION

Monitor B/P, pulse, serum electrolytes, renal function. Monitor for hypotension when initiating therapy.

### PATIENT/FAMILY TEACHING

• Avoid tasks that require alertness, motor skills until response to drug is established (possible dizziness effect). • Maintain proper hydration. • Avoid pregnancy. • Immediately report suspected pregnancy. • Report any sign of infection (sore throat, fever). • Avoid excessive exertion during hot weather (risk of dehydration, hypotension).

## temazepam

te-**maz**-e-pam
(Apo-Temazepam ✦, Restoril)
**Do not confuse Restoril with Risperdal, Vistaril, or Zestril, or temazepam with flurazepam, lorazepam, or clonazepam.**

**T**

## ◆CLASSIFICATION

**PHARMACOTHERAPEUTIC:** Benzodiazepine **(Schedule IV). CLINICAL:** Sedative-hypnotic.

## USES

Short-term treatment of insomnia.

## PRECAUTIONS

**Contraindications:** Hypersensitivity to temazepam. Narrow-angle glaucoma, CNS depression, pregnancy, breastfeeding, severe, uncontrolled pain, sleep apnea. **Cautions:** Mental impairment, elderly, pts with drug dependence potential.

## ACTION

Enhances action of inhibitory neurotransmitter gamma-aminobutyric acid (GABA), resulting in CNS depression. **Therapeutic Effect:** Induces sleep.

## PHARMACOKINETICS

Well absorbed from GI tract. Protein binding: 96%. Widely distributed. Crosses blood-brain barrier. Metabolized in liver. Primarily excreted in urine. Not removed by hemodialysis. **Half-life:** 9.5–12.4 hrs.

## ⧗ LIFESPAN CONSIDERATIONS

**Pregnancy/Lactation:** Crosses placenta. May be distributed in breast milk. Chronic ingestion during pregnancy may produce withdrawal symptoms, CNS depression in neonates. **Children:** Not recommended in pts younger than 18 yrs. **Elderly:** Use small initial doses with gradual dosage increases to avoid ataxia, excessive sedation.

## INTERACTIONS

**DRUG:** Alcohol, other **CNS depressants** (e.g., lorazepam, morphine, zolpidem) may increase CNS depression. **HERBAL: St. John's wort** may decrease concentration. **Gotu kola, kava kava, St. John's wort, valerian** may increase CNS depression. **FOOD:** None known. **LAB VALUES:** None significant.

## AVAILABILITY (Rx)

**Capsules:** 7.5 mg, 15 mg, 22.5 mg, 30 mg.

## ADMINISTRATION/HANDLING

**PO**
• Give without regard to meals. • Capsules may be emptied and mixed with food.

## INDICATIONS/ROUTES/DOSAGE

**Insomnia**
**PO: ADULTS:** 15–30 mg at bedtime. **ELDERLY, DEBILITATED:** 7.5–15 mg at bedtime.

**Dosage in Renal/Hepatic Impairment**
No dose adjustment.

## SIDE EFFECTS

**Frequent:** Drowsiness, sedation, rebound insomnia (may occur for 1–2 nights after drug is discontinued), dizziness, confusion, euphoria. **Occasional:** Asthenia, anorexia, diarrhea. **Rare:** Paradoxical CNS excitement, restlessness (particularly in elderly, debilitated pts).

## ADVERSE EFFECTS/ TOXIC REACTIONS

Abrupt or too-rapid withdrawal may result in pronounced restlessness, irritability, insomnia, hand tremor, abdominal/muscle cramps, vomiting, diaphoresis, seizures. Overdose results in drowsiness, confusion, diminished reflexes, respiratory depression, coma. **Antidote:** Flumazenil (see Appendix J for dosage).

## NURSING CONSIDERATIONS

### BASELINE ASSESSMENT

Question for possibility of pregnancy before initiating therapy. Assess B/P, pulse, respirations immediately before administration. Raise bed rails. Provide environment conducive to sleep (back rub, quiet environment, low lighting). Assess mental status, sleep patterns.

T

---

◆ Canadian trade name     ⬛ Non-Crushable Drug     **HIGH ALERT** High Alert drug

### INTERVENTION/EVALUATION

Assess elderly or debilitated pts for paradoxical reaction, particularly during early therapy. Monitor respiratory, cardiovascular, mental status. Evaluate for therapeutic response: decrease in number of nocturnal awakenings, increase in length of sleep.

### PATIENT/FAMILY TEACHING

• Avoid alcohol, other CNS depressants. • Avoid tasks that require alertness, motor skills until response to drug is established. • May cause daytime drowsiness. • Take approximately 30 min before bedtime. • Inform physician if pregnant or planning to become pregnant.

---

## temozolomide HIGH ALERT

tem-oh-**zoe**-loe-myde
(Temodal , Temodar)
**Do not confuse Temodar with Tambocor.**

### ◆CLASSIFICATION

**PHARMACOTHERAPEUTIC:** Imidazotetrazine derivative, alkylating agent. **CLINICAL:** Antineoplastic.

### USES

Treatment of adults with refractory anaplastic astrocytoma, newly diagnosed glioblastoma multiforme (concomitantly with radiotherapy, then as maintenance therapy). **OFF-LABEL:** Malignant glioma, metastatic melanoma, metastatic CNS lesions, cutaneous T-cell lymphomas, advanced neuroendocrine tumors, soft tissue sarcoma, pediatric neuroblastoma. Ewing's sarcoma (recurrent or progressive).

### PRECAUTIONS

**Contraindications:** Hypersensitivity to temozolomide, dacarbazine. **Cautions:** Severe renal/hepatic impairment, pregnancy.

### ACTION

Produces cytotoxic effect through alkylation of DNA causing DNA double strand breaks and apoptosis. **Therapeutic Effect:** Inhibits DNA replication, causing cell death.

### PHARMACOKINETICS

Rapidly, completely absorbed after PO administration. Protein binding: 15%. Peak plasma concentration: 1 hr. Penetrates blood-brain barrier. Eliminated in urine (38%), feces (19%). **Half-life:** 1.6–1.8 hrs.

###  LIFESPAN CONSIDERATIONS

**Pregnancy/Lactation:** May cause fetal harm. May produce malformation of external organs, soft tissue, skeleton. If possible, avoid use during pregnancy. Unknown if drug is distributed in breast milk. **Children:** Safety and efficacy not established. **Elderly:** Pts older than 70 yrs may experience higher risk of developing grade 4 neutropenia, grade 4 thrombocytopenia.

### INTERACTIONS

**DRUG: Medications causing blood dyscrasias** (altering blood cell counts) may increase leukopenic, thrombocytopenic effects. **Valproic acid** may decrease oral clearance. **Bone marrow depressants** may increase myelosuppression. **Live virus vaccines** may potentiate virus replication, increase vaccine side effects, decrease pt's antibody response to vaccine. **HERBAL: Echinacea** may decrease effects. **FOOD: All foods** decrease rate, extent of drug absorption. **LAB VALUES:** May decrease Hgb, neutrophils, platelets, WBC count, lymphocytes.

### AVAILABILITY (Rx)

**Capsules:** 5 mg, 20 mg, 100 mg, 140 mg, 180 mg, 250 mg. **Injection, Powder for Reconstitution:** 100 mg.

### ADMINISTRATION/HANDLING

**IV**

• Reconstitute each 100-mg vial with 41 ml Sterile Water for Injection to provide concentration of 2.5 mg/ml. • Swirl gently; do not shake. • Do NOT further

---

dilute. • Infuse over 90 min. • Stable for 14 hrs (includes infusion time).

## PO

• Food reduces rate, extent of absorption; increases risk of nausea, vomiting. • For best results, administer at bedtime. • Give capsule whole with glass of water. Do not break, open, or crush capsules.

## INDICATIONS/ROUTES/DOSAGE

### Anaplastic Astrocytoma (Refractory)

**IV Infusion, PO: ADULTS, ELDERLY:** Initially, 150 mg/m²/day for 5 consecutive days of 28-day treatment cycle. Subsequent doses of 100–200 mg/m²/day based on platelet count, absolute neutrophil count (ANC) during previous cycle. **ANC greater than 1,500/mm³ and platelets more than 100,000/mm³ Maintenance:** 200 mg/m²/day for 5 days q4wks. Continue until disease progression is observed. Minimum: 100 mg/m²/day for 5 days q4wks.

### Glioblastoma Multiforme

**Note:** *Pneumocystis carinii* pneumonia (PCP) prophylaxis required during concomitant phase and continue in pts who develop lymphocytopenia until recovery to grade 1 or less. **IV Infusion, PO: ADULTS, ELDERLY:** 75 mg/m² daily for 42 days (with focal radiotherapy). **Maintenance: (begin 4 wks after concomitant phase): (Cycle 1):** 150 mg/m² once daily for 5 days followed by 23 days without treatment. **(Cycles 2–6):** May increase to 200 mg/m² once daily for 5 days followed by 23 days without treatment if ANC greater than 1,500/mm³, platelets greater than 100,000/mm³, and nonhematologic toxicity with previous cycle.

### Dosage in Renal/Hepatic Impairment

No dose adjustment. Use caution in severe hepatic impairment.

## SIDE EFFECTS

**Frequent (53%–33%):** Nausea, vomiting, headache, fatigue, constipation, seizure. **Occasional (16%–10%):** Diarrhea, asthenia, fever, dizziness, peripheral edema, incoordination, insomnia. **Rare (9%–5%):** Paresthesia, drowsiness, anorexia, urinary incontinence, anxiety, pharyngitis, cough.

## ADVERSE EFFECTS/TOXIC REACTIONS

Myelosuppression is characterized by neutropenia and thrombocytopenia, with elderly and women showing higher incidence of developing severe myelosuppression. Usually occurs within first few cycles; is not cumulative. Nadir occurs in approximately 26–28 days, with recovery within 14 days of nadir. May increase occurrence of pneumocystis carinii pneumonia, myelodysplastic syndrome including myeloid leukemia, or secondary malignancies.

## NURSING CONSIDERATIONS

### BASELINE ASSESSMENT

Obtain baseline CBC. Before dosing, ANC must be greater than 1,500/mm³ and platelet count greater than 100,000/mm³. Potential for nausea, vomiting (readily controlled with antiemetic therapy).

### INTERVENTION/EVALUATION

Obtain CBC on day 22 (21 days after first dose) or within 48 hrs of that day, and wkly, until ANC is greater than 1,500/mm³ and platelet count is greater than 100,000/mm³. Monitor for hematologic toxicity (fever, sore throat, signs of local infection, unusual bruising/bleeding from any site), symptoms of anemia (excessive fatigue, weakness).

### PATIENT/FAMILY TEACHING

• To reduce nausea/vomiting, take on an empty stomach. • Promptly report fever, sore throat, signs of local infection, unusual bruising/bleeding from any site, or difficulty breathing. • Avoid crowds, those with infection. • Do not have immunizations without physician's approval. • Avoid pregnancy.

T

---

✤ Canadian trade name        🗡 Non-Crushable Drug        🔲 High Alert drug

# temsirolimus

tem-sir-**oh**-li-mus
(Torisel)
**Do not confuse temsirolimus with everolimus, sirolimus, or tacrolimus.**

## ◆CLASSIFICATION

**PHARMACOTHERAPEUTIC:** Kinase inhibitor. **CLINICAL:** Antineoplastic.

## USES

Treatment of advanced renal cell carcinoma.

## PRECAUTIONS

**Contraindications:** Hypersensitivity to temsirolimus. Moderate-severe hepatic impairment; bilirubin greater than 1.5 times upper limit of normal (ULN). **Cautions:** Hypersensitivity to sirolimus, mild hepatic impairment, diabetes mellitus, hyperlipidemia. Concurrent use with other medication that may cause angioedema (e.g., ACE inhibitors).

## ACTION

Prevents activation of mTOR (mammalian target of rapamycin), preventing tumor cell division. **Therapeutic Effect:** Inhibits tumor cell growth, produces tumor regression.

## PHARMACOKINETICS

Metabolized in liver. Eliminated primarily in feces. **Half-life:** 17 hrs.

## ⌛ LIFESPAN CONSIDERATIONS

**Pregnancy/Lactation:** May cause fetal harm. Unknown if distributed in breast milk. **Children:** Safety and efficacy not established. **Elderly:** No age-related precautions noted.

## INTERACTIONS

**DRUG:** CYP3A4 inhibitors (e.g., <u>atazanavir</u>, <u>clarithromycin</u>, <u>ketoconazole</u>, <u>ritonavir</u>) may increase concentration. CYP3A4 inducers (e.g., <u>carbamazepine</u>, <u>rifampin</u>) may decrease concentration. **FOOD: Grapefruit products** may increase plasma concentration. **HERBAL: St. John's wort** may decrease plasma concentration. Herbs with hypoglycemic properties (**e.g., garlic, ginger, ginseng**) may increase risk for hypoglycemia. **LAB VALUES:** May increase serum bilirubin, alkaline phosphatase, AST, creatinine, glucose, cholesterol, triglycerides. May decrease WBCs, neutrophils, Hgb, platelets, serum phosphorus, potassium.

## AVAILABILITY (Rx)

**Injection Solution Kit:** 25 mg/ml supplied with 1.8-ml diluent vial.

## ADMINISTRATION/HANDLING

 **IV**

**Reconstitution •** Inject 1.8 ml of diluent into vial. • The vial contains an overfill of 0.2 ml (30 mg/1.2 ml). • Due to the overfill, the drug concentration of resulting solution will be 10 mg/ml. • A total volume of 3 ml will be obtained, including the overfill. • Mix well by inverting the vial. Allow sufficient time for air bubbles to subside. • Mixture must be injected rapidly into 250 ml 0.9% NaCl. • Invert bag to mix; avoid excessive shaking (may cause foaming).
**Rate of Administration •** Administer through an in-line filter not greater than 5 microns; infuse over 30–60 min. • Final diluted infusion solution should be completed within 6 hrs from the time drug solution and diluent mixture is added to the 250 ml 0.9% NaCl.
**Storage •** Refrigerate kit. • Reconstituted solution appears clear to slightly turbid, colorless to yellow, and free from visible particulates. • The 10 mg/ml drug solution/diluent mixture is stable for up to 24 hrs at room temperature. • Solutions diluted for infusion (in 250 ml 0.9% NaCl) must be infused within 6 hrs of preparation.

## 🔲 IV INCOMPATIBILITIES

Both acids and bases degrade solution; combinations of temsirolimus with agents capable of modifying solution pH should be avoided.

## INDICATIONS/ROUTES/DOSAGE

◀ALERT▶ Pretreat with IV diphenhydramine 25–50 mg, 30 min before infusion.

**Renal Cancer**
**IV: ADULTS/ELDERLY:** 25 mg once wkly. Treatment should continue until disease progresses or unacceptable toxicity occurs.

**Dosage with Concomitant CYP3A4 Inhibitors/Inducers**
**Inhibitors:** Consider dosage of 12.5 mg/wk. **Inducers:** Consider dosage of 50 mg/wk.

**Dosage in Renal Impairment**
No dose adjustment.

**Dosage in Hepatic Impairment**
**Mild impairment:** Reduce dose to 15 mg/wk. **Moderate to severe impairment:** Contraindicated.

## SIDE EFFECTS

**Common (51%–32%):** Asthenia, rash, mucositis, nausea, edema (facial edema, peripheral edema), anorexia. **Frequent (28%–20%):** Generalized pain, dyspnea, diarrhea, cough, fever, abdominal pain, constipation, back pain, impaired taste. **Occasional (19%–8%):** Weight loss, vomiting, pruritus, chest pain, headache, nail disorder, insomnia, nosebleed, dry skin, acne, chills, myalgia.

## ADVERSE EFFECTS/ TOXIC REACTIONS

UTI occurs in 15% of pts, hypersensitivity reaction in 9%, pneumonia in 8%, upper respiratory tract infection, hypertension, conjunctivitis in 7%.

## NURSING CONSIDERATIONS

### BASELINE ASSESSMENT

Question possibility of pregnancy. Obtain baseline CBC, serum chemistries, renal function, LFT routinely thereafter.

### INTERVENTION/EVALUATION

Offer antiemetics to control nausea, vomiting. Monitor daily pattern of bowel frequency, stool consistency. Assess skin for evidence of rash, edema. Monitor CBC, particularly Hgb, platelets, neutrophil count; LFT, renal function tests. Monitor for shortness of breath, fatigue, hypertension. Assess oropharynx for stomatitis, mucositis.

### PATIENT/FAMILY TEACHING

• Avoid crowds, those with known infection. • Avoid contact with anyone who recently received live virus vaccine. • Do not have immunizations without physician's approval (drug lowers body resistance). • Promptly report fever, unusual bruising/bleeding from any site.

## *tenecteplase* HIGH ALERT

ten-**eck**-te-plase
(TNKase)
**Do not confuse TNKase with tPA.**

### ◆CLASSIFICATION

**PHARMACOTHERAPEUTIC:** Tissue plasminogen activator. **CLINICAL:** Thrombolytic.

## USES

Management of ST-elevation myocardial infarction (STEMI) for lysis of thrombi to restore perfusion and reduce mortality.

## PRECAUTIONS

**Contraindications:** Hypersensitivity to tenecteplase. Active internal bleeding, cerebral aneurysm, AV malformation, bleeding diathesis, history of CVA, intracranial or intraspinal surgery or trauma within past 2 mos, intracranial neoplasm, severe uncontrolled hypertension. **Cautions:** Recent major surgery, GI or genitourinary (GU) bleeding, trauma, acute pericarditis, subacute bacterial endocarditis, pregnancy, severe hepatic impairment, hemorrhagic ophthalmic conditions, concurrent use of anticoagulants, elderly, cerebrovascular disease, hemostatic defects.

## ACTION

Produced by recombinant DNA that binds to fibrin and converts plasminogen to plasmin. Initiates fibrinolysis by degrading fibrin clots, fibrinogen, other plasma proteins. **Therapeutic Effect:** Exerts thrombolytic action (dissolves clots).

## PHARMACOKINETICS

Extensively distributed to tissues. Completely eliminated by hepatic metabolism. **Half-life:** 90–130 min.

## ⊠ LIFESPAN CONSIDERATIONS

**Pregnancy/Lactation:** Unknown if distributed in breast milk. **Children:** Safety and efficacy not established. **Elderly:** May have increased risk of intracranial hemorrhage, stroke, major bleeding; caution advised.

## INTERACTIONS

**DRUG:** Anticoagulants (e.g., **heparin, warfarin**), **aspirin, dipyridamole, glycoprotein IIb/IIIa inhibitors** increase risk of bleeding. **HERBAL:** Cat's claw, dong quai, evening primrose, feverfew, garlic, ginkgo biloba, ginseng, red clover may increase risk of bleeding. **FOOD:** None known. **LAB VALUES:** Decreases plasminogen, fibrinogen levels during infusion, decreasing clotting time (confirms presence of lysis). May decrease Hgb, Hct.

## AVAILABILITY (Rx)

Injection, Powder for Reconstitution: 50 mg.

## ADMINISTRATION/HANDLING

 **IV**

**Reconstitution** • Add 10 ml Sterile Water for Injection without preservative to vial to provide concentration of 5 mg/ml. • Gently swirl until dissolved. Do not shake. • If foaming occurs, leave vial undisturbed for several min.

**Rate of Administration** • Administer as IV push over 5 sec.

**Storage** • Store at room temperature. • If possible, use immediately, but may refrigerate up to 8 hrs after reconstitution. • Appears as colorless to pale yellow solution. • Do not use if discolored or contains particulates. • Discard after 8 hrs.

## ⊠ IV INCOMPATIBILITIES

Do not mix with dextrose-containing solutions or any other medications.

## INDICATIONS/ROUTES/DOSAGE

◄**ALERT**► Give as single IV bolus over 5 sec. Precipitate may occur when given in IV line containing dextrose. Flush line with saline before and after administration.

**Acute MI**
**IV: ADULTS:** Dosage is based on pt's weight. Treatment should be initiated as soon as possible after onset of symptoms.

| Weight (kg) | (mg) | (ml) |
|---|---|---|
| 90 or more | 50 | 10 |
| 80–less than 90 | 45 | 9 |
| 70–less than 80 | 40 | 8 |
| 60–less than 70 | 35 | 7 |
| Less than 60 | 30 | 6 |

**Dosage in Renal/Hepatic Impairment**
No dose adjustment.

## SIDE EFFECTS

**Frequent:** Bleeding (minor, 21.8%; major, 4.7%).

## ADVERSE EFFECTS/ TOXIC REACTIONS

Internal bleeding, including intracranial, retroperitoneal, GI, GU, respiratory sites, may occur. Lysis of coronary thrombi may produce atrial or ventricular arrhythmias, stroke.

**T**

## NURSING CONSIDERATIONS

### BASELINE ASSESSMENT

Obtain baseline B/P, apical pulse. Record weight. Evaluate 12-lead EKG, cardiac enzymes, serum electrolytes. Assess Hgb, Hct, platelet count, thrombin time, aPTT, PT, fibrinogen level before therapy is instituted. Type and hold blood. Screen for contraindications (e.g., history of CVA, bleeding of any kind, uncontrolled hypertension).

### INTERVENTION/EVALUATION

Monitor continuous EKG for arrhythmias, B/P, pulse, respirations q15min until stable, then hourly or per protocol. Check peripheral pulses, heart and lung sounds. Monitor for chest pain relief; notify physician of continuation/recurrence (note location, type, intensity). Assess for overt or occult blood in any body substance. Monitor aPTT per protocol. Maintain B/P. Avoid any trauma that might increase risk of bleeding (e.g., injections, shaving). Assess neurologic status with vital signs.

---

## tenofovir

TOP 100

ten-**oh**-foe-veer
(Vemlidy, Viread)

■ **BLACK BOX ALERT** ■ Lactic acidosis, severe hepatomegaly with steatosis (fatty liver), including fatalities, have occurred.

### FIXED-COMBINATION(S)

**Atripla:** tenofovir (TDF)/efavirenz/emtricitabine (antiretroviral agents): 300 mg/600 mg/200 mg. **Complera:** tenofovir (TDF)/emtricitabine/rilpivirine (antiretroviral agents): 300 mg/200 mg/25 mg. **Descovy:** tenofovir (TAF)/emtricitabine: 25 mg/200 mg. **Genvoya:** tenofovir (TAF)/elvitegravir/cobicistat/emtricitabine: 10 mg, 150 mg/150 mg/200 mg. **Odefsey:** tenofovir (TAF)/emtricitabine/rilpivirine: 25 mg/200 mg/25 mg. **Stribild:** tenofovir (TDF)/elvitegravir (an integrase inhibitor)/cobicistat (a pharmacokinetic enhancer)/emtricitabine (a nucleoside reverse transcriptase inhibitor): 300 mg/150 mg/150 mg/200 mg. **Truvada:** tenofovir (TDF)/emtricitabine (an antiretroviral agent): 300 mg/200 mg.

### ◆CLASSIFICATION

**PHARMACOTHERAPEUTIC:** Nucleotide analogue (reverse transcriptase inhibitor). **CLINICAL:** Antiretroviral.

## USES

Treatment of HIV-1 infection in combination with at least two other antiretroviral agents. Treatment of chronic hepatitis B virus infection in pts with hepatic disease. **Vemlidy:** Treatment of chronic hepatitis B virus infection in adults with compensated liver disease.

## PRECAUTIONS

**Contraindications:** Hypersensitivity to tenofovir. **Cautions:** Hepatic/renal impairment, pts at risk for hepatic disease (e.g., obesity); concurrent nephrotoxic medications, pts with low body weight, risk factors or prior history of pancreatitis, elderly.

## ACTION

Inhibits HIV reverse transcriptase by interfering with HIV viral RNA–dependent DNA polymerase. Inhibits replication of hepatitis B virus (HBV) by inhibiting HBV polymerase. **Therapeutic Effect:** Slows HIV replication, reduces HIV RNA levels (viral load). Inhibits HBV replication.

## PHARMACOKINETICS

Bioavailability in fasted pts is approximately 25%. High-fat meals increase bioavailability. Protein binding: 0.7%–7.2%. Excreted in urine. Removed by hemodialysis. **Half-life:** 17 hrs.

## ⧖ LIFESPAN CONSIDERATIONS

**Pregnancy/Lactation:** Unknown if drug crosses placenta or is distributed in breast milk. **Children:** Safety and

T

efficacy not established. **Elderly:** No age-related precautions noted.

## INTERACTIONS

**DRUG:** May increase **didanosine** concentration. May decrease concentrations of **atazanavir, indinavir, lamivudine, lopinavir, ritonavir. HERBAL:** None significant. **FOOD: High-fat food** increases bioavailability. **LAB VALUES:** May increase serum ALT, AST, creatinine, phosphate, protein; urinary glucose. May decrease neutrophils.

## AVAILABILITY (Rx)

**Tablets:** *(Vemlidy):* 25 mg. *(Viread):* 150 mg, 200 mg, 250 mg, 300 mg. **Oral Powder:** 40 mg per 1 g of oral powder.

## ADMINISTRATION/HANDLING

### PO

• (Vemlidy) Give with food. (Viread) May be given without regard to meals.
• Give oral powder with soft food. Do not mix in liquid; use only the supplied dosing scoop to measure power.

## INDICATIONS/ROUTES/DOSAGE

**Hepatitis B**
PO: *(Vemlidy):* **ADULTS, ELDERLY:** 25 mg once daily with food. *(Viread):* **ADULTS, ELDERLY, CHILDREN 12 YRS AND OLDER:** 300 mg once daily.

**HIV (in Combination with Other Antiretroviral Agents)**
PO: **ADULTS, ELDERLY, CHILDREN 12 YRS AND OLDER (WEIGHT 35 KG OR GREATER):** 300 mg once daily. **CHILDREN 2 YRS AND OLDER (WEIGHT LESS THAN 35 KG):** 8 mg/kg/dose once daily. **Maximum:** 300 mg/day.

**Dosage in Renal Impairment**

| Creatinine Clearance | Dosage |
|---|---|
| 30–49 ml/min | 300 mg q48h |
| 10–29 ml/min | 300 mg q72–96h |
| Hemodialysis | 300 mg q7days or after approximately 12 hrs of dialysis |

**Dosage in Hepatic Impairment**
No dose adjustment.

## SIDE EFFECTS

**Occasional:** GI disturbances (diarrhea, flatulence, nausea, vomiting).

## ADVERSE EFFECTS/ TOXIC REACTIONS

Lactic acidosis, hepatomegaly with steatosis (excess fat in liver) occur rarely; may be severe.

## NURSING CONSIDERATIONS

### BASELINE ASSESSMENT

Obtain baseline laboratory testing, esp. serum renal function, triglycerides, LFT and at periodic intervals during therapy. Offer emotional support.

### INTERVENTION/EVALUATION

Closely monitor for evidence of GI discomfort. Monitor daily pattern of bowel activity, stool consistency. Monitor CBC, reticulocyte count, serum renal function, LFT, CD4 cell count, HIV, RNA plasma levels.

### PATIENT/FAMILY TEACHING

• Continue therapy for full length of treatment. • Tenofovir is not a cure for HIV infection, nor does it reduce risk of transmission to others. • Take with a high-fat meal (increases absorption). • Report persistent abdominal pain, nausea, vomiting.

# terbinafine

ter-**bin**-a-feen
(Apo-Terbinafine ✦, Lamisil, Lamisil AT, Terbinex)
**Do not confuse Lamisil with Lamictal, or terbinafine with terbutaline.**

## ◆CLASSIFICATION

**PHARMACOTHERAPEUTIC:** Synthetic allylamine antifungal. **CLINICAL:** Antifungal.

## USES

**Systemic:** Treatment of onychomycosis (fungal disease of nails due to dermatophytes). Treatment of tinea capitis. **Topical:** Treatment of tinea cruris (jock itch), tinea pedis (athlete's foot), tinea corporis (ringworm), tinea versicolor.

## PRECAUTIONS

**Contraindications:** Hypersensitivity to terbinafine. **Cautions:** Preexisting hepatic or renal impairment (CrCl 50 ml/min or less), sensitivity to allylamine antifungals (e.g., butenafine). Not recommended in pts with active or chronic hepatic disease.

## ACTION

Inhibits the enzyme squalene epoxidase, thereby interfering with fungal biosynthesis. **Therapeutic Effect:** Results in death of fungal cells.

## PHARMACOKINETICS

Well absorbed following PO administration. Protein binding: 99%. Metabolized in liver. Primarily excreted in urine; minimal elimination in feces. **Half-life:** PO, 36 hrs; topical, 22–26 hrs.

## ⧗ LIFESPAN CONSIDERATIONS

**Pregnancy/Lactation:** Distributed in breast milk. **Children:** Safety and efficacy not established. **Elderly:** Age-related renal impairment may require dosage adjustment.

## INTERACTIONS

**DRUG: Alcohol, other hepatotoxic medications (e.g., acetaminophen, amiodarone, ketoconazole, isoniazid)** may increase risk of hepatotoxicity. **CYP3A inducers (e.g., rifampin)** may increase clearance. **CYP3A inhibitors (e.g., cimetidine, fluconazole)** may decrease clearance. **HERBAL:** None significant. **FOOD:** None known. **LAB VALUES:** May increase serum ALT, AST.

## AVAILABILITY (Rx)

**Cream (Lamisil AT):** 1%. **Gel (Lamisil Advanced):** 1%. **Oral Granules (Lamisil):** 125 mg/packet. **Tablets (Lamisil,** Terbinex): 250 mg. **Topical Solution (Lamisil, Lamisil AT):** 1%.

## ADMINISTRATION/HANDLING

• Tablets may be given without regard to food. • Granules should be sprinkled on a spoonful of nonacidic food (e.g., mashed potatoes). Instruct pt to swallow without chewing.

## INDICATIONS/ROUTES/DOSAGE

**Tinea Pedis**
**Topical: ADULTS, ELDERLY, CHILDREN 12 YRS AND OLDER:** (Cream): Apply once or twice daily for at least 1 wk. (Gel/Solution): Apply once daily for at least 1 wk.

**Tinea Cruris, Tinea Corporis**
**Topical: ADULTS, ELDERLY, CHILDREN 12 YRS AND OLDER:** Apply once daily for at least 1 wk until signs/symptoms significantly improve; not to exceed 4 wks.

**Onychomycosis**
**Note:** Continue for 6 wks. **PO: ADULTS, ELDERLY, CHILDREN 12 YRS AND OLDER:** 250 mg/day for 6 wks (fingernails) or 12 wks (toenails).

**Tinea Versicolor**
**Topical Solution: ADULTS, ELDERLY:** Apply to the affected area once or twice daily for 7 days.

**Tinea Capitis**
**Note:** Continue for 6 wks.
**PO: ADULTS, ELDERLY:** 250 mg once daily. **CHILDREN 4 YRS AND OLDER:** (Use granules). **WEIGHING GREATER THAN 35 KG:** 250 mg once daily. **WEIGHING 25–35 KG:** 187.5 mg once daily. **WEIGHING LESS THAN 25 KG:** 125 mg once daily.

**Dosage in Renal Impairment**
No dose adjustment.

**Dosage in Hepatic Impairment**
Not recommended in pts with active or chronic hepatic disease.

## SIDE EFFECTS

**Frequent (13%): PO:** Headache. **Occasional (6%–3%): PO:** Abdominal pain, flatulence, urticaria, visual disturbance. **Rare: PO:** Diarrhea, rash, dyspepsia, pruritus, altered taste, nausea. **Topical:** Irritation, burning, pruritus, dryness.

## ADVERSE EFFECTS/ TOXIC REACTIONS

Hepatobiliary dysfunction (including cholestatic hepatitis), serious skin reactions, severe neutropenia occur rarely. Ocular lens, retinal changes have been noted.

## NURSING CONSIDERATIONS

### BASELINE ASSESSMENT

Serum LFT should be obtained in pts receiving treatment for longer than 6 wks.

### INTERVENTION/EVALUATION

Check for therapeutic response. Discontinue medication, notify physician if local reaction occurs (irritation, redness, swelling, pruritus, oozing, blistering, burning). Monitor LFT in pts receiving treatment for longer than 6 wks.

### PATIENT/FAMILY TEACHING

• Keep areas clean, dry; wear light clothing to promote ventilation. • Avoid topical cream contact with eyes, nose, mouth, other mucous membranes. • Rub well into affected, surrounding area. • Do not cover with occlusive dressing. • Report rash, dark urine, abdominal pain, anorexia, yellowing of skin.

# terbutaline

ter-**bue**-ta-leen
(Bricanyl ✤)
**Do not confuse Brethine with methergine, or terbutaline with terbinafine. Should not be used for prolonged tocolysis (longer than 48–72 hrs).**

## ◆CLASSIFICATION

**PHARMACOTHERAPEUTIC:** Sympathomimetic (adrenergic agonist). **CLINICAL:** Bronchodilator, premature labor inhibitor.

## USES

Symptomatic relief of reversible bronchospasm due to bronchial asthma, bronchitis, emphysema. **OFF-LABEL:** Delays premature labor in pregnancies between 20 and 34 wks.

## PRECAUTIONS

**Contraindications:** Hypersensitivity to terbutaline. Cardiac arrhythmias associated with tachycardia, tachycardia caused by digoxin toxicity. **(Additional) Injection:** Prolonged prevention or management of preterm labor. **Oral:** Prevention or treatment of preterm labor. **Cautions:** Cardiac impairment, diabetes mellitus, glaucoma, hypertension, hyperthyroidism, history of seizures.

## ACTION

Stimulates beta$_2$-adrenergic receptors, resulting in relaxation of uterine, bronchial smooth muscle. **Therapeutic Effect:** Inhibits uterine contractions. Relieves bronchospasm, reduces airway resistance.

## PHARMACOKINETICS

Partially absorbed in GI tract following PO administration. Protein binding: 14%–25%. Metabolized in liver. Excreted in urine (30%–50%), feces (unspecified). **Half-life:** 11–16 hrs.

## ⧗ LIFESPAN CONSIDERATIONS

**Pregnancy/Lactation:** Crosses placenta; distributed in breast milk. **Children:** Safety and efficacy not established in pts younger than 6 yrs. **Elderly:** Increased risk of tremors, tachycardia due to sympathomimetic sensitivity.

# INTERACTIONS

**DRUG:** May decrease effects of **beta blockers (e.g., labetolol, metoprolol). Digoxin, sympathomimetics** may increase risk of arrhythmias. **MAOIs** may increase risk of hypertensive crisis. **Tricyclic antidepressants (e.g., amitriptyline, nortriptyline)** may increase cardiovascular effects. **HERBAL:** Ephedra, yohimbe may cause CNS stimulation. **FOOD:** None known. **LAB VALUES:** May decrease serum potassium. May increase serum glucose.

# AVAILABILITY (Rx)

**Injection Solution:** 1 mg/ml. **Tablets:** 2.5 mg, 5 mg.

# ADMINISTRATION/HANDLING

IV

• May administer undiluted, direct IV over 5–10 min or continuous infusion diluted in D₅W or 0.9% NaCl.

**SQ**

• Do not use if solution appears discolored. • Inject subcutaneously into lateral deltoid region.

**PO**

• Give without regard to food (give with food if GI upset occurs). • Tablets may be crushed.

# INDICATIONS/ROUTES/DOSAGE

**Bronchospasm**

**PO: ADULTS, ELDERLY, CHILDREN 15 YRS AND OLDER:** Initially, 2.5–5 mg 3 times/day. **Maintenance:** 2.5–5 mg 3 times/day q6h while awake. **Maximum:** 15 mg/day. **CHILDREN 12–14 YRS:** 2.5 mg 3 times/day. **Maximum:** 7.5 mg/day. **CHILDREN YOUNGER THAN 12 YRS:** Initially, 0.05 mg/kg/dose q8h. May increase up to 0.15 mg/kg/dose. **Maximum:** 5 mg/24 hr. **SQ: ADULTS, CHILDREN 12 YRS AND OLDER:** Initially, 0.25 mg. Repeat in 15–30 min for 3 doses. Total dose of 0.75 mg should not be exceeded. **CHILDREN**

**YOUNGER THAN 12 YRS:** 0.005–0.01 mg/kg/dose to a maximum of 0.4 mg/dose q15–20min for 3 doses. May repeat q2–6h as needed.

**Preterm Labor**

◀ALERT▶ IV form should be used with caution in pregnancy; do not administer for longer than 48–72 hrs.

**IV: ADULTS:** Acute: 2.5–10 mcg/min. May increase gradually q15–20min up to 17.5–30 mcg/min. **SQ:** 0.25 mg q20min–3 hrs.

**Dosage in Renal/Hepatic Impairment**
No dose adjustment.

# SIDE EFFECTS

**Frequent (38%–23%):** Tremor, anxiety. **Occasional (11%–10%):** Drowsiness, headache, nausea, heartburn, dizziness. **Rare (3%–1%):** Flushing, asthenia, oropharyngeal dryness, irritation (with inhalation therapy).

# ADVERSE EFFECTS/ TOXIC REACTIONS

Too-frequent or excessive use may lead to decreased drug effectiveness and/or severe, paradoxical bronchoconstriction. Excessive sympathomimetic stimulation may cause palpitations, extrasystoles, tachycardia, chest pain, slight increase in B/P followed by a substantial decrease, chills, diaphoresis, skin blanching.

# NURSING CONSIDERATIONS

## BASELINE ASSESSMENT

**Bronchospasm:** Offer emotional support (high incidence of anxiety due to difficulty in breathing, sympathomimetic response to drug). **Preterm labor:** Assess baseline maternal pulse, B/P, frequency and duration of contractions, fetal heart rate. Question history of cardiac arrhythmias, narrow-angle glaucoma, hypertension, seizures.

## INTERVENTION/EVALUATION

**Bronchospasm:** Monitor rate, depth, rhythm, type of respiration; quality, rate of

T

pulse. Assess lung sounds for rhonchi, wheezing, rales. Monitor ABGs. Observe lips, fingernails for cyanosis. Observe for clavicular retractions, hand tremor. Evaluate for clinical improvement (quieter, slower respirations, relaxed facial expression, cessation of clavicular retractions). **Preterm labor:** Monitor for frequency, duration, strength of contractions. Diligently monitor maternal and fetal heart rate.

### PATIENT/FAMILY TEACHING

• Report persistent palpitations, chest pain, muscle tremor, dizziness, headache, flushing, breathing difficulties. • May cause nervousness, anxiety, shakiness. • Avoid excessive use of caffeine derivatives (chocolate, coffee, tea, cola, cocoa).

---

# teriflunomide

ter-i-**floo**-noe-myde
(Aubagio)
**Do not confuse teriflunomide with leflunomide.**

■ **BLACK BOX ALERT** ■ May result in major birth defects. Pregnancy must be excluded before initiating therapy, and must be avoided during treatment or prior to completion of an accelerated elimination procedure. Severe hepatic injury may occur. Do not initiate with acute/chronic liver disease or ALT greater than 2 times upper limit of normal.

### ◆CLASSIFICATION

**PHARMACOTHERAPEUTIC:** Pyrimidine synthesis inhibitor, immunomodulatory agent. **CLINICAL:** Multiple sclerosis agent.

## USES

Treatment of relapsing forms of multiple sclerosis.

## PRECAUTIONS

**Contraindications:** Hypersensitivity to teriflunomide. Pregnant women or women of childbearing potential who are not using reliable contraception, severe hepatic impairment, concurrent use of leflunomide. **Cautions:** Concomitant neurotoxic medications, diabetes, pulmonary disease, severe immunodeficiency or bone marrow dysplasia, history of significant hematologic abnormalities, uncontrolled infection, history of new/recurrent infections, pts older than 60 yrs.

## ACTION

Inhibits pyrimidine synthesis, exhibiting anti-inflammatory and antiproliferative properties. **Therapeutic Effect:** May slow progression of multiple sclerosis.

## PHARMACOKINETICS

Well absorbed following PO administration. Peak concentration: 1–4 h. Protein binding: greater than 99%. Metabolized by hydrolysis. Eliminated in urine (23%), feces (38%). **Half-life:** 18–19 days.

## ⌛ LIFESPAN CONSIDERATIONS

**Pregnancy/Lactation:** May produce embryo-fetal toxicity. Pregnancy contraindicated. Avoid breastfeeding. Detected in human semen. **Children:** Safety and efficacy not established in pts younger than 18 yrs of age. **Elderly:** No age-related precautions noted.

## INTERACTIONS

**DRUG:** May increase concentration/effects of **CYP2C8 substrates (e.g., repaglinide, paclitaxel, pioglitazone, or rosiglitazone), oral contraceptives.** May decrease concentration/effects of **warfarin, CYP1A2 substrates (e.g., duloxetine, tizanidine). HERBAL:** None significant. **FOOD:** None known. **LAB VALUES:** May increase serum potassium, ALT, AST, alkaline phosphatase, bilirubin. May decrease WBCs, neutrophil count.

## AVAILABILITY (Rx)

**Tablets:** 7 mg, 14 mg.

## ADMINISTRATION/HANDLING

**PO**
• Give without regard to food.

---

## INDICATIONS/ROUTES/DOSAGE

**Multiple Sclerosis**
**PO: ADULTS, ELDERLY:** 7 mg or 14 mg once daily.

**Dosage in Renal Impairment**
No dose adjustment.

**Dosage in Hepatic Impairment**
**Mild to moderate impairment:** No dose adjustment. **Severe impairment:** Contraindicated.

## SIDE EFFECTS

**Frequent (19%–6%):** Headache, diarrhea, nausea, alopecia, paresthesia, upper abdominal pain. **Occasional (4%–3%):** Hypertension, oral herpes, anxiety, hypertension, toothache, musculoskeletal pain. **Rare (2%–1%):** Seasonal allergy, sciatica, burning sensation, carpal tunnel syndrome, blurred vision, acne, pruritus, myalgia, abdominal distention, conjunctivitis.

## ADVERSE EFFECTS/ TOXIC REACTIONS

Influenza occurs in 12% of pts, upper respiratory infection with sinusitis, bronchitis, in 9%. Cystitis, sinusitis, viral gastroenteritis may occur. Neutropenia, leukopenia occur rarely.

## NURSING CONSIDERATIONS

### BASELINE ASSESSMENT

Because of high potential for birth defects/fetal death, female pts must avoid pregnancy. Obtain baseline PPD for latent TB. Obtain CBC, hepatic function test results prior to treatment, and for 6 mos thereafter. Obtain baseline pregnancy test. Assess limitations for activities of daily living due to multiple sclerosis.

### INTERVENTION/EVALUATION

Monitor for signs/symptoms of infection. Treatment should not be initiated if pt has active infection; discontinuation of treatment must be considered. If drug-induced hepatic impairment, peripheral neuropathy, severe skin reaction occur,

discontinue medication, begin accelerated elimination procedure (cholestyramine or charcoal for 11 days).

### PATIENT/FAMILY TEACHING

• Women of childbearing potential must be counseled regarding fetal risk, use of reliable contraceptives confirmed, possibility of pregnancy excluded. • May take without regard to food.

# teriparatide

**ter**-i-**par**-a-tide
(Forteo)
■ **BLACK BOX ALERT** ■ Increased risk of osteosarcoma; risk dependent on dose and duration.

## ◆ CLASSIFICATION

**PHARMACOTHERAPEUTIC:** Parathyroid hormone. **CLINICAL:** Osteoporosis agent.

## USES

Treatment of postmenopausal women with osteoporosis who are at increased risk for fractures. Treatment of men with primary or hypogonadal osteoporosis who are at high risk for fractures. High-risk pts include those with a history of osteoporotic fractures, who have failed previous osteoporosis therapy, or were intolerant of previous osteoporosis therapy. Treatment of glucocorticoid-induced osteoporosis in men and women.

## PRECAUTIONS

**Contraindications:** Hypersensitivity to teriparatide. **Cautions:** Conditions that increase risk of osteosarcoma (e.g., Paget's disease, unexplained elevations of alkaline phosphatase level, open epiphyses, prior skeletal radiation therapy, implant therapy), hypercalcemia, hypercalcemic disorders (e.g., hyperparathyroidism), bone metastases, history of skeletal malignancies, metabolic bone diseases other than osteoporosis, cardiac disease, renal/hepatic impairment, pts at risk for orthostasis, active or recent urolithiasis.

**T**

## ACTION

Stimulates osteoblast function. Increases calcium absorption from GI tract/renal tubular reabsorption. **Therapeutic Effect:** Increases bone mineral density, bone mass/strength, reduces osteoporosis-related fractures.

## PHARMACOKINETICS

Extensively absorbed following SQ injection. Metabolized in liver. Excreted in urine. **Half-life:** 1 hr.

## LIFESPAN CONSIDERATIONS

**Pregnancy/Lactation:** Unknown if drug crosses placenta or is distributed in breast milk. **Children:** Safety and efficacy not established. **Elderly:** No age-related precautions noted.

## INTERACTIONS

**DRUG:** None significant. **HERBAL:** None significant. **FOOD:** None known. **LAB VALUES:** May increase serum calcium (transient), uric acid.

## AVAILABILITY (Rx)

**Injection Solution:** 250 mcg/ml (2.4 ml) delivers 20 mcg/dose.

## ADMINISTRATION/HANDLING

### SQ

• Refrigerate, but minimize time out of refrigerator. Do not freeze; discard if frozen. • Administer into thigh, abdominal wall.

## INDICATIONS/ROUTES/DOSAGE

**Osteoporosis**
**SQ: ADULTS, ELDERLY:** 20 mcg once daily into thigh, abdominal wall.

**Dosage in Renal/Hepatic Impairment**
No dose adjustment.

## SIDE EFFECTS

**Occasional:** Leg cramps, nausea, dizziness, headache, orthostatic hypotension, tachycardia.

## ADVERSE EFFECTS/ TOXIC REACTIONS

Angina pectoris has been reported.

## NURSING CONSIDERATIONS

### BASELINE ASSESSMENT

Check urinary, serum calcium, ionized calcium levels, serum parathyroid hormone levels.

### INTERVENTION/EVALUATION

Monitor bone mineral density, urinary/serum calcium levels, serum parathyroid hormone levels. Observe for symptoms of hypercalcemia. Monitor B/P for hypotension, pulse for tachycardia.

### PATIENT/FAMILY TEACHING

• Go from lying to standing slowly. • Report persistent symptoms of hypercalcemia (nausea, vomiting, constipation, lethargy, asthenia).

---

## testosterone     TOP 100

tes-**tos**-te-rone
(Andriol ✦, Androderm, <u>AndroGel Pump</u>, Andropository ✦, Aveed, Axiron, Delatestryl, Depotest ✦, Depo-Testosterone, Everone ✦, FIRST-Testosterone, FIRST-Testosterone MC, Fortesta, Natesto, Striant, Testim, Testopel, Vogelxo Pump)

■ **BLACK BOX ALERT** ■ Virilization in children and women may occur following secondary exposure to testosterone gel. Aveed: Serious pulmonary oil microembolism reaction and anaphylaxis reported during or immediately after administration.

**Do not confuse testosterone with testolactone, Testoderm with Estraderm.**

◆ **CLASSIFICATION**

**PHARMACOTHERAPEUTIC:** Androgen. **CLINICAL:** Sex hormone.

---

## USES

Androgen replacement therapy in treatment of delayed male puberty, male hypogonadism (congenital or acquired), inoperable female breast cancer pts who are 1–5 yrs postmenopausal.

## PRECAUTIONS

**Contraindications:** Hypersensitivity to testosterone. Breastfeeding, pregnant or who may become pregnant, prostate or breast cancer in males. Depo-Testosterone: Severe cardiac hepatic/renal disease. **Cautions:** Renal/hepatic/cardiac dysfunction, pts with history of MI or CAD; conditions influenced by edema (e.g., seizure disorder, migraines).

## ACTION

Promotes growth, development of male sex organs, maintains secondary sex characteristics in androgen-deficient males. **Therapeutic Effect:** Relieves androgen deficiency.

## PHARMACOKINETICS

Well absorbed after IM administration. Protein binding: 98%. Metabolized in liver. Primarily excreted in urine. Unknown if removed by hemodialysis. **Half-life:** 10–100 min.

## ⌛ LIFESPAN CONSIDERATIONS

**Pregnancy/Lactation:** Contraindicated during lactation. **Children:** Safety and efficacy not established; use with caution. **Elderly:** May increase risk of hyperplasia, stimulate growth of occult prostate carcinoma.

## INTERACTIONS

**DRUG:** May decrease serum glucose, requiring **insulin** adjustments. **HERBAL:** **St. John's wort** may decrease concentration/effects. **FOOD:** None known. **LAB VALUES:** May increase Hgb, Hct, LDL, serum alkaline phosphatase, bilirubin, calcium, potassium, sodium, AST. May decrease HDL.

## AVAILABILITY (Rx)

**Cream (First Testosterone, MC):** 2%. **Ointment (First Testosterone):** 2% **Gel, Topical (AndroGel, Testim):** 1%, 1.62%. **(Vogelxo):** 50-mg packet or tube, 12.5 mg/actuation metered dose pump. **(Fortesta):** 10 mg/actuation. **Injection (Cypionate [Depo-Testosterone]):** 100 mg/ml, 200 mg/ml. **(Enanthate [Delatestryl]):** 200 mg/ml. **(Aveed [undecanoate]):** 750 mg/3 ml. **Mucoadhesive, for Buccal Application (Striant):** 30 mg. **Nasal Gel (Natesto):** 5.5 mg/actuation. **Pellet, for Subcutaneous Implantation (Testopel):** 75 mg. **Solution (Metered Dose Pump [Axiron]):** 30 mg/activation. **Transdermal System (Androderm):** 2 mg/day or 4 mg/day.

## ADMINISTRATION/HANDLING

### IM

• Give deep in gluteal muscle. • Do not give IV. • Warming or shaking redissolves crystals that may form in long-acting preparations. • Wet needle of syringe may cause solution to become cloudy; this does not affect potency.

### Buccal

**(Striant):** • Apply to gum area (above incisor tooth). • Hold firmly in place for 30 sec to ensure adhesion. Instruct pt to not chew or swallow. • Not affected by food, toothbrushing, gum, chewing, alcoholic beverages. • Remove before placing new system.

### Transdermal

**(Androderm):** • Apply to clean, dry area on skin on back, abdomen, upper arms, thighs. • Do not apply to bony prominences (e.g., shoulder) or oily, damaged, irritated skin. Do not apply to scrotum. • Rotate application site with 7-day interval to same site.

### Transdermal Gel

**(AndroGel, Testim, Vogelxo):** • Apply (morning preferred) to clean, dry, intact skin of shoulder, upper arms (AndroGel 1% may also be applied to abdomen). • Upon opening packet(s),

T

squeeze entire contents into palm of hand, immediately apply to application site. • Allow to dry. • Do not apply to genitals. **(Fortesta):** Apply to skin of front and inner thighs.

**Topical Solution**

**(Axiron):** • Apply using applicator to axilla at same time each morning. • Avoid washing site for 2 hrs after application.

## INDICATIONS/ROUTES/DOSAGE

**Male Hypogonadism**

**IM: ADULTS:** 50–400 mg q2–4wks or 75–100 mg/wk or 150–200 mg q2wks. *(Aveed):* 750 mg at initiation, 4 wks and q10 wks thereafter. **ADOLESCENTS:** Initiation of pubertal growth: 25–75 mg q3–4wks, titrate q6–9mos to 100–150 mg. Duration: 3–4yrs. **Maintenance Virilizing Dose:** 100 mg/m$^2$/dose twice monthly. **SQ:** *(Pellets):* **ADULTS:** 150–450 mg q3–6mos.
**Topical Gel:** *(Fortesta):* 40 mg once daily in morning. Range: 10–70 mg. *(Vogelxo):* 50 mg once daily (one tube or one packet or 4 pump actuations).
**Topical Solution:** *(Axiron):* **ADULTS, ELDERLY:** 60 mg once daily (1 pump activation of 30 mg to each axilla). Range: 30–120 mg.
**Transdermal Patch:** *(Androderm):* **ADULTS, ELDERLY:** Start therapy with 4 mg/day patch applied at night. Apply patch to abdomen, back, thighs, upper arms. Dose adjustment based on testosterone levels.
**Transdermal Gel:** *(AndroGel):* **ADULTS, ELDERLY:** **(AndroGel 1%):** Initial dose of 5 g delivers 50 mg testosterone and is applied once daily to abdomen, shoulders, upper arms. May increase to 7.5 g, then to 10 g, if necessary. **(AndroGel 1.62%):** Initial dose of 40.5 mg applied once daily in the morning to shoulder and upper arms. May increase to 81 mg. Further adjustments based on testosterone levels.
**Transdermal Gel:** *(Testim):* **ADULTS, ELDERLY:** Initial dose of 5 g delivers 50 mg testosterone and is applied once daily to the shoulders, upper arms. May increase to 10 g (100 mg testosterone).
**Buccal:** *(Striant):* **ADULTS, ELDERLY:** 30 mg q12h.
**Nasal Gel:** *(Natesto):* **ADULTS ELDERLY:** 11 mg (2 actuations, 1 per each nostril) 3 times/day.

**Delayed Male Puberty**

**IM:** *(Cypionate or enanthate):* **ADOLESCENTS:** 50–200 mg q2–4wks for limited duration.
**SQ:** *(Pellets):* **ADULTS:** 150–450 mg q3–6mos.

**Breast Carcinoma**

**IM:** *(Testosterone Cypionate, Testosterone Ethanate):* **ADULTS:** 200–400 mg q2–4wks.

**Dosage in Renal/Hepatic Impairment**
Use caution.

## SIDE EFFECTS

**Frequent:** Gynecomastia, acne. **Females:** Hirsutism, amenorrhea, other menstrual irregularities; deepening of voice; clitoral enlargement (may not be reversible when drug is discontinued). **Occasional:** Edema, nausea, insomnia, oligospermia, priapism, male-pattern baldness, bladder irritability, hypercalcemia (in immobilized pts, those with breast cancer), hypercholesterolemia, inflammation/pain at IM injection site. **Transdermal:** Pruritus, erythema, skin irritation. **Rare:** Polycythemia (with high dosage), hypersensitivity.

## ADVERSE EFFECTS/ TOXIC REACTIONS

Peliosis hepatitis (presence of blood-filled cysts in parenchyma of liver), hepatic neoplasms, hepatocellular carcinoma have been associated with prolonged high-dose therapy. Anaphylactic reactions occur rarely. Venous thromboembolism (e.g., DVT, PE) reported.

## NURSING CONSIDERATIONS

### BASELINE ASSESSMENT

Establish baseline weight, B/P, Hgb, Hct. Check serum hepatic function, electrolytes, cholesterol. Wrist X-rays may be ordered to determine bone maturation in children.

### INTERVENTION/EVALUATION

Weigh daily, report wkly gain of more than 5 lb; evaluate for edema. Monitor I&O. Monitor B/P. Assess serum electrolytes, cholesterol, Hgb, Hct (periodically for high dosage), LFT, radiologic exam of wrist, hand (when using in prepubertal children). With breast cancer or immobility, check for hypercalcemia (lethargy, muscle weakness, confusion, irritability). Ensure adequate intake of protein, calories. Assess for virilization. Monitor sleep patterns. Check injection site for redness, swelling, pain.

### PATIENT/FAMILY TEACHING

• Regular visits to physician and monitoring tests are necessary. • Do not take any other medication without consulting physician. • Maintain diet high in protein, calories. • Food may be better tolerated in small, frequent feedings. • Weigh daily, report 5 lb/wk gain. • Report nausea, vomiting, acne, pedal edema. • **Females:** Promptly report menstrual irregularities, hoarseness, deepening of voice. • **Males:** Report frequent erections, difficulty urinating, gynecomastia.

## tetracycline

tet-ra-**sye**-kleen
(Apo-Tetra ✦, Nu-Tetra ✦)

### FIXED-COMBINATION(S)

**Pylera:** tetracycline/bismuth/metronidazole (an anti-infective): 125 mg/ 140 mg/125 mg.

### ◆CLASSIFICATION

**PHARMACOTHERAPEUTIC:** Tetracycline. **CLINICAL:** Antibiotic.

## USES

Treatment of susceptible infections due to *Rickettsiae, M. pneumoniae, C. trachomatis, C. psittaci, H. ducreyi, Yersinia pestis, Francisella tularensis, Vibrio cholerae, Brucella* spp.; treatment of susceptible infections due to gram-negative organisms including inflammatory acne vulgaris, Lyme disease, mycoplasma disease, *Legionella*, Rocky Mountain spotted fever, chlamydial infection in pts with gonorrhea. Part of multidrug regimen of *H. pylori* eradication to reduce risk of duodenal ulcer recurrence.

## PRECAUTIONS

**Contraindications:** Hypersensitivity to tetracycline. **Cautions:** Sun, ultraviolet light exposure (severe photosensitivity reaction). Renal, hepatic impairment. Avoid use during tooth development (children 8 yrs or younger). Do not use during pregnancy.

## ACTION

Inhibits bacterial protein synthesis by binding to ribosomes. **Therapeutic Effect:** Bacteriostatic.

## PHARMACOKINETICS

Readily absorbed from GI tract. Protein binding: 30%–60%. Widely distributed. Excreted in urine; eliminated in feces through biliary system. Not removed by hemodialysis. **Half-life:** 6–11 hrs (increased in renal impairment).

## ⌛ LIFESPAN CONSIDERATIONS

**Pregnancy/Lactation:** Readily crosses placenta. Distributed in breast milk. Avoid use in women during last half of pregnancy. **Children:** Not recommended in pts 8 yrs or younger; may cause permanent staining of teeth, enamel hypoplasia, decreased linear skeletal growth rate. **Elderly:** No age-related precautions noted.

T

---

## INTERACTIONS

**DRUG:** May decrease effects of **oral contraceptives. Antacids, calcium or iron supplements, laxatives containing magnesium** may form nonabsorbable, undigestible complexes. **HERBAL: Dong quai, St. John's wort** may increase risk of photosensitivity. **FOOD: Dairy products** inhibit absorption. **LAB VALUES:** May increase serum BUN, alkaline phosphatase, amylase, bilirubin, ALT, AST.

## AVAILABILITY (Rx)

**Capsules:** 250 mg, 500 mg.

## ADMINISTRATION/HANDLING

**PO**
• Give with full glass of water 1 hr before or 2 hrs after meals. • Avoid antacids, dairy products within 3 hrs of tetracycline.

## INDICATIONS/ROUTES/DOSAGE

◄**ALERT**► Space doses evenly around the clock.

**Usual Dosage**
PO: **ADULTS, ELDERLY:** 250–500 mg q6–12h. **CHILDREN OLDER THAN 8 YRS:** 25–50 mg/kg/day in 4 divided doses.

**Dosage in Renal Impairment**
Dosage interval is modified based on creatinine clearance.

| Creatinine Clearance | Dosage |
|---|---|
| 50–80 ml/min | Usual dose q8–12h |
| 10–49 ml/min | Usual dose q12–24h |
| Less than 10 ml/min | Usual dose q24h |

**Dosage in Hepatic Impairment**
No dose adjustment.

## SIDE EFFECTS

**Frequent:** Dizziness, light-headedness, diarrhea, nausea, vomiting, abdominal cramps, photosensitivity (may be severe). **Occasional:** Pigmentation of skin or mucous membranes, anal/genital pruritus, stomatitis, discoloration of teeth.

## ADVERSE EFFECTS/ TOXIC REACTIONS

Superinfection (esp. fungal), anaphylaxis, elevated intracranial pressure (ICP) may occur. Bulging fontanelles occur rarely in infants.

## NURSING CONSIDERATIONS

### BASELINE ASSESSMENT
Question for history of allergies, esp. tetracyclines, sulfite.

### INTERVENTION/EVALUATION
Assess skin for rash. Monitor daily pattern of bowel activity, stool consistency. Monitor food intake, tolerance. Be alert for superinfection (diarrhea, stomatitis, anal/genital pruritus). Monitor B/P, level of consciousness (potential for elevated ICP).

### PATIENT/FAMILY TEACHING
• Continue antibiotic for full length of treatment. • Space doses evenly. • Take oral doses on empty stomach (1 hr before or 2 hrs after food, beverages). • Avoid antacids, dairy products within 3 hrs of tetracycline. • Drink full glass of water with capsules; avoid bedtime doses. • Report diarrhea, rash, other new symptoms. • Protect skin from sun, ultraviolet light exposure. • Consult physician before taking any other medication. • Avoid tasks that require alertness, motor skills until response to drug is established (may cause dizziness, light-headedness).

## thiamine (vitamin B₁)

thy-a-min
(Betaxin ✲)
**Do not confuse thiamine with Thorazine.**

◆**CLASSIFICATION**
**PHARMACOTHERAPEUTIC:** Water-soluble vitamin. **CLINICAL:** Vitamin B complex.

## USES

Prevention/treatment of thiamine deficiency (e.g., beriberi, Wernicke's encephalopathy syndrome, peripheral neuritis associated with pellagra, alcoholic pts with altered sensorium), metabolic disorders.

## PRECAUTIONS

**Contraindications:** Hypersensitivity to thiamine. **Cautions:** Wernicke's encephalopathy.

## ACTION

Combines with adenosine triphosphate in liver, kidneys, leukocytes to form thiamine diphosphate, a coenzyme necessary for carbohydrate metabolism. **Therapeutic Effect:** Prevents, reverses thiamine deficiency.

## PHARMACOKINETICS

Rapidly and completely absorbed from GI tract, primarily in duodenum, after IM administration. Widely distributed. Primarily excreted in urine.

## ⧗ LIFESPAN CONSIDERATIONS

**Pregnancy/Lactation:** Crosses placenta. Unknown if drug is distributed in breast milk. **Children/Elderly:** No age-related precautions noted.

## INTERACTIONS

**DRUG:** None significant. **HERBAL:** None significant. **FOOD:** None known. **LAB VALUES:** None significant.

## AVAILABILITY

**Injection Solution (Vitamin B₁):** 100 mg/ml. **Tablets (OTC):** 50 mg, 100 mg, 250 mg, 500 mg.

## ADMINISTRATION/HANDLING

◀ALERT▶ V, IM administration used only in acutely ill or those unresponsive to PO route (GI malabsorption syndrome). IM route preferred to IV use. Give by IV push, or add to most IV solutions and give as infusion.

**PO**
• May take without regard to food.

## ▓ IV INCOMPATIBILITIES

None known.

## ▓ IV COMPATIBILITIES

Famotidine (Pepcid), multivitamins, folic acid magnesium.

## INDICATIONS/ROUTES/DOSAGE

**Dietary Supplement**
PO: **ADULTS, ELDERLY:** 1–2 mg/day. **CHILDREN:** 0.5–1 mg/day. **INFANTS:** 0.3–0.5 mg/day.

**Thiamine Deficiency (Beriberi)**
PO: **ADULTS, ELDERLY:** 5–30 mg/dose IM or IV 3 times/day (if critically ill), then 5–30 mg/day orally, as a single dose or in 3 divided doses, for 1 mo. **CHILDREN:** 10–25 mg IM or IV (if critically ill) or 10–50 mg/dose orally every day for 2 wks, then 5–10 mg/day for 1 mo.

**Alcohol Withdrawal Syndrome**
IV, IM: **ADULTS, ELDERLY:** 100 mg/day for several days, then PO: 50–100 mg/day.

**Metabolic Disorders**
PO: **ADULTS:** 10–20 mg/day.

**Wernicke's Encephalopathy**
IV: **ADULTS, ELDERLY:** Initially, 100 mg then IV/IM: 50–100 mg/day until consuming a regular, balanced diet.

**Dosage in Renal/Hepatic Impairment**
No dose adjustment.

## SIDE EFFECTS

**Frequent:** Pain, induration, tenderness at IM injection site.

## ADVERSE EFFECTS/ TOXIC REACTIONS

IV administration may result in rare, severe hypersensitivity reaction marked by feeling of warmth, pruritus, urticaria, weakness, diaphoresis, nausea, restlessness, tightness in throat, angioedema,

T

cyanosis, pulmonary edema, GI tract bleeding, cardiovascular collapse.

## NURSING CONSIDERATIONS

### INTERVENTION/EVALUATION

Assess for clinical improvement (improved sense of well-being, weight gain). Observe for reversal of deficiency symptoms (**neurologic:** altered mental status, peripheral neuropathy, hyporeflexia, nystagmus, ophthalmoplegia, ataxia, muscle weakness; **cardiac:** venous hypertension, bounding arterial pulse, tachycardia, edema).

### PATIENT/FAMILY TEACHING

• Discomfort may occur with IM injection. • Foods rich in thiamine include pork, organ meats, whole grain and enriched cereals, legumes, nuts, seeds, yeast, wheat germ, rice bran. • Urine may appear bright yellow.

---

# *tiaGABine

tye-a-ga-been
(Gabitril)
**Do not confuse tiagabine with tizanidine.**

### ◆CLASSIFICATION

**PHARMACOTHERAPEUTIC:** Anticonvulsant. **CLINICAL:** Anticonvulsant.

## USES

Adjunctive therapy for treatment of partial seizures in adults and children 12 yrs or older.

## PRECAUTIONS

**Contraindications:** Hypersensitivity to tiagabine. **Cautions:** Hepatic impairment. Pts at risk for suicidal behavior/thoughts.

## ACTION

Enhances activity of gamma-aminobutyric acid (GABA), the major inhibitory neurotransmitter in the CNS. **Therapeutic Effect:** Inhibits seizures.

## PHARMACOKINETICS

Rapidly absorbed from GI tract. Protein binding: 96%. Metabolized in liver. Primarily eliminated in feces. **Half-life:** 2–5 hrs.

## ⬛ LIFESPAN CONSIDERATIONS

**Pregnancy/Lactation:** May produce teratogenic effects. Distributed in breast milk. **Children:** Safety and efficacy not established in pts younger than 12 yrs. **Elderly:** Age-related hepatic impairment may require dosage adjustment.

## INTERACTIONS

**DRUG: Carbamazepine, phenobarbital, phenytoin** may increase clearance. May alter effects of **valproic acid.** **HERBAL: Evening primrose** may decrease seizure threshold. **St. John's wort** may decrease concentration. **Gotu kola, kava kava, St. John's wort, valerian** may increase CNS depression. **FOOD:** None known. **LAB VALUES:** None significant.

## AVAILABILITY (Rx)

**Tablets:** 2 mg, 4 mg, 12 mg, 16 mg.

## ADMINISTRATION/HANDLING

• Give with food.

## INDICATIONS/ROUTES/DOSAGE

**Note:** Pts not taking enzyme-inducing antiepileptic drugs (AEDs). Lower doses required, slower titration may be needed.

**Partial Seizures**
**PO: ADULTS, ELDERLY: (Pts receiving enzyme-inducing AED regimens):** Initially, 4 mg once daily. May increase by 4–8 mg/day at wkly intervals. **Maintenance:** 32–56 mg/day. **CHILDREN 12–18 YRS:** Initially, 4 mg once daily for 1 wk. May increase by 4 mg in 2 divided doses for 1 wk, then may increase by 4–8 mg at wkly intervals thereafter. **Maximum:** 32 mg/day in 2–4 divided doses.

**Dosage in Renal Impairment**
No dose adjustment.

---

**Dosage in Hepatic Impairment**
Use caution.

## SIDE EFFECTS

**Frequent (34%–20%):** Dizziness, asthenia (loss of strength, energy), drowsiness, nervousness, confusion, headache, infection, tremor. **Occasional:** Nausea, diarrhea, abdominal pain, impaired concentration.

## ADVERSE EFFECTS/ TOXIC REACTIONS

Overdose characterized by agitation, confusion, hostility, weakness. Full recovery occurs within 24 hrs of discontinuation.

## NURSING CONSIDERATIONS

### BASELINE ASSESSMENT

Review history of seizure disorder (intensity, frequency, duration, LOC). Observe frequently for recurrence of seizure activity. Initiate seizure precautions.

### INTERVENTION/EVALUATION

For pts on long-term therapy, serum hepatic/renal function tests, CBC should be performed periodically. Assist with ambulation if dizziness occurs. Assess for clinical improvement (decrease in intensity, frequency of seizures). Monitor for depression, unusual behavior, suicidal ideation or thoughts.

### PATIENT/FAMILY TEACHING

• Go from lying to standing slowly.
• Avoid tasks that require alertness, motor skills until response to drug is established.
• Avoid alcohol. • Report worsening seizure activity, thoughts of suicide, increased depression.

## ticagrelor

tye-**ka**-grel-or
(Brilinta)

■ **BLACK BOX ALERT** ■ May cause significant, sometimes fatal bleeding. Do not use with active bleeding or history of intracranial bleeding.

Do not initiate in pts planning urgent coronary artery bypass graft (CABG) surgery. Discontinue at least 5 days prior to any surgery. Suspect bleeding in any pt who is hypotensive and has had recent percutaneous coronary intervention (PCI), CABG, or other surgical procedures. If possible, manage bleeding without discontinuing therapy to decrease risk of cardiovascular events. Aspirin maintenance doses greater than 100 mg/day may reduce effectiveness and should be strictly avoided.

## ◆CLASSIFICATION

**PHARMACOTHERAPEUTIC:** $P2Y_{12}$ platelet aggregation inhibitor. **CLINICAL:** Antiplatelet.

## USES

Reduce rate of cardiovascular death, MI, stroke in pts with acute coronary syndrome (ACS) or history of MI. Reduce rate of stent thrombosis in pts who have been stented for treatment of ACS.

## PRECAUTIONS

**Contraindications:** Hypersensitivity to ticagrelor. History of intracranial hemorrhage, active pathologic bleeding, severe hepatic impairment. **Cautions:** Moderate hepatic impairment, renal impairment, history of hyperuricemia or gouty arthritis. Pts at increased risk of bradycardia, concurrent use of strong CYP3A4 inhibitors or inducers, elderly. (Recommend holding dose 5 days before planned surgery if applicable.) Pts with risk factors for bleeding (e.g., trauma, peptic ulcer disease).

## ACTION

Reversibly inhibits platelet $P2Y_{12}$ ADP receptor to prevent signal transduction and platelet activation. **Therapeutic Effect:** Reduces platelet aggregation.

## PHARMACOKINETICS

Readily absorbed after PO administration. Protein binding: 99%. Metabolized in liver. Primarily excreted in feces (58%), urine (26%). **Half-life:** 7–9 hrs.

## ⌛ LIFESPAN CONSIDERATIONS

**Pregnancy/Lactation:** Unknown if distributed in breast milk. Must either discontinue breastfeeding or discontinue drug therapy. **Children:** Safety and efficacy not established. **Elderly:** No age-related precautions noted.

## INTERACTIONS

**DRUG: Aspirin** greater than 100 mg/day may decrease effectiveness. **CYP3A4 inhibitors (e.g., atazanavir, clarithromycin, ketoconazole, nefazodone, ritonavir, saquinavir)** may increase concentration/effects. **CYP3A4 inducers (e.g., carbamazepine, dexamethasone, phenytoin, rifampin)** may decrease concentration/effects. **Anticoagulants (e.g., warfarin), antiplatelets, NSAIDs** may increase risk of bleeding. May increase concentration of **digoxin, simvastatin, lovastatin. HERBAL: St. John's wort** may decrease effectiveness. **Fenugreek, feverfew, flaxseed, garlic, ginger, ginkgo biloba, ginseng, omega-3, red clover** with anticoagulant/antiplatelet activity may increase risk of bleeding. **FOOD: Grapefruit products** may increase potential for bleeding. **LAB VALUES:** May increase serum uric acid, creatinine.

## AVAILABILITY (Rx)

**Tablets:** 60 mg, 90 mg.

## ADMINISTRATION/HANDLING

**PO**
• Give without regard to meals. • May be crushed, mixed with water, and drunk immediately (refill glass with water, stir and drink contents).

## INDICATIONS/ROUTES/DOSAGE

**Acute Coronary Syndrome**
**PO: ADULTS:** Initially, 180 mg once, then 90 mg twice daily. Give with aspirin 325 mg once (loading dose), then maintain with aspirin 75–100 mg daily. Continue for up to 12 mos, then decrease dose to 60 mg twice daily.

**Dosage in Renal Impairment**
No dose adjustment.

**Dosage in Hepatic Impairment**
**Mild impairment:** No dose adjustment. **Moderate impairment:** Use caution. **Severe impairment:** Avoid use.

## SIDE EFFECTS

**Occasional (13%–7%):** Dyspnea, headache. **Rare (5%–3%):** Cough, dizziness, nausea, diarrhea, back pain, fatigue.

## ADVERSE EFFECTS/ TOXIC REACTIONS

Life-threatening events including intracranial bleeding, epistaxis, intrapericardial bleeding with cardiac tamponade, hypovolemic shock requiring vasopressive support, or blood transfusion reported. Pts with history of sick sinus syndrome, second- or third-degree AV block, bradycardic syncope have increased risk of bradycardia. May induce episodes of atrial fibrillation, hypotension, hypertension. Gynecomastia reported in less than 1% of men.

## NURSING CONSIDERATIONS

### BASELINE ASSESSMENT

Obtain CBC, serum chemistries, renal function, LFT. Question for history of bleeding, stomach ulcers, colon polyps, head trauma, cardiac arrhythmias, unstable angina, recent MI, hepatic impairment, hypertension, stroke. Receive full medication history including herbal products. Question for history of COPD, chronic bronchitis, emphysema, asthma, exertional dyspnea.

### INTERVENTION/EVALUATION

Routinely screen for bleeding. Assess skin for bruising, hematoma. Monitor renal function, uric acid, digoxin levels if applicable. Report hematuria, epistaxis, coffee-ground emesis, black/tarry stools. Monitor EKG for chest pain, shortness of breath, syncope.

### PATIENT/FAMILY TEACHING

• It may take longer to stop bleeding during therapy. • Do not vigorously blow nose. • Use soft toothbrush, electric razor to decrease risk of bleeding. • Immediately report bloody stool, urine, or nosebleeds. • Report all newly prescribed medications. • Inform physician of any planned dental procedures or surgeries.

## tigecycline

**tye-gee-sye-kleen**
(Tygacil)

■ **BLACK BOX ALERT** ■ Use reserved where alternative treatments not appropriate.

### ◆CLASSIFICATION

**PHARMACOTHERAPEUTIC:** Glycylcycline. **CLINICAL:** Antibiotic.

## USES

Treatment of susceptible infections due to *E. coli, E. faecalis, S. aureus, S. agalactiae, S. anginosus* group (includes *S. anginosus, S. intermedius, S. constellatus), S. pyogenes, B. fragilis, Citrobacter freundii, E. cloacae, K. oxytoca, K. pneumoniae, B. thetaiotaomicron, B. uniformis, B. vulgatus, C. perfringens, Peptostreptococcus micros* including complicated skin/skin structure infections, complicated intra-abdominal infections, community-acquired bacterial pneumonia.

## PRECAUTIONS

**Contraindications:** Hypersensitivity to tigecycline. **Cautions:** Hypersensitivity to tetracyclines, pregnancy, hepatic impairment, monotherapy for pts with intestinal perforation. Do not use for diabetic foot infections, healthcare-acquired pneumonia, or ventilator-associated pneumonia.

## ACTION

Inhibits protein synthesis by binding to ribosomal receptor sites of bacterial cell wall. **Therapeutic Effect:** Bacteriostatic effect.

## PHARMACOKINETICS

Extensive tissue distribution, minimally metabolized. Eliminated by biliary/fecal route (59%), urine (33%). Protein binding: 71%–89%. **Half-life:** Single dose: 27 hrs; following multiple doses: 42 hrs.

## 🕱 LIFESPAN CONSIDERATIONS

**Pregnancy/Lactation:** May cause fetal harm. May be distributed in breast milk. Permanent discoloration of the teeth (brown-gray) may occur if used during tooth development. **Children:** Safety and efficacy not established in pts younger than 18 yrs. **Elderly:** No age-related precautions noted.

## INTERACTIONS

**DRUG:** May decrease effects of **oral contraceptives** may be decreased. May increase concentration of **warfarin;** increase bleeding time. **HERBAL:** None significant. **FOOD:** None known. **LAB VALUES:** May increase serum alkaline phosphatase, amylase, BUN, bilirubin, glucose, LDH, ALT, AST. May decrease Hgb, WBCs, thrombocytes, serum potassium, protein.

## AVAILABILITY (Rx)

**Injection, Powder for Reconstitution** (Tygacil): 50-mg vial.

## ADMINISTRATION/HANDLING
### 📥 IV

**Reconstitution** • Add 5.3 ml 0.9% NaCl or $D_5W$ to each 50-mg vial. • Swirl gently to dissolve. • Resulting solution is 10 mg/ml. • Immediately withdraw 5 ml reconstituted solution and add to 100 ml 0.9% NaCl or $D_5W$ bag for infusion (final concentration should not exceed 1 mg/ml).

**Rate of Administration** • Administer over 30–60 min every 12 hrs. • May be given through a dedicated line or piggyback. If same line is used for sequential infusion of several different drugs, line should be flushed before and after infusion of tigecycline with either 0.9% NaCl or $D_5W$.

T

---

**Storage** • Reconstituted solution is stable for up to 6 hrs at room temperature or up to 24 hrs if refrigerated. • Reconstituted solution appears yellow to red-orange. • Discard if solution is discolored (green, black) or precipitate forms.

### ▨ IV INCOMPATIBILITIES

Amphotericin B, methylprednisolone, voriconazole.

### ▨ IV COMPATIBILITIES

Amikacin, azithromycin, aztreonam, cefepime, ceftazidime, ciprofloxacin, doripenem, ertapenem, fluconazole, gentamicin, linezolid, piperacillin-tazobactam, potassium chloride, telavancin, tobramycin, vancomycin.

### INDICATIONS/ROUTES/DOSAGE

**Systemic Infections**
**IV: ADULTS OVER 18 YRS, ELDERLY:** Initially, 100 mg, followed by 50 mg every 12 hrs for 5–14 days.

**Dosage in Renal Impairment**
No dose adjustment.

**Dosage in Hepatic Impairment**
No dose adjustment in mild to moderate impairment.

**Dosage in Severe Hepatic Impairment**
**IV: ADULTS OVER 18 YRS, ELDERLY:** Initially, 100 mg, followed by 25 mg every 12 hrs.

### SIDE EFFECTS

**Frequent (29%–13%):** Nausea, vomiting, diarrhea. **Occasional (7%–4%):** Headache, hypertension, dizziness, increased cough, delayed healing. **Rare (3%–2%):** Peripheral edema, pruritus, constipation, dyspepsia, asthenia (loss of strength, energy), hypotension, phlebitis, insomnia, rash, diaphoresis.

### ADVERSE EFFECTS/ TOXIC REACTIONS

Dyspnea, abscess, pseudomembranous colitis (abdominal cramps, severe watery diarrhea, fever) ranging from mild to life-threatening may result from altered bacterial balance in GI tract.

## NURSING CONSIDERATIONS

### BASELINE ASSESSMENT

Obtain baseline CBC, hepatic function test. Question for history of allergies, esp. tetracyclines, before therapy.

### INTERVENTION/EVALUATION

Monitor daily pattern of bowel activity, stool consistency. Be alert for superinfection: fever, anal/genital pruritus, oral mucosal changes (ulceration, pain, erythema). Nausea, vomiting may be controlled by antiemetics.

### PATIENT/FAMILY TEACHING

• Report diarrhea, rash, mouth soreness, other new symptoms.

# tiotropium

tye-oh-**trope**-ee-yum
(Spiriva HandiHaler, Spiriva Respimat)
**Do not confuse Spiriva with Inspra, or tiotropium with ipratropium.**

## FIXED-COMBINATION(S)

**Stiolto Respimat:** tiotropium/olodaterol (a bronchodilator): 2.5 mcg/2.5 mcg.

## ◆CLASSIFICATION

**PHARMACOTHERAPEUTIC:** Anticholinergic. **CLINICAL:** Bronchodilator.

## USES

Long-term maintenance treatment of bronchospasm associated with COPD, including chronic bronchitis, emphysema, and for reducing COPD exacerbations. Maintenance treatment of asthma in pts 12 yrs and older.

## PRECAUTIONS

**Contraindications:** Hypersensitivity to tiotropium. History of hypersensitivity to ipratropium. **Cautions:** Narrow-angle glaucoma, prostatic hypertrophy, bladder neck obstruction, moderate to severe renal impairment, history of hypersensitivity to atropine, myasthenia gravis.

## ACTION

Binds to recombinant human muscarinic receptors at smooth muscle, resulting in long-acting bronchial smooth muscle relaxation. **Therapeutic Effect:** Relieves bronchospasm.

## PHARMACOKINETICS

Binds extensively to tissue. Protein binding: 72%. Metabolized by oxidation. Excreted in urine. **Half-life:** 5–6 days.

## ⧗ LIFESPAN CONSIDERATIONS

**Pregnancy/Lactation:** Unknown if distributed in breast milk. **Children:** Safety and efficacy not established. **Elderly:** Higher frequency of dry mouth, constipation, UTI noted with increasing age.

## INTERACTIONS

**DRUG:** Concurrent administration with **anticholinergics (e.g., ipratropium)** may increase adverse effects. **HERBAL:** None significant. **FOOD:** None known. **LAB VALUES:** None significant.

## AVAILABILITY (Rx)

**Inhalation Spray (Spiriva Respimat):** 1.25 mcg/actuation, 2.5 mcg/actuation.
**Powder for Inhalation (Spiriva):** 18 mcg/capsule (in blister packs).

## ADMINISTRATION/HANDLING

**Inhalation (Spiriva)**
• Open dustcap of HandiHaler by pulling it upward, then open mouthpiece. • Place capsule in center chamber and firmly close mouthpiece until a click is heard, leaving the dustcap open. • Hold HandiHaler device with mouthpiece upward, press piercing button completely in once, and release. • Instruct pt to breathe out completely before breathing in slowly and deeply but at rate sufficient to hear the capsule vibrate. • Have pt hold breath as long as it is comfortable until exhaling slowly. • Instruct pt to repeat once again to ensure full dose is received.
**Spiriva Respimat** • Refer to manufacturer's pt instructions.
**Storage** • Store at room temperature. Do not expose capsules to extreme temperature, moisture. • Do not store capsules in HandiHaler device. • Use immediately once foil is peeled back or removed.

## INDICATIONS/ROUTES/DOSAGE

**COPD (Maintenance Treatment, Reduction of COPD Exacerbations)**
**Inhalation:** *(Spiriva):* **ADULTS, ELDERLY:** 18 mcg (1 capsule)/day via HandiHaler inhalation device. **(Spiriva Respimat):** 2 inhalation (2.5 mg/inhalation) once daily.

**Asthma**
**Inhalation:** *(Spiriva Respimat):* **ADULTS, ELDERLY, CHILDREN 12 YRS AND OLDER:** 2 inhalations of 1.25 mcg once daily.

**Dosage in Renal Impairment**
**CrCl 50 ml/min or less:** Use caution in moderate to severe impairment.

**Dosage in Hepatic Impairment**
No dose adjustment.

## SIDE EFFECTS

**Frequent (16%–6%):** Dry mouth, sinusitis, pharyngitis, dyspepsia, UTI, rhinitis. **Occasional (5%–4%):** Abdominal pain, peripheral edema, constipation, epistaxis, vomiting, myalgia, rash, oral candidiasis.

## ADVERSE EFFECTS/ TOXIC REACTIONS

Angina pectoris, depression, flu-like symptoms, glaucoma, increased intraocular pressure occur rarely.

**T**

---

## NURSING CONSIDERATIONS

### BASELINE ASSESSMENT

Offer emotional support (high incidence of anxiety due to difficulty in breathing, sympathomimetic response to drug). Auscultate lung sounds.

### INTERVENTION/EVALUATION

Monitor rate, depth, rhythm, type of respiration; quality, rate of pulse. Assess lung sounds for rhonchi, wheezing, rales. Monitor ABGs. Observe for clavicular retractions, hand tremor. Evaluate for clinical improvement (quieter, slower respirations, relaxed facial expression, cessation of clavicular retractions).

### PATIENT/FAMILY TEACHING

• Increase fluid intake (decreases lung secretion viscosity). • Do not use more than 1 capsule for inhalation at any one time. • Rinsing mouth with water immediately after inhalation may prevent mouth/throat dryness, thrush. • Avoid excessive use of caffeine derivatives (chocolate, coffee, tea, cola, cocoa). • Report eye pain/discomfort, blurred vision, visual halos.

# tipiracil/trifluridine

trye-**flure**-i-deen/tye-**pir**-a-sil
(Lonsurf)
**Do not confuse trifluridine with floxuridine, or tipiracil with tipifarnib or Pipracil.**

## ◆CLASSIFICATION

**PHARMACOTHERAPEUTIC:** Nucleoside metabolic inhibitor/thymidine phosphorylase inhibitor. **CLINICAL:** Antineoplastic.

## USES

Treatment of pts with metastatic colorectal cancer who have been previously treated with fluoropyrimidine-, oxaliplatin-, and irinotecan-based chemotherapy, an anti–vascular endothelial growth factor (VEGF) biological therapy, and if RAS wild-type, an anti–epidermal growth factor (EGFR) therapy.

## PRECAUTIONS

**Contraindications:** Hypersensitivity to trifluridine or tipiracil. **Cautions:** Baseline anemia, leukopenia, neutropenia, thrombocytopenia; active infection, pts at increased risk of infection (e.g., diabetes, indwelling catheters), pts with high tumor burden. History of pulmonary embolism.

## ACTION

Trifluridine interferes with DNA synthesis and cell proliferation of cancer cells. Tipiracil increases exposure of trifluridine by inhibiting metabolism via thymidine phosphorylase. **Therapeutic Effect:** Inhibits tumor cell growth and metastasis.

## PHARMACOKINETICS

Rapidly absorbed. Metabolized by thymidine phosphorylase (not metabolized in liver). Protein binding: trifluridine: 96%; tipiracil: 8%. Peak plasma concentration: 2 hrs. Eliminated primarily in urine (50%). **Half-life:** trifluridine: 1.4 hrs (2.1 hrs at steady state); tipiracil: 2.1 hrs (2.4 hrs at steady state).

## ⏳ LIFESPAN CONSIDERATIONS

**Pregnancy/Lactation:** Avoid pregnancy; may cause fetal harm. Female pts of reproductive potential must use effective contraception during treatment. Unknown if distributed in breast milk. Must either discontinue drug or discontinue breastfeeding. **Males:** Due to risk of potential exposure, male pts must use condoms during sexual activity during treatment and up to 3 mos after discontinuation. **Children:** Safety and efficacy not established. **Elderly:** May have increased risk of neutropenia, thrombocytopenia.

## INTERACTIONS

**DRUG:** Not specified (no formal studies have been conducted). **HERBAL:** None

---

underlined – top prescribed drug

significant. **FOOD:** None known. **LAB VALUES:** Expected to decrease Hct, Hgb, platelets, neutrophils, RBC, WBC.

## AVAILABILITY (Rx)

**Fixed-Dose Combination Tablets:** trifluridine/tipiracil: 15 mg/6.14 mg, 20 mg/8.19 mg.

## ADMINISTRATION/HANDLING

**PO**

• Give within 1 hr of completion of morning and evening meals. Do not give on empty stomach.

## INDICATIONS/ROUTES/DOSAGE

**Note:** Do not initiate the cycle until ANC is 1,500/mm³ or greater; febrile neutropenia is resolved; platelet count is 75,000/mm³ or greater; grade 3 or 4 nonhematologic toxicity is resolved to grade 1 or 0.

**Colorectal Cancer**
**PO: ADULTS, ELDERLY:** (Dose based on trifluridine component) 35 mg/m² (rounded to nearest 5-mg increment) twice daily on days 1–5 and days 8–12 of 28-day cycle. Continue until disease progression or unacceptable toxicity. **Maximum:** 80 mg/dose (based on trifluridine component).

**Dose Modification**
Based on Common Terminology Criteria for Adverse Events (CTCAE).

**Hematological/Nonhematologic Toxicity**
Interrupt treatment for ANC less than 500/mm³; febrile neutropenia; platelet count less than 50,000/mm³; grade 3 or 4 nonhematologic toxicity. Do not restart until ANC is 1,500/mm³ or greater; febrile neutropenia is resolved; platelet count is 75,000/mm³ or greater; grade 3 or 4 nonhematologic toxicity is resolved to grade 1 or 0 (except grade 3 nausea and/or vomiting controlled by antiemetic therapy; grade 3 diarrhea responsive to antidiarrheal medication). Once resolved, resume at decreased incremental dose of 5 mg/m² from previous dose. A maximum of 3 dose reductions is allowed to dosage minimum of 20 mg/m² twice daily. Do not increase dose after it has been reduced.

**Dosage in Renal Impairment**
**Mild to moderate impairment:** No dose adjustment. **Severe impairment:** Not studied; use caution.

**Dosage in Hepatic Impairment**
**Mild impairment:** No dose adjustment. **Moderate to severe impairment:** Not studied; use caution.

## SIDE EFFECTS

**Frequent (52%–19%):** Asthenia, fatigue, nausea, diarrhea, decreased appetite, vomiting, abdominal pain, pyrexia. **Occasional (8%–7%):** Stomatitis, dysgeusia, alopecia.

## ADVERSE EFFECTS/TOXIC REACTIONS

Severe and/or life-threatening myelosuppression including anemia (77% of pts), grade 3 anemia (18% of pts), neutropenia (67% of pts), grade 3 or 4 neutropenia (27% and 11% of pts), thrombocytopenia (42% of pts), grade 3 or 4 thrombocytopenia (5% and 1% of pts), febrile neutropenia (3.8% of pts) may occur. Infectious processes including nasopharyngitis, urinary tract infection reported in 2%–4% of pts. Pulmonary embolism occurred in 2% of pts. Interstitial lung disease occurs rarely.

## NURSING CONSIDERATIONS

### BASELINE ASSESSMENT

Obtain baseline CBC and screen for anemia, neutropenia, thrombocytopenia. Obtain vital signs. Verify pregnancy status before start of each cycle. Screen for active infection; history of pulmonary embolism. Assess hydration status. Question pt's usual stool characteristics (color, frequency, consistency).

### INTERVENTION/EVALUATION

Follow proper handling and disposal procedures for cytotoxic drugs. Monitor

**T**

ANC, CBC on day 15 of each cycle. If any grade 3 or 4 hematologic toxicity occurs, repeat ANC, CBC more frequently. If chest pain, dyspnea, tachycardia occurs, provide supplemental $O_2$ and obtain radiologic testing to rule out pulmonary embolism. Diligently monitor for infection. Monitor daily stool pattern, consistency. Encourage PO intake. Monitor for bleeding if thrombocytopenia occurs.

**PATIENT/FAMILY TEACHING**

• Blood levels will be monitored regularly. • Treatment may cause fetal harm. Female pts of childbearing potential should use effective contraception during treatment. Immediately report suspected pregnancy. Do not breastfeed. • Male pts must use condoms during sexual activity. • Immediately report chest pain, difficult breathing, fast heart rate, rapid breathing; may indicate life-threatening blood clot in the lungs. • Report symptoms of bone marrow suppression or infection such as bruising easily, chills, cough, dizziness, fainting, fever, shortness of breath, weakness, or burning with urination. • Avoid crowds; those with active infection. • Take within 1 hr of breakfast and evening meal. • Drink plenty of fluids. • Report diarrhea, nausea, vomiting that is not controlled by antinausea, antidiarrheal medication. • Report bleeding of any kind.

# tipranavir

tye-**pran**-a-veer
(Aptivus)

■ **BLACK BOX ALERT** ■ May cause hepatitis (including fatalities), hepatic dysfunction. Intracranial hemorrhage has occurred (in combination with ritonavir).

## ◆CLASSIFICATION

**PHARMACOTHERAPEUTIC:** Protease inhibitor. **CLINICAL:** Antiretroviral.

## USES

Treatment of HIV infection in combination with ritonavir and other antiretroviral agents (limited to highly treatment experienced or multi–protease inhibitor resistant pts).

## PRECAUTIONS

**Contraindications:** Hypersensitivity to tipranavir. Moderate to severe hepatic impairment, medications dependent on CYP3A for clearance, concurrent use of tipranavir/ritonavir with strong CYP3A inducers: alfuzosin, amiodarone, bepridil, dihydroergotamine, ergonovine, ergotamine, flecainide, lovastatin, methylergonovine, midazolam (oral), propafenone, quinidine, rifampin, sildenafil (pulmonary arterial hypertension), simvastatin, St. John's wort, triazolam. **Cautions:** Hemophilia, known sulfonamide allergy, mild hepatic impairment, pts at increased risk for bleeding from trauma, surgery, concurrent antiplatelet/anticoagulant therapy.

## ACTION

Binds to HIV-1 protease activity sites. Inhibits cleavage of viral protein precursors into functional proteins necessary for infectious HIV. **Therapeutic Effect:** Prevents formation of mature infectious viral cells.

## PHARMACOKINETICS

Incompletely absorbed following PO administration. Protein binding: 98%–99%. Metabolized in liver. Eliminated in feces (82%), urine (4%). **Half-life:** 6 hrs.

## ☒ LIFESPAN CONSIDERATIONS

**Pregnancy/Lactation:** Unknown if drug crosses placenta or is distributed in breast milk. **Children:** Safety and efficacy not established. **Elderly:** Age-related hepatic impairment may require dosage adjustment.

## INTERACTIONS

**DRUG:** May interfere with metabolism of **amiodarone, bepridil, ergotamine,**

midazolam, oral contraceptives. **Carbamazepine, phenobarbital, phenytoin, rifampin** may decrease concentration. May increase concentration of **colchicine, HMG-CoA reductase inhibitors, fluoxetine, paroxetine, sertraline. HMG-CoA reductase inhibitors** may increase risk of myopathy including rhabdomyolysis. **HERBAL:** St. **John's wort** may lead to loss of virologic response, potential resistance to tipranavir. **FOOD: High-fat meals** may increase bioavailability. **LAB VALUES:** May increase serum cholesterol, triglycerides, amylase, ALT, AST. May decrease WBC count.

## AVAILABILITY (Rx)

**Capsules:** 250 mg. **Oral Solution:** 100 mg/ml.

## ADMINISTRATION/HANDLING

### PO

• May take without regard to food. When taken with ritonavir tablets, must be taken with meals. • Store unopened bottles of capsules in refrigerator. • Do not freeze/refrigerate oral solution. • Once bottle is opened, capsules may be stored at room temperature for 60 days. Use oral solution within 60 days after opening.

## INDICATIONS/ROUTES/DOSAGE

**Note:** Must be taken with ritonavir.

### HIV Infection

**PO: ADULTS, ELDERLY:** 500 mg administered with 200 mg of ritonavir twice daily. **CHILDREN 2–18 YRS:** 14 mg/kg with 6 mg/kg ritonavir twice daily. **Maximum:** 500 mg with 200 mg ritonavir twice daily.

### Dosage in Renal Impairment

No dose adjustment.

### Dosage in Hepatic Impairment

**Mild impairment:** Use caution. **Moderate to severe impairment:** Contraindicated.

## SIDE EFFECTS

**Frequent (11%):** Diarrhea. **Occasional (7%–2%):** Nausea, fever, fatigue, headache, depression, vomiting, abdominal pain, weakness, rash. **Rare (Less Than 2%):** Abdominal distention, anorexia, flatulence, dizziness, insomnia, myalgia.

## ADVERSE EFFECTS/ TOXIC REACTIONS

Bronchitis occurs in 3% of pts. Anemia, neutropenia, thrombocytopenia, diabetes mellitus, hepatic failure, hepatitis, peripheral neuropathy, pancreatitis occur rarely.

## NURSING CONSIDERATIONS

### BASELINE ASSESSMENT

Obtain baseline LFT before beginning therapy and at periodic intervals during therapy. Offer emotional support. Obtain full medication history and screen for interactions.

### INTERVENTION/EVALUATION

Closely monitor for evidence of GI discomfort. Monitor daily pattern of bowel activity, stool consistency. Assess skin for evidence of rash. Monitor serum chemistry tests for marked laboratory abnormalities, particularly hepatic profile, CD4 cell count, HIV RNA plasma levels. Assess for opportunistic infections (onset of fever, oral mucosa changes, cough, other respiratory symptoms).

### PATIENT/FAMILY TEACHING

• Eat small, frequent meals to offset nausea, vomiting. • Continue therapy for full length of treatment. • Doses should be evenly spaced. • Tipranavir is not a cure for HIV infection, nor does it reduce risk of transmission to others. • Pt may continue to experience illnesses, including opportunistic infections. • Diarrhea can be controlled with OTC medication.

**T**

 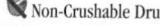

# *tiZANidine

tye-**zan**-i-deen
(Apo-Tizanidine ✦, Zanaflex)
**Do not confuse tizanidine with
tiagabine.**

## ◆CLASSIFICATION

**PHARMACOTHERAPEUTIC:** Skeletal
muscle relaxant. **CLINICAL:** Antispastic.

## USES

Acute and intermittent management of
muscle spasticity (spasms, stiffness, rigidity), spasticity associated with multiple
sclerosis or spinal cord injury.

## PRECAUTIONS

**Contraindications:** Hypersensitivity to tizanidine. Concurrent use with strong CYP1A2
inhibitors. **Cautions:** Renal/hepatic disease,
pts at risk for severe hypotensive effects,
cardiac disease, psychiatric disorders, elderly.

## ACTION

Increases presynaptic inhibition of spinal
motor neurons mediated by alpha$_2$-
adrenergic agonists, reducing facilitation
to postsynaptic motor neurons. **Therapeutic Effect:** Reduces muscle spasticity.

## PHARMACOKINETICS

Metabolized in liver. Primarily excreted
in urine. **Half-life:** 2 hrs.

## INTERACTIONS

**DRUG: Alcohol, other CNS depres-
sants (e.g,. lorazepam, morphine,
zolpidem)** may increase CNS depressant effects. **Antiarrhythmics (e.g.,
amiodarone, sotalol), cimetidine,
oral contraceptives, acyclovir** may
increase risk of bradycardia, hypotension, or **CNS** depression. **Strong
CYP1A2 inhibitors (e.g., ciprofloxacin, fluvoxamine)** may increase
concentration/adverse effects (contraindicated). **HERBAL: Gotu kola, kava
kava, St. John's wort, valerian** may
increase CNS depression. **Black cohosh,**
**hawthorn, periwinkle** may increase
hypotensive effect. **FOOD:** None known.
**LAB VALUES:** May increase serum alkaline phosphatase, ALT, AST.

## AVAILABILITY (Rx)

**Capsules:** 2 mg, 4 mg, 6 mg. **Tablets:**
2 mg, 4 mg.

## ADMINISTRATION/HANDLING

**PO**
• Capsules may be opened and sprinkled on food. • May give without regard to food. • Administration should
be consistent and not switched between
giving with or without food.

## INDICATIONS/ROUTES/DOSAGE

**Muscle Spasticity**
**PO: ADULTS, ELDERLY:** Initially, 2 mg 3
times/day at 6- to 8-hr intervals as needed.
Can be gradually increased in 2- to 4-mg
increments with a minimum of 1–4 days
between dosage increases. **Maximum:** 36
mg/24 hrs in divided doses.
**Discontinuation of Therapy:** Gradually
taper dose by 2–4 mg daily.

**Dosage in Renal Impairment**
May require dose reduction/less frequent
dosing. **CrCl less than 25 ml/min:** Reduce dose by 50%. If higher doses needed,
increase dose instead of frequency.

**Dosage in Hepatic Impairment**
Avoid use if possible. If used, monitor for
adverse effects (e.g., hypotension).

## SIDE EFFECTS

**Frequent (49%–41%):** Dry mouth, drowsiness, asthenia. **Occasional (16%–4%):**
Dizziness, UTI, constipation. **Rare (3%):**
Nervousness, amblyopia, pharyngitis, rhinitis, vomiting, urinary frequency.

## ADVERSE EFFECTS/
TOXIC REACTIONS

Hypotension may be associated with bradycardia, orthostatic hypotension, and, rarely,
syncope. Risk of hypotension increases as
dosage increases; hypotension is noted
within 1 hr after administration.

T

## NURSING CONSIDERATIONS

### BASELINE ASSESSMENT

Record onset, type, location, duration of muscular spasm. Check for immobility, stiffness, swelling. Obtain LFT.

### INTERVENTION/EVALUATION

Assist with ambulation at all times. For those on long-term therapy, serum hepatic/renal function tests should be performed periodically. Evaluate for therapeutic response (decreased intensity of skeletal muscle pain/tenderness, improved mobility, decrease in spasticity). Go from lying to standing slowly.

### PATIENT/FAMILY TEACHING

• Avoid tasks that require alertness, motor skills until response to drug is established. • Avoid sudden changes in posture. • May cause hypotension, sedation, impaired coordination. • Avoid alcohol.

---

# tobramycin

**toe-bra-mye-sin**
(TOBI, Tobrex)

■ **BLACK BOX ALERT** ■ May cause neurotoxicity, nephrotoxicity, ototoxicity. Ototoxicity usually is irreversible. Increased risk of neuromuscular blockade, including respiratory paralysis, particularly when given after anesthesia or muscle relaxants. May cause fetal harm.
**Do not confuse tobramycin with vancomycin, or Tobrex with TobraDex.**

### FIXED-COMBINATION(S)

**TobraDex:** tobramycin/dexamethasone (a steroid): 0.3%/0.1% per ml or per g. **Zylet:** tobramycin/loteprednol: 0.3%/0.5%.

### ◆CLASSIFICATION

**PHARMACOTHERAPEUTIC:** Aminoglycoside. **CLINICAL:** Antibiotic.

## USES

Treatment of susceptible infections due to *P. aeruginosa,* other gram-negative organisms including skin/skin structure, bone, joint, respiratory tract infections; postop, burn, intra-abdominal infections; complicated UTI; septicemia; meningitis. **Ophthalmic:** Superficial eye infections: blepharitis, conjunctivitis, keratitis, corneal ulcers. **Inhalation:** Bronchopulmonary infections *(Pseudomonas aeruginosa)* in pts with cystic fibrosis.

## PRECAUTIONS

**Contraindications:** Hypersensitivity to tobramycin, other aminoglycosides (cross-sensitivity) and their components. **Cautions:** Renal impairment, preexisting auditory or vestibular impairment, conditions that depress neuromuscular transmission, Parkinson's disease, myasthenia gravis, hypocalcemia, preganancy, elderly.

## ACTION

Irreversibly binds to protein on bacterial ribosomes. **Therapeutic Effect:** Interferes with protein synthesis of susceptible microorganisms.

## PHARMACOKINETICS

Rapid, complete absorption after IM administration. Protein binding: less than 30%. Widely distributed (does not cross blood-brain barrier; low concentrations in CSF). Excreted unchanged in urine. Removed by hemodialysis. **Half-life:** 2–4 hrs (increased in renal impairment, neonates; decreased in cystic fibrosis, febrile or burn pts).

## ⌛ LIFESPAN CONSIDERATIONS

**Pregnancy/Lactation:** Drug readily crosses placenta; distributed in breast milk. May cause fetal nephrotoxicity. Ophthalmic form should not be used in breastfeeding mothers and only when specifically indicated in pregnancy. **Children:** Immature renal function in neonates, premature infants may increase risk of toxicity. **Elderly:** Age-related renal impairment

T

---

may increase risk of toxicity; dosage adjustment recommended.

## INTERACTIONS

**DRUG: Nephrotoxic medications (e.g., NSAIDs, IV contrast, lisinopril, furosemide), ototoxic medications (e.g., bumetanide, furosemide)** may increase risk of nephrotoxicity, ototoxicity. **Neuromuscular blockers (e.g., cisatracurium, vercuronium)** may increase neuromuscular blockade. **HERBAL:** None significant. **FOOD:** None known. **LAB VALUES:** May increase serum BUN, bilirubin, creatinine, alkaline phosphatase, LDH, ALT, AST. May decrease serum calcium, magnesium, potassium, sodium. Therapeutic peak serum level: 5–20 mcg/ml; therapeutic trough serum level: 0.5–2 mcg/ml. Toxic peak serum level: greater than 20 mcg/ml; toxic trough serum level: greater than 2 mcg/ml.

## AVAILABILITY (Rx)

**Infusion, Premix:** 60 mg/50 ml, 80 mg/100 ml. **Inhalation Powder (TOBI Podhaler):** 28 mg in a capsule. **Injection, Powder for Reconstitution:** 1.2 g. **Injection, Solution:** 10 mg/ml, 40 mg/ml. **Ointment, Ophthalmic (Tobrex):** 0.3%. **Solution, Nebulization (TOBI):** 60 mg/ml. **Solution, Ophthalmic (Tobrex):** 0.3%.

## ADMINISTRATION/HANDLING

**◀ALERT▶** Coordinate peak and trough lab draws with administration times.

 **IV**

**Reconstitution** • Dilute with 50–100 ml D₅W or 0.9% NaCl. Amount of diluent for infants, children depends on individual need.
**Rate of Administration** • Infuse over 30–60 min.
**Storage** • Store vials at room temperature. • Solutions may be discolored by light or air (does not affect potency). • Reconstituted solution stable for 24 hrs at room temperature or 96 hrs if refrigerated.

**IM**
• To minimize discomfort, give deep IM slowly. • Less painful if injected into gluteus maximus rather than lateral aspect of thigh.

**Inhalation**
• Refrigerate. • May store at room temperature up to 28 days after removing from refrigerator. • Do not use if cloudy or contains particulates. • **Podhaler:** • Pt must not swallow capsules. • Doses should be as close as possible to 12 hrs apart and not less than 6 hrs apart. • Use Podhaler device supplied.

**Ophthalmic**
• Place gloved finger on lower eyelid, pull out until pocket is formed between eye and lower lid. • Place correct number of drops (¼–½ inch ointment) into pocket. • **Solution:** Apply digital pressure to lacrimal sac for 1–2 min (minimizes drainage into nose/throat, reducing risk of systemic effects). • **Ointment:** Instruct pt to close eye for 1–2 min, rolling eyeball (increases contact area of drug to eye). • Remove excess solution/ointment around eye.

## ⚕ IV INCOMPATIBILITIES

Amphotericin B complex (Abelcet, AmBisome, Amphotec), heparin, indomethacin (Indocin), piperacillin-tazobactam (Zosyn), propofol (Diprivan), sargramostim (Leukine, Prokine).

## ⚕ IV COMPATIBILITIES

Amiodarone (Cordarone), calcium gluconate, cefepime, ceftaroline, ceftazidime, dexmedetomidine (Precedex), diltiazem (Cardizem), furosemide (Lasix), hydromorphone (Dilaudid), insulin, linezolid (Zyvox), magnesium sulfate, midazolam (Versed), morphine, nicardipine (Cardene), tigecycline (Tygacil).

## INDICATIONS/ROUTES/DOSAGE

**◀ALERT▶** Space parenteral doses evenly around the clock. Dosage based on ideal body weight. Peak, trough levels

T

determined periodically to maintain desired serum concentrations (minimizes risk of toxicity). Recommended peak level: 4–10 mcg/ml; trough level: 0.5–2 mcg/ml.

**Usual Parenteral Dosage**
IV: ADULTS, ELDERLY: 3–7.5 mg/kg/day in 3 divided doses. Once-daily dosing: 4–7 mg/kg every 24 hrs. CHILDREN 5 YRS AND OLDER: 2–2.5 mg/kg/dose q8h. CHILDREN YOUNGER THAN 5 YRS: 2.5 mg/kg/dose q8h. NEONATES LESS THAN 1 KG (14 DAYS OR YOUNGER): 5 mg/kg/dose q48h; (15–28 DAYS): 4–5 mg/kg/dose q24–48hrs. 1–2 KG (7 DAYS OR YOUNGER): 5 mg/kg/dose q48h; (8–28 DAYS): 4–5 mg/kg/dose q24–48hrs. GREATER THAN 2 KG (7 DAYS OR YOUNGER): 4 mg/kg q24h; (8–28 DAYS): 4 mg/kg q12–24hrs.

**Usual Ophthalmic Dosage**
Ophthalmic Ointment: ADULTS, ELDERLY, CHILDREN 2 MOS AND OLDER: Apply ½ inch to conjunctiva q8–12h (q3–4h for severe infections).
Ophthalmic Solution: ADULTS, ELDERLY, CHILDREN 2 MOS AND OLDER: 1–2 drops in affected eye q4h (2 drops/hr for severe infections).

**Usual Inhalation Dosage (Cystic Fibrosis)**
Inhalation High Dose: ADULTS, CHILDREN 6 YRS AND OLDER: 300 mg q12h 28 days on, 28 days off. Podhaler: Four 28-mg capsules twice daily for 28 days followed by 28 days off.

**Dosage in Renal Impairment**
Dosage and frequency modified based on degree of renal impairment, serum drug concentration. After loading dose of 1–2 mg/kg, maintenance dose and frequency are based on serum creatinine levels, creatinine clearance.

| Creatinine Clearance | Dosing Interval |
|---|---|
| 41–60 ml/min | q12h |
| 21–40 ml/min | q24h |
| 10–20 ml/min | q48h |
| Less than 10 ml/min | q72h |

| Creatinine Clearance | Dosing Interval |
|---|---|
| Hemodialysis | Loading dose 2–3 mg/kg then 1–2 mg/kg q48–72h |
| Continuous renal replacement therapy | Loading dose 2–3 mg/kg then 1–2.5 mg/kg q24–48h |

**Dosage in Hepatic Impairment**
No dose adjustment.

## SIDE EFFECTS

Occasional: IM: Pain, induration. IV: Phlebitis, thrombophlebitis. Topical: Hypersensitivity reaction (fever, pruritus, rash, urticaria). Ophthalmic: Tearing, itching, redness, eyelid swelling. Rare: Hypotension, nausea, vomiting.

## ADVERSE EFFECTS/ TOXIC REACTIONS

Nephrotoxicity (acute kidney injury, acute tubular necrosis, renal failure) may be reversible if drug is stopped at first sign of symptoms. Irreversible ototoxicity (dizziness, ringing/roaring in ears, hearing loss), neurotoxicity (headache, dizziness, lethargy, tremor, visual disturbances) occur occasionally. Risk increases with higher dosages or prolonged therapy or if solution is applied directly to mucosa. Superinfections, particularly fungal infections, may result from bacterial imbalance with any administration route. Anaphylaxis may occur.

## NURSING CONSIDERATIONS

### BASELINE ASSESSMENT

Dehydration must be treated before beginning parenteral therapy. Question for history of allergies, esp. aminoglycosides, sulfite (and parabens for topical, ophthalmic routes). Establish baseline for hearing acuity. Obtain baseline lab tests, esp. renal function.

### INTERVENTION/EVALUATION

Monitor I&O (maintain hydration), urinalysis, renal function. Monitor results of

T

peak/trough blood tests. **Therapeutic serum level:** peak: 5–20 mcg/ml; trough: 0.5–2 mcg/ml. **Toxic serum level:** peak: greater than 20 mcg/ml; trough: greater than 2 mcg/ml. Be alert to ototoxic, neurotoxic symptoms. Evaluate IV site for phlebitis (heat, pain, red streaking over vein). Assess for rash. Be alert for superinfection, particularly anal/genital pruritus, changes of oral mucosa, diarrhea. When treating pts with neuromuscular disorders, assess respiratory response carefully. **Ophthalmic:** Assess for redness, swelling, itching, tearing.

### PATIENT/FAMILY TEACHING

• Report any hearing, visual, balance, urinary problems, even after therapy is completed. • **Ophthalmic:** Blurred vision, tearing may occur briefly after application. • Report persistent tearing, redness, irritation.

## tocilizumab

toe-si-**liz**-oo-mab
(Actemra)

■ **BLACK BOX ALERT** ■ Tuberculosis, serious, invasive fungal infections, other opportunistic infections have occurred. Test for tuberculosis prior to and during treatment, regardless of initial result.

### ◆CLASSIFICATION

**PHARMACOTHERAPEUTIC:** Interleukin (IL)-6 receptor inhibitor. **CLINICAL:** Antirheumatic arthritis agent.

### USES

Treatment of moderate to severe rheumatoid arthritis in adults who had inadequate response to disease-modifying antirheumatic drugs (DMARDs). Treatment of active systemic juvenile idiopathic arthritis (SJIA) in pts 2 yrs of age and older. Treatment of active polyarticular juvenile idiopathic arthritis (PJIA) in pts 2 yrs and older.

## PRECAUTIONS

**Contraindications:** Hypersensitivity to tocilizumab. **Cautions:** Platelet count 100,000/mm³ or less, ANC less than 2,000/mm³, ALT, AST greater than 1.5 times upper limit of normal (ULN) prior to treatment. Do not administer to pts with active infection. Preexisting or recent-onset CNS demyelinating disorders, including multiple sclerosis; pts with chronic or recurrent infection or who have been exposed to tuberculosis; hematologic cytopenia, hepatic impairment, elderly, pts at increased risk of GI perforation. Avoid live vaccinations.

## ACTION

Binds to IL-6 receptors, inhibiting signals of proinflammatory cytokines. **Therapeutic Effect:** Inhibits/slows structural joint damage, improves physical function.

## PHARMACOKINETICS

Distributed in steady state of plasma and tissue compartments. Undergoes biphasic elimination from circulation. **Half-life:** 11–13 days.

## ⧖ LIFESPAN CONSIDERATIONS

**Pregnancy/Lactation:** Unknown if distributed in breast milk. **Children:** Safety and efficacy not established. **Elderly:** Cautious use due to increased risk of serious infections, malignancy.

## INTERACTIONS

**DRUG:** Anakinra, abatacept, **corticosteroids, methotrexate** may increase risk of infection. **Live vaccines** not recommended. May decrease effects of **lovastatin, simvastatin, oral contraceptives, warfarin, phenytoin.** **HERBAL: Echinacea** may alter levels/effects. **FOOD:** None known. **LAB VALUES:** May increase serum ALT, AST, lipids. May decrease platelets, neutrophils.

## AVAILABILITY (Rx)

**Injection Solution:** 20 mg/ml (80 mg/ 4 ml, 200 mg/10 ml, 400 mg/20 ml).

**Syringe for Subcutaneous Administration:** 162 mg/0.9 ml.

## ADMINISTRATION/HANDLING

◀ **ALERT** ▶ Do not infuse IV push or bolus.

 **IV**

**Reconstitution** • Dilute in 100 ml 0.9% NaCl (50 ml 0.9% NaCl for SJIA pts weighing less than 30 kg). • Prior to mixing, withdraw and discard volume of NaCl equal to volume of patient-dosed solution. • Invert bag to avoid foaming. • Inject solution and dilute for mixture that equals 50 ml or 100 ml in NaCl bag.

**Rate of Administration** • Infuse over 1 hr.

**Storage** • Refrigerate vials; do not freeze. • Diluted solutions may be stored for 24 hrs at room temperature or refrigerated. • Protect from light until time of use. • Solution appears colorless. Discard solution if appears cloudy, discolored, or contains particulate.

## INDICATIONS/ROUTES/DOSAGE

**Note:** Do not infuse concomitantly in same IV line with other drugs. Do not begin if ANC less than 2,000/mm³, platelets less than 100,000/mm³, or ALT or AST more than 1.5 times ULN.

**Moderate to Severely Active Rheumatoid Arthritis**

**IV Infusion: ADULTS, ELDERLY:** 4 mg/kg every 4 wks initially. May increase to 8 mg/kg every 4 wks. **Maximum:** 800 mg per dose.

**SQ: ADULTS, ELDERLY (100 KG OR GREATER):** 162 mg/wk. **(LESS THAN 100 KG):** 162 mg every other wk. May increase to every wk based on clinical response.

**Dosage Modification**
Hepatic enzyme levels greater than ULN.

| Lab Value | Recommendation |
|---|---|
| 1–3 times ULN | Dose modify concomitant DMARDs or reduce dose to 4 mg/kg until ALT, AST normalized |
| Greater than 3–5 times ULN | Interrupt treatment until ALT, AST less than 3 times ULN, then follow guidelines for 1–3 times ULN |
| Greater than 5 times ULN | Discontinue treatment |

**SJIA**
**IV: CHILDREN MORE THAN 30 KG:** 8 mg/kg q2wks. **CHILDREN 30 KG OR LESS:** 12 mg/kg q2wks.

**PJIA**
**IV: CHILDREN MORE THAN 30 KG:** 8 mg/kg q4wks. **CHILDREN 30 KG OR LESS:** 10 mg/kg q4wks.

**Dosage in Renal Impairment**
**Mild impairment:** No dose adjustment. **Moderate to severe impairment:** Use caution (not studied).

**Dosage in Hepatic Impairment**
Not recommended.

## SIDE EFFECTS

**Occasional (8%–6%):** Upper respiratory tract infection, nasopharyngitis, headache, hypertension. **Rare (5%–3%):** Infusion reaction, dizziness, bronchitis, rash, oral ulceration.

## ADVERSE EFFECTS/ TOXIC REACTIONS

Up to 48% of pts experience elevated ALT, AST. Neutropenia, thrombocytopenia occur in 4% of pts. Serious infections, including sepsis, pneumonia, tuberculosis, invasive fungal infections, hepatitis B have occurred. Anaphylactic reaction, rash, pruritus, urticaria, bronchospasm, swelling, dyspnea occur in less than 0.2% of pts; hypersensitivity reactions (hypertension, headaches, flushing) occur more frequently. Increased risk of lymphoma, melanoma. New onset or exacerbation of CNS demyelinating disorders, including multiple sclerosis. Risk of

**T**

gastric perforation with concomitant use of NSAIDs, corticosteroids.

## NURSING CONSIDERATIONS

### BASELINE ASSESSMENT

Evaluate pt for active tuberculosis and test for latent infection prior to initiating treatment and periodically during therapy. Induration of 5 mm or greater with tuberculin skin testing should be considered a positive test result when assessing for latent tuberculosis. Antifungal therapy should be considered for pts who reside or travel to regions where mycoses are endemic. Do not initiate therapy during an active infection. Viral reactivation can occur in cases of herpes zoster, HIV. Assess baseline lab results (hepatic enzymes, cholesterol, triglycerides, platelets, neutrophils) q4–8wks during treatment. Pts should report history of diverticulitis, weakened immune system, HIV, hepatic disease, GI bleeding, hemoptysis, diarrhea, weight loss, cancer, prior cancer treatment, use of NSAIDs, glucocorticosteroids.

### INTERVENTION/EVALUATION

Monitor hepatitis B carriers during and several months following therapy. If reactivation occurs, consider interrupting treatment. Monitor pts for signs/symptoms of tuberculosis regardless of baseline PPD. Discontinue treatment if pt develops acute infection, opportunistic infection, or sepsis and initiate appropriate antimicrobial therapy. Monitor warfarin, theophylline, cyclosporine levels for therapeutic ranges. Modify, interrupt, or discontinue treatment if ALT, AST is 1–5 times ULN.

### PATIENT/FAMILY TEACHING

• Inform pt that therapy may lower immune system response. • Detail any concomitant immunosuppressive therapy, methotrexate. • Report any history of HIV, fungal infections, hepatitis B, multiple sclerosis, hemoptysis, tuberculosis, or close relatives with active tuberculosis. • Report any travel plans to possible endemic areas. • Report signs/symptoms of stomach pain to evaluate risk of gastric perforation or history of taking NSAIDs, corticosteroids, methotrexate. • Pt will need blood levels drawn q4–8wks during treatment along with routine tuberculosis screening. • Seek immediate medical attention if adverse reaction occurs. • Do not receive live vaccines during therapy. • Notify physician if pregnant or planning on becoming pregnant. • During treatment, report any signs of liver problems, such as stomach pains, yellowing of skin/eyes, dark-amber urine, clay-colored or bloody stools, fatigue, reduced appetite, coffee ground emesis. • Pt must adhere to strict dosing schedule. • Decreased platelet count may lead to risk of bleeding.

# tofacitinib

toe-fa-**sye**-ti-nib
(Xeljanz, Xeljanz XR)
**Do not confuse tofacitinib with tipifarnib or Xeljanz with Xeloda.**

■ **BLACK BOX ALERT** ■ Increased risk for developing bacterial, viral, invasive fungal, other opportunistic infections including tuberculosis, cryptococcosis, pneumocystosis that may lead to hospitalization or death; infections often occurred in combination with other immunosuppressants (methotrexate, corticosteroids). Test for latent tuberculosis prior to treatment and during treatment, regardless of initial result. Malignancies including lymphoma, nonmelanoma skin cancer reported. Increased rate of Epstein-Barr virus–associated post-transplant lymphoproliferative disorder observed in renal transplant pts who are treated with tofacitinib and other immunosuppressive therapy drugs.

## ◆CLASSIFICATION

**PHARMACOTHERAPEUTIC:** Janus kinase (JAK) inhibitor. **CLINICAL:** Antirheumatic agent.

## USES

Treatment of adult pts with moderate to severe active rheumatoid arthritis with previous inadequate response or intolerance to methotrexate. May be used as monotherapy or in combination with methotrexate or other nonbiologic disease-modifying antirheumatic drugs (DMARDs). Do not use in combination with other biologic DMARDs or with potent immunosuppressants (e.g., azathioprine, cyclosporine).

## PRECAUTIONS

**Contraindications:** Hypersensitivity to tofacitinib. **Cautions:** Pts exposed to TB, history of serious opportunistic infections, conditions that predispose to infections (e.g., diabetes), pts at risk for GI perforation (e.g., diverticulitis), pts who resided or traveled in areas where TB is endemic, moderate to severe renal impairment, elderly, hepatic impairment, history of anemia, hyperlipidemia, hepatitis, Asian ancestry, pts with history of interstitial lung disease, heart rate less than 60 bpm, conduction abnormalities, ischemic heart disease, HF.

## ACTION

Inhibits JAK enzymes which are involved in stimulating hematopoiesis and immune cell functioning. **Therapeutic Effect:** Reduces inflammation, tenderness, swelling of joints; slows or prevents progressive joint destruction in rheumatoid arthritis (RA).

## PHARMACOKINETICS

Rapidly absorbed following PO administration. Protein binding: 40%. Peak concentration: 30–60 min. Metabolized in liver. Eliminated primarily in urine. **Half-life:** 3 hrs.

## ⌛ LIFESPAN CONSIDERATIONS

**Pregnancy/Lactation:** Not recommended in nursing mothers. Must either discontinue drug or discontinue breastfeeding. Unknown if distributed in breast milk. **Children:** Safety and efficacy not established. **Elderly:** Increased risk for serious infections, malignancy.

## INTERACTIONS

**DRUG:** May alter effects of **live virus vaccines. Immunosuppressants (e.g., azathioprine, cyclosporine)** may increase risk for added immunosuppression, infection. **CYP3A4 inhibitors (e.g., ketoconazole), CYP2C19 inhibitors (e.g., fluconazole)** may increase concentration/effects. **CYP3A4 inducers (e.g., rifampin, phenytoin)** may decrease concentration/effects. **HERBAL: St. John's wort** may decrease concentration/effect. **FOOD:** None known. **LAB VALUES:** May increase ALT, AST, bilirubin, lipids, creatinine. May decrease Hgb, neutrophils, lymphocytes.

## AVAILABILITY (Rx)

**Tablets, Film-Coated:** (Xeljanz): 5 mg. **(Xeljanz XR):** 11 mg.

## ADMINISTRATION/HANDLING

### PO

• Give without regard to food. • Do not cut, split, crush, or chew XR tablet.

## INDICATIONS/ROUTES/DOSAGE

**◀ALERT▶** Do not initiate treatment in pts with baseline active infection (systemic/localized), severe hepatic impairment, lymphocytes less than 500/mm³, ANC less than 1,000/mm³, Hgb less than 9 g/dL.

**Moderate to Severe Rheumatoid Arthritis**
**PO: ADULTS/ELDERLY:** (Xeljanz): 5 mg twice daily. **(Xeljanz XR):** 11 mg once daily.

**Dose Modification**
Reduce to 5 mg once daily for any of the following: moderate to severe renal impairment, moderate hepatic impairment, concurrent use of potent CYP3A4 inhibitors, concurrent use of one or more moderate CYP3A4 or potent CYP2C19 inhibitors.

**Lymphopenia**
Interrupt treatment until lymphocytes greater than or equal to 500/mm³. Discontinue if lymphocytes less than 500/mm³ after repeat testing.

### Neutropenia
Interrupt treatment until neutrophils greater than 1,000/mm³. Discontinue if neutrophils less than 500/mm³ after repeat testing.

### Anemia
Interrupt treatment until Hgb greater than or equal to 9 g/dL or baseline Hgb decreases less than or equal to 2 g/dL after repeat testing.

### Hepatotoxicity
Interrupt treatment until diagnosis of drug-induced hepatic injury has been excluded.

### Dosage in Renal Impairment
**Mild impairment:** No dose adjustment. **Moderate to severe impairment:** 5 mg once daily.

### Dosage in Hepatic Impairment
**Mild impairment:** No dose adjustment. **Moderate impairment:** 5 mg once daily. **Severe impairment:** Not recommended.

## SIDE EFFECTS

**Rare (4%–2%):** Upper respiratory tract infection, diarrhea, nasopharyngitis, headache, hypertension.

## ADVERSE EFFECTS/ TOXIC REACTIONS

Neutropenia, lymphopenia may increase risk for infection. Serious infections may include aspergillosis, BK virus, cellulitis, coccidioidomycosis, cryptococcus, cytomegalovirus, esophageal candidiasis, histoplasmosis, invasive fungal infections, listeriosis, pneumocystosis, pneumonia, tuberculosis, UTI, sepsis. Increased risk for various malignancies. May induce viral reactivation of hepatitis B or C virus infection, herpes zoster, HIV. Epstein-Barr virus–associated post-transplant lymphoproliferative disorder reported in 2% of pts with renal transplant. Increased risk for GI perforation.

## NURSING CONSIDERATIONS

### BASELINE ASSESSMENT
Obtain vital signs, CBC, BMP, LFT, lipid panel, urine pregnancy test results. Evaluate for active tuberculosis (TB) and test for latent infection prior to and during treatment. Induration of 5 mm or greater with purified protein derivative (PPD) is considered positive result when assessing for latent TB. Question possibility of pregnancy or breastfeeding. Screen for history/comorbidities. Obtain full medication history including vitamins, herbal products.

### INTERVENTION/EVALUATION
Obtain CBC every 4–8 wks, then every 3 mos, lipid panel 4–8 wks after initiation; hepatic function panel if hepatic impairment suspected. Monitor for TB regardless of baseline PPD. Consider discontinuation if pt develops acute infection, opportunistic infection, sepsis; initiate appropriate antimicrobial therapy. Immediately report any hemorrhaging, melena, abdominal pain, hemoptysis (may indicate GI perforation).

### PATIENT/FAMILY TEACHING
• Routinely monitor blood levels. • Therapy will lower immune system response. • Do not receive live virus vaccines. • Other immunosuppressant drugs may increase risk for infection. • Expect routine TB screening. • Fever, cough, burning with urination, body aches, chills, skin changes may indicate infection. • Report history of HIV, recent infections, hepatitis B or C, TB or close relatives who have active TB. • Report any travel plans to possible endemic areas. • Notify physician if pregnant or planning pregnancy. • Do not breastfeed. • Immediately report bleeding of any kind. • Yellowing of skin or eyes, right upper quadrant abdominal pain, bruising, clay-colored stool, dark urine may indicate liver problem. • Avoid grapefruit products.

# tolterodine

tol-**ter**-oh-deen
(Detrol, Detrol LA, Unidet ✦)
**Do not confuse Detrol with Ditropan, or tolterodine with fesoterodine.**

## ◆CLASSIFICATION

**PHARMACOTHERAPEUTIC:** Muscarinic receptor antagonist. **CLINICAL:** Antispasmodic.

## USES

Treatment of overactive bladder in pts with symptoms of urinary frequency, urgency, incontinence.

## PRECAUTIONS

**Contraindications:** Hypersensitivity to tolterodine or fesoterodine. Gastric retention, uncontrolled narrow-angle glaucoma, urinary retention. **Cautions:** Renal impairment, clinically significant bladder outflow obstruction (risk of urinary retention), GI obstructive disorders (e.g., pyloric stenosis [risk of gastric retention]), treated narrow-angle glaucoma, myasthenia gravis, prolonged QT interval (congenital/medications, hypokalemia, hypomagnesemia), hepatic impairment, elderly.

## ACTION

Antagonist of muscarinic receptors mediating urinary bladder contraction. Increases residual urine volume, reduces detrusor muscle pressure. **Therapeutic Effect:** Decreases urinary frequency, urgency.

## PHARMACOKINETICS

Immediate-release form rapidly, well absorbed after PO administration. Protein binding: 96%. Metabolized in liver. Primarily excreted in urine. Unknown if removed by hemodialysis. **Half-life:** Immediate-release: 2–10 hrs. Extended-release: 7–18 hrs.

## ⧗ LIFESPAN CONSIDERATIONS

**Pregnancy/Lactation:** Unknown if drug is distributed in breast milk. Breastfeeding not recommended. **Children:** Safety and efficacy not established. **Elderly:** No age-related precautions noted.

## INTERACTIONS

**DRUG:** CYP3A4 inhibitors (e.g., **clarithromycin, erythromycin, ketoconazole**) may increase concentration. **Fluoxetine** may inhibit drug metabolism. **HERBAL: St. John's wort** may decrease concentration/effects. **FOOD:** None known. **LAB VALUES:** None known.

## AVAILABILITY (Rx)

**Tablets (Detrol):** 1 mg, 2 mg.

⧗ **Capsules (Extended-Release [Detrol LA]):** 2 mg, 4 mg.

## ADMINISTRATION/HANDLING

**PO**
• May give without regard to food.
• Give extended-release capsules whole; do not break, crush, or open.

## INDICATIONS/ROUTES/DOSAGE

**Overactive Bladder**
**PO: ADULTS, ELDERLY (IMMEDIATE-RELEASE):** 1–2 mg twice daily **(WITH CYP3A4 INHIBITORS):** 1 mg twice daily. **(EXTENDED-RELEASE):** 2–4 mg once daily. **(WITH CYP3A4 INHIBITORS):** 2 mg once daily.

**Dosage in Renal/Hepatic Impairment**
**Mild to moderate impairment: (IMMEDIATE-RELEASE):** 1 mg twice daily. Use caution. **(EXTENDED-RELEASE):** 2 mg once daily. Use caution. **Severe impairment:** Not recommended.

## SIDE EFFECTS

**Frequent (40%):** Dry mouth. **Occasional (11%–4%):** Headache, dizziness, fatigue, constipation, dyspepsia, upper respiratory tract infection, UTI, dry eyes, abnormal vision (accommodation problems), nausea, diarrhea. **Rare (3%):** Drowsiness,

T

---

chest/back pain, arthralgia, rash, weight gain, dry skin.

## ADVERSE EFFECTS/ TOXIC REACTIONS

Overdose can result in severe anticholinergic effects, including abdominal cramps, facial warmth, excessive salivation/lacrimation, diaphoresis, pallor, urinary urgency, blurred vision, prolonged QT interval.

## NURSING CONSIDERATIONS

### BASELINE ASSESSMENT

Assess degree of overactive bladder (urinary urgency, frequency, incontinence). Question history as listed in Precautions.

### INTERVENTION/EVALUATION

Assist with ambulation if dizziness occurs. Question for visual changes. Monitor incontinence, postvoid residuals.

### PATIENT/FAMILY TEACHING

• May cause blurred vision, dry eyes/ mouth, constipation. • Report any confusion, altered mental status. • Avoid tasks that require alertness, motor skills until response to drug is established.

# tolvaptan

tol-**vap**-tan
(Samsca)

■ **BLACK BOX ALERT** ■ Osmotic demyelination (dysphagia, lethargy, slurred speech or inability to speak, seizures, coma, death) may occur with too-rapid correction of hyponatremia; slow rate of correction is essential. Should be initiated and reinitiated only in a hospital where serum sodium is monitored closely.

## ◆CLASSIFICATION

**PHARMACOTHERAPEUTIC:** Vasopressin antagonist. **CLINICAL:** Hyponatremia adjunct.

## USES

Treatment of symptomatic hypervolemic or euvolemic hyponatremia resistant to correction with fluid restriction, including pts with HF, cirrhosis, and syndrome of inappropriate antidiuretic hormone (SIADH).

## PRECAUTIONS

**Contraindications:** Hypersensitivity to tolvaptan. Hypovolemic hyponatremia, concurrent use with strong CYP3A4 inhibitors (clarithromycin, indinavir, itraconazole, ketoconazole, nefazodone, nelfinavir, ritonavir, saquinavir), pts with urgent need to raise sodium level, inability to sense or respond to thirst, pts who are anuric. **Cautions:** Hyperkalemia, concurrent use of medications that increase serum potassium, GI bleeding in pts with cirrhosis, dehydration, hypovolemia, concurrent use with hypertonic saline.

## ACTION

Promotes excretion of free water (without loss of serum electrolytes), resulting in net fluid loss, increased urine output, decreased urine osmolarity and increase in serum sodium concentration. **Therapeutic Effect:** Restores normal serum sodium levels.

## PHARMACOKINETICS

Readily absorbed following oral administration. Metabolized in liver. Protein binding: 99%. Eliminated in feces. **Half-life:** 5 hrs.

## ⧖ LIFESPAN CONSIDERATIONS

**Pregnancy/Lactation:** Systemic exposure to fetus likely. Potential for decreased neonatal viability, delayed growth/development. Unknown if distributed in breast milk. **Children:** Safety and efficacy not established. **Elderly:** No age-related precautions noted.

## INTERACTIONS

**DRUG:** CYP3A4 inhibitors (e.g., clarithromycin, diltiazem, fluconazole, ketoconazole, nefazodone, saquinavir, verapamil) may increase concentration, effects. **CYP3A4 inducers (e.g., carbamazepine, phenytoin, rifabutin, rifampin)** may decrease concentration. **Cyclosporine** may increase concentration. **HERBAL: St. John's wort** may decrease concentration. **FOOD: Grapefruit products** may increase absorption, concentration. **LAB VALUES:** May increase serum potassium, magnesium. May alter serum glucose.

## AVAILABILITY (Rx)

**Tablets:** 15 mg, 30 mg, 60 mg.

## ADMINISTRATION/HANDLING

• Give without regard to meals.

## INDICATIONS/ROUTES/DOSAGE

**Usual Dosage**
**PO: ADULTS, ELDERLY:** 15 mg once daily. Increase dose to 30 mg once daily, after at least 24 hrs (**maximum:** 60 mg once daily), to achieve desired level of serum sodium.

**Dosage in Renal Impairment**
Not recommended with CrCl less than 10 ml/min.

**Dosage in Hepatic Impairment**
Avoid use.

## SIDE EFFECTS

**Frequent (16%–13%):** Thirst, dry mouth. **Occasional (11%–4%):** Increase in urine output/urgency, asthenia, nausea, constipation, hyperglycemia, anorexia.

## ADVERSE EFFECTS/ TOXIC REACTIONS

Dysphagia, lethargy, slurred speech or inability to speak, affective changes, spastic quadriparesis, seizures, coma, death may occur with too-rapid correction of hyponatremia.

# NURSING CONSIDERATIONS

### BASELINE ASSESSMENT

Initiate only in hospital setting with serum sodium monitoring. Obtain baseline CBC, BMP, LFT, renal function test. Assess for increased pulse rate, poor skin turgor, nausea, diarrhea (signs of hyponatremia).

### INTERVENTION/EVALUATION

During initiation and titration, frequently monitor for changes in serum electrolytes and volume. Avoid fluid restriction during first 24 hrs of therapy. Monitor for improvement in signs/symptoms of hyponatremia, hypernatremia (flushing, edema, restlessness, dry mucous membranes, fever).

### PATIENT/FAMILY TEACHING

• Continue ingesting fluids in response to thirst. • Report urinary changes, loss of strength, unusual fatigue. • Report immediately symptoms of osmotic demyelination (e.g., trouble speaking/ swallowing, confusion, mood changes, trouble controlling body movements, seizures).

# topiramate

toe-**peer**-a-mate
(Apo-Topiramate ✦, Qudexy XR, Topamax, Topamax Sprinkle, Trokendi XR)
**Do not confuse Topamax or topiramate with Tegretol, Tegretol XR, or Toprol XL.**

## ◆CLASSIFICATION

**PHARMACOTHERAPEUTIC:** Carbonic anhydrase inhibitor. **CLINICAL:** Anticonvulsant.

## USES

Monotherapy for treatment of partial-onset or primary generalized tonic-clonic seizures in pts 2 yrs and older (immediate-release, Qudexy XR) or 10 yrs and older (Trokendi XR). Adjunctive therapy for partial-onset, primary generalized tonic-clonic seizures or seizures associated with Lennox-Gastaut syndrome in pts 2 yrs and older (immediate-release, Qudexy XR) or 6 yrs and older (Trokendi XR). Prevention of migraine headache (immediate-release only). **OFF-LABEL:** Neuropathic pain, diabetic neuropathy, prophylaxis of cluster headaches, infantile spasms.

## PRECAUTIONS

**Contraindications:** Hypersensitivity to topiramate. (Extended-Release): Recent alcohol use (within 6 hrs prior to or after); pts with metabolic acidosis who are taking metformin. **Cautions:** Hepatic/renal impairment, elderly, pts who are high risk for suicide, respiratory impairment, pts with congenital metabolism dysfunction or decreased mitochondrial activity. During strenuous exercise, exposure to high environmental temperature, concomitant use of medications with anticholinergic activity.

## ACTION

Blocks neuronal sodium channels, enhances GABA activity; antagonizes glutamate receptors. **Therapeutic Effect:** Decreases seizure activity.

## PHARMACOKINETICS

Rapidly absorbed after PO administration. Protein binding: 15%–41%. Metabolized in liver. Primarily excreted unchanged in urine. Removed by hemodialysis. **Half-life:** 21 hrs.

## ⧖ LIFESPAN CONSIDERATIONS

**Pregnancy/Lactation:** Unknown if distributed in breast milk. **Children:** No age-related precautions noted in pts older than 2 yrs. **Elderly:** Age-related renal impairment may require dosage adjustment.

## INTERACTIONS

**DRUG:** Alcohol, other CNS depressants (e.g., lorazepam, morphine, zolpidem) may increase CNS depression. Carbamazepine, phenytoin, valproic acid may decrease concentration/effects. Carbonic anhydrase inhibitors may increase risk of kidney stone formation and severity of metabolic acidosis. May decrease effectiveness of oral contraceptives. **HERBAL:** Evening primrose may decrease seizure threshold. **FOOD:** None known. **LAB VALUES:** May reduce serum bicarbonate, increase ALT, AST.

## AVAILABILITY (Rx)

**Capsules (Sprinkle):** 15 mg, 25 mg.

⧆ **Tablets:** (Topamax, Topiragen) 25 mg, 50 mg, 100 mg, 200 mg. ⧆ **Capsules, Extended-Release (Trokendi XR):** 25 mg, 50 mg, 100 mg, 200 mg. **Qudexy XR:** 25 mg, 50 mg, 100 mg, 150 mg, 200 mg.

## ADMINISTRATION/HANDLING

**PO**

• Do not break, crush, dissolve, or divide tablets (bitter taste). • Give without regard to meals. • Sprinkle capsules may be swallowed whole or contents sprinkled on teaspoonful of soft food and swallowed immediately; do not chew. • **Trokendi XR:** • Give whole. Do not sprinkle on food, chew, or crush. **Qudexy XR:** Swallow whole; may open and sprinkle on spoonful of soft food.

## INDICATIONS/ROUTES/DOSAGE

**Adjunctive Treatment of Partial-Onset Seizures, Lennox-Gastaut Syndrome (LGS), Tonic-Clonic Seizures**

**PO: ADULTS, ELDERLY, CHILDREN 17 YRS AND OLDER:** *(Immediate-Release):* Initially, 25 mg once or twice daily for 1 wk. May increase by 25–50 mg/day at wkly intervals. Usual maintenance dose: 100–200 mg twice daily (partial-onset) or 200 mg 2 times/day (primary tonic-clonic). **Maximum:** 1,600 mg/day. **CHILDREN 2–16 YRS:** Initially, 1–3 mg/kg/day to maximum of 25 mg at night for 1 wk. May increase by 1–3 mg/kg/day at wkly intervals given in 2 divided doses. **Maintenance:** 5–9 mg/kg/day in 2 divided doses. **ADULTS, ELDERLY:** *(Extended-Release):* Initially, 25–50 mg/day. Increase by 25–50 mg/day at wkly intervals, up to 400 mg/day. **CHILDREN 2 YRS AND OLDER:** Initially, 25 mg (based on range of 1–3 mg/kg) once daily at bedtime for 1 wk. Increase dose by 1–3 mg/kg at 1–2 wk intervals up to 5–9 mg/kg once daily.

## Monotherapy with Partial-Onset, Tonic-Clonic Seizures

**PO: ADULTS, ELDERLY, CHILDREN 10 YRS AND OLDER:** *(Immediate-Release):* Initially, 25 mg twice daily. Increase at wkly intervals up to 400 mg/day according to the following schedule: Wk 1, 25 mg twice daily. Wk 2, 50 mg twice daily. Wk 3, 75 mg twice daily. Wk 4, 100 mg twice daily. Wk 5, 150 mg twice daily. Wk 6, 200 mg twice daily. **CHILDREN 2–9 YRS:** Initially, 25 mg/day. Then 25 mg 2 times/day wk 2; then increase by 25–50 mg/day at wkly intervals up to minimum dose. (see table below) **ADULTS, ELDERLY, CHILDREN 10 YRS OR OLDER:** *(Extended-Release):* **(Qudexy XR, Trokendi XR):** Initially, 50 mg once daily. Increase by 50 mg/day at wkly intervals for first 4 wks, then by 100 mg/day for wks 5 and 6, up to 400 mg/day. **CHILDREN 2–9 YRS:** (Qudexy XR only): Initially, 25 mg once daily in evening. May increase to 50 mg once daily in wk 2, then 25–50 mg/day at wkly intervals over 5–7 wks up to **minimum daily dose (32 KG OR MORE):** 250 mg; **(12–31 KG):** 200 mg; **(11 KG OR LESS):** 150 mg. **Maximum daily dose: (38 KG OR MORE):** 300 mg; **(23–38 KG):** 350 mg; **(12–22 KG):** 300 mg; **(11 KG OR LESS):** 250 mg.

| Wgt. | Minimum | Maximum |
|---|---|---|
| 11 kg or less | 150 mg/day in 2 divided doses | 250 mg/day in 2 divided doses |
| 12–22 kg | 200 mg/day in 2 divided doses | 300 mg/day in 2 divided doses |
| 23–31 kg | 200 mg/day in 2 divided doses | 350 mg/day in 2 divided doses |
| 32–38 kg | 250 mg/day in 2 divided doses | 350 mg/day in 2 divided doses |
| 39 or more kg | 250 mg/day in 2 divided doses | 400 mg/day in 2 divided doses |

## Migraine Prevention

**PO: ADULTS, ELDERLY, CHILDREN 12 YRS and OLDER:** Initially, 25 mg/day. May increase by 25 mg/day at 7-day intervals up to a total daily dose of 100 mg/day in 2 divided doses.

## Dosage in Renal Impairment

Reduce drug dosage by 50% and titrate more slowly in pts who have CrCl less than 70 ml/min.

## Dosage in Hepatic Impairment

Use with caution.

## SIDE EFFECTS

**Frequent (30%–10%):** Drowsiness, dizziness, ataxia, nervousness, nystagmus, diplopia, paresthesia, nausea, tremor. **Occasional (9%–3%):** Confusion, breast pain, dysmenorrhea, dyspepsia, depression, asthenia, pharyngitis, weight loss, anorexia, rash, musculoskeletal pain, abdominal pain, difficulty with coordination, sinusitis, agitation, flu-like symptoms. **Rare (3%–2%):** Mood disturbances (e.g., irritability, depression), dry mouth, aggressive behavior, impaired heat regulation.

## ADVERSE EFFECTS/ TOXIC REACTIONS

Psychomotor slowing, impaired concentration, language problems (esp. word-finding difficulties), memory disturbances occur occasionally. Metabolic acidosis, suicidal ideation occur rarely.

## NURSING CONSIDERATIONS

### BASELINE ASSESSMENT

**Seizures:** Review history of seizure disorder (intensity, frequency, duration, level of consciousness). Initiate seizure precautions. Provide quiet, dark environment. Question for sensitivity to topiramate, pregnancy, use of other anticonvulsant medication (esp. carbamazepine, valproic acid, phenytoin). **Migraine:** Assess pain location, duration, intensity. Assess renal function.

T

---

✦ Canadian trade name        🚫 Non-Crushable Drug        �high Alert⎯ High Alert drug

**INTERVENTION/EVALUATION**

Observe frequently for recurrence of seizure activity. Assess for clinical improvement (decrease in intensity/frequency of seizures). Monitor renal function tests, LFT. Assist with ambulation if dizziness occurs.

**PATIENT/FAMILY TEACHING**

• Avoid tasks that require alertness, motor skills until response to drug is established (may cause dizziness, drowsiness, impaired concentration). • Drowsiness usually diminishes with continued therapy. • Avoid use of alcohol, other CNS depressants. • Do not abruptly discontinue drug (may precipitate seizures). • Strict maintenance of drug therapy is essential for seizure control. • Do not chew, crush, dissolve, or divide tablets (bitter taste). • Maintain adequate fluid intake (decreases risk of renal stone formation). • Report blurred vision, eye pain. • Report suicidal ideation, depression, unusual behavior. • Use caution with activities that may increase core temperature (exposure to extreme heat, dehydration). • Instruct pt to use alternative/additional means of contraception (topiramate decreases effectiveness of oral contraceptives).

---

## topotecan    HIGH ALERT

toe-poe-**tee**-kan
(Hycamtin)

■ **BLACK BOX ALERT** ■ Must be administered by personnel trained in administration/handling of chemotherapeutic agents. Potent immunosuppressant; severe neutropenia (absolute neutrophil count [ANC] less than 500 cells/mm$^3$) occurs in 60% of pts. Do not administer with baseline neutrophils less than 1,500/mm$^3$ and platelets less than 100,000/mm$^3$.

**Do not confuse Hycamtin with Hycomine, Mycamine, or topotecan with irinotecan.**

◆**CLASSIFICATION**

**PHARMACOTHERAPEUTIC:** DNA topoisomerase inhibitor. **CLINICAL:** Antineoplastic.

## USES

Treatment of metastatic ovarian cancer, relapsed or refractory small cell lung cancer, recurrent or resistant cervical cancer (in combination with cisplatin). **OFF-LABEL:** Treatment of central nervous system lesions/lymphoma, Ewing's sarcoma, rhabdomyosarcoma, neuroblastoma, acute myeloid leukemia.

## PRECAUTIONS

**Contraindications:** Hypersensitivity to topotecan. Baseline neutrophil count less than 1,500 cells/mm$^3$ and platelet count less than 100,000/mm$^3$, severe myelosuppression. **Cautions:** Mild myelosuppression, renal impairment, breastfeeding, pregnancy, elderly. Pts at risk for developing interstitial lung disease (e.g., lung cancer, pulmonary fibrosis).

## ACTION

Interacts with topoisomerase I, an enzyme that relieves torsional strain in DNA by inducing reversible single-strand breaks. Prevents religation of DNA strand, resulting in damage to double-strand DNA, cell death. **Therapeutic Effect:** Produces cytotoxic effect.

## PHARMACOKINETICS

Hydrolyzed to active form after IV administration. Protein binding: 35%. Excreted in urine. **Half-life:** 2–3 hrs (increased in renal impairment).

## ⊠ LIFESPAN CONSIDERATIONS

**Pregnancy/Lactation:** May cause fetal harm. Avoid pregnancy; breastfeeding not recommended. **Children:** Safety and efficacy not established. **Elderly:** Age-related renal impairment may require dosage adjustment.

---

## INTERACTIONS

**DRUG: Live virus vaccines** may potentiate virus replication, increase vaccine side effects, decrease pt's antibody response to vaccine. **Other bone marrow depressants** may increase risk of myelosuppression. **HERBAL: Echinacea** may decrease effectiveness. **FOOD:** None known. **LAB VALUES:** May increase serum bilirubin, ALT, AST, alkaline phosphatase. May decrease RBC, leukocyte, neutrophil, platelet counts, Hgb, Hct.

## AVAILABILITY (Rx)

**Injection, Powder for Reconstitution:** 4 mg (single-dose vial). **Injection, Solution:** 1 mg/ml (4 ml).

 **Capsule:** 0.25 mg, 1 mg.

## ADMINISTRATION/HANDLING

◀**ALERT**▶ Because topotecan may be carcinogenic, mutagenic, teratogenic, handle drug with extreme care during preparation/administration.

**PO**
• May take with or without food.
• Swallow whole; do not break, crush, dissolve, or divide capsule. • Do not take replacement dose if vomiting occurs.

🗓 **IV**

**Reconstitution** • Reconstitute each 4-mg vial (lyophilized powder) with 4 ml Sterile Water for Injection. • Further dilute with 50–100 ml 0.9% NaCl or D₅W. **Rate of Administration** • Administer as IV infusion over 30 min. • Extravasation associated with only mild local reactions (erythema, ecchymosis).
**Storage** • Store vials (lyophilized powder) at room temperature; refrigerate diluted solution. Diluted solution for infusion stable for 24 hrs at room temperature.

## 🔲 IV INCOMPATIBILITIES

Dexamethasone (Decadron), 5-fluorouracil, mitomycin (Mutamycin).

## 🔲 IV COMPATIBILITIES

Carboplatin (Paraplatin), cisplatin (Platinol AQ), cyclophosphamide (Cytoxan), doxorubicin (Adriamycin), etoposide (VePesid), gemcitabine (Gemzar), granisetron (Kytril), ondansetron (Zofran), paclitaxel (Taxol), palonosetron (Aloxi), vincristine (Oncovin).

## INDICATIONS/ROUTES/DOSAGE

◀**ALERT**▶ Do not give topotecan if baseline neutrophil count is less than 1,500 cells/mm³ and platelet count is less than 100,000/mm³. For retreatment, neutrophils should be greater than 1,000/mm³, platelets greater than 100,000/mm³, and Hgb 9 g/dL or greater.

**Ovarian Carcinoma, Small Cell Lung Cancer**
**IV: ADULTS, ELDERLY:** 1.5 mg/m²/day over 30 min for 5 consecutive days, beginning on day 1 of 21-day course. Minimum of 4 courses recommended. If severe neutropenia (neutrophil count less than 1,500/mm³) occurs during treatment, reduce dose for subsequent courses by 0.25 mg/m² or administer filgrastim (G-CSF) no sooner than 24 hrs after last dose of topotecan.
**PO (Small Cell Lung Cancer): ADULTS, ELDERLY:** 2.3 mg/m²/day for 5 days; repeat q21days (dose rounded to nearest 0.25 mg). **For severe neutropenia or prolonged neutropenia, platelets less than 25,000/mm³, recovery from grade 3 or 4 diarrhea:** Reduce dose by 0.4 mg/m²/day for subsequent cycles.

**Cervical Cancer**
**IV: ADULTS, ELDERLY:** 0.75 mg/m²/day for 3 days (followed by cisplatin 50 mg/m² on day 1 only). Repeat q21days (baseline neutrophil count greater than 1,500/mm³ and platelet count greater than 100,000/mm³). For severe febrile neutropenia (neutrophils less than 1,000/mm³ with temperature of 38°C) or platelet count less than 25,000/mm³: Reduce dose to 0.6 mg/m²/day for

**T**

---

subsequent cycles. If necessary, further decrease dose to 0.45 mg/m²/day.

**Dosage in Renal Impairment**

**IV:** No dosage adjustment is necessary in pts with mild renal impairment (CrCl 40–60 ml/min). For moderate renal impairment (CrCl 20–39 ml/min), give 0.75 mg/m².

**PO: CrCl 30–49 ml/min:** 1.5 mg/m²/day. May increase by 0.4 mg/m²/day following first cycle if no GI/hematologic toxicities occur. **CrCl less than 30 ml/min:** Decrease dose to 0.6 mg/m²/day. May increase by 0.4 mg/m²/day following first cycle if no GI/hematologic toxicities occur.

**Dosage in Hepatic Impairment**

No dose adjustment.

## SIDE EFFECTS

**Frequent (77%–21%):** Nausea, vomiting, diarrhea, total alopecia, headache, dyspnea. **Occasional (9%–3%):** Paresthesia, constipation, abdominal pain. **Rare:** Anorexia, malaise, arthralgia, asthenia, myalgia.

## ADVERSE EFFECTS/ TOXIC REACTIONS

Severe neutropenia (absolute neutrophil count [ANC] less than 500 cells/mm³) occurs in 60% of pts (develops at median of 11 days after day 1 of initial therapy). Thrombocytopenia (platelet count less than 25,000/mm³) occurs in 26% of pts. Severe anemia (RBC count less than 8 g/dL) occurs in 40% of pts (develops at median of 15 days after day 1 of initial therapy).

## NURSING CONSIDERATIONS

### BASELINE ASSESSMENT

Offer emotional support. Assess CBC with differential before each dose. Myelosuppression may precipitate life-threatening hemorrhage, infection, anemia. If platelet count drops, minimize trauma to pt (e.g., IM injections, pt positioning). Premedicate with antiemetics on day of treatment, starting at least 30 min before administration.

### INTERVENTION/EVALUATION

Assess for bleeding, signs of infection, anemia. Monitor hydration status, I&O, serum electrolytes (diarrhea, vomiting are common side effects). Monitor CBC for evidence of myelosuppression. Monitor renal function, LFT. Assess response to medication; provide interventions (e.g., small, frequent meals; antiemetics for nausea/vomiting). Question for complaints of headache. Assess breathing pattern for evidence of dyspnea.

### PATIENT/FAMILY TEACHING

• Hair loss is reversible but new hair may have different color, texture. • Diarrhea may cause dehydration, electrolyte depletion. • Antiemetic and antidiarrheal medications may reduce side effects. • Notify physician if diarrhea, vomiting, persistent fever, bruising/bleeding, yellowing of eyes/skin occur. • Do not have immunizations without physician's approval (drug lowers resistance). • Avoid contact with those who have recently received live virus vaccine.

# torsemide

**tore**-se-myde
(Demadex)
**Do not confuse torsemide with furosemide.**

## ◆CLASSIFICATION

**PHARMACOTHERAPEUTIC:** Loop diuretic. **CLINICAL:** Antihypertensive, diuretic.

## USES

Treatment of hypertension either alone or in combination with other antihypertensives. Edema associated with HF, hepatic/renal impairment.

## PRECAUTIONS

**Contraindications:** Hypersensitivity to torsemide. Anuria, other sulfonylureas.

**Cautions:** Pts with cirrhosis, hypotension, hypokalemia.

## ACTION

Enhances excretion of sodium, chloride, potassium, water at ascending limb of loop of Henle. Reduces plasma, extracellular fluid volume. **Therapeutic Effect:** Produces diuresis; lowers B/P.

## PHARMACOKINETICS

| Route | Onset | Peak | Duration |
|---|---|---|---|
| PO, IV (diuresis) | 30–60 min | 1–2 hrs | 6–8 hrs |

Rapidly, well absorbed from GI tract. Protein binding: 97%–99%. Metabolized in liver. Primarily excreted in urine. Not removed by hemodialysis. **Half-life:** 2–4 hrs.

## ⌛ LIFESPAN CONSIDERATIONS

**Pregnancy/Lactation:** Unknown if drug is distributed in breast milk. **Children:** Safety and efficacy not established. **Elderly:** No age-related precautions noted.

## INTERACTIONS

**DRUG: NSAIDs, aspirin** may increase risk of renal impairment. May increase risk of **digoxin** toxicity associated with torsemide-induced hypokalemia. May increase risk of **lithium** toxicity. **Other hypokalemia-causing medications (e.g., HCTZ)** may increase risk of hypokalemia. **HERBAL: Ephedra, ginseng, yohimbe, licorice** may worsen hypertension. **Black cohosh** may increase antihypertensive effect. **FOOD:** None known. **LAB VALUES:** May increase serum BUN, creatinine, uric acid. May decrease serum calcium, chloride, magnesium, potassium, sodium.

## AVAILABILITY (Rx)

**Injection Solution:** 10 mg/ml. **Tablets:** 5 mg, 10 mg, 20 mg, 100 mg.

## ADMINISTRATION/HANDLING

### 💧 IV

**Rate of Administration**
**◀ALERT▶** Flush IV line with 0.9% NaCl before and following administration. • May give undiluted as IV push over minimum of 2 min.
**Storage** • Store at room temperature.

### PO
• Give without regard to food. Give with food to avoid GI upset, preferably with breakfast (prevents nocturia).

## 🔲 IV COMPATIBILITY

Milrinone (Primacor).

## INDICATIONS/ROUTES/DOSAGE

**Hypertension**
**PO: ADULTS, ELDERLY:** Initially, 2.5–5 mg/day. May increase to 10 mg/day if no response in 4–6 wks. If no response, add additional antihypertensive. Range: 5–10 mg/day.

**Edema Associated with HF**
**PO, IV: ADULTS, ELDERLY:** Initially, 10–20 mg/day. May increase by approximately doubling dose until desired therapeutic effect is attained. **Maximum dose:** PO: 200 mg; IV: 100–200 mg.

**Edema Associated with Chronic Renal Failure**
**PO, IV: ADULTS, ELDERLY:** Initially, 20 mg/day. May increase by approximately doubling dose until desired therapeutic effect is attained. **Maximum dose:** 200 mg/day.

**Hepatic Cirrhosis**
**PO: ADULTS, ELDERLY:** Initially, 5–10 mg/day given with aldosterone antagonist or potassium-sparing diuretic. May increase by approximately doubling dose until desired therapeutic effect is attained. **Maximum single dose:** 40 mg.

**Dosage in Renal/Hepatic Impairment**
No dose adjustment.

T

## SIDE EFFECTS

**Frequent (10%–4%):** Headache, dizziness, rhinitis. **Occasional (3%–1%):** Asthenia insomnia, nervousness, diarrhea, constipation, nausea, dyspepsia, edema, EKG changes, pharyngitis, cough, arthralgia, myalgia. **Rare (Less Than 1%):** Syncope, hypotension, arrhythmias.

## ADVERSE EFFECTS/ TOXIC REACTIONS

Ototoxicity may occur with too-rapid IV administration or with high doses; must be given slowly. Overdose produces acute, profound water loss, volume/electrolyte depletion, dehydration, decreased blood volume, circulatory collapse.

## NURSING CONSIDERATIONS

### BASELINE ASSESSMENT

Check serum electrolyte levels, esp. potassium. Obtain baseline weight; check for edema. Assess for rales in lungs, signs of HF.

### INTERVENTION/EVALUATION

Monitor B/P, serum electrolytes (esp. potassium), I&O, weight. Notify physician of any hearing abnormality. Note extent of diuresis. Assess lungs for rales. Check for signs of edema, particularly of dependent areas. Although less potassium is lost with torsemide than with furosemide, assess for signs of hypokalemia (change of muscle strength, tremor, muscle cramps, altered mental status, cardiac arrhythmias).

### PATIENT/FAMILY TEACHING

• Take medication in morning to prevent nocturia. • Expect increased urinary volume, frequency. • Report palpitations, muscle weakness, cramps, nausea, dizziness. • Do not take other medications (including OTC drugs) without consulting physician. • Eat foods high in potassium such as whole grains (cereals), legumes, meat, bananas, apricots, orange juice, potatoes (white, sweet), raisins.

# trabectedin

tra-**bek**-te-din
(Yondelis)

◆CLASSIFICATION

**PHARMACOTHERAPEUTIC:** Alkylating agent. **CLINICAL:** Antineoplastic.

## USES

Treatment of unresectable or metastatic liposarcoma or leiomyosarcoma in pts who have received a prior anthracycline-containing regimen.

## PRECAUTIONS

**Contraindications:** Hypersensitivity reaction, anaphylactic reaction to trabectedin. **Cautions:** Baseline anemia, neutropenia, thrombocytopenia; chronic liver disease, cirrhosis, hepatic impairment, hepatitis; renal impairment; history of DVT, pulmonary embolism; recent MI, cardiomyopathy, HF. Concomitant use of strong CYP3A inducers, strong CYP3A inhibitors not recommended.

## ACTION

Binds to guanine residues in the minor groove of DNA, leading to cell cycle disruption and cellular death. **Therapeutic Effect:** Inhibits tumor cell growth and metastasis.

## PHARMACOKINETICS

Widely distributed. Metabolized in liver. Protein binding: 97%. Eliminated in feces (58%), urine (6%). Hemodialysis not expected to enhance elimination. **Half-life:** 175 hrs.

## ⧗ LIFESPAN CONSIDERATIONS

**Pregnancy/Lactation:** Avoid pregnancy; may cause fetal harm/malformations. Female pts of reproductive potential should use effective contraception during treatment and up to 2 mos after discontinuation. Breastfeeding not recommended. **Males:** Male pts with female partners of reproductive potential should use barrier methods, abstinence during treatment and up to 5 mos after discontinuation. May impair fertility in both females and males. **Children:** Safety and efficacy not established. **Elderly:** Safety and efficacy not established.

## INTERACTIONS

**DRUG: Strong CYP3A inducers (e.g., carbamazepine, phenobarbital, rifampin)** may decrease concentration/effect. **Strong CYP3A inhibitors (e.g., clarithromycin, ketoconazole, ritonavir)** may increase concentration/effects. **HERBAL: St. John's wort** may decrease concentration/effect. **FOOD: Grapefruit products** may increase concentration/effect. **LAB VALUES:** May decrease Hgb, Hct, platelets, neutrophils, RBCs; serum albumin, phosphate. May increase serum alkaline phosphatase, ALT, AST, bilirubin, CPK, creatinine. May reduce diagnostic effect of *Coccidioides immitis* skin test.

## AVAILABILITY (Rx)

**Powder for Reconstitution:** 1 mg.

## ADMINISTRATION/HANDLING

 IV

**Reconstitution •** Contents are hazardous; use cytotoxic precautions during handling and disposal. • Reconstitute with 20 ml Sterile Water for Injection for final concentration of 0.05 mg/ml. • Shake until fully dissolved. • Visually inspect solution for particulate matter or discoloration. Solution should appear clear, colorless to pale brownish-yellow in color. Discard if solution is discolored or particles are observed. • Dilute in 500 ml 0.9% NaCl or D₅W bag. • See manufacturer guidelines for materials/containers that are compatible with diluted solution.
**Infusion Guidelines •** Premedicate with dexamethasone 20 mg IV (or appropriate corticosteroid) 30 mins prior to each infusion. • Infuse diluted solution immediately after reconstitution.

• Use an inline, 0.2-micron polyethersulfone filter. • Infuse via dedicated central venous line using an infusion pump.
**Rate of Administration •** Infuse over 24 hrs.
**Storage •** Refrigerate unused vials. • Diluted solution must be administered within 30 hrs of reconstitution.

## ⧗ IV INCOMPATIBILITIES

Do not mix or infuse with other medications.

## INDICATIONS/ROUTES/DOSAGE

**Liposarcoma, Leiomyosarcoma**
**IV: ADULTS, ELDERLY:** 1.5 mg/m² once q3wks until disease progression or unacceptable toxicity.

**Dosage in Renal Impairment**
**CrCl greater than or equal to 30 ml/min:** No dose adjustment.
**CrCl greater less than 30 ml/min or end-stage renal disease:** Not specified; use caution.

**Dosage in Hepatic Impairment**
**Mild impairment:** No dose adjustment.
**Moderate impairment:** 0.9 mg/m² once q3wks. **Severe impairment:** Not recommended.

**Dose Reduction for Normal Hepatic Function or Mild Hepatic Impairment**
**Initial dose:** 1.5 mg/m² once q3wks.
**First dose reduction:** 1.2 mg/m² once q3wks. **Second dose reduction:** 1 mg/m² once q3wks.

**Dose Reduction for Moderate Hepatic Impairment**
**Initial dose:** 0.9 mg/m² once q3wks.
**First dose reduction:** 0.6 mg/m² once q3wks. **Second dose reduction:** 0.3 mg/m² once q3wks.

**Dose Modification**
**Hepatotoxicity**
**Serum ALT/AST greater than 2.5 times upper limit of normal (ULN):** Delay next dose for up to 3 wks.

T

---

Alkaline phosphatase greater than 2.5 times ULN; serum ALT/AST greater than 5 times ULN; total serum bilirubin greater than ULN: Delay next dose for up to 3 wks, then resume at reduced dose level.

**Hematologic Toxicity**

Absolute neutrophil count (ANC) less than 1,500/mm³: Delay next dose for up to 3 wks.

ANC less than 1,000/mm³ with fever or infection; ANC less than 500/mm³ lasting more than 5 days: Delay next dose for up to 3 wks, then resume at reduced dose level.

Platelet count less than 100,000/mm³: Delay next dose for up to 3 wks.

Platelet count less than 25,000/mm³: Delay next dose for up to 3 wks, then resume at reduced dose level.

**Nonhematologic Toxicity**

CPK greater than 2.5 times ULN: Delay next dose for up to 3 wks.

CPK greater than 5 times ULN: Delay next dose for up to 3 wks, then resume at reduced dose level.

Decreased LVEF less than lower limit of normal or clinical evidence of cardiomyopathy: Delay next dose for up to 3 wks.

Decreased LVEF with an absolute decrease of 10% or more from baseline and less than lower limit of normal, or clinical evidence of cardiomyopathy: Delay next dose for up to 3 wks, then resume at reduced dose level.

Any other grade 3 or 4 reaction: Delay next dose for up to 3 wks, then resume at reduced dose level.

**Permanent Discontinuation**

Permanently discontinue for persistent adverse effects requiring a delay of treatment for more than 3 wks; continued adverse effects after reducing dose to 1 mg/m² in pts with normal hepatic function, or 0.3 mg/m² in pts with preexisting moderate hepatic impairment; severe hepatic dysfunction with bilirubin 2 times ULN, and ALT/AST 3 times ULN, and alkaline phosphatase less than 2 times ULN in prior treatment cycle in pts with baseline normal hepatic function; exacerbation of hepatic dysfunction in pts with preexisting moderate hepatic impairment.

## SIDE EFFECTS

**Frequent (75%–25%):** Nausea, fatigue, asthenia, malaise, vomiting, decreased appetite, constipation, diarrhea, peripheral edema, dyspnea, headache. **Occasional (15%–11%):** Insomnia, arthralgia, myalgia, paresthesia.

## ADVERSE EFFECTS/TOXIC REACTIONS

Anemia, neutropenia, thrombocytopenia is an expected response to therapy. Life-threatening, sometimes fatal, neutropenic sepsis (3% of pts) may occur. Grade 3 or 4 neutropenia (43% of pts), febrile neutropenia (5% of pts) were reported. Fatal rhabdomyolysis, muscular toxicity may result in renal failure. CPK elevation occurred in 32% of pts; grade 3 or 4 CPK elevation occurred in 6% of pts. Hepatotoxicity, including hepatic failure, may occur. LFT elevation occurred in 70%–90% of pts. Cardiomyopathy including decreased ejection fraction, diastolic dysfunction, HF, right ventricular dysfunction reported in 6% of pts; grade 3 or 4 cardiomyopathy reported in 4% of pts. Drug extravasation may result in tissue necrosis requiring debridement. Other adverse effects may include phlebitis (15% of pts), pulmonary embolism (less than 10% of pts), hypersensitivity reaction.

## NURSING CONSIDERATIONS

### BASELINE ASSESSMENT

Obtain ANC, CBC, CPK, BMP, LFT; vital signs prior to each dose and periodically thereafter. Obtain baseline echocardiogram to assess LVEF. Verify placement of central venous line. Receive full medication history. Assess nutritional status. Question history of DVT, pulmonary embolism, cardiac disease, recent MI;

renal/hepatic impairment; prior hypersensitivity reaction. Screen for active infection. Offer emotional support.

### INTERVENTION/EVALUATION

Monitor ANC, CBC for anemia, neutropenia, thrombocytopenia; CPK, serum creatinine for rhabdomyolysis, renal failure; LFT for hepatotoxicity; BMP for electrolyte imbalance (esp. in pts with diarrhea, vomiting, malnutrition); vital signs. Assess LVEF by echocardiogram at 2- to 3-mo intervals (or more frequently in pts with cardiomyopathy). Diligently screen for infections, sepsis. Monitor for DVT (leg or arm pain/swelling), rhabdomyolysis (decreased urinary output, amber-colored urine, fatigue, muscle pain/weakness), pulmonary embolism (sudden chest pain, dyspnea, hypoxia, tachycardia), HF (dyspnea, fatigue, palpitations, edema, exercise intolerance); hypersensitivity reaction; side effects of dexamethasone (e.g., hyperglycemia, weight loss, decreased appetite). Monitor I&Os. Monitor daily pattern bowel activity, stool consistency.

### PATIENT/FAMILY TEACHING

• Treatment may depress your immune system and reduce your ability to fight infection. Report symptoms of infection such as body aches, chills, cough, fatigue, fever. Avoid those with active infection. • Blood levels, echocardiograms will be routinely monitored. • Life-threatening events such as heart failure (shortness of breath, fast or slow heart rate, exercise intolerance, swelling of the ankles or legs), liver injury or failure (abdominal pain, easy bruising, clay-colored stools, dark-amber urine, fatigue, loss of appetite, yellowing of skin or eyes), muscle toxicity (muscle pain/weakness, kidney failure), blood clots in lungs (difficulty breathing, fast heart rate, chest pain). • Avoid pregnancy. Female pts of childbearing potential should use effective contraception during treatment and for at least 2 mos after last dose. Do not breastfeed. Male pts with female partners of reproductive potential should use condoms during sexual activity for at least 5 mos after last dose. • Treatment may impair fertility. • Avoid grapefruit products, herbal supplements. • Do not receive live vaccines.

## *traMADol

tram-a-dol
(Apo-Tramadol ♣, ConZip, Synapryn FusePaq, Ultram, Ultram ER)
**Do not confuse tramadol with tapentadol, Toradol, Trandate or Ultram with Ultracet.**

### FIXED-COMBINATION(S)

**Ultracet:** tramadol/acetaminophen (a non-narcotic analgesic): 37.5 mg/325 mg.

### ◆CLASSIFICATION

**PHARMACOTHERAPEUTIC:** Centrally acting synthetic opioid analgesic. **CLINICAL:** Analgesic.

## USES

**Immediate-Release:** Management of moderate to moderately severe pain. **Extended-Release:** Around-the-clock management of moderate to moderately severe pain for extended period.

## PRECAUTIONS

**Contraindications:** Hypersensitivity to tramadol, opioids. **(Additional) Ultram, Ultram ER:** Acute alcohol intoxication, concurrent use of centrally acting analgesics, hypnotics, opioids, psychotropic drugs, hypersensitivity to opioids. **(Additional) ConZip,** Severe/acute bronchial asthma, hypercapnia, significant respiratory depression. **Caution:** CNS depression, anoxia, advanced hepatic cirrhosis, respiratory depression, elevated ICP, history of seizures or risk for seizures, hepatic/renal impairment, treatment of acute abdominal conditions, opioid-dependent pts, head injury, myxedema, hypothyroidism, hypoadrenalism, pregnancy. Avoid use in pts who are suicidal or addiction prone, emotionally disturbed, depressed, heavy alcohol users, elderly, debilitated pts.

## ACTION

Binds to mu-opioid receptors, inhibits reuptake of norepinephrine, serotonin, inhibiting ascending and descending pain pathways. **Therapeutic Effect:** Reduces pain.

## PHARMACOKINETICS

| Route | Onset | Peak | Duration |
|-------|-------|------|----------|
| PO | Less than 1 hr | 2–3 hrs | 9 hrs |

Rapidly, almost completely absorbed after PO administration. Protein binding: 20%. Metabolized in liver (reduced in pts with advanced cirrhosis). Primarily excreted in urine. Minimally removed by hemodialysis. **Half-life:** 6–7 hrs (increased in renal/hepatic failure).

## ⌛ LIFESPAN CONSIDERATIONS

**Pregnancy/Lactation:** Crosses placenta. Distributed in breast milk. **Children:** Safety and efficacy not established. **Elderly:** Age-related renal impairment may require dosage adjustment.

## INTERACTIONS

**DRUG:** Alcohol, other CNS depressants (e.g., lorazepam, morphine, zolpidem) may increase CNS depression. Carbamazepine decreases concentration/effects. CYP2D6 inhibitors (e.g., paroxetine), CYP3A4 inhibitors (e.g., erythromycin), triptans, selective serotonin reuptake inhibitors (SSRIs), tricyclic antidepressants (e.g., amitriptyline, doxepin) may increase risk of seizures, risk of serotonin syndrome. **HERBAL:** Gotu kola, kava kava, St. John's wort, valerian may increase CNS depression. St. John's wort may increase risk of serotonin syndrome. **FOOD:** None known. **LAB VALUES:** May increase serum creatinine, ALT, AST. May decrease Hgb. May cause proteinuria.

## AVAILABILITY (Rx)

**Tablets (Immediate-Release) (Ultram):** 50 mg. **Capsule (Variable-Release):** ConZip: 100 mg (25 mg immediate/75 mg extended), 200 mg (50 mg immediate/150 mg extended), 300 mg (50 mg immediate/250 mg extended). **Suspension, Oral (Synapryn FusePaq):** 10 mg/ml.

**Tablets (Extended-Release) (Ultram ER):** 100 mg, 200 mg, 300 mg.

## ADMINISTRATION/HANDLING

**PO**
• Give without regard to meals but consistently with or without meals.
• Extended-Release: Swallow whole; do not break, crush, dissolve, or divide.

## INDICATIONS/ROUTES/DOSAGE

**Moderate to Moderately Severe Pain**
**PO (Immediate-Release): ADULTS, ELDERLY:** 50–100 mg q4–6h. **Maximum:** 400 mg/day for pts 75 yrs and younger; 300 mg/day for pts older than 75 yrs.
**PO (Extended-Release): ADULTS, ELDERLY:** Initially, 100 mg once daily. Titrate q5days. **Maximum:** 300 mg once daily.

**Dosage in Renal Impairment**
**Immediate-Release:** For pts with CrCl less than 30 ml/min, increase dosing interval to q12h. **Maximum:** 200 mg/day. Do not use extended-release.

**Dosage in Hepatic Impairment**
**Immediate-Release:** Cirrhosis: Dosage is decreased to 50 mg q12h. Do not use extended-release with severe hepatic impairment.

## SIDE EFFECTS

**Frequent (25%–15%):** Dizziness, vertigo, nausea, constipation, headache, drowsiness. **Occasional (10%–5%):** Vomiting, pruritus, CNS stimulation (e.g., nervousness, anxiety, agitation, tremor, euphoria, mood swings, hallucinations), asthenia, diaphoresis, dyspepsia, dry mouth, diarrhea. **Rare (less than 5%):** Malaise, vasodilation, anorexia, flatulence, rash, blurred vision, urinary retention/frequency, menopausal symptoms.

## ADVERSE EFFECTS/ TOXIC REACTIONS

Seizures reported in pts receiving tramadol within recommended dosage range. May have prolonged duration of action, cumulative effect in pts with hepatic/renal impairment, serotonin syndrome (agitation, hallucinations, tachycardia, hyperreflexia).

## NURSING CONSIDERATIONS

### BASELINE ASSESSMENT

Assess onset, type, location, duration of pain. Assess drug history, esp. carbamazepine, analgesics, CNS depressants, MAOIs. Review past medical history, esp. epilepsy, seizures. Assess renal function, LFT.

### INTERVENTION/EVALUATION

Monitor pulse, B/P, renal/hepatic function. Assist with ambulation if dizziness, vertigo occurs. Dry crackers, cola may relieve nausea. Palpate bladder for urinary retention. Monitor daily pattern of bowel activity, stool consistency. Sips of water may relieve dry mouth. Assess for clinical improvement, record onset of relief of pain.

### PATIENT/FAMILY TEACHING

• May cause dependence. • Avoid alcohol, OTC medications (analgesics, sedatives). • May cause drowsiness, dizziness, blurred vision. • Avoid tasks requiring alertness, motor skills until response to drug is established. • Report severe constipation, difficulty breathing, excessive sedation, seizures, muscle weakness, tremors, chest pain, palpitations.

## trametinib

tra-**me**-ti-nib
(Mekinist)
**Do not confuse trametinib with imatinib or tipifarnib.**

## ◆CLASSIFICATION

**PHARMACOTHERAPEUTIC:** Kinase inhibitor. **CLINICAL:** Antineoplastic.

## USES

Used as a single agent or in combination with dabrafenib for treatment of unresectable or metastatic melanoma with BRAF V600E or V600L mutations, as detected by FDA-approved test. Single-agent regimen is not indicated in pts who have received prior BRAF-inhibitor therapy.

## PRECAUTIONS

**Contraindications:** Hypersensitivity to trametinib. **Cautions:** Cardiac/pulmonary impairment, preexisting diabetes or diabetes.

## ACTION

Inhibits mitogen-activated extracellular kinase (MEK). **Therapeutic Effect:** Inhibits tumor cell growth, causing apoptosis.

## PHARMACOKINETICS

Rapidly absorbed after PO administration. Protein binding: 97.4%. Peak plasma concentration: 1.5 hrs. Metabolized in liver. Excreted in feces (80%), urine (20%). **Half-life:** 3.9–4.8 days.

## ⧗ LIFESPAN CONSIDERATIONS

**Pregnancy/Lactation:** Avoid pregnancy. May cause fetal harm. Must use effective nonhormonal contraception during treatment and for at least 4 wks after discontinuation (intrauterine device, barrier methods). Unknown if distributed in breast milk. Must either discontinue breastfeeding or discontinue treatment. **Children:** Safety and efficacy not established. **Elderly:** May have increased risk of adverse effects, skin lesions, primary malignancies. **Males:** May decrease sperm count.

## INTERACTIONS

**DRUG:** May decrease levels/effect of **aripiprazole, ibrutinib, saxagliptin, simeprevir. HERBAL:** None known. **FOOD: High-fat meals** may decrease absorption/effect. **LAB VALUES: SINGLE REGIMEN:** May increase serum alkaline phosphatase, ALT, AST. May decrease serum albumin; Hgb, Hct. **COMBINATION**

T

**REGIMEN:** May increase serum alkaline phosphatase, ALT, AST, bilirubin, calcium, creatinine, glucose, GGT, potassium. May decrease Hgb, Hct, leukocytes, lymphocytes, neutrophils, platelets; serum albumin, calcium, magnesium, phosphorus, potassium, sodium.

## AVAILABILITY (Rx)

**Tablets:** 0.5 mg, 2 mg.

## ADMINISTRATION/HANDLING

**PO**

• Administer at least 1 hr before or 2 hrs after meal.

## INDICATIONS/ROUTES/DOSAGE

**Melanoma**

**PO: ADULTS/ELDERLY:** 2 mg once daily (either as a single agent or in combination with dabrafenib). Continue until disease progression or unacceptable toxicity occurs.

**Dose Reduction Schedule**

**Trametinib Regimen: FIRST DOSE REDUCTION:** 1.5 mg once daily. **SECOND DOSE REDUCTION:** 1 mg once daily. Discontinue if unable to tolerate 1-mg dose.
**Dabrafenib Combination Regimen: FIRST DOSE REDUCTION:** 100 mg twice daily. **SECOND DOSE REDUCTION:** 75 mg twice daily.
**THIRD DOSE REDUCTION:** 50 mg twice daily. Discontinue if unable to tolerate 50-mg dose.

**Dose Modification**

Based on Common Terminology Criteria for Adverse Events (CTCAE) grading 1–4.
**Cardiac: ASYMPTOMATIC DECREASE IN LEFT VENTRICULAR EJECTION FRACTION (LVEF) GREATER THAN 10% FROM BASELINE:** Withhold trametinib up to 4 wks. If LVEF improved, resume at lower dose level. Discontinue if not improved. Do not modify dabrafenib dose. **SYMPTOMATIC HF OR DECREASE IN LVEF GREATER THAN 20% FROM BASELINE:** Discontinue trametinib. Withhold dabrafenib until improved, then resume at lower dose level.

**CUTANEOUS EVENTS: INTOLERABLE GRADE 2 SKIN TOXICITY OR GRADE 3–4 TOXICITY:** Withhold both regimens for up to 3 wks. If improved, resume both at lower dose level. Discontinue both regimens if not improved. **FEBRILE EVENTS: FEVER OF 101.3°F–104°F:** Do not modify trametinib dose. Withhold dabrafenib until fever resolved, then resume at either same dose or lower dose level.

**FEVER GREATER THAN 104°F OR FEVER COMPLICATED BY DEYDRATION, HYPOTENSION, RENAL FAILURE:** Withhold trametinib until resolved, then resume at either same dose or lower dose level. Withhold dabrafenib until resolved, then resume at either lower dose level or discontinue.
**New Primary Malignancies: CUTANEOUS:** No changes required for either regimen. **NONCUTANEOUS:** Do not change trametinib dose. Discontinue dabrafenib in pts who develop RAS mutation-positive malignancies.
**Nonspecific Adverse Reactions: INTOLERABLE GRADE 2 OR ANY GRADE 3:** Withhold both regimens until resolved to grade 0–1, then resume at lower dose level. Discontinue both regimens if not improved. **FIRST OCCURRENCE OF ANY GRADE 4 REACTIONS:** Withhold both regimens until resolved to grade 0–1, then resume at lower dose level or discontinue.
**Ocular Toxicities: GRADE 2–3 RETINAL PIGMENT EPITHELIAL DETACHMENTS:** Withhold trametinib up to 3 wks. If improved to grade 0–1, resume at lower dose level. Discontinue if not improved. Do not modify dabrafenib. **RETINAL VEIN OCCLUSION:** Discontinue trametinib. Do not modify dabrafenib.
**UVEITIS OR IRITIS:** Do not modify trametinib. Withhold dabrafenib for up to 6 wks. If improved to grade 0–1, then resume at same dose level. Discontinue if not improved.
**Pulmonary: INTERSTITIAL LUNG DISEASE:** Discontinue trametinib. Do not modify dabrafenib.
**Venous Thromboembolism: UNCOMPLICATED (DVT) OR (PE):** Withhold trametinib for up to 3 wks. If improved to

grade 0–1, then resume at lower dose level. Discontinue if not improved. Do not modify dabrafenib. **LIFE-THREATENING PE:** Discontinue both regimens.

**Dosage in Renal/Hepatic Impairment**
No dose adjustment.

## SIDE EFFECTS

*Single Regimen:*
**Frequent (57%–32%):** Rash, diarrhea, lymphedema, peripheral edema. **Occasional (19%–10%):** Dermatitis acneiform, hypertension, stomatitis, mouth ulceration, mucosal ulceration, abdominal pain, dry skin, pruritus, paronychia, folliculitis, cellulitis, dizziness, dysgeusia, blurred vision, dry eye.
*Combination Regimen:*
**Frequent (71%–40%):** Pyrexia, chills, fatigue, rash, nausea, vomiting. **Occasional (36%–11%):** Diarrhea, abdominal pain, peripheral edema, headache, cough, arthralgia, night sweats, myalgia, constipation, decreased appetite, back pain, dry skin, insomnia, dermatitis acneiform, dizziness, muscle spasm, extremity pain, actinic keratosis, erythema, oral/throat pain, urinary tract infection, pruritus, dry mouth, dehydration.

## ADVERSE EFFECTS/ TOXIC REACTIONS

Primary malignancies including basal or squamous cell carcinoma, keratoacanthoma, pancreatic adenocarcinoma, glioblastoma (brain cancer) reported. DVT, PE reported in 9% of pts. May increase cell proliferation of wild-type BRAF melanoma or new malignant melanomas. Serious, sometimes fatal intracranial or gastric bleeding occurred in 5% of pts. Other hemorrhagic events may include conjunctival/gingival/rectal/hemorrhoidal/vaginal bleeding; epistaxis (nosebleed); melena (bloody stools). Cardiomyopathy, HF, decreased LVEF reported in 7%–9% of pts. Ocular toxicities such as retinal vein occlusion, retinal detachment, vision loss, glaucoma, uveitis, iritis reported. Cough, dyspnea, hypoxia,

pleural effusion, infiltrates may indicate interstitial lung disease. Serious febrile reactions may lead to renal failure, severe dehydration, hypotension, rigors. Skin toxicities including palmar-plantar erythrodysesthesia syndrome (PPES), papilloma have occurred. Hyperglycemia reported in 2%–5% of pts. Other effects may include hypertension, rhabdomyolysis. May prolong QT interval of cardiac cycle.

## NURSING CONSIDERATIONS

### BASELINE ASSESSMENT

Obtain baseline CBC, serum metabolic panel (with LFT), magnesium, phosphate, ionized calcium, capillary glucose level, vital signs. Obtain BRAF V600E mutation history, negative pregnancy status, ophthalmologic exam with visual acuity, echocardiogram, EKG before initiating treatment. Assess skin for moles, lesions, papillomas. Question current breastfeeding status. Receive full medication history including herbal products. Question any history as listed in PRECAUTIONS.

### INTERVENTION/EVALUATION

Offer emotional support. Monitor CBC, serum electrolytes, capillary blood glucose, stool characteristics routinely. Monitor for signs of hyperglycemia (thirst, polyuria, confusion, dehydration). Assess skin for new lesions, toxicities every 2 mos during treatment and at least 6 mos after discontinuation. Obtain LVEF by echocardiogram 1 mo after initiation, then every 2–3 mos; ophthalmologic exam with any vision changes. Immediately report any altered mental status, bleeding events, vision changes, eye pain/swelling/infection, fever, urinary changes. Screen for bleeding of any kind. If dyspnea or leg swelling occurs, contact physician and initiate appropriate medical therapy (may require oxygen therapy, EKG, or radiologic test to rule out DVT, PE, or ILD).

**T**

### PATIENT/FAMILY TEACHING

• Blood work, cardiac function tests, eye exams will be performed routinely. • Treatment may lead to heart failure, vision changes, lung complications, difficulty breathing, fever, skin toxicities (such as severe rash, peeling), high blood pressure, severe diarrhea. • Report bloody stools/urine, heavy menstruation, or nosebleeds. • Do not breastfeed. • Avoid pregnancy; nonhormonal contraception should be used during treatment and up to 4 wks after treatment. • Take medication at least 1 hr before or at least 2 hrs after meal (food reduces absorption). • Report any increased urination, thirst, confusion (may indicate high blood sugar); chest pain, eye pain, fever, leg swelling, new skin moles or lesions, vision changes. • Minimize sunlight exposure. • Males may experience a decreased sperm count. • Report any newly prescribed medications.

---

## *trastuzumab*

tras-**too**-zoo-mab
(Herceptin)

■ **BLACK BOX ALERT** ■ Anaphylactic reaction, infusion reaction, acute respiratory distress syndrome have been associated with fatalities. Reduction in left ventricular ejection fraction, severe heart failure may result in thrombus formation, stroke, cardiac death. Exposure during pregnancy may result in pulmonary hypoplasia, skeletal malformations, neonatal death.

### ◆CLASSIFICATION

**PHARMACOTHERAPEUTIC:** Monoclonal antibody. **CLINICAL:** Antineoplastic.

### USES

Treatment of *HER2* overexpressing breast cancer (adjuvant), metastatic breast cancer, metastatic gastric or gastro-esophageal junction adenocarcinoma (in pts without prior treatment). **OFF-LABEL:** Treatment of *HER2*–positive metastatic breast cancer in pts who have not received prior anti-*HER2* therapy or in pts whose cancer has progressed on prior trastuzumab therapy (in combination with lapatinib).

### PRECAUTIONS

**Contraindications:** Hypersensitivity to trastuzumab. **Cautions:** Preexisting cardiac disease or dysfunction, preexisting pulmonary disease or extensive pulmonary tumor involvement, preganancy.

### ACTION

Binds to *HER2* protein, overexpressed in 25%–30% of primary breast cancers, inhibiting proliferation of tumor cells. **Therapeutic Effect:** Inhibits growth of tumor cells, mediates antibody-dependent cellular cytotoxicity.

### PHARMACOKINETICS

Half-life: 11–23 days.

### ☒ LIFESPAN CONSIDERATIONS

**Pregnancy/Lactation:** Unknown if distributed in breast milk. **Children:** Safety and efficacy not established. **Elderly:** Age-related cardiac dysfunction may require dosage adjustment.

### INTERACTIONS

**DRUG:** None significant. **HERBAL:** None significant. **FOOD:** None known. **LAB VALUES:** None significant.

### AVAILABILITY (Rx)

**Injection, Powder for Reconstitution:** 440 mg.

### ADMINISTRATION/HANDLING

 IV

**Reconstitution** • Reconstitute with 20 ml Bacteriostatic Water for Injection to yield concentration of 21 mg/ml.

• Add calculated dose to 250 ml 0.9% NaCl (do not use D5W). • Gently mix contents in bag.

**Rate of Administration** • Do not give IV push or bolus. • Give loading dose (4 mg/kg) over 90 min. Give maintenance infusion (2 mg/kg) over 30 min.

**Storage** • Refrigerate. • Reconstituted solution appears colorless to pale yellow. • Reconstituted solution in vial is stable for 28 days if refrigerated after reconstitution with Bacteriostatic Water for Injection (if using Sterile Water for Injection without preservative, use immediately; discard unused portions). • Solution diluted in 250 ml 0.9% NaCl stable for 24 hrs if refrigerated.

### 🔳 IV INCOMPATIBILITIES

Do not mix with D5W or any other medications.

## INDICATIONS/ROUTES/DOSAGE

### Breast Cancer (Adjuvant)

**IV: ADULTS, ELDERLY: (with concurrent paclitaxel or docetaxel):** Initially, 4 mg/kg as 90-min infusion, then 2 mg/kg wkly as 30-min infusion for 12 wks followed 1 wk later (when concurrent chemotherapy completed) by 6 mg/kg infusion over 30–90 min q3wks for total therapy duration of 52 wks. **(with docetaxel/carboplatin):** Initially, 4 mg/kg as 90-min infusion, then 2 mg/kg wkly as 30-min infusion for a total of 18 wks, followed 1 wk later (when concurrent chemotherapy completed) by 6 mg/kg infused over 30–90 min q3wks for total therapy duration of 52 wks **(follow multimodality chemotherapy):** Initially, 8 mg/kg over 90 min, then 6 mg/kg over 30–90 min q3wks for total of 52 wks.

### Breast Cancer (Metastatic)

**IV: ADULTS, ELDERLY: (Either as single agent or in combination with paclitaxel):** Initially, 4 mg/kg as 90-min infusion, then 2 mg/kg as 30-min infusion wkly until disease progression.

### Gastric Cancer

**IV: ADULTS, ELDERLY: (In combination with cisplatin and either capecitabine or fluorouracil for 6 cycles, then as monotherapy):** Initially, 8 mg/kg over 90 min, then 6 mg/kg over 30–90 min q3wks until disease progression.

### Dosage Adjustment in Cardiotoxicity

Left ventricular ejection fraction (LVEF) 16% or greater decrease from baseline WNL (within normal limits) or LVEF below normal limits and 10% or greater decrease from baseline: Hold treatment for 4 wks. Repeat LVEF q4wks. Resume therapy if LVEF returns to normal limits in 4–8 wks and remains at 15% or less decrease from baseline.

### Dosage in Renal/Hepatic Impairment

No dose adjustment.

## SIDE EFFECTS

**Frequent (Greater Than 20%):** Pain, asthenia, fever, chills, headache, abdominal pain, back pain, infection, nausea, diarrhea, vomiting, cough, dyspnea. **Occasional (15%–5%):** Tachycardia, HF, flu-like symptoms, anorexia, edema, bone pain, arthralgia, insomnia, dizziness, paresthesia, depression, rhinitis, pharyngitis, sinusitis. **Rare (Less Than 5%):** Allergic reaction, anemia, leukopenia, neuropathy, herpes simplex.

## ADVERSE EFFECTS/ TOXIC REACTIONS

Cardiomyopathy, ventricular dysfunction, HF occur rarely. Pancytopenia may occur.

## NURSING CONSIDERATIONS

### BASELINE ASSESSMENT

Evaluate left ventricular function. Obtain baseline echocardiogram, EKG, multigated acquisition (MUGA) scan. Obtain CBC at baseline and at regular intervals during therapy.

T

### INTERVENTION/EVALUATION

Frequently monitor for deteriorating cardiac function. Assess for asthenia (loss of strength, energy). Assist with ambulation if asthenia occurs. Monitor for fever, chills, abdominal pain, back pain. Offer antiemetics if nausea, vomiting occur. Monitor daily pattern of bowel activity, stool consistency.

### PATIENT/FAMILY TEACHING

• Do not have immunizations without physician's approval (lowers resistance). • Avoid contact with those who have recently taken oral polio vaccine. • Avoid crowds, those with infection.

---

## *traZODone

traz-o-done
(Apo-Trazodone ✦,
Novo-Trazodone ✦, Oleptro)

■ **BLACK BOX ALERT** ■ Increased risk of suicidal ideation and behavior in children, adolescents, young adults 18–24 yrs with major depressive disorder, other psychiatric disorders.
**Do not confuse trazodone with tramadol or ziprasidone.**

### ◆ CLASSIFICATION

**PHARMACOTHERAPEUTIC:** Serotonin reuptake inhibitor. **CLINICAL:** Antidepressant.

### USES

Treatment of depression. **OFF-LABEL:** Insomnia.

### PRECAUTIONS

**Contraindications:** Hypersensitivity to trazodone. Use of MAOIs (concurrently or within 14 days of discontinuing trazodone or MAOI); initiation in pt receiving linezolid or methylene blue. **Cautions:** Cardiac disease, arrhythmias, cerebrovascular disease, hepatic/renal impairment, pts at high risk of suicide. Conditions predisposing to priapism (e.g., sickle cell anemia); concurrent use of antihypertensives; history of seizure disorder or conditions predisposing to seizures (e.g., alcoholism); elderly.

### ACTION

Blocks reuptake of serotonin at neuronal presynaptic membranes, increasing its availability at postsynaptic receptor sites. **Therapeutic Effect:** Relieves depression.

### PHARMACOKINETICS

Well absorbed from GI tract. Protein binding: 85%–95%. Metabolized in liver. Primarily excreted in urine. Unknown if removed by hemodialysis. **Half-life:** 5–9 hrs (increased in elderly).

### ⌛ LIFESPAN CONSIDERATIONS

**Pregnancy/Lactation:** Drug crosses placenta; minimally distributed in breast milk. **Children:** Safety and efficacy not established in pts younger than 6 yrs. **Elderly:** More likely to experience sedative, hypotensive effects; lower dosage recommended.

### INTERACTIONS

**DRUG:** CYP3A4 inhibitors (e.g., ritonavir, ketoconazole) increase concentration/effects. May increase concentration of **digoxin, phenytoin. HERBAL:** Gotu kola, kava kava, St. John's wort, valerian may increase CNS depression and serotonin syndrome. **FOOD:** None known. **LAB VALUES:** May decrease WBC, neutrophil counts.

### AVAILABILITY (Rx)

**Tablets:** 50 mg, 100 mg, 150 mg, 300 mg.

🌠 **Tablets:** (Extended-Release [Oleptro]): 150 mg, 300 mg.

### ADMINISTRATION/HANDLING

**PO**

• Give shortly after snack, meal (reduces risk of dizziness). • Tablets may be crushed. • Do not crush or divide extended-release tablets. Give whole or break in half along score line. • Best taken at bedtime.

---

## INDICATIONS/ROUTES/DOSAGE

◄ **ALERT** ► Therapeutic effect may take up to 6 wks to occur.

### Depression

**PO: ADULTS:** *(Immediate-Release):* Initially, 150 mg/day in 3 equally divided doses. Increase by 50 mg/day at 3- to 4-day intervals until therapeutic response is achieved. **Maximum:** 600 mg/day (inpatients); 400 mg/day (outpatients). **ELDERLY:** Initially, 25–50 mg at bedtime. May increase by 25–50 mg every 3–7 days. Range: 75–150 mg/day. *Tablets (Extended-Release):* **ADULTS, ELDERLY:** Initially, 150 mg once daily. May increase by 75 mg q3days. **Maximum:** 375 mg/day. **ADOLESCENTS 13–18 YRS:** *(Immediate-Release):* Initially, 25–50 mg/day. May increase to 100–150 mg/day in divided doses. **CHILDREN 6–12 YRS:** *(Immediate-Release):* Initially, 1.5–2 mg/kg/day in divided doses. May increase gradually q3–4 days to 6 mg/kg/day in 3 divided doses.

### Dosage in Renal/Hepatic Impairment
Use caution.

## SIDE EFFECTS

**Frequent (9%–3%):** Drowsiness, dry mouth, light-headedness, dizziness, headache, blurred vision, nausea, vomiting. **Occasional (3%–1%):** Nervousness, fatigue, constipation, myalgia/arthralgia, mild hypotension. **Rare:** Photosensitivity reaction.

## ADVERSE EFFECTS/ TOXIC REACTIONS

Priapism, altered libido, retrograde ejaculation, impotence occur rarely. Appears to be less cardiotoxic than other antidepressants, although arrhythmias may occur in pts with preexisting cardiac disease.

## NURSING CONSIDERATIONS

### BASELINE ASSESSMENT
Assess mental status, mood, behavior. For pts on long-term therapy, serum hepatic/renal function tests, blood counts should be performed periodically. Elderly are more likely to experience sedative, hypotensive effects.

### INTERVENTION/EVALUATION
Monitor for suicidal ideation (esp. at beginning of therapy or dosage change). Assess appearance, behavior, speech pattern, level of interest, mood. Monitor WBC, neutrophil count, hepatic enzymes. Assist with ambulation if dizziness, lightheadedness occurs.

### PATIENT/FAMILY TEACHING
• Immediately discontinue medication, consult physician if priapism occurs. • May take after meal, snack. • May take at bedtime if drowsiness occurs. • Change positions slowly to avoid hypotensive effect. • Avoid tasks that require alertness, motor skills until response to drug is established. • Tolerance to sedative, anticholinergic effects usually develops during early therapy. • Photosensitivity to sun may occur. • Dry mouth may be relieved by sugarless gum, sips of water. • Report visual disturbances, worsening depression, suicidal ideation, unusual changes in behavior. • Do not abruptly discontinue medication. • Avoid alcohol.

---

## *tretinoin*    HIGH ALERT

**tret**-i-noyn
(Atralin, Avita, Refissa, Rejuva-A ✦, Renova, Retin-A, Retin-A Micro, Tretin X, Vesanoid ✦)

■ **BLACK BOX ALERT** ■ High risk for teratogenicity; major fetal abnormalities, spontaneous abortions. Pts with acute promyelocytic leukemia (APL) are at severe risk for reactions (fever, dyspnea, acute respiratory distress syndrome [pulmonary infiltrates, pleural effusions, pericardial effusions]), edema, hepatic, renal, and/or multiorgan failure; 40% develop leukocytosis.

**Do not confuse tretinoin with isotretinoin, phenytoin, or triamcinolone.**

T

---

## FIXED-COMBINATION(S)

With octyl methoxycinnamate and oxybenzone, moisturizers, and SPF-12, a sunscreen (Retin-A Regimen Kit).

## ◆CLASSIFICATION

PHARMACOTHERAPEUTIC: Retinoid. CLINICAL: Antiacne, transdermal, antineoplastic.

## USES

Topical: Treatment of acne vulgaris, photodamaged skin. PO: Induction of remission in pts with acute promyelocytic leukemia (APL). OFF-LABEL (PO): Maintenance therapy in APL, combination therapy (arsenic trioxide) for remission induction in APL. Topical: Some skin cancers.

## PRECAUTIONS

Contraindications: Hypersensitivity to tretinoin. Sensitivity to parabens (used as preservative in gelatin capsule). Extreme Caution: Topical: Eczema, sun exposure. Cautions: Topical: Those with considerable sun exposure in their occupation, hypersensitivity to sun. PO: Elevated serum cholesterol/triglycerides, concurrent use of antifibrinolytic agents.

## ACTION

Antiacne: Decreases cohesiveness of follicular epithelial cells. Increases turnover of follicular epithelial cells. Therapeutic Effect: Causes expulsion of blackheads. Bacterial skin counts are not altered. Transdermal: Exerts effects on growth/differentiation of epithelial cells. Therapeutic Effect: Alleviates fine wrinkles, hyperpigmentation. Antineoplastic: Induces maturation, decreases proliferation of acute promyelocytic leukemia (APL) cells. Therapeutic Effect: Repopulation of bone marrow, and peripheral blood with normal hematopoietic cells.

## PHARMACOKINETICS

Topical: Minimally absorbed. PO: Well absorbed following PO administration. Protein binding: greater than 95%. Metabolized in liver. Primarily excreted in urine. Half-life: 0.5–2 hrs.

## ⏳ LIFESPAN CONSIDERATIONS

Pregnancy/Lactation: Topical: Use during pregnancy only if clearly necessary. Unknown if distributed in breast milk. PO: Teratogenic, embryotoxic effect. Children/Elderly: Safety and efficacy not established.

## INTERACTIONS

DRUG: TOPICAL: Retinoids (e.g., acitretin, oral tretinoin) may increase drying, irritative effects. PO: Tetracyclines may increase risk of pseudotumor cerebri, intracranial hypertension. Aminocaproic acid may increase risk of thrombotic complications. CYP3A4 inducers (e.g., phenobarbital, rifampin) may decrease concentration/effects. CYP3A4 inhibitors (e.g., ketoconazole) may increase concentration, risk of toxicity. HERBAL: St. John's wort may decrease concentration/effects. Dong quai, St. John's wort may increase photosensitization. Vitamin A supplementation may increase vitamin A toxicity. FOOD: None known. LAB VALUES: PO: Leukocytosis occurs commonly (40%). May elevate serum hepatic function tests, cholesterol, triglycerides.

## AVAILABILITY (Rx)

Cream: 0.02% (Renova), 0.025% (Avita, Retin-A, Tretin X), 0.05% (Refissa, Retin-A, Tretin X), 0.1% (Retin-A). Gel: 0.01% (Retin-A, Tretin X), 0.025% (Avita, Retin-A, Tretin X), 0.04% (Retin-A Micro), 0.1% (Retin-A Micro).

Capsules: (Vesanoid): 10 mg.

## ADMINISTRATION/HANDLING

PO
• Do not crush/break capsule. • Administer with a meal.

**Topical**
• Thoroughly cleanse area before applying tretinoin. • Lightly cover only affected area. Liquid may be applied with fingertip, gauze, cotton; do not rub onto unaffected skin. • Keep medication away from eyes, mouth, angles of nose, mucous membranes. • Wash hands immediately after application.

## INDICATIONS/ROUTES/DOSAGE

### Acne
**Topical: ADULTS, CHILDREN 12 YRS AND OLDER:** Apply once daily at bedtime or in the evening.

### Remission Induction in Acute Promyelocytic Leukemia (APL)
**PO: ADULTS:** 45 mg/m²/day given as 2–3 evenly divided doses until complete remission is documented. Discontinue therapy 30 days after complete remission or after 90 days of treatment, whichever comes first.

### Remission Maintenance in APL
**PO: ADULTS, ELDERLY:** 45 mg/m²/day in 2 divided doses for 15 days q3mos for 2 yrs. **CHILDREN:** 25 mg/m²/day in 2 divided doses for 15 days q3mos for 2 yrs.

### Dosage in Renal/Hepatic Impairment
No dose adjustment.

## SIDE EFFECTS

**Topical:** Temporary change in pigmentation, photosensitivity. Local inflammatory reactions (peeling, dry skin, stinging, erythema, pruritus) are to be expected and are reversible with discontinuation of tretinoin. **Frequent: PO (87%–54%):** Headache, fever, dry skin/oral mucosa, bone pain, nausea, vomiting, rash. **Occasional: PO (26%–6%):** Mucositis, earache or feeling of fullness in ears, flushing, pruritus, diaphoresis, visual disturbances, hypotension/hypertension, dizziness, anxiety, insomnia, alopecia, skin changes. **Rare (Less Than 6%):** Altered visual acuity, temporary hearing loss.

## ADVERSE EFFECTS/ TOXIC REACTIONS

**PO:** Retinoic acid syndrome (fever, dyspnea, weight gain, abnormal chest auscultatory findings [pulmonary infiltrates, pleural/pericardial effusions], episodic hypotension) occurs commonly (25%), as does leukocytosis (40%). Syndrome generally occurs during first month of therapy (sometimes after first dose). High-dose steroids (dexamethasone 10 mg IV) at first suspicion of syndrome reduce morbidity, mortality. Pseudotumor cerebri may be noted, esp. in children (headache, nausea, vomiting, visual disturbances). **Topical:** Possible tumorigenic potential when combined with ultraviolet radiation.

## NURSING CONSIDERATIONS

### BASELINE ASSESSMENT
**PO:** Inform women of childbearing potential of risk to fetus if pregnancy occurs. Instruct on need for use of 2 reliable forms of contraceptives concurrently during therapy and for 1 mo after discontinuation of therapy, even in infertile women. Pregnancy test should be obtained within 1 wk before institution of therapy. Obtain initial serum LFT, cholesterol, triglyceride levels.

### INTERVENTION/EVALUATION
**PO:** Monitor LFT, hematologic, coagulation profiles, cholesterol, triglycerides. Monitor for signs/symptoms of pseudotumor cerebri in children.

### PATIENT/FAMILY TEACHING
• **Topical:** Avoid exposure to sunlight, tanning beds; use sunscreens, protective clothing. • Protect affected areas from wind, cold. • If skin is already sunburned, do not use drug until fully healed. • Keep tretinoin away from eyes, mouth, angles of nose, mucous membranes. • Do not use medicated, drying, abrasive soaps; wash face no more than 2–3 times/day with gentle soap. • Avoid use of preparations containing

T

alcohol, menthol, spice, lime (e.g., shaving lotions, astringents, perfume). • Mild redness, peeling are expected; decrease frequency or discontinue medication if excessive reaction occurs. • Nonmedicated cosmetics may be used; however, cosmetics must be removed before tretinoin application. • Improvement noted during first 24 wks of therapy. • **Antiacne:** Therapeutic results noted in 2–3 wks; optimal results in 6 wks. **Oral:** • Avoid tasks requiring motor skills, alertness until response to drug is established. • Avoid alcohol. • Avoid exposure to sunlight, tanning beds. • Report persistent vomiting, diarrhea, unusual bleeding/bruising, acute abdominal pain, vision changes, or if pregnancy is suspected.

# triamcinolone

trye-am-**sin**-oh-lone

# triamcinolone acetonide

(Kenalog, Kenalog-10, Kenalog-40, Nasacort AQ, Triderm)

# triamcinolone hexacetonide

(Aristospan)
**Do not confuse Nasacort with Nasalcrom.**

## FIXED-COMBINATION(S)

**Myco-II, Mycolog II, Myco-Triacet:** triamcinolone/nystatin (an antifungal): 0.1%/100,000 units/g.

## ◆ CLASSIFICATION

**PHARMACOTHERAPEUTIC:** Adrenocortical steroid. **CLINICAL:** Anti-inflammatory.

## USES

**Nasal inhalation:** Management of seasonal, perennial rhinitis in adults and children 2 yrs and older. **(OTC):** Relief of hay fever, other upper respiratory allergies. **Intra-articular:** Acute gouty arthritis, bursitis, tenosynovitis, epicondylitis, rheumatoid arthritis, synovitis of osteoarthritis. **Intralesional:** Alopecia areata, discoid lupus erythematosus, keloids, lichen plaques, psoriatic plaques. **Topical:** Relief of inflammation, pruritus associated with corticoid-responsive dermatoses.

## PRECAUTIONS

**Contraindications:** Hypersensitivity to triamcinolone. Systemic fungal infections, cerebral malaria, serious infections. **IM:** Idiopathic thrombocytopenic purpura. **Topical:** Local fungal, viral, bacterial infections. **Cautions:** Administration of live virus vaccines, following acute MI, elderly, hepatic impairment, myasthenia gravis, pts at risk for osteoporosis/seizures/GI disease, history of tuberculosis (may reactivate disease), hypothyroidism, cirrhosis, HF, hypertension, renal insufficiency, diabetes, cardiovascular disease. Prolonged therapy should be discontinued slowly.

## ACTION

Inhibits accumulation of inflammatory cells at inflammation sites, phagocytosis, lysosomal enzyme release, synthesis/release of mediators of inflammation. **Therapeutic Effect:** Prevents/suppresses cell-mediated immune reactions. Decreases/prevents tissue response to inflammatory process.

## INTERACTIONS

**DRUG: Amphotericin, diuretics** may worsen hypokalemia. May increase risk of **digoxin** toxicity (due to hypokalemia). May decrease effects of **insulin, oral hypoglycemics. CYP3A inducers (e.g., phenytoin, rifampin)** may decrease effects. May reduce response to **vaccines**

due to inhibition of antibody response. **HERBAL: Echinacea** may decrease effects. **FOOD:** None known. **LAB VALUES:** May increase serum glucose, lipid, amylase, sodium. May decrease serum calcium, potassium, thyroxine.

## AVAILABILITY (Rx)

**Cream:** 0.025%, 0.1%. **Injection, Suspension (Kenalog-10):** 10 mg/ml. (Kenalog-40): 40 mg/ml. **Ointment:** 0.025%, 0.1%, 0.5%. **Paste, Oral, Topical:** 0.1%. **Suspension, Spray Nasal Inhalation (Nasacort AQ):** 55 mcg/inhalation.

## ADMINISTRATION/HANDLING

**Topical**
• Gently cleanse area before application.
• Use occlusive dressings only as ordered.
• Apply sparingly, rub into area thoroughly.

## INDICATIONS/ROUTES/DOSAGE

**Triamcinolone Hexacetonide**
**Intralesional:** Up to 0.5 mg/square inch. Range: 2–48 mg.
**Intra-articular:** Average dose: 2–20 mg q3–4 wks.

**Triamcinolone Acetonide**
**Intra-articular: ADULTS, ELDERLY:** Initially: 2–20 mg/day. Doses can be adjusted between 20–80 mg as needed.

**Rhinitis**
**Note:** Discontinue if symptomatic relief not observed within 3 wks (1 wk of OTC use). **Intranasal: ADULTS, ELDERLY, CHILDREN 12 YRS AND OLDER:** Initially, 220 mcg/day as 2 sprays in each nostril once daily. **CHILDREN 6–11 YRS:** Initially, 110 mcg/day as 1 spray in each nostril once daily. May increase to 2 sprays in each nostril once daily. **CHILDREN 2–5 YRS:** 110 mcg/day as 1 spray in each nostril once daily.

**Usual Topical Dosage**
**Topical: ADULTS, ELDERLY, CHILDREN:** 2–3 times/day. May give 1–2 times/day or as intermittent therapy.

**Dosage in Renal/Hepatic Impairment**
No dose adjustment.

## SIDE EFFECTS

**Frequent:** Insomnia, dry mouth, heartburn, nervousness, abdominal distention, diaphoresis, acne, mood swings, increased appetite, facial flushing, delayed wound healing, increased susceptibility to infection, diarrhea, constipation. **Occasional:** Headache, edema, change in skin color, frequent urination. **Rare:** Tachycardia, allergic reaction (rash, urticaria), altered mental status, hallucinations, depression. **Topical:** Allergic contact dermatitis.

## ADVERSE EFFECTS/ TOXIC REACTIONS

**Long-term therapy:** Muscle wasting (arms, legs), osteoporosis, spontaneous fractures, amenorrhea, cataracts, glaucoma, peptic ulcer, HF. **Abrupt withdrawal following long-term therapy:** Anorexia, nausea, fever, headache, arthralgia, rebound inflammation, fatigue, weakness, lethargy, dizziness, orthostatic hypotension. Anaphylaxis occurs rarely with parenteral administration. Sudden discontinuation may be fatal. Blindness has occurred rarely after intralesional injection around face, head.

## NURSING CONSIDERATIONS

### BASELINE ASSESSMENT
Question for hypersensitivity to any corticosteroids. Obtain baselines for height, weight, B/P, serum glucose, electrolytes.

### INTERVENTION/EVALUATION
**Oral inhalation, intranasal:** Check mucous membranes for signs of fungal infection. Monitor growth in children. Monitor B/P.

### PATIENT/FAMILY TEACHING
• Report if condition being treated persists or worsens. • Avoid exposure to chickenpox or measles. • Avoid alcohol. • **Inhalation:** Do not take for acute asthma attack. • Rinse mouth to decrease risk of

**T**

mouth soreness. • Report oropharyngeal lesions or soreness (stomatitis). • **Nasal:** Report unusual cough/spasm, persistent nasal bleeding, burning, infection.

# trimethoprim

trye-**meth**-oh-prim
(Apo-Trimethoprim ✤, Primsol)

## FIXED-COMBINATION(S)

**Bactrim, Septra:** trimethoprim/sulfamethoxazole (a sulfonamide): 16 mg/80 mg/ml (injection), 40 mg/200 mg/5 ml (suspension), 80 mg/400 mg, 160 mg/800 mg (tablets).

## ◆CLASSIFICATION

**PHARMACOTHERAPEUTIC:** Folate antagonist. **CLINICAL:** Antibacterial.

## USES

Treatment of UTI caused by susceptible strains of *E. coli, P. mirabilis, K. pneumoniae*. Treatment of acute otitis media due to *H. influenzae, S. pneumoniae*. **OFF-LABEL:** Treatment of pneumonia caused by *Pneumocystis jiroveci* (in combination with dapsone).

## PRECAUTIONS

**Contraindications:** Hypersensitivity to trimethoprim. Megaloblastic anemia due to folic acid deficiency. **Cautions:** Renal/hepatic impairment, pts with folic acid deficiency, elderly.

## ACTION

Inhibits folic acid reduction to tetrahydrofolate, inhibiting microbial growth. **Therapeutic Effect:** Bacteriostatic.

## PHARMACOKINETICS

Rapidly, completely absorbed from GI tract. Protein binding: 42%–46%. Widely distributed, including to CSF. Metabolized in liver. Primarily excreted in urine. Moderately removed by hemodialysis. **Half-life:** 8–10 hrs (increased in renal impairment, newborns; decreased in children).

## ⧗ LIFESPAN CONSIDERATIONS

**Pregnancy/Lactation:** Drug readily crosses placenta; is distributed in breast milk. **Children:** Safety and efficacy not established. **Elderly:** No age-related precautions noted. May increase incidence of thrombocytopenia.

## INTERACTIONS

**DRUG: Folate antagonists (e.g., methotrexate)** may increase risk of megaloblastic anemia. May increase concentration, side effects of **phenytoin. HERBAL:** None significant. **FOOD:** None known. **LAB VALUES:** May increase serum BUN, bilirubin, creatinine, ALT, AST.

## AVAILABILITY (Rx)

**Oral Solution (Primsol):** 50 mg/5 ml. **Tablets:** 100 mg.

## ADMINISTRATION/HADLING

**PO**
• Space doses evenly to maintain constant therapeutic level. • Give with milk or food.

## INDICATIONS/ROUTES/DOSAGE

**UTI**
**PO: ADULTS, ELDERLY, CHILDREN 12 YRS AND OLDER:** 100 mg q12h or 200 mg once daily for 10–14 days. **CHILDREN YOUNGER THAN 12 YRS:** 4–6 mg/kg/day in 2 divided doses for 10 days.

**Otitis Media**
**PO: CHILDREN, 6 MOS AND OLDER:** 10 mg/kg/day in divided doses q12h for 10 days. **Maximum:** 400 mg/day.

***Pneumocystis jiroveci* Pneumonia (PCP)**
**ADULTS, ELDERLY, CHILDREN 12 YRS AND OLDER:** 15–20 mg/kg/day in 3 divided doses for 21 days in combination with dapsone.

**Dosage in Renal Impairment**
Dosage and frequency are modified based on creatinine clearance.

| Creatinine Clearance | Dosage |
|---|---|
| Greater than 30 ml/min | No change |
| 15–30 ml/min | 50 mg q12h or 100 mg once daily |
| Less than 15 ml/min | Avoid use |

**Dosage in Hepatic Impairment**
No dose adjustment.

## SIDE EFFECTS

**Occasional:** Nausea, vomiting, diarrhea, decreased appetite, abdominal cramps, headache. **Rare:** Hypersensitivity reaction (pruritus, rash), methemoglobinemia (bluish fingernails, lips, skin; fever; pale skin; sore throat; asthenia, photosensitivity.

## ADVERSE EFFECTS/ TOXIC REACTIONS

Stevens-Johnson syndrome, erythema multiforme, exfoliative dermatitis, anaphylaxis occur rarely. Hematologic toxicity (thrombocytopenia, neutropenia, leukopenia, megaloblastic anemia) more likely to occur in elderly, debilitated, alcoholics, those with renal impairment or receiving prolonged high dosage.

## NURSING CONSIDERATIONS

### BASELINE ASSESSMENT

Assess hematology baseline reports, serum renal function tests.

### INTERVENTION/EVALUATION

Assess skin for rash. Evaluate food tolerance. Monitor serum hematology reports, renal function, LFT. Check for developing signs of hematologic toxicity (pallor, fever, sore throat, malaise, bleeding/bruising).

### PATIENT/FAMILY TEACHING

• Space doses evenly. • Complete full length of therapy (10–14 days). • May take on empty stomach or with food if stomach upset occurs. • Avoid sun, ultraviolet light; use sunscreen, wear protective clothing. • Immediately report pallor, fatigue, sore throat, bruising/bleeding, discoloration of skin, fever, rash.

# triptorelin

**trip**-toe-**rel**-in
(Trelstar, Trelstar Depot, Trelstar LA)

## ◆CLASSIFICATION

**PHARMACOTHERAPEUTIC:** Gonadotropin-releasing hormone analogue. **CLINICAL:** Antineoplastic.

## USES

Palliative treatment of advanced prostate cancer.

## PRECAUTIONS

**Contraindications:** Hypersensitivity to triptorelin, luteinizing hormone-releasing hormone (LHRH), LHRH agonists, pregnancy. **Cautions:** None known.

## ACTION

Through a negative feedback mechanism, inhibits gonadotropin hormone secretion. Circulating levels of luteinizing hormone (LH), follicle-stimulating hormone (FSH), testosterone, estradiol rise initially, then subside with continued therapy. **Therapeutic Effect:** Suppresses growth of abnormal prostate tissue.

## ⏳ LIFESPAN CONSIDERATIONS

**Pregnancy/Lactation:** Unknown if distributed in breast milk. **Children:** Safety and efficacy not established. **Elderly:** No age-related precautions noted.

## INTERACTIONS

**DRUG:** None significant. **HERBAL:** None significant. **FOOD:** None known. **LAB VALUES:** May alter serum pituitary-gonadal function test results. May cause transient increase in serum testosterone, usually during first wk of treatment.

---

## AVAILABILITY (Rx)

Injection, Powder for Reconstitution (Trelstar Depot): 3.75 mg. Injection, Powder for Reconstitution (Trelstar LA): 11.25 mg, 22.5 mg.

## ADMINISTRATION/HANDLING

**IM**

• Reconstitute with 2 ml Sterile Water for Injection. • Administer into large muscle mass, esp. gluteus muscle, alternating injection sites.

## INDICATIONS/ROUTES/DOSAGE

**Prostate Cancer**

**IM: ADULTS, ELDERLY:** 3.75 mg once q4wks, 11.25 mg q12 wks, or 22.5 mg q24 wks.
**IM (Trelstar LA): ADULTS, ELDERLY:** 11.25 mg q12wks, 22.5 mg q24wks.

**Dosage in Renal/Hepatic Impairment**
No dose adjustment.

## SIDE EFFECTS

**Frequent (Greater Than 5%):** Hot flashes, skeletal pain, headache, impotence. **Occasional (5%–2%):** Insomnia, vomiting, leg pain, fatigue. **Rare (Less Than 2%):** Dizziness, emotional lability, diarrhea, urinary retention, UTI, anemia, pruritus.

## ADVERSE EFFECTS/ TOXIC REACTIONS

Bladder outlet obstruction, skeletal pain, hematuria, spinal cord compression with weakness, paralysis of lower extremities may occur.

## NURSING CONSIDERATIONS

### INTERVENTION/EVALUATION

Obtain serum testosterone, prostate-specific antigen (PSA), prostatic acid phosphatase (PAP) levels periodically during therapy. Serum testosterone, PAP levels should increase during first wk of therapy. Testosterone level then should decrease to baseline level or less within 2 wks, PAP level within 4 wks. Monitor pt closely for worsening signs and symptoms of prostatic cancer, esp. during first wk of therapy (due to transient increase in testosterone).

### PATIENT/FAMILY TEACHING

• Do not miss monthly injections. • May experience increased skeletal pain, blood in urine, urinary retention initially (subsides within 1 wk). • Hot flashes may occur. • Report tachycardia, persistent nausea or vomiting, numbness of arms/legs, pain/swelling of breasts, difficulty breathing, infection at injection site.

# trospium

**tro**-spee-um
(Trosec ✦)

## ◆CLASSIFICATION

**PHARMACOTHERAPEUTIC:** Anticholinergic. **CLINICAL:** Antispasmotic.

## USES

Treatment of overactive bladder with symptoms of urge urinary incontinence, urgency, urinary frequency.

## PRECAUTIONS

**Contraindications:** Hypersensitivity to trospium. Gastric retention, uncontrolled narrow-angle glaucoma, urinary retention. **Cautions:** Decreased GI motility, renal/hepatic impairment, obstructive GI disorders, ulcerative colitis, intestinal atony, myasthenia gravis, controlled narrow-angle glaucoma, bladder flow obstruction, Alzheimer's disease, hot weather/exercise, elderly.

## ACTION

Antagonizes effect of acetylcholine on muscarinic receptors, producing parasympatholytic action. **Therapeutic Effect:** Reduces smooth muscle tone in bladder.

## PHARMACOKINETICS

Minimally absorbed after PO administration. Protein binding: 50%–85%. Distributed in plasma. Excreted in feces (82%), urine (6%). **Half-life:** 20 hrs.

## ⌛ LIFESPAN CONSIDERATIONS

**Pregnancy/Lactation:** Unknown if drug crosses placenta or is distributed in breast milk. **Children:** Safety and efficacy not established. **Elderly:** Higher incidence of dry mouth, constipation, dyspepsia, UTI, urinary retention in pts 75 yrs and older.

## INTERACTIONS

**DRUG: Other anticholinergic agents** increase severity, frequency of side effects, may alter absorption of other drugs due to anticholinergic effects on GI motility. **Morphine, procainamide, tenofovir, vancomycin** may increase concentration. **HERBAL:** None significant. **FOOD: High-fat meals** may reduce absorption. **LAB VALUES:** None significant.

## AVAILABILITY (Rx)

🗡 Tablets (Sanctura): 20 mg. 🗡 Capsules, Extended-Release (Sanctura XR): 60 mg.

## ADMINISTRATION/HANDLING

### PO

• Store at room temperature. • Give at least 1 hr before meals or on an empty stomach. • Do not break, crush, dissolve, or divide tablets or extended-release capsules; swallow whole. • Administer tablets at bedtime, capsules in morning with full glass of water, 1 hr before eating.

## INDICATIONS/ROUTES/DOSAGE

**Overactive Bladder**
**PO: ADULTS:** *(Immediate-Release):* 20 mg twice daily. **ELDERLY 75 YRS AND OLDER:** 20 mg once daily at bedtime. *(Extended-Release):* 60 mg once daily.

**Dosage in Renal Impairment**
For pts with CrCl less than 30 ml/min, immediate-release dosage reduced to 20 mg once daily at bedtime. Extended-release not recommended.

**Dosage in Hepatic Impairment**
**Mild impairment:** No dose adjustment. **Moderate to severe impairment:** Use with caution.

## SIDE EFFECTS

**Frequent (20%):** Dry mouth. **Occasional (10%–4%):** Constipation, headache. **Rare (Less Than 2%):** Fatigue, upper abdominal pain, dyspepsia (heartburn, indigestion, epigastric pain), flatulence, dry eyes, urinary retention.

## ADVERSE EFFECTS/TOXIC REACTIONS

Overdose may result in severe anticholinergic effects, characterized by nervousness, restlessness, nausea, vomiting, confusion, diaphoresis, facial flushing, hypertension, hypotension, respiratory depression, irritability, lacrimation. Supraventricular tachycardia and hallucinations occur rarely.

## NURSING CONSIDERATIONS

### BASELINE ASSESSMENT

Assess for presence of dysuria, urinary urgency, frequency, incontinence.

### INTERVENTION/EVALUATION

Monitor for symptomatic relief. Monitor I&O; palpate bladder for retention. Monitor daily pattern of bowel activity, stool consistency. Dry mouth may be relieved by sips of tepid water.

### PATIENT/FAMILY TEACHING

• Report nausea, vomiting, diaphoresis, increased salivary secretions, palpitations, severe abdominal pain. • Swallow tablets, extended-release capsules whole.

T

---

# umeclidinium

ue-**mek**-li-**din**-ee-um
(Incruse Ellipta)
**Do not confuse umeclidinium
with aclidinium or clidinium.**

### FIXED COMBINATION(S)

**Anoro Ellipta:** umeclidinium/
vilanterol (long-acting beta₂-adrenergic agonist): 62.5 mcg/25 mcg.

### ◆CLASSIFICATION

**PHARMACOTHERAPEUTIC:** Anticholinergic. **CLINICAL:** Bronchodilator.

## USES

Long-term, once daily, maintenance treatment of airflow obstruction in pts with COPD including chronic bronchitis and/or emphysema.

## PRECAUTIONS

**Contraindications:** Hypersensitivity to umeclidinium. Severe hypersensitivity to milk proteins or any drug components. **Cautions:** Bladder neck obstruction, myasthenia gravis, narrow-angle glaucoma, prostatic hypertrophy, urinary retention. Not recommended in pts with acutely deteriorating COPD requiring emergent relief of acute symptoms.

## ACTION

Inhibits muscarinic M3 receptor in lungs, resulting in relaxation of bronchial smooth muscle. **Therapeutic Effect:** Relieves bronchospasm, reduces airway resistance, improves bronchodilation.

## PHARMACOKINETICS

Rapidly absorbed following inhalation. Primarily metabolized by enzyme cytochrome P4502D6. Protein binding: 89%. Peak concentration: 5–15 min. Steady state reached within 14 days. **Half-life:** 11 hrs.

## ⌛ LIFESPAN CONSIDERATIONS

**Pregnancy/Lactation:** Unknown if distributed in breast milk. Must either discontinue drug or discontinue breast-feeding. **Children:** Not indicated in this pt population. **Elderly:** No age-related precautions noted.

## INTERACTIONS

**DRUG: Anticholinergics** (e.g., atropine, dicyclomine, glycopyrrolate, scopolamine), **medications with anticholingeric properties** (e.g., **diphenhydramine**) may increase effects/risk of toxicity. **HERBAL:** None significant. **FOOD:** None known. **LAB VALUES:** None known.

## AVAILABILITY (Rx)

**Inhalation Powder:** 62.5 mcg/capsule (in blister packs containing 7 or 30 doses).

## ADMINISTRATION/HANDLING

**Inhalation**

**Administration** • Follow instructions for preparation according to manufacturer guidelines. • Fully exhale with inhaler away from mouth and place mouthpiece between lips. • Do not block air vent with fingers. • Take one long, steady, deep breath and continue inhalation for as long as possible. • Remove mouthpiece and hold breath for 3–4 sec. Do not inhale another dose if medication not tasted or felt (dose was delivered). • Close lid cover.
**Storage** • Store at room temperature up to 6 wks after opening tray. • Do not refrigerate or freeze. • Protect from sunlight and moisture. • Discard after counter reaches 0. • Do not reuse inhaler.

## INDICATIONS/ROUTES/DOSAGE

**COPD**
**Inhalation: ADULTS, ELDERLY:** One inhalation (62.5 mcg) once daily, at same time each day. **Maximum:** 1 inhalation/24 hrs.

**Dose Modification**
**Deterioration of COPD**: Discontinue treatment. Institute short-acting bronchodilators and supportive pulmonary therapy.

**Dosage in Renal Impairment**
No dose adjustment.

**Dosage in Hepatic Impairment**
**Mild to moderate impairment:** No dose adjustment. **Severe impairment:** Use caution.

## SIDE EFFECTS

**Occasional (8%–5%):** Nasopharyngitis, upper respiratory tract infection. **Rare (3%–1%):** Cough, arthralgia, viral respiratory tract infection, pharyngitis, myalgia, abdominal pain, toothache, tachycardia.

## ADVERSE EFFECTS/ TOXIC REACTIONS

Life-threatening asthma-related events, bronchospasm, worsening of COPD-related symptoms have been reported. Hypersensitivity reactions may occur (esp. in pts with undiagnosed, severe milk protein allergy or allergy to products containing lactose). Worsening of narrow-angle glaucoma (eye pain, blurry vision, visual halos, colored images in association with red eyes from conjunctival congestion and corneal edema) may occur. May cause worsening of urinary retention, esp. in pts with prostatic hypertrophy or bladder neck obstruction.

## NURSING CONSIDERATIONS

**BASELINE ASSESSMENT**
Obtain baseline $O_2$ saturation, vital signs; pulmonary function test, if applicable. Assess respiratory rate, depth, rhythm. Assess lung sounds for wheezing, rales. Screen for concomitant use of anticholinergic medications. Question history of asthma, BPH, bladder neck obstruction. Teach proper inhaler priming and administration techniques. Conduct ophthalmologic exam in pts with narrow-angle glaucoma.

**INTERVENTION/EVALUATION**
Routinely monitor $O_2$ saturation, vital signs. Auscultate lung sounds and monitor for symptom improvement. Recommend discontinuation of short-acting beta$_2$-agonists while on long-term therapy. Monitor for COPD deterioration, narrow-angle glaucoma, urinary retention/obstruction. Monitor for increased use of rescue inhaler; may indicate worsening of respiratory status.

**PATIENT/FAMILY TEACHING**
• Report fever, productive cough, body aches, paradoxical bronchospasm, difficulty breathing; may indicate lung infection, worsening of COPD. • Therapy not intended for acute COPD symptom relief, and extra doses are not advised. • Report symptoms of acute narrow-angle glaucoma, urinary retention, bladder distention. • Refill prescription when counter on left of inhaler reaches red area of scale. • Follow manufacturer guidelines for proper use of inhaler. • Drink plenty of fluids (decreases lung secretion viscosity). • Rinse mouth with water after inhalation to decrease mouth/throat irritation.

---

# ustekinumab   TOP 100

yoo-ste-**kin**-ue-mab
(Stelara)
**Do not confuse Stelara with Aldara, or ustekinumab with infliximab or rituximab.**

## ◆CLASSIFICATION

**PHARMACOTHERAPEUTIC:** Monoclonal antibody. **CLINICAL:** Antipsoriasis agent.

U

## USES

Treatment of adults 18 yrs or older with moderate to severe plaque psoriasis who are candidates for systemic therapy or phototherapy. Treatment of adults with active psoriatic arthritis alone or in combination with methotrexate. Treatment of adults with moderate to severe active Crohn's disease.

---

## PRECAUTIONS

**Contraindications:** Hypersensitivity to ustekinumab. **Cautions:** History of chronic infection, recurrent infection, active tuberculosis, prior malignancy, renal/hepatic impairment. Avoid use of live vaccines.

## ACTION

Strongly binds with cellular components involved in responses to inflammation and immune system, thereby decreasing likelihood of aggravating psoriatic eruptions. **Therapeutic Effect:** Significantly slows growth, migration of circulating total lymphocytes (predominant in psoriatic lesions).

## PHARMACOKINETICS

Following subcutaneous injections, clearance is affected by body weight, is not affected by gender or race. Degraded into small peptides and amino acids via catabolic pathways. Serum concentration reaches steady state at 28 wks. **Half-life:** 10–126 days.

## ⌛ LIFESPAN CONSIDERATIONS

**Pregnancy/Lactation:** Unknown if distributed in breast milk. **Children:** Not indicated for use in this pt population. **Elderly:** Age-related increased incidence of infection requires cautious use.

## INTERACTIONS

**DRUG: Immunosuppressive agents (e.g., abatacept, cyclosporine, fingolimod, methotrexate, sirolimus)** increase risk of infection. **Abciximab, trastuzumab** may increase concentration/effects. May decrease therapeutic effects of **vaccines;** increase risk of adverse effects of **live vaccines. HERBAL:** Echinacea may decrease concentration/effects. **FOOD:** None known. **LAB VALUES:** May increase lymphocyte count.

## AVAILABILITY (Rx)

**Injection Solution (Prefilled Syringes):** 45 mg/0.5 ml, 90 mg/ml.

## ADMINISTRATION/HANDLING

### SQ

• Do not inject into areas where skin is tender, bruised, erythematous, indurated. • Administer into thigh, abdomen, buttocks, upper arm. • Refrigerate unopened vial. • Solution appears colorless to light yellow. Discard if solution contains more than a few small translucent or white particles or is cloudy.

## INDICATIONS/ROUTES/DOSAGE

**Plaque Psoriasis**
**SQ: ADULTS, ELDERLY WEIGHING 100 KG OR LESS:** Initially, 45 mg, then 45 mg 4 wks later, followed by 45 mg every 12 wks. **WEIGHING MORE THAN 100 KG:** Initially, 90 mg, then 90 mg 4 wks later, followed by 90 mg every 12 wks. **Note:** 45 mg also efficacious; however, 90 mg is recommended due to greater efficacy.

**Psoriatic Arthritis**
**SQ: ADULTS, ELDERLY:** Initially, 45 mg repeated in 4 wks followed by 45 mg q12wks. **PTS WITH COEXISTENT MODERATE TO SEVERE PLAQUE PSORIASIS WEIGHING MORE THAN 100 KG:** Initially, 90 mg repeated in 4 wks, then 90 mg q12wks.

**Crohn's Disease**
**IV INFUSION: ADULTS, ELDERLY:** Initially, 520 mg (greater than 85 kg); 390 mg (56–85 kg); 260 mg (up to 54 kg), then a subcutaneous 90-mg dose 8 wks after initial IV dose, then q8wks thereafter.

**Dosage in Renal/Hepatic Impairment**
No dose adjustment.

## SIDE EFFECTS

**Occasional (8%–4%):** Nasopharyngitis, upper respiratory tract infection, headache. **Rare (3%–1%):** Fatigue, diarrhea, back pain, dizziness, pruritus, injection site erythema, myalgia, depression.

## ADVERSE EFFECTS/ TOXIC REACTIONS

Worsening of psoriasis, thrombocytopenia, malignancies, serious infections (cellulitis, diverticulitis, gastroenteritis, pneumonia, osteomyelitis, UTI, postoperative wound infection) have been noted. Reversible posterior leukoencephalopathy syndrome (headache, seizures, confusion, visual disturbances) occurs rarely.

## NURSING CONSIDERATIONS

### BASELINE ASSESSMENT

Pts should not receive live vaccines during treatment, 1 yr prior to initiating treatment, or 1 yr following discontinuation of treatment. Inform pt of duration of treatment and required monitoring procedures. Assess skin prior to therapy; document extent and location of psoriasis lesions. Test pt for tuberculosis infection prior to initiating treatment.

### INTERVENTION/EVALUATION

Closely monitor for signs/symptoms of active tuberculosis during and after treatment. Assess skin throughout therapy for evidence of improvement of psoriasis lesions. Monitor for worsening of lesions.

### PATIENT/FAMILY TEACHING

• If appropriate, pt may self-inject after proper training in preparation and injection technique. • Report any signs of infection. • If new diagnosis of malignancy occurs, inform physician of current treatment with ustekinumab.

# *valACYclovir

val-a-**sye**-kloe-veer
(Apo-Valacyclovir ✤, Valtrex)
**Do not confuse valacyclovir with
acyclovir or valganciclovir, or
Valtrex with Valcyte.**

## ◆CLASSIFICATION
**PHARMACOTHERAPEUTIC:** Antiviral.
**CLINICAL:** Antiviral.

## USES

Treatment of herpes zoster (shingles)
in immunocompetent pts. Treatment of
initial and recurrent genital herpes in
immunocompetent adults. Prevention of
recurrent genital herpes and reduction of
transmission of genital herpes in immunocompetent pts. Suppression of genital
herpes in HIV-infected pts. Treatment of
cold sores, chickenpox in immunocompetent children. **OFF-LABEL:** Prophylaxis
and treatment of cancer-related HSV, VZV.

## PRECAUTIONS

**Contraindications:** Hypersensitivity to
acyclovir, valacyclovir. **Cautions:** Renal
impairment, concurrent use of nephrotoxic agents, elderly.

## ACTION

Converted to acyclovir by intestinal/
hepatic metabolism. Competes for viral
DNA polymerase; inhibits incorporation
into viral DNA. **Therapeutic Effect:** Inhibits DNA synthesis and viral replication.

## PHARMACOKINETICS

Rapidly absorbed after PO administration.
Protein binding: 13%–18%. Rapidly converted by hydrolysis to active compound
acyclovir. Widely distributed to tissues,
body fluids (including CSF). Primarily
eliminated in urine. Removed by hemodialysis. **Half-life:** (acyclovir) 2.5–3.3 hrs
(increased in renal impairment).

## ⧗ LIFESPAN CONSIDERATIONS
**Pregnancy/Lactation:** May cross placenta. May be distributed in breast milk.
**Children:** Safety and efficacy not established. **Elderly:** Age-related renal impairment may require dosage adjustment.

## INTERACTIONS
**DRUG: Nephrotoxic medications (e.g.,
ACE inhibitors, aminoglycosides, IV
contrast media)** may increase risk of
nephrotoxicity, renal impairment. **HERBAL:**
None significant. **FOOD:** None known. **LAB
VALUES:** None significant.

## AVAILABILITY (Rx)
**Tablets:** 500 mg, 1,000 mg.

## ADMINISTRATION/HANDLING
**PO**
• Give without regard to meals. • If GI
upset occurs, give with meals.

## INDICATIONS/ROUTES/DOSAGE
**Herpes Zoster (Shingles)**
**PO: ADULTS, ELDERLY:** 1 g 3 times/day
for 7 days.

**Herpes Simplex (Cold Sores)**
**PO: ADULTS, ELDERLY:** 2 g twice daily for
1 day (separate by 12 hrs).

**Initial Episode of Genital Herpes**
**PO: ADULTS, ELDERLY:** 1 g twice daily for
10 days.

**Recurrent Episodes of Genital Herpes**
**PO: ADULTS, ELDERLY:** 500 mg twice daily
for 3 days.

**Suppressive Therapy of Genital Herpes**
**PO: ADULTS, ELDERLY: (HIV infected):**
500 mg twice daily. **(Immunocompetent):** 1 g once daily (500 mg once daily
in pts with 9 or fewer recurrences/yr).

V

---

**Genital Herpes**

| Creatinine Clearance | Initial Episode | Recurrent Episode | Suppressive Therapy |
|---|---|---|---|
| 10–29 ml/min | 1 g q24h | 500 mg q24h | 500 mg q24–48h |
| Less than 10 ml/min | 500 mg q24h | 500 mg q24h | 500 mg q24–48h |

**Chickenpox**

PO: **CHILDREN 2–17 YRS:** 20 mg/kg/dose 3 times/day for 5 days. **Maximum:** 1 g 3 times/day.

**Dosage in Renal Impairment**

Dosage and frequency are modified based on creatinine clearance. **HD:** Give dose postdialysis.

**Cold Sores/Herpes Zoster**

| Creatinine Clearance | Herpes Zoster | Cold Sores |
|---|---|---|
| 30–49 ml/min | 1 g q12h | 1 g q12h × 2 doses |
| 10–29 ml/min | 1 g q24h | 500 mg q12h × 2 doses |
| Less than 10 ml/min | 500 mg q24h | 500 mg as single dose |

**Dosage in Hepatic Impairment**

No dose adjustment.

## SIDE EFFECTS

**Frequent: Herpes zoster (17%–10%):** Nausea, headache. **Genital herpes (17%):** Headache. **Occasional: Herpes zoster (7%–3%):** Vomiting, diarrhea, constipation (50 yrs and older), asthenia, dizziness (50 yrs and older). **Genital herpes (8%–3%):** Nausea, diarrhea, dizziness. **Rare: Herpes zoster (3%–1%):** Abdominal pain, anorexia. **Genital herpes (3%–1%):** Asthenia, abdominal pain.

## ADVERSE EFFECTS/ TOXIC REACTIONS

Neutropenia, thrombocytopenia, renal failure occur rarely.

## NURSING CONSIDERATIONS

### BASELINE ASSESSMENT

Question for history of allergies, particularly to valacyclovir, acyclovir. Tissue cultures for herpes zoster, herpes simplex should be obtained before giving first dose (therapy may proceed before results are known). Assess medical history, esp. HIV infection, bone marrow or renal transplantation, renal/hepatic impairment.

### INTERVENTION/EVALUATION

Monitor CBC, LFT, renal function, urinalysis. Evaluate cutaneous lesions. Provide analgesics, comfort measures for herpes zoster (esp. exhausting to elderly). Encourage fluids. Keep pt's fingernails short, hands clean.

### PATIENT/FAMILY TEACHING

• Drink adequate fluids. • Do not touch lesions with fingers to avoid spreading infection to new site. • **Genital herpes:** Continue therapy for full length of treatment. • Space doses evenly. • Avoid sexual intercourse during duration of lesions to prevent infecting partner. • Valacyclovir does not cure herpes. • Report if lesions recur or do not improve. • Pap smears should be done at least annually due to increased risk of cervical cancer in women with genital herpes. • Initiate treatment at first sign of recurrent episode of genital herpes or herpes zoster (early treatment within first 24–48 hrs is imperative for therapeutic results).

---

# *valGANciclovir

val-gan-**sye**-kloe-veer
(Apo-Valganciclovir ✦, Valcyte)
■ **BLACK BOX ALERT** ■ May adversely affect spermatogenesis, fertility. Risk for granulocytopenia, anemia, thrombocytopenia.
**Do not confuse Valcyte with Valium or Valtrex, or valganciclovir with valacyclovir.**

**V**

---

## ◆CLASSIFICATION

**PHARMACOTHERAPEUTIC:** Synthetic nucleoside. **CLINICAL:** Antiviral.

## USES

**Adults:** Treatment of cytomegalovirus (CMV) retinitis in AIDS. Prevention of CMV disease in high-risk renal, cardiac, renal-pancreas transplant pts. **Children:** Prevention of CMV disease in high-risk renal and cardiac transplant pts.

## PRECAUTIONS

**Contraindications:** Hypersensitivity to valganciclovir, ganciclovir. **Cautions:** Use extreme caution in children due to long-term carcinogenicity, reproductive toxicity. Renal impairment, concurrent nephrotoxic medications, preexisting bone marrow suppression or cytopenias, history of cytopenic reactions to other drugs, elderly (at greater risk for renal impairment).

## ACTION

Inhibits binding of deoxyguanosine triphosphate to DNA polymerase. **Therapeutic Effect:** Inhibits viral DNA synthesis.

## PHARMACOKINETICS

Well absorbed, rapidly converted to ganciclovir by intestinal mucosal cells and hepatocytes. Widely distributed including CSF, ocular tissue. Slowly metabolized intracellularly. Primarily excreted in urine. Removed by hemodialysis. **Half-life:** Ganciclovir: 4 hrs (increased in renal impairment).

## ⧗ LIFESPAN CONSIDERATIONS

**Pregnancy/Lactation:** Avoid pregnancy; may cause fetal harm/malformations. Female pts of reproductive potential should use effective contraception during treatment. Avoid breastfeeding; may be resumed no sooner than 72 hrs after last dose. May impair fertility in both females and males. **Children:** Safety and efficacy not established in pts younger than 12 yrs. **Elderly:** Age-related renal impairment may require dosage adjustment.

## INTERACTIONS

**DRUG: Bone marrow depressants** may increase myelosuppression. May increase risk of toxicity of **didanosine, mycophenolate. Probenecid** may decrease renal clearance, increase concentration. **Zidovudine (AZT)** may increase risk of hematologic toxicity. **HERBAL:** None significant. **FOOD: All foods** maximize drug bioavailability. **LAB VALUES:** May decrease creatinine clearance, platelet count, neutrophils, Hgb, Hct. May increase serum creatinine.

## AVAILABILITIES (Rx)

**Powder for Oral Solution:** 50 mg/ml (100 ml).

**◆ Tablets:** 450 mg.

## ADMINISTRATION/HANDLING

**PO**

• Take with meals. • Do not break, crush, dissolve, or divide tablets; give whole (potential carcinogen). • Avoid contact with skin. • Wash skin with soap, water if contact occurs. • Store oral suspension in refrigerator. Discard after 49 days.

## INDICATIONS/ROUTES/DOSAGE

**Note:** Do not use if absolute neutrophil count (ANC) less than 500/mm$^3$, platelets less than 25,000/mm$^3$, or Hgb less than 8 g/dl.

**Cytomegalovirus (CMV) Retinitis**
**PO: ADULTS:** Initially, 900 mg (two 450-mg tablets) twice daily for 21 days. **Maintenance:** 900 mg once daily.

**Prevention of CMV After Transplant**
**PO: ADULTS, ELDERLY:** 900 mg once daily beginning within 10 days of transplant and continuing until 100 days (heart, kidney, or pancreas transplant) or 200 days (kidney transplant) posttransplant. **CHILDREN 4 MOS–16 YRS:** Once daily based on body surface area (BSA) and CrCl using formula: (Dose = 7 × BSA × CrCl). **Maximum:** 900 mg/day.

V

**Dosage in Renal Impairment**
Dosage and frequency are modified based on creatinine clearance.

| Creatinine Clearance | Induction Dosage | Maintenance Dosage |
| --- | --- | --- |
| 60 ml/min or higher | 900 mg twice daily | 900 mg once daily |
| 40–59 ml/min | 450 mg twice daily | 450 mg once daily |
| 25–39 ml/min | 450 mg once daily | 450 mg every 2 days |
| 10–24 ml/min | 450 mg every 2 days | 450 mg twice wkly |

**Dosage in Hepatic Impairment**
No dose adjustment.

## SIDE EFFECTS

**Frequent (16%–9%):** Diarrhea, neutropenia, headache. **Occasional (8%–3%):** Nausea. **Rare (Less Than 3%):** Insomnia, paresthesia, vomiting, abdominal pain, fever.

## ADVERSE EFFECTS/ TOXIC REACTIONS

Hematologic toxicity, including severe neutropenia (most common), anemia, thrombocytopenia, leukopenia, aplastic anemia, pancytopenia, bone marrow suppression may occur. Retinal detachment occurs rarely. Overdose may result in renal toxicity. May decrease sperm production, fertility.

## NURSING CONSIDERATIONS

### BASELINE ASSESSMENT

Obtain baseline CBC, serum chemistries, renal function, urinalysis; pregnancy test. Receive full medication history.

### INTERVENTION/EVALUATION

Monitor I&O, ensure adequate hydration (minimum 1,500 ml/24 hrs). Diligently evaluate CBC for decreased WBCs, Hgb, Hct, platelets; changes in urinary characteristics, consistency. Question pt regarding vision, therapeutic improvement, complications.

### PATIENT/FAMILY TEACHING

• Valganciclovir provides suppression, not cure, of CMV retinitis. • Frequent blood tests are necessary during therapy because of toxic nature of drug. • Ophthalmologic exam q4–6wks during treatment is advised. • Report any new symptom promptly. • May temporarily or permanently inhibit sperm production in men, suppress fertility in women. • Barrier contraception should be used during and for 90 days after therapy (mutagenic potential). • Swallow whole; do not chew, crush, dissolve, or divide. • Avoid handling broken/crushed tablets, oral solution. • Report fever, chills, unusual bleeding/bruising, urinary changes.

# valproic acid

val-**pro**-ick **as**-id
(Apo-Divalproex ✦, Depacon, Depakene, Depakote, Depakote ER, Depakote Sprinkle, Novo-Divalproex ✦, Stavzor)

■ **BLACK BOX ALERT** ■ Embryo, fetal neural tube defects (spina bifida) have occurred. Life-threatening pancreatitis, complete hepatic failure have occurred.

**Do not confuse Depakene with Depakote.**

## ◆CLASSIFICATION

**PHARMACOTHERAPEUTIC:** Carboxylic acid derivative. **CLINICAL:** Anticonvulsant, antimanic, antimigraine.

## USES

Monotherapy/adjunctive therapy of complex partial seizures, simple and complex absence seizures. Adjunctive therapy of multiple seizures **Additional uses for Depakote, Depakote ER, Stavzor:** Treatment of manic episodes with bipolar disorder, prophylaxis of migraine headaches. **OFF-LABEL:** Refractory status epilepticus, diabetic neuropathy. Mood stabilizer for behaviors in dementia.

**V**

## PRECAUTIONS

**Contraindications:** Hypersensitivity to valproic acid. Active hepatic disease, urea cycle disorders, known mitocondrial disorders; migraine prevention in pregnant women. **Cautions:** Children younger than 2 yrs. Pts at risk for hepatotoxicity. History of hepatic impairment, bleeding abnormalities, pts at high risk for suicide, elderly.

## ACTION

Directly increases concentration of inhibitory neurotransmitter gamma-aminobutyric acid (GABA). **Therapeutic Effect:** Produces anticonvulsant effect, stabilizes mood, prevents migraine headache.

## PHARMACOKINETICS

Well absorbed from GI tract. Protein binding: 80%–90%. Metabolized in liver. Primarily excreted in urine. Not removed by hemodialysis. **Half-life:** 9–16 hrs (may be increased in hepatic impairment, elderly, children younger than 18 mos).

## ⧖ LIFESPAN CONSIDERATIONS

**Pregnancy/Lactation:** Drug crosses placenta; is distributed in breast milk. **Children:** Increased risk of hepatotoxicity in pts younger than 2 yrs. **Elderly:** No age-related precautions, but lower dosages recommended.

## INTERACTIONS

**DRUG: Carbapenems** (e.g., **meropenem**), **CYP3A4 inducers** (e.g., **carbamazepine, phenytoin**) may decrease concentration/effects. May alter effect of **warfarin**. May increase concentration of **lamotrigine. Topiramate** may increase risk of elevated serum ammonia levels. **HERBAL: Evening primrose** may decrease seizure threshold. **FOOD:** None known. **LAB VALUES:** May increase serum LDH, bilirubin, ALT, AST. **Therapeutic serum level:** 50–100 mcg/ml; **toxic serum level:** greater than 100 mcg/ml.

## AVAILABILITY (Rx)

**Capsules (Depakene):** 250 mg. **Capsules, Sprinkle (Depakote Sprinkle):** 125 mg.

**Injection, Solution (Depacon):** 100 mg/ml. **Syrup (Depakene):** 250 mg/5 ml.

 **Capsules, Delayed-Release (Stavzor):** 125 mg, 250 mg, 500 mg.  **Tablets, Delayed-Release (Depakote):** 125 mg, 250 mg, 500 mg.  **Tablets, Extended-Release (Depakote ER):** 250 mg, 500 mg.

## ADMINISTRATION/HANDLING
### 💉 IV

**Reconstitution** • Dilute each single dose with at least 50 ml D₅W, 0.9% NaCl, or lactated Ringer's.
**Rate of Administration** • Infuse over 60 min at rate of 20 mg/min or less. • Alternatively, single doses of up to 45 mg/kg given over 5–10 min (1.5–6 mg/kg/min).
**Storage** • Store vials at room temperature. • Diluted solutions stable for 24 hrs. • Discard unused portion.

### PO
• May give without regard to food. Do not mix oral solution with carbonated beverages (may cause mouth/throat irritation). • May sprinkle capsule (Depakote Sprinkle) contents on applesauce and give immediately (do not chew sprinkle beads). • Give delayed-release/extended-release tablets whole. Do not crush, break, open delayed-release capsule (Stavzor). • Regular-release and delayed-release formulations usually given in 2–4 divided doses/day. Extended-release formulation (Depakote ER) usually given once daily.

## ▦ IV INCOMPATIBILITIES
None known.

## ▦ IV COMPATIBILITIES
Cefepime, ceftazidime.

## INDICATIONS/ROUTES/DOSAGE

**Seizures**
**PO: ADULTS, ELDERLY, CHILDREN 10 YRS AND OLDER:** Initially, 10–15 mg/kg/day in 1–3 divided doses. May increase by 5–10 mg/kg/day at wkly intervals up to

**V**

60 mg/kg/day. **Usual adult dosage:** 1,000–2,500 mg/day.

**IV: ADULTS, ELDERLY, CHILDREN:** Same frequency as oral dose.

**Manic Episodes**
**PO:** *(Depakote):* **ADULTS, ELDERLY:** Initially, 750 mg/day in divided doses. **Maximum:** 60 mg/kg/day.
**PO:** *(Extended-Release [Depakote ER]):* Initially, 25 mg/kg/day once daily. **Maximum:** 60 mg/kg/day. *(Delayed-Release [Stavzor]):* Initially, 750 mg/day in divided dose. Titrate to lowest therapeutic dose. **Maximum:** 60 mg/kg/day.

**Prevention of Migraine Headaches**
**PO:** *(Extended-Release [Depakote ER]):* **ADULTS, ELDERLY:** Initially, 500 mg/day for 7 days. May increase up to 1,000 mg/day.
**PO:** *(Delayed-Release [Depakote]):* **ADULTS, ELDERLY, CHILDREN 16 YRS AND OLDER:** Initially, 250 mg twice daily. May increase up to 1,000 mg/day. **ADULTS, ELDERLY, CHILDREN 12 YRS AND OLDER:** *(Stavzor):* 250 mg twice daily. May increase to 1,000 mg/day.

**Dosage in Renal Impairment**
No dose adjustment.

**Dosage in Hepatic Impairment**
**Mild to moderate impairment:** Not recommended. **Severe impairment:** Contraindicated.

## SIDE EFFECTS

**Frequent: Epilepsy:** Abdominal pain, irregular menses, diarrhea, transient alopecia, indigestion, nausea, vomiting, tremors, fluctuations in body weight. **Mania (22%–19%):** Nausea, drowsiness. **Occasional: Epilepsy:** Constipation, dizziness, drowsiness, headache, skin rash, unusual excitement, restlessness. **Mania (12%–6%):** Asthenia, abdominal pain, dyspepsia, rash. **Rare: Epilepsy:** Mood changes, diplopia, nystagmus, spots before eyes, unusual bleeding/bruising.

## ADVERSE EFFECTS/ TOXIC REACTIONS

Hepatotoxicity may occur, particularly in first 6 mos of therapy. May be preceded by loss of seizure control, malaise, weakness, lethargy, anorexia, vomiting rather than abnormal LFT results. Blood dyscrasias may occur.

## NURSING CONSIDERATIONS

### BASELINE ASSESSMENT

**Anticonvulsant:** Review history of seizure disorder (intensity, frequency, duration, level of consciousness). Initiate safety measures, quiet dark environment. CBC should be performed before and 2 wks after therapy begins, then 2 wks following maintenance dose. Obtain baseline LFT. **Antimanic:** Assess behavior, appearance, emotional status, response to environment, speech pattern, thought content. **Antimigraine:** Question pt regarding onset, location, duration of migraine, possible precipitating symptoms.

### INTERVENTION/EVALUATION

Monitor CBC, LFT, serum ammonia. **Anticonvulsant:** Observe frequently for recurrence of seizure activity. Assess skin for ecchymoses, petechiae. Monitor for clinical improvement (decrease in intensity/frequency of seizures). **Antimanic:** Question for suicidal ideation. Assess for therapeutic response (interest in surroundings, increased ability to concentrate, relaxed facial expression). **Antimigraine:** Evaluate for relief of migraine headache and resulting photophobia, phonophobia, nausea, vomiting. **Therapeutic serum level:** 50–100 mcg/ml; **toxic serum level:** greater than 100 mcg/ml.

### PATIENT/ FAMILY TEACHING

• Do not abruptly discontinue medication after long-term use (may precipitate seizures). • Strict maintenance of drug therapy is essential for seizure control. • Avoid tasks that require alertness, motor skills until response to drug is

**V**

---

established. • Drowsiness usually disappears during continued therapy. • Avoid alcohol. • Carry identification card, bracelet that notes anticonvulsant therapy. • Report liver problems such as nausea, vomiting, lethargy, altered mental status, weakness, loss of appetite, abdominal pain, yellowing of skin, unusual bruising/bleeding. • Report if seizure control worsens, suicidal ideation (depression, unusual changes in behavior, suicidal thoughts) occurs.

# valsartan

val-**sar**-tan
(Apo-Valsartan ✹, Diovan)
■ **BLACK BOX ALERT** ■ May cause fetal injury, mortality. Discontinue as soon as possible once pregnancy is detected.
**Do not confuse Diovan with Zyban, or valsartan with losartan or Valstar.**

## FIXED-COMBINATION(S)

**Diovan HCT:** valsartan/hydrochlorothiazide (a diuretic): 80 mg/12.5 mg, 160 mg/12.5 mg, 160 mg/25 mg, 320 mg/12.5 mg, 320 mg/25 mg. **Byvalson:** valsartan/nebivolol (a beta blocker): 80 mg/5 mg. **Exforge:** valsartan/amlodipine (a calcium channel blocker): 160 mg/5 mg, 160 mg/10 mg, 320 mg/5 mg, 320 mg/10 mg. **Exforge HCT:** valsartan/amlodipine (a calcium channel blocker)/hydrochlorothiazide (a diuretic): 160 mg/5 mg/12.5 mg, 160 mg/5 mg/25 mg, 160 mg/10 mg/12.5 mg, 160 mg/10 mg/25 mg, 320 mg/10 mg/25 mg. **Valturna:** valsartan/aliskiren (a direct renin inhibitor): 160 mg/150 mg, 320 mg/300 mg.

## ◆CLASSIFICATION

**PHARMACOTHERAPEUTIC:** Angiotensin II receptor antagonist. **CLINICAL:** Antihypertensive.

## USES

Treatment of hypertension alone or in combination with other antihypertensives. Treatment of HF (NYHA Class II–IV). Reduce mortality in high-risk pts (left ventricular failure/dysfunction) following MI.

## PRECAUTIONS

**Contraindications:** Hypersensitivity to valsartan. Concomitant use with aliskiren in pts with diabetes. **Cautions:** Concurrent use of potassium-sparing diuretics or potassium supplements, mild to severe hepatic impairment, unstented bilateral/unilateral renal artery stenosis, renal impairment, significant aortic/mitral stenosis, elderly.

## ACTION

Directly antagonizes angiotensin II receptors. Blocks vasoconstrictor, aldosterone-secreting effects of angiotensin II, inhibiting binding of angiotensin II to $AT_1$ receptors. **Therapeutic Effect:** Produces vasodilation, decreases peripheral resistance, decreases B/P.

## PHARMACOKINETICS

Poorly absorbed after PO administration. Food decreases peak plasma concentration. Protein binding: 95%. Metabolized in liver. Eliminated in feces (83%), urine (13%). Unknown if removed by hemodialysis. **Half-life:** 6 hrs.

## ☒ LIFESPAN CONSIDERATIONS

**Pregnancy/Lactation:** May cause fetal harm. Unknown if distributed in breast milk. **Children:** Safety and efficacy not established. **Elderly:** No age-related precautions noted.

## INTERACTIONS

**DRUG:** NSAIDs may decrease antihypertensive effects. **Potassium-sparing drugs (e.g., spironolactone, triamterene), potassium supplements** may increase serum potassium. **Diuretics (e.g., furosemide, HCTZ)** may produce additive hypotensive effects. **HERBAL: Ginger, ginseng, licorice** may worsen

V

hypertension. **Black cohosh, periwinkle** may increase antihypertensive effects. **FOOD:** None known. **LAB VALUES:** May increase serum bilirubin, ALT, AST, BUN, creatinine, potassium. May decrease Hgb, Hct, WBC.

## AVAILABILITY (Rx)

**Tablets:** 40 mg, 80 mg, 160 mg, 320 mg.

## ADMINISTRATION/HANDLING

**PO**
• Give without regard to meals.

## INDICATIONS/ROUTES/DOSAGE

**Hypertension**
**PO: ADULTS, ELDERLY:** Initially, 80–160 mg/day in pts who are not volume depleted. **Maximum:** 320 mg/day. **CHILDREN 6–16 YRS:** Initially, 1.3 mg/kg once daily (**maximum:** 40 mg). May increase up to 2.7 mg/kg once daily (**maximum:** 160 mg/day).

**HF**
**PO: ADULTS, ELDERLY:** Initially, 20–40 mg twice daily. May increase up to 160 mg twice daily. **Maximum:** 320 mg/day.

**Post-MI, Left Ventricular Dysfunction**
**PO: ADULTS, ELDERLY:** May initiate 12 hrs or longer following MI. Initially, 20 mg twice daily. May increase within 7 days to 40 mg twice daily. May further increase up to target dose of 160 mg twice daily.

**Dosage in Renal Impairment**
**CrCl greater than 30 ml/min:** No dose adjustment. **CrCl 30 ml/min or less: ADULTS:** Safety/efficacy not established. **CHILDREN 6–16 YRS:** Not recommended.

**Dosage in Hepatic Impairment**
No dose adjustment.

## SIDE EFFECTS

**Rare (2%–1%):** Insomnia, fatigue, heartburn, abdominal pain, dizziness, headache, diarrhea, nausea, vomiting, arthralgia, edema.

## ADVERSE EFFECTS/ TOXIC REACTIONS

Overdosage may manifest as hypotension, tachycardia. Bradycardia occurs less often. Viral infection, upper respiratory tract infection (cough, pharyngitis, sinusitis, rhinitis) occur rarely.

## NURSING CONSIDERATIONS

### BASELINE ASSESSMENT

Obtain CBC, BMP, LFT. Obtain B/P, apical pulse immediately before each dose, in addition to regular monitoring (be alert to fluctuations). If excessive reduction in B/P occurs, place pt in supine position, feet slightly elevated. Question for possibility of pregnancy. Assess medication history (esp. diuretic). Question for history of hepatic/renal impairment, renal artery stenosis, history of severe HF.

### INTERVENTION/EVALUATION

Maintain hydration (offer fluids frequently). Assess for evidence of upper respiratory infection. Monitor serum electrolytes, renal function, LFT, Hgb, Hct, urinalysis, B/P, pulse. Observe for symptoms of hypotension.

### PATIENT/ FAMILY TEACHING

• Females of childbearing potential must use effective contraception during treatment. • Inform physician as soon as possible if pregnancy occurs. • Report any sign of infection (sore throat, fever). • Do not stop taking medication. • Report swelling of extremities, chest pain, palpitations; decreased urine output, amber-colored urine, fatigue, yellowing of the skin or eyes.

## vancomycin

van-koe-**mye**-sin
(Vancocin)
**Do not confuse vancomycin with clindamycin, gentamicin, tobramycin, or Vibramycin.**

**V**

---

## ◆CLASSIFICATION

**PHARMACOTHERAPEUTIC:** Tricyclic glycopeptide antibiotic. **CLINICAL:** Antibiotic.

## USES

**Systemic:** Treatment of infections caused by staphylococcal, streptococcal spp. bacteria. **PO:** Treatment of *C. difficile*–associated diarrhea and treatment of enterocolitis caused by *Staphylococcus aureus* (including MRSA). **OFF-LABEL:** Treatment of infections caused by gram-positive organisms in pts with serious allergies to beta-lactam antibiotics; treatment of beta-lactam–resistant gram-positive infections. Surgical prophylaxis, treatment of prosthetic joint infection.

## PRECAUTIONS

**Contraindications:** Hypersensitivity to vancomycin. **Cautions:** Renal impairment; concurrent therapy with other ototoxic, nephrotoxic medications, elderly, dehydration.

## ACTION

Binds to bacterial cell walls, altering cell membrane permeability, inhibiting RNA synthesis. **Therapeutic Effect:** Bactericidal.

## PHARMACOKINETICS

**PO:** Poorly absorbed from GI tract. Primarily eliminated in feces. **Parenteral:** Widely distributed (except CSF). Protein binding: 10%–50%. Primarily excreted unchanged in urine. Not removed by hemodialysis. **Half-life:** 4–11 hrs (increased in renal impairment).

## ⌛ LIFESPAN CONSIDERATIONS

**Pregnancy/Lactation:** Drug crosses placenta. Unknown if distributed in breast milk. **Children:** Close monitoring of serum levels recommended in premature neonates, young infants. **Elderly:** Age-related renal impairment may increase risk of ototoxicity, nephrotoxicity; dosage adjustment recommended.

## INTERACTIONS

**DRUG: Aminoglycosides (e.g., gentamicin, tobramycin), amphotericin B, cisplatin** may increase risk of ototoxicity, nephrotoxicity of parenteral vancomycin. **HERBAL:** None significant. **FOOD:** None known. **LAB VALUES:** May increase BUN. **Therapeutic peak serum level:** (Not routinely obtained) 20–40 mcg/ml; **therapeutic trough serum level:** 10–20 mcg/ml. **Toxic peak serum level:** greater than 40 mcg/ml; **toxic trough serum level:** greater than 20 mcg/ml.

## AVAILABILITY (Rx)

**Capsules (Vancocin):** 125 mg, 250 mg. **Infusion (Premix [Vancocin HCl]):** 500 mg/100 ml, 750 mg/150 ml, 1 g/200 ml. **Injection, Powder for Reconstitution (Vancocin HCl):** 500 mg, 750 mg, 1 g. **Solution, Oral:** 25 mg/ml, 50 mg/ml. **Suspension, Oral:** 50 mg/ml.

## ADMINISTRATION/HANDLING

 **IV**

**◀ALERT▶** Give by intermittent IV infusion (piggyback) or continuous IV infusion. Do not give IV push (may result in exaggerated hypotension or "red man" syndrome). **Reconstitution** • For intermittent IV infusion (piggyback), reconstitute each 500-mg vial with 10 ml Sterile Water for Injection (20 ml for 1-g vial) to provide concentration of 50 mg/ml. • Further dilute with D₅W or 0.9% NaCl to final concentration not to exceed 5 mg/ml. **Rate of Administration** • Administer over 60 min or longer (30 min for each 500 mg recommended). • Monitor B/P closely during IV infusion.
**Storage** • Reconstituted vials are stable for 14 days at room temperature or if refrigerated. • Diluted solutions are stable for 14 days if refrigerated or 7 days at room temperature. • Discard if precipitate forms.

**PO**
• May give with food. • Powder for injection may be reconstituted and diluted for oral administration.

---

## ▦ IV INCOMPATIBILITIES

Albumin, amphotericin B complex (Abelcet, AmBisome, Amphotec), aztreonam (Azactam), cefazolin (Ancef), cefotaxime (Claforan), cefoxitin (Mefoxin), ceftazidime (Fortaz), ceftriaxone (Rocephin), cefuroxime (Zinacef), foscarnet (Foscavir), heparin, nafcillin (Nafcil), piperacillin and tazobactam (Zosyn).

## ▦ IV COMPATIBILITIES

Amiodarone (Cordarone), calcium gluconate, dexmedetomidine (Precedex), diltiazem (Cardizem), hydromorphone (Dilaudid), insulin, lorazepam (Ativan), magnesium sulfate, midazolam (Versed), morphine, nicardipine (Cardene), potassium chloride, propofol (Diprivan).

## INDICATIONS/ROUTES/DOSAGE

**Usual Parenteral Dosage**
**IV: ADULTS, ELDERLY:** 10–30 mg/kg/dose q8–12h. Dosage requires adjustment in renal impairment. **CHILDREN OLDER THAN 1 MO:** 10–15 mg/kg/dose q6h. **Maximum:** 2,000 mg/dose. **NEONATES:** 15 mg/kg q24h up to 10–15 mg/kg/dose q6–24h.

**Staphylococcal Enterocolitis, Antibiotic-Associated Pseudomembranous Colitis Caused by *Clostridium difficile***
**PO: ADULTS, ELDERLY:** 125–500 mg 4 times/day for 7–10 days. **CHILDREN:** 40 mg/kg/day in 3–4 divided doses for 7–10 days. **Maximum:** 2 g/day.

**Dosage in Renal Impairment**
After loading dose, subsequent dosages and frequency are modified based on creatinine clearance, severity of infection, and serum concentration of drug.

**Dosage in Hepatic Impairment**
No dose adjustment.

## SIDE EFFECTS

**Frequent: PO:** Bitter/unpleasant taste, nausea, vomiting, mouth irritation (with oral solution). **Rare: Parenteral:** Phlebitis, thrombophlebitis, pain at peripheral IV site, dizziness, vertigo, tinnitus, chills, fever, rash, necrosis with extravasation. **PO:** Rash.

## ADVERSE EFFECTS/ TOXIC REACTIONS

Nephrotoxicity (acute kidney injury, acute tubular necrosis, renal failure), ototoxicity (temporary or permanent hearing loss) may occur. Too-rapid infusion may cause "Red man syndrome," a common adverse reaction characterized by pruritus, urticaria, erythema, angioedema, tachycardia, hypotension, myalgia, maculopapular rash (usually appears on face, neck, upper torso). Cardiovascular toxicity (cardiac depression, arrest) occurs rarely. Onset usually occurs within 30 min of start of infusion, resolves within hrs following infusion. May result from too-rapid rate of infusion.

## NURSING CONSIDERATIONS

### BASELINE ASSESSMENT

Avoid other ototoxic, nephrotoxic medications if possible. Obtain culture, sensitivity test before giving first dose (therapy may begin before results are known).

### INTERVENTION/EVALUATION

Monitor serum renal function tests, I&O. Assess skin for rash. Check hearing acuity, balance. Monitor B/P carefully during infusion. Evaluate IV site for phlebitis (heat, pain, red streaking over vein). Obtain vancomycin peak/trough level as ordered by physician or pharmacist. **Therapeutic serum level: peak:** 20–40 mcg/ml; **trough:** 10–20 mcg/ml. **Toxic serum level: peak:** greater than 40 mcg/ml; **trough:** greater than 20 mcg/ml.

### PATIENT/ FAMILY TEACHING

• Continue therapy for full length of treatment. • Doses should be evenly spaced. • Report ringing in ears, hearing loss, changes in urinary frequency or consistency. • Lab tests are important part of total therapy.

V

# vandetanib

van-**det**-a-nib
(Caprelsa)

■ **BLACK BOX ALERT** ■ Can prolong QT interval (torsades de pointes and sudden cardiac death reported). Do not use in pts with hypokalemia, hypocalcemia, hypomagnesemia, congenital long QT syndrome. Electrolyte imbalances must be corrected prior to initiating therapy. If medication that prolongs QT interval is needed, more frequent EKG monitoring is recommended. EKGs should be obtained during wks 2–4 and wks 8–12 after starting therapy and 3 mos thereafter. Any dose reduction or interruption related to QT prolongation greater than 2 wks must have frequent EKG monitoring as noted above. Only certified prescribers and pharmacies with a restricted distribution program are able to prescribe and dispense.

## ◆CLASSIFICATION

**PHARMACOTHERAPEUTIC:** Tyrosine kinase inhibitor. **CLINICAL:** Antineoplastic.

## USES

Treatment of symptomatic or progressive medullary thyroid cancer in pts with unresectable locally advanced or metastatic disease.

## PRECAUTIONS

**Contraindications:** Hypersensitivity to vandetanib. Congenital long QT syndrome. **Cautions:** Pregnancy, concurrent medications that prolong QT interval, hypokalemia, hypomagnesemia, hypothyroidism, cerebrovascular disease, moderate to severe renal/hepatic impairment, hypertension, uncompensated HF, history of torsades de pointes.

## ACTION

Inhibits tyrosine kinases including epidermal growth factor (EGF) and vascular endothelial growth factor (VEGF). Inhibits cell migration, proliferation, survival, and angiogenesis (new blood vessel formation). **Therapeutic Effect:** Inhibits thyroid tumor cell growth and metastasis.

## PHARMACOKINETICS

Slowly absorbed following PO administration. Peak concentration: 4–10 hrs. Metabolized in liver. Protein binding: 90%. Excreted in feces (44%), urine (25%). **Half-life:** 19 days.

## ⊠ LIFESPAN CONSIDERATIONS

**Pregnancy/Lactation:** May cause fetal harm. Avoid pregnancy. Must use effective contraception during treatment and for at least 4 mos after treatment. Unknown if distributed in breast milk. **Children:** Safety and efficacy not established. **Elderly:** No age-related precautions noted.

## INTERACTIONS

**DRUG:** Medications prolonging QT interval (e.g., **amiodarone, azithromycin, ciprofloxacin, clarithromycin, erythromycin, haloperidol**) may increase risk of QT prolongation. **CYP3A4 inducers** (e.g., **carbamazepine, oxcarbazepine, phenytoin, rifampin**) may decrease concentration/effects. **HERBAL:** **St. John's wort** may decrease concentration/effect. **FOOD:** **Grapefruit products** may increase risk of torsades de pointes, myelotoxicity. **LAB VALUES:** May decrease WBC, Hgb, neutrophils. May increase serum bilirubin, ALT, AST, creatinine; urine protein. May alter serum calcium, glucose, magnesium, potassium.

## AVAILABILITY (Rx)

**Tablets:** 100 mg, 300 mg.

## ADMINISTRATION/HANDLING

**PO**

• Give without regard to food. • Do not crush. • May disperse in 2 oz of noncarbonated water and stir for 10 min until tablet is evenly dispersed (will not completely dissolve). May administer dispersion immediately. Can be given via feeding tube. • Direct contact of crushed tablets with skin or mucous

V

membranes should be strictly avoided. If contact occurs, wash thoroughly.

**Storage** • Contact pharmacy to properly discard out-of-date tablets.

## INDICATIONS/ROUTES/DOSAGE

**Thyroid Cancer**
**PO: ADULTS, ELDERLY:** 300 mg once daily. Continue until disease progression or unacceptable toxicity.

**Dosage Adjustment for QT Prolongation or Toxicity**
Interrupt therapy until resolved or improved, then restart at 100–200 mg once daily.

**Dosage in Renal Impairment**
**CrCl less than 50 ml/min:** 200 mg once daily. Closely monitor QT interval.

**Dosage in Hepatic Impairment**
**Mild impairment:** No dose adjustment.
**Moderate to severe impairment:** Not recommended.

## SIDE EFFECTS

**Frequent (57%–21%):** Diarrhea/colitis, rash, dermatitis acneiform/acne, nausea, headache, fatigue, anorexia, abdominal pain. **Occasional (15%–10%):** Dry skin, vomiting, asthenia, photosensitivity, insomnia, nasopharyngitis, dyspepsia, cough, pruritus, weight decrease, depression.

## ADVERSE EFFECTS/
## TOXIC REACTIONS

Prolonged QT interval resulting in torsades de pointes, ventricular arrhythmias, sudden cardiac death have been reported. Frequent diarrhea may result in electrolyte imbalances. Severe skin reactions, including Stevens-Johnson syndrome, have been reported. Interstitial lung disease (ILD) or pneumonitis reported (may result in respiratory-related death). Consider ILD in pts with hypoxia, pleural effusion, cough, dyspnea. Ischemic cerebrovascular events have been reported. Life-threatening events including hypertensive crisis, reversible posterior leukoencephalopathy syndrome (RPLS) have

been noted. Adverse reactions resulting in death included respiratory failure/arrest, aspiration pneumonia, cardiac failure, sepsis, GI bleeding.

## NURSING CONSIDERATIONS

### BASELINE ASSESSMENT

Obtain CBC with differential, serum chemistries, magnesium, ionized calcium, TSH, UA, EKG, vital signs. Obtain negative urine pregnancy before therapy. Question for history of congenital long QT syndrome, HF, arrhythmias, hepatic/renal impairment, seizures, CVA, hemorrhagic events, HTN. Obtain full medication history including contraception. Perform full head-to-toe exam including visual acuity, thorough skin assessment.

### INTERVENTION/EVALUATION

Monitor blood levels including electrolytes esp. during episodes of diarrhea. Obtain EKG during wks 2–4, wks 8–12, then every 3 mos thereafter. Obtain EKG for palpitations, chest pain, hypokalemia, hyperkalemia, hypocalcemia, bradycardia, ventricular arrhythmias, syncope. Report any respiratory changes including dyspnea, cough (may indicate ILD). Reversible posterior leukoencephalopathy syndrome should be considered in pts with seizures, headache, visual disturbances, confusion, altered mental status. Ophthalmologic exams including slit lamp recommended in pts with visual disturbances.

### PATIENT/FAMILY TEACHING

• Blood levels, EKGs will be routinely monitored. • Strictly avoid pregnancy. Contraception should be taken during treatment and 4 mos after discontinuation. • Changes in mental status, seizures, headache, blurry vision, trouble speaking, one-sided weakness may indicate stroke, high blood pressure crisis, or life-threatening brain swelling. Immediately report any newly prescribed medications. • Do not take herbal products. • Limit exposure to sunlight. • Report any yellowing of skin or eyes, abdominal pain, bruising, black/tarry stools, dark urine, decreased urine output, skin changes. • Report palpitations, chest pain, shortness of breath, dizziness, fainting (may indicate arrhythmia).

# varenicline

var-**en**-i-kleen
(Champix ✦, Chantix)
■ **BLACK BOX ALERT** ■ Risk of psychiatric symptoms and suicidal behavior. Agitation, hostility, depressed mood have been reported.

## ◆CLASSIFICATION

**PHARMACOTHERAPEUTIC:** Selective partial nicotine agonist. **CLINICAL:** Smoking deterrent.

## USES

Aid to smoking cessation treatment.

## PRECAUTIONS

**Contraindications:** Hypersensitivity to varenicline. **Cautions:** Renal impairment, history of suicidal ideation or preexisting psychiatric illness, bipolar disorder, depression, schizophrenia. History of seizures or factors that lower seizure threshold.

## ACTION

Prevents nicotine stimulation of mesolimbic system associated with nicotine addiction. **Therapeutic Effect:** Decreases desire to smoke.

## PHARMACOKINETICS

Completely absorbed following PO administration. Absorption unaffected by food, time of day dosing. Maximum plasma concentration: 3–4 hrs. Steady state reached within 4 days. Protein binding: 20%. Minimal metabolism. Removed by hemodialysis. Primarily excreted unchanged in urine. **Half-life:** 24 hrs.

## ⧖ LIFESPAN CONSIDERATIONS

**Pregnancy/Lactation:** Unknown if distributed in breast milk. **Children:** Not recommended. **Elderly:** Age-related renal impairment may require dosage adjustment.

## INTERACTIONS

**DRUG: Cimetidine** may increase effect. **HERBAL:** None significant. **FOOD:** None known. **LAB VALUES:** None significant.

## AVAILABILITY

▧ Tablets (Film-Coated): 0.5 mg, 1 mg.

## ADMINISTRATION/HANDLING

• Give after meal and with full glass of water. • Do not break, crush, dissolve, or divide film-coated tablets.

## INDICATIONS/ROUTES/DOSAGE

◀ALERT▶ Therapy should start 1 wk before stopping smoking.

**Smoking Deterrent**
**PO: ADULTS, ELDERLY: Days 1–3:** 0.5 mg once daily. **Days 4–7:** 0.5 mg twice daily. **Day 8–end of treatment:** 1 mg twice daily. Therapy should last for total of 12 wks. Pts who have successfully stopped smoking at the end of 12 wks should continue with an additional 12 wks of treatment to increase likelihood of long-term abstinence.

**Dosage in Renal Impairment**
**CrCl less than 30 ml/min:** 0.5 mg once daily. **Maximum:** 0.5 mg twice daily.
**End-stage renal disease, undergoing hemodialysis: Maximum:** 0.5 mg once daily.

**Dosage in Hepatic Impairment**
No dose adjustment.

## SIDE EFFECTS

**Frequent (30%–13%):** Nausea, insomnia, headache, abnormal dreams. **Occasional (8%–5%):** Constipation, abdominal discomfort, fatigue, dry mouth, flatulence,

V

altered taste, dyspepsia, vomiting, anxiety, depression, irritability. **Rare (3%–1%):** Drowsiness, rash, increased appetite, lethargy, nightmares, gastroesophageal reflux disease, rhinorrhea, agitation, mood swings.

## ADVERSE EFFECTS/ TOXIC REACTIONS

Abrupt withdrawal may cause irritability, sleep disturbances in 3% of pts. Hypertension, angina pectoris, arrhythmia, bradycardia, coronary artery disease, gingivitis, anemia, lymphadenopathy occur rarely. May cause bizarre behavior, suicidal ideation.

## NURSING CONSIDERATIONS

### BASELINE ASSESSMENT

Screen, evaluate for coronary heart disease (history of MI, angina pectoris), cardiac arrhythmias, suicidal ideation.

### INTERVENTION/EVALUATION

Discontinue use if cardiovascular symptoms occur or worsen. Monitor for psychiatric symptoms (changes in behavior, mood, level of interest, appearance).

### PATIENT/FAMILY TEACHING

• Initiate treatment 1 wk before quit smoking date. • Take with food and with full glass of water. • With twice-daily dosing, take 1 tablet in morning, 1 in evening. • Report persistent nausea, insomnia. • Report change in behavior, mood, level of interest, appearance.

# vasopressin

vay-soe-**pres**-in
(Pressyn ✦, Pressyn AR ✦, Vasostrict)
**Do not confuse Pitressin with Pitocin.**

## ◆CLASSIFICATION

**PHARMACOTHERAPEUTIC:** Posterior pituitary hormone. **CLINICAL:** Vasopressor, antidiuretic.

## USES

Prevention/control of polydipsia, polyuria, dehydration in pts with neurogenic diabetes insipidus or differential diagnosis of diabetes insipidus. **Vasostrict:** To increase blood pressure in adults with vasodilatory shock who remain hypotensive despite fluids and catecholamines. **OFF-LABEL:** Adjunct in treatment of acute massive GI hemorrhage or esophageal varices.

## PRECAUTIONS

**Contraindications:** Hypersensitivity to vasopressin. **Cautions:** Seizures, migraine, asthma, vascular disease, renal/cardiac disease, goiter (with cardiac complications), arteriosclerosis, nephritis, elderly.

## ACTION

Increases reabsorption of water by renal tubules. Directly stimulates smooth muscle in GI tract. **Therapeutic Effect:** Causes peristalsis, vasoconstriction.

## PHARMACOKINETICS

| Route | Onset | Peak | Duration |
|---|---|---|---|
| IV | N/A | N/A | 0.5–1 hr |
| IM, SQ | 1–2 hrs | N/A | 2–8 hrs |

Distributed throughout extracellular fluid. Metabolized in liver, kidney. Primarily excreted in urine. **Half-life:** 10–20 min.

## ⧗ LIFESPAN CONSIDERATIONS

**Pregnancy/Lactation:** Caution in giving to breastfeeding women. **Children/ Elderly:** Caution due to risk of water intoxication/hyponatremia.

## INTERACTIONS

**DRUG:** Alcohol, demeclocycline, **lithium, norepinephrine** may decrease antidiuretic effect. **Carbamazepine, chlorpropamide, clofibrate** may increase antidiuretic effect. **HERBAL:** None significant. **FOOD:** None known. **LAB VALUES:** None significant.

**V**

---

## AVAILABILITY (Rx)

Injection Solution: 20 units/ml.

## ADMINISTRATION/HANDLING

 IV

**Reconstitution** • Dilute with D₅W or 0.9% NaCl to concentration of 0.1–1 unit/ml (usual concentration: 100 units/500 ml D₅W).
**Rate of Administration** • Give as IV infusion.
**Storage** • Store at room temperature.

**IM, SQ**
• Give with 1–2 glasses of water to reduce side effects.

## 🔃 IV INCOMPATIBILITIES

Furosemide (Lasix), phenytoin (Dilantin).

## 🔃 IV COMPATIBILITIES

Amiodarone, argatroban, diltiazem (Cardizem), dobutamine (Dobutrex), dopamine (Intropin), heparin, insulin, milrinone (Primacor), nitroglycerin, norepinephrine (Levophed), pantoprazole (Protonix), phenylephrine.

## INDICATIONS/ROUTES/ DOSAGE

**Diabetes Insipidus**
◀ALERT▶ May be administered intranasally by nasal spray or on cotton pledgets; dosage is individualized.
**IV Infusion: ADULTS, CHILDREN:** 0.5 milliunits/kg/hr. May double dose q30min. **Maximum:** 10 milliunits/kg/hr.
**IM, SQ: ADULTS, ELDERLY:** 5–10 units 2–4 times/day. **CHILDREN:** 2.5–10 units, 2–4 times/day.

**GI Hemorrhage**
**IV Infusion: ADULTS, ELDERLY:** Initially, 0.2–0.4 unit/min progressively increased to 0.8 unit/min. **CHILDREN:** 0.001–0.01 unit/kg/min. Titrate as needed. **Maximum:** 0.01 unit/kg/min.

**Vasodilatory Shock**
**IV Infusion: ADULTS, ELDERLY:** Initially, 0.01 units/min. Titrate by 0.005 units/min at 10–15 min intervals. **Maximum:** 0.07 units/min.

**Dosage in Renal/Hepatic Impairment**
No dose adjustment.

## SIDE EFFECTS

**Frequent:** Pain at injection site (with vasopressin tannate). **Occasional:** Abdominal cramps, nausea, vomiting, diarrhea, dizziness, diaphoresis, pale skin, circumoral pallor, tremors, headache, eructation, flatulence. **Rare:** Chest pain, confusion, allergic reaction (rash, urticaria, pruritus, wheezing, difficulty breathing, facial/peripheral edema), sterile abscess (with vasopressin tannate).

## ADVERSE EFFECTS/ TOXIC REACTIONS

Anaphylaxis, MI, water intoxication have occurred. Elderly, very young are at higher risk for water intoxication.

## NURSING CONSIDERATIONS

**BASELINE ASSESSMENT**
Establish baselines for weight, B/P, pulse, serum electrolytes, Hgb, Hct, urine specific gravity.

**INTERVENTION/EVALUATION**
Monitor I&O closely, restrict intake as necessary to prevent water intoxication. Weigh daily if indicated. Check B/P, pulse frequently. Monitor serum electrolytes, Hgb, Hct, urine specific gravity. Evaluate injection site for erythema, pain, abscess. Report side effects to physician for dose reduction. Be alert for early signs of water intoxication (drowsiness, listlessness, headache, seizures). Observe for evidence of GI bleeding. Withhold medication, report immediately any chest pain, allergic symptoms.

V

## PATIENT/FAMILY TEACHING

• Promptly report headache, chest pain, shortness of breath, other symptoms. • Stress importance of I&O. • Avoid alcohol. • Report confusion, seizure activity.

# vedolizumab

ve-doe-**liz**-ue-mab
(Entyvio)
**Do not confuse vedolizumab with certolizumab, eculizumab, natalizumab, omalizumab, tocilizumab.**

## ◆CLASSIFICATION

**PHARMACOTHERAPEUTIC:** Integrin receptor antagonist. **CLINICAL:** Monoclonal antibody.

## USES

Treatment of adults pts with moderately to severely active ulcerative colitis (UC) who have had an inadequate response with, lost response to, or were intolerant to a tumor necrosis factor (TNF) blocker or immunomodulator; or had an inadequate response with, were intolerant to, or demonstrated dependence on corticosteroids: inducing and maintaining clinical response and clinical remission; improving endoscopic appearance of the mucosa; achieving corticosteroid-free remission. Treatment of adults pts with moderately to severely active Crohn's disease (CD) who have had an inadequate response with, lost response to, or were intolerant to a TNF blocker or immunomodulator; or had an inadequate response with, were intolerant to, or demonstrated dependence on corticosteroids: achieving clinical response and clinical remission; achieving corticosteroid-free remission.

## PRECAUTIONS

**Contraindications:** Hypersensitivity to vedolizumab. **Cautions:** Hepatic impairment, immunocompromised pts, live vaccine administration. Pts with history of severe infections (not recommended during active infection), conditions predisposing to infections (e.g., diabetes, renal failure, open wounds, indwelling catheters). Preexisting or recent-onset CNS demyelinating disorders including multiple sclerosis.

## ACTION

Binds to T-lymphocyte integrin receptors and blocks the interaction with mucosal addressin cell adhesion molecule-1 (MAdCAM-1). Inhibits migration and homing of memory T-lymphocytes into inflamed GI tissue. **Therapeutic Effect:** Reduces chronic inflammation of colon.

## PHARMACOKINETICS

Metabolism not specified. Elimination not specified. **Half-life:** 25 days.

## ⧗ LIFESPAN CONSIDERATIONS

**Pregnancy/Lactation:** Unknown if distributed in breast milk. Use caution when administering to nursing women. **Children:** Safety and efficacy not established. **Elderly:** No age-related precautions noted.

## INTERACTIONS

**DRUG:** **Natalizumab** may increase risk of progressive multifocal leukoencephalopathy (PML). **Other TNF blockers (e.g., infliximab)** may increase risk of infection. **HERBAL:** None significant. **FOOD:** None known. **LAB VALUES:** May increase serum ALT, AST, bilirubin.

## AVAILABILITY (Rx)

**Lyophilized Powder for Injection:** 300 mg.

## ADMINISTRATION/HANDLING
💉 IV

• Do not administer IV push or bolus. • Reconstitute with Sterile Water for injection and subsequently dilute with 0.9% NaCl only. • After infusion completed, flush IV line with 30 ml of 0.9% NaCl.

**V**

---

**Reconstitution** • Remove flip cap and swab with alcohol. • Reconstitute vial with 4.8 ml Sterile Water for Injection. Direct stream toward glass wall to avoid excessive foaming. • Gently swirl contents for at least 15 sec until completely dissolved. • Do not shake or invert vial. • Allow solution to sit at room temperature for up to 20 min to allow remaining foam to settle and powder to dissolve. If not fully dissolved after 20 min, allow additional 10 min for dissolution. Do not use if product not dissolved within 30 min. • Visually inspect for particulate matter and discoloration. Do not use discolored or particle matter observed. • Prior to withdrawing solution, invert vial 3 times to ensure mixing. • Withdraw 5 ml and further dilute in 250 ml 0.9% NaCl bag. • Infuse immediately.
**Rate of Administration** • Infuse over 30 min.
**Storage** • Reconstituted solution should appear clear to opalescent, colorless to light brownish yellow and free of particles. • May refrigerate diluted solution for up to 4 hrs.

## INDICATIONS/ROUTES/DOSAGE

**Ulcerative Colitis and Crohn's Disease**
**IV: ADULTS, ELDERLY:** 300 mg once at wk 0, wk 2, and wk 6, then every 8 wks thereafter. Discontinue in pts who do not show evidence of therapeutic benefit by wk 14.

**Dosage in Renal Impairment**
Use caution.

**Dosage in Hepatic Impairment**
Use caution. Discontinue for jaundice or signs/symptoms of hepatic injury.

## SIDE EFFECTS

**Occasional (13%–4%):** Nasopharyngitis, headache, arthralgia, nausea, pyrexia, upper respiratory tract infection, fatigue, cough, bronchitis, influenza, back pain.
**Rare (3%):** Rash, pruritus, sinusitis, oropharyngeal pain, extremity pain.

## ADVERSE EFFECTS/ TOXIC REACTIONS

Infusion-related reactions, including anaphylaxis, characterized by bronchospasm, dyspnea, flushing, hypotension, laryngeal edema, nausea, pyrexia, tachycardia, wheezing, vomiting, reported in less than 1% of pts. May increase risk of severe infections such as anal abscess, cytomegaloviral colitis, giardiasis, *Listeria* meningitis, *Salmonella* sepsis, TB, UTI, which may lead to fatal sepsis. PML (weakness, paralysis, vision loss, aphasia, cognition impairment) has occurred rarely; however, immunocompromised pts are at increased risk for development. Drug-induced hepatotoxicity with ALT, AST greater than 3 times upper limit of normal reported in less than 2% of pts. Malignancies including B-cell lymphoma, breast cancer, colon cancer, lung cancer of primary neuroendocrine carcinoma, lung neoplasm, malignant hepatic neoplasm, melanoma, renal cancer, squamous cell carcinoma, transitional cell carcinoma occur rarely. Immunogenicity (antivedolizumab antibodies) occurred in 4%–13% of pts.

## NURSING CONSIDERATIONS

### BASELINE ASSESSMENT

Obtain CBC, LFT. Prior to initiating treatment, all pts should be up to date with all immunizations according to proper guidelines. Continuously screen for active infection. Evaluate for active TB and test for latent infection prior to and during treatment. Induration of 5 mm or greater with tuberculin skin test should be considered a positive result when assessing for latent TB. Antifungal therapy should be considered for those who reside in or travel to regions where mycoses are endemic. Have supplemental oxygen, anaphylaxis kit readily available. Conduct full neurologic exam. Question history of malignancies.

### INTERVENTION/EVALUATION

Routinely monitor LFT. Withhold treatment if acute infection, opportunistic infection, sepsis occurs and initiate appropriate antimicrobial therapy. Monitor for hypersensitivity reaction. Infusion-related reactions generally occur within 2 hrs after infusion. Consider administration of antihistamine, antipyretic, and/or if corticosteroid if mild to moderate hypersensitivity reaction occurs. If anaphylaxis occurs, provide immediate resuscitation support. Monitor for new onset or worsening of neurologic symptoms, esp. in pts with CNS disorders; may indicate PML.

### PATIENT/FAMILY TEACHING

• Blood levels, TB screening will be routinely monitored. • Therapy may lower immune system response. Report travel plans to possible endemic areas. • Do not receive live vaccines unless approved by your doctor. • Report history of fungal infections, multiple sclerosis, TB or close relatives who have active TB. • Infusion may cause severe allergic reactions such as face/tongue swelling, hives, itching, low blood pressure, trouble breathing, or, in some cases, anaphylaxis. • Do not breastfeed. • Abdominal pain, bruising, clay-colored stools, dark-amber urine, fatigue, loss of appetite, yellowing of skin or eyes may indicate liver problem. • Paralysis, vision changes, impaired speech, altered mental status may indicate life-threatening neurologic event called progressive multifocal leukoencephalopathy (PML).

## vemurafenib

vem-ue-**raf**-e-nib
(Zelboraf)

### ◆CLASSIFICATION

**PHARMACOTHERAPEUTIC:** BRAF kinase inhibitor. **CLINICAL:** Antineoplastic.

## USES

Treatment of unresectable or metastatic melanoma with a BRAF V600E mutation as detected by FDA-approved test.

## PRECAUTIONS

**Contraindications:** Hypersensitivity to vemurafenib. **Cautions:** Avoid sun exposure. Prolonged QT syndrome, concurrent use of medications that prolong QT interval, hepatic impairment, uncorrected electrolyte imbalance (hypokalemia, hypomagnesemia), elderly.

## ACTION

Inhibits kinase activity of certain mutated forms of BRAF. **Therapeutic Effect:** Blocks tumor cell proliferation in melanoma with the mutation.

## PHARMACOKINETICS

Readily absorbed after PO administration. Protein binding: 99%. Minimally metabolized in liver. Primarily excreted in feces (94%). **Half-life:** 57 hrs. Range: 30–120 hrs.

## ⧗ LIFESPAN CONSIDERATIONS

**Pregnancy/Lactation:** Avoid pregnancy. May cause fetal harm. Must use effective contraception during treatment and for at least 2 mos after discontinuation. Unknown if distributed in breast milk. Must either discontinue breastfeeding or discontinue therapy. **Children:** Safety and efficacy not established. **Elderly:** May have increased risk of adverse reactions, side effects.

## INTERACTIONS

**DRUG:** Antiarrhythmics (e.g., amiodarone, procainamide, quinidine, sotalol), azithromycin, barbiturates, ciprofloxacin, dexamethasone, fluconazole, haloperidol, phenothiazines, phenytoins, trazodone, tricyclic antidepressants, vardenafil, voriconazole may prolong QT interval. CYP3A4 inhibitors (e.g., atazanavir, clarithromycin, ketoconazole, phenobarbital, rifampin) may alter concentration. May increase bleeding effect with **warfarin**. **HERBAL:** None significant. **FOOD:** None known. **LAB VALUES:** May increase serum alkaline phosphatase, ALT, AST, gamma-glutamyl transferase (GGT), bilirubin.

## AVAILABILITY (Rx)

**Film-Coated Tablets:** 240 mg.

## ADMINISTRATION/HANDLING

**PO**
• Give in morning and evening approximately 12 hrs apart. • Give without regard to food. • Do not break, crush, dissolve, or divide tablets; swallow whole. • Give with full glass of water.

## INDICATIONS/ROUTES/DOSAGE

**Note:** Management of adverse drug reactions may require dose reduction, treatment interruption, or discontinuation.

**Melanoma**
**PO: ADULTS, ELDERLY:** 960 mg twice daily (in morning and evening about 12 hrs apart). Continue until disease progression or unacceptable toxicity.

**Dosage Modification**
Based on Common Terminology Criteria for Adverse Events (CTCAE). **Grade 1 or grade 2 (tolerable):** No dose adjustment. **Grade 2 (intolerable) or grade 3:** *First incident:* Interrupt treatment until toxicity returns to grade 0 or 1, then resume at 720 mg twice daily. *Second incident:* Interrupt treatment, then resume at 480 mg twice daily. *Third incident:* Discontinue. **Grade 4:** *First incident:* Interrupt treatment, then resume at 480 mg twice daily. *Second incident:* Discontinue.

**Dosage in Renal/Hepatic Impairment**
**Mild to moderate impairment:** No dose adjustment.
**Severe impairment:** Use with caution.

## SIDE EFFECTS

**Frequent (53%–33%):** Arthralgia, alopecia, fatigue, rash, nausea. **Occasional (28%–11%):** Diarrhea, hyperkeratosis, headache, pruritus, pyrexia, dry skin, extremity pain, anorexia, vomiting, peripheral edema, erythema, dysgeusia, myalgia, constipation, asthenia. **Rare (8%–5%):** Maculopapular rash, actinic keratosis, musculoskeletal pain, back pain, cough, papular rash.

## ADVERSE EFFECTS/ TOXIC REACTIONS

Cutaneous squamous cell carcinoma (cuSCC) and keratoacanthomas reported in 24% of pts. Pts at increased risk of cuSCC include elderly, pts with prior skin cancer, chronic sun exposure. Hypersensitivity reactions including erythema, hypotension, anaphylaxis reported. Mild to severe photosensitivity were reported. Serious dermatologic reactions include Stevens-Johnson syndrome, epidermal necrolysis. Ophthalmologic reactions including uveitis reported. Increased LFT may lead to discontinuation.

## NURSING CONSIDERATIONS

### BASELINE ASSESSMENT
Obtain serum chemistries, renal function test, magnesium, ionized calcium, EKG, PT/INR if taking warfarin. Assess skin for moles, lesions, papilloma and perform full dermatologic exam. Obtain baseline ophthalmologic exam, visual acuity. Assess medication history for QT-prolonging drugs. Obtain negative urine pregnancy before initiating treatment.

### INTERVENTION/EVALUATION
Monitor EKG 15 days after initiation, then monthly for first 3 mos, then every 3 mos thereafter. Routinely assess skin and for 6 mos after discontinuation. Immediately report any new skin lesions. Obtain EKG for palpitations, chest pain, hypokalemia, hyperkalemia, hypocalcemia, bradycardia, ventricular arrhythmias, syncope. Monitor PT/INR while pt is on warfarin. Pruritus, difficulty breathing, erythema, hypotension may indicate anaphylaxis.

### PATIENT/FAMILY TEACHING
• Blood levels, EKG, eye examinations are routinely ordered. • Strictly avoid pregnancy. Contraception should be used during treatment and 2 mos after discontinuation. • Avoid sunlight exposure.

• Report any skin changes including new warts, sores, reddish bumps that bleed or do not heal, change in mole size or color. • Report any yellowing of skin or eyes, abdominal pain, bruising, black/tarry stools, dark urine, decreased urine output, skin changes. • Report palpitations, chest pain, shortness of breath, dizziness, fainting (may indicate arrhythmia).

# venetoclax

ven-**et**-oh-klax
(Venclexta)
**Do not confuse venetoclax or Venclexta with Venelex.**

## ◆CLASSIFICATION

**PHARMACOTHERAPEUTIC:** B-cell lymphoma-2 inhibitor. Antiapoptotic protein. **CLINICAL:** Antineoplastic.

## USES

Treatment of pts with chronic lymphocytic leukemia (CLL) with 17p deletion, as detected by an FDA-approved test, who have received at least one prior therapy.

## PRECAUTIONS

**Contraindications:** Hypersensitivity to venetoclax. Concomitant use of strong CYP3A inhibitors at initiation and during ramp-up phase. **Cautions:** Baseline anemia, leukopenia, neutropenia, thrombocytopenia; concomitant use of moderate CYP3A inhibitors, P-gp inhibitors; active infection or pts at increased risk of infection (diabetes, kidney failure, indwelling catheters, open wounds), hepatic/renal impairment, electrolyte imbalance; history of gout; pts at high risk for tumor lysis syndrome (high tumor burden).

## ACTION

Binds to and inhibits B-cell lymphoma-2 protein and displaces proapoptotic proteins, restoring process of apoptosis. **Therapeutic Effect:** Inhibits tumor cell growth and metastasis.

## PHARMACOKINETICS

Widely distributed. Metabolized in liver. Protein binding: highly bound (unspecified). Peak plasma concentration: 5–8 hrs. Eliminated in feces (greater than 99%). **Half-life:** 26 hrs.

## ⧗ LIFESPAN CONSIDERATIONS

**Pregnancy/Lactation:** Avoid pregnancy; may cause fetal harm/malformations. Female and male pts of reproductive potential should use effective contraception during treatment and for at least 30 days after discontinuation. Unknown if distributed in breast milk. Breastfeeding not recommended. May impair fertility in males. **Children:** Safety and efficacy not established. **Elderly:** No age-related precautions noted.

## INTERACTIONS

**DRUG: Strong CYP3A inhibitors (e.g., clarithromycin, ketoconazole, ritonavir)** may significantly increase concentration/effect; use contraindicated. **Moderate CYP3A inhibitors (e.g., erythromycin, ciprofloxacin, diltiazem, dronedarone, fluconazole, verapamil), P-gp inhibitors (e.g., amiodarone, azithromycin, captopril, carvedilol, cyclosporine, felodipine, ranolazine, ticagrelor)** may increase concentration/effect; consider alternative therapy. **Strong CYP3A inducers (e.g., carbamazepine, phenytoin, rifampin)** may decrease concentration/effect. **HERBAL: St. John's wort** may decrease concentration/effect. **FOOD: Grapefruit products, Seville oranges, starfruit** may increase concentration/effect. Low-fat meals, high-fat meals increase exposure/concentration. **LAB VALUES:** May decrease Hgb, Hct, neutrophils, platelets, RBCs; serum calcium, potassium. Tumor lysis syndrome may result in elevated serum phosphate, potassium, uric acid.

## AVAILABILITY (Rx)

**Tablets:** 10 mg, 50 mg, 100 mg.

## ADMINISTRATION/HANDLING

### PO
• Give with food and water at same time each day. • Administer tablets whole; do not cut, crush, or divide. • If a dose is missed by no more than 8 hrs, administer as soon as possible. If dose is missed by more than 8 hrs or if vomiting occurs after dosing, skip dose and administer the next dose on schedule.

## INDICATIONS/ROUTES/DOSAGE

### CLL
**PO: ADULTS, ELDERLY: Week 1:** 20 mg once daily for 7 days. **Week 2:** 50 mg once daily for 7 days. **Week 3:** 100 mg once daily for 7 days. **Week 4:** 200 mg once daily for 7 days. **Week 5 and beyond:** 400 mg once daily. Continue until disease progression or unacceptable toxicity.

### Dose Modification
Based on Common Terminology Criteria for Adverse Events (CTCAE). For pts with dose interruption greater than 1 wk during 5-wk ramp-up phase or greater than 2 wks at 400 mg daily dose, reassess risk of tumor lysis syndrome to determine if reinitiation with a reduced dose is needed. Consider discontinuation in pts who require reduced dosage of less than 100 mg for more than 2 wks.

### Dose Reduction Schedule
**Note:** During ramp-up phase, continue reduced dose for 1 wk before increasing dose.
**Dose interruption at 400 mg:** Resume at 300 mg.
**Dose interruption at 300 mg:** Resume at 200 mg.
**Dose interruption at 200 mg:** Resume at 100 mg.
**Dose interruption at 100 mg:** Resume at 50 mg.
**Dose interruption at 50 mg:** Resume at 20 mg.
**Dose interruption at 20 mg:** Resume at 10 mg.

### Tumor Lysis Syndrome
**Any occurrence of blood chemistry abnormalities:** Withhold next dose, then resume at same dose if resolved within 24–48 hrs of last dose. If not resolved within 48 hrs, resume at reduced dose.
**Any event of tumor lysis syndrome:** Resume at reduced dose once resolved.

### Grade 3 or 4 Nonhematologic Toxicity
**First occurrence:** Withhold treatment until resolved to grade 1 or baseline, then resume at same dose.
**Second and subsequent occurrences:** Withhold treatment until resolved, then follow dose reduction schedule (or reduce dose at prescriber's discretion).

### Hematologic Toxicity
**First occurrence of grade 3 or 4 neutropenia with infection or fever; grade 4 hematologic toxicity (except lymphopenia):** Withhold treatment until resolved to grade 1 or baseline, then resume at same dose.
**Second and subsequent occurrences:** Withhold treatment until resolved, then follow dose reduction schedule (or reduce dose at prescriber's discretion).

### Concomitant Use CYP3A Inhibitors, P-gp Inhibitors
**Strong CYP3A inhibitors:** Avoid inhibitor or reduce venetoclax dose by at least 75%.
**Moderate CYP3A inhibitors or P-gp inhibitors:** Avoid inhibitor or reduce venetoclax dose by at least 50%.

### Dosage in Renal/Hepatic Impairment
**Mild to moderate impairment:** No dose adjustment.
**Severe impairment:** Not specified; use caution.

## SIDE EFFECTS

**Frequent (35%–14%):** Diarrhea, nausea, fatigue, pyrexia, vomiting, headache, constipation. **Occasional (13%–10%):** Cough, peripheral edema, back pain.

---

## ADVERSE EFFECTS/TOXIC REACTIONS

Anemia, neutropenia, thrombocytopenia is an expected response to therapy. Grade 3 or 4 neutropenia reported in 41% of pts. Pts with high tumor burden, renal impairment; concomitant use of strong or moderate CYP3A inhibitors, P-gp inhibitors may experience life-threatening tumor lysis syndrome, which mainly occurs during the 5-wk ramp-up phase and as early as 6–8 hrs after dose (hospitalization may be necessary). Tumor lysis syndrome may cause renal failure requiring emergent dialysis. Other reactions may include upper respiratory tract infection, pneumonia, autoimmune hemolytic anemia.

## NURSING CONSIDERATIONS

### BASELINE ASSESSMENT

Obtain ANC, CBC, BMP, renal function test; serum phosphate, calcium; vital signs prior to initiation and periodically thereafter. Obtain pregnancy test in female pts of reproductive potential. Question history of hepatic/renal impairment, gout. Assess all pts for high risk of tumor lysis syndrome and provide adequate hydration and antihyperuricemics (according to manufacturer guidelines) prior to first dose. Conduct tumor burden assessments including blood chemistries, radiologic testing (e.g., CT scan). Replete electrolytes prior to initiation. Receive full medication history (esp. CYP3A inhibitors, P-gp inhibitors, drugs with narrow therapeutic index). Screen for active infection. Offer emotional support.

### INTERVENTION/EVALUATION

Monitor ANC, CBC for anemia, leukopenia, neutropenia, thrombocytopenia. Diligently monitor for tumor lysis syndrome (acute renal failure, electrolyte imbalance, cardiac arrhythmias, seizures). Monitor for infection and provide appropriate antimicrobial therapy if indicated. To reduce risk of neutropenia-associated infection, consider administration of granulocyte-colony stimulating factor (e.g., filgrastim). Monitor for toxicities if discontinuation of CYP3A inhibitors, P-gp inhibitors is unavoidable. Monitor I&Os. Assess hydration status.

### PATIENT/FAMILY TEACHING

• Treatment may depress your immune system and reduce your ability to fight infection. Report symptoms of infection such as body aches, chills, cough, fatigue, fever. Avoid those with active infection. • Therapy may cause tumor lysis syndrome (a condition caused by the rapid breakdown of cancer cells), which can cause kidney failure and may lead to death. Report decreased urination, amber-colored urine; confusion, difficulty breathing, fatigue, fever, muscle or joint pain, palpitations, seizures, vomiting. • Drink at least 6–8 glasses of water every day. • Avoid pregnancy. Female and male pts of childbearing potential should use effective contraception during treatment and for at least 2 mos after last dose. Do not breastfeed. • Treatment may impair fertility. • Avoid grapefruit products, Seville oranges, starfruit, herbal supplements. • Do not take newly prescribed medications unless approved by prescriber who originally started therapy. • Do not receive live vaccines.

# venlafaxine

ven-la-**fax**-een
(Apo-Venlafaxine XR* Effexor XR)

■ **BLACK BOX ALERT** ■ Increased risk of suicidal ideation and behavior in children, adolescents, young adults 18–24 yrs with major depressive disorder, other psychiatric disorders.

## ◆CLASSIFICATION

**PHARMACOTHERAPEUTIC:** Phenethylamine derivative. **CLINICAL:** Antidepressant.

---

## USES

Treatment of depression. Treatment of generalized anxiety disorder (GAD), social anxiety disorder (SAD). Treatment of panic disorder, with or without agoraphobia. **OFF-LABEL:** Treatment of attention-deficit hyperactivity disorder (ADHD), obsessive-compulsive disorder (OCD), hot flashes, diabetic neuropathy, post-traumatic stress disorder (PTSD).

## PRECAUTIONS

**Contraindications:** Hypersensitivity to venlafaxine. Use of MAOIs intended to treat psychiatric disorders concurrently or within 14 days of discontinuing MAOI. Initiation of MAOI to treat psychiatric disorder within 7 days of discontinuing venlafaxine, initiation in pts receiving linezolid or methylene blue. **Cautions:** Seizure disorder, renal/hepatic impairment, pts at high risk for suicide, recent MI, mania, volume-depleted pts, narrow-angle glaucoma, HF, hyperthyroidism, abnormal platelet function. Pts with increased intraocular pressure, elderly.

## ACTION

Potentiates CNS neurotransmitter activity by inhibiting reuptake of serotonin, norepinephrine, and, to lesser degree, dopamine. **Therapeutic Effect:** Relieves depression.

## PHARMACOKINETICS

Well absorbed from GI tract. Protein binding: 25%–30%. Metabolized in liver. Primarily excreted in urine. Not removed by hemodialysis. **Half-life:** 3–7 hrs; metabolite, 9–13 hrs (increased in hepatic/renal impairment).

## ⧗ LIFESPAN CONSIDERATIONS

**Pregnancy/Lactation:** Unknown if distributed in breast milk. **Children:** Children, adolescents are at increased risk for suicidal ideation and behavior, worsening depression, esp. during first few mos of therapy. **Elderly:** No age-related precautions noted.

## INTERACTIONS

**DRUG:** CYP3A4 inhibitors (e.g., **clarithromycin, ketoconazole**) may increase concentration/effects. **MAOIs** may cause neuroleptic malignant syndrome, autonomic instability (including rapid fluctuations of vital signs), extreme agitation, hyperthermia, altered mental status, myoclonus, rigidity, coma. **Triptans (e.g., almotriptan, sumatriptan), selegiline, SSRIs, trazodone, tricyclic antidepressants (e.g., amitripyline, doxepin)** may increase risk of serotonin syndrome. May increase risk of bleeding with **NSAIDs, aspirin, warfarin. HERBAL: Gotu kola, kava kava, St. John's wort, valerian** may increase CNS depression. **St. John's wort** may increase risk of serotonin syndrome. **FOOD: Grapefruit products** may increase concentration/effect. **LAB VALUES:** May increase serum cholesterol CPK, LDH, prolactin, GGT.

## AVAILABILITY (Rx)

**Tablets:** 25 mg, 37.5 mg, 50 mg, 75 mg, 100 mg.

🐾 **Capsules (Extended-Release [Effexor XR]):** 37.5 mg, 75 mg, 150 mg. 🐾 **Tablets (Extended-Release):** 37.5 mg, 75 mg, 150 mg, 225 mg.

## ADMINISTRATION/HANDLING

**PO**
• Give with food. • Scored tablet may be crushed. • Do not break, crush, dissolve, or divide extended-release tablets. • May open capsule, sprinkle on applesauce. Give immediately without chewing and follow with full glass of water.

## INDICATIONS/ROUTES/DOSAGE

**Depression**
**PO:** *(Immediate-Release):* **ADULTS, ELDERLY:** Initially, 37.5–75 mg/day in 2–3 divided doses. May increase up to 75 mg/day at intervals of 4 days or longer. Usual dose: 75–225 mg/day. **Maximum:** 375 mg/day in 3 divided doses.
**PO:** *(Extended-Release):* **ADULTS, ELDERLY:** Initially, 37.5–75 mg/day as

single dose with food. May increase by 75 mg/day at intervals of 4 days or longer. Usual dose: 75–225 mg once daily. **Maximum:** 225 mg/day.

### Generalized Anxiety Disorder (GAD)
**PO:** *(Extended-Release):* **ADULTS, ELDERLY:** Initially, 37.5–75 mg/day. May increase by 75 mg/day at 4-day intervals up to 225 mg/day.

### Panic Disorder
**PO:** *(Extended-Release):* Initially, 37.5 mg/day. May increase to 75 mg after 7 days followed by increases of 75 mg/day at 7-day intervals up to 225 mg/day.

### Social Anxiety Disorder (SAD)
**PO:** *(Extended-Release):* **ADULTS, ELDERLY:** 75 mg once daily.

### Dosage in Renal/Hepatic Impairment
Consider decreasing venlafaxine dosage by 50% in pts with moderate hepatic impairment, 25% in pts with mild to moderate renal impairment, 50% in pts on dialysis (withhold dose until completion of dialysis). When discontinuing therapy, taper dosage slowly over 2 wks.

## SIDE EFFECTS

**Frequent (greater than 20%):** Nausea, drowsiness, headache, dry mouth. **Occasional (20%–10%):** Dizziness, insomnia, constipation, diaphoresis, nervousness, asthenia, ejaculatory disturbance, anorexia. **Rare (less than 10%):** Anxiety, blurred vision, diarrhea, vomiting, tremor, abnormal dreams, impotence.

## ADVERSE EFFECTS/ TOXIC REACTIONS

Sustained increase in diastolic B/P of 10–15 mm Hg occurs occasionally. Serotonin syndrome (agitation, confusion, hallucinations, hyperreflexia), neuroleptic malignant syndrome (muscular rigidity, fever, cognitive changes), suicidal ideation have occurred.

## NURSING CONSIDERATIONS

### BASELINE ASSESSMENT
Obtain initial weight, B/P. Assess appearance, behavior, speech pattern, level of interest, mood. Assess risk of suicide.

### INTERVENTION/EVALUATION
Monitor signs/symptoms of depression, B/P, weight. Assess sleep pattern for evidence of insomnia. Check during waking hours for drowsiness, dizziness, anxiety; provide assistance as necessary. Assess appearance, behavior, speech pattern, level of interest, mood for therapeutic response. Monitor for suicidal ideation (esp. at initiation of therapy or changes in dosage).

### PATIENT/ FAMILY TEACHING
• Take with food to minimize GI distress. • Do not increase, decrease, suddenly stop medication. • Avoid tasks that require alertness, motor skills until response to drug is established. • Report if breastfeeding, pregnant, or planning to become pregnant. • Avoid alcohol. • Report worsening depression, suicidal ideation, unusual changes in behavior.

# verapamil

ver-**ap**-a-mil
(Apo-Verap ✦, Calan, Calan SR, Isoptin SR, Novo-Veramil SR ✦, Verelan, Verelan PM)
**Do not confuse Calan with Covera-HS or Verelan with Voltaren.**

## FIXED-COMBINATION(S)

**Tarka:** verapamil/trandolapril (an ACE inhibitor): 240 mg/1 mg, 180 mg/2 mg, 240 mg/2 mg, 240 mg/4 mg.

## ◆CLASSIFICATION

**PHARMACOTHERAPEUTIC:** Calcium channel blocker. **CLINICAL:** Antihypertensive, antianginal, antiarrhythmic, hypertrophic cardiomyopathy therapy adjunct.

**V**

---

 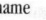

## USES

**Parenteral:** Management of supraventricular tachyarrhythmias (SVT), temporary control of rapid ventricular rate in atrial flutter/fibrillation. **PO:** Treatment of hypertension, angina pectoris, supraventricular tachyarrhythmias (SVT), atrial fibrillation/flutter (rate control).

## PRECAUTIONS

**Contraindications:** Hypersensitivity to verapamil. Atrial fibrillation/flutter in presence of accessory bypass tract (e.g., Wolff-Parkinson-White, Lown-Ganong-Levine syndromes), severe left ventricular dysfunction, cardiogenic shock, second- or third-degree heart block (except with pacemaker), hypotension (SBP less than 90 mm Hg), sick sinus syndrome (except with pacemaker). **IV (additional):** IV beta-blocking agents, ventricular tachycardia. **Cautions:** Renal/hepatic impairment, concomitant use of beta blockers and/or digoxin, myasthenia gravis, elderly, hypertrophic cardiomyopathy. Avoid use in HF.

## ACTION

Inhibits calcium ion entry across cardiac, vascular smooth-muscle cell membranes, dilating coronary arteries, peripheral arteries, arterioles. **Therapeutic Effect:** Decreases heart rate, myocardial contractility; slows SA, AV conduction. Decreases total peripheral vascular resistance by vasodilation.

## PHARMACOKINETICS

Well absorbed from GI tract. Protein binding: 90% (60% in neonates). Metabolized in liver. Primarily excreted in urine. Not removed by hemodialysis. **Half-life: (single dose):** 2–8 hrs, **(multiple doses):** 4.5–12 hrs.

## ⧗ LIFESPAN CONSIDERATIONS

**Pregnancy/Lactation:** Drug crosses placenta; distributed in breast milk. Breastfeeding not recommended. **Children:** No age-related precautions noted. **Elderly:** Age-related renal impairment may require dosage adjustment.

## INTERACTIONS

**DRUG: Beta-adrenergic blockers (e.g., carvedilol, metoprolol)** may have additive negative effects on heart rate, AV conduction, or contractility. **Statins (e.g., simvastatin)** may increase risk of myopathy, rhabdomyolysis. May increase concentration of **cyclosporine, carbamazepine.** May increase **digoxin** concentration. **CYP3A4 inducers (e.g., rifampin)** may decrease concentration/effects. **HERBAL: St. John's wort** may decrease concentration/effects. **Ephedra, ginseng, ginger, licorice, yohimbe, black cohosh, periwinkle** may worsen hypertension. **FOOD: Grapefruit products** may increase concentration. **LAB VALUES:** EKG may show prolonged PR interval. **Therapeutic serum level:** 0.08–0.3 mcg/ml; **toxic serum level:** N/A.

## AVAILABILITY (Rx)

**Injection Solution:** 2.5 mg/ml. **Tablets (Calan):** 40 mg, 80 mg, 120 mg.

🍃 **Capsules (Extended-Release):** 100 mg, 120 mg, 180 mg, 200 mg, 240 mg, 300 mg, 360 mg. 🍃 **Tablets (Extended-Release):** 120 mg, 180 mg, 240 mg.

## ADMINISTRATION/HANDLING

### 💉 IV

**Reconstitution** • May give undiluted. **Rate of Administration** • Administer IV push over 2 min for adults, children; give over 3 min for elderly. • Continuous EKG monitoring during IV injection is required for children, recommended for adults. • Monitor EKG for rapid ventricular rate, extreme bradycardia, heart block, asystole, prolongation of PR interval. Notify physician of any significant changes. • Monitor B/P q5–10min. • Pt should remain recumbent for at least 1 hr after IV administration. **Storage** • Store vials at room temperature.

### PO

• Do not give with grapefruit products. • Do not crush or cut extended-release tablets, capsules. Give extended-release tablets with food. • Sustained-release capsules may be opened and sprinkled on applesauce, then swallowed immediately (do not chew).

### ▦ IV INCOMPATIBILITIES

Albumin, amphotericin B complex (Abelcet, AmBisome, Amphotec), nafcillin (Nafcil), propofol (Diprivan), sodium bicarbonate.

### ▦ IV COMPATIBILITIES

Amiodarone (Cordarone), calcium chloride, calcium gluconate, dexamethasone (Decadron), digoxin (Lanoxin), dobutamine (Dobutrex), dopamine (Intropin), furosemide (Lasix), heparin, hydromorphone (Dilaudid), lidocaine, magnesium sulfate, metoclopramide (Reglan), milrinone (Primacor), morphine, multivitamins, nitroglycerin, norepinephrine (Levophed), potassium chloride, potassium phosphate, procainamide (Pronestyl), propranolol (Inderal).

## INDICATIONS/ROUTES/DOSAGE

**Supraventricular Tachyarrhythmias (SVT)**
**IV:** **ADULTS, ELDERLY:** Initially, 2.5–5 mg over 2 min. May give 5–10 mg 15–30 min after initial dose. **Maximum total dose:** 20–30 mg. **CHILDREN 1–15 YRS:** 0.1–0.3 mg/kg over 2 min. **Maximum initial dose:** 5 mg. May repeat in 30 min. **Maximum second dose:** 10 mg.

**Angina, Unstable Angina, Chronic Stable Angina**
**PO:** *(Immediate-Release):* **ADULTS:** Initially, 80–120 mg 3 times/day. For elderly pts, those with hepatic dysfunction, 40 mg 3 times/day. Titrate to optimal dose. **Maintenance:** 240–480 mg/day in 3–4 divided doses. Usual range: 80–160 mg 3 times/day.

**Atrial Fibrillation (rate control)**
**IV:** **ADULTS, ELDERLY:** Initially, 0.075–0.15 mg/kg (usual: 5–10 mg) over 2 min. May repeat with 10 mg after 15–30 min. **PO:** *(Immediate-Release):* 240–480 mg/day in 3–4 divided doses.

**Hypertension**
**PO:** *(Immediate-Release):* **ADULTS, ELDERLY:** Initially, 80 mg 3 times/day. Range: 240–480 mg/day in divided doses.
**PO:** *(Sustained-Release [Calan SR, Isoptin SR]):* **ADULTS, ELDERLY:** Initially, 120–180 mg once daily. May increase at wkly intervals to 240 mg once daily, then 180 mg twice daily. **Maximum:** 240 mg twice daily.
*[Verelan]:* Initially, 120–180 mg once daily. May increase dose at wkly intervals to 240 mg/day, then 360 mg/day, then 480 mg/day maximum.
**PO:** *(Extended-Release [Verelan PM]):* **ADULTS, ELDERLY:** Initially, 100–200 mg once daily at bedtime. May increase dose at wkly intervals to 300 mg once daily, then 400 mg once daily maximum.

**Chronic Atrial Fibrillation (Rate Control), SVT**
**PO:** *(Immediate-Release):* **ADULTS, ELDERLY:** 240–480 mg/day in 3–4 divided doses. Usual range: 120–360 mg/day.

**Dosage for Renal Impairment**
**CrCl less than 10 ml/min:** Dose reduction (50%–75%) of normal dose recommended.

**Dosage in Hepatic Impairment**
Dose reduction (20%–50%) of normal dose recommended.

## SIDE EFFECTS

**Frequent (7%):** Constipation. **Occasional (4%–2%):** Dizziness, light-headedness, headache, asthenia, nausea, peripheral edema, hypotension. **Rare (less than 1%):** Bradycardia, dermatitis, rash.

## ADVERSE EFFECTS/ TOXIC REACTIONS

Rapid ventricular rate in atrial flutter/fibrillation, marked hypotension, extreme bradycardia, HF, asystole, second- or third-degree AV block occur rarely. **Antidote:** Glucagon 5–10 mg over 1 min, then infuse 1–10 mg over 1 hour.

**V**

---

## NURSING CONSIDERATIONS

### BASELINE ASSESSMENT

Record onset, type (sharp, dull, squeezing), radiation, location, intensity, duration of anginal pain, precipitating factors (exertion, emotional stress). Check B/P for hypotension, pulse for bradycardia immediately before giving medication.

### INTERVENTION/EVALUATION

Assess pulse for quality, rate, rhythm. Monitor B/P. Monitor EKG for cardiac changes, particularly prolongation of PR interval. Notify physician of any significant EKG interval changes. Assist with ambulation if dizziness occurs. Assess for peripheral edema. For those taking oral form, monitor daily pattern of bowel activity, stool consistency. **Therapeutic serum level:** 0.08–0.3 mcg/ml; **toxic serum level:** N/A.

### PATIENT/FAMILY TEACHING

• Do not abruptly discontinue medication. • Compliance with therapy regimen is essential to control anginal pain. • Go from lying to standing slowly. • Avoid tasks that require alertness, motor skills until response to drug is established. • Limit caffeine. • Avoid or limit alcohol. • Report continued, persistent angina pain, irregular heartbeats, shortness of breath, swelling, dizziness, constipation, nausea, hypotension. • Avoid grapefruit products.

---

## vilazodone

vil-**az**-oh-done
(Viibryd)

■ **BLACK BOX ALERT** ■ Increased risk of suicidal ideation and behavior in children, adolescents, and young adults 18–24 yrs of age with major depressive disorder, other psychiatric disorders.

### ◆ CLASSIFICATION

**PHARMACOTHERAPEUTIC:** Selective serotonin reuptake inhibitor. **CLINICAL:** Antidepressant.

## USES

Treatment of major depressive disorder.

## PRECAUTIONS

**Contraindications:** Hypersensitivity to vilazodone. Use of MAOIs intended to treat psychiatric disorders (with or within 14 days of stopping vilazodone or MAOI), starting vilazodone in pts receiving linezolid or methylene blue. **Cautions:** History of seizures; pts at risk for suicide, hepatic impairment, elderly.

## ACTION

Enhances serotonergic activity in CNS by selectively inhibiting reuptake of serotonin. **Therapeutic Effect:** Relieves depression.

## PHARMACOKINETICS

Readily absorbed from GI tract. Peak concentration: 4–5 hrs. Widely distributed. Protein binding: 96%–99%. Metabolized in liver. **Half-life:** 25 hrs.

## ⌛ LIFESPAN CONSIDERATIONS

**Pregnancy/Lactation:** Unknown if drug crosses placenta or is excreted in breast milk. **Children:** Safety and efficacy not established. **Elderly:** No age-related precautions noted.

## INTERACTIONS

**DRUG: Aspirin, NSAIDs, warfarin** may increase risk of bleeding. **Strong CYP3A4 inhibitors (e.g., ketoconazole, nefazodone, ritonavir)** may increase concentration. **Almotriptan, buspirone, eletriptan, naratriptan, SNRIs (e.g., venlafaxine), SSRIs (e.g., sertraline), sumatriptan, tramadol, tryptophan** may increase risk of serotonin syndrome. **HERBAL: St. John's wort** may increase risk of serotonin syndrome. **FOOD:** None known. **LAB VALUES:** None significant.

## AVAILABILITY (Rx)

**Tablets:** 10 mg, 20 mg, 40 mg.

## ADMINISTRATION/HANDLING

### PO

• Give with food (administration without food can result in inadequate drug concentration, may diminish effectiveness).

## INDICATIONS/ROUTES/DOSAGE

### Depression

PO: **ADULTS, ELDERLY:** Initially, 10 mg once daily for 7 days, followed by 20 mg once daily. May increase to 40 mg once daily after a minimum of 7 days. **Note:** When discontinuing treatment, reduce dose gradually. From 40 mg/day: taper to 20 mg/day for 4 days, then 10 mg/day for 3 days. From 20 mg/day: taper to 10 mg/day for 7 days.

### Concomitant Moderate/Strong CYP3A4 Inhibitors

PO: **ADULTS, ELDERLY:** 20 mg/day.

### Concomitant Strong CYP3A4 Inducers

May increase dose to 80 mg/day when used concomitantly for more than 14 days.

### Dosage in Renal/Hepatic Impairment

No dose adjustment.

## SIDE EFFECTS

**Frequent (28%–23%):** Diarrhea, nausea. **Occasional (9%–3%):** Dizziness, dry mouth, insomnia, vomiting, decreased libido, abnormal dreams, fatigue, sweating. **Rare (2%):** Dyspepsia, flatulence, paresthesia, restlessness, arthralgia, abnormal orgasm, delayed ejaculation, increased appetite, palpitations, tremor.

## ADVERSE EFFECTS/ TOXIC REACTIONS

Serotonin syndrome (agitation, confusion, hallucinations, hyperreflexia), neuroleptic malignant syndrome (fever, muscular rigidity, cognitive changes).

## NURSING CONSIDERATIONS

### BASELINE ASSESSMENT

Assess behavior, appearance, emotional status, response to environment, speech pattern, thought content, risk of suicide.

### INTERVENTION/EVALUATION

Monitor B/P, heart rate, weight. Monitor for suicidal ideation (esp. at initiation of therapy or changes in dosage). Assess for therapeutic response (greater interest in surroundings, improved self-care, increased ability to concentrate, relaxed facial expression).

### PATIENT/FAMILY TEACHING

• Avoid tasks that may require alertness, motor skills until response to drug is established (may cause dizziness). • Slowly go from lying to standing. • Take with food. • Do not suddenly stop taking medication; withdraw gradually. • Report suicidal ideation, signs of mania/hypomania. Avoid alcohol.

---

# *vinBLAStine

vin-**blas**-teen

■ **BLACK BOX ALERT** ■ Must be administered by personnel trained in administration/handling of chemotherapeutic agents. Fatal if given intrathecally (ascending paralysis, death). Vesicant; avoid extravasation.

**Do not confuse vinblastine with vincristine or vinorelbine.**

## ◆CLASSIFICATION

**PHARMACOTHERAPEUTIC:** Vinca alkaloid. **CLINICAL:** Antineoplastic.

## USES

Treatment of Hodgkin's lymphoma, lymphocytic lymphoma, histiocytic lymphoma, advanced stage of mycosis fungoides, advanced testicular carcinoma, Kaposi's sarcoma, Letterer-Siwe disease, breast carcinoma, choriocarcinoma. **OFF-LABEL:** Treatment of bladder, ovarian cancer; non–small-cell lung cancer; soft tissue sarcoma, melanoma.

## PRECAUTIONS

**Contraindications:** Hypersensitivity to vinblastine. Bacterial infection, significant

V

---

 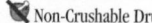

granulocytopenia. **Cautions:** Hepatic impairment, severe leukopenia, neurotoxicity, recent exposure to radiation therapy, chemotherapy, ischemic heart disease, preexisting pulmonary disease.

## ACTION

Binds to tubulin, inhibiting microtubule formation; may interfere with nucleic acid, protein synthesis. **Therapeutic Effect:** Inhibits cell division by disrupting mitotic spindle.

## PHARMACOKINETICS

Does not cross blood-brain barrier. Protein binding: 99%. Metabolized in liver. Primarily eliminated in feces. **Half-life:** 24.8 hrs.

## ⌛ LIFESPAN CONSIDERATIONS

**Pregnancy/Lactation:** If possible, avoid use during pregnancy, esp. during first trimester. Breastfeeding not recommended. **Children/Elderly:** No age-related precautions noted.

## INTERACTIONS

**DRUG:** May decrease concentration/anticonvulsant effects of **phenytoin. CYP3A4 inhibitors (e.g., erthromycin, ketoconazole)** may increase level/toxicity. **Bone marrow depressants** may increase myelosuppression. **Live virus vaccines** may potentiate virus replication, increase vaccine side effects, decrease pt's antibody response to vaccine. **HERBAL: St. John's wort** may decrease concentration. Avoid **black cohosh, dong quai** in estrogen-dependent tumors. **FOOD:** None known. **LAB VALUES:** May increase serum uric acid.

## AVAILABILITY (Rx)

**Injection, Powder for Reconstitution:** 10 mg. **Injection Solution:** 1 mg/ml.

## ADMINISTRATION/HANDLING

**◄ALERT►** May be carcinogenic, mutagenic, teratogenic. Handle with extreme care during preparation and administration. Give by IV injection. Leakage from IV site into surrounding tissue may produce extreme irritation. Avoid eye contact with solution (severe eye irritation, possible corneal ulceration may result). If eye contact occurs, immediately irrigate eye with water.

 **IV**

**Reconstitution** • Reconstitute 10-mg vial with 10 ml 0.9% NaCl to provide concentration of 1 mg/ml. May further dilute in 50 ml $D_5W$ or 0.9% NaCl.
**Rate of Administration** • Inject into tubing of running IV infusion or directly into vein over 1 min (IV infusion over 5–15 min). • Do not inject into extremity with impaired, potentially impaired circulation caused by compression or invading neoplasm, phlebitis, varicosity. • Rinse syringe, needle with venous blood before withdrawing needle (minimizes possibility of extravasation). • Extravasation may result in cellulitis, phlebitis. Large amount of extravasation may result in tissue sloughing. If extravasation occurs, give local injection of hyaluronidase, apply warm compresses.
**Storage** • Refrigerate unopened vials. • Solution appears clear, colorless. • Following reconstitution, solution is stable for 30 days if refrigerated. • Discard if solution is discolored or precipitate forms.

## ▩ IV INCOMPATIBILITY

Furosemide (Lasix).

## ▩ IV COMPATIBILITIES

Allopurinol (Aloprim), cisplatin (Platinol AQ), cyclophosphamide (Cytoxan), doxorubicin (Adriamycin), etoposide (VePesid), 5-fluorouracil, gemcitabine (Gemzar), granisetron (Kytril), heparin, leucovorin, methotrexate, ondansetron (Zofran), paclitaxel (Taxol), vinorelbine (Navelbine).

## INDICATIONS/ROUTES/DOSAGE

**◄ALERT►** Dosage individualized based on clinical response, tolerance to adverse effects. When used in combination therapy,

V

consult specific protocols for optimum dosage, sequence of drug administration.

### Usual Dosage

**IV: ADULTS, ELDERLY:** Initially, 3.7 mg/m² (adjust dose q7days based on WBC response) up to 5.5 mg/m² (second wk), 7.4 mg/m² (third wk), 9.25 mg/m² (fourth wk), and 11.1 mg/m² (fifth wk). **Maximum:** 18.5 mg/m². **CHILDREN:** 3–6 mg/m² q7–14days. **Maximum:** 12.5 mg/m²/wk.

### Dosage in Renal Impairment

No dose adjustment.

### Dosage in Hepatic Impairment

**Direct serum bilirubin concentration 1.5–3 mg/dL:** Reduce dose by 50%. **Greater than 3 mg/dL:** Avoid use.

## SIDE EFFECTS

**Frequent:** Nausea, vomiting, alopecia. **Occasional:** Constipation, diarrhea, rectal bleeding, headache, paresthesia (occur 4–6 hrs after administration, persist for 2–10 hrs), malaise, asthenia, dizziness, pain at tumor site, jaw/face pain, depression, dry mouth. **Rare:** Dermatitis, stomatitis, phototoxicity, hyperuricemia.

## ADVERSE EFFECTS/ TOXIC REACTIONS

Hematologic toxicity manifested most commonly as leukopenia, less frequently as anemia. WBC reaches its nadir 4–10 days after initial therapy, recovers within 7–14 days (high dosage may require 21-day recovery period). Thrombocytopenia is usually mild and transient, with recovery occurring in few days. Hepatic insufficiency may increase risk of toxicity. Acute shortness of breath, bronchospasm may occur, particularly when administered concurrently with mitomycin.

## NURSING CONSIDERATIONS

### BASELINE ASSESSMENT

Nausea, vomiting easily controlled by antiemetics. Discontinue therapy if WBC, platelet counts fall abruptly (unless drug is clearly destroying tumor cells in bone marrow). Obtain CBC wkly or before each dosing.

### INTERVENTION/EVALUATION

If neutrophils fall below 2,000/mm³, assess diligently for signs of infection. Assess for stomatitis; maintain strict oral hygiene. Monitor for hematologic toxicity: infection (fever, sore throat, signs of local infection), unusual bruising/bleeding from any site, symptoms of anemia (excessive fatigue, weakness). Monitor daily pattern of bowel activity, stool consistency. Avoid constipation.

### PATIENT/FAMILY TEACHING

• Immediately report any pain/burning at injection site during administration. • Pain at tumor site may occur during or shortly after injection. • Do not have immunizations without physician approval (drug lowers resistance). • Avoid crowds, those with infection. • Promptly report fever, sore throat, signs of local infection, unusual bruising/bleeding from any site. • Hair loss is reversible, but new hair growth may have different color, texture. • Report persistent nausea/vomiting. • Avoid constipation by increasing fluids, bulk in diet, exercise as tolerated.

---

## *vinCRIStine          HIGH ALERT

vin-**cris**-teen
(Marqibo, Vincasar PFS)

■ **BLACK BOX ALERT** ■ Must be administered by personnel trained in administration/handling of chemotherapeutic agents. Fatal if given intrathecally (ascending paralysis, death). Vesicant; avoid extravasation. Marqibo and Vincasar are not interchangeable.
**Do not confuse vincristine with vinblastine.**

## ◆ CLASSIFICATION

**PHARMACOTHERAPEUTIC:** Vinca alkaloid. **CLINICAL:** Antineoplastic.

V

---

## USES

**Vincasar:** Treatment of acute lymphocytic leukemia (ALL), Hodgkin's lymphoma, advanced non-Hodgkin's lymphomas, neuroblastoma, rhabdomyosarcoma, Wilms tumor. **Marqibo:** Relapsed Philadelphia chromosome negative (Ph⁻) ALL in adults whose disease has progressed after 2 or more antileukemic therapies. **OFF-LABEL: Vincasar:** Treatment of multiple myeloma, chronic lymphocytic leukemia (CLL), brain tumors, small cell lung cancer, ovarian germ cell tumors, Ewing's sarcoma, gestational trophoblastic tumors, retinoblastoma.

## PRECAUTIONS

**Contraindications:** Hypersensitivity to vincristine. Demyelinating form of Charcot-Marie-Tooth syndrome. Intrathecal administration. **Caution:** Hepatic impairment, pts receiving radiation therapy through ports (including liver), neurotoxicity, preexisting neuromuscular disease, hepatobiliary dysfunction, elderly.

## ACTION

Binds to tubulin, inhibiting microtubule formation; may interfere with nucleic acid/protein synthesis. **Therapeutic Effect:** Inhibits cell division by disrupting mitotic spindle.

## PHARMACOKINETICS

Does not cross blood-brain barrier. Protein binding: 75%. Metabolized in liver. Primarily eliminated in feces by biliary system. **Half-life:** 24 hrs. Marqibo: 45 hrs.

## ⌛ LIFESPAN CONSIDERATIONS

**Pregnancy/Lactation:** If possible, avoid use during pregnancy, esp. first trimester. May cause fetal harm. Breastfeeding not recommended. **Children:** No age-related precautions noted. **Elderly:** More susceptible to neurotoxic effects.

## INTERACTIONS

**DRUG:** May decrease concentration/anticonvulsant effects of **phenytoin.** **Itraconazole** may increase severity of neuromuscular side effects. **Live virus vaccines** may potentiate virus replication, increase vaccine side effects, decrease pt's antibody response to vaccine. **HERBAL:** St. John's wort, echinacea may decrease concentration. **FOOD:** None known. **LAB VALUES:** May increase serum uric acid.

## AVAILABILITY (Rx)

**Injection Solution (Vincasar):** 1 mg/ml. **Injection Suspension (Marqibo):** 5 mg/31 ml.

## ADMINISTRATION/HANDLING

### 💧 IV

**◀ALERT▶** May be carcinogenic, mutagenic, teratogenic. Handle with extreme care during preparation and administration. Give by IV injection. Use extreme caution in calculating, administering vincristine. Overdose may result in serious or fatal outcome.

*Vincasar*

**Reconstitution** • May give undiluted or diluted in 25–50 ml D₅W or 0.9% NaCl.

**Rate of Administration** • Inject dose into tubing of running IV infusion or directly into vein over 1 min. May be administered as 5–10 min infusion (preferred). • Do not inject into extremity with impaired, potentially impaired circulation caused by compression or invading neoplasm, phlebitis, varicosity. • Extravasation produces stinging, burning, edema at injection site. Terminate injection immediately, locally inject hyaluronidase, apply heat (disperses drug, minimizes discomfort, cellulitis).

**Storage** • Refrigerate unopened vials. • Solution appears clear, colorless. • Discard if solution is discolored or precipitate forms.

*Marqibo*

**Note:** See manufacturer supply kit. Once prepared, concentration will equal 5 mg/31 ml. • Calculate dose of vincristine and remove volume equal to volume of

intended solution from 100 ml 0.9% NaCl or D₅W infusion bag. Inject vincristine into infusion bag (total volume: 100 ml).
**Rate of Administration** • Administer over 60 min.
**Storage** • Solution must be administered within 12 hrs of preparation.

## 🏵 IV INCOMPATIBILITIES

Furosemide (Lasix), idarubicin (Idamycin).

## 🏵 IV COMPATIBILITIES

Allopurinol (Aloprim), cisplatin (Platinol AQ), cyclophosphamide (Cytoxan), cytarabine (Ara-C, Cytosar), doxorubicin (Adriamycin), etoposide (VePesid), 5-fluorouracil, gemcitabine (Gemzar), granisetron (Kytril), leucovorin, methotrexate, ondansetron (Zofran), paclitaxel (Taxol), vinorelbine (Navelbine).

## INDICATIONS/ROUTES/DOSAGE

**Usual Dosage (Vincasar)**
**IV: ADULTS, ELDERLY:** 1.4 mg/m², frequency may vary based on protocol. **CHILDREN WEIGHING MORE THAN 10 KG:** 1.5–2 mg/m², frequency may vary based on protocol. **CHILDREN WEIGHING LESS THAN 10 KG:** 0.05 mg/kg once wkly. **Maximum:** 2 mg.

**Dosage in Renal Impairment**
No dose adjustment.

**Dosage in Hepatic Impairment**

| Bilirubin | Dosage |
|---|---|
| Bilirubin greater than 3 mg/dL | 50% of normal |

**ALL (Marqibo)**
**IV: ADULTS, ELDERLY:** 2.25 mg/m² q7days. Infuse over 1 hr.

**Dosage in Renal/Hepatic Impairment (Marqibo)**
No dose adjustment.

## SIDE EFFECTS

**Expected:** Peripheral neuropathy (occurs in nearly every pt; first clinical sign is depression of Achilles tendon reflex). **Frequent:** Peripheral paresthesia, alopecia, constipation/obstipation (upper colon impaction with empty rectum), abdominal cramps, headache, jaw pain, hoarseness, diplopia, ptosis/drooping of eyelid, urinary tract disturbances. **Occasional:** Nausea, vomiting, diarrhea, abdominal distention, stomatitis, fever. **Rare:** Mild leukopenia, mild anemia, thrombocytopenia.

## ADVERSE EFFECTS/ TOXIC REACTIONS

Acute dyspnea, bronchospasm may occur, esp. when administered concurrently with mitomycin. Prolonged or high-dose therapy may produce foot/wrist drop, difficulty walking, slapping gait, ataxia, muscle wasting. Acute uric acid nephropathy may occur.

## NURSING CONSIDERATIONS

### BASELINE ASSESSMENT

Obtain baseline CBC, LFT. Offer pt/family emotional support.

### INTERVENTION/EVALUATION

Monitor serum uric acid levels, renal/hepatic function studies, CBC. Assess Achilles tendon reflex. Monitor daily pattern of bowel activity, stool consistency. Monitor for ptosis, diplopia, blurred vision. Question pt regarding urinary changes.

### PATIENT/FAMILY TEACHING

• Immediately report any pain/burning at injection site during administration. • Hair loss is reversible, but new hair growth may have different color/texture. • Report persistent nausea/vomiting. • Report signs of peripheral neuropathy (burning/numbness of bottom of feet, palms of hands). • Report fever, sore throat, unusual bleeding/bruising, shortness of breath.

**V**

# vinorelbine

HIGH ALERT

vin-oh-**rel**-been
(Navelbine)

**■ BLACK BOX ALERT ■** Must be administered by personnel trained in administration/handling of chemotherapeutic agents. Fatal if given intrathecally (ascending paralysis, death). Extravasation produces thrombophlebitis, local tissue necrosis. May produce severe granulocytopenia.
**Do not confuse vinorelbine with vinblastine or vincristine.**

## ◆CLASSIFICATION

**PHARMACOTHERAPEUTIC:** Vinca alkaloid. **CLINICAL:** Antineoplastic.

## USES

Single agent or in combination with cisplatin for treatment of unresectable, advanced, non–small-cell lung cancer (NSCLC). **OFF-LABEL:** Treatment of metastatic breast cancer, cervical carcinoma, ovarian carcinoma, malignant pleural mesothelioma, soft tissue sarcoma, small-cell lung cancer.

## PRECAUTIONS

**Contraindications:** Hypersensitivity to vinorelbine. Granulocyte count before treatment of less than 1,000/mm³. **Cautions:** Compromised marrow reserve due to prior chemotherapy/radiation therapy; hepatic impairment, neurotoxicity; neuropathy, pulmonary impairment.

## ACTION

Binds to tubulin, inhibiting microtubule formation; may interfere with nucleic acid protein synthesis. **Therapeutic Effect:** Prevents cellular division by disrupting formation of mitotic spindle.

## PHARMACOKINETICS

Widely distributed after IV administration. Protein binding: 80%–90%. Metabolized in liver. Primarily eliminated in feces by biliary system. **Half-life:** 28–43 hrs.

## ⏳ LIFESPAN CONSIDERATIONS

**Pregnancy/Lactation:** If possible, avoid use during pregnancy, esp. during first trimester. May cause fetal harm. Unknown if distributed in breast milk. Breastfeeding not recommended. **Children:** Safety and efficacy not established. **Elderly:** No age-related precautions noted.

## INTERACTIONS

**DRUG: Bone marrow depressants** may increase risk of myelosuppression. **Cisplatin** significantly increases risk of granulocytopenia. **Live virus vaccines** may potentiate virus replication, increase vaccine side effects, decrease pt's antibody response to vaccine. **Mitomycin** may produce an acute pulmonary reaction. **Paclitaxel** may increase neuropathy. **CYP3A4 inhibitors (e.g., erythromycin, ketoconazole)** may increase concentration/effects. **HERBAL: St. John's wort** may decrease concentration. **FOOD:** None known. **LAB VALUES:** May increase serum bilirubin, alkaline phosphatase, ALT, AST.

## AVAILABILITY (Rx)

**Injection Solution:** 10 mg/ml (1-ml, 5-ml vials).

## ADMINISTRATION/HANDLING

 IV

**◄ALERT►** IV needle, catheter must be correctly positioned before administration. Leakage into surrounding tissue produces extreme irritation, local tissue necrosis, thrombophlebitis. Handle drug with extreme care during administration; wear protective clothing per protocol. If solution comes in contact with skin/mucosa, immediately wash thoroughly with soap, water.
**Reconstitution •** Must be diluted and administered via syringe or IV bag.

V

**SYRINGE DILUTION** • Dilute calculated vinorelbine dose with D₅W or 0.9% NaCl to concentration of 1.5–3 mg/ml.

**IV BAG DILUTION** • Dilute calculated vinorelbine dose with D₅W, 0.45% or 0.9% NaCl, 5% dextrose and 0.45% NaCl, Ringer's or lactated Ringer's to concentration of 0.5–2 mg/ml.

**Rate of Administration** • Administer diluted vinorelbine over 6–10 min into side port of free-flowing IV closest to IV bag followed by flushing with 75–125 ml of one of the solutions. • If extravasation occurs, stop injection immediately; give remaining portion of dose into another vein.

**Storage** • Refrigerate unopened vials. • Protect from light. • Unopened vials are stable at room temperature for 72 hrs. • Do not administer if particulate has formed. • Diluted vinorelbine may be used for up to 24 hrs under normal room light when stored in polypropylene syringes or polyvinyl chloride bags at room temperature.

## 🔲 IV INCOMPATIBILITIES

Acyclovir (Zovirax), allopurinol (Aloprim), amphotericin B (Fungizone), amphotericin B complex (Abelcet, AmBisome, Amphotec), ampicillin (Omnipen), cefazolin (Ancef), ceftriaxone (Rocephin), cefuroxime (Zinacef), 5-fluorouracil (5-FU), furosemide (Lasix), ganciclovir (Cytovene), methylprednisolone (Solu-Medrol), sodium bicarbonate.

## 🔲 IV COMPATIBILITIES

Calcium gluconate, carboplatin (Paraplatin), cisplatin (Platinol AQ), cyclophosphamide (Cytoxan), cytarabine (ARA-C, Cytosar), dacarbazine (DTIC), daunorubicin (Cerubidine), dexamethasone (Decadron), diphenhydramine (Benadryl), doxorubicin (Adriamycin), etoposide (VePesid), gemcitabine (Gemzar), granisetron (Kytril), hydromorphone (Dilaudid), idarubicin (Idamycin), methotrexate, morphine, ondansetron (Zofran), vinblastine (Velban), vincristine (Oncovin).

## INDICATIONS/ROUTES/DOSAGE

**◀ ALERT ▶** Dosage adjustments should be based on granulocyte count obtained on the day of treatment, as follows:

| Granulocyte Count (cells/mm³) on Day of Treatment | Dosage |
|---|---|
| 1,500 or higher | 100% of starting dose |
| 1,000–1,499 | 50% of starting dose |
| Less than 1,000 | Do not administer |

**NSCLC Monotherapy**
**IV Injection: ADULTS, ELDERLY:** 30 mg/m² administered wkly over 6–10 min.

**NSCLC Combination Therapy with Cisplatin**
**IV Injection: ADULTS, ELDERLY:** 25–30 mg/m² every wk.

**Dosage in Renal Impairment**
No dose adjustment. **HD:** Decrease dose to 20 mg/m²/wk given post-HD or on non-HD days.

**Dosage in Hepatic Impairment**

| Bilirubin | Dosage |
|---|---|
| 2 mg/dL or less | 100% of dose |
| 2.1–3 mg/dL | 50% of dose |
| Greater than 3 mg/dL | 25% of dose |

## SIDE EFFECTS

**Frequent (35%–12%):** Asthenia, nausea, constipation, erythema, pain, vein discoloration at injection site, fatigue, peripheral neuropathy manifested as paresthesia, hyperesthesia, diarrhea, alopecia. **Occasional (10%–5%):** Phlebitis, dyspnea, loss of deep tendon reflexes. **Rare:** Chest pain, jaw pain, myalgia, arthralgia, rash.

## ADVERSE EFFECTS/TOXIC REACTIONS

Bone marrow depression is manifested mainly as granulocytopenia (may be severe). Other hematologic toxicities

**V**

 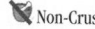

(neutropenia, thrombocytopenia, leukopenia, anemia) increase risk of infection, bleeding. Acute shortness of breath, severe bronchospasm occur infrequently, particularly in pts with preexisting pulmonary dysfunction.

## NURSING CONSIDERATIONS

### BASELINE ASSESSMENT

Review medication history. Obtain CBC prior to each dose. Granulocyte count should be at least 1,000 cells/mm³ before vinorelbine administration. Granulocyte nadirs occur 7–10 days following dosing. Do not give hematologic growth factors within 24 hrs before administration of chemotherapy or earlier than 24 hrs following cytotoxic chemotherapy. Advise women of childbearing potential to avoid pregnancy during drug therapy.

### INTERVENTION/EVALUATION

Diligently monitor injection site for swelling, redness, pain. Frequently monitor for myelosuppression during and following therapy (infection [fever, sore throat, signs of local infection], unusual bleeding/bruising, anemia [excessive fatigue, weakness]). Monitor pts developing severe granulocytopenia for evidence of infection, fever. Crackers, dry toast, sips of cola may help relieve nausea. Monitor daily pattern of bowel activity, stool consistency. Question for tingling, burning, numbness of hands/feet (peripheral neuropathy). Pt complaint of "walking on glass" is sign of hyperesthesia.

### PATIENT/FAMILY TEACHING

• Immediately report redness, swelling, pain at injection site. • Avoid crowds, those with infection. • Do not have immunizations without physician's approval. • Promptly report fever, signs of infection, unusual bruising/bleeding from any site, difficulty breathing. • Avoid pregnancy. • Hair loss is reversible, but new hair growth may have different color, texture.

# vismodegib

**vis**-moe-**deg**-ib
(Erivedge)

■ **BLACK BOX ALERT** ■ May result in embryo-fetal death or severe birth defects including missing digits, midline defects, irreversible malformations due to embryotoxic and teratogenic properties. Verify pregnancy status prior to initiation. Advise use of effective contraception in female pts. Advise male pts of potential exposure risk through seminal fluid.

## ◆CLASSIFICATION

**PHARMACOTHERAPEUTIC:** Hedgehog pathway inhibitor. **CLINICAL:** Antineoplastic.

## USES

Treatment of adult pts with metastatic basal cell carcinoma, locally advanced basal cell carcinoma with recurrence after surgery, or pts who are not candidates for surgery or radiation.

## PRECAUTIONS

◀**ALERT**▶ Do not donate blood products for at least 7 mos after discontinuation. **Contraindications:** Hypersensitivity to vismodegib. **Cautions:** Hepatic/renal impairment. History of significant cardiac disease.

## ACTION

An inhibitor of Hedgehog pathway, binding to and inhibiting smoothened, a transmembrane protein involved in hedgehog signal transduction. **Therapeutic Effect:** Inhibits tumor cell growth and metastasis of basal cell carcinoma.

## PHARMACOKINETICS

Metabolized in liver. Protein binding: 99%. Excreted in feces (82%), urine (4%). **Half-life:** 4 days (daily dosing), 12 days (single dose).

## ⌛ LIFESPAN CONSIDERATIONS

**Pregnancy/Lactation:** May cause fetal harm. Not recommended in nursing mothers. Must either discontinue drug or discontinue breastfeeding. Unknown if distributed in breast milk. Contraception recommended during treatment and up to 7 mos after discontinuation. **Children:** Safety and efficacy not established. **Elderly:** Safety and efficacy not established.

## INTERACTIONS

**DRUG: P-glycoprotein inhibitors (e.g., clarithromycin, erythromycin)** may increase concentration/effects. **Antacids, H₂ blockers (e.g., famotidine), proton pump inhibitors (e.g., pantoprazole)** may decrease concentration/effect. **HERBAL:** None significant. **FOOD:** None known. **LAB VALUES:** May decrease potassium, sodium, GFR. May increase serum BUN, creatinine.

## AVAILABILITY (Rx)

🔖 **Capsules:** 150 mg.

## ADMINISTRATION/HANDLING

### PO

• Give without regard to food. • Give whole. Do not break, crush, or open capsule.

## INDICATIONS/ROUTES/DOSAGE

**Advanced or Metastatic Basal Cell Carcinoma**

**PO: ADULTS/ELDERLY:** 150 mg once daily. Continue until disease progression or unacceptable toxicity.

**Dosage in Renal/Hepatic Impairment**
No dose adjustment.

## SIDE EFFECTS

**Frequent (71%–40%):** Muscle spasm, alopecia, dysgeusia, weight loss, fatigue. **Occasional (30%–11%):** Nausea, amenorrhea, diarrhea, anorexia, constipation, vomiting, arthralgia, loss of taste.

## ADVERSE EFFECTS/ TOXIC REACTIONS

May cause spontaneous abortion, fetal demise, birth defects. Azotemia (renal impairment) reported in 2% of pts.

## NURSING CONSIDERATIONS

### BASELINE ASSESSMENT

Obtain negative pregnancy test (urine/ serum) before initiation, BMP. Question current breastfeeding status. Assess skin, moles for other possible malignancies.

### INTERVENTION/EVALUATION

Obtain STAT human chorionic gonadotropin (HCG) level if pregnancy suspected, BMP if electrolyte imbalance or renal impairment suspected. Offer emotional support. Encourage PO intake if diarrhea occurs. Offer antiemetics for nausea/vomiting. Report oliguria, dark or concentrated urine.

### PATIENT/FAMILY TEACHING

• Avoid pregnancy. • May cause birth defects or miscarriage. • Do not breastfeed. • Male pts must use condoms with spermicide during sexual activity, despite history of vasectomy. • Female pts must use contraception for at least 7 mos after stopping treatment. • Immediately report suspected pregnancy. • Do not donate blood for at least 7 mos after stopping treatment. • Swallow capsules whole; do not break, crush, or open. • Hair loss is an expected side effect. • Strictly monitor menstrual cycle. • Report dark-colored urine or decreased urine output despite hydration.

---

# vitamin D (vitamin D analogues)

# calcitriol

kal-si-**trye**-ole
(Calcijex ✦, Rocaltrol, Vectical)

**V**

---

# doxercalciferol

**dox**-er-kal-**sif**-e-role
(Hectorol)

# ergocalciferol

**er**-goe-kal-**sif**-e-role
(Drisdol)

# paricalcitol

**par**-i-**kal**-si-tol
(Zemplar)

## ◆CLASSIFICATION

**PHARMACOTHERAPEUTIC:** Fat-soluble vitamin. **CLINICAL:** Vitamin D analogue.

## USES

**Calcitriol:** Manage hypocalcemia in pts on chronic renal dialysis, secondary hypoparathyroidism in chronic kidney disease (CKD), manage hypocalcemia in hypoparathyroidism. **(Topical):** Treatment of mild to moderate plaque psoriasis. **Doxercalciferol:** Treatment of secondary hyperparathyroidism in CKD. **Ergocalciferol:** Treatment of refractory rickets, hypophosphatemia, hypoparathyroidism, dietary supplement. **Paricalcitol: (Intravenous):** Treatment/prevention of secondary hyperparathyroidism associated with stage 5 CKD. **(PO):** Treatment/prevention of secondary hyperparathyroidism associated with stage 3 and 4 CKD and stage 5 CKD pts on hemodialysis or peritoneal dialysis. **OFF-LABEL: Calcitriol:** Vitamin D–dependent rickets. **Ergocalciferol:** Prevention/treatment of vitamin D deficiency in pts with CKD, osteoporosis prevention.

## PRECAUTIONS

**Contraindications:** Hypersensitivity to cholecalciferol, ergocalciferol. Vitamin D toxicity, hypercalcemia. **Cautions:** Pts with malabsorption syndrome. Concurrent use with digoxin.

## ACTION

**Calcitriol:** Stimulates calcium transport in intestines, resorption in bones, and tubular reabsorption in kidney; suppresses parathyroid hormone (PTH) secretion/synthesis. **Doxercalciferol:** Regulates blood calcium levels, stimulates bone growth, suppresses PTH secretion/synthesis. **Ergocalciferol:** Promotes active absorption of calcium and phosphorus, increasing serum levels to allow bone mineralization; mobilizes calcium and phosphate from bone, increases reabsorption of calcium and phosphate by renal tubules. **Paricalcitol:** Suppresses PTH secretion/synthesis. **Therapeutic Effect:** Essential for absorption, utilization of calcium, phosphate, control of PTH levels.

## PHARMACOKINETICS

**Calcitriol:** Rapidly absorbed. Protein binding: 99.9%. Metabolized to active metabolite (ergocalciferol). Excreted in feces (49%), urine (16%). **Half-life:** 5–8 hrs. **Doxercalciferol:** Metabolized in liver. **Half-life:** 32–37 hrs. **Ergocalciferol:** Metabolized in liver. **Paricalcitol:** Readily absorbed. Protein binding: 99.8%. Metabolized in liver. Primarily excreted in feces. **Half-life:** 5–7 hrs.

## ⧗ LIFESPAN CONSIDERATIONS

**Pregnancy/Lactation:** Unknown if drug crosses placenta. Infant risk cannot be excluded. **Children/Elderly:** No age-related precautions noted.

## INTERACTIONS

**DRUG: Magnesium-containing antacids** may increase risk of hypermagnesemia. **Calcium-containing products, concurrent vitamin D (or derivatives)** may increase risk of hypercalcemia. May increase **digoxin** toxicity due to hypercalcemia (may cause arrhythmias). **HERBAL:** None

V

significant. **FOOD:** None known. **LAB VALUES:** May increase serum cholesterol, calcium, magnesium, phosphate, ALT, AST, BUN, creatinine.

## AVAILABILITY (Rx)

**Calcitriol**
Capsules, Softgel (Rocaltrol): 0.25 mcg, 0.5 mcg. Injection Solution: 1 mcg/ml. Oral Solution (Rocaltrol): 1 mcg/ml.

**Doxercalciferol**
Capsules, Softgel (Hectorol): 0.5 mcg, 1 mcg, 2.5 mcg. Injection Solution (Hectorol): 2 mcg/ml.

**Ergocalciferol**
Capsules (Drisdol): 50,000 units (1.25 mg). Liquid, Oral (Drisdol): 8,000 units/ml (200 mcg/ml). Tablets: 400 units.

**Paricalcitol**
Capsules, Gelatin (Zemplar): 1 mcg, 2 mcg, 4 mcg. Injection Solution (Zemplar): 2 mcg/ml.

## ADMINISTRATION/HANDLING

**Calcitriol**
**PO**
• May take without regard to food.

 **IV**

• May give as IV bolus at end of dialysis.

**Doxercalciferol**
**PO**
• May take without regard to food.

 **IV**

• May give as IV bolus via catheter at end of dialysis.

**Ergocalciferol**
**PO**
• May take without regard to food.

**Paricalcitol**
**PO**
• May take without regard to food.
• For 3 times/wk dosing, give no more frequently than every other day.

 **IV**

• Give bolus anytime during dialysis.
• Do not give more frequently than every other day.

## INDICATIONS/ROUTES/DOSAGE

**Calcitriol**
**Hypocalcemia on Chronic Renal Dialysis**
**PO: ADULTS, ELDERLY: (ROCALTROL):** Initially, 0.25 mcg/day or every other day. May increase by 0.25 mcg/day at 4- to 8-wk intervals. Range: 0.5–1 mcg/day.
**IV: ADULTS, ELDERLY:** 1–2 mcg 3 times/wk. Adjust dose at 2- to 4-wk intervals. Range: 0.5–4 mcg 3 times/wk.

**Hypocalcemia in Hypoparathyroidism**
**PO: ADULTS, CHILDREN 6 YRS AND OLDER: (ROCALTROL):** Initially, 0.25 mcg/day. May increase at 2- to 4-wk intervals. Range: 0.5–2 mcg/day. **CHILDREN 1–5 YRS:** 0.25–0.75 mcg once daily. **CHILDREN YOUNGER THAN 1 YR:** 0.04–0.08 mcg/kg once daily. **NEONATES:** 1 mcg once daily first 5 days of life.

**Secondary Hyperparathyroidism Associated with Moderate to Severe CKD Not on Dialysis**
**PO: ADULTS, ELDERLY, CHILDREN 3 YRS AND OLDER: (ROCALTROL):** Initially, 0.25 mcg/day. May increase to 0.5 mcg/day. **CHILDREN YOUNGER THAN 3 YRS:** Initially, 0.01–0.015 mcg/kg/day.

**Doxercalciferol**
**Secondary Hyperparathyroidism (Dialysis)**
**PO: ADULTS, ELDERLY:** Initial dose (intact parathyroid hormone [iPTH] greater than 400 pg/ml): 10 mcg 3 times/wk at dialysis. Dose titrated to lower iPTH to 150–300 pg/ml, with dosage adjustments made at 8-wk intervals. **Maximum:** 20 mcg 3 times/wk.
**IV: ADULTS, ELDERLY:** Initial dose (iPTH greater than 400 pg/ml): 4 mcg 3 times/wk after dialysis, given as bolus dose. Dose titrated to lower iPTH to

**V**

150–300 pg/ml, with dosage adjustments made at 8-wk intervals. **Maximum:** 18 mcg/wk.

### Secondary Hyperparathyroidism (Predialysis)

**PO: ADULTS, ELDERLY:** Initially, 1 mcg/day. Titrate dose to lower iPTH to 35–70 pg/ml for stage 3 CKD and 70–110 pg/ml for stage 4 CKD. **Maximum:** 3.5 mcg/day.

### Ergocalciferol
### Dietary Supplement

**PO: ADULTS, ELDERLY, CHILDREN:** 10 mcg (400 units)/day. **NEONATES:** 10–20 mcg (400–800 units)/day.

### Hypoparathyroidism

**PO: ADULTS, ELDERLY:** 625 mcg–5 mg (25,000–200,000 units)/day (with calcium supplements). **CHILDREN:** 1.25–5 mg (50,000–200,000 units)/day (with calcium supplements).

### Nutritional Rickets, Osteomalacia

**PO: ADULTS, ELDERLY, CHILDREN:** 25–125 mcg (1,000–5,000 units)/day for 8–12 wks. **ADULTS, ELDERLY (WITH MALABSORPTION SYNDROME):** 250–7,500 mcg (10,000–300,000 units)/day. **CHILDREN (WITH MALABSORPTION SYNDROME):** 250–625 mcg (10,000–25,000 units)/day.

### Vitamin D–Dependent Rickets

**PO: ADULTS, ELDERLY:** 250 mcg–1.5 mg (10,000–60,000 units)/day. **CHILDREN:** 75–125 mcg (3,000–5,000 units)/day. **Maximum:** 1,500 mcg (60,000 units)/day.

### Vitamin D–Resistant Rickets

**PO: ADULTS, ELDERLY, CHILDREN:** 300 mcg–12.5 mg (12,000–500,000 units)/day.

### Hypophosphatemia

**PO: ADULTS, ELDERLY:** 250–1,500 mcg (10,000–60,000 units)/day with phosphate supplements. **CHILDREN:** 1,000–2,000 mcg (40,000–80,000 units)/day with phosphate supplements.

### Plaque Psoriasis
**Topical: ADULTS, ELDERLY:** Apply to affected area twice daily.

### Paricalcitol
### Secondary Hyperparathyroidism in Stage 5 CKD

**IV: ADULTS, ELDERLY, CHILDREN 5 YRS AND OLDER:** Initially, 0.04–0.1 mcg/kg given as bolus dose no more frequently than every other day at any time during dialysis. May increase by 2–4 mcg every 2–4 wks. Dose is based on serum iPTH levels.

### Secondary Hyperparathyroidism in Stages 3 and 4 CKD

**Note:** Initial dose based on baseline serum iPTH levels. Dose adjusted q2wks based on iPTH levels relative to baseline. **PO: ADULTS, ELDERLY: (iPTH 500 PG/ML OR LESS):** 1 mcg/day or 2 mcg 3 times/wk. **(iPTH GREATER THAN 500 PG/ML):** 2 mcg/day or 4 mcg 3 times/wk.

### Dosage in Renal/Hepatic Impairment
No dose adjustment.

## SIDE EFFECTS

Frequencies not defined. **Calcitriol:** Cardiac arrhythmias, headache, pruritus, hypercalcemia, polydipsia, abdominal pain, metallic taste, nausea, vomiting, myalgia, soft tissue calcification. **Doxercalciferol:** Edema, pruritus, nausea, vomiting, headache, dizziness, dyspnea, malaise, hypercalcemia. **Ergocalciferol:** Hypercalcemia, hypervitaminosis D, decreased renal function, soft tissue calcification, bone demineralization, nausea, constipation, weight loss. **Paricalcitol:** Edema, nausea, vomiting, hypercalcemia.

## ADVERSE EFFECTS/ TOXIC REACTIONS

Early signs of overdose manifested as weakness, headache, drowsiness, nausea, vomiting, dry mouth, constipation, muscle/bone pain, metallic taste. Later signs of overdose evidenced by polyuria, polydipsia, anorexia, weight loss, nocturia, photophobia, rhinorrhea, pruritus, disorientation, hallucinations, hyperthermia, hypertension, cardiac dysrhythmias.

## NURSING CONSIDERATIONS

### BASELINE ASSESSMENT

Obtain baseline serum calcium, ionized calcium, phosphorus, alkaline phosphatase, creatinine, PTH.

### INTERVENTION/EVALUATION

Monitor serum, urinary calcium levels, serum phosphate, magnesium, BUN, creatine, alkaline phosphatase determinations (therapeutic calcium level: 9–10 mg/dL), PTH measurements. Estimate daily dietary calcium intake. Encourage adequate fluid intake. Monitor for signs/symptoms of vitamin D intoxication.

### PATIENT/FAMILY TEACHING

• Adequate calcium intake should be maintained. • Dietary phosphorus may need to be restricted (foods high in phosphorus include beans, dairy products, nuts, peas, whole-grain products). • Oral formulations may cause hypersensitivity reactions. Avoid excessive doses. • Report signs/symptoms of hypercalcemia (headache, weakness, drowsiness, nausea, vomiting, dry mouth, constipation, metallic taste, muscle or bone pain). • Maintain adequate hydration. • Avoid changes in diet or supplemental calcium intake (unless directed by health care professional). • Avoid magnesium-containing antacids in pts with renal failure.

---

## vorapaxar

vor-a-**pax**-ar
(Zontivity)

■ **BLACK BOX ALERT** ■ Avoid use in pts with history of CVA, intracranial hemorrhage (ICH), TIA or with active pathologic bleeding. Antiplatelet agents increase risk of bleeding, including ICH and fatal bleeding.

## ◆CLASSIFICATION

**PHARMACOTHERAPEUTIC:** Protease-activated receptor-1 antagonist. **CLINICAL:** Antiplatelet.

## USES

To reduce thrombotic cardiovascular events in pts with history of MI or peripheral artery disease (PAD). Reduces rate of a combined endpoint of cardiovascular death, CVA, MI, and urgent coronary revascularization.

## PRECAUTIONS

**Contraindications:** Hypersensitivity to vorapaxar. History of CVA, ICH, TIA; active bleeding. **Cautions:** Hepatic impairment, pts at increased risk of bleeding (anticoagulant use, elderly, low body weight, trauma) or with history of bleeding disorders.

## ACTION

Inhibits thrombin-induced and thrombin receptor agonist peptide (TRAP)–induced platelet aggregation. **Therapeutic Effect:** Inhibits platelet aggregation, reduces incidence of thrombus.

## PHARMACOKINETICS

Readily absorbed. Widely distributed. Metabolized in liver. Protein binding: greater than 99%. Peak plasma concentration: 1 hr. Steady state reached in 21 days. Eliminated in feces (58%), urine (25%). **Half-life:** 5–13 days.

## ⌛ LIFESPAN CONSIDERATIONS

**Pregnancy/Lactation:** Unknown if distributed in breast milk. **Children:** Safety and efficacy not established. **Elderly:** May have increased risk of bleeding.

## INTERACTIONS

**DRUG:** Aspirin, anticoagulants (e.g., warfarin), fibrinolytics (e.g., tissue plasminogen activator), NSAIDs, serotonin norepinephrine reuptake

V

---

inhibitors (e.g., **duloxetine**), SSRIs (e.g., **paroxetine**) may increase risk of bleeding. **Strong CYP3A4 inducers (e.g., rifampin)** may decrease concentration/effects; **CYP3A4 inhibitors (e.g., clarithromycin, ketoconazole)** may increase concentration/effects. **HERBAL:** St. John's wort may decrease concentration/effects. **FOOD:** None known. **LAB VALUES:** May decrease Hbg, Hct; serum iron.

## AVAILABILITY (Rx)

**Tablets:** 2.08 mg.

## ADMINISTRATION/HANDLING

**PO**
• Give without regard to meals.

## INDICATIONS/ROUTES/DOSAGE

**Reduction of Thrombotic Cardiovascular Events (Pts with PAD, MI)**
**PO: ADULTS, ELDERLY:** 2.08 mg once daily (in combination with aspirin and/or clopidogrel).

**Dosage in Renal Impairment**
No dose adjustment.

**Dosage in Hepatic Impairment**
**Mild to moderate impairment:** No dose adjustment.
**Severe impairment:** Not recommended.

## SIDE EFFECTS

**Rare (2%):** Depression, rash, skin eruptions, exanthemas.

## ADVERSE EFFECTS/ TOXIC REACTIONS

Hemorrhagic events (25% of pts) including fatal bleeding (less than 1%), GI bleeding (4%), ICH (less than 1%) have been reported. Vorapaxar increases risk of moderate to severe bleeding by 55%.

## NURSING CONSIDERATIONS

### BASELINE ASSESSMENT

Obtain baseline CBC, PFA level. Question history of CVA, intracranial hemorrhage (ICH), transient ischemic attack (TIA) (therapy contraindicated); anemia, bleeding ulcers, GI/genitourinary (GU) bleeding, recent surgery, spinal punctures, open wounds; hepatic impairment. Receive full medication history including herbal products.

### INTERVENTION/EVALUATION

Monitor CBC. Question for increased menstrual bleeding/discharge. Monitor for confusion, headache, hemiparesis, vision change (may indicate ICH); hematuria, GI bleeding. Assess peripheral pulses; skin for ecchymosis, petechiae. Check for excessive bleeding from minor cuts, scratches, skin tears. Consider transfusion of platelets or RBCs if severe bleeding occurs.

### PATIENT/FAMILY TEACHING

• It may take longer to stop bleeding.
• Bruising may occur more easily.
• Report unexpected, prolonged, excessive bleeding of any kind, or blood in sputum, stool, urine, or vomitus. • Avoid alcohol, over-the-counter anti-inflammatories such as aspirin, ibuprofen, or naproxen. • Consult doctor before any planned surgery, dental work. • Use electric razor, soft toothbrush to prevent bleeding. • Report confusion, headache, one-sided weakness, trouble speaking, or vision problems; may indicate life-threatening bleeding of brain.

# voriconazole

vor-i-**kon**-a-zole
(Vfend)
**Do not confuse voriconazole with fluconazole.**

## ◆CLASSIFICATION

**PHARMACOTHERAPEUTIC:** Triazole derivative. **CLINICAL:** Antifungal.

## USES

Treatment of invasive aspergillosis, esophageal candidiasis. Treatment of serious fungal infections caused by *Scedosporium apiospermum, Fusarium* spp. Treatment of candidemia in non-neutropenic pts. Treatment of disseminated *Candida* infections of skin and viscera. **OFF-LABEL:** Empiric treatment of fungal meningitis or osteoarticular, infections, coccidioidomycosis in HIV pts, fungal endophthalmitis, infection prophylaxis of graft vs host disease or pts with allogenic hematopoietic stem cell transplant.

## PRECAUTIONS

**Contraindications:** Hypersensitivity to voriconazole. Concurrent administration of carbamazepine, efavirenz (400 mg/day or greater), ergot alkaloids, pimozide, quinidine (may cause prolonged QT interval, torsades de pointes), rifabutin, rifampin, ritonavir (800 mg/day or greater), sirolimus, St. John's wort. **Cautions:** Severe renal/hepatic impairment, hypersensitivity to other azole antifungal agents. Pts at risk for acute pancreatitis, pts with fructose intolerance, glucose-galactose malabsorption; concomitant nephrotoxic medications; hypokalemia, hypomagnesemia, hypocalcemia. May prolong QT interval; use caution in pts with history of QT syndrome, concomitant medications that prolong QT interval, electrolyte imbalance.

## ACTION

Interferes with fungal cytochrome activity, decreasing ergosterol synthesis, inhibiting fungal cell membrane formation. **Therapeutic Effect:** Damages fungal cell wall membrane.

## PHARMACOKINETICS

Rapidly, completely absorbed after PO administration. Widely distributed. Protein binding: 58%. Metabolized in liver. Primarily excreted as metabolite in urine. **Half-life:** Variable, dose dependent.

## LIFESPAN CONSIDERATIONS

**Pregnancy/Lactation:** May cause fetal harm. **Children:** Safety and efficacy not established in pts younger than 12 yrs. **Elderly:** No age-related precautions noted.

## INTERACTIONS

**DRUG:** May increase concentration, risk of toxicity of **alprazolam, calcium channel blockers** (e.g., **diltiazem, verapamil**), **cyclosporine, efavirenz, ergot alkaloids, HMG-CoA reductase inhibitors** (e.g., **lovastatin**), **methadone, midazolam, protease inhibitors** (e.g., **amprenavir, saquinavir**), **rifabutin, sirolimus, tacrolimus, triazolam, warfarin. Carbamazepine, rifabutin, rifampin, ritonavir** may decrease concentration/effect. **HERBAL: St. John's wort** may significantly decrease concentration. **FOOD: Grapefruit products** may increase concentration. **LAB VALUES:** May increase serum alkaline phosphatase, ALT, AST, bilirubin, creatinine. May decrease potassium.

## AVAILABILITY (Rx)

**Injection, Powder for Reconstitution:** 200 mg. **Powder for Oral Suspension:** 200 mg/5 ml. **Tablets:** 50 mg, 200 mg.

## ADMINISTRATION/HANDLING

 **IV**

**Reconstitution** • Reconstitute 200-mg vial with 19 ml Sterile Water for Injection to provide concentration of 10 mg/ml. Further dilute with 0.9% NaCl or D$_5$W to provide concentration of 0.5–5 mg/ml. **Rate of Administration** • Infuse over 1–2 hrs at a rate not to exceed 3 mg/kg/hr. **Storage** • Store powder for injection at room temperature. • Use reconstituted solution immediately. • Do not use after 24 hrs when refrigerated.

### PO
• Give 1 hr before or 1 hr after a meal. • Do not mix oral suspension with any other medication or flavoring agent. • Shake suspension for about 10 sec before use.

## IV INCOMPATIBILITY

Tigecycline (Tygacil).

---

 Canadian trade name     Non-Crushable Drug     HIGH ALERT High Alert drug

## ❖ IV COMPATIBILITIES

Anidulafungin, caspofungin, ceftaroline, doripenem.

## INDICATIONS/ROUTES/DOSAGE

**Invasive Aspergillosis**
**IV: ADULTS, ELDERLY, CHILDREN 12 YRS AND OLDER:** Initially, 6 mg/kg q12h for 2 doses, then 4 mg/kg q12h, then oral maintenance dose. **(LESS THAN 40 KG):** 100 mg q12h (**maximum:** 300 mg/day). **(40 KG OR GREATER):** 200 mg q12h (**maximum:** 400 mg/day). **CHILDREN 3–11 YRS OF AGE: (HIV exposed):** Initially, 6–8 mg/kg (**maximum:** 400 mg) q12h for 2 doses, then 7 mg/kg (**maximum:** 200 mg) q12h. **(Non–HIV exposed):** 5–7 mg/kg/dose q12h.
**PO: (HIV exposed):** Initially, 8 mg/kg (**maximum:** 400 mg) q12h for 2 doses, then 7 mg/kg (**maximum:** 200 mg) q12h. **(Non–HIV exposed):** 9 mg/kg/dose q12h.

**Candidemia, Other Deep Tissue Candida Infections**
**IV: ADULTS, ELDERLY, CHILDREN 12 YRS AND OLDER:** Initially, 6 mg/kg q12h for 2 doses, then 3–4 mg/kg q12h, then oral maintenance dose. **LESS THAN 40 KG:** 100 mg q12h (**maximum:** 300 mg/day). **40 KG OR GREATER:** 200 mg q12h (**maximum:** 600 mg/day).

**Esophageal Candidiasis**
**PO: ADULTS, ELDERLY WEIGHING 40 KG OR MORE:** 200 mg q12h for minimum of 14 days, then at least 7 days following resolution of symptoms. **Maximum:** 600 mg/day. **ADULTS, ELDERLY WEIGHING LESS THAN 40 KG:** 100 mg q12h for minimum of 14 days, then at least 7 days following resolution of symptoms. **Maximum:** 300 mg/day.

**Dosage in Pts Receiving Phenytoin**
**IV:** Increase maintenance dose to 5 mg/kg q12h.
**PO:** Increase 200 mg q12h to 400 mg q12h (pts weighing 40 kg or more) or 100 mg q12h to 200 mg q12h (pts weighing less than 40 kg).

**Dosage in Pts Receiving Efavirenz**
Increase dose to 400 mg q12h and reduce efavirenz to 300 mg/day.

**Dosage in Renal Impairment**
No dose adjustment. IV dosing not recommended in pts with CrCl 50 ml/min or less.

**Dosage in Hepatic Impairment**
**Mild to moderate impairment:** Reduce maintenance dose by 50%.
**Severe impairment:** Use only if benefits outweigh risks. Monitor closely for toxicity.

## SIDE EFFECTS

**Frequent (20%–6%):** Abnormal vision, fever, nausea, rash, vomiting. **Occasional (5%–2%):** Headache, chills, hallucinations, photophobia, tachycardia, hypertension.

## ADVERSE EFFECTS/ TOXIC REACTIONS

Hepatotoxicity (jaundice, hepatitis, hepatic failure), acute renal failure have occurred in severely ill pts.

## NURSING CONSIDERATIONS

### BASELINE ASSESSMENT

Obtain baseline serum hepatic/renal function tests. Receive full medication history and screen for interactions. Question medical history as listed in Precautions.

### INTERVENTION/EVALUATION

Monitor serum renal function, LFT. Monitor visual function (visual acuity, visual field, color perception) for drug therapy lasting longer than 28 days.

### PATIENT/FAMILY TEACHING

• Take at least 1 hr before or 1 hr after a meal. • Avoid grapefruit products. • Avoid driving at night. • Report visual changes (blurred vision, photophobia, yellowing of skin/eyes). • Avoid performing hazardous tasks if changes in vision occur. • Avoid direct sunlight. • Women of childbearing potential should use effective contraception.

# vorinostat

vor-**in**-o-stat
(Zolinza)
**Do not confuse vorinostat with Votrient.**

## ◆CLASSIFICATION

**PHARMACOTHERAPEUTIC:** Histone deacetylase inhibitor. **CLINICAL:** Antineoplastic.

## USES

Treatment of cutaneous manifestations in pts with cutaneous T-cell lymphoma (CTCL) with progressive, persistent, or recurrent disease, on or following two systemic therapies.

## PRECAUTIONS

**Contraindications:** Hypersensitivity to vorinostat. **Cautions:** History of deep vein thrombosis (DVT), diabetes mellitus, hepatic impairment, preexisting hypokalemia, hypomagnesemia, pts with history of QT prolongation or medications that prolong QT interval. Use caution during perioperative period in pts requiring bowel surgery.

## ACTION

Inhibits activity of histone deacetylase enzymes that catalyze removal of acetyl groups of proteins, causing accumulation of acetylated histones. **Therapeutic Effect:** Terminates cell growth, causes apoptosis.

## PHARMACOKINETICS

Protein binding: 71%. Metabolized to inactive metabolites. Excreted in urine. **Half-life:** 2 hrs.

## LIFESPAN CONSIDERATIONS

**Pregnancy/Lactation:** May cause fetal harm. Unknown if distributed in breast milk. **Children:** Safety and efficacy not established. **Elderly:** No age-related precautions noted.

## INTERACTIONS

**DRUG:** May increase effect of **warfarin. Valproic acid** increases risk of GI bleeding, thrombocytopenia. **HERBAL:** None significant. **FOOD:** None known. **LAB VALUES:** May decrease serum calcium, potassium, sodium, phosphate, platelet count. May increase serum glucose, creatinine; urine protein.

## AVAILABILITY (Rx)

Capsules: 100 mg.

## ADMINISTRATION/HANDLING

**PO**
• Do not break, crush, dissolve, or divide capsules. • Give with food. • Maintain adequate hydration during treatment.

## INDICATIONS/ROUTES/DOSAGE

**Cutaneous T-Cell Lymphoma (CTCL)**
**PO: ADULTS, ELDERLY:** 400 mg once daily with food. Continue until disease progression or unacceptible toxicity. Dosage adjustment for toxicity: Dose may be reduced to 300 mg once daily with food. May be further reduced to 300 mg once daily with food for 5 consecutive days each wk.

**Dosage in Renal Impairment**
Use caution.

**Dosage in Hepatic Impairment**
**Mild to moderate impairment:** 300 mg once daily.
**Severe impairment:** 100–200 mg once daily.

## SIDE EFFECTS

**Frequent (50%–24%):** Fatigue, diarrhea, nausea, altered taste, anorexia. **Occasional (21%–11%):** Weight decrease, muscle spasms, alopecia, dry mouth, chills, vomiting, constipation, dizziness, peripheral edema, headache, pruritus, cough, fever.

## ADVERSE EFFECTS/ TOXIC REACTIONS

Thrombocytopenia occurs in 25% of pts, anemia in 15%. Pulmonary embolism occurs in 4% of pts. Deep vein thrombosis (DVT) occurs rarely.

## NURSING CONSIDERATIONS

### BASELINE ASSESSMENT

Baseline PT, INR, CBC, serum chemistry tests, esp. serum potassium, calcium, magnesium, glucose, creatinine should be obtained prior to therapy and every 2 wks during first 2 mos of therapy and monthly thereafter. Inform women of childbearing potential of risk to fetus if pregnancy occurs.

### INTERVENTION/EVALUATION

Monitor CBC, serum electrolytes; PT/INR q2wks for 2 mos, then monthly. Monitor signs/symptoms of DVT. Encourage fluid intake, approximately 2 L/day input. Assess for evidence of dehydration. Provide antiemetics to control nausea/vomiting. Monitor daily pattern of bowel activity, stool consistency.

### PATIENT/FAMILY TEACHING

• Drink at least 2 L/day of fluids to prevent dehydration. • Report persistent vomiting, diarrhea. • Report shortness of breath, pain in any extremity.

---

# vortioxetene

vor-tye-**ox**-e-teen
(Trintellix)
**Do not confuse vortioxetene with fluoxetine, paroxetine, or venlafaxine.**

■ **BLACK BOX ALERT** ■ Antidepressants have an increased risk of suicidal ideation and behavior in children, adolescents, and young adults. Monitor closely for worsening or emergence of suicidal thoughts and behaviors.

## ◆CLASSIFICATION

**PHARMACOTHERAPEUTIC:** Selective serotonin reuptake inhibitor (SSRI). **CLINICAL:** Antidepressant.

## USES

Treatment of major depressive disorder.

## PRECAUTIONS

**Contraindications:** Hypersensitivity to vortioxetene. Monoamine oxidase inhibitors (MAOIs). Do not use MAOIs within 21 days of stopping vortioxetene; do not use vortioxetene within 14 days of stopping an MAOI. Concomitant use of linezolid or intravenous methylene blue. **Cautions:** History of angioedema, dehydration, hyponatremia, pts at risk for bleeding, elderly, pts at high risk of suicide; family history of bipolar disorder, mania, hypomania; hepatic impairment, seizure disorder, elderly.

## ACTION

Blocks reuptake of neurotransmitter serotonin at CNS presynaptic membranes, increasing availability at postsynaptic receptor sites. **Therapeutic Effect:** Relieves depression.

## PHARMACOKINETICS

Readily absorbed following PO administration. Metabolized in liver, primarily through oxidation. Protein binding: 98%. Peak plasma concentration: 7–11 hrs. Steady state reached within 2 wks. Excreted in urine (59%), feces (26%). **Half-life:** 66 hrs.

## ⏳ LIFESPAN CONSIDERATIONS

**Pregnancy/Lactation:** May cause fetal harm when administered in third trimester. Unknown if distributed in breast milk. Exposed neonates are at increased risk of apnea, cyanosis, prolonged hospitalization, pulmonary hypertension,

V

seizures, serotonin syndrome. **Children:** Safety and efficacy not established in pediatric population. **Elderly:** May have increased risk of dehydration, hyponatremia.

## INTERACTIONS

**DRUG: Strong CYP inducers (e.g., carbamazepine, phenytoin, rifampin)** may decrease concentration/effects. **Strong CYP2D6 inhibitors (e.g., bupropion, fluoxetine, paroxetine)** may increase concentration/effect. **MAOIs** contraindicated; may cause malignant hyperthermia, hypertensive crisis, hyperreflexia, seizures, serotonin syndrome. **Serotonergic drugs (e.g., buspirone, fentanyl, linezolid, tramadol, tricyclic antidepressants, triptans)** may increase risk of serotonin syndrome. **Anticoagulants, antiplatelets, NSAIDs** may increase risk of bleeding. **Diuretics** may increase risk of hyponatremia. **HERBAL: St. John's wort** may increase risk of serotonin syndrome. **FOOD:** None known. **LAB VALUES:** May decrease serum sodium.

## AVAILABILITY (Rx)

**Tablets:** 5 mg, 10 mg, 20 mg.

## ADMINISTRATION/HANDLING

**PO**
• Give without regard to meals. May administer with milk or food if GI upset occurs.

## INDICATIONS/ROUTES/DOSAGE

**Major Depressive Disorder**
**PO: ADULTS/ELDERLY:** Initially, 10 mg once daily. May increase to 20 mg as tolerated. **Maintenance:** 5–20 mg once daily.

**Dose Modification**
**Concomitant Use of Strong CYP2D6 Inhibitors:** Reduce dose by half of intended therapy. **Maximum:** 10 mg once daily. **Concomitant Use of Strong CYP Inducers:** If co-administered for more than 14 days, consider increasing vortioxetene dose. **Maximum:** Do not exceed more than 3 times original dose. **CYP2D6 poor metabolizers: Maximum:** 10 mg once daily.

**Dosage in Renal Impairment**
No dose adjustment.

**Dosage in Hepatic Impairment**
**Mild to moderate impairment:** No dose adjustment. **Severe impairment:** Not recommended.

## SIDE EFFECTS

**Frequent (32%–22%):** Nausea, sexual dysfunction. **Occasional (10%–3%):** Diarrhea, dizziness, dry mouth, constipation, vomiting, flatulence, abnormal dreams, pruritus.

## ADVERSE EFFECTS/ TOXIC REACTIONS

Life-threatening serotonin syndrome may include mental status changes (agitation, hallucinations, delirium, coma), autonomic instability (tachycardia, labile blood pressure, dizziness, sweating, flushing, hyperthermia), neuromuscular symptoms (tremor, rigidity, myoclonus [localized muscle twitching], hyperactive reflexes, incoordination), seizures, GI symptoms (nausea, vomiting, diarrhea). May increase risk of bleeding events such as ecchymosis, hematoma, epistaxis (nosebleed), petechiae. Mania/hypomania may indicate baseline bipolar disorder. Syndrome of inappropriate antidiuretic hormone (SIADH), also known as water intoxication or dilutional hyponatremia, may induce seizures, coma, or death. Angioedema, dyspnea, rash may indicate allergic reaction. May increase risk of suicidal ideation and behavior once treatment is therapeutic. May alter sexual drive, ease of arousal, ease of reaching orgasm, or cause erectile dysfunction in men or decreased lubrication in women.

V

## NURSING CONSIDERATIONS

### BASELINE ASSESSMENT

Obtain baseline electrolytes. Note serum sodium level. Assess appearance, behavior, speech pattern, level of interest, mood. Screen for history of bipolar disorder, bleeding events, SIADH, prior allergic reactions to drug class. Receive full medication history including herbal products.

### INTERVENTION/EVALUATION

Monitor serum sodium levels. Screen for signs of SIADH (confusion, seizures). Offer emotional support. Assess mental status for depression, suicidal ideation (esp. during first few mo of therapy or with dosage change), anxiety, social function. Monitor daily pattern of bowel activity, stool consistency. Assist with ambulation if dizziness occurs. Monitor pt for symptoms of serotonin syndrome, mania/hypomania. Offer antiemetic for nausea, vomiting. Monitor for allergic reactions.

### PATIENT/FAMILY TEACHING

• Dry mouth may be relieved with sugarless gum, sips of water. • Report neurologic changes: confusion, excessive talking, hallucinations, headache, hyperactivity, insomnia, racing thoughts, seizure-like activity, tremors; sexual dysfunction; fever; or any type of allergic reaction • Avoid tasks that require alertness, motor skills until response to drug is established (may cause dizziness, drowsiness). • Take with food if nausea occurs. • Report pregnancy. • Avoid alcohol. • Do not take OTC medications such as aspirin or ibuprofen without consulting physician. • Immediately report thoughts of suicide, self-destructive behavior, or violence. • Sexual dysfunction such as inability to reach orgasm, difficulty maintaining an erection, or lack of sexual drive may occur.

V

# warfarin

 TOP 100 · HIGH ALERT

war·far·in
(Apo-Warfarin ✦, Coumadin, Jantoven, Novo-Warfarin ✦)

■ **BLACK BOX ALERT** ■ May cause major or fatal bleeding. Risk factors include history of GI bleeding, hypertension, cerebrovascular disease, heart disease, malignancy, trauma, anemia, renal insufficiency, age 65 yrs and older, high anticoagulation factor (INR greater than 4). Consider cardiac/hepatic function, age, nutritional status, concurrent medications, risk of bleeding when dosing warfarin. Genetic variations have been identified as factors associated with dosage and bleeding risk. Genotyping tests are available.

**Do not confuse Coumadin with Kemadrin, or Jantoven with Janumet or Januvia.**

## ◆CLASSIFICATION

**PHARMACOTHERAPEUTIC:** Coumarin derivative. **CLINICAL:** Anticoagulant.

## USES

Prophylaxis, treatment of thromboembolic disorders and embolic complications arising from atrial fibrillation or valve replacement. Risk reduction of systemic embolism following MI (e.g., recurrent MI, stroke). **OFF-LABEL:** Adjunct treatment in transient ischemic attacks.

## PRECAUTIONS

**Contraindications:** Hypersensitivity to warfarin. Hemorrhagic tendencies (e.g., cerebral aneurysms, bleeding from GI tract), recent or potential surgery of eye or CNS, neurosurgical procedures, open wounds, severe uncontrolled or malignant hypertension, spinal puncture procedures, uncontrolled bleeding, ulcers, unreliable or noncompliant pts, unsupervised pts, blood dyscrasias, pericarditis or pericardial effusion, pregnancy (except in women with mechanical heart valves at high risk for thromboembolism), bacterial endocarditis, threatened abortion. Major regional lumbar block anesthesia or traumatic surgery, eclampsia/preeclampsia. **Cautions:** Active tuberculosis, acute infection, diabetes, heparin-induced thrombocytopenia and deep vein thrombosis, pts at risk for hemorrhage, moderate to severe renal impairment, moderate to severe hypertension, thyroid disease, polycythemia vera, vasculitis, open wound, menstruating and postpartum women, indwelling catheters, trauma, prolonged dietary deficiencies, disruption of GI normal flora, history of peptic ulcer disease, protein C deficiency, elderly.

## ACTION

Interferes with hepatic synthesis of vitamin K–dependent clotting factors, resulting in depletion of coagulation factors II, VII, IX, X. **Therapeutic Effect:** Prevents further extension of formed existing clot; prevents new clot formation, secondary thromboembolic complications.

## PHARMACOKINETICS

| Route | Onset | Peak | Duration |
|-------|-------|------|----------|
| PO | 1.5–3 days | 5–7 days | 2–5 days |

Well absorbed from GI tract. Protein binding: 99%. Metabolized in liver. Primarily excreted in urine. Not removed by hemodialysis. **Half-life:** 20–60 hrs.

## ⧗ LIFESPAN CONSIDERATIONS

**Pregnancy/Lactation:** Contraindicated in pregnancy (fetal, neonatal hemorrhage, intrauterine death). Crosses placenta; distributed in breast milk. **Children:** More susceptible to effect. **Elderly:** Increased risk of hemorrhage; lower dosage recommended.

## INTERACTIONS

**DRUG: Amiodarone, azole antifungals, cimetidine, disulfiram, fluvoxamine, sulfamethoxazole-trimethoprim, levothyroxine, metronidazole, NSAIDs,**

W

omeprazole, platelet aggregation inhibitors (e.g., clopidogrel), salicylates (e.g., aspirin), thrombolytic agents (e.g., alteplase), thyroid hormones may increase effect. Griseofulvin, hepatic enzyme inducers (e.g., rifampin), vitamin K may decrease effects. Alcohol may enhance anticoagulant effect. HERBAL: Cat's claw, dong quai, evening primrose, feverfew, garlic, ginger, ginkgo biloba, ginseng possess antiplatelet activity, may increase risk of bleeding. Ginseng, St. John's wort may decrease effect. FOOD: None known. LAB VALUES: None known.

## AVAILABILITY (Rx)

Tablets (Coumadin, Jantoven): 1 mg, 2 mg, 2.5 mg, 3 mg, 4 mg, 5 mg, 6 mg, 7.5 mg, 10 mg.

## ADMINISTRATION/HANDLING

### PO

• Give without regard to food. Give with food if GI upset occurs. • Give at same time each day.

## INDICATIONS/ROUTES/DOSAGE

◀ALERT▶ Initial dosing must be individualized.

### Anticoagulant

PO: ADULTS, ELDERLY: Initially, 2–5 mg/daily for 2 days OR 5–10 mg daily for 1–2 days, adjusting the dose based on INR results. Usual maintenance dose: 2–10 mg/day, but may vary outside these guidelines. CHILDREN: Initially, 0.05–0.2 mg/kg/day. Maximum: 10 mg. Maintenance: Adjust based on INR.

### Dosage in Renal/Hepatic Impairment

No dose adjustment. Closely monitor INR.

## SIDE EFFECTS

Occasional: GI distress (nausea, anorexia, abdominal cramps, diarrhea). Rare: Hypersensitivity reaction (dermatitis, urticaria), esp. in those sensitive to aspirin.

## ADVERSE EFFECTS/TOXIC REACTIONS

Bleeding complications ranging from local ecchymoses to major hemorrhage may occur. Antidote: Vitamin K. Amount based on INR, significance of bleeding. Range: 2.5–10 mg given orally or slow IV infusion (see Appendix J for dosage). Hepatotoxicity, blood dyscrasias, necrosis, vasculitis, local thrombosis occur rarely.

## NURSING CONSIDERATIONS

### BASELINE ASSESSMENT

Cross-check dose with coworker. Obtain CBC, PT/INR before administration and daily following therapy initiation. When stabilized, follow with INR determination q4–6wks. Obtain genotyping prior to initiating therapy if available.

### INTERVENTION/EVALUATION

Monitor INR diligently. Assess CBC for anemia; urine/stool for occult blood. Be alert to complaints of abdominal/back pain, severe headache, confusion, seizures, hemiparesis, aphasia (may be sign of hemorrhage). Decrease in B/P, increase in pulse rate may be sign of hemorrhage. Question for increase in amount of menstrual discharge. Assess peripheral pulses; skin for ecchymoses, petechiae. Check for excessive bleeding from minor cuts, scratches. Assess gums for erythema, gingival bleeding.

### PATIENT/ FAMILY TEACHING

• Take medication at same time each day. • Blood levels will be monitored routinely. • Do not take, discontinue any other medication except on advice of physician. • Avoid alcohol, aspirin, drastic dietary changes. • Consult with physician before surgery, dental work. • Urine may become red-orange.

W

• Avoid, minimize significant bodily trauma. • Report bleeding, bruising, red or brown urine, black stools. • Use electric razor, soft toothbrush to prevent bleeding. • Report coffee-ground vomitus, blood-tinged mucus from cough. • Do not use any OTC medication without physician approval (may interfere with platelet aggregation). • Seek immediate medical attention for stroke–like symptoms (confusion, difficulty speaking, headache, one-sided weakness); bloody stool or urine.

W

# zafirlukast

za-**fir**-loo-kast
(Accolate)
**Do not confuse Accolate
with Accupril, Accutane, or
Aclovate.**

## ◆CLASSIFICATION

**PHARMACOTHERAPEUTIC:** Leukotriene receptor antagonist. **CLINICAL:** Antiasthma.

## USES

Prophylaxis, chronic treatment of bronchial asthma in adults and children 5 yrs and older.

## PRECAUTIONS

**Contraindications:** Hypersensitivity to zafirlukast. Hepatic impairment. **Cautions:** Elderly. Not approved for acute asthma attacks, status asthmaticus.

## ACTION

Competitive antagonist of leukotriene receptor. Leukotriene production and receptor occupation are associated with pathophysiology of asthma. **Therapeutic Effect:** Reduces airway edema, smooth muscle constriction; alters cellular activity associated with inflammatory process. Reduces signs/symptoms of asthma.

## PHARMACOKINETICS

Rapidly absorbed after PO administration (food reduces absorption). Protein binding: 99%. Metabolized in liver. Primarily excreted in feces. Unknown if removed by hemodialysis. **Half-life:** 10 hrs.

## ☒ LIFESPAN CONSIDERATIONS

**Pregnancy/Lactation:** Drug is distributed in breast milk. Do not administer to breastfeeding women. **Children:** Safety and efficacy not established in pts younger than 5 yrs. **Elderly:** No age-related precautions noted.

## INTERACTIONS

**DRUG: Erythromycin, theophylline** may decrease concentration/effect. **Aspirin** may increase concentration/effects. May increase effects of **warfarin** (increases INR). **HERBAL:** None significant. **FOOD: Food** decreases bioavailability by 40%. **LAB VALUES:** None significant.

## AVAILABILITY (Rx)

**Tablets:** 10 mg, 20 mg.

## ADMINISTRATION/HANDLING

**PO**
• Give 1 hr before or 2 hrs after meals.

## INDICATIONS/ROUTES/DOSAGE

**Bronchial Asthma**
**PO: ADULTS, ELDERLY, CHILDREN 12 YRS AND OLDER:** 20 mg twice daily. **CHILDREN 5–11 YRS:** 10 mg twice daily.

**Dosage in Renal Impairment**
No dose adjustment.

**Dosage in Hepatic Impairment**
Contraindicated.

## SIDE EFFECTS

**Frequent (13%):** Headache. **Occasional (3%):** Nausea, diarrhea. **Rare (Less Than 3%):** Generalized pain, asthenia, myalgia, fever, dyspepsia, vomiting, dizziness.

## ADVERSE EFFECTS/
## TOXIC REACTIONS

Concurrent administration of inhaled corticosteroids increases risk of upper respiratory tract infection.

## NURSING CONSIDERATIONS

**BASELINE ASSESSMENT**
Obtain medication history. Assess LFT.

**INTERVENTION/EVALUATION**
Monitor rate, depth, rhythm, type of respiration; quality, rate of pulse. Assess lung sounds for rhonchi, wheezing, rales. Monitor LFT.

## PATIENT/FAMILY TEACHING

• Increase fluid intake (decreases lung secretion viscosity). • Take as prescribed, even during symptom-free periods. • Do not use for acute asthma episodes. • Do not alter, stop other asthma medications. • Do not breastfeed. • Report nausea, jaundice, abdominal pain, flu-like symptoms, worsening of asthma.

# zanamivir

zan-**am**-i-veer
(Relenza Diskhaler)

## ◆CLASSIFICATION

**PHARMACOTHERAPEUTIC:** Antiviral. **CLINICAL:** Antiviral, anti-influenza.

## USES

Treatment of uncomplicated acute illness due to influenza virus A and B in adults, children 7 yrs and older who have been symptomatic for less than 2 days. Prevention of influenza A and B in adults and children 5 yrs and older.

## PRECAUTIONS

**Contraindications:** Hypersensitivity to zanamivir. **Cautions:** Not recommended in respiratory disease (e.g., COPD, asthma), renal/hepatic impairment.

## ACTION

Inhibits influenza virus enzyme neuraminidase, essential for viral replication. **Therapeutic Effect:** Prevents viral release from infected cells.

## PHARMACOKINETICS

Systemically absorbed, approximately 4%–17%. Protein binding: less than 10%. Not metabolized. Excreted unchanged in urine. **Half-life:** 2.5–5.1 hrs.

## ⏳ LIFESPAN CONSIDERATIONS

**Pregnancy/Lactation:** Unknown if drug crosses placenta or is distributed in breast milk. **Children:** Safety and efficacy not established in pts younger than 7 yrs. **Elderly:** No age-related precautions noted.

## INTERACTIONS

**DRUG:** None significant. **HERBAL:** None significant. **FOOD:** None known. **LAB VALUES:** None significant.

## AVAILABILITY (Rx)

**Powder for Inhalation:** 5 mg/blister.

## ADMINISTRATION/HANDLING

**Inhalation**

• Instruct pt to use Diskhaler device provided, exhale completely; then, holding mouthpiece 1 inch away from lips, inhale and hold breath as long as possible before exhaling. • Rinse mouth with water immediately after inhalation (prevents mouth/throat dryness). • Store at room temperature.

## INDICATIONS/ROUTES/DOSAGE

**Treatment of Influenza Virus**
**Inhalation: ADULTS, ELDERLY, CHILDREN 7 YRS AND OLDER:** 2 inhalations (one 5-mg blister per inhalation for total dose of 10 mg) twice daily (approximately 12 hrs apart) for 5 days.

**Prevention of Influenza Virus**
**Inhalation: ADULTS, ELDERLY, CHILDREN 5 YRS AND OLDER:** 2 inhalations (10 mg) once daily for duration of exposure period (10 days for household exposure, 28 days for community exposure).

**Dosage in Renal/Hepatic Impairment**
No dose adjustment.

## SIDE EFFECTS

**Occasional (3%–2%):** Diarrhea, sinusitis, nausea, bronchitis, cough, dizziness, headache. **Rare (Less Than 1.5%):** Malaise, fatigue, fever, abdominal pain, myalgia, arthralgia, urticaria.

## ADVERSE EFFECTS/ TOXIC REACTIONS

May produce neutropenia. Broncho-spasm may occur in those with history of COPD, bronchial asthma.

## NURSING CONSIDERATIONS

### BASELINE ASSESSMENT

Pts requiring an inhaled bronchodilator at same time as zanamivir should use the bronchodilator before zanamivir administration.

### INTERVENTION/EVALUATION

Provide assistance if dizziness occurs. Monitor daily pattern of bowel activity, stool consistency.

### PATIENT/FAMILY TEACHING

• Follow manufacturer guidelines for use of delivery device. • Avoid contact with those who are at high risk for influenza. • Continue treatment for full 5-day course. • Doses should be evenly spaced. • In pts with respiratory disease, an inhaled bronchodilator should be readily available.

## zidovudine

zye-**doe**-vue-deen
(Apo-Zidovudine ✤, Novo-AZT ✤, Retrovir)

■ **BLACK BOX ALERT** ■ Neutropenia, severe anemia may occur. Lactic acidosis, severe hepatomegaly with steatosis (fatty liver), including fatalities, have occurred. Symptomatic myopathy, myositis associated with prolonged use.

**Do not confuse Retrovir with acyclovir or ritonavir.**

### FIXED-COMBINATION(S)

**Combivir:** zidovudine/lamivudine (an antiviral): 300 mg/150 mg. **Trizivir:** zidovudine/lamivudine/abacavir (an antiviral): 300 mg/150 mg/300 mg.

## ◆CLASSIFICATION

**PHARMACOTHERAPEUTIC:** Nucleoside reverse transcriptase inhibitors. **CLINICAL:** Antiretroviral.

## USES

Treatment of HIV infection in combination with at least two other antiretroviral agents. Prevention of maternal/fetal HIV transmission. **OFF-LABEL:** Prophylaxis in health care workers at risk for acquiring HIV after occupational exposure (part of multi–drug regimen).

## PRECAUTIONS

**Contraindications:** Potentially life-threatening allergic reactions to zidovudine or its components. **Cautions:** Bone marrow compromise, renal/hepatic dysfunction. Combination with interferon with or without ribavirin in HIV/hepatitis C virus (HCV) co-infection.

## ACTION

Interferes with viral RNA-dependent DNA polymerase, an enzyme necessary for viral HIV replication. **Therapeutic Effect:** Slows HIV replication, reducing progression of HIV infection.

## PHARMACOKINETICS

Rapidly, completely absorbed from GI tract. Protein binding: 25%–38%. Metabolized in liver. Crosses blood-brain barrier and is widely distributed, including to CSF. Primarily excreted in urine. Minimal removal by hemodialysis. **Half-life:** 0.5–3 hrs (increased in renal impairment).

## ▧ LIFESPAN CONSIDERATIONS

**Pregnancy/Lactation:** Unknown if drug crosses placenta or distributed in breast milk. Unknown if fetal harm or effects on fertility can occur. **Children:** No age-related precautions noted. **Elderly:** Information not available.

## INTERACTIONS

**DRUG:** **Bone marrow depressants, ganciclovir** may increase myelosuppression. May be antagonistic with **doxorubicin.** Hematologic toxicities may occur with **interferon alfa.** **HERBAL:** None significant. **FOOD:** None known. **LAB VALUES:** May increase mean corpuscular volume (MCV).

## AVAILABILITY (Rx)

Capsules (Retrovir): 100 mg. Injection Solution (Retrovir): 10 mg/ml. Syrup (Retrovir): 50 mg/5 ml. Tablets: 300 mg.

## ADMINISTRATION/HANDLING

 IV

**Reconstitution** • Must dilute before administration. • Remove calculated dose from vial and add to $D_5W$ to provide concentration no greater than 4 mg/ml.
**Rate of Administration** • Infuse over 1 hr. May infuse over 30 min in neonates.
**Storage** • After dilution, IV solution is stable for 24 hrs at room temperature; 48 hrs if refrigerated. • Use within 8 hrs if stored at room temperature or 24 hrs if refrigerated to minimize potential for microbial-contaminated solution. • Do not use if solution is discolored or precipitate forms.

### PO

• Keep capsules in cool, dry place. Protect from light. • May administer without regard to food. • Space doses evenly around the clock. • Pt should maintain an upright position when given medication to prevent esophageal ulceration.

### ⊞ IV INCOMPATIBILITIES

None known.

### ⊞ IV COMPATIBILITIES

Dexamethasone (Decadron), dobutamine (Dobutrex), dopamine (Intropin), heparin, lorazepam (Ativan), morphine, potassium chloride.

## INDICATIONS/ROUTES/DOSAGE

### HIV Infection

**PO: ADULTS, ELDERLY:** 300 mg q12h. **CHILDREN 4 WKS TO 18 YRS WEIGHING 30 KG OR MORE:** 300 mg q12h. **WEIGHING 9–29 KG:** 9 mg/kg q12h. **WEIGHING 4–8 KG:** 12 mg/kg q12h. **PREMATURE NEONATES, GA 35 WKS OR GREATER:** 4 mg/kg q12h, increase to 12 mg/kg q12h after 4 wks of age. **GA 30–34 WKS:** 2 mg/kg q12h for 2 wks, then 3 mg/kg q12h, then 12 mg/kg q12h after 6-8 wks. **GA LESS THAN 30 WKS:** 2 mg/kg q12h, then 3 mg/kg q12h at 4 wks of age, then 12 mg/kg q12h after 8–10 wks of age.
**IV: ADULTS, ELDERLY, CHILDREN OLDER THAN 12 YRS:** 1 mg/kg/dose q4h around the clock. **CHILDREN 12 YRS AND YOUNGER: FULL-TERM NEONATES:** 3 mg/kg/dose q12h. **PREMATURE NEONATES:** 1.5–2.3 mg/kg/dose q12h based on gestation at birth.

### Prevention of Maternal/Fetal HIV Transmission

**PO: ADULTS:** 300 mg 2 times/day. Begin at 14–34 wks' gestation and continue until start of labor.
**IV** *(During Labor and Delivery):* 2 mg/kg loading dose, then IV infusion of 1 mg/kg/hr until delivery. **NEONATAL:** Begin 6–12 hrs after birth and continue for first 6 wks of life. Use IV route only until oral therapy can be administered.
**PO: FULL-TERM INFANTS:** 4 mg/kg/dose q12h (IV: 3 mg/kg/dose q12h). **INFANTS 30–34 WKS' GESTATION:** 2 mg/kg/dose q12h; increase to 3 mg/kg/dose at 2 wks of age (IV: 1.5 mg/kg/dose q12h; increase to 2.3 mg/kg/dose q12h at 2 wks of age). **INFANTS LESS THAN 30 WKS' GESTATION:** 2 mg/kg/dose q12h; increase to 3 mg/kg/dose q12h at 4 wks of age (IV: 1.5 mg/kg/dose q12h; increase to 2.3 mg/kg/dose q12h at 4 wks of age).

### Dosage in Renal Impairment

**ADULTS, ELDERLY: CrCl less than 15 ml/min, including hemodialysis or peritoneal dialysis: PO:** 100 mg q8h or 300 mg once daily. **IV:** 1 mg/kg q6–8hr.

---

**INFANTS OLDER THAN 6 WKS, CHILDREN, ADOLESCENTS: GFR 10 ml/min/1.73m² or greater:** No adjustment. **GFR less than10 ml/min/1.73m²:** Administer 50% of dose q8h.

**Dosage in Hepatic Impairment**
No dose adjustment.

## SIDE EFFECTS

**Expected (46%–42%):** Nausea, headache. **Frequent (20%–16%):** Abdominal pain, asthenia, rash, fever, acne. **Occasional (12%–8%):** Diarrhea, anorexia, malaise, myalgia, drowsiness. **Rare (6%–5%):** Dizziness, paresthesia, vomiting, insomnia, dyspnea, altered taste.

## ADVERSE EFFECTS/ TOXIC REACTIONS

Anemia (occurring most commonly after 4–6 wks of therapy), granulocytopenia are particularly significant in pts with pretherapy low baselines. Neurotoxicity (ataxia, fatigue, lethargy, nystagmus, seizures) may occur.

## NURSING CONSIDERATIONS

### BASELINE ASSESSMENT

Avoid drugs that are nephrotoxic, cytotoxic, myelosuppressive; may increase risk of toxicity. Obtain specimens for viral diagnostic tests before starting therapy (therapy may begin before results are obtained). Check hematology reports for accurate baseline.

### INTERVENTION/EVALUATION

Monitor CBC, reticulocyte count, CD4 cell count, HIV RNA plasma levels. Check for bleeding. Assess for headache, dizziness. Monitor daily pattern of bowel activity, stool consistency. Evaluate skin for acne, rash. Be alert to development of opportunistic infections (fever, chills, cough, myalgia). Monitor I&O, serum renal function, LFT. Check for insomnia.

### PATIENT/FAMILY TEACHING

• Doses should be evenly spaced around the clock. • Zidovudine is not a cure for HIV infection, nor does it reduce risk of transmission to others. Acts to reduce symptoms and slows or arrests progress of disease. • Do not take any medications without physician's approval. • Bleeding from gums, nose, rectum may occur and should be reported to physician immediately. • Blood counts are essential because of bleeding potential. • Dental work should be done before therapy or after blood counts return to normal (often wks after therapy has stopped). • Inform physician if muscle weakness, difficulty breathing, headache, inability to sleep, unusual bleeding, rash, signs of infection occur.

# ziprasidone

zi-**prah**-si-done
(Geodon, Zeldox ✦)
■ **BLACK BOX ALERT** ■ Increased risk of mortality in elderly pts with dementia-related psychosis, mainly due to pneumonia, HF.
**Do not confuse Ziprasidone with trazodone.**

## ◆CLASSIFICATION

**PHARMACOTHERAPEUTIC:** Piperazine derivative. **CLINICAL:** Antipsychotic.

## USES

Treatment of schizophrenia, acute agitation in pts with schizophrenia. Treatment of acute mania or mixed episodes associated with bipolar disorder with or without psychosis. Maintenance treatment of bipolar disorder as adjunct to lithium or valproic acid. **OFF-LABEL:** Psychosis/agitation related to Alzheimer's dementia.

## PRECAUTIONS

**Contraindications:** Hypersensitivity to ziprasidone. Conditions associated with risk of prolonged QT interval, congenital long QT syndrome, concurrent use of other QT prolongation medications (e.g., class IA and III antiarrhythmics, moxifloxacin, tacrolimus, thioridazine). Uncompensated HF. Recent MI. **Cautions:** Pts with bradycardia, hypokalemia, hypomagnesemia may be at greater risk for torsades de pointes. History of MI or unstable heart disease, seizures, cardiac arrhythmias, disorders where CNS depression is a feature, elderly; pts at risk for aspiration pneumonia, hepatic impairment, pts at high risk for suicide, hypotensive episodes, breast cancer, or other prolactin-dependent tumors, Parkinson's disease, diabetes. History of cardiac arrhythmias, disorders where CNS depression is a feature; elderly.

## ACTION

Exact mechanism unknown. Antagonizes alpha-adrenergic, dopamine, histamine, serotonin receptors; inhibits reuptake of serotonin, norepinephrine. **Therapeutic Effect:** Diminishes symptoms of schizophrenia, depression.

## PHARMACOKINETICS

Well absorbed after PO administration. Food increases bioavailability. Protein binding: 99%. Metabolized in liver. Eliminated in feces. Not removed by hemodialysis. **Half-life: PO:** 7 hrs; **IM:** 2–5 hrs.

## ⧗ LIFESPAN CONSIDERATIONS

**Pregnancy/Lactation:** Unknown if drug crosses placenta or is distributed in breast milk. **Children:** Safety and efficacy not established. **Elderly:** No age-related precautions noted.

## INTERACTIONS

**DRUG: Alcohol, other CNS depressants (e.g., lorazepam, morphine, zolpidem)** may increase CNS depression. **Carbamazepine** may decrease concentration.

**Ketoconazole** may increase concentration. **Medications causing prolongation of QT interval (e.g., amiodarone, dofetilide, haloperidol, sotalol)** may increase effects on cardiac conduction leading to malignant arrhythmias (e.g., torsades de pointes). **HERBAL: Gotu kola, kava kava, St. John's wort, valerian** may increase CNS depression. **St. John's wort** may decrease concentration. **FOOD: All foods** enhance bioavailability. **LAB VALUES:** May prolong QT interval. May increase serum glucose, prolactin levels.

## AVAILABILITY (Rx)

**Capsules:** 20 mg, 40 mg, 60 mg, 80 mg.
**Injection, Powder for Reconstitution:** 20 mg.

## ADMINISTRATION/HANDLING

### IM

• Store vials at room temperature; protect from light. • Reconstitute each vial with 1.2 ml Sterile Water for Injection to provide concentration of 20 mg/ml. • Reconstituted solution stable for 24 hrs at room temperature or 7 days if refrigerated.

### PO

• Give with food (increases bioavailability).

## INDICATIONS/ROUTES/DOSAGE

◀ALERT▶ Dosage greater than 80 mg twice daily are not recommended in most pts.

**Schizophrenia**
**PO: ADULTS, ELDERLY:** Initially, 20 mg twice daily with food. Titrate at intervals of no less than 2 days based on response and tolerability. **Maintenance:** 40–100 mg twice daily.

**Acute Agitation (Schizophrenia)**
**IM: ADULTS, ELDERLY:** 10 mg q2h or 20 mg q4h. **Maximum:** 40 mg/day.

**Bipolar Disorder (acute and maintenance as adjunct to lithium or valproate)**
**PO: ADULTS, ELDERLY (Acute):** Initially, 40 mg twice daily. May increase to 60–80 mg

---

✦ Canadian trade name     🍃 Non-Crushable Drug     🔲 High Alert drug twice daily on second day of treatment. **Maintenance:** 40–80 mg twice daily.

**Dosage in Renal Impairment**

**Oral:** No dose adjustment. **IM:** Use caution.

**Dosage in Hepatic Impairment**

Use caution.

## SIDE EFFECTS

**Frequent (30%–16%):** Headache, drowsiness, dizziness. **Occasional:** Rash, orthostatic hypotension, weight gain, restlessness, constipation, dyspepsia. **Rare:** Hyperglycemia, priapism.

## ADVERSE EFFECTS/ TOXIC REACTIONS

Prolongation of QT interval (as seen on EKG) may produce torsades de pointes, a form of ventricular tachycardia. Pts with bradycardia, hypokalemia, hypomagnesemia are at increased risk.

## NURSING CONSIDERATIONS

### BASELINE ASSESSMENT

Assess pt's behavior, appearance, emotional status, response to environment, speech pattern, thought content. EKG should be obtained to assess for QT prolongation before instituting medication. Blood chemistry for serum magnesium, potassium should be obtained before beginning therapy and routinely thereafter.

### INTERVENTION/EVALUATION

Assess for therapeutic response (greater interest in surroundings, improved self-care, increased ability to concentrate, relaxed facial expression). Monitor weight.

### PATIENT/FAMILY TEACHING

• Avoid tasks that require alertness, motor skills until response to drug is established. • Avoid alcohol.

# zoledronic acid

zoe-le-**dron**-ik **as**-id
(Aclasta ✿, Reclast, Zometa)
**Do not confuse Zometa with Zofran or Zoladex.**

## ◆CLASSIFICATION

**PHARMACOTHERAPEUTIC:** Bisphosphonate. **CLINICAL:** Calcium regulator, bone resorption inhibitor.

## USES

**Zometa:** Treatment of hypercalcemia of malignancy, bone metastases of solid tumors. Treatment of multiple myeloma. **Reclast:** Treatment and prevention of postmenopausal osteoporosis, glucocorticoid-induced osteoporosis, treatment of Paget's disease. Treatment of osteoporosis in men to increase bone mass. **OFF-LABEL:** Prevention of bone loss associated with aromatase inhibitor therapy in postmenopausal women with breast cancer or androgen deprivation therapy in men with prostate cancer.

## PRECAUTIONS

**Contraindications:** Hypersensitivity to zolendronic acid, other bisphophonates (e.g., alendronate, risedronate). **Reclast Only:** CrCl less than 35 ml/min, acute renal impairment, hypocalcemia. **Cautions:** Elderly. **(Oncology Indications):** History of aspirin-sensitive asthma, mild to moderate renal impairment. **(Non-Oncology Indications):** Pts with disturbances of calcium and mineral metabolism (e.g., hypoparathyroidism, malabsorption syndrome).

## ACTION

Inhibits bone resorption by action on osteoclasts. Inhibits osteoclast activity/ skeletal calcium release induced by tumors; inhibits osteoclast-mediated resorption. **Therapeutic Effect: (Tumor):** Increases urinary calcium,

Z

phosphorus excretion; decreases serum calcium, phosphorus levels. **(Osteoporosis):** Reduces bone turnover.

## ⌛ LIFESPAN CONSIDERATIONS

**Pregnancy/Lactation:** Unknown if drug crosses placenta or is distributed in breast milk. **Children:** Safety and efficacy not established. **Elderly:** Age-related renal impairment may require dosage adjustment.

## INTERACTIONS

**DRUG: Loop diuretics (e.g., furosemide)** may increase risk for hypocalcemia. **Nephrotoxic drugs (e.g., IV contrast dye, furosemide, lisinopril, rifampin)** may increase risk for nephrotoxicity. **HERBAL:** None significant. **FOOD:** None known. **LAB VALUES:** May decrease serum magnesium, calcium, phosphate.

## AVAILABILITY (Rx)

**Injection Solution (Zometa):** 4 mg/5 ml vial, 4 mg/100 ml single-use ready-to-use bottle. **(Reclast):** 5 mg diluted in 100 ml ready-to-infuse solution.

## ADMINISTRATION/HANDLING

◄**ALERT**► Pt should be adequately rehydrated before administration of zoledronic acid.

 **IV (Zometa)**

**Reconstitution** • Further dilute Zometa with 100 ml 0.9% NaCl or D₅W. **Rate of Administration** • Adequate hydration is essential in conjunction with zoledronic acid. • Administer as IV infusion over not less than 15 min (increases risk of deterioration in renal function). **Storage** • Store intact vials at room temperature. • Infusion of solution must be completed within 24 hrs.

 **IV (Reclast)**

• Administer as IV infusion over not less than 15 min. • Follow infusion with a 10-ml 0.9% NaCl flush of IV line.

## 🔲 IV INCOMPATIBILITIES

Do not mix with other medications.

## INDICATIONS/ROUTES/DOSAGE

**Hypercalcemia (Zometa)**
**IV Infusion: ADULTS, ELDERLY:** 4 mg IV infusion given over no less than 15 min. Retreatment may be considered, but at least 7 days should elapse to allow for full response to initial dose.

**Multiple Myeloma, Bone Metastases of Solid Tumors (Zometa)**
**IV: ADULTS, ELDERLY:** 4 mg q3–4wks.

**Paget's Disease (Reclast)**
**IV: ADULTS, ELDERLY:** 5 mg as a single dose. Data about retreatment not available (seldom required within 5 yrs).

**Osteoporosis Treatment (Reclast)**
**IV: ADULTS, ELDERLY:** 5 mg once yearly. Consider discontinuing after 3–5 yrs in pts with low risk of fractures.

**Treatment/Prevention of Glucocorticoid-Induced Osteoporosis (Reclast)**
**IV: ADULTS, ELDERLY:** 5 mg once yearly.

**Prevention of Postmenopausal Osteoporosis (Reclast)**
**IV: ADULTS, ELDERLY:** 5 mg once q2yrs.

**Dosage in Renal Impairment**
**(Reclast): CrCl less than 35 ml/min:** Contraindicated.
**(Zometa):** (Multiple Myeloma, Metastatic Bone Lesions of Solid Tumors)

| Creatinine Clearance | Dosage |
|---|---|
| 50–60 ml/min | 3.5 mg |
| 40–49 ml/min | 3.3 mg |
| 30–39 ml/min | 3 mg |
| Less than 30 ml/min | Not recommended |

**(Zometa):** (Hypercalcemia of Malignancy)
**Mild to moderate impairment:** No adjustment. **Severe impairment: (SCr greater than 4.5 mg/dL):** Use caution only after considering risk versus benefit.

**Dosage in Hepatic Impairment**
No dose adjustment.

## SIDE EFFECTS

**Frequent (44%–26%):** Fever, nausea, vomiting, constipation. **Occasional (15%–10%):** Hypotension, anxiety, insomnia, flu-like symptoms (fever, chills, bone pain, myalgia, arthralgia). **Rare:** Conjunctivitis.

## ADVERSE EFFECTS/ TOXIC REACTIONS

Renal toxicity may occur if IV infusion is administered in less than 15 min.

### NURSING CONSIDERATIONS

#### BASELINE ASSESSMENT

Prior to initiation, obtain dental exam for pts at risk for osteonecrosis. Establish baseline serum electrolytes, renal function test.

#### INTERVENTION/EVALUATION

Monitor serum renal function, CBC. Assess vertebral bone mass (document stabilization, improvement). Monitor serum calcium, phosphate, magnesium, creatinine levels. Assess for fever. Monitor food intake, daily pattern of bowel activity, stool consistency. Check I&O, serum BUN, creatinine in pts with renal impairment.

---

## *ZOLMitriptan

zole-mi-**trip**-tan
(Zomig, Zomig Rapimelt ✶,
Zomig-ZMT)
**Do not confuse zolmitriptan with sumatriptan.**

### ◆CLASSIFICATION

**PHARMACOTHERAPEUTIC:** Serotonin receptor agonist. **CLINICAL:** Antimigraine.

## USES

Treatment of acute migraine attack with or without aura. **OFF-LABEL:** Short-term prevention of menstrual migraines.

## PRECAUTIONS

**Contraindications:** Hypersensitivity to zolmitriptan. Arrhythmias associated with conduction disorders (e.g., Wolff-Parkinson-White syndrome), basilar or hemiplegic migraine, coronary artery disease, ischemic heart disease (including angina pectoris, history of MI, silent ischemia, Prinzmetal's angina), uncontrolled hypertension, use within 24 hrs of ergotamine-containing preparations or another serotonin receptor agonist, MAOI used within 14 days. Additional for nasal spray: Cerebrovascular syndromes (e.g., stroke), peripheral vascular disease. **Cautions:** Mild to moderate renal/hepatic impairment, pt profile suggesting cardiovascular risks (e.g., hypertension, hypercholesterolemia, smoker, obesity, diabetes), elderly.

## ACTION

Binds selectively to serotonin receptors, producing vasoconstrictive effect on cranial blood vessels. **Therapeutic Effect:** Relieves migraine headache.

## PHARMACOKINETICS

Well absorbed after PO administration. Protein binding: 25%. Metabolized in liver. Eliminated in urine (60%), feces (30%). **Half-life:** 2.8–3.7 hrs.

## ⌛ LIFESPAN CONSIDERATIONS

**Pregnancy/Lactation:** Unknown if drug is distributed in breast milk. **Children:** Safety and efficacy not established in pts younger than 12 yrs. **Elderly:** No age-related precautions noted.

## INTERACTIONS

**DRUG: Ergotamine-containing medications** may produce vasospastic reaction. **Fluoxetine, fluvoxamine, paroxetine, sertraline** may produce hyperreflexia, incoordination, weakness. **MAOIs** may dramatically increase concentration. **HERBAL:** None significant. **FOOD:** None known. **LAB VALUES:** None significant.

## AVAILABILITY (Rx)

Nasal Spray (Zomig): 2.5 mg, 5 mg.
Tablets (Zomig): 2.5 mg, 5 mg.

🔖 Tablets (Orally Disintegrating [Zomig-ZMT]): 2.5 mg, 5 mg.

## ADMINISTRATION/HANDLING

### PO
• Give without regard to food. Tablets may be broken.

### Orally Disintegrating Tablet (ODT)
• Give whole; do not break, crush, cut.
• Place on pts tongue, allow to dissolve.
• Not necessary to administer with liquid.

### Nasal
• Instruct pt to clear nasal passages as much as possible before use. • With head upright, pt should close one nostril with index finger, breathe out gently through mouth. • Instruct pt to insert nozzle into open nostril about ½ inch, close mouth, and while taking a breath through nose, release spray dosage by firmly pressing plunger. • Have pt remove nozzle from nose, gently breathe in through nose and out through mouth for 15–20 sec. Tell pt to avoid breathing in deeply.

## INDICATIONS/ROUTES/DOSAGE

### Acute Migraine Attack
**PO: ADULTS, ELDERLY, CHILDREN OLDER THAN 18 YRS:** Initially, 1.25–2.5 mg (**Maximum:** 5 mg). If headache returns, may repeat dose after 2 hrs. **Maximum:** 10 mg/24 hrs.
**Orally Disintegrating Tablet: ADULTS, ELDERLY:** Initially, 2.5 mg (**Maximum:** 5 mg) at onset of migraine headache. If headache returns, may repeat dose after 2 hrs. **Maximum:** 10 mg/24 hrs.
**Intranasal: ADULTS, ELDERLY, CHILDREN 12 YRS AND OLDER:** Initially, 2.5 mg (**Maximum:** 5 mg). If headache returns, may repeat dose after 2 hrs. **Maximum:** 10 mg/24 hrs.

### Dosage in Renal Impairment
No dose adjustment.

### Dosage in Hepatic Impairment
**Nasal/ODT: Mild impairment:** No dose adjustment. **Moderate to severe impairment:** Not recommended. **Tablet: Mild:** No dose adjustment. **Moderate to severe impairment:** Initially, 1.25 mg. (**Maximum daily dose:** 5 mg in severe impairment.)

## SIDE EFFECTS

**Frequent (8%–6%): PO:** Dizziness, paresthesia, neck/throat/jaw pressure, drowsiness. **Nasal:** Altered taste, paresthesia. **Occasional (5%–3%): PO:** Warm/hot sensation, asthenia, chest pressure. **Nasal:** Nausea, drowsiness, nasal discomfort, dizziness, asthenia, dry mouth. **Rare (2%–1%):** Diaphoresis, myalgia.

## ADVERSE EFFECTS/TOXIC REACTIONS

Cardiac events (ischemia, coronary artery vasospasm, MI), noncardiac vasospasm-related reactions (hemorrhage, stroke) occur rarely, particularly in pts with hypertension, diabetes, strong family history of coronary artery disease; pts who are obese; smokers; males older than 40 yrs; postmenopausal women.

## NURSING CONSIDERATIONS

### BASELINE ASSESSMENT
Question for history of peripheral vascular disease, coronary artery disease, renal/hepatic impairment, MAOI use. Question pt regarding onset, location, duration of migraine, possible precipitating factors.

### INTERVENTION/EVALUATION
Monitor for evidence of dizziness. Monitor B/P, esp. in pts with hepatic impairment. Assess for relief of migraine headache, migraine potential for photophobia, phonophobia (sound sensitivity, light sensitivity, nausea, vomiting).

### PATIENT/FAMILY TEACHING
• Take single dose as soon as symptoms of actual migraine attack appear. • Medication is intended to relieve migraine, not

to prevent or reduce number of attacks. • Lie down in quiet dark room for additional benefit after taking medication. • Avoid tasks that require alertness, motor skills until response to drug is established. • Report chest pain; palpitations; tightness in throat; edema of face, lips, eyes; rash; easy bruising; blood in urine or stool; pain or numbness in arms or legs.

## zolpidem

zole-pi-dem
(Ambien, Ambien CR, Edluar, Intermezzo, Sublinox ✤, Zolpimist)
**Do not confuse Ambien with ativan, or zolpidem with zaleplon.**

### ◆CLASSIFICATION

**PHARMACOTHERAPEUTIC:** Nonbenzodiazepine **(Schedule IV). CLINICAL:** Sedative-hypnotic.

### USES

**Ambien, Edluar, Zolpimist:** Short-term treatment of insomnia (with difficulty of sleep onset). **Ambien CR:** Treatment of insomnia (with difficulty of sleep onset and/or sleep maintenance). **Intermezzo:** Treatment of insomnia characterized by middle-of-the-night awakening followed by difficulty returning to sleep in pts with 4 or more hrs of sleep time remaining.

### PRECAUTIONS

**Contraindications:** Hypersensitivity to zolpidem. **Cautions:** Hepatic/renal impairment, pts with depression, history of drug dependence, sleep apnea, COPD, respiratory disease, myasthenia gravis, debilitated pts, elderly.

### ACTION

Enhances action of inhibitory neurotransmitter gamma-aminobutyric acid (GABA). **Therapeutic Effect:** Induces sleep with fewer nightly awakenings, improves sleep quality.

### PHARMACOKINETICS

| Route | Onset | Peak | Duration |
|---|---|---|---|
| PO | 30 min | N/A | 6–8 hrs |

Rapidly absorbed from GI tract. Protein binding: 92%. Metabolized in liver; excreted in urine. Not removed by hemodialysis. **Half-life:** 1.4–4.5 hrs (increased in hepatic impairment).

### ⌛ LIFESPAN CONSIDERATIONS

**Pregnancy/Lactation:** Unknown if drug crosses placenta or is distributed in breast milk. **Children:** Safety and efficacy not established. **Elderly:** More likely to experience falls or confusion; decreased initial doses recommended. Age-related hepatic impairment may require dosage adjustment.

### INTERACTIONS

**DRUG: Alcohol, other CNS depressants (e.g., gabapentin, lorazepam, morphine)** may increase CNS depression. **HERBAL: Gotu kola, kava kava, valerian** may increase CNS depression. **St. John's wort** may decrease concentration/effect. **FOOD:** None known. **LAB VALUES:** None significant.

### AVAILABILITY (Rx)

**Oral Solution (Zolpimist):** 5 mg/actuation. **Tablets (Ambien):** 5 mg, 10 mg. **Tablets (Sublingual [Edluar]):** 5 mg, 10 mg. **(Intermezzo):** 1.75 mg, 3.5 mg.

🏷 **Tablets (Extended-Release [Ambien CR]):** 6.25 mg, 12.5 mg.

### ADMINISTRATION/HANDLING

**PO**
• For faster sleep onset, do not give with or immediately after a meal. • Do not break, crush, dissolve, or divide Ambien CR tablets; give whole. • Edluar sublingual tablets to be placed under tongue and allowed to disintegrate. Do not swallow or administer with water. • Spray

Zolpimist directly into mouth over tongue.

## INDICATIONS/ROUTES/DOSAGE

**Note:** Dosage adjustment is recommended for female pts.

**Insomnia**

**PO, Spray, Sublingual:** *(Edluar, Zolpimist):* **ADULTS:** (males) 10 mg, (females) 5 mg immediately before bedtime. **ELDERLY, DEBILITATED:** 5 mg immediately before bedtime.

*(Intermezzo):* **ADULTS, ELDERLY:** 1.75 mg (females) 3.5 mg (males) taken once in middle of night with 4 or more hrs of expected sleep yet to come.

**PO:** *(Extended-Release):* **ADULTS:** (males) 6.25–12.5 mg, (females) 6.25 mg immediately before bedtime. **ELDERLY, DEBILITATED:** 6.25 mg immediately before bedtime.

**Dosage in Renal Impairment**

No dose adjustment; use caution.

**Dosage in Hepatic Impairment**

**PO:** *(Immediate-Release Tablet, Spray, Sublingual Tablet):* 5 mg. *(Extended-Release Tablet):* 6.25 mg. *(Intermezzo):* 1.75 mg.

## SIDE EFFECTS

**Occasional (7%):** Headache, change in appetite. **Rare (less than 2%):** Dizziness, nausea, diarrhea, muscle pain, sleepwalking.

## ADVERSE EFFECTS/ TOXIC REACTIONS

Overdose may produce severe ataxia (clumsiness, unsteadiness), bradycardia, diplopia, severe drowsiness, nausea, vomiting, difficulty breathing, unconsciousness. Abrupt withdrawal following long-term use may produce weakness, facial flushing, diaphoresis, vomiting, tremor. Drug tolerance/dependence may occur with prolonged use of high dosages. May cause amnesic events that include cooking, sleepwalking, sexual activity, driving.

## NURSING CONSIDERATIONS

### BASELINE ASSESSMENT

Assess B/P, pulse, respirations, mental status, sleep patterns. Raise bed rails, provide call light. Provide environment conducive to sleep (back rub, quiet environment, low lighting). Do not give unless a full night of sleep is planned.

### INTERVENTION/EVALUATION

Monitor sleep pattern of pt. Evaluate for therapeutic response to insomnia: decrease in number of nocturnal awakenings, increase in length of sleep. Monitor daytime alertness, respiratory rate, behavior profile.

### PATIENT/FAMILY TEACHING

• Do not abruptly discontinue medication after long-term use. • Avoid alcohol and tasks that require alertness, motor skills until response to drug is established. • Tolerance, dependence may occur with prolonged use of high dosages. • Do not break, chew, crush, dissolve, or divide Ambien CR tablets; swallow whole. • Therapy may need to be discontinued if cooking, driving, sleepwalking occurs without recollection. • Do not take unless a full 8 hrs of sleep is planned.

# zonisamide

zoe-**nis**-a-mide
(Zonegran)
**Do not confuse Zonegran with Sinequan, or zonisamide with lacosamide.**

## ◆CLASSIFICATION

**PHARMACOTHERAPEUTIC:** Succinimide. **CLINICAL:** Anticonvulsant.

## USES

Adjunctive therapy in treatment of partial seizures in adults, children older than 16 yrs with epilepsy. **OFF-LABEL:** Bipolar disorder.

## PRECAUTIONS

**Contraindications:** Hypersensitivity to zonisamide. Allergy to sulfonamides. **Cautions:** Renal/hepatic impairment, pts at high risk for suicide or metabolic acidosis (e.g., severe respiratory disease).

## ACTION

Exact mechanism unknown. May stabilize neuronal membranes, suppress neuronal hypersynchronization by blocking sodium, calcium channels. **Therapeutic Effect:** Reduces seizure activity.

## PHARMACOKINETICS

Well absorbed after PO administration. Metabolized in liver. Extensively bound to RBCs. Protein binding: 40%. Primarily excreted in urine. **Half-life:** 63 hrs (plasma), 105 hrs (RBCs).

## ⌛ LIFESPAN CONSIDERATIONS

**Pregnancy/Lactation:** Unknown if distributed in breast milk. **Children:** Safety and efficacy not established in pts younger than 16 yrs. **Elderly:** No age-related precautions noted, but lower dosages recommended.

## INTERACTIONS

**DRUG: Alcohol, other CNS depressants** (e.g., **lorazepam, morphine, zolpidem**) may increase sedative effect. **CYP3A4 inducers** (e.g., **carbamazepine, phenobarbital, phenytoin, valproic acid**) may increase metabolism, decrease effect. **HERBAL:** None significant. **FOOD:** None known. **LAB VALUES:** May increase serum BUN, creatinine.

## AVAILABILITY (Rx)

🐾 **Capsules:** 25 mg, 50 mg, 100 mg.

## ADMINISTRATION/HANDLING

**PO**

• May give with or without food. • Do not crush, break capsules. Give capsules whole. • Do not give to pts allergic to sulfonamides.

## INDICATIONS/ROUTES/DOSAGE

**Note:** Do not use if CrCl is less than 50 ml/min.

**Partial Seizures**
**PO: ADULTS, ELDERLY, CHILDREN OLDER THAN 16 YRS:** Initially, 100 mg/day. May increase to 200 mg/day after 2 wks. Further increases to 300 mg/day and 400 mg/day can be made with minimum of 2 wks between adjustments. Range: 100–600 mg/day.

**Dosage in Renal Impairment**
Not recommended with CrCl less than 50 ml/min.

**Dosage in Hepatic Impairment**
Use with caution.

## SIDE EFFECTS

**Frequent (17%–9%):** Drowsiness, dizziness, anorexia, headache, agitation, irritability, nausea. **Occasional (8%–5%):** Fatigue, ataxia, confusion, depression, impaired memory/concentration, insomnia, abdominal pain, diplopia, diarrhea, speech difficulty. **Rare (4%–3%):** Paresthesia, nystagmus, anxiety, rash, dyspepsia, weight loss.

## ADVERSE EFFECTS/ TOXIC REACTIONS

Overdose characterized by bradycardia, hypotension, respiratory depression, coma. Leukopenia, anemia, thrombocytopenia occur rarely.

## NURSING CONSIDERATIONS

### BASELINE ASSESSMENT

Review history of seizure disorder (intensity, frequency, duration, LOC). Initiate seizure precautions. CBC, LFT should be performed before therapy begins and periodically during therapy.

### INTERVENTION/EVALUATION

Observe frequently for recurrence of seizure activity. Assess for clinical improvement (decrease in intensity, frequency of seizures). Assist with ambulation if dizziness occurs.

### PATIENT/FAMILY TEACHING

• Strict maintenance of drug therapy is essential for seizure control. • Avoid tasks that require alertness, motor skills until response to drug is established. • Avoid alcohol. • Report if rash, back/abdominal pain, blood in urine, fever, sore throat, ulcers in mouth, easy bruising occur. • Report worsening depression, unusual behavior, suicidal ideation.

# CALCULATION OF DOSES

Frequently, dosages ordered do not correspond exactly to what is available and must be calculated.

## RATIO/PROPORTION:

A pt is to receive 65 mg of a medication. It is available as 80 mg/2 ml. What volume (ml) needs to be administered to the patient?

STEP 1: Set up ratio.

$$\frac{80 \text{ mg}}{2 \text{ ml}} = \frac{65 \text{ mg}}{x \text{ (ml)}}$$

STEP 2: Cross multiply and divide each side by the number with x to determine volume to be administered.

$$80 \text{ mg} \times (x) \text{ ml} = 65 \text{ mg} \times 2 \text{ ml}$$
$$80 \, x = 130$$
$$x = \frac{130}{80} = 1.625 \text{ ml}$$

## CALCULATIONS IN MICROGRAMS PER KILOGRAM PER MINUTE (mcg/kg/min):

A 63-year-old pt (weight 165 lb) is to receive medication A at a rate of 8 mcg/kg/min. Given a solution containing medication A in a concentration of 500 mg/250 ml, at what rate (ml/hr) would you infuse this medication?

STEP 1: Convert to same units. In this problem, the dose is expressed in mcg/kg; therefore, convert weight to kg (2.2 lb = 1 kg) and drug concentration to mcg/ml (1 mg = 1,000 mcg).

$$165 \text{ lb divided by } 2.2 = 75 \text{ kg}$$
$$\frac{500 \text{ mg}}{250 \text{ ml}} = \frac{2 \text{ mg}}{\text{ml}} = \frac{2,000 \text{ mcg}}{\text{ml}}$$

STEP 2: Number of mcg/hr.

$$(75 \text{ kg}) \times 8 \text{ mcg/kg/min} = 600 \text{ mcg/min or } 36,000 \text{ mcg/hr}$$

STEP 3: Number of ml/hr.

$$36,000 \text{ mcg/hr divided by } 2,000 \text{ mcg/ml} = 18 \text{ ml/hr}$$

# CONTROLLED DRUGS (UNITED STATES)

**Schedule I:** Medications having no legal medical use. These substances may be used for research purposes with proper registration (e.g., heroin, LSD).

**Schedule II:** Medications having a legitimate medical use but are characterized by a very high abuse potential and/or potential for severe physical and psychic dependency. Emergency telephone orders for limited quantities of these drugs are authorized, but the prescriber must provide a written, signed prescription order (e.g., morphine, amphetamines, hydrocodone, oxycodone).

**Schedule III:** Medications having significant abuse potential (less than Schedule II). Telephone orders are permitted (e.g., codeine in combination with other substances such as butalbital).

**Schedule IV:** Medications having a low abuse potential. Telephone orders are permitted (e.g., benzodiazepines, tramadol, zolpidem).

**Schedule V:** Medications having the lowest abuse potential of the controlled substances. Some Schedule V products may be available without a prescription (e.g., certain cough preparations containing limited amounts of an opiate).

# WOUND CARE

A wound is any process that disrupts the normal structure and function of tissues. Wounds can be closed (e.g., bruise, sprain) or open (e.g., abrasion, surgical wound). The most common chronic wounds are nonhealing surgical wounds, pressure ulcers, diabetic foot ulcers, and venous ulcers.

## TYPES OF OPEN WOUNDS

| | |
|---|---|
| Superficial | Damage only to the epithelium; heals rapidly via regeneration of epithelial cells. |
| Partial thickness | Involves the dermal layer and is associated with blood vessel damage. |
| Full thickness | Involves subcutaneous fat and deeper layers (e.g., muscle, bone). |
| | Requires the longest time to heal. |
| | Connective tissue needs to regenerate; contraction occurs during the healing process. |

## WOUND HEALING

Wound healing is a complex process resulting in restored cell structure and tissue layers after an injury. When skin is damaged, it begins to heal from the bottom layer up and from the outside inward. Wound healing involves cellular, physiologic, biochemical, and molecular processes. They are interdependent and overlapping. An acute wound usually heals within several wks, whereas chronic wounds take 6 wks or longer to heal. Additionally, other factors can delay the healing process. These include trauma/edema, infection, necrosis, lack of oxygen delivery to the tissues, advanced age, obesity, chronic diseases (e.g., diabetes, anemia), vascular insufficiency, and immunodeficiency.

Wound healing can be divided into three phases: inflammation, proliferation, and maturation.

| | |
|---|---|
| Inflammation | Occurs within seconds of the injury and can last up to 3 days. |
| | Associated with redness, heat, swelling, and pain. |
| | Immediate vasoconstriction of damaged blood vessels and coagulation limiting blood loss occurs. |
| | Following vasoconstriction, histamine and other chemical mediators are released from damaged cells, causing vasodilation and release of growth factors essential for wound healing (e.g., increased capillary permeability and release of exudate). |
| Proliferation | Granulation tissue composed of macrophages, fibroblasts, immature collagen, blood vessels, and ground substance is formed. |
| | Fibroblasts stimulate production of collagen and elastin, increasing the strength of the wound and stimulating growth of new blood vessels. |
| | As granulation fills the wound site, the edges of the wound pull together, decreasing the surface of the wound. |

| | |
|---|---|
| | Epithelialization then occurs: Epithelial cells migrate from the wound edge, covering the wound and resulting in scar formation. |
| | This phase usually lasts 2 to 3 wks. |
| Maturation | Collagen fibers cross link and reorganize, increasing the strength of scar. This process can take anywhere from 3 wks to 2 yrs. |

## WOUND DRESSINGS

Dressings play a major role in wound management. They protect the wound, keeping it moist and thus promote healing (only diabetic, dry, gangrenous toes require a moisture-free environment for effective healing).

Hydrocolloid, hydrogel, film, and foam dressing can handle large amounts of exudate and promote auto-debridement. Alginate and collagen-based dressings promote granulation of tissue. Silver and iodine dressings are used to avoid infections, which may delay wound healing.

## WOUND CARE PRODUCTS

| Description | General Uses | Comments |
|---|---|---|
| **Alginate dressings:** Spun fibers of brown seaweed that act as ion exchange mechanisms to absorb serous fluid or exudate, forming a gel-like covering that conforms to the shape of the wound. Facilitate autolytic debridement and maintain a moist wound environment. **Products:** Algicell, Carra Sorb. Available as ropes, pads. | Abrasions/lacerations/skin tears Arterial/venous ulcers Deep and tunneling wounds Diabetic ulcers Pressure ulcers Second-degree burns Odorous wounds Contaminated and infected wounds | Good for moderately to heavily exudative wounds and hemorrhagic wounds Can be left in place until soaked with exudate Requires a secondary dressing (e.g., transparent film, foam, hydrocolloids) Do not moisten prior to use Nonadhesive, nonocclusive Contraindicated in third-degree burns; not recommended for dry or minimally exudative wounds |
| **Collagenase ointment:** Sterile enzymatic debriding ointment that possesses the ability to digest collagen in necrotic tissue. **Products:** Santyl. | Debriding chronic dermal ulcers and severely burned areas | Can be used for infected wounds Gauze is used as a secondary dressing Discontinue when granulation tissue is present Optimal pH for enzymatic action is 6–8 Avoid acidic agents for cleansing; avoid detergents and agents containing heavy metal (e.g., mercury or silver), which may adversely affect enzymatic activity |

*Continued*

| Description | General Uses | Comments |
|---|---|---|
| **Trypsin, castor oil, Peru balsam: Trypsin** is a mild debriding agent that helps shed damaged skin cells. **Castor oil** acts as a lubricant to protect tissue. **Peru balsam** increases blood flow to a wound area, reduces wound odor. **Products:** Granulex, Xenaderm. Available as gel, ointment, spray. | Promotes healing/ treatment of decubitus ulcers, varicose ulcer, and dehiscent wounds | Can be used for infected wounds<br>Avoid concurrent use of silver-containing products (may reduce efficacy)<br>Promotes healing and relieves pain caused by bed sores and other skin ulcers |
| **Hydrophilic polyurethane foam:** Also called open cell foam dressings. Sheets of foamed solutions of polymers containing variably sized open cells that can hold wound exudate away from wound bed. Maintains moist wound environment. **Products:** Curafoam, Lyofoam. Available as sheets in a wide variety of formulations. | Moderate to heavy exudative wounds with or without a clean granular wound bed<br>Diabetic ulcers, pressure ulcers, venous stasis ulcers<br>Draining surgical incisions<br>Superficial burns<br>Tube and drain sites | Contraindicated for use in third-degree burns<br>Not recommended for wounds with little to no exudate or when tunneling is present<br>Good for cavitating wounds<br>Highly absorbent, semi-occlusive dressing<br>Usual dressing change is up to 3 times/wk<br>Can be worn during bathing |
| **Hydrocolloids:** Formulations of elastomeric, adhesive, and gelling agents; the most common absorbent ingredient is carboxymethylcellulose. Most hydrocolloids are backed with a semi-occlusive film layer. The wound side of the dressing is adhesive, adhering to a moist surface as well as to dry skin but not to the moist wound bed. As wound fluid is absorbed, the hydrocolloid forms a viscous gel in the wound bed, enhancing a moist wound environment. **Products:** Hydrocol, Tegasorb. Available as dressings, granules, patches, paste. | Minimal to moderate exudate in partial and full thickness wounds<br>Cuts and abrasions<br>First- and second-degree burns<br>Pressure ulcers<br>Stasis ulcers | Not for wounds producing heavy exudate, infected wounds, dry eschar-covered wounds<br>May provide pain relief<br>Good for chronic wounds that are epithelializing<br>Can be left in place for up to 7 days<br>Contraindicated for third-degree burns<br>Can shower while wearing |

| Description | General Uses | Comments |
|---|---|---|
| **Hydrogels:** Glycerin- or water-based dressings designed to hydrate the wound. May absorb small amounts of exudate. **Products:** Curacel, Duo Derm, Intra Site. Available as gel, sheets, gauze. | Partial and full thickness wounds Dry to minimal exudate Cuts and abrasions First- and second-degree burns Pressure ulcers Stasis ulcers | Not for wounds producing moderate to heavy exudate Not for infected wounds May provide pain relief Good for wounds that are debriding Good for keeping a dry wound moist Can be left in place for 1–3 days |
| **Iodine compounds: Cadexomer iodine:** Iodine is complexed with a polymeric cadexomer starch vehicle, forming a topical gel or paste. The cadexomer moiety absorbs exudate and debris and releases iodine for antimicrobial activity. **Products:** Iodosorb, Iodoflex. Available as gel, dressing, ointment, powder. | Chronic nonhealing, exuding wounds including pressure or leg ulcers and exuding, infected wounds | Requires use of a secondary dressing Contraindicated in pts with iodine sensitivity, Hashimoto's thyroiditis, nontoxic nodular goiter, children Dressing to be changed when it turns white, indicating that the iodine has been depleted Do not use on dry necrotic tissue |
| **Silver compounds Silver sulfadiazine cream:** Silver possesses bactericidal properties. Has been shown to reduce bacterial density, vascular margination, migration of inflammatory cells. Enhances rate of re-epithelialization. **Products:** Silvadene, SSD, Thermazene. | Prevent infection in second- and third-degree burns Prevent or treat infection in chronic wounds | May have cytotoxic effects that could delay wound healing Allergic reactions may occur Use should be limited to a 2- to 4-wk period Bacteria may become resistant with prolonged use Avoid use with collagenase- or trypsin-containing debriding agents |
| **Transparent film dressings:** Polyurethane sheets coated on one side with an adhesive that is inactivated by moisture and will not adhere to a moist surface such as the wound bed. Have no absorbent capacity and are impermeable to fluids and bacteria but are semipermeable to oxygen and water vapor. **Products:** Bioclusive, CarraFilm, Tegaderm HP. Available in a variety of sizes and features. | Prophylaxis on high-risk intact skin Superficial wounds with minimal or no exudate Wounds on elbows, heels, or flat surfaces; covering of blisters; and retention of primary dressing | Prevents wound desiccation and contamination by bacteria Contraindicated in third-degree burns Promotes autolysis of necrotic tissue in the wound; maintains moist environment Avoid in arterial ulcers and infected wounds requiring frequent monitoring Do not use as primary dressing on wounds with depth or tunneling May provide pain relief Usually changed up to 3 times/wk |

*Continued*

| Description | General Uses | Comments |
|---|---|---|
| **Becaplermin gel:** Recombinant formulation of platelet-derived growth factor that promotes cell mitogenesis and proliferation of cells involved in wound repair. Enhances formation of granulation tissue. **Products:** Regranex. | Diabetic foot ulcers that extend into subcutaneous tissue or beyond and have an adequate blood supply | Usually applied daily Adequate blood supply and absence of necrotic tissue are needed for efficacy Repeated use (3 or more tubes) may increase risk of cancer-related death Use cautiously in pts with known malignancy |

# DRUGS OF ABUSE

| Substance | Brand/Street Names | Administered | Effects of Intoxication | Potential Health Consequences |
|---|---|---|---|---|
| Amphetamine | Adderall, Dexedrine; bennies, black beauties, hearts, speed, truck drivers, uppers | Injection, smoked, snorted | Increased heart rate, blood pressure, body temperature, metabolism; increased energy, mental alertness; tremors; reduced appetite; irritability; anxiety; panic; violent behavior; psychosis | Weight loss, insomnia, cardiac or cardiovascular complications, stroke, seizures, addiction, tremor, irritability |
| Barbiturates | Nembutal, Seconal, Phenobarbital; barbs, reds, phennies, yellows, yellow jackets | Injection, oral | Reduction of pain and anxiety; feeling of well-being; lowered inhibitions; slowed pulse/breathing; lowered blood pressure; poor concentration; sedation, drowsiness | Confusion, fatigue; impaired coordination, memory, judgment; respiratory depression or arrest; addiction; depression; unusual excitement; fever; irritability; slurred speech; dizziness |
| Benzodiazepines | Ativan, Librium, Valium, Xanax; candy, downers, tranks | Oral | Reduction of pain and anxiety; feeling of well-being; lowered inhibitions; slowed pulse/breathing; lowered blood pressure; poor concentration; sedation, drowsiness | Confusion, fatigue; impaired coordination, memory, judgment; respiratory depression or arrest; addiction; dizziness |

Continued

| Substance | Brand/ Street Names | Administered | Effects of Intoxication | Potential Health Consequences |
|---|---|---|---|---|
| Bupropion | *Wellbutrin;* poor man's cocaine | Oral | Increased heart rate, B/P, and temperature; mental alertness; feel euphoric, exhilarated, energetic | Seizures, tachycardia, arrhythmias, loss of consciousness |
| Cocaine | Blow, bump, candy, coke, crack, rock, snow, toot | Injection, smoked, snorted | Increased heart rate, blood pressure, body temperature, metabolism; increased energy, mental alertness; tremors; reduced appetite; irritability; anxiety; panic; violent behavior; psychosis | Weight loss, insomnia, cardiac or cardiovascular complications, stroke, seizures, addiction, nasal damage from snorting, rapid or irregular heartbeat, headaches, malnutrition |
| Codeine | *Fiorinal with codeine, Tylenol with codeine;* Captain Cody, schoolboy, loads, pancakes and syrup | Injection, oral | Pain relief, euphoria, drowsiness | Respiratory depression and arrest, nausea, confusion, constipation, sedation, unconsciousness, coma, tolerance, addiction |
| Dextromethorphan | Found in some cough and cold medications; poor man's PCP, velvet, Robo, Triple C | Oral | Impaired motor function, feeling of being separated from one's body and environment; euphoria; slurred speech; confusion; dizziness; distorted visual perceptions | |

| Substance | Brand/ Street Names | Administered | Effects of Intoxication | Potential Health Consequences |
|---|---|---|---|---|
| Flunitraze- pam | Rohypnol; for- get-me pill, Mexican Va- lium, roofies, roofinol, rope, rophies | Oral, snorted | Sedation, mus- cle relaxation, confusion, memory loss, dizziness, impaired coordination, reduced pain/ anxiety, feeling of well-being | Addiction; confusion, fatigue, memory loss, respiratory depression |
| Gabapentin | Neurontin, Lyrica, Lycia; gabbie | Oral | Self-treatment of alcohol, co- caine, or opi- oid craving; euphoria, relaxation | Diarrhea, double vi- sion, drowsi- ness, lethar- gic, slurred speech |
| GHB | Georgia home boy, grievous bodily harm, liquid ecstasy, goop, liquid X | Oral | Drowsiness, nausea, head- ache, disorien- tation, loss of coordination, memory loss | Uncon- sciousness, seizures, coma, confu- sion, nausea, vomiting, headache |
| Heroin | Smack, brown sugar, dope, junk, white horse, China white | Injection, smoked, snorted | Euphoria, drowsiness, impaired coor- dination, dizzi- ness, confu- sion, nausea, sedation, feel- ing of heavi- ness in the body, slowed breathing | Constipation, confusion, sedation, re- spiratory de- pression, coma, addic- tion |
| Hydroco- done | Vicodin, Lortab; vike, watson-387 | Oral | Pain relief, euphoria, drowsiness | Respiratory depression and arrest, nausea, confusion, constipation, sedation, un- conscious- ness, coma, tolerance, addiction |

Continued

| Substance | Brand/ Street Names | Administered | Effects of Intoxication | Potential Health Consequences |
|---|---|---|---|---|
| Inhalants | Solvents (paint thinner, glues), nitrites (laughing gas, snappers, poppers) | Inhaled through nose or mouth | Stimulation, loss of inhibition, headache, nausea or vomiting, slurred speech, loss of motor coordination, wheezing | Cramps, muscle weakness, depression, memory impairment, damage to cardiovascular and nervous systems, unconsciousness, sudden death |
| Ketamine | Ketalar; cat Valium, Special K, kit kat, vitamin K | Injection, snorted, smoked | Increased heart rate and blood pressure, impaired motor function, feelings of being separated from one's body and environment; at high doses: delirium, depression, respiratory depression or arrest; death | Memory loss, numbness, nausea/vomiting, anxiety, tremors, respiratory depression |
| Loperamide | Imodium; poor man's methadone | Oral | Reducing symptoms of opioid withdrawal | CNS depression, intestinal blockage |

| Substance | Brand/ Street Names | Administered | Effects of Intoxication | Potential Health Consequences |
|---|---|---|---|---|
| LSD | Acid, cubes, microdot, yellow sunshine, blotter, bloomers | Oral, absorbed through mouth tissues | Altered states of perception and feeling; hallucinations; nausea; increased body temperature, heart rate, blood pressure; loss of appetite; sweating; sleeplessness; numbness; dizziness; weakness; tremors; impulsive behavior; rapid shifts in emotion | Flashbacks, hallucinogen persisting perception disorder |
| Marijuana | Blunt, ganja, grass, joint, Mary Jane, pot, reefer, sinsemilla, skunk, weed | Oral, smoked | Euphoria, relaxation, slowed reaction time, impaired balance and coordination, increased heart rate and appetite, impaired learning and memory, anxiety, panic attacks, psychosis | Cough, impaired memory and learning, anxiety, panic attacks, frequent respiratory infections, possible mental health decline, addiction |
| MDMA | Ecstasy, Adam, clarity, Eve, lover's speed, peace, Molly | Injection, oral, snorted | Mild hallucinogenic effects, increased tactile sensitivity, empathic feelings, lowered inhibition, anxiety, chills, sweating, teeth clenching, muscle cramping | Reduced appetite, irregular heartbeat, heart failure, impaired memory, hyperthermia, addiction |

*Continued*

| Substance | Brand/Street Names | Administered | Effects of Intoxication | Potential Health Consequences |
|---|---|---|---|---|
| Mescaline | Buttons, cactus, peyote | Oral, smoked | Altered states of perception and feeling; hallucinations; nausea; increased body temperature, heart rate, blood pressure; loss of appetite; sweating; sleeplessness; numbness; dizziness; weakness; tremors; impulsive behavior; rapid shifts in emotion | Loss of appetite, nausea, weakness, chronic mental disorders |
| Methamphetamine | Desoxyn; meth, ice, crank, crystal, go fast, speed | Oral, injection, smoked, snorted | Increased heart rate, blood pressure, body temperature, metabolism; increased energy, mental alertness; tremors; reduced appetite; irritability; anxiety; panic; violent behavior; psychosis | Weight loss, insomnia, cardiac or cardiovascular complications, stroke, seizures, addiction, severe dental problems, behavior/memory loss, impaired memory and learning, tolerance, addiction |
| Methylphenidate | Ritalin; JIF, MPH, Skippy, smart drug, vitamin R | Injection, oral, snorted | Increase or decrease in blood pressure; psychotic episodes | Digestive problems, loss of appetite, weight loss, reduced appetite, rapid irregular heartbeat, heart failure, seizures, stroke |

| Substance | Brand/ Street Names | Administered | Effects of Intoxication | Potential Health Conse- quences |
|---|---|---|---|---|
| Morphine | *Roxanol, Du- ramorph;* M, Miss Emma, monkey, white stuff | Injection, oral, smoked | Pain relief, eu- phoria, drowsi- ness | Respiratory depression and arrest, nausea, confusion, constipation, sedation, un- conscious- ness, coma, tolerance, addiction |
| Oxycodone | *OxyContin, Percodan;* oxycotton, oxycet, hillbilly heroin, killers, OCs | Injection, oral | Pain relief, eu- phoria, drowsi- ness | Respiratory depression and arrest, nau- sea, confu- sion, consti- pation, sedation, un- conscious- ness, coma, tolerance, addiction |
| PCP | *Phencyclidine;* angel dust, boat, hog, love boat, peace pill | Injection, oral, smoked | Impaired mo- tor function, feelings of be- ing separated from one's body and environment, analgesia, psy- chosis, ag- gression, vio- lence, slurred speech, loss of coordination, hallucinations | Memory loss, loss of appetite, panic, aggression, violence |
| Psilocybin | Magic mush- rooms, purple passion, shrooms | Oral | Altered states of perception and feeling, hallucinations, nausea, ner- vousness, paranoia, panic | Chronic mental disorders |
| Quetiapine | *Seroquel;* baby heroin, Suzie-Q, Q-ball | Oral | Reduced anxi- ety, sedation | Arrhythmias, coma, death (with over- dose) |

# EQUIANALGESIC DOSING

Guidelines for equianalgesic dosing of commonly used analgesics are presented in the following table. The dosages are approximate to 10 mg of morphine intramuscularly. These guidelines are for the management of acute pain in the opioid-naïve pt. Dosages may vary for the opioid-tolerant pt and for the management of chronic pain. Dosing adjustments for renal or hepatic insufficiency may also be necessary. Clinical response is the criterion that must be applied for each pt with titration to desired response.

| Name | Equianalgesic Oral Dose | Equianalgesic Parenteral Dose (IV, IM, SQ) |
|------|------|------|
| Codeine | 200 mg | 100–130 mg |
| Fentanyl | Not available | 0.1 mg (100 mcg) |
| Hydrocodone | 30–45 mg | Not available |
| Hydromorphone (Dilaudid) | 7.5–8 mg | 1.5–2 mg |
| Hydromorphone (Dilaudid) (Controlled-Release) | 7.5 mg | N/A |
| Meperidine (Demerol) | 300 mg | 75 mg |
| Methadone (Dolophine) | 10–20 mg | 10 mg |
| Morphine | 30 mg | 10 mg |
| Oxycodone (OxyContin) | 20–30 mg | Not available |
| Oxymorphone | 10 mg | 1 mg |
| Oxymorphone (Extended-Release) | 10 mg | N/A |

# HERBALS: COMMON NATURAL MEDICINES

The use of herbal therapies is increasing in the United States. Because of the rise in the use of herbal therapy, the following is presented to provide some basic information on some of the more popular herbs. Please note this is not an all-inclusive list, which is beyond the scope of this handbook.

| Name | Uses | Comments |
|---|---|---|
| Aloe vera | Orally: osteoarthritis, inflammatory bowel diseases (e.g., ulcerative colitis), fever, itching, inflammation.<br>Topically: burns, wound healing, psoriasis, sunburn, frostbite, cold sores. | Well tolerated. Orally can cause abdominal pain, cramps; topically can cause burning, itching, contact dermatitis.<br>May lower blood glucose levels and have additive effects with antidiabetic medications. |
| Bilberry | Orally: improve visual acuity (e.g., night vision, cataracts), atherosclerosis, chronic fatigue syndrome, venous insufficiency, varicose veins, hemorrhoids.<br>Topically: mild inflammation of mouth and throat mucous membranes. | Can inhibit platelet aggregation, increase risk of bleeding when combined with antiplatelet or anticoagulant medications (e.g., aspirin, clopidogrel, enoxaparin, warfarin).<br>May lower blood glucose. |
| Bitter orange | Orally: appetite stimulant, dyspepsia.<br>Topically: inflammation of the eyelid, conjunctiva, retina. | May cause hypertension, cardiovascular toxicity.<br>May increase concentration/effects of midazolam; concurrent use with MAOIs may increase blood pressure (avoid use); combination with caffeine can increase blood pressure, heart rate. |
| Black cohosh | Orally: symptoms of menopause, premenstrual syndrome (PMS), dysmenorrhea, dyspepsia, inducing labor in pregnant women, anxiety, fever, cough, cardiovascular disease, cognitive function, infertility, osteoarthritis, osteoporosis, rheumatoid arthritis.<br>Topically: acne, mole, and wart removal; improve skin appearance. | Can cause GI upset, rash, headache, dizziness, increased weight, cramping, breast tenderness, vaginal spotting/bleeding.<br>May decrease effects of cisplatin; may increase risk of hepatic damage with hepatotoxic medications. |

*Continued*

| Name | Uses | Comments |
|------|------|----------|
| Capsicum (cayenne pepper) | Orally: dyspepsia, flatulence, diarrhea, cramps, toothache, hyperlipidemia.<br>Topically: pain of shingles, osteoarthritis, rheumatoid arthritis, postherpetic neuralgia, diabetic neuralgia, trigeminal neuralgia. | Orally can cause upper abdominal discomfort (e.g., gas, bloating, nausea, diarrhea, belching); topically can cause burning, stinging, erythema. May increase effects/adverse effects of antiplatelet medications. |
| Chamomile | Prepared as a tea and used as a mild sedative, relaxant, and sleeping aid; used for indigestion, itching, and inflammation. | Large amounts may cause vomiting. |
| Chastberry | Orally: menstrual irregularities (e.g., dysmenorrhea, amenorrhea, metrorrhagia). | Can cause GI upset, headache, diarrhea, nausea, itching, urticaria, rash, insomnia, increased weight, irregular menstrual bleeding.<br>Can interfere with efficacy of oral contraceptives, hormone replacement therapy. |
| Clove (clove oil) | Orally: dyspepsia, expectorant, diarrhea, halitosis, flatulence, nausea, vomiting.<br>Topically: toothache, mouth and throat inflammation. | Topically can cause tissue irritation, allergic dermatitis. |
| Co-enzyme Q-10 | Heart failure, angina, diabetes, hypertension. | Can cause GI side effects (e.g., nausea, vomiting, diarrhea, appetite suppression, heartburn, epigastric discomfort).<br>Can decrease blood pressure and have an additive effect with antihypertensive medications; may reduce anticoagulant effects of warfarin. |
| Cranberry | Prevention/treatment of urinary tract infections, neurogenic bladder, urinary deodorizer in incontinence, kidney stones, prevention of urinary catheter blockage. | Usually well tolerated. Large amounts can cause GI upset, diarrhea, nausea, vomiting. Greater than 1,000 ml daily can increase risk of uric acid, kidney stone formation. |
| DHEA | Slow or reverse aging, weight loss, metabolic syndrome, increase immune and cognitive function. | At high dose can cause acne, hirsutism, hair loss, voice deepening, insulin resistance, altered menstrual pattern.<br>May interfere with antiestrogen effects of anastrozole, letrozole, or other aromatase inhibitors; may overcome estrogen receptor antagonist activity of tamoxifen in estrogen receptor positive cancer cells. |

| Name | Uses | Comments |
|------|------|----------|
| Dong quai | Dysmenorrhea, premenstrual syndrome, menopausal symptoms. | May cause photosensitivity and photodermatitis.<br>May increase effect/risk of bleeding with antiplatelet and anticoagulant medications (e.g., aspirin, warfarin). |
| Echinacea | Treat/prevent common cold, influenza, other upper respiratory tract infections. | Usually well tolerated. Can cause GI effects (e.g., nausea, abdominal pain, diarrhea, vomiting). Stimulates immune function—may exacerbate autoimmune diseases (e.g., multiple sclerosis, rheumatoid arthritis, systemic lupus erythematosis). |
| Eucalyptus | Orally: infections, fever, dyspepsia, expectorant for coughs. Topically: inflammation of respiratory tract mucous membranes, rheumatoid arthritis, nasal stuffiness. | Orally: GI effects (e.g., nausea, vomiting, diarrhea). Topically (prolonged exposure/large amounts): agitation, drowsiness, muscle weakness, ataxia. |
| Evening primrose oil | Premenstrual syndrome (PMS), endometriosis, symptoms of menopause (e.g., hot flashes). | May increase risk of bruising/bleeding with antiplatelet/anticoagulant medications (e.g., aspirin, clopidogrel, enoxaparin, warfarin). |
| Feverfew | Orally: fever, headaches, prevention of migraines, menstrual irregularities. Topically: toothaches, antiseptic. | Orally: GI effects (e.g., heartburn, nausea, diarrhea, constipation, abdominal pain, bloating, flatulence). Topically: contact dermatitis. May have additive effects, increase risk of bleeding with antiplatelet medications. |
| Fish oil | Hyperlipidemia, hypertriglyceridemia, hypertension, stroke, depression, rheumatoid arthritis, osteoporosis, psoriasis, Crohn's disease. | Can cause a fishy aftertaste, halitosis, heartburn, dyspepsia, nausea, loose stools, rash. May have additive effect with antihypertensive medication. |
| Garlic | Hypertension, hyperlipidemia, age-related vascular changes, atherosclerosis, chronic fatigue syndrome, menstrual disorders, coronary heart disease, peripheral arterial disease. | Dose-related effects including breath/body odor, mouth and GI burning/irritation, heartburn, flatulence, nausea, vomiting, diarrhea. May increase effects of antiplatelets (e.g., aspirin, clopidogrel, enoxaparin), anticoagulants (e.g., warfarin); may decrease effects of oral contraceptives, cyclosporine, protease inhibitors, and non-nucleoside reverse transcriptase inhibitors (NNRTIs). |

*Continued*

| Name | Uses | Comments |
|------|------|----------|
| Ginger | Motion sickness, morning sickness, dyspepsia, rheumatoid arthritis, osteoarthritis, loss of appetite, migraine headache, diarrhea, flatulence, irritable bowel syndrome, dysmenorrhea. | Usually well tolerated. At high doses of 5 g/day may cause abdominal discomfort, heartburn, diarrhea, irritant effect in mouth and throat.<br>May increase risk of bleeding with antiplatelet medications and anticoagulants (e.g., aspirin, clopidogrel, enoxaparin, warfarin). |
| Ginkgo | Dementia (including Alzheimer's), vascular dementia, mixed dementia. | Mild GI upset, headache, dizziness, constipation, palpitations, allergic skin reactions. Large doses can cause diarrhea, nausea, vomiting, weakness. Decreases platelet aggregation; may increase risk of bleeding with antiplatelet and anticoagulants (e.g., aspirin, clopidogrel, enoxaparin, warfarin). |
| Ginseng | Increases resistance to environmental stress, improves well-being, boosts energy, diuretic. | May cause insomnia, vaginal bleeding, headache, hypertension, hypotension, decreased appetite, edema.<br>May decrease effectiveness of warfarin. |
| Glucosamine | Osteoarthritis, glaucoma, temporomandibular joint arthritis. | May cause mild GI effects (e.g., nausea, heartburn, diarrhea, constipation).<br>May increase risk of bleeding with anticoagulants (e.g., warfarin). |
| Gotu kola | Reduce fatigue, anxiety, depression, improve memory and intelligence. | May cause GI upset, nausea, drowsiness.<br>May cause additive sedative effects/side effects with CNS depressants (e.g., clonazepam, lorazepam, zolpidem). |
| Grapefruit | Hyperlipidemia, atherosclerosis, weight loss and obesity. | May increase concentrations/effects of benzodiazepines, calcium channel blockers, carbamazepine, carvedilol, clomipramine, cyclosporine, estrogens, lovastatin, simvastatin, atorvastatin. |
| Green tea | Improves cognitive performance and mental alertness. | Can cause nausea, vomiting, abdominal bloating, dyspepsia, flatulence, diarrhea. Higher doses can cause dizziness, insomnia, fatigue, agitation.<br>May increase effects of amphetamines, caffeine. |

| Name | Uses | Comments |
|------|------|----------|
| Hawthorn | Congestive HF, coronary heart disease, angina, arrhythmias. | Generally well tolerated. Can cause vertigo, dizziness, nausea, GI complaints, fatigue, sweating, rash. |
| Kava kava | Anxiety disorders, stress, attention-deficit hyperactivity disorder (ADHD), insomnia, restlessness. | GI upset, headache, dizziness, drowsiness, enlarged pupils and disturbances of oculomotor equilibrium and accommodation, dry mouth, allergic skin reactions. May increase drowsiness, motor reflex depression with alcohol, benzodiazepines, other CNS depressants. |
| L-carnitine | Treatment of primary L-carnitine deficiency, acute myocardial infarction, supplement to total parenteral nutrition, L-carnitine deficiency in those requiring hemodialysis. | Can cause nausea, vomiting, abdominal cramps, heartburn, gastritis, diarrhea, body odor, seizures. |
| Licorice | Gastric and duodenal ulcers, sore throat, bronchitis, dyspepsia, cough, osteoarthritis, chronic gastritis, menopausal symptoms, osteoporosis, bacterial/viral infections. | Excessive ingestion can cause pseudohyperaldosteronism with sodium and water retention, hypokalemia, alkalosis. May lead to hypertension, edema, arrhythmias. May reduce effect of antihypertensive medication therapy, warfarin. |
| Melatonin | Jet lag, insomnia, shift-work disorder. | Can cause daytime drowsiness, headache, dizziness. May increase effect of antiplatelets, anticoagulants (e.g., aspirin, clopidogrel, enoxaparin, warfarin). May cause additive sedation with CNS depressants (e.g., alcohol, benzodiazepines). |
| Milk thistle | Liver disorders, chronic inflammatory liver disease, hepatic cirrhosis, chronic hepatitis. | Usually well tolerated. Can cause nausea, diarrhea, dyspepsia, flatulence, abdominal bloating, anorexia. |
| Nettle | Urinary disorders associated with benign prostatic hyperplasia (e.g., nocturia, frequency, dysuria, urinary retention). | Generally well tolerated. May cause GI complaints, sweating, allergic skin reactions. May decrease effects of warfarin. |
| Peppermint | Common cold, cough, inflammation of mouth and pharynx, sinusitis, fever, cramps of upper GI tract, dyspepsia, flatulence, irritable bowel syndrome (IBS), fever, tension headache. | Can cause heartburn, nausea, vomiting, allergic reactions including flushing and headache. May increase concentration/effects of cyclosporine. |

*Continued*

| Name | Uses | Comments |
|------|------|----------|
| Red yeast | Maintain desirable cholesterol levels in healthy people; reduce cholesterol in hyperlipidemia; indigestion; diarrhea; improve blood circulation. | Can cause abdominal discomfort, heartburn, flatulence, dizziness. May increase cyclosporine concentration. |
| SAMe | Depression, anxiety, heart disease, fibromyalgia, osteoarthritis, tendonitis, dementia, Alzheimer's disease, Parkinson's disease. | Higher doses can cause flatulence, nausea, vomiting, diarrhea, constipation, headache, mild insomnia, anorexia, sweating, dizziness, nervousness. May have additive adverse effects with MAOIs including hypertension, hyperthermia, agitation, confusion, coma. May have additive serotonergic effects and serotonin syndrome-like effects (e.g., agitation, tremors, tachycardia, diarrhea, hyperreflexia, shivering, diaphoresis) with antidepressants. |
| Saw palmetto | Symptoms of benign prostatic hyperplasia (BPH). | Can cause dizziness, headache, GI complaints (e.g., nausea, vomiting, constipation, diarrhea). May increase effect of antiplatelets, anticoagulants (e.g., aspirin, clopidogrel, enoxaparin, warfarin). May interfere with contraceptives. |
| St. John's wort | Depression, anxiety, heart palpitations; mood disturbances associated with menopause, ADHD, obsessive-compulsive disorder (OCD), seasonal affective disorder (SAD), premenstrual syndrome (PMS), social phobia. | Usually well tolerated. Can cause insomnia, vivid dreams, restlessness, agitation, irritability, GI discomfort, diarrhea, fatigue, dry mouth, dizziness, headache. May decrease effect of alprazolam, amitriptyline, oral contraceptives, cyclosporine, imatinib, irinotecan, NNRTIs, phenytoin, protease inhibitors, tacrolimus, warfarin. May cause additive serotonergic effects with antidepressants, paroxetine, sertraline, tramadol. |
| Turmeric | Osteoarthritis, rheumatoid arthritis, dyspepsia, abdominal pain, Crohn's disease, ulcerative colitis, diarrhea, flatulence, loss of appetite, hepatitis, *H. pylori*, peptic ulcers, irritable bowel syndrome. | Usually well tolerated. Can cause dyspepsia, diarrhea, distention, GERD, nausea, vomiting. May increase risk of bleeding with antiplatelets/anticoagulants. May increase risk of hypoglycemia with antidiabetic drugs. |

| Name | Uses | Comments |
|------|------|----------|
| Valerian | Insomnia, anxiety-associated restlessness, sleeping disorders. | Can cause headache, excitability, insomnia, gastric discomfort, dry mouth, vivid dreams, morning drowsiness.<br>May have additive sedative effects with alcohol, benzodiazepines, other CNS depressants. |
| Yohimbe | Aphrodisiac, impotence, exhaustion, angina, hypertension, diabetic neuropathy, postural hypotension. | Can cause excitation, tremors, insomnia, anxiety, hypertension, tachycardia, dizziness, irritability, headache, fluid retention, rash, nausea, vomiting. High doses can cause respiratory depression.<br>May have additive effects with MAOIs. Tyramine-containing foods increase risk of hypertensive crisis. |

# LIFESPAN, CULTURAL ASPECTS, AND PHARMACOGENOMICS OF DRUG THERAPY

## LIFESPAN

Drug therapy is unique to pts of different ages. Age-specific competencies involve understanding the development and health needs of the various age groups. Pregnant pts, children, and elderly people represent different age groups with important considerations during drug therapy.

## CHILDREN

In pediatric drug therapy, drug administration is guided by the age of the child, weight, level of growth and development, and height. The dosage ordered is to be given either by kilogram of body weight or by square meter of body surface area, which is based on the height and weight of the child. Many dosages based on these calculations must be individualized based on pediatric response.

If the oral route of administration is used, often syrup or chewable tablets are given. Additionally, sometimes medication is added to liquid or mixed with foods. Remember to never force a child to take oral medications because choking or emotional trauma may ensue.

If an intramuscular injection is ordered, the vastus lateralis muscle in the midlateral thigh is used because the gluteus maximus is not developed until walking occurs and the deltoid muscle is too small. For intravenous medications, administer very slowly in children. If given too quickly, high serum drug levels will occur with the potential for toxicity.

## PREGNANCY

Women of childbearing years should be asked about the possibility of pregnancy before any drug therapy is initiated. Advise a woman who is either planning a pregnancy or believes she may be pregnant to inform her physician immediately. During pregnancy, medications given to the mother pass to the fetus via the placenta. Teratogenic (fetal abnormalities) effects may occur. Breastfeeding while the mother is taking certain medications may not be recommended due to the potential for adverse effects on the newborn.

The choice of drug ordered for pregnant women is based on the stage of pregnancy because the fetal organs develop during the first trimester. Cautious use of drugs in women of reproductive age who are sexually active and who are not using contraceptives is essential to prevent the potential for teratogenic or embryotoxic effects.

## ELDERLY

Elderly people are more likely to experience an adverse drug reaction owing to physiologic changes (e.g., visual, hearing, mobility changes, chronic diseases) and cognitive changes (short-term memory loss or alteration in the thought process) that may lead to multiple medication dosing. In chronic disease states such as hypertension, glaucoma, asthma, or arthritis, the daily ingestion of multiple medications increases the potential for adverse reactions and toxic effects.

Decreased renal or hepatic function may lower the metabolism of medications in the liver and reduce excretion of medications, thus prolonging the half-life of the drug and the potential for toxicity. Dosages in elderly people should initially be smaller than for the general adult population and then slowly titrated based on pt response and therapeutic effect of the medication.

## CULTURE

The term *ethnopharmacology* was first used to describe the study of medicinal plants used by indigenous cultures. More recently, it is being used as a reference to the action and effects of drugs in people from diverse racial, ethnic, and cultural backgrounds. Although there are insufficient data from investigations involving people from diverse backgrounds that would provide reliable information on ethnic-specific responses to all medications, there is growing evidence that modifications in dosages are needed for some members of racial and ethnic groups. There are wide variations in the perception of side effects by pts from diverse cultural backgrounds. These differences may be related to metabolic differences that result in higher or lower levels of the drug, individual differences in the amount of body fat, or cultural differences in the way individuals perceive the meaning of side effects and toxicity. Nurses and other health care providers need to be aware that variations can occur with side effects, adverse reactions, and toxicity so that pts from diverse cultural backgrounds can be monitored.

Some cultural differences in response to medications include the following:

**African Americans:** Generally, African Americans are less responsive to beta blockers (e.g., propranolol [Inderal]) and angiotensin-converting enzyme (ACE) inhibitors (e.g., enalapril [Vasotec]).

**Asian Americans:** On average, Asian Americans have a lower percentage of body fat, so dosage adjustments must be made for fat-soluble vitamins and other drugs (e.g., vitamin K used to reverse the anticoagulant effect of warfarin).

**Hispanic Americans:** Hispanic Americans may require lower dosages and may experience a higher incidence of side effects with tricyclic antidepressants (e.g., amitriptyline).

**Native Americans:** Alaskan Eskimos may suffer prolonged muscle paralysis with the use of succinylcholine when administered during surgery.

There has been a desire to exert more responsibility over one's health and, as a result, a resurgence of self-care practices. These practices are often influenced by folk remedies and the use of medicinal plants. In the United States, there are several major ethnic population subgroups (white, black, Hispanic, Asian, and Native Americans). Each of these ethnic groups has a wide range of practices that influence beliefs and interventions related to health and illness. At any given time, in any group, treatment may consist of the use of traditional herbal therapy, a combination of ritual and prayer with medicinal plants, customary dietary and environmental practices, or the use of Western medical practices.

## AFRICAN AMERICANS

Many African Americans carry the traditional health beliefs of their African heritage. Health denotes harmony with nature of the body, mind, and spirit, whereas illness is seen as disharmony that results from natural causes or divine punishment. Common practices to the art of healing include treatments with herbals and rituals known empirically to restore health. Specific forms of healing include using home remedies, obtaining medical advice from a physician, and seeking spiritual healing.

Examples of healing practices include the use of hot baths and warm compresses for rheumatism, the use of herbal teas for respiratory illnesses, and the use of kitchen condiments in folk remedies. Lemon, vinegar, honey, saltpeter, alum, salt, baking soda, and Epsom salt are common kitchen ingredients used. Goldenrod, peppermint, sassafras, parsley, yarrow, and rabbit tobacco are a few of the herbals used.

## HISPANIC AMERICANS

The use of folk healers, medicinal herbs, magic, and religious rituals and ceremonies are included in the rich and varied customs of Hispanic Americans. This ethnic group believes that God is responsible for allowing health or illness to occur. Wellness may be viewed as good luck, a reward for good behavior, or a blessing from God. Praying, using herbals and spices, wearing religious objects such as medals, and maintaining a balance in diet and physical activity are methods considered appropriate in preventing evil or poor health.

Hispanic ethnopharmacology is more complementary to Western medical practices. After the illness is identified, appropriate treatment may consist of home remedies (e.g., use of vegetables and herbs), use of over-the-counter patent medicines, and use of physician-prescribed medications.

## ASIAN AMERICANS

For Asian Americans, harmony with nature is essential for physical and spiritual well-being. Universal balance depends on harmony among the elemental forces: fire, water, wood, earth, and metal. Regulating these universal elements are two forces that maintain physical and spiritual harmony in the body: the *yin* and the *yang*. Practices shared by most Asian cultures include meditation, special nutritional programs, herbology, and martial arts.

Therapeutic options available to traditional Chinese physicians include prescribing herbs, meditation, exercise, nutritional changes, and acupuncture.

## NATIVE AMERICANS

The theme of total harmony with nature is fundamental to traditional Native American beliefs about health. It is dependent on maintaining a state of equilibrium among the physical body, the mind, and the environment. Health practices reflect this holistic approach. The method of healing is determined traditionally by the medicine man, who diagnoses the ailment and recommends the appropriate intervention.

Treatment may include heat, herbs, sweat baths, massage, exercise, diet changes, and other interventions performed in a curing ceremony.

## EUROPEAN AMERICANS

Europeans often use home treatments as the front-line interventions. Traditional remedies practiced are based on the magical or empirically validated experience of ancestors. These cures are often practiced in combination with religious rituals or spiritual ceremonies.

Household products, herbal teas, and patent medicines are familiar preparations used in home treatments (e.g., saltwater gargle for sore throat).

## PHARMACOGENOMICS

Traditionally, medications are prescribed using a "one size fits all" philosophy. In general, the genetic makeup is similar in all humans, regardless of race or sex. However, people inherit variations in their genes, which can affect the way a person responds to a medication. A genetic variation may make a medication stay in the body longer, causing serious side effects, or a variation may make the medication less potent.

For example, two people taking the same cancer medication may have very different responses. One may have severe, life-threatening side effects, whereas the second may have few, if any, side effects. The drug may shrink a tumor in one person but not in another.

**Pharmacogenomics** examines how a person's genetic makeup affects response to medications. Although widespread application still lies in the future, pharmacogenomics has the potential to personalize medical therapies. Physicians eventually will be able to prescribe medications based on an individual's genotype, thereby maximizing effectiveness and minimizing side effects.

## PHARMACOGENOMICS

Pharmacogenomics is an expanding field that explores the effect of inter-individual genetic differences on pharmacokinetics, pharmacodynamics, drug efficiency, and safety of drug treatments. Pharmacogenomic biomarkers (proteins) can provide predictive tools for improving drug response and reducing adverse drug reactions. These biomarkers mainly originate from genes encoding drug-metabolizing enzymes, drug transporters, drugs targets, and human leukocyte antigens. Currently, more than 100 drugs contain pharmacogenomic information in the package labeling. The goal is to develop personalized genetic-based strategies that will optimize therapeutic outcomes.

Personalized treatments are especially warranted when prescribing medications with a narrow therapeutic index or when toxicity can be life threatening. Antineoplastics, anticoagulants, and anti-HIV therapies are often administered at maximum tolerated doses. This approach can result in toxicity and/or produce a poor response to therapy. Severe adverse drug reactions are one of the most common reasons for hospital admissions. Genetic testing for drug responses is expected to decrease hospitalizations by as much as 30%.

**Carbamazepine (Tegretol)** has been linked to dose-dependent side effects and life-threatening adverse effects. It is metabolized by enzymes encoded by the CYP3A4 gene to its active metabolite. An association has been found between the HLA-B*1502 allele and risk of Stevens-Johnson syndrome/toxic epidermal necrolysis, particularly in Asians. Before initiating carbamazepine treatment in high-risk patients, genetic testing for the HLA-B*1502 allele is recommended by the Food and Drug Administration (FDA).

Tumor cells carry the same genetic polymorphins of normal cells. However, malignant cells are genetically unstable and can produce genetic changes that can alter disposition of active drug at the tumor site. Genetic analysis of tumors can help predict therapeutic benefit (or lack thereof) of targeted biologics such as **trastuzumab (Herceptin)** for ERBB2 *(HER2)*–amplified breast cancers or **erlotinib (Tarceva)** for epidermal growth factor receptor (EGFR)–overexpressing lung cancers.

Genetic mutations in tumors can also predict resistance to treatment, as noted in colorectal cancers, where activating mutations in *KRAS* are known to be a predictive marker for resistance to the EGFR-specific monoclonal antibodies **cetuximab (Erbitux)** and **panitumumab (Vectibix)**.

By utilizing the information provided by pharmacogenomic testing, drug therapy is changing to a more individualized approach. Anticipated benefits of pharmacogenomics include creation of better vaccines, safer medications targeted to specific diseases, and more appropriate dosing of medications at the onset of therapy. Ultimately, we may see a decrease in health care costs due to more efficient clinical trials, reduced adverse drug reactions, and less time needed to find effective therapy for patients.

# NORMAL LABORATORY VALUES

## HEMATOLOGY/COAGULATION

| Test | Normal Range |
| --- | --- |
| Activated partial thromboplastin time (aPTT) | 25–35 sec |
| Erythrocyte count (RBC count) | M: 4.5–5.5 million cells/mm$^3$<br>F: 4.0–4.9 million cells/mm$^3$ |
| Hematocrit (HCT, Hct) | M: 41%–50%<br>F: 36%–44% |
| Hemoglobin (Hb, Hgb) | M: 13.5–16.5 g/dL<br>F: 12.0–15.0 g/dL |
| Leukocyte count (WBC count) | 4.5–10.0 thousand cells/mm$^3$ |
| Leukocyte differential count | |
|   Basophils | 0%–0.75% |
|   Eosinophils | 1%–3% |
|   Lymphocytes | 25%–33% |
|   Monocytes | 3%–7% |
|   Neutrophils—bands | 3%–5% |
|   Neutrophils—segmented | 54%–62% |
| Mean corpuscular hemoglobin (MCH) | 26–34 pg/cell |
| Mean corpuscular hemoglobin concentration (MCHC) | 31%–37% Hb/cell |
| Mean corpuscular volume (MCV) | 80–100 fL |
| Partial thromboplastin time (PTT) | 60–85 sec |
| Platelet count (thrombocyte count) | 100–450 thousand/mm$^3$ |
| Prothrombin time (PT) | 11–13.5 sec |
| RBC count (see Erythrocyte count) | |

## CLINICAL CHEMISTRY (SERUM PLASMA, URINE)

| Test | Normal Range |
| --- | --- |
| Alanine aminotransferase (ALT) | 8–36 units/L<br>8–78 units/L (children 0–2 mos) |
| Albumin | 3.2–5 g/dl |
| Alkaline phosphatase | 33–131 (adults 25–60 yrs)<br>51–153 (adults older than 60 yrs) |
| Amylase | 30–110 units/L |
| Aspartate aminotransferase (AST) | 5–35 units/L |
| Bilirubin (direct) | 0–0.3 mg/dL |
| Bilirubin (total) | 0.1–1.2 mg/dL |
| BUN | 7–20 mg/dL |
| Calcium, ionized | 2.24–2.46 mEq/L |

| Test | Normal Range |
| --- | --- |
| Calcium (total) | 8.6–10.3 mg/dL |
| Carbon dioxide ($CO_2$) total | 23–30 mEq/L |
| Chloride | 95–108 mEq/L |
| Cholesterol (total) | Less than 200 mg/dL |
|    HDL cholesterol | 40–60 mg/dL |
|    LDL cholesterol | Less than 160 mg/dL |
| Creatinine | 0.5–1.4 mg/dl |
| Creatinine clearance | M: 80–125 ml/min/1.73 m$^2$<br>F: 75–115 ml/min/1.73 m$^2$ |
| Creatine kinase (CK) isoenzymes | |
|    CK-BB | 0% |
|    CK-MB (cardiac) | 0%–3.9% |
|    CK-MM (muscle) | 96%–100% |
| Creatine phosphokinase (CPK) | 8–150 units/L |
| Ferritin | 13–300 ng/ml |
| Glucose (preprandial) | Less than 115 mg/dL |
| Glucose (fasting) | 60–110 mg/dL |
| Glucose (nonfasting, 2 hrs postprandial) | Less than 120 mg/dL |
| Hemoglobin A1c | Less than 8 |
| Iron | 66–150 mcg/dL |
| Iron-binding capacity, total (TIBC) | 250–420 mcg/dL |
| Lactate dehydrogenase (LDH) | 56–194 units/L |
| Lipase | 23–208 units/L |
| Magnesium | 1.6–2.5 mg/dL |
| Osmolality | 289–308 mOsm/kg |
| Oxygen saturation | 90–95 (arterial)<br>40–70 (venous) |
| pH | 7.35–7.45 (arterial)<br>7.32–7.42 (venous) |
| Phosphorus, inorganic | 2.8–4.2 mg/dL |
| Potassium | 3.5–5.2 mEq/L |
| Protein (total) | 6.5–7.9 g/dL |
| Sodium | 134–149 mEq/L |
| Thyroid-stimulating hormone (TSH) | 0.7–6.4 milliunits/L (adults 20 yrs<br>or younger)<br>0.4–4.2 milliunits/L (adults 21–54 yrs)<br>0.5–8.9 milliunits/L (adults 55–87 yrs) |
| Transferrin | Greater than 200 mg/dL |
| Triglycerides (TG) | 45–155 mg/dL |
| Urea nitrogen | 7–20 mg/dL |
| Uric acid | M: 2–8 mg/dL<br>F: 2–7.5 mg/dL |

# CYTOCHROME P450 (CYP) ENZYMES

Most drugs are eliminated from the body, at least in part, by being changed chemically to a less lipid-soluble product (i.e., metabolized) and thus more likely to be excreted from the body via the kidney or bile. Drugs may go through two different metabolic processes: phase 1 and phase 2 metabolism.

In phase 1 metabolism, hepatic microsomal enzymes found in the endothelium of liver cells metabolize drugs via hydrolysis and oxidation and reduction reactions. These chemical reactions make the drug more water soluble. In phase 2 metabolism, large water-soluble substances (e.g., glucuronic acid, sulfate) are attached to the drug, forming inactive, or significantly less active, water-soluble metabolites. Phase 2 processes include glucuronidation, sulfation, conjugation, acetylation, and methylation.

Virtually any of the phase 1 and phase 2 enzymes can be inhibited, and some of these enzymes can be induced by drugs. Inhibiting the activity of metabolic enzymes results in increased concentrations of the drug (substrate), whereas inducing metabolic enzymes results in decreased concentrations of the drug (substrate).

The term "cytochrome P450" (CYP enzymes) refers to a family of more than 100 enzymes in the human body that modulate various physiologic functions. First identified in the 1950s, the CYP enzyme system contains two large subgroups: steroidogenic and xenobiotic enzymes. Only the xenobiotic group is involved in the metabolism of drugs. The xenobiotic group includes four major enzyme families: CYP1, CYP2, CYP3, and CYP4. The primary role of these families is the metabolism of drugs. These families are further subdivided into subfamilies designated by a capital letter and given a specific enzyme number (1, 2, 3, etc.) according to the similarity in amino acid sequence it shares with other enzymes (e.g., CYP1A2).

The key CYP450 enzymes include CYP1A2, CYP2C9, CYP2C19, CYP2D6, and CYP3A4 and may be responsible for metabolism of 75% of all drugs, with the CYP3A subfamily responsible for nearly half of this activity.

The CYP enzymes are found in the endoplasmic reticulum of cells in a variety of human tissue but are primarily concentrated in the liver and intestine. CYP enzymes can be both inhibited and induced, leading to increased or decreased serum concentration of the drug (along with its effects).

The following tables of CYP substrates, inhibitors, and inducers provide a perspective on drugs that are affected by, or affect, cytochrome P450 (CYP) enzymes. **CYP substrate** includes drugs reported to be metabolized, at least in part, by one or more CYP enzymes. **CYP inhibitor** includes drugs reported to inhibit one or more CYP enzymes. **CYP inducer** contains drugs reported to induce one or more CYP enzymes.

## P450 ENZYMES: SUBSTRATES, INHIBITORS, INDUCERS
### CYP1A2 ENZYME

| CYP1A2 SUBSTRATES | CYP1A2 INHIBITORS | CPY1A2 INDUCERS |
| --- | --- | --- |
| Caffeine | Cimetidine (Tagamet) | Barbiturates |
| Clozapine (Clozaril) | Ciprofloxacin (Cipro) | Carbamazepine (Tegretol) |
| Mirtazapine (Remeron) | Fluvoxamine | Rifampin (Rifadin) |
| Olanzapine (Zyprexa) | Zileuton (Zyflo) | Smoking |
| Ramelteon (Rozerem) | | |
| Ropinirole (Requip) | | |
| Tizanidine (Zanaflex) | | |

- CYP1A2 enzyme is increasingly involved in drug interactions.
- More potent inhibitors include cimetidine, ciprofloxacin, and fluvoxamine.
- Smoking is the most important inducer, but rifampin and barbiturates also can increase enzyme activity.
- Example of reaction: Tizanidine plasma concentrations increased more than 30-fold when the inhibitor fluvoxamine was given concurrently.

### CYP2C9 ENZYME

| CYP2C9 SUBSTRATES | CYP2C9 INHIBITORS | CYP2C9 INDUCERS |
| --- | --- | --- |
| Candesartan (Atacand) | Amiodarone (Cordarone) | Barbiturates |
| Celecoxib (Celebrex) | Clopidogrel (Plavix) | Carbamazepine (Tegretol) |
| Diclofenac (Voltaren) | Fluconazole (Diflucan) | Rifampin (Rifadin) |
| Glipizide (Glucotrol) | Metronidazole (Flagyl) | St. John's wort |
| Glyburide (DiaBeta) | Sulfamethoxazole | |
| Ibuprofen (Advil, Motrin) | Valproic acid (Depakote) | |
| Irbesartan (Avapro) | | |
| Meloxicam (Mobic) | | |
| Warfarin (Coumadin) | | |

- More potent inhibitors include amiodarone, metronidazole, and sulfamethoxazole.
- All of the inducers can substantially increase enzyme activity.
- Both warfarin and oral hypoglycemics are of serious concern with regard to drug interactions. Substrates warranting attention include warfarin and oral hypoglycemics.

### CYP2C19 ENZYME

| CYP2C19 SUBSTRATES | CYP2C19 INHIBITORS | CYP2C19 INDUCERS |
| --- | --- | --- |
| Citalopram (Celexa) | Cimetidine (Tagamet) | Barbiturates |
| Diazepam (Valium) | Clopidogrel (Plavix) | Carbamazepine (Tegretol) |
| Escitalopram (Lexapro) | Esomeprazole (Nexium) | Rifampin (Rifadin) |
| Omeprazole (Prilosec) | Fluconazole (Diflucan) | St. John's wort |
| Pantoprazole (Protonix) | Fluvoxamine | |
| Sertraline (Zoloft) | Modafinil (Provigil) | |

- Inhibition by itself does not frequently cause adverse effects compared with other CYP enzymes because many of the substrates do not have serious toxicity.
- Inhibition or induction of the enzyme nonetheless may result in an adverse drug interaction.

- Racial background is important in the likelihood of being deficient in this enzyme (e.g., 3%–5% of Caucasians and 12%–23% of Asians are poor metabolizers of this enzyme).

## CYP2D6 ENZYME

| CYP2D6 SUBSTRATES | CYP2D6 INHIBITORS | CYP2D6 INDUCERS |
| --- | --- | --- |
| Amitriptyline (Elavil) | Amiodarone (Cordarone) | See comment below |
| Atomoxetine (Strattera) | Bupropion (Wellbutrin) | |
| Duloxetine (Cymbalta) | Fluoxetine (Prozac) | |
| Fluoxetine (Prozac) | Paroxetine (Paxil) | |
| Metoclopramide (Reglan) | | |
| Metoprolol (Lopressor) | | |
| Paroxetine (Paxil) | | |
| Risperidone (Risperdal) | | |
| Tamoxifen (Nolvadex) | | |
| Tolterodine (Detrol) | | |
| Tramadol (Ultram) | | |
| Venlafaxine (Effexor) | | |

- Potent inhibitors include fluoxetine and paroxetine.
- Evidence suggests that this enzyme is not very susceptible to enzyme induction.
- Genetics, rather than drug therapy, accounts for most ultra-rapid metabolizers (e.g., Greeks, Portuguese, Saudis, and Ethiopians have high enzyme activity).

## CYP3A4 ENZYME

| CYP3A4 SUBSTRATES | CYP3A4 INHIBITORS | CYP3A4 INDUCERS |
| --- | --- | --- |
| Alfuzosin (Uroxatral) | Amiodarone (Cordarone) | Carbamazepine (Tegretol) |
| Alprazolam (Xanax) | Clarithromycin (Biaxin) | Efavirenz (Sustiva) |
| Budesonide (Entocort EC) | Diltiazem (Cardizem) | Phenobarbital |
| Carbamazepine (Tegretol) | Erythromycin (Ery-Tab) | Rifampin (Rifadin) |
| Cyclosporine (Neoral) | Fluconazole (Diflucan) | St. John's wort |
| Fluticasone (Flovent) | Fluoxetine (Prozac) | |
| Lovastatin (Mevacor) | Itraconazole (Spoiranox) | |
| Repaglinide (Prandin) | Ketoconazole (Nizoral) | |
| Sildenafil (Viagra) | Verapamil (Calan, Isoptin) | |
| Simvastatin (Zocor) | | |
| Tadalafil (Cialis) | | |

- This enzyme metabolizes about half of all medications on the market.
- Drug toxicity of CYP3A4 substrates due to inhibition of CYP3A4 is relatively common.
- This enzyme is very sensitive to induction, tending to lower plasma concentrations of substrates, resulting in reduced efficacy of the substrate.
- Most potent inhibitors include clarithromycin, itraconazole, and ketoconazole.
- Rifampin is a potent inducer and may reduce serum concentrations of substrates by as much as 90%.

# POISON ANTIDOTE CHART

| Poisoning Agent | Antidote | Dosage |
|---|---|---|
| Acetaminophen | Acetylcysteine (Acetadote, Mucomyst) | PO: ADULTS, CHILDREN: Loading dose: 140 mg/kg, then 70 mg/kg q4h for a total of 18 doses. Total dose delivered: 1,330 mg/kg. IV: ADULTS, CHILDREN: Loading dose: 150 mg/kg over 60 min, then 50 mg/kg for 4 hrs, then 100 mg/kg over 16 hrs. Total dose delivered: 300 mg/kg. |
| Anticholinergic agents (e.g., atropine) | Physostigmine | IM/IV/SQ: ADULTS: Initially, 0.5–2 mg, then repeat q20min until response occurs or adverse effects occur. Repeat 1–4 mg q30–60min as life-threatening symptoms recur. IV: CHILDREN (Reserve for life-threatening situation only): 0.01–0.03 mg/kg/dose. May repeat after 15–20 min to maximum total dose of 2 mg, or until response occurs or adverse cholinergic effects occur. |
| Arsenic | Dimercaprol (BAL in oil) | Mild Poisoning IM: ADULTS, CHILDREN: 2.5 mg/kg/dose q6h for 2 days, then q12h for 1 day, then once daily for 10 days. Severe Poisoning IM: ADULTS, CHILDREN: 3 mg/kg/dose q4h for 2 days, then q6h for 1 day, then q12h for 10 days. |
| Benzodiazepines (e.g., midazolam) | Flumazenil (Romazicon) | IV: ADULTS: 0.2 mg over 30 sec. May give 0.3-mg dose after 30 sec if desired LOC not obtained. Additional doses of 0.5 mg can be given over 30 sec at 1-min intervals up to cumulative dose of 3 mg. CHILDREN: 0.01 mg/kg (**maximum:** 0.2 mg) with repeat doses of 0.01 mg/kg (**maximum:** 0.2 mg) given every minute to maximum total cumulative dose of 1 mg. |
| Beta blockers (e.g., propranolol) | Glucagon | IV: ADULTS: 5–10 mg over 1 min, followed by infusion of 1–10 mg/hr. |
| Calcium channel blockers (e.g., verapamil) | Glucagon | IV: ADULTS: 5–10 mg over 1 min, followed by infusion of 1–10 mg/hr. |

*Continued*

| Poisoning Agent | Antidote | Dosage |
|---|---|---|
| Carbamate pesticides | Atropine | IV: ADULTS: Initially, 1–5 mg doubled q5min until signs of muscarinic excess abate.<br>IV INFUSION: ADULTS: 0.5–1 mg/hr.<br>IM: ADULTS (Mild symptoms): 2 mg. If severe symptoms develop after first dose, 2 additional doses should be repeated in 10 min. (Severe symptoms): Immediately administer three 2-mg doses.<br>IV: CHILDREN: 0.02–0.05 mg/kg q10–20min until atropine effect observed, then q1–4h for at least 24 hrs.<br>IM: 0.5–2 mg/dose based on weight (0.5 mg: 15–40 lb, 1 mg: 41–90 lb, 2 mg: greater than 90 lb). (Mild symptoms): 1 injection. (Severe symptoms): 2 additional injections given in rapid succession 10 min after receiving first injection. |
| Digoxin (Lanoxin) | Digoxin immune FAB (Digibind) | **ADULTS**<br>Unknown amount of ingestion: 800 mg IV infusion if acute ingestion, 240 mg IV infusion if chronic ingestion.<br>**Dosing for Ingestion of Single Large Dose**<br>Dose (in no. of vials) = (Total digitalis body load in mg)/(0.5 mg of digitalis bound per vial).<br>Total digitalis body load in mg = (No. of tablets/capsules ingested) $\times$ (mg strength of tablet/capsule) $\times$ (bioavailability of tablet/capsule). Digoxin tablets and elixir are 80% bioavailable. Digoxin capsules and injection are 100% bioavailable.<br>**Dosing Based on Serum Level**<br>Digoxin: Dose (in no. of vials) = (Serum digoxin level in ng/mL) $\times$ (weight in kg)/(100).<br>Digitoxin: Dose (in no. of vials) = (Serum digitoxin level in ng/mL) $\times$ (weight in kg)/(1,000).<br><br>**CHILDREN**<br>**Dosing for Ingestion of Single Large Dose**<br>Dose (in no. of vials) = (Total digitalis body load in mg)/(0.5 mg of digitalis bound per vial).<br>Total digitalis body load in mg = (No. of tablets/capsules ingested) $\times$ (mg strength of tablet/capsule) $\times$ (bioavailability of tablet/capsule). Digoxin tablets and elixir are 80% bioavailable. Digoxin capsules and injection are 100% bioavailable.<br>WEIGHING 20 kg or less: Dilution of reconstituted vial to 1 mg/ml may be desirable for doses of 3 mg or less.<br>Dose (in no. of mg) = Dose (in no. of vials) $\times$ 38 mg/vial.<br>Dose (in no. of vials) = (Serum digoxin level in ng/ml) $\times$ (weight in kg)/(100). |

| Poisoning Agent | Antidote | Dosage |
|---|---|---|
| Ethylene glycol | Fomepizole (Antizol) | IV: ADULTS, CHILDREN: Loading dose 15 mg/kg, then 10 mg/kg q12h for 4 doses, then 15 mg/kg q12h thereafter until ethylene glycol levels reduced to less than 20 mg/dl and patient is asymptomatic with normal pH. |
| Extravasation vasoconstrictive agents (e.g., dopamine) | Phentolamine (Regitine) | ADULTS, CHILDREN: Infiltrate area with small amount of solution made by diluting 5–10 mg in 10 ml 0.9% NaCl within 12 hrs of extravasation. In general, do not exceed 0.1–0.2 mg/kg (5 mg total). |
| Heparin | Protamine | IV: ADULTS, CHILDREN: Dosage is determined by most recent dosage of heparin or low molecular weight heparin (LWH): 1 mg protamine neutralizes 90–115 units of heparin and 1 mg (100 units) of LWH. **Maximum:** 50 mg. |
| Iron | Deferoxamine (Desferal) | Acute<br>IM: ADULTS: Initially, 1,000 mg, then 500 mg q4h for 2 doses. Additional doses of 0.5 g q4–12h. **Maximum:** 6 g/24 hrs.<br>CHILDREN 3 YRS AND OLDER: 90 mg/kg/dose q8h (not to exceed 1 g/dose). **Maximum:** 6 g/24 hrs.<br>IV: ADULTS, CHILDREN: 15 mg/kg/hr. **Maximum:** 6 g/24 hrs.<br><br>Chronic<br>IM: ADULTS: 500–1,000 mg/day.<br>IV: ADULTS, CHILDREN: 15 mg/kg/hr. **Maximum:** 12 g/24 hrs. |
| Isoniazid | Pyridoxine (vitamin $B_6$) | IV: ADULTS, CHILDREN: Total dose of pyridoxine equal to amount of isoniazid ingested as first dose of 1–4 g IV, then 1 g IM q30min until total dose completed. If not known, give 5 g at rate of 1 g/min. May repeat q5–10min. |
| Lead | Calcium EDTA | Symptomatic<br>Treat for 3–5 days; give in conjunction with dimercaprol.<br>IM: ADULTS, CHILDREN: 167 mg/m² q4h.<br>IV: ADULTS, CHILDREN: 1 g/m² as 8- to 24-hr infusion or divided q12h.<br><br>Lead Encephalopathy<br>Treat for 5 days; give concurrently with dimercaprol.<br>IM: ADULTS, CHILDREN: 250 mg/m² q4h.<br>IV: ADULTS, CHILDREN: 50 mg/kg/day as 24-hr continuous infusion. |

*Continued*

| Poisoning Agent | Antidote | Dosage |
|---|---|---|
| Lead | Dimercaprol (BAL in oil) | **Mild** IM: ADULTS, CHILDREN: Loading dose 4 mg/kg, then 3 mg/kg/dose q4h for 2–7 days. Begin calcium EDTA with second dose.<br><br>**Severe and Lead Encephalopathy** IM: ADULTS, CHILDREN: 4 mg/kg/dose q4h for 3–5 days. Begin calcium EDTA with second dose. |
| Lead | Succimer (Chemet) | PO: ADULTS, CHILDREN: 10 mg/kg/dose q8h for 5 days, then q12h for 14 days. **Maximum:** 500 mg/dose. Note: For children younger than 5 yrs, dose based on mg/m$^2$. |
| Methanol | Fomepizole (Antizol) | IV: ADULTS, CHILDREN: Loading dose 15 mg/kg, then 10 mg/kg q12h for 4 doses, then 15 mg/kg q12h thereafter until ethylene glycol levels reduced to less than 20 mg/dl and patient is asymptomatic with normal pH. |
| Opioids (e.g., morphine) | Naloxone (Narcan) | IV/IM/SQ: ADULTS: 0.4–2 mg/dose. May repeat every 2–3 min as needed. Therapy may need to be reassessed if no response is seen after cumulative dose of 10 mg.<br>CHILDREN (5 YRS OR OLDER or WEIGHING 20 KG OR GREATER): 2 mg/dose IV/IM/SQ. May repeat every 2–3 min as needed. Therapy may need to be reassessed if no response is seen after cumulative dose of 10 mg.<br>CHILDREN (WEIGHING LESS THAN 20 KG): 0.1 mg/kg/dose. May repeat every 2–3 min as needed. |
| Organophosphate pesticides | Atropine | IV: ADULTS: Initially, 1–5 mg doubled q5min until signs of muscarinic excess abate.<br>IV INFUSION: ADULTS: 0.5–1 mg/hr.<br>IM: ADULTS (Mild symptoms): 2 mg. If severe symptoms develop after first dose, 2 additional doses should be repeated in 10 min. (Severe symptoms): Immediately administer three 2-mg doses.<br>IV: CHILDREN: 0.02–0.05 mg/kg q10–20min until atropine effect observed, then q1–4h for at least 24 hrs.<br>IM: 0.5–2 mg/dose based on weight (0.5 mg: 15–40 lb, 1 mg: 41–90 lb, 2 mg: greater than 90 lb). (Mild symptoms): 1 injection. (Severe symptoms): 2 additional injections given in rapid succession 10 min after receiving first injection. |

| Poisoning Agent | Antidote | Dosage |
|---|---|---|
| Organophosphate pesticides | Pralidoxime (Protopam) | IM/IV: ADULTS: 1–2 g. Repeat in 1–2 hrs if muscle weakness has not been relieved, then at 10- to 12-hr intervals if cholinergic signs recur.<br>CHILDREN: 20–50 mg/kg/dose. Repeat in 1–2 hrs if muscle weakness is not relieved, then at 10- to 12-hr intervals if cholinergic signs recur. |
| Warfarin (Coumadin) | Phytonadione (vitamin K) | PO/IV/SQ: ADULTS: 2.5–10 mg/dose. May repeat in 12–48 hrs if given PO, 6–8 hrs if given by IV or SQ route.<br>CHILDREN: 0.5–5 mg depending on need for further anticoagulation, severity of bleeding. |

# PREVENTING MEDICATION ERRORS AND IMPROVING MEDICATION SAFETY

Medication safety is a high priority for the health care professional. Prevention of medication errors and improved safety for the pt are important, esp. in today's health care environment when today's pt is older and sometimes sicker and the drug therapy regimen can be more sophisticated and complex.

A medication error is defined by the National Coordinating Council for Medication Error Reporting and Prevention (NCC MERP) as "any preventable event that may cause or lead to inappropriate medication use or pt harm while the medication is in the control of the health care professional, pt, or consumer."

Most medication errors occur as a result of multiple, compounding events as opposed to a single act by a single individual.

Use of the wrong medication, strength, or dose; confusion over sound-alike or look-alike drugs; administration of medications by the wrong route; miscalculations (esp. when used in pediatric pts or when administering medications intravenously); and errors in prescribing and transcription all can contribute to compromising the safety of the pt. The potential for adverse events and medication errors is definitely a reality and is potentially tragic and costly in both human and economic terms.

Health care professionals must take the initiative to create and implement procedures to prevent medication errors from occurring and implement methods to reduce medication errors. The first priority in preventing medication errors is to establish a multidisciplinary team to improve medication use. The goal for this team would be to assess medication safety and implement changes that would make it difficult or impossible for mistakes to occur. Some important criteria in making improved medication safety successful include the following:

- Promote a nonpunitive approach to reducing medication errors.
- Increase the detection and the reporting of medication errors, near misses, and potentially hazardous situations that may result in medication errors.
- Determine root causes of medication errors.
- Educate about the causes of medication errors and ways to prevent these errors.
- Make recommendations to allow organization-wide, system-based changes to prevent medication errors.
- Learn from errors that occur in other organizations and take measures to prevent similar errors.

Some common causes and ways to prevent medication errors and improve safety include the following:

**Handwriting:** Poor handwriting can make it difficult to distinguish between two medications with similar names. Also, many drug names sound similar, esp. when the names are spoken over the telephone, poorly enunciated, or mispronounced.

- Take time to write legibly.
- Keep phone or verbal orders to a minimum to prevent misinterpretation.

- Repeat back orders taken over the telephone.
- When ordering a new or rarely used medication, print the name.
- Always specify the drug strength, even if only one strength exists.
- Express dosages for oral liquids only in metric weights or volumes (e.g., mg or ml), not by teaspoon or tablespoon.
- Print generic and brand names of look-alike or sound-alike medications.

**Zeros and decimal points:** Hastily written orders can present problems even if the name of the medication is clear.

- Never leave a decimal point "naked." Place a zero before a decimal point when the number is less than a whole unit (e.g., use 0.25 mg or 250 mcg, **not** .25 mg).
- Never have a trailing zero following a decimal point (e.g., use 2 mg, **not** 2.0 mg).

**Abbreviations:** Errors can occur because of a failure to standardize abbreviations. Establishing a list of abbreviations that should never be used is recommended.

- Never abbreviate unit as "U"; spell out "unit."
- Do not abbreviate "once daily" as OD or QD or "every other day" as QOD; spell it out.
- Do not use D/C, as this may be misinterpreted as either discharge or discontinue.
- Do not abbreviate drug names; spell out the generic and/or brand names.

**Ambiguous or incomplete orders:** These types of orders can cause confusion or misinterpretation of the writer's intention. Examples include situations when the route of administration, dose, or dosage form has not been specified.

- Do not use slash marks—they may be read as the number one (1).
- When reviewing an unusual order, verify the order with the person writing the order to prevent any misunderstanding.
- Read over orders after writing.
- Encourage that the drug's indication for use be provided on medication orders.
- Provide complete medication orders—do not use "resume preop" or "continue previous meds."
- Provide the age and, when appropriate, the weight of the pt.

**High-alert medications:** Medications in this category have an increased risk of causing significant pt harm when used in error. Mistakes with these medications may or may not be more common but may be more devastating to the pt if an error occurs. A list of high-alert medications can be obtained from the Institute for Safe Medication Practices (ISMP) at www.ismp.org.

**Technology** available today that can be used to address and help solve potential medication problems or errors includes the following:

- Electronic prescribing systems—This refers to computerized prescriber order entry systems. Within these systems is the capability to incorporate medication safety alerts (e.g., maximum dose alerts, allergy screening). Additionally, these systems should be integrated or interfaced with pharmacy and laboratory systems to provide drug–drug and drug–disease interactions alerts and include clinical order screening capability.
- Bar codes—These systems are designed to use bar-code scanning devices to validate identity of pts, verify medications administered, document administration, and provide safety alerts.

- "Smart" infusion pumps—These pumps allow users to enter drug infusion protocols into a drug library along with predefined dosage limits. If a dosage is outside the limits established, an alarm is sounded and drug delivery is halted, informing the clinician that the dose is outside the recommended range.
- Automated dispensing systems; point-of-use dispensing system—These systems should be integrated with information systems, esp. pharmacy systems.
- Pharmacy order entry system—This should be fully integrated with an electronic prescribing system with the capability of producing medication safety alerts. Additionally, the system should generate a computerized medication administration record (MAR), which would be used by the nursing staff while administering medications.

**Medication reconciliation:** Medication errors generally occur at transition points in the pt's care (admission, transfer from one level of care to another [e.g., critical care to general care area], and discharge). Incomplete documentation can account for up to 60% of potential medication errors. Therefore, it becomes necessary to accurately and completely reconcile medication across the continuum of care. This includes the name, dosage, frequency, and route of medication administration.

Medication reconciliation programs are a process of identifying the most accurate list of all medications a pt is taking and using this list to provide correct medications anywhere within the health care system. The focus is on not only compiling a list but using the list to reduce medication errors and provide quality pt care.

### Additional Strategies to Reduce Medication Errors

The ISMP, FDA, and other agencies have identified high-risk areas associated with medication errors. They include the following:

**At-risk population:** At-risk populations primarily include pediatric and geriatric pts. For both, this risk is due to altered pharmacokinetic parameters with little published information regarding medication use in these groups. Additionally, in the pediatric population, the risk is due to the need for calculating doses based on age and weight, lack of available dosage forms, and concentrations for smaller children.

In a USP report, more than one-third of medication errors reaching the pt occurred in pts 65 yrs of age and older. Almost 40% of people 60 yrs and older take at least five medications. More than 50% of fatal hospital medication errors involve seniors. In the senior population, age-related physiologic changes (e.g., decreased renal function, reduced muscle mass) increase the risk for adverse events.

**Avoid abbreviations and nomenclature:** The confusion caused by abbreviations has prompted the ISMP to develop a list of abbreviations that should be avoided (see back cover of handbook).

**Recognize prescription look-alike and sound-alike medications:** The ISMP has developed an extensive list of confused drug names (see www.jointcommission. org). See individual monographs for **DO NOT CONFUSE** information.

**Focus on high alert medications:** High alert medications are medications that bear a heightened risk of causing significant pt harm if incorrectly used. High alert medications in the handbook have a colored background for the entire monograph.

**Look for duplicate therapies and interactions:** Drug interactions and duplicate therapies can increase risk of adverse reactions. Refer to individual monographs for significant interaction information (drug, herbal, food).

**Report errors to improve process:** This action plays an important role in preventing further errors. The intent is to identify system failures that can be altered to prevent further errors.

# PARENTERAL FLUID ADMINISTRATION

Replacing fluids in the body is based on body fluid needs. Water comprises approximately 60% of the adult body. Approximately 40% is intracellular fluid and 20% is extracellular fluid, of which 15% is interstitial (tissues) and 5% is intravascular. The walls separating these compartments are porous, allowing water to move freely between them. Small particles such as sodium and chloride can pass through the walls, but larger molecules such as proteins and starches usually are unable to pass through the walls.

Hydrostatic and osmotic pressures are forces that move water and regulate the body's water. Intravenous fluid manipulates these two pressures. Hydrostatic pressure reflects the weight and volume of water. The greater the volume, the higher the blood pressure.

**Effects of Osmotic Pressure:** *Osmosis* is the diffusion of water across a semipermeable membrane from an area of high concentration to an area of low concentration (water moves into the compartment of higher concentration of particles, or solute). This is similar to the action of a sponge soaking up water. This pull is referred to as *osmotic pressure*. It is the number of particles in each compartment that keeps water where it is supposed to be. By administering fluids with more (or fewer) particles than blood plasma, fluid is pulled into the compartment where it is needed the most.

How do we know where the water is needed? To assess water balance, measure the *osmolality* of blood plasma (number of particles [osmoles] in a kilogram of fluid). *Osmolarity* is the number of particles in a liter of fluid. Normal serum osmolality is approximately 300 milliosmoles (mOsm) per liter.

Crystalloids are made of substances that form crystals (e.g., sodium chloride) and are small, so easy movement between compartments is possible. Crystalloids are categorized by their tonicity (a synonym for osmolality). An isotonic solution has the same number of particles (osmolality) as plasma and will not promote a shift of fluids into or out of cells. Examples of isotonic crystalloid solutions are 0.9% sodium chloride and lactated Ringer's solution. Dextrose 5% in water is another isotonic crystalloid. However, it is quickly metabolized, and the fluid quickly becomes hypotonic. Hypotonic solutions (e.g., $D_5W$, 0.45% sodium chloride) are a good source of free water, causing a shift out of the vascular bed and into cells by way of osmosis. Hypotonic solutions are given to correct cellular dehydration and hypernatremia. Hypertonic solutions have more particles than body water and pull water back into the circulation, which can shrink cells.

## SODIUM CHLORIDE

### USES

- Extracellular fluid replacement when chloride loss is greater than or equal to sodium loss
- Treatment of metabolic alkalosis in the presence of fluid loss; chloride ions cause a compensatory decrease of bicarbonate ions
- Sodium depletion, extracellular fluid volume deficit with sodium deficit
- Initiation and termination of blood transfusion, preventing hemolysis of RBCs (occurs with dextrose in water solutions)

## SIDE EFFECTS/ABNORMALITIES

* Hypernatremia
* **Acidosis:** 0.9% sodium chloride contains one-third more chloride ions than is present in extracellular fluid; excess chloride ions cause loss of bicarbonate, resulting in acidosis
* **Hypokalemia:** Increased potassium excretion at the same time extracellular fluid is increasing, which further decreases potassium concentration in extracellular fluid
* Circulatory overload

## DEXTROSE (GLUCOSE)
### EFFECTS

* Provides calories for essential energy
* Improves hepatic function because it is converted into glycogen
* Spares body protein, preventing unnecessary breakdown of protein tissue
* Prevents ketosis
* Stored in the liver as glycogen, causing a shift of potassium from extracellular to intracellular fluid compartment

## USES

* Dehydration
* Hyponatremia
* Hyperkalemia
* Vehicle of drug delivery and nutrition

**Note:** Once infused, dextrose is rapidly metabolized to water and carbon dioxide, becoming hypotonic rather than isotonic.

## SIDE EFFECTS/ABNORMALITIES

* Dehydration: Osmotic diuresis occurs if dextrose is given faster than the pt's ability to metabolize it
* Hypokalemia (see Effects)
* Hyperinsulinism due to rapid infusion of hypertonic solution
* Water intoxication due to an imbalance based on increase in extracellular fluid volume from water alone

### SELECTED PARENTERAL FLUIDS

| Solution | Comments |
|---|---|
| Dextrose 5% in water (D$_5$W) | Supplies approximately 170 cal/L and free water to aid in renal excretion of solutes<br>Avoid excessive volumes in pts with increased antidiuretic hormone activity or to replace fluids in hypovolemic pts |
| 0.9% Sodium chloride (0.9% NaCl) | Isotonic fluid commonly used to expand extracellular fluid in presence of hypovolemia<br>Can be used to treat mild metabolic alkalosis |

| Solution | Comments |
| --- | --- |
| 0.45% Sodium chloride (0.45% NaCl) | Hypotonic solution that provides sodium, chloride, and free water; sodium and chloride allow kidneys to select and retain needed amounts<br>Free water is desirable as aid to kidneys in elimination of solutes |
| 3% Sodium chloride | Used only to treat severe hyponatremia |
| Lactated Ringer's solution | Isotonic solution that contains sodium, potassium, calcium, and chloride in approximately the same concentrations as found in plasma<br>Used to treat hypovolemia, burns, and fluid loss as bile or diarrhea |

# COMMON TERMINOLOGY CRITERIA FOR ADVERSE EVENTS (CTCAE)

The Common Terminology Criteria for Adverse Events (CTCAE) is descriptive terminology used for reporting an adverse event (AE) in a concise and standardized manner. It is supported by the U.S. Department of Health and Human Services, National Institutes of Health, and National Cancer Institute. An AE term is a unique representation of a specific event that can be used for medical documentation and scientific analyses. Along with cancer medications, other drugs may use the CTCAE system for dose and treatment modifications.

CTCAE terms are grouped by system organ classes, such as *Blood/Lymphatic, GI, Nervous, Renal,* and *Respiratory* disorders. Within each system organ class, AEs are listed and accompanied by a brief description. A grading scale is then provided for each AE term, and each grade refers to a specific severity.

The CTCAE grading scale displays grades 1–5 with particular descriptions and/or recommendations. The severity for each AE is based on the following generalized guidelines: **Grade 1:** Asymptomatic or mild symptoms; clinical or diagnostic observations only; intervention not indicated. **Grade 2:** Moderate; minimal, local, or noninvasive intervention indicated; limiting age-appropriate instrumental activity of daily living (ADL). **Grade 3:** Severe or medically significant but not immediately life threatening; hospitalization or prolonged hospitalization indicated; disabling; limiting self-care ADL. **Grade 4:** Life-threatening consequences; urgent intervention indicated. **Grade 5:** Death related to AE.

## CTCAE EXAMPLES

| Adverse Event | Grade | | | | |
|---|---|---|---|---|---|
| | 1 | 2 | 3 | 4 | 5 |
| *Blood/ Lymphatic* **Anemia** | Hgb < lower limit of normal– 10 g/dL | Hgb 8–10 g/dL | Hgb <8 g/ dL; transfusion indicated | Life-threatening consequences Urgent intervention indicated | Death |
| *Gastrointestinal* **Diarrhea** | Increase of <4 stools/day over baseline Mild ostomy output | Increase of 4–6 stools/day over baseline Moderate ostomy output | Increase of 7 stools/ day over baseline Severe ostomy output Hospitalization required | Life-threatening consequences Urgent intervention indicated | Death |
| *General* **Fever** | 38–39°C (100.4– 102.2°F) | >39–40°C (102.3–104° F) | >40°C (>104° F) for less than 24 hrs | >40°C (>104°F) for more than 24 hrs | Death |

| Adverse Event | Grade | | | | |
|---|---|---|---|---|---|
| | 1 | 2 | 3 | 4 | 5 |
| *Infections* **UTI** | N/A | Localized; local intervention indicated (topical, antifungal, antiviral) | IV antibiotic, antifungal, antiviral intervention indicated. Radiologic or surgical intervention indicated | Life-threatening consequences Urgent intervention indicated | Death |
| *Investigations* **Lipase increased** | >ULN–1.5 times ULN | >1.5–2 times ULN | >2–5 times ULN | >5 times ULN | N/A |
| *Metabolism/ Nutrition* **Hyperkalemia** | >ULN–5.5 mmol/L | >5.5–6 mmol/L | >6–7 mmol/L | >7 mmol/L; life-threatening consequences | Death |

*ULN,* Upper limit of normal.

# Index

---

**bold** – generic drug name                                    regular type – trade name

---

**bold** – generic drug name                         regular type – trade name

**bold page #** – main drug entry

---

**bold** – generic drug name                              regular type – trade name

---

**bold page #** – main drug entry

**bold page #** – main drug entry

# COMMONLY USED ABBREVIATIONS

**ABG(s)**—arterial blood gas(es)
**ACE**—angiotensin-converting enzyme
**ADHD**—attention-deficit hyperactivity disorder
**AIDS**—acquired immunodeficiency syndrome
**ALT**—alanine aminotransferase, serum
**ANC**—absolute neutrophil count
**aPTT**—activated partial thromboplastin time
**AST**—aspartate aminotransferase, serum
**AV**—atrioventricular
**bid**—twice per day
**B/P**—blood pressure
**BSA**—body surface area
**BUN**—blood urea nitrogen
**CBC**—complete blood count
**Ccr**—creatinine clearance
**CNS**—central nervous system
**CO**—cardiac output
**COPD**—chronic obstructive pulmonary disease
**CPK**—creatine phosphokinase
**CSF**—cerebrospinal fluid
**CT**—computed tomography
**CVA**—cerebrovascular accident
**D$_5$W**—dextrose 5% in water
**dl**—deciliter
**DNA**—deoxyribonucleic acid
**EEG**—electroencephalogram
**EKG**—electrocardiogram
**esp.**—especially
**g**—gram
**GGT**—gamma glutamyl transpeptidase
**GI**—gastrointestinal
**GU**—genitourinary
**H$_2$**—histamine
**Hct**—hematocrit
**HDL**—high-density lipoprotein
**HF**—heart failure
**Hgb**—hemoglobin
**HIV**—human immunodeficiency virus
**HMG-CoA**—3-hydroxy-3-methylglutaryl-coenzyme A (HMG-CoA) reductase inhibitors (statins)
**hr/hrs**—hour/hours
**HTN**—hypertension
**I&O**—intake and output
**ICP**—intracranial pressure
**ID**—intradermal
**IgA**—immunoglobulin A

**IM**—intramuscular
**IOP**—intraocular pressure
**IV**—intravenous
**K**—potassium
**kg**—kilogram
**LDH**—lactate dehydrogenase
**LDL**—low-density lipoprotein
**LOC**—level of consciousness
**MAC**—*Mycobacterium avium* complex
**MAOI**—monoamine oxidase inhibitor
**mcg**—microgram
**mEq**—milliequivalent
**mg**—milligram
**MI**—myocardial infarction
**min**—minute(s)
**mo/mos**—month/months
**N/A**—not applicable
**Na**—sodium
**NaCl**—sodium chloride
**NG**—nasogastric
**NSAID(s)**—nonsteroidal anti-inflammatory drug(s)
**OD**—right eye
**OS**—left eye
**OTC**—over the counter
**OU**—both eyes
**PCP**—*Pneumocystis jiroveci* pneumonia
**PO**—orally, by mouth
**prn**—as needed
**PSA**—prostate-specific antigen
**pt/pts**—patient/patients
**PT**—prothrombin time
**PTCA**—percutaneous transluminal coronary angiography
**q**—every
**qid**—four times daily
**RBC**—red blood cell count
**REM**—rapid eye movement
**RNA**—ribonucleic acid
**SA**—sinoatrial node
**sec**—second(s)
**SSRI**—selective serotonin reuptake inhibitor
**tbsp**—tablespoon
**tid**—three times daily
**TNF**—tumor necrosis factor
**tsp**—teaspoon
**UTI**—urinary tract infection
**VLDL**—very-low-density lipoprotein
**WBC**—white blood cell count
**wk/wks**—week/weeks
**yr/yrs**—year/years